PRAISE FOR THE FIRST EDITION

"The best such publication to date."

—C. NORMAN SHEALY, M.D., Ph.D.,
Founder, American Holistic Medical Association

"An excellent resource on a wide range of subjects that will be helpful to everyone."

—BERNIE S. SIEGEL, M.D.,
Author, *Love, Medicine & Miracles*

". . . this is the book that is needed right now."

—MARGARET MASON, *Washington Post*

"Essential to the future of medicine."

—BRUCE LOUIS ERICKSON, Consultant,
World Health Organization

"Those wanting to understand the rationale and therapeutic approach of the diverse natural healing arts will find this book a welcome resource."

—JOSEPH PIZZORNO, N.D.,
Co-Founder and President Emeritus, Bastyr University, and
Co-Author, *Encyclopedia of Natural Medicine*

PRAISE FROM OUR READERS

"All of my adult life, I've suffered from severe intestinal problems. That is, until I found the information in Alternative Medicine. *Then I discovered an enzyme therapist featured in the book. After four weeks of treatment, I started feeling better; after four months, my condition was completely resolved. This information changed my life."*

—GENE LAW, Colorado

"When my thumbs became very painful and stiff, I knew I was in for another bout of osteoarthritis. In Alternative Medicine, *a dentist explains that dental mercury amalgams can set off arthritis. I had a new mercury amalgam filling replaced with a non-mercury filling and my thumbs returned to normal."*

—ROGER SMITH, Virginia

"I was diagnosed with incurable lymphedema in 1995. My failing health inspired an urgent health quest. I tried everything without success. Then I began the exploration of numerous alternative books. My breakthrough came with the discovery of Alternative Medicine, *which provided pivotal information resulting in the restoration of my health."*

—MUFFY E. VAN NOSTRAND, Pennsylvania

Alternative Medicine

THE DEFINITIVE GUIDE

Second Edition

LARRY TRIVIERI, JR., and JOHN W. ANDERSON, Editors

Introduction by Burton Goldberg

www.naturalsolutionsmag.com

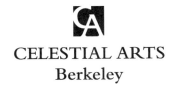

CELESTIAL ARTS
Berkeley

Library of Congress Cataloging-in-Publication Data
on file with the Publisher

ISBN: 978-1-58761-141-4

Printed in the United States of America

Design by Toni Tajima and Felipe Lujan-Bear

17 16 15 14 13 12 11 10 9

Second Edition

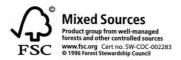

Mixed Sources
Product group from well-managed
forests and other controlled sources
www.fsc.org Cert no. SW-COC-002283
© 1996 Forest Stewardship Council
FSC

CREDITS FOR THE SECOND EDITION

President: Rick Prill

Editor: Larry Trivieri, Jr., and John W. Anderson

Medical Advisors: Leon Chaitow, N.D., D.O., W. Lee Cowden, M.D., and Rima Laibow, M.D.

Writers: Larry Trivieri, Jr., and John W. Anderson

Contributing Editors: Gerri C. Borenstein, Ellen Cavalli, Russ DiCarlo, Elaine Gavalas, Lew Kahler, Tom Klaber, Richard Leviton, Blake More

Researcher: Louise Phelps

Production: Felipe Lujan-Bear

Design: Toni Tajima and Felipe Lujan-Bear

A special thanks to Blair Kellison of Alternative-Medicine.com and Veronica Randall of Celestial Arts for all their help in making this project a reality.

CONTENTS

Quick Reference A-Z Section of Additional Health Conditions

Appendices

IMPORTANT INFORMATION

THIS BOOK IS intended as an educational tool to acquaint the reader with alternative methods for the maintenance of good health and the treatment of illness. The publisher hopes the book will enable the reader to improve his or her well-being and to better understand, assess, and choose the appropriate course of treatment for an illness or health condition.

Because the methods described in this book are, by definition, alternative methods, many of them have not been investigated and/or approved by any government or regulatory agency. National, state, and local laws vary regarding the use and application of many of the treatments that are discussed. Accordingly, this book should not be substituted for the advice and treatment of a physician or other licensed health-care professional, but rather should be used in conjunction with professional care. Pregnant women, in particular, are especially urged to consult with their physician before using any therapy.

All of the factual information in this book has been drawn from the scientific literature. To protect privacy, all patient names have been changed. Branded products and services discussed in the book are evaluated solely on the independent and direct experience of the health-care practitioners quoted. Reference to them does not imply an endorsement or superiority over other branded products and services, which may provide similar or superior results.

Your health is important. Use this book wisely. Discuss the alternative treatment options described herein with your doctor. Ultimately, you, the reader, must take full responsibility for your health and how you use this book. The publisher expressly disclaims responsibility for any adverse effects resulting from the use of the information contained herein.

USER'S GUIDE

This book is interactive. Use these icons to find more information and get the most out of this book.

 Turn to another place in this book for more information.

 Here are additional books on the same subject worth reading.

 Many times the text mentions a medical term that requires explanation. Instead of interrupting the text, the explanation is put under this Quick Definition icon.

 Contact information of organizations, professionals, and publications for more information on a particular subject.

 There may be some risks, uncertainties, side effects, or special contraindications regarding a procedure or substance.

 Please give this point your special attention.

 Indicates a promising area that needs more scientific reseach and medical testing.

 Alternative medicine saves money—here is another example of its cost-saving ability.

EDITORIAL BOARD

Robert S. Ivker, D.O., Author of six books, including *Sinus Survival;* President-elect, American Board of Holistic Medicine, Littleton, Colorado

Bernard Jensen, D.C., Lecturer; Author of *Nature Cures;* Founder and Director, Valley Ranch, Escondido, California

Konrad Kail, N.D., Member of the Advisory Council to the National Center for Complementary and Alternative Medicine (NCCAM); past President of the American Association of Naturopathic Physicians, Phoenix, Arizona

Vasant Lad, M.A.Sc., Ayurvedic Physician; Director, The Ayurvedic Institute, Albuquerque, New Mexico

Susana Alcázar Leyva, M.D., President of the Albert Szent-Gyorgy Gerontological Center; Vice President of the Hans Selye Institute of Scientific Research, Mexico City, Mexico

Evarts Loomis, M.D., F.A.C.S., Co-founder, American Holistic Medical Association; Founder, Meadowlark Holistic Health Retreat, Hemet, California

Wolfgang Ludwig, Sc.D., Ph.D., Director, Institute for Biophysics, Horb, Germany

Marshall Mandell, M.D., F.A.C.A.I., F.A.A.E.M., Fellow of the American College of Allergists; Author of *5-Day Allergy Relief System;* Medical Director, New England Foundation for Allergic and Environmental Diseases, Norwalk, Connecticut

Gaston Naessens, Director, Center for Experimental Research and Biologics, Rock Forest, Quebec, Canada

Maoshing Ni, D.O.M., Ph.D., L.Ac., President, Yo San University of Traditional Chinese Medicine, Marina del Rey, California

Patricia A. Norris, Ph.D., Co-founder, Life Sciences Institute of Mind-Body Health, Topeka, Kansas

Richard Passwater, Ph.D., Executive Vice President, Solgar Nutritional Research Center, Berlin, Maryland

Kenneth R. Pelletier, Ph.D., M.D. (Hon), Senior Clinical Fellow, Stanford Center for Research in Disease Prevention, Department of Medicine, Stanford University School of Medicine, Palo Alto, California

Joseph E. Pizzorno, N.D., Author of *Total Wellness;* President Emeritus, Bastyr University, Kenmore, Washington

Martin L. Rossman, M.D., Founder, Academy for Guided Imagery, Mill Valley, California

Anthony Scott-Morley, D.Sc., Ph.D., B.A., B.Ac., M.D. (Alt. Med.), Director, Institute of Bioenergetic Medicine; Member of the World Research Foundation, Dorset, England

Hari Sharma, M.D., F.R.C.P.C., Professor of Pathology, Director, Cancer Prevention and Natural Products Research, The Ohio State University College of Medicine, Columbus, Ohio

C. Norman Shealy, M.D., Ph.D., Co-founder and first President, American Holistic Medical Association; Director, Shealy Institute for Comprehensive Health Care; Professor of Psychology, Forest Institute of Professional Psychology, Springfield, Missouri

Bernie Siegel, M.D., Founder of ECaP (Exceptional Cancer Patients), New Haven, Connecticut

Carl Simonton, M.D., Board Certified, Director, Simonton Cancer Center, Pacific Palisades, California; Director, Psychoneuroimmunology Counseling Program, Cancer Treatment Centers of America, Brea, California

Lendon H. Smith, M.D., Author of 13 books including *Feed Your Kids Right*, Portland, Oregon

Virender Sodhi, M.D. (Ayurveda), N.D., Founder and Director, Ayurvedic and Naturopathic Medical Clinic, Bellevue, Washington

Hector Solorzano Del Rio, M.D., D.Sc., President of the Society of Investigation of Acupuncture and Oriental Medicine; Coordinator, Alternative Medical Studies Program; Professor of Pharmacology, University of Guadalajara, Mexico

Michael Stern, D.C., Founder and Director, Research for Alternative Medicine (RAM) Foundation, Minneapolis, Minnesota

William Tiller, Ph.D., Author of *Science and Human Transformation;* Professor Emeritus, Stanford University, Palo Alto, California

CONTRIBUTORS
AND CONSULTANTS

We gratefully acknowledge each of these health experts, who contributed material for and/or reviewed the chapters that follow. To locate a contributor within the text, please see the Index.

Ernesto Adler, M.D., D.D.S., Clinica Dental, Lloret de Mars, Spain

Lauri Aesoph, N.D., Sioux Falls, South Dakota

Moses Albalas, O.D., O.M.D., H.M.D., Ph.D., L.Ac., Los Angeles, California

Majid Ali, M.D., Dipl., Consulting Physician, Institute of Preventive Medicine, Denville, New Jersey; Associate Professor (Adj.), Columbia University Medical School; Director, Department of Pathology, Immunology, and Laboratories, Holy Name Hospital, Teaneck, New Jersey

Norman Allan, Ph.D., D.C., Toronto, Ontario, Canada

Ted Allen, M.D., Nassau, The Bahamas

Connie Allred, President, International Association of Colon Therapy, Los Angeles, California

Robert A. Anderson, M.D., Founding President, American Board of Holistic Medicine

Connierae Andreas, Co-director, NLP Comprehensive, Boulder, Colorado

Nancy Appleton, Ph.D., Santa Monica, California

Ed Arana, D.D.S., Co-founder and President, American Academy of Biological Dentistry, Carmel Valley, California

Judith Aston, M.F.A., Founder and Director, The Aston Training Center, Incline Village, Nevada

Robert C. Atkins, M.D., Author, *Dr. Atkins' Health Revelations;* Founder and Medical Director, The Atkins Center for Complementary Medicine, New York, New York

Laurence Badgley, M.D., Foster City, California

Steven Bailey, N.D., Graduate Assistant Professor, National College of Naturopathic Medicine; Director, Northwest Naturopathic Clinic, Portland, Oregon

Rudolph M. Ballentine, M.D., Author, *Radical Healing;* Board of Trustees, Medical Staff, Himalayan Institute; Director, Center for Holistic Medicine, Bronx, New York

Julian Barnard, Author of *Guide to the Bach Flower Remedies* and *Healing Herbs of Edward Bach,* Hereford, England

Beatrice Barnett, N.D., D.C., Director, Lifestyle Institute, Margate, Florida

John Baron, D.O., Director, Baron Clinic and Associates, Cleveland, Ohio

Richard Barrett, N.D., Associate Academic Dean, National College of Naturopathic Medicine, Portland, Oregon

Fereydoon Batmanghelidj, M.D., Author, *Your Body's Many Cries for Water,* Falls Church, Virginia

Abram Ber, M.D., Founding Member, American Holistic Medical Association, Phoenix, Arizona

Guy Berard, E.N.T., Les Ollieres, France

D. Lindsey Berkson, M.A., D.C., Santa Fe, New Mexico

Jean Berry, President and CEO, LifeCell Technologies, Inc., Coconut Grove, Florida

Ann Berwick, B.S.C., Founder and President of the National Association for Holistic Aromatherapy, Boulder, Colorado

Rita Bettenburg, N.D., Research Director, Clinical Faculty, National College of Naturopathic Medicine, Portland, Oregon

David R. Bierman, L.Ac., President, Safe Environments, Berkeley, California

Harvey Bigelson, M.D., Medical Director, Center for Progressive Medicine, Scottsdale, Arizona

Robert Bingham, M.D., former Medical Director, Desert Arthritis and Medical Clinic, Desert Hot Springs, California

Timothy C. Birdsall, N.D., Technical Director, Thorne Research, Inc., Sandpoint, Idaho

Leyardia Black, N.D., former Professor of Gynecology, Bastyr University, Lopez Island, Washington

Robert Blaich, D.C., D.I.B.A.K., Diplomate, International Board of Applied Kinesiology, Denver, Colorado

Jeffrey Bland, Ph.D., President, HealthComm, Inc., Gig Harbor, Washington

Mark Blumenthal, Founder and Executive Director, American Botanical Council; Editor, *HerbalGram*, Austin, Texas

Dean Bonlie, D.D.S., President, MagnetiCo Inc., Calgary, Alberta, Canada

Helen L. Bonny, Ph.D., R.M.T., Director, The Bonny Foundation, Philadelphia, Pennsylvania

Michael Borkin, N.M.D., Westlake Village, California

Joan Borysenko, Ph.D., Author of ten books, including *Minding the Body/Mending the Mind*; Mind-Body Health Sciences, Boulder, Colorado

Mary Bove, N.D., L.M., former Chair, Botanical Medicine Department, Bastyr University, Kenmore, Washington

Randall Bradley, N.D., D.H.A.N.P., Lincoln, Nebraska

James Braly, M.D., Author, *Dr. Braly's Food Allergy and Nutrition Revolution*, Hollywood, Florida

Eric Braverman, M.D., Director, Princeton Associates for Total Health (PATH), Princeton, New Jersey

Arline and Harold Brecher, Co-authors, *40-Something Forever*, Herndon, Virginia

David E. Bresler, Ph.D., L.Ac., Author, *Free Yourself From Pain*; former Director, U.C.L.A. Pain Center; Co-Director, Academy for Guided Imagery, Mill Valley, California

Barbara Brewitt, M.Div., Ph.D., Biomed Comm, Inc., Seattle, Washington

Phyllis J. Bronson, Ph.D., Aspen Clinic for Preventive and Environmental Medicine, Aspen, Colorado

Donald J. Brown, N.D., Author, *Herbal Prescriptions for Health and Healing*; former Professor of Botanical Medicine, Bastyr University, Kenmore, Washington

Erma Brown, B.S.N., P.H.N., Co-director, Foundation for Environmental Health Research, Beaverton, Oregon

Jane Buckle, R.N., Author, *Clinical Aromatherapy in Nursing*, London, England

Annemarie Buhler, Phyto-Aromatherapy Institute, South Pasadena, California

Helen Varney Burst, C.N.M., M.S.N., D.H.L. (Hon), F.A.C.N.M., Professor, Nurse Midwifery Program, Adult Health Division, Yale University School of Nursing, New Haven, Connecticut

Dwight Byers, Author of *Better Health with Foot Reflexology*; President, Ingham Publishing, International Institute of Reflexology, St. Petersburg, Florida

Chanchal Cabrera, M.N.I.M.H., Vancouver, British Columbia, Canada

Cherie Calbom, M.S., C.N., Author, *Juicing for Life, Cooking for Life*, and *Nutrition and Cancer*, Kirkland, Washington

Etienne Callebout, M.D., London, England

Don G. Campbell, B.M.Ed., Author, *The Mozart Effect*; Director of the Institute for Music, Health & Education, Boulder, Colorado

Eve Campanelli, Ph.D., Nutritional Consultant, Master Herbalist, Beverly Hills, California

Patricia Cane, Ph.D., Research Associate in Obstetrics/Gynecology, Cedars Sinai Hospital, Los Angeles, California

William M. Cargile, B.S., D.C., F.I.A.C.A., past Chairman of Research, American Association of Oriental Medicine

James A. Carlson, D.O., F.A.O.A.S., past President, American Association of Orthopedic Medicine, Knoxville, Tennessee

James Carter, M.D., Professor of Nutrition, Tulane University School of Public Health and Tropical Diseases, New Orleans, Louisiana

Joseph Carter, L.Ac., C.M.T., Berkeley, California

Robert Cathcart III, M.D., Los Altos, California

Leon Chaitow, N.D., D.O., Editor, *Journal of Alternative and Complementary Medicine;* Author of over 60 books; Director, Nutrition and Health Research Associates, London, England

Emanuel Cheraskin, M.D., D.M.D., Professor Emeritus, University of Alabama Medical Center, Birmingham, Alabama

Nalini Chilkov, Lic.Ac., O.M.D., Santa Monica, California

Eleanor Chin, D.C., Mill Valley, California

Deepak Chopra, M.D., Author of numerous books, including *Quantum Healing* and *Ageless Body, Timeless Mind*; Founder and Director, The Chopra Center for Well-Being, La Jolla, California

James Hoyt Clark, Orem, Utah

Walter Jess Clifford, M.S., President and Director, Clifford Consulting and Research, Colorado Springs, Colorado

John C. Cline, M.D., B.Sc., C.C.F.P., A.B.C.T., Medical Director, Cline Medical Centre and Oceanside Medicine Research Institute, Vancouver Island, British Columbia, Canada

Drew Collins, N.D., Director, Oasis Naturopathic Medical Clinic, Prescott Valley, Arizona

Trevor Cook, Ph.D., D.I.Hom., past President, British Homeopathic Medical Association, Middlesex, England

Vaughn Cook, L.Ac., Dipl.Ac. (NCCA), Director, Utah Acupuncture Clinic, Salt Lake City, Utah

Mark Cooper, N.D., L.Ac., Portland, Oregon

Ignacio Coronel, M.D., Mexico City, Mexico

Serafina Corsello, M.D., Director, Corsello Centers for Nutritional Complementary Medicine, Huntington and New York, New York

Harris L. Coulter, Ph.D., Author, *Divided Legacy*; Founder and Director, Center for Empirical Medicine, Washington, D.C.

W. Lee Cowden, M.D., Co-Author of *Alternative Medicine Definitive Guide to Cancer, Cancer Diagnosis: What Steps to Take*, and *Longevity*, Fort Worth, Texas

Elmer M. Cranton, M.D., Author, *Bypassing Bypass*, Troutdale, Virginia

Walter Crinnion, N.D., Kirkland, Washington

William Crook, M.D., F.A.A.P., F.A.C.A., F.A.C.A.I., Author, *The Yeast Connection* and *Help for the Hyperactive Child*; President, International Health Foundation, Jackson, Tennessee

Pat Culliton, M.A., Dipl.Ac. (NCCA), Director, Acupuncture and Alternative Medicine, Hennepin County Medical Center, Minneapolis, Minnesota

Michael Cummings, D.O., F.N.T.O.S., London, England

Ralph Alan Dale, Ed.D., Ph.D., C.A., Dipl.Ac., Director, Acupuncture Education Center, North Miami Beach, Florida

Inez d'Arcy-Francis, Ph.D., Kentfield, California

Marc Darrow, M.D., Author, *The Collagen Revolution*; Co-director, Joint Rehabilitation and Sports Medical Center, Los Angeles, California

Katie Data, N.D., Fife, Washington

Stephen Davies, B.M., B.Ch., London, England

Don G. Davis, D.C., Director, Davis Chiropractic Group, Hayward, California

Rena Davis, M.S., President, Davis Nutritional Consultants, St. Helens, Oregon

Christopher Day, M.A., Vet.M.B., M.R.C.V.S., Vet.F.F.Hom., England

Martin Dayton, M.D., D.O., B.S., H.M.D., F.H.F.P., Director, Medical Center Sunny Isles, Miami Beach, Florida

Sandra C. Denton, M.D., Alaska Alternative Medicine Center, Anchorage, Alaska

Kathleen DesMaisons, Ph.D., Author, *The Sugar Addict's Total Recovery Program*; Albuquerque, New Mexico

Ravi Devgan, M.D., Toronto, Canada

Subhuti Dharmananda, Ph.D., Director, Institute for Traditional Medicine, Portland, Oregon

W. John Diamond, M.D., Co-author of *Alternative Medicine Definitive Guide to Cancer*; Medical Director, Triad Medical Center, Reno, Nevada

Darius Dinshaw, S-CN., President, Dinshaw Health Society, Malaga, New Jersey

Roy Dittman, L.Ac., O.M.D., Director, Bodymind Systems Medical Center, Santa Monica, California

Patrick Donovan, R.N., N.D., Fellow, Health Studies Collegium Academic Faculty, Bastyr University, Kenmore, Washington

William C. Douglass, M.D., Clayton, Georgia

Frederich Douwes, M.D., Klinik St. Georg, Munich, Germany

John Downing, O.D., Ph.D., Director, Light Therapy Institute, Santa Rosa, California

Suzannah Doyle, Certified Fertility Educator, Director of Fertility Awareness Services, Corvallis, Oregon

Daniel D. Dugi, Jr., M.D., Cuero, Texas

James Duke, Ph.D., Author, *The Green Pharmacy*; former Economic Botanist, United States Department of Agriculture, Beltsville, Maryland

Lindsey Duncan, C.N., Santa Monica, California

Nancy Dunne, N.D., President, Montana Association of Naturopathic Physicians, Missoula, Montana

Daniel Dunphy, P.A.-C., San Francisco, California

Charmane Eastman, Ph.D., Director, Biological Rhythms Research Laboratory; Associate Professor, Psychology Department, Rush Presbyterian, St. Luke's Medical Center, Chicago, Illinois

Stephen B. Edelson, M.D., Edelson Center for Environmental and Preventive Medicine, Atlanta, Georgia

James D. Edwards, D.C., Board of Governors, American Chiropractic Association, Austin, Texas

Sharry Edwards, M.Ed., founding Director, Sound Health Research Institute, Athens, Ohio

Jason Elias, M.A., L.Ac., Co-author, *Chinese Medicine for Maximum Immunity*; Integral Health Associates, New Paltz, New York

Gary Emerson, D.C., OptiHealth, Santa Ana, California

Donald Epstein, D.C., Founder and President of Association for Network Chiropractors, Boulder, Colorado

Samuel S. Epstein, M.D., Author, *Politics of Cancer Revisited*; Professor of Occupational and Environmental Medicine, School of Public Health, University of Illinois Medical Center, Chicago, Illinois

Robert Erdman, M.A., Ph.D., Kent, England

David Essel, M.S., Fort Myers Beach, Florida

William T, Evans, M.D., Roaring Fork Valley, Colorado

William Faber, D.O., Co-author, *Pain, Pain Go Away*; Director, Milwaukee Pain Clinic, Milwaukee, Wisconsin

Steven Fahrion, Ph.D., Co-founder, Life Sciences Institute of Mind-Body Health, Topeka, Kansas

Charles Farr, M.D., Ph.D., Founder, International Bio-Oxidative Medicine Association; Medical Director, Genesis Medical Center, Oklahoma City, Oklahoma

J. Herbert Fill, M.D., former New York City Commissioner of Mental Health, New York, New York

Ray Fisch, N.D., Ph.D., C.H., Los Angeles, California

Richard D. Fischer, D.D.S., F.A.G.D., F.I.A.O.M.T., Executive Vice President, International Academy of Oral Medicine and Toxicology, Annandale, Virginia

Barbara Loe Fisher, Co-author, *A Shot in the Dark*; Co-founder, National Vaccine Information Center, Vienna, Virginia

Bob Flaws, Dipl.Ac., Dipl. C.H., F.N.A.A.O.M., Iris Acupuncture Health Associates, Boulder, Colorado

Bill Flocco, Director, American Academy of Reflexology, Burbank, California

David Frawley, O.M.D., Author, *Ayurvedic Healing*; Director, American Institute of Vedic Studies, Santa Fe, New Mexico

Joyce Frye, D.O., F.A.C.O.G., Founder, The Women's Group; Chairman, Gynecology Department, Presbyterian Medical Center, Philadelphia, Pennsylvania

Charles Gabelman, M.D., Diplomate, American Board of Allergy and Immunology, Director, Comprehensive Medical Center, Encinitas, California

Alan R. Gaby, M.D., past President, American Holistic Medical Association, Seattle, Washington

Michael Reed Gach, Ph.D., Author, *Acu-Yoga*; Director, The Acupressure Institute, Berkeley, California

Daniel Gagnon, Medical Herbalist, Botanical Research and Educational Institute, Santa Fe, New Mexico

Michael Galitzer, M.D., Co-founder, American Health Institute, Los Angeles, California

Martin Gallagher, D.C., Director, Medical Wellness Associates, Pittsburgh, Pennsylvania

Leo Galland, M.D., Author, *Four Pillars of Healing*, New York, New York

Stuart Garber, D.C., Director, Westside Chiropractic Center, West Los Angeles, California

Zane Gard, M.D., Co-director, Foundation for Environmental Health Research, Beaverton, Oregon

Michael Gerber, M.D., H.M.D., Reno, Nevada

Larrian Gillespie, M.D., Director, Pelvic Pain Treatment Center and the Women's Clinic for Interstitial Cystitis, Beverly Hills, California

Ann Louise Gittleman, M.S., Author, *Guess What Came to Dinner* and *Beyond Pritikin*, Bozeman, Montana

Jochen Gleditsch, M.D., D.D.S., Honorary President, German Acupuncture Association, Munich, Germany

Nicholas Gonzalez, M.D., New York, New York

George Goodheart, D.C., F.I.C.C., D.I.B.A.K., Author, *You'll Be Better: The Story of Applied Kinesiology*; Research Director, International College of Applied Kinesiology, Grosse Point Woods, Michigan

Garry F. Gordon, M.D.(H.), Co-founder, American College of Advancement in Medicine; Founder and Director, Gordon Research, Inc., Payson, Arizona

James Gordon, M.D., Clinical Professor, Departments of Psychiatry and Community and Family Medicine, Georgetown University School of Medicine; Chair, National Advisory Council to the National Center for Complementary and Alternative Medicine, National Institutes of Health; Director, The Center for Mind-Body Studies, Washington, D.C.

Jay N. Gordon, M.D., F.A.A.P., Santa Monica, California

Ray Gottlieb, O.D., Ph.D., Madison, New Jersey

Frances Gough, M.D., Sound Weight Solutions, Bellevue, Washington

Jay Gould, Ph.D., Radiation and Public Health Project, Miami Beach, Florida

Robert N. Grove, Ph.D., Medical Psychologist, Center for Neurofeedback, Culver City, California

Scott J. Gregory, O.M.D., Pacific Palisades, California

Warren S. Grundfest, M.D., Medical Director, Laser Research and Technology Development, Cedars Sinai Medical Center, Los Angeles, California

Eduardo Guerrero, M.D., P.A., Houston, Texas

H.C. Gurney, Jr., D.V.M., Conifer, Colorado

Elson M. Haas, M.D., Author, *Staying Healthy with Nutrition*; Director, Preventive Medical Center of Marin, San Rafael, California

Leonard Haimes, M.D., Medical Director, Medicine and Lifestyle, Environmental and Internal Medicine, Chelation Therapy, Boca Raton, Florida

Tim Hallbom, M.S.W., Partner, Western States Training Associates, NLP of Utah LC, Salt Lake City, Utah

Grace Halloran, Ph.D., Integrated Visual Healing, San Leandro, California

Steven Halpern, Ph.D., Author, *Sound Health*; President, SOUND Rx Records and Tapes; Director, Sound Health Research Institute, San Anselmo, California

Milton Hammerly, M.D., Medical Director, American Whole Health, Littleton, Colorado

Richard T. Hansen, D.M.D., F.A.C.A.D., Co-author, *The Key to Ultimate Health*; Director, Center for Advanced Dentistry, Fullerton, California

Jeff Harris, N.D., Seattle, Washington

Joseph Hattersley, M.A., Olympia, Washington

Ross Hauser, M.D., Co-author, *Prolo Your Pain Away*; founding Medical Director, Caring Medical and Rehabilitation Services, Oak Park, Illinois

Christopher J. Hegarty, Novato, California

Jane Heimlich, Author of *What Your Doctor Won't Tell You*, Cincinnati, Ohio

Joseph Heller, Founder and Director, Hellerwork, Mt. Shasta, California

Eileen Henry, L.Ac., Director, Institute of Psycho-Structural Balancing, Santa Monica, California

Silena Heron, N.D., R.N., Sedona, Arizona

John Hibbs, N.D., Natural Health Clinic, Seattle, Washington

Roger C. Hirsh, O.M.D., L.Ac., Dipl. (NCCA), Santa Monica, California

Christopher Hobbs, L.Ac., Author, *Foundations of Health: Healing With Herbs and Foods*

Philip Hoekstra, Ph.D., Thermoscan, Inc., Huntington Woods, Michigan

Abram Hoffer, M.D., Ph.D., F.R.C.P., Founder of the Canadian Schizophrenia Foundation; Editor-in-Chief, *Journal of Orthomolecular Medicine*, Victoria, British Columbia, Canada

David Hoffmann, B.Sc., M.N.I.M.H., past President, American Herbalists Guild, Sebastopol, California

Jay M. Holder, M.D., D.C., Ph.D., 1991 Winner, Albert Schweitzer Prize in Medicine; Director, Holder Research Institute, Miami, Florida

Joy Holm, Ph.D., University of California at Santa Cruz, Santa Cruz, California

Mark Holmes, O.M.D., L.Ac., Dipl.Ac. (NCCA), Director, Center for Regeneration, Beverly Hills, California

Leonard G. Horowitz, D.M.D., M.A., M.P.H., Co-author, *Emerging Viruses: AIDS and Ebola—Nature, Accident, or Intentional?*

Susanne Houd, M.D., midwife, Program Director, Department of Midwifery, The Michener Institute, Toronto, Ontario, Canada

Janet Hranicky, Ph.D., Founder and President, American Health Institute, Los Angeles, California

Tori Hudson, N.D., Co-author, *Women's Encyclopedia of Natural Medicine*; former Academic Dean, National College of Naturopathic Medicine, Portland, Oregon

Richard P. Huemer, M.D., Medical Director, Cascade Park Health Center, Vancouver, Washington

Vicki Hufnagel, M.D., Beverly Hills, California

Hal A. Huggins, D.D.S., M.S., Author, *Uninformed Consent: The Hidden Dangers of Dental Care*; President, Matrix, Inc., Colorado Springs, Colorado

David Hughes, Ph.D., The Hyperbaric Oxygen Institute, San Bernardino, California

Bonnie Humiston, R.N., M.S., Director, The Feldenkrais Guild, Salem, Oregon

Karl Humiston, M.D., Salem, Oregon

Valerie Hunt, Ph.D., Professor Emeritus, University of California at Los Angeles, Los Angeles, California

Corazon Ibarra-Ilarina, M.D., H.M.D., Biomedical Health Center, Reno, Nevada

Robert S. Ivker, D.O., Author of six books, including *Sinus Survival*; President-Elect, American Board of Holistic Medicine, Littleton, Colorado

Christine Jackson, Editor, *Explore* magazine, Mt. Vernon, Washington

Jennifer Jacobs, M.D., M.P.H., Director, Evergreen Center for Homeopathic Medicine, Edmonds, Washington

Robert H. Jacobs, N.M.D., D.Hom. (Med), Society for Complementary Medicine, London, England

Terry S. Jacobs, N.M.D., D.Hom. (Med), Director, College of Homeopathy, Santa Monica, California

Roger Jahnke, L.Ac., O.M.D., Author, *The Healing Promise of Qi*; Chairperson, National Qigong Association; Director, Health Action, Santa Barbara, California

Philip A. Jenkins, D.D.S., Los Gatos, California

Bernard Jensen, D.C., Ph.D., Author, *Nature Cures*; Founder and Director, Valley Ranch, Escondido, California

Carol Jessup, M.D., El Cerrito, California

Kris Johnson, Director of Public Relations and Marketing, Western States Training Associates, NLP of Utah, Salt Lake City, Utah

Eric Jones, N.D., Dean of Academic Affairs, Bastyr University, Kenmore, Washington

Deane Juhan, Author of *Job's Body*; Trager Instructor, Mill Valley, California

James J. Julian, M.D., Los Angeles, California

Jon Kabat-Zinn, Ph.D., Associate Professor of Medicine; Founder and Director, Stress Reduction Clinic, University of Massachusetts Medical Center, Worcester, Massachusetts

Konrad Kail, N.D., Author, *Allergy Free*; Member of the Advisory Council to the National Center for Complementary and Alternative Medicine (NCCAM); past President of the American Association of Naturopathic Physicians, Phoenix, Arizona

Jon Kaiser, M.D., Author, *Immune Power: A Comprehensive Treatment Program for HIV*; San Francisco, California

Harvey Kaltsas, Ac.Phys. (FL), D.Ac. (RI), Dipl.Ac. (NCCA), Sarasota, Florida

Ellen Kamhi, Ph.D., R.N., H.N.C., Co-author, *Arthritis: An Alternative Medicine Definitive Guide*, New York, New York

Patricia Kaminski, Co-author, *Flower Essence Repertory*; Co-founder, Flower Essence Society, Nevada City, California

Patricia Kane, Ph.D., Millville, New Jersey

Leslie J. Kaslof, Author of *Wholistic Dimensions in Healing*

Richard Kaye, D.C., Director, Quantum Healing Center, San Diego, California

Raphael Kellman, M.D., New York, New York

Julian Kenyon, M.D., M.B., Ch.B., Southhampton, Hampshire, England

Dharma Singh Khalsa, M.D., Author, *Brain Longevity*; Director, Alzheimer's Prevention Foundation, Tucson, Arizona

Glenn King, Director, King Institute for Better Health, Dallas, Texas

Robert King, past President, American Massage Therapy Association; Co-director, Chicago School of Massage Therapy, Chicago, Illinois

Patrick Kingsley, M.B.B.S., L.R.C.P., D.Obst., R.C.O.G., Leicestershire, England

Dietrich Klinghart, M.D., Ph.D., President, American Academy of Neural Therapy, Seattle, Washington

Janet Konefal, Ph.D., M.P.H., C.A., Associate Professor, University of Miami School of Medicine, Miami, Florida

Constantine A. Kotsanis, M.D., Grapevine, Texas

Eugene Kozhevnikov, M.D., O.M.D., St. Petersburg, Russia

A .M. Krasner, Ph.D., Founder, American Board of Hypnotherapy, Santa Ana, California

Dolores Krieger, R.N., Ph.D., Author, *Living the Therapeutic Touch: Healing as Lifestyle*; Professor Emeritus, New York University Graduate School of Nursing; Founder of Therapeutic Touch, Port Chester, New York

Daniel F. Kripke, M.D., Department of Psychiatry, University of California at San Diego, San Diego, California

Fredi Kronenberg, Ph.D., Columbia University Department of Rehabilitation Medicine, College of Physicians and Surgeons, New York, New York

Tom Kruzel, N.D., Scottsdale, Arizona

Paul J. Kulkosky, Ph.D., Professor of Psychology, University of Southern Colorado

Richard A. Kunin, M.D., Orthomolecular Medicine and Psychiatry, San Francisco, California

Roy Kupsinel, M.D., Editor and Publisher, *Health Consciousness*, Oviedo, Florida

Marc LaBel, O.M.D., L.Ac., Los Angeles, California

Vasant Lad, M.A.Sc., Author, *Ayurveda: The Science of Self-Healing*; Director, The Ayurvedic Institute, Albuquerque, New Mexico

Rima Laibow, M.D., founding Medical Director, Alexandria Institute, Croton-on-Hudson, New York

Gary LaLonde, C.Ht., President, Premiere Performance Inc., Wales, Michigan

Raymond W. Lam, M.D., Department of Psychiatry, University of British Columbia

Susan Lange, O.M.D., Co-director, Meridian Health Center, Santa Monica, California

Susan Lark, M.D., Author, *Dr. Susan Lark's Menopause Self-Help Book*; Director, Menopause and PMS Self-Help Center, Los Altos, California

Tim Leasenby, D.C., Aurora, Illinois

John R. Lee, M.D., Author, *What Your Doctor May Not Tell You About Menopause*, Sebastopol, California

Lita Lee, Ph.D., Author of *The Enzyme Cure*, Lowell, Oregon

Martin Lee, Ph.D., Director, Great Smokies Diagnostic Laboratory, Asheville, North Carolina

Michael Lesser, M.D., Berkeley, California

Buck Levin, Ph.D., R.D., Assistant Professor of Nutrition, Bastyr University, Kenmore, Washington

Emil Levin, M.D., Medical Director, Holistic Medical Center, West Hollywood, California

Warren Levin, M.D., F.A.A.F.P., F.A.C.N., F.A.C.A.I., Medical Director, World Health Medical Group, New York, New York

Stephen Levine, Ph.D., Founder and President, Allergy Research Group, San Leandro, California

Thomas E. Levy, M.D., J.D., Peak Energy Performance, Colorado Springs, Colorado

Douglas C. Lewis, N.D., former Chairperson of Physical Medicine, Bastyr University Natural Health Clinic, Seattle, Washington

Susana Alcázar Leyva, M.D., President of the Albert Szent-Gyorgy Gerontological Center; Vice President of the Hans Selye Institute of Scientific Research, Mexico City, Mexico

Jacob Liberman, O.D., Ph.D., past President, College of Syntonic Optometry; Director, Aspen Center for Energy Medicine, Aspen, Colorado

Edward Lichten, M.D., Southfield, Michigan

Molly Linton, N.D., L.M., Seattle, Washington

Andrew H. Lockie, M.R.C.G.P., M.F. Hom., Dip. Obst., R.C.O.G., Guildford, Surrey, England

Nancy Lonsdorf, M.D., Medical Director, Maharishi Ayurveda Medical Association, Washington, D.C.

Evarts Loomis, M.D., F.A.C.S., Co-founder, American Holistic Medical Association; Founder, Meadowlark Holistic Health Retreat, Hemet, California

Howard F. Loomis, Jr., D.C., Madison, Wisconsin

Nicholas J. Lowe, M.D., Director, Skin Research Foundation of California; Clinical Professor, Department of Dermatology, U.C.L.A. School of Medicine, Los Angeles, California

Wolfgang Ludwig, Sc.D., Ph.D., Director, Institute for Biophysics, Horb, Germany

Jeff Maitland, Faculty Chair, The Rolf Institute, Boulder, Colorado

Marshall Mandell, M.D., F.A.C.A.I., F.A.A.E.M., Fellow of the American College of Allergists; Author, *5-Day Allergy Relief System;* Medical Director, New England Foundation for Allergies and Environmental Diseases, Norwalk, Connecticut

Peter Guy Manners, M.D., D.O., Ph.D., Director, Bretforton Hall Clinic, Bretforton, Worcestershire, England

Rick Marinelli, N.D., M.Ac.O.M., President, Naturopathic Physicians Acupuncture Association, Beaverton, Oregon

Jeffrey L. Marrongelle, D.C., C.C.N., Schuylkill Haven, Pennsylvania

Hugh McGrath, Jr., M.D., Associate Professor, Department of Rheumatology, Louisiana State University Medical Center, New Orleans, Louisiana

Paul McTaggart, President and Founder, Progressive Nutrition, Ventura, California

Faizi Medeiros, N.D., Director, Upper Valley Naturopathic Clinic, Norwich, Vermont

Bruce Milliman, N.D., Associate Professor of Medicine, Bastyr University, Kenmore, Washington

Robert D. Milne, M.D., Co-author, *Alternative Medicine Definitive Guide to Headaches*, Las Vegas, Nevada

Gerald Montgomery, M.D., Director, New Mexico Orthopedic Medicine and Pain Treatment Clinic, Albuquerque, New Mexico

Warwick L. Morrison, M.D., Associate Professor of Dermatology, Johns Hopkins University, Baltimore, Maryland

Richard Moskowitz, M.D., Watertown, Massachusetts

Gowri Motha, M.D., London, England

Filibert Muñoz, M.D., Instituto Medico Biologico, Tijuana, Mexico

Robin Munro, Ph.D., Director, Yoga Biomedical Trust, Cambridge, England

Michael T. Murray, N.D., Co-author, *Encyclopedia of Natural Medicine*, Issaquah, Washington

Gaston Naessens, Director, Center for Experimental Research and Biologics, Rock Forest, Quebec, Canada

Margaret Naesser, Ph.D., Dipl.Ac. (NCCA), Associate Research Professor of Neurology, Boston University School of Medicine, Boston, Massachusetts

Robert A. Nagourney, M.D., Long Beach, California

Devi S. Nambudripad, D.C., L.Ac., R.N., Ph.D., Author, *Say Goodbye to Illness*, Buena Park, California

Richard A. Neubauer, M.D., Author, *Hyperbaric Oxygen Therapy*; Director, Ocean Hyperbaric Center, Lauderdale-by-the-Sea, Florida

Randall Neustaedter, O.M.D., L.Ac., C.C.H., Author, *The Vaccine Guide: Making an Informed Choice*; Redwood City, California

Rex E. Newnham, Ph.D., D.O., M.D., Director, Arthritis and Rheumatism Natural Health Association, North Yorkshire, England

Daoshing Ni, D.O.M., Ph.D., L.Ac., Tao of Wellness Center, Santa Monica, California

Maoshing Ni, D.O.M., Ph.D., L.Ac., Co-author, *Tao of Nutrition*; President, Yo San University of Traditional Chinese Medicine, Marina del Rey, California

Robert Norett, D.C., Director, Stillpoint Health Center, Venice, California

Patricia A. Norris, Ph.D., Co-founder, Life Sciences Institute of Mind-Body Health, Topeka, Kansas

Christiane Northrup, M.D., F.A.C.O.G., Author, *Women's Bodies, Women's Wisdom*; past President, American Holistic Medical Association, Yarmouth, Maine

Gary Null, Ph.D. Author, *Gary Null's Ultimate Lifetime Diet*, New York, New York

Gary R. Oberg, M.D., F.A.A.P., F.A.A.E.M., past President, American Academy of Environmental Medicine; Medical Director, Crystal Lake Center for Allergy and Environmental Medicine, Crystal Lake, Illinois

Katherine O'Hanlan, M.D., Co-author of *Natural Menopause: Guide to a Woman's Most Misunderstood Passage*; Associate Director of Stanford University's Gynecologic Cancer Section, Palo Alto, California

Mary Olsen, D.C., Huntington, New York

David W. Orme-Johnson, Ph.D., Chairman, Department of Psychology, Maharishi International University, Fairfield, Iowa

Humphrey Osmond, M.D., M.R.C.P., F.R.C. Psy., Bryce Nova Program, Tuscaloosa, Alabama

Frank Ottiwell, Director, Alexander Training Institute, San Francisco, California

Sujata Owens, R.S.Hom., Northfield, Minnesota

Tonis Pai, M.D., Kivimae Hospital, Tallin, Estonia

Hazel Parcells, N.D., D.C., Ph.D., Founder, Parcells Center, Santa Fe, New Mexico

Richard Passwater, Ph.D., Executive Vice President, Solgar Nutritional Research Center, Berlin, Maryland

Terry Patten, President, Tools for Exploration, San Rafael, California

David Paul, M.D., Medical Director, Vail Valley Medical Center, Vail, Colorado

Linus Pauling, Ph.D., (1901-1994), Two-time Nobel laureate: Chemistry (1954), Peace (1962); Director, Linus Pauling Institute of Science and Medicine, Palo Alto, California

Larry Payne, Ph.D., Director, Samata Yoga Center, President, International Association of Yoga Therapy, Los Angeles, California

Meyrick J. Peak, Ph.D., Senior Scientist, Argonne National Laboratory, Center of Mechanistic Biology, Argonne, Illinois

Raymond Peat, Ph.D., President, International College, Eugene, Oregon

Kenneth R. Pelletier, Ph.D., M.D. (Hon), Senior Clinical Fellow, Stanford Center for Research in Disease Prevention, Department of Medicine, Stanford University School of Medicine, Palo Alto, California

Gene Peniston, Ed.D., A.B.M.P., Chief, Psychology Service, Sam Rayburn Memorial Veterans Center, Bonham, Texas

Marvin Penwell, D.O., Director, Linden Medical Center, Linden, Michigan

Erik Peper, Ph.D., Associate Director, Institute for Holistic Healing Studies, San Francisco State University, San Francisco, California

Candace Pert, Ph.D., visiting Professor, Center for Molecular and Behavioral Neuroscience, Rutgers University, New Jersey

Janice K. Phelps, M.D., Author of *The Hidden Addiction and How to Get Free From It*, Sagle, Idaho

Harry H. Philibert, M.D., Metairie, Louisiana

William H. Philpott, M.D., Co-author, *Magnet Therapy: An Alternative Medicine Definitive Guide* and *Brain Allergies*; Chairman, Bio-Electro-Magnetics Institute Institutional Review Board, Choctaw, Oklahoma

Richard Pitcairn, D.V.M., Ph.D., Eugene, Oregon

John Pittman, M.D., Medical Director, CURE AIDS NOW, Salisbury, North Carolina

Joseph E. Pizzorno, N.D., Author of *Total Wellness;* President Emeritus, Bastyr University, Kenmore, Washington

Kent L. Pomeroy, M.D., Founder and past President, American Association of Orthopedic Medicine, Scottsdale, Arizona

Michelle Pouliot, N.D., Torrington, Connecticut

Maile Pouls, Ph.D., Co-author, *The Supplement Shopper*, Santa Cruz, California

John Powers, (1916-1999), past President, Prentice Hall, Aspen, Colorado

Marvin Prescott, D.M.D., Los Angeles, California

Joan Priestley, M.D., Anchorage, Alaska

James Privitera, M.D., Medical Director, NutriScreen, Inc., Covina, California

Gus J. Prosch, Jr., M.D., Biomed Associates, P.C., Birmingham, Alabama

Bonnie Prudden, C.B.P.M., Author, *Pain Erasure*; Director, Institute for Physical Fitness and Myotherapy, Stockbridge, Massachusetts

Fernando C. Ramirez del Rio, M.D., International Head and Spinal Injury Center, Tijuana, Mexico

Theron G. Randolph, M.D., (1906-1995), President, Human Ecology Research Foundation, Batavia, Illinois; Founder of the field of environmental medicine

Karl Ransberger, M.D., Medizinische, Enzymeforschungsgesellschaft, Geretstried, Germany

Doris J. Rapp, M.D., F.A.A.A., F.A.A.P., F.A.A.E.M., Clinical Assistant Professor of Pediatrics, State University of New York at Buffalo; past President, American Academy of Environmental Medicine, Buffalo, New York

Matthias Rath, M.D., Author, *Eradicating Heart Disease*; former Director, Linus Pauling Institute of Science and Medicine, Palo Alto, California

Thomas Rau, M.D., Medical Director, Paracelsus Clinic, Switzerland

Harold Ravins, D.D.S., Los Angeles, California

William Rea, M.D., Dallas, Texas

William Reed, M.D., Vice President, California Homeopathic Medical Association; Center for Health, Santa Monica, California

Michelle Reillo, B.S.N., R.N., Author, *AIDS Under Pressure*; Lifeforce Hyperbaric Oxygen Institute, Baltimore, Maryland

Joseph Riccioli, C.Ht. NBCDCH, Director, Hypnosis Healing Center, Totowa, New Jersey

Bernard Rimland, Ph.D., Director, Autism Research Institute, San Diego, California

Douglas Ringrose, M.D., Director, Ringrose Wellness Institute, Edmonton, Alberta, Canada

Hugh D. Riordan, M.D., Director, Center for the Improvement of Human Functioning, Wichita, Kansas

Neil Riordan, M.S., P.A.-C., President, Aidan Inc., Tempe, Arizona

Berndt Rohrmann, M.D., Heidelberg, Germany

Terry Rondberg, D.C., Author, *Chiropractic First*; President, World Chiropractic Alliance, Chandler, Arizona

Gary S. Ross, M.D., San Francisco, California

Harvey M. Ross, M.D., Los Angeles, California

Herbert Ross, D.C., Co-author, *Sleep Disorders: An Alternative Medicine Definitive Guide*, Aspen, Colorado

Martin L. Rossman, M.D., Author, *Guided Imagery for Self-Healing*; Co-founder, Academy for Guided Imagery, Mill Valley, California

Jonathan Rothschild, President, Cardiovascular Research, Concord, California

Robert Jay Rowen, M.D., Director, Omni Medical Center, Anchorage, Alaska

Daniel F. Royal, D.O., The Nevada Clinic, Las Vegas, Nevada

F. Fuller Royal, M.D., Medical Director, The Nevada Clinic, Las Vegas, Nevada

Theodore Rozema, M.D., F.A.A.F.P., President, Great Lake Association of Clinical Medicine; Sec., American Board of Chelation Therapy, Landrum, South Carolina

Dante Ruccio, N.D., Adjunct Professor, La Salle University, Newark, New Jersey

Mary Kay Ryan, Dipl.Ac. NCCA, Co-founder, AIDS Alternative Health Project and Northside HIV Treatment Center, Chicago, Illinois

Billie Jay Sahley, Ph.D., Director, Pain and Stress Center, San Antonio, Texas

Debra Nuzzi St. Claire, M.H., Boulder, Colorado

Trevor K. Salloum, N.D., Kelowna, British Columbia, Canada

Michael B. Schachter, M.D., Suffern, New York

Mary Pullig Schatz, M.D., Author, *Back Care Basics*; President, Medical Staff, Centennial Medical Center, Nashville, Tennessee

Alexander Schauss, Ph.D., former Executive Director, Citizens for Health, Washington, D.C.

Luc De Schepper, M.D., Ph.D., Lic.Ac., C.Hom., D.I. Hom., Santa Fe, New Mexico

Michael A. Schmidt, B.S., D.C., C.C.N., Director, Brookview Health Sciences, Anoka, Minnesota

Kurt Schnaubelt, Ph.D., Author, *Advanced Aromatherapy*; Director, Pacific Institute of Aromatherapy, San Rafael, California

Therese Schroder-Sheker, Executive Director, The Chalice of Repose Project; Professor of Music-Thanatology, St. Patrick Hospital, Missoula, Montana

Anthony Scott-Morley, D.Sc., Ph.D., B.A., B.Ac., M.D. (Alt. Med.), Director, Institute of Bioenergetic Medicine; Member of the World Research Foundation, Dorset, England

K. Warner Shaie, Ph.D., Pennsylvania State University, State College, Pennsylvania

Frank Shallenberger, M.D., H.M.D., Director, Nevada Center of Alternative and Anti-Aging Medicine, Carson City, Nevada

Deane Shapiro, Ph.D., Professor in Residence, Department of Psychiatry and Human Behavior, California College of Medicine, University of California at Irvine, Irvine, California

Hari Sharma, M.D., F.R.C.P.C., Professor Emeritus, Ohio State University College of Medicine and Public Health, Columbus, Ohio

C. Norman Shealy, M.D., Ph.D., Author, *Sacred Healing*; Co-founder and first President, American Holistic Medical Association; Director, Shealy Institute for Comprehensive Health Care; Professor of Psychology, Forest Institute of Professional Psychology, Springfield, Missouri

David K. Shefrin, N.D., Beaverton, Oregon

John A. Sherman, N.D., Seattle, Washington

Benjamin Shield, Ph.D., Certified Rolfer, Craniosacral Therapist, Pacific Health Resources, Santa Monica, California

Bernie Siegel, M.D., Author, *Love, Medicine, and Miracles*; Founder of ECaP (Exceptional Cancer Patients), New Haven, Connecticut

Charles Siemers, Certified Rolfer, Manhattan Beach, California

Penny Simkin, P.T., Co-author, *Pregnancy, Childbirth and the Newborn*; Seattle, Washington

David Simon, M.D., Medical Director, Chopra Center for Well-Being, La Jolla, California

Carl Simonton, M.D., Board Certified, Director, Simonton Cancer Center, Pacific Palisades, California; Director, Psychoneuroimmunology Counseling Program, Cancer Treatment Centers of America, Brea, California

Stephen T. Sinatra, M.D., New England Heart Center, Manchester, Connecticut

Alicia Sirkin, B.F.R.P., Miami, Florida

Solomon Slobins, O.D., Director, College of Syntonic Optometry, Fall River, Massachusetts

Marian Small, N.D., L.Ac., Seattle, Washington

C. Tom Smith, M.D., Ph.D., H.M.D., D.Hom. (Med.), Director, International Clinic of Biological Regeneration (North American Office), Florissant, Missouri

Lendon H. Smith, M.D., Author of 13 books, including *Feed Your Kids Right*, Portland, Oregon

Michael Smith, M.D., Medical Director, Lincoln Hospital, Substance Abuse Division, New York, New York

Virender Sodhi, M.D. (Ayurveda), N.D., Founder and Director, Ayurvedic and Naturopathic Medical Clinic, Bellevue, Washington

Pierre Sollier, M.F.C.C., Lafayette, California

Hector Solorzano Del Rio, M.D., D.Sc., President, Society of Investigation of Acupuncture and Oriental Medicine; Coordinator, Program for Studies of Alternative Medicine; Professor of Pharmacology, University of Guadalajara, Mexico

Nick Soloway, L.M.T., D.C., L.Ac., Portland, Oregon

Anne H. Spencer, Ph.D., C.Ht., Founder and Executive Director, International Medical and Dental Hypnotherapy Association

Ralph Sprintge, M.D., Head, Interdisciplinary Pain Clinic and Music Medicine Research Labs at Sport-Krankenhaus Hellersen; Executive Director, International Society for Music in Medicine, Germany

William H. Stager, M.S., D.O., The Upledger Institute, Palm Beach Gardens, Florida

Leana Standish, N.D., Ph.D., Director of Research, Bastyr University, Kenmore, Washington

Jill Stansbury, N.D., Battle Ground, Washington

John Steele, Ph.D., Lifetree Aromatix, Sherman Oaks, California

David A. Steenblock, M.S., D.O., Mission Viejo, California

Joanne Stefanatos, D.V.M., Animal Kingdom Veterinary Hospital; President, American Holistic Veterinary Medical Association, Las Vegas, Nevada

Zannah Steiner, C.M.P., R.M.T., Soma Therapy Centre, Vancouver, British Columbia, Canada

Peter M. Stephan, M.D. (Hom.), M.Sc., Kt. Comm., O.S.J.J., Founder, The Stephan Clinic, London, England

Michael Stern, D.C., Founder and Director, Research for Alternative Medicine (RAM) Foundation

Jesse Stoff, M.D., Tuscon, Arizona

Ralph Strauch, Ph.D., certified Feldenkrais practitioner, Los Angeles, California

Gerard V. Sunnen, M.D., Associate Clinical Professor of Psychiatry, New York University Bellevue Hospital Medical Center, New York, New York

Murray R. Susser, M.D., Medical Director, Omnidox Medical Group, Santa Monica, California

Roy Swank, M.D., Ph.D., Director, Swank Multiple Sclerosis Clinic, School of Medicine, Oregon Health Sciences University, Portland, Oregon

John M. Sward, Ph.D., Director of Counseling, Center for the Improvement of Human Functioning, Wichita, Kansas

Glen M. Swartwout, O.D., F.I.C.A.N., F.S.C.O., Founder, Achievement of Excellence Research Academy International; President, Starfire International, Hilo, Hawaii

Joyal Taylor, D.D.S., Author, *Complete Guide to Mercury Toxicity from Dental Fillings*; President, The Environmental Dental Association, Rancho Santa Fe, California

Michael Terman, Ph.D., Director, Light Therapy Unit, New York State Psychiatric Institute, New York, New York

Dick Thom, D.D.S., N.D., Beaverton, Oregon

Billie M. Thompson, Ph.D., Director, Sound, Listening, and Learning Center, Phoenix, Arizona

Kay Thompson, D.D.S., Pittsburgh, Pennsylvania

Carvel Tiekert, D.V.M., Bel Air, Maryland

William Tiller, Ph.D., Author, *Science and Human Transformation*; Professor Emeritus, Stanford University, Palo Alto, California

Robert Tisserand, Editor, *International Journal of Aromatherapy*, Hove, East Sussex, England

Desmond Tivy, M.D., Lee, Massachusetts

Marjorie K. Toomim, Ph.D., Director, Biofeedback Institute of Los Angeles, Los Angeles, California

Joseph Trachtman, O.D., Ph.D., Brooklyn, New York

Elias Tsambis, M.D., A.B.P.N., Director of Medicine, New York Institute of Medical Research, Nyack, New York

Dennis Tucker, Ph.D., L.Ac., Sierra Acupuncture Clinic, Nevada City, California

Dana Ullman, M.P.H., Author, *Discovering Homeopathy*; Director, Homeopathic Educational Services, Berkeley, California

Joseph F. Unger, Jr., D.C., D.I.C.S., Chairman, SacroOccipital Research Society International (SORSI), Prairie Village, Kansas

John E. Upledger, D.O., O.M.M., Author, *Your Inner Physician and You*; Fellow of the American Academy of Osteopathy; Medical Director, Upledger Institute, Upledger Foundation, Palm Beach Gardens, Florida

Matt Van Benschoten, O.M.D., M.A., C.A., Reseda, California

Joseph Vargas, Ph.D., Founder and Director, Wholistic Health Center, Houston, Texas

Gary Verigan, D.D.S., Escalon, California

Anne Vermilye, M.S., C.C.H.T., C.M.T., Mill Valley, California

George von Hilsheimer, Ph.D., Diplomate of the American Academy of Pain Management, Maitland, Florida

Marika von Viczay, N.D., Ph.D., Asheville, North Carolina

Dietrich Wabner, Dr. (rer. nat.), Hon. I.F.A. and Forum Essenzia; President, Natural Oils Research Association, Windsor, England; Professor, Technical University, Munich, Germany

Scott Walker, D.C., Encinitas, California

Charles Wallach, D.Sc., Ph.D., President, Behavioral Research Association; Director, AIDS Policy Research Center, Canoga Park, California

William Walsh, Ph.D., Carl Pfeiffer Treatment Center, Naperville, Illinois

Dale Walters, Ph.D., Director of Education, Center of Applied Psychophysiology, Menninger Clinic, Topeka, Kansas

Gunther M. Weil, Ph.D., Aspen, Colorado

Melvyn R. Werbach, M.D., Author, *Nutritional Influences on Illness*; former Assistant Clinical Professor at the School of Medicine, University of California at Los Angeles; retired Director of the Biofeedback Medical Clinic, Tarzana, California

Toni Weschler, M.P.H., Founder, FACTS (Fertility Awareness Counseling and Training Seminars), Seattle, Washington

Bill Wesson, D.D.S., Aspen, Colorado

Jo Anne Whitaker, M.D., F.A.A.P., Director, Bowen Research and Training Institute, Palm Harbor, Florida

Julian Whitaker, M.D., Founder, American Preventive Medical Association; Editor, *Health & Healing*; Director, Whitaker Wellness Institute, Newport Beach, California

Harold Whitcomb, M.D., Director, Aspen Clinic for Preventive and Environmental Medicine, Aspen, Colorado

Richard S. Wilkinson, M.D., Director, Yakima Allergy Clinic, Yakima, Washington

Jacquelyn J. Wilson, M.D., D.Ht., past President, American Institute of Homeopathy, Escondido, California

Rex Wilson, N.D., Beverly Hills, California

Honora Lee Wolfe, Dipl.Ac., Author, *Managing Menopause Naturally With Chinese Medicine*; Iris Acupuncture Health Care Associates, Boulder, Colorado

Helen M. Wood, L.M.T., Director, Wood Hygenic Institute, Kissimmee, Florida

Jonathan Wright, M.D., Director, Tahoma Clinic, Kent, Washington

Jing-Nuan Wu, O.M.D., L.Ac., Director, Taoist Center, Washington, D.C.

Ray C. Wunderlich, Jr., M.D., Preventive/Nutritional Medicine, St. Petersburg, Florida

Paul Yanick, Jr., Ph.D., Woodbridge, New Jersey

Judy Zacharski, P.T., Director, Facial Pain and TMJ Clinic, Menomonee Falls, Wisconsin

Eugene Zampieron, N.D., A.H.G., Co-author, *Arthritis: An Alternative Medicine Definitive Guide*, Woodbury, Connecticut

Jared L. Zeff, N.D., L.Ac., Academic Dean, National College of Naturopathic Medicine, Portland, Oregon

Qingcai Zhang, M.D. (China), Lic.Ac., New York, New York

Rong-Rong Zheng, M.D., Director of Research, Qi-Gong Institute of Shanghai Academy of Traditional Chinese Medicine, San Francisco, California

Michael F. Ziff, D.D.S., Co-author, *Dentistry Without Mercury*; Foundation for Toxic-Free Dentistry, Orlando, Florida

Sam Ziff, Ph.D., Co-author, *Dental Mercury Detox*; Foundation for Toxic-Free Dentistry, Orlando, Florida

John Zimmerman, Ph.D., Diplomate, American Board of Sleep Medicine; Director, Bio-Electro-Magnetics Institute; Mountain Medical Sleep Center, Carson City, Nevada

INTRODUCTION TO THE SECOND EDITION

BY BURTON GOLDBERG

TWO SYSTEMS OF health care exist in the United States today: conventional Western medicine and alternative medicine. The first is the world of the American Medical Association—medical doctors who rely on drugs and surgery to treat disease symptoms and who inadvertently align themselves with the multi-billion-dollar pharmaceutical industry. Conventional medicine is superb in dealing with acute medical conditions and traumatic injury, and in providing emergency treatment. But there's no question that alternative medicine works better for just about everything else, especially for chronic degenerative diseases like cancer, heart disease, and rheumatoid arthritis, and for more common ailments such as asthma, gastrointestinal disorders, and headaches.

Alternative medicine is more cost-effective in the long term, because it emphasizes prevention and goes after causes rather than symptoms. Many alternative methods work by assisting your body to heal itself. It doesn't trap people on the merry-go-round that begins with one drug and requires them to take others to compensate for the side effects each one causes. You probably know someone who has had the experience of getting rid of one illness, only to come down with another from the procedure used by the doctor. Maybe that someone is you. People I love, including my son and both of my parents, have suffered through medical procedures that were unnecessarily traumatic because their physicians neglected the basics.

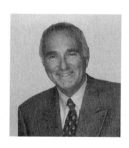

Everything you'll read about in the pages that follow has been rigorously verified by the health experts themselves, in order to give you what you need to achieve optimal health.

Alternative medicine has a lot to offer you. But our government is ignoring its well-established methods and federal funds are not being sufficiently allocated to study them. This was true when the first edition of this book was published in 1993 and it remains true today. But alternative medicine has made great strides over the last decade and interest in alternative therapies continues to skyrocket. More than two-thirds of all Americans now employ some form of alternative medicine to prevent and treat disease, and research is increasingly validating the effectiveness of alternative modalities for a variety of health conditions. We can continue to change the system by channeling our consumer medical dollars toward a more humane and effective medicine.

I never expected the study of alternative medicine to become the passion of my life. But when the 19-year-old daughter of a friend tried to commit suicide, I had to find a way to help. Most people would send her to a psychologist and figure that's the answer. But it wasn't the answer. Her therapist finally threw his hands up and suggested vitamin therapy, so we pursued it. We found out that the daughter's mental distress was caused by hypoglycemia, an imbalance created by food allergies, problems in her pancreas, and an overgrowth of harmful bacteria in her gastrointestinal tract. When she was treated for hypoglycemia, her mental illness disappeared. She is now a healthy mother of eight children.

That's how it started for me—seeing people who had a serious illness being cured just by changing their lifestyle and diet and taking nutritional supplements. The amazing success I saw got me hooked. One Connecticut doctor, Marshall Mandell, M.D., dramatically showed me how a person's state of mind could be affected when exposed to a substance to which they were allergic. He brought a very bright woman in and out of depression simply by placing different substances under her tongue. A single dose of one allergenic substance caused her to put her head between her knees and cry. When she was given a relieving dose, she experienced instantaneous release.

This episode sparked my interest in environmental medicine, the study of how substances affect the body. From there, I looked into such alternatives as homeopathy, electromagnetic diagnosing and treatment, mind/body medicine, and the newest protocols for cancer. My interest in new concepts in health care led me to Europe, Russia, and Israel. There I discovered people being cured of diseases, even the most serious, by methods never even heard of in the U.S.

It is possible to reverse chronic disease. Many of the health problems you face can be solved simply, directly, and inexpensively without toxic side effects. The alternatives in this book are sound, based on science, and really work. Many are natural as opposed to drug-based therapies. I've seen dramatic healing in a wide range of serious cases, without the disturbing side effects mainstream medicine so often creates. The procedures are available and being used now, but you won't hear about them from your doctor.

Your well-being—and that of your family—depends on knowing about these alternatives. That's why a team of over 400 leading medical doctors, naturopaths, osteopaths, homeopaths, chiropractors, acupuncturists, scientists, researchers, and reporters were assembled to produce this work. With this new edition, we have continued our investigation into the most current discoveries in alternative medicine to create a thoroughly revised and updated version. As always, our goal is to provide you with the latest and most credible information on the widest range of viable alternative health-care options.

In light of the burgeoning interest alternative medicine is now receiving from patients and doctors alike, having such information at your disposal is more critical than ever before. In order to benefit from unconventional medical techniques, you must be able to distinguish between what works and what doesn't. Empowering you to do so is the reason this book exists. It represents the collective wisdom of alternative physicians and researchers worldwide, and you can be assured that everything you'll read about in the pages that follow has been rigorously verified by the health experts themselves, in order to give you what you need to achieve optimal health.

Let me conclude by saying that I'm not against mainstream, conventional medicine. The Chinese have a saying about the wisdom of "walking on both feet," which means in this context using the best of Eastern and Western procedures. There is no single approach that works for all people or with all conditions. This goes for alternative medicine as well. Experience shows that you're likely to get the best results with a practitioner who has trained in a number of modalities. There may be many underlying factors influencing your health—nutritional deficiency, poor digestion, toxicity from environmental pollutants, or mental and emotional stress. You want a practitioner who is capable of determining exactly what needs to be done to help you regain health and vitality. You also want an open-minded practitioner who treats you as an individual. What's good for Harry is not necessarily good for Mary—you are biochemically unique.

Let your journey to health begin with the information in this book. Here is an optimistic and totally realistic thought to carry with you: most everything is reversible—you need only find the right therapies. Be well and God bless!

My dear Kepler, what do you say of the leading philosophers here, to whom I have offered a thousand times of my own accord to show my studies, but who, with the lazy obstinacy of a serpent who has eaten his fill, have never consented to look at the planets or moon, or telescope? Verily, just as serpents close their ears, so do men close their eyes to the light of truth.

—GALILEO IN A LETTER TO JOHANNES KEPLER, CIRCA 1630

Part One

Medicine for the 21st Century

UNDERSTANDING
ALTERNATIVE MEDICINE

I N THE FACE OF AN increasingly inadequate system of conventional medicine, a growing number of people are turning to alternative medicine to address their needs. Growing numbers of Americans now recognize the effectiveness of alternative medicine's approach to health, which blends body and mind, science and experience, and traditional and cross-cultural avenues of diagnosis and treatment. In 1993, a study published in the *New England Journal of Medicine* found that over a third of those surveyed chose alternative medicine over conventional methods, because of the medical establishment's emphasis on diagnostic testing and treatment with drugs without focusing on the patient as a whole.[1] More recent studies show that more than two-thirds of people in the United States and Canada now employ some form of alternative medicine to prevent and treat disease.[2] Moreover, in 1997 alone, $27 billion was spent by U.S. citizens for this purpose, most of which was paid for out-of-pocket since the majority of the treatments within the field of alternative medicine are not covered by health insurance, despite their proven efficacy.[3]

But perhaps the most telling statistic related to alternative medicine's growing popularity is a study that estimates that the per capita supply of alternative physicians will increase by 124% by 2010, compared to a growth rate of only 16% for conventional physicians. The study, conducted by the Health Policy Institute at the Medical College of Wisconsin, in Milwaukee, examined trends in three alternative therapies (acupuncture, chiropractic, and naturopathic medicine) that are currently

> *The doctor of the future will give no medicine, but will interest his patients in the care of the human frame, in diet, and in the cause and prevention of disease.*
>
> —THOMAS EDISON

licensed and regulated in the U.S. By 2010, a 230% growth rate is predicted for the supply of classical acupuncturists (excluding those who are M.D.s), while the number of chiropractors (D.C.s) and naturopaths (N.D.s) will double and triple, respectively.[4] It is obvious that what was once considered a "fringe" interest is well on its way to becoming the primary medical approach of the new millennium.

 See Acupuncture, Chiropractic, Naturopathic Medicine.

To fully appreciate this growing shift towards a new medical paradigm, however, it is important to understand what alternative medicine is and, just as importantly, *is not;* the current crisis in modern medicine and how it occurred; the various factors that contribute to both health and disease; and the steps we as individuals and as a nation must take in order to return to health.

What "Alternative Medicine" Means

In its broadest sense, the term *alternative medicine* is used simply to denote approaches to health and healing that do not rely on drugs, surgery, and/or other conventional medical procedures for treating illness. However, such a definition, accurate though it may be, fails to fully address the true scope of what alternative medicine is, how it works, and how its underlying philosophy differs from that of conventional medicine.

The Origins of Conventional Medicine

The roots of conventional medicine, meaning the drug- and surgery-based mainstream medical procedures that came into dominance in the early 20th century, can be traced back to the time of Rene Descartes (1596-1650), the famous scientist and philosopher whose work led certain of his followers to develop Cartesianism, a philosophy characterized by its rationalistic, dualistic worldview. A perhaps unintended consequence of Cartesianism was the separation of the "mind" from the "body." This ultimately led to the various fields of specialization that now comprise conventional medicine, each one of which focuses exclusively upon its particular branch of medicine and the organ system it treats, usually without regard for how the human organism and life itself are interwoven.

In the mid-19th century, the discovery of disease-causing microbes further added to the bedrock of conventional medical theory. At that time, there were two opposing theories concerning the cause of disease— one theory held that infecting microbes known as germs (bacteria, viruses, and fungi) caused illness, while the other maintained that such microbes only became infectious if conditions inside the body were right for them, due to imbalances in various body systems. According to the latter theory, keeping the body's internal environment healthy was the key to ensuring exposure to such microbes did not result in infection, and thus illness. But the former "germ theory of disease," which was advocated by Louis Pasteur (1822-1895), became dominant. This heralded the birth of modern medicine, with its emphasis on infectious causes of disease rather than on the creation and maintenance of physiological harmony and balance. As a result, modern medical science greatly expanded its role in the treatment of illness.

This was followed by the rapid development of microscopy, bacterial cultures, vaccines, X rays, and, in the 1930s, the discovery of antibacterial drugs (antibiotics) such as penicillin and sulfa drugs. However, the more that medical science embraced the germ theory of disease, the more it focused only on treating specific aspects of illness (symptoms) and superseded the individual's role in his or her own health. In the process, the role of conventional doctors increasingly moved away from that of teacher (*doctor* is derived from the Latin verb *docere*, meaning "to teach") to that of authoritarian figures whose advice patients are expected to unquestioningly follow.

It has also led to the organization of medical schools into various departments of specialty, such as cardiology, nephrology, neurology, dermatology, orthopedics, and psychiatry. This forces students to focus their study on one organ system at a time, as if each bodily organ functioned independently of all the others, or to choose one for exclusive study in preparation for a career in medicine as a specialist in that organ system.

"Our system of disease classification is based on specific organs as well," notes John R. Lee, M.D., of Sebastopol, California. "We name our diseases by the organ that is being affected. Thus we have arthritis, tonsillitis, appendicitis, heart or gallbladder disease, colitis, prostatitis, and many other examples. We even name the cancer we get by the organ it affects. This diverts attention away from the intrinsic interrelatedness of all parts of the body and the complex dynamism of life forces. It is no wonder that our 'modern' doctors understand so little of holistic concepts of health."

During his lifetime, German physician and chemist Samuel Hahnemann (1755-1843), the developer of homeopathy, recognized the inherent limitations of such a symptom-based approach to medicine, as well as its potential to cause harm (side effects) to patients. He coined the term *allopathy* (meaning "other suffering") to describe what, in his view, was a misguided and inadequate method of disease care and prevention.[5] From his term is derived the phrase *allopathic medicine* used to describe modern conventional medical methods.

The Philosophy of Alternative Medicine

The underlying concepts of alternative medicine are far older than those of conventional, allopathic medicine, and have, in fact, infused various healing traditions around the world since the dawn of recorded history. As early as 5,000 B.C.E., for example, "physician-sages" formulating the healing traditions of both traditional Chinese medicine (TCM) and Ayurvedic medicine (from India) recognized that human beings were comprised of body, mind, and spirit, and that health represented a harmonious balance within all three of these aspects of existence, as well as the free flow of invisible vital energy (known in China as *qi* and in India as *prana*) throughout the various body systems. Since that time, in healing traditions worldwide, medical wisdom evolved with a framework that linked health to this state of harmony and disease to a state of disharmony or imbalance, and took into account the multiple factors that contributed to both.

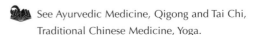 See Ayurvedic Medicine, Qigong and Tai Chi, Traditional Chinese Medicine, Yoga.

THE PURPOSE OF MEDICINE: WAR OR REPAIR?

The thrust of modern conventional medicine can be described by the metaphor of war. Disease is considered an invasion by an enemy and treatment is aimed at developing "magic bullets" in the form of drugs and vaccines to eliminate that enemy. We have seen, for example, a failed "war on cancer," a proliferation of antibiotics, and a growing number of surgical procedures, cell-killing radiation treatments, and chemical medications (such as chemotherapy), all of which do harm to the body, in one form or another, in their attempts to restore health.

Lost in this approach is the concept of repairing the imbalances that allow the illnesses to occur in the first place. Medical science has become one-sided in its focus, increasingly losing sight of the whole person in its attempt to treat the body's individual parts.

"A more useful metaphor for medicine would be repair, not war," says John R. Lee, M.D., of Sebastopol, California. "If we think of the body as a house, we see that problems lie in the gaps and breakdowns that occur in the foundation, allowing various pests to make their way inside. The contemporary physician addresses this problem by selling you poisons or traps to kill or catch the pests. But this still doesn't prevent other undesirables from coming in through the gaps in the future. How much better it would be for your physician to learn where the holes are and help you to repair them, while teaching you how to prevent them from occurring again."

Such a view also informed the philosophy of the ancient Greek physician Hippocrates (477-360 B.C.E.), the father of Western medicine. "The genius of Hippocrates," Dr. Lee points out, "was not in the drugs he used or his diagnostic skills, but in his insight that the elements which were needed to produce and maintain health were natural and that they included hygiene, a calm and balanced mental state, proper diet, a sound work and home environment, and physical conditioning. In addition, he recognized the life forces that pervade all of nature and which have multiple expressions, some known, some theorized, and many unknown. He taught that health depended upon living in harmony with these forces."

 See Diet, Environmental Medicine, Holistic Self-Care, Mind/Body Medicine.

These same tenets were also present in the healing traditions of ancient Africa, Amerindian cultures, and the cultures of other indigenous peoples. The primary role of healers and physicians in each of these traditions was to instruct others in the art and practice of living harmoniously with themselves and their environment, with emphasis placed on each of the above mentioned categories related to health. Only within the last few centuries has that emphasis changed, to the point where modern medicine has now become "increasingly one-sided in its focus, seeking out ever more powerful drugs to treat bacteria, viruses, fungi, and other microorganisms, while focusing on body parts and specialization to the point where the individual being treated is altogether forgotten."[6]

Recognizing the health risks and other dangers inherent in such a one-sided focus, alternative physicians have for the last few decades been in the vanguard among those educating health-care professionals and laypeople alike in the way in which alternative medicine can more safely and comprehensively deal with the modern health-care crisis. Among the leaders in this movement is C. Norman Shealy, M.D., Ph.D., of Springfield, Missouri, a world-renowned neurosurgeon who, in 1978, founded the American Holistic Medical Association (AHMA), the goal of which is "to provide a 'common community' for physicians committed to treating the 'whole person' according to the philosophy of holistic medicine."[7]

"Holistic medicine's comprehensive definition of health is at odds with our predominant health-care system, which is based almost entirely upon the diagnosis and treatment of disease symptoms," according to *The American Holistic Medical Association Guide to Holistic Health.* "While conventional medicine is unsurpassed in treating acute life-threatening illness and injuries, its reliance on pharmaceutical drugs and surgery has left it largely a failure in terms of handling chronic conditions."[8]

This view is shared by alternative physicians in general, all of whom recognize that the most effective form of health care treats the patient's entire being— body, mind, and spirit—and at the same time empowers patients by educating them in the many ways to take personal responsibility for their health. "The result," according to Robert S. Ivker, D.O., past President of the AHMA, and President-elect of the

American Board of Holistic Medicine, "is that their patients learn to safely and effectively treat any physical, mental, and spiritual condition that may be impeding the flow of vital energy in their lives, so that they not only start to get better, they also begin to thrive and experience more energy and joy in being alive. When this happens, there is a sense of harmony and balance in the physical, environmental, mental, emotional, spiritual, and social aspects of their lives." Ultimately, Dr. Ivker adds, the goal of holistic medical approaches is not simply to prevent and cure disease, but to help patients create and maintain optimal health, which he describes as "the unlimited and unimpeded free flow of life force energy throughout your body, mind, and spirit."[9]

The Best of Both Worlds

It is important to recognize that practitioners of alternative medicine are not opposed to conventional medical practices, and do not hesitate to employ them (either in their own practice or through referrals to conventional M.D.s) when appropriate. This is particularly true when dealing with patients faced with acute, life-threatening illnesses or injuries. Both systems of medicine have much to offer, and the wisest form of health care is one which makes use of each of them in an integrated manner that most fully meets patient needs.

The strengths and weaknesses of both systems are outlined in the table on page 8, created by Dr. Ivker.

Holistic Healing Principles

The following 12 principles, established by the board of trustees of the American Holistic Medical Association, lie at the heart of the new paradigm of health care that is emerging in the 21st century.[10]

1. Holistic physicians embrace a variety of safe, effective diagnostic and treatment options. These include education for lifestyle changes and self-care, complementary diagnostic and treatment approaches, and conventional drugs and surgery.

2. Searching for the underlying causes of disease is preferable to treating symptoms alone.

3. Holistic physicians expend as much effort in establishing what kind of patient has a disease as they do in establishing what kind of disease a patient has.

4. Prevention is preferable to treatment and is usually more cost-effective. The most cost-effective approach evokes the patient's own innate healing capacities.

5. Illness is viewed as a manifestation of a dysfunction of the whole person, not as an isolated event.

6. A major determining factor in the healing process

OTHER NAMES FOR ALTERNATIVE MEDICINE

Since the publication of the first edition of *Alternative Medicine: The Definitive Guide* in 1993, alternative medicine has increasingly begun to be referred to by other terms: *complementary medicine, integrative medicine,* and *holistic medicine.* In essence, all of these terms point to the same medical goal—treating patients from the most comprehensive perspective by addressing all of the multiple factors (physical, environmental, mental/emotional, social, and spiritual) that play a role in both health and disease. Such a holistic, "whole person" approach to health care is the opposite of symptom-care, which is the focus of conventional, allopathic medicine. Nonetheless, alternative physicians do not discount the many benefits that conventional medicine can provide, especially in cases of acute, life-threatening disease.

---

is the quality of the relationship established between physician and patient, in which the patient is encouraged to take responsibility for his or her health.

7. The ideal physician-patient relationship considers the needs, desires, awareness, and insight of the patient, as well as of the physician.

8. Physicians significantly influence patients by their example.

9. Illness, pain, and the dying process can be learning opportunities for both patients and physicians.

10. Holistic physicians encourage their patients to evoke the healing power of love, hope, humor, and enthusiasm, and to release the toxic consequences of hostility, shame, greed, depression, and prolonged fear, anger, and grief.

11. Unconditional love is life's most powerful medicine. Holistic physicians strive to adopt an attitude of unconditional love for patients, themselves, and other practitioners.

12. Optimal health is much more than the absence of sickness. It is the conscious pursuit of the highest qualities of the physical, environmental, mental, emotional, spiritual, and social aspects of human experience.

	HOLISTIC MEDICINE	CONVENTIONAL MEDICINE
Philosophy	Based on the integration of allopathic (M.D.), osteopathic (D.O.), naturopathic (N.D.), energy, and ethnomedicine.	Based on allopathic medicine.
Primary Objective of Care	To promote optimal health and, as a by-product, to prevent and treat disease.	To cure or mitigate disease.
Primary Method of Care	Empower patients to heal themselves by addressing the causes of their disease and facilitating lifestyle changes.	Focus on the elimination of physical symptoms.
Diagnosis	Evaluate the whole person through holistic medical history, holistic health score sheet, physical exam, lab data (including nonconventional medical testing).	Evaluate the body with history, physical exam, lab data.
Primary Care Treatment Options	Love applied to the body, mind, and spirit through diet, exercise, attitudinal and behavioral modifications, relationship and spiritual counseling, bioenergy enhancement.	Drugs and surgery.
Secondary Care Treatment Options	Botanical (herbal) medicine, homeopathy, acupuncture, manual medicine (bodywork, chiropractic, osteopathic medicine), biomolecular therapies, physical therapy, drugs, and surgery.	Diet, exercise, physical therapy, and stress management.
Weaknesses	Shortage of holistic physicians and training programs; time-intensive, requiring a commitment to a healing process, not a quick fix.	Ineffective in preventing and curing chronic disease; expensive.
Strengths	Teaches patients to take responsibility for their own health, and in so doing is cost-effective in treating both acute and chronic illness; therapeutic in preventing and treating chronic disease; essential in creating optimal health.	Highly effective in treating both acute and life-threatening illness and injuries.

Courtesy of Robert S. Ivker, D.O. Used with permission.

The Crisis in Modern Medicine

It is no secret that our contemporary conventional medical system is in a state of terrible disarray. Though conventional medicine excels in the management of medical emergencies, certain bacterial infections, trauma care, and many often heroically complex surgical techniques, it has failed miserably in the areas of disease prevention and the management of the myriad new and chronic illnesses presently filling our hospitals and physicians' offices. In addition, as a nation we pay more for our medical care and accomplish less than most other nations of comparable living standards, while health-care costs continue to spiral out of control.

Treatment of chronic disease currently accounts for 85% of the national health-care bill.[11] This state of affairs is due to the fact that we spend almost nothing to treat the causes of chronic disease before major illness develops, according to a report from the American Association of Naturopathic Physicians. "We wait for illness to develop and then spend huge sums on heroic measures, even then ignoring the underlying lifestyle-related causes. This is the equivalent of waiting for a leaky roof to destroy the infrastructure of a house and then repairing the damage without fixing the leak. This is naturally expensive and ineffective.

"Perhaps the greatest evidence of the depth of the crisis is that we have come to accept such levels of chronic disease as normal, despite evidence that much of it is preventable. Former Surgeon General C. Everett Koop, in his 1988 *Report on Nutrition and Health*, points out that 'dietary imbalances' are the leading preventable contributors to premature death in the U.S. and recommends the expansion of nutrition and lifestyle-modification education for all health-care professionals."[12] This is borne out by the U.S. Centers for Disease Control and Prevention, which states that 54% of heart disease, 37% of cancer, 50% of cerebrovascular disease, and 49% of atherosclerosis (hardening of the arteries) is preventable through lifestyle modification.[13]

The changes that are necessary, however, will not be implemented as long as physicians earn their living and win renown primarily by delivering rescue medicine (interventions that simply treat symptoms), since it is in this area and not prevention that they benefit most. If the U.S. is to be saved from catastrophic health-care costs, which are currently over $1 trillion annually,[14] it is time to take a good look at the wisdom and cost-effectiveness of alternative medicine.

Doctors are confronted daily with patients suffering from illnesses for which conventional medicine offers only superficial treatment of symptoms. The magic of antibiotics is vanishing as a host of resistant infections emerge. Diseases such as AIDS and chronic fatigue syndrome have shown us clearly that our present treatments are simply not effective and hint at new health problems that may lie ahead. The metaphor of a modern plague may be appropriate. Growing numbers of people lack vitality and suffer from a host of complaints difficult to define. Most adults, and many children, today suffer from complaints including allergies, headaches, lack of energy, excessive fatigue, and various digestive and respiratory disorders, along with a variety of emotional states ranging from mild depression to mood swings and anxiety.

They are manifesting what Jeffrey Bland, Ph.D., of Gig Harbor, Washington, calls a state of "vertical ill health." "They are not sick enough to lie down (in which case they would become 'horizontally ill') and yet consider themselves 'normal' because most of the people they know are equally unhealthy," explains Leon Chaitow, N.D., D.O., of London, England. "They derive only limited benefit from the flood of tranquilizers, antidepressants, analgesics, and anti-inflammatory drugs they are commonly prescribed, while the side effects they develop from these drugs just add to their list of woes."

Thoughtful physicians are becoming increasingly aware that something is wrong with their patients' immune systems, since they continue to suffer from illnesses that normal immune function should be able to deal with. Yet this decline in immune efficiency is something contemporary medical treatments seem unable to do anything about. Doctors and patients alike are perplexed by this failure of drug-based therapies to bring relief. As a result, patients often become trapped in a cycle of dependency on physicians to monitor and constantly adjust their medications rather than becoming empowered to change lifestyle factors that might allow their body to regain its healthful potential.

"Most over-the-counter and almost all prescribed drug treatments merely mask symptoms or control health problems, or in some way alter the way organs or systems work," Dr. Lee states. "Drugs almost never deal with the reasons why these problems exist, while they frequently create new health problems as side effects of their activities.

> *Most over-the-counter and almost all prescribed drug treatments merely mask symptoms or control health problems, or in some way alter the way organs or systems work. Drugs almost never deal with the reasons why these problems exist, while they frequently create new health problems as side effects of their activities.*
> —JOHN R. LEE, M.D.

"People realize that their headaches are not due to aspirin deficiency or that their hypertension is not being properly addressed by prescriptions of drugs that merely induce diuresis [excessive urine excretion]. They are seeking answers that address the root causes of their health problems and aid in restoring normal, healthy body function. This is not to say that treatment of the symptoms of a condition is wrong. What would be wrong would be to think that by eliminating the symptom we have dealt with the problem itself."

Why We Become Ill

Health is far more than the absence of disease. When we are healthy all our bodily systems and functions are harmoniously balanced and integrated with each other and we are also in balance with our environment. In this state of equilibrium, our defense mechanisms and our immune system can efficiently handle most of the

WHY CONVENTIONAL DOCTORS THINK THE WAY THEY DO

When people first hear about alternative medical treatments, they often ask the obvious question: "If this treatment is so effective, why doesn't my doctor know about it?" According to John R. Lee, M.D., of Sebastopol, California, there are a number of reasons for this. "The first reason lies in the fact that the selection process of medical students depends in large part on college grades," Dr. Lee says. "Students get high grades when they simply repeat in their tests exactly what the teacher wants them to say. Students who question what they are being taught, on the other hand, usually do not get the higher grades. Medical schools therefore are filled with students who are good at adopting given 'wisdom' but not necessarily good at thinking and questioning, because they have learned to follow precepts handed to them by presumed authorities."

The second reason that accounts for the way many doctors think is that medical schools tend to be organized into organ-specific departments. "The idea of an underlying link between these different departmentalized diseases is non-existent within this framework," Dr. Lee says. "Furthermore, the influence of nutrition on the way cells function is ignored or derided by many department heads who defend their own orthodox concepts."

The third reason is one of simple economics. "When leaving medical school, the young doctor finds him- or herself in a system that rewards what is called 'rescue' medicine, or interventions that treat symptoms," Dr. Lee explains. "There is no reward, and there may well be scorn from fellow doctors, for those who take the time and trouble to try and prevent illness or attempt to correct nutritional deficiencies that may be causing the patient's condition. Medical record keeping and billing for insurance also require doctors to adhere to this superficial, organ classification of disease. Economic rewards follow only from sticking to this particular model of ill health and treatment."

Malpractice is another great fear among doctors. "People should note that the definition of malpractice is not whether the practice is 'good' or 'bad' for the patient, but rather if the practice in question is what other doctors in the given locality normally do or prescribe," Dr. Lee states. He adds that doctors also, quite naturally, seek the professional and social approval of their peers. "Both of these factors conspire to 'keep the doctor in line,' limiting the likelihood of a doctor adopting unconventional practices."

---

hazards that life presents, whether these are pathogenic (disease-causing) organisms, toxic substances, or stress factors of various kinds.

Foundations of Health

According to Dr. Chaitow, positive health depends upon three interconnected factors. The first is the body's structural system, including all of the muscles, bones, ligaments, nerves, blood vessels, and organs, and their functions. The second factor is the body's biochemical processes, which involve the absorption and utilization of nutrients and the elimination of wastes, along with the complicated biochemical relationships that are the key to cellular function and health. The third factor comprises the mind and emotions, as well as the spiritual dimension of each person.

"When there is a balanced, energetic, interplay among these three components, we have health," Dr. Chaitow says. "But when imbalances exist within any of these factors, or in their relationships with each other, ill health occurs."

Homeostasis

In a state of health, if we cut ourselves, we heal. If we are bruised, strained, or suffer a broken bone, healing starts immediately. If we are exposed to infection, our immune system deals with it. These are illustrations of the body's natural tendency towards repairing itself. This tendency is known as homeostasis, the maintenance of the body's internal organs and defenses to compensate for external health hazards.

When homeostasis is called into play to handle a "crisis," its activity is usually experienced as "symptoms." For example, when you are exposed to an infection, your body will mount an aggressive defensive response that might result in fever. Or, should you injure yourself, the healing process, which starts immediately, might involve inflammation and swelling of the traumatized area. In other words, under normal conditions, the body will attempt to heal itself without help and the symptoms produced will indicate what sort of healing process is going on. Unfortunately many people, including all too many physicians, rather than respecting these homeostatic processes and simply waiting for them to finish their tasks, will actively try to suppress the symptoms of self-repair, whether this be a raised temperature or inflammation in an injured area. When this occurs, we are in effect saying that we know more than our body's innate intelligence about what is good for it.

In order to maintain good health, therefore, it is important to recognize that many symptoms are evidence that healing is under way and that, unless they are actually unbearable or dangerous, the symptoms should be left alone so that the repair processes can be completed.

Stress Adaptation

The late Canadian physiologist Hans Selye, M.D., developed a model of how the body copes with stress, which he called the general adaptation syndrome (GAS). The three stages of GAS offer a clear explanation of how and why nearly all forms of illness develop. In Dr. Selye's model, the initial acute reaction to any irritant or stress factor is called the Alarm Stage. An example of this stage occurs when a muscle in the body is overworked. Soreness will follow and the muscle may even become inflamed. In a state of health, such symptoms will quickly pass and the muscle will return to its normal state within a day or two, as the self-regulating, balancing mechanisms of homeostasis do their work.

However, if the muscle is continuously overworked, or exposed to additional strains from other stress factors, it will eventually start to adapt and accommodate itself to the repetitive stress factor in order to cope with the demands of the stress in ways beyond those of the Alarm Stage. Eventually, the body as a whole will also begin adapting itself in this same manner, at which point, the second, or Resistance Stage, comes into play.

This stage is usually without symptoms at first and it can last for many years. In fact, Resistance Stage adaptation lasts for as many years as the body's resources and reserves will allow, while the body continues its attempts at repair. Depending on individual genetic makeup as well as factors such as nutritional deficiencies, trauma, illnesses, medications, and surgeries that have been acquired in life, the ability to continue to adapt and resist will vary significantly from person to person. This explains why two people faced with apparently identical challenges will respond quite differently. One might meet the challenge with no sign of difficulty, while the other might collapse into serious illness.

Most people will display the collection of minor symptoms that become the norm of Dr. Bland's "vertically ill" as they cope with life's stresses, whether these be structural, biochemical, or emotional. It is at the end of the Resistance Stage, when a person's adaptive mechanisms begin to fail, that the final stage of GAS results, known as the Exhaustion Stage. At this point, the person's inability to cope with repetitive, and often multiple, stress factors will inevitably lead to actual disease, usually of a chronic nature.

Returning to the example of the overworked muscle, one can clearly see how each of these stages would progress. When a muscle is first overworked, the Alarm Stage reaction manifests as pain, stiffness, and perhaps inflammation. If this stress of overwork becomes chronic, during the Resistance Stage the muscle becomes increasingly less elastic and more fibrous, placing stress on the points where it is anchored into bone. This creates additional problems of pain, coordination difficulties, and stress on the joints. Left untreated, the muscle will eventually enter into the Exhaustion Stage, with the fibrousness and inflammation possibly degenerating into fibrositis (muscular rheumatism) and the joints, due to the uneven wear and tear caused by muscular imbalances, would show signs of arthritis.

It is the interaction between what is being adapted to and the individual's reserves and resources which determines when, and at what level, illness will result. To use another example, treating high blood pressure by prescribing a drug could possibly be effective in momentarily lowering blood pressure, but if it is being caused by emotional stress or improper diet, the underlying causes would be unaffected and could soon result in additional problems elsewhere in the body. Helping the person learn to better deal with stressful emotions, or providing instructions on the role proper diet and nutrition plays in overall health, would be far more effective long-term approaches.

"The same principles apply to all health problems," states Dr. Chaitow. "If we can remove the cause of the problem, increase the powers of adaptation and resistance, or ideally do both of these, we restore the opportunity for the self-regulating mechanisms of homeostasis to operate again and healing can begin."

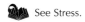 See Stress.

Other Factors Contributing to Illness

As a growing number of patients struggle with illnesses involving depressed immune function and overstressed hormonal and nervous systems, physicians must cope with the fact that these illnesses simply do not respond to the types of treatments being offered by conventional medicine today. To better understand this situation, we must first look at some of the factors influencing our health.

GENETICS

From our parents, we receive our genetic inheritance and are born with constitutional strengths and weaknesses over which we have no control. External factors provide additional layers of influence, which act on our genetically acquired ability to adapt and cope.

DIET

The late Emanuel Cheraskin, M.D., D.M.D., of Birmingham, Alabama, pictured the sick individual as a layered "onion" whose signs and symptoms serve as the onion's outer layers, with layers of biochemical imbalance lying underneath. At the core of the onion, according to Dr. Cheraskin's research, lies poor diet. That diet is so essential to health is not surprising. The foods and liquids we consume, along with the air we breathe, have a fundamental effect on our well-being.

A healthy diet of pesticide-free fruits and vegetables, whole grains, seeds, and nuts, along with organically raised, free-range poultry and certain types of fish, can supply us with all of the essential nutrients our bodies require for optimum efficiency, energy, and freedom from disease. Such a diet is rare today, however, having been replaced by foods high in unhealthy levels of fat, preservatives, chemical additives, and, in the case of most of the meat available in the U.S., antibiotics and hormones, due to the way our livestock is raised. These factors alone can contribute to much of the chronic illnesses besetting people today.

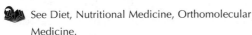 See Diet, Nutritional Medicine, Orthomolecular Medicine.

MENTAL AND EMOTIONAL STRESS

Research in the field of mind/body medicine has revealed that there is a direct link between mental and emotional distress and the body's ability to resist illness. It has also been discovered that unresolved or unexpressed thoughts and feelings are translated in the body as neurochemicals. These chemicals communicate with other systems of the body, particularly the autonomic nervous system, causing the body to react in a manner similar to when physical stress is present. Fear, for example, arouses the nervous system and triggers a flood of adrenal (stress) hormones, causing an accelerated heart rate and intensified breathing. Under healthy conditions, such reactions soon subside, but chronic fear, anger, grief, and other powerful emotions can keep the nervous system in a constant state of arousal. This allows stress to build up in the body, eventually attacking the body's organs and resulting in depressed immunity.

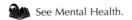 See Mental Health.

ENVIRONMENTAL POLLUTION

Pollutants in the air, water, soil, and the foods we eat can contribute to illnesses ranging from birth defects and cancer to Alzheimer's disease. They also can create a severe toll on the immune system, leading to many other chronic conditions, such as allergies.

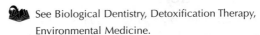 See Biological Dentistry, Detoxification Therapy, Environmental Medicine.

DENTAL FACTORS

The relationship between common dental 'silver' amalgam fillings and chronic illness is now recognized by a growing number of dentists, physicians, and researchers. The problem lies with the fact that calling the fillings "silver" is a misnomer, because they are actually composed of 50% mercury, one of the metals most toxic to the body. Over time, mercury can slowly leech out of the fillings. When this happens, damage may occur to the nervous system, leading to symptoms resembling multiple sclerosis, chronic fatigue syndrome, and senile dementia. Infections in the gums can diminish health by suppressing immune function and increasing the susceptibility to disease elsewhere in the body. The misalignment between the skull and jaw caused by temporomandibular joint syndrome can also create various types of stress, resulting in depression, insomnia, headaches, fatigue, chronic pain, and low back pain.

INAPPROPRIATE USE OF ANTIBIOTICS

Antibiotics are valuable drugs when used appropriately, but the evidence today points to massive overuse. Antibiotics are often prescribed for medical conditions that do not warrant them. For instance, they are routinely given for colds, but many colds are the result of viral infections, and while antibiotics kill bacteria, they have no effect on viruses.

The use of antibiotics can also result in a variety of side effects due to the way their powerful actions interfere with the delicate balance of the body's systems. This can result in the destruction of the "friendly" bacteria in the body, leading to yeast overgrowth, both locally (vaginal infections) and systemically (candidiasis); interference with nutrient absorption; the development of food allergies; recurrent ear infections; and immune suppression, as evidenced by the large percentage of adults suffering from chronic fatigue syndrome who have histories of recurrent antibiotic treatment as children or adolescents.[15]

 See Antibiotics (Appendix), Candidiasis, Chronic Fatigue Syndrome, Holistic Self-Care.

ELECTROMAGNETIC FIELDS

Electromagnetic fields (EMFs) are invisible yet active forces produced by electrical appliances (including computers, microwave ovens, and even electric razors), power lines, and electrical wiring. Researchers have only recently begun to realize the effects EMFs can have on health. In 1990, the Special Epidemiology Studies Program of the California Department of Health Services noted that EMFs can, in fact, change biological tissue, although the full range of their health effects remains unknown.[16] Additional studies by the U.S. Environmental Protection Agency have found possible associations between EMFs and miscarriages, birth defects, leukemia, brain cancers, and lymphomas.[17]

 See Energy Medicine, Magnetic Field Therapy.

GEOPATHIC STRESS

Geopathic refers to illnesses that are caused, or contributed to, by areas of harmful radiation from the earth itself. That such a possibility exists has been known to traditional cultures for thousands of years. The Chinese art of *feng shui* (the study of subtle earth energies and their relation to human life), for instance, takes into account the effects of harmful radiation from the earth to safeguard against building over the locations from which they emanate. According to Anthony Scott-Morley, D.Sc., Ph.D., M.D. (alt. med.), of Dorset, England, as many as 30% to 50% of the chronically ill exhibit some signs of geopathic stress. These include excessive sleeping, cold extremities, respiratory difficulties, and unexplained mood changes and depression. "While geopathic stress may not be the cause of these conditions, it certainly seems likely that it is a contributing factor," Dr. Scott-Morley says.

 For a more in-depth discussion of the implications of geopathic stress to health, see section on geopathic stress in the Cancer chapter.

All of the above factors can contribute to a decline in organ and body system function, resulting in illness. Even so, the pathway back to health does exist.

The Return to Health

The vast majority of illnesses are self-limiting, meaning that they get better all on their own. Alternative medicine recognizes this fact, realizing that health will usually arise spontaneously when the conditions for health exist. Therefore, once you are ill, getting healthy again requires the very same inputs that were needed to keep you healthy in the first place.

This may seem obvious but it's a message worth restating. As Dr. Chaitow says, "To regain health once it has been lost, we need to begin to reverse some, and ideally all, of those processes which may be negatively impacting us and over which we have some degree of control. This includes taking responsibility for stopping those lifestyle choices that we know are harmful, whether this be smoking, excessive alcohol intake, or using drugs. In addition, we need to start to positively address the real needs that such behavior masks."

Depending on the nature of our health problems, this might involve starting to eat more nutritiously, sleeping and exercising in a more regular and balanced way, and making sure of receiving reasonable exposure to fresh air and sunlight. It may also include hygienic considerations, detoxifying and cleansing our bodies, addressing any structural or mechanical imbalances, as well as learning how to properly cope with stress, and deal with our mental and emotional needs. "That sounds like a vast prescription," Dr. Chaitow says. "However, even if only some of it can be addressed, such as diet and relaxation, a remarkable phenomenon occurs as homeostasis begins to function more efficiently and health begins to return."

In beginning the journey back to health, we may require help, especially if our bodies have been overloaded and compromised for some time. According to Dr. Chaitow, the help should come from the treatment that is most appropriate for the individual. "This might involve alternative treatments aimed at helping restore nutritional balance or treatments geared toward the removal of toxic burdens in the body. Or it might involve restoring normal nerve and circulatory supply by addressing structural imbalances. One of the advantages of alternative medicine is that it affords the individual the broadest range of health treatment options. Of course, preventive care is always a better choice than waiting to restore health once it has been lost."

Our bodies are not designed to become ill—they are designed to heal and remain healthy. "Even if conventional medicine tells you that your condition is incurable or that your only option is to live a life dependent on drugs with troublesome side effects, there is hope for improving or reversing your condition," Dr. Chaitow says.

One of the advantages of alternative medicine is that it affords the individual the broadest range of health treatment options.

Treatment

When, for any of a variety of reasons, our homeostatic potential is limited, or when we are more vulnerable and susceptible because of a decline in immune system efficiency, it is time to seek treatment to encourage the recovery processes. The treatment chosen should seek to eliminate causes, remove the obstacles to recovery, or encourage normal homeostasis. "All alternative healing methods focus on one or more of these key elements," says Dr. Chaitow, "which explains why there are so many different forms of treatment in the field of alternative medicine. The treatments themselves do not 'cure' the condition, they simply restore the body's self-healing ability. Some treatments focus on biochemistry, others address structural imbalances, while some deal with a person's energetic or emotional requirements. Whatever treatment approach works will effectively help homeostasis to function more efficiently and will not have added to the body's burden by increasing toxicity or weakening any element of the body's ability to function."

Selecting the Appropriate Treatment: Many Roads to Rome

Alternative medicine offers a wide variety of treatment options. Some of these, such as chiropractic, osteopathy, craniosacral therapy, and the various systems of bodywork, address structural imbalances within the body. Others focus on maintaining the body's biochemical balance of hormones, enzymes, and nutrients in order to maintain proper cellular function. These include diet, nutritional supplements, herbal medicine, and enzyme therapy. Still others seek to restore mental and emotional balance, including mind/body medicine, biofeedback training, meditation, hypnotherapy, guided imagery, and Neuro-Linguistic Programming. Finally,

systems such as acupuncture, homeopathy, energy medicine, magnetic field therapy, and neural therapy address the energetic levels of the body.

Some systems of alternative medicine, such as Ayurvedic medicine, naturopathic medicine, and traditional Chinese medicine, incorporate a wide range of these methods to offer complete systems of health care. While the treatment methods of alternative medicine may vary in their approach, all of them are linked by a common philosophy that:

- Focuses on empowering the individual to accept responsibility for at least a part of the task of recovery and future health maintenance

- Emphasizes sound nutrition as a core requirement for health

- Recommends a balanced lifestyle, adequate and appropriate exercise, rest, and emotional tranquillity as prerequisites for a state of health

- Attempts to ensure detoxification and the efficiency of the organs and systems of the body

- Recognizes the importance of the musculoskeletal system as a potential source of interference with nerve transmission and the body's energy pathways, and as a reflection of the individual's internal physical and emotional state

- Most importantly, treats the individual instead of his or her symptoms

 See Biofeedback Training and Neurotherapy, Bodywork, Craniosacral Therapy, Enzyme Therapy, Guided Imagery, Hypnotherapy, Neural Therapy.

Individuality

The late Roger Williams, Ph.D., of the University of Texas, showed that, in any group of 15 to 20 people, there can be a range of nutritional requirements from person to person that varies by as much as 700%.[18] "Your actual need for a particular vitamin is almost certain to be different from mine," says Dr. Chaitow, "and our requirements for this vitamin will also vary depending upon our age and any emotional, biochemical, or physical stresses with which we may be coping. What this illustrates is that there is no uniform prescription as to what any of us require nutritionally. Our bodies know what we need, however, and as long as they

SELECTING AN ALTERNATIVE PRACTITIONER

The choice to explore alternative medicine can be a crucial turning point in one's life, affecting physical as well as mental and emotional health. With the help of an alternative practitioner, it is possible to take control of one's personal health, and thereby eliminate the sense of frustration and helplessness that many feel when dealing with conventional medicine.

But how does one go about selecting an alternative practitioner? Not surprisingly, many of the same criteria used to choose a conventional doctor are important in seeking out an expert in natural medicine. Yet because the very nature of the alternative approach is far more encompassing than the conventional one, there are a number of other critical factors that should be taken into account in the selection process. The following suggestions offer basic guidelines for choosing an alternative practitioner:

- **Educate yourself about the general principles of alternative health care.** The success of alternative care is dependent upon an informed patient as well as a knowledgeable practitioner. Even after selecting a practitioner, the education process must continue, becoming an ongoing aspect of a person's approach to alternative care. As Garry F. Gordon, M.D., co-founder of the American College of Advancement in Medicine, notes, "I encourage people to learn to become their own doctor and use health practitioners as 'educators,' realizing that we can learn something from everyone."

- **If you are selecting a general practitioner, choose someone with a diverse background and expertise in a wide variety of disciplines.** "I think you want to find someone who has a relatively eclectic background," says Elson Haas, M.D., Director of the Preventive Medical Center of Marin, in San Rafael, California. "A great limitation of conventional medicine is that the only choice is really drugs or surgery. Ideally, you want someone who can use both natural approaches as well as pharmaceutical ones, someone who can balance their rational approach with a more intuitive approach, so that they are not just operating from their own bias."

- **Find a practitioner with whom you can communicate openly and with whom you have a good rapport.** "If you do not have a doctor who will sit back and listen to what you have to say for 20 minutes to a half-hour," says John R. Lee, M.D., of Sebastopol, California, "you do not have a doctor who is going to find the cause." Adds Dr. Gordon: "If you don't feel you can communicate adequately and get your questions answered, you need to shop some more, because any anxiety over the doctor-patient selection puts a negative damper on the healing process."

- **Select a physician who is sensitive to your particular needs and circumstances.** Dr. Haas stresses the importance of what he calls "patient-centered" health care. "This means you really take the person as the primary mode and really work around what their needs are," he says.

- **Choose an alternative approach in which you have confidence.** In alternative medicine, the mental and emotional aspects of healing cannot be separated from the physical. It is vital, therefore, that one believe in the alternative method one has chosen. As Dr. Gordon explains, "If I could show you stacks of evidence about homeopathy, but you tell me that you will never understand how it works, I'm going to get half the effect from you than I would from a person that had a neighbor whose life was saved by homeopathy, was well-informed about therapy, and was ready to take a homeopathic remedy when they walked in the door."

There are numerous ways to locate alternative practitioners. In the "Where to Find Help" sections at the back of each chapter in Parts Two and Three of this book, you will find listings of organizations that can provide nationwide referrals for practitioners of more than 50 alternative healing modalities. Referrals to physicians (M.D.s and D.O.s) who practice holistic medicine can also be obtained by contacting the American Holistic Medical Association or the American Board of Holistic Medicine. Or visit the practitioner directory located on our companion website: www.alternativemedicine.com.

remain healthy and we supply them with the benefits of a healthy diet, in their own innate wisdom they will automatically take what they need from the food we eat."

Since, even in terms of nutritional requirements, each person is unique, it follows that what is required to return to health also can vary drastically from individual to individual. It is with this in mind that alternative physicians begin their diagnosis and subsequent treatments. Understanding all of the factors that play a role in both health and illness, their focus is on meeting the specific needs of each of their patients, rather than attempting to superimpose any one particular model or approach to health as the answer for every person.

"All too often, this understanding is lacking in conventional medicine, however," Dr. Chaitow says. "For example, the conventional doctor who has 12 patients with asthma will often provide each of them with the same recommendations and prescription drugs, in effect treating the condition and not the patients themselves.

"An alternative practitioner, on the other hand, will realize that asthma has numerous causes. Some of his patients might be experiencing an allergic reaction to foods or something in their environment, others might have succumbed to a viral infection, while still others might be asthmatic because of diminished nerve supply due to a misaligned spine. Such a practitioner will therefore seek to determine the underlying cause for his patients' conditions and treat each of them differently, using the method that will best stimulate their bodies to heal themselves. This distinction between approaches is a cornerstone of alternative medicine."

The return to health, therefore, is a road that each person must walk according to his or her own unique individuality. It is also a road that needs to address one's entire being, taking into account one's mental, emotional, and physical aspects, as well as the structural, biochemical, and energetic components that shape each of us. It is precisely because alternative medicine honors and understands these concepts that it is now positioned to become a valuable and necessary path-

way for meeting the medical crisis we, as a planet, are currently facing.

Where to Find Help

To locate a physician (M.D. or D.O.) trained in the practice of alternative, holistic healing methods, contact the following organizations.

American Holistic Medical Association
6728 Old McLean Village Drive
McLean, Virginia 22101
(703) 556-9245
Website: www.holisticmedicine.org

American Board of Holistic Medicine
P.O. Box 5388
Lynnwood, Washington 98043
(425) 741-2996

Recommended Reading

The American Holistic Medical Association Guide to Holistic Health. Larry Trivieri, Jr. New York: John Wiley & Sons, 2001.

Divided Legacy: A History of the Schism in Medical Thought, Vols. 1-4. Harris L. Coulter, Ph.D. Berkeley, CA: North Atlantic Books, 1975, 1982, 1988, 1994.

Radical Healing. Rudolph Ballentine, M.D. New York: Three Rivers Press, 2000.

HOW THE BODY WORKS

UNDERSTANDING HOW the body works can help you better appreciate alternative medicine's underlying philosophy of health and healing and empower you to take practical responsibility for your own well-being. Recognizing the importance of the body's systems allows alternative physicians to focus on the source of disease instead of merely treating symptoms. It is becoming increasingly clear that to arrive at an adequate understanding of the disease process, we must acknowledge the intricate web of relations that exists within the body. Hormone production, nutrition, stress, toxic load, immune system competence, and brain function influence one another and modify genetic and cellular activities associated with health and overall life expectancy. Such an understanding also makes it easier to promote overall good health, improve underlying systemic weaknesses or imbalances, and prevent disease from recurring.

The body's primary health systems are the nervous system, the musculoskeletal system, the immune system, the lymphatic system, the detoxification system, the gastrointestinal (digestive) system, the endocrine system, the cardiovascular system, the respiratory system, and the reproductive system.

The Nervous System

The nervous system, comprised of the brain, spinal cord, nerves, and all the chemical messengers that ensure communication throughout the body, controls and regulates all of the other body systems. The billions of cells that make up the brain are housed in the cerebellum and in two large lobes known as the left and right hemispheres. These hemispheres float in a pool of cerebrospinal fluid and are further safeguarded against outside danger by the skull (cranium) and by the meninges, protective coverings that rest just above the wrinkled layer of brain (the cerebral cortex) nearest the skull. The brain itself sits on a pillar of tissue known as the brain stem. The oldest part

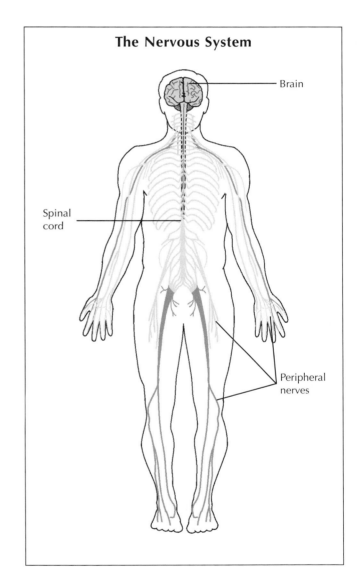

The Nervous System

Brain

Spinal cord

Peripheral nerves

of the brain, the brain stem controls the basic functions of the body, including consciousness, heartbeat, blood pressure, and respiration.

The brain stem descends through an opening in the skull and connects to the bundle of nerves known as the spinal cord. Besides being protected by the vertebrae, the spinal cord, like the brain, is covered by meninges and

The Skeletal System

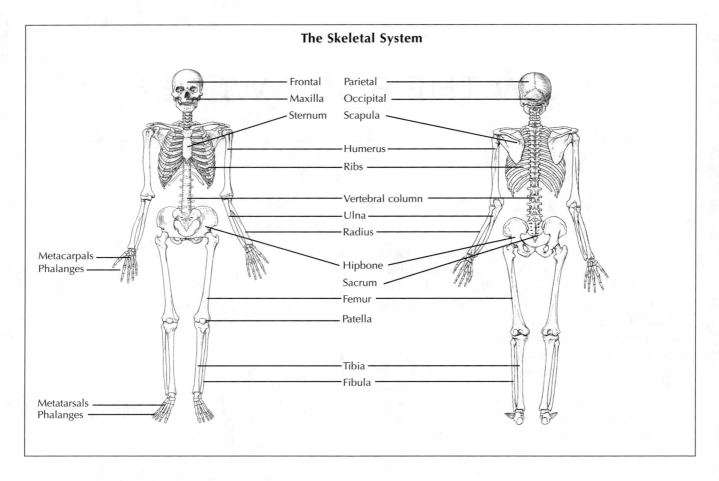

Frontal
Maxilla
Sternum
Parietal
Occipital
Scapula
Humerus
Ribs
Vertebral column
Ulna
Radius
Metacarpals
Phalanges
Hipbone
Sacrum
Femur
Patella
Tibia
Fibula
Metatarsals
Phalanges

surrounded by cerebrospinal fluid. Two types of nerves are believed to pass between the spinal cord and the brain: large bundled nerve fibers carrying the sense of touch and the smaller bundles carrying sensations of pain.

The brain and the nerves speak to each other, nerve cell by nerve cell, via a distinctive group of chemicals called neurotransmitters. Neurotransmitters are the doorway to a functioning nervous system—they facilitate sensory perception, muscle contraction, emotions, thoughts, and the awareness of pain. Most neurotransmitters carry out multiple tasks throughout the brain and nervous system and can be likened to words whose meanings change to suit the needs of their users.

The nervous system as a whole is comprised of three overlapping systems: the central nervous system (CNS), which includes the brain and spinal cord; the autonomic nervous system (ANS), which controls involuntary functions such as heart rate, digestion, and glandular function; and the peripheral nervous system (PNS), which connects the CNS to all the body tissues and voluntary muscles. Health and healing rely upon the equilibrium of these three interrelated nerve systems and the unimpeded nerve flow that is essential for the proper function of the body's other systems.

Because pairs of spinal nerves exit between the vertebra of the spinal column and extend to every part of

the body (muscles, bones, organs, glands, etc.), nerve function can become impeded when the spinal system (including the cranium) and the body's musculoskeletal structures become misaligned due to injury or other causes. For this reason, alternative physicians check for such misalignments as part of their overall comprehensive health program. Should such misalignments be present, a number of alternative therapies can be used to correct them, including certain forms of bodywork, chiropractic, craniosacral therapy, neural therapy, osteopathic medicine, and prolotherapy. Acupuncture and yoga may also help improve nerve function, and biofeedback training and neurotherapy can be used to improve brain function.

 See Acupuncture, Biofeedback Training and Neurotherapy, Bodywork, Chiropractic, Craniosacral Therapy, Neural Therapy, Osteopathic Medicine, Prolotherapy, Yoga.

The Musculoskeletal System

The musculoskeletal system, which consists of the bones, joints, muscles, and connective tissue, helps support the

The Superficial Muscles

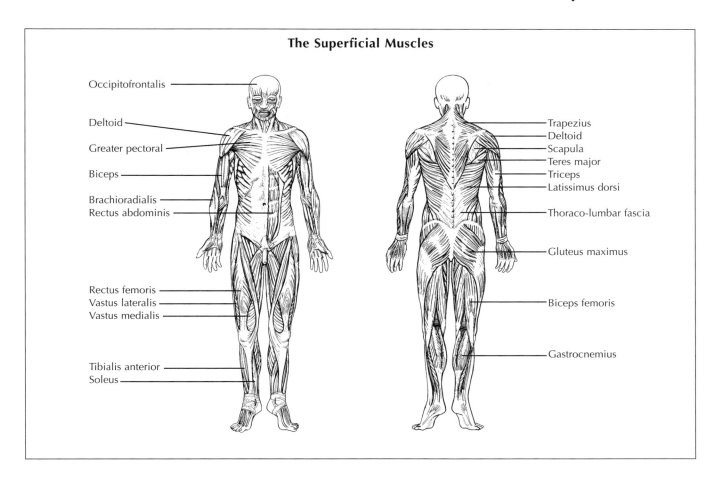

Occipitofrontalis

Deltoid

Greater pectoral

Biceps

Brachioradialis
Rectus abdominis

Rectus femoris
Vastus lateralis
Vastus medialis

Tibialis anterior
Soleus

Trapezius
Deltoid
Scapula
Teres major
Triceps
Latissimus dorsi

Thoraco-lumbar fascia

Gluteus maximus

Biceps femoris

Gastrocnemius

nervous system and is vital for optimum health. When musculoskeletal misalignments occur, we become prone to a wide range of health problems. Although such misalignments are usually associated with external factors such as prolonged stress, poor posture, ill-fitting footwear, or a traumatic injury, they can also be due to internal dysfunction, such as allergy/sensitivity problems, gastrointestinal disturbances, and hormonal imbalances.

Everyone carries some degree of stress in the muscles of the face, skull, upper shoulders, or back at some point in life. If such stress is prolonged, it can lead to chronically contracted muscles, which cause the underlying structure of the body to pull and contract. Over time, this results in adaptive compensation strategies by the body, leading to asymmetrical posture and other musculoskeletal imbalances. Alternative physicians realize that many people today are walking around with one side of their body longer than the other side, or with their head tilted to one side, and seek to correct such imbalances. Bodywork, chiropractic, craniosacral therapy, osteopathic medicine, and yoga are some of the therapeutic approaches that can be helpful.

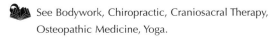 See Bodywork, Chiropractic, Craniosacral Therapy, Osteopathic Medicine, Yoga.

Generally, the musculoskeletal system has a cause-and-effect relationship with the entire body. When either the spine or the musculature are misaligned, the blood supply and the nervous system signals cannot circulate freely to all parts of the body. This forces the spine and the muscles to further compensate for the resulting reduced energy in ways for which they were not designed.

A good example of this mechanism is seen when looking at musculoskeletal imbalances that originate in the head and neck. As the most mobile part of the spine, the head and neck affect the way weight comes through the feet. Head and neck misalignments can throw off the hips, forcing the spine to compensate. This, in turn, may cause the shoulder muscles that run upward along the base of the skull to shorten, the back tissues of the neck to become overstretched, and the jaw to become contracted, all of which pinch or place increased pressure on the nerves running through the base of the skull, down the neck and shoulders, and at the junction where the skull and jaw meet.

Over time, the neck and head become like the pole that tightrope walkers use to keep their balance, struggling against all of these other holding patterns, blocking energy, and causing further muscle strain, blood vessel constriction, nerve irritation, and headaches. This can compromise other functions of the body, bringing about chronic disturbances such as increased emotional tension, digestive problems, hormonal imbalances, and toxicity.

Other results of unhealthy musculoskeletal structure include tightness or restriction in cranial bone movement or in the dura, the membrane surrounding the brain and spinal cord; imbalances in cerebrospinal fluid pressure; fibrosis (in which fibrous connective tissue replaces normal tissue in the muscles or organs); scar formation in the sub-occipital area, the region where the top of the neck meets the base of the skull; and restrictions in the movement of the back of the skull and the first two cervical vertebrae (the atlas and the axis).

Musculoskeletal misalignments can not only negatively influence the tone of the muscles that attach to the neck and head, but also shut off blood supply to the brain. This is because 30% of the blood delivered to the brain comes through the vertebral artery. If the neck is out of alignment due to poor posture or trauma, the brain can actually go into partial asphyxiation as the oxygen level decreases and the carbon dioxide level increases. Headaches, especially tension headaches, are symptoms of this occurrence.

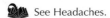 See Headaches.

Poor Posture

Hunching over your desk, slouching on the couch, and wearing ill-fitting footwear all put undue pressure on the spinal column, pinching nerves and muscles and leading to head pain. The trapezius, the triangle-shaped muscle that covers each shoulder blade, is one of the major muscles associated with pain arising from bad posture. Tense or fatigued people tend to roll their shoulders forward, contracting the trapezius, pulling on the pain sensors in the muscle tissue and causing these muscles to pull and strain the scalp. This, in turn, jams the cranial bones and puts extra pressure on the artery that runs up the back of the skull, reducing blood circulation to the brain.

Poor posture is closely related to digestive function. Eating poorly by consuming devitalized, processed foods, for instance, decreases digestive function, and the resultant drop in energy can cause difficulty in keeping good posture.

The Immune System

The immune system is a complex network of specialized organs, cells, and substances that acts as the body's primary defense against disease and a wide variety of bacterial, viral, and fungal infections, all of which we come in contact with simply by breathing, eating, and the acts of everyday living. In addition, on a daily basis many cells are damaged or killed due to trauma, toxins, microbial attack, and other processes in the body. The immune system is responsible for removing such cells, a task it can only perform if healthy.

To protect us against infectious agents and the development of disease, the immune system employs three basic defensive strategies. Its first line of defense is the skin and gastrointestinal tract, which act as physical barriers, coupled with millions of immune cells to prevent infection. The second line of defense is the bloodstream and inflammatory response, which cause exposed body tissue to redden, become warm, and/or swell in an attempt to contain infectious agents and prevent them from spreading further. However, if this response is too great or occurs over a prolonged period, further damage to tissues and cells may ensue. The final line of defense occurs within various organs of the body, particularly the spleen, liver, and lymph nodes.

Primary Organs of the Immune System

Skin: Along with mucous membranes, the skin is the body's first line of defense against microbial infection. Together, they form a protective barrier to keep harmful organisms from penetrating deeper into the body.

Stomach: Stomach acid is another barrier employed by the body to destroy harmful organisms.

Pancreas: The pancreas, when healthy, produces various enzymes that help digest foods. Certain of these enzymes, especially chymotrypsin, are absorbed intact into the bloodstream to be carried to distant body sites, where they digest the fibrin coating on the surface of microbes, cancer cells, and other diseased cells. This allows immune cells to recognize and destroy such cells once their protective coating is destroyed.

Bone Marrow: Bone marrow within the red, fleshy portion of the thigh bones produces infant stem cells, which ultimately develop into several types of immune cells.

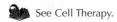 See Cell Therapy.

Spleen: The spleen houses immune cells that manufacture antibodies. It also contains white pulp filled with lymphocytes and macrophage cells, and acts like a large lymph node, except that it filters blood rather than lymph fluid.

Liver: The liver is the primary filtering and waste-processing plant of the body. It breaks down and disposes of dead immune cells and the waste products they have accumulated. It is lined with immune cells that help eliminate microorganisms from the bloodstream.

Thymus Gland: The thymus gland secretes thymosin, a hormone that strengthens immune response. It also instructs certain lymphocytes to specialize their function. The thymus is also an essential part of the endocrine system.

Lymphatic System: The lymphatic system acts as the body's master drainage system and is comprised of lymph nodes, clusters of immune tissue that detect and filter foreign and potentially harmful substances in the lymph fluid. Lymph fluid flows in the lymphatic system throughout the body, helping to maintain the fluid level of cells and carrying various substances from body tissues to the blood. The primary concentrations of lymph nodes are in the neck, armpits, chest, groin, and abdomen.

Types of Immune Cells

The body's immune response is carried out by various immune cells that support each other, including one trillion lymphocytes and 100 million trillion antibodies, which the lymphocytes produce and secrete. A lymphocyte is a specialized white blood cell that represents 25% to 40% of the body's total blood count. Lymphocytes increase during infection and when a person is fighting immune diseases such as cancer. Produced in the bone marrow, they are found in high concentrations in lymph nodes, the spleen, and the thymus gland.

They occur in three forms: B cells, T cells, and natural killer (NK) cells. B cells mature in the lymph nodes and produce antibodies to neutralize antigens (harmful microorganisms or foreign cells). T cells mature in the thymus gland and react to and destroy specific invading antigens, cancerous cells, or infectious agents. Helper T cells (also known as T4 or CD4 cells) secrete immune proteins (particularly the interleukins and interferon) to stimulate B cells and macrophages and activate killer T cells. Suppressor T cells prevent excessive immune reactions by suppressing antibody activity.

NK cells are a type of nonspecific, free-ranging lymphocyte. Unlike other lymphocytes, NK cells are not activated by a specific antigen, but recognize and quickly destroy any foreign invader on first contact. They contain an estimated 100 different biochemical substances for destroying foreign cells. Their primary role is surveillance—to rid the body of aberrant or foreign cells before they can mature and produce cancer and infection.

Macrophages are a form of white blood cell that can engulf germs and foreign proteins and then damage or destroy them by releasing enzymes. Macrophages act as the immune system's vacuum cleaners and filter feeders, ingesting everything that is not normal healthy tissue, including old blood cells. Neutrophils are a type of leukocyte formed in the bone marrow and released into the bloodstream. Their principle activity is to ingest foreign particles, especially harmful bacteria and fungi.

Interferon, familiar to many as a cancer treatment, is a natural protein produced by cells in response to a virus or other foreign substance. Vitamin C and certain herbs can also stimulate its production. Interleukin is a class of immune messenger protein with various functions, including T-cell activation.

Antibodies are protein molecules set in motion by the immune system against a specific antigen. Also referred to as immunoglobulins, antibodies occur in the blood, lymph, colostrum, saliva, and gastrointestinal and urinary tracts, usually within three days of the first encounter with an antigen. The antibody binds tightly with the antigen as a preliminary for removing it from the body or destroying it.

The Antigen–Specific Immune Response

The immune response begins when a macrophage encounters a foreign invader and consumes it. As it does so, it displays pieces of the invader (antigens) on its surface. Helper T cells recognize the antigen displayed and bind to the macrophage. This union stimulates the production of chemical substances, such as interleukin-1 by the macrophage and interleukin-2 by the T cell, that allow for intercellular communication between immune cells.

Interleukin-2 signals helper T cells and NK cells to multiply. The proliferating helper T cells release substances that cause B cells to multiply and produce antibodies. NK cells now begin shooting holes in host cells that have been infected by the invading microorganism. At the same time, the antibodies released by the B cells bind to antigens on the surfaces of free-floating foreign material. This makes it easier for macrophages or NK cells to destroy antigens and signals other blood components to puncture holes in the invaders.

Finally, as infection is brought under control, the activated T and B cells are turned off by suppressor T cells. However, a few "memory cells" remain to quickly respond if the same microorganisms attack again.

Fever can also be involved as part of the immune response, further helping the body to heal. When body temperature rises, antibodies are manufactured at a faster rate and blood and lymph more quickly move to their destinations. In some cases, invading microbes are killed by the higher body temperature. Similarly, inflammation and swelling of tissue also help to localize infection so that the body can heal faster.

Causes of Immune Dysfunction

An overactive or underactive immune system can lead to a variety of disease conditions. Although immunity can decline with age, this is not inevitable and impaired immunity is more often due to a variety of other factors. According to Joseph Pizzorno, N.D., founder and President Emeritus of Bastyr University, in Kenmore, Washington, and author of *Total Wellness*, such factors (ranked in descending order of importance) include: intake of sugar and other concentrated carbohydrates, food allergy, obesity, excess alcohol consumption, nutritional deficiencies, heavy metals, pesticides, drugs (especially aspirin, acetaminophen, ibuprofen, and corticosteroids), toxic chemicals, excessive exercise, stress, inadequate rest, frequent exposure to infectious agents (bacteria, viruses, fungi, parasites), *Candida* overgrowth in the bowel, excessive fish oil supplementation, air pollution, vaccinations, severe trauma (including major surgery), chronic antibiotic use, and perimenopausal hormone imbalances in women.[1]

Among the disease conditions associated with impaired immunity are allergies, autoimmune diseases (such as lupus, rheumatoid arthritis, thyroiditis), cancer, chronic fatigue syndrome, heart disease, and multiple sclerosis.

 See Addictions, Allergies, Arthritis, Cancer, Candidiasis, Chronic Fatigue Syndrome, Heart Disease, Multiple Sclerosis, Parasitic Infections, Sleep Disorders, Stress.

The Lymphatic System

The lymphatic system is a subset of the immune system and acts as the body's "master drain." It includes a vast network of capillaries that transport lymph, a series of lymph nodes throughout body (primarily in the neck, groin, and armpits) that collect the lymph, and three organs (the tonsils, spleen, and thymus) that produce white blood cells known as lymphocytes to scavenge for toxins and microbes. The lymphatic network parallels that of the blood vessels and can be likened to a tree in the body, with the branches extending up into the head, the roots going down to the feet, and the thoracic duct, or "trunk," located in the chest.

Since 1930, it has been known that lymphatic vessels have the ability to remove blood proteins and excess water from the spaces around the body's cells, allowing

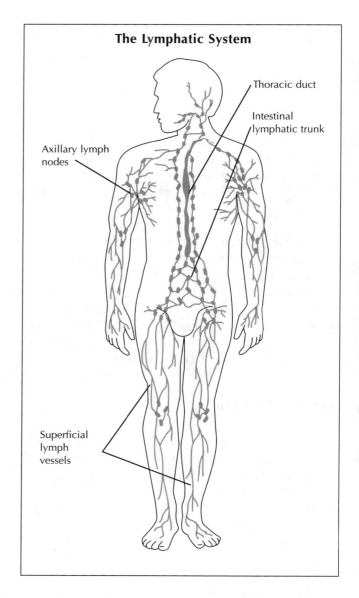

The Lymphatic System

Thoracic duct

Intestinal lymphatic trunk

Axillary lymph nodes

Superficial lymph vessels

the cells to receive life-supporting oxygen.[2] When the lymphatic system becomes congested, the cells become oxygen-deprived. Over time, this can result in the onset of pain and disease.

Lymph is the fluid that fills the spaces between the cells, containing nutrients to be delivered to the cells, and cellular debris (bacteria, dead cells, fatty globules, heavy metals, and other waste products) to be removed. The lymphatic system's primary purpose is to carry toxins away from the cells by collecting and filtering lymph, neutralizing and disposing of bacteria, other microbes, and toxins, and then returning its contents to the bloodstream.

The lymph flows slowly through the body to the thoracic duct (at the rate of three quarts per day), where it drains into the bloodstream. Once in the blood, the toxins are transported to the liver and kidneys, where they are broken down and excreted. Some of the lymph also empties directly into the colon, where it is eliminated with the feces. Unlike blood circulation, the lymphatic system does not have a pump like the heart to move it along. Rather, its movement depends on muscle contractions, general body activity, lymphatic massage and other forms of compression, and gravity. Research has shown that deep breathing each day is one of the most effective methods of activating the lymphatic system and keeping lymph flowing.[3]

The lymphatic system becomes most active during times of illness such as the flu, when the lymph nodes, particularly at the throat, visibly swell with collected waste products. By reactivating the flow of lymph as part of an overall treatment program, alternative physicians are often able to quickly reverse such disease conditions. By providing instruction in the various ways proper lymph flow can be maintained, they also empower people to more effectively prevent disease from occurring.

The Detoxification System

In healthy individuals, the body's detoxification system is able to neutralize and eliminate toxins, thereby minimizing tissue damage and preventing illness. But the detoxification system, including the liver, the intestines, and the lymphatic system, can become overwhelmed by toxins. Toxic overload causes congestion in the lymphatic system, in which thickened lymph accumulates in the nodes without being emptied into the blood for removal from the body, and may also involve chronic intestinal constipation and liver dysfunction.[4] The body's inability to remove toxins is a major cause of accelerated aging and a primary contributor to chronic, degenerative disease processes.

The detoxification system has two lines of defense. Specific organs prevent toxins from entering the body, while others neutralize and excrete the poisonous compounds that get through this initial line of defense. Key components of the detoxification system include the gastrointestinal barrier, including the small and large intestines; the lymphatic system; kidneys, bladder, and other components of the urinary system; skin, including sweat and sebaceous glands; and the lungs.

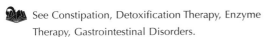 See Constipation, Detoxification Therapy, Enzyme Therapy, Gastrointestinal Disorders.

The gastrointestinal tract usually serves as the first line of defense against toxins entering the body. When it becomes compromised, it also affords disease-causing agents a place to fester, sometimes to the point where they eventually break through the intestinal membrane and enter the bloodstream. Once the bowel is toxic, the entire body soon follows. When undigested food parti-

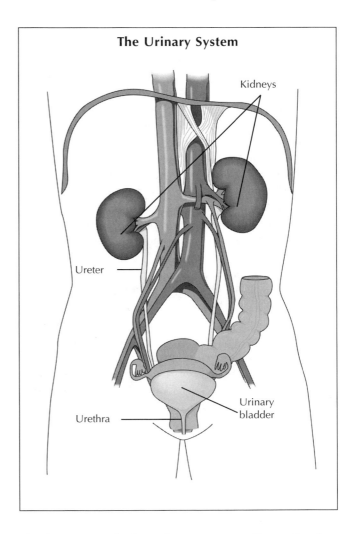

The Urinary System

Kidneys

Ureter

Urethra

Urinary bladder

cles, bacteria, and other substances normally confined to the intestines escape into the bloodstream, they trigger the immune system and inflammation ensues. If the intestines continue letting toxins through, then the liver, lymph, kidneys, skin, and other organs involved in detoxification become overwhelmed.

The liver bears most of the burden for eliminating toxins once they have entered the bloodstream. All foreign substances are carried to the liver to be filtered and expelled from the body. Using enzymes and antioxidants (see Quick Definition), the liver chemically transforms toxins into harmless substances that can be excreted via the urine or stool. Other toxins are eliminated through the lymphatic system, the kidneys, the skin (through perspiration), and the respiratory system.

An **antioxidant** is a natural biochemical substance that protects living cells against harmful free radicals. Antioxidants readily react with oxygen breakdown products and neutralize them before oxidative damage occurs.

HOW THE LIVER HANDLES TOXINS

The largest internal organ, the liver is one of the body's most important components, performing over 500 functions and filtering virtually everything we take into our bodies. Working to maintain stability and harmony between various body systems, the liver functions as a nutrient warehouse and processing facility, supplying and regulating thousands of essential substances in the body, and dismantling the millions of toxic compounds that enter the body each day.

The liver performs this last function by collecting toxic waste from the blood, which flows through it at a rate of approximately 1½ quarts per minute. As the blood enters the liver, specialized immune cells and enzymes remove and destroy harmful bacteria and other foreign matter. Cells known as hepatocytes are able to manufacture new enzymes for every new waste that enters the liver. This ability to "customize" enzymes is what makes the liver such a potent detoxifier.

In addition to harmful chemicals, the hepatocytes break down excess hormones, such as estrogen, cortisol, and adrenaline, circulating in the blood. The hepatocyte's enzyme system works in a two-phase cycle, first deactivating toxins, then "packaging" them in a molecular structure that allows them to dissolve in water, making it easier for toxins to be excreted in urine or feces. When the liver's ability to detoxify becomes impaired due to toxic overload, it becomes more difficult for toxins to be eliminated. This causes them to circulate in the blood and accumulate in fat and muscle tissue.

QD **Enzymes** are specialized living proteins fundamental to all living processes in the body. They are necessary for every chemical reaction and the normal activity of the organs, tissues, and cells, and are also essential for the production of energy required to run cellular functions. Certain enzymes also enable the body to digest and assimilate food, while others assist in ridding the body of toxins and cellular debris.

When imbalances occur in the detoxification system, the result can be poor digestion, poor assimilation of nutrients, constipation, bloating and gas, immune dysfunction, reduced liver function, and a host of degenerative diseases. For this reason, alternative physicians often employ detoxification therapies to reduce or eliminate the body's "toxic load," restore the proper function of the immune and other body systems, and help alleviate age-related illnesses.

The Gastrointestinal (Digestive) System

The gastrointestinal system is comprised of a 30-foot hollow tube called the alimentary canal. Its job is to absorb nutrients while trying to prevent the absorption of abnormal substances. This is accomplished by the coordinated efforts of three processes: the nerve-controlled muscles that push food through the canal; gastric juice secretions by the stomach, pancreas, and liver, which allow for the subsequent breakdown of the food; and the absorption of fluids and nutrients by the small and large intestines.

Digestion starts the moment food enters your mouth. As you begin chewing, alkaline enzymes secreted from the salivary and parotid glands begin to break down the food. As you swallow, the food is moved rapidly through the esophagus and lands in the stomach reservoir, where it is stored, liquified and processed by the acidic gastric juices. The stomach—under the careful control of the nervous system by way of the vagus nerve and stomach-secreted hormones gastrin and histamine—releases enzymes (pepsinogens) and hydrochloric acid to reduce proteins to medium-sized fragments called polypeptides.

Once the food is thoroughly broken down, it passes into the small intestine, where it is met with an intense secretion of digestive enzymes from the pancreas and bile from the liver. The intestinal wall of the small intestine is essentially the front line of the digestive defense, because it safeguards against the absorption of toxic molecules. This task is carried out by the microvilli, tiny hair-like "fingers" that sift through all partially digested particles and selectively soak up proteins, carbohydrates, fats, vitamins, and minerals as they pass along. Over the ensuing 4–6 hours, most of these nutrients are assimilated as the food travels through the first 40 inches of the small intestine, leaving the remaining 20 feet to absorb the leftover water, electrolytes, bile salts, and vitamin B_{12}.

A healthy intestinal wall, one coated primarily with "friendly" bacterial microorganisms, provides the protective lining that is necessary to keep damaging substances out of the body's circulation while letting helpful ones in. However, repeated exposure to harmful substances sends the white blood cells living alongside the microvilli into attack mode. Although intended to help, this effort irritates the intestinal lining even more because these white blood cells begin to explode shortly after

The Gastrointestinal System

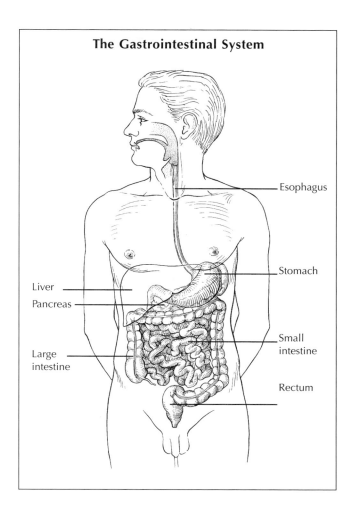

Esophagus

Stomach

Liver

Pancreas

Small intestine

Large intestine

Rectum

bloodstream and, in time, the body goes into "oxidative stress," eventually overloading the system and causing chronic illnesses such as autoimmune diseases, chronic fatigue syndrome, premenstrual syndrome, irritable bowel syndrome, and headaches.

The cells of the liver also produce bile (which is stored in the gallbladder), another essential tool of digestive defense, which performs two important functions. First, bile helps to eliminate unfilterable breakdown products (called bilirubin) from the blood before they are passed to the kidneys. Second, bile neutralizes stomach acid and eases the intestinal absorption of fats and fat-soluble vitamins. If the liver becomes overloaded with toxins or too much stored glucose, the gallbladder's canals become compressed, which decreases bile flow and impairs digestion.

An overloaded, swollen liver also reduces the flow of blood from the pelvic and abdominal regions. This blood pooling may putrefy in time, setting the stage for a host of problems including hemorrhoids, bowel irritation, uterine/ovarian or prostate irritation, neck pain and stiffness, and, in severe cases, heart palpitations. Once the liver becomes unable to dilute toxins and keep the blood clear, the gastrointestinal system becomes exhausted.

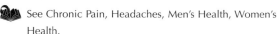 See Chronic Pain, Headaches, Men's Health, Women's Health.

The Endocrine System

The endocrine system is comprised of the pineal, pituitary, hypothalamus, thyroid, parathyroid, adrenals, pancreas, gonads or sex glands, and other glandular tissue located in the intestines, kidneys, lungs, heart, and blood vessels. Controlled by the higher centers of the brain and the nervous system, these glands secrete hormones directly into the bloodstream in an attempt to maintain balance and harmony within the body.

Hormones act as powerful electrochemical messengers, even when released in minute amounts. Among other functions, they guide and regulate most of the body's subtle biochemistry, normalize substances that maintain homeostasis, integrate bodily functions, and determine your size, stature, fat and hair distribution, the sound of your voice, your emotions, and the occurrence of head pain. Scientists have identified hundreds of hormones, with new ones still being discovered.

The endocrine glands release their hormones via a complex interplay between higher brain glands (the hypothalamus and the pituitary) and their end-organ glands (the thymus, thyroid, parathyroid, adrenals, pancreas, and the gonads). This process serves as a sensitive messenger service, with individual hormone carriers spe-

absorbing the abnormal particles, thus releasing a round of inflammatory hormones, like histamine, with which the intestinal wall must also contend.

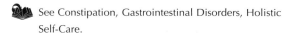 See Constipation, Gastrointestinal Disorders, Holistic Self-Care.

At this point, the front line of digestive defense has fallen, and abnormal proteins and toxic particles begin passing through the intestinal membrane into the bloodstream, causing what is called "leaky gut syndrome." To address this situation, the body calls upon the liver. Nothing enters the bloodstream without first passing through the liver. Normally, this giant blood filter ensures that all useful elements of food undergo interchange, synthesis, oxidation, and storage, and that all toxins are metabolized and processed into safe by-products that the kidneys can eliminate.

But when the body is repeatedly exposed to pollutants and toxins, thorough detoxification is no longer guaranteed. Problems such as leaky gut, bacterial overgrowth (dysbiosis), alcoholism, and drug abuse increase the load on the liver, causing oxidation reactions to produce free radicals faster than enzymatic reactions can process them. This allows free radicals to escape into the

cially programmed to communicate only with specific hormone receptors.

 See Natural Hormone Replacement Therapy.

An Overview of the Endocrine Glands

Hypothalamus and Pituitary: The hypothalamus and pituitary govern the release of the body's hormones and set in motion the entire biochemical chain of events. The hypothalamus, which is a section of brain tissue rather than a true gland, exerts direct control over the pituitary by releasing hormones that activate it. The pituitary then sends special messages, relayed by hormones called gonadotropins, to all the other endocrine glands, telling them what hormones to make and when to make or stop making them.

The pituitary, a pea-sized gland that hangs below the brain and directly behind the eyes, is divided into three parts or lobes. The anterior lobe, or front portion, produces and secretes six hormones: prolactin, which initiates the production of breast milk; adrenocorticotrophin (ACTH), which stimulates the adrenal cortex hormones; thyrotrophin, which stimulates the production of thyroid hormones and regulates the breakdown of fat; somatotropin, a growth hormone that stimulates all body tissues and fat cells to control the growth of long bones and prevent aging; follicle-stimulating hormone (FSH), which stimulates the maturation of ovarian follicles; and luteinizing hormone (LH), which stimulates the production of estrogen and progesterone in females and testosterone in males.

The intermediate lobe of the pituitary contains cells called melanocytes that produce melatonin. The posterior lobe, or back portion, is an extension of the brain. Rich in specialized nerve cells, it produces two hormones: oxytocin, which determines breast milk ejection and smooth-muscle contractions in the uterus; and vasopressin, which helps the kidneys and arteries control water reabsorption, controls smooth-muscle contraction in the arteries, and aids in circulation.

Pineal Gland: Shaped like a pinecone (hence its name) the pineal gland is located in a pocket at the rear of the brain near what is known as the splenium of the corpus collosum. The pineal gland's primary function is the biosynthesis of the hormone melatonin, which controls skin pigmentation and the circadian rhythm (sleep/wake cycle). Melatonin can also initiate defensive responses to toxins in the blood.

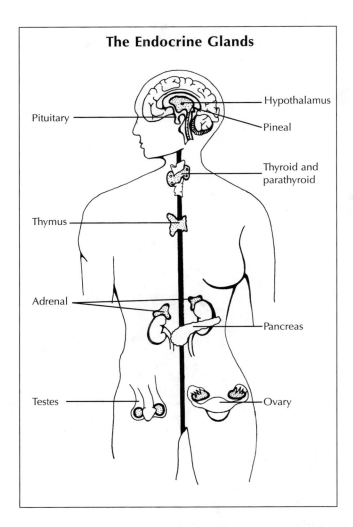

The Endocrine Glands

Thymus Gland: This tiny gland, located in the center of the chest directly behind the breastbone, is a key producer of immune cells.

Thyroid Gland: The thyroid gland acts as the body's thermostat, the chief pacesetter of metabolism. It also determines the rate at which the body uses energy and, like the adrenals, helps run and regulate nearly every organ and system in the body—cell reproduction and growth, tissue repair, circulation, heart rate, nerve tissue sensitivity, hair, skin, and nail growth, sex hormone regulation, and both cholesterol and sugar metabolism in the liver.

Parathyroid Glands: The parathyroid glands are small, saucer-shaped knobs on the back and side of each thyroid lobe. These tiny glands secrete a hormone called parahormone that allows more calcium to enter the bloodstream. If the parathyroid malfunctions, calcium levels may fall too low, which can lead to problems in muscles and nerves.

Pancreas: The pancreas lies in the upper abdomen and performs a hormonal function in addition to a digestive one. As the producer of insulin, this vital gland is responsible for balancing blood sugar (glucose) levels in the body. A sufficient supply of glucose to the cells in the body is essential—without this, the cells starve.

Adrenal Glands: The adrenals act as the body's energy reserve tank. These two triangular glands perched above the kidneys are responsible for overall health and vitality, since they supervise all hormone functioning. Each of these glands is divided into two parts, an inner section called the medulla and an outer layer called the cortex.

The adrenal medulla produces a set of hormones called catecholamines—the stress hormone adrenaline (also known as epinephrine), noradrenaline (or norepinephrine), and dopamine—all of which play an important role in the way we respond to danger, intense emotion, low blood sugar, extreme temperatures, oxygen shortages, low blood pressure, and stress.

The adrenal cortex manufactures three categories of steroidal hormones: mineralocorticoids, which help control the body's fluid balance by regulating the kidney's reabsorption of sodium and potassium; glucocorticoids, which affect the metabolism of carbohydrates, proteins, sugar, and fats, maintain blood pressure, and enable the body to respond to physical stress; and sex hormones, androgens and estrogens, which are responsible for male and female characteristics.

The chemistry of life depends on the ability of the adrenals to control the body's internal fire: if there is too little oxidation, the internal fire will not burn, yet too much will cause burnout. Therefore, the adrenals must constantly monitor glandular activity, nerve energy, physical energy, and oxidation throughout the entire body. In addition, the adrenals support immunity, determine red and white blood cell counts, aid in blood clotting, and control voluntary muscles, bodily strength, the heart muscles, blood pressure, uterine tone, and involuntary muscle contractions (peristalsis).

Sex Glands: The sex glands (gonads), the ovaries and testes, are the most difficult glands to regulate. Sex hormones, such as estrogen, progesterone, DHEA, and testosterone, have a delicate function and require constant fluctuations in the glandular balance to stay in tune. For proper coordination between the sex glands and the sex hormones, the pituitary must be doing its job exactly as it should. If this fails to occur, the biofeedback mechanism by which the ovaries or testes self-regulate is thrown out of kilter, as are the hypothalamus and the pituitary, causing the entire endocrine system to become imbalanced.

Health Effects of Hormonal Imbalance

As people age, the endocrine glands may begin to shrink in size, causing hormone production to also decline (some hormone production may increase in an attempt to stimulate failing glands). This affects the activity of a multitude of processes throughout the body. The pineal gland, for example, produces melatonin, an antioxidant that affects sleep, body rhythms, and emotional well-being. Melatonin levels decline with age. So does DHEA, produced by the adrenal gland. At age 70, an individual produces just 10% of the DHEA produced at age 25. Reduced levels of DHEA have been linked to heart disease, lupus, skin cancer, and diabetes. Women are well aware of the effects of shifting hormone levels with age, particularly the symptoms of menopause. But hormone imbalances can also contribute to a number of other health problems, including weight gain, yeast infections, fibroids, and breast cancer. And in males, lower levels of testosterone lead to diminished sex drive, impotence, and loss of bone tissue and muscle mass.

The Cardiovascular System

Also known as the circulatory system, the cardiovascular system consists of the heart and blood vessels, which work together to transport blood throughout the body, carrying oxygen and nutrients to the cells and tissues and carrying away cellular waste products for filtration and elimination.

The heart is a hollow, muscular organ in the chest that contracts rhythmically to circulate blood throughout the body. It both sends blood rich with oxygen and nutrients out to the body's tissues and pumps blood from the rest of the body to the lungs to be re-oxygenated. At rest, the heart normally beats 60-80 times per minute (100,000 beats per day) and during exercise or stress may beat up to 200 times per minute. The average amount of blood pumped per heartbeat (at rest) is 2.5 ounces (1,980 gallons per day).

Completing the cardiovascular system are the blood vessels. These consist of the aorta (the body's largest artery), the arteries, the arterioles, the capillaries, the venules, the veins, and the vena cava. The arteries carry blood away from the heart and, except for the pulmonary artery, blood passing through the arteries is usually oxygenated. As arteries become progressively smaller, they are called arterioles.

The body's smallest blood vessels are the capillaries, which serve as the interface between the arterioles and the venules. Capillary membranes are extremely thin and

BLOOD FLOW THROUGH THE HEART

The heart is actually two pumps side by side, each consisting of two chambers—the left and right atria, and the left and right ventricles. These chambers are connected by valves that allow blood flow in one direction only. The rhythm of each heartbeat is regulated by a part of the heart muscle known as the sinoatrial node, connected to the central nervous system, which acts as a natural pacemaker.

Blood flows through the heart as follows: Blood that has been oxygenated in the lungs flows into the left atrium, then is pumped through the aorta to replenish the entire body. Oxygen-depleted blood returns from all parts of the body to the right atrium, where it is pumped through the right ventricle via the pulmonary artery to the lungs.

Each heartbeat has two phases: diastole (resting) and systole (contracting). During the diastolic phase, the left atrium fills with oxygenated blood from the lungs, and the right atrium fills with oxygen-depleted blood from the body. The systolic, or contraction, phase begins from the top of the heart as both atria squeeze the blood into the ventricles: the right atrium through the tricuspid valve into the right ventricle, the left atrium through the mitral valve into the left ventricle.

The contraction then continues from the bottom of the heart, squeezing both ventricles upward. The right ventricle moves blood through the pulmonary valve into the pulmonary artery, and then into the lungs. Blood from the left ventricle is pumped through the aortic valve and into the aorta, then out to all parts of the body.

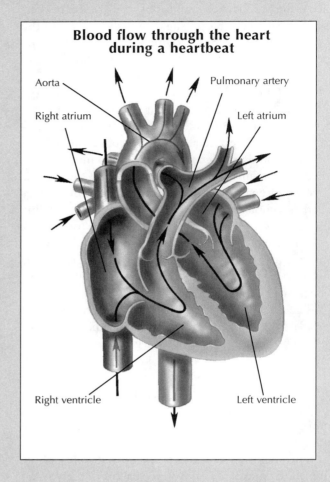

Blood flow through the heart during a heartbeat

Aorta

Pulmonary artery

Right atrium

Left atrium

Right ventricle

Left ventricle

The diastolic, or resting phase, then restarts as all valves close and the atria begin to refill.

---

permeable, allowing for the exchange of gases. The venules are tiny vessels that continue from the capillaries until they eventually merge and form veins, the blood vessels that carry blood back to the heart. All the body's veins come together to form the superior and inferior vena cava, which is connected to the heart's right atrium.

Heart function and overall circulation can be negatively impacted by a variety of factors, especially the buildup of "vulnerable plaque," which can occur in response to microbial infection and accounts for an estimated 85% of all cases of heart attack and stroke; atherosclerosis due to oxidized cholesterol and/or elevated homocysteine levels; poor diet and nutritional deficiencies; lack of exercise; chronic stress; and other factors that are often not considered by conventional M.D.s, such as

mercury exposure, low thyroid function, environmental pollution, and poorly managed emotions (especially anger and rage).

 See Biological Dentistry, Diet, Environmental Medicine, Heart Disease, Holistic Self-Care, Hypertension, Mind/Body Medicine, Stress.

The Respiratory System

The respiratory system is comprised of the nose, sinuses, larynx, trachea, bronchi, and the lungs, and provides oxygen to every cell in the body while also expelling carbon dioxide. "To accomplish this, the average person inhales about 22,000 pints of air per day," says Robert S.

The Circulatory System

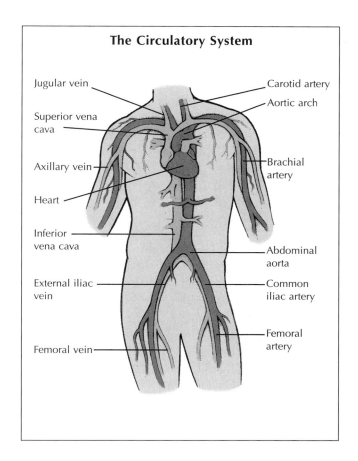

Jugular vein
Carotid artery
Aortic arch
Superior vena cava
Axillary vein
Brachial artery
Heart
Inferior vena cava
Abdominal aorta
External iliac vein
Common iliac artery
Femoral artery
Femoral vein

The Respiratory System

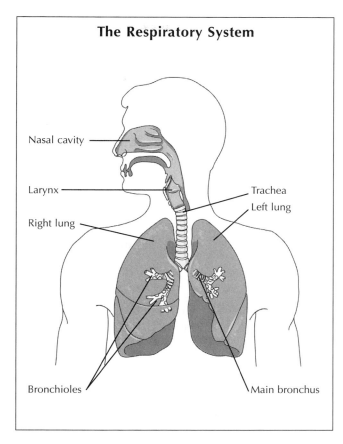

Nasal cavity
Larynx
Right lung
Trachea
Left lung
Bronchioles
Main bronchus

Ivker, D.O., President-elect of the American Board of Holistic Medicine and author of *Sinus Survival*. "Nothing is more important to optimal physical well-being than the quality of our air and our ability to breathe it. During the past 20 years, both of these critical aspects of health have drastically diminished."[5]

The nose and the sinuses (four sets of air-filled cavities around the nose and eyes) act as the body's primary air filter and protect the lungs from invading microorganisms and particulates (dust, sand, soot, smoke, etc.). Each sinus connects to the nasal passage by thin ducts, which is what makes mucus drainage and air exchange possible. Both the nose and sinuses also act as humidifiers and temperature regulators, moistening dry air and cooling hot air and warming cool air that would otherwise shock and harm the lungs.

A single, continuous tissue known as the respiratory epithelium serves as the outermost lining of the entire respiratory tract, extending from just inside the nostrils to the alveolar sacs in the lungs. The epithelium's outer tissue is the mucous membrane, also known as the mucosa, which acts as a first line of defense against foreign microbes and particulates, a task primarily performed by the cilia, microscopic hair-like filaments. When the mucous membrane breaks down, sinus infections, colds, and other respiratory ailments can occur.

The respiratory tract extends down from the nose and mouth to the trachea, or windpipe, in the neck, and then into the thorax, which divides into the main bronchi of the left and right lungs. The bronchi subdivide into smaller bronchi and bronchioles, ending up in the alveoli, small air sacs where gaseous exchange occurs. The lungs themselves are divided into lobes—three on the right and two on the left (to accommodate the heart).

There are two types of respiration: external respiration, or breathing, which refers to the intake of oxygen and exhalation of carbon dioxide; and internal, or cellular, respiration, during which glucose and other small molecules are oxidized to produce energy. Internal respiration requires adequate supplies of oxygen and creates carbon dioxide as a by-product. Both of these processes have been compromised in many people today, primarily due to environmental pollution, which has created what Dr. Ivker terms "America's first environmental epidemic—respiratory disease."[6] Other contributing factors to diminished respiratory capacity, according to Dr. Ivker, include cigarette smoke, impaired immunity, emotional stress (repressed anger or sadness), poor diet, food allergies and sensitivities, overuse of antibiotics, dental problems, and genetic inheritance.[7]

 See Addictions, Allergies, Biological Dentistry, Diet, Mental Health, Mind/Body Medicine, Stress.

The Reproductive System

The male and female reproductive systems, in addition to generating new life, are viewed by many alternative practitioners as a gauge of one's overall health and longevity. Men and women who have healthy reproductive organs also tend to be healthy in general, and men and women who enjoy healthy sexual relations throughout their lifetimes on average exhibit fewer overall health problems as they age.

The Female Reproductive System

Throughout her life, a woman's reproductive system follows rhythmic patterns of change, monthly cycles, and the completion of those cycles with menopause. By becoming acquainted with the needs, characteristics, and problems of each phase, a woman can make informed choices about lifestyle and health care.

The female reproductive organs—the uterus (womb), two ovaries (connected to the uterus by the Fallopian tubes), the cervix, vagina, and clitoris—mature during puberty, the stage during which a girl becomes a woman and menstruation begins. Like the male reproductive system, it is activated and regulated by sex hormones (estrogen, progesterone, and, in lesser amounts, testosterone) produced by the ovaries during the menstrual cycle.

A woman menstruates an average of 400 to 500 times during her lifetime. Yet there are many misconceptions about menstruation and some have been repeated so often that they are considered fact. Most notable is the assumption that the average menstrual cycle is 28 days, neatly paralleling the cycles of the moon. While women's bodies do have an observable rhythm, the menstrual cycle actually has a wide range of lengths that can be considered normal. In addition, while two or three generations ago women began to menstruate at around 15 or 16 years of age, today puberty begins at 12 or 13.

The monthly menstrual cycle results from coordinated hormonal interplay among the hypothalamus, pituitary gland, and the ovaries. Each month at the start of the cycle, estrogen is secreted by the 10-20 eggs growing in the ovaries. The estrogen triggers the thickening of the lining of the uterus (the endometrium) with blood vessels, glands, and cells in anticipation of new life. It also causes the production of a cervical fluid that facilitates the passage of sperm through the cervical opening and enhances its survival. Once the mature egg has left the ovaries, it can be fertilized in the fallopian tubes.

Next, estrogen production subsides and progesterone production increases. This second hormone forms a thick mucus plug in the cervix to prevent sperm or bacteria from entering and maintains the endometrium in a nutri-

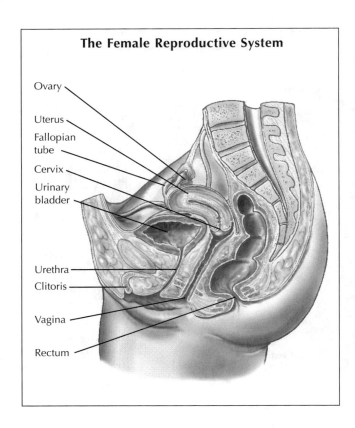

The Female Reproductive System

Ovary
Uterus
Fallopian tube
Cervix
Urinary bladder
Urethra
Clitoris
Vagina
Rectum

tious, blood-rich stage in anticipation of the egg's fertilization by the sperm (conception). If conception does not occur, all hormone levels drop and some of the endometrial layer is released, or "shed." This is called menstruation. The cycle then starts over. If fertilization does occur, progesterone secretion continues to increase, maintaining the uterine lining and pregnancy until the placenta takes over secreting progesterone and other hormones at about three months' gestation.

By becoming aware of her menstrual cycle, a woman is better able to plan her days accordingly. The monthly cycle can also be used as a guide in maintaining general health, because, as research is now suggesting, a woman's immune system peaks before ovulation and decreases afterward.[8] In addition, as Suzannah Doyle, a certified fertility educator from Corvallis, Oregon, points out, research shows that vaccinations, surgery, and prescription drugs have fewer harmful side effects when women use them before ovulation. "In the future, a woman's own observed fertility signs will enable doctors to actually adjust drug dosages for their patients," Doyle says. "Fertility signs are already being used by some health-care providers to increase the effectiveness and accuracy of surgeries, drug therapies, and procedures such as PAP smears and diaphragm fittings."

During the course of her life, a woman will eventually stop menstruating and enter menopause. Generally, this occurs between the ages of 48 and 52, but some women cease menstruating as early as their late thirties and early forties, while others don't stop until their mid-fifties. Because women are healthier now, menopause no longer indicates the onset of old age, and women can expect to live a third of their adult lives after menopause.[9]

Menopause commences when the ovaries stop producing estrogen. Perimenopause is the period commonly thought of as the 5-10 years before menopause (approximately between the ages of 35 and 50). It is characterized by several years of irregular cycles with no ovulation since the ovaries are at the end of their egg supply. Without an egg's presence, progesterone is no longer produced and therefore perimenopause is frequently characterized by estrogen dominance, with side effects ranging from water retention, weight gain, and mood swings to fibrocystic breasts, breast cancer, fibroids, or endometrial cancer.

The onset of menopause, however, does not mean that estrogen levels drop to zero. Some estrogen is still produced in fat cells, the supporting tissue around the ovaries, and in the intestinal tract using precursors produced by the adrenals. Weight gain after menopause can be the body's attempt to take advantage of this situation. Estrogen is also made through other chemical pathways in the body.[10] It is this reserve of estrogen that many natural therapies draw on for their effectiveness.

In addition to premenstrual syndrome (PMS) and menopausal problems (hot flashes, vaginal dryness), other common health complaints associated with the female reproductive system include hormonal imbalances, infertility and other problems associated with pregnancy, excessive or absence of menstruation (menorrhagia and amenorrhea), dysmenorrhea (menstrual cramps), bladder infections (cystitis), endometriosis, uterine fibroids, ovarian cysts, and cancer of the cervix or ovaries. Since many of these conditions are often chronic, alternative medicine is generally more effective than conventional medicine in treating them, and far more noninvasive.

 See Natural Hormone Replacement Therapy, Pregnancy and Childbirth, Women's Health.

The Male Reproductive System

The male reproductive system consists of the penis, testicles (testes), epididymis (a tube along the back of the testicles where sperm is stored), prostate gland, urethra, vas deferens (a tube connecting the testicles to the urethra), the seminal vesicles (which secrete a thick fluid that forms part of the semen), and bladder. The primary function of the male reproductive system is to produce testosterone, the male sex hormone, and to produce and store sperm.

The penis is composed of spongy tissue and a network of nerves and blood vessels. When men become sexually aroused, the spongy tissue becomes engorged

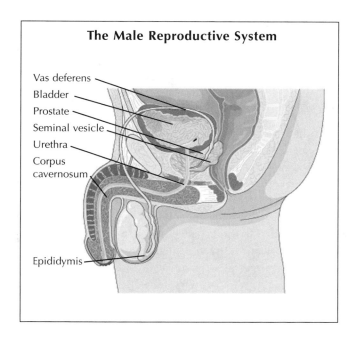

The Male Reproductive System

Vas deferens
Bladder
Prostate
Seminal vesicle
Urethra
Corpus cavernosum
Epididymis

with blood, causing an erection. Arousal can occur due to either physical or psychological (sexual thoughts, daydreams, or fantasies) factors or a combination of the two. The testicles, supported by the scrotum, contain hundreds of tubules, within which millions of sperm are produced daily. Testosterone is also manufactured in the testicles and influences male characteristics such as body hair, voice, and whether or not a man will experience male-pattern baldness. Testosterone levels also influence how fat is distributed in a man's body.

Sperm is collected from the testicles by the epididymis, where they mature and are stored. Prior to the moment of ejaculation, the sperm exit the epididymis to travel along the vas deferens, toward the base of the bladder. There, they mix with secretions produced by the prostate gland. As arousal continues, contractions of the prostate and seminal vesicles cause the sperm to mix with prostatic and seminal fluids and enter the urethra. As the urethra fills, further arousal causes rhythmic contraction of the penis's erectile tissues, eventually culminating in orgasm and ejaculation.

As men enter midlife, levels of their male hormones, known as androgens, decline and can become unbalanced. When this occurs, a variety of symptoms begin to manifest, including fatigue, less endurance and muscle strength, loss of libido, weight gain (especially around the midriff), and impotence. Such symptoms are indications of the andropause complex, also referred to as "male menopause," a diagnosis that is increasingly gaining acceptance among physicians. According to Gary S. Ross, M.D., of San Francisco, California, the andropause complex of symptoms is usually noticeable by the time a man is in his fifties, although they can appear much earlier. All such symptoms are signs that a man's hormones, both

THE PROSTATE GLAND'S RELATIONSHIP TO HEALTH

The prostate gland lies at the base of the bladder, surrounding the urethra, and weighs less than an ounce. The size of a walnut, it is bordered by the rectum, bladder, pubic bone, and pelvic muscles. Its purpose is to secrete substances that protect or enhance the functional properties of sperm cells and to provide a fluid support system for the sperm cells. It does this by secreting a thin, milky alkaline fluid during ejaculation to enhance delivery and fertility of the sperm. In addition, the prostate acts as the genitourinary system's first line of defense against infection and disease.

Prostate fluid consists of zinc (in the male body, the prostate has the highest concentration of this mineral and zinc may be largely responsible for the prostate's ability to defend against infection and disease), citric acid, potassium, fructose, prostaglandins, proteolytic enzymes, prostate specific antigen (PSA), and acid phosphatase. Levels of these last two substances, when elevated, are considered reliable indicators of prostate cancer.

Some of the more common problems associated with the prostate are benign prostatic hypertrophy (BPH), prostatitis, and prostate cancer. All of these conditions are greatly influenced and accelerated by the aging process and therefore need to be monitored regularly, especially as men move through middle age into older age.

other alternative physicians, their success in doing so is increasingly possible.

 See Detoxification Therapy, Diet, Herbal Medicine, Homeopathy, Men's Health, Natural Hormone Replacement Therapy, Nutritional Medicine.

Recommended Reading

Atlas of the Human Body. Takeo Takahashi. New York: HarperCollins, 1994.

Illustrated Guide to the Human Body. Charles Clayman, ed. New York: DK Publishing, 1995.

Longevity: An Alternative Medicine Definitive Guide. W. Lee Cowden, M.D., Ferre Akbarpour, M.D., and Russ DiCarlo, with Burton Goldberg. Tiburon, CA: AlternativeMedicine.com Books, 2001.

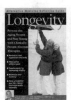

in terms of their levels and their ratios to one another, are in a state of flux, shifting into a new, midlife configuration.

Declining hormone levels, and the resultant symptoms that accompany them, are not inevitable, however, and may be slowed or reversed by a number of alternative therapies, including natural hormone replacement therapy and the use of glandular extracts. Other important approaches (often used together) include proper diet, nutritional supplementation, detoxification, exercise, herbal medicine, and homeopathy. "Men today are very active and want to stay at their best rather than letting themselves go, getting old and fat," Dr. Ross says. "They want to keep going at the same pace and have a proactive attitude about resolving symptoms of male menopause as they appear." Thanks to the comprehensive treatment approaches employed by Dr. Ross and

HOLISTIC SELF-CARE

It's supposed to be a professional secret, but I'll tell you anyway. We doctors do nothing. We only help and encourage the doctor within.

—ALBERT SCHWEITZER (1875-1965)

PRACTITIONERS OF alternative medicine approach healing from a holistic perspective whose primary goal is the creation and maintenance of optimum health in body, mind, and spirit. In addition to the comprehensive care they provide to achieve that goal, they also serve as teachers, instructing their patients in effective methods of self-care. Such methods not only assist patients in their journey back to wellness, but also help them prevent disease from occurring in the first place. What follows is an overview of these self-care principles, divided into three categories—physical health, mental health, and spiritual health—all of which must be addressed in order to truly achieve a state of abundant well-being.

CAUTION This information is not intended as a substitute for professional care. Although these measures can play a significant role in helping to reverse disease, if you suffer from chronic or serious illness, seek immediate professional medical assistance.

Physical Health

Being healthy physically means not only having a healthy body, but also having a healthy environment in which to live and work. To help heal the body, alternative physicians encourage their patients to become responsible for their diet and nutritional needs, to exercise regularly and to get adequate sleep, and to take steps to ensure their home and work environments are free of potentially harmful toxic chemicals and pollutants.

Diet and Nutrition

Proper diet is a cornerstone of optimum physical health and can also positively influence mood and mental function. Since the mid-20th century, however, the typical American diet has become increasingly devoid of essential nutrients, due to several factors:

- The advent of commercial farming methods, which have resulted in minerally deficient soil and an overreliance on pesticides used to grow crops, and antibiotics, hormones, and other drugs used in raising livestock.

- The burgeoning popularity of the fast-food industry and processed "junk foods," which contain unhealthy chemical additives, saturated fats and trans-fatty oils, and white flour and refined starches.

- Environmental pollutants, which continue to poison our air, land, and sea, to the point where even certain, once healthy kinds of seafood are now unsafe to eat due to the levels of mercury and other harmful substances they contain.

Making matters worse, this pervasive contamination of our food supply is in many ways abetted by the U.S. Food and Drug Administration (FDA) and other government agencies, which continue to permit the multi-billion-dollar food industry to grow, harvest, and process its products with hundreds of questionably safe chemicals, industrial pollutants, dyes, stabilizers, and preservatives, despite the mounting evidence that such ingredients play a major role in the many degenerative diseases that have become so widespread since their use began.

The first rule of diet, therefore, is to eliminate, or at least minimize, your intake of processed, commercially grown food. Instead, emphasize a whole-foods diet rich in organic fruits and vegetables, complex carbohydrates, nuts, seeds, fiber, pure water, and, if possible, organically raised meat and poultry products. Also, reduce or elimi-

THE IMPORTANCE OF PURE WATER

"The most important life-giving substance in the body, and the one that the body desperately depends on, is water," states Fereydoon Batmanghelidj, M.D., an expert on the role chronic dehydration can play in disease and author of *Your Body's Many Cries for Water*. Comprising approximately 75% of the body, water is found both outside and inside the cells and is the basis for all bodily fluids: blood, lymph, saliva, digestive juices, urine, and perspiration. Because water is the regulator of all of the body's functions, it is equated with life. It is the main source of energy transport for every cell in the body, conducting electrical and magnetic energy that supplies the power to live.

Water also facilitates energizing the skin's many photo-sensitive and energy-sensitive nerve endings that receive and transmit signals, making them more responsive and enhancing the skin's vitality. It also protects both the skin and mucous membrane barrier functions and acts as an antioxidant by flushing oxidants and other toxins out through the kidneys. This is the basic way the brain cells maintain an alkaline environment. In addition, the sinuses drain better when they are well hydrated and their mucous membrane is more resistant to infection.

According to Dr. Batmanghelidj, most people unknowingly suffer from chronic dehydration. Dehydration contributes to toxic overload in the body, which can lead to a hyper-active immune system and cause or contribute to a variety of diseases, including arthritis, asthma, colitis, depression, diabetes, dyspeptic ulcer, duodenitis, gastritis, heartburn, headaches, high blood pressure, high cholesterol, low back pain, neck pain, and osteoporosis. Chronic dehydration is also a cause of kidney stones and other kidney problems.

In place of water, many people drink alcohol, coffee, non-herbal teas, soda, and other caffeine-containing beverages. Such liquids, rather than hydrating the body, further exacerbate dehydration. Dr. Batmanghelidj and alternative physicians in general recommend avoidance of such beverages and that water be used in their place. "Your body needs an absolute minimum of six to eight 8-ounce glasses of water a day," Dr. Batmanghelidj says. "Thirst should be satisfied at all times. With increase in water intake, the thirst mechanism becomes more efficient."

The best times to drink water, according to Dr. Batmanghelidj, are one 8-ounce glass 30 minutes before taking food (breakfast, lunch, dinner) and a similar amount 2½ hours after each meal. "This is the very minimum amount of water that your body needs," he says. "For the sake of not shortchanging your body, two more glasses of water should be taken around the heaviest meal or before going to bed."

After a few days of drinking six to ten 8-ounce glasses of water, Dr. Batmanghelidj also recommends adding some salt to your diet. This is particularly necessary if you begin to experience muscle cramps at night, a sign of salt-deficiency, according to Dr. Batmanghelidj. The reason for this is because the body "is under a constant drive to retain salt to keep water inside the system" and increased water intake alone causes the body to lose salt. To balance salt content once you add it to your diet, Dr. Batmanghelidj recommends 1-2 glasses of orange juice be consumed each day for its potassium content.

Because tap water all too often contains a variety of unhealthy contaminants, including microorganisms, heavy metals, chlorine, fluoride, and other impurities, it is recommended that you have your water tested. If it tests positive for such contaminants, you should consider filtering your water, using either a charcoal or ceramic filter or a reverse osmosis system. Ordinary tap water is acceptable, however, if testing does not show contamination, Dr. Batmanghelidj says.[1]

---

nate your intake of red meats, fats, and milk and dairy products.

For many people, adopting a whole foods diet alone will produce significant health benefits. For others, however, further attention needs to be given to the foods they eat, especially if their health problems persist after following such a diet for a reasonable amount of time (1-2 months). Such people may unknowingly suffer from food allergies or sensitivities, or require the professional assistance of a skilled physician or nutritionist, who can help tailor a diet specific to their unique metabolic type and biochemical individuality. This is an area of expertise that is far more common among practitioners of alternative medicine than among conventional doctors, who receive little training in diet and nutrition during their medical education. Naturopathic physicians and practitioners of Ayurvedic and traditional Chinese medicine (TCM) can also provide valuable dietary advice.

See Allergies, Ayurvedic Medicine, Diet, Environmental Medicine, Naturopathic Medicine, Traditional Chinese Medicine.

Diet also affects the acid-alkaline balance of the cells, which plays a role in your level of health and well-being. Hazel Parcells, N.D., who was 106 years old when she died, observed that all decay and disease occurs in highly acidic states. The body of a person who is chronically tired and sleepy is usually acidic and will age quickly. But when the cells in a body are more alkaline, the person ages less quickly and has more energy and drive. An individual can alter this chemical balance to favor a more balanced pH by changing how and what they eat (in accordance with their metabolic type).

NUTRITIONAL SUPPLEMENTS

Due the increasing prevalence of environmental pollution, the stresses of modern living, and the spread of virulent pathogens, nutritional supplementation is another important self-care health option. Few Americans obtain the minimum, recommended amounts of vitamins and minerals from their diet. And there are many reasons to believe that the Recommended Dietary Allowances (RDAs) are arbitrary, set too low in many cases, and do not begin to address unique nutritional needs. Although each of us requires the same nutrients for proper health, the amount of each can vary considerably, due to a host of factors, such as age, genetics, stress levels, lifestyle, and exposure to toxins. Pregnant women and people who regularly smoke or consume alcohol also have different nutritional requirements, as do people who are ill or suffer from allergies. In order to tailor a nutritional supplementation program that ideally suits your needs, consider consulting with a nutritionally oriented physician or clinical nutritionist.

See Addictions, Nutritional Medicine, Orthomolecular Medicine, Pregnancy and Childbirth.

For general purposes, the following list of supplements, created by Robert A. Anderson, M.D., and Robert S. Ivker, D.O., founding President and President-elect, respectively, of the American Board of Holistic Medicine, provides a suggested dosage range for the most common antioxidant vitamins and minerals:

- Vitamin C (polyascorbate): 1,000–2,000 mg three times daily

- Beta carotene: 25,000 IU once or twice daily

- Vitamin E: 400 IU once or twice daily

- B-complex vitamins: 50–100 mg of each per day

- Folic acid: 400–800 mcg daily

- Selenium: 100–200 mcg daily

- Zinc picolinate: 20–40 mg per day

- Calcium citrate or apatite: 1,000 mg daily

- Magnesium citrate or aspartate: 500 mg daily

- Chromium polynicotinate: 200 mcg per day

- Manganese: 10–15 mg per day

- Copper: 2 mg per day

- Iron: 10–18 mg daily

"People who are exposed to higher levels of stress and increased exposure to pollutants, or who are not feeling well or experiencing diminished sleep, should use the higher doses," Dr. Ivker advises. "Otherwise, take at least the minimum dose of each nutrient every day, preferably with your meals."[2]

PROBIOTICS

Inside each of us live vast numbers of bacteria without which we could not remain in good health. There are several thousand billion in each person (more than all the cells in the body) divided into over 400 species, most of them living in the digestive tract. Certain of these bacteria help to maintain good health, while others have a definite value in helping us regain health once it has been upset. The use of friendly bacteria supplements is known as probiotics, meaning "for life."

Lactobacillus acidophilus is the predominant friendly bacteria in the upper intestinal tract. It helps reduce the levels of harmful bacteria and yeasts in the small intestine and also produces lactase, an enzyme important in the digestion of milk. Acidophilus is also involved in the production of B vitamins (niacin, folic acid, pyridoxine) during the digestive process.

Bifidobacterium bifidum and *B. longum* are the primary friendly bacteria in the large intestine. *Bifidobacteria* protect the large intestine from invading bacteria and yeasts, and also manufacture B vitamins and help the body detoxify bile. *B. infantis* is the prevalent friendly bacteria in the intestines of infants.

Streptococcus thermophilus and *L. bulgaricus* are most commonly found in yogurt and exist only transiently in the digestive tract. They produce lactic acid, which encourages the growth of other friendly bacteria, and they also synthesize bacteriocins (natural antibiotic-like substances) that kill harmful bacteria.

Lactobacilli, *Bifidobacteria*, and *Streptococci* are the bacteria most commonly found in probiotic supplements. Other beneficial species that may be included are *L. casei*,

L. plantarum, L. sporogenes, L. brevis, and *Saccharomyces boulardii.* Without bacteria like acidophilus, you would be unable to properly digest your food and absorb vitamins and other nutrients. But digestion is only the beginning of the health benefits probiotics can provide. Other benefits include:

- The manufacture of certain B vitamins, including niacin (B₃), pyridoxine (B₆), folic acid, and biotin.[3]

- Enhanced immune system activity.[4]

- Manufacture of the milk-digesting enzyme lactase, which helps digest calcium-rich dairy products.[5]

- Production of antibacterial substances that kill or deactivate hostile disease-causing bacteria.[6] Friendly bacteria do this by changing the local levels of acidity, by depriving pathogenic bacteria of their nutrients, or by actually producing their own antibiotic substances.[7]

- Anticarcinogenic effect, since probiotics are active against certain tumors.[8]

- Improved efficiency of the digestive tract.[9]

- Reduction of high cholesterol levels.[10]

- Protection against radiation damage and deactivation of many toxic pollutants.[11]

- Recycling of estrogen (a female hormone), which reduces the likelihood of menopausal symptoms and osteoporosis.[12]

Friendly bacteria have been shown to be useful in treatment of acne, psoriasis, eczema, allergies, migraines, gout (by reducing uric acid levels), rheumatic and arthritic conditions, cystitis, candidiasis, colitis, irritable bowel syndrome, and some forms of cancer.[13]

Many factors influence the health of the intestinal flora. While the type of friendly bacteria living in a region may seem much the same in health and disease, the tasks they perform change according to circumstances. For example, when *Bifidobacteria* are in a good state of health, they will detoxify pollutants and carcinogens, as well as manufacture various B vitamins. When in a poor state of health, however, they cannot do these jobs as well or at all.

Local acidity is one major influence on the function of the friendly bacteria. This is affected by diet, digestive function, and stress.[14] Another important influence is the speed of peristalsis (the wavelike contraction of the intestines), which moves food along the digestive tract. If it is too rapid (as in diarrhea, irritable bowel syndrome, or colitis) or too slow (as in constipation), this causes changes in their function. The bacteria are healthier on a diet rich in complex carbohydrates (vegetables, whole grains, legumes) and low in animal fats, fatty meat, sugars, and cultured dairy products.[15] Not surprisingly, the diet that is best for people is also ideal for healthy bacteria.

Intestinal flora are also influenced to a major extent by the degree of infection by yeasts and bacteria in the bowel. Certain drugs, especially antibiotics, can severely upset this delicate balance—penicillin will kill friendly bacteria just as efficiently as it will kill disease-causing bacteria.[16] Steroids (cortisone, ACTH, prednisone, and birth control pills) also cause great damage to the bowel flora.

The difficulty with probiotics is getting them into your intestines in an active form. *L. acidophilus* and other bacteria can easily be destroyed during the manufacturing process or by heat and light while being stored. They can also be dissolved by acids in the stomach when probiotics are taken orally. When selecting a supplement, therefore, it is important to find one that will deliver viable (live) bacterial cultures to where they can do you some good. Yogurt, which many people consume for its probiotic content, is generally not as good as a supplement in re-colonizing the intestines. The reason is that yogurt contains primarily *L. bulgaricus* and *S. thermophilus,* friendly bacteria that only temporarily inhabit the colon. Supplements contain a sufficient variety of bacteria and in great enough numbers to aid in repopulating the intestines.

Most probiotic supplements contain *Lactobacilli* intended to colonize the small intestine and *Bifidobacteria* for the colon. Some products carry "cocktails" of bacteria that should not be together in a container and are only minutely a part of the total flora picture, such as *Bacillus laterosporus* and *Streptococcus faecium,* which should be avoided. Even cocktails of the best friendly bacteria should not be kept in the same container since they are destined to inhabit different regions of the digestive tract. Encapsulating beneficial bacteria in vitamin E or wheat germ oil (known as oil-matrix delivery), will solve this problem.

When being separated from the "soup" in which they are cultured, some manufacturers spin the bacteria in a centrifuge. This damages the delicate chains of bacteria, which does not happen when a slower (and therefore more expensive) filtration process is used. It is preferable to take the friendly bacteria as a powder, as similar damage can occur if the bacteria are in capsule or tablet form. The bacteria should be stored in a dark glass (never plastic) container. Viable cultures of the par-

WHEN TO USE PROBIOTIC SUPPLEMENTS

- Under professional guidance if there are chronic bowel problems or ongoing infections such as candidiasis.

- As a preventive against food poisoning when traveling (*Bifidobacteria* and acidophilus kill most food-poisoning bacteria).

- After (and during) any period when antibiotics are taken.

- By all premenopausal and menopausal women to reduce chances of osteoporosis.

- By anyone with high cholesterol problems.

- By anyone with chronic health problems (acne, skin problems, allergies, arthritis, cancer) under professional guidance.

- By anyone receiving radiation treatment.

- By anyone having recurrent vaginal or bladder infections (thrush or cystitis).

- *Bifidobacteria infantis* should be given to all babies.

ticular bacteria you want, as a rule, need to be refrigerated after the opening of their container. They should not be taken at meal times to avoid the extreme acidity of the stomach when it has food in it. All good products should carry a guarantee of viable colonizing bacteria up to a specific expiration date.

A recommended dosage is between one billion and ten billion bacteria per day (check the label of each particular probiotic supplement for details of the number of organisms it contains). If you're currently taking antibiotics, the dosage can be increased to 15–20 billion organisms. Other than mild gastrointestinal upset, the use of probiotics does not produce any side effects; however, if you are taking antibiotics, consult with your physician before supplementing with probiotics as they can affect the metabolism of some antibiotics.

Exercise

Next to diet, exercise is the most important factor for achieving and maintaining optimum physical health. It provides health benefits for people of all ages and can also prolong life. A Finnish study of nearly 8,000 men and women, for instance, found that those who did not exercise increased their risk of dying by 400% compared to individuals in the high-activity group.[17] Here are some tips to help you get started:

- Frequency and duration of activity are more important than intensity. Moderately intense exercise, such as brisk walking, is enough for health benefits if done most days of the week. Normal daily activities as well as formal exercise sessions add up. You get health benefits from walking up stairs and carrying out the trash, gardening, cleaning, shopping, vacuuming, making the bed, and mowing the lawn.

- If you can, engage in moderate to vigorous exercise using the large muscles for 30–60 minutes three or more times a week; you're likely to gain even more health benefits in addition to greater fitness.

- You don't have to do all your exercise at one time during the day. You can accumulate short periods of moderately intense activity, such as mowing a patch of lawn or walking up hills, in 5- to 10-minute intervals that total 30 minutes throughout the day. The key is the total amount of energy expended not the intensity.

- Strengthening exercises (such as weight training) at least twice a week help counteract muscle loss due to aging. And since calories are burned more quickly by muscle tissue, muscle mass is a key factor in helping maintain a healthful weight. The more lean muscle mass you can preserve, the bigger the "engine" in which to burn calories.

- Ideally, you should have four goals for your exercise regimen: aerobic capacity, strength, flexibility, and weight control (exercise plus optimal nutrition).

- Plan a logical progression. If you have unstable joints from injury or arthritis, or you're in a weakened condition, start by improving your muscle strength and flexibility. Build strength using lighter weights and gently exercising the weakest parts of your body

- When you're ready to add an aerobic exercise, start at a comfortable level, such as walking 5-10 minutes over a short distance indoors. Increase one to five minutes per session, as tolerated.

- Remember that for your fitness to improve, you need to exercise regularly. Try for a minimum of 30 minutes of low to moderately intense physical activity on most days of the week. Over time, you may be able to build up to 30-60 minutes of moderate to vigorous exercise.

- Include variety. Combine three types of exercise—stretching (flexibility), endurance (aerobic), and strengthening (weight training)—with three levels of intensity—warm-up, workout level, and cool-down—in each exercise session. When you're fit, a typical session might include a five-minute warm-up (stretching or slow walking), 20-40 minutes of aerobic activity (brisk walking, bicycling, or rowing), 10-15 minutes of weight training, and a five-minute cool-down of stretching.

- Mixed training (cross training) reduces your chance of injury to or overuse of one specific muscle or joint. Alternate among exercises that emphasize different parts of your body.

- Schedule time for recovery. Many people start with frenzied zeal, exercising too long or too intensely, and give up when muscles and joints become sore or injured. Start slowly and build up gradually, allowing time between sessions for your body to rest and recover.

- For most older people, brisk walking becomes a mainstay exercise. Walking for 20-30 minutes or more at least three but preferably five times a week offers health benefits. If one of your goals is losing weight, you may want to walk about 40 minutes several times a week. That's because you burn more fat during longer-duration, lower-intensity exercise than you do during shorter exercise periods.

Precautions: Before beginning any exercise program, consult your physician and have a thorough exam to rule out any health conditions that may need attention. If you have heart disease, diabetes, or are at high risk for these or other serious illnesses, begin an exercise program only with your physician's approval. Inactive men over the age of 40 and women over 50 should also consult their physician. If you have been physically inactive for some time, it is important to consult with your physician to determine if you may need to undergo an accelerated detoxification program before you begin exercising. Ask your doctor how your medications may affect your exercise plan. Drugs for diabetes, high blood pressure, and heart disease, as well as sedatives, anti-histamines and cold medications, can cause dehydration, impaired balance, and blurred vision; in addition, some medications can affect the way your body reacts to exercise.

Sleep

One of the key elements for physical health is adequate sleep. "It's while we are sleeping that the body's regenerative processes are at work," explains leading alternative physician Joseph Pizzorno, N.D., founder and President Emeritus of Bastyr University and author of *Total Wellness*. "But in our society today, adequate sleep is becoming lost. If you look at the amount of sleep we get now compared to our grandparents, we are averaging almost two hours less sleep a night. And even when we are getting sleep, we aren't sleeping as deeply. We're sleeping later at night and bypassing the normal circadian rhythm that's created by nature."[18]

Lack of sleep can contribute to a host of health risks, including impaired immunity and susceptibility to disease, impaired mental function, increased accident risk, stress, and anxiety and depression. Becoming aware of your sleep patterns is therefore a vital tool in maintaining your physical health.

The following guidelines can help you achieve deeper, more satisfying sleep:

- Be aware of how many hours of sleep you require in order to function optimally and then make sure you get enough sleep each night.

- Get up at the same time each day and avoid the temptation to wake up early or sleep late, especially on weekends and holidays.

- Avoid daytime naps.

- Eat a healthy diet and avoid food substances that affect serotonin levels, such as chocolate, caffeine, alcohol, and cheese.

- Exercise during the day to reduce stress levels, which is conducive to better sleep.

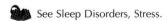 See Sleep Disorders, Stress.

Creating a Healthy Home and Work Environment

Ensuring that your home and work environments are healthy is another essential self-care precaution that can improve your physical health. Many office environments, especially those that are new and air-conditioned, lack clean, fresh air because their windows are sealed. Such buildings are also at risk for "sick building syndrome," due to the chemical nature of the materials used to build and furnish them. Indoor plants at home and in the office can help counteract such risks, due to their ability to oxygenate the air and filter out carbon dioxide and organic chemicals. Plants also help to keep indoor air moist, which makes for healthier breathing. The use of humidifiers (especially during winter months to help prevent dry air caused by indoor heating and unopened windows) and a negative ion generator, which acts as an efficient air cleaner, is also recommended.[19]

Many household products, such as synthetic particleboard, plastics, polyester, and carpets, can add to the risk of indoor environmental pollution and should particularly be avoided by people who are highly allergic or chemically sensitive. Products made of wood, cotton, wool, and metal are more advisable. If your home or office has carpets or rugs, make sure they are cleaned regularly to avoid build-up of molds and bacteria. Also replace commercial cleaning products with nontoxic products free of chemical additives. And during winter months, reduce the use of coal- and wood-burning stoves and fireplaces and have your furnace filter checked for efficiency.

If you work at a computer, take regular breaks during the day and, if possible, try to spend time each day outdoors in a natural setting. To further protect against the effects of electromagnetic fields (EMFs) caused by computer screens and other devices, consider using various energy devices that can safeguard against EMF pollution.

Avoiding secondhand smoke is also recommended. Finally, at night during sleep, keep a bedroom window open to allow for fresh air.[20]

 See Energy Medicine, Environmental Medicine.

Other Self-Care Approaches for Physical Well-Being

The following professional care therapies contain aspects that can be adapted to your physical self-care protocol: Aromatherapy, Ayurvedic Medicine, Bodywork, Detoxification Therapy, Enzyme Therapy, Herbal Medicine, Homeopathy, Hydrotherapy, Hyperthermia, Light Therapy, Magnetic Field Therapy, Naturopathic Medicine, Qigong and Tai Chi, Sound Therapy, Traditional Chinese Medicine, Yoga. See the individual chapters for more details.

Mental Health

Mental health is defined as a "condition of peace of mind, contentment, and positive beliefs and attitudes."[21] The field of psychoneuroimmunology (PNI) has provided us with startling insights into how our central nervous system and brain, immune system, and endocrine systems are all linked by way of nerves and chemical messengers called neurotransmitters. As a result of this mind-body connection, there is interplay between what we think and feel (consciously and subconsciously) and the condition of our bodies.

In our response to stress, free-radical production is increased dramatically; at the same time, our adrenal glands secrete cortisol, adrenaline, and other hormones. This flood of stress hormones has a cascading adverse effect on other hormones related to longevity, such as DHEA, growth hormone, and insulin. This affects the body's ability to repair cells, tissues, and organs. It is in this way that negative mental and emotional states dampen immune system function and deplete organ reserve, predisposing us toward age-related illnesses.

The following are a number of self-care approaches that can be used to relieve stress, improve your mental/emotional outlook, and lead to greater self-understanding.

Affirmations

Affirmations, also known as autosuggestions, are positive statements that can be used to change the way you think about yourself and your health. Since the unconscious cannot tell the difference between a real or imagined idea, it responds to whatever suggestions you give it, eventually helping to create the reality that matches your most predominant beliefs, attitudes, and thoughts. By repeating a positive affirmation each time a negative, self-defeating thought comes to mind, you can retrain your mind and learn to respond more confidently to the world around you, as well as improve your overall health. Over time, old, limited thoughts and mental patterns that contributed to anxiety, depression, or stress will lose their charge and eventually stop arising altogether.

Using affirmations does not mean suppressing any thought that is not "good," however. Instead, affirmations are used as a reshaping tool that you can call upon to rid yourself of thoughts that serve no positive purpose. For example, if you are prone to headaches and your thoughts keep informing you that you haven't had a headache in a while and are therefore due for one, instead of giving in and feeding such thoughts, you can overcome them by using an affirmation, such as "I am headache free and I deserve to stay that way." Initially, this may seem to be silly or an attempt to fool yourself, but if you pay attention and keep repeating the affirmation, before long you will say it and mean it and the results you expect will follow.

Affirmations can be used in any area of your life. To be most effective, choose one or two affirmations that feel most comfortable and memorize them, so that you can say them whenever a negative thought enters your mind. You might also consider mentally repeating your affirmation 10-20 times once or twice a day. Useful affirmations include:

- I am healthy, relaxed, and free of pain and disease.

- I love myself, and I deserve to feel healthy and alive.

- I approve of myself, and I am safe to be who I am.

- I am flexible, open, and loving towards myself and the world around me.

- Every day in every way, I am getting better and better.

- I am in the flow of life, and I am grateful for the gift of being alive.

- In every way, I am healing and learning to accept the joy life offers.

- My life is my own and I easily resolve my conflicts.

Breathwork

Breath not only keeps the body alive with vital oxygen, it also has the power to alter consciousness and affect your mental and emotional health. Most of us, however, pay little attention to the way we breathe, taking short, shallow breaths, releasing the air we inhale before it comes close to reaching the bottoms of our lungs. In addition, particularly when overwhelmed by pain or stress, we forget to breathe altogether.

Once you recognize the influence your emotions and thoughts have on your breath, you can begin to use your breath to influence these states and to reconnect with the natural flow of life. By regularly practicing one or more of the following exercises, you will become more aware of the breaths you take and will find it easier to breathe more deeply. Breathe through your nose as you practice the exercises. When you breathe in, initiate the action from deep inside your diaphragm to allow your lungs a full range of motion.

THREE-PART BREATH

This technique is designed to draw air deep into the diaphragm so it can oxygenate the entire system. To perform it, divide each deep inhalation into three parts, the first part lifting the belly, the second part filling the lungs, and the third part extending into the upper chest. Hold for three seconds, then release in one long exhalation. Repeat five times.

TWENTY-CYCLE BREATH

This exercise was developed by Leonard Orr, considered the modern father of breathwork therapy. It can be performed anywhere and can serve as a pleasant way to alter your mood or thought process. It is performed by taking four short, continuous breaths (no pause between the inhalation and the exhalation), followed by one extended long breath. Repeat this cycle five times.

WU BREATHING

Wu is a Chinese breathing technique. Lie down in a relaxed position with your head on a little pillow and your arms resting at your sides, your feet a little more than hip-width apart. Place the tip of your tongue on the roof of your mouth, just behind where your front teeth meet the gums, and begin to breathe naturally through your nose. Imagine the breath coming through your nose to the top of your head and then down to the center of your belly. Continue breathing and visualizing in this manner for 20-30 minutes, concentrating on the breath coming in through your head. Do this in the morning and at night.

PULSE BREATHING

This technique combines diaphragmatic breathing with a pulsed, hard exhalation. To begin, take a deep breath and exhale, then inhale and exhale forcefully (called a pulse breath). Then take two deep-breathing cycles and a pulse breath; three deep-breathing cycles and a pulse breath; four deep-breathing cycles and a pulse breath; five deep-breathing cycles and a pulse breath. Perform this exercise twice daily or any time you are under stress.

Flower Essences

Developed in the 1930s by British physician Edward Bach, D.Hom., flower essence therapy is a form of healing that influences emotional states in order to help bring about physical and psychological well-being. Although not intended to treat physical conditions directly, flower essences have a wide range of applications, working to balance the negative feelings and stress that often impede health and recovery. As emotions stabilize, a more positive outlook is achieved, triggering an immune system response that stimulates physical healing. Although initial treatments are best administered under the supervision of a health practitioner trained in their use, flower essences are ideally suited as a self-care protocol once their use and application is understood. Completely nontoxic and nonaddictive, they are administered according to individual need.

Journal Writing

Journal writing, or "journaling," is an excellent way to release the frustrations that can accompany illness and can often provide valuable insights about life issues, including steps you it can take to more effectively resolve them. Since journal writing is performed alone and in private, you will not be rejected for whatever you express on paper. This gives you the opportunity to better express how you feel and to learn to accept whatever comes up, without judgment. Over time, keeping a journal can provide new perspectives that help you better understand and resolve the emotions, patterns, images, and "dramas" that may be linked to the issues you are exploring and provide new information that you otherwise might not have considered.

All that is required to keep a journal is a pen, paper, and your thoughts. Write without worrying about whether you are saying anything important or not, and without being concerned about grammar or punctuation. All that matters when keeping a journal is that you are open and honest about your thoughts and feelings. As your writing connects you to your "healer within," you may be surprised at how much you have to express and how good it feels to write it down.

Relaxation Exercises

Like meditation, biofeedback, and creative visualization, relaxation exercises help to relax blood flow, decrease muscle pain and tension, ease emotional stress, improve sleep, and positively alter brain chemistry. The following exercises are both effective and easy to perform and can be done nearly anywhere.

PROGRESSIVE RELAXATION

Lie on the floor, couch, or bed, with your shoes off. If you wish, you can play soft music or light candles to set the stage for relaxation. Spend a few moments observing your breath, paying attention to each inhalation and exhalation. Take at least five full diaphragmatic breaths. Now begin relaxing the muscles of your body, group by group, starting with your feet and working up to your neck, face, and head. To aid in this process, mentally tell yourself what body area is now relaxing: "My toes and feet are now relaxed, my shins and calf muscles are now relaxed, my knees are now relaxed," and so forth. Unless you wish to fall asleep, don't do this exercise immediately after meals or in the morning.

CUE-CONTROLLED RELAXATION

Either sit with your back straight or lie on your back with your arms next to your sides. Become aware of your breath and begin to breathe in through your nose and out through your mouth, entirely emptying your lungs as you exhale and allowing your stomach to rise as you inhale. Place one hand on your stomach and the other hand on your chest, making sure that only your stomach is moving. Breathe at a slow and regular rate, inhaling to a count of four, holding your breath for a count

of one, exhaling to a count of four, holding your breath for a count of one, and then repeating the cycle. As you breathe, mentally repeat the statement "I am relaxed," saying "I am" as you inhale, and "relaxed" as you exhale. Do this for five minutes or longer.

OTHER RELAXATION TIPS

If you sit at a desk all day and start to feel yourself becoming "tight," sometimes simply closing your eyes and scanning your body for possible muscle tension can be enough to relax stiff muscles. Also, be sure to take breaks during the day, standing up to stretch. When you do so:

- Breathe deeply, rolling your head in clockwise and counterclockwise circles.

- Roll your shoulders, front and back, up and down, until you feel the blood tingling in your hands.

- Take both hands and massage the back of your neck, pressing beneath the bony ridges at the back until you feel your muscles becoming softer and more responsive.

Other Self-Care Approaches for Mental Well-Being

The following professional care therapies contain aspects that can be adapted to your self-care protocol for mental well-being: Aromatherapy, Biofeedback Training and Neurotherapy, Flower Essences, Guided Imagery, Hypnotherapy, Light Therapy, Magnetic Field Therapy, Mind/Body Medicine, Qigong and Tai Chi, Sound Therapy, Yoga. See the individual chapters for more details.

Spiritual Health

Being spiritually healthy means consciously cultivating a connection with spirit, the divine life force that makes all life possible, and being healthy socially in terms of your relationships with your family, friends, and community. "Spiritual and social health are interconnected, since it is through our committed relationships that we find the greatest opportunities for spiritual growth and for learning how to receive and impart unconditional love," Dr. Ivker says.[22] This aspect of health, although often neglected or ignored, holds the key to achieving lasting peace of mind. Self-care approaches such as prayer and the observance of spiritual or religious traditions, meditation, practicing gratitude, and spending time in volunteerism help deepen your awareness of yourself as a spiritual, socially connected human being.

Prayer

Prayer is the oldest and most popular form of spiritual self-care and has been shown to result in greater feelings of well-being, reduced stress, and the rapid triggering of the "relaxation response."[23] In addition to traditional prayers from the world's great religions, prayer can take the form of a personal conversation between yourself and your deity. Simply taking time to acknowledge the blessings of the day can also be an effective form of prayer. What is important is that the form of prayer be comfortable for you and that you pray sincerely on a regular basis. Many people find that the effectiveness of their prayers are bolstered in a group setting and during the observance of religious services, such as in a church, mosque, or temple.

Meditation

Like prayer, mediation is also part of the world's spiritual and religious traditions. For more than 30 years, Western science has been verifying the numerous physical and psychological benefits that the regular practice of meditation can provide. Traditional meditation practices are ideally taught by an accomplished spiritual teacher, but once learned, it is a practice that easily lends itself to self-care. It can also be practiced at any time, simply by focusing the attention on your breathing and observing what is occurring around you in the present moment, without judgment or regard for the past or future.

Practicing Gratitude

According to Dr. Anderson, the regular practice of gratitude "produces feelings of joy and self-acceptance, and is an attitude that anyone can choose to have, just as we can choose to see the glass half full or half empty." Dr. Anderson adds that choosing to practice gratitude makes it easier to let go of negative thoughts and emotions.[24] The easiest way of practicing gratitude is to cultivate an awareness of all you have to be grateful for during the course of each day. Acknowledging the kindness, help, and other forms of support you receive from others will further increase your sense of gratitude. You can also keep a gratitude journal by taking time each night to write down the blessings that came your way during the day. Doing so will help you move beyond taking your life for granted and transform the way you perceive and live your life.

Volunteerism

During the last decade, many Americans became part of a growing trend toward volunteerism, seeking to participate in ways of "giving back" to their communities. "Such selfless acts of giving go to the essence of spirit, which is always with us supporting our lives while asking for nothing in return," Dr. Ivker says. "Sharing with others your time, help, and special gifts and talents in ways that benefit them provides you with perhaps the most powerful means of engaging and expressing spirit and enhancing social health."[25]

Volunteering can take many forms, such as donating money or clothes to charity, spending time helping out at a homeless shelter or soup kitchen, providing tutoring services to after-school or adult literacy programs, or simply taking time to listen to the needs and concerns of your family members, friends, neighbors, or co-workers. Another form of volunteerism that is regaining popularity is tithing, the practice of donating a percentage of one's salary to charity.

Research has shown that taking the time to help others not only results in your own increased positive emotions, but also significantly increases longevity. One study conducted at the University of Michigan's Survey Research Center, in Tecumseh, Michigan, followed over 2,700 men for 14 years. At the end of that period, it was found that those who did regular volunteer work had death rates 2 ½ times lower than those who didn't volunteer. "It may be that the highest form of selfishness is selflessness," says Dr. Ivker, commenting on the study. "When we freely choose to help others, we seem to get as much as, or more than, what we give."[26]

 See Mind/Body Medicine.

Recommended Reading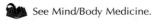

The American Holistic Medical Association Guide to Holistic Health. Larry Trivieri, Jr. New York: John Wiley & Sons, 2001.

The Complete Self-Care Guide to Holistic Medicine. Robert S. Ivker, D.O., Robert A. Anderson, M.D., and Larry Trivieri, Jr. New York: Tarcher/Putnam, 1999.

Longevity: An Alternative Medicine Definitive Guide. W. Lee Cowden, M.D., Ferre Akbarpour, M.D., and Russ DiCarlo, with Burton Goldberg. Tiburon, CA: AlternativeMedicine.com Books, 2001.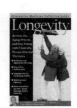

Total Wellness. Joseph Pizzorno. Rocklin, CA: Prima Publishing, 1996.

Physical Health

Body for Life. Bill Phillips and Michael D'Orso. New York: HarperCollins, 1999.

Gary Null's Ultimate Lifetime Diet. Gary Null. New York: Broadway Books, 2000.

Home Safe Home: Protecting Yourself and Your Family from Everyday Toxics and Harmful Household Products. Debra Dadd-Redalia and Debra Lynn Dadd. New York: Tarcher/Putnam, 1997.

Staying Healthy with Nutrition. Elson Haas. Berkeley, CA: Celestial Arts, 1992.

The Supplement Shopper. Gregory Pouls, D.C., and Maile Pouls, Ph.D., with Burton Goldberg. Tiburon, CA: Future Medicine Publishing, 1999.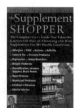

Your Body's Many Cries for Water. Fereydoon Batmanghelidj. Falls Church, VA: Global Health Solutions, 1992.

Mental Health

Bach Flower Therapy: Theory and Practice. Mechthild Scheffer. Rochester, VT: Healing Arts Press, 1988.

Deep Healing: The Essence of Mind/Body Medicine. Emmett Miller. Carlsbad, CA: Hay House, 1997.

You Can Heal Your Life. Louise Hay. Carlsbad, CA: Hay House, 1984, 1987.

Spiritual Health

Sacred Healing. C. Norman Shealy. Boston: Element Books, 1999.

MEDICAL FREEDOM

Unless we put medical freedom into the Constitution, the time will come when medicine will organize into an undercover dictatorship. To restrict the art of healing to one class of men and deny equal privileges to others will constitute the Bastille of medical science. All such laws are un-American and despotic and have no place in a republic. The Constitution of this republic should make special privilege for medical freedom as well as religious freedom.

—BENJAMIN RUSH, M.D., SIGNER OF DECLARATION OF INDEPENDENCE, PHYSICIAN TO GEORGE WASHINGTON

FREEDOM IS AT THE heart of American society. We have freedom of speech, freedom of worship, and freedom of the press. But Americans lack one freedom that seems increasingly more vital for a truly free society—the freedom to choose the health care of their choice. This basic freedom is being suppressed by state and federal agencies, as well as the vested financial interests of the "medical/pharmaceutical complex," comprised of the conventional medical establishment and the multinational pharmaceutical companies. Despite the fact that conventional treatments are often ineffective, simply mask symptoms, and are subject to troubling side effects, Americans who seek better and more effective medicine must struggle to win the right to open access to alternative practitioners and treatments. In recent decades:

- Government regulatory agencies have made a concerted effort to punish and harass medical professionals who recommend or practice nutritional and herbal medicine and other alternative therapies to maintain health and prevent and treat illness.

- State medical boards have censured and revoked the licenses of conscientious physicians who practice alternative medicine, simply because their treatments are not conventional and do not conform to accepted "standards of care." These actions are taken despite the fact that many of these treatments work.

- Insurance companies have routinely refused to pay for alternative treatments, labeling them "unapproved therapies," regardless of the benefit received by the patients. This stance denies tens of millions of Americans their basic right to the health care of their choice.

- The general public has been denied free access to information concerning the documented health benefits of nutritional supplements and herbs by restrictive labeling regulations established by the U.S. Food and Drug Administration (FDA). This restriction of information comes despite the fact that large-scale independent studies have shown that many Americans, especially the elderly, are suffering from nutritional deficits that could be corrected by dietary supplementation.

- Manufacturers of nutritional supplements and herbs, as well as health food stores, have been the target of FDA seizures in an attempt to block the manufacture and sale of numerous natural substances whose therapeutic effects have been scientifically validated.

These strong-arm tactics are being used despite the estimate of former Surgeon General C. Everett Koop that, out of 2.1 million deaths a year in the U.S., 1.6 million are related to poor nutrition.[1] The bias against alternative medicine on both the state and federal level has

PRICE GOUGING BY THE PHARMACEUTICAL INDUSTRY

The U.S. Food and Drug Administration's process for approval of a drug costs as much as $250 million and 5-10 years of development time. Yet the profits of pharmaceutical companies are among the highest of any industry in the world and often come at the expense of human health. For example, a recent cancer drug, Levamisole, taken in combination with another drug, Fluorouacil, was shown to reduce the recurrence rate of advanced colon cancers by 41% when taken following surgery, according to a study conducted at the Mayo Clinic, in Rochester, Minnesota. But this same drug, which costs $15 annually when used as a treatment for worms in animals, has a price tag of $1,200 when used to treat cancer patients for the same period.[2]

American pharmaceutical prices are also much higher than those of other nations, especially those with national health insurance and centralized purchasing and price negotiation. And if drug companies wish to peddle their medicines in countries with national health insurance, they are told that they must lower their price. In Mexico, for example, the price of the common prescription pain reliever Naprosyn is less than a fourth of that in the U.S. Indeed, many drug prices in the U.S. are much higher than in Mexico and many other countries.[3]

become clearly established and has links to the campaign of the medical establishment to squelch the emergence of alternative medicine in the United States.

The Uneven Playing Field

Despite the growing popularity of alternative medicine, including its acceptance by increasing numbers of conventional health-care practitioners, its full integration into America's overall health-care system remains seriously impeded by a number of unfair advantages conventional medicine currently retains. Chief among these are the FDA's overt antagonism to alternative healing methods; the existing conflict of interest among the FDA, the pharmaceutical industry it is supposed to regulate, and conventional medical journalists; the inherent fallacies of the controlled clinical trial (CCT), relied upon by pharmaceutical and other conventional medical companies and the FDA before new medical substances and procedures are allowed to enter the marketplace; the con-

tinued suppression of unorthodox research; and the unfair tactics employed by the American Medical Association in tandem with state medical boards.

The Food and Drug Administration: Medical Establishment Cops

The FDA's suppression of alternative medicine, and especially of nutritional supplements, constitutes a war for power with billions of dollars and American's health at stake, according to Julian Whitaker, M.D., past President of the American Preventive Medical Association and editor of *Health and Healing*. "This is not a reasonable debate on public safety or honesty in labeling," says Dr. Whitaker. "It is an ugly struggle for power."

The FDA is a branch of the Department of Health and Human Services, funded annually through the U.S. Congress. It has the authority to regulate foods, drugs, cosmetics, and medical devices that are sold between states or imported. The FDA is also responsible for ensuring that products are pure and unadulterated and not misrepresented through false labeling, declarations of ingredients, or net weight statements. The FDA regulates certain manufacturing processes, holding jurisdiction over a product from the initial shipment of its raw materials across state lines to the shipment of the finished product from a manufacturing distribution facility outside the state. In addition, some drugs, medical devices, food additives, and food coloring require premarketing FDA approval. If someone markets a product without such approval, the FDA can take regulatory action.

"The FDA has very wide-ranging regulatory powers that are restricted only by the courts. However, the FDA is rarely restricted because it is considered to be an agency of experts dealing with expert issues," notes attorney Jay Geller, of Santa Monica, California, an authority on FDA law and a former employee in the general counsel's office of the FDA. This lack of restriction allows the FDA to investigate alternative medicine practitioners with a relative lack of accountability. "There are two ways that the FDA is able to harass alternative physicians," says Alan R. Gaby, M.D., past President of the American Holistic Medical Association. "They can raid their clinics or restrict the availability of effective medicinal substances. Whether or not the FDA has overstepped their legal boundary is unclear, but I do believe that what they are doing is improper. If there were unbiased individuals running the FDA, this would not be happening, as I think it has much to do with their own bias and attitudes."

Konrad Kail, N.D., past President of the American Association of Naturopathic Physicians, holds a similar view. "The FDA's plan is to remove the agents used by alternative physicians, such as supplements and herbs, since they cannot remove the physicians," he says. "They are using the brute force of their power to unfairly police a specific group of individuals who tend to practice alternative medicine. As far as I am concerned, this is a politically motivated move by conventional medicine in order to remove the competition from the marketplace. They are using the FDA to accomplish their own political motivations."

The FDA's bias in favor of conventional medicine may stem from the informal but very real connection it has with the pharmaceutical industry. One study, for instance, found that half of the high-ranking FDA officials have been formerly employed as key executives in pharmaceutical companies immediately prior to joining the FDA. In addition, the study found that half of these officials would then serve in an executive capacity in a pharmaceutical company immediately upon leaving the FDA.[4]

Freedom of Information and FDA Regulation of Nutritional Supplements and Herbs

"The FDA has always had a perceived bias against dietary supplements and has historically looked on them with a jaundiced eye," says attorney Geller. "The agency has expressed virtually no interest in trying to find a balance between the requirements necessary to approve prescription drugs and those appropriate to allow preventive health claims for naturally occurring substances such as vitamins, minerals, enzymes, amino acids, and herbs. Even with the studies that have come out on the potential benefits of vitamin E for preventing heart disease, the FDA's position is that there are not going to be any claims allowed for dietary supplements that do not meet the standards applied to prescription drugs."

The FDA has also seized safe and effective natural remedies, such as coenzyme Q10 and evening primrose oil, from health food stores and distributors because they did not approve of the statements being made about these supplements, according to Dr. Gaby, despite the fact that extensive scientific literature supports their use. "Coenzyme Q10 has been shown to be valuable in treating congestive heart failure, cardiomyopathy [a disease of the heart muscle], and high blood pressure; and evening primrose oil has proven effective in the treatment of eczema, high blood pressure, and arthritis," he notes. Dr. Gaby finds that FDA policies make it extremely difficult for consumers to learn about the health benefits of any natural substance, including nutritional supplements and herbs. "According to the FDA's interpretation of the law," he says, "any substance for which a health claim is made

THE PERILS OF PRESCRIPTION DRUGS

Injury, even death, from prescription drugs has now become routine. That is the view of Thomas J. Moore, senior fellow in health policy at the George Washington University Medical Center and author of *Prescription for Disaster: The Hidden Dangers in Your Medicine Cabinet.* Prescription drugs are responsible for over 100,000 deaths in the United States each year, Moore points out, while one million users are severely injured and another two million are harmed as a result of hospitalization for prescription drug–related problems. So serious is the problem that the use of properly prescribed prescription drugs now ranks as the fourth leading cause of death in the U.S. But according to Moore, the extent of the harm is even greater than that, due to the lack of figures on the number of patients whose drug-related injuries are sufficient to consult a physician but do not require hospitalization. Moore estimates such cases total in the millions as well. These facts justify his conclusion that prescription drugs "rank as one of the greatest man-made dangers in modern society."

Ritalin, which is routinely prescribed for 10% of all male U.S. schoolchildren to control their behavior, is an example of this danger. Not only does Ritalin commonly cause side effects (including loss of appetite, insomnia, Tourette's syndrome, and stomachache), but its long-term effects are unknown. Even Ritalin's manufacturer admits that "sufficient data on the safety and efficacy of long-term use of Ritalin are not yet available." In addition, only after Ritalin was approved by the U.S. Food and Drug Administration (FDA) was data published showing that it could cause cancer in mice.

"In fact, prescription drugs are seldom evaluated for long-term effects," Moore says, "and the public health consequences of this glaring failure are truly frightening." Despite this fact, Moore adds that the public should not expect drug companies to be looking out for their safety, since they are now spending more than $10 billion a year to persuade you (and your physician) to buy their products.

becomes a drug, subject to the same strict rules and regulations as prescription pharmaceuticals."

Dr. Kail feels that such rules are unnecessary. "We don't need to have more restrictions on supplements and herbs," he says. "This will only act to benefit the pharmaceutical companies and doctors who are already making enormous profits in this field and make it more expensive for people to take care of themselves. Health care will be taken out of the hands of the people and put back into the hands of institutions. People can do a lot to take care of themselves if they are taught how to do it."

One such example of FDA bias and its damaging effects on national health concerns the use of saw palmetto berries for prostate disease. "The extract of the saw palmetto berry has been shown in scientific studies to be about three times more effective than the Merck prostate drug, Proscar, for alleviating symptoms of prostate enlargement," Dr. Whitaker reports. "Furthermore, saw palmetto extract has no toxicity." On the other hand, Proscar causes impotence, ejaculation dysfunction, decreased libido, and birth defects.[5] Yet, the FDA recommended that saw palmetto berry be removed from the market while allowing Proscar to remain available. Fortunately, this recommendation has not been implemented.

The bias against natural cures is alarming. For example, according to summaries from the nation's poison control centers, one death was associated with the use of a nutritional supplement from 1983 to 1990 and that was due to regular overuse of niacin by a mentally disturbed individual. On the other hand, properly prescribed medical drugs cause about 130,000 deaths per year, or roughly 356 deaths every day.[6] "So as not to alarm the public or hurt the pharmaceutical industry, the FDA looks the other way when prescription drugs kill hundreds of thousands and harm millions," says Dr. Whitaker.

Science in the Interest of Profit

The FDA's bias is further shown by its selective implementation of policy directives. Its duty, by law, is to set standards for drug advertisements. Yet, according to a study conducted at the University of California and published in *The Wall Street Journal,* 60% of the pharmaceutical ads from medical journals violated FDA guidelines. But the FDA, to this day, has done nothing about these violations.[7]

Another connection between the FDA and the pharmaceutical industry is through the Pharmaceutical Advertising Council (PAC). In 1985, the PAC teamed up with the FDA to solicit funds from the pharmaceutical industry for the purpose of combating medical quackery. "The Pharmaceutical Advertising Council and the FDA also issued a joint statement addressed to the presidents of advertising and PR agencies nationwide asking them to cooperate with a joint venture anti-fraud and quackery campaign," according to Mark Blumenthal, Executive Director of the American Botanical Council. "The letter has joint letterhead from the FDA and the PAC and

is signed by the directors of both organizations. On the surface it appears to be patently illegal. The FDA is supposed to regulate the pharmaceutical industry, but instead they are teaming up to work on an anti-fraud campaign against an industry that some could construe to be an economic competitor."

Further evidence of the FDA's bias toward drugs as opposed to nutritional supplements is demonstrated by the FDA's Dietary Supplements Task Force Final Report, which reads in part, "The Task Force considered various issues in its deliberations, including what steps are necessary to ensure that the existence of dietary supplements on the market does not act as a disincentive for drug development."[8]

Such conflicts of interest also exist within the prestigious world of medical journals. The next time you read a scientific article in one of the major conventional medical magazines touting the benefits of a drug or medical procedure, bear in mind that the authors may have a vested financial interest in the success of that drug or procedure. This caution is based on the research of Stanley Krimsky, Ph.D., of the Department of Urban and Environmental Policy at Tufts University, in Medford, Massachusetts. Dr. Krimsky analyzed 1,105 university-based authors in Massachusetts and 789 articles published in 1992 in 14 scientific and medical journals, including the *New England Journal of Medicine (NEJM)* and *Science.* His analysis revealed that 15.3% of the authors had at least one financial interest in their published articles. In addition, Dr. Krimsky reported that 10% of journal authors were inventors or held patent applications related to their article's subject matter; 6.2% were members of the scientific advisory boards for biotechnology companies associated with the article; and 1.4% were major shareholders or officers in such companies.

Writing about an example of such a conflict of interest, the *NEJM* reported on the financial relationship between the authors of medical articles supporting the use of calcium channel-blockers for treating high blood pressure and the companies that manufacture them. *NEJM* researchers checked the medical literature from March 1995 to September 1996 for articles (70 were selected) on safety issues surrounding calcium channel-blockers. They then questioned the authors of the articles (all of whom were doctors) about any possible financial ties they had to the drug companies whose drugs they were writing about. In doing so, they discovered that doctors who provided "scientific" evidence in support of calcium channel-blocker safety were 96% more likely to have financial relationships with the manufacturers compared to 37% who wrote critically. In addition, supportive physicians were 100% more likely to have financial links to a drug company, compared to 67%

L-TRYPTOPHAN: BANNING A VALUABLE NATURAL TREATMENT FOR ANXIETY AND INSOMNIA

Much has been written about the ban of L-tryptophan, an essential amino acid widely used for more than 30 years as a dietary supplement to treat depression, insomnia, premenstrual syndrome, stress, and hyperactivity in children. At its core, however, the L-tryptophan story is a textbook case in how the government and private industry conspire to keep safe and effective natural remedies out of the hands of the public.

In December 1989, the U.S. Food and Drug Administration (FDA), responding to an outbreak of a rare blood disorder among some individuals taking L-tryptophan, pulled the substance off the market pending investigation. The disorder, eosinophilia-myalgia syndrome (EMS), was linked to impurities in the supplements as well as immune system weaknesses that increased susceptibility to the illness. Among the 1,550 known cases in the U.S. as of May 1990, 24 deaths were reported. The outbreak was traced to a contaminated batch of L-tryptophan produced by one Japanese manufacturer (Showa Denko K.K.). Despite the fact that the FDA and the U.S. Centers for Disease Control and Prevention both concluded that virtually all EMS patients used L-tryptophan from Showa Denko K.K., the amino acid was banned by the FDA in capsule or tablet shortly thereafter. The FDA's double standard continued, however, since this same substance was freely added to baby foods, tube feedings, and pet products. Then FDA Commissioner David Kessler, under attack by his critics for authorizing the ban, told Congress in July 1993, "Despite recent intense research, the exact cause of EMS and an understanding of how it develops have not been established."

"This is an obvious lie," counters Julian Whitaker, M.D., past President of the American Preventive Medical Association. "You do not allow babies, the elderly, and the infirm to have access to a supplement that is too toxic for the healthy adult population."

According to Garry F. Gordon, M.D., Co-founder of the American College of Advancement in Medicine, the agency's crusade against L-tryptophan dated back at least a decade. When Dr. Gordon served as a medical expert for the National Nutritional Food Association, which opposed the FDA's original effort to remove L-tryptophan from the market, he recalls that, "As we left the courtroom, they said, 'Well, you beat us this time, but we have lots of other avenues and we will get it stopped'." The FDA's ban on L-tryptophan, asserts Dr. Gordon, was directly linked to the power of the pharmaceutical industry. Because of L-tryptophan's effectiveness in combating insomnia, depression, and other health problems, it was impacting the pharmaceutical market for prescription drugs. "People didn't need their Valium, they didn't need their Librium, they didn't need their Prozac," Dr. Gordon says. "Therefore, physicians who use L-tryptophan, along with other dietary supplements, are harassed by the FDA acting on behalf of the pharmaceutical industry."

After protest of the FDA's action continued to mount, the FDA finally rescinded its ban a few years later, but with the restriction that L-tryptophan supplements are only available through a prescription.

among those who wrote neutral reviews and 43% among those who expressed critical views.[9]

The rate of published voluntary disclosures of financial interest by scientists in the 14 leading journals analyzed by Dr. Krimsky was "virtually zero." He noted that it seems increasingly evident that the goal of objective, financially unentangled research is "challenged by the perception that someone stands to benefit from the research in a way that could bias the manuscript or its findings." As a result of the discoveries made by Dr. Krimsky, the *NEJM,* and other investigators, some peer-reviewed journals are now beginning to require financial disclosure statements from their article contributors.[10]

Controlled Clinical Trials: Keeping Alternative Medicine at Bay

Critics of alternative medicine disparage many of its therapeutic approaches as being "unproven," due to the lack of controlled clinical trials (CCTs) that attest to their efficacy. This argument is fallacious for two reasons. First, an entire body of CCTs does in fact exist, supporting the merits of alternative medicine. For the most part, however, such studies rarely see publication in conventional medical journals, in large part due to the financial pressure that is brought to bear on journal editors by the medical/pharmaceutical complex, which is the primary source of advertising revenues for such publications. As a result, assuming they are published at all, CCTs that validate alternative medicine often go unnoticed, appearing in journals outside the scope of conventional M.D.s and the mainstream media. Moreover, CCTs can be extremely expensive to conduct (in many cases, costing millions of dollars). Although the National Center for Complementary and Alternative Medicine (part of the National Institutes of Health) annually allocates $150 million for research into alternative healing approaches, such a sum is a mere fraction compared to the billions of tax dollars spent on conventional medical research each year. In addition, alternative researchers lack the additional billions of dollars supplied to conventional researchers each year by the pharmaceutical companies.

But the more serious problem regarding CCTs, according to Harris Coulter, Ph.D., Founder and Director of the Center for Empirical Medicine, in Washington, D.C., and author of the report *The Controlled Clinical Trial: An Analysis*, lies in the fact that, by their inherent nature, CCTs cannot guarantee safety or efficacy, yet are nonetheless "used as a stick to beat alternative medicine with for failing to perform these trials."[11]

According to Dr. Coulter, although conventional physicians and researchers consider the CCT to be the "gold standard" of medicine, no controlled clinical trial matching its textbook definition has ever been performed, since its theoretical requirements are unrealistic and unscientific. "How can you test a drug on 12 or 100 or 1,000 identical, or 'homogenous' people, all with the same thing wrong with them?" Dr. Coulter asks. "Allopaths [conventional physicians] can't even find five homogenous patients. You'll always find things that are different between people, because we are all chemically, physically, structurally, and emotionally unique. The CCT can never tell a doctor how a given patient will react to any given drug at any given time. The findings from the so-called controlled clinical trial are useless in one-on-one doctor-patient interactions."

Dr. Coulter claims that the popularity of the CCT is due primarily to political reasons and used to keep alternative medicine at bay. "Since these trials are very expensive—it costs about $200 million today to get a new drug on the market—the controlled clinical trial is really an instrument for limiting competition in medicine and for raising the costs of medicines to the public," he says.[12]

In addition to the medical monopoly the CCT helps perpetuate, Dr. Coulter points out that fraud in safety testing is another possibility where CCTs are involved, due to the enormous sums of money researchers are paid by the manufacturers of the very drugs they are researching. "Frightful examples of dishonesty, fraud, negligence, and other kinds of wrongdoing in clinical trials have been staple fare for readers of the daily press since the 1970s,

when Congressional committees and subcommittees renewed their interest in the topic," he says.

One of the many examples of such fraud occurred in 1976, when the General Accounting Office (GAO) found that clinical trials of a drug designed to prevent rejection of kidney transplants had led to 85 deaths among 650 participating patients, yet not one of these deaths was reported to the FDA prior to the drug's approval. "In 1990," Dr. Coulter writes, "the GAO reported that over half the drugs approved as 'safe' by the FDA between 1976 and 1985 caused such serious side effects as to require re-labeling of the drug or its withdrawal from the market. These side effects were described as 'common' and resulted in hospitalization, permanent disability, and even death." He adds that "there is no reason to assume that these practices have ceased. And even when adverse reactions are reported, they are not properly incorporated into the evaluation of the drug."

Although his extensive analysis of the CCT caused him to conclude that it "has little or no medical justification," Dr. Coulter does ascribe one definite socioeconomic function to it: "that of restricting the flow of new knowledge into medicine and of new medicines into commerce." In this way, he says, the CCT helps perpetuate the monopoly and quasi-monopoly position of the medical industrial complex.

"In the not-too-distant past, medical innovation was due precisely to scientists working with patients and coming forward with new suggestions for treatment, but this avenue has now been closed off almost completely. While articles are still published detailing the experience and ideas of an individual practitioner, they are not regarded as sources of new discoveries. They do not appear in reputable journals and are not taken seriously by anyone. The practitioner has been relegated to the sidelines."

In their stead, Dr. Coulter claims, the drug manufacturers have become the agents of innovation and change in the medical arena, with the power to dictate which medicines become available to the public. "The clinical trial, with its accompanying financial pressure, favors large corporations over small, established businesses over new entries," he observes. "And since the FDA's requirements are stricter than those of any other country, foreigners wishing to sell in the U.S. market must comply with these more rigid standards. The monopoly position of U.S. drug manufacturers is thereby extended beyond this country's borders."[13]

The Medical Establishment and the Suppression of Unorthodox Research

The FDA is not the only force that practitioners of alternative medicine must contend with. In order to receive grants for medical research and be published in the major medical and scientific journals, physicians and researchers are compelled not to stray far from conventional views. Otherwise, they run the risk of being shut out of the mainstream and find themselves without the funding they need to carry on their work. The American Society for Clinical Nutrition, for example, publishers of the *American Journal of Clinical Nutrition*, acknowledges at the front of each issue of their journal the "generous support" of certain organizations for selected educational activities of the society. Among the companies that provide this support are Coca-Cola, General Foods Corporation, General Mills, Gerber Products Company, the NutraSweet® Group, Pillsbury, and numerous pharmaceutical companies. "Would these organizations support research about the damaging effects of the processed foods they are selling?" Dr. Gaby asks, pointing out the unlikelihood of such a scenario.

Furthermore, physicians who abide by a conventional Western medical perspective are more likely to publish papers and be on editorial boards of scientific journals than their peers who hold to different philosophies. "There is kind of a self-selection process where physicians who are against alternative medicine end up being on the editorial boards of the journals," Dr. Gaby says. It's important to bear in mind that many medical journals receive a substantial amount of revenue from the advertising dollars they get from the pharmaceutical industry, whose interests would not be served by articles and studies that recommended the use of alternative medicine over drugs and surgery.

The ideal of clinical trials is another weapon the medical establishment wields to suppress unconventional modes of therapy and research, according to Dr. Coulter, especially with regard to physician-inventors who may not be willing to sell the fruits of their research to large corporations. "These physicians are told blandly by the FDA that their therapies do not measure up to 'scientific' standards, even though these standards are not attained by anyone else," he says. "At the same time, drugs from more favored suppliers can be exempted from the testing requirements by a letter from the FDA Commissioner."[14]

One area where this is particularly true is cancer research. As Dr. Coulter points out, researchers and practitioners of alternative treatments for cancer are censured for their failure to perform clinical trials, then branded as "quacks" and, in some instances, even turned over to the police. "But the discerning critics in the FDA and the American Cancer Society apply a more stringent rule to 'unorthodox' physicians than they do to their own grant recipients," he says. "Cancer is known to be a highly heterogeneous disease, with any sample composed of numerous subsets differing significantly from each other.

Conventional drug trials in cancer are nearly always conducted with very small patient samples and, in fact, are criticized for this. But unorthodox practitioners are cited as 'unscientific' for doing the same thing." The ire directed at unorthodox cancer therapies has little to do with the supposed scientific inadequacies of these therapies. Rather, the contrary: the more promising the idea, the more likely it is to end up on the American Cancer Society's list of "Unproven Methods of Cancer Management."

"The ordinary observer might assume that the treatments on this list have been demonstrated to be ineffective," continues Dr. Coulter. "That is not the case: they have not been subjected to any testing at all—neither by the American Cancer Society nor by any other agency, public or private. They merely seem ineffective in the light of prevailing theories of cancer etiology and therapy." Dr. Coulter doubts that any procedure on the "Unproven Methods" list will ever obtain the financing or bureaucratic approval needed to establish its therapeutic value. "Hence," he says, "characterizing a cancer therapy as 'unproven' is a self-fulfilling prophecy in the truest sense of the word. Competition by maverick researchers is effectively suppressed."

The National Cancer Institute (NCI) has shown an equal bias against alternative practitioners. Despite the apparent failure of the costly "war on cancer," the NCI continues to wage a campaign against nutritionally based cancer treatments, which may be one of the keys to halting and even reversing cancerous growths. An example of this can be found in the case of Joe Gold, M.D., of Syracuse, New York.

A veteran of NASA's medical corps, Dr. Gold discovered that an easily synthesized substance called hydrazine sulfate could help cancer patients reverse their disease by preventing the wasting-away process that accompanies cancer and which inhibits the body's normal processing of nutrients. In fact, a significant percentage of those with cancer die of the malnutrition caused by this inhibition, rather than the cancer itself.

Hydrazine sulfate is inexpensive and was first developed by Dr. Gold at the Syracuse Cancer Research Institute in the early 1970s. It subsequently underwent more than 15 years of controlled testing at both U.C.L.A. Harbor Hospital, in Los Angeles, and at the Petrov Research Institute, in St. Petersburg, Russia. Results showed that hydrazine sulfate was able to stop, and even reverse, tumor growth in many cancer patients and were published in leading medical journals, including *The Lancet*, *Cancer*, and the *Journal of Clinical Oncology*. And in a 1991 multi-institutional study, scientists from the Petrov Institute reported that hydrazine sulfate stopped tumors in roughly half their patients, including those tumors that attack the breast, ovaries, cervix, endometrium, and vulva. A smaller but significant number of patients had even more profound results, with their tumors disappearing altogether.[15]

The NCI has not followed up on the Russian study, which American cancer officials have dismissed as "poorly done work not up to our standards." Compounding the NCI's omission is the fact that national U.S. clinical trials conducted in 1992 and 1993 were allowed to occur without heeding Dr. Gold's warnings that hydrazine sulfate is not effective when used in conjunction with incompatible substances such as alcohol, sleeping pills, and tranquilizers. Patients (94%) were allowed to ingest these substances, in effect scuttling the test results, which were inconclusive. Instead of initiating further tests and conducting them according to Dr. Gold's established protocol, NCI officials continue to reject hydrazine sulfate as a viable cancer treatment, informing physicians that its use is little more than "quackery."[16] In sabotaging the trials, the NCI not only managed to discredit the use of hydrazine sulfate in the minds of most of the world's doctors, but also undoubtedly added to the suffering and shortened the lives of many of the trial's patients.

In 1994, an investigation was begun under the leadership of GAO Assistant Director Barry Tice, whose group compiled a report that scathingly criticized the NCI for ignoring Dr. Gold's protocol. On June 5, 1995, the report was sent to the FDA, the Public Health Service, and the NCI for review. When top officials at the NCI read the report, their reaction was characterized by eyewitnesses as "going ballistic." The NCI then went on a campaign to have the GAO change the report, and they succeeded. In-house politicians at the GAO altered or deleted damning portions of the text and retitled it "Contrary to Allegations, NIH Studies of Hydrazine Sulfate Were Not Flawed."

"You can imagine how upset I was, and still am, about that title," Tice said in a subsequent interview. "The impact of the changes and a few key deletions was tremendous. Those changes took the NCI almost completely off the hook." In a later interview, Jeffrey Robbins, acting Chief Counsel of the Senate Subcommittee on Investigation, which looked into the matter further, stated that the NCI studies "are flawed to the point of being meaningless" and admitted that the final GAO report did not tell the truth about the NCI. "I am not a doctor," he added. "I do not know if hydrazine sulfate cures cancer, but I do know that the American people did not get what they paid for in all this: an unbiased report on the conduct of the NCI. That is wrong and should not stand." As of this writing, however, it has.

The American Medical Association and State Medical Boards: Does Conformity Equal Competence?

The American Medical Association (AMA) was formed in 1847 ostensibly to protect the public from charlatans, since at that time anyone could offer medical services and drugs uncontested. For the remainder of the 19th century, the AMA successfully lobbied states to require licensing of all physicians. Eventually, the AMA set up a Council on Medical Education to oversee all medical schools. The AMA was so successful that the number of medical schools in the U.S. actually decreased by half from the early 1900s to 1944, from 160 in 1904 to just 77 in 1940.[17]

"Throughout the past century, physicians and medical educators labored to improve the practice of medicine in the U.S. by making it more dependent on scientific research," notes Karl E. Humiston, M.D., of Salem, Oregon. "By controlling the accreditation of medical schools, the AMA aggressively played a major role in this. However, in building this system of medical research and teaching, they naturally relied heavily on those forms of research for which they were able to get financial support, which is mainly the clinical testing of drugs." Today, the AMA is able to prevent doctors who do not subscribe to its views from serving on hospital staffs and it also controls medical boards on the state level. The purpose of such medical boards is to protect the public against incompetent and unscrupulous doctors. But, as Dr. Gaby notes, "They often inappropriately extend that function to eliminating doctors that deviate from the arbitrary standards of care that are based on what they understand. The excuse for censuring a doctor or revoking his license is that he is incompetent, and the proof is that he deviates from the standards of care. Therefore, by definition, if you deviate, you are incompetent."

A telling example of the power of state medical boards to censure and harass competent physicians who deviate from conventional therapies is the case of Warren Levin, M.D., of New York City. The medical establishment so strenuously objected to Dr. Levin's effective use of chelation therapy, vitamin supplements, exercise, and counseling that it waged a 16-year campaign against him at a cost of approximately $1 million.

Despite its efforts, the Office of Professional Medical Conduct of the New York State Health Department was unable to come up with a single allegation of patient injury attributed to Dr. Levin. Nevertheless, the state medical board's hearing officers managed to ignore and insult a parade of highly respected physicians and scientists who came to Dr. Levin's defense, including the late Linus Pauling, Ph.D., a two-time Nobel laureate. At the same time, the hearing officers did accept and honor the testimony of a doctor who denounced chelation therapy as useless. And although the prosecution witness in question admitted under cross-examination that he had never read anything about chelation therapy, met a doctor who used it, or even seen a patient who received it, the panel found him to be a "credible and authoritative witness." The panel therefore recommended that Dr. Levin be stripped of his license to practice.

It is ironic that at the same time the government is searching for effective, lower-cost approaches to the nation's health-care needs, a physician like Dr. Levin, who for years was providing his patients with exactly such an approach and achieving impressive results, could be prevented from practicing his profession.

Positive Developments in Protecting Your Medical Freedom of Choice

Despite the clear advantages the powers-that-be within the medical establishment have over alternative medicine, the tide is starting to turn. Since 1990, for instance, 11 states—Alaska, Colorado, Georgia, Massachusetts, New York, North Carolina, Ohio, Oklahoma, Oregon, Texas, and Washington—have passed freedom of practice statutes, allowing physicians the freedom to practice alternative forms of medicine (and patients to have access to alternative therapies) without fear of retribution from state medical boards. The statutes say that failure to conform to standards of care shall not by itself be considered incompetence unless patients are harmed or exposed to unreasonable risk. These new laws are paving the way for medical freedom throughout the U.S., providing citizens with a true choice in their medical treatment.

The U.S. Congress is also beginning to recognize the validity of alternative medicine. In 1992, Congress established the Office of Alternative Medicine at the National Institutes of Health (NIH), with an annual budget of $2 million to be used to investigate the potential of promising alternative therapies. Subsequently designated the National Center for Complementary and Alternative Medicine (NCCAM), it now has an annual budget of $150 million. Although this remains inadequate funding for such an important task, it is clearly a step in the right direction. Both developments are in the spirit of the World Health Organization's call for integration of the various forms of "traditional medi-

ROBERT JAY ROWEN, M.D., AND ALASKA'S LEGISLATIVE MIRACLE

When Robert Jay Rowen, M.D., took on a new patient in the spring of 1989, he did not know that he would soon be taking on Alaska's medical establishment as well. Little more than a year later, however, Dr. Rowen's battle would culminate in a historic victory for practitioners of alternative medicine.

A family practitioner based in Anchorage, Dr. Rowen founded the Omni Medical Center in 1986, which offers a range of alternative treatments, including acupuncture, homeopathy, and chelation therapy. Though he often publicly addressed the benefits of such treatments, he was anything but a political activist. All this changed after a meeting with Patrick Rodey, Alaska's Senate majority leader, who came to Dr. Rowen as a patient. After a discussion about the dangers facing alternative physicians in this country, Senator Rodey agreed to sponsor a bill protecting freedom of choice in medicine.

With the help of another of Dr. Rowen's patients, former state Attorney General Edgar Paul Boyko, a bill was drafted. But the state medical board and Department of Occupational Licensing testified against the measure, and it languished in the Senate. When a similar version of the bill was attached to a piece of House legislation supported by the medical establishment, the House finance committee removed the entire provision protecting alternative medicine due to pressure from lobbies for the Alaska State Medical Association. But the bill was reintroduced as an amendment and passed in the House by a two-to-one margin. Despite additional pressure from the medical lobby, it finally passed the Senate and the governor signed the bill into law on June 14, 1990.

cine," such as homeopathy, naturopathic medicine, traditional Chinese medicine, Ayurvedic medicine, and herbal medicine, with conventional modern medicine in order to help meet the global health-care needs of the 21st century.

In order for change to take place in the practice of medicine in America, it is important to have alternative physicians on state medical boards. In fact, certain laws already on the books may help put this into action. In 1993, for instance, Vincent Speckhart, M.D., of Norfolk, Virginia, reported that in dealing with the state medical board of Virginia, he discovered a 100-year-old state law that required that two homeopaths always sit on the board, a law that had been ignored for over 20 years.

The state of Alaska, meanwhile, is taking the lead in this area. On July 23, 1992, Alaska Governor Walter J. Hickel appointed Robert Jay Rowen, M.D., to the state medical board. Dr. Rowen is an alternative physician from Anchorage, Alaska, whose dedicated efforts led to the passage of the landmark legislation on freedom of practice, making Alaska the first state to adopt such a measure. The governor of Alaska announced his bold move in the following press release: "I am putting Dr. Rowen on the medical board not to be controversial but to be helpful. He is a strong advocate of prevention as the first line of defense. And as the costs of traditional medical care continue to go up, it will be those who care for themselves through prevention who will live better lives. He believes prevention simply costs society less. Dr. Rowen has a sound medical background, yet he is open minded about new ideas that can help heal. I think we need that now more than ever. I believe a balanced perspective in this seven-member board is best for Alaskans and best for the future of health care."

Actions We Can Take to Restore Our Medical Freedom

A combination of grassroots activity, market forces, and public awareness about the full benefits of alternative medicine will do much to restore medical freedom in America. Because people can feel powerless in the face of large, influential institutions such as the FDA or Congress, it is essential that they are able to find a common vehicle through which they can empower themselves and effect change.

Alexander Schauss, Ph.D., former Executive Director of the nonprofit health-care advocacy groups Citizens for Health and the American Preventive Medical Association (APMA), cites the effect grassroots movements can have on legislation: "A U.S. senator was trying to introduce an amendment that would delay restrictive labeling laws for dietary supplements. It was predicted to be defeated. Through our network, we initiated 1,800 phone calls through our national phone tree, and we reached an additional 15,000 people through a fax network. Within 48 hours, the Senate was receiving approximately 10,000 phone calls per hour. That helped the bill easily pass by a margin of 94 to one and shows that people really can make a difference."

In North Carolina, grassroots forces also demonstrated their ability to effect change. Doctors statewide were losing their licenses as a result of alternative health-care modalities that they incorporated into their standard practices. The movement started out as 12 people fed up with government interference in their freedom to make health choices, but soon grew to a core group of 3,000 people. The group ended up having a dramatic impact on state legislators.

As Dr. Schauss points out, people often underestimate the power of grassroots organizations. "The average congressional district has around 200,000 people and only 10% or 15% of those people vote," he says. "So you only need half of those voters to keep a person in Congress." Therefore, one of the most practical ways citizens can hasten the acceptance of alternative medicine is to organize letter-writing campaigns to Congress and the President demanding that research into these methods be conducted and that persecution of practitioners, manufacturers, and researchers of alternative medicine cease.

It is important to note that this is not to imply that any new medicines should be approved without proper testing, as reasonable safeguards are always desirable. Nonetheless, it is essential to promote freedom of choice in both gaining access to information on new treatments as well as access to the treatments themselves once they are established as viable alternatives.

"If everyone in this country wrote a truthful and honest letter to all their representatives and senators at both state and federal levels expressing their feelings about the medical industry and demanding a choice in health care, we could see a big change," states Dr. Kail. "Tell them that you want to be able to choose health practitioners—an acupuncturist, chiropractor, naturopath, or an M.D.—who can practice alternative therapies without fear of losing their licenses."

Citizens must also mobilize to overcome the refusal of insurance companies to pay for established alternative treatments. For more than a decade, through the auspices of both the APMA and Citizens for Health, grassroots organizations have been contacting medical insurance companies, urging them to pay for preventive, nutritional, and exercise programs, with some success. Mutual of Omaha, for instance, a major insurance company in the U.S., is now reimbursing people who follow Dean Ornish's program for preventing and reversing heart disease, which involves exercise, stress management techniques such as meditation, and dietary and lifestyle changes.

As alternative medicine continues to wage its battle against the seemingly unyielding forces of government and conventional medicine, grassroots organizations will play perhaps the most important role in raising public awareness and in initiating both legislative and societal change. If alternative medicine is to gain its proper place

GETTING ALTERNATIVE MEDICINE COVERED BY MEDICAL INSURANCE

—by Burton Goldberg

Insurance pays over $100 billion every year for ineffectual or even harmful conventional medical treatments. It is time to make proven alternative therapies affordable and available to everyone.

Would you join me in helping to rectify one of the great inequities of our time? This is the disparity between medical insurance coverage of alternative therapies compared with conventional treatments. One of the questions I am asked most frequently has nothing to do with how to treat any one particular health condition—it is how to get medical insurance to cover alternative therapies.

Every day I learn about exciting advances in alternative medicine and hear inspiring stories of patients who have been cured of diseases conventional medicine calls "incurable." But what good are these medical miracles if people do not have the money to pay for them? Therefore, to make alternative medicine available to more people, I have started a nonprofit foundation with the purpose of getting every state in the U.S. to pass legislation that requires insurance companies to cover alternative treatments on an equal footing with mainstream medicine.

In general, alternative medicine costs less than conventional treatments, but, ironically, it is more expensive to individuals because they must pay for it out-of-pocket. This is a tragedy. To see why, we have to look no further than the number one and two killers in this country: heart disease and cancer.

If you get cancer, your medical insurance or Medicare will pay thousands of dollars for surgery, radiation, or chemotherapy—whatever is the standard of practice for your particular kind of cancer. This in spite of the fact that after spending more than $2 billion annually for research over the last quarter century, the incidence and mortality for most kinds of cancer remain unchanged or continue to rise.

However, if you want to get treated at an alternative clinic, where the success rate is upwards of ten times higher than conventional treatments (with the subsequent quality of life also immeasurably better), the cost could run $5,000 per week for an in-patient program. This is still less than the cost of conventional treatment, for which hospitalization can cost $5,000 per day, but this would all have to come out of your pocket. And presently, it might have to occur outside of the U.S., because many therapies proven effective abroad are not allowed to be practiced within our borders.

With heart disease, if you have a blocked artery, you can be one of the 500,000 people in this country every year who have a bypass operation, which costs between $50,000 and $100,000, and it will cost you little, if anything, because it is probably covered by your HMO or Medicare. However, it is an entirely different story if you want to prevent or reverse heart disease by going to an alternative physician, who would likely prescribe lifestyle changes, supplements, and chelation therapy. A full examination, follow-ups, laboratory work, and a year's complete treatment could cost between $5,000 and $7,500. This is a fraction of what conventional treatment costs, but the chances are that you would be responsible for paying all of it. That is, if you are lucky enough to live in one of 11 states in which doctors can perform chelation therapy without risk of losing their medical license.

Yet, according to the General Accounting Office, less than 10% of bypass operations are necessary and studies in the medical literature show no significant difference in the death rates between heart attack victims who receive bypass surgery and those who do not. Still, approximately $4 billion is spent on bypass surgery every year.

Here, of course, is where the difficulty lies: the people to whom these billions of dollars are being paid do not want a change in the status quo. Those industries that have the most to lose include insurance carriers, which make their money as a percentage of their gross revenues. From a business point of view, insurance companies would be most profitable insuring lots of sick people employing ineffective, expensive medicines.

Also threatened by alternative medical insurance coverage would be conventional medical doctors. There are, unfortunately, a significant portion who don't want to go back to school to learn an entirely new medical paradigm and

GETTING ALTERNATIVE MEDICINE COVERED BY MEDICAL INSURANCE, continued

others who don't want to face the fact that, in their ignorance or arrogance, they have let many of their patients suffer or die unnecessarily. People now make more visits to alternative practitioners than to primary care conventional doctors and spend more out-of-pocket for alternative services than for hospitalization services. Without the insurance "subsidy," conventional doctors would lose even more of their patients.

Pharmaceutical companies would be the biggest losers. Expensive patented drugs that only suppress symptoms and have toxic side effects would only be used in the rarest circumstances in alternative medicine. If there was a major shift in this country from sick-care to real health-care, the drug giants would have to do what the tobacco companies have done to survive: once it became common knowledge that their main product was poison, they would have to diversify into entirely different businesses.

There is formidable opposition, then, to getting alternative medical therapies covered by insurance—the pharmaceutical and insurance industries are among the top political contributors on national and state levels. Physicians' trade organizations are also major players. The monetary stakes are huge: $37 billion is spent annually on direct medical costs for cancer treatment and an equivalent amount is spent treating heart disease. Conventional medicine in this country is an industry with annual revenues of billions of dollars.

On the other hand, much of the public—and many doctors—do want more access to alternative medicine. The following statistics were compiled and documented by health activist Monica Miller of HealthLobby.com:

- 80% of medical students and 70% of family physicians want training in complementary and alternative medicine (CAM)

- 69% of Americans use unconventional medical therapies

- 67% of HMOs offer at least one form of CAM care

- 64% of U.S. medical schools offer courses in CAM

- 60% of physicians have referred patients to CAM practitioners

- 56% of Americans surveyed believe their health plans should cover alternative therapies

- 29 health insurers and HMOs already cover some CAM therapies

So, it is possible to get alternative therapies covered by medical insurance—in fact, it has been done in one state. In 1993, the state of Washington passed a law requiring insurance policies to provide coverage for treatments and services by every category of licensed health-care providers, starting in 1996. Washington currently licenses naturopathic doctors, acupuncturists, chiropractors, certified dietitians and nutritionists, massage therapists, and midwives. A coalition of insurance providers immediately initiated a legal challenge to the legislation, but the law was upheld in 2001 by the Washington State Supreme Court.

Washington is an exception, however. And before we can get medical coverage for alternative therapies, we have to make alternative therapies themselves available. Presently, only Alaska, Colorado, Georgia, Massachusetts, New York, North Carolina, Ohio, Oklahoma, Oregon, Texas, and Washington have laws that protect patient access to alternative therapies. Individual states vary widely in the licensing of health-care practitioners other than M.D.s. Providers such as naturopaths, acupuncturists, and homeopaths must also be recognized and their services included in insurance coverage. In addition, insurance law and policy has to be defined by statute, so that, for example, "medical necessity" is something determined by the physician on a case-by-case basis instead of by an insurance underwriter.

Making alternative medicine available for everyone is more than a matter of money—it is no exaggeration to say that it's a matter of life and death. There is much work to do and we are just getting started. To find out how you can help by volunteering your time or contributing to the foundation, please contact me: Burton Goldberg, AlternativeMedicine.com, Inc., 1650 Tiburon Blvd., Tiburon, California 94920; e-mail: foundation@alternativemedicine.com. Together, we can make a difference.

in preventing and alleviating health problems, citizens must organize, mobilize, and act. To become involved and to receive more information, contact the APMA, Citizens for Health, and the other organizations listed at the end of this chapter, which are leading the way in securing what should be a basic human right—medical freedom.

The Power of Procedures: A Game Plan for Victory

In tandem with grassroots activity, much can be achieved to secure medical freedom via the legislatures of the remaining 39 states that have yet to safeguard the practice of and unencumbered access to alternative medicine, according to Dr. Humiston, who serves as Oregon's state coordinator for Citizens for Health. The key to doing so, he believes, lies in the proper use of regulating procedures. "Procedures are the life of the bureaucrat," Dr. Humiston explains. "They control him and he uses them to control others." Clinic and hospital staffs are also governed by what is written in their procedure books, Dr. Humiston notes, with all procedures typically determined by conventional medicine. "There are no words to allow them to use alternative medicine, no matter how much some of them may wish to do," he says.

Recognizing that fact is important, according to Dr. Humiston. "Just as the financial supporters of research influence medical education, the payers of medical services [insurance companies and HMOs] influence our medical practice," he observes. "When they realize how much the right procedures can save them money, they may start requiring them of their providers." To that end, he recommends that citizens actively seek to have politicians, labor unions, and anyone else involved in the payment for organized health care demand that the following be included in the clinic and hospital procedure books:

"Based on the fact that, according to orthodox medical research, typically a third of patients are not helped by the treatments proven by that research, proper and effective medical care for the entire populace requires: (1) procedures to identify those individuals not helped by orthodox treatment for their illnesses; and (2) procedures for selecting alternatives for them."

"Having these words in their procedure books, the staff performing actual care of patients will consider treatments that otherwise do not occur to them," Dr. Humiston says. "Alternatives will then become safe to think about and use." This tactic was successfully used in 1995 by proponents of alternative medicine to get Oregon to amend its medical practice law so that the Oregon licensing board could no longer punish doctors for using alternative medicine. "Already frustrated by the arrogance of the [Oregon] medical board in other matters, the legislators heard from voters protesting the board's recent revocation of the medical license of a very popular and competent M.D. whose only offenses were to use chelation therapy, clinical ecology allergy testing, and other alternative medical methods," Dr. Humiston recounts.

"The proponents of alternative medicine used only one argument in support of this bill: that by allowing only orthodox medicine to be practiced by Oregon M.D.s, the Board of Medical Examiners was depriving a third of the legislators' constituents of the alternatives they needed. Each legislator was given photocopies of graphs from recent medical literature showing clearly that the best drugs were proven to help only two-thirds of patients. The bill passed unanimously in spite of Oregon Medical Association opposition."

Dr. Humiston advises proponents of alternative medicine in states where its practice is not yet freely guaranteed by law to notice how Oregon's law now defines alternative medicine so as to allow physicians to do whatever works, no longer limited to the scope of orthodox medical school research. The law says: "Alternative medical treatment means: (1) a treatment that the treating physician, based on the physician's professional experience, has an objective basis to believe has a reasonable probability for effectiveness in its intended use even if the treatment is outside recognized scientific guidelines, is unproven, is no longer used as a generally recognized or standard treatment or lacks the approval of the U.S. Food and Drug Administration; (2) a treatment that is supported for specific usages or outcomes by at least one other physician licensed by the Board of Medical Examiners; and (3) a treatment that poses no greater risk to a patient than the generally recognized or standard treatment."

"However much we may personally believe that alternative medicine is safer, cheaper, and generally more effective, years of saying so has not changed much in our health-care system for the better," Dr. Humiston says. He believes a more effective course of action to ensure medical freedom lies in following the method that succeeded with the Oregon legislature. "Refer to the fact that orthodox medical research typically proves that their best treatments fail to help a third of people, who therefore need an alternative," Dr. Humiston advises. "This is plainly true and no one disputes it.

"Orthodox medicine is fundamentally impersonal, because it relies on scientific research in a coldly impersonal way," Dr. Humiston adds. "The procedure books that guide their treatment of patients (standards of practice, clinical guidelines, hospital and clinic policies) use impersonal language. That is why policy and procedure books have such a powerful effect on medical practice.

An Open Letter to the President of the United States

President _____
The White House
1600 Pennsylvania Avenue, N.W.
Washington, D.C. 20500

Dear Mr. President:

To realize effective health care with cost reduction requires unlocking the strangulation hold of the pharmaceutical companies, the American Medical Association (AMA), and the U.S. Food and Drug Administration (FDA) on all forms of fully effective, low-cost alternative, complementary, integrative, holistic medicine. No group can be expected to surrender a profitable monopoly position, even in the national interest, unless forced to do so.

Nowhere has conventional Western medicine produced more dismal results than in the quest to defeat cancer and AIDS. After more than 50 years of government-sponsored research, the rate of cancer has increased in America while the death rate remains unchanged. Incredibly, the pharmaceutical medical establishment is persecuting those who are succeeding at reversing these scourges. In contrast, Germany sponsors alternative therapies and is having extraordinary success.

It didn't take 50 years to usher in the Atomic Age once President Roosevelt decided it should be done. It didn't take 50 years to usher in the Space Age once President Kennedy decided it should be done. Beyond any health-care plan lies the Health Age. Rapid, giant strides in improving health care and lowering its costs can be made if you will:

- Place a strong leader, free of entanglements with any form of medicine, in charge of the fight against cancer and AIDS.

- Instruct that person to allocate resources to those alternative approaches that produce the most objectively favorable results.

- Expand the National Center for Complementary and Alternative Medicine and increase public funding for research into alternative medical therapies, especially for the treatment of cancer and other chronic degenerative diseases.

- Curb the FDA from protecting the medical establishment by blindly attacking alternative medicine and the physicians who practice it.

- Change FDA procedure so that cost-effective, natural compounds can win approval to make health claims, not just expensive, highly synthesized, often-toxic patentable drugs.

- Stop toxic chemicals and pollutants from getting into our air, water, food, homes, schools, workplaces, and Earth. Stop the abundant studies implicating these toxins in cancer from being silenced by those who profit from their use.

To bring about the Health Age, you will have to reclaim the many innovative minds that have been driven underground by powerful forces. You will have to refocus funds for research into areas that threaten these powerful forces. We want you to go down in history as the President who ushered America into the Health Age.

For Medical Freedom,

_____

"There is probably nothing more profitable to the drug companies than interminable treatment of patients with drugs that do not work. Yet countless patients, at great cost to our nation, are kept on these treatments because they have been proven to help two-thirds of people and health-care providers have no policies or procedures to do otherwise. When those who pay the bills realize how much of their money is being wasted, and how much can be saved by requiring policies and procedures to identify patients not helped by standard treatment and select alternatives for them, it may happen."

Writing Your Elected Representatives

A grassroots letter-writing campaign to the President and elected representatives is an effective means of applying public pressure to incorporate legislation favoring alternative medicine as an essential component to reforming our nation's health-care system. We urge everyone to write to the President and your local representatives and senators to express your desire for medical freedom. A personal letter is best, but you can also copy and send the "Open Letter to the President" and create a variation of it to send to your local legislators. Be sure to sign it and include your full name and address to better ensure that your letter is read. A mailed letter is best, but you can also send e-mail. To find the names and addresses of your local senators and representatives, visit these websites:

- Senate —
  www.senate.gov/contacting/index_by_state.cfm

- House of Representatives —
  www.house.gov/writeup

Where to Find Help

The following organizations are leading the way in the fight for medical freedom. We urge all readers to contact them for more information and to donate time and/or money to the important causes they support.

American Preventive Medical Association (APMA)
9912 Georgetown Pike, Suite D-2
P.O. Box 458
Great Falls, Virginia 22066
(800) 230-APMA
Website: www.apma.net

APMA was established in 1993 to serve as an advocate for health-care freedom for individual consumers, companies, and health practitioners, as well as state governments and policy-setting boards at hospitals, HMOs, and health/medical organizations. The APMA also seeks to help expand the body of case law in support of health freedom.

Center for Empirical Medicine
4221 45th Street N.W.
Washington, D.C. 20016
(877) 297-4343
Website: www.empiricaltherapies.com

Founded by Dr. Harris Coulter, the Center is a publishing and lobbying organization providing an alternative to the way medicine is conceptualized and practiced today by the interlocking directorate of allopathic physicians and pharmaceutical manufacturers.

Citizens for Health
5 Thomas Circle N.W., Suite 500
Washington, D.C. 20005
(202) 483-1652
Website: www.citizens.org

Citizens for Health is a national nonprofit, grassroots consumer advocacy group committed to empowering individuals to make informed health choices about, and protecting and advancing consumer access to, natural health products and therapies.

Foundation for the Advancement of Innovative Medicine (FAIM)
Health Lobby/Monica Miller
Two Executive Boulevard
Suffern, New York 10601
(877) 634-3246
Websites: www.faim.org and www.healthlobby.com

FAIM was incorporated in 1989 as a voice for innovative medicine's health professionals, patients, and medical suppliers. Among its goals are the education of those within the health field and the general public as to the benefits and issues of innovative, alternative medicine and to secure the freedom of choice and guaranteed reimbursements for patients who seek to use such medicine. Health Lobby, administered by health consumer advocate Monica Miller, is a sister organization of FAIM and shares its goals.

Institute for Health Freedom (IHF)
1155 Connecticut Avenue N.W., Suite 300
Washington, D.C. 20036
(202) 429-6610
Website: www.ForHealthFreedom.org

IHF was established to bring the issues of personal health freedom to the forefront of America's health policy debate. Its mis-

KEEP INFORMED

To keep abreast of the latest developments in alternative medicine, visit our website **www.alternativemedicine.com** and consider subscribing to *Alternative Medicine* magazine. For information on subscribing, call (800) 333-HEAL.

sion is to present the ethical and economic case for strengthening personal health freedom. It is a nonpartisan, nonprofit research center that, through its research, publications, and public policy debates, provides a forum for exchanging ideas about health freedom. IHF publishes a bimonthly newsletter, Health Freedom Watch, to keep the public informed about important health freedom issues.

Physicians Committee for Responsible Medicine (PCRM)
5100 Wisconsin Avenue, Suite 400
Washington, D.C. 20016
(202) 686-2210
Website: www.pcrm.org

Founded in 1985, PCRM is a nonprofit organization supported by over 5,000 physicians and 100,000 laypersons. PCRM programs combine the efforts of medical experts and grassroots individuals to promote preventive medicine through research programs, reforms of federal nutrition policies, and the advocacy of higher ethics and effectiveness in the use and research of drugs, synthetic hormones, and other mainstream medical approaches.

Recommended Reading

Bitter Pills: Inside the Hazardous World of Legal Drugs. Stephen M. Fried. New York: Bantam Doubleday, 1999.

Alternative Medicine Definitive Guide to Cancer. W. John Diamond, M.D., and W. Lee Cowden, M.D., with Burton Goldberg. Tiburon, CA: Future Medicine Publishing, 1997. (See specifically Chapter 26: "How Cancer Politics Have Kept You in the Dark Regarding Successful Alternative Treatments.")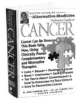

Overdose: The Case Against the Drug Companies. Jay S. Cohen, M.D. New York: Tarcher/Putnam, 2001.

Politics in Healing: The Suppression and Manipulation of American Medicine. Daniel Haley. Washington, DC: Potomac Valley Press, 2000.

Prescription for Disaster: The Hidden Dangers in Your Medicine Cabinet. Thomas J. Moore. New York: Simon & Schuster, 1999.

The highest ideal of cure is the speedy, gentle, and enduring restoration of health by the most trustworthy and least harmful way.

—SAMUEL HAHNEMANN (1755-1843), FOUNDER OF HOMEOPATHY

Part Two

Alternative Therapies

ACUPUNCTURE

Acupuncture alleviates pain and can increase immune response by balancing the flow of vital life energy throughout the body. It is an element of traditional Chinese medicine that in the West is often used as a stand-alone treatment for a wide range of disease conditions, from the common cold and flu to addiction and chronic fatigue syndrome. It is also effective as an adjunct treatment for AIDS.

ACUPUNCTURE ORIGINATED IN China over 5,000 years ago. It is based on the belief that health is determined by a balanced flow of *qi* (also referred to as *chi*), the vital life energy present in all living organisms. According to acupuncture theory, *qi* circulates in the body along 12 major energy pathways called meridians, each linked to specific internal organs and organ systems. According to William M. Cargile, B.S., D.C., F.I.A.C.A., past Chairman of Research for the American Association of Oriental Medicine, there are over 1,000 acupoints within the meridian system that can be stimulated to enhance the flow of *qi*. When special needles are inserted into these acupoints (just under the skin), they help correct and rebalance the flow of energy and consequently relieve pain and restore health.

 See Qigong and Tai Chi, Traditional Chinese Medicine.

How Acupuncture Works

In the 1960s, Professor Kim Bong Han and a team of researchers in Korea attempted to document the existence of meridians in the human body using microdissection techniques. They found evidence that there exists an independent series of fine ductlike tubes corresponding to the paths of traditional acupuncture meridians. Fluids in this system sometimes travel in the same direction as the blood and lymph, but at other times flow in the opposite direction. They realized that these ducts are different from the vascular and lymphatic systems that Western science had previously identified, and that the meridians themselves might exist within them.[1]

The existence of the meridian system was further established by French researcher Pierre de Vernejoul, who injected radioactive isotopes into the acupoints of humans and tracked their movement with a special gamma imaging camera. The isotopes traveled 12 inches along acupuncture meridians within four to six minutes. Vernejoul then challenged his work by injecting isotopes into blood vessels at random areas of the body rather than into acupoints. The isotopes did not travel in the same manner at all, further indicating that the meridians do indeed comprise a system of separate pathways within the body.[2]

In 1997, acupuncture's credibility as a viable medical treatment was bolstered by the U.S. Food and Drug Administration (FDA), which reclassified the acupuncture needle from "experimental" to "medical device" status, thereby acknowledging that the acupuncture needle is a safe and effective medical instrument. Also in 1997, the National Institutes of Health (NIH) released an efficacy statement endorsing acupuncture for a variety of conditions, including post-operative pain, dental pain following surgery, nausea associated with chemotherapy, morning sickness, tennis elbow, and carpal tunnel syndrome. The FDA estimates that Americans make 9-12 million visits per year to acupuncturists and spend as much as $500 million on acupuncture treatments annually.[3]

The Electrical Properties of Acupuncture

Current research suggests that there is a specific relationship between acupuncture points, meridians, and the electrical currents of the body. Since the 1950s, numerous studies have been conducted using electrical devices to measure the galvanic skin response (GSR) of both meridians and specific acupoints. These studies not only verify the existence of the meridian system, but also indicate that the acupoints themselves have a higher level of electrical conductance than non-acupuncture sites.[4]

In the 1970s, under a grant from the NIH, Robert O. Becker, M.D., and biophysicist Maria Reichmanis were able to prove that electrical currents did indeed flow along the ancient Chinese meridians and that 25% of the acupuncture points existed along those scientifically measurable lines. They reasoned that these points acted as amplifiers to boost the minute electrical signals as they traveled along the body, and that the insertion of a needle could interfere with that flow and thus block the stimulus of pain.[5] The other acupuncture points, Dr. Becker suggests, "may simply be weaker or a different link than the ones our instruments revealed."[6]

Conditions Benefited by Acupuncture

The World Health Organization has cited over 40 conditions that acupuncture can treat, including migraines, sinusitis, the common cold, tonsillitis, asthma, inflammation of the eyes, addictions, myopia, duodenal ulcer and other gastrointestinal disorders, trigeminal neuralgia (severe facial pain), Meniere's disease (ringing in the ears coupled with dizziness), tennis elbow, paralysis from stroke, speech aphasia (loss of language abilities due to brain damage), sciatica, and osteoarthritis.[7] Acupuncture has also been found to be effective in the treatment of a variety of rheumatoid conditions and brings relief in 80% of those who suffer from arthrosis.[8] There is also evidence to suggest that acupuncture is valuable in the treatment of environmentally induced illnesses due to radiation,[9] pesticide poisoning,[10] toxic compounds, and air pollution.

According to Maoshing Ni, D.O.M., Ph.D., L.Ac., President of Yo San University of Traditional Chinese Medicine, in Marina Del Rey, California, other conditions for which acupuncture can be effective, either alone or when used in conjunction with contemporary conventional medicine, include stroke rehabilitation, headaches, addiction, menstrual cramps, fibromyalgia, low back pain, and asthma. Dr. Ni treats many conditions with acupuncture, and reports, "Even in acute abdominal problems such as appendicitis or kidney stone and gallstone attacks, acupuncture can be used before surgery to arrest the condition before it progresses further." Dr. Ni also treats immune system dysfunction, respiratory disease, and hormonal imbalances that lead to menstrual irregularities and menopause-related problems, and he helps many people with depression, anxiety, and sleep disorders, sometimes in conjunction with but often without having to resort to psychiatric drugs.

Jay Holder, M.D., D.C., Ph.D., Director of the Holder Research Institute, in Miami, Florida, states that there are literally thousands of conditions that acupuncture is appropriate to treat. He recalls children in the emergency

ACUPUNCTURE IN THE WESTERN WORLD

Chinese immigrants brought acupuncture to America in the mid-1800s, but it was largely ignored until 1971 when James Reston, a respected *New York Times* columnist, underwent an emergency appendectomy while in China. Reston reported on the amazing post-surgical pain relief he enjoyed via a few well-placed acupuncture needles. This report attracted the attention of the American medical community and many physicians traveled to China to observe the use of acupuncture for pain relief. They discovered that acupuncture is part of a complex, integrated healing system that goes far beyond pain relief and can treat a variety of conditions, including diseases of the eyes, nerves, muscles, heart, and the organs of digestion and reproduction. By the end of the 1970s, acupuncture schools and practitioners could be found throughout America, supported by dozens of professional associations and publications.

room on the verge of asthmatic asphyxiation being relieved in less than 30 seconds solely with the use of acupuncture. Dr. Holder believes that acupuncture should be considered an essential life support measure for emergency room medicine.

Pain

Acupuncture has proven to be a successful treatment for pain relief, as it appears to stimulate the release of endorphins and enkephalins, the body's natural painkilling chemicals.[11] David Eisenberg, M.D., Clinical Research Fellow at Harvard Medical School states, "There is evidence that acupuncture influences the production and distribution of a great many neurotransmitters (substances that transmit nerve impulses to the brain) and neuromodulators (substances produced by neurons that affect neurotransmitters) and that this in turn alters the perception of pain."[12] The medical journal *Pain* reviewed a number of studies that provided further evidence of acupuncture's importance as an alternative to conventional analgesic (pain-relieving) medication.[13] Acupuncture can reduce the need for conventional painkilling drugs (and their attendant side effects).[14] Patients treated with acupuncture after oral surgery had less intense pain than those who received a placebo treatment.[15]

Acupuncture is more effective than massage for neck pain, according to a recent study. Almost 200 patients with chronic neck pain received a 30-minute treatment, five times a week, for three weeks. Those treated with

Acupuncture meridians

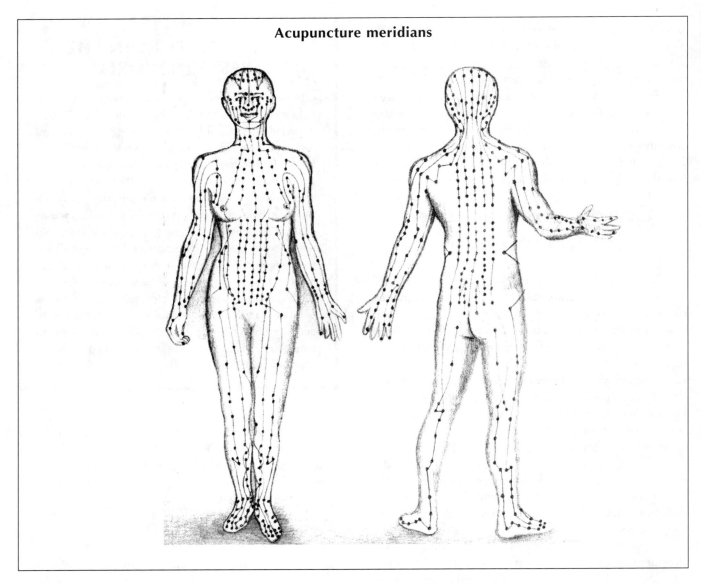

acupuncture had a greater reduction in pain than those treated with massage. Acupuncture proved most effective in those who had suffered with neck pain for over five years and those with myofascial pain syndrome (muscle pain due to physical or mental tension).[16]

In one study of over 20,000 patients at the University of California at Los Angeles, acupuncture reduced both the frequency and severity of muscle tension headaches and migraines.[17] Another study, involving 204 patients suffering from chronic painful conditions, resulted in 74% experiencing significant pain relief for over three months after acupuncture treatment.[18] Younger patients are particularly helped by acupuncture for the treatment of various types of pain.[19]

The NIH has also touted acupuncture's ability to trigger the release of endogenous painkillers, based on clinical evidence that shows opioids are released during acupuncture treatments and that the analgesic effects of acupuncture are at least partially explained by these

actions.[20] Other studies have also demonstrated that acupuncture can dramatically decrease brain activities associated with pain as monitored by using magnetic resonance imaging.[21]

Addiction

In 1989, the British medical journal *The Lancet* documented a study noting that when acupuncture was added to the treatment program of chronic alcoholics, it significantly increased the percentage of those who completed the program. Furthermore, it reduced their need for alcohol, with fewer relapses and readmissions to a detoxification center.[22]

In another study conducted at the Lincoln Substance Abuse/Acupuncture Clinic in New York City, 68 pregnant women addicted to cocaine participated in a program in which they received acupuncture treatments in conjunction with a detoxification regimen, counseling, and daily urinalysis tests. Those who attended the program for ten visits or more showed significantly higher infant birth weights than those who attended less than ten times.[23]

Other studies have documented the effectiveness of acupuncture in the treatment of opium and heroin addictions, with a 100% success rate in alleviating the symptoms of withdrawal.[24] "Acupuncture also claims good success rates with cigarette addiction, where a newly discovered acupoint called *Tien Mi* is used in conjunction with other traditional acupoints, particularly those located on the ear," says Dr. Ni.

Dr. Holder, who is also the Founder and Director of Exodus, a residential treatment hospital for addicts in Miami, Florida, has had success in the research and treatment of addictions relating to work, sex, gambling, food disorders, as well as substance abuse (chemical dependency), and has developed a form of auriculotherapy (ear acupuncture) for addiction treatment.

According to Dr. Holder, every addiction corresponds to a different set of ear acupoints. "Every drug of choice has a receptor site mechanism that is very specific. What we do is meet the needs of that receptor site by supplying and directing the endorphins or enkephalins through acupuncture." Using auriculotherapy, Dr. Holder reports success rates of over 80% for nicotine, alcohol, cocaine, heroin, and other mood-altering substances among addicts.[25] For this work, Dr. Holder was the first American to be awarded the Albert Schweitzer prize in medicine.

 The government should examine the wealth of existing studies on the efficacy of acupuncture and fund further studies to speed the integration of this valuable form of treatment into America's health-care system.

Today, there are approximately 300 acupuncture-based substance abuse programs in the United States. Because of the success of these programs, many state judiciary systems and legislators have encouraged their development. According to the National Acupuncture Detoxification Association:

- Several methadone programs in New York City noted that using acupuncture as a part of their treatment program resulted in major reductions in client tension and increased compliance with the program.

- In treatment programs begun in the state of Washington, acupuncture participation correlated with reduced drug use (as much as 50% compared with patients who did not use acupuncture).

- Women incarcerated in the Santa Barbara, California, county jail who received 32 or more acupunc-

ture treatments while in custody had an overall reincarceration rate 26% lower than the control group that received no acupuncture. Those who received fewer than 32 treatments had a 17% lower rate of incarceration during the first four months after release from jail.[26]

- Acupuncture detoxification programs have also been established in countries around the world, including Canada, Mexico, Great Britain, Sweden, Germany, Hungary, Romania, Spain, Saudi Arabia, and Trinidad.

ACUPUNCTURE: A SUBSTITUTE FOR SURGICAL ANESTHESIA

In 1979, David Eisenberg, M.D., was invited to the Beijing Neurosurgical Institute, in China, to witness and assist in a major surgical operation carried out using only acupuncture for the relief of pain. The patient was a 58-year-old university professor with a brain tumor located near his pituitary gland. The neurosurgeon, Dr. Wang Zhong-Cheng, recommended acupuncture analgesia because it had significantly fewer side effects than other anesthetic treatments. Throughout a four-hour operation that included the removal of a portion of the skull to reach the tumor, the patient remained fully conscious, alert, and relaxed. He received only a mild preoperative sedative and the acupuncture consisted of the insertion of five needles attached to a low-voltage battery. He felt no pain, and his pulse and blood pressure remained stable. When the surgery was completed, the patient stood up, thanked the surgeon, and walked out of the operating room without help.[27]

More than 90% of all head and neck surgeries performed at the Beijing Neurosurgical Institute are performed using acupuncture analgesia. Dr. Eisenberg has also reported on its use for thyroid operations, where treatment consisted of inserting two needles in the hand. It has also been used successfully for open-chest surgery and tonsillectomies. It does not however, always provide adequate pain relief for abdominal, gynecological, or heart and lung surgery, according to the Beijing Institute. And because not all patients respond well to acupuncture analgesia, traditional anesthesia is kept available during all surgeries.

Mental Disorders

Professor Pierre Huard of the Medical Faculty of Paris and Dr. Ming Wong of the Medical Faculty of Rennes, both in France, report that acupuncture "is equivalent to the effect of tranquilizers in cases of depression, worry, insomnia, and nervous disorders, and its action is swift and lasting."[28]

In a six-month study conducted by Tom Atwood, M.S.W., Director of Mental Health Care Management at Heart of Texas Region Mental Health Mental Retardation Center, in Waco, Texas, 16 patients in a residential care home received auriculotherapy for a variety of conditions, including paranoid schizophrenia and borderline personality disorders. Hospitalization stays dropped from 27 days to eight days following the initiation of acupuncture, compared to records of the previous year. Hypertensive patients experienced reduced blood pressure, and patients generally reported sleeping better. In addition, they became more productive.[29] According to Atwood, other responses were:

- Less agitation and calmer behavior

- Improved clarity of thought

- Reduced aggression

- Improved social interaction

- Improvement in facial complexion

Atwood notes, "These patients who are normally the most resistant, and the most likely to be readmitted for hospitalization, were also more willing to have acupuncture as opposed to other treatments offered at our center."

Alzheimer's disease is the most common cause of mental decline and dementia among the elderly in the U.S., affecting approximately 10% of all Americans over the age of 65, and approximately 50% of those 85 years old or older. It is characterized by the shrinkage of the brain and the death of nerve cells, leading to loss of mental functions such as memory, learning, and concentration. "In my professional experience, acupuncture can be effective in early stages of Alzheimer's disease, helping to slow down its progression and improving its accompanying symptoms," Dr. Ni states. Dr. Ni's clinical findings in this regard are supported by two recent studies presented at the 2000 World Alzheimer's Conference, in Washington, D.C., which reported that acupuncture can increase patients' verbal and motor skills, and improve mood and cognitive function.[30]

Acupuncture has also proved beneficial for treating hyperactive children. In a controlled clinical trial, nearly 50% of children with attention deficit hyperactivity disorder (ADHD) who underwent acupuncture treatment showed improvement in their symptoms. Researchers concluded that acupuncture was a useful alternative to conventional medications for some hyperactive children.[31]

AIDS

Although acupuncture does not cure AIDS, it is often used with Chinese herbs to improve a patient's immune function and to reduce uncomfortable or dangerous symptoms, including night sweats, fatigue, and digestive disturbances. At an international conference held by the European associations for acupuncture detoxification, Dr. Wu Bo Ping of China reported on his work in Tanzania where he treated 160 AIDS patients with Chinese herbology. In addition to noting considerable improvement among them, seven of the patients converted from HIV (human immunodeficiency virus) positive to HIV negative.[32]

A recent study used acupuncture to treat HIV patients experiencing sleep disturbances, a common side effect of the condition. The study involved 21 HIV-infected men and women, 29-50 years old, who experienced sleep disturbances three or more times per week. Acupuncture was individualized to address insomnia and other symptoms reported by the participants. Sleep activity and sleep quality significantly improved after five weeks of acupuncture treatments.[33]

Along with his associate Harvey Grossbard, O.M.D., D.Hom., Dr. Holder has used acupuncture to significantly extend the life span and improve the quality of life in AIDS patients. Dr. Grossbard predicts that the final result of research in this area will be statistically significant and will establish acupuncture as beneficial in the treatment of HIV and AIDS patients. Drs. Holder and Grossbard describe the case of a man with AIDS, who was suffering from Kaposi's sarcoma, whose T-cell count returned to normal within three months of treatment with acupuncture and Chinese herbs. Additionally, the patient's lesions disappeared.

Dr. Ni also cites research that is being conducted with HIV patients at the Kuan Yin Clinic, in San Francisco, California. Overseen by acupuncturist Misha Cohen, the studies show acupuncture to be beneficial in increasing immune function and white blood cell (T cell) production, as well as alleviating many of the symptoms related to HIV infection and AIDS. "Community outreach programs such as Being Alive in West Hollywood, California, where interns from Yo San University provide acupuncture treatments free of charge, have also helped many HIV patients," Dr. Ni says.

Dr. Cargile has worked with AIDS patients for many years and has increased T-cell counts from 210 to 270 with just three acupuncture treatments. "One of these patients had a T-cell count of 30 to 40," Dr. Cargile says, "We eventually brought it up to 270, and although that is half the level a person needs, he's been doing great for the last six months." He adds that the key to understanding acupuncture's influence on blood values and cell counts lies in its ability to minimize stress and strengthen the body's adaptive mechanisms. "I think that if we had more acupuncture and less AZT [an AIDS medication] and protease inhibitors, we would see a qualitative improvement in these patients' health."

Studies show acupuncture to be beneficial in increasing immune function and white blood cell production, as well as alleviating many of the symptoms related to HIV infection and AIDS.

Infertility

As more and more women postpone childbearing until later in life, the rate of infertility has risen sharply in the U.S., and this trend is estimated to continue. "Conventional allopathic medicine employs hormonal and technological methods to treat infertility," Dr. Ni says. "Acupuncture, on the other hand, focuses on normalizing and enhancing fertility functions." According to Dr. Ni's brother, Daoshing Ni, D.O.M., Ph.D., L.Ac., a specialist in fertility medicine at the Tao of Wellness Center, in Santa Monica, California, "Acupuncture is a viable procedure for improving age-related infertility and any other infertility conditions due to weakened function. Its efficacy can be applied to situations of substandard semen perimeter, poor follicular recruitment, weak follicular quality, poor vaginal lubrication, sluggish or quickened ovulation, luteal phase defect, decreased thyroid and adrenal functions, and hypothalamic dysfunction." A recent study found that acupuncture increased sperm counts in ten of 15 male patients with very poor sperm density, especially those with a history of genital tract inflammation.[34] Though acupuncture is the main procedure, its effectiveness can be maximized with the combination of Chinese herbal medicine, moxibustion, Qigong, and dietary and lifestyle modification.

Side Effects Related to Conventional Cancer Treatments

Conventional medicine treats cancer conditions in three ways: surgery, chemotherapy, and radiation. "These methods often produce debilitating side effects and leave patients weakened and dispirited," says Dr. Ni. Symptoms can include nausea, loss of appetite, diarrhea, dizziness, fatigue, hair loss, muscle and joint pain, neuropathy, swelling, depression, weight loss, anemia, and low white blood cell counts. In one study of patients with breast cancer receiving high-dose chemotherapy, adjunct electroacupuncture was more effective in controlling nausea and vomiting than conventional medications.[35]

"Acupuncture has been demonstrated to be very effective in countering the adverse effects of chemotherapy and radiation," says Dr. Ni, who reports that 90% of his cancer patients are referrals from oncologists who have seen the often dramatic results of acupuncture for their patients. "When combined with Chinese herbal medicine and dietary adjustments, acupuncture can help increase production of red and white blood cells, as well as platelet counts, and increase patients' vitality tremendously," Dr. Ni adds. "It gives patients a new lease on life."

A Typical Acupuncture Treatment

First-time patients generally fill out a questionnaire regarding their medical history and are then interviewed by the acupuncturist, who will study the patient, observing the color of the face and any coating on the tongue. Practitioners take into account body language and tone of voice, and will ask about urine color, the menstrual cycle, sensitivity to temperature and seasons, digestive problems, eating and sleeping habits, and emotional stress. Finally, the practitioner will use the wrist to diagnose and test the 12 radial pulses commonly used in Chinese medical diagnosis.

After diagnosis, specific needles are placed in any of over 1,000 locations on the body. Acupuncture, however, calls for no more than 10-12 needles per treatment. In fact, the more skillful the acupuncturist, the fewer the needles he or she will need to use. Essentially, acupuncture is painless. Although a slight pricking sensation may be felt when needles are inserted, a competent acupuncturist will cause no pain. Any slight tugging or aching sensation passes quickly. As a patient, it is important to tell the acupuncturist if any acupoint is uncomfortable, as a slight change of needle position or pressure can instantly eliminate the discomfort.

EAR ACUPUNCTURE

Auriculotherapy, or ear acupuncture, was developed in France shortly after World War II by Paul Nogier, M.D. As a young physician in Lyon, Dr. Nogier observed a tiny peculiar scar in the auricula, or outer ear, of certain patients. The scar, he discovered, was the result of cauterization performed by a local healer as a treatment for sciatica. In most of the cases, Dr. Nogier learned, the procedure had cured the condition.

Dr. Nogier investigated this phenomenon and found that certain points on the outer ear formed a reflex system that could affect other areas when the points were properly stimulated. By 1957 he had worked out 30 basic auricular points that could neurologically affect the body's different layers of skin tissue. Dr. Nogier presented a paper on his discoveries at the Munich Acupuncture Convention. This led to further research on the subject in China and Japan that corroborated Dr. Nogier's findings. Today, Chinese ear acupuncture charts are adapted from Dr. Nogier's work and he has been officially recognized by the Chinese government as the father of modern ear acupuncture. In 1989, auriculotherapy was officially recognized by the World Health Organization as a viable medical modality.

Auriculotherapy is used in the treatment and control of pain, dyslexia, and other functional imbalances. It is applied through the use of acupuncture needles, ear massage, and, in certain cases, electrical stimulation or infrared treatment. In the U.S., it has also become known as a successful treatment for alcohol, cigarette, and drug addiction and is used in treatment centers throughout the country.

Auriculotherapy is used in the treatment and control of pain, dyslexia, and other functional imbalances.

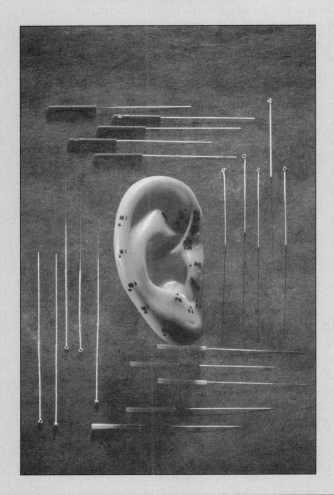

Acupuncture needles are of different lengths and gauges, but are generally hair-thin, solid, and made of stainless steel. To protect both the acupuncturist and patients from AIDS and hepatitis, most acupuncturists use pre-sterilized, disposable needles.

Some treatments last only a few seconds, while others take 45 minutes or longer. Sometimes, an ear needle is used that lies flush against the skin of the ear and, after being covered with tape, is allowed to remain in the ear for more than a week. Generally, however, needles are left in place for 20-30 minutes.

Chinese herbs in the form of teas, pills, and capsules are often given to supplement acupuncture therapy. Finally, the acupuncturist may also recommend changes in diet, lifestyle, and physical activity.

Non-Needle Stimulation of Acupoints

In addition to the use of needles, other forms of treatment are applied to acupoints. Heat is used by burning an herb called moxa (mugwort, or *Artemisia vulgaris*) above the point to be treated. Studies from China have suggested that this particular herb is unique in that it stimulates acupoints and hastens the body's self-healing. The acupuncturist burns a pinch of moxa on a slice of ginger atop an acupoint, or alternatively, the moxa is placed directly on the point and removed as soon as it feels too warm to the patient. There are certain points where a needle can't be used, according to Dr. Cargile, for example, the navel, nipples, or penis. Moxibustion is useful for treating these points.

"A common example of the use of moxa is the highly effective method of remedying the breech position of the fetus in pregnant mothers by burning moxa over an acupoint in the little toes of both feet," Dr. Ni says. When used for this purpose, moxibustion can also be an effective alternative to cesarean births, as evidenced by a recent study conducted by researchers in Italy and China. In the study, 260 women who were pregnant for the first time, and whose babies were in a breech position after 33 weeks, were divided into two groups. The first group received daily moxibustion treatments for one to two weeks, while the other group received conventional pregnancy care. The babies whose mothers received moxa treatments became "measurably more active" and 75% of them were able to then move into proper position for a normal delivery, compared to less than half of the babies whose mothers received conventional care.[36]

Another traditional treatment, especially for large muscle pain, is cupping, which utilizes a glass or bamboo cup to create suction on the skin above a painful muscle or acupuncture point. In place of needles, the acupuncturist may substitute electrostimulation, ultrasound waves, laser beams, or heat to acupuncture points. In China, experiments have included the use of synthetic needles, sonar rays, and injections of water or steroids into acupuncture points.

Tui Na, a form of acupressure, is another method of stimulating acupoints without needles. It is employed by applying steady finger pressure to specific acupoints, and manual manipulation of the joints and muscle tissue. "*Tui Na* is appropriate for very young children and for those who suffer from musculoskeletal conditions," Dr. Ni says.

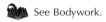 See Bodywork.

The Future of Acupuncture

A growing understanding and greater respect for acupuncture, resulting from tests being conducted worldwide, leads Dr. Cargile to feel that acupuncture will increasingly be integrated into a system of overall health care in the United States. "Not only is acupuncture effective as a primary modality, it also can play a vital role as an adjunctive therapy due to how effective the meridian system is as a means of proper diagnosis," says Dr. Cargile. "Because the meridians influence every cell in the body and pass through every organ and organ system, acupuncture provides health practitioners with an

---

ACUPUNCTURE AND PET CARE

H.C. Gurney, D.V.M., a Colorado-based veterinarian, is one of a growing number of veterinarians in the U.S. who has discovered the benefits of acupuncture for animals. Dr. Gurney has found it an effective alternative for conditions not amenable to conventional therapy, such as behavioral problems, chronic pain, allergies, and autoimmune diseases. Dr. Gurney is a member of the International Veterinary Acupuncture Society (IVAS), under whose auspices veterinarians are trained to become pet acupuncturists. The director of IVAS, Meredith Snader, D.V.M., reports using acupuncture to successfully treat dolphins, birds, monkeys, horses, and livestock, as well as dogs and cats.

Acupuncture is recognized as a valid veterinary medical procedure used mainly for surgical anesthesia and for the alleviation of chronic pain; it has been shown to be clinically effective in relieving symptoms in 84% of those animals suffering from arthritic pain and other degenerative joint diseases. It is also effective in eliminating certain forms of epileptic convulsions.[37]

---

accurate and noninvasive means of determining health deficiencies, as well as a method of reestablishing balance. In short, it provides maximum benefits without the dangerous side effects associated with many of the approaches of conventional medicine."

Acupuncture's growing acceptance by the conventional medical establishment is attested to by the fact that nearly a third of all conventional medical schools in the U.S. now include content related to acupuncture as part of a required course. According to Dennis Tucker, Ph.D., L.Ac., of Nevada City, California, "While acupuncture represents a legacy of concepts that predate Western civilization, as a contemporary health-care system it also represents a synthesis of continuously evolving scientific and technological developments, which provides us with new tools to meet current clinical challenges. The future of acupuncture will to some degree depend upon our ability to reconcile the old and the new within a new science of energy medicine. This can only be accomplished if we honor both our traditional roots and the challenge of building on the foundation provided by scientific research."

Where to Find Help

As with other forms of alternative health care, the legality of practicing acupuncture varies between states. In some states, there is no licensing, while others limit practice to physicians such as medical doctors and chiropractors. In other states, such as Maryland, nonphysician licensed acupuncturists are allowed to practice, provided their patients have been referred to them by a physician. In California and a few other states, acupuncturists are considered primary health-care professionals and can see any patient without a physician's referral. Where acupuncture is legal, the acupuncturist must have graduated from an approved school and passed a state licensing examination. The following organizations will help you find a qualified acupuncturist:

American Association of Oriental Medicine
433 Front Street
Catasauqua, Pennsylvania 18032
(888) 500-7999
Website: www.aaom.org

The AAOM is a national professional trade organization of acupuncturists who meet acceptable standards of competency and can provide you with the names and locations of local members.

American Academy of Medical Acupuncture
4929 Wilshire Blvd., Suite 428
Los Angeles, California 90010
(323) 937-5514
Website: www.medicalacupuncture.org

The purpose of the AAMA is to promote the integration of concepts from traditional and modern forms of acupuncture with conventional Western medicine in order to create a more comprehensive approach to health care. Membership is comprised of M.D.s and D.O.s (osteopathic physicians) with at least two years of experience practicing medical acupuncture.

National Commission for the Certification of Acupuncturists
P.O. Box 97075
Washington, D.C. 20090
(202) 232-1404

The NCCA offers a test that some states use to verify basic competency in acupuncture.

The American College of Addictionology and Compulsive Disorders
975 Arthur Godfrey Road, Suite 500
Miami Beach, Florida 33140
(305) 534-3635

This is the official agency that board certifies doctors of all specialties in acupuncture treatment of addiction and compulsive disorders.

National Acupuncture Detoxification Association
P.O. Box 1927
Vancouver, Washington 98668
(888) 765-NADA
Website: www.acudetox.com

NADA offers literature in eight languages, plus videotapes, dealing with their program. Training is also provided for both practitioners and the lay public. Certification is available.

Recommended Reading

Acupuncture: Everything You Ever Wanted to Know. Gary F. Fleischman. Barrytown, NY: Barrytown Ltd., 1998.

Acupuncture for Everyone. Ruth Kidson. Rochester, VT: Healing Arts Press, 2000.

Acupuncture: Is It for You? J.R. Worsley. New York: Harper & Row, 1973.

The American Association of Oriental Medicine's Complete Guide to Chinese Herbal Medicine. David Molony and Ming Ming Pan Molony. New York: Berkley Books, 1998.

Between Heaven and Earth: A Guide to Chinese Medicine. Harriet Beinfield, L.Ac., and Efrem Korngold, L.Ac., O.M.D. New York: Ballantine Books, 1992.

Clinical Acupuncture: Scientific Basis. Gabriel Stux and R. Hammerschlag. New York: Springer, 2000.

The Web That Has No Weaver: Understanding Chinese Medicine. Ted J. Kaptchuk. Chicago: Contemporary Books, 2000.

The Yellow Emperor's Classic of Medicine. Maoshing Ni. Boston: Shambhala, 1995.

APPLIED KINESIOLOGY

Applied kinesiology can determine health imbalances in the body's organs and glands by identifying weaknesses in specific muscles. By stimulating or relaxing these key muscles, an applied kinesiologist can diagnose and resolve a variety of health problems.

APPLIED KINESIOLOGY employs a simple strength resistance test on a specific indicator muscle that is related to the organ or part of the body that is being tested. If the muscle tests strong (maintaining its resistance), it indicates health. If it tests weak, it can mean infection or dysfunction. "Because of the close clinical relationship between specific muscle dysfunction and related organ or gland dysfunction, applied kinesiology can be used to identify and treat a wide variety of health problems, whether the problem originates in a muscle, gland, or organ," says Robert Blaich, D.C., of Denver, Colorado, a leading expert in applied kinesiology. "In applied kinesiology, the muscle-gland-organ link can indicate the cause of the health problem and lead to further diagnostic tests for confirmation. Once the problem is identified, it can be treated by a variety of techniques to strengthen the muscles involved and restore health."

> *Because of the close clinical relationship between specific muscle dysfunction and related organ or gland dysfunction, applied kinesiology can be used to identify and treat a wide variety of health problems, whether the problem originates in a muscle, gland, or organ.*
>
> —ROBERT BLAICH, D.C.

siologist studies the activity of muscles and the relationship of muscle strength to health. To illustrate this relationship, Dr. Blaich contrasts the approach taken by applied kinesiology with that of conventional medicine in treating asthma. Conventionally, asthma is treated with adrenal hormones or their derivatives, but is still considered to be a problem related to the lungs. By contrast, an applied kinesiologist looks for a weakness in specific muscles in the low back and legs that, although normally associated with low-back pain or knee problems, share a connection with the adrenal glands. The applied kinesiologist would both strengthen these muscles and help the adrenal glands produce their own bronchodilators (chemicals that relax or open the air passages in the lungs).

 See Acupuncture, Chiropractic, Osteopathic Medicine.

"Muscle testing is often the key to balancing mechanically opposed muscles, since a muscle spasm usually exists secondary to and opposite a weak muscle," Dr. Blaich explains. "If you want to bend your elbow, the bicep muscle must 'turn on' and the tricep muscle 'turn off'. If both muscles are either 'on' or 'off', the elbow will not bend.

"When you realize that muscles turn on and off during all normal activities, it is easy to understand how an injury may leave a particular muscle stuck on or off. For example, when you step forward with your left leg, the right arm also goes forward because the extensor muscles that pull back on the right arm are 'turned off'.

How Applied Kinesiology Works

Developed by chiropractic physician George Goodheart, Jr., D.C. (see "The Origin of Applied Kinesiology"), applied kinesiology incorporates the principles of a variety of holistic therapies, including chiropractic, osteopathic medicine, and acupuncture, and involves manual manipulation of the spine, extremities, and cranial bones as the structural basis of its procedures. An applied kine-

This 'turning off' is controlled by and dependent upon getting the correct messages from the nerve endings in the left foot. When you step down on the left foot, the joint receptors there send a message that shuts off the right shoulder. So, if a patient comes to me with a right shoulder problem, it may actually be due to a misaligned bone in the left foot that is causing the shoulder to be stuck on or off. The person's nervous system is acting as if he's taking a step with his left foot when, in fact, he is not."

A muscle that is stuck 'on' acts like a tense muscle spasm, such as a 'charley horse.' A muscle that is stuck 'off' may appear flaccid. Diagnostic evaluation by the applied kinesiologist determines whether muscles are on or off as they should be during normal activity. Dr. Blaich adds that "this knowledge gives us an entirely new mechanism for the understanding of muscle spasm."

Muscle dysfunction in an otherwise healthy person can be corrected through the use of various reflexes or by performing a manual procedure on the muscle, such as deep massage, goading pressure on the attachment points, or realignment. By this method, according to Dr. Blaich, muscles can be reset to function smoothly.

The goals of applied kinesiology are to:

- Determine patient health status and correlate findings with standard diagnostic procedures

- Restore postural balance, correct gait impairment, improve range of motion

- Restore normal nerve function

- Achieve normal endocrine, immune, digestive, and other internal organ functions

- Intervene early in degenerative processes to prevent or delay pathological conditions

Strong and Weak Muscles

Recent research has demonstrated a neurologic difference between "strong" and "weak" muscles, as identified through applied kinesiology testing. Weak muscles will commonly exhibit as much actual force as normal muscles. However, there are other dynamics to a weak muscle besides the actual force it generates. Studies suggest that part of this other quality lies in the timing of the electrical activity in the muscle. Research also shows that "clear, consistent, and predictable differences" occur in the way the brain and central nervous system function when muscles test strong compared to when they test weak.[1] Additional research has also shown that there is a

THE ORIGIN OF APPLIED KINESIOLOGY

George Goodheart, Jr., D.C., a chiropractic physician and the founder of applied kinesiology, first observed in 1964 that, in the absence of skeletal deformity, postural distortion is often associated with muscle dysfunction. A delivery boy who frequently came to Dr. Goodheart's office exhibited "winged scapulae" (flaring of the shoulder blades). This deformity occurs if a specific muscle is weakened by being slightly separated from the bone and is not doing its job of holding the shoulder blades in their proper position. Dr. Goodheart was aware of the development and utilization of manual muscle tests for the purpose of disability evaluation (developed at Johns Hopkins University in the 1940s), and he experimented with the boy by doing a manual procedure of firm, goading pressure on the attachment points of the weak (serratus anterior) muscles. An immediate response was that the muscles "turned on" and the boy's shoulder blades adopted a normal position.

Dr. Goodheart saw that these noninvasive, manipulative treatments restored neuromuscular function, and today they are the core approach to a therapy that encompasses joint manipulation and mobilization, myofascial (muscle sheath) therapies, cranial adjustments, meridian therapy, clinical nutrition, dietary management, and various reflex procedures.

Over the years, Dr. Goodheart discovered and developed many other procedures that returned injured, strained, or otherwise disabled muscles to their normal state. He taught his techniques to others, and eventually applied kinesiology was born. In 1974, a group of practitioners founded the International College of Applied Kinesiology, and today applied kinesiology is a widely practiced method of diagnosis and treatment that is currently being used by many chiropractors, osteopathic physicians, homeopaths, and other practitioners of alternative medicine.

fundamental neurological difference between "weak" muscles and muscles that are normally fatigued.[2]

Muscles become weak for many reasons, including immobility (such as when an arm is in a cast), lack of exercise, poor posture, gland or organ dysfunction, or injury. A weak muscle, notes Dr. Blaich, will often have a delayed reaction to stimulus. According to Dr. Blaich, some of the common internal causes of muscle weakness are:

- Dysfunction of the nerve supply (nerve interference between the spine and the muscles)

- Impairment of lymphatic drainage

- Reduced blood supply

- Abnormal pressure in the cerebrospinal fluid affecting the nerve-to-muscle relationship

- Blockage of an acupuncture meridian

- Chemical imbalance

- Organ or gland dysfunction

If one or more of these conditions exist, a muscle may exhibit abnormal function when tested. The abnormality usually manifests as muscle weakness. The bones that should be supported by that muscle may be misaligned or inflamed, or may exhibit signs of premature wear and tear, commonly in the form of osteoarthritis.

Conditions Benefited by Applied Kinesiology

Muscles perform the critical function of supporting and moving the bones. According to Dr. Goodheart, if a muscle is not functioning properly, the bones and joints that it supports will function poorly, or not at all. This is why people with structural imbalances, musculoskeletal imbalances, and joint problems can benefit from applied kinesiology, and why applied kinesiology is so popular with the chiropractic profession, which many patients consult because of physical pain or dysfunction.

Muscle-Organ Relationships in Applied Kinesiology

While developing his theory and practice of applied kinesiology, Dr. Goodheart concluded that specific muscles are universally related to specific organs. Because of this relationship, a wide variety of nonmuscular conditions (problems with organs or systems) are often benefited. For example, because the deltoid muscle in the shoulder shares a relationship to the lungs, the muscle test can be an indicator of the state of the lungs and can serve as an excellent monitor of their condition.

Reflex areas that stimulate either the deltoid or the lungs stimulate both. If an individual has a lung infection or an abnormal function in one or both lungs, he or she will probably exhibit weakness of one or both deltoid muscles. Not only would there be a lung infection, but because of deltoid weakness a problem may develop in the shoulder. Under normal circumstances, once the lung infection clears or if the body adapts to the infection, the deltoid muscle will return to its normal state. However, if a chronic, low-grade infection lingers, the patient can be left with a weakened deltoid muscle. The applied kinesiologist evaluating the patient will likely need to stimulate the nerve and blood supply, as well as lymphatic drainage and acupuncture energy to the lungs in order for them to clear. Once the lung problem is resolved, deltoid muscle function can return to normal.

Interestingly, toxic fumes inhaled into the lungs can conceivably stimulate the brain to produce an immediate weakening of a deltoid muscle, as its link to the lungs can serve to monitor lung toxicity. Inhalation of the same fumes may also weaken a muscle related to the liver, such as the pectoralis major (a large fan-shaped muscle of the upper chest that acts to flex and rotate the arm), because of the increased demands placed on the liver to detoxify the harmful substances.

 Applied kinesiology procedures are not intended as a single method of diagnosis. They should enhance standard diagnosis, not replace it.

Nutrition in Applied Kinesiology

Specific vitamins or nutrients are sometimes needed to help a patient with a particular condition, such as an upper respiratory tract infection. One way to identify nutritional substances of value to this specific ailment is to test the patient's weak deltoid muscle while putting the substance on the tongue to stimulate nerve endings, which, in turn, trigger certain areas in the brain to make changes in the body. If the correct nutrient is applied, there should be an immediate strengthening of the deltoid muscle.

Dr. Blaich tells of a conductor who came to him because severe pains in his shoulder were inhibiting his ability to conduct. After four hours in front of the orchestra, he could not raise his shoulder. Dr. Blaich evaluated the shoulder area and determined the main problem to be a specific muscle, the pectoralis major. He reset the muscle by correcting a specific cranial fault through minute manipulation of the bones in the head. The problem recurred, and through detailed testing, Dr. Blaich determined that the problem was caused by eating wheat. The patient was found to have a gluten allergy, and as long as he avoided eating wheat, he had no problems with his shoulder.

A TYPICAL VISIT TO AN APPLIED KINESIOLOGIST

What happens on a visit to an applied kinesiologist depends entirely on the particular problem, and whether it is acute or chronic. Patient history is recorded, including diet and lifestyle. Inquiries are made about changes in either that could relate to the problem. The patient's posture, gait, and any obvious physical problems (such as a dropped shoulder, a limp, or a lean to one side) are carefully examined. In addition, before muscle testing is performed, blood tests may be ordered if organ dysfunction or infection are suspected.

The results of muscle testing may indicate the need for stimulation of acupuncture points or it may indicate the need to test nutrients on the tongue to see if these strengthen the weak muscle. The spine may be adjusted and reflexes may be stimulated to aid in lymphatic drainage to a particular organ. Further blood tests may be indicated or specific therapies suggested to strengthen a particular organ.

Applied Kinesiology and Food Allergies

Recent research indicates that applied kinesiology can be an effective and inexpensive way to detect hidden food allergies. Foods that cause an allergic reaction usually also affect neuromuscular function, resulting in patterns of reversible muscle weakness. In order to detect food allergies, practitioners of applied kinesology employ oral provocative testing (having patients place suspected food samples in their mouth), while specific muscle tests are performed. Weakened or inhibited muscle function that occurs during this procedure is often an indication that the patient is allergic or sensitive to the food in question.

In 1998, a pilot study was conducted to determine the accuracy of applied kinesiology for food allergy screening compared to radio-allergosorbent test (RAST) and immune complex testing for blood levels of antibodies (immunoglobulin E and IgG). The study involved 17 subjects, each of whom tested positive in oral provocative testing of one or two foods while applied kinesiology was employed. Test subjects were found to be allergic or hypersensitive to a total of 21 foods, including cornmeal, whole-wheat flour, soy flour, brewer's yeast, powdered egg, and potato flour. Follow-up RAST and immune complex testing confirmed 19 of the 21 (90.5%)

suspected food allergies indicated by applied kinesiology muscle testing.[3]

Applied Kinesiology and Sports

Because it deals so effectively with the interaction of muscles during activity, applied kinesiology is a superb approach to any type of athletic ailment or injury. It is so effective at improving muscle interaction and stabilization that it is often used not only for rehabilitation but also as a way to prevent injury and improve athletic performance.

A football player running down the field with a weak knee-stabilizing muscle is an "accident looking for a place to happen," notes Dr. Blaich. If he moves the wrong way, the knee joint could give out and conceivably cause serious injury. If he is evaluated and treated by an applied kinesiologist, the weak knee muscle will be recognized and treated, and serious injury avoided.

The muscle/organ link can be helpful in identifying "rate limiting factors" or "weak links" in the performance of top athletes. In 1983 and 1984, Dr. Blaich identified adrenal weakness accompanying other structural and chemical imbalances in a bicyclist named Alexi Grewal. Alexi was a talented young athlete, full of promise and motivation, but with a history of asthma. He was treated by Dr. Blaich, who worked to improve Alexi's adrenal gland and diaphragm muscle function as well as structural balance. Alexi's health and performance improved enough to win a gold medal in the 1984 Olympics.

CAUTION Applied kinesiology is a highly specialized technique and should only be performed by a licensed health professional trained in differential diagnosis (a systematic method for diagnosing a disorder that lacks unique signs or symptoms). There have been many sincere attempts to teach laypeople to use manual muscle testing as a method of home health care, but there are definite limitations to diagnostic conclusions made by someone not properly trained in manual muscle testing. The skill of the practitioner in the accuracy of performing manual muscle testing, and the diagnostic conclusions that one makes regarding the outcome of a muscle test, are very significant. A manual muscle test can be a valuable indicator of some function in the body, but the interpretation of the test is complex and should be handled by trained professionals.

The Future of Applied Kinesiology

Applied kinesiology is rapidly gaining acceptance among health practitioners and the public, due to the nonintrusive nature of this diagnostic technique and therapy. As a result, growing numbers of health-care professionals, including M.D.s, chiropractors, and osteopaths, now incorporate applied kinesiology into their overall treatment programs.

Where to Find Help

For more information on applied kinesiology, or for help in locating an applied kinesiology professional, contact:

International College of Applied Kinesiology
6405 Metcalf Avenue, Suite 503
Shawnee Mission, Kansas 66202-3929
(913) 384-5336
Website: www.icak.com

Referral service for those seeking an applied kinesiologist. Supplies written information on various aspects of health and nutrition as well as a newsletter on request.

Recommended Reading

Applied Kinesiology: Muscle Response in Diagnosis, Therapy, and Preventive Medicine. Tom and Carol Valentine. Rochester, VT: Inner Traditions, 1989.

You'll Be Better: The Story of Applied Kinesiology. George Goodheart, Jr., D.C. Geneva, OH: AK Printing, 1989. Distributed by Dr. Goodheart; call (313) 882-4868.

Your Body Can Talk: How to Use Simple Muscle Testing to Learn What Your Body Knows and Needs. Susan L. Levy and Carol Lehr. Prescott, AZ: Hohm Press, 1996.

AROMATHERAPY

Aromatherapy uses the essential oils extracted from plants and herbs to treat conditions ranging from infections and skin disorders to immune deficiencies and stress. Essential oils have been used throughout Europe for over 120 years, and a system of medical aromatherapy is currently practiced in France. Used in conjunction with other alternative healing modalities, aromatherapy is gaining ground in the United States as well.

AROMATHERAPY IS a unique branch of herbal medicine that utilizes the medicinal properties found in the essential oils of various plants. Through different processes of distillation—using steam, water and steam, or cold pressing—the volatile constituents of the plant's oil (its essence) are extracted from its flowers, leaves, branches, or roots. (The overall manufacture of essential oils, from growing plants to distilling the oil, is labor intensive and requires large amounts of plant material and manpower, both of which can make certain essential oils expensive.) According to Kurt Schnaubelt, Ph.D., Director of the Pacific Institute of Aromatherapy, in San Rafael, California, the term *aromatherapy* is somewhat misleading, as it can suggest an exclusive role for the aroma in the healing process. "In actuality," Dr. Schnaubelt says, "the oils exert much of their therapeutic effect through their pharmacological properties and their small molecular size, making them one of the few therapeutic agents to easily penetrate bodily tissues."

Aromatherapy is very effective for bacterial infections of the respiratory system,[1] immune deficiencies such as Epstein-Barr virus (a form of herpes virus believed to be the causative agent in infectious mononucleosis), and numerous skin disorders.[2] It is also useful for other infections such as cystitis[3] and herpes simplex.[4] The immediate and often profound effect that essential oils have on the central nervous system also makes aromatherapy an excellent method for stress management.[5]

 See Herbal Medicine for a description of pharmacological properties of essential oils.

How Aromatherapy Works

According to Dr. Schnaubelt, "The chemical makeup of essential oils gives them a host of desirable pharmaco-

> **Aromatherapy is a unique branch of herbal medicine that utilizes the medicinal properties found in the essential oils of various plants.**

logical properties, ranging from antibacterial, antiviral, and antispasmodic, to uses as diuretics (promoting production and excretion of urine), vasodilators (widening blood vessels), and vasoconstrictors (narrowing blood vessels). Essential oils also act on the adrenal glands, ovaries, and the thyroid, and can energize or pacify, detoxify, and facilitate the digestive process." The oils' therapeutic properties also make them effective for treating infections, interacting with the various branches of the nervous system, modifying immune response, and harmonizing moods and emotions.

Essential oil preparations are generally broad spectrum, meaning that they benefit multiple areas of the body simultaneously. "Essential oils, unlike pharmaceutical drugs, are in a complete and balanced form that our bodies are designed to absorb and use beneficially," states aromatherapist Anne Vermilye, M.S., C.C.H.T., C.M.T., of Mill Valley, California. "Hundreds of different molecules assist in the activity of each oil, not just a 'most active ingredient'."

Essential oils, unlike pharmaceutical drugs, are in a complete and balanced form that our bodies are designed to absorb and use beneficially.

—ANNE VERMILYE,
M.S., C.C.H.T., C.M.T.

The Physiological Effects of Fragrance

Aromatic molecules that interact with the top of the nasal cavity emit signals that are modified by various biological processes before traveling to the limbic system, the emotional switchboard of the brain.[6] There they create impressions associated with previous experiences and emotions. Because the limbic system is directly connected to those parts of the brain that control heart rate, blood pressure, breathing, memory, stress levels, and hormone balance, scientists have learned that inhalation of oil fragrances may be one of the fastest ways to achieve physiological or psychological effects. "Through inhalation, essential oil vapors are absorbed into the bloodstream through the tissues of the lungs while they pass through the olfactory nerves," Vermilye explains. "As these vapors pass through the olfactory nerves, they affect the following areas of the brain: the cortex, which governs all the intellectual processes; the pituitary, which oversees all hormonal activity, including adrenal hormones; and the hypothalamus, which plays a direct role in controlling anger and aggression."

John Steele, Ph.D., of Sherman Oaks, California, and Robert Tisserand, of London, England, leading researchers in the field of aromatherapy, have studied the effects on brain-wave patterns when essential oils are inhaled or smelled. Their findings show that oils such as orange, jasmine, and rose have a tranquilizing effect and work by altering the brain waves into a rhythm that produces calmness and a sense of well-being. In the same way, the so-called stimulating oils—basil, black pepper, rosemary, and cardamom—work by producing a heightened energy response.[7]

Inhaling the fragrance of certain essential oils can help clear sinuses or free congestion in the chest, as well as alter the neurochemistry of the brain to produce

changes in mental and emotional behavior. Even aromas too subtle to be consciously detected can have significant effects on central nervous system activity, sometimes to the point of cutting in half the amount of time needed to perform a visual search task.[8]

How to Use Aromatherapy

Aromatherapy uses essential oils to affect the body in several ways. The benefits of essential oils can be obtained through inhalation, external application, or orally by ingestion.

Inhalation Methods

- **Diffusers** disperse microparticles of the essential oil into the air. They can be used to achieve beneficial results in respiratory conditions or to simply change the air with the mood-lifting or calming qualities of the fragrance.

- **Steam tents** are an efficient way to deliver concentrated doses of essential oils into the respiratory tract, according to Vermilye. "They can eliminate a cold or flu at the onset and may be useful as a preventive measure when exposed to someone with an illness," she says. To employ this method, boil a pot of water in a stainless steel or glass pot. Remove from the stove and add two to three drops of essential oil. "Rosemary, lavender, tea tree, eucalyptus, Ravensara aromatica, palmarosa, and chamomile are ideal oils for steaming," Vermilye says. Quickly tent your face over the pot by covering your head with a towel. Be sure to raise yourself high enough to keep from getting burned. Keep your eyes shut and breathe deeply for five minutes.

- **Nose cone** is a method Vermilye has found to be highly useful for treating respiratory ailments (except asthma). "Take a napkin or tissue and make a 2 ½ inch square," Vermilye instructs. "Use a blend of the following oils: Ravensara aromatica, *Eucalyptus radiata*, and either chamomile, thyme-linalol, palmarosa, niaouli, or tea tree. Place two drops in the center of the paper. Fold in half and roll up to fit into the nostril. Place the dry end, with no oil, into the nostril and keep it there for 20 minutes."

- **Floral waters** are easily made and can be sprayed into the air or directly onto skin that is too sensitive to the touch. Use about ten drops of essential oils and the rest pure water to fill a 4-ounce glass bottle with spray. As a room disinfectant, use five drops lavender, three drops palmarosa, eucalyptus, or Ravensara aromatica, and three drops of Roman chamomile. Or try a mixture of seven drops of neroli with five drops of lavender to refresh and relax.

External Applications

Oils are readily absorbed through the skin. Convenient applications are baths, massages, hot and cold compresses, floral water sprays, or a simple topical application of diluted oils.[9]

- **Baths** are beneficial as well as cleansing. Essential oils in a hot bath can stimulate the skin, induce relaxation, and energize the body. The heat of the bath helps the oils penetrate the skin faster and enhances circulation. Certain essential oils, such as rosemary, can stimulate the elimination of toxins through the skin. When you get out of a bath, you should wrap yourself quickly in a flannel sheet and warm blanket. Lie down and try to fall asleep. The sweating this will promote is extremely beneficial. Be sure to drink plenty of water and wash off afterwards in a shower so you do not reabsorb the toxins. Essential oils can also be used in foot and sitz baths.

  See Hydrotherapy.

- **Massage** works the oils into the skin and, depending on the oil and the massage technique used, can either calm or stimulate an individual. "Since massage oil blends are quite potent, they should be kept within a range of 10 drops to 30 drops of essential oil per ounce of carrier oil," Vermilye says. Good carrier oils include sweet almond, avocado, sesame, hazelnut, soy (be careful of genetically altered soy products), safflower, jojoba, and sunflower. Although it is preferable to use a fresh blend for each application, some blends will keep for up to two months. To further enhance the absorption rate, once the massage is finished cover the body in a flannel sheet or warm blanket.

  CAUTION Cancerous tissues and lymph nodes should not be massaged with essential oils.

- **Compresses** soothe minor aches and pains, reduce swelling, and treat sprains.

Internal Application

For certain conditions (such as organ dysfunction or disorder), it can be advantageous to take oils internally. It is essential to receive proper medical guidance for internal use of oils. However, such professional guidance is difficult to obtain in the United States.

"The easiest way to get the oils into the stomach and/or small intestines is to put a tiny bit of cocoa butter with a drop or two of essential oil in a gelatin capsule," Vermilye explains. "To administer oils directly to the throat like a lozenge, put a drop or two of oil into a teaspoon of honey, onto a sugar cube, or onto a charcoal tablet. To make a mouthwash, put a few drops of peppermint, sage, anise, or thyme in a glass of water."

Essential oils can also be applied via suppositories, a method that is quite common in France, according to Vermilye. "By being absorbed into the rectal veins, essential oils bypass the liver and reach the heart and other organs without alteration," she says.

CAUTION In their pure state, certain oils, such as clove and cinnamon, can cause irritation or skin burn. These oils call for careful and expert application. It is recommended that they be diluted with a less irritating essential oil before being applied to the skin. Essential oils can cause a toxic reaction if ingested. Consult a physician before taking any oils internally, especially if you are pregnant.

Conditions Benefited by Aromatherapy

The value of aromatherapy in the treatment of infectious diseases has gained increased attention in recent years. Its use for this purpose is widespread in France, where a system of aromatherapeutic medicine has been developed.[10] French physicians routinely prescribe aromatherapy preparations and French pharmacies stock essential oils alongside the more conventional drugs. In England, aromatherapy is used mainly for stress-related health issues. Hospital nursing staffs administer essential oil massage to relieve pain and to induce sleep.[11] This type of massage has proven particularly effective in relieving stress associated with surgery, cancer,[12] and AIDS.

"For nurses, aromatherapy is an excellent communication tool," says Jane Buckle, R.N., author of *Clinical Aromatherapy in Nursing*. "Touch and the providing of pleasing aromas are a means of interacting with patients, many of whom, if they are in intensive care, are not able to relate their discomfort in words to their care providers. Aromatherapy, delivered through touch, can give great comfort and may alter patient perceptions of pain."

English hospitals also use a variety of vaporized essential oils (including lemon, lavender, and lemongrass) to help combat the transmission of airborne infectious diseases.[13] Essential oils are also used topically on wound sites to counter infection.

Bacterial and Viral Infections

Essential oils are powerful antimicrobial agents.[14] These oils lack the negative side effects (kidney toxicity, anemia, lowered white blood cell count) of conventional antibiotics and do not destroy intestinal bacteria, the loss of which can lead to secondary infections. In a hallmark study conducted in 1973, a blend of the essential oils clove, cinnamon, melissa, and lavender was found to be as effective in treating bronchial conditions as commercial antibiotics.[15]

"Because the oils work in a different way from antibiotics, they do not have the usual side effects and they tend to stimulate the immune system instead of depressing it," says Tisserand. "Oils of cinnamon and eucalyptus are as powerful against some microorganisms as conventional antibiotics and are especially effective against flu viruses. Sandalwood oil is not only a classic perfume oil, but also a traditional remedy for sore throats and laryngitis. Lavender oil, so often used in toilet waters and scented sachets, has a dramatic healing action on burns."[16]

In November 1995, research on the broad range of antimicrobial effects of essential oils and essential oil components was presented at the First Wholistic and Scientific Conference on the Therapeutic Uses of Essential Oils, in San Francisco, California. Conducted by Rolf Deininger, M.D., of Cologne, Germany, the study found that aromatherapy was effective in treating "conditions of the upper respiratory tract, skin, gastrointestinal tract, urogenital tract, nervousness, and arterial conditions" caused by bacteria, viruses, or fungi.[17] Commenting on the study, Dr. Schnaubelt states, "Given the extremely favorable track record of essential oils in treating viral diseases, one would expect researchers to jump on this opportunity to study cures that could be effective and available to all. But again, since oils cannot be patented and scientists are economically dependent, these potential cures elicit mostly yawns from the scientific establishment." Dr. Schnaubelt also points out that, in addition to inhibiting pathogens, essential oils improve overall metabolic activity and immune response, and enhance the healing of the immuno-psychological aspects of infectious disease.[18]

According to Vermilye, the antimicrobial effects of essential oils are due to the oils' ability to enter the cell walls of microbes and cut off oxygen. "This stops the formation of energy within the cells of microbes and kills them," she says. "In addition, essential oils attack the whole pathogen, not just a specific aspect of the organism. This is commonly thought to be why we do not develop resistance to the effects of essential oils, as

can happen with prolonged use of conventional drugs." Among the most beneficial essential oils for dealing with infectious diseases, Vermilye recommends bay laurel, German and Roman chamomile, clove bud, ginger, lavender, oregano, rosemary, thyme, *Eucalyptus radiata*, helichrysum, neroli, niaouli, palmarosa, and Ravensara aromatica. "These are all essential oils that I have had positive and exciting results with, and scientific studies have proven their effectiveness for inhibiting pathogens," she says.

> *Given the extremely favorable track record of essential oils in treating viral diseases, one would expect researchers to jump on this opportunity to study cures that could be effective and available to all. But again, since oils cannot be patented and scientists are economically dependent, these potential cures elicit mostly yawns from the scientific establishment.*
>
> —KURT SCHNAUBELT, PH.D.

Herpes Simplex

Due to their strong antiviral properties, many essential oils are highly effective against the herpes simplex virus, according to a study presented at the First Congress on Aromatherapy, in Cologne, Germany, in 1987.[19] Jean Valnet, M.D., a French physician, recommends a blend of lemon and geranium;[20] Tisserand suggests *Eucalyptus radiata* and bergamot. Dr. (rer. nat.) Dietrich Wabner, a professor at the Technical University of Munich, reports that a single application of either true rose oil or melissa oil led to complete remission of herpes simplex lesions.

The most effective treatment is to apply the oils at the first sign of an outbreak. If herpes lesions have already appeared, the oil is applied directly on the lesions and, in most cases, the lesions dry within a day or two and are in complete remission within three to five days. If the drying process creates discomfort, a 10% dilution of the essential oil(s) can be mixed in a high-quality vegetable base oil. "We have documented this pattern of remission in almost all the cases we were able to observe over the years," reports Dr. Schnaubelt. "Whenever the specific

HISTORY OF AROMATHERAPY

Plants and their essential oils have been used therapeutically from ancient times in countries as diverse as Egypt, Italy, India, and China.[22] In Europe, essential oils were first used in ritualistic healing practices during the Middle Ages as a means of combating illness, and burning incense to prevent the spread of cholera and plague was commonly used in the 17th and 18th centuries. "Aromatic plants and essential oils were supposed to control the impurity of the air, so their use grew as well," says aromatherapist Anne Vermilye, M.S., C.C.H.T., C.M.T. "It was common practice to inhale from sponges soaked in vinegar or a lemon stuck with cloves to ward off disease, and candles scented with rose petals, cloves, and musk were burnt in sick rooms as a preventive measure." In most of the world, plant essences remain popular today as therapeutic agents and are utilized in everything from antiseptic creams and skin ointments to liniments for arthritic pain.

The term *aromatherapy* was coined in 1937 by the French chemist Rene-Maurice Gattefosse. While working in his family's perfume laboratory, Dr. Gattefosse burned his hand. He knew lavender was used in medicine for treating burns and inflammation, and he immediately immersed his hand in a container of pure lavender oil on his workbench. When the burn quickly lost its redness and began to heal, he was impressed enough by the oil's regenerative ability to begin researching the curative powers of other essential oils. This marked the beginning of the modern-day science of aromatherapy for the treatment of common ailments. In the U.S., the popularity of aromatherapy has grown rapidly over the last two decades, fueled by the increasing demand for non-toxic and non-threatening restorative therapies.

pain indicating the recurrence of the lesions occurs, oils are applied before the outbreak of the lesion and more often than not the outbreak is prevented. After repeating this procedure three to four times, herpes simplex typically stops recurring."

Among the essential oils Dr. Schnaubelt recommends for treating herpes are may chang (*Litsea cubeba*), tea tree, melissa, creeping hyssop (*Hyssophus officinalis* var. *decumbens*), or a mixture of geranium, *Eucalyptus radiata*, and *E. citriodora* oils. He advises applying the oils undiluted to the affected area.[21]

Shingles (Herpes Zoster Infection)

"Another effective use of essential oils is the topical treatment of shingles, a painful skin virus," says Dr. Schnaubelt. "Our greatest success in the treatment of shingles is by applying a blend of 50% Ravensara aromatica and 50% *Calophyllum inophyllum* (related to St. John's wort). Drastic improvements and complete remission occur within seven days."

Skin Conditions

Essential oils are also utilized for skin problems based on their skin-friendly properties. Examples are thyme oil, whose highly antiseptic properties are nonirritating; neroli oil, whose rejuvenating properties produce an effect similar to hormones (neroli is also used to prevent stretch marks); rosemary oil, known to regenerate cells and improve metabolic activity in the inner layer of the skin; and everlast, possibly the most effective anti-inflammatory agent in aromatherapy. Thyme-linalol and rosewood oil are effective when used topically for acne.

Other effective essential oils for skin conditions are carrot seed oil (an effective tissue revitalizer excellent for use on the face) and eucalyptus oil (commonly used to regulate over-productive sebaceous glands, which help to retain body heat and prevent sweat evaporation). In cases of bites or stings, Dr. Valnet points out that the essential oils basil, cinnamon, garlic, lavender, lemon, onion, sage, savory, and thyme are effective due to their antitoxic and antivenomous properties.[23]

Muscular Disorders

There have been many studies outlining the effects of various essential oils on the nervous system and their ability to relieve muscle spasm.[24] Combinations of essential oils with high proportions of ester compounds (clary sage, Roman chamomile, and lavender) are especially effective in this regard and are used in massage as well as in advanced spa treatments.

Arthritis

Studies by Dr. Hildebret Wagner, Chair of the Institute of Pharmaceutical Biology at Ludwig Maximilian University, in Munich, Germany, show that the essential oils that are stimulatory, such as clove, cinnamon, and thyme, can have anti-inflammatory effects in treating arthritis. Dr. Wagner suggests that the irritation caused by these oils stimulates the adrenal glands and triggers the release of anti-inflammatory substances, the body's natural cortisone-like material.[25] The more practical and effective application of everlast and eucalyptus to relieve arthritis pain comes out of French medical aromatherapy. "Because of their very strong local anti-inflammatory action, these oils often reduce arthritis symptoms within moments of application," says Dr. Schnaubelt.

Imbalances of the Autonomic Nervous System

Research conducted in Germany has shown that an aromatherapeutic formula known as Klosterfrau Melissengeist (KMG) can alleviate a variety of disease conditions caused by imbalances of the autonomic nervous system (ANS, the body's "automatic pilot," which controls breathing, heart rate, and digestion). KMG, which has been used in Germany for nearly 200 years, is an alcohol co-distillate of eight essential oils: *Folia melissae, Flores caryophylli, Rhizoma zingiberis, Rhizoma heleni, Rhizoma galangae, Fructus piperis nigri, Radix angelicae,* and *Radix gentianae.*

ANS imbalances can be caused by stress, environmental toxins, poor diet, lack of relaxation, and various mental/emotional factors and, if left untreated, can result in ultimately severe physical disease. Conditions related to ANS imbalances are numerous and include arrhythmia (irregular heartbeat), anxiety, coldness in the extremities, depression, dizziness, headaches and migraines, hot flashes, and nervousness. Yet, as Dr. Schnaubelt points out, "Imbalances of the autonomic nervous system do not appear to be a recognized condition in North America."[26]

A multicentered, double-blind study on the effects of KMG found that it resulted in significant improvement in the symptoms and conditions related to ANS imbalances among all participants in the study. According to Dr. Schnaubelt, a closer analysis revealed improvements in nervousness, inner restlessness, unaccountable excitability, blushing, palpitations, headaches, and other psychological factors, as well as a "significant improvement in the area of ego strength according to standardized psychological profiles" and "immense improvements in emotional stability."[27] Another study of KMG found that it increased the patient's ability to concentrate, reduced the incidence of depression, and improved physical conditions such as heart pain, dizziness, lack of appetite, headache, and gastrointestinal disorders caused by ANS imbalances.[28]

Among the other health conditions for which Dr. Schnaubelt has found essential oils to be effective are allergies, bladder infections, bruises, burns, conjunctivitis, cystitis, diarrhea, earache, fatigue, women's health conditions (menopause, PMS, vaginitis), fever, hemorrhoids, insomnia, motion sickness, respiratory conditions (asthma, bronchitis, colds and flu, sinusitis), sexually transmitted diseases (chlamydia, genital warts), sprains, tendinitis, and wounds and scars.[29]

PURCHASING ESSENTIAL OILS

Selecting essential oils from the many different varieties in the marketplace can be confusing. Vast differences in price exist for what seems to be one and the same oil. Inquiries are practically always met with a universal assurance that the oil is absolutely pure and natural. This is not always the case: many suppliers do not verify the purity of the oils they distribute. When purchasing essential oils, it is important to take note of their purity, quality, and price.

"Pure essential oils are expensive," according to Kurt Schnaubelt, Ph.D. "Often, 1,000 pounds of plant are needed to produce one pound of essence. This process involves manpower to cultivate and harvest the plant and the energy cost for distillation. Because of the variations in these factors, the prices of essential oils can differ. If every oil in a line carries the same price tag, this is a sure sign of large-scale homogenization and adulteration for the production of sheer fragrance oils as opposed to essential oils."

Essential oils should be called "essential oils" on the label. If names are used that sound evasive, such as "pure botanical perfume" or "pure fragrance essence," this is an indication that the supplier is aware that the oils are not true essential oils, adds Dr. Schnaubelt.

Oil essences are most commonly produced to create fragrances and to process food. The quality requirements of these oils are substantially lower than those used for aromatherapy. Companies that concern themselves solely with aromatherapy will go to great lengths to ensure purity.

While pure, natural essential oils may seem expensive, one or two drops will go far, and this makes them cost-effective. In contrast, the effectiveness of lower grade oils, or oils that are diluted, drastically diminishes over time due to a loss of their essential properties. The best way to purchase essential oils for aromatherapy applications is from a supplier who specializes in essential aromatherapy oils.

Some Essential Oils and Their Applications

According to Dr. Schnaubelt and Anne Vermilye, the following essential oils are among the most widely used therapeutically:

Eucalyptus (Eucalyptus radiata): This particular form of eucalyptus, also called *Eucalyptus australiana,* is a classic antiviral and expectorant agent.[30] It is best used through a diffuser or topically as a chest rub for rheumatism, muscular pains, or neuralgia.

Everlast (Helichrysum italicum): Skin care professionals use everlast in dilutions of 2% or lower for its tissue-regenerating qualities on scars. Applied topically, it is a powerful anti-inflammatory agent and can prevent hemorrhaging and swelling after sports injuries or bruising. Because of its ketone (an organic chemical derived by oxidation of alcohol) content, this oil should only be used topically and in concentrations not exceeding 2%.

Geranium (Pelargonium x asperum): A fragrant oil with antifungal and antiviral properties.[31] It is gentle on the skin and gives body to the fragrance of many essential oil compositions.

German Chamomile (Matricicaria chamomilia): Chamomile is effective when used in the bath or in a massage oil blend. Can also reduce a fever as it rids the body of bacteria.

Ginger (Zingiber officinale): When used internally, ginger relieves diarrhea, gas, and other digestive discomforts. A ginger/cardamom stomach pack applied externally soothes abdominal pain and tension.

Lavender (Lavendula angustifolia): The classic oil of aromatherapy has the broadest spectrum of benefits—it can be used undiluted on burns, small injuries, skin ulcers, eczema, and insect bites. Lavender's high ester content gives it a calming, almost sedative quality.

Mandarin (Citrus reticulata): Mandarin's calming properties and universally pleasing fragrance make this oil a top choice to release anxiety. It is typically dispersed in a room with a diffuser.

Neroli (Citrus aurantium): Mix this with any carrier oil to use as a perfume or spray. Will ease anxiety, tension, and menopausal upsets.

Niaouli (Melaleuca quinquenervia viridiflora): Niaouli calms respiratory allergies, is a vitalizing and balancing agent for overactive and oily skin, and helps with hemorrhoids (in the non-acute stage). It is also effective on bacterial and fungal infections.

Palmarosa (Cymbopogon martinii): A staple in many homemade aromatherapy compositions, palmarosa's pleasant fragrance and excellent antiseptic/antiviral activity have uses in skin care and in the treatment of herpes.

Peppermint (Mentha piperita): A drop of this oil on the tongue provides relief for nausea and travel sickness. It is also effective for irritable bowel syndrome. In France, small doses of peppermint oil (50 mg) are given three times a day as a stimulant for the liver during convalescence.

Ravensara aromatica (Cinnamomum camphora): This oil is commonly used as an inhalation remedy for bronchitis and respiratory infections. If applied topically, it can also be used to treat shingles and other sores.

Roman Chamomile (Anthemis nobilis): Recommended to calm an upset mind or body. A drop rubbed on the solar plexus can bring rapid relief of mental or physical stress. It may also help with liver engorgement.

Rosemary (Rosmarinus officinalis): There are a number of varieties of rosemary that have different chemical compositions. The softest and most expensive type is rosemary verbenon, which is a staple in aromatherapy skin care, as it activates the metabolism in the outer layer of the skin and improves cell regeneration. This is especially helpful on sore joints and muscles.

Spikenard (Nardostachys jatamansii): This oil is from the root of a plant from the Himalayan mountains. One belief is that the spikenard oil embodies the life energy of the plant.[32] For that reason, it is often used at the core of aromatherapy blends that are aimed toward benefiting the psyche.

Tea Tree (Melaleuca alternifolia): A nonirritating antiseptic, tea tree has antibacterial, antiviral, and antifungal properties. Applied topically, it is useful in healing pus-filled wounds or acne and for treating many types of mild or chronic infections that occur in the mouth and genital area.

Thyme (Thymus vulgaris or linalol): Considered a powerful broad-spectrum antibiotic oil, it has shown positive results treating urinary infections and eliminating parasites and *Candida*. Best used internally, but not recommended for daily use.

Aromatherapy in the Home

Aromatherapy is ideally suited for home use. While it is true that irresponsible use of essential oils may pose certain risks, these risks are small compared to the potential gain. Typical problems are caused by excessive use of potentially irritating or allergenic oils such as clove, cinnamon, oregano, or savory, but with proper knowledge these pitfalls are easily avoided. Most health-food stores now carry essential oils, and many even carry starter kits with selections of the most widely used oils. Following are some typical applications of essential oils in the home:

- **Daily hygiene:** Gentle antiviral essential oils, such as *Eucalyptus radiata*, Ravensara aromatica, and niaouli can be spread over the skin before, during, or after the morning shower. This practice strengthens the body's resistance to sickness during the cold or flu season.

- **Digestive and stress-related discomfort:** A drop of anise seed oil, mixed with a spoon of honey or by itself, helps to release gastrointestinal cramping. Tarragon stimulates digestion and calms a nervous digestive tract.

- **Bruises and sports injuries:** Everlast relieves pain after injuries and prevents hemorrhaging and swelling.

- **Mosquito and other insect bites:** Lavender is unsurpassed in treating itching or stinging from mosquito bites or bee stings.

- **Burns:** The restorative powers of lavender oil on burnt skin inspired the very emergence of aromatherapy.

- **Energy:** Essential oils of black spruce and peppermint are effective stimulants that work by strengthening the adrenal cortex.[34]

- **Relaxation:** Essential oils like citronella and *Eucalyptus citriodora* can be diffused in the air, or rubbed on the wrists, solar plexus, and temples, for quick and effective relaxation. Mandarin is a fragrance favored by children and its calming qualities can slow down highly active children. Lavender oil added to the bath

PRECAUTIONS WHEN USING ESSENTIAL OILS

Certain essential oils, such as those derived from thuja, wormwood, mugwort, tansy, hyssop, and sage, can cause a toxic reaction if taken internally. However, their toxicity is much lower when applied externally. Other essential oils with a high-phenol (disinfectant) content, such as oregano and savory, should not be taken internally for any prolonged period of time (exceeding 10-21 days), as doing so might have negative implications on certain aspects of liver metabolism.

Clove and cinnamon should also be used with caution, as they are known allergenics. Approximately 5% of the population will exhibit a dermatitis reaction to these two oils when they are applied to the skin. Interestingly, the toxicity of these oils is a factor when applied to the skin, but comparatively low when ingested in moderate doses.[33] Occasionally, irritation can also occur from overuse of a particular oil; this is not hazardous and will disappear when use of the oil is discontinued.

or sprayed on bed sheets reduces tension and enhances relaxation.[35]

- **Nausea:** Peppermint is the classic oil for alleviating nausea and travel sickness. Its beneficial uses for irritated colon are clearly documented.[36]

Therapeutic and Easy-to-Use Preparations

The following preparations are recommended by Vermilye as easy-to-use, self-care methods. When mixing preparations, use glass, ceramic, or stainless steel utensils.

- **Nose drops to moisten and disinfect:** 5-7 drops of either Ravensara aromatica, palmarosa, or Roman chamomile, added to five drops each of lavender and helichrysum in ½ oz of base oil.

- **Air spray to disinfect:** Fill a 4-oz glass spray bottle with pure water, then add five drops of lavender and three drops each of Roman chamomile, palmarosa, eucalyptus, and Ravensara aromatica.

- **Air spray for relaxation:** Fill a 4-oz glass spray bottle with pure water, then add ten drops neroli and five drops lavender. (Vermilye recommends taking a 1-oz spray bottle in carry-on luggage to use as a relaxation aid when traveling.)

- **Shingles ointment:** Combine 1 oz each of aloe vera gel and witch hazel with ten drops palmarosa and 20 drops each of Ravensara aromatica and laurelwood. Apply generously.

- **Hemorrhoid ointment:** Combine ½ oz each of aloe gel and witch hazel with 5 oz each of lavender, German chamomile, and helichrysum, and dab on with a cotton ball. Refrigerate for added relief.

- **Genital herpes:** Dab on undiluted palmarosa with a cotton swab at the first sensation of an outbreak or on a lesion. Repeat up to five times per day.

- **Herpes on mouth:** Dab on undiluted palmarosa until lesions have dried. Then add vitamin E to palmarosa, tea tree, or ravensara oil and apply.

- **Nerve pain:** To 2 oz of base oil, add five drops each of clove bud, ginger, rosemary, *Eucalyptus citridora*, and helichrysum. (Use only from the knees down, on feet, or with muscle and joint injuries.)

- **Chest rub for colds and flu:** To 1 tbsp of base oil, add five drops of either Ravensara, eucalyptus, tea tree, niaouli, Roman chamomile, palmarosa, rosemary, or elemi.

- **Oil for bruises:** To ½ oz of base oil, add ten drops each of helichrysum and rosemary, two drops clove, and five drops *Eucalyptus citridora*.

- **Steam tents for colds:** Boil a pot of water, then add two drops of either tea tree, niaouli, calophyllum, eucalyptus, rosemary, Roman chamomile, Ravensara aromatica, palmarosa, helichrysum, or lavender. Tent your head with a towel, keeping your face high enough so you don't get burned, close your eyes and breathe for five minutes as necessary. Avoid when colds are compounded by asthma.

- **Baths:** To boost immunity, to a hot bath add one cup of salt base mixed with four drops each of bay laurel and palmarosa (or tea tree), plus seven drops lavender. To improve your mood, to a hot bath add one cup of salt base mixed with seven drops each of neroli and lavender. To soothe tired muscles, to a hot bath add one cup of salt base mixed with seven drops rosemary, three drops helichrysum, and five drops each of eucalyptus and lavender.

- **Antifungal foot soaks:** To a hot foot bath, add one cup of salt base mixed with ten drops each of tea tree and palmarosa, plus five drops clove bud.

The Future of Aromatherapy

"While aromatherapy is practiced by medical doctors in France, this has not been the case in England and the United States," says Tisserand. "With the increasing demand for holistic health care and the 'green revolution,' the demand for aromatherapy will increase and I hope we will reach the point where medical doctors incorporate it into their repertoire. It will become routine for doctors to send culture samples to the pharmacist for testing, and identify the relevant aromatherapy for the patient. The stress-relieving properties associated with aromatherapy make it an indispensable part of health care."

Dr. Schnaubelt also believes that the use of aromatherapy will become increasingly widespread. "For many common infectious diseases, aromatherapy offers more effective and more wholesome solutions than conventional medicine," he says. "If aromatherapy was allowed to compete only on its merits, it would be a great competitor for a variety of aspects of conventional medicine. Much of the future of aromatherapy will be determined through political processes. The powers in place in the medical market will try to keep aromatherapy out, because it threatens profits to the conventional medical establishment. However, the demand of the consumer for more and better access to alternative methods will continue to offset such vested interests and should do much to make aromatherapy more popular as a healing modality."

For many common infectious diseases, aromatherapy offers more effective and more wholesome solutions than conventional medicine.

—KURT SCHNAUBELT, PH.D.

 The federal government should examine the wealth of existing studies worldwide on the efficacy of aromatherapy and fund further studies to speed the integration of this valuable form of treatment into America's health-care system.

Where to Find Help

For more information on aromatherapy, or help in locating aromatherapy products, contact:

Bio Excel
775 E. Blithedale #337
Mill Valley, California 94941
(415) 482-0555

A source for aromatherapy information and products.

Lotus Light
P.O. Box 1008
Wilmot, Wisconsin 53170
(414) 889-8501
Website: www.lotuspress.com/lotuslight.html

Provides mail-order distribution of aromatherapy videotapes, books, and materials.

National Association for Holistic Aromatherapy (NAHA)
2000 Second Avenue, Suite 206
Seattle, Washington 98121
(888) ASK-NAHA
Website: www.naha.org

NAHA offers aromatherapy courses and they distill and sell their own aromatherapy products. NAHA also acts as a referral service for aromatherapists and publishes The Aromatherapy Journal.

The Pacific Institute of Aromatherapy
P.O. Box 6723
San Rafael, California 94903
(415) 479-9121
Website: www.pacificinstituteofaromatherapy.com

The Pacific Institute of Aromatherapy offers courses to individuals and companies interested in learning about, or becoming certified in, the practice of aromatherapy. Call for a brochure and course listing.

Recommended Reading

Advanced Aromatherapy: The Science of Essential Oil Therapy. Kurt Schnaubelt. Rochester, VT: Healing Arts Press, 1995.

Aromatherapy for Healing the Spirit. Gabriel Mojay. New York: Henry Holt, 1996.

Aromatherapy to Heal and Tend the Body. Robert Tisserand. Santa Fe, NM: Lotus Light Press, 1988.

The Art of Aromatherapy. Robert B. Tisserand. Rochester, VT: Destiny Books, 1987.

Clinical Aromatherapy in Nursing. Jane Buckle, R.N. London: Arnold/Hodder Headline Group, 1997.

Medical Aromatherapy: Healing with Essential Oils. Kurt Schnaubelt. Berkeley, CA: Frog Ltd., 1999.

The Practice of Aromatherapy. Jean Valnet. Rochester, VT: Inner Traditions, 1990.

AYURVEDIC MEDICINE

Practiced in India for the past 5,000 years, Ayurvedic medicine (meaning "science of life") is a comprehensive system of medicine that combines natural therapies with a highly personalized approach to maintaining health and to the treatment of disease. Ayurvedic medicine places equal emphasis on body, mind, and spirit, and strives to restore the innate harmony of the individual.

THE FIRST QUESTION an Ayurvedic physician asks is not "What disease does my patient have?" but "Who is my patient?" explains Deepak Chopra, M.D., a Western-trained endocrinologist who has introduced Ayurvedic medicine to the general reader through a number of popular books. "By 'who'," adds Dr. Chopra, "the physician does not mean your name, but how you are constituted."

"Constitution" is the keystone of Ayurvedic medicine and refers to the overall health profile of the individual, including strengths and susceptibilities. The subtle and often intricate identification of a person's constitution is the first critical step in the process. Once established, it becomes the foundation for all clinical decisions.

To determine an individual's constitution, Ayurvedic doctors first identify the patient's metabolic body type. A specific treatment plan is then designed to guide the individual back into harmony with his or her environment, which may include dietary changes, exercises, yoga, meditation, massage, herbal tonics, herbal sweat baths, medicated enemas, and medicated inhalations. Rather than focusing on treating specific disease conditions, Ayurveda's main goal is to help maintain balance in the person's body, mind, and spirit. However, practitioners have found it effective for a wide variety of conditions, including heart disease, respiratory conditions, gastrointestinal problems, stress, and allergies, among others.[1]

Metabolic Body Types

Underlying Ayurveda is the view that everything is composed of five basic elements: ether/space, air, fire, water, and earth. These are similar to the elements in traditional Chinese medicine. The elements combine to form the metabolic body types, or *doshas*. The three metabolic body types are *vata* (ether/space and air), *pitta* (fire and

water), and *kapha* (water and earth). They include distinctions of physique similar to the Western view of body types as thin, muscular, and fat, but Ayurvedic medicine also includes mental and spiritual aspects and considers the body types to have far greater influence on a person's health and well-being than do physical attributes alone.

Dr. Chopra describes the Ayurvedic body type as a blueprint that outlines all of the innate tendencies built into a person's system. One's *dosha* and the characteristics that reveal it clarify why one person, for example, will have no reaction to milk, chili, loud noise, or humidity, while another will not be able to tolerate them. Most people are a mixture of *dosha* characteristics (such as *vata-pitta*), with one usually more predominant than another. Each of the body types flourishes under a specific diet, exercise plan, and lifestyle.

The *Vata* Body Type

According to Dr. Chopra, the primary characteristic of the *vata* metabolic type is changeability. Unpredictability and variability—in size, shape, mood, and action—is the *vata* trademark. *Vatas* tend to be slender with prominent features, joints, and veins, along with cool, dry skin. Moody, enthusiastic, imaginative, and impulsive, the *vata* type is quick to grasp ideas and is good at initiating things but poor at finishing them. *Vata* energy fluctuates, with jagged peaks and valleys. *Vatas* eat and sleep erratically and are prone to anxiety, insomnia, premenstrual syndrome, and constipation.

The *Pitta* Body Type

The *pitta* metabolic type is relatively predictable. The *pitta* person is of medium build, strength, and endurance, well-proportioned, and easily maintains a stable weight. Often fair, the *pitta* type will frequently have red or blond hair, freckles, and a ruddy complexion. *Pittas* have a quick, articulate, biting intelligence, and can be critical or passionate with a short, explosive temper. Efficient and moderate in daily habits, the *pitta* type eats and sleeps regularly—eating three meals a day and sleeping eight hours at night. *Pitta* types tend to perspire heavily and are warm and often thirsty. They suffer from acne, ulcers, hemorrhoids, and stomach ailments.

The *Kapha* Body Type

"The basic theme of the *kapha* metabolic type is relaxed," says Dr. Chopra. The *kapha* person is solid, heavy, and strong. With a tendency to be overweight, *kaphas* have slow digestion and somewhat oily hair, and cool, damp, pale skin. Everything *kapha* is slow—*kapha* types are slow to anger, slow to eat, slow to act. They sleep long and heavily. *Kaphas* tend to procrastinate and be obstinate. A *kapha* body type will be prone to high cholesterol, obesity, allergies, and sinus problems.

The Three *Doshas* and Health

Although each person's metabolic type is determined by a predominant *dosha*, all three *doshas* are present in varying degrees in every cell, tissue, and organ of the body. According to Vasant Lad, M.A.Sc., an Ayurvedic physician and Director of the Ayurvedic Institute, in Albuquerque, New Mexico, the *doshas* are located in and govern specific areas/tissues (*dhatus*) of the body:

- *Vata* is motion that activates the physical systems, physical activity, and nerve force, and allows the body to breathe and circulate blood. The seats of *vata* are the large intestine, pelvic cavity, bones, skin, ears, and thighs.

- *Pitta*, the metabolism, processes food, air, and water and is responsible for charging the hundreds of endocrine and enzymatic activities throughout the body. The seats of *pitta* are the small intestine, stomach, sweat glands, blood, skin, and eyes.

- *Kapha*, the structure of bones, tendons, muscle, and fat that holds the body together, offers nourishment and protection. The chest, the lungs, and the fluid surrounding the spinal cord are the seats of *kapha* in the body.

When the *doshas* are balanced in accordance with an individual's constitution, the result is vibrant health and energy. But when the delicate balance is disturbed, the

CHARACTERISTICS OF AYURVEDIC BODY TYPES

Vata
- Thin
- Prominent features, joints, veins
- Cool, dry skin
- Eats and sleeps at all hours
- Enthusiastic, infectious energy
- Intuitive
- Imaginative
- Vivacious
- Hyperactive
- Moody
- Anxiety and nervous disorders
- Constipation
- Cramps

Pitta
- Medium build
- Fair, thin hair
- Warm, ruddy, perspiring skin
- Doesn't miss a meal
- Lives by the clock
- Intelligent and articulate
- Orderly, efficient
- Intense and passionate
- Warm, loving
- Short temper, perfectionist
- Ulcers, heartburn
- Hemorrhoids
- Acne

Kapha
- Heavyset
- Thick, wavy hair
- Cool, thick, pale, oily skin
- Eats slowly
- Sleeps long, heavily
- Compassionate, forgiving, and tolerant
- Slow, graceful, relaxed
- Slow to anger
- Affectionate
- Procrastination
- Obesity
- Allergies, sinus problems
- High cholesterol

RESEARCH SHOWS THE EFFECTIVENESS OF AYURVEDIC TREATMENT

An increasing number of clinical studies are verifying the efficacy of Ayurvedic medicine, particularly herbal preparations, as modern science catches up with this ancient healing tradition.

- The powdered bark of the *Terminalia arjuna* tree has antioxidant (free-radical scavenging) properties comparable to vitamin E.[2]

- A number of Ayurvedic herbs and dried fruits, such as ginger and *Prunus amygdalus,* have shown the ability to stimulate the immune system.[3]

- *Ashwagandha* protects the heart and has anticoagulant properties.[4] It has also demonstrated significant antitumor effects.[5]

- The gum resin of *Boswellia serrata* has been shown effective in the treatment of bronchial asthma. In one study, 70% of patients showed improvement in symptoms and number of attacks.[6]

- Thyme *(Thymus vulgaris)* extract has shown antibacterial activity.[7]

- Ginger *(Zingiber officinale)* may help relieve migraine headaches, without the side effects common to the standard drugs for this condition.[8]

- In a study of 16 patients with diabetes, ten patients showed improved glucose tolerance after six weeks of taking the herb *Coccinia indica.*[9]

- Curcumin, an antioxidant isolated from the spice turmeric *(Curcuma longa),* stimulates enzymes involved in the detoxification of free radicals, which may be responsible for its anti-inflammatory and anticancer activities.[10]

types, they can take appropriate measures, through changes in diet, lifestyle, and environment, to restore *dosha* balance, which will prevent disease and ensure continued good health.

Ayurveda defines health as soundness and balance among body, mind, and soul, and equilibrium among the *doshas.* According to Ayurvedic medicine, there are seven major factors that can disrupt physiological harmony—genetic, congenital, internal, seasonal, and magnetic/electrical influences; external trauma; and natural tendencies/habits. "Disease is the result of a disruption of the spontaneous flow of Nature's intelligence within our physiology," says Virender Sodhi, M.D. (Ayurveda), N.D., Director of the Ayurvedic & Naturopathic Medical Clinic, in Bellevue, Washington. "When we violate Nature's law and cannot adequately rid ourselves of the results of this disruption, then we have disease." Ayurvedic medicine sees poor digestion and poor elimination of wastes from the body as key factors in most diseases.

There are pathologies recognized as being genetically based. For example, when placed in a particular environment, a predisposed individual may have a tendency to develop a health problem prompted by the surroundings. This genetic susceptibility can be triggered in the womb by the mother's lifestyle, diet, habits, activities, and emotions. Accordingly, individuals possess natural tendencies to adopt certain habits, such as overeating and smoking. From birth, stressors—both inner and outer—challenge an individual's health. For example, hot, spicy food can induce an ulcer or damage the liver. Disease can also have an emotional cause, such as deep-seated, unresolved anger, fear, anxiety, grief, or sadness. External traumas and injuries can also play an influential role.

Ayurveda also takes into account how the seasons and time of day influence health. Dietary and other therapeutic suggestions are often prescribed with this in mind. To say that summer is a *pitta* season means that *pitta* qualities are at their height during this time. Summer's bright light and heat can induce inflammatory conditions such as hives, rash, acne, biliary (pertaining to bile) disorders, diarrhea, or conjunctivitis in *pitta* individuals. The *vata* season is autumn and, because autumn reflects windy, dry, and cold qualities, *vata* people tend to develop neurological, muscular, and rheumatic problems such as constipation, sciatica, arthritis, and rheumatism. Winter's deep cold and biting winds bring out more *kapha* characteristics and stresses the *kapha* individual's respiratory system with colds, hay fever, cough, congestion, sneezing, and sinus disorders. Spring is both *pitta* and *kapha*: the coolness, budding leaves, and beautiful flowers of early spring enhance the *kapha* constitution, while late spring promotes *pitta.*

body becomes susceptible to outside stressors, which may range from viruses and bacteria to poor nutrition and overwork. Imbalance in the *doshas* is the first sign that the mind and body are not perfectly coordinated, notes Dr. Chopra. He points out that once people understand the characteristics and qualities ascribed to their body

The Art of Ayurvedic Diagnosis

Ayurvedic physicians have traditionally relied on the powers of observation rather than equipment and laboratory testing to diagnose disease. Diagnosis is based on physical observation, questioning the patient as to personal and family history, palpation (feeling the body), and listening to the heart, lungs, and intestines. This approach is changing, however, as physicians integrate Ayurvedic traditions with modern diagnostic methods.

Ayurvedic physicians pay special attention to the pulse, tongue, eyes, and nails. Whereas Western medical doctors use the pulse to determine heart rate, Ayurvedic doctors describe three distinct types of pulses: *vata*, *pitta*, and *kapha*. They can distinguish 12 radial (or wrist) pulses: six on the right wrist (three superficial and three deep) and six on the left wrist. By focusing on the relationship between the pulses and the internal organs, combined with knowledge of *dosha*/organ relationships, a skillful practitioner can feel the strength, vitality, and normal physiological tone of specific organs at each of the 12 sites.

The tongue is another diagnostic site. By observing the surface of the tongue and looking for discoloration and/or sensitivity of particular areas, an adept practitioner can gain insight into the functional status of internal organs. For example, a whitish tongue indicates a disruption of *kapha* and accumulation of mucus, while a black to brown discoloration indicates a *vata* disturbance. A dehydrated tongue is symptomatic of a decrease in the plasma, while a pale tongue indicates a decrease in red blood cells.

The eyes can also indicate a person's *dosha* and health status: small and unsteady eyes indicate a *vata* type; sharp and reddish eyes indicate *pitta*; and wide and white eyes are *kapha*. Thin, brittle fingernails are typically found in *vata* types; medium, pink-colored nails are *pitta*; and wide, white nails suggest a *kapha* type. Spots on the nails can also indicate nutrient deficiencies.[11]

Ayurvedic physicians routinely perform urine examinations to help them diagnose *dosha* imbalance in a patient. An early morning midstream sample of urine is collected and its color observed. Blackish-brown indicates a *vata* disorder; dark yellow, an imbalance with *pitta*. If the urine is cloudy, there is a *kapha* disorder. When a person is constipated or is not drinking adequate amounts of water, the urine will be dark yellow. Red urine indicates a blood disorder. Normal urine has a typical uremic, or musty, smell. A foul odor, however, indicates toxins in the system. Acidic urine, which creates a burning sensation, indicates excess *pitta*. A sweet smell to the urine indicates a diabetic condition; an individual with this condition may experience goose bumps on the skin surface while passing urine. Gravel in the urine indicates stones in the urinary tract.

 With its strong emphasis on prevention and education, Ayurvedic medicine can help to provide long-term savings to consumers.

Disease Management in Ayurvedic Medicine

Ayurvedic medicine holds that in order to restore health, one must first understand and correctly diagnose the disease or bodily imbalance. After diagnosis, there are four main methods by which an Ayurvedic physician manages disease: cleansing and detoxifying, palliation, rejuvenation, and mental hygiene.

Cleansing and Detoxifying (*Shodan*)

Cleansing in Ayurvedic medicine takes on a far more encompassing role than in Western medicine, where a physician rarely has a patient release material from the stomach, sinuses, or bowels. In contrast, the purifying techniques of vomiting, bowel purging and enemas, blood cleansing, and nasal douching, collectively called *pancha karma,* are commonly used by Ayurvedic physicians to remove toxins from different areas of the body. In Ayurvedic medicine, toxins are considered the root of disease and are often the result of undigested, unabsorbed, and unassimilated food.

In preparation for cleansing, notes Dr. Sodhi, an herbal oil massage may be performed. The oil is a liquid form of fat that is well absorbed through the skin. Once in the system, it can pick up various toxins, such as pesticides, viruses, and bacteria, which are eventually disposed of through normal channels of elimination. To further elimination, an herbal steam sauna often follows the massage treatment.

Once cleansing begins, purgative therapy eliminates *vata*, *pitta,* and *kapha* impurities from the body. Blood cleansing is accomplished by removing blood or donating blood to the blood bank and by using certain cleansing and blood-thinning herbs. "It's a known scientific fact," says Dr. Sodhi, "that whenever you give blood, the bone marrow gets stimulated. They have found that the blood volume is restored in 30-45 minutes."

Ghee (clarified butter) and buttermilk yogurt are used to reestablish intestinal flora, especially if it has been washed away during the cleansing process. Inserting herbs through various routes other than the mouth (nose, anus, and skin) ensures that the medicinal qualities are not bro-

AYURVEDA AND CANCER

"According to Ayurveda, cancer arises in the body when one acts against nature, or against the natural healthful balance of the body," states Virender Sodhi, M.D. (Ayurveda), N.D., Director of the Ayurvedic & Naturopathic Medical Clinic, in Bellevue, Washington. Ayurveda seeks to balance the mental, physical, and emotional aspects of life, paving the way to health.

In the Ayurvedic tradition, foods, herbs, and spices are the pharmacy. The basic diet is made up of natural foods free of chemicals and pesticides. "Our food should be harvested when ripe and consumed while still fresh, so it can provide us with its full range of benefits," says Dr. Sodhi. Strong digestion is fundamental to good health, ensuring the absorption of needed nutrients and preventing the build-up of toxins in the body. Leafy greens, fresh fruits and vegetables, whole grains, nuts, seeds, beans and legumes, along with limited amounts of animal products, are all part of a well-rounded diet. Fruits and vegetables also contain an abundance of antioxidants, vitamins, minerals, and other valuable nutrients.

"A high-fat diet has been associated with disease, which could be due, in part, to the fat solubility of toxins, which increases the likelihood of ingesting high amounts of toxins by eating a high-fat diet," says Dr. Sodhi. Healthy fats include fish oils (be sure they are fresh and contain no heavy metals or pollutants), ghee or butter, olive oil, and high quality nut, seed, and vegetable oils. A diet high in fiber has protective actions against some types of cancer and fermented milk products, such as yogurt, have been shown to inhibit cancer cell growth.

Dr. Sodhi recommends supplementing the diet with vitamin E (400 IU or more daily), selenium (200 mcg daily), and vitamin C (up to 2,000 mg daily). The *amla* fruit is the richest food source of vitamin C and contains a wealth of bioflavonoids. Coenzyme Q10 and fish or flax oils are also important. *Ashwagandha*, also known as Indian ginseng or winter cherry, is a powerful adaptogen, helping the body to cope with stress and maintain its natural equilibrium. Turmeric *(Curcuma longa)* is an antioxidant with strong anti-inflammatory and anti-infective properties.

A strong immune system is important for overall health. Cancerous cells arise in the body daily. The immune system's role is first detecting foreign elements or abnormal cell growth, then making sure these elements are not allowed to gain a foothold and grow in the body. Diet, herbs, and exercise all play a role in maintaining healthy immune system function. Some useful herbs include *amla*, *ashwagandha*, *neem*, *triphala*, and turmeric, according to Dr. Sodhi. Stress can profoundly weaken the immune system; therefore, activities such as meditation, yoga, and other exercises to help alleviate stress are highly recommended.

Ayurveda has long noted that exercise supports and promotes good health. "Researchers in the last several years have noted that exercise increases the ability of the immune system's natural killer cells to fight emerging cancer cells," states Dr. Sodhi. "Performing yoga postures, as well as breathing exercises *(pranayama)* are excellent ways to reduce the potentially harmful impact of daily stress and can be beneficial for patients with cancer."

Liver cleansing is an important part of maintaining health and an optimally functioning immune system. The liver is the body's main detoxifying organ, mitigating the potential harm from toxins produced naturally within our bodies as well as those encountered in the environment. If we are exposed to a toxic chemical and the liver is unable to excrete it, then the chemical may cause damage in the body. Ayurveda prescribes several liver-tonifying herbs, including *Andrographis paniculata*, *Picrorhiza kurroa*, and *Eclipta alba*. Additionally, an Ayurvedic cleansing treatment called *pancha karma* has been shown to have powerful detoxification effects.

"Ayurveda's principles of health, and its preventative measures for dealing with cancer as well as myriad other life-threatening illnesses, teach us that we can play an active and critical role in preserving and enhancing our well-being," concludes Dr. Sodhi.

ken down by stomach enzymes. Certain herbal concoctions, medicated oils, and *ghee* are often administered into the nose to increase mental clarity.

Palliation (*Shaman*)

The next step in Ayurvedic disease management is palliation, or *shaman*, used to balance and pacify the bodily *doshas*. *Shaman* focuses more on the spiritual dimension of healing and uses a combination of herbs, fasting, chanting, yoga stretches, breathing exercises, meditation, and lying in the sun for a limited time. These techniques are useful for those with a dysfunctional immune system or for those who are too ill or emotionally weak to undergo the more strenuous forms of physical cleansing in *pancha karma*. Because of its curative and preventative aspects, *shaman* can also be utilized by the healthy person. Like all enlightened healing methods, Ayurveda emphasizes prevention above curing disease.

One method of *shaman*, called "kindling the fire," is absolutely necessary in *kapha* and *vata* disorders with patients who have low gastric fire. The patient consumes honey with certain herbs like *pippili* (long pepper), ginger, cinnamon, and black pepper. (This should be done cautiously with *pitta* people, however.)

 Many of the chapters in Part Three: Health Conditions contain information on the application of Ayurvedic medicine to specific illnesses.

Rejuvenation (*Rasayana*)

After the cleansing regimen, a program of tonification called *rasayana* begins. Tonification means enhancing the body's inherent ability to function, and *rasayana* is similar to a physiological tune-up. It is used to restore vitality to the reproductive system, countering sterility and infertility, bringing forth healthier progeny, and improving sexual performance. In addition, it is said that *rasayana* promotes longevity by slowing down the biological clock.

Ayurvedic medicine uses three subcategories of *rasayana* treatments to rejuvenate and restore the body's tissues and organs: special herbs prepared as pills, powders, jellies, and tablets; mineral preparations specific to a person's condition and *dosha*; and exercises (specifically, yoga positions and breathing exercises).

Mental Hygiene and Spiritual Healing (*Satvajaya*)

Satvajaya is a method of improving the mind to reach a higher level of spiritual/mental functioning and is accomplished through the release of psychological stress, emo-

---

TREATMENTS IN AYURVEDIC MEDICINE

- Diet: Prescribed according to *dosha* and season. The taste of the food (sweet, sour, salty, pungent, bitter, or astringent), its hot- or cold-producing abilities, and whether the food is light or heavy, solid or liquid, and oily or dry are primary considerations. Also, certain foods should not be eaten together.

- Exercise: Vigorous exercise and yoga stretching are encouraged in Ayurveda to "kindle the internal fire"—improve circulation, stimulate metabolism, and sharpen the mind. Exercises are prescribed according to an individual's constitution.

- Meditation: Considered a form of mental cleansing, meditation enhances both self-awareness and awareness of one's environment, family, friends, and work.

- Herbs: Ayurvedic physicians use an extensive number of herbs in treating illness. Depending on their innate qualities, herbs are used to rebuild and rejuvenate the body and its various systems. Research is now confirming the effectiveness of Ayurvedic herbs for a variety of conditions, including asthma, cardiovascular disease, hepatitis B, and eye disorders, among others.[12]

- Massage: Massage that uses herbal oils is an important part of Ayurvedic treatment. Upon absorption through the skin, the medicated oils help to remove toxins from the system.

- Sun: Ayurvedic philosophy states that the sun is not only a source of heat and light but also of higher consciousness. It improves circulation, aids absorption of vitamin D, and strengthens the bones. Each of the three *doshas* benefits from different lengths of time spent in the sun; however, proper protection and care is a must. Because of the risk of developing skin cancer, no one who has multiple moles should lie in the sun for extended periods of time.

- Breathing: Breathing exercises, or *pranayama*, can be learned from an experienced teacher. Depending on the *dosha* type, *pranayama* can bring a sense of tranquility and peace and alleviate stress.

SUCCESS STORY: AYURVEDA AND HEART DISEASE

"The most common disease in the United States is heart disease," says Virender Sodhi, M.D. (Ayurveda), N.D., Director of the Ayurvedic & Naturopathic Medical Clinic, in Bellevue, Washington. One of Dr. Sodhi's most interesting heart cases involved a 55-year-old male with chest pain (angina) so severe that he could not walk more than ten steps before having to sit down. He came to Dr. Sodhi's office after receiving word that he needed immediate bypass surgery. Refusing the surgery, doctors told him, would mean certain death.

Before beginning treatment, Dr. Sodhi ordered a battery of tests. "I do lab tests before and after a cleansing program," asserts Dr. Sodhi. Angiographic studies showed that his patient's coronary arteries were blocked—the left main coronary artery was 90% narrowed, the anterior descending was 80% narrowed, and the right coronary was 30% blocked. Blood tests indicated elevated cholesterol levels at 278 and decreased HDLs (high-density lipoproteins, the good cholesterol) at a low 38. Dr. Sodhi determined that his patient was a *pitta-kapha* individual and started him on an appropriate cleansing program that included a change of diet and appropriate herbs.

After three months, the man's cholesterol levels dropped more than 30% and HDLs rose to 48. More importantly, though, his exercise tolerance had dramatically improved. "He was doing treadmill exercise at the speed of five miles per hour for 45 minutes without any angina," reports Dr. Sodhi. Dr. Sodhi says his patient continues to do fine: he now jogs up and down hills with no symptoms and his heart readings have shown improvement. "There is a hospital in Bombay," continues Sodhi, "which has done about 3,300 cases with this method for treating coronary heart diseases. All of them with about 99% success."

"*Satvajaya* can decondition the mind so we can see things fresh, with the eyes of a child," says David Frawley, O.M.D., Director of the American Institute of Vedic Studies, in Santa Fe, New Mexico. "*Satvajaya* techniques rid us of negative emotions, thought patterns, and prejudices that may weigh us down like undigested food."

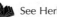 See Herbal Medicine, Meditation, Yoga.

The Future of Ayurvedic Medicine

Although the advent of Western medical practices temporarily loosened the roots of Ayurvedic medicine in India, Ayurveda has since that time made a comeback in its country of origin and has spread around the world to Europe, Japan, and North and South America. There are 108 Ayurvedic colleges in India that grant degrees after a five-year program, and 300,000 Ayurvedic physicians are represented by the All India Ayur-Veda Congress.

Ayurvedic conferences, sponsored by governments and/or medical associations, have taken place in Brazil, Poland, Czechoslovakia, and Hungary. In the Soviet Union, the Soviet Research Center for Preventive Medicine oversees the Institute of Maharishi Ayur-Veda. Furthermore, in the U.S., the National Institutes of Health is researching Ayurveda and its integration with other healing practices, such as naturopathic, chiropractic, and allopathic medicine.[13] In 2001, the American University of Complementary Medicine (AUCM), in West Los Angeles, California, began offering an M.S. degree and a combined scholarly-clinical Ph.D. program in Ayurvedic medicine, the first programs of their kind in the nation.

Dr. Sodhi devotes much of his time to seeking out medical studies that support Ayurvedic treatments. He observes that "considerable modern research has proven the efficacy of Ayurvedic herbal preparations and research has now moved to elucidating their mechanisms and sites of action."[14] In Dr. Sodhi's opinion, combining modern medical diagnostic procedures with traditional methods makes for more effective use of Ayurvedic treatments.

Groups outside of the Ayurvedic community have also taken steps to recognize this established healing tradition. The World Health Organization recognizes Ayurvedic medicine and supports research and the integration of the Ayurvedic system of health care into modern medicine. Even the *Journal of the American Medical Association* has printed a short article on Ayurveda, followed by a lively response—both pro and con—from its readers.[15]

tional distress, and unconscious negative beliefs. The categories of *satvajaya* include: mantra or sound therapy to change the vibratory patterns of the mind; *yantra,* or concentrating on geometric figures, to take the mind out of ordinary modes of thinking; *tantra* to direct energies through the body; meditation to alter states of consciousness; and gems, metals, and crystals for their subtle vibratory healing powers.

In light of this renewed interest, Dr. Lad reminds us of all that Ayurvedic medicine has to offer. "According to Ayurvedic principles, by understanding oneself—by identifying one's constitution and recognizing sources of *doshic* aggravation—one can not only follow the proper guidelines to cleanse, purify, and prevent disease, but also uplift oneself into a realm of awareness previously unknown."

Where to Find Help

For more information on Ayurvedic treatments, or to locate an Ayurvedic physician, contact the organizations below. Often, Ayurvedic medical centers throughout the U.S. are associated with yoga institutes. Check local phone listings for other sources of Ayurvedic medical care.

Ayurvedic & Naturopathic Medical Clinic
2115 112th Avenue N.E.
Bellevue, Washington 98004
(425) 453-8022
Website: www.ayurvedicscience.com

Dr. Virender Sodhi's clinic provides medical training for physicians and health-care practitioners, as well as individual courses for laypeople.

Ayurvedic Institute
11311 Menaul Blvd. N.E.
Albuquerque, New Mexico 87112
(505) 291-9698
Website: www.ayurveda.com

The institute, directed by Dr. Vasant Lad, trains people from all walks of life in most of the aspects of Ayurveda.

Canadian Association of Ayurvedic Medicine
P.O. Box 749 Station B
Ottawa, Ontario, Canada K1P 5P8
(613) 837-5737

This professional organization maintains a referral list of Canadian Ayurvedic doctors, supports university-based research, and advocates research and practice in Ayurveda. CAAM provides training in Ayurveda for physicians and the general public. It also offers primary courses in French.

The Maharishi Ayur-Veda Health Center
R.R. #2
Huntsville, Ontario, Canada P0A 1K0
(705) 635-2234

This residential treatment center offers Ayurvedic treatments and education.

The Raj, Maharishi Ayur-Veda Health Center
1734 Jasmine Avenue
Fairfield, Iowa 52556
(641) 472-9580
Website: www.theraj.com

This residential treatment center offers Ayurvedic treatments and education.

Sharp Institute for Human Potential and Mind-Body Medicine
8010 Frost Street, Suite 300
San Diego, California 92123
(800) 82-SHARP
Website: www.sharp.com

The Sharp Institute has three components: patient care at the Center for Mind-Body Medicine, where Ayurvedic and other complementary therapies are offered; courses in mind-body and Ayurvedic medicine for the general public and health-care providers; and research to validate the effectiveness of Ayurvedic therapies.

Recommended Reading

Ageless Body, Timeless Mind. Deepak Chopra, M.D. New York: Three Rivers Press, 1998.

The Ayurveda Encyclopedia. Swami Sada Shiva Tirtha. Bayville, NY: Ayurveda Holistic Center Press, 1998.

Ayurvedic Healing. David Frawley, O.M.D. Twin Lakes, WI: Lotus Press, 2000.

Ayurveda: The Science of Self-Healing. Vasant Lad, M.D. Santa Fe, NM: Lotus Press, 1984.

The Complete Book of Ayurvedic Home Remedies. Vasant Lad, M.D. New York: Three Rivers Press, 1999.

Contemporary Ayurveda. Hari Sharma, M.D., and Christopher Clark, M.D. London: Churchill Livingstone, 1998.

Perfect Health. Deepak Chopra, M.D. New York: Three Rivers Press, 2001.

Quantum Healing. Deepak Chopra, M.D. New York: Bantam Books, 1990.

BIOFEEDBACK TRAINING AND NEUROTHERAPY

Biofeedback training teaches a person how to change and control the body's vital functions through the use of information supplied by electronic devices. Biofeedback is particularly useful for learning to reduce stress, eliminate headaches, control asthmatic attacks, recondition injured muscles, and relieve pain. Neurotherapy is a type of biofeedback that optimizes brain function, thereby helping to improve cognitive abilities and regulate immune and emotional functions. Because neurotherapy positively impacts the nervous system at many levels, it can be beneficial for a wide variety of health conditions and also has a high success rate as a treatment for addiction.

THE IDEA THAT A PERSON can learn to modify his or her own vital functions is relatively new. Before the 1960s, most scientists believed that autonomic functions, such as heart rate and pulse, digestion, brain waves, and muscle behavior, could not be voluntarily controlled. Recently, biofeedback, along with other methods of self-regulation, such as guided imagery, progressive relaxation, and meditation, has found widespread acceptance among physicians, physiologists, and psychologists alike.

Biofeedback training is a method of learning how to consciously regulate bodily functions that are normally unconscious (such as breathing, heart rate, and blood pressure) in order to improve overall health. It refers to any process that measures and reports back information immediately about the biological system of the person being monitored so he or she can learn to consciously influence that system.

📖 See Guided Imagery, Mind/Body Medicine.

Neurotherapy, also known as neurofeedback therapy or brain-wave therapy, is a sophisticated form of biofeedback used to normalize and optimize brain-wave patterns (beta, alpha, theta, delta). This is accomplished through the use of a computerized system connected to electroencephalograph (EEG) sensors applied to the scalp. The EEG readings are rapidly analyzed by the

> *The self-regulation skills acquired through biofeedback training are retained by the individual even after the feedback device is dispensed with.*
>
> —PATRICIA NORRIS, PH.D.

computer and the brain is then encouraged to recognize normal, healthy brain waves. The computer produces audio and visual feedback and positive reinforcements when the desired brain wave states are achieved. Once the brain learns how to change its habitual wave patterns into those that are more appropriate for overall psychophysiological functioning, the changes tend to be permanent and often continue to improve even after the treatment ends. Demonstrated benefits of neurotherapy include improvements in short-term memory, concentration, speech, motor skills, energy levels, sleep patterns, and overall emotional well-being.

How Biofeedback Works

A person seeking to regulate heart rate would train with a biofeedback device set up to transmit one blinking light or one audible beep per heartbeat. By learning to alter the rate of the flashes and beeps, the subject would learn how to control the heart rate. "The self-regulation skills acquired through biofeedback training are retained by the individual even after the feedback device is dispensed with," explains Patricia Norris, Ph.D., former Clinical Director of the Biofeedback and Psychophysiology Clinic at the Center for Applied Psychophysiology at the Menninger Clinic and a current founding member of Life Sciences Institute of Mind-Body Health, both in Topeka,

Kansas. "In fact, with practice, biofeedback skills continue to improve. It is like taking tennis lessons. If you stop taking the lessons but continue playing, your game will improve. With biofeedback, it works the same way. The more you practice, the better you get."

Electrodes are placed on the patient's skin (a simple, painless process) and the patient is then instructed to use various techniques such as meditation, relaxation, and visualization to effect the desired response (muscle relaxation, lowered heart rate, or lowered temperature). The biofeedback device reports the patient's progress by a change in the speed of the beeps or flashes, the pitch or quality of the tone, or success in a video game program.

The effects of biofeedback can be measured in a variety of ways: monitoring skin temperature influenced by blood flow beneath the skin; monitoring galvanic skin response (GSR), the electrical conductivity of the skin; observing muscle tension with an electromyograph (EMG); tracking heart rate with an electrocardiograph (EKG); and using an electroencephalograph to monitor brain-wave activity. Normal, healthy, "relaxed" readings include fairly warm skin, low sweat gland activity (this keeps the skin's conductivity low), and a slow, even heart rate. Biofeedback technologies utilize computers to provide a rapid and detailed analysis of activities within the complex human system. Biofeedback practitioners interpret changes in these readings to help the patient learn to stabilize erratic and unhealthy biological functions.

Conditions Benefited by Biofeedback Training

Biofeedback training has a vast range of applications for health and prevention, particularly in cases where psychological, immunological, and neurological factors play a role. Sleep disorders, hyperactivity and attention deficit in children, and other behavioral disorders respond well to biofeedback training, as do dysfunctions stemming from inadequate control over muscles or muscle groups, autoimmune diseases, and all diseases related to stress. Incontinence, postural problems, back pain, temporomandibular joint (TMJ) syndrome, and even loss of control due to brain or nerve damage have all shown improvement when patients undergo biofeedback training.

Biofeedback has also been shown to help other problems such as heart dysfunction, gastrointestinal disorders (acidity, constipation, ulcers, irritable bowel syndrome), difficulty swallowing, esophageal dysfunction, ringing in the ears, twitching of the eyelids, fatigue, Raynaud's disease (uncomfortably cold hands due to circulatory problems), and cerebral palsy. Severe structural problems like

HISTORY OF BIOFEEDBACK

Instrumented biofeedback was pioneered by O. Hobart Mowrer in 1938, when he used an alarm system triggered by urine to stop bed-wetting in children. But it was not until the late 1960s, when Barbara Brown, Ph.D., at the Veterans Administration Hospital, in Sepulveda, California, and Elmer Green, Ph.D., and Alyce Green of the Menninger Foundation, in Topeka, Kansas, used EEG biofeedback to observe and record the altered states/self-regulation of yogis that biofeedback began to attract widespread attention.

"The Greens' work with yogis, and the work of Joe Kamiya to teach subjects to experience a 'drugless high,' is what really brought biofeedback to public notice," says Melvyn Werbach, M.D., retired Director of the Biofeedback Medical Clinic, in Tarzana, California. "There started to be tremendous interest, articles on biofeedback in national newspapers and magazines, and the idea of higher states of consciousness being related to something that could be scientifically measured really caught on."

broken bones and slipped discs are among the only conditions that don't respond to biofeedback.

 See Addictions, Back Pain, Gastrointestinal Disorders, Headaches, Hypertension, Respiratory Disorders, Sleep Disorders, Stress.

Stress-Related Disorders

One of the most common uses for biofeedback training is the treatment of stress and stress-related disorders, including insomnia, TMJ syndrome, migraines, asthma, hypertension, gastrointestinal disorders, and muscular dysfunction.

 By teaching self-regulation skills, biofeedback can allow patients to take more control of their health and help prevent disorders that can result in costly medical procedures.

Insomnia: Biofeedback can often successfully treat insomnia as long as the appropriate form of biofeedback is used with the specific, corresponding type of insomnia. "Biofeedback is appropriate when insomnia is due to over-activation of the autonomic nervous system," says Melvyn Werbach, M.D., former Assistant Clinical Professor at the School of Medicine, University of California at Los Angeles, and retired Director of the Biofeedback Medical Clinic in Tarzana, California. "In this case, we use biofeedback of muscle tension and skin dampness in conjunction with general relaxation techniques."

EEG biofeedback, however, seems useful when insomnia is due to a mental/emotional problem, not a physical problem. "I use it with people who have a problem with obsessive thinking when they try to sleep," Dr. Werbach continues. "Their bodies relax very nicely, but they just can't get their minds off of whatever it is that their minds go to. This is when EEG biofeedback is most effective."

Temporomandibular Joint Syndrome: Dr. Werbach also reports using biofeedback to successfully treat TMJ syndrome. "The most dramatic case I can think of," he says, "is a patient who came to the U.C.L.A. Pain Control Unit after using bite plates in his mouth to stop the teeth from grinding together. His last bite plate had been a metal one, prescribed by a dentist who thought it would finally solve the problem. Instead, he bit through the metal. He had severe pain in all the typical areas associated with TMJ and was quite depressed about the whole thing. He had tried everything. Working with him, we took biofeedback readings from the masseter muscle (the muscle involved in closing the jaw) and using them, trained him to relax his jaw. Since he was so preoccupied with his mouth, we also worked on reducing general muscle tension in the rest of his body by teaching him relaxation techniques through control of his breathing and surface finger temperature. It was strikingly effective."

Migraines: The use of biofeedback to treat migraines began as a chance discovery at the Menninger Clinic (previously Menninger Foundation) in the early 1960s. Elmer Green, Ph.D., and Alyce Green were measuring a woman's skin temperature to track her physiological changes while undergoing a series of relaxation exercises. They noticed a sudden 10° F increase in the woman's hand temperature. When asked, she reported that a headache she had been experiencing had disappeared at that very moment.

The Greens pioneered a biofeedback temperature device and went on to teach patients how to alleviate migraines simply by using relaxation techniques to elevate the temperature of their hands. Biofeedback can also reduce the dosages of drugs needed to combat migraines, and sometimes eliminate them altogether, according to a report by Steven L. Fahrion, Ph.D., former Director of the Center for Applied Psychophysiology at the Menninger Clinic, and current founding member of Life Sciences Institute of Mind-Body Health.[1] In addition, biofeedback training has been shown to provide marked benefits for children who suffer from migraines, with improvement of symptoms ranging from 81% to 95% among children between the ages of 7 and 15.[2]

Asthma: Asthma responds especially well to biofeedback training. A recent 15-month follow-up study of 17 asthmatics, trained with biofeedback to increase their inhalation volume, found that all reported fewer emergency room visits, a lowered need for medication, and decreased incidence and severity of wheezing attacks. "By learning to increase their inhalation volume the subjects knew they had control over their breathing," concluded the authors of the study, Erik Peper, Ph.D., and Vicci Tibbets, of San Francisco State University. "This experience reduced their fear so that they could continue to exhale and inhale air during the onset of wheezing. As one participant reported: 'It gave me a sense of control and hope that I never had before.'"[3]

Hypertension: Biofeedback training is an effective tool for teaching people self-regulation and relaxation to help lower blood pressure.[4] This was confirmed in a recent meta-analysis of randomized clinical trials, which found that biofeedback training resulted in a reduction of both systolic and diastolic blood pressure levels. The researchers recommended that biofeedback be considered by practitioners as an appropriate therapy for hypertensive patients.[5] The greatest successes in controlling hypertension are with patients who combine biofeedback training with other forms of relaxation, visualization, exercise, and a healthy diet.

Gastrointestinal Disorders: Robert Grove, Ph.D., of Culver City, California, is a specialist in the application of biofeedback to gastrointestinal disorders. He reports great success in treating irritable bowel syndrome, colitis, a wide variety of eating disorders (including bulimia and anorexia), heartburn, and functional dyspepsia (a digestive disorder marked by stomachache, heartburn, and nausea). Dr. Grove uses movement retraining, wherein special sensors are able to pick up movement in the digestive tract and alter it. "Gastrointestinal disorder is a specialty area," explains Dr. Grove, "and other forms of biofeedback will fail under these conditions. For one thing, gastrointestinal patients seem to be hyper-reactive to all types of stimuli such as a light being turned on or a telephone ringing—things that normally don't bother other patients. The gastrointestinal tract responds to these stimuli by shutting down, and biofeedback helps focus on creating a protection from the arousal." The Menninger Clinic also successfully treats people for gastrointestinal disorders, including Crohn's disease (a chronic inflammatory condition affecting the colon or terminal part of the small intestine) and ulcerative colitis.

Biofeedback is also effective for treating constipation and has been proven to help patients with chronic constipation exacerbated by pelvic dysfunction avoid surgery. In one study, four patients with constipation and pelvic dysfunction received biofeedback training after being advised that surgery would be necessary to correct their condition. After only four outpatient sessions, all of the patients improved in terms of bowel movement frequency, incidence of bloating and straining, and reduction in laxative use, and were able to avoid surgery. Moreover, follow-up showed that they maintained the improvements for approximately nine months without the need for further treatment.[6]

Muscular Dysfunctions: Marjorie K. Toomim, Ph.D., Director of the Biofeedback Institute of Los Angeles, uses EMG biofeedback to detect muscle imbalances in order to prevent and correct injuries. For example, a runner with problem knee muscles was hooked to the EMG and Dr. Toomim was immediately able to see that the runner was placing a disproportionate amount of her weight to one side. The muscles on the inside of the leg were stronger than those on the outside. To correct the imbalance, the patient needed to exercise only the outer thigh muscles. While hooked up to the EMG feedback device, the patient could see exactly when the weaker outside muscles were exercising and when the stronger inner muscles were at rest. "In this case, the EMG gave us information we couldn't have gotten in any other way," says Dr. Toomim, "and it empowered the patient to take control of her own muscular re-education."

Dr. Werbach believes biofeedback training is sometimes more effective than surgery for patients with back problems. By teaching patients both relaxation techniques and control over their muscle spasms, biofeedback helps them reduce or eliminate back pain.

Psychologist Bernard Brucker, Ph.D., of the University of Miami Medical School uses EMG biofeedback to teach patients with serious spinal injuries to walk again. Sophisticated EMG feedback replaces the sensation of motion lost by spinal cord injury, reduces muscle spasm, detects activity in muscles mistakenly believed to lack energy, and strengthens muscles so they function once again.[7]

Yale University research affiliate and Professor Emeritus at Rockefeller University, Neal E. Miller, Ph.D., along with Barry Dworkin, Ph.D., of Penn State University, developed a small biofeedback device worn on the body to treat curvature of the spine. When the wearer slouches forward, a soft beep is emitted; if he or she does not straighten up, a piercing alarm goes off. Several studies have shown it to be especially effective in treating kyphosis, a front-to-back curvature.[8]

Incontinence: Biofeedback can successfully treat incontinence. A $13-billion-a-year problem among institutionalized elderly, incontinence results when people lose the ability to control the muscles used for urination or defecation.[9] One report from the U.S. Department of

---

UNUSUAL SUCCESS STORIES: BIOFEEDBACK AND COMA

Melvyn Werbach, M.D., retired Director of the Biofeedback Medical Clinic, in Tarzana, California, was once approached by a woman whose husband had been in a coma for several months. Dr. Werbach and an associate arranged to hook the man up to various biofeedback devices in an attempt to communicate with him. While Dr. Werbach monitored the biofeedback equipment, his associate asked the comatose patient to concentrate on specific areas of his body. To everyone's surprise, the galvanic skin response monitor began to move with the request. Although he was in a coma, the patient was able to hear. At the end of the session, the family and staff were shocked to hear him moan loudly. Perhaps catalyzed by the biofeedback communication, the patient came out of his coma within a month of this initial session. Almost two years later, Dr. Werbach got a call from the patient. "Hearing his voice was one of the most rewarding moments I have ever had in the practice of medicine," says Dr. Werbach.[12]

California therapist Margaret Ayers has also had success bringing patients out of level-two coma, using Neuropathways EEG Imaging, a form of neurotherapy that she invented. Level-two coma means the patient is unable to respond to sound, verbal commands, light, touch, or pressure. Peter, 30, had been in a coma for three months, following eight brain surgeries to remove a baseball-sized tumor. After a one-hour session with Ayers, during which time Peter's brain was trained to make small responses to electrical stimulation, he snapped out of his coma, opened his eyes, and kissed his wife. After four more sessions, spaced a month apart, Peter was able to speak, eat, and move one side of his body. Another of Ayers's patients, Collin, 21, had spent two years in a coma following a motorcycle accident, but regained consciousness after only two 1-hour neurotherapy treatments.

Health and Human Services analyzed 22 different studies and concluded that muscular reeducation through biofeedback training had a success rate ranging from 54% to 95%, depending on the patient group.[10] In another study, 55 otherwise healthy women between the ages of 25 and 81 with symptoms of stress, urgency, and mixed urinary incontinence underwent a 16-week self-directed biofeedback training program. Of the 44 women who completed the training, 43% were completely free of

HEART RATE VARIABILITY: USING BIOFEEDBACK TO ACCESS ANSWERS FROM THE NERVOUS SYSTEM

Physicians at the Nevada Clinic, in Las Vegas, report that a test called Heart Rate Variability (HRV) acts as a dependable indicator of how the nervous system responds to any type of medical treatment. According to Daniel F. Royal, D.O., HRV testing has the capacity to objectively demonstrate and thus prove the effectiveness of any given remedy. "HRV could supply the alternative medical community with a common testing procedure by which different medical approaches could be uniformly evaluated and compared," he states.

"Heart rate is largely determined by the autonomic nervous system (ANS)," explains William T. Evans, of Roaring Fork Valley, Colorado, who is actively involved in using HRV studies to evaluate the ANS. "Contrary to what is popularly believed, a healthy heart does not beat with a regular rhythm but has a continuously varying rate. The range of heart variability is an indicator of a person's resilience and correlates with longevity and balance."

HRV provides a computerized graph of the shape of the pulse wave of the heart's left and right carotid arteries. The approach is called "noncognitive" biofeedback, because it works without the patient's conscious participation or awareness. Instead, the HRV device "talks" directly with the patient's nervous system. When the heart rate shifts, this change is routed by computer into audio-visual signals (light flashes and intermittent sounds) that the patient

becomes aware of through the use of headphones and a TV screen. Frequency information obtained by HRV is then returned to the patient through light and sound waves generated in accordance with the specific rhythm of the heart, which in turn help to rebalance the ANS.

HRV testing can also reveal imbalances in the patient's ANS even when he or she reports feeling well. This is valuable because an imbalance in the ANS will eventually produce physical symptoms. If imbalances are caught early, steps can be taken to prevent the onset of symptoms.

Among HRV's other advantages are its speed and specificity in evaluating medical approaches. Homeopathic remedies, for instance, produce changes in the ANS and heart rate. HRV can measure these subtle but important changes immediately after ingestion of the homeopathic remedy to help better determine its efficacy. In addition to homeopathic remedies, HRV can evaluate a patient's response to pharmaceutical drugs, nutritional supplements, herbs, acupuncture treatments, chiropractic adjustments, and dental amalgam removal, among other treatment approaches. In addition, Dr. Evans notes, "The life-sustaining and life-protecting aspects of the ANS and HRV offer a form of biofeedback information which can be used to assist people in learning how to evoke and maintain a healthy balance."

symptoms while another 36% reported at least a 50% improvement of their condition.[11]

Biofeedback Training as a Healing Visualization Tool

Because biofeedback training empowers patients by teaching them to control one or more of their body processes, it is proving a useful adjunct to conventional therapies for cancer and other chronic diseases. Dr. Norris uses biofeedback training to teach cancer patients and patients with AIDS and other immune system disorders to reduce stress (which simultaneously increases immune function). Using imagery and visualization, she helps patients become confident in the capacity for self-regulation of their bodies. Her first cancer patient, Garrett Porter, 9, overcame an inoperable brain tumor with the help of biofeedback-assisted visualization.[13] More than a decade later, over 300 cancer patients who used

biofeedback-assisted visualization have been studied at the Menninger Clinic, with results ranging from increased comfort and reduced stress to a complete recovery from cancer.

How Neurotherapy Works

The outgrowth of pioneering biofeedback studies conducted in the 1960s and 1970s, neurotherapy involves the use of computerized EEG biofeedback equipment to normalize brain-wave states and to increase the abundance of alpha and theta waves associated with heightened states of optimal mental functioning, pleasure, insight, and creativity. "Everything we do and are physiologically, and most of what we do and are psychologically, is mediated through the brain," explains Rima Laibow, M.D., founding Medical Director of the Alexandria Institute, in Croton-on-Hudson, New York, where neurotherapy is an integral part of the comprehensive treatment options offered to patients. "Any process that the body engages in can be modified on a voluntary basis if information about what the body is doing is fed back to the individual in a way that's usable." Neurotherapy allows practitioners to gather information from the brain about how it is functioning and then, through feedback of light and sound signals, to train it to more regularly produce the brain-wave states associated with healthy psychophysiological functioning.

Any process that the body engages in can be modified on a voluntary basis if information about what the body is doing is fed back to the individual in a way that's usable.

—RIMA LAIBOW, M.D.

During a neurotherapy session, sensors placed on the patient's scalp register the electrical signals (brain waves) produced by the brain. "It's important to note that there is no electrical current introduced into the brain," Dr. Laibow says. "Neurotherapy is entirely a passive receptor system, much like a radio receiver, yet it provides people with the opportunity to master the control of their brain-wave states. This often leads to improved self-regulation of processes at many levels, from the physical to the meditative. It's an extremely empowering process."

During a neurotherapy session, the brain's EEG signals are read through the scalp sensors and then fed into a computer that assesses the efficacy of the EEG. When a desirable brain-wave state is reached, the computer responds with light and sound signals that reward the brain. "In effect, the light and sound tell the brain to do whatever it just did again," Dr. Laibow explains. "And the brain listens: it learns to change the rhythm of its communications and repair follows." Functional states are impacted by changing the way the brain functions and returning it to a more efficient level of integration.

According to Dr. Laibow, "Neurotherapy offers a much more profound level of mastery than conventional biofeedback can provide. Additionally, once the brain is trained to achieve a fine level of discrimination and control, it often seems to continue to improve its ability to do so."

People who undergo neurotherapy learn how to self-regulate their brain waves to produce and increase alpha-and theta-wave activity (or other wave forms, if appropriate), allowing them to experience regular states of contentment and well-being, concentration, and attention. This is "a very big biological correction that occurs in the treatment process," says Dr. Fahrion, a leading researcher in the neurotherapy field. "You're literally changing personal biology, the way someone functions." Both Drs. Fahrion and Norris note that, concurrent with such changes, there are positive changes in brain chemistry, posture, overall health, and tension levels. "We see people looking differently, standing differently, being different in their bodies, and being healthier," Dr. Norris reports.[14]

Drs. Fahrion and Norris stress that the positive results produced by neurotherapy are not simply due to, in Dr. Fahrion's words, "just buying EEG devices and hooking people up," but part of a comprehensive treatment plan that requires psychological expertise in order to effectively deal with the various emotions, beliefs, and memories that can arise during the process. Dr. Laibow concurs. "Because a 'new' brain needs to process old information in a new way, we see patients for neurotherapy in combination with reintegrative psychotherapy," she says. "That's a requirement, because the results of applying a technological solution to these problems without a perceptual and emotional solution are not very satisfying over the long run. When patients integrate psychotherapy with neurotherapy, the results tend to be much more durable."

Conditions Benefited by Neurotherapy

Because of the way neurotherapy positively impacts brain function, and thus most other psychophysiological functions, it offers benefit for a wide variety of disease conditions, as well as serving as a powerful tool for personal growth and awareness. Among its current applications are alcoholism and addiction, autism, brain disorders and injuries (including early- and mid-stage Alzheimer's disease, attention deficit hyperactivity disorder, coma, and closed head injury), cancer, psychiatric disorders (including anxiety or panic attacks, bipolar and unipolar depression, mood swings, obsessive-compulsive disorder, post-traumatic stress disorder, rage, and schizophrenia), chronic pain, and strokes. Other demonstrated benefits include improvements in short-term memory, concentration, speech, motor skills, sleep patterns, and emotional balance.

In a study conducted by Dr. Laibow and fellow researchers, neurotherapy was shown to provide a wide range of benefits for patients with brain injuries. The study involved 27 patients who suffered from brain injuries and exhibited a list of 48 clinical symptoms. After receiving neurotherapy sessions, the conditions of 25 of the patients improved by 61% to 100%, while the remaining two patients, whose injuries were related to vascular accidents, also achieved some improvement. In another study, researchers found that both normal test subjects and subjects suffering from brain injury experienced increases in memory function after receiving neurotherapy, with overall improvements among those with brain injuries ranging from 68% to 181%.[15]

Among other conditions for which Dr. Laibow reports neurotherapy has benefit are allergies, arthritis (both rheumatoid and osteoarthritis), asthma, autoimmune disorders, chronic fatigue syndrome, chronic pain, eating disorders, fibromyalgia, headaches (atypical, cluster, migraine, and tension), hyper- and hypotension, insomnia, irritable bowel syndrome, learning disabilities, Lyme disease, muscle spasms, myofascial pain syndrome, optic neuritis, post-polio syndrome, spinal cord injury, and Tourette's syndrome.

Neurotherapy is also effective as a treatment for alcoholism and addiction, as demonstrated by a three-year study conducted by Drs. Fahrion and Norris at the Ellsworth Correctional Facility, in Kansas, in the mid-1990s. Participants in the study were convicted felons diagnosed with alcohol or drug problems, almost all of whom had previously failed other treatment programs. Each participant received three weeks of neurotherapy, along with visualization and psychological intervention, just prior to being released back into society. After release, they were followed closely by parole officers, which allowed for detailed follow-up information. Preliminary results after two years showed that 63% of the participants remained drug- and alcohol-free (tested by frequent urinalysis), with no failure of terms of parole. Just as impressively, recidivism for new crimes was only 4% among all participants, prompting the district court administrative judge to say that neurotherapy could become "the model of addiction treatment for the entire country."[16]

Drs. Fahrion and Norris also offer neurotherapy to patients suffering from cancer and other life-threatening conditions. "With cancer patients, the aim is always to be as well as possible for as long as possible and to get entirely well if possible," Dr. Norris says. She reports that between 10% and 12% of patients who were considered terminal have recovered while receiving neurotherapy and that most people "have greatly extended their longevity."[17]

The Future of Biofeedback Training and Neurotherapy

The latest developments in both biofeedback training and neurotherapy concern the self-regulation of bodily functions that, until now, were considered inaccessible. "The most exciting innovation in biofeedback would be to provide people with moment-to-moment feedback of changes in the levels of chemicals within the bloodstream," says Dr. Werbach. "In other words, to have equipment that can monitor, for example, hormone levels as they are at the moment and give feedback that will in turn enable a person to learn to influence his or her hormonal levels. Now that has incredible potential."

In the future, Drs. Fahrion and Norris expect that neurotherapy will become widely used in psychotherapy, for group problem solving and in the area of personal growth, in addition to its current medical applications. "I believe that self-regulation, which is what we're talking about with biofeedback and neurotherapy, and the psycho-neuro-immune physiological restoration of wellness is a profound movement forward," adds Dr. Laibow. "The great breakthrough is that there is now a technological mirror of the self, if you will, which we are applying to help people find out more about their wholeness. As they do, the opportunities for self-regulation and empowerment are extraordinary."

 Additional research into biofeedback training and neurotherapy could help people better understand mind/body interaction and its importance in maintaining health.

Where to Find Help

When undertaking biofeedback training, it is important to find a qualified practitioner with a firm grasp of both physiology and psychology. Practitioners should be certified by the Biofeedback Certification Institute of America. Most major cities have a biofeedback association. Check your local phone book or contact an organization below for more information.

Association for Applied Psychophysiology and Biofeedback
10200 West 44th Avenue, Suite 304
Wheat Ridge, Colorado 80033
(303) 422-8436
Website: www.aapb.org

Provides contact information for certified biofeedback practitioners nationwide.

Biofeedback Certification Institute of America
10200 West 44th Avenue, Suite 304
Wheat Ridge, Colorado 80033
(303) 420-2902
Website: www.bcia.org

Conducts the certification program for biofeedback practitioners and offers a nationwide directory of practitioners.

Center for Applied Psychophysiology
Menninger Clinic
(800) 351-9058
Website: www.menninger.edu

One of the pioneering groups in biofeedback, this organization has research, treatment, and workshops in all areas of mind/body medicine, and extensive work with biofeedback; includes the Biofeedback and Psychophysiology Clinic.

Life Sciences Institute of Mind-Body Health
4636 S.W. Wanamaker Road
Topeka, Kansas 66610
(785) 271-8686
Website: www.cjnetworks.com/~lifesci

A leading treatment and research facility for biofeedback and neurotherapy, as well as other forms of mind/body medicine, founded by leading pioneers in the field, including Drs. Steven Fahrion and Patricia Norris.

Neurotherapy and Biofeedback Certification Board
1973 N. Nellis Blvd., PMB 264
Las Vegas, Nevada 89115
(800) 838-1931

For information on biofeedback training and neurotherapy and referrals to therapists trained in their use.

Medi-Tec Systems, Inc.
3720 Howard Hughes Parkway, Suite 270
Las Vegas, Nevada 89108
(702) 732-9153

Provides HRV equipment and training.

Tools for Wellness
9755 Independence Avenue
Chatsworth, California 91311
(800) 456-9887
Website: www.toolsforwellness.com

A leading resource for home biofeedback devices and other wellness products. Call for a catalog.

Recommended Reading

A Symphony in the Brain: The Evolution of the New Brain Wave Biofeedback. Jim Robbins. New York: Atlantic Monthly Press, 2000.

Biofeedback: An Introduction and Guide. David G. Danskin and Mark Crow. Palo Alto, CA: Mayfield Publishing, 1981.

The Future of the Body: Explorations into the Further Evolution of the Human Species. Michael Murphy. Los Angeles: Jeremy P. Tarcher, 1992.

The High Performance Mind: Mastering Brain Waves for Insight, Healing, and Creativity. Anna Wise. New York: Jeremy P. Tarcher, 1997.

Third Line Medicine. Melvyn R. Werbach, M.D. New York: Third Line Press, 1988.

Why Me? Harnessing the Healing Power of the Human Spirit. Patricia Norris, Ph.D. and Garrett Porter. Walpole, NH: Stillpoint Publishing, 1985.

BIOLOGICAL DENTISTRY

Biological dentistry stresses the use of nontoxic restorative materials for dental treatment and focuses on the impact that dental toxins and hidden dental infections can have on overall health.

THERE IS A growing recognition among alternative dentists and physicians that dental health has a tremendous impact on the overall health of the body. European researchers estimate that perhaps as much as half of all chronic degenerative illness can be linked either directly or indirectly to dental problems and the traditional techniques of modern dentistry used to treat them. The well-publicized dangers associated with the use of silver/mercury fillings (amalgams) are only the tip of the iceberg as far as the negative impact that dentistry can have on health.

"One of the problems in the United States is that dentists are trained to practice with only the most meager of diagnostic equipment," says Gary Verigan, D.D.S., of Escalon, California. "These instruments, consisting primarily of X rays, are incapable of detecting enough about the tooth and its surrounding environment, giving the dentist only a superficial understanding of the problem and the impact it may be having on the patient's overall health." People often go through many doctors and therapies in search of answers for their problems, never realizing that their chronic conditions may be traceable to dental complications.

In contrast, biological dentistry treats the teeth, jaw, and related structures with specific regard to how treatment will affect the entire body. According to Hal Huggins, D.D.S., M.S., of Colorado Springs, Colorado, a pioneer in this field, "Dental problems, such as cavities, infections, toxic or allergy-producing filling materials, root canals, and misalignment of the teeth or jaw, can have far-reaching effects throughout the body."

> *Dental problems, such as cavities, infections, toxic or allergy-producing filling materials, root canals, and misalignment of the teeth or jaw, can have far-reaching effects throughout the body.*
>
> —HAL HUGGINS, D.D.S., M.S.

How Dental Problems Contribute to Illness

"Dental infections and disturbances can cause pain and dysfunction throughout the body," states Edward Arana, D.D.S., President of the American Academy of Biological Dentistry, "including limited motion and loose tendons, ligaments, and muscles. Structural and physiological dysfunction can also occur, impairing organs and glands." Dr. Arana cites several major types of dental problems that can cause illness and dysfunction in the body:

- Infections under and around teeth

- Problems with specific teeth related to the acupuncture meridians and the autonomic nervous system

- Root canals

- Toxicity from dental restoration materials

- Bio-incompatability to dental restoration materials

- Electrogalvanism and ion migration

- Temporomandibular joint (TMJ) syndrome, a painful condition of the jaw, usually caused by stress or injury

Some of the more common causes of these dental problems are unerupted teeth (teeth that have not broken through the gum), wisdom teeth (both impacted and

YOUR TEETH ARE ALIVE

"Most people, including dentists, are rather ambivalent about teeth," observes Hal Huggins, D.D.S., M.S. "Pull them, fill them, crown them—what does it matter? Well, it does matter." Dr. Huggins bases this claim on the work of Ralph Steinman, M.D., a researcher for Loma Linda University, in California, who investigated the life of the tooth for several decades. "His research was the most important about how a tooth actually lives," Dr. Huggins says. "I'm talking about the complex biochemical life of enzymes, mineral catalysts, and energy production that we, as people, can disturb, and we, as dentists, can destroy, depending on how we treat our teeth."

In nearly 70 scientific publications, Dr. Steinman described radioactive isotopes moving from the pulp chamber, through the dentin, to the surface of the tooth in one hour. "This occurred when there was no decay," Dr. Huggins emphasizes. "Fluid transfer from the surface of the tooth through the enamel, through the dentin, into the pulp chamber could also be seen with the same radioisotopes where there was decay. His research proved that dental decay is an active, biological process under the direction of endocrine glands in our body.

"In turn, the endocrine glands that control decay are under the influence of how much protein, fat, and carbohydrate we consume. Dr. Steinman showed that a high-sugar diet created decay at the same rate in animals fed through a stomach tube, where food never touched the teeth, as when they ate the food normally. This should open the eyes of dentists and toothpaste manufacturers who tell us that it is food sitting on a tooth that causes decay. In other words, decay is not a mechanical process, but an active, biological one."

Dr. Huggins laments the fact that Dr. Steinman's work is not taught today in any dental school. "Most professors of cariology, the science of dental decay, report never

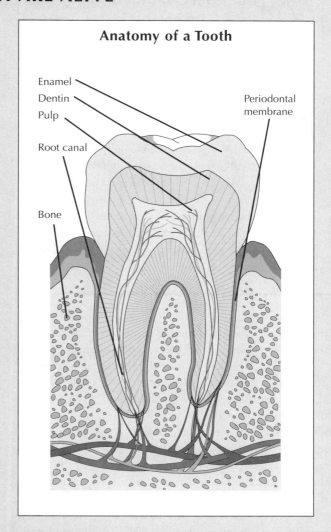

Anatomy of a Tooth

Enamel
Dentin
Pulp
Root canal
Bone
Periodontal membrane

having heard of him," Dr. Huggins says. "They teach what the American Dental Association dictates: cleaning your teeth with a fluoridated toothpaste is preferred over cleaning up your diet. Yet, Dr. Steinman was one of the most respected researchers of the last half of the 20th century and taught the most significant material on how diet controls dental decay."

unimpacted), amalgam-filled cavities and root canals, cysts, bone cavities, and areas of bone condensation due to inflammation. These conditions can be diagnosed using methods such as blood tests, applied kinesiology, electrodermal screening (EDS), and, in some cases, X rays. A thorough review of the patient's medical and dental histories is also essential.

 See Acupuncture, Applied Kinesiology, Biofeedback Training and Neurotherapy, Energy Medicine.

Infections Under the Teeth

Pockets of infection can exist under the teeth and be undetectable on X rays. This is particularly true for teeth that have had root canals, as it is very difficult to eliminate all the bacteria and toxins from the roots during this procedure. These infections may persist for years without the patient's knowledge. When infections are present, toxins can leak out and depress the function of the immune system, leading to chronic degenerative diseases

ELECTRODERMAL SCREENING

Developed by Reinhold Voll, M.D., of Germany in the 1940s, electroacupuncture biofeedback, or electrodermal screening, makes use of the acupuncture meridian system to screen for infections and dysfunction in the body. Today, it is employed as a screening tool by alternative health practitioners worldwide, including biological dentists. As employed in biological dentistry, it involves placing an electrode on an individual tooth, then applying a small electrical current and recording the response. Any deviation from the normal reading indicates that there is an infection or disturbance in the vicinity of that particular tooth.[1] This deviation can also indicate a similar unhealthy state in the organ that shares the same meridian as the tooth.

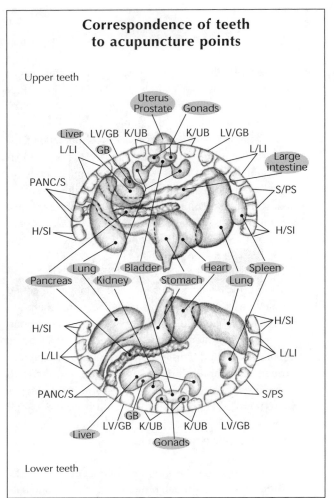

Correspondence of teeth to acupuncture points

Upper teeth

Uterus Prostate · Gonads

Liver · LV/GB · K/UB · K/UB · LV/GB
L/LI · GB · L/LI
Large intestine
PANC/S
S/PS
H/SI · H/SI

Lung · Bladder · Heart · Spleen
Pancreas · Kidney · Stomach · Lung

H/SI · H/SI
L/LI · L/LI
PANC/S · S/PS
GB
Liver · LV/GB · K/UB · K/UB · LV/GB
Gonads

Lower teeth

©1983 Ralph Alan Dale

throughout the body. Once the infection is eliminated, many of the symptoms of disease will disappear.

Infections near the root of the tooth can also travel into the bone and destroy it, according to Harold Ravins, D.D.S., of Los Angeles, California. "One way to detect this is to stick a needle into the bone—if it is too soft, there is infection," he says. "Another way is with neural therapy, which involves the injection of an anesthetic around a suspected tooth. If this relieves the problems in other parts of the body, it means there is a disturbance under the tooth."

Some dentists use applied kinesiology to identify these hidden infections. Applied kinesiology employs a simple strength resistance test on a specific indicator muscle that is related to the organ or part of the body being tested. If the muscle tests strong (maintains its resistance), it indicates health. If it tests weak, it can mean infection or dysfunction.

Electrodermal screening (EDS) is another method used to screen for hidden dental infections. Philip Jenkins, D.D.S., of Los Gatos, California, uses EDS testing to find infections, identify them, and then determine the appropriate homeopathic remedies with which to treat them. Any determinations using EDS should always be confirmed by a physician.

Relationship Between Specific Teeth and Illness

In the 1950s, Reinhold Voll, M.D., of Germany, discovered that each tooth in the mouth relates to a specific acupuncture meridian. Using electroacupuncture biofeedback, he found that if a tooth became infected or diseased, the organ on the same meridian could also become unhealthy. He also found that the opposite held true, that dysfunction in a specific organ could lead to a problem in the corresponding tooth. For example, Dr. Ravins has observed that people who hit their front teeth too hard often have kidney disturbances, as there is a specific relationship between the kidneys and the front teeth.

Ernesto Adler, M.D., D.D.S., of Spain, reports that many diseases can be caused by the wisdom teeth, which have a relationship to almost all organs of the body. When wisdom teeth are impacted, Dr. Adler points out, they press upon the nerves of the mandible (the large bone that makes up the lower jaw), which can result in disturbances in other areas of the body, including stammering, epilepsy, pain in the joints, muscle cramps, depression, headaches, and heart problems.

Poor dental health can also affect sexual vitality and the reproductive organs, according to Michael Gerber, M.D., H.M.D., of Reno, Nevada. "Many of my patients who have had cancer or other diseases of the reproductive organs, urogenital tract, or breast, have had decay, disease, or root canals in the corresponding teeth," he says.

LASER DENTISTRY: THE HEALTHY ALTERNATIVE TO ROOT CANALS

It is estimated that over 30 million root canals are performed in the U.S. each year, and this number is expected to double within five years. However, a growing number of physicians, as well as dentists, now believe that root canals can cause or contribute to a wide range of illnesses and degenerative diseases. According to Richard T. Hansen, D.M.D., F.A.C.A.D., Director of the Center for Advanced Dentistry, in Fullerton, California, root canals may soon become a thing of the past due to the latest generation of laser equipment and techniques, which provide patients with a healthier alternative, repairing previously performed dental work and preventing the need for root canals in the future.

A conventional dental drill, according to Dr. Hansen, "basically grinds away everything in its path," and creates heat friction and vibration that traumatize the teeth's nerves. "A laser, on the other hand, works very specifically on only the diseased part of the tooth," Dr. Hansen explains. "A decayed tooth has an extremely high water content compared to a healthy tooth. Because of that, the laser can be selectively targeted to vaporize only the decay area. Using a laser, you can pinpoint the target area and remove the decay, inject a liquid composite or ceramic composite, and keep most of the tooth intact. In addition, the laser works in such a way that, in almost all cases, you never need anesthetic, since it doesn't cause any reaction to the nerve of the tooth. The laser also automatically sterilizes the decay area while it's working, whereas the dental drill not only cannot sterilize, it pushes bacteria deeper into the tooth."

Although the cost of laser dentistry is typically 30%-50% higher than a conventional filling, Dr. Hansen maintains that it is still more cost-effective in the long-term. "A regular filling, especially a silver filling, will probably have to be replaced with larger fillings later on, whereas you may never need to replace a laser filling," he says. "But the real cost savings is that, by not traumatizing the tooth, you're avoiding further dental work and possibly serious health conditions in the future, as well as the need for root canals."

Dr. Hansen has also pioneered a laser technique for treating infected nerves, which typically result in root canals. "Instead of doing a root canal, we can do laser nerve treatment on the bleeding, infected nerve and make it healthy again," he says. His method enables dentists to selectively clean the infected part of the nerve while still keeping most of it intact. Laser dentistry is also useful for treating cavities and tooth fracture, as well as poor blood supply to the tissue surrounding the teeth. "We have a laser to stimulate lymphatic drainage and stimulate the reduction of inflammation to help with circulation in the tissue," Dr. Hansen says. "It's a low-level laser stimulation that penetrates deep enough to get into the bone and around the teeth."

Since only a few hundred dentists in the U.S. currently use the new generation of lasers, Dr. Hansen established the Advanced Health Research Institute, a nonprofit organization to help individuals locate laser dentistry practitioners nationwide.

Other common symptoms associated with dental disease are neurological disorders (numbness or tingling in the face, head, or extremities, and visual disturbances), chronic sinus infections, facial pain (trigeminal neuralgia), panic and anxiety, and, most commonly, chronic fatigue.

 Although electroacupuncture biofeedback is used worldwide, especially in Europe, in the U.S. it is employed only as an experimental device. More studies are needed to verify its importance in the field of biological dentistry and as a general diagnostic tool for all health practitioners.

Root Canals as a Cause of Illness

The late Weston Price, D.D.S., M.S., F.A.C.D., former Director of Research for the American Dental Association, made the astonishing claim that if teeth that have had root canals are removed from patients suffering from kidney and heart disease, these diseases will resolve in most cases. Moreover, implanting these teeth in animals results in the animals developing the same kind of disease found in the person. Dr. Price found that toxins seeping out of root canals may cause systemic diseases of the heart, kidney, uterus, and nervous and endocrine systems.[2]

Michael Ziff, D.D.S, of Orlando, Florida, points out that research has demonstrated that 100% of root canals result in residual infection. This may be due to the imperfect seal that allows bacteria to penetrate. The oxygen-lacking environment of a root canal can cause the bacteria to undergo changes, adds Dr. Huggins, producing potent toxins that then leak out into the body. Nutrient materials are able to seep into the root canal through the porous channels in the tooth, allowing bacteria to flourish. Susceptibility to these types of reactions is usually genetic, but stresses to the system (abuse of alcohol, drugs, caffeine) can induce them in normal individuals. Pregnancy and influenza also increase susceptibility to leakage of toxins from root canals, according to Dr. Huggins.

Research has demonstrated that 100% of root canals result in residual infection.

Dr. Huggins states that when a tooth with a root canal is removed, the periodontal ligament that attaches the tooth to the underlying bone should also be removed, otherwise a pocket of infection can remain. Full removal of the tooth and ligament stimulates the old bone to produce new bone for healing. "Extraction of root canal teeth should be the first thought when considering the health of the patient," he adds.

Toxicity from Dental Restoration Materials

"Dental amalgam fillings can release mercury, tin, copper, silver, and sometimes zinc into the body," says Dr. Arana. These metals have various degrees of toxicity and, when placed as fillings in the teeth, can corrode or disassociate into metallic ions (charged atoms). These metallic ions can then migrate from the tooth into the root of the tooth, the mouth, the bone, the connective tissues of the jaw, and finally into the nerves. From there, they can travel into the central nervous system, where the ions will reside, permanently disrupting the body's normal functioning if nothing is done to remove them.

Other types of metal-based dental restorations can similarly release toxic metals into the body. According to David E. Eggleston, D.D.S., of the Department of Restorative Dentistry at the University of Southern California, in Los Angeles, a patient undergoing dental work developed kidney disease due to nickel toxicity from the dental crowns that were being placed in the patient's mouth. As each successive crown was placed, the disease intensified, verified by blood and urine tests and physical examination. Once the nickel crowns were removed, the patient gradually became symptom free.[3]

The late Theron Randolph, M.D., founder of the field of environmental medicine, believed that both the medical and dental professions have become too lax in dealing with the scope and potential danger of toxic metals. "Although it is not clear whether dental amalgams

and other metals used in dental work are the primary or secondary cause of many health problems," he said, "both doctors and dentists have to be concerned with evaluating the clinical implications of using toxic metals in the body." Dr. Randolph believed part of the problem stems from American dental schools ignoring the mounting evidence on toxicity from dental restorations, especially amalgams, despite clear documentation shown in European studies.

In September 1992, then California governor Pete Wilson requested that the State Board of Dental Examiners develop a fact sheet on dental materials to be distributed to dentists. California is the first state to pass such legislation, notes Joyal Taylor, D.D.S., of Rancho Santa Fe, California, President of the Environmental Dental Association. He hopes this will pave the way for a total ban on the use of mercury in dental restorations, adding that up to 3,000 dentists across the country are now calling for such a ban.

MERCURY DENTAL AMALGAMS

While all metals used for dental restoration can be toxic, the most harmful are the mercury dental amalgams (silver/mercury) used for fillings. According to Dr. Taylor, "These so-called 'silver fillings' actually contain 50% mercury and only 25% silver." Mercury has been recognized as a poison since the 1500s, yet mercury amalgams have been used in dentistry since the 1820s. They are still being used today, even though the Environmental Protection Agency (EPA) declared scrap dental amalgam a hazardous waste in 1988. Even the American Dental Association, which has so far refused to ban amalgams, now instructs dentists to "know the potential hazards and symptoms of mercury exposure, such as the development of sensitivity and neuropathy," to use a no-touch technique for handling the amalgam, and to store it under liquid, preferably glycerin or radiographic fixer solution, in unbreakable, tightly sealed containers.[4]

For some dentists, such as Richard D. Fischer, D.D.S., of Annandale, Virginia, these measures are not enough. Since becoming aware of the health risks amalgams pose, he has refused to work with them and had his own silver fillings removed. "I don't feel comfortable using a substance designated by the EPA to be a waste disposal hazard," he says. "I can't throw it in the trash, bury it in the ground, or put it in a landfill, but they say it's okay to put it in people's mouths. That doesn't make sense."

According to the German Ministry of Health, "Amalgam is considered a health risk from a medical viewpoint due to the release of mercury vapor."[5] Everyday activities such as chewing and brushing the teeth have been shown to release mercury vapors from amalgams.[6] Amalgams can also erode and corrode with time (ideally they should be replaced after 7-10 years), adding to their toxic output.

I don't feel comfortable using a substance [mercury amalgams] designated by the EPA to be a waste disposal hazard. I can't throw it in the trash, bury it in the ground, or put it in a landfill, but they say it's okay to put it in people's mouths. That doesn't make sense.

—RICHARD D. FISCHER, D.D.S.

Studies by the World Health Organization show that a single amalgam can release 3-17 micrograms of mercury per day,[7] making dental amalgam a major source of mercury exposure.[8] A Danish study of 100 men and 100 women showed that increased blood mercury levels were related to the presence of more than four amalgam fillings.[9] American, Swedish, and German scientists examining cadavers have also found a clear relationship between the number of fillings and the amount of mercury in the brain and kidneys.[10]

In Germany the sale and manufacture of amalgams has been prohibited since March 1992.[11] In Sweden, after a special commission determined that amalgam was a toxic material, that country's Social Welfare and Health Administration issued an advisory against its use in the dental treatment of pregnant women. Furthermore, Sweden has promised to ban amalgams entirely as soon as a suitable replacement is found.[12] Until then, the government pays 50% of the cost for removal of amalgams. In the U.S., however, little is being done to deal with the effects of mercury amalgams because most dentists still maintain that they are safe. They continue to place mercury in their patients' mouths even though the metal is more toxic than arsenic.[13]

The problem is so widespread that Dr. Taylor now devotes his entire practice to the removal of amalgams. "There have been no studies [in the United States] on the safety of mercury in dental work, but when it leaks from the teeth it can cause both physical and mental problems," he states.[14] Numbness and tingling, paralysis, tremors, and pain are just some of the symptoms of chronic metal intoxication associated with the use of mercury dental amalgams.

TEN WAYS MERCURY IS TOXIC TO THE BODY

1. It inhibits the repair of DNA, our basic genetic material.

2. It alters the ability of cells to selectively allow materials through their membranes.

3. It changes the three-dimensional shape of molecules, producing nonfunctional chemicals.

4. It alters the activities of enzymes, which are needed for all biochemical reactions in the body.

5. It interferes with the transmission of nerve impulses from the brain to the rest of the body, producing tremors, shaking, tingling, and numbness.

6. It can provoke the immune system to mount an autoimmune response against the body.

7. It interferes with endocrine gland function and hormone secretion.

8. It can displace and deactivate vital minerals, such as calcium, magnesium, zinc, and chromium.

9. It kills "friendly" bacteria in the digestive tract, preventing absorption of nutrients.

10. By creating new strains of bacteria, it may create resistance to antibiotics.

Though the ideal replacement for mercury amalgams has not yet been found, there are some less toxic alternatives that biological dentists are working with. These include "composite fillings," which are a combination of resins, metals, or other ingredients. Containing no mercury, they are less toxic and slower to break down than conventional amalgams.

Dr. Huggins recommends that people who choose to have their amalgams removed ask their dentists to use a rubber dam, a thin sheet of rubber that slips over the teeth. "Dams prevent over 95% of the mixture of mercury and water produced by the drilling out of old fillings from going down your throat," he says. "They also reduce the amount of mercury that you might absorb from your cheeks and under your tongue." Dr. Huggins also suggests that people consider early morning appoint-

SYMPTOM ANALYSIS OF PATIENTS WHO ELIMINATED MERCURY FILLINGS

The following represents a summary of 1,569 patients in six different studies evaluating the health effects of replacing mercury-containing dental fillings with non-mercury fillings. The data was derived from the following sources: 762 Patient Adverse Reaction Reports submitted to the U.S. Food and Drug Administration by patients and 807 patient reports from Sweden, Denmark, Canada, and the U.S.[15]

Symptom	Number Reporting	Number Cured/Improved	Percent Cured/Improved
Allergy	221	196	89
Anxiety	86	80	93
Bad temper	81	68	84
Bloating	88	70	80
Blood pressure problems	99	53	54
Chest pains	79	69	87
Depression	347	315	91
Dizziness	343	301	88
Fatigue	705	603	86
Intestinal problems	231	192	83
Gum problems	129	121	94
Headaches	531	460	87
Insomnia	187	146	78
Irregular heartbeat	159	139	87
Irritability	132	119	90
Lack of concentration	270	216	80
Lack of energy	91	88	97
Memory loss	265	193	73
Metallic taste	260	247	95
Multiple sclerosis	113	86	76
Muscle tremor	126	104	82

ments for amalgam removal, rather than later in the day, because the mercury vapor from other patients' sessions can linger in the air for hours and be absorbed by breathing. Some dentists use mercury vapor filter systems, he points out, but those who do are rare.

Charles Gableman, M.D., of Encinitas, California, always advises the removal of his patients' amalgam fillings. According to Dr. Gableman, patients with chronic fatigue syndrome or with a lack of resistance to infections, allergies, and thyroid dysfunction, all improve after their fillings are properly removed. He believes it is possible that these patients have suffered from allergies their entire lives and that the mercury toxicity from the fillings simply adds to the body's toxic load and "pushes them over the edge," resulting in chronic medical problems.

Extensive clinical evidence based on patient case histories attests to the effects of mercury amalgam toxicity. Dr. Taylor cites an example of a woman who came to him suffering from rheumatoid arthritis. After having her amalgam fillings removed, she not only had relief from her arthritis, but her allergies abated to a large extent.

Another patient of Dr. Taylor's was suffering from numerous symptoms of environmental illness. She exhibited multiple sclerosis–type symptoms, could only tolerate four or five foods, and developed sensitivities to chemicals, noise, light, and electromagnetic radiation. She also had jaundice and had been diagnosed with yeast overgrowth. After having her amalgam fillings

CALIFORNIA AND MAINE DENTISTS REQUIRED TO WARN OF MERCURY HAZARDS

On November 15, 2000, the judge of the Superior Court of California, in San Francisco, signed a consent decree that marks a true milestone in California's dental treatments. In a landmark decision, the judge ruled that, beginning on February 15, 2001, patients must be informed of the link between birth defects and silver-mercury dental fillings, in order to be in compliance with Proposition 65. "This is a turnaround from the American Dental Association's policy (which is still current) that silver-mercury amalgams are safe and that any dentist who suggests otherwise to his patients can have his license revoked," comments Hal Huggins, D.D.S., M.S.

Officially called "The Safe Drinking Water and Toxic Enforcement Act of 1986," Proposition 65 was overwhelmingly passed by California voters in order to address growing concerns about exposure to toxic chemicals. As a result of the Superior Court's ruling, California dentists with more than ten employees must clearly post a sign in their office that reads "Warning: Amalgam Fillings Contain a Chemical Element Known to the State of California to Cause Birth Defects or Other Reproductive Harm."

"In spite of the proven connection between mercury and birth defects, the California Dental Association and allied industries fought to be exempted from having to post this warning," Dr. Huggins reports. Only after being sued, and then engaging in a series of legal battles, have they finally ceded the issue, due to the judge's ruling. Dr. Huggins points out that since the ruling only affects dentists with

ten or more employees, the law does provide a loophole. To address this problem, he advises that patients in California "ask if your dentist has fewer than ten employees, has posted the warning, or is hiding behind the loophole. This is a good way to determine your dentist's integrity."

On August 30, 2001, Maine Governor Angus King signed into law an even more comprehensive bill that requires all Maine dentists to display a poster and provide a brochure informing patients about the presence of mercury in amalgam fillings and about mercury's negative health effects. Maine Senate President Michael Michaud, who spearheaded the bill, said upon its passage, "We hope that the U.S. will take Maine's lead and move forward with legislation at the national level." Pam Anderson, a consumer advocate who played a leading role in mustering grassroots support of the bill, added that she hopes Maine will follow the law by banning the use of dental amalgams in all women of child-bearing age and in children.

As a result of these rulings, "Dentistry is bracing itself for a major change in the philosophy and methodology of randomly placing toxic substances in non-informed patients," Dr. Huggins says. "They are finding themselves potentially abandoned by the American Dental Association, their state organizations, their schools, their insurance companies, their patients, and even their own employees. The enforcement of these rules will almost certainly result in some dental group or organization being served up on a 'silver-mercury' platter."

removed, she found that she was able to eat many different foods again, enabling her to regain the 60 pounds she lost. Her sensitivities to noise, light, and electromagnetic radiation also diminished and her yeast infection and jaundice cleared up.

Bio-incompatibility to Dental Restoration Materials

In the same way that some people have adverse reactions to prescription drugs, some people also react negatively to specific dental materials. A person can already have been sensitized to dental restoration materials through previous exposure from the environment and foods, even breast milk. This bio-incompatibility (incompatibility of the body) to the dental material can lead to severe allergic reactions, including food allergies, and can contribute

to chronic fatigue syndrome, chronic sinusitis and headaches, neurological illnesses, disturbances of the immune system, chronic inflammatory changes (rheumatoid arthritis, phlebitis, and fibromyalgia), and intractable pain syndrome. However, dentists often don't test for sensitivity to dental restoration materials before placing them in their patients' mouths. The most common reactions are produced by the various metal components that make up mercury amalgams used for fillings, including mercury, copper, tin, zinc, and silver.[16]

Patients can be screened for sensitivity by a blood test based on the work of Douglas Swartzendruber, Ph.D., of the University of Colorado, at Colorado Springs. Working with Dr. Huggins in the 1980s to determine which dental materials were the most hazardous for health, Dr. Swartzendruber developed a technique

MERCURY POISONING

Because mercury is a cumulative poison, building up in the body with repeated exposure, its effects can be devastating.[17] Mercury can bind to the DNA (deoxyribonucleic acid) of cells, as well as to the cell membranes, distorting the cell surface markers and thus interfering with normal cell functions.[18] When this happens, the immune system no longer recognizes the cell as part of the body and will attack it. This can be the basis of many autoimmune diseases, such as multiple sclerosis and arthritis.

Mercury poisoning can also lead to symptoms such as anxiety, depression, confusion, irritability, and the inability to concentrate. It can cause kidney disease and cardiac and respiratory disorders. Multiple sclerosis patients have been found to have eight times higher levels of mercury in their cerebrospinal fluid (the fluid that surrounds the brain and spinal cord) as compared to neurologically healthy patients.[19]

Mercury poisoning often goes undetected for years because the symptoms do not necessarily suggest mercury as the initiating cause. For example, it is capable of producing symptoms indistinguishable from those of multiple sclerosis (MS)[20] and can mimic the symptoms of Lou Gehrig's disease (amyotrophic lateral sclerosis, or ALS, a syndrome marked by muscular weakness and atrophy due to degeneration of motor neurons of the spinal cord, medulla, and cortex).

Mercury can also produce allergic reactions with symptoms such as urticaria (an itchy rash), eczema, headaches, asthma, and digestive problems. The Environmental Protection Agency states that women chronically exposed to mercury vapor experience an increased frequency of menstrual disturbances and spontaneous abortions. A high mortality rate has also been observed among infants born to women who displayed symptoms of mercury poisoning.[21]

According to Hal Huggins, D.D.S., M.S., among the more common diseases related to mercury poisoning from dental amalgams are Alzheimer's disease, arthritis, cancer, diabetes, heart disease, leukemia, lupus, Parkinson's disease, and reproductive problems (including birth defects). "Mercury can pass through any tissue in the body," Dr. Huggins says. "It disrupts normal metabolism anywhere it goes, crossing the placental barrier and the blood-brain barrier; therefore, it can be involved in almost any disorder."

In the 1990s, Dr. Huggins interviewed 1,320 patients who were suffering from mercury toxicity. What follows is a list of symptoms and the percentage that responded to proper dental amalgam removal and mercury detoxification treatment: unexplained irritability (73.3%); frequent periods of depression (72%); numbness and tingling in arms and legs (67.3%); frequent urination (64.5%); chronic fatigue (63.1%); digestive problems (60.6%); memory problems (58%); unexplained rashes, skin irritation, or itching (40.4%); insomnia (36.4%); painful joints (35.5%); tachycardia (32.4%); and headaches (20.1%). "Contrary to patients with common medical diseases, mercury toxic patients may have 20 to 40 presenting symptoms and diseases," Dr. Huggins says. "This combination of multiple symptoms and diseases is one of the first things that differentiates mercury toxicity from other diseases. For this reason, successful treatment lies in a multidisciplined approach."

Dr. Huggins also points out that the same symptoms can be the result of exposure to nickel, which is found in removable partial dentures, crowns and bridges, orthodontic braces, children's "chrome crowns," and as a base under porcelain crowns. Exposure to toxins formed in root canals and cavitations (areas in the bone that did not heal after teeth were removed) can also create such symptoms, according to Dr. Huggins.

Dr. Huggins has also found that there is a clear relationship between mercury levels in patients and dramatic changes in their white blood cell (WBC) counts. White blood cells are the key operatives in the immune system's defense against foreign substances and disease-provoking agents. "Overly high WBC levels tend to come down and depressed levels tend to come up when mercury fillings are removed," Dr. Huggins reports. "Bear in mind that the normal range for WBCs is 4,500 to 10,500, with 5,500 being optimal. However, this level is increasingly achieved only by those who have no mercury fillings. For the rest of us, the highs are climbing and the lows are dropping. The norm for WBCs has been changing in the last 30 years and it may be due to increased mercury exposure. The evidence now shows that mercury amalgam fillings are the major source of mercury exposure for the general public, at rates six times higher than found in fish and seafood. In fact, the new copper dental amalgams, first introduced in 1976, release 50 times more mercury than the 'conventional' dental amalgams previously in use."

that identified each material's relative toxicity. Today, this test, which screens for the reactivity of approximately 1,000 dental materials, is available from Thomas Levy, M.D., J.D., at Peak Energy Performance, in Colorado Springs.

In this test, the patient's blood is exposed to the various components and by-products of dental materials to see if they provoke an immune reaction (antibody production). This information is then matched through a computer database to various dental products, enabling the dentist or physician to select safe products for each patient. Bio-incompatible and toxic materials already in the mouth can then be replaced with nonreactive materials. Applied kinesiology can also be used to test all materials and anesthetics before using them on patients. "Kinesiology tests for electrical compatibility of materials and the blood test measures immune compatibility," Dr. Huggins says.

After any dental material is removed, Dr. Huggins always recommends a thorough detoxification, since simply removing the fillings is not enough to rid the body of accumulated toxic materials that may continue to cause allergic reactions. He places his patients on a detoxification regimen that can include nutritional support, acupressure, and massage treatments. Chelating agents, such as EDTA (ethylenediaminetetraacetic acid) and vitamin C, can be used intravenously or in tablet form. He cautions, however, that any detoxification therapy should only be administered under the supervision of a qualified health professional and that detoxification procedures occur slowly. "Successful detoxification has a maximum speed and it simply cannot operate any faster," he says. "When toxins are released within the body, they do not disappear, but must be processed by the liver, kidneys or a removal procedure that bypasses these organs."

Dr. Huggins likens rapid detoxification to ramming a bulldozer at an apple tree and then trying to catch all of the falling apples. "Suppose 100 apples fall down, maybe you'll be able to catch two, while the rest fall everywhere," he says. "That is what happens with detoxification that proceeds too rapidly. Mercury comes out all over the body, and the body cannot get rid of it. The result is that you become re-toxified." Patients and physicians need to realize that detoxification is related to the ability of the body to eliminate, not to the dosage of detoxifying agents. To ensure that detoxification is occurring properly, Dr. Huggins recommends that patients be screened every few days with appropriate blood tests to monitor their red and white blood cell counts.

Electrogalvanism

Due to its mineral content, saliva in the mouth is electrically conductive. As a result, when saliva interacts with a dental restoration containing metal, a battery is created, causing an effect known as electrogalvanism. "Electrogalvanism is literally the electricity generated by a person's fillings," says Dr. Arana. "The saliva acts as a conductant and the dissimilar metal fillings then try to neutralize each other to balance out the electrical charge. This has the effect of causing toxic material from the fillings to erode, like the terminals of a battery, and leak into the body." Dr. Arana points out that even two similar amalgam fillings, if they were not placed on the same day, are likely to be of different compositions and therefore generate an electrical current between them. Even gold fillings or crowns are usually put over old fillings of a different metal, so electrogalvanism can even occur within a single tooth.

Since the teeth, the mouth, and the bone root all contain fluid, there are a variety of combinations that can determine where this electrical current flows. "It can go from a tooth to a muscle, a joint, an organ, and even to part of the brain, to the point where it can change the permeability of the blood-brain barrier," Dr. Arana states. "Electrogalvanism is frequently the cause of lack of concentration and memory, insomnia, psychological problems, tinnitus, vertigo, epilepsy, hearing loss, and eye problems, to name but a few." Since high dental currents lead to erosion of the restoration materials, this problem rarely exists without coexisting problems of heavy metal toxicity, which can act synergistically with multiple chemical sensitivities to cause environmental illness.

Electrogalvanism can be identified by an instrument known as an electrogalvanometer, which measures the electrical current and voltage generated by the dental amalgam. Applied kinesiology can also be used to test for electrogalvanism between the upper and lower teeth. If the indicator muscle becomes weak when the patient gently touches the upper teeth to the lower teeth, then metal fillings from the top are forming a circuit with metal fillings on the bottom. Since high dental currents create neurological stress, the muscle becomes weak as soon as one metal touches another. Likewise, when the teeth are apart, and the circuit is broken, the indicator muscle will become strong again.

"We suspect that the reason why many dental splints, even bad ones, often improve a patient's TMJ dysfunction problem is that these splints are made out of plastic and work like a circuit-breaker whenever they are in place," Dr. Arana says. "The TMJ problems that improve are really problems created by high dental currents."

Temporomandibular Joint (TMJ) Syndrome

TMJ dysfunction is caused by the misalignment of the teeth, jaws, and muscles. The symptoms of TMJ dys-

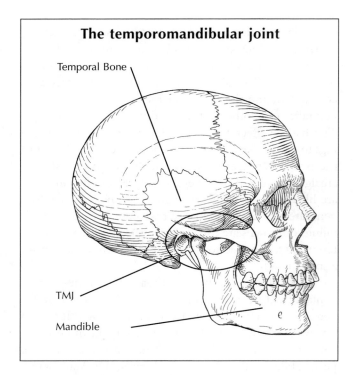

The temporomandibular joint

Temporal Bone

TMJ

Mandible

function vary and include pain, clicking or grating sounds when the mouth opens, and difficulty opening the mouth very wide. TMJ dysfunction can occur for three reasons. First, the patient loses teeth through decay or trauma, or loses height of some teeth through bruxism (grinding) or age. Or there are iatrogenic (treatment-induced) problems such as dental restorations that make the teeth either too high or too low. The other cause can be developmental problems. "In the last 200 years, developmental abnormalities of the upper and/or lower jaw have become very common. This has been directly linked to the intake of processed foods, especially sugar and flour," noted Dr. Price.[22]

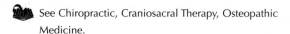 See Chiropractic, Craniosacral Therapy, Osteopathic Medicine.

Because chewing is the primary mechanism necessary for supplying nutrients to the body, if the jaws or teeth are out of alignment, the entire cranium will distort in order to chew properly. The structural compensations necessary for this readjustment can be responsible for such varied symptoms as depression, loss of concentration, insomnia, headaches, neck pain, and low back pain—all caused by TMJ dysfunction.

TMJ dysfunction is diagnosed by observation of symmetry of facial features, midline shift of teeth, asymmetric wear of dental surfaces, asymmetry of jaw movement, tenderness over joints, and tenderness in associated muscles. It can also be diagnosed by X rays, arthrograms (joint X rays), MRI (magnetic resonance imaging), computerized motion studies, applied kinesiology, and electrodermal screening.

Dr. Ravins believes balancing the jaw is essential to relieving TMJ dysfunction. Using computerized technology, he can measure movements of the jaw and determine where irregularities lie. By using orthopedic appliances (similar to braces) worn in the mouth at night, the jaw can be realigned, relieving the symptoms. Other dentists use craniosacral therapy or cold laser therapy to help correct TMJ syndrome.

Biological Treatment of Dental Problems

Biological dentists treat dental problems in a variety of ways. In addition to stressing the use of nontoxic restoration materials for dental work, they focus on the impact of dental toxins and hidden dental infections on health. As we've seen, biological dentists are concerned with the safe removal of mercury amalgam fillings. They also investigate cavitations as a source of bodywide illness and seek to safely correct the misalignment of teeth and jaw structures. They emphasize the conservation of all healthy tooth material and employ the latest techniques of bioenergetic medicine, including neural therapy, oral acupuncture, cold laser therapy, homeopathy, mouth balancing, and diet and nutrition.

Neural Therapy

According to the principles of neural therapy, the body is charged with electricity or biological energy. This energy flows throughout the body, with every cell possessing its own specified frequency range. As long as this energy flow is unimpeded and stays within its normal range, the body will remain healthy. However, if this balance breaks down, disruptions in the normal function of cells can occur, eventually leading to chronic disorders.

When injury, inflammation, or infection is present in the mouth, there is usually a corresponding blockage in the body's normal energy flow. "Neural therapy allows the dentist to confirm if the problem in the tooth is causing illness elsewhere in the body," says Dr. Arana. The problem may lie in the tooth itself or in a distant organ on the same energy meridian as the tooth. Injection of a local anesthetic (such as procaine) around the tooth to remove the energy blockage will often resolve the problem.

 See Neural Therapy, Traditional Chinese Medicine.

Oral Acupuncture

Oral acupuncture, according to Jochen Gleditsch, M.D., D.D.S., of Munich, Germany, has been taught to dentists since 1976 and its use is expanding rapidly. It involves

THE HEALTH RISKS OF FLUORIDATION

Fluoride is commonplace today in toothpaste, mouthwash, and drinking water. In the U.S., over 121 million people are now drinking fluoridated water. Many experts argue that it poses a serious health risk. Fluoride is a known poison and is classified as very toxic to extremely toxic in the National Library of Medicine's computerized data service on toxic substances. Numerous studies have demonstrated that fluorides are retained in the body and can build up to poisonous concentrations.[23] "An enormous body of research documenting the toxic effects of acute and prolonged fluoride ingestion can readily be found in the medical library," says Thomas E. Levy, M.D., J.D., co-author of *Uninformed Consent: The Hidden Dangers of Dental Care.* "However, no amount of data seems to impress the fluoride proponents to even consider that fluoride's toxic effects need to be taken seriously." Researchers in Holland found that fluoride increases the frequency of genetic damage in sperm cells of animals exposed to X rays and inhibits the repair of DNA.[24]

Fluoride was first introduced into the public water systems in the U.S. in 1945 through an experiment based on research by H. Trendley Dean, D.D.S., the father of fluoridation, for the Public Health Service. Dr. Dean was trying to determine the reason some people had higher than normal levels of staining of their teeth. He cited fluoride as the cause of the staining, but also credited fluoride as the reason these same people had fewer cavities.[25] In 1950, the Public Health Service recommended using artificial fluoridation in the public water systems to fight tooth decay. Since the time fluoride entered the water system, there have been many health-related problems linked to its use but no statistically significant reduction in tooth decay. Dr. Dean himself has twice been forced to admit in court that his original statistics favoring fluoridation were invalid.[26]

Christa Danielson, M.D., found an increased risk of hip fracture in men and women over age 65 who had been exposed to fluoride in their drinking water for 20 years. At least 10% of fluoride in adults is deposited in bones and studies have shown a positive correlation between higher fluoride intake and decreased bone mass and strength.[27] In 1975, John Yiamouyiannis, M.D., and Dean Burk, M.D., compared ten large U.S. cities that fluoridated their water with ten cities that did not. They discovered a link between fluoride and a 10% increase in cancer deaths over a period of 13-17 years. Further tests confirmed that fluoride added to water causes cancer in laboratory animals.[28]

In spite of these findings, fluoride is still commonplace in the U.S. today. It has, however, been banned in Austria, Denmark, France, Greece, Italy, Luxembourg, the Netherlands, Norway, and Spain. Recently, Canada's foremost promoter of fluoridation, Dr. Hardy Limeback, head of Preventive Dentistry, University of Toronto, and President of the Canadian Association of Dental Research, told his colleagues and students that he had unintentionally misled them. "For the past 15 years," he stated, "I had refused to study the toxicology information readily available to anyone. Poisoning our children was the furthest thing from my mind."

Among the findings that finally opened Dr. Limeback's eyes was a study at the University of Toronto that confirmed that "residents of cities that fluoridate have double the fluoride in their hip bones vis-a-vis the balance of the population. Worse, we discovered that fluoride is actually altering the basic structure of bones." Skeletal fluorosis is a debilitating condition that occurs when fluoride accumulates in bones, making them extremely weak and brittle. According to Dr. Limeback, the earliest symptoms of the condition are mottled and brittle teeth. "In Canada, we are now spending more money treating dental fluorosis than we do treating cavities," he says.

Dr. Levy adds that dental fluorosis is the one toxic side effect of fluoride that even its proponents acknowledge as real. "This condition reliably occurs whenever a large enough and long enough exposure to fluoride and its associated compounds occurs during the period when tooth enamel is actively forming," he says. "Teeth can become mottled and spotted, discolored, pitted, or even completely disfigured, depending upon the degree of fluoride exposure."

In 1985, the American Dental Association's Council on Scientific Affairs recommended that no fluoride supplementation should be given to babies from birth to six months of age, even if the local public water supply had not been fluoridated.[29] "This begs a very important question," Dr. Levy says. "How can any community fluoridate its public water supply and still protect all the babies under six months of age, as currently advised by the ADA?" Another official recommendation by the Council is that children younger than age six should be advised not to use a toothpaste containing more than 1,100 parts per million of fluoride.[30] "Yet, there are few pro-fluoride dentists who exhibit any restraint in promoting fluoride intake," Dr. Levy points out.

"It is of the utmost importance in America that the science of fluoridation gets introduced to the politics of fluoridation," he adds. "New research is not really needed to expose the many dangers of water fluoridation. Instead, following the current published recommendations in the mainstream dental literature would go a long way toward resolving the continuing insanity of fluoridating everybody's water."

the injection of saline water, weak local anesthetics, or sterile complex homeopathic remedies into specific acupuncture points of the oral mucous membrane. It can also be combined with neural therapy. Drs. Arana and Ravins use oral acupuncture to relieve pain during dental procedures with great success. Some dentists also use it to relax patients before any dental procedure. Toothaches, tooth sensitivities, jaw pain, gingivitis, and other local problems often respond to oral acupuncture.

Dr. Gleditsch discovered that there are specific oral acupuncture points related to each tooth. "The total of these oral acupuncture points forms a complete microsystem," he explains, "with a clear reference to the system of acupuncture meridians." When a particular acupuncture meridian is under stress, the corresponding oral acupuncture point(s) become very sensitive to localized pressure. This phenomenon can be used for both diagnostic and treatment purposes, according to Dr. Gleditsch. He commonly uses acupoints in the mouth to treat neuralgia, sinusitis, pain in distant parts of the body, allergic conditions, and digestive disorders. Since needle acupuncture is impractical within the oral cavity due to the danger of choking, Dr. Gleditsch uses injections of saline or local anesthetic into the points. Laser stimulation can also be used.

Cold Laser Therapy

Cold laser therapy is an alternative form of acupuncture that is especially useful for treating patients who object to the use of needles. The "cold laser" gets its name from the fact that its power output and the light spectrum it uses are incapable of causing any thermal damage to tissues. This therapy kills bacteria, aids in wound healing, reduces inflammation, and helps to rebalance the flow of energy in the body's meridian system. It has also been used to treat TMJ dysfunction[31] and to promote healing and reduce muscle spasm after removal of impacted wisdom teeth, according to Dr. Ravins.

 See Homeopathy, Light Therapy, Nutritional Medicine.

Homeopathy

"Homeopathic remedies can help alleviate the pain or discomfort of dental emergencies, at least temporarily, until proper dental care can be received," according to Dr. Fischer. "They are not intended to replace regular dental care, but rather to serve as a safe and effective complement."

- Abscesses can be treated with homeopathic dilutions of *Belladonna, Hepar sulph., Silicea, Myristica,* and *Calendula.*

- *Gelsemium, Aconite, Coffea cruda,* and *Chamomilla* can be used to allay the apprehension of a visit to the dentist.

- Post-surgical bleeding is treated with *Phosphorous* and, if accompanied by bruising and soreness, with *Arnica.*

- *Chamomilla* is good for a dry socket after an extraction.

- A toothache can be treated with *Belladonna, Magnesium phos., Coffea cruda,* or *Chamomilla.*

Mouth Balancing

Dr. Ravins specializes in balancing the mouth to improve a wide range of health problems, including TMJ dysfunction. He believes that structural deformities of the skull influence the entire body. "With new computerized technology, I can diagnose muscle dysfunction and pick up vibrations from the jaw and movement of the mandible," he says. Often the misalignment has been caused by a prior accident. By analyzing this data and making special orthopedic braces to be worn in the mouth, Dr. Ravins can realign the jaw and remove pain and other symptoms such as headaches, shoulder pain, and back problems.

Many patients who come to Dr. Ravins complain of eye problems such as blurred vision (often occurring after eating) and pressure and pain behind the eyes. Since the bones around the eyes are close to those of the jaw, a misaligned jaw can easily put pressure on the eyes themselves. Stress in the mouth can also affect the nerves and blood supply to the eyes, and infections in the mouth can cause muscle spasms that will affect the eyes. According to Dr. Ravins, once any misalignments in the mouth are corrected with orthopedic braces, the eye problems usually dissipate. The problems often return though, when the appliances are removed. While eye problems should always be checked by an eye doctor first, if the problem is not uncovered by an eye examination, a biological dentist may be able to help.

Diet and Nutrition

Diet is an important factor in dental health, a fact proven by Dr. Price at the beginning of the 20th century. During that time, he visited aboriginal people and photographed their dental arches, noting their rate of tooth decay before and after going off their native diet and consuming refined foods and sugars. Within two generations following this dietary change, the dental arch went from wide jaws with perfect tooth alignment to narrow jaws

DENTAL HEALTH AND AGING

"If you want to live a long, healthy life, then you should try your best to keep as many of your natural teeth as you can," states Harold Ravins, D.D.S., who has observed during more than 30 years of dental practice that his healthiest patients are those who have the most natural teeth. "I know for a fact that missing your natural teeth is one of the greatest causes of premature aging." The reason for this, according to Dr. Ravins, is that life flows from the teeth. "When any of your 32 original teeth are lost, a small bit of your life is lost also," he says. "If there is a 'master plan' for the human body, surely it includes a life lived with all 32 teeth intact, and not for people to be wearing dentures at age 40."

Dr. Ravins's golden rule of dentistry is to save a tooth at all costs. Dr. Ravins likens the teeth to the keys on a typewriter operating 24 hours a day as the terminal endings of sensory nerve pathways. "When you extract a tooth, you leave a pathway with no terminal ending, and this alters nerve reflexes for the worse," he says. "On the other hand, when you restore the tooth's enamel surface with a filling or crown, you also alter the way this tooth works as a sensory receptor for the body. This means any change you make to a tooth must be physiologically compatible with the patient's nervous system."

Dr. Ravins also points out that the teeth are connected to the brain and, as a consequence, are constantly stimulating it, something that false teeth cannot do. "The fewer natural teeth, the less stimulation to the central nervous system—the less neural stimulation, the more aging," he says. "I contend that the relationship between teeth and the brain is one of the most important areas in all dentistry."

The teeth help support facial structure as well, especially around the lips. Poor dental structure (worn-down, crooked, or missing teeth) or a poor bite can often result in facial lines and wrinkles. "When your teeth are missing or excessively worn down, you will lack what dentists call sufficient 'vertical dimension' to support the facial skin," Dr. Ravins explains. "This means your face may develop lines and wrinkles and that 'caved-in' look so prevalent in the elderly."

The stress caused to the entire body from missing teeth is often the most severe kind of stress your body can experience, according to Dr. Ravins. "When natural teeth are missing, your face may experience less than adequate blood circulation, which is why many people with excessive dental problems sport a pale and pasty look to their facial skin." Dr. Ravins's advice is simple: the more natural teeth you have, and the more missing teeth you have replaced (so there are no gaps), the better the skin and facial structure will look and the better you will feel. He recommends that patients who need to replace a tooth that has been out for many years be sure to have their dentists first pretreat the mouth by repositioning any teeth that may have moved from their original position.

He believes in doing everything possible to save existing teeth, even if it's inconvenient. "If a person had a tooth pulled instead of saving it with a full crown, she would lose not only the tooth, but the tooth's root," he says. "When a root is extracted from the jaw, the jaw will become that much smaller and narrower as it fills in the area from the extracted root. One of the ways to live a longer life is to have as wide a jaw as possible. Dentally speaking, the big mouths live the longest."

---

with crooked teeth. The decay rate went from one cavity for every ten people to ten cavities per person.

Dr. Huggins, like many other biological dentists, makes nutritional supplementation part of his overall protocol for dealing with dental conditions, especially for the patient recovering from mercury amalgam toxicity. "There is a standard regimen we use to help correct basic chemistry problems," he says. "From there, we might use additional supplementation based on what the patient's chemistry dictates." According to Dr. Huggins, the basic supplementation program aids in the excretion of mercury from the cells, prevents the exacerbation of symp-

toms, and provides the patient with a nutrient base for rebuilding damaged tissues.

Dr. Huggins relies upon blood chemistries, complete blood count, urinalysis, hair analysis, and other biological testing to determine what supplements a patient might require to attain a balanced chemistry. He then uses follow-up tests to determine if the supplement doses are correct or need to be adjusted.

A proper diet is important for patients suffering from mercury toxicity if the body is to undertake repair. "Blood chemistries can be used to determine the amount of carbohydrate, fat, and protein each individual requires in their diet for maximum efficiency," Dr. Huggins says.

THE POLITICS OF DENTISTRY

Although many new techniques of biological dentistry are available, only 2,000 to 3,000 dentists across the U.S. are using them in practice. This is due to a deliberate effort by the American Dental Association (ADA) to suppress such practices, even to the point of rescinding the licenses of practitioners using them. Electrodermal screening by dentists is not allowed in some states and dentists may lose their license for using it, despite its proven effectiveness for screening hidden infections under teeth. Dental acupuncture is also banned in some states.

In 1987, the ADA wrote a provision into their code to declare the removal of clinically serviceable mercury amalgams from patients' teeth to be unethical, according to Michael Ziff, D.D.S., of Orlando, Florida. Any dentist doing so is in violation of the code and the ADA is assisting state boards in prosecuting these dentists, despite all the evidence of mercury toxicity.

The financial and legal implications of an admission by the ADA that mercury is toxic and harmful to health may be a possible motive behind this move. If the ADA admitted that mercury amalgams are a health hazard, insurance companies or the government would possibly have to pay for the removal of mercury amalgams from practically the entire population of the U.S. Another possibility is raised by Hal Huggins, D.D.S., M.S., who asks, "Could the fact that the ADA owns the patents for amalgam have anything to do with their resistance to admitting that mercury may have caused most of the incurable diseases of the past century?"

Another interesting point, Dr. Huggins continues, "is that, until 1984, the ADA code of ethics stated that if any dentist discovered something that was either beneficial or detrimental to dentists or patients, he or she was obligated to inform both the profession and the public. Following a talk I gave in July 1984 to dental scientists at the ADA's headquarters about the damaging effects of mercury fillings, that portion of the code was removed and replaced with the new ethics code, which says that if a dentist removes mercury fillings due to the health risk aspect, he or she is unethical and subject to license revocation. Since then, many dentists have lost their licenses or been put on probation for suggesting that mercury could be hazardous. In addition, just before I made my presentation, the ADA issued a press release describing the meeting and claiming that the ADA had 'reaffirmed the safety of amalgam.' Despite this assurance, after my presentation all dental amalgam manufacturers increased their product liability insurance by 1,000%."

At present, according to Dr. Huggins, "No dental publication will carry articles on mercury toxicity, no dentist is allowed to tell a patient that mercury is toxic, and no lecturer is allowed to mention it in front of dentists. How does this constitute interest in patients' or dentists' health, permit freedom of speech and opinion, advance the science of dentistry, or allow dentists, in the ADA's own words, to 'know the potential hazards and symptoms of mercury exposure'?"

Despite this ominous situation, the growing number of research studies on biological dental techniques, the information coming out of Europe and Canada on mercury toxicity,[32] and increasing public awareness of the dangers of traditional dental practices are combining to build support for the small number of dentists risking their livelihood to practice safe dentistry in the U.S.

"Periodic blood tests can then be used to tell how the body is progressing in its healing ability and when supplements or the diet itself need to be altered again."

The Future of Biological Dentistry

Mercury and other dental materials contribute to many of the degenerative diseases for which patients seek medical help today. Traditional dentistry and medicine have not yet recognized this growing danger, but biological dentistry is confronting it head-on. Using all the knowledge and skills of conventional dental medicine along with alternative health therapies, biological dentists are striving to provide individuals with biocompatible, aesthetic, comfortable, functional, and enduring dental work.

While much research has already been done on mercury toxicity from dental amalgams, and on the creation of safe, nontoxic alternatives, much more still needs to be done, especially in the U.S. Dr. Randolph believed that medicine and dentistry must come together to solve the mercury problem and make dentistry a health-enhancing endeavor that eliminates, instead of promotes, disease.

"The emphasis must be more in the way of prevention," says Dr. Arana. "So when people in the anti-amalgam movement say we're going to have to retrain the dentists, they're right, but it can be done. I think the materials used now are very close to being able to fix teeth so they're white and beautiful without any danger of toxicity problems."

Toxic-free, biological dental treatment has the possibility of an overall stress reduction so great that patients could lose all or many of their distressing chronic disease symptoms. "The next great advancement in medicine will come from dentists," says Dr. Arana. "Biological dentistry will, out of necessity, become the dental medicine of the 21st century."

Where to Find Help

Many organizations and dentists are involved in promoting the practice of biological dentistry. Contact an organization below for more information.

Advanced Health Research Institute

211 South State College Blvd., Suite 316
Anaheim, California 92806
(888) 792-1102
Website: www.ahrinstitute.com

AHRI is a nonprofit organization founded by Richard Hansen, D.M.D., to help individuals obtain information about laser dentistry and to locate a laser dentistry practitioner in their area.

American Academy of Biological Dentistry (AABD)

P.O. Box 856
Carmel Valley, California 93924
(831) 659-5385
Website: www.biologicaldentistry.org

The purpose of the AABD is to promote biological dental medicine, which uses nontoxic diagnostic and therapeutic approaches. They publish a quarterly journal and hold regular seminars on biological diagnosis and therapy.

DAMS

P.O. Box 7249
Minneapolis, Minnesota 55407-0249
(800) 311-6265

DAMS (Dental Amalgam Mercury Syndrome) is a support and educational organization designed to help those suffering from mercury amalgam toxicity, to raise public awareness of the problem, and to provide documentation of the condition to the U.S. Food and Drug Administration.

Environmental Dental Association

9974 Scripps Ranch Blvd., Suite 36
San Diego, California 92131
(800) 388-8124

The EDA is an organization of alternative dentists who are concerned about the potential toxic effects of various dental procedures and materials. Member dentists believe that the most important environment of all is the human body and that some dentistry can cause harmful side effects. The EDA provides a referral service for patients seeking alternative dentists in their area and also offers books and products on alternative dentistry for the public.

Fluoride Action Network

Website: www.fluoridealert.org

An online international coalition that seeks to end water fluoridation and alert people to fluoride's health and environmental risks.

Holistic Dental Association

P.O. Box 5007
Durango, Colorado 81301
(970) 259-1091
Website: www.holisticdental.org

Advocacy group promoting holistic approaches to dentistry. Membership is open to dentists, physicians, and other healthcare practitioners, as well as the general public.

International Academy of Oral Medicine and Toxicology (IAOMT)

P.O. Box 608531
Orlando, Florida 32860-8531
(407) 298-2450
Website: www.iaomt.org

A professional organization of dentists, physicians, and research scientists worldwide dedicated to scientifically investigating the biocompatibility of materials used in dentistry.

Matrix, Inc.

P.O. Box 49145
Colorado Springs, Colorado 80949
(866) 948-4638 or (719) 522-0566
Website: www.hugnet.com

The official information center for Dr. Huggins's research on multidisciplinary approaches for treating dentally toxic patients and autoimmune diseases. Also makes available all of Dr. Huggins's books, audio and videotapes, educational booklets, and recommended nutritional supplements.

Peak Energy Performance, Inc. (PEP)
4680 Edison Avenue, Suite A
Colorado Springs, Colorado 80915
(800) 331-2303 or (719) 548-1600
Website: www.peakenergy.com

PEP offers help to people who are seeking to avoid toxins and reach better states of health. In particular, PEP seeks to increase awareness of the effects of dental toxicity on health. For those who decide to minimize their exposure to dental toxins, PEP assists in finding the safest way to achieve this goal.

Safe Water Coalition
5615 West Lyons Court
Spokane, Washington 99208
(509) 328-6704

The purpose of this organization is to educate legislators and the public on the hazards of fluoridation.

Recommended Reading

The Complete Guide to Mercury Toxicity from Dental Fillings. Joyal Taylor. San Diego, CA: Scripps Publishing, 1988.

Dental Mercury Detox. Sam and Michael Ziff. Orlando, FL: Bio-Probe, 1993.

Dentistry Without Mercury. Sam and Michael Ziff. Orlando, FL: Bio-Probe, 1993.

Fluoride, The Aging Factor. John Yiamouyiannis, Ph.D. Delaware, OH: Health Action Press, 1986.

Infertility and Birth Defects: Is Mercury from Silver Dental Fillings a Hidden Cause? Sam and Michael Ziff. Orlando, FL: Bio-Probe, 1987.

It's All in Your Head: The Link Between Mercury Amalgams and Illness. Hal Huggins, D.D.S. New York: Avery/Penguin Putnam, 1993.

The Key to Ultimate Health. Ellen Hodgson Brown and Richard Hansen. Fullerton, CA: Advanced Health Research Publishing, 2000.

Mercury Poisoning from Dental Amalgam: A Hazard to the Human Brain. Patrick Stortebecker, M.D., Ph.D. Orlando, FL: Bio-Probe, 1986.

The Missing Link. Sam and Michael Ziff. Orlando, FL: Bio-Probe, 1992.

Silver Dental Fillings: The Toxic Time Bomb. Sam Ziff. Santa Fe, NM: Aurora Press, 1986.

Uninformed Consent: The Hidden Dangers of Dental Care. Hal Huggins, D.D.S., and Thomas Levy, M.D., J.D. Charlottesville, VA: Hampton Roads Publishing, 1999.

BODYWORK

The term bodywork *refers to a wide range of therapies, such as massage, deep tissue manipulation, movement awareness, and bioenergetic therapies, which are employed to improve the structure and functioning of the body. The benefits of bodywork in all its forms include pain reduction, relief of musculoskeletal tension, improved blood and lymphatic circulation, and promoting deep relaxation.*

FOR CENTURIES, the therapeutic use of touch has been applied to heal the body and reduce the tensions of daily life. Today, there are over 100 schools of bodywork, from therapeutic massage to structural bodywork therapies like Rolfing® and Hellerwork that employ deep tissue techniques to restructure the body. Movement therapies, such as the Feldenkrais Method™ and the Alexander Technique, help realign the body through the correction of postural imbalances to promote more efficient function of the nervous system. Pressure point therapies apply pressure on various areas of the body to relieve pain and restore proper energy flow. Bioenergetic systems of bodywork, such as acupressure, polarity therapy, Therapeutic Touch™, and Reiki, help balance energy in the body and bring about enhanced health and well-being. Bodywork approaches within the field of somatic psychology focus on the interrelationship between body (soma) and mind (psyche). The majority of bodywork practitioners employ a combination of bodywork methods.

 See Energy Medicine, Mind/Body Medicine.

Therapeutic Massage

Within the past two decades, an overwhelming accumulation of scientific evidence has supported the claim that massage therapy is beneficial.[1] According to John Yates, Ph.D., author of *A Physician's Guide to Therapeutic Massage,* massage can benefit conditions such as muscle spasms and pain, spinal curvature (lordosis, scoliosis), soreness related to injury and stress, headaches, whiplash, temporomandibular joint (TMJ) syndrome, and tension-related respiratory disorders (bronchial asthma or emphysema). Massage can also help reduce swelling, help correct posture, improve body motion, and facilitate the elimination of toxins from the body.[2] Lymphatic massage, for example, can move metabolic wastes through the body to promote a rapid recovery from illness or disease.

Other studies show that massage can be used as an adjunct in the treatment of cardiovascular disorders and neurological and gynecological problems and can often be used in place of pharmacological drugs.[3] Other conditions for which therapeutic massage has shown benefit include arthritis, carpal tunnel syndrome, gastrointestinal disorders, and insomnia.[4] According to the Quebec Task Force on Spinal Disorders, massage is the most frequently used therapy for musculoskeletal problems and is particularly useful in controlling pain.[5]

Because of its many benefits, therapeutic massage is an increasingly popular part of physical therapy practices, nursing practices, and sports medicine clinics. It is also the most commonly used form of bodywork in the U.S., used by an estimated 20 million Americans each year.[6] In addition, a survey of conventional primary care physicians and family practitioners conducted in 1998 found that 54% encouraged their patients to pursue therapeutic massage as a treatment.[7]

Gertrude Beard, R.N., R.P.T., former Associate Professor of Physical Therapy at Northwestern University Medical School, in Chicago, Illinois, summarizes the findings of numerous research studies on the therapeutic effects of massage. Studies indicate that massage:

- Has a sedative effect upon the nervous system and promotes voluntary muscle relaxation.

- Is effective in promoting recovery from fatigue produced by excessive exercise.

119

Because of its many benefits, therapeutic massage is an increasingly popular part of physical therapy practices, nursing practices, and sports medicine clinics.

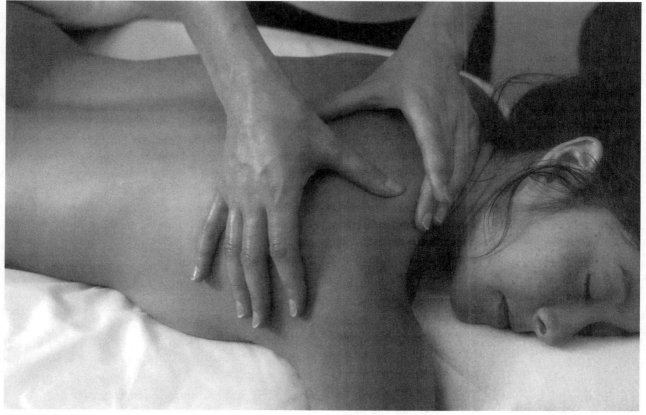

- Can help break up scar tissue and lessen fibrosis and adhesions, which develop as a result of injury and immobilization.

- Can relieve certain types of pain.

- Provides effective treatment of chronic inflammatory conditions by increasing lymphatic circulation.

- Helps reduce swelling from fractures.

- Affects circulation through the capillaries, veins, and arteries, and increases blood flow through the muscles.

- Can loosen mucus and promote drainage of fluids from the lungs by using percussive and vibratory techniques.

- Can increase peristaltic action (muscular contractions) in the intestines to promote fecal elimination.[8]

Researchers have also found that certain massage techniques can trigger reflex actions in the body to stimulate organs. Beard adds that these should only be applied under the direction of a knowledgeable physician or physical therapist.

How Massage Releases Tension and Promotes Relaxation

Muscle tension, whether from normal activity or from awkward movement or stress, contributes to muscle fatigue and pain by compressing nerve fibers in the muscle. Prolonged contraction interferes with the elimination of chemical wastes in the muscles and surrounding tissues and can cause frequent nerve and muscle pain. If not properly addressed, these body tensions have a tendency to build into chronic patterns of stress.

Prolonged tension can often cause pain in other parts of the body. For example, headaches are often caused by overly tense muscles in the neck, shoulders, and lower back. Even contracted abdominal muscles can trigger headaches in certain people (a common complaint of women with menstrual difficulties).

For these tension-related conditions, Robert D. Milne, M.D., of Las Vegas, Nevada, an expert on headache relief, finds that massage can break up muscular waste deposits and stimulate circulation. He adds that accumulated metabolic wastes often form "trigger points" within muscles. These are specific areas that are painful to the touch. "They feel like knots or rope within the muscle and perpetuate muscle tension," explains Dr. Milne. By applying deep pressure to these points, the tension or spasm can often be eliminated.

Common Types of Therapeutic Massage

Swedish Massage—Swedish massage is the most common form of massage therapy in the U.S. Swedish massage therapists use a combination of stroking, kneading, and friction techniques over the full body, working specifically on the superficial skin layers of muscles. Practitioners and clients determine which areas of the body to focus on and which elements to employ. The primary benefits of Swedish massage are numerous: it promotes general relaxation, improved circulation, relief from muscle tension, restored flexibility, and the elimination of waste products in the tissues. Sessions usually last an hour and can be done in conjunction with hydrotherapy to enhance the benefits.

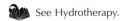 See Hydrotherapy.

Deep Tissue Massage—Deep tissue massage employs more direct pressure on deeper muscle layers. Therapists use slow strokes and friction techniques as they work against the grain of the muscles. Although clients often feel sore immediately following sessions, deep tissue massage is highly effective on lower back pain and on chronically tight muscles.

Sports Massage—Sports massage is no longer the luxury of elite athletes. Today, it is an effective way to remain healthy and injury free whether you are a professional athlete or just a weekend exerciser. Sports therapists are readily available in health clubs, spas, and exercise facilities, as well as on college campuses. Sessions combine deep tissue with Swedish massage techniques. Sports massage has many benefits, from easing muscle aches and pains to enhancing performance before sporting events. It can also restore muscle tone and mobility after vigorous workouts and eliminate the buildup of lactic acid, which causes pain and stiffness.

Lymphatic Massage—Lymphatic massage focuses on improving the circulation of the lymphatic system, a body-wide network of vessels and lymph nodes. By stimulating lymph flow by lightly stroking the primary areas of the body through which lymph fluid is filtered (neck, armpits, upper torso, and groin), practitioners help prevent lymph congestion, thereby ensuring that the body's cells receive adequate levels of life-enriching oxygen. Some massage therapists may also employ energy devices, such as the Light Beam Generator, to further stimulate lymph flow.

 See Energy Medicine.

 Therapeutic massage may be contraindicated for certain forms of cancer, some forms of heart disease, infectious diseases, certain skin conditions, and phlebitis. If you suffer from such conditions, consult with your physician before receiving massage therapy.

Bodywork: A New Approach to Awareness and Physical Health

The contemporary systems of bodywork are as concerned with relaxation and physical therapy as are the traditional schools of massage. Designations such as neuromuscular therapy, connective tissue massage, myofascial therapy, trigger point massage, and soft tissue manipulation further distinguish these contemporary systems. However, most are based on one or more of the following principles or techniques:

- The use of pressure or deep friction to alter the muscular and soft tissue structures

- The use of movement to affect physiological structure and functioning

- The use of education and awareness to change or enhance physiological functioning

- The use of breathing and emotional expression to eliminate tension and to change physiological functioning

The following categories of bodywork represent some of the most influential practitioners, theories, and techniques in the field today.

 By addressing tension, stress, and structural imbalances in the body, bodywork can be an important part of a health maintenance program and can reduce long-term health costs.

Movement Reeducation Therapies

Bodywork approaches in this category can help improve body function by addressing the way habitual movement patterns (walking, standing, sitting) impact health. By training people to become more aware of their bodies and the way they move, practitioners help to improve posture, balance, and ease of movement, resulting in enhanced feelings of well-being.

ALEXANDER TECHNIQUE

Frederick Matthias Alexander was one of the first people to notice how faulty posture in daily activities (sitting, standing, moving) is connected with serious physical and emotional problems. Alexander pioneered a simple, effective approach to rebalancing the body through awareness, movement, and touch. A Shakespearean actor, Alexander began to experience a recurring loss of his voice while on stage. When he studied himself in a mirror, he discovered that he unconsciously and habitually moved his head back and down, tensed his neck and throat, and sucked in his breath whenever he thought of using his voice. From his observations, Alexander developed a method that used his breath to alter this habitual muscular response, and he eventually recovered his voice. This marked the beginning of the Alexander Technique.

Alexander was aware that the correct relationship of one's head, neck, and back is essential for proper movement and functioning. He observed that people habitually misuse their bodies for such mundane activities as sitting or standing, and Alexander helped his students become conscious of these faulty habits and postures. He taught how to interrupt or inhibit familiar postural "sets" that corresponded to these recurring habits so that the body could be guided to allow improved motion, balance, and posture. "Most people have lost good use of their bodies by the time they are past early childhood," states Wilfred Barlow, author of *The Alexander Technique.* Poor or inhibited use of the body can contribute to many diseases, including debilitating curvatures of the spine, rheumatism, arthritis, and a variety of gastrointestinal and breathing disorders.[9] According to Barlow, all of these can be positively affected by learning how to properly hold and use the body.

> *Most people have lost good use of their bodies by the time they are past early childhood.*

In the early 1970s, experiments conducted by Frank Pierce Jones at Tufts University, in Boston, Massachusetts, concluded that the Alexander Technique could effectively interrupt or inhibit habitual and learned responses that interfere with proper body functioning. By doing so, it allows for a restoration of natural balance and responsiveness during movement.[10] In a more recent study, women over the age of 65 who were taught the Alexander Technique showed improved balance, leading researchers to conclude that it could help reduce the incidence of falls in women of that age group.[11]

Preliminary research also indicates that the Alexander Technique is useful in helping patients cope with Parkinson's disease. In one study, seven patients with Parkinson's received an average of 12 sessions of instruction in the Alexander Technique. Following their training, all of them reported that they were significantly less depressed. In addition, they had "a significantly more positive body concept and had significantly less difficulty in performing daily activities."[12] Other research has shown that the Alexander Technique is beneficial for treating chronic back pain when incorporated as part of a multidisciplinary approach that also includes chiropractic, acupuncture, and psychological intervention.[13]

 See Acupuncture, Chiropractic.

In a typical session, a student may lie on a table, sit on a stool, or remain standing. The student may be given instructions such as "Let your head move forward and up to allow your torso to lengthen and widen." While saying this, the teacher gently prevents the old habit and encourages a new improved response of the head/neck/back relationship. During this time, the student is told to "do nothing"—the student simply thinks about the instruction given by the teacher. Eventually, the student constructs a new body image and by doing so retrains and reorganizes the way he or she moves.

Although the number of instructors trained in the Alexander Technique is comparatively small (fewer than 2,000), its popularity has spread around the world, including Australia, Europe, South America, South Africa, Canada, and Israel, in addition to the U.S. In Europe, there are many Alexander Technique teachers at various colleges, particularly in the departments of drama, speech, dance, and music. Athletes find the Alexander Technique helpful for improving their performance skills and for relief of chronic pain. Many well-known actors have also received training in the Alexander Technique because of the benefits it provides.

FELDENKRAIS METHOD

Moshe Feldenkrais was a physicist involved with nuclear radiation research and antisubmarine technology in

France and England. Like Alexander, personal trauma in the form of a sports-related injury drove him to explore the functioning of the body. Rather than submitting to the recommended surgery, he sought an alternative solution through the study of the nervous system and human behavior. Applying his experience of martial arts, physiology, anatomy, psychology, and neurology, Feldenkrais succeeded in reversing his impairment and taught himself how to walk without pain.

The notion of "self-image" is central to the theory and technique of Feldenkrais and his method. According to Feldenkrais, "Each one of us speaks, moves, thinks, and feels in a different way, each according to the image of himself that he has built up over the years. In order to change our mode of action, we must change the image of ourselves that we carry within us."[14]

Each one of us speaks, moves, thinks, and feels in a different way, each according to the image of himself that he has built up over the years. In order to change our mode of action, we must change the image of ourselves that we carry within us.

—MOSHE FELDENKRAIS

Feldenkrais viewed the human organism as a complex system of intelligence and function in which all movement reflects the state of the nervous system and is also the basis of self-awareness. We become accustomed to our movements, good or bad, and this can lead to physical and emotional problems. Feldenkrais reasoned that if the negative habitual patterns of movement are interrupted, the body will learn to function with greater ease, fluidity, and motion. This improves one's self-image and simultaneously increases awareness and health.

Feldenkrais recognized the importance of breath and viewed it as an integral form of movement. Poor movement and poor functioning impairs breathing and improper breathing interferes with the proper functioning of the body. He found that even the movement of the eyes could seriously interfere with how other parts of the body function.

Feldenkrais developed two approaches for working with students and clients: one implements group lessons

AWARENESS THROUGH MOVEMENT

Ralph Strauch, Ph.D., a certified Feldenkrais practitioner in Los Angeles, California, suggests the following simple method taken from a typical Awareness Through Movement lesson. This particular lesson is designed to improve how the neck and head turn.

- Sit comfortably with your body upright and your feet on the floor. Close your eyes and turn your head slowly to the right until it stops. Notice if the movement is smooth and fluid or somewhat stiff and jerky. Open your eyes and notice how far you turned and then bring your head back to the center.

- Slowly repeat the movement another 20-25 times. Do not turn as far as you can and do not "try" hard to do it; simply move slowly and easily, noticing what you feel. Pay attention to the parts of your body that take part in the turning; be aware of how far down your spine you feel the movement. Let your eyes move in unison with your head, looking to the right then coming back to the center. Allow your shoulders to take part in the movement as well.

- Now sit quietly and notice how you feel. After a few moments, close your eyes and again turn your head to the right. Does it go farther this time? Has the quality of the movement changed? Turn your head to both the left and the right and notice any differences in movement or ease. Most people will notice an improvement in the quality of movement to the right. The process of watching the movement, not the movement itself, produces this change. It is an increase in awareness that allows the movement to improve.

To test this, try the following: Close your eyes and imagine doing the same movement to the left. Imagine the movement becoming smoother and easier over 10-15 times. Feel the imaginary movement in the spine, the shoulders, and the eyes, just as if you had done the actual movement. Now actually turn the head to the left and the right and notice how the movement has improved.

(called Awareness Through Movement®) and the other focuses on individualized hands-on touch and movement (called Functional Integration®). Participants of Awareness Through Movement are guided through a slow and gentle sequence designed to replace old patterns of movement with new ones. As the client learns how to listen to these lessons, he or she develops an awareness of subtle changes in habit and movement. Feldenkrais wrote that the lessons are designed to improve mobility, "to turn the impossible into the possible, the possible into the easy, and the easy into the elegant."[15]

With Functional Integration, learning occurs through touch. The practitioner actively directs the client's body through movements individualized to their particular needs. The Feldenkrais Method differs from most other schools of bodywork in that there is no attempt to structurally alter the body. Instead, it is through touch that the practitioner attempts to communicate to the person a sense of improved self-image and movement. Feldenkrais viewed forcefully imposed "posture" as rigid and inflexible and shunned the idea of imposing rules of proper form and function. His teaching imparts a sense of exploration, experimentation, and innovation that allows each person to find the optimal style of movement.

The Feldenkrais Method helps people move more easily and is also useful for those who have limitations of movement caused by stress, accidents, back problems, or other physically debilitating illnesses, including stroke. It has also been shown to reduce perceived stress and lower anxiety levels associated with multiple sclerosis.[16] "But," adds Ralph Strauch, Ph.D., a certified Feldenkrais practitioner, "our primary concern is with the person, not the disorder." Performers and athletes have praised Feldenkrais for improving their levels of performance and many have utilized the work as a means of enhancing personal growth.

THE TRAGER APPROACH

Beginning in 1927, Milton Trager, M.D., developed this intuitive and playful approach to movement reeducation that uses a method of gentle, rhythmical touch combined with a series of movement exercises.[17] Although the techniques are very different from Feldenkrais work, the purpose is largely the same: to help the client recognize and release habitual patterns of tensions that are present in posture and movement. He established the Trager Institute with Betty Fuller in 1980.

The Trager® Approach uses no specific techniques of movement or massage. Instead, the practitioner is taught to feel how the client is holding his or her body and, by applying various rocking, pulling, and rotational movements to the client's head, torso, and appendages, the therapist gently loosens tense muscles and stiff joints.

"The concern of the Trager Approach is not with moving particular muscles or joints per se," says Deane

Juhan, an instructor at the Trager Institute, "but with using motion in muscles and joints to produce particular sensory feelings, namely positive, pleasurable feelings that enter the central nervous system and begin to trigger tissue changes by means of the many sensory-motor feedback loops between the mind and the muscles."[18] These gentle movements provoke a sense of deep relaxation and help increase flexibility and range of motion in the joints and limbs. Dr. Trager believed that the unconscious mind will always mimic movements that result in an improved sense of pleasure and freedom, and that it is the practitioner's responsibility to help plant this sense of well-being in the person's body. As he said, "The Trager Approach consists of the use—not the laying on—of the hands to influence deep-seated psycho/physiological patterns of the mind and to interrupt their projection into the body's tissues."[19]

Mentastics® is a term coined by Dr. Trager to mean "mental gymnastics." These exercises are free-flowing, dance-like movements designed to increase awareness of how the body moves for the purpose of learning how to move more effortlessly. An exercise may be as simple as letting the arms or legs drop to one side or adding a small shaking or swinging motion to a foot and leg while walking. Dr. Trager designed the exercises to reinforce the relaxation awareness established from hands-on bodywork.

Dr. Trager took a particular interest in applying his approach to people suffering from severe neuromuscular disturbances resulting from injury, disease, and aging, including disorders such as polio, muscular dystrophy, and multiple sclerosis. In addition, many athletes have found that the work has increased their efficiency of movement and stamina.

Structural Bodywork

Bodywork in this category is concerned with improving physical functioning by releasing musculoskeletal tensions, misalignments, and imbalances caused by the effects of gravity and habitual patterns of stress-reaction.

ROLFING®

Biochemist Ida P. Rolf, Ph.D., gained her first exposure to therapeutic manipulation when, as a young woman, she was successfully treated by an osteopath for a respiratory condition. The doctor performed manipulations to reposition a rib that had been displaced by a kick from a horse. Dr. Rolf began to glimpse the operating premise that would become the cornerstone of her work: the body's structure profoundly affects all physiological and psychological processes.

Dr. Rolf was also influenced by her exposure to yoga, which led her to the principle that "bodies need to lengthen and be balanced, and a balanced body will give rise to a better human being."[20] She founded the Rolf Institute for Structural Integration in 1970, which has since trained bodyworkers from around the world in her methods.

 See Yoga.

Rolfing, the popular name for Structural Integration, is based on the idea that human function is improved when the segments of the body (head, torso, pelvis, legs, feet) are properly aligned. Most people are not aware if and when their bodies are out of balance. For example, when standing, many people put most of their weight on their heels, but doing so throws the balance backward. In order to compensate, the upper body must lean too far forward, throwing the pelvis out of alignment. In addition, in order to see, the head has to be tilted back. To hold this position, the muscles of the neck, back, and legs must remain overly contracted and stressed. After maintaining this posture for months or years, the fascial tissues (fibrous layers covering muscles) of the body have to compensate to hold everything in this out-of-balance position. Movement becomes impaired and this reduces mental clarity and increases emotional stress.

Dr. Rolf believed that manually manipulating and stretching the fascial tissues could reestablish balance and poise. The fascia is a thin, elastic, semi-fluid membrane that envelops every muscle in the body and unites the skin with underlying tissue. Fascia also plays an integral role in maintaining posture and proper movement. Dr. Rolf defined fascia as "the organ of change" and stated that injury, chronic stress, or other trauma can lead to its deterioration. According to Dr. Rolf, when fascia becomes increasingly more solid, rigid, and sticky, it begins to restrict the movement of muscles and joints.

Practitioners of Structural Integration, known as "Rolfers," use pressure applied with the fingers, knuckles, and elbows to release fascial adhesion. Doing so helps to reorganize the tissue back to its proper geometric planes by lifting, lengthening, and balancing the body segments. Balance is an essential fact in Rolfing. "If the head is supported and balanced by the shoulders, the shoulders by the chest, the chest by the pelvis, and so on, then gravity can only reinforce balance," noted Dr. Rolf.[21] Typically, Rolfing sessions are spaced one week apart for a period of ten weeks, resulting in significant, noticeable improvement in posture, musculoskeletal alignment, and overall well-being. Clients also have the option of receiving four or more advanced sessions, which are usually offered one to two years after the initial sequence.

Depending on the depth and degree of tissue adhesion, pain may be felt when pressure is applied. Dr. Rolf

pointed out that it could hardly be expected that profound tissue changes such as changes in position or tone could be accomplished without a dramatic reaction. "People often call this reaction pain, but it is not the pain we associate with injury or hurt," she stated.[22]

Over the years, in order to enhance the effectiveness of the physical manipulations, a system of movement education called Rolfing Movement Integration has developed. Weekly sessions allow the teacher and client to explore the possibilities for developing free, more balanced movements. These movements can then be applied to all aspects of daily living: sitting, standing, breathing, running, and housework.

Valerie Hunt, Ed.D., and Wayne Massey have conducted research on the effects of Rolfing at the Department of Kinesiology, University of California, at Los Angeles. The study concluded that: movements were smoother, larger, and less constrained; there were less extraneous movements; body movements were more dynamic and energetic; carriage was more erect; and there was less obvious strain to maintain a held position.[23] A similar study conducted at the University of Maryland indicates that Rolfing reduces chronic stress, promotes changes in body structure, and enhances neurological function. In addition, those who suffered from lordosis, or sway back, experienced a reduction in the curvature of the spine.[24]

 See Applied Kinesiology, Craniosacral Therapy, Osteopathic Medicine.

Dr. Rolf's work has profoundly influenced contemporary bodywork. Her research into fascia and the role of gravity in determining balance has added tangible credibility to the structural approach to body therapy. Nearly everyone can benefit from Rolfing, and those who suffer from pain and stiffness related to mechanical imbalances and poor posture will be particularly rewarded.

 Rolfing is contraindicated for anyone suffering from acute pain related to bone weakness (fracture, osteoporosis) and is also not advisable for conditions such as cancer, rheumatoid arthritis, acute skin inflammation, and chronic addiction.

MYOFASCIAL RELEASE

This form of structural bodywork, developed by physical therapist John Barnes, takes a whole-body approach to healing. Like Rolfing, Myofascial Release attempts to improve body structure by releasing tension in the fascia and the muscles. Practitioners work with their fingers, the palms of their hands, and elbows to apply slow, deliberate strokes to the body lasting between 90 seconds and three or more minutes. Individual sessions are 30-90 minutes, with initial sessions occurring with short intervals between visits in order to achieve maximum benefit. Tension and chronic pain relief, improved body alignment, and faster recovery from injury are the most common benefits of Myofascial Release. Over 20,000 health-care providers from the fields of medicine, physical therapy, and therapeutic massage employ Myofascial Release as part of their practice, making it one of the most common forms of structural bodywork.

⚠️**CAUTION** Myofascial Release is contraindicated for cases of aneurysm, rheumatoid arthritis, or malignant tumors, and practitioners should avoid areas of the body with bruises, fractures, or wounds until they have healed.

ASTON-PATTERNING

Several years after completing her graduate studies in dance and fine arts at the University of California, at Los Angeles, Judith Aston was involved in back-to-back car accidents that left her with debilitating injuries. After conventional medical treatment failed, a physician recommended that she see Dr. Rolf. As a result of Dr. Rolf's technique, Aston's condition improved dramatically. Because of her background in teaching dance, and her ability to train people to see and perform movements, Dr. Rolf asked her to develop a movement education system for Rolfing to help maintain the structural alignment achieved in the treatment sessions. This system was called Rolf-Aston Structural Patterning. Aston began training people in 1971 and, during the next seven years, she trained Rolfers in movement analysis and the basics of movement education.

She went on to develop Aston-Patterning in its current form in 1977. Unlike Dr. Rolf's model and its focus on body symmetry and alignment, Aston noted that all movement is naturally asymmetrical and that a healthy body develops asymmetrically through adaptation to the kinds of work, recreation, sports, and other daily activities it performs. In addition, Aston focuses on how to distinguish what is changeable and what is a true asymmetrical limitation. Aston's work also has an individual focus since, as she says, "people aren't recipes." Aston also teaches students a technique she calls "spiraling" to work the deep tissues without pain.

Aston-Patterning work focuses on four areas: movement reeducation, massage and soft tissue bodywork, fitness training, and environmental "design" (for example, altering the height of an office chair and furniture to suit a particular body). Participants learn to integrate Aston's principles of movement with specific methods for strengthening and stretching the body.

Neshama Franklin, a health journalist, describes a demonstration session she received from an Aston-Patterner. "We started with an evaluation of the way I walk. The practitioner noted that my weight distribution was off balance—heavy on the heels with my feet pointed at different angles. Then, she explored my body with massage. Any resistance or tension was dutifully marked on a chart. I liked the specific, graphic way the chart helped me see the patterns of tension in my body. After the massage, we returned to walking and I explored ways to distribute my weight more evenly. The result was a new stride that felt springy and light. Six months later, I could still recapture that ease of movement when I focused on what I learned at the demonstration session."[25]

Aston-Patterning can be used to develop better movement and coordination or for managing painful conditions such as backaches, headaches, and tennis elbow. Physical therapists also use Aston-Patterning as an adjunct for those suffering from neck and back pain and for working with adolescents with postural dysfunction.[26]

HELLERWORK

Developed by Joseph Heller, the first president of the Rolf Institute, Hellerwork combines deep touch, movement education, and verbal dialogue. This approach works to structurally realign the body as well as facilitate an awareness of the mind/body relationship. Hellerwork specifically addresses the interwoven complexity of the mechanical, psychological, and energetic functioning of the human body.

The mechanical aspect of Hellerwork, patterned after Rolfing, is designed to properly align the body with the Earth's gravitational field. Heller felt that the physical changes achieved by manual manipulation were not sufficient to bring about permanent change in the body. He incorporated a thematic approach to each of the 11 Hellerwork sessions in order to provide a basis for organizing the emotional content of the work. For example, the first Hellerwork session is designed to unlock tension and unconscious holding patterns in the chest to allow for more natural breathing. The practitioner engages the client in a dialogue intended to call attention to emotions and attitudes that affect the physiological process of breathing.

Hellerwork uses movement and awareness to teach clients how to sit, stand, walk, run, or lift in ways that are appropriate to the natural design of their bodies. The process is designed to minimize mechanical stress and create more efficient use of the body's energy. In a unique experiment, Hellerwork was administered to the staff of a computer software company in Portland, Oregon. At the completion of the series, employees were surveyed regarding their experiences. Every employee reported a reduction in physical stress and an improvement in posture. Additionally, 84% noticed less back pain, 81% felt that their job effectiveness had increased, and 94% experienced an improvement in their work relationships and an improved ability to communicate.[27]

Hellerwork can improve body alignment and flexibility and can offer increased vitality and greater emotional clarity and freedom of expression. It is beneficial for anyone suffering painful and stiff muscles due to structural imbalances or for conditions that may be the result of injury, emotional trauma, or sustained stress.

BARRAL VISCERAL MANIPULATION

Developed by French osteopathic physician Jean Pierre Barral, D.O., the goal of Barral Visceral Manipulation is to release restrictions and tensions in the body by gently manipulating the internal organs and their connective tissues. According to Zannah Steiner, C.M.P., R.M.T., of the Soma Therapy Centre, in Vancouver, British Columbia, Canada, the therapy enhances organ function and mobility, improves fluid circulation, increases hormonal secretion, strengthens immune function, eases muscle spasms, and can also facilitate the release of unexpressed emotions.

Dr. Barral developed his technique following years of research, which showed that the internal organs have a distinct biological rhythm of 5-8 cycles per minute. Each organ moves, or rotates, subtly with respect to the orientation it originally had when it was developing in the fetus, which Dr. Barral defines as the organ's "embryogenic axis." When tissue surrounding the organ becomes damaged, fixed, or adhered, it becomes a point of chronic irritation that can interfere with the organ's mobility and visceral rhythm.

According to Steiner, if an organ, such as the liver, cannot "move" with respect to its surrounding tissues, it will start working contrary to neighboring organs (in this case, the gallbladder or stomach) as well as the surrounding muscles, membranes, fascia, and bones. For example, adhesions around the lungs or a thickening of its tissues can eventually destabilize vertebrae in the spinal column.

Practitioners of Barral therapy use "light, precise, mechanical force" to relieve these abnormal tissue tensions. This rebalances the affected organ on its desired axis, thereby correcting its dysfunction. Because of its ability to improve the function and mobility of all major organs in the body, Barral Visceral Manipulation can provide benefit for a wide range of disease conditions.

BOWEN THERAPY

Bowen therapy was developed in the 1950s by Thomas Bowen, a lay healer from Australia, who possessed a keen knowledge of human structure and nerve function and their relationship to health. Over time, Bowen developed a reputation for being able to "cure the incurable" and, at one point in his career, he was treating over 13,000 patients per year, most of whom required only two or three sessions with him in order to become well. Although little known in the U.S., Bowen therapy is a popular form of bodywork in Australia, New Zealand, and western Europe.

Jo Anne Whitaker, M.D., F.A.A.P., Director of the Bowen Research and Training Institute, in Palm Harbor, Florida, describes Bowen therapy as "a unique, gentle, hands-on therapy that has minimal side effects and works on the whole person—body, mind, and spirit." Dr. Whitaker's research indicates that Bowen therapy's ability to relieve the pain of a wide range of acute and chronic disease conditions is due to its ability to stimulate the body to balance the autonomic nervous system (ANS). "The ANS regulates 80% to 90% of our physiological and emotional functions and governs such things as digestion, respiration, heart and circulatory function, blood pressure, muscles, glands, immune function, and motor skills," she explains. "Bowen therapy, because of its ability to positively effect the ANS, allows the body to adjust physiologically and psychologically to bring itself into a balanced state."

Unlike other forms of structural bodywork, Bowen therapy is extremely gentle and noninvasive. "A typical Bowen session involves an interview to assess the person's history and problems," Dr. Whitaker says. "The technique is performed on a padded table or bed with the person initially lying prone and fully clothed. The treatment involves a series of moves consisting of pulling the skin away from an underlying muscle or tendon, applying gentle pressure against its side, then holding and releasing it while allowing the underlying structure to spring back to its normal position." The moves are performed in a specific pattern and the basic treatments involve three sets of moves on the lower back, upper back, and neck. Other moves, specific to the client's health problem, can also be added.

A typical treatment lasts 20-45 minutes. Following treatment, the client is assisted to a sitting position, then to stand, putting weight equally on both feet, before walking briefly around the room to help the body absorb the full effect of the changes that have been made. "Post-treatment instructions include drinking plenty of water, not sitting for longer than 30 minutes without walking around for a short time on the day of treatment, and avoiding other therapies for 5-7 days," Dr. Whitaker says.

The effects of treatment can be immediate or may occur over the next few days. "Occasionally, clients experience a residual soreness or flu-like symptoms on the day following treatment, but that will subside with more water intake and walking," Dr. Whitaker says. "Emotional release may also occur during treatment or afterwards." In the majority of cases, client symptoms are completely relieved in one to three sessions, according to Dr. Whitaker, although chronic conditions may require more long-term therapy.

Among the conditions for which Bowen therapy can provide benefit are acute and chronic pain; arm, shoulder, back, neck and cranial problems; digestive and gastrointestinal disorders; acute and chronic fatigue; frozen shoulder; fibromyalgia; headaches and migraines; leg problems, including hamstrings, knees, and ankles; respiratory conditions; sports and work-related injuries; stress; and temporomandibular joint (TMJ) syndrome. In addition, clients typically report greater energy, enhanced positive moods, and improved cognitive function, as well as reduced feelings of anger, depression, and tension.

In 1995, a variation of Bowen therapy known as Neurostructural Integration Technique (NST) was developed by Michael Nixon-Livy, based on his desire to systematize the techniques Bowen developed into a training format that could be easily and quickly learned by health professionals. It works in much the same way as Bowen therapy and provides essentially the same benefits.

Pressure Point Therapies

Pressure point therapies apply pressure on various areas of the body to relieve pain and restore proper energy flow. Some of these therapies are based on the concept of vital life energy, or *qi* (see Quick Definition), which flows through energy channels, called meridians, running throughout the body.

 QD   ***Qi*** (pronounced CHEE) is a Chinese word variously translated to mean "vital energy," "essence of life," and "living force." In Chinese medicine, the proper flow of *qi* along energy channels (meridians) within the body is crucial to a person's health and vitality. There are many types of *qi* classified according to source, location, and function (such as activation, warming, defense, transformation, and containment). Within the body, *qi* and blood are closely linked, as each is considered to flow along with the other. *Qi* may be stagnant (non-moving), deficient (partially absent), or excessive (inappropriately abundant) from a given organ system. The manipulation and readjustment of *qi* to treat disease and ensure maximum health benefit is the basic principle of acupuncture and acupressure, although other remedies and therapies can be used to influence *qi*.

 See Acupuncture, Qigong and Tai Chi, Traditional Chinese Medicine.

ACUPRESSURE

Over 5,000 years ago, the Chinese discovered that when certain points on the body are pressed, punctured, or heated, certain ailments are relieved. The beneficial effects are thought to be due to the release of energy blocks in the meridians. As the art developed, more and more points were discovered that not only alleviated pain, but also influenced the functioning of internal organs and body systems.

Whereas acupuncture uses needles, acupressure uses the pressure of the fingers and hands. Acupressure is older than acupuncture and, once learned, can serve as an effective self-care and preventive treatment for tension-related ailments. Its underlying theory considers symptoms as an expression of the condition of the whole person and focuses on relieving pain and discomfort. It is also concerned with responding to tensions and toxicities in the body before they develop into illnesses.

Two types of self-acupressure techniques are Acu-Yoga and *Do-In*. Acu-Yoga utilizes the whole body for breathing, finger pressure, yogic postures, meditation, and stretches. *Do-In* also incorporates body awareness, stretching, and breathing, but focuses on vigorous techniques that stimulate the body through the acupoints and meridians.

Acupressure massage techniques and practices (referred to as *Tui Na* in China and *Amma* in Japan) use rubbing, kneading, percussion, and vibration to improve circulation and to stimulate stale blood and lymph from tissues. Acupressure provides many of the same health benefits common to acupuncture treatments. Recent research has found that it is effective as a preventive measure against post-operative nausea and vomiting, both of which are common side effects of general anesthesia. In one randomized, double-blind study, involving 200 otherwise healthy patients who required short surgical procedures, 108 patients were supplied with acupressure bands (to apply pressure to a specific acupoint on the forearm) prior to the application of anesthesia and kept in place for six hours following surgery. The remaining 92 patients served as a control group, with bands placed inappropriately on a different part of the forearm. In the first group, only 23% of the patients experienced nausea or vomiting as a result of receiving anesthesia compared to 41% in the control group.[28]

ORIENTAL BODYWORK

Oriental bodywork has developed primarily through a combination of instinct and hands-on experience. Its principles and healing techniques integrate acupressure techniques with breathing meditation, herbal remedies, and massage. Contemporary practitioners continue to incorporate these traditional principles along with the discovery of new treatment protocols and bodywork styles. While traditional acupoints are common to all styles of Oriental bodywork, each style has distinctive characteristics that incorporate unique ways of touching and interacting with clients. These systems can positively regulate and harmonize the body and can be used to relieve pain and muscular discomfort, correct imbalances, and prevent illness.

The following descriptions focus on the primary styles or methods currently in practice:

- *Shiatsu* means "finger pressure" in Japanese. This well-known method uses a firm sequence of rhythmic pressure held on specific points for 3-10 seconds and is designed to awaken the acupuncture meridians. Michael Reed Gach, Ph.D., Director of the Acupressure Institute, in Berkeley, California, recalls a highly athletic patient, who often complained of pain in his back and leg muscles. He had found no relief with massage therapy, but *shiatsu* produced excellent results on his back and legs, the deep pressure releasing the stiffness and improving the muscle tone and circulation.

- *Jin Shin Jyutsu* was developed in Japan by Jiro Murai, who rediscovered the ancient *qi* flow in his own body and mapped a powerful system of healing points, which he then used to cure himself of a life-threatening illness. Combinations of points are held with the fingertips for a minute or more, usually with the clients lying on their back. Various schools of the *Jin Shin* style have evolved, including *Jin Shin Do* and *Jin Shin* acupressure. *Jin Shin Do*, meaning "the way of compassionate spirit," was developed during the 1980s by psychotherapist Iona M. Teeguarden, M.A., L.M.F.C.C. This gentle system is a synthesis of acupuncture/acupressure techniques, Taoist breathing exercises, and Western psychotherapeutic theory. A typical 90-minute session focuses on applying the appropriate finger pressure to acupoints in and near tension areas of the body while the client lies fully clothed on a massage table. As physical and emotional tensions are released, clients often experience deep relaxation close to euphoria.

REFLEXOLOGY

Reflexology states that there are reflex areas in the hands and feet that correspond to every part of the body, including organs and glands, and that these parts can be affected by stimulating the appropriate reflex areas. Reflexology is used to relieve stress and tension, stimulate deep relaxation, improve the blood supply, and promote the

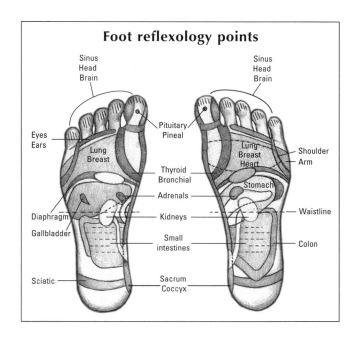

Foot reflexology points

unblocking of nerve impulses to normalize and balance the entire body.

Reflexology evolved out of an earlier European system known as zone therapy and was introduced to America by William Fitzgerald, M.D., a laryngologist at St. Francis Hospital in Connecticut. Dr. Fitzgerald discovered he could induce numbness and alleviate certain symptoms in the body by applying finger pressure to specific points on the hands and mouth. Eunice Ingham, a physiotherapist, used Dr. Fitzgerald's work as the basis for what is known today as reflexology. Ingham mapped organ reflexes on the feet and developed techniques for inducing a stimulating, healing effect in those areas.

Reflexologists apply precise pressure to release blockages that inhibit energy flow and cause pain and disease. This pressure is believed to affect internal organs and glands by stimulating reflex points of the body. Practitioners often target the breakup of lactic acid and calcium crystals accumulated around the 7,200 nerve endings in each foot. "Perhaps this is why we feel so much better when our feet are treated," writes Ray Wunderlich, Jr., M.D., of Florida. "Nerve endings in the feet have extensive interconnection through the spinal cord and brain to all areas of the body." Dr. Wunderlich believes that even though reflexology is medically unproven, it still deserves wide usage as a valuable adjunct to the medical care of patients in need.[29]

Modern reflexologists continue to witness startling effects from their treatments. Bill Flocco, founder of the American Academy of Reflexology, in conjunction with Terrence Oleson, Ph.D., Associate Professor of Research at the University of California, at Los Angeles, conducted a study of the effects of reflexology in alleviating premenstrual syndrome (PMS). Results indicated a 62% reduction in the PMS symptoms of those undergoing reflexology treatment.[30] Dr. Wunderlich notes that reflexology is also helpful for people with hypertension, anxiety, or painful conditions of the body.

One study examined the effects of reflexology on anxiety and pain in 23 female patients suffering from lung or breast cancer. All of the patients were also regularly receiving medications. After receiving 30 minutes of treatment by a certified reflexologist, researchers observed that all of the women experienced a significant decrease in anxiety and that the women with breast cancer also experienced a significant decrease in pain. Based on their findings, the researchers concluded that reflexology has a place as a self-care protocol alongside conventional medical care for such patients.[31]

Another study found that reflexology can be effective as a treatment for chronic migraines and tension headaches. In the study, 220 patients who suffered from frequent headaches or migraine attacks received reflexology treatments for up to six months. A follow-up survey of the patients conducted three months later found that 81% were helped by the treatments or completely cured. In addition, 19% of patients who previously had to take medication to control their headaches or migraine attacks were able to discontinue their use.[32]

BONNIE PRUDDEN MYOTHERAPY™

Bonnie Prudden is a leading authority on physical fitness and exercise therapy. Her research helped create the President's Council on Physical Fitness and Sports in the 1950s. From her experience, she developed a technique for relieving pain that is simple enough to be taught to a child.

Prudden's work is based on the application of manual pressure to sensitive spots known as "trigger points." Her work grew out of the pioneering medical discipline called trigger point injection therapy, developed by Janet Travell, M.D., in which sensitive and often painful muscular spots are injected with a saline or procaine solution. In 1976, while working with Desmond Tivy, M.D., another advocate of trigger point injection therapy, Prudden discovered that a relatively deep pressure applied to these same points for 5-7 seconds could relieve pain for roughly 90% of all muscle-related cases, without the use of invasive and often painful injections. "At first, we worked mainly with backs," Prudden writes. "Instead of taking weeks to get rid of pain with exercise and injections, it was taking only a few sessions, often only one. Arm, shoulder, and neck pain all surrendered. We even had several stroke patients who had severely contracted arm muscles. Soon, they too were free of pain and their limbs free of contracture."[33]

Trigger points can be caused by trauma at any age, including prenatal injury, accidents, childhood and sexual abuse, sports injuries, the repetitive motions connected with work or hobbies, and any invasive procedure, from injections to surgery. Trigger points are often exacerbated by disease, substance abuse, and aging. They are highly irritable spots that may lie quietly for years within a muscle and can be "fired" as a result of certain physical or emotional conditions. Muscle spasm is the result. This, in turn, causes more pain and creates a spasm-pain-spasm cycle.

To relieve the pain, the cycle must be broken. Although medication can interrupt the cycle, the underlying cause—the resident trigger point—remains. Once medication wears off, another bout with physical or emotional stress can reactivate the painful cycle. This is the cause of most recurring or chronic pain. Once a trigger point is created, others often form in the immediate and surrounding area. For treatment to be successful, these satellite points must also be addressed.

Prudden's books on pain, *Pain Erasure* and *Myotherapy*, include charts for locating the major trigger points. These points can be found easily by touch, as pressing on a trigger point may be relatively painful. Press each muscle with your finger at one-inch intervals. When a tender spot is found, apply pressure until the first sign of discomfort. Because the tension underlying these trigger points is of a chronic nature, several sessions will be needed to eliminate the trigger points and their satellites. This specific exercise, designed to reeducate the muscle to return to normal function, is the key to success with Bonnie Prudden Myotherapy. It is also important to do three-minute sessions five times a day to prevent old tensing habits from taking over. After the session, stretching exercises are needed to retrain the muscles to relax.

Bonnie Prudden Myotherapy can be effective in relieving muscle pain, strains, sprains, dislocations, tension headaches, and migraines. Numerous pain clinics now use the technique. It also treats TMJ syndrome and neck, shoulder, arm, hand, back, chest, and abdominal pain. Hemorrhoids, spasms in the muscles surrounding the prostate, as well as impotence and incontinence (when resulting from spasms in the muscles of the pelvic floor) can also benefit. Myotherapy is invaluable in knee and foot pain and leg cramps caused by aging. Diseases such as arthritis, lupus, and multiple sclerosis also respond, as they all affect muscles that house trigger points.

Bioenergetic Systems of Bodywork

Bodywork therapies in this category are based on an underlying philosophy which recognizes that the physical bodies of all living beings are surrounded by an invisible bioenergy field and that health depends on the coherence of this field and the proper flow of vital energy throughout the body's bioenergetic pathways (meridians). Bioenergetic healing approaches have been a part of religious and indigenous healing traditions worldwide for millennia and, in recent decades, a number of modern techniques based on these ancient methods have also been developed. All such "laying on of hands" methods of energy medicine involve a process of transferring healing energies from one individual to another.

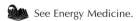 See Energy Medicine.

THERAPEUTIC TOUCH

Therapeutic Touch (TT) was developed in 1971 by Dolores Krieger, Ph.D., R.N., Professor Emeritus of New York University (NYU) Graduate School of Nursing, and her mentor, the late Dora Kunz, a widely respected healer. Together, they originated a nonreligious, secular form of healing that combined the laying on of hands with a number of other ancient bioenergetic techniques, which was initially taught at NYU as an extension of professional nursing care.

During a TT session, there is generally no physical contact between patient and practitioner, although touch may be employed when treating fractures and parts of the body affected by physical trauma. TT practitioners begin each session by quieting themselves through a process known as "going on center." This enables them to become better aware of and more deeply connect with the specific bioenergetic needs of their patients. A brief assessment period follows in which the practitioner places his or her hands 2-6 inches away from the patient and, using slow, rhythmic hand motions, locates blockages in the patient's biofield. The practitioner then works to replenish the flow of subtle life force energy where necessary, while releasing any congestion or obstruction that may be present. This is accomplished by smoothing the biofield itself, using hand motions, usually beginning at the crown of the patient's head and moving toward the feet, while the practitioner visualizes the biofield's energies becoming more coherent and organized. Sessions typically last 20-30 minutes and patients commonly report a variety of benefits, including noticeable feelings of relaxation, improved energy levels, pain reduction, diminished stress, and general well-being.

John Zimmerman, Ph.D., Assistant Professor of Psychiatry at the University of Colorado, has conducted studies to measure the body's magnetic field during TT sessions. Dr. Zimmerman was able to quantify several distinct changes in the biofield—signals up to several hundred times larger than background noise appeared while the practitioner worked. Other researchers have documented additional physiologic changes within the human body and in animals during TT treatments, including changes in brain wave patterns.[34]

Today, Therapeutic Touch provides the greatest amount of credibility for bioenergetic forms of energy medicine. An estimated 40,000 doctors, nurses, and other health professionals in the U.S. and throughout the world use Therapeutic Touch as an integral part of their practice. It is also included as a viable technique in a number of nursing textbooks. According to Dr. Krieger, TT is also available in over 200 hospitals and taught in more than 100 fully accredited colleges and universities nationwide, as well as in over 75 other nations.[35]

TT has proven effective in treating a variety of medical conditions. The proper use of TT can decrease anxiety, reduce pain, and ease problems associated with autonomic nervous system dysfunction.[36] TT has been shown to alter enzyme activity, increase hemoglobin levels, and accelerate the healing of wounds.[37] However, the technique is primarily known for its ability to relieve pain and reduce stress and anxiety.[38] Studies have shown that patients receiving Therapeutic Touch experienced a significant reduction of headache pain.[39] Further evidence supports the use of TT technique to calm crying babies, ease asthmatic breathing, reduce pain in postoperative patients, and reduce fever and inflammation.[40] It is now commonly practiced and taught in Lamaze classes, due to its ability to reduce anxiety and discomfort among pregnant women.[41]

HEALING TOUCH

A variant of Therapeutic Touch, Healing Touch was developed by Janet Mentgen, R.N., in 1981. Like TT practitioners, practitioners of Healing Touch seek to assess and then rectify bioenergetic blockages and disruptions. Besides employing TT methods, practitioners use a number of other bioenergetic techniques that are mastered over four certified levels of training. Healing Touch is used by a growing number of holistically oriented nurses and, since 1989, has been sanctioned by the American Holistic Nurses Association (which also endorses TT), due to its ability to hasten the healing process, relieve pain, reduce anxiety, and improve overall well-being.[42]

REIKI

Meaning "the free passage of universal life energy," Reiki involves transference of energy between Reiki practitioners and their clients in order to restore harmony to the biofield and bolster the body's inherent healing processes. Reiki practitioners claim that its principles evolved from ancient Tibetan Buddhist healing practices that were transmitted from teacher to disciple. Dr. Mika Usui, a Japanese scholar and Christian minister, is said to have rediscovered these principles in the late 1800s. One of his pupils, Saichi Takata, then introduced Reiki to the U.S. in 1937.

Reiki treatments vary according to individual need and are generally administered with clients lying down as the practitioner lays hands on various areas of the body. Prior to becoming a practitioner, students of Reiki undergo a number of training levels in which they are initiated by a "Reiki master" and attuned to healing symbols, which are then focused upon as Reiki practitioners send healing energy to their clients. Although Reiki has not received the same degree of scientific study as Therapeutic Touch, evidence of its efficacy does exist. In one published study on the adjunctive use of Reiki to manage pain, it was found that when Reiki treatments where administered by a Reiki therapist to patients who were also receiving conventional pain medication, there was a "highly significant reduction in pain following the Reiki treatment." The study involved 20 volunteers who were experiencing pain for a variety of reasons, including cancer.[43] In the last decade, Reiki has become popular as a form of bioenergetic healing, and there are an estimated 200,000 Reiki practitioner worldwide.

POLARITY THERAPY

Randolph Stone, D.C., D.O., N.D., who was deeply interested in the electromagnetic energy currents of the human body, developed polarity therapy. Dr. Stone explored the world's healing systems for an understanding of their underlying essence. He based his work on the Eastern concept that illness originates from blockages in energy flow.

Polarity hands-on techniques include manipulation of pressure points and joints, massage, breathing techniques, hydrotherapy, exercise, reflexology, and even simply holding pressure points on the body. Both hands are used—one is considered electromagnetic positive, the other negative—to release energy blockages in the body and help to restore a natural flow. Polarity bodywork is both invigorating and rejuvenating and can result in positive changes on the physical, mental, and emotional levels.

The stretches and other exercises used in polarity therapy are simple techniques that anyone can employ to release energy blockages and restore a balanced energy flow in the body. These techniques, combined with dietary and nutritional counseling based upon traditional Chinese medicine, as well as emotional balancing work, help clients achieve a heightened level of well-being. The benefits of polarity therapy may include improvement in physical health, increased energy, and a deeper understanding of oneself.

Polarity therapy is taught by individuals and at various schools worldwide. In 1984, the American Polarity

Therapy Association was formed to assist in networking, research, maintaining quality of practice, and to certify practitioners.

Somatic Psychology

Bodywork approaches within the field of somatic psychology focus on the interrelationship between body (soma) and mind (psyche). While this notion of a connection among mind, body, and emotion began in many of the ancient healing traditions of the Greeks, Chinese, and Indians, modern somatic psychology derives its theories from Wilhelm Reich, M.D., a former student of Sigmund Freud, who coupled his own interest in the movement of energy throughout the body with Freud's concepts of psychology and theorized that psychological disorders are directly caused by suppressed energy in the body.

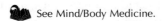 See Mind/Body Medicine.

REICHIAN THERAPY

People who undergo bodywork often experience powerful emotional releases. Dr. Reich, the founder of Reichian therapy, realized that feelings and emotions are reflected in the body posture and behavior of the individual. During the first half of the 20th century, he developed a system of bodywork and breathing that is capable of bringing these often buried emotions to the surface. Unlike Freud, who was more interested in the concepts that led him to develop psychoanalysis, Dr. Reich's primary interest was in how and why energy in the body became blocked. Based on extensive research, he came to view psychological disorders as the direct result of blocked or suppressed vital energy (which he termed *orgone*), which over time caused habitual patterns of muscle tension and postural misalignments. Dr. Reich called such chronic patterns "armoring." Although he used his techniques for the purposes of psychological intervention, Dr. Reich's work left a deep impression on many who later developed their own bodywork techniques, including Dr. Rolf.

Dr. Reich's techniques were deceptively simple, foremost being the act of breathing. By asking his patients to breathe deeply and continuously, he was able to unlock chronic physical tensions and release pent-up and unconscious feelings and memories. The power of the breath has led many bodywork practitioners to incorporate deep breathing techniques into their work. Dr. Reich also paid close attention to how patients held themselves and would occasionally apply deep pressure to tense muscle groups in the face, neck, back, torso, and legs. Additionally, he would ask his patients to kick, hit, or move in various ways that were designed to release the musculature and free hidden emotions.

Today, many other bodywork systems have adapted Dr. Reich's techniques in some form into their own theory and practice. Psychotherapists also recognize the importance the body plays in maintaining psychological health and many have integrated bodywork and massage into their practices.

BIOENERGETICS

Developed by Alexander Lowen, M.D., a former student of Dr. Reich, Bioenergetics, an offshoot of Reichian therapy, similarly employs breathing and physical exercises to alleviate stress and resolve emotional armoring patterns. In Dr. Lowen's view, there are five distinct patterns of armoring, each of which can be determined by observing a person's physical structure and movement. Bioenergetic practitioners help their clients become more conscious of their emotions and beliefs and how they influence musculoskeletal constrictions.

During sessions, clients perform various exercises developed by Dr. Lowen, which enable them to become aware of where and how they store tension in their bodies. In the process, repressed feelings may surface, accompanied by the release of muscular tension. Typically, clients are shown how to breathe deeply and continuously throughout the exercise process in order to further facilitate the healing process. Massage and deep tissue work is sometimes employed as well, and clients may also be encouraged to vocalize the emotions and memories that surface during the course of treatment.

Although the primary intent of Bioenergetics is psychotherapeutic, many clients also report that the therapy results in the resolution of a variety of physical conditions. These include headaches and migraines, gastrointestinal disorders, insomnia, respiratory conditions, and stress-related ulcers.

HAKOMI

The word *hakomi* comes from the Hopi language and means "Who are you and how do you stand in relation to these many realms?" Developed by Ron Kurtz, Hakomi combines various body-centered psychotherapeutic methods with systems theory and Eastern concepts of mindful awareness and nonviolence. It is a noninvasive technique that employs touch, massage therapy, structural alignment, movement exercises, and energy work.

Throughout each Hakomi session, clients are taught how to maintain self-awareness and be alert to what is occurring in their bodies, which can result in a heightened state of consciousness and vulnerability. While in this state, the Hakomi practitioner uses positive statements, or "probes," intended to evoke insights, memo-

ries, emotions, and personal issues relevant to the client's life. Typically, as this occurs, the client will fall back on the habitual coping mechanisms (armoring, postural shifts, voice inflections) he or she normally employs to manage such experiences. As the coping mechanisms surface, the practitioner encourages them through a process called "taking over," offering verbal or physical support for their further unfoldment. The end result, according to Kurtz, is that clients find themselves relaxing their coping mechanisms, gaining deeper insights and feelings of greater security. They also learn to recognize physiological clues (posture, breathing, movement, tone of voice) related to their core beliefs. Hakomi is characterized by its compassionate, spiritual approach to healing.

THE ROSEN METHOD

Developed by German physical therapist Marion Rosen, the Rosen Method employs breathing exercises, relaxation techniques, massage, and psychotherapy to resolve chronic tension due to limiting, and usually unconscious, belief patterns and memories stored in the body. The client lies on a massage table while the practitioner uses light, gentle touch to locate areas of chronic tension, paying close attention to changes in body tone and breathing patterns. As the unconscious patterns that have contributed to their condition are detected, clients are taught how to release them. To enhance the work and help clients retain their gains, movement and stretching exercises specific to the Rosen Method may also be employed. Benefits of the Rosen Method include reduced anxiety and physical tension, improved circulation, and greater self-awareness. It may also help with certain physical conditions, such as joint immobility and dementia.

RUBENFELD SYNERGY METHOD

The Rubenfeld Synergy Method was developed by somatic psychology pioneer Ilana Rubenfeld, who has spent the last four decades refining it. An outgrowth of Rubenfeld's background as a former practitioner of Gestalt therapy, Ericksonian hypnosis, Alexander Technique, and the Feldenkrais Method, the Rubenfeld Synergy Method incorporates touch and movement therapy with verbal expression and is concerned with healing and integrating all aspects of a person's being. Synergists, as practitioners are called, regard the body, mind, emotions, and spirit as part of a dynamically interrelated whole and view awareness as the first key to positive change.

During a session, the practitioner employs a variety of gentle touch approaches in order to determine where tension is being held in the client's body. As each area is uncovered, the Synergist will often speak with their client, helping him or her to better understand the tension's underlying causes. At times, focus may also be

ENERGY PSYCHOLOGY METHODS

The newest approach to healing in somatic psychology is known as "energy psychology." Central to the therapies that comprise such methods is the theory that mental and emotional dysfunctions, as well as addictive behaviors, are due to stored or blocked energetic patterns in the individual's subtle energy field. Practitioners of energy psychology employ specific sequences of acupoint tapping to access and release these blocked energies, often resulting in complete relief of long-standing psychological issues, phobias, and self-destructive behavioral patterns in as little as a single session. Certain therapies in this category also make use of applied kinesiology and breathing techniques. Among the therapies in this category are Callahan Thought Field Therapy, Energy Diagnostic Treatment Methods (EDxTM), Emotional Freedom Techniques (EFT), Neuro-Emotional Technique (NET), and Quantum Emotional Clearing.

placed on the client's breathing or movement patterns and, when appropriate, the Synergist may also employ Gestalt therapy or visualization techniques to further clarify for the client the issues related to their distress.

The Rubenfeld Synergy Method is a gradual process and primarily concerned with leading clients to greater levels of self-awareness as they begin to integrate their physical, mental, emotional, and spiritual energies into a greater expression of wholeness. Depending on the needs of each client, treatments can range from six weeks to several years. Commonly reported benefits of the Rubenfeld Synergy Method include greater self-esteem and self-confidence, improved levels of relaxation, and an overall reduction of tension-related physical symptoms.

 See Mind/Body Medicine.

The Future of Bodywork

Numerous systems of bodywork have been reviewed in this chapter. Some are based on the physical manipulation of body structures, while others focus on the manipulation of the body's energy fields. Others use awareness and learning as the basis for improving body movement and functioning. Importantly, most recognize the value of emotions and have integrated a mind/body philosophy into their practice.

According to Michael Murphy, author of *The Future of the Body* and co-founder of the Esalen Institute in Big Sur, California, these disciplines, when properly applied, have the potential for bringing about transformations of the human personality. He suggests that these systems of bodywork "promote attributes beyond those to which they are primarily addressed." These include increased somatic awareness and self-regulation, improvement of communication abilities, increased vitality, and an improved sense of self. "Somatic disciplines can contribute to balanced programs for growth," Murphy maintains, leading ultimately to extraordinary functioning and then to the possibility for self-transcendence. This, says Murphy, is the future of the body.[44]

Where to Find Help

If you live in a large community, you should be able to find publications that list sources for bodywork and massage therapies. Holistic practitioners are also a good source for referrals. Many massage therapy schools also offer training in various bodywork techniques and are a good source for information and referrals. Check your bookstore for literature on massage techniques.

Massage

American Massage Therapy Association
820 Davis Street, Suite 100
Evanston, Illinois 60201
(847) 864-0123
Website: www.amtamassage.org

Offers comprehensive information on most areas of massage and bodywork, including an extensive review of scientific research. They also publish the Massage Therapy Journal, *available at many newsstands and health food stores.*

American Bodywork and Massage Professionals
28677 Buffalo Park Road
Evergreen, Colorado 80349
(800) 458-2267
Website: www.abmp.com

For information, referrals, and training.

Esalen Institute
Highway 1
Big Sur, California 93920
(408) 667-3000
Website: www.esalen.org

Offers weekend and more extensive programs in holistic health. Many of the systems mentioned in this chapter were introduced and popularized at Esalen, which, under the direction of Michael Murphy, offers a unique training program in integrative body therapy.

Movement Reeducation Therapies

American Society for the Alexander Technique
P.O. Box 60008
Florence, Massachusetts 01062
(800) 473-0620
Website: www.alexandertech.com

For information, referrals, and training in the Alexander Technique.

Feldenkrais Guild of North America
3611 S.W. Hood Avenue, Suite 100
Portland, Oregon 97201
(800) 775-2118
Website: www.feldenkrais.com

For information, practitioner training, and certification in the Feldenkrais Method.

The Trager Institute
3800 Park East Drive, Suite 100, Room 1
Beachwood, Ohio 44122
(216) 896-9383
Website: www.trager.com

For practitioner directory, information, training, and certification in the Trager Approach.

Structural Bodywork

International Rolf Institute
205 Canyon Road
Boulder, Colorado 80306
(303) 449-5903
Website: www.rolf.org

For information, practitioner training, and certification in Rolfing.

The Aston Training Center
P.O. Box 3568
Incline Village, Nevada 89450
(775) 831-8228
Website: www.AstonEnterprises.com

The center trains health-care professionals and laypeople to become certified Aston-Patterning practitioners.

Hellerwork International
3435 M Street
Eureka, California 95503
(800) 392-3900
Website: www.hellerwork.com

For information, referral directory, training, and certification in Hellerwork.

International Alliance of Healthcare Educators (IAHE)
11211 Prosperity Farms Road, Suite D-325
Palm Beach Gardens, Florida 33410
(800) 311-9204
Website: www.iahe.org

For information, referrals, and training in Barral Visceral Manipulation.

Bowen Research and Training Institute, Inc.
P.O. Box 627
Palm Harbor, Florida 34682
(727) 937-9077

For information, referrals, and training in Bowen Therapy.

Pressure Point Therapies

Acupressure Institute
1533 Shattuck Avenue
Berkeley, California 94709
(800) 442-2232
Website: www.acupressure.com

For information on acupressure, career training, and mail-order catalog.

American Oriental Bodywork Therapy Association (AOBTA)
Laurel Oak Corporate Center, Suite 408
1010 Haddonfield-Berlin Road
Voorhees, New Jersey 08043
(856) 782-1616
Website: www.healthy.net/associations/pa/bodywork/about1.htm

For information on acupressure and Oriental bodywork, professional membership, practitioner directory, and referrals.

The International Alliance of Healthcare Educators (IAHE)
11211 Prosperity Farms Road, Suite D-325
Palm Beach Gardens, Florida 33410
(800) 311-9204
Website: www.iahe.com

For information on Oriental bodywork, professional membership, practitioner directory, and referrals.

International Institute of Reflexology
5650 First Avenue North
P.O. Box 12462
St. Petersburg, Florida 33733
(727) 343-4811

Website: www.reflexology-usa.net

For information on reflexology, seminars, publications, and referrals.

Bonnie Prudden Pain Erasure
P.O. Box 65240
Tucson, Arizona 85719
(800) 221-4634
Website: www.bonnieprudden.com

For a list of certified Bonnie Prudden myotherapy practioners and clinics where myotherapy is offered. Offers programs for babies, children, nursing homes, industry, and for the handicapped.

Bioenergetic Systems of Bodywork

Nurse Healers–Professional Associates International
3760 South Highland Drive, Suite 429
Salt Lake City, Utah 84106
(801) 273-3399
Website: www.therapeutic-touch.org

For information, referrals, and training in Therapeutic Touch.

Healing Touch International
12477 W. Cedar Drive, Suite 202
Lakewood, Colorado 80228
(303) 989-7982
Website: www.healingtouch.net

For information, referrals, and training in Healing Touch.

International Center for Reiki Training
29209 Northwestern Highway, Suite 592
Southfield, Michigan 48034
(800) 332-8112
Website: www.reiki.org

For information, referrals, and training in Reiki.

American Polarity Therapy Association
P.O. Box 19858
Boulder, Colorado 80308
(303) 545-2080
Website: www.polaritytherapy.org

For information on Polarity Therapy, publications, and referral directory.

Somatic Psychology

The Naropa Institute
Somatic Psychology Department
2130 Arapahoe Avenue
Boulder, Colorado 80302
(303) 444-0202 or (303) 546-5284

Website: www.naropa.edu

Provides information and training in various somatic psychology approaches.

The Hakomi Institute
P.O. Box 1873
Boulder, Colorado 80306
(888) 421-6699
Website: www.hakomiinstitute.com

For information, referrals, and training in Hakomi.

The Rosen Method
Website: www.rosenmethod.org

Provides links to the various regional Rosen centers throughout the U.S., plus further information on the Rosen Method.

The Rubenfeld Synergy Center
(877) 776-2468
Website: www.rubenfeldsynergy.com

For information, referrals, and training in the Rubenfeld Synergy Method.

Recommended Reading

Bodywork. Thomas Claire. New York: Quill/William Morrow, 1995.

The Future of the Body. Michael Murphy. New York: Tarcher/Putnam, 1992.

Massage

The Book of Massage. Lucinda Lidell. New York: Fireside, 1984.

Massage for Common Ailments. Sara Thomas. New York: Fireside, 1989.

Alexander Technique

The Alexander Technique. Wilfred Barlow. New York: Alfred A. Knopf, 1991.

The Alexander Technique. John Gray. New York: St. Martin's Press, 1991.

Feldenkrais Method

Awareness Through Movement. Moshe Feldenkrais. New York: Harper & Row, 1972.

The Potent Self: A Guide to Spontaneity. Moshe Feldenkrais and M. Kimmey. San Francisco: Harper & Row, 1992.

Trager Approach

Trager Mentastics: Movement as a Way to Agelessness. Milton Trager and Cathy Guadagno. Barrytown, NY: Station Hill Press, 1987.

Rolfing

Rolfing: The Integration of Human Structures. Ida P. Rolf. New York: Harper & Row, 1977.

Aston–Patterning

Aston Postural Assessment Workbook. Judith Aston. San Antonio, TX: Psychological Corporation, 1999.

Hellerwork

Bodywise. Joseph Heller and William Henkin. Berkeley, CA: Wingbow Press, 1991.

Acupressure and Oriental Bodywork

Acupressure's Potent Points. Michael R. Gach. New York: Bantam Books, 1990.

Acupressure Way of Health: Jin Shin Do. Iona M. Teeguarden. New York: Kodansha International, 1978.

Acu-Yoga: The Acupressure Stress Management Book. Michael Gach. New York: Kodansha International, 1981.

The Complete Book of Shiatsu Therapy. Toru Namikoshi. New York: Kodansha International, 1981.

Reflexology

Better Health with Foot Reflexology. Dwight Byers. St. Petersburg, FL: Ingham Publishing, 1987.

Body Reflexology: Healing at Your Fingertips. Mildred Carter. West Nyack, NY: Parker Publishing, 1986.

Hand and Foot Reflexology: A Self-Help Guide. Kevin and Barbara Kunz. New York: Simon & Schuster, 1987.

Bonnie Prudden Myotherapy

Myotherapy. Bonnie Prudden. New York: Ballantine, 1985.

Pain Erasure. Bonnie Prudden. New York: Ballantine, 1985.

Therapeutic Touch

Accepting Your Power to Heal: Personal Practice of Therapeutic Touch. Dolores Krieger. Santa Fe, NM: Bear and Company, 1993.

Living the Therapeutic Touch: Healing as Lifestyle. Dolores Krieger. Wheaton, IL: Quest Books, 1988.

Therapeutic Touch: A Practical Guide. Janet McCrae. New York: Alfred A. Knopf, 1992.

Reiki

Reiki: Universal Life Energy. Bodo Baginski. Mendocino, CA: LifeRhythm, 1988.

Polarity Therapy

Esoteric Anatomy: The Body as Consciousness. Bruce Burger. Berkeley, CA: North Atlantic Books, 1998.

A Guide to Polarity Therapy: The Gentle Art of Hands-On Healing. Maruti Seidman. Boulder, CO: Elan Press, 1991.

Your Healing Hands: The Polarity Experience. Richard Gordon. Santa Cruz, CA: Wingbow Press, 1978.

Hakomi Method

Body-Centered Psychotherapy: The Hakomi Method. Ron Kurtz. Mendocino, CA: LifeRhythm, 1990.

Rubenfeld Synergy Method

Listening Hands: Self-Healing Through the Rubenfeld Synergy Method of Talk and Touch. Ilana Rubenfeld. New York: Bantam, 2000.

Somatic Psychology

Getting in Touch: The Guide to New Body-Centered Therapies. Christine Caldwell. Wheaton, IL: Quest Books, 1997.

Bodies in Revolt: A Primer in Somatic Thinking. Thomas Hanna. New York: Freeperson Press, 1997.

CELL THERAPY

Cell therapy promotes physical regeneration through the injection of healthy cellular material into the body. It is used to stimulate healing, counteract the effects of aging, and treat a variety of degenerative diseases, such as arthritis, Parkinson's disease, atherosclerosis, and cancer.

CELL THERAPY WAS developed by the late Paul Niehans, M.D., a noted Swiss specialist in the field of gland and organ transplants. He is given credit for discovering the process in 1931, even though there are studies in the United States dating back to 1929. His first attempt was actually due to necessity while performing an emergency operation on a woman whose parathyroid glands had been damaged during thyroid surgery. Dr. Niehans intended to transplant fresh parathyroid glands from a steer calf (an accepted practice at the time), but as there was no time to perform a transplant, he mixed a finely minced portion of the gland with a saline solution and injected it into the patient. Her convulsions stopped and she recovered fully. Following the success of this first procedure, Dr. Niehans administered cellular injections to thousands of people including Pope Pius XII, the Duke and Duchess of Windsor, Emperor Hirohito, and former President Dwight D. Eisenhower.

A more recent development, human stem cells may also play an important role in the future of cell therapy. These cells offer the possibility of providing the capacity to repair damaged tissues by supplying a renewable source of new cells. While controversial and yet to be conclusively proven, the use of human stem cells holds great promise for Parkinson's disease, Alzheimer's, heart disease, and other conditions.

What is Cell Therapy?

The broadest definition of cell therapy includes the use of human blood transfusions and bone marrow transplants as well as injections of cellular materials. Cell therapy, as it is discussed here, refers to the injection of cellular material from organs, fetuses, or embryos of animals, or the transplantation of human stem cells, to stimulate healing and treat a variety of degenerative diseases. The main

countries practicing cell therapy, or organotherapy, are Germany, Switzerland, and France.

Several schools of thought exist as to the ideal practice of cell therapy. The various methods include the use of live cells, freeze-dried cells, cells from specific organs, homeopathic formulations, and embryonic preparations. All of these techniques have been used successfully, with different methods targeting different conditions.

- The first cell therapy method was the "fresh" process, in which freshly killed sheep organs were processed and injected into patients. However, the cells survived for only 20 minutes and large amounts needed to be given for the therapy to be effective, which made patients sore for long periods of time. According to cell therapy expert Ted Allen, M.D., of Nassau, the Bahamas, "Initially live cells from organs of freshly killed sheep were used, but the time from the extraction of organs and cells to their subsequent injection was too short to allow for adequate sterility testing. With live cells, there is also the possibility of an immune reaction rejecting the transplant, as often happens with organ transplants."

- Also in use are German opotherapy products, which have been altered by a sterilization process (lyophilization, pasteurization, etc.). The effect of the therapy is substitutional, working at the tissue level without bringing about intrinsic stimulation of the organ itself.

In 1949, Swiss scientists at Nestlé developed the freeze-drying method of processing coffee. Dr. Niehans worked with Nestlé to adapt this technique to conserve biological matter without damage. The result was a process in which sterility could be regulated and cell material could be conserved for longer periods of time. In the cell therapy treatments, the injected cellular material contains a lesser amount of foreign protein than when an entire organ is transplanted, substantially reducing the rejection risk. When whole cells are used in the freeze-drying procedure, the cell surface is still present. This surface is antigenic, meaning it may cause an immune response. For this reason, patients who receive freeze-dried whole cells should be warned of the possibility of an allergic reaction, although the likelihood of this occurring is rare. However, the injection of freeze-dried or lyophylized cells is very painful.

The process of ultrafiltration (the fine filtering of homogenized whole cells down to cell components called ultrafiltrates) removes the cell surface coat and its antigenic material in order to reduce the risk of rejection. The use of freeze-dried cell ultrafiltrates also allows for better quality control and prolonged storage.

- Homeopathic cell therapy, which was widespread in France prior to the introduction of embryo organotherapy, has the effect of restoring functional balance.

- Embryo organotherapy is the use of cells taken from embryos. At one time cells from mature animals were used, today animal embryo cells are the preferred choice. They do not induce immune sensitization or rejection because they do not yet bear the surface antigens. Today, most cell therapy employs embryonic tissues. According to studies by Eberhard Amtmann, of the Institute for Virus Research, in Heidelberg, Germany, cell therapy using embryonic cells may be able to extend the life of the cells by as much as a third. However, in cases involving the parathyroid glands, adult tissues are sometimes used, as these glands are difficult to extract from embryos. More recently, cells from pigs have been found to work very efficiently, according to Peter Stephan, M.D., of the Stephan Clinic, in London, England.

Human Stem Cells

Stem cells are the "mother cells" of all the cells in our body. They have the capacity to repair any tissue damage, which is why researchers are excited about their potential to extend life span and retain the healthy nature of organs in the body. There are three types of stem cells—fetal, umbilical, and adult.

After a very few cycles of replication following fertilization of the egg by a sperm, a structure called a blastocyst is formed. The center of this structure is filled with thousands of "pluripotent" stem cells, or cells that can differentiate into any tissue in the body. The number of pluripotent stem cells expands throughout the early development of the fetus, while simultaneously differentiating into the organs that make up the body. There are intermediate cells between pluripotent stem cells and final specialized cells such as red blood cells or heart cells, called "multipotent" stem cells. Eventually, the number of stem cells peaks and finally begins to decline as the developing embryo reaches the second trimester.

Preliminary research indicates that these cells may have the potential capacity to repair organs composed of a large number of cell types, such as the liver and brain. Multipotent stem cells secrete substances that enable them to identify damaged or deficient cells and repair or augment them. This approach is particularly exciting for conditions that involve cells that do not repair or regenerate well, such as the brain and heart, offering new hope for persons suffering from extensive damage in those organs, as well as offering a supply of cells to replace those lost through the aging process.

Cell therapy is particularly exciting for conditions that involve cells that do not repair or regenerate well, such as the brain and heart, offering new hope for persons suffering from extensive damage in those organs.

Although the number of stem cells declines with age, they are found in children and adults. Obviously, the use of fetal stem cells for human therapy is fraught with ethical and moral issues. Therefore, work with umbilical cord stem cells has begun, as well as studies with adult stem cells. However, 12-week-old fetal stem cells are 27 times more potent than adult cells and nine times more potent than umbilical cells for tissue repair. Furthermore, umbilical and adult stem cells may develop self-antigens, which may result in immune system rejection when used therapeutically. Stem cells harvested from a particular individual and then frozen until later use have shown promising results.[1]

In 1988, former President Ronald Reagan, responding to anti-abortion activists, placed a ban on any new research involving human fetal tissue. In 1993, former President Bill Clinton lifted the ban, enabling scientists to resume work in this field. But controversy continues

SUCCESS STORY: SHARK EMBRYO CELLS FOR SPINAL INJURIES

When Isreal Romero's pickup truck flipped over, breaking several vertebrae in his spine, he lost all sensation from his chest to his feet. He was only 30 years old, a Mexican fisherman who made his living diving for abalone and lobster off the Baja coast, but now it looked like he'd be spending the rest of his life in a wheelchair. That has been the almost guaranteed fate for most people who damage their spinal cord. In America, an estimated 200,000 people suffer partial or complete paralysis from spinal cord injuries and about 10,000 new accidents happen every year, leaving the victims close to totally disabled. Yet, thanks to a combination of highly skilled surgery and a medical breakthrough, five years after his seemingly life-ruining accident, Isreal is not only walking again, but back at work diving.

Isreal was shunted from doctor to clinic to rehabilitation center, but nobody held out much hope for him. Then, he visited the International Head and Spinal Injury Center, in Tijuana, Mexico, under the direction of orthopedic surgeon Fernando C. Ramirez del Rio, M.D., and German physician Wolfram Kühnau, M.D. Dr. Ramirez and his surgical team undertook a series of delicate operations to release, decompress, and remodel the dura sac (the membrane containing the spinal nerves). Using live cell therapy in a procedure developed by Dr. Kühnau, Dr. Ramirez injected living cells (not cartilage) from shark embryos into Isreal's dura sac to regrow the damaged nerves in the spinal cord. The shark embryo cells, before they have differentiated into specific immune or organ-building cells, represent "the highest quality cells available," Dr. Kühnau says. Once inside the human body, they act as pure raw material for regrowing tissue.

Isreal began to regain sensation within a week. He stayed at Dr. Ramirez's clinic for two months, receiving more injections and physical rehabilitation. Two years later, he was able to move about with a walker. Five years after his accident, Isreal is 80%-90% recovered, says Dr. Ramirez, and is diving for abalone once more. The remaining 10%-20% recovery will happen after a few more live cell injections have been completed.

The fact that Isreal is walking again, or even feeling sensation in his limbs, after his accident is highly remarkable. What is even more surprising is Dr. Ramirez's calm statement that had Isreal been able to remain for longer stays at the clinic, his recovery time could have been dramatically reduced. "There is a direct relationship between the frequency of the applications of shark embryo cells and the speed of recovery of the spinal cord," says Dr. Ramirez. "The more frequent the treatments, the faster the mobility is restored."

Dr. Ramirez has treated several more patients with spinal cord injuries and their recovery time has been charted in months, not years. Results of this caliber are unheard of in the annals of neurosurgery and physical rehabilitation. According to conventional medicine, Dr. Ramirez's successes should not be possible. "We are the first clinic I know of to do this anywhere," he comments. "Most doctors will not touch the spinal cord, with surgery or any direct treatment. They say nothing can be done. We say something can be done, and we do it."

Recently, Dr. Ramirez added two new materials to his spine-regrowing injections: nerve growth factor and live cells from the brains of sharks. He found this to be especially effective in his work with quadriplegics, patients who have lost movement in all four limbs. Embryonic shark brain cells seem to speed the recovery process by regrowing spinal tissue faster. Today, four of Dr. Ramirez' patients are walking again, two with a walker, two on their own.

---

to swirl around the use of human embryos for stem cell research, with restrictions on federal research funding proposed in 2001 by President George W. Bush.

Recent research has found that stem cells can also be obtained from the placenta, bone marrow, and even fat, and cloning techniques may one day be used to grow them from adult cells as well, but embryos remain the preferred source for stem cells. Embryonic stem cells can transform into virtually every type of cell, whereas adult stem cells are more limited and also less plentiful in the body.[2]

The Practice of Cell Therapy

There are a variety of methods for employing cell therapy. According to Dr. Allen, "Cells injected into the body find their way to the patient's weak or damaged organ and stimulate the body's healing process. Cells do not actually travel whole, but are broken down to their molecular levels and incorporated in similar structures. This is supported by studies from the Universities of Vienna and Heidelberg, where the movement of cells labeled with dyes or radioactive material was traced after injection.[3] Without fail, kidney cells migrated to the kidney, liver cells to the liver, and so forth."

Dr. Allen employs cell therapy mainly for revitalization purposes. He uses a combination of five different cell types: pituitary, liver, connective tissue, male or female gonads, and one that varies based on the needs of the patient. If the patient has problems with a certain organ, then additional cells specific to that organ can be used. Three to five injections are given in one session. For general revitalization purposes, the patient returns for further injections as necessary. This may continue for six months, one year, or even two years. Dr. Allen believes cell therapy stimulates the immune system, helping it either to prevent disease or to fight it when necessary. In the case of cancer, Dr. Allen feels that cell therapy enhances the overall health of cancer patients and helps them withstand the rigors of chemotherapy and radiation.

"The main benefit of cell therapy is an overall stimulation of the body and its processes," says Tom Smith, M.D., Ph.D., H.M.D., D.Hom. He views cell therapy as an adjunct to other forms of therapy and feels it gives the body a basic support system that allows other therapeutic measures to work more successfully. At Dr. Smith's International Clinic for Biological Regeneration, which has branches in England and the Bahamas, patients are first screened to assess if cell therapy is an appropriate treatment for them. Following this screening, an initial test injection is given to ensure that the patient will not suffer from an allergic reaction. For patients who exhibit a reaction, especially those with a history of allergies, cell therapy may not be advisable.

Dr. Stephan developed a form of cell therapy called Therapeutic Immunology, in which cell extracts are administered along with antibodies raised in animals. Therapeutic Immunology is distinguished from traditional cell therapy in that it is a gentler process and has no side effects. "It is more of a vaccination approach to regeneration," Dr. Stephan explained. "Cells of various organs, glands, and other parts of the body are taken from specially raised animals known to be healthy and free of disease. The cells are placed in solution and filtered to remove the unwanted protein elements, and then introduced into a secondary mammal. The injected antigens react with the cells of this mammal and produce antibodies, which appear in the mammal's bloodstream and can be measured. When the antibodies reach the desired level, blood is taken in the same way as it is for vaccines. The serum is then separated and the antibodies are prepared and tested for purity and effectiveness, before being given to the patient to regenerate the immune system."

Dr. Stephan also used a technique known as Bio-Nutritional Therapy. In this therapy, cells, cell extracts,

---

STAGES OF THERAPEUTIC EFFECT

According to Ted Allen, M.D., of Nassau, the Bahamas, the therapeutic effect of cell therapy appears in three stages. First, there is the immediate reaction in which the patient experiences increased vitality. For example, when Dr. Allen treated a patient with hepatitis, his blood and liver profile tests returned to nearly normal within 36 hours. His symptoms disappeared and follow-up tests confirmed a restored level of health.

In some cases, this response is followed by an immune reaction that can cause slight fatigue and last for several weeks. The third stage is the long-term healing phase. Cellular and organ regeneration will take a minimum of 4-6 months, with the patient's condition continuing to improve over the next few years by way of increased stamina, better blood supply and skin tone, and an overall sense of well-being.

---

and antibodies are combined with nutrients and ATP (adenosine triphosphate, a compound involved in the storage and transfer of energy in cells) to promote tissue regeneration. The mixture is administered either under the tongue or via the nasal or rectal passages, allowing the body to absorb only as much as it needs.

Research into the proper application of human stem cells is still in its infancy. Stem cell therapy holds great promise in the area of organ transplants. In the future, it is hoped that instead of whole organ transplants, cell therapy will allow physicians to transplant healthy replacement cells (generated from stem cells) to repopulate and regenerate the failing organ. For example, healthy heart muscle cells could be used to treat a failing heart. Transplantation of replacement cells for the pancreas could someday be used as a treatment for Type I diabetes. Other conditions that could potentially benefit from transplanting stem cells include Parkinson's disease, Alzheimer's disease, burns, spinal cord injuries, and arthritis.[4]

Conditions Benefited by Cell Therapy

Although the reason cell therapy promotes healing is not fully understood, its practice has been successful with a number of health conditions. Early in his practice, Dr. Niehans noticed that cancer rarely developed in the over 1,000 women he treated for menopausal difficulties with

DENDRITIC CELL THERAPY FOR CANCER

Virtually every major cancer center in the U.S. is involved in clinical trials with dendritic cell therapy, a type of cancer vaccine showing remarkable results. But it is already available and proving its worth outside the U.S. The new approach seeks to stimulate the immune system to destroy cancer sites and cells. Researchers are attempting to create cancer vaccines through a number of techniques, experimenting with a variety of substances that stimulate different types of immune responses.

Presently, the National Cancer Institute has 100 active cancer vaccine trials—15 of these are devoted to dendritic cell therapy. Dendritic cells (DCs) are a rare type of white blood cell, generally accounting for less than 0.2% of total blood cells. Dendritic cells were identified only in 1973, by Ralph Steinman, M.D., head of Rockefeller's Laboratory of Immunology and Cellular Physiology, and the late Zanvil Cohn. The critical role DCs play in immunity wasn't appreciated until the early 1990s, when their use in immunotherapy studies first began appearing.

Cancer's causes and the immune system's failure to effectively deal with it are related. Cancer cells have unique and potent defenses that can make them undetectable by the immune system and disrupt our normal immune responses, weakening or preventing an attack on them. Specifically, they secrete substances called cytokines (some cytokines increase immune response and some suppress it). If we think of the cells of the immune system as an army, cytokines are the spies and scouts, alerting the main forces to the number, whereabouts, and vulnerable points of the enemy. The T cells are the main forces. Thus, the actions of cancer cell–produced cytokines have the effect of leaving our immune "army" without the knowledge of where the enemy is or how to effectively attack it.

Dendritic cell therapy is designed to overcome these defenses and stimulate the body to mount an effective attack on tumor cells—with no toxic side effects. A crucial discovery was made in 1996, when Drs. Michael Roth and Sylvia Kiertscher of the Jonsson Cancer Center at the University of California at Los Angeles, reported that DCs could be created outside the body from more common blood cells called monocytes. This made the creation of a vaccine more practical. To create the vaccine, DCs in culture are exposed to all or part of cancer cells from the patient's tumor. The DCs incorporate this material, break it down into protein fragments, and present them on their surface as antigens. These antigen-loaded DCs are injected into the patient's body, usually far from the tumor site. This stimulates the T cells to proliferate, each T cell producing many clones containing the same tumor-specific antigen. This creates a new army of T cells able to recognize and effectively attack the patient's cancer.

Dendritic cell therapy is being researched at the University of Heidelberg in Germany, the Institute Curie in France, and hospitals throughout Europe. Practically every major medical center in the U.S. is involved in this work, including Memorial Sloan-Kettering, Cedars-Sinai, Dana Farber/Harvard Medical School, M.D. Anderson, and Johns Hopkins University. They have been conducting clinical trials with dendritic cell therapy for melanoma (skin cancer) and prostate, kidney, breast, colon, and other cancers with encouraging outcomes.[5] One private company that has been deeply involved with dendritic cell therapy research is Aidan Incorporated, in Tempe, Arizona. Like other biotechnology firms, Aidan has developed proprietary dendritic cell therapy cancer protocols that are showing remarkable results. And this therapy is available now, not as a clinical trial but as part of an integrated anticancer program at the BioPulse Clinic, in Tijuana, Mexico. "They have just started using it in combination with their other protocols, but the responses have been very positive," says Neil Riordan, M.S., P.A.-C., president of Aidan.

---

ovarian follicular cells taken from sheep. Whereas the number of registered deaths from cancer averaged 25%, the rate for Dr. Niehans' patients was 4%. In the 1960s, Dr. Stephan carried out a similar survey of his own patients and found the same 4% rate. Although these documented facts do not constitute a scientific study, the results suggest the need for further research.

Dr. Niehans considered cancer to be an immunological problem. He believed that cell injections from cancer-resistant animals could increase resistance to cancer in humans and even induce regression of cancer cells in certain cases. This theory is gaining support due to research showing that RNA from healthy cells injected into cancerous tissues retards cancer growth and reduces malignancy.[6] Dr. Niehans used cell therapy to stimulate the regeneration of underdeveloped, diseased, and age-damaged organs. He was successful at treating sexual dysfunction and discovered that sexual vitality could be restored through his therapy. His ultimate aim was to "make all the organs struck by old age capable once more of functioning properly."[7]

Dr. Stephan used cell therapy to treat male impotence. He has had great success with a combination treatment he developed consisting of erectile tissue and cells from the testicle, prostate, the pituitary gland, diencephalon (the area of the brain that includes the thalamus and hypothalamus), and the neurovascular system. A trial experiment using Dr. Stephan's protocol was conducted on 3,500 people who had volunteered for help with sexual revitalization. The study found a 76% success rate among the patients, who ranged from 22 to 76 years old.

Dr. Stephan used cell therapy in the treatment of more than 30,000 patients. Among the conditions he treated are arthritis, heart and circulatory problems, menopause, painful menstruation, and infertility and sterility. Dr. Stephan's treatments have also been successful with cystitis, prostate problems, herpes, lung and bronchial problems, and premature aging.

CAUTION Cell therapy is not recommended for those with severe kidney disease, liver failure, or acute (short-term) infections and inflammatory diseases. Patients who show an allergic reaction to the test injection should not receive the treatment.

Franz Schmid, M.D., of Aschaffenberg, Germany, reports on extensive studies with cell therapy in a wide range of diseases. In one study, 72 patients with arteriosclerosis were treated with a mixture of placenta, liver, and testes. Fifty-eight of them showed marked improvement with a lowering of cholesterol levels and improvement in walking distance.[8] In another study, one year after cell therapy, five of nine heart patients had improved EKG (electrocardiogram) readings and the remaining four were free of complaints.[9] Hepatitis is another disease successfully treated by cell therapy.

For skin problems, particularly burns and scars, Dr. Schmid uses a topical cream prepared with cell extracts. In one case, a young child with second and third degree burns from a gas explosion showed almost complete healing within 19 days. Eighteen months later, no scarring was visible. Certain skin problems may require cell therapy to be given intravenously.[10]

 Additional research into cell therapy could provide valuable information on immunological disorders such as AIDS and cancer, which could save many lives.

Research with Human Stem Cells

Because fetal tissue is especially adaptive to transplantation, scientists are hopeful that transplanted fetal cells will

---

CELL THERAPY AND AIDS

The late Peter Stephan, M.D., of the Stephan Clinic, in London, England, saw cell therapy becoming more widely used to treat AIDS. "My belief is that the answer to the AIDS problem lies not with a specific vaccine or treatment," he said, "but with a therapy that improves the natural function of the total immune system." In cell therapy, this is accomplished by injecting new cells of the spleen, bone marrow, and lymph, together with those of the thymus gland. The injections improve the efficiency of these cell groups and thus increase the body's own ability to fight infection.

"This approach applies not only to AIDS but to other viral infections, since viruses have the ability to change form," according to Dr. Stephan. "A healthy immune system is able to adapt to this change by producing a whole range of antibodies to attack any viral form. Maintaining health lies in the enhancement of the body's natural functions, not in overdosing it with unnatural chemicals."

---

be able to assume the functions of cells that have been destroyed or damaged. A study published in the *New England Journal of Medicine* in 1992 reported that the transplantation of human fetal cells had been successfully used to treat patients with Parkinson's disease. In the case of Parkinson's, cells that normally produce the neurotransmitter dopamine die off, resulting in a loss of muscle control. When fetal cells from a corresponding area of the brain are injected into the brain of a Parkinson's patient, many of the symptoms, such as tremors and paralysis, have been known to disappear, allowing the patient to lead a normal life. The studies cited constant improvement in the patients' motor skills and reported diminished symptoms and signs of Parkinson's as a result of these transplants.[11] However, a recent study involving 40 patients with Parkinson's left many of them worse off, as the transplanted cells started producing excessive amounts of dopamine.[12]

Fetal cell transplants are also being investigated as a possible therapy for Alzheimer's disease, a chronic mental disorder involving progressive, irreversible loss of intellectual functions including comprehension, memory, and speech. Preliminary animal studies have shown that transplanted stem cells migrated to damaged areas of the brain needing repair. This is potentially also helpful for stroke victims.[13]

Stem cells may be helpful for treating heart disease by rebuilding damaged heart muscle and blood vessels.

In one study, injected stem cells (from bone marrow) migrated to the damaged areas and transformed into heart muscle cells. After nine days, new heart muscle cells covered 68% of the damaged area of the heart and they also stimulated the formation of new blood vessels.[14]

The Future of Cell Therapy

Stem cells may play an important role in the future of medicine. These cells, manipulated to develop into specialized cells, offer the possibility of providing the capacity to continually repair damaged tissues or prolong the life span of important organ systems such as the brain and immune system by supplying a renewable source of new cells. Research needs to continue to find the best and most reliable source for these cells and to develop new therapies using stem cells.

> *The process of the regeneration of the human system must be done within the laws of biological science. It is a matter of helping things happen rather than forcing them upon the body.*
>
> —PETER STEPHAN, M.D.

Dr. Stephan coined the phrase "body servicing" to explain his approach to medicine because, according to him, people today service everything but their bodies. "We are living longer, but we are wearing out," he said. "Medical science and better food and hygiene have given us more years to our lives. Cell therapy is concerned with giving more life to those years. I feel that the future of this type of therapy has never been more secure, due to the recent research and development programs exploring the use of new tissues to repair worn out or damaged tissues in the body. And obviously it is better to repair an organ than to replace it, since introducing new cells in the body is better tolerated than introducing whole new organs."

Cell therapy as a practice can contribute greatly to the servicing of the body because of its ability to work in accordance with the body's natural system. "The process of the regeneration of the human system must be done within the laws of biological science," Dr.

Stephan said. "It is a matter of helping things happen rather than forcing them upon the body."

Where to Find Help

For more information on cell therapy, contact an organization below.

Aidan Incorporated
621 South 48th Street
Tempe, Arizona 85281
(800) 529-0269 or (480) 446-8181
Website: www.aidan-az.com

For information on dendritic cell therapy.

BioPulse Clinics
10421 South Jordan Gateway, Suite 500
South Jordan, Utah 84095
(888) 552-2855
Website: www.alternativemedicine.com/healthcenter/biopulse

For information on dendritic cell therapy.

International Clinic of Biological Regeneration (ICBR)
North American Information Office
P.O. Box 509
Florissant, Missouri 63032
(800) 826-5366 or (314) 921-3997
Website: www.icbr.com

International Clinic of Biological Regeneration has offices in England and the Bahamas. They also have an American information office where they can be reached for referrals and other information.

International Head and Spinal Injury Center
Wolfram Kühnau, M.D.
Paseo Tijuana No. 406
Desp. 104, Primer Piso, Edificio Allen Lloyd
Tijuana, B.C., Mexico 22320
(011) 526-683-5151

For information on cell therapy using shark embryo cells.

The Stephan Clinic
27 Harley Place, Harley Street
London, England W1N 1HB
(020) 7-636-6196

The Stephan Clinic was founded in 1965 and has treated more than 30,000 patients. It has been in the forefront of research and development of cell therapy and associated techniques.

Recommended Reading

Forever Young: A Practical Guide to Youth Extension. E. Michael Molnar. West Hartford, CT: Witkower Press, 1985.

Introduction to Cellular Therapy. Paul Niehans, M.D. Savage, MD: Cooper Square Publishers, 1960.

Options: The Alternative Cancer Therapy Book. Richard Walters. New York: Avery Penguin Putnam, 1992.

Stem Cell Biology and Gene Therapy. Peter J. Quesenberry, Gary S. Stein, and Bernard Forget, eds. New York: Wiley-Liss, 1998.

CHELATION THERAPY

Chelation therapy is a safe and effective method for drawing toxins and metabolic wastes from the bloodstream. Chelating agents administered intravenously increase blood flow and may in some cases remove arterial plaque. Chelation therapy, if used in a total program where all risk factors are managed, can potentially help reverse atherosclerosis and prevent heart attacks and strokes, and may be used as an alternative to bypass surgery and angioplasty. It is also useful for treating a variety of disease conditions and, most importantly, regular chelation therapy appears to provide a strong anti-aging effect and remarkably increases energy.

CHELATION (KEY–LAY–SHUN) comes from the Greek word *chele,* meaning "to claw" or "to bind." Chelation therapy is used to rid the body of unnecessary and toxic metals and is employed by a growing number of physicians to improve circulation and help reverse the process of atherosclerosis (hardening of the arteries). The reversal, when it occurs, is accomplished in part through the removal of the calcium content of plaque from the artery walls through the injection of chelating agents. By restoring good circulation to all the tissues of the body, chelation therapy can help to avoid bypass surgery, reverse gangrene, alleviate intermittent claudication (cramps) of the legs, and restore memory.

Due to its ability to remove toxic metal ions, chelation therapy reduces internal inflammation caused by free radicals (highly reactive, destructive molecules) and as a result can ease the discomfort and disability from most degenerative diseases, including arthritis, scleroderma (a hardening that occurs in skin and certain organs), and lupus. It also holds promise for treating the early stages of senile dementia and Alzheimer's disease. Best results are seen when chelation therapy is administered in conjunction with a program of oral supplements, such as *Ginkgo biloba* and phosphatidyl serine, which act as oral chelators in the body.

Chelation therapy has been used safely on more than one million patients in the United States over the past 50 years,[1] but EDTA (ethylenediaminetetraacetic acid), the drug used during the infusions, has yet to receive U.S.

According to current drug safety standards, aspirin is nearly three-and-a-half times more toxic than EDTA.

Food and Drug Administration (FDA) approval for anything other than lead and heavy metal toxicity and the treatment of hypercalcemia. Even so, numerous alternative physicians in the U.S. recommend and use chelation therapy for cardiovascular disease and related health problems, based on their own clinical experience, which has shown that chelation consistently improves blood flow and relieves symptoms associated with vascular disorders caused by arteriosclerosis in more than 80% of patients.[2] Such physicians follow the treatment protocol established by the American College of Advancement in Medicine (ACAM) and the American Board of Chelation Therapy (ABCT), the two leading advocacy organizations for EDTA chelation therapy in the U.S.

How Chelation Therapy is Administered

Chelation therapy is performed on an outpatient basis, is painless, and takes approximately 3 ½ hours. For optimal results, physicians who use chelation therapy recommend 20-30 treatments given at an average rate of one to three per week, with patient evaluations being made at regular intervals.[3]

The patient reclines comfortably and is given an intravenous (I.V.) solution of EDTA with vitamins and minerals. To monitor the patient's progress, James Julian, M.D., of Los Angeles, California, recommends that the following tests be taken before, during, and after chelation:

- Blood pressure and circulation check on all four extremities

- Cholesterol and other blood components

- Vascular studies

- Blood sugar and general nutritional assessment

- Kidney and other detoxification organ function

- Tissue minerals and heavy metals, if indicated

A whole foods, low-fat diet and appropriate exercise are normally recommended as part of a full treatment program. According to Garry F. Gordon, M.D., of Payson, Arizona, the father of the modern-day chelation therapy movement and co-founder of both ACAM and ABCT, a carefully tailored program of vitamin and nutritional supplements should also be part of the treatment and may include ascorbic acid (vitamin C), heparin, selenium, chromium, copper, zinc, and manganese. Smoking is strongly discouraged and alcohol should be consumed only in moderation.

The cost per treatment can vary, depending in part on the nutritional ingredients the doctor may use. As a member of Board of Homeopathic Medical Examiners for Arizona in charge of chelation peer review, Dr. Gordon requires that all newly recognized cardiovascular risk factors, including C-reactive protein, homocysteine, and lipoprotein Lp(a), are tested and treated on any patient having chelation therapy for any vascular problem.

Conditions Benefited by Chelation Therapy

By 1948, the U.S. Navy had begun using EDTA to safely and successfully treat lead poisoning. At the same time, EDTA was being used to remove calcium from pipes and boilers. Norman Clarke, Sr., M.D., Director of Research at Providence Hospital, in Detroit, Michigan, hypothesized that because calcium plaque is a prominent component in atherosclerosis, EDTA would be an effective treatment for heart conditions. His experiments with EDTA chelation for heart patients provided support for his theory. Patients with angina reported dramatic relief from chest pain. Healing was also reported by patients with gangrene. For many patients, memory, sight, hear-

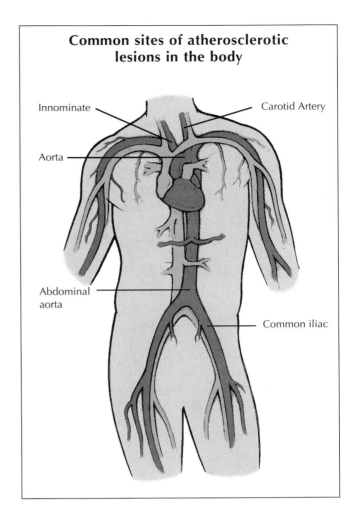

Common sites of atherosclerotic lesions in the body

Innominate

Carotid Artery

Aorta

Abdominal aorta

Common iliac

ing, and sense of smell improved, and most reported increased vigor.[4]

EDTA chelation therapy has since proven to be a safe and effective adjunct in the treatment and prevention of ailments linked to atherosclerosis, such as coronary artery disease (heart attacks), strokes, peripheral vascular disease (leading to pain in the legs and ultimately gangrene and amputation), and arterial blockages elsewhere in the body. According to current drug safety standards, aspirin is nearly three-and-a-half times more toxic than EDTA.[5]

Warren Levin, M.D., of New York City, once administered chelation therapy to a psychoanalyst on the staff of a major New York medical center. "He was in his fifties and looked remarkably healthy, except that he was in a wheelchair. He had awakened that morning to discover his lower leg was cold, numb, mottled, and blue, with two black-looking toes. He rushed to his hospital and consulted the chief of vascular surgery, who recommended an immediate amputation above the knee. He asked this world-renowned surgeon about the possibility of using chelation in this situation and was told 'Don't bother me with that voodoo'." He decided to get a second opinion, but that physician also urged him to have an imme-

CHELATION THERAPY VS. BYPASS SURGERY AND ANGIOPLASTY

Cardiovascular disease is the number one killer in the U.S. Each year, 500,000 Americans die from heart attacks and there are an estimated 1,500,000 new and recurrent cases.[6] Nearly 300,000 bypass surgeries and 250,000 angioplasties are performed in the U.S. every year. Nearly 20,000 deaths occur each year as a result of these procedures.[7]

In 1992, Nortin Hadler, M.D., Professor of Medicine at the University of North Carolina School of Medicine, wrote that none of the 250,000 balloon angioplasties performed the previous year could be justified and that only 3% to 5% of the 300,000 coronary artery bypass surgeries done the same year were actually indicated. Yet a cost comparison study prepared for the Great Lakes Association of Clinical Medicine in 1993 estimated that $10 billion was spent in the U.S. in 1991 on bypass surgery alone.[8] At a symposium of the American Heart Association, Henry McIntosh, M.D., stated that bypass surgery should be limited to patients with crippling angina who do not respond to more conservative treatment.[9]

Chelation therapy offers a viable alternative. In a study of 2,870 cases, Efrain Olszewer, M.D., and James Carter, M.D., head of nutrition at the Department of Applied Health Science, School of Public Health and Tropical Medicine at Tulane University, documented that EDTA chelation therapy brought about significant symptomatic improvement in 93.9% of patients suffering from ischemic heart disease (coronary artery blockage).[10] Elmer Cranton, M.D., of Troutdale, Virginia, estimates chelation therapy can help avoid bypass surgery in 85% of cases. He points out that during all the time that chelation therapy has been administered according to established protocol, not one serious side effect has been reported.

Garry F. Gordon, M.D., of Payson, Arizona, points out that EDTA chelation can be beneficial for bypass candidates even when the therapy appears unsuccessful in reducing the amount of calcification in coronary arteries. The reason for this, according to Dr. Gordon, has to do with the fact that 85% of heart attacks, strokes, and other types of cardiovascular disease are caused by the rupture of vulnerable, non-calcified arterial plaque and subsequent clot formation. "It is now widely accepted that the underlying cause of death in heart attacks and strokes is from a blood clot related to this vulnerable, soft (non-calcified) plaque due to an active infection in the arterial wall," Dr. Gordon explains. "Unfortunately, most patients are unaware of this

new information about vulnerable plaque or that it is not readily detected by any of the currently widely available vascular tests, including angiograms. This means that most surgical procedures on blood vessels are operating on the wrong plaque."

The popular CAT scan test has revealed that many people who have no known risk factors nonetheless have a serious accumulation of calcium in their coronary arteries. "Some of these patients are told to get angiograms, which in nearly everyone over the age of 40 shows some significant narrowing," says Dr. Gordon. "If the patient is lucky, they see a chelation physician, but not everyone (perhaps only 50%) actually get reversal of this calcium in their coronary vessels. Those who do not show improvement on the repeat CAT scan are very disappointed. Some may mistakenly opt for surgery, despite the fact that their so-called unsuccessful chelation treatments have enabled them to easily sustain a far higher level of physical activity than they were capable of prior to beginning treatment."

Dr. Gordon adds that improved oxygenation of ischemic tissues usually results from intravenous chelation. "This, in and of itself, is a reasonable goal for patients with cardiovascular conditions, and simple exercise tolerance testing is very useful in evaluating this," he says. "Those who are still showing serious calcium in their blood vessels may be candidates for a new approach using EDTA rectal suppositories combined with antibiotics or other substances to maintain high levels of EDTA. Or they may respond to special enzymes, such as Wobenzymes, designed to treat this kind of problem. Such enzymes do not break down in the stomach and can lower the C-reactive protein levels and help eliminate the pathogens now believed to be contributing to many cases of coronary artery calcification."

 See Enzyme Therapy, Heart Disease.

Because of the failure of conventional procedures to detect and treat vulnerable plaque, Dr. Gordon considers the standard vascular tests relied upon by conventional physicians to sell bypass and other invasive techniques to patients as being unreliable and misleading. "Since the vulnerable plaque involved in the vast majority of heart attacks and strokes cannot be detected by modern technology, heart surgery is generally attacking the wrong plaque and thus is providing little, if any, long-term benefit at great expense and risk," he concludes.

diate amputation. When asked about chelation therapy, the second doctor's response was "You can try it if you want, but it's a waste of time."

"Through his own tenacity, the psychoanalyst showed up in my office," continues Dr. Levin. "We started emergency chelation and after nine treatments—one every other day—he was pain free and picking up. After 17 chelation treatments, he was walking on the leg again. He never had an amputation and he lived the rest of his life without any further complications."

Anecdotal stories of patient success tend to mean little to a medical researcher like Morton Walker, D.P.M. "But," he writes, "what must an investigative medical journalist do when exposed to story after story of potentially imminent death, blindness, amputation, paralysis, and other problems, and upon visiting these people to check their stories, finds them presently free of all signs of their former health problems? About 200 individuals who were victims of hardening of the arteries are [now] vibrant, productive, youthful looking, vigorous, and enthusiastically endorse chelation therapy as the cause of their prolonged good health. I have turned up not a single untruth."[11]

Medical journalists Harold and Arline Brecher, who have written extensively about chelation therapy, note that physicians who use it not only advise it for their patients, but also use it for themselves. "We have yet to find a physician who offers chelation to his patients who does not chelate himself, his family, and friends," they report.

 Chelation therapy could save millions of dollars each year by preventing unnecessary coronary bypass surgeries, angioplasties, and other expensive procedures related to vascular disorders.

One study documented significant improvement in 99% of patients suffering from peripheral vascular disease and blocked arteries of the legs. Plus, 24% of those patients with cerebrovascular and other degenerative cerebral diseases also showed marked improvement, with an additional 30% having good improvement. Overall, nearly 90% of all treated patients had marked or good improvement as a result of chelation therapy.[12]

One double-blind study revealed that every patient suffering from peripheral vascular disease who was treated with chelation therapy showed a statistically significant improvement after only ten treatments.[13] In another study, 88% of the patients receiving chelation showed improvement in cerebrovascular blood flow.[14] Additional studies found that 58 of 65 patients whose physicians had recommended bypass surgery were able to forgo the procedure following chelation and that chelation also enabled another 24 of 27 patients scheduled to receive

amputations to avoid such drastic measures.[15] Other documented benefits of chelation therapy include:

- Normalization of 50% of cardiac arrhythmias[16]
- Improved cerebrovascular arterial occlusion[17]
- Improved memory and concentration when diminished circulation is a cause[18]
- Improved vision (with vascular-related vision difficulties)[19]
- Significantly reduced cancer mortality rates (as a preventive measure)[20]
- Protection against iron poisoning and iron storage disease[21]
- Detoxification of snake and spider venoms[22]
- Improvement in brain and kidney function[23]

However, recent developments that have led to a new understanding of the role inflammation plays in cardiovascular disease indicate that chelation therapy should no longer be considered as a primary or "single complete therapy" for the long-term management of cardiovascular disease.[24] Dr. Gordon shares this view: "I believe that intravenous EDTA chelation therapy for cardiovascular disease should never be employed without concurrent aggressive and effective pharmacological or nutritional therapy for all the newly recognized cardiovascular risk factors." These include replenishment of deficient minerals and dealing with the infectious and hypercoagulability (excessive blood clotting) aspects.

EDTA chelation therapy still offers many dramatic benefits for patients with cardiovascular disease, and it deserves far greater recognition as part of any cardiovascular support program. In addition, with the recent recognition that some heart conditions show increased levels of toxic heavy metals (some as much as 20,000 times normal), chelation therapy should be far more routinely employed.

According to Elmer Cranton, M.D., of Troutdale, Virginia, chelation therapy can also have a profound effect on overall health. "In my clinical experience, there is no doubt that chelation therapy to some extent slows the aging process," says Dr. Cranton. "Allergies and chemical sensitivities also seem to improve somewhat due to a better functioning of the immune system. All types of arthritis and muscle and joint pains seem to be more easily controlled after chelation, although it is not a cure. In most cases, the progression of Alzheimer's disease will be slowed and, in some cases, the improvement is quite remarkable and the disease does not seem to progress. Macular degeneration, a major cause of visual loss in the elderly, is often improved and almost always arrested or slowed in its progression by chelation therapy."

Rima Laibow, M.D., founding Medical Director of the Alexandria Institute of Natural and Integrative Medicine, in Croton-on-Hudson, New York, confirms that chelation therapy offers benefits for patients suffering from senile dementia and Alzheimer's disease. One of Dr. Laibow's patients was a 68-year-old woman who had suffered from increasing forgetfulness during the previous 15 months. "Prior to the onset of her symptoms, the woman had always been spry and independent," Dr. Laibow says. "She consulted with me after visits to several other doctors, who diagnosed her condition as early dementia of the Alzheimer's type."

Dr. Laibow treated her with a series of chelation treatments to eliminate the toxins that had accumulated in her brain and body. In addition, she supplemented the woman's diet with crucial nutrients and eliminated harmful foods. "Before long, the woman's memory and personality slowly began to re-emerge as the chelation took effect," Dr. Laibow says, "and eventually mental status exams confirmed that she had regained her former level of functioning, enabling her to continue her independent lifestyle without limitation or disability." In addition, her intermittent claudication (lameness after walking or exercise), which she had also been suffering from, was completely corrected by chelation therapy.

Other conditions that Dr. Laibow has successfully treated using chelation therapy include acute and chronic viral infections, asthma, autoimmune conditions, chemical sensitivity and environmental disease, chronic fatigue syndrome, chronic pain, Crohn's disease, emphysema, macular degeneration, tendinitis, ulcerative colitis, and hives, in addition to arteriosclerotic and coronary artery disease. She has also successfully used chelation to protect against the side effects of chemotherapy and radiation treatments.

 Research is needed to validate the effectiveness of chelation therapy in reversing atherosclerosis and related circulatory conditions. If approved by the FDA as a treatment for atherosclerosis, chelation therapy could save thousands of lives annually.

Oral Chelation

There are a variety of substances that act as oral chelating agents, according to Dr. Gordon. "Oral chelation is a well-documented, firmly established medical practice," he says. He points out that penicillamine, a drug used to treat heavy metal poisoning, rheumatoid arthritis, and Wilson's disease (a rare metabolic disorder resulting in an excess accumulation of copper in the liver, red blood cells, and brain), works in a fashion very similar to EDTA. "Some of the benefits derived from penicillamine in the treatment of rheumatoid arthritis are undoubtedly related to the control and removal of excess free radicals. And EDTA itself, when taken orally, provides most of its chelating activities in the body, even though only about 5%-18% of it is actually absorbed." The chelating effects are less dramatic and slower than when received intravenously, but the oral approach has several major advantages, including convenience, potential long-term continuous health maintenance, and low cost. In addition, more than 300 references to oral chelators exist in scientific literature[25] and research published in 2000 has established the safety of the oral use of EDTA.[26]

Dr. Gordon uses many nutritionally based substances as oral chelators, such as garlic, vitamin C, bromelain, carrageenan, *Ginkgo biloba*, malic acid, rutin, selenium, zinc, and certain amino acids such as cysteine and methionine. "Cysteine is effective in the treatment of nickel toxicity," he says, "and it seems to also increase glutathione in the body, which helps to control free radicals." However, he does not find that cysteine-containing supplements are entirely safe in larger quantities, since they have been shown to increase the level of mercury that enters the brain, and thus are only safely used in low levels, unless for a short time under careful supervision to treat a specific problem.

In his patients who use oral chelation formulas, Dr. Gordon has consistently observed a reduction of cholesterol by an average of 20% or more, which he feels significantly decreases the likelihood of atherosclerosis. "The thousands of patients who follow our recommended oral chelation program have all successfully avoided strokes and heart attack rates were also greatly diminished," he says. "We've never had more than two heart attacks per year among all of our patients, even those with a history of severe heart disease. An oral chelation program can do more for overall longevity than you can do even with the most prudent lifestyle possible, because of the continuous nutritional protection chelation offers against a stressful and polluted world. In fact, we probably could so improve brain functioning that Ritalin and tranquilizer sales would plummet if everyone simply realized we have 1,000 times more lead in our bones today than before the industrial age. We are not able to cope with this level of toxic metals and need more metal detoxification than ever before."

Dr. Gordon does not recommend oral chelation as a complete substitute for intravenous chelation therapy, however. "There is a significant difference in both the rapidity and degree of benefits achieved with intravenous chelation over any currently available oral chelation agents," he says. "And the intravenous approach is clearly the proper choice for patients who have only a few months to get well before facing surgery or worse." But for patients whose conditions are not as drastic, as well as for those who want to optimally safeguard themselves against free radicals and plaque buildup, Dr. Gordon views oral chelation as an effective, noninvasive, inexpensive choice.

An oral chelation program can do more for overall longevity than you can do even with the most prudent lifestyle possible, because of the continuous nutritional protection chelation offers against a stressful and polluted world.

—GARRY F. GORDON, M.D.

He also recommends oral chelation as a follow-up maintenance program to I.V. chelation. "Generally, the toxic metals that are removed by I.V. EDTA chelation will start to reaccumulate once treatment is discontinued," he explains. "For this reason, a number of oral chelators can help maintain chelation benefits more effectively over a lifetime." Since no single oral chelator exists that is capable of effectively dealing with the wide range of potentially toxic metals and infectious agents associated with degenerative illness, Dr. Gordon has formulated a broad-spectrum oral chelation formula to address such concerns. "The dosage can be adjusted to permit patients to bring their cardiac risk factors, including platelet aggregation, fibrinogen, and homocysteine, into safe ranges, as confirmed by independent laboratory testing," he says. "Based on these tests, I routinely take patients off of aspirin, coumadin, and other dangerous and ineffective medications."

Dr. Gordon reports that oral EDTA is also safe and effective for treating mercury toxicity, which can be caused by dental amalgams. "More than 1,000,000 patients with mercury toxicity have been safely treated with EDTA therapy in the past 40 years," he says, "and there is no report of anything but enhanced mental functioning in these patients." Many people have been told they cannot do chelation as long as any amalgam fillings are in the mouth. This is not true in Dr. Gordon's experience. Because of its effectiveness in this regard, he states that "regular long-term use of oral chelators such as garlic, alginic acid, L-methionine, ferulic and fulvic acid, selenium, and, to some extent, EDTA, can provide a less expensive alternative for patients with dental amalgams who cannot afford the expense of having them replaced."

CHELATION THERAPY AND CANCER

Beginning in 1958, a lengthy study was conducted in Switzerland on 231 adults who lived near a well-traveled highway and had a higher rate of cancer mortality than other people of the same city who lived in traffic-free areas. The study group also suffered from a higher incidence of nervous disorders, headaches, fatigue, gastrointestinal disorders, depression, and substance abuse. The researchers suggested that their symptoms might be due to a higher level of exposure to lead from automobile exhaust.

Three years later, 59 patients from this group received ten or more EDTA chelation treatments plus vitamins B₁ and C, while the remaining 172 members of the group were untreated. An 18-year follow-up study of the group conducted by Walter Blumer, M.D., of Nestal, Switzerland, revealed that only one of the 59 treated patients died of cancer (1.7%) as compared to 30 deaths (17.6%) from cancer among the nontreated subjects. This is a 90% reduction of mortality from cancer. Dr. Blumer found that death from atherosclerosis was also reduced among the treated patients. His findings were based upon Swiss death certificates and statistical evidence showing that EDTA chelation therapy was the only significant difference between the treated group and the other patients.[27]

Commenting on Dr. Blumer's study, Garry F. Gordon, M.D., says, "Anything that reduces your burden of toxic metals, which stimulates free radicals, sufficiently safeguards your immune system so that your body can more efficiently handle early cancers." Dr. Gordon prefers to view chelation therapy in terms of cancer prevention and not as a treatment in itself. "Cancer has been linked to free-radical pathology and EDTA chelation removes elements, such as iron, that can accelerate this pathology," he says. "Therefore, chelation treatments can minimize one's risk of developing cancer."

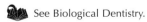 See Biological Dentistry.

Dr. Gordon is currently involved in educating physicians and patients alike about the remarkable benefits that oral chelating agents, including oral EDTA, can offer. "Since we now live on a poisoned planet, there is no one alive today that does not have more toxic metals than they can safely manage," he says. "Thus, lowering toxic metals in patients, from birth on, will result in greater health and less degenerative disease." Dr. Gordon believes that oral chelation should be as routine as taking vitamin C supplements and at a comparative cost. "This would help the treatment of virtually every known health problem and allow most of us to live years longer while maintaining a far higher level of health," he says.

> **CAUTION** EDTA normally should not be used during pregnancy, severe kidney failure, and hypoparathyroidism.

How to Find the Right Doctor

Patients interested in chelation therapy should choose a doctor who follows the protocol of the American Board of Chelation Therapy or the American College of Advancement in Medicine (ACAM). Dr. Gordon notes that physicians who specialize in the field of chelation therapy will also have a diplomate status with the ABCT.

- Prior to chelation, a complete physical examination that includes a heart function test, hair mineral analysis, an electrocardiogram, a stress test, and Doppler flow analysis should be conducted. Kidney function must also be checked.

- EDTA dosage should be individualized for each patient according to age, sex, weight, and kidney function, and should be administered slowly over a period of three or more hours.

- Treatments should be administered by well-trained staff who are readily available to deal with any symptoms that might occur during the process, such as weakness or dizziness from low blood sugar levels.

If a patient decides to have chelation therapy, it should be performed by an experienced doctor, who has completed the training conducted by ACAM. If the therapy is administered by a nurse or nonphysician, a qualified physician must be on the premises at all times during the procedure.

The Future of Chelation Therapy

Because the patent for EDTA has expired, it is unlikely that any pharmaceutical company will invest the money

necessary to fund studies for FDA approval of chelation therapy, despite the overwhelming evidence of its effectiveness for improving blood flow and its anti-aging benefits. Robert Haskell, M.D., writes, "Of all the regimens you can use to help a patient combat degenerative disease and restore health, chelation therapy is the most powerful. It produces the greatest number of benefits to the body, far beyond improved blood flow. If you want to get your prescribed nutrition to those parts of the body in which they must work, chelation therapy is the way to do it."[28]

Dr. Gordon, while remaining a strong advocate of both I.V. and oral chelation therapy, believes that the role of EDTA in clinical practice needs to be reevaluated and foresees it being used primarily as an adjunctive therapy, since its primary function is eliminating excess levels of heavy metals. "I fear negative outcomes from currently proposed or ongoing chelation cardiovascular studies where removal of the wrong plaque is the focus," he says. "If, on the other hand, long-term outcomes and quality-of-life data are compared to standard conventional therapies, these data should offset any detected failure to remove plaque. Combined with treatment of all the newly recognized risk factors, a comprehensive chelation protocol will be shown to produce exceptional long-term medical benefits."

Dr. Gordon's position is that chelation therapy is clearly not reversing plaque in everyone who receives it, yet "over 80% of chelation patients state that it is one of the best things they ever did." Dr. Gordon warns that the heart surgery and cardiovascular drug industries, threatened by the loss of revenue when people elect chelation therapy (oral or I.V.), will set up studies that will prove chelation therapy does not work for the thing they will ask it to do—reverse obstructing plaque. "Yet plaque has been in man for the past 5,000 years and we now know it is not involved in 85% of heart attacks," he points out. "We die of a blood clot induced by an inflammatory process in our blood vessels. Both I.V. and oral chelation allow patients to achieve dramatic symptomatic relief, yet that will not count in any proposed study financed by the special interests that seek to discredit such approaches. Thus, we have a therapy that can help everyone achieve higher energy and higher health and improved IQ, yet it will be loudly proclaimed a failure with the large government-funded studies that are set to begin soon."

To prevent such an outcome, patients and physicians need to better educate themselves about the already established efficacy of both oral and I.V. chelation therapy, as well as the actual basis as to why and how they can be so effective.

Where to Find Help

As in all the specialties of medicine, board certification assures that a particular physician has been trained and his or her knowledge has been demonstrated to be at the highest level. For more information on chelation therapy, contact one of the following organizations:

American Board of Chelation Therapy
Great Lakes College of Clinical Medicine
1407-B North Wells Street
Chicago, Illinois 60610
(800) 286-6013
Website: www.glccm.org

ABCT established the protocol for chelation therapy in 1983 and has been certifying physicians trained in the specialty of chelation therapy. Write or call for the names of board-certified physicians.

American College of Advancement in Medicine (ACAM)
23121 Verdugo Drive, Suite 204
Laguna Hills, California 92654
(800) 532-3688
Website: www.acam.org

ACAM seeks to establish certification and standards of practice for chelation therapy. It provides training and education and sponsors semi-annual conferences for physicians and scientists. It provides referrals and informational material, including a directory (updated monthly) of physicians worldwide trained in preventive medicine as well as in the ACAM protocol. The organization also provides a copy of the ACAM protocol for chelation to the public. For more information, send a stamped, self-addressed envelope.

Gordon Research Institute (GRI)
708 E. Highway 260
Payson, Arizona 85541
(520) 474-3684
Website: www.gordonresearch.com

Founded by Garry F. Gordon, M.D., GRI has compiled over 40 years of scientific research related to I.V. and oral EDTA chelation therapy and provides information for anyone considering either form of the therapy or wanting to know more about Dr. Gordon's proprietary oral chelation products.

Recommended Reading

Bypassing Bypass. Elmer Cranton. Troutdale, VA: Hampton Roads, 1997.

Chelation Extends Life. James Julian, M.D. Hollywood, CA: Wellness Press, 1982.

The Chelation Way. Morton Walker, D.P.M. Garden City Park, NY: Avery Publishing Group, 1990.

40-Something Forever. Harold and Arline Brecher. New York: Health Savers Press, 1992.

The Healing Powers of Chelation Therapy. John P. Trowbridge, M.D., and Morton Walker, D.P.M. Stamford, CT: New Way of Life, 1992.

Questions from the Heart. Terry Chappell, M.D. Troutdale, VA: Hampton Roads, 1995.

Scientific Basis of EDTA Chelation Therapy. Bruce Halstead. Colton, CA: Golden Quill Publishers, 1979.

A Textbook on EDTA Chelation Therapy (Special Issue, Journal of Advancement in Medicine, Volume 2, Numbers 1 & 2). Elmer Cranton, ed. New York: Human Sciences Press, 1989.

CHIROPRACTIC

Recognizing the importance of a properly functioning nervous system, chiropractors use safe adjustments of the spine to allow the body's innate intelligence to reach and maintain the highest possible level of health. An estimated 23-28 million people visit chiropractors each year in the United States to receive drugless and surgery-free care.

SINCE ITS FOUNDING as a profession in 1895, chiropractic has become the second largest primary health-care field in the world and one of the fastest growing. The popularity of chiropractic can be traced to several factors, including a general increased interest in wellness and holistic health, an awareness of the dangers posed by many conventional medical procedures and drugs, and the very high patient satisfaction that is a hallmark of the profession. The search for a non-medical approach that respects the body's innate healing abilities has led millions of people directly to chiropractic. Although many people still associate chiropractic only with back and neck pain, it has also been shown to be safe and effective in improving function and enhancing performance of the body's healing powers. With chiropractic's emphasis on wellness, patients have also recovered from a variety of injuries, illnesses, and many other serious health problems.

How Chiropractic Works

The practice of chiropractic focuses on the relationship between the structure of the spine and the function coordinated by the nervous system, and how this relationship affects the preservation and restoration of health. When there is nerve interference caused by misalignments in the spine, known as subluxations, tension and/or pain can occur and the body's defenses can be diminished. By adjusting the spine to remove subluxations, normal nerve function can be restored.

The spinal column, or backbone, consists of 24 small bones called vertebrae and extends from the back of the skull to below the small of the back. The vertebrae form a protective "tunnel" for the spinal cord. Pairs of spinal nerves branch off the spinal cord between each of the vertebra and extend to every part of the body, including

muscles, bones, organs, and glands. Over this complex highway of nerves, the brain sends messages that regulate all bodily functions and receives feedback about the health and functioning of each part of body.

"When subluxation occurs, it can result in tension in the tissues of the nervous system," explains chiropractic researcher and educator Michael Stern, D.C., of Minneapolis, Minnesota. "This, in turn, can impede the functioning of the nervous system, resulting in diminished or distorted communication between the brain and the rest of the body, and contributing to a wide variety of health problems." For instance, tension in the lower back may force a person to compensate by bending forward, which can interfere with the movement of the ribs and restrict the functioning of the lungs. It may also cause the neck muscles to contract, which in many cases can lead to muscle spasms, headaches, strained vision, or balance and coordination problems.

One of the most obvious results of subluxations can be a decrease in spinal mobility. Dr. Stern relates the case of an 80-year-old woman who suffered from osteoporosis, was "bent over like a pretzel," and could not even see ahead of her as she walked. "After several sessions in which I gently adjusted her, her ability to stand upright and see ahead of her was noticeably improved," Dr. Stern says. "She was also able to walk more easily and reported improvements in her digestion and elimination, as well as her overall level of stress. As her case demonstrates, neither age nor osteoporosis are contraindications for chiropractic."

Although the impact of a subluxation isn't always as dramatic as in the case above, usually symptoms related to spinal misalignment are quite clear and can include muscle spasms, pain, headaches, stiffness, or digestive difficulties. These symptoms are actually valuable messages from the body to alert the person that a problem already

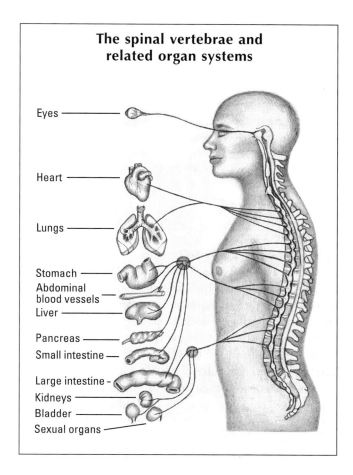

The spinal vertebrae and related organ systems

Eyes

Heart

Lungs

Stomach
Abdominal
blood vessels
Liver

Pancreas
Small intestine

Large intestine
Kidneys
Bladder
Sexual organs

Dr. Blaich, the woman had a long history of severe, almost monthly, bladder infections. She had been through years of medical treatment, but nothing had helped her problem. In addition to her chronic infections, she also experienced severe bladder pain if she were under any stress at all, which indicated to Dr. Blaich that there was a direct link between her condition and her nervous system. "By identifying the subluxations of the lower vertebrae that were irritating the nerves to the bladder, and by correcting those subluxations, we were able to reduce the irritation to the bladder," Dr. Blaich says. "After only four treatments, she got over the infections and had no more recurrences of either the infections or the pain."

Millions of patients who have suffered for years report finding relief from back pain, asthma, headaches, hearing problems, and a long list of other disease conditions after receiving chiropractic care and discovering the role that subluxation played in their illness.

—TERRY A. RONDBERG, D.C.

exists. The effects of subluxation can also be far more subtle or even completely imperceptible, however, and can slowly undermine one's health. The distorted nerve flow caused by the vertebral subluxation can cause long-term damage to organs, which does not become obvious until the condition has progressed.

When the vertebrae are properly aligned, the spine remains mobile, allowing the electrical impulses from the brain to travel freely along the spinal cord to the organs, thus maintaining healthy function. When subluxations occur, they impede this normal flow in the nerve structures, which in turn affects normal organ function.

"The vertebral subluxation is often referred to as the silent killer if it is not causing a symptom or warning signal, since it will still rob you of your vitality and weaken your immune system," notes Terry A. Rondberg, D.C., President of the World Chiropractic Alliance. "Millions of patients who have suffered for years report finding relief from back pain, asthma, headaches, hearing problems, and a long list of other disease conditions after receiving chiropractic care and discovering the role that subluxation played in their illness."

An example of this is a patient treated by Robert Blaich, D.C., of Denver, Colorado. Prior to coming to

The goal of chiropractic is to correct vertebral subluxations and allow the body to repair and restore itself the way it was designed to do. As Dr. Rondberg says, "The chiropractic philosophy is based on common sense, and was best summed up by Dr. Albert Schweitzer when he said, 'Each patient carries his own doctor inside him—we are at our best when we give the doctor who resides within each patient a chance to work.' That's precisely what chiropractors do. They help give the 'doctor within' each patient a chance to work by correcting vertebral subluxations that may be interfering with the natural flow of life energy over the spinal nerves to all the tissue cells and other parts of the body." When nerve interference is reduced, the body has a better chance of reaching its goal of better health. That's why chiropractic is used as an integral part of wellness and preventive care as well as a way to help overcome particular health problems.

HISTORY OF CHIROPRACTIC

Spinal adjustment has been practiced in every civilization, from the early Egyptians onward. In 1895, Daniel David Palmer, a longtime student of physiology and anatomy, founded the modern-day system and theory of chiropractic. Palmer had encountered a janitor who had been deaf for 17 years, following an injury to his upper spine. While examining the janitor's spine, Palmer found a misaligned vertebra (subluxation) that corresponded to the spot the man had injured just prior to losing his hearing. By administering a specific thrust or adjustment to the vertebra, Palmer restored the man's hearing.

Fundamental to Palmer's philosophy of health is the idea that all living beings are endowed with what he termed *innate intelligence*. Palmer believed that this intelligence regulates all the vital functions of the body as it flows through the central nervous system.[1] Because of this belief, Palmer felt that the primary task of the chiropractor was not to treat conditions but to remove nerve interference caused by subluxations so that the innate intelligence could carry out its role of maintaining the body's health and equilibrium without obstruction.

In contrast to the growing popularity of medication and surgical intervention, Palmer's approach appealed to patients interested in natural methods of healing. Chiropractic, he said, embraces "the science of life, the knowledge of how organisms act in health and disease, and also the art of adjusting the neuroskeleton."

The Advantages of Chiropractic Care

Numerous scientific and medical research projects have demonstrated that chiropractic care has several major advantages over conventional medical treatment for many patients. Chiropractic is significantly safer than conventional care, has been shown to be either as effective or more effective than conventional treatments for certain conditions such as back pain, and is usually less expensive.

"Safety is a primary advantage and one that has attracted millions of people to chiropractic," Dr. Rondberg says. "Since the beginning of the industrial age, most people have turned to medical disciplines for answers to health problems. This has created a multibillion-dollar disease industry, but according to almost every study done in the past few decades, it hasn't helped make us any healthier. Major life-threatening diseases like cancer, heart disease, and diabetes are striking more people than ever. At the same time, the overuse, misuse, and abuse of drugs and surgical procedures are actually adding to the death toll. Chiropractic, on the other hand, does not introduce anything foreign into the body."

Because it does not involve drugs or invasive procedures, chiropractic is far safer than conventional medicine, a claim that has been supported by numerous scientific research projects. One measure of the relative risk involved in any health discipline is the cost of malpractice insurance. The higher the risk, the higher the insurance premiums. In 1992, medical doctors in the U.S. paid nearly $42 billion in malpractice premiums, while chiropractors paid only $62 million.[2]

A study known as *The Manga Report* conducted under the auspices of the Ministry of Health, in Ontario, Canada, reviewed all available international evidence on the use of chiropractic for back pain. Pran Manga, Ph.D., the lead researcher, concluded that "many medical therapies are of questionable validity or are clearly inadequate. Chiropractic care is greatly superior to medical treatment in terms of scientific validity, safety, cost effectiveness, and patient satisfaction."[3] Another major research project, known as *The New Zealand Report,* came to a similar conclusion in 1979, noting that "modern chiropractic is a soundly based and valuable branch of health care." Among the many case histories the report documented was that of a woman who had medical treatment for several years after being seriously injured in a car accident. The medical treatment never fully repaired the damage and after wearing a stabilizing brace for nearly ten years, she consulted a chiropractor. According to the report, "After the first adjustment, she walked out of his room without the brace and without pain. She was able to enjoy a healthy, active pain-free body."[4]

Although the overall safety of chiropractic is unquestioned, some medical critics have claimed that chiropractic adjustments have been linked to strokes. However, scientific evidence indicates that there is no validity to that claim. Over a ten-year period, for example, Danish researchers found only five cases of "irreversible CVA [cerebrovascular accidents] after chiropractic treatment." Based on their findings, they estimated a risk of one stroke per 1,320,000 neck adjustments, an extremely rare occurrence.[5]

Chiropractic's cost-saving benefits have also been documented. This is particularly evident with regard to treatment for low-back pain. In 1995, an analysis of insurance claim records showed that the mean outpatient cost for conventional medical treatment of low-back pain was $1,027 compared to a mean cost of $647 incurred by patients who received chiropractic care. Research also shows that chiropractic patients with low-back pain require an average of 6.3 days of compensation pay due to work loss compared to 25.6 days of compensation pay for patients who receive conventional care.[6] Furthermore, according to records from the Worker's Compensation Fund, the average medical patient was paid ten times more compensation than the average chiropractic patient for the treatment of low-back pain. Even though the chiropractic patient tends to pay a little more for individual treatments than the medical patient, the conventional medical costs were more extreme because patients required more treatments.[7]

Types of Chiropractic Care

Although there is fairly widespread agreement on the definition and purpose of chiropractic, individual chiropractors can vary in how they view their role as health-care providers. Since chiropractic's inception, some chiropractors made broad and, at times, unsubstantiated claims that chiropractic could 'cure' any number of ailments. They viewed vertebral subluxations as the cause of diseases and, by correcting the spinal misalignments, felt they were treating the diseases themselves. This differs from the standard concept of correcting subluxations in order to allow the body to function properly and repair or restore itself—a subtle difference, but an important one.

While some doctors of chiropractic limit their practice to detection and correction of vertebral subluxations, others employ a variety of complementary treatments in conjunction with manual spinal alignment techniques. These range from exercise and lifestyle recommendations, nutritional counseling, and massage, to traction, extremity adjusting, hot and cold packs, orthotics, and various diagnostic instruments, such as X rays and surface electromyography (EMG). Other treatment modalities, such as electrical stimulation, ultrasound, diathermy, cryotherapy, and neurologic and orthopedic tests, may also be employed, as well as a number of full-body medical diagnostic procedures, such as blood tests, urinalysis, and full-body X rays.

Acupuncture, herbal medicine, homeopathy, colonic irrigation, fasting, galvanic stimulation, and other techniques are used by some chiropractors as well. A small percentage of chiropractors, depending on their licensing and the state in which they practice, may also perform gynecological and breast exams, perform minor surgery, cast fractures, give manipulation under anesthesia, prescribe drug and vitamin injections, and use magnetic resonance imaging (MRI) and computerized tomography (CT) scans, invasive electromyography, and other medical procedures allowed by law.

The Benefits of Chiropractic Treatment

Early chiropractors believed that subluxations were the cause of all disease. Today, the profession understands much more clearly the multifactorial nature of health and illness. Yet, while subluxations may not be the sole cause of a given disease, they are still a major predisposing factor because they prevent the nervous system from working optimally to help keep the body healthy. By correcting vertebral subluxations, the chiropractic adjustment can help maintain the overall health of the nervous system and the body's organs.

Chiropractic adjustments are also helpful in preventing everyday wear and tear on joints and ligaments by maintaining the proper mobility of the joints. It can also help decrease accumulation of scar formation after serious injury, thus preventing later weakness or stiffness of the affected joints. During a chiropractic session, if localized areas of dysfunction are apparent, treatment will usually focus on increasing spinal motion. This can be accomplished through the use of a combination of touch, active motion (having the patient bend or stretch in precise ways), and passive movement (in which the chiropractic physician assists the patient) in order to initiate a specific adjustment.

One of the most common complaints from patients seeking chiropractic care is low-back pain. In a two-year study by Britain's Medical Research Council, chiropractic treatment was found more effective than hospital outpatient care for low-back pain. Years later, those patients treated with chiropractic care continued to suffer less pain than those treated by medical doctors.[8] Studies conducted by the Florida Department of Labor and the Rand Corporation, in Los Angeles, California, came to similar conclusions.[9] Along with these landmark studies, there is also a general shift of attitude within the medical community that supports chiropractic's new role and acknowledges the vital importance of the nervous system in relation to the normal functioning and relative health of the body.

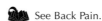 See Back Pain.

According to the American Chiropractic Association, chiropractic is also an effective treatment for neck injuries, whiplash, scoliosis (curvature of the spine), carpal tunnel syndrome, repetitive stress disorders, certain sports injuries (particularly those that limit range of motion), and as an aid for dealing with the physiological changes experienced by women during and after pregnancy.[10] The following ailments have also responded well to chiropractic care: respiratory conditions, gastrointestinal disorders, sinusitis, bronchial asthma, heart disease, high blood pressure, and the common cold.[11]

Patients visiting chiropractic physicians often discover that the underlying causes of their illnesses are not what they expected them to be. A man who had been experiencing extreme pain after ejaculation for a number of years came to Dr. Blaich. The man assumed that the problem stemmed from his vasectomy and his medical doctors had not reached any other conclusion. After a series of tests, Dr. Blaich was able to determine that the man's condition was actually caused by a misalignment in his lower back, which was affecting his prostate and had nothing to do with his vasectomy. In a matter of three or four treatments with Dr. Blaich, the man's discomfort disappeared completely.

In a case published in the *Journal of Manipulative and Physiological Therapeutics*, a man whose speech was impaired due to a spastic constriction of his vocal chords, sought help from two university hospitals. When nothing could be found, he was prescribed psychiatric therapy. The man visited a chiropractor instead, who diagnosed a subluxation in the upper spine. His speech began to return after the second adjustment and, by the fifth adjustment, he was completely free of any speech impediments. When he became hoarse several months later, additional adjustments cleared up the problem, which never returned.[12]

Chiropractic has also been successful in treating various disturbances of the body, including peripheral joint injuries (hands, knees, elbows, hips, shoulders), sprains, arthritis, bursitis, and menstrual difficulties, plus a wide range of emotional problems, from mild depression to schizophrenia. Evidence also shows that chiropractic adjustment combined with proper nutrition can improve and, in some cases, reverse osteoarthritis.[13] Just as significantly, research shows that the long-term benefits of regular chiropractic care helps to maintain the health of the body as we age and prevent decline in physical capabilities among the elderly. In a study published in 1996, researchers found that elderly chiropractic users were "less likely to have been hospitalized, less likely to have used a nursing home, more likely to report a better health status, more likely to exercise vigorously, and more likely to be mobile in the community. In addition, they were less likely to use prescription drugs."[14]

Chiropractic for Children

Correcting subluxations may be particularly important for infants and children, according to many chiropractic experts. "Starting with the birthing process itself, our bodies are subjected to many spinal traumas," say Drs. Stuart and Theresa Warner, D.C., founders of the World Children's Wellness Foundation. "Even the most 'natural' of births can cause stress and strain to the developing spine. This initial damage can be compounded when developing proper head support for the child, and as the child learns to sit up, crawl, and walk. During this time of rapid spinal growth, tiny bumps and falls can be the cause of many unexplained health problems."[15]

Chiropractic adjustments have been shown to have a positive result with many common childhood illnesses, including otitis media, or ear infections. Most pediatricians treat ear infections with an antibiotic or oral decongestant or even with a surgical procedure called a tympanotomy (during which tubes are inserted into the ear canals). However, all of these treatments have been shown to be either ineffective or risky. Several studies show that chiropractic, on the other hand, is both safe and effective for ear infections. In one study of 46 children (age 5 and under) with otitis media, 93% of all episodes improved, 75% in ten days or less.[16] In another study, five children with chronic recurrent otitis media all responded favorably to chiropractic care.[17]

The same is true for another common childhood ailment, asthma, which has reached epidemic proportions in the U.S. and many other nations. A study of 81 asthmatic children (ages one to 17) reported an improvement in 90.1% after they had been under chiropractic care for 60 days. The study's authors concluded, "Chiropractic care, for correction of vertebral subluxation, is a safe, nonpharmaceutical health-care approach, which may also be associated with significant decreases in asthma-related impairment as well as a decreased incidence of asthmatic attacks."[18]

Chiropractic and Addiction

Jay Holder, M.D., D.C., Ph.D., of Miami, Florida, working with the University of Miami School of Medicine and the Florida Chiropractic Society, conducted the first large-scale human study to prove the effectiveness of the chiropractic adjustment in dealing with chemical addiction. Dr. Holder has seen dramatic preliminary results from the triple-blind study showing that a person receiving chiropractic care is ten times more likely to complete a drug program. "This equates to about a 97% retention rate," he says.

Retention rate, or how long a person stays in a treatment program, is extremely important. "The longer a drug addict is in a treatment center, the better the end results will be and the more likely the person will be successful staying drug-free the rest of his or her life," Dr. Holder explains. "By removing subluxations that interfere with the normal functioning of the nervous system, a person is more likely to complete their term of stay, because the person now can meet the needs of the other modalities offered as treatment. We have fewer people with drug detoxification or withdrawal symptoms, their physical complaints are almost eliminated, and they can now concentrate on dealing with their addiction."

The American College of Addictionology and Compulsive Disorders (ACACD), in Miami, Florida, has chosen chiropractic as the profession of choice in training for board certification in addictionology. "The ACACD targeted the chiropractic community because chiropractic is a drugless approach," states Dr. Holder. "People who are chemically dependant must stay away from mood-altering substances their entire lives. What type of primary-care physician is going to be best able to meet the needs of the recovery community? Obviously, someone who isn't going to use mood-altering substances."

When to See a Chiropractor

Subluxations rarely take care of themselves and, according to Dr. Blaich, most people have subluxations they aren't even aware of that are causing problems. "When someone takes a fall and ends up with a misalignment of the lower spine, typically he or she will just ignore it after a few days, when the pain has gone away," he says. "Then, the person finds out years later that the hip has been deteriorating more rapidly than it should have been."

Dr. Blaich laments that people often pay more attention to the maintenance of their cars than they do to the care of their bodies. "People can see the premature wear and tear on their car's tires that occurs if the wheels are misaligned, yet the same holds true for the human body if the spine is misaligned," he says. A chiropractor can quickly show people where these subluxations are and teach patients how and when to recognize the warning signs that may eventually lead to serious health problems.

"It is essential for a person to have the spine aligned on a regular basis, just as the person would go to a dentist to have his or her teeth cleaned to prevent disease," contends Dr. Holder. "This keeps the spine free from subluxation and is the best preventative measure the person can take against disease." According to Dr. Holder, subluxations can be caused by five factors: physical, which includes trauma; mental, such as stress; genetic predisposition; chemical (imbalance or toxicity); and thermal, which includes extreme changes in temperature.

Dr. Holder advocates that a person see a chiropractor once every month to six weeks, on average, though it really depends on how long an individual can hold the adjustment. Certain cases, adds Dr. Holder, require more attention, such as alcohol and drug addiction, recurring injuries due to sports and work, and pregnancy. "If a woman is pregnant, her needs are increased, because the

nervous system of a woman directs the creation of the embryo and the fetus," says Dr. Holder. "When a woman receives adjustments during her pregnancy, there is also better delivery, less back pain, healthier children, and less chance of a miscarriage."

Dr. Holder's assertions are echoed by Dr. Stern. "Chiropractic care, by keeping the nervous system and the pathways between the brain and every cell of the body as healthy and tension-free as possible, is an ideal form of primary, preventive, and restorative care that ensures a patient's body is operating at its optimum state of healing and wellness," he says.

> *Chiropractic care, by keeping the nervous system and the pathways between the brain and every cell of the body as healthy and tension-free as possible, is an ideal form of primary, preventive, and restorative care that ensures a patient's body is operating at its optimum state of healing and wellness.*
>
> —MICHAEL STERN, D.C.

The Chiropractic Visit

A typical first visit to a chiropractor usually consists of a consultation and complete spinal examination. Most doctors will also provide some patient education if the individual is not familiar with chiropractic care. After obtaining personal information and a health history, the doctor will conduct a thorough chiropractic examination. The most common examination is called palpation. The doctor carefully feels, or palpates, the entire spinal region to detect vertebral misalignments. Other methods or instruments, including spinal X ray, may be used to verify the findings and to rule out pathology, such as cancer. All of the examination techniques are safe, painless, and noninvasive. After the spinal examination, the chiropractor reviews their findings and recommends a course of treatment.

At the heart of chiropractic care is the adjustment. "The spinal adjustment is a precise and specific means of correcting subluxation, misalignment, tension, and nerve interference," Dr. Stern explains. "Chiropractors spend many hours of their education learning how to properly diagnose and treat subluxation and often utilize different

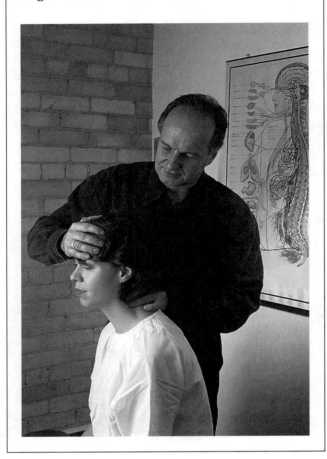

The spinal adjustment is a precise and specific means of correcting subluxation, misalignment, tension, and nerve interference.

techniques and different force applications when adjusting patients during the course of treatment." Although instruments are sometimes used, most adjustments are by hand (*chiropractic* means "done by hand"). Most adjustments of the lower back are applied with the patient lying in a side posture, while adjustments to the mid- and upper back occur with the patient lying prone and face-down. Cervical and neck adjustments are usually given with the patient in a supine, upright position. Adjustments may also be made while the patient is sitting.

It is impossible to predict how many adjustments a person will require to obtain maximum restoration of proper nerve flow. Numerous factors, including the length of time the nerves have been affected by subluxations, as well as the patient's lifestyle and general fitness level, all play a part in the process. In all cases, though, the chiropractor will recommend a treatment plan with appropriate re-evaluations after an initial period of care.

There are three levels of chiropractic care: acute care, the restorative phase, and the wellness phase. During the acute level of care, the chiropractor's objective is to reduce stress damage to the spine and nervous system. At this level, which is common when a patient is seeking help for specific health problems or is suffering from pain or other symptoms, adjustments can be as frequent as several times a week.

The restorative phase begins after the spine is nearly or completely aligned, when it must be monitored to make sure it holds the adjustment for longer periods of time. After being misaligned for months or even years, the body may have a tendency to resume the habitual alignment and periodic adjustments may be required. During the wellness phase, the patient has periodic examinations or adjustments to ensure that the nerve flow is not encountering interference from new subluxations. "This phase is useful as part of an optimal wellness, prevention, and maintenance program, and is an effective form of stress management," Dr. Stern says. "It is also used by many athletes to ensure optimal performance."

The Future of Chiropractic

Chiropractic now enjoys wide acceptance by the medical community, with large increases in patient numbers. More and more chiropractors are on staff at hospitals, appointed to workers' compensation medical examination boards, and commissioned to the armed forces as health-care providers. Chiropractors are now used for expert testimony in the legal arena and are often part of the physician team in sports medicine. In some states, chiropractors are being designated as primary-care physicians in health-care plans. The communication between chiropractic and medical physicians has greatly improved as well, and it is likely that these trends will continue to blossom in America and abroad.

Where to Find Help

American Chiropractic Association
1701 Clarendon Boulevard
Arlington, Virginia 22209
(800) 986-4636
Website: www.acatoday.com

A major source for chiropractic information. Monthly publication and newsletter. Clinical councils with specialization in sports injuries and physical fitness, mental health, neurology, diagnosis and internal disorders, nutrition, orthopedics, physiological therapeutics, diagnostic imaging, and occupational health.

International Chiropractors Association
1110 North Glebe Road, Suite 1000
Arlington, Virginia 22201
(703) 528-5000
Website: www.chiropractic.org

The original chiropractic association founded by B.J. Palmer, the son of the founder of chiropractic, Daniel David Palmer. Programs and services to meet the needs of chiropractors, patients, students, and the public. Concerned with legislation, health-care policy, continuing education, skills development, publications, and interprofessional relations.

World Chiropractic Alliance
2950 N. Dobson Road, Suite 1
Chandler, Arizona 85224
(800) 347-1011
Website: www.worldchiropracticalliance.org

An international association of chiropractors with the purpose of promoting and advancing the profession. Offers guidance and assistance to professionals. Emphasis on correction of vertebral subluxation. Provides public education and information. Publishes two newspapers for professionals and provides referrals for chiropractors nationwide.

The American College of Addictionology and Compulsive Disorders
975 Arthur Godfrey Road, Suite 500
Miami, Florida 33140
(305) 534-3635

Trains and board certifies chiropractors as addictionologists. Also provides referrals to chiropractors certified as addiction specialists worldwide.

Recommended Reading

Chiropractic: Compassion and Expectation. Terry Rondberg and Timothy Feuling. Chandler, AZ: *The Chiropractic Journal,* 1999.

Chiropractic First. Terry Rondberg. Chandler, AZ: *The Chiropractic Journal,* 1998.

The Chiropractor's Health Book. Leonard McGill. New York: Crown, 1997.

Today's Health Alternative. Raquel Martin. Tehachapi, CA: America West Publishers, 1992.

CRANIOSACRAL THERAPY

Craniosacral therapy manipulates the bones of the skull and the base of the spine and tailbone in order to treat a range of conditions, from headache and ear infection to stroke, spinal cord injury, and cerebral palsy. For decades, various forms of cranial manipulation have been used to improve overall body functioning, and today craniosacral therapy is gaining acceptance by health professionals worldwide as a successful treatment modality.

EACH OF US IS FAMILIAR with the body's cardiac rhythm (heartbeat) and respiratory rhythm (breathing). Yet there is a third and equally important body rhythm known as the craniosacral rhythm that results from the increase and decrease in the volume of cerebrospinal fluid within and around the craniosacral system.

Cranio refers to the cranium, or head, and *sacral* refers to the base of the spine and tailbone. The craniosacral system is comprised of the brain and spinal cord (the central nervous system); the cerebrospinal fluid that bathes the brain and spinal cord as well as their cellular components; the surrounding meninges (membranes) that enclose the brain, spinal cord, and cerebrospinal fluid; and the bones of the spine and skull that house these membranes.

There is a rhythmic motion in the craniosacral system created by the rise and fall of cerebrospinal fluid pressure. An increase in this pressure occurs as cerebrospinal fluid filters from the bloodstream and enters the craniosacral system, causing a predictable movement of the cranial bones. The pressure diminishes as the cerebrospinal fluid is reabsorbed into the bloodstream through the inner membranes of the brain, allowing the bones to return to their original position. The cranial therapist monitors this wavelike motion to determine any restriction or dysfunction in the craniosacral system. This subtle rhythm ranges from six to ten cycles per minute and is for the most part unaffected by the heart and respiratory rhythms, except in severe disease states.

A cranial therapist is trained to "palpate," or feel with his or her hands, the motion of the craniosacral system as a unified, integrated movement. The touch is extremely gentle and sensitive, and one is able to diagnose the move-

> *The craniosacral system has a profound effect on health and well-being.*

ment of the system as a whole by locating critical points of restriction in the cranium and the base of the spine and tailbone.

Restrictions that result from injury, inflexibility of the joints of the spine and cranium, or dysfunction in other parts of the body, can all cause abnormal motion in the craniosacral system. The abnormal motion leads to stresses in the cranial mechanism that can contribute to dysfunction and poor health, especially in the brain, the spinal cord, and the glands of the head (pituitary and pineal, hence the entire endocrine system). The purpose of craniosacral therapy is to enhance the functioning of these important systems.

How Craniosacral Therapy Works

There are three major approaches to craniosacral therapy: sutural, meningeal, and reflex. Each differs slightly in its therapeutic approach and application.

The Sutural Approach

The sutural approach was popularized by Dr. William Garner Sutherland, an early 20th-century osteopathic physician. In this technique, the therapist manipulates the sutures (where the bones meet) of the skull to ease pressure and increase mobility of the cranial bones. By removing the stress between the cranial bones, the sutural approach normalizes the relationship of one bone to another. This allows for a remodeling of the entire craniosacral system and an enhancement of its function.

While still a medical student, Dr. Sutherland observed that the bones of the skull are designed to move in accor-

SomatoEmotional Release

SomatoEmotional Release® (SER) is a term coined by John E. Upledger, D.O., O.M.M., developer of CranioSacral Therapy (CST), to describe a phenomenon that he and fellow practitioners observed as they became increasingly proficient in the use of CST—the release of tissue memories and energy cysts, foreign or disruptive energies lodged within the patient's body. "In the late 1970s, joint research conducted by biophysicist Zvi Karni and myself led to our discovery that the body often retains the imprint of physical forces from accidents, injuries, and emotional shocks," Dr. Upledger explains. "These dysfunctional areas are frequently isolated in what I call 'energy cysts'. SomatoEmotional Release provides CST practitioners with the manual and verbal skills they require to help release these destructive patterns from their patients' bodies."

According to Dr. Upledger, although reasonably healthy people can adapt to energy cysts and traumatic tissue memories, their continued presence can interfere with the body's ability to perform its normal functions without requiring additional energy. "As time passes, these adaptive patterns can lose their effectiveness," Dr. Upledger says. "That's when symptoms and dysfunctions may appear and become increasingly difficult to ignore. You may even become less resistant to other illnesses."

SER sessions begin with the practitioner gently placing his or her hands on the patient, silently inviting the body to do whatever it deems appropriate at the time. "When the therapist offers a comforting and trustworthy attitude, we find that the patient is encouraged on some nonconscious level," Dr. Upledger says. "It usually takes only a few minutes for the patient to assume the body position of their choice. The body position allows a generalized release of stored-up emotion that seems to come from the body tissues and is most often expressed through the nervous system, the vocal apparatus, etc. There may be crying, shaking, laughing, pain, almost anything you can imagine. It all depends on what it is that the patient has nonconsciously decided to deal with during that session."

According to Dr. Upledger, SER has the capacity to dramatically change people's lives, enabling them to see objectively what they are doing with their lives as they recall traumas, accidents, and other experiences that they have been holding beneath the surface of their awareness, often for years. "Once these suppressed experiences break through the surface, the problems can be dealt with and resolved," Dr. Upledger says. "When the problems remain suppressed, they can cause trouble, but you don't know what the cause of the trouble may be, nor do you know the reasons for the symptoms."

Practitioners trained by Dr. Upledger often combine SER with CST in order to afford their patients the fullest opportunity to heal, addressing both the underlying physical and mental/emotional causes of their conditions.

dance with one another. At the time, his theory was considered ridiculous, as prevailing scientific opinion stated that the bones of the skull become fused together around the age of 35. Despite both scientific and clinical evidence to support Dr. Sutherland's view,[1] debate continues to this day within the scientific community, and many anatomical texts still teach that the bones of an adult human skull are fused and immobile. Dr. Sutherland spent years experimenting with his hypothesis, and eventually developed a sophisticated system of diagnosis and treatment known as cranial osteopathy.

The Meningeal Approach

In the late 1970s, John Upledger, D.O., O.M.M., an osteopathic physician, led a multidisciplinary research team of anatomists, physiologists, biophysicists, and bioengineers at Michigan State University in an attempt to determine the scientific basis of the craniosacral system. Their work produced a practical model of the dynamic movement of the cranium and craniosacral system. Dr. Upledger applied his research to develop CranioSacral Therapy (CST), an approach that focuses primarily on manipulating the underlying membranes, or meninges. He has taught this approach to thousands worldwide.

Tension or restriction in the meninges creates disturbances in the craniosacral system. A meningeal approach, such as Dr. Upledger's CranioSacral Therapy, focuses on releasing restrictions of the cranial sutures and the underlying membranes through gentle hands-on contact with the bones of the craniosacral system, the ribs, and the vertebral column. The therapist monitors the rhythmical movement in the craniosacral system resulting from the increase and decrease in cerebrospinal fluid pressure. When abnormal motion is detected in the craniosacral system, the therapist locates the point of restricted movement and brings about a release by gently tractioning and elongating the meningeal membranes.

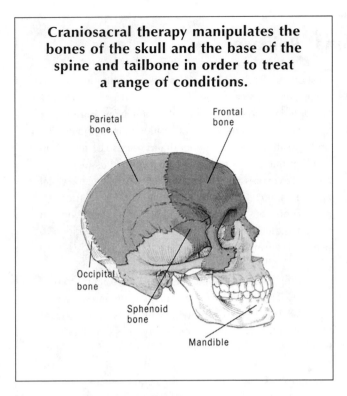

Craniosacral therapy manipulates the bones of the skull and the base of the spine and tailbone in order to treat a range of conditions.

Parietal bone

Frontal bone

Occipital bone

Sphenoid bone

Mandible

The Reflex Approach

The reflex approach relieves stress in the craniosacral system and in other structures and organs of the body. By stimulating nerve endings in the scalp or between cranial sutures, this approach triggers the nervous system to turn off stress signals. As a result, stress patterns and consequent cranial restrictions are released. Applied kinesiology, developed by George Goodheart, D.C., utilizes the reflex approach in conjunction with specific cranial adjustments to locate and treat distortions in the craniosacral system.

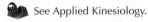 See Applied Kinesiology.

A system of craniosacral therapy that combines the sacral, meningeal, and reflex approaches is Sacro-Occipital Technique (S.O.T.), developed by Dr. Major B. DeJarnette, a chiropractor who studied with Dr. Sutherland in the 1920s. Also known as "craniopathy," S.O.T. removes restrictions between the cranial bones and in the craniosacral system. S.O.T. strives to reestablish structural stability and improve neurological function. Dr. DeJarnette produced positive clinical results with S.O.T. in the treatment of conditions related to the central nervous system. He also found that disorders such as diabetes, constipation, anxiety, impotence, asthma, cataracts, and inflammation, when associated with specific restrictions between sutures of the cranium, could be alleviated with a precise cranial technique.

Restrictions of motion of a particular cranial bone can pose serious consequences to the function of the body. Marc Pick, D.C., D.I.C.S., a widely acclaimed researcher and teacher of S.O.T., recalls a woman in her late seventies who had complete deafness in one ear for 25 years. After Dr. Pick corrected the restricted motion of the temporal bone (which houses the inner and outer ear) on the affected side, the woman's hearing immediately returned.

Conditions Benefited by Craniosacral Therapy

Imbalances in the craniosacral mechanism often begin before birth. Inadequate prenatal nutrition can result in underdevelopment of the facial and jaw bones, which can later impair smooth functioning of the craniosacral system. Difficult delivery, extended periods of engagement (the time the baby's head is in the birth canal), or the incorrect application of forceps, even suction, can produce severe stresses and distortion to the growing cranial tissues. This consequently can affect the baby's general health. Many of these stresses to the newborn's craniosacral system are normally considered untreatable by conventional medicine and often go unnoticed. Left untreated, such stresses can later contribute to a wide range of seemingly unrelated health problems.

Among the range of problems commonly addressed by physicians proficient in cranial osteopathy are pediatric problems, such as birth trauma, cerebral palsy, colic, developmental problems, and ear infections; somatic pain, such as back and neck pain, headache, joint pain syndrome, pleurisy, sciatica, and traumatic injury; systemic problems, such as chronic infectious diseases, edema, and fatigue; dental problems, such as malocclusion, orthodontic problems, and temporomandibular joint (TMJ) syndrome; scoliosis; genitourinary problems; respiratory conditions; neurological syndromes, such as Down syndrome, head trauma, post-concussion syndrome, and seizures; ear, nose, and throat problems; digestive disorders; and conditions related to pregnancy, including prevention of labor problems.[2]

According to Dr. Upledger, craniosacral therapy can also provide benefit for numerous health conditions. These include acute systemic infectious conditions (chicken pox, fever, flu, measles), allergies, osteoarthritis and rheumatoid arthritis, attention deficit disorders (ADD and ADHD), autism, back and neck pain, Bell's palsy, cerebral ischemic episodes (small strokes), cerebral palsy, chronic pain syndrome, dyslexia, ear and hearing problems, endocrine imbalances, headache, hypertension, mental retardation, neuromusculoskeletal conditions, post-traumatic stress disorder, premenstrual syndrome (PMS), postpartum depression, seizures, and visual problems.[3]

Through its ability to improve the general functioning of the central nervous system and address many difficult conditions, craniosacral therapy can offer substantial long-term cost savings to consumers.

Treating Infants and Children

Some of the most successful craniosacral treatments are performed on newborns and infants. At this stage, the cranial bones are primarily cartilage and the membranes are growing and changing very rapidly, so they are very responsive to the gentle corrections of the therapist's fingers. Newborns can be treated immediately after birth.

For many years, cranial osteopaths have successfully treated infants for common conditions such as earaches, sinus congestion, vomiting, irritability, and hyperactivity, using only craniosacral therapy. In these cases, craniosacral therapists commonly find compression at the base of the skull, which they maintain is related to the birthing process, and particularly the extreme backward extension of the baby's head during delivery.

For many years, cranial osteopaths have successfully treated infants for common conditions such as earaches, sinus congestion, vomiting, irritability, and hyperactivity, using only craniosacral therapy.

Specific conditions that relate to the overall function of the craniosacral system also benefit from craniosacral therapy. Robert C. Fulford, a retired osteopathic physician and instructor of craniosacral therapy, had great success in using craniosacral therapy to treat problems other doctors could not solve. Dr. Fulford regularly cured children of recurring ear infections by simply, in his words, "freeing up their breathing and getting their tailbone unstuck," allowing the craniosacral rhythm to return to normal. When the respiratory motion of the craniosacral system is restricted, fluid backs up into the ear, providing a breeding ground for bacterial infections.[4]

Effects on the Central Nervous System

Decreased efficiency of the central nervous system contributes to many chronic and nonspecific conditions, and problems within the craniosacral system are responsible for tremendous suffering and loss of potential vigor and health. The proper alignment of the craniosacral system allows the nervous system to rest at a more stress-free level. Individuals who experience craniosacral treatment describe profound states of relaxation, of feeling lighter and more integrated. "When there is synchronous movement in the craniosacral system, the physiology of the central nervous system functions more efficiently and the nerve tissue is, in general, healthier," says Robert Norett, D.C., Director of the Stillpoint Health Center, in Venice, California.

When there is synchronous movement in the craniosacral system, the physiology of the central nervous system functions more efficiently and the nerve tissue is, in general, healthier.

—ROBERT NORETT, D.C.

Craniosacral therapy is used to evaluate and treat problems involving the brain and spinal cord, especially direct trauma to the head and spine. Other treatable conditions include chronic pain, headache, temporomandibular joint (TMJ) syndrome, mood disorders, dyslexia, autism, stroke, epilepsy, cerebral palsy, dizziness, and tinnitus (ringing in the ears). Also benefited are systemic conditions such as edema (swelling), recurrent infections, hypertension, hypotension, and some muscular conditions.

According to Dr. Norett, the entrapments and compressions around the nerve and blood vessels that pass in and out of the cranium and spine can be alleviated through craniosacral therapy. Hundreds of small holes that carry these vessels can become thick with connective tissue and effectively "choke" the vessels. He cites the case of the owner and chef of a French restaurant who had slipped and hit the back of his head against a stove. "As a result of the trauma, he lost his sense of smell, vital to his work as a chef," says Dr. Norett. "We found significant restriction of the area inside the cranium where the olfactory nerves (affecting the sense of smell) pass through, and within about five treatments, he had improved dramatically."

Dr. Upledger has had great success treating chronic, severe, and disabling headaches. He reports that up to 85% of resistant long-term headaches respond favorably to craniosacral therapy. The benefit of this treatment is that once the headaches are gone, they do not return, and the patient is not dependent upon a lifetime of periodic therapy sessions.[5]

Dr. Upledger cites the story of a U.S. naval officer who had been on active duty during World War II. Recurring headaches accompanied by a loud noise in his ears began after he stood next to a cannon as it was being fired. Although he tried every kind of treatment available through the Navy, he found no relief. When he visited Dr. Upledger, he had been living with the pain for 25 years. After evaluating his craniosacral system, Dr. Upledger found the skull bones on the left side of his head were jammed inward and stuck. Dr. Upledger manually released the compression of the cranial bones and the left side of the head expanded immediately. His pain vanished on the spot. By the third visit, his ear noise had stopped.[6]

Joseph F. Unger, D.C., F.I.C.S., reports of a patient in continual pain from a two-year-old radical mastectomy scar. She also had swelling and pains in the arm on the side of the surgery. Using a S.O.T. cranial technique, Dr. Unger was able to eradicate the pain from the scar. Over the next 2-3 weeks, the swelling in her arm diminished almost to normal.

 Research into the function of the craniosacral system could help provide a broader understanding of human anatomy, physiology, and the role of the craniosacral system in health.

The Future of Craniosacral Therapy

Craniosacral therapy is rapidly gaining acceptance among health practitioners and the public. This is due in part to the nonintrusive nature of this therapy and how it works with the entire structure, physiology, mind, and spirit. As a result, growing numbers of health-care professionals, including M.D.s, chiropractors, holistic dentists, osteopaths, physical therapists, and registered nurses, now incorporate craniosacral techniques into their overall treatment programs. In 1994, the nonprofit American Craniosacral Therapy Association was founded by Dr. Upledger, other therapists, and concerned laypersons, in order to increase public awareness of Craniosacral Therapy and ultimately develop CST into an independently licensed profession. To that end, Dr. Upledger and his associates continue to offer nationally certified training in CST, while continuing to research its health-care applications.

Where to Find Help

For further information about craniosacral therapy, and for referrals, contact:

American CranioSacral Therapy Association
Upledger Institute
11211 Prosperity Farms Road
Palm Beach Gardens, Florida 33410
(407) 622-4706
Website: www.upledger.com

The association promotes increased awareness and acceptance of CranioSacral Therapy among both laypersons and health professionals, and oversees the development of certification training for CST practitioners nationwide. The Upledger Institute offers certification training in CranioSacral Therapy, SomatoEmotional Release, and related techniques worldwide and teaches to cross-disciplinary health professionals. Offers information to the public and has a referral network of more than 2,000 members.

The Cranial Academy
8202 Clearvista Parkway, Suite 9-D
Indianapolis, Indiana 46256
(317) 594-0411
Website: www.cranialacademy.com

The Cranial Academy teaches cranial therapy to osteopaths according to the work of Dr. William Sutherland. Call for referrals to osteopaths trained in cranial therapy.

Sacro-Occipital Research Society International (SORSI)
P.O. Box 6067
Leawood, Kansas 66206
(888) 245-1011
Website: www.sorsi.com

SORSI teaches postgraduate courses and certifies chiropractors in Sacro-Occipital Technique (S.O.T.) according to Dr. Major B. DeJarnette. Trains and certifies chiropractors in craniopathy. Call for a referral to a certified chiropractor in craniopathy.

Recommended Reading

A Brain is Born: Exploring the Birth and Development of the Central Nervous System. John E. Upledger, D.O., F.A.A.O. Berkeley, CA: North Atlantic Books, 1997.

The Discovery and Practice of SomatoEmotional Release. John E. Upledger, D.O., F.A.A.O. Berkeley, CA: North Atlantic Books, 2001.

Dr. Fulford's Touch of Life. Robert C. Fulford with Gene Stone. New York: Pocket Books, 1996.

An Introduction to Craniosacral Therapy. Don Cohen and John E. Upledger, D.O., F.A.A.O. Berkeley, CA: North Atlantic Books, 1996.

Your Inner Physician and You: CranioSacral Therapy and SomatoEmotional Release. John E. Upledger, D.O., F.A.A.O. Berkeley, CA: North Atlantic Books, 1992.

DETOXIFICATION THERAPY

Each year, people are exposed to thousands of toxic chemicals and pollutants in the Earth's atmosphere, water, food, and soil. These toxins manifest themselves in the body in a variety of symptoms, including decreased immune function, neurotoxicity, hormonal dysfunction, psychological or mood disturbances, and even cancer. Detoxification therapy helps to rid the body of chemicals and pollutants and can facilitate a return to health.

DETOXIFICATION IS the body's natural process of eliminating or neutralizing toxins via the liver, kidneys, and lungs, as well as in urine, feces, and through the sweat. Yet, as a result of the industrial revolution and the post–World War II petrochemical revolution, toxins have accumulated in the human system faster than they can be eliminated.

People now carry within their bodies a modern-day chemical cocktail derived from industrial chemicals, pesticides, food additives, heavy metals (like lead), and anesthetics, plus the residues of pharmaceuticals, legal drugs (alcohol, tobacco, caffeine), and illegal drugs (heroin, cocaine, marijuana).

Today, people are exposed to chemicals in far greater concentrations than were previous generations: over 69 million Americans live in areas that exceed smog standards;[1] most drinking water contains over 700 chemicals, including excessive levels of lead;[2] some 3,000 chemicals are added to the food supply; and as many as 10,000 chemicals in the form of solvents, emulsifiers, and preservatives are used in food processing and storage, which can remain in the body for years.[3] To make matters worse, food and product labels do not always list every ingredient. When people consume these foods—especially seafood, meat, dairy products, and poultry—they ingest all the chemicals and pesticides that have remained as contaminants accumulating in the food chain.

Everyday products such as gasoline, paint, household cleansers, cosmetics, pesticides, and dry cleaning fluid also

> *People now carry within their bodies a modern-day chemical cocktail derived from industrial chemicals, pesticides, food additives, heavy metals, and anesthetics, plus the residues of pharmaceuticals, and legal and illegal drugs.*

pose a serious threat, because the body cannot easily break them down. At the same time, ecological changes in the environment are occurring faster than the human organism can adapt to them. As the Earth becomes more and more polluted, the body inadvertently becomes a filter that "traps" these pollutants.

"The current level of chemicals in the food and water supply, and the indoor and outdoor environment, has lowered our threshold of resistance to disease and has altered our body's metabolism, causing enzyme dysfunction, nutritional deficiencies, and hormonal imbalances," says Marshall Mandell, M.D., father of the field of bio-ecologic medicine.

Bio-accumulation, a buildup in the body of foreign substances, seriously compromises physiological and psychological health. Over the last ten years, hundreds of studies have demonstrated the dangers to health from toxic bio-accumulation.[4]

"A body with a healthy immune system, efficient organs of elimination and detoxification, and a sound circulatory and nervous system can handle a great deal of toxicity," states Leon Chaitow, N.D., D.O., of London, England. "But if the body has been damaged from chronic exposure to environmental pollutants, restoring these functions, organs, and systems can be accomplished only through detoxification therapies, including fasting, chelation, and nutritional, herbal, and homeopathic methods, which accelerate the body's own natural cleansing processes. These therapies will dominate medical thinking in the years ahead."

Benefits of Detoxification

"The process of detoxification, through special cleansing diets as well as juice and water fasts, is the missing link to rejuvenating the body and preventing such chronic diseases as cancer, cardiovascular problems, arthritis, diabetes, and obesity," says Elson Haas, M.D., Director of the Preventive Medical Center of Marin, in San Rafael, California, and author of *The Detox Diet*. "The modern diet, with excess animal proteins, fats, caffeine, alcohol, and chemicals, inhibits the optimum function of our cells and tissues. The cleansing of toxins and waste products will restore function and vitality."

Dr. Haas has practiced juice fasting regularly for over 25 years and advises his patients to undertake some form of detoxification periodically to clear wastes and dead cells and to revitalize the body's natural functions and healing capacities. He points out that the most important and longest lasting effect of detoxification therapy is the reduction of stress on the immune system, along with greater mental clarity. Other benefits can include increased vitality, reduced blood pressure and blood fats (cholesterol and triglycerides), and an improved assimilation of vitamins and minerals. Detoxification is instrumental for maintenance of the normal function and integrity of the intestinal flora and can enhance the natural ability of the body to resist infections, allergies, and skin disorders. Dr. Haas adds that most people will feel mentally and physically rejuvenated after detoxification therapy, with a corresponding reduction in symptoms and disease.

Does Your Body Need Detoxification?

The "loading theory" of toxicity, according to its formulator, Serafina Corsello, M.D., Director of the Corsello Centers for Nutritional Complementary Medicine in New York City and Huntington, New York, states that no single factor causes a disease, such as exposure to infectious agents or psychological traumas that lower immune resistance. Rather, the cumulative load of multiple poisons creates an illness. Everyone has a specific level of tolerance that cannot be exceeded if good health is to be maintained. If the amount of toxins within the body stays below that level, the body can usually adapt and rid itself of these.

You don't suddenly get sick—it takes a long time for the body to break down. This process is compounded of layers of toxicity, malnutrition, and dysfunction, she notes. All these factors impinge on the immune system's natural vitality to resist the downhill slide into illness. When the system is overwhelmed, the body's defense mechanisms malfunction and symptoms, such as fatigue, confusion, aggression, or mental disorder, may occur.

Indications that the body may need detoxification are headaches, joint pain, recurrent respiratory problems, back pain, allergy symptoms, insomnia, mood changes, digestive problems, and food reactions. Conditions such as arthritis, constipation, hemorrhoids, sinus congestion, ulcers, psoriasis, and acne can also indicate the need for detoxification.

Laboratory tests can shed light on the need for detoxification. Tests can involve analysis of stool, urine, and blood, liver function, and hair analysis. However, physicians who are not familiar with detoxification may be reluctant to perform such tests. People considering a detoxification program will want to find a doctor who understands the concepts of detoxification.

 See Arthritis, Candidiasis, Constipation, Parasitic Infections.

 Great care must be taken to insure the safe and effective removal of toxins. Any detoxification therapy should be administered only after consultation with a qualified health professional.

Some Preliminary Cautions

According to Dr. Chaitow, a key question to ask yourself is: "Am I well enough to undertake rapid and active detoxification or should I go through the process more slowly?" If a person is robust and vital, a more vigorous program may be required than if the person is unwell and somewhat fragile in health. Dr. Chaitow recommends that each individual seek the advice of a qualified health professional to help select the appropriate degree of intensity. People who are recovering drug users, alcoholics, diabetics, or who have eating disorders should not apply any detoxification method without strict medical supervision.

It is also important to note that detoxification may not be appropriate for individuals who are underweight or physically weak, or for those people with a hypothyroid or a hypoglycemic condition. Anyone with a cancerous condition, or who is just recovering from surgery, should always consult a qualified health professional before any detoxification program is carried out. And women who are pregnant or nursing should generally avoid detoxification practices.

Finally, people should know what to expect during detoxification. Dr. Chaitow states, "Early on, you could develop a headache and furred tongue. As the weeks pass, your skin should become clearer, although it may be spotty for a while. Your eyes will become clearer, your brain sharper, digestion more efficient, energy levels high, and you may well regain a sense of youthful clarity."

Forms of Detoxification

Several methods of detoxification are currently available. These include fasting and specific diets, colon hydrotherapy, liver flush, vitamin C therapy, chelation therapy, and hyperthermia or sauna therapy. It is advisable to seek professional advice when choosing a detoxification program.

Before getting started on a detoxification program, it is important to make fundamental lifestyle and dietary changes so that you do not introduce more toxins into your body. Here are some basic steps that you can take to reduce your toxic load:

- Use Only Organically Raised Foods—Take this recommendation as a mandatory general guideline in your food choices. Eat foods that are certified organic. They will be free of contaminants, synthetic pesticides and herbicides, hormones, preservatives, dyes, artificial colorings, and antibiotics. Many health food and grocery stores offer organic produce and meat as do some farmers markets.

- Get the Poisons Off Your Vegetables—Since the Food and Drug Administration tests only about 1% of produce for pesticide residues, cleaning your food is the only way to ensure that you are not eating agricultural poisons. The solution to this problem may be naturally derived produce washes, now available to consumers concerned about preventing food-borne illnesses.

- Maintain a Household Free of Toxic Chemicals— It is advisable to remove chemical contaminants and toxic household cleansers from your home, or at least to limit your exposure to them. Substitute natural cleaning products, such as distilled white vinegar, baking soda, Borax, lemon juice, citrus cleaners (non-petroleum-based), Castille soaps, and safe commercial products, for the toxic ones. These products are available in many health food stores or through mail-order services provided by environmentally concerned companies.

- Breathe Clean Air—As the average American spends most of their time indoors, the quality of indoor air becomes crucial. Toxic substances such as pollens, dust mites, mold spores, tobacco smoke residues, benzene, chloroform, chemical gases, and formaldehyde are now commonly found in tightly sealed indoor environments. Ozone and ionizing air-filters are now

available for home use. Common houseplants can be used as filters to remove pollution from indoor air, an idea that first came out of NASA space research in the 1970s. Scientists discovered that not only could plants recycle oxygen, but they seemed to be able to remove air pollutants too.

- Filter Your Water—Tap water is a major source of the toxic chemicals that the liver is required to process. The practical solution is to get a water filter for the home and office, or at least to start using commercially purified and bottled water.

Fasting

Fasting is one of the easiest, most inexpensive, and effective methods of detoxification. There are basically two types of fasts, water and juice. Results depend upon both the health of the individual and the length of the fast. Fasting is often combined with enemas and colon therapy for the purpose of ridding the body of stagnation and toxins trapped in the bowels. For many people, fasting can be used as an adjunct to the healing process and is an invaluable aid for those seeking enhancement of their overall physical, mental, and spiritual health. Short fasts (two to five days) can be performed at home as part of a personal health-maintenance program. Longer fasts, undertaken with medical supervision, can serve to strengthen the immune system, alleviate food allergies, and reduce or eliminate medications for certain health conditions.

> **IMPORTANT** Long fasts require medical supervision as well as prior assessment of nutrient levels to insure that deficiency does not occur. Short weekend fasts are safe for most people, although advice from an appropriate health-care professional experienced in detoxification is advisable.

Fasting aids most health concerns because during a fast:

- The body continues its natural process of excreting stored toxins, while the intake of new toxins is decreased. In this way, total body toxicity is reduced.

- With the elimination of food and its allergens, the immune system's workload is also greatly reduced and the digestive tract is spared the constant inflammation due to allergic reactions.

- With the lowering of blood fats (after the fourth day of the fast), the thinner blood affords increased oxygenation of tissues and enhanced delivery of white blood cells (boosting immune function) throughout the body.

- Significantly less energy is directed at food digestion (which involves the use of blood, oxygen, and nutrients). This allows for greater reserves of energy and nutrients for use by the systems of self-regulation (immune function, cell growth, eliminatory processes).

- The metabolizing (burning) of fat and its conversion to energy-yielding molecules releases many fat-stored chemicals (pesticides, drugs) into the bloodstream at a time when the body has enhanced eliminatory capabilities.

- The innate ability of the body to recognize old, nonessential tissues and subsequently dissolve them, while recycling their important nutrients for new cell production, furthers elimination and leads to broadly enhanced physiological function.

- A person's awareness and sensitivity to diet and surroundings are elevated. Fasting has been used as a spiritual practice in many cultures to enhance health and well-being.

There are differing ideas about what constitutes an ideal fast. In any case, it is essential to consult a health professional before undertaking a fast to ascertain your physical condition and to determine the length and type of fast that is most appropriate. During a prolonged fast (more than a couple of days), vitamin or mineral supplements may be necessary, as well as changes in dosage of any medication. Periodic blood tests are recommended during the fast to monitor one's condition.

Trevor Salloum, N.D., of Kelowna, British Columbia, Canada, favors water fasting and stresses the use of only pure water (distilled, spring, or purified by reverse osmosis). He considers juice to be a food since it supplies carbohydrates, which inhibit the development of ketone metabolism (breakdown of fats), and maintains that a juice fast is, in effect, a restricted diet. Dr. Salloum believes that during a fast, water should be consumed according to thirst, with a minimum of three glasses a day.

Certain practitioners recommend a juice fast because of the withdrawal symptoms water fasting causes when nutrients and drugs (prescription and recreational) are released into the bloodstream for elimination. This detoxification process is much less severe on a juice fast.

WATER FASTING

True fasting is done by consuming only filtered water and/or herbal teas, with zero caloric intake. Fasting on water causes rapid release of toxins in the body, where they have been buried in the fat for long periods of time. Dr. Chaitow recommends a water-only fast (24-36 hours) starting Friday evening and ending Sunday morning (or as an alternative, just all day Saturday). Make sure that not less than four and not more than eight pints of water are consumed during the fast. On Sunday, have a day of raw foods—fruit and salad only, well chewed, plus the recommended amounts of drinking water.

For many patients, fasting on water can create health issues if the body is not adequately prepared for this shock. While water fasting is the best method of detoxification, it should be done only under the guidance of a health-care practitioner who has experience in supervising fasts of this type.

JUICE FASTING

Evarts G. Loomis, M.D., of Hemet, California, Cofounder of the American Holistic Medical Association, prescribes vegetable juices (equal parts carrot and celery, diluted with water in a 1:1 ratio) for detoxification. If desired, green vegetables such as green beans, zucchini, watercress, and parsley can be added. Dr. Loomis also prescribes a detoxifying cocktail that combines garlic, lemon juice, grapefruit juice, and olive oil. This is given at bedtime because the liver, a major organ for detoxification, is most active between 11 p.m. and 1 a.m., according to traditional Chinese medicine.

In addition, juice therapy offers a balanced way to supplement the diet, according to Steven Bailey, N.D., of the Northwest Naturopathic Clinic, in Portland, Oregon. "One of the most convenient therapies available is the use of raw fruit and vegetable juices to augment the typical diet. Juice therapy can also aid in a treatment program by stimulating the immune system, reducing blood pressure, aiding in detoxification, and protecting the body from harmful environmental factors. It is also used to help diagnose and treat food allergies and is the ideal nutritional remedy for individuals suffering from nausea or digestive problems."

Vegetable juices are used extensively in fasting and as nutritional supplements because of their high vitamin and mineral content. Fruit juices, however, provide a quicker pick-me-up as they are immediately absorbed. Fruit juices also remain stable for a longer period of time and "travel" better than vegetable juices, which oxidize quickly, breaking down the protective enzymes and vitamins. It is always preferable to juice fresh, organic fruits and vegetables oneself just prior to drinking in order to maximize nutritional value. If this isn't possible, juices should be purchased from a health food store the same day that they are made.

Dr. Haas recalls a man who, at 5′9″ and 231 pounds, had high blood pressure, an elevated cholesterol level,

MEDICINAL QUALITIES OF FRUITS AND VEGETABLES

Many fruits and vegetables have scientifically proven medicinal qualities. So far, studies have documented the medicinal effects of fruit juices, with very little research applied to vegetable juices. Cherie Calbom, M.S., C.N., a nutritionist from Seattle, Washington, and co-author of *Juicing for Life*, recommends the following juice remedies:

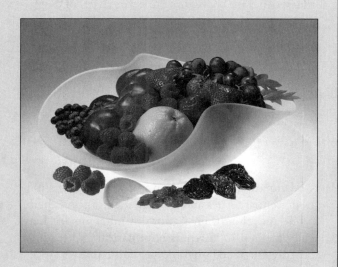

- Apple: Apples are rich in sorbitol, a form of sugar and a gentle laxative.

- Apple, grape, and blueberry: These fruits are a source of polyphenols, antioxidants that have been shown to kill viruses.[5]

- Beet: Beet greens are rich in magnesium, beta carotene, and vitamins C and E. Beetroot is rich in potassium, folic acid, and the antioxidant glutathione. Beet juice is valued for its vitamin, mineral, and nutrient content. Due to its strong taste, it should be mixed with other juices.

- Blueberry and cranberry: When consumed on a regular basis, these juices can help prevent recurrent urinary tract infections.[6]

- Cabbage: Cabbage juice is famous for its ulcer-healing capabilities,[7] but should be used only in conjunction with a doctor's prescribed therapy for ulcer treatment.

- Cantaloupe: Cantaloupe has a blood-thinning effect that can help prevent heart attacks and strokes.[8]

- Carrot: Carrot juice is an excellent source of beta carotene, potassium, trace minerals, and antioxidants. Yellowish coloration of the skin may occur when large amounts are consumed. This coloration is harmless, and will fade when consumption is reduced.

- Celery: Celery juice contains antioxidants, potassium, and sodium, and helps lower blood pressure. Celery juice can be diluted with water and used as a sports drink to replace fluid and mineral loss due to sweating. It contains the same ulcer-healing factors found in cabbage juice.

- Cherry: A traditional remedy for gout pain.

- Garlic: This herb is a treasure house of healing compounds. It acts as a natural antibiotic and blood thinner and can reduce cholesterol levels.[9] Juice a clove and add it to your favorite vegetable juice mix.

- Ginger: The root of the ginger plant has anti-inflammatory properties and will also protect the stomach from irritation caused by nonsteroidal, anti-inflammatory drugs (such as aspirin).[10] Migraines and motion sickness can also be relieved with ginger juice.[11]

- Lemon: Lemon juice is a traditional appetite stimulant. Place 1-2 tablespoons of fresh, unsweetened lemon juice in a glass of water and drink 30 minutes before meals to stimulate the flow of saliva and digestive juices.

- Pineapple: Raw pineapple juice contains the enzyme bromelain, which has been shown to have gentle anti-inflammatory properties.[12] Swish the raw juice around the site of a tooth extraction to reduce swelling.

and a marked inability to handle stress. After going on a ten-day juice cleansing diet supervised by Dr. Haas, he dropped 18 pounds and was inspired to make major and permanent changes to his diet. He followed a vegetarian-oriented, whole foods regimen. Consequently, his blood pressure and cholesterol normalized and he found a more comfortable body weight of about 195 pounds.

EXPERIENCES DURING A FAST

Patients report a spectrum of feelings as they proceed through a fast. Most encounter physiological and psychological withdrawal effects during the first three days and, in some cases, for longer periods. The more prepared your body is, the fewer and less intense the side effects. Transient headaches, energy fluctuations, hypoglycemia, halitosis (bad breath), increased body odor, constipation, nausea, rectal mucus discharge, acne, and a temporary aggravation of many conditions are common.

Serious side effects are very rare and usually occur in people on long fasts, who should be under medical supervision. Symptoms can include fainting/dizziness, dangerously low blood pressure, cardiac arrhythmia, severe vomiting or diarrhea, and kidney problems. It is important to consult with a practitioner skilled in fasting before you execute this vital aspect of detoxification.

> **CAUTION** Certain conditions contraindicate fasting, including diabetes, eating disorders, epilepsy, hypoglycemia, kidney disease, malnutrition, pregnancy, lactation, severe bronchial asthma, terminal illness, tuberculosis, and ulcerative colitis. Long-term fasts should be done under professional supervision.

Diets

Diets are another effective method of detoxification. They involve very little cost other than the purchase of healthy food. And while a detoxification program is not primarily concerned with weight loss, by introducing a more efficient and healthier way to eat, detoxification often results in weight loss. It is important to note again that, before embarking on any kind of fast or diet, one should always consult with a doctor or a qualified health professional.

WEEKEND MONO DIET

Dr. Chaitow often suggests a full weekend mono diet, beginning Friday night and extending through to Sunday evening, relying on a single food such as grapes, apples, pears (best choices if you have a history of allergy); papaya (ideal if digestive problems are present); or brown rice, buckwheat, millet, or potatoes (skin included), boiled and eaten whenever desired. Up to a pound (dry weight) of any grain such as rice or millet may be eaten daily; taste can be made palatable with the addition of a little lemon juice and olive oil. Or one may eat up to three pounds of potatoes daily.

According to Dr. Chaitow, "Whichever type of detoxification modality you choose, make sure you rest, keep warm, and don't have a very strenuous schedule; this should be a time in which you allow all available energy to focus on the cleansing and repairing processes of detoxification." On the other hand, Dr. Haas does suggest that people continue to exercise as tolerated because it supports the detoxification process, as does taking steams and saunas.

When the tongue no longer becomes furred during detoxification and headaches no longer appear, these intensive detoxification weekends can be spaced apart—three a month, then two, and then, as maintenance, once a month thereafter.

In between weekend detoxification intensives, Dr. Chaitow recommends a milder program of detoxification be employed:

- Breakfast: Fresh fruit (raw or lightly cooked, no sweetening) and yogurt with live bacterial cultures, homemade muesli (seeds, nuts, grains) and yogurt, or cooked grains (buckwheat, millet, linseed, barley, rice) and yogurt. Herbal tea is recommended, especially linden blossom, chamomile, mint, sage, lemon verbena, or a lemon and hot water drink.

- Lunch/Supper: One of the meals should be a raw salad with potato or brown rice and one of the following: bean curd (tofu), low-fat cheese, nuts, or seeds. If raw food is difficult to digest, stir-fried vegetables and tofu or steamed vegetables eaten with a potato or rice and low-fat cheese, nuts, or seeds will suffice. The other main meal should consist of fish, chicken, or game, or be vegetarian (bean and grain combination and/or vegetables lightly steamed or stir-fried). Seasoning can include garlic and herbs, but avoid salt as much as possible.

- Desserts: Lightly stewed fruit with added apple or lemon juice (not sugar) or live natural yogurt.

Remember to eat slowly, chew well, and don't drink with meals (consume at least two pints of liquid daily between meals). Also, take one high-potency multivitamin/mineral capsule daily, three garlic capsules, and a daily acidophilus supplement for bowel detoxification support.

THE DETOX DIET

Developed by Dr. Haas, this three-week plan helps to detoxify the body tissues of protein and acid wastes that

THE DETOX DIET MENU

Morning (upon arising): Two glasses of water (filtered, spring, or reverse osmosis)—one of these mixed with the juice of half a lemon. After a little stretching, have one serving of fresh fruit such as apple, pear, banana, grapes, or citrus. Then, 15-30 minutes later, eat one bowl of cooked whole grains (millet, brown rice, amaranth, quinoa, or buckwheat). Flavor with two tablespoons of fruit juice for a sweeter taste or use the "better butter" mixture (mentioned below) with a little salt or tamari for a deeper flavor.

Lunch (12 p.m. to 1 p.m.) and Dinner (5 p.m. to 6 p.m.): One to two medium bowls of steamed vegetables; use a variety, including roots, stems, and greens.[13] A seasoning—"better butter"— can be made by mixing 1/2 cup of cold-pressed canola oil (or olive or flaxseed oils) into a soft (room temperature) 1/2 pound of organic butter; then place in dish and refrigerate. Use about one teaspoon per meal or a maximum of three teaspoons daily.

11 a.m. and 3 p.m.: One to two cups of vegetable water, saved from the steamed vegetables. Add a little sea salt or kelp and drink slowly, mixing each mouthful with saliva.

Evening: Herbal teas—peppermint, chamomile, pau d'arco, or blends.

DETOXIFICATION SUPPORT

A person undergoing detoxification therapy can do a number of things during the process to help aid the natural cleansing ability of the body, according to Leon Chaitow, N.D., D.O. His suggestions include:

Hydrotherapy: Epsom salt baths or wet sheet packs, once weekly.

Skin brushing: To assist the skin elimination function, daily.

Stretching and relaxation exercises: Practice daily.

Aerobic exercise (if appropriate): Brisk walking, jogging, dancing, etc., daily except during the fast period.

Massage and manual lymphatic drainage: As often as available; twice weekly if possible.

Aromatherapy: Use of appropriate (to your condition) essential aromatherapy oils, in baths or massage.

Breathing, relaxation, and meditation methods: Once or twice daily for at least 10-15 minutes.

---

can create both inflammatory and degenerative changes when interacting in the body. This diet plan is a gentle and safe way to detoxify, notes Dr. Haas, and can also help to reduce weight, increase vitality, and promote healing. Dr. Haas adds that when foods oxidize in the body, they leave a residue or ash. If the foods are acidic, they leave an acid residue (acidic ash, sulfur, phosphorus, chlorine, or free radicals), which can be harmful. Success with this method is achieved by the elimination of acid-forming foods from your diet. This makes the question not only what to eat, but also what *not* to eat.

Essentially this diet consists of fruits and vegetables (mostly vegetables), plus fresh sprouts and millet and other grains, avoiding wheat. The diet also focuses on particular eating principles, including exceptional chewing (30-50 times per mouthful), drinking quality water plus the steamed vegetable water, and eating all food prior to nightfall, generally before 6:30 p.m. Dr. Haas recommends the following guidelines:

- Relax a few minutes before and after each meal.

- Eat in a comfortable sitting position.

- Eat primarily steamed fresh vegetables and some fresh greens.

- Chew very well and take your time when you eat.

- Take only herbal teas after dinner.

Precautions: Dr. Haas points out that you may feel a little weak or have a few symptoms (fatigue, headaches, or irritability) the first couple of days, but notes that this will pass. Clarity and a feeling of well-being should appear by the third or fourth day, if not before. If during this diet you start to feel weak or hungry, assess your water intake and elimination; if needed, you can eat a small portion of protein (3-4 ounces) in the mid-afternoon. This could be fish; free-range, organic chicken; or some beans, such as lentils, garbanzo, mung, or black beans. Remember that even in a clean and healthy body, the full effects of an alkaline diet do not begin to be felt for 5-7 days.

Colon Therapy

Making sure that the bowels are consistently active is important to healthy detoxification. At least two bowel movements daily is ideal. When this doesn't occur, it is likely the individual needs detoxification. Drew Collins, N.D., of Prescott Valley, Arizona, states, "When the colon becomes burdened with an accumulation of waste material—impacted feces, bacteria, fungi, viruses, parasites, and dead cellular material—the result is bowel toxemia. This condition causes inflammation and swelling of the bowel surface and can lead to a host of other health problems. Normal absorption of nutrients, secretory functions, and normal muscular function of the colon are disrupted. Irregular and inefficient bowel movement is the result, further suppressing recovery and encouraging other problems." Bowel toxemia and improper digestion can cause a buildup in the intestines of pathological bacteria, viruses, and fermented and putrefactive gases that become dangerous to the body and can lead to other illnesses.

Colonic irrigation is one of the most effective ways to cleanse the large intestine of accumulated toxins and waste products. It functions to draw toxins from the blood and lymph back into the colon for excretion. In a typical session, a trained colon therapist gently guides an applicator, or speculum, into the rectum. Filtered water, which may contain vitamins, herbs, friendly bacteria, or oxygen (as prescribed by a physician), is gradually introduced into and released from the colon using a colonic machine, in order to remove fecal material and gas buildup. Colon therapy helps to dislodge fecal material trapped in the pockets and folds of the colon. In this way, conditions that favor normal flora are restored.

A single session lasts 30-45 minutes and uses two to six liters of water. Colonic irrigation cleans the entire five feet of the colon, unlike an enema, which cleanses only the sigmoid colon, the lower 8-12 inches of the bowel. It is advisable to eat and drink lightly prior to colon therapy. An enema beforehand will empty the rectum and increase the efficiency of the colon therapy. After colon therapy, gentle, nourishing food should be taken, such as vegetable soups and broths and fruit or vegetable juices.

One colon therapy session may not be enough to produce major benefits. It may be necessary to have several if you have long-standing complaints or a serious problem with constipation. Dr. Collins points out that toxic residues are often released into both the bloodstream and the lumen (inside of the bowel) during colon therapy. Although colonic irrigation is usually a soothing and refreshing experience, release of these toxins can bring about a temporary "healing crisis."

Colon therapy can be combined with massage, nutritional programs, and special diets to help cleanse the bowels and aid in the treatment of poor digestion or yeast and parasitic infections. It can also be used prior to other detoxification programs. There are certain contraindications for colon therapy, including ulcerative colitis (ulceration of the colon lining), diverticulitis (inflammation of a sac or pouch in the intestinal tract), Crohn's disease (in the acute inflammatory stage), severe hemorrhoids, spasms in the muscles surrounding the prostate, and tumors of the large intestine or rectum. Patients in a weakened state should avoid colon therapy without direct medical supervision.

Natural Liver Flush

The healthy and efficient functioning of the liver is central to detoxification and disease prevention, which explains why it is advisable to periodically flush the organ clean using natural substances, says master herbalist and acupuncturist Christopher Hobbs, L.Ac. "Liver flushes are used to stimulate elimination of wastes from the body, to open and cool the liver, to increase bile flow, and to improve overall liver functioning," says Dr. Hobbs. "I have taken liver flushes for many years now and can heartily recommend them." Here are Dr. Hobbs' instructions for preparing and administering a liver flush:[14]

- Citrus Juice—Squeeze enough fresh lemons or limes to produce one cup of juice. A small amount of distilled or spring water may be added to dilute the juice, but the more sour it tastes, the better it will perform as a liver cleanser. Orange and grapefruit juices may also be used, provided they are blended with some lemon or lime juice.

- Garlic and Ginger—To the citrus juice mixture, add the juice of 1-2 cloves of garlic, freshly squeezed in a garlic press, and a small amount of freshly grated raw ginger juice. Grate the raw ginger on a cheese or vegetable grater, then put the shreds into a garlic press and squeeze out the juice.

- Olive Oil—Add one tablespoon of high-quality olive oil (such as extra virgin) to the citrus, garlic, and ginger juice. Either blend or shake the ingredients to guarantee complete mixing.

- Taking the Flush—The liver flush is best taken in the morning, preferably after some stretching and breathing exercises, says Dr. Hobbs. Do not eat any foods for one hour following the flush, he adds.

- Cleansing Herbal Tea—After an hour has elapsed, Dr. Hobbs recommends taking two cups of an herbal blend he calls "Polari Tea." It consists of dry portions

COFFEE ENEMA TO PURGE THE LIVER

A coffee enema can be a useful option for detoxifying the liver. It causes the blood vessels in the large intestine to expand, helping to purge the liver and colon of accumulated toxins and waste products. The enema is prepared by brewing organic caffeinated coffee and letting it cool to body temperature, then delivering it via an enema bag. Coffee contains choleretics, substances that increase the flow of toxin-rich bile from the gallbladder. The coffee enema may be among the only pharmaceutically effective choleretics noted in the medical literature that can be safely used many times daily without toxic effects. "The coffee enema is capable of purging toxins because it dilates the bile ducts and stimulates enzymes capable of removing toxins from the blood," says Etienne Callebout, M.D., a London-based physician and homeopath. Caffeine also stimulates dilation of blood vessels and relaxation of smooth muscles, which further increases bile flow; this effect does not happen when the coffee is consumed as a beverage.[15]

HYPERBARIC OXYGEN FOR DETOXIFICATION

Hyperbaric oxygen therapy (HBOT) is another highly effective means of removing toxins from the body. In HBOT, a person is placed in a sealed chamber that is filled with pure oxygen. Oxygen "burns up" disease-producing microorganisms and toxins in the body. The use of oxygen under pressure to treat serious health conditions including stroke is well established medically, though not yet widely used in this country. There are only 300 hyperbaric oxygen chambers in the U.S., while in Russia, for example, there are 2,000.

In HBOT, a patient sits or lies on a stretcher for 30-120 minutes in a sealed chamber, which is pressurized at up to two-and-a-half atmospheres (the pressure of air at sea level) with pure oxygen. The increased pressure makes it possible to breathe oxygen at a concentration higher than allowed by any other means. After treatment, the chamber is depressurized slowly with the patient resting inside. Most of the hyperbaric facilities in the U.S. are affiliated with hospitals or the military.

of fennel (1 part), flax (1 part), burdock (¼ part), fenugreek (1 part), licorice (¼ part), and peppermint (1 part). Simmer the herbs (except the peppermint) for 20 minutes, then add the peppermint and steep for ten minutes. For convenience, you may prepare several quarts of the tea in advance.

- Continuing the Flush—Dr. Hobbs suggests doing the liver flush twice yearly, in the spring and fall, for two full cycles each. A cycle consists of ten consecutive days of taking the flush ingredients, followed by three days off, then another ten days on. "I have never seen anyone experience negative side effects from this procedure."

Vitamin C Therapy

Each year, more and more studies on vitamin C confirm its importance in healing and maintaining health. The relationship between vitamin C and body toxicity is complex. For example, people deficient in vitamin C are far more susceptible to environmental pollutants. Conversely, exposure to various toxins, like lead or benzene, will deplete a person's vitamin C stores. Evidence also suggests that vitamin C deficiency hampers the body's own detoxification process.

As a detoxification agent, vitamin C combines with certain toxins in the body and destroys them.[16] According to Robert Cathcart III, M.D., of Los Altos, California, vitamin C functions as a free-radical scavenger, neutralizing the immunosuppressive toxins produced by infectious diseases. Dr. Cathcart has successfully treated over 11,000 patients with vitamin C therapy, and his results have been widely published in professional journals.

Chelation Therapy

Since the late 1940s, chelation therapy has been routinely used to draw lead, mercury, and other heavy metals out of the body, if a person has been exposed to life-threatening levels. It has also been used for years by alternative therapists as a way of detoxifying individuals who, simply through normal everyday exposures, have accumulated levels of toxins that impair optimal health. Chelation therapy refers to a method of binding up ("chelating") toxins (such as heavy metals) and metabolic wastes and removing them from the body while at the same time increasing blood flow.

In chelation therapy, a synthetic amino acid known as EDTA (ethylenediaminetetraacetic acid) is administered intravenously and binds to various toxic metals in the blood, such as lead, mercury, cadmium, and alu-

UNCLOGGING THE LYMPHATIC SYSTEM

Lymph is a clear fluid containing lymphocytes (T cells and B cells of the immune system) that circulates through the channels of the lymphatic system carrying waste away from all parts of the body to the lymph nodes. The lymph nodes filter out the wastes in the lymph, particularly bacteria, and eliminate them, while at the same time allowing the lymphocytes to pass through.

Lymphatic circulation can be enhanced by lymphatic massage as well as osteopathic and chiropractic lymphatic drainage techniques, according to Jared Zeff, N.D., L.Ac., Academic Dean of the Naturopathic College of Natural Medicine, in Portland, Oregon. There are now devices, such as the Light Beam Generator (LBG), that stimulate the lymphatic system. An LBG emits photons of light and a high-frequency electrostatic field to correct the electromagnetic charge on cells. This stimulates the lymphatic system by breaking open sealed and calcified vessels, increasing blood circulation, reducing edema, and carrying away waste products that have built up in the tissues, thereby inducing detoxification.

Dry skin brushing, if done correctly, also helps to physically move toxic lymph fluid through the lymph vessels. It improves the skin's ability to eliminate toxins, oxygenates the tissues, and reduces cellulite. One session of light, but brisk, stimulation of the skin is equivalent to 20 minutes of exercise for encouraging the healthy movement of fluid through the lymphatic channels.

Jack Shields, M.D., a lymphologist from Santa Barbara, California, conducted a study on the effects of breathing on the lymphatic system. He found that deep, diaphragmatic breathing stimulated the cleansing of the lymph system by creating a vacuum effect that sucked the lymph through the channels. This increased the rate of toxic elimination by as much as 15 times the normal pace.[19] Exercise is another effective treatment for unclogging the lymph and restoring its flow. Any vigorous aerobic exercise causes lymphatic flow to accelerate.

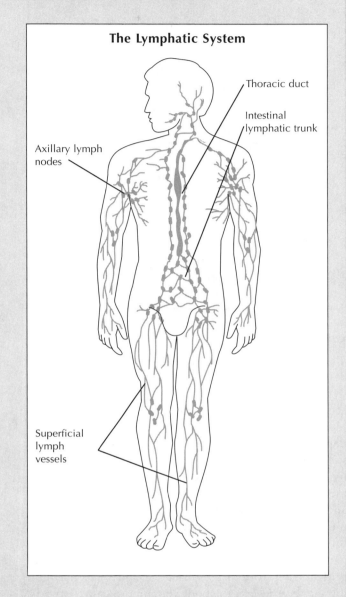

The Lymphatic System

Thoracic duct

Intestinal lymphatic trunk

Axillary lymph nodes

Superficial lymph vessels

minum. The toxins are then flushed from the body through the kidneys. EDTA is three times less toxic than common aspirin.[17] Chelation therapy has been tested and used safely for the past 30 years on an estimated 500,000 patients.[18] EDTA has FDA (Food and Drug Administration) approval for lead and heavy metal tox-

icity and over 1,000 physicians offer chelation therapy in the U.S.

 See Biological Dentistry, Chelation Therapy, Environmental Medicine, Hydrotherapy, Hyperthermia, Oxygen Therapies.

DETOXIFICATION BATHS

The late Hazel Parcells, N.D., D.C., Ph.D., recommended the following detoxification baths at The Parcells' System of Scientific Living, in Albuquerque, New Mexico.

- For poisoning from irradiated food: Dissolve two pounds of baking soda in a tub of very hot water and sit in it. As the water begins to cool, toxins pass through the skin by osmosis.

- For general radiation: Add one pound each of sea salt and baking soda to hot water and sit in the bath until the water has cooled.

- For heavy metals, insecticides, and carbon monoxide: Add one cup of Clorox to a hot bath and soak in it until the temperature cools.

Hyperthermia

The only detoxification program that has proven successful in removing fat-stored toxins from the body is hyperthermia, or heat stress detoxification (saunas), according to Zane Gard, M.D., and Erma Brown, P.H.N. Heat stress, says Dr. Gard, can also remove calcium deposits from the blood vessels and break down scar tissue from their walls. Other studies demonstrate that hyperthermia can remove chemicals such as DDE (a metabolite of DDT), PCBs (polychlorinated biphenyls), and dioxin from fat cells.[20] Practitioners of alternative medicine have long recognized hyperthermia as a useful technique in detoxification therapy.

The body uses its own internally generated heat to protect itself from viruses, bacteria, and other harmful substances. A fever is the body's attempt to destroy invading organisms and to sweat impurities out through the skin. A state of natural hyperthermia exists when body temperature rises above its normal level of 98.6° F. Fever is an effective natural process of curing disease and restoring health—hyperthermia represents a way to recreate this natural healing process. An increase in body temperature causes many physiological responses to occur. Particularly, by increasing the production of antibodies and interferon, it stimulates the immune system.

Saunas are a useful form of hyperthermia because they induce copious sweating. The heat forces toxic materials out of fat cells to be excreted through the sweat glands. Initiate sweating and increased circulation by exercising 20-30 minutes on a stationary bicycle, mini trampoline, or treadmill. Immediately following the exercise, sit in the sauna for up to 30 minutes, followed by a cool (but not cold) shower. The temperature from a "low heat" sauna should be between 140° –180° F, in contrast to the 200° –210° F for a non-therapeutic standard sauna. The sauna may be repeated again followed by a plunge into a bath or under a shower whose temperature is 65° F. Over a period of three to four days, increase your time in the sauna to a total of up to two hours, divided into 30-minute periods with a short cooling-off period in between. It's important to shower and towel dry, because the removal of sweat prevents reabsorption of toxins. While doing the sauna program, consume adequate amounts of water to avoid dehydration (a minimum of two quarts before and after entering the sauna).

According to Dr. Gard, studies show that hyperthermia can affect numerous body systems, including the cardiovascular, endocrine, neurological, neuromuscular, respiratory, blood, skin, and immune.[21] Hyperthermia can be combined with other detoxification therapies. However, proper medical supervision and laboratory evaluations are necessary, because the removal of certain toxins can have a potentially adverse effect on the body, particularly on the kidneys and liver.

The Future of Detoxification Therapy

"I believe that detoxification is a way to clear potential acute and chronic disease out of the body. It's a way to heal many early conditions," Dr. Haas states. Detoxification today has become a cornerstone for many doctors like Dr. Haas, who stress preventative measures rather than just disease control. "My idea is to create healing hospital environments," adds Dr. Haas. "People can check in and, if they have a certain condition, still be provided with medicine or surgery, if necessary. But it will also be a place where people can go to learn how to make changes in their life so they can clear up the problems that they already have and avoid those they don't. Detoxification is a major part of that process."

Dr. Chaitow states, "The need to tackle toxic burdens before they manifest themselves as disease has never been greater. It is clear that the future of health care will have at its very core an absolute requirement for safe and effective detoxification procedures, hopefully instituted before the individual's immune system and vital organs have ceased to operate adequately."

Where to Find Help

There are many modalities that address detoxification of the body. Contact the organizations below for information and referrals.

Chelation Therapy

American College for Advancement in Medicine (ACAM)
23121 Verdugo Drive, Suite 204
Laguna Hills, California 92653
(800) 532-3688
Website: www.acam.org

This pioneering organization seeks to establish certification and standards of practice for chelation therapy. They provide training and education, and sponsor semi-annual conferences for physicians and scientists. ACAM provides referrals and informational material, including a listing of all physicians worldwide trained in preventive medicine as well as in the ACAM protocol for chelation therapy.

Colon Therapy

International Association for Colon Therapy
2051 Hilltop Drive, Suite A-11
Redding, California 96002
(916) 222-1498

Referrals to a nationwide network of colon therapists. Holds seminars on colon therapy for both professionals and the general public. Funds a national certification panel for colon therapists.

Fasting

International Association of Professional Natural Hygienists
Regency Health Resort and Spa
2000 South Ocean Drive
Hallandale, Florida 33009
(305) 454-2220

A professional organization of doctors who specialize in therapeutic fasting. They all follow the same protocol for fasting. Doctors available in the U.S., Canada, Australia, England, Greece, Israel, Japan, and Poland.

American Association of Naturopathic Physicians
601 Valley Street, Suite 105
Seattle, Washington 98109
(206) 298-0126
Website: www.naturopathic.org

Provides referrals to a nationwide network of accredited or licensed naturopathic physicians.

Hyperbaric Oxygen Therapy

American College of Hyperbaric Medicine (ACHM)
P.O. Box 25914-130
Houston, Texas 77265
(713) 528-0657

ACHM has worked to develop hyperbaric oxygen therapy as a distinct medical specialty. They provide protocols, training, and other information to practitioners and the general public.

Hyperthermia

International Clinical Hyperthermia Society (ICHS)
1502 East Country Line Road South
Indianapolis, Indiana 46227
(317) 887-7651
Website: www.hyperthermia-ichs.org

The ICHS provides a forum for researchers and physicians to discuss the use of hyperthermia and to share their clinical findings. Active members include surgeons, medical and radiation oncologists, medical physicists (including basic scientists), nurses, and administrators.

Bastyr University Natural Health Clinic
1307 North 45th Street, Suite 200
Seattle, Washington 98103
(206) 632-0354
Website: www.bastyr.edu

The physical medicine department of the Natural Health Clinic of Bastyr University uses hyperthermia treatment for detoxification and in conditions ranging from upper respiratory infection to chronic fatigue syndrome and HIV.

Laboratory Testing

Accu-Chem Laboratories
990 North Bowser Road, Suite 800
Richardson, Texas 75081
(972) 234-5412

This laboratory performs a complete array of pesticide and industrial chemical analyses on blood, urine, and body tissues.

MetaMetrix Medical Laboratory
5000 Peachtree Industrial Blvd., Suite 110
Norcross, Georgia 30071
(800) 221-4640 or (770) 446-5483

The ToxMet screen from MetaMetrix Medical Laboratory provides an inexpensive but detailed analysis of the levels of specific heavy metals in a patient's system, based on a urine sample.

Great Smokies Diagnostic Laboratory
63 Zillicoa Street
Asheville, North Carolina 28801
(800) 522-4762 or (704) 253-0621
Website: www.gsdl.com

Offers over 125 specialized diagnostic assessments that cover a wide range of physiological areas, including digestive, immune, nutritional, endocrine, and metabolic function.

Recommended Reading

Body/Mind Purification Program. Leon Chaitow, N.D., D.O. New York: Simon and Schuster, 1990.

The Complete Book of Juicing. Michael T. Murray. Rocklin, CA: Prima Publishing, 1997.

The Detox Diet. Elson Haas, M.D. Berkeley, CA: Celestial Arts, 1998.

Detoxification and Healing. Sidney M. Baker, M.D. New Canaan, CT: Keats, 1997.

Diet for a Poisoned Planet. David Steinman. New York: Harmony Books, 1990.

Dr. Jensen's Guide to Diet and Detoxification. Bernard Jensen. Los Angeles: Keats Publishing, 2000.

Juice Fasting and Detoxification. Steve Meyerowitz. Great Barrington, MA: Sproutman Publications, 1999.

Juicing for Life. Cherie Calbom and Maureen B. Keane. Garden City Park, NY: Avery Publishing Group, 1992.

Natural Detoxification. Jacqueline Krohn and Frances Taylor. Point Roberts, WA: Hartley & Marks, 2000.

The 7-Day Detox Miracle. Peter Bennett, N.D., Stephen Barrie, and Sara Faye. Roseville, CA: Prima Publishing, 2001.

Staying Healthy with Nutrition. Elson Haas, M.D. Berkeley, CA: Celestial Arts, 1992.

DIET

Diet plays a central role in a person's overall health, but achieving a good diet is not as simple as it sounds. Eating the right foods no longer insures proper health due to over-farming the land where food is grown (causing nutrient loss), excessive food processing, the use of additives and other chemicals, and toxins contaminating the food supply. Therefore, it is important to pay attention not only to what foods are eaten, but also to how that food was grown before it reached the table. Americans should consume far less fat, animal protein, and processed foods, and eat more complex carbohydrates, fruits, and vegetables.

THE TYPICAL AMERICAN diet of the past few decades has increasingly included more processed and contaminated foods than ever before. At the same time, Americans now suffer from more degenerative diseases, causing many physicians to suggest a strong link between what one eats and how one feels. Over the years, medical research has shown that saturated fats, white flour, refined starches, feedlot-fattened beef and pork, and chemical additives and pesticides—all common elements of the American diet—are major contributors to poor health and disease.

The *Surgeon General's Report on Nutrition and Health* acknowledged, "What we eat may affect our risk for several of the leading causes of death for Americans, notably, degenerative diseases such as atherosclerosis, heart disease, stroke, diabetes, and some types of cancer. These disorders, together, now account for more than two-thirds of all deaths in the United States."

More Food, Less Nutrients

Little more than a century ago, food was unprocessed and unrefined, grown on clean, living (often virgin) soil, with fresh air and pure water. It contained no preservatives, chemicals, or pesticides. Today, most Americans gulp down pesticide-laden coffee and pastries concocted of refined flour, sugar, and margarine for breakfast, rush to fast-food restaurants for a high-fat lunch, and grab canned or frozen sauces and soups, chemically treated vegetables, hormone-laden meats, and hybridized, genetically engineered grains to microwave for dinner. "The truth

is, with the crippled condition of our national diet, we are compelled to overfeed ourselves to get a little nourishment," said the late Hazel Parcells, N.D., D.C., Ph.D., former Director of the Parcells Center, in Santa Fe, New Mexico. "We may look well-fed, but I believe we are basically undernourished."[1]

Over the past century, commercial farmers have adopted intensive cropping methods that rely on large quantities of synthetic chemical fertilizers. The fertilizers, which consist mostly of nitrogen salts that encourage rapid plant growth, return only a fraction (or none) of the vital minerals to the soil that growing plants remove. Consequently, the mineral content of American soils, along with the nutritive value of the plants grown in them, has steadily declined.

Paul Bergner, Clinical Director of the Rocky Mountain Center for Botanical Studies, in Boulder, Colorado, has charted the mineral content of plants grown in the U.S. over the past 50 years. His data show that, since 1948, levels of the essential minerals iron, manganese, and copper have declined significantly in a variety of crops. The iron content of lettuce, for example, has dropped from an average of 51.6 mg per 100 g of food in 1948 to a mere 0.5 mg today. This serious depletion of nutrients from the country's food supply is "leading our entire nation down the road to malnutrition and disease," according to Bergner.[2]

Americans now eat fewer nutrient-rich foods, such as whole grains, unrefined cereals, fruits, and vegetables. It's little wonder that the leading nutritional problem in the U.S. is "overconsumptive undernutrition," or the eating of too many empty-calorie foods, says Jeffrey Bland, Ph.D., a nutrition expert based in Gig Harbor, Washington. Although people consume plenty of food, it is not the right kind of food. Studies have concluded that almost two-thirds of an average American's diet is made up of fats and refined sugars having low to no nutrient density. Consequently, the remaining third of the average diet is relied on for the essential nutrients needed to maintain health, which may or may not be from nutrient-dense foods. The result is nutrient deficiencies that can rob the body of its natural resistance to disease, lead to premature aging, and weaken overall physiological and psychological performance.[3]

Too Much Sugar

In 1922, the U.S. consumption of sugar was five pounds per person per year; in 1990, that figure had skyrocketed to 135 pounds. "Refined sugars do not contain the essential nutrients necessary to even metabolize them properly," says James Braly, M.D. "Sugary processed foods are also unlikely to contain much fiber, so the high consumption of sugar-laden foods contributes to a harmful, low-fiber diet."[4] While cookies, cakes, candies, ice cream, and soft drinks predictably contain high amounts of sugar, surprisingly so do salad dressings, cereals, yogurt, catsup, and relish. In general, food that is frozen, canned, cured, and processed is likely to be high in sugar. Sucrose is sugar (cane sugar to be specific), so is lactose (milk sugar), and maltose (grain sugar). Other sugar derivatives, including fructose and corn syrup, contribute to the excessive sugar load.

Sugar provides empty calories and is a cheap way to get a boost of energy, since it is metabolized by the body into glucose. But too much sugar swamps the body, which is incapable of processing the sugar effectively. With continued overuse of sugar, the pancreas eventually wears out and is no longer able to clear sugar from the blood efficiently. The blood sugar level rises and diabetes may result.

Thirty minutes after consuming sugar, the immune system is measurably suppressed, losing as much as 50% of its capacity.[5] Sugar consumption is linked to a variety of health problems, such as mood swings, heart disease, gallbladder disease, ulcers, colitis, overeating, and addictive behaviors such as alcoholism.[6]

Repetition vs. Variety in the Diet

Nutritionist D. Lindsey Berkson, M.A., D.C., of Santa Fe, New Mexico, sees today's typical American diet as containing too few foods. "Unfortunately, most Americans tend to avoid variety and commit the dietary sin of monotony," she says, "eating the same foods meal after meal, only disguised by different names." They also consume food not according to what is best for them but according to what tastes best.

According to Dr. Berkson, the American menu is actually made of various combinations of the same foods, usually wheat, beef, eggs, potatoes, and milk products. For example, she points out, a breakfast of eggs, sausage, toast, and hash browns is the same as a lunch of a hamburger on a bun and fries, which is the same as a dinner of steak and potatoes or pasta. All of these meals, besides the fact that they are high-fat, high-calorie, low-fiber, and filled with toxins, are strikingly devoid of fruits and vegetables and are low in many essential nutrients. Such repetition can build deficiencies into the body.

Daily consumption of the same foods also tends to produce allergies and hypersensitivities to those foods, according to experts in environmental medicine. Instead of nourishing the body, these foods may start to act against it. Eating a varied diet minimizes these problems. The optimal diet should consist of more vegetables, fruits, and whole grains than any other foods.

 The *Dietary Guidelines for Americans* (jointly issued by the U.S. Department of Agriculture and the Department of Health and Human Services) puts at the top of its dietary recommendations the suggestion that one "eat a variety of foods" in order to get the widest variety of nutrients.

Toxins in the Food Chain

One of the greatest long-term problems that health-conscious individuals face is the pervasive contamination of America's food supply. For decades, the U.S. Food and Drug Administration (FDA) and other government agencies have allowed the multibillion-dollar food industry to grow and process its products with hundreds of questionably safe chemicals such as pesticides, herbicides, dyes, stabilizers, and preservatives, as well as antibiotics, hormones, and other drugs given to animals. The long-term consequences of ingesting these chemicals are still not well understood. Many experts now believe that lifetime ingestion of these chemicals can play a major role in causing cancer, neurotoxicity (destruction of nerve tissue by toxic substances), birth defects, decreased immune function, food allergies, and chemical sensitivity.

 See Environmental Medicine.

In his book *Diet for a Poisoned Planet,* David Steinman, former representative of the public interest at the National Academy of Sciences, makes an exhaustive study of chemical residues in the food chain. As a solution, he recommends the general principle of eating food as low on the food chain as possible. Animal products, high on the food chain, are laden with pesticides from the foods the animals consume, as well as antibiotics and various hormones. Plants, on the other hand, are relatively less contaminated, usually only by what's been sprayed on them. Although many believe that the first step toward a healthy diet is knowing what to eat, it is more important to know what to avoid.

Pesticides

Over 400 pesticides are currently licensed for use on America's foods and, every year, over 2.5 billion pounds are dumped on croplands, forests, lawns, and fields. A person can get several types of pesticides with a salad, different ones in meat or fish, still others in the vegetables on the side, and a separate dose with dessert. Wine has pesticides and, in many areas, water as well. In a single meal, a person would easily consume residues of a dozen different neurotoxic or carcinogenic chemicals.

> *Over 400 pesticides are currently licensed for use on America's foods and, every year, over 2.5 billion pounds are dumped on croplands, forests, lawns, and fields.*

Yet, the Office of Pesticide Programs at the Environmental Protection Agency (EPA) does not include the potential for multiple exposures to the same pesticide when calculating permitted residue levels of a given compound. The agency sets these levels with "blinders" to the fact that people eat more than one product that might have residues. EPA scientists have found that, at times, if these residues were totaled, they would exceed 500% of the allowed daily intake.[7]

Furthermore, many chemicals in food have not been adequately tested for human safety. And they have certainly not been tested with the "chemical cocktail syndrome" (or multiple chemical exposure) in mind. The EPA does not have a scientifically acceptable method for determining the risk for multiple exposures. Yet, when scientists have done studies, it seems quite clear that the chemicals act synergistically. In one study, a scientific team used three chemicals on animals. The chemicals were tested one at a time without ill effect. When the scientists gave the animals two at a time, a decline in health was noted. When the animals were given all three chemicals at once, they all died within two weeks.[8]

Growth Hormones

Recombinant bovine growth hormone (BGH) is a genetically engineered, synthetic version of a hormone naturally produced by cows. Its purpose is to increase a cow's milk production by as much as 25%. This is economically absurd, since American dairy farmers already produce a surplus of dairy products. Twice per month, BGH is injected into three million cows (30% of all milk-producing cows).

The FDA's approval of BGH was in large part due to a Monsanto Corporation (the manufacturer of BGH) study of rats that had been fed milk laced with BGH. Originally, the FDA reported that no traces of BGH were found in the rats' blood, but it was later disclosed that officials from the FDA never read the entire report. It was found that 20%-30% of the rats did, in fact, have traces of BGH in their bloodstream and some of the rats developed thyroid cysts. Other researchers are suggesting a possible link between BGH and prostate and breast cancers, though there is not yet any direct and conclusive evidence.[9]

However, it's difficult to avoid BGH unless you buy organic dairy products and beef, because the FDA does not require labeling of BGH-laced products (which include yogurt, cheese, and other dairy products), despite surveys showing that the majority of consumers favor labeling. In fact, Monsanto helped sponsor federal legislation (which passed) that prevents milk producers from labeling their products as being free of BGH even when they are.

Additives

Approximately 2,000 food additives—artificial colors and flavors, stabilizing agents, texturizers, sweeteners, antimicrobials, and antioxidants—are currently permitted in America's food supply. Studies show that some additives may be carcinogenic, such as Blue Dye No. 1, Blue Dye No. 2, and Green Dye No. 3, while others pose different hazards. In 1981, researchers at the National Institutes of Health reported that Red Dye No. 3 may interfere with brain neurotransmitters.[10] Meanwhile, aspirin-sensitive people have developed life-threatening asthmatic symptoms when ingesting Yellow Dye No. 5, which is found in breakfast cereals, soft drinks, ice cream, candy, bakery products, and pasta.[11]

Food additives can also have profound effects on behavior. Authorities at Tehama County Juvenile Hall, in Red Bluff, California, had positive results in curbing antisocial behavior when they used honey in place of sugar and eliminated meats cured with nitrites and other foods with additives.[12] U.S. Naval Correction Center officials in Seattle, Washington, discovered that removing white bread and refined sugar from the diet of inmates reduced the incidence of violent behavior.[13]

In 1979, the New York City public schools ranked in the 39th percentile on standardized scholastic achieve-

FOOD ADDITIVES TO AVOID

Aspartame: chemical sweetener used in NutraSweet® and Equal®

Bromated Vegetable Oil: emulsifier in foods and clouding agent in soft drinks

Butylated Hydroxyanisole (BHA) and Butylated Hydroxytoluene (BHT): prevents fats, oils, and fat-containing foods from going rancid

Citrus Red Dye No. 2: used to color orange skins

Monosodium Glutamate (MSG): flavor-enhancer used in processed, packaged, and fast foods

Nitrites: used as preservatives in cured meats to prevent spoilage

Saccharin: artificial sweetener, used in Sweet 'n' Low®

Sulfur Dioxide, Sodium Bisulfite, Sulfites: preserves dried fruits, shrimp, frozen potatoes

Tertiary Butylhydroquinone: used to spray the inside of cereal and cheese packages

Yellow Dye No. 6: used in candy and carbonated beverages as a coloring

ment test scores, meaning that 61% of the nation's public schools scored higher. That same year, the New York City Board of Education ordered a reduction of the sugar content of foods served in the schools and banned two synthetic food colorings. In 1980, New York's achievement test scores went up to the 47th percentile. Next, the schools banned all synthetic colorings and flavorings. Test scores increased again, bringing New York City schools up to the 51st percentile. By 1983, when the additives BHA and BHT were removed from foods, New York City schools scored in the 55th percentile. Prior to the dietary changes, the academic performance of the students never varied more than 1% in the course of a year.[14]

Irradiation

This process exposes food to radioactive materials, such as cesium-137 and cobalt-60, to kill insects, bacteria, molds, and fungi, prevent sprouting, and extend shelf life.

Irradiation may not be as dangerous as its harshest critics charge; however, this process leads to the formation of additional toxic substances in foods, including benzene and formaldehyde. Irradiation of foods may also have other hazardous consequences. For example, a study conducted for the U.S. Army and the U.S. Department of Agriculture found that mice fed a diet rich in irradiated chicken died sooner and had a higher incidence of tumors.[15]

Furthermore, foods that have been irradiated lose much of their nutritional value. The vitamin C content of potatoes can be reduced by as much as 50%, according to a Japanese study.[16] In cooked pork, a dose of irradiation equal to one-third the level permitted by the FDA reduced thiamin (vitamin B_1) levels by 17%.[17] Finally, irradiation plants pose hazards to workers as well as to the communities where they are located.

Unfortunately for consumers, while foods irradiated as a whole must be labeled with the flowerlike radura symbol, irradiated ingredients within foods are not identified. For example, commercially prepared spaghetti sauces may contain irradiated ingredients, but do not have to carry any warning.

Genetic Engineering

The proliferation of genetically engineered organisms (GEOs) or "Frankenfoods" is another example of the devastating effect agribusiness has had on our food supply. Frankenfoods are foods that have been genetically engineered, which breaks down fundamental genetic barriers and permanently alters the genetic code of plants by combining them with the genes of dissimilar and unrelated species. This procedure is radically different from traditional plant breeding, which works within, not across, species boundaries.

Scores of companies are now using gene-splicing technology to produce never-before-seen genetic combinations. Over 90% of current genetic research in agriculture is for the purpose of creating plants that are cheaper to grow and transport and have an indefinite shelf life without losing the appearance of freshness—in other words, for bigger profits. According to a survey of field-tested food crops conducted by the Union of Concerned Scientists, 93% of genetic changes are performed to make food production and processing easier and more profitable, and only 7% are done to improve nutrition or taste.[18]

The danger is that if you have food sensitivities, your next serving of corn, soybeans, potatoes, or tomatoes may be a kind of Trojan horse, bringing unsuspected allergens and toxins (from the unnatural gene combinations) into your body. It's even more alarming to know that there has been almost no safety testing and, since the altered substances are not listed on food labels, no way of knowing which foods contain them. As a consumer, you are now deprived of your right to make an informed choice when you select foods. As things stand today, GEOs are all but unavoidable.

The Milk Controversy

Milk has traditionally been viewed as just about the most perfect food, especially for children. More recently, however, experts have begun to question the safety of milk. Child-care expert Benjamin Spock, M.D., shocked the nation by warning parents about the dangers of milk.[19] According to the Physicians' Committee for Responsible Medicine (PCRM), milk may cause diabetes, ovarian cancer, cataracts, iron deficiency, and allergies in both children and adults.[20] Additional medical research associates milk consumption with a greater frequency of cancer of the lymph system.[21]

The statements of the PCRM may have some merit, but much more research will be required before a final verdict. Until then, keep these guidelines in mind:[22]

- Breast milk is best for babies up to at least age 2. Efficient breast pumps can be obtained from hospitals (or purchased) to extract breast milk and make life easier for working mothers.

- Mothers who are breast-feeding infants whose siblings or parents had childhood diabetes should avoid drinking large amounts of cow's milk, as proteins from the cow's milk that can trigger this condition may be absorbed intact and end up in mother's breast milk.

- Persons with blood type O should not consume milk and other dairy products at all.

- Other adults and children over the age of 2 should drink only skim or 1% low-fat milk in moderation.

- People who suffer from recurring bouts of diarrhea, bronchitis, eczema, asthma, or runny nose, should be tested for a milk or cheese allergy and should avoid all allergens in their diet.

- People who get gas, diarrhea, or cramps after eating cheese or drinking milk, should not consume these dairy products at all or should consume smaller quantities with meals, switch to a lactose-reduced milk, or try lactase pills (containing the enzyme for digesting milk).

Most milk is pasteurized. In the pasteurization process, milk is heated at high temperatures, much higher than necessary to kill any bacteria. High heat destroys all the enzymes in the milk. In addition, whole milk and whole dairy products, such as ice cream and cheese, may contain concentrated fat-soluble pesticides. They can also contain sulfa drugs and antibiotics as a result of mixing milk from healthy cows with the milk from ill or medicated cows. For reduction in toxins from dairy products, rely on nonfat products. Another option is milk substitutes such as soy, almond, rice, or goat's milk. Health food stores and many supermarkets sell these products, which are frequently made with organic ingredients.

Problems with Eating Red Meat

The combination of a high-fat diet and toxic overload may have a harmful synergistic effect on human health. Fatty foods, particularly red meat, can increase the toxicity of the chemicals that are lodged in them. In several animal studies, chemical carcinogens were more likely to produce tumors in the group that was fed fatty foods than in the group fed low-fat foods.[23] Thus, a high-fat diet of animal-derived foods can be especially troublesome, because the most potent pesticides are concentrated in fat and the chemical properties of fat itself may actually increase their carcinogenicity. Worldwide, a clear association consistently appears between the highest rates of breast, colon, and prostate cancers and nations that have the fattiest diets.[24]

The link between cancer and meat-eaters' exposure to toxic chemicals goes even deeper. All fried and broiled foods contain mutagens, chemicals that can damage cellular reproductive material. But fried and broiled meats have far more mutagens than similarly prepared plant foods. One study indicates that 20% of American meat-eaters may have toxic mutagens in their digestive tracts that can be absorbed into the bloodstream. The same study indicates that vegetarians are unlikely to have any mutagens in their digestive tracts.[25]

Fishing in Polluted Waters?

The industrial and agricultural pollution of rivers, lakes, and seas has led to widespread environmental contamination. Many of the most popular seafood dishes today are contaminated with pesticides and industrial chemicals that have been shown to cause cancer and birth defects. Industrial chemicals such as PCBs (polychlorinated biphenyls) and methyl mercury tend to accumulate in significant amounts in some fish and crustaceans.

Studies in Michigan indicate that PCB exposure during pregnancy causes a delay of infant brain development, resulting in slower neuromuscular development, as well as causing decreased head circumference, birth

MAD COW DISEASE

The specter of mad cow disease increasingly overshadows the beef industry in the U.S., Canada, and Europe. Mad cow disease, clinically known as bovine spongiform encephalopathy (BSE), is a deadly illness resulting in a slow and painful deterioration of the brain, turning it into a mushy sponge. BSE was born of the agricultural practice of feeding farm animals the rendered parts of other farm animals (ground-up brain tissue and spinal cords from sheep, chickens, cows, and other animals). The practice of using rendered animal parts for feed started as a cost-saving measure, a way to recycle dead and diseased animals and provide a source of protein for the live ones.

BSE is not supposed to cross the "inviolable" barrier between species (cattle to human), but apparently it has. In 1996, ten people died in England due to a new strain of Creutzfeldt-Jakob Disease (CJD, the human equivalent of BSE), which the British government linked to eating meat from cows infected with BSE. CJD has now killed a total of 100 people in Britain.[26] Researchers at Yale University suggest the disease is capable of mutating into different forms. They also speculate that CJD/BSE might be more widespread than originally thought. BSE first started showing up in England in the mid-eighties. In 1988, the government required that all cattle showing symptoms of BSE be destroyed. Then, in 1989, the British government banned the feeding of rendered animal parts to cows.

In spite of these warning signs and recent outbreaks of mad cow disease, U.S. agriculture still permits the feeding of rendered animal parts to cattle, claiming that U.S. cattle are "safe" from the disease. Of the approximately 44 million beef cattle in the U.S., 75% are regularly fed this diet of animal parts. This amounts to about 3.3 million tons of rendered animal feed per year, a $3 billion business in the U.S.

Rendered feed from countries whose herds were infected with mad cow has been prohibited from being imported into the U.S. However, at the height of the mad cow epidemic in Britain, at least 500,000 tons of bovine by-products were exported from Britain to 70 countries around the world. Thirty-seven tons were exported to the U.S. as recently as 1997, in spite of the ban. Further, the U.S. still imports huge quantities of dairy products, gelatin, collagen, fat, and other beef by-products from Britain and Europe. These are used in cosmetics, pharmaceutical drugs, vaccines, supplements, and processed foods.[27] All of these can potentially contain the infectious agent that causes mad cow.

The U.S. Food and Drug Administration (FDA) has only recently begun to take action by instituting a "mammal to mammal feeding ban." However, the voluntary "ban" still allows blood, gelatin, some beef parts, pigs, horses, and chickens to be used in animal feed, so BSE molecules (called prions) can still be transmitted to humans.

Both the testing procedures and regulations regarding cattle feed are ineffective. Federal meat inspectors examine less than 1% of the carcasses being processed for consumption. Out of 900 million head of cattle, the U.S. Department of Agriculture has tested only 12,000 sick cows for mad cow disease.[28] Of 5,000 feed handlers already inspected, 700 were not in compliance with regulations designed to keep rendered feed from cattle. Up to 40% of the companies were not using the required labels to identify rendered feed. And another 5,000 companies have yet to be inspected.[29]

The fact that as yet there have been no confirmed cases of mad cow disease in the U.S. means nothing. "The only thing that stands between us and an epidemic," says Robert Rowher, Director of Molecular Virology at the V.A. Medical Center, in Baltimore, Maryland, "is unmitigated luck."[30] In the meantime, the prudent will avoid all meats unless they are certified organically raised without rendered animal parts as feed.

Mad cow disease originated from "factory farming" practices. After 15 years of dealing with this crisis, scientists advising European governments have come to the conclusion that ending factory farming is the only way to eradicate the disease. One way to bring this about is to get involved politically. Support activist and consumer groups and vote for politicians whose priority is to stop the poisoning of ourselves and our planet.

SAFE AND UNSAFE SEAFOOD

The lists below, compiled by David Steinman, author of *Diet for a Poisoned Planet*, indicate the safest (green light) and the highest risk (red light) seafood choices.

Green Light Seafood	Red Light Seafood	
Abalone	Bass (freshwater)	Mullet
Arctic char	Black cod (California black cod,	Northern pike
Crawfish	butterfish, and sablefish)	Ocean perch
Dungeness crab	Bluefish	Rock cod
Grouper	Buffalo fish, Carp	Rockfish
Haddock	Catfish	Sablefish
Halibut	Caviar	Sea herring
Mahi mahi	Chub	Shark
Marlin	Cod	Sheepshead
Octopus	Coho salmon, Great Lakes salmon,	Striped bass, White bass
Orange roughy	Norwegian salmon	Sturgeon
Pacific salmon (wild)	Croaker	Swordfish
Red snapper	Drum	Walleye
Scallops	Eel	Weakfish
Sea bass	Lake trout	Whitefish
Shrimp	Maine lobster	White perch, Yellow perch
Sole	Mackerel	
Spiny lobster		
Squid		
Talapia		
Tuna		
Wahoo		
Whiting		
Yellowtail		

---

weight, and gestation period.[31] Such severe birth defects were seen among infants whose mothers ate only two or three Great Lakes fish a month over several years, long before they ever considered the effects that such toxins could have on their pregnancies. Methyl mercury has also been shown to cause birth defects.

As a rule, it is safest to avoid all freshwater fish, including farm-raised catfish, as well as swordfish and shark. Deep-water fish such as red snapper, grouper, halibut, and orange roughy are generally safe.

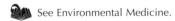 See Environmental Medicine.

Exploring Your Biochemical Individuality

"Whether a food—even one that is whole and natural—acts to irritate or nourish your body depends largely on your biological makeup," says Buck Levin, Ph.D., R.D., Assistant Professor of Nutrition at Bastyr University, in Kenmore, Washington. Each person is a unique product of genetics and environment—pioneering biochemist Roger Williams, Ph.D., referred to this concept as "biochemical individuality." Body types are used by many alternative medicine practitioners as a guide to help patients tailor their own diet plan. By eating in a way that works best with your particular metabolism, you may notice improved energy levels and not experience as many cravings between meals. "Dietary needs are different for each of us and, in order to develop your ideal diet, you will need to explore your own biochemical individuality," says Dr. Levin.

Just like fingerprints, each of us has a unique metabolism, that is, how we convert food into energy for running all of the body's processes. In fact, many chronic illnesses may be simply symptoms of an underlying disturbance in metabolism. Your body type could be the key

A BRIEF SURVEY OF BODY TYPING

The idea that each of us has a specific body type is not a new one. Ayurvedic medicine, the 5,000-year-old traditional medicine of India, describes three metabolic, constitutional body types *(doshas)*, in association with the basic elements of nature—*vata* (air and ether, rooted in the intestines), *pitta* (fire and water/stomach), and *kapha* (water and earth/lungs). Ayurvedic physicians use these categories (which also have psychological aspects) as the basis for prescribing individualized programs of herbs, diet, massage, breathing exercises, meditation, yoga postures, and detoxification techniques.

Traditional Chinese medicine (TCM) originated in China over 5,000 years ago and is a comprehensive system of medical practice that heals the body according to the principles of nature and balance. A Chinese medicine physician considers the flow of vital energy *(qi)* in a patient through close examination of the patient's pulse, tongue, eyes, ears, fingernails, body odor, voice tone and strength, and general demeanor, among other elements. Underlying imbalances and disharmony in the body are described in terminology analogous to the natural world (heat, cold, dryness, or dampness). TCM employs a body-typing paradigm called the Five Element Theory, which holds that each individual expresses the energy of the elements of fire, wood, air, water, and metal in different measures and that an interplay of *yin* (passive, watery, stationary, dark, calming) and *yang* (active, fiery, moving, bright, energizing) energies influences one's health.

Modern science is now catching up with these concepts. One recent body-typing system is glandular types, developed in the early 1980s by Eliot D. Abravanel, M.D., of Los Angeles, California, author of *Dr. Abravanel's Body Type Diet*. This approach is based upon the idea that each one of us has a "dominant" endocrine gland that controls the workings of our internal chemistry, namely how our bodies process and use proteins, carbohydrates, and fats. It also determines our general body shape, fat distribution, food preferences, and energy level, and is associated with a distinctive set of personality traits and behavior patterns, according to Dr. Abravanel. The main types are adrenal, pituitary, thyroid, and gonadal.

Another body-typing system was developed by James D'Adamo, N.D., founder of the Institute for the Advancement of Natural Therapy, in Toronto, Canada, who pioneered the idea that blood type is a determinant of individual nutritional requirements. His observations of more than 3,000 patients led him to conclude that the four basic blood groups—O, A, B, and AB—have different physiological and nutritional needs. Dr. D'Adamo's work on blood type and diet has been continued by his son, Peter D'Adamo, N.D., author of *Eat Right for Your Type*.

Although wide-ranging in their origins and principles, all these systems share a belief that everyone has a distinct physiological fingerprint that cannot be ignored.

---

to your health. The way to discover this biochemical "fingerprint" is metabolic typing. One of the most detailed and reliable body-typing systems is called "metabolic typing," based on research done by George Watson, Ph.D., William Donald Kelley, D.D.S., Francis Pottenger, M.D., and others. Your type is determined from a series of questions or diagnostic tests that reveal which physiological systems tend to drive your body.

Determining Your Type

The first step in looking at one's biochemistry is determining the acid/alkaline state, or pH, of the blood. Ideal arterial blood pH is slightly alkaline at 7.35 to 7.45. A blood pH above this is considered alkaline and below is acidic. Blood pH indicates your state of health and your body type will predispose you to being more acidic or more alkaline. Saliva pH can be measured at home (just before meals) as a daily guide and should range from 6.5

to 6.8. When you are too acid or too alkaline, your body doesn't absorb or use nutrients as well, which can lead to an array of problems, including weight gain, fatigue, allergies, high blood pressure, and many other chronic illnesses. Each body type requires specific foods and dietary supplements to help rebalance the pH.

To further understand this typing system, it is important to understand its two primary criteria: the autonomic nervous system and oxidation rate. One of these systems will be dominant and influence all of your body's processes. This concept of dominance in metabolic typing was first described by William L. Wolcott, author of *The Metabolic Typing Diet* and founder of the Metabolic Typing Education Center, in Winthrop, Washington, an organization that performs metabolic typing evaluations.

- Autonomic Nervous System—Each of our bodies has a unique way of functioning, determined by genetics and controlled by the autonomic nervous system (ANS). The ANS can be likened to your body's automatic pilot—it keeps you alive through breathing, heart rate, and digestion. The ANS has two divisions: the sympathetic and the parasympathetic. The sympathetic nervous system expends energy and is associated with action, arousal, and stress. It energizes us by increasing our heart rate, blood pressure, and muscle tension; the thyroid, pituitary, and adrenal glands are sympathetic-influenced. The parasympathetic nervous system conserves body energy, slows heart rate, and increases the activity of the intestines, liver, and pancreas. People who are ANS dominant tend to be dominant in either sympathetic function or parasympathetic function.

- Oxidation Rate—Oxidation refers to the process of converting food into energy. All foods—proteins, fats, and carbohydrates—are converted into energy (measured in calories), which are then burned off by the body. Ideally, your calorie intake matches the amount of calories you use as energy. But if your carbohydrate oxidation rate is too fast, it tends to acidify the blood or saliva, and if your carbohydrate oxidation is too slow, it alkalinizes your blood and saliva pH. An imbalance will also tend to convert foods into fat instead of using it as energy.

Wolcott has refined metabolic body typing after working for eight years with Dr. Kelley and continuing to research its applications for over 20 years. He uses a number of tests to identify an individual's biochemistry before creating a program of appropriate diet and exercise to bring a person to optimal health. These tests provide information that, taken together and analyzed by an experienced health practitioner, can more accurately identify your type.

- Blood Typing—Blood is classified into four blood types or groups according to the presence of type A and type B antigens on the surface of red blood cells. These antigens are also called agglutinogens and pertain to the blood cells' ability to agglutinate, or clump together. Type O blood (containing neither type) is found in 47% of the Caucasian population; type A, 41%; type B, 9%; type AB, 3%. Blood type is considered relevant to metabolic typing because agglutination also occurs in the body in response to a type of protein called lectin. Lectins are found in 30% of the foods we eat; they have characteristics similar to blood antigens and can thus sometimes become "an enemy" when they enter the body.

- Glucose Metabolism—During the glucose tolerance test, a drink rich in sugars is given and blood or saliva and urine samples are taken and measured to determine how quickly or slowly the body is "burning off" or oxidizing the sugars.

- Oxidative or Autonomic—Your blood pressure, heart rate, pulse, and respiratory rate will be recorded at the beginning of testing to determine levels in a fasting state and again after the glucose test is administered. Changes in the readings will show if you are oxidative or autonomic.

- Body Temperature—Known as the basal temperature, this shows whether your metabolism, essentially the internal "furnace" that burns the calories you are consuming, is operating efficiently.

- Food Diary—The diary provides a detailed list of all the foods consumed over a 3-day period.

- Hair Analysis—Your hair is analyzed to reveal what minerals you may be lacking.

- *Candida*—The presence of the yeast-like fungus *Candida albicans* will provide information regarding food allergies and the resulting symptoms of fatigue or incomplete digestion and absorption of foods.

- Photos of Your Body—Photos are used to record what parts of your body tend to store fat.

- General Health—An extensive survey with questions regarding what you eat, what snacks you crave, sleeping habits, and general outlook on life is also given. An electrodermal screening test can determine if any of your organs are underactive or overstimulated.

With this information, an experienced health practitioner can determine each person's metabolic type and then make specific dietary recommendations. For instance, some people have a tendency to burn off their carbohydrates too quickly and, at the same time, are poor at converting fats to fuel that can be used by the body. They have acidic blood and do best on a whole foods diet including whole (preferably sprouted) grains, extensive animal protein, and full-fat dairy foods. Wheat is to be avoided as it is too acid-forming. Others are alkaline because of slow carbohydrate metabolism and do well eating a diet that limits high-fat, high-purine animal proteins. Low-fat dairy foods and whole grains are allowable, but sprouted wheat should be favored as it is more acid-forming.

Depending on your metabolic type, you may thrive on a low-protein, relatively low-fat diet or on a diet including full-fat dairy foods with more animal protein. By eating in a way that works with your metabolism, you may notice improved energy levels, a natural balancing of body weight, and relief from chronic health problems due to an underlying imbalance in your metabolism.

 See Allergies, Detoxification Therapy.

The Whole Foods Diet

Americans should consume far less animal fat, hydrogenated oils, and processed foods, and eat more complex carbohydrates, especially raw salads and whole grains, preferably sprouted that are rich in fiber, and several servings daily of fruits and vegetables. Dr. Levin offers a simple prescription for a healthy diet: one of natural, whole foods. "By whole foods, we mean consuming a diet that is as high in foods as whole as possible, with the least amount of processed, adulterated, fried, or sweetened additives," says Dr. Levin.

A whole foods diet (preferably guided by metabolic typing and blood typing) is generously filled with a wide variety of vegetables, fruits, and grains; raw seeds and nuts and their butters; beans; fermented milk products such as yogurt and kefir; and fish, poultry, and bean products like tofu. It should also be lower in animal meats, fats, and fatty cheeses as opposed to low-fat milk products. A sense of balance is important in approaching one's diet. If the majority of meals are comprised of whole, fresh foods, then a little junk food, some alcohol, and a piece of candy here or there won't hurt. But when too few whole foods are consumed, as compared to "stressor" foods (those lacking in nutritional value), the body's physiology is damaged.

 According to Buck Levin, Ph.D., the average U.S. supermarket stocks over 24,000 items whose true 'natures' have often been drastically altered and ultimately devitalized.

Eating Lower on the Food Chain

While it is preferable that a whole foods diet be as plant-based as possible for those who metabolically tolerate such a diet, it may not be necessary to become a complete vegetarian, thus eliminating meats and other animal foods from the diet totally. Today, many kinds of dairy products are completely fat-free and many animal foods are low in fat. Even so, unless your metabolic type

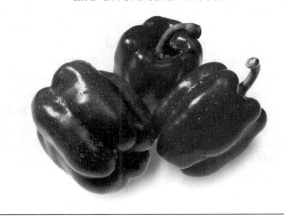

A vegetarian lifestyle can reduce the risk of heart disease, diabetes, colon cancer, hypertension, obesity, osteoporosis, and diverticular disease.

requires more animal-derived food for ideal health, meats and other animal products should be eaten as a specialty rather than a staple, to add variety to one's diet once or twice a week. Always choose the leanest meats possible (range fed or wild game), as this will cut down effectively on calories, weight gain, and toxic exposure.

There are many reasons to stick to a more plant-based diet. First, important antioxidant nutrients including vitamin C, beta carotene, vitamin E, and cancer-fighting substances known as phytochemicals, are found in fruits, vegetables, and grains. These antioxidant nutrients are considered the best protection against age- and environment-related diseases, from dandruff, bad breath, and wrinkling to cataracts, cancer, diabetes, and heart attacks. A recent study found that a diet rich in fruits and vegetables reduces a woman's risk of getting breast cancer, perhaps by a factor of two-to-one.[32] Also, the high fiber content of plant foods helps keep the digestive tract clean by binding to and causing bowel elimination of many potentially dangerous toxins. Plant foods tend to have a lower toxicity than animal foods to begin with, because they are lower on the food chain and have had less exposure to accumulating toxins.

Medical evidence points to the benefits of moving toward a vegetarian-based diet, if one's metabolic type allows it. Dean Ornish, M.D., of the University of California at San Francisco, demonstrates that a diet free of animal protein, along with exercise and stress-reduction measures, can reverse heart disease.[33] The American Dietetic Association has published research showing that a vegetarian lifestyle can reduce the risk of heart disease, diabetes, colon cancer, hypertension, obesity, osteoporosis, and diverticular disease.[34]

Therapeutic Foods

All whole, natural foods have regenerative and restorative powers, says Dr. Levin. Indeed, meeting the health needs of the body is the aim of a balanced diet. Some foods, however, are unusually rich in nutrients and contain unique beneficial chemical components.

Garlic: Garlic has well-documented health effects, including reduction of cholesterol and triglycerides, preventing abnormal clot formation, reducing blood pressure, and enhancing immune capacity. Garlic contains sulfur-rich compounds—allin and allicin, chromium, phosphorus, and sulfur-containing amino acids. Raw garlic swallowed in small pieces with water (like tablets) is a great flu remedy, or its cloves can be roasted whole and brushed lightly with oil. If you are worried about bad breath, chew a sprig of parsley.

Ginger: The roots of this reed-like plant contain compounds called gingerols and shogaols, which relax the intestinal tract, prevent motion sickness, and relieve nausea and vomiting (especially during pregnancy). Ginger is an excellent source of minerals, especially manganese. Ginger ale can be a delicious bottled form of this food, but buy only natural brands at health food stores and avoid the overprocessed, sugar-sweetened, grocery store brands. A word of caution: ginger can aggravate problems associated with elevated estrogen levels in women.

Soy: Substituting soy protein for animal protein may decrease high total cholesterol by as much as 10%, LDL cholesterol by 13%, and triglycerides by more than 10%, but without decreasing the "good" HDL cholesterol. Soy helps reduce blood fats by boosting thyroid hormone levels. Soybeans are excellent for reducing cancer risk since they contain five types of anti-cancer agents. For example, the soy isoflavone genistein diminishes the growth of new blood vessels in cancerous tissues, thus inhibiting proliferation. Studies have shown that genistein and daidzein protect against estrogen-related cancers.[35]

Carrots: When eaten raw, carrots are efficient colon-cleansers, which tone the bowel, reduce the re-absorption of estrogen, and lower cholesterol. Two carrots every day supply enough beta carotene to cut the risk of stroke in half among men who have signs of heart disease, according to one study.[36] In another study, women who ate five or more servings of carrots per week had a stroke rate 68% lower than those who ate only one serving. However, diabetics may want to limit the amount of carrots they consume since they contain high amounts of natural sugars.

Cruciferous Vegetables: Bok choy, collards, kale, broccoli, cabbage, cauliflower, mustard greens, Brussels sprouts, radishes, and turnips contain a type of flavonoid that activates liver detoxification enzymes. The crucifers are noteworthy due to their wide array of sulfur-containing compounds, but they also contain anti-cancer and antioxidant vitamins. They should be eaten lightly cooked so as not to adversely affect thyroid function.

Citrus Fruits: Oranges, grapefruits, lemons, and limes contain large amounts of vitamin C, bioflavonoids, fiber, and phytochemicals such as coumarins known to help prevent abnormal blood clots from forming. The potassium in citrus fruits helps lower blood pressure and pectin from grapefruit pulp helps lower cholesterol levels.

Tomatoes: Tomatoes contain lycopene (the substance that gives the tomato its deep red color), which belongs to a family of natural pigments (carotenoids) found in plants. According to current research, lycopene is a top-flight antioxidant, capable of protecting the body against many degenerative diseases, including prostate, cervical, and gastrointestinal cancers.

Mushrooms: A mainstay in Chinese medicine and cuisines, mushrooms help to promote health and longevity. They have an immune-boosting effect, which helps reduce the risk of cancer and enhances heart health. Shiitake has been found to enhance immune system function, ward off infection, and neutralize cancerous cells.[37] Reishi is a variety of mushroom that also fights infection and has traditionally been used to treat heart disease and lower blood pressure and cholesterol.[38] Maitake mushroom lowers blood pressure and may help in the control of diabetes.[39]

Nuts: In a recent report, it was revealed that people eating nuts (peanuts, walnuts, almonds) at least five times per week lived, on average, seven years longer. Nut eaters also benefited by experiencing a lower incidence of heart attacks.[40] Nuts are high in fat, but it's the good types of fat, polyunsaturated and monounsaturated. Some nuts are good sources of alpha-linolenic acid (an omega-3 EFA) and vitamin E.

Legumes: Peas and beans, such as kidney, lima, soybean, navy, black, and lentils, are loaded with protein, folic acid, and amino acids. Lima beans are also a rich source of fiber, containing 10 g per cup. Legumes are effective at reducing cholesterol levels and help fight against the development of diabetes.

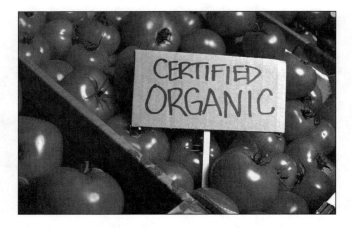

Blackstrap Molasses: Drop for drop, it contains more calcium than milk, more iron than beef, and more potassium than bananas. It's easily used as a sugar substitute or eaten in place of jam and jelly.

Yeasts: These single-celled organisms contain high concentrations of B vitamins and many minerals. Yeasts can be purchased in dried form and sprinkled on top of foods. Baker's, brewer's, and torula yeast are the three forms of "nutritional" yeasts most commonly available. Do not eat yeast or yeast products if you have candidiasis, the overgrowth of the fungus *Candida albicans*. *Candida* may overgrow when the immune system is weakened and this may contribute to other immune deficiency health conditions such as chronic fatigue syndrome.

See Candidiasis, Chronic Fatigue Syndrome, Herbal Medicine.

Fermented Foods: Cheese, yogurt, buttermilk, sauerkraut, and beer are familiar examples of fermented foods. These foods are processed with enzymes from bacteria, yeasts, and molds that create gradual chemical changes in the structure of the foods. Fermented foods can aid in digestion and balance bacterial populations in the gut. They also have a naturally long shelf life and retain their vitamin content much longer than nonfermented foods.

Raw Foods: While raw foods have a greater risk of contamination by microorganisms than cooked foods, this risk is minimal with high-quality foods and is more than offset by the gain in nutrients and enzymes that would otherwise be lost in cooking. Also, high-fiber raw foods have water-absorbing properties that make them especially effective in absorbing digestive juices from the gastrointestinal tract, thus helping to regulate the digestive process. None of these benefits are possible, though, unless the raw foods are well chewed.

Raw Juice: There is no better way to get nutrients from fresh, organic vegetables than to run them through a juicer. The bioflavonoids in the pulp of peppers, for example, will be in the juice along with the vitamin C. Experiment with different combinations like parsley, spinach, and cucumber, or carrot, celery, and beet. Add fresh garlic and ginger for an immune boost.

Green Tea: Tea contains high levels of flavonoids, which stop the development of LDL or "bad" cholesterol and discourage it from sticking to the artery walls. Loaded with active phytochemicals called catechins, lightly processed green tea can help lower blood cholesterol levels and reduce the chances of developing cancer.

Benefits of a Whole Foods Diet

According to Dr. Levin, a whole foods diet promotes health by decreasing fat and sugar intake and increasing fiber and nutrient intake. Ideally, it means more satisfaction and less overeating.

- **More Fiber**—Most animal products, such as meat, cheese, milk, eggs, and butter, contain no fiber, compared to brown rice, broccoli, oatmeal, or almonds, which have 6-15 g per serving. Fiber is the transport system of the digestive tract, moving food wastes out of the body before they have a chance to form potentially cancer-causing chemicals. These toxic chemicals can cause colon cancer or pass through the gastrointestinal membrane into the bloodstream and damage other cells.

- **Less Fat**—On a percentage-of-calories basis, most vegetables contain less than 10% fat and most grains contain 16%-20% fat. By comparison, whole milk and cheese contain 74% fat. A rib roast is 75% fat and eggs are 64% fat. Low-fat milk or a skinned, baked chicken breast still have 38% fat. Not only do animal foods have more fat, but most of these fats are saturated fats, which research has shown raise cholesterol levels. In addition, a lower fat, whole foods diet means fewer calories, since an ounce of fat contains twice as many calories as an ounce of complex carbohydrates. Studies have shown that a diet containing fewer calories can increase health and extend life.[41]

- **Decreased Sugar Consumption**—Eating a diet high in natural complex carbohydrates tends to be more filling and decreases the desire to consume processed sugars. Lower sugar consumption also decreases overall food intake. As with fat, sugar is a hidden and unwelcome ingredient in many processed foods.

- **More Nutrients**—Plant foods are richer sources of nutrients than their animal counterparts. Compare wheat germ to round steak. Ounce for ounce, wheat germ contains twice the vitamin B$_2$, vitamin K, potassium, iron, and copper; three times the vitamin B$_6$, molybdenum, and selenium; 15 times as much magnesium; and over 20 times the vitamin B$_1$, folate, and inositol. The steak has only three nutrients in greater amounts—vitamin B$_{12}$, chromium, and zinc.

- **Increased Variation**—A greater variety of vegetables also exposes the consumer to, literally, more colorful foods—red beets, chard, yellow squash, red peppers, cabbage. "This is more important than you may have imagined," says Dr. Berkson. "Variations in color are due to various minerals, vitamins, and other nutrients that perform important health-promoting functions in the body."

- **More Food Satisfaction and Less Over-Eating**—Foods such as vegetables, whole grains, and beans that are dense in nutrients and fiber require more eating (chewing) time and often result in consumption of fewer calories. Eating whole foods makes a person satisfied more quickly, which means he or she eats less. Eating less is associated with longevity and optimal health.[42]

Dietary Fats— The Whole Story

Certain fats, particularly the essential fatty acids (EFAs), are vital for the healthy functioning of our bodies—for the smooth running of the gastrointestinal system, the formation of cell membranes and hormones, and for balance in the nervous system. Fatty acids are the chemical molecules that make up most fats. Since the body cannot synthesize EFAs from other nutrients, it must obtain them directly from food.

Unfortunately, many individuals today do not obtain the EFAs that they need. Dr. Bland says that an increasing number of Americans suffer from an essential fatty acid deficiency. Even though Americans now consume about 40% more fats per day than our ancestors did in 1909, the "mass commercial refinement of fats, oil products, and the foods containing them has effectively eliminated the essential fatty acids from our food chain," observes Michael T. Murray, N.D., of Issaquah, Washing-

ton. Because of this, he estimates that Americans may be consuming only 10% of the EFAs required for good health.

Omega-3 and omega-6 oils are the two principal types of EFAs. The primary omega-3 oil is alpha-linolenic acid (ALA), found in flaxseed and walnut oils, as well as pumpkin seeds, walnuts, and soybeans. Fish oils, such as salmon, cod, and mackerel, contain the other important omega-3 oils, DHA (docosahexaenoic acid) and EPA (eicosapentaenoic acid). Linoleic acid is the main omega-6 oil and is found in most vegetable oils, including safflower, corn, peanut, and sesame. The most therapeutic form of omega-6 oil is gamma-linolenic acid (GLA), found in evening primrose, black currant, and borage oils. A balance of these oils in the diet is required for good health. Once in the body, omega-3 and omega-6 are converted to prostaglandins, locally produced, hormone-like substances that regulate many metabolic functions, particularly inflammatory processes.

Benefits of increasing your intake of EFAs include reduced risk of heart attack through decreased blood clotting, lower triglyceride levels, and lower blood pressure. Certain fatty acids, especially oleic acid (present in milk, butter, and extra-virgin olive oil) are vital in the transport of calcium from the blood to the tissues. Omega-3 and omega-6 oils may also prevent certain forms of cancer.[43] In therapeutic doses, EFAs can help lessen the pain of arthritis and prevent abnormal heart rhythms.[44]

Choosing the Right Fats

The current recommendation from groups such as the American Heart Association and the American Cancer Society is to reduce daily fat consumption to 30% of total caloric intake, with an emphasis on substituting unsaturated fats like olive oil for saturated ones such as butter. While this is a step in the right direction, many healthcare experts believe that for long-term health and weight control, fats should constitute 15%-20% of your daily calories. They should also be selected carefully, making sure to exclude all harmful fats.

In general, choose vegetable and seed oils that are cold-pressed. This means that the oils were extracted from their sources with a minimum of heat, a process that protects the oils from damage. Always check the expiration date of any oil you buy; many high-quality oils have a short shelf life (3-4 months). In addition, look for dairy products that have not been homogenized. Most butters available on your supermarket shelf are made from homogenized milk, but in response to increased consumer demand, many stores are also beginning to carry raw butter, made from nonhomogenized milk.

A QUICK GUIDE TO FATS

Fat or oil (*lipid* is the biochemical term) is one of the six basic food groups. Fats and oils are made of building blocks called fatty acids. Structurally, a fatty acid is a chain of carbon atoms with a certain quantity of hydrogen atoms attached. The more hydrogen atoms attached to the carbon atoms, the more "saturated" a fat is. Fats come in three natural forms (saturated, monounsaturated, and polyunsaturated) and one man-made form (called hydrogenated or trans fats).

Saturated Fats—Saturated fats are solid at room temperature and are primarily found in animal foods and tropical oils, such as coconut and palm oil. A fatty acid that has its full quota of hydrogen atoms is a saturated fatty acid. The body produces saturated fats from sugar, which is one reason why low-fat foods do not decrease body fat—their high sugar and starch content is converted into stored fat in the body. Although high fat intake from animal sources has been associated with heart disease, some amount of saturated fat in the diet is necessary to help the body's cells remain healthy and resistant to disease.

Unsaturated Fats—Unsaturated fatty acids tend to be liquid at room temperature. Most vegetable oils (coconut and palm oils are exceptions) are unsaturated. Unsaturated means some of the atoms of the fatty acid are not filled with hydrogen.

- Monounsaturated Fats: When a fatty acid lacks only two hydrogen atoms, it is a monounsaturated fatty acid. Monounsaturated fats are considered important to health because of their ability to lower levels of "bad" cholesterol and maintain or raise levels of "good" cholesterol. Olive oil is naturally high in monounsaturated fats and is probably the most widely used oil, both for cooking and raw on salads, on a worldwide basis.

- Polyunsaturated Fats: Oils high in polyunsaturated fats include flaxseed and canola oils, as well as oils from pumpkin seeds, sunflower seeds, walnuts, and soybeans. A fatty acid lacking four or more hydrogen atoms is a polyunsaturated fatty acid.

Hydrogenated and Trans Fats—These fats are created using a synthetic process in which natural oils are broken down into a semi-solid fat by adding hydrogen atoms to an unsaturated fat molecule. This process is widely used to prolong the shelf life of commercial baked goods, packaged foods, most salad dressings, margarine, and cooking oils such as corn and safflower. The molecules that make up a large percentage of these fats, called trans-fatty acids, are known to interfere with the healthy functioning of our bodies due to their unusual molecular shape.

Here are some dietary recommendations from nutritional biochemist Patricia Kane, Ph.D., of Millville, New Jersey, for supplying the body with nourishing, healthy fats:

- Use liberal amounts of cold-processed flaxseed oil; similarly, use cold-pressed walnut, avocado, sesame, almond, or grapeseed oils.

- Reduce carbohydrate intake and avoid all refined sugars, processed foods, margarine, hydrogenated oils, and gluten-containing foods such as wheat, oats, and barley.

- For better mineral density, increase consumption of ground raw nuts and seeds (especially sesame), seaweeds, fish, tempeh (fermented soybeans), poultry, avocado, and legumes.

- Incorporate certain spices and herbs into the diet such as fresh ground black or cayenne pepper, thyme oil, and ginger; these foods contain substances that will help stabilize fats in the cell membranes.

- Avoid all fats and oils containing very-long-chain fatty acids, such as mustard, peanut butter, peanut oil, and canola oil; cook only with coconut oil.

Making the Transition to a Whole Foods Diet

Eating better means living better. The types of dietary changes that you make should not be threatening, limiting, or difficult to live with. Most Americans were raised eating meat and the transition to a vegetarian-oriented, whole foods diet may seem daunting. However, this change may be easier and more pleasurable than imag-

VEGETABLE OILS: THE GOOD AND THE BAD FATS

All vegetable oils contain levels of unsaturated and saturated fats. Generally, oils with a higher percentage of unsaturated fats are more healthful.

Oil	Monounsaturated	Polyunsaturated	Saturated
Olive	72%	9%	14%
Flax	72%	19%	9%
Pumpkinseed	57%	34%	9%
Hempseed	80%	12%	8%
Safflower	12%	75%	9%
Peanut	46%	32%	17%
Corn	24%	59%	13%
Soybean	23%	59%	14%
Sunflower	20%	66%	10%
Sesame seed	40%	40%	18%
Butter	29%	4%	62%
Coconut	6%	2%	87%

ined and, considering the enormous health benefits, worth it. Here are some tips:

- Eat more high-protein plant foods like grains, legumes, nuts, and seeds.

- When dining out, try more exotic, foreign vegetarian foods. Most ethnic restaurants—Indian, Chinese, Thai, Japanese, Mexican, Latin American, African, Middle Eastern—offer wonderful dishes with vegetables and grains. You can also prepare many of these at home.

- Experiment with spices and seasonings. For secrets to the exotic flavors found in vegetarian cooking, pick up several vegetarian or ethnic cookbooks.

- Choose range-fed, hormone-free, additive-free meats available at health food stores and quality markets.

- If your metabolic type requires more protein and/or fats, consider using more healthy oils on your salads or vegetables, eating more miso and tofu, and supplementing with free-form mixed amino acids.

- Don't be rigid about your diet—allow yourself some meat and dairy. Move toward a whole foods diet gradually. "Don't become so worried about your diet that it becomes a burden," says Dr. Berkson. "It is not what you eat once in a while that builds your optimal body, but what you eat most of the time."

- Achieve rhythm in your diet. As important as what you eat is how and when you eat, adds Dr. Berkson. Eating regularly provides your body with a consistent intake of nutrients and avoids the stress associated with not knowing when your next meal will come or of going all day without food and then overeating in the evening.

At the Market

Choosing the ingredients for an ideal diet in today's markets requires a healthy dose of skepticism, diligence, and a certain amount of fortitude to resist slipping into old patterns. But the improvements in your food choices will pay off in better health for you and your family. Nutritionists recommend that you adopt a dual shopping strategy, buying some foods at major supermarkets and other foods at health food stores, obtaining the best from both.

- Read labels. The cover of the package is the last place one is apt to find the truth about a product. Bold statements like "100% Natural" or "98% Fat-Free" might be legal, but may be inaccurate. Go directly to the ingredient list and nutritional analysis. Fortunately, new labeling regulations will mean better and more accurate information for consumers.

- Concentrate on vegetables, salads, and complex carbohydrates. The "main dish" approach centering on protein and a high-fat sauce is out. Replace fat-laden meat loaf and pork ribs with some whole grains or whole-grain pastas, beans, and fresh vegetables, plus enough olive oil, nuts, nut oils, seeds, or seed oils to balance the metabolism.

- Shop at your local health food store, where the emphasis is on quality and health. On the other hand, not all fresh fruits and vegetables sold in the health food store are organic. Look for labels that identify organically grown foods.

- Buy organic foods. Organic farming is a system of cultivation that doesn't use artificial fertilizers, pesticides, herbicides, growth regulators, and livestock feed additives. Crop rotations, crop residues, animal manures, green manures, legumes, organic wastes, mineral-bearing rock, and biological pest controls are used by organic farmers to raise whole, natural foods. If you cannot buy all organic produce, buy the organic produce that substitutes for the most pesticide-contaminated crops, such as grapes, carrots, and apples, and buy the non-organic fruits and vegetables that are less likely to be laden with pesticides (bananas, pineapple, watermelon, oranges, and tangerines tend to be relatively pesticide-free). If funds are limited, buy all meats and dairy products as organic, because nonorganic meats and dairy have up to 20 times more pesticides than nonorganic vegetables.

- Buy seasonal foods. By definition, foods grown out of season must be treated or manipulated to grow. Perhaps they were grown in greenhouse environments with artificial lights or induced to grow through chemical treatment. Often, the nonseasonal foods are imported from Third World nations where pesticides, banned in the U.S., continue to be used, poisoning the food, the land, and farm workers. Seasonal foods are healthier, more abundant, and less expensive.

- Eat colorfully. Instead of being concerned with getting all the "right" vitamins and minerals in perfect ratios, Dr. Berkson suggests focusing on eating a colorful diet. By making an effort to get at least three different-colored vegetables or fruits at both lunch and dinner, you will insure the best exposure to appropriate nutrients.

In the Kitchen

By its very nature, food has limitations—it needs to be stored and prepared with care. Overcooking vegetables can cut their vitamin B_1 content in half and destroy their enzymes; exposing milk to light can do the same thing to its vitamin B_2 content. You can take a number of steps to preserve the freshness, cleanliness, and nutrient value of your foods.

Cleaning and Storing Foods

Since the FDA tests only about 1% of produce for pesticide residues, cleaning your food is the only way to ensure that you are not eating agricultural poisons. Even organic foods may have residues of potentially harmful substances. Thoroughly wash produce in cold water, preferably filtered, says Dr. Levin. Use a vegetable brush with natural bristles to scrub the skins of sturdier vegetables such as potatoes to remove dirt and any residual surface toxins, but don't remove the skins as they contain vital nutrients. You may also want to consider naturally derived produce washes now available to consumers, such as grapefruit seed extract.

The main vitamin thieves in your kitchen are heat, air, and light. Vitamins A, B complex, C, and D are susceptible to damage by UV light. Vitamin E is damaged by oxygen. In general, the less exposure your food has to air, light, and heat, the better.

- Garlic, onions, potatoes, carrots, beets, and other root vegetables store well in cool, dark, dry places.

- Spices hold up well under refrigeration or even in the freezer, especially if purchased in large quantities and used over a period of months. Purchasing spices in whole seed form and then grinding with a mortar and pestle when ready for use is highly recommended. Better yet, grow your own. Parsley, basil, oregano, and thyme grow well in small pots on the windowsill and will provide fresh spices every night.

- Oils tend to store best under refrigeration and dark-glass containers are recommended to minimize exposure of fat-soluble vitamins to light.

 See Enzyme Therapy, Nutritional Medicine.

Choosing Cookware

Glass (or Pyrex®), ceramics (including clay, terra-cotta, enamel, and porcelain), cast iron, and stainless steel should head your list for cookware materials. At the bottom of the list should be aluminum, plastic, and cookware featuring synthetic nonstick surfaces. According to Dr. Levin, here's why:

- Glass is your best choice. It does not interact with the food prepared in it and works well in the refrigerator or freezer, on the stovetop, and in the oven.

- Ceramics are porcelain-covered metals, like cast iron, that combine the excellent heating capacities of metal with the friendly cooking surface of porcelain. Clay or "earthenware" pots are excellent for oven baking, but be careful about the glazes, as some contain lead or cadmium, both known to be hazardous.

- Cast iron is heavy and requires the extra step of curing before use (to cure cast iron, wash in hot, soapy water, rinse, towel dry, rub with refined oil, and place in an oven preheated to 300° F for three hours). In exchange for the extra weight and care, cast iron cookware may help prevent you from becoming anemic, if you are a menstruating woman. One-half cup of spaghetti sauce prepared in a stainless steel skillet will provide you with less than 1 mg of iron. Prepared in a cast iron skillet, the same sauce gives you 6 mg of iron.

- Stainless steel adds neither the potentially positive nutrient value of cast iron nor any of the negative elements found in aluminum or plastic. However, stainless steel offers the chef an excellent and easy cooking surface along with hassle-free cleaning.

- Aluminum cookware can release traces of aluminum into the food, which may make their way into the bone matrix and create changes in cognitive functioning.[45] Exactly how much aluminum is able to migrate from aluminum cookware into your food? Studies have shown that foods cooked in aluminum pans can pick up the element, but the quantity is disputable.[46] This debate is particularly fierce with respect to anodized aluminum. Anodized cookware is constructed of aluminum that has been placed in an electrolytic solution and subjected to an electrical current, which changes its molecular structure. This process seals the pores of the aluminum and lessens—and some say eliminates—its interaction with food. Nevertheless, there's at least a question mark associated with aluminum and its stability in cookware.

MICROWAVING FOODS

A microwave oven cooks by generating heat in the food itself. It contains a magnetron tube, which converts electricity into electromagnetic radiation. Microwaves tend to diminish the formation of nitrosamine chemicals that can be formed when cooking nitrate-cured meats such as bacon and ham.[47] If you intend to eat these meats, cooking them in the microwave may be better than baking them in a conventional oven or frying.

Microwave oven radiation is not very powerful and it drops off quickly as one moves away from the appliance. Yet, medical science has uncovered disturbing news about the effects of microwave radiation on health—including eye damage and carcinogenic effects.

There may be another more disturbing side to this modern convenience. Microwaving may cause chemical changes in foods beyond those associated with being exposed to heat.[48] For example, researchers have discovered that microwaving infant formula for ten minutes alters the structure of its component amino acids, possibly resulting in functional, structural, and immunological abnormalities.[49]

- Plastics for food preparation, particularly in the microwave, are controversial at best and they could be dangerous, as many of the resins used in plastics are cancer-causing substances. Molecules from polyvinyl chloride (PVC), polyethylene, polyvinylidene chloride, and plasticizers in plastic wraps have been conclusively shown to migrate into foods at the high temperatures achieved in microwave ovens. The worst culprit in this regard is cyclic polyethylene terephthalate (PET) trimmer—the thin, mirrorlike, grey stripping that absorbs microwave energy and is often used to make microwave pizza crusts brown and microwave popcorn crunchy. Avoid microwave cookware containing these materials; stick with glass and unleaded ceramics instead.

 The results of studies that explore the immediate risks associated with food cooked in microwave ovens indicate the need for further research into the health risks of repeated microwave use.

Kitchen Cleansers

Many dishwashing liquids, bleaches, chlorinated scouring powders, all-purpose cleansers, and drain cleaners contain petrochemicals that do not belong in the kitchen. Nontoxic, environmentally safe alternatives are available in every category of cleanser and detergent. In general, look for products that are water-based, free of phosphates and propellants, and biodegradable. Baking soda makes an excellent scouring powder, and vinegar added to water can be used for cleaning windows.

Water and Water Filters

Drinking pure water is very important for health. It is also important to use pure water in the preparation and cleaning of food. Unfortunately, the public water supply is not always capable of providing optimally pure water. According to the EPA, the tap water of 30 million people in the U.S. contains potentially hazardous levels of lead.[50] In addition, one out of every four public water systems has violated federal standards for tap water.[51]

America's water can contain many contaminants, including pathogenic bacteria, radioactive particles, heavy metals, industrial wastes, and chemical residues. Even chlorine and fluoride, intentionally added to public water supplies, are considered by many to pose a risk to health. While adding chlorine-type compounds to drinking water protects the public from several kinds of potentially deadly bacteria such as typhus, chlorine has been proven to form cancer-causing compounds in drinking water. Fluoride, added to water to prevent tooth decay, seems to also have negative effects on bones and even the teeth. Studies suggest that fluoride can cause mottling of the teeth and make bones more brittle in the elderly, leading to an increased rate of fracture.[52]

 See Biological Dentistry, Osteoporosis.

Drinking water containing lead can create health problems for both children and adults, including hypertension, mental deterioration, impotency, birth defects, and learning difficulties. Unless a house has newer copper water lines, lead can leach out of the older water pipes and plumbing into the water. In determining the quality of water in the home, ask the local water department for standards and analysis. It is also important to verify your home's water quality yourself. Easy-to-run tests are usually inexpensive as well.

Bottled water is a viable alternative, but be careful about the source. Many bottled waters are simply repackaged city supplies. Choose only those products that provide a full analysis of their contents upon request. Also, look for waters that have been purified through deionization (many such brands are known as reverse-osmo-sis purified or distilled). Bottled waters often contain molecules of plastic that have leached out of the bottles in which the water is stored.

The best step is to buy a water filter. The cost can range from $150 for an under-the-sink model, combining carbon filtration with reverse osmosis, to $1,500 for a whole-house filter that will purify even the water for your shower. There are four basic types of filtration:

- Solid block carbon filters appear to be much more effective in removing organic chemicals, such as solvents and trihalomethanes, than activated carbon filters, which use granulated or powdered carbon. If you prefer to leave dissolved minerals in your water, carbon block filters are a recommended choice since they do not remove these inorganic compounds.

- Reverse osmosis systems force water under pressure through a membrane. They are most effective against inorganic pollutants like nitrates and metals such as lead. Deionization resins are also used to accomplish this purpose.

- Distillation purifies water by boiling and condensing it. Metals and inorganic compounds are effectively removed in this way because they are heavier than water, but some organic compounds have a boiling point close to that of water and therefore may not be removed.

- Ultraviolet rays can also be employed to purify water, by killing bacteria and other microorganisms that may be present. However, it is not able to remove chemical contaminants.

The best systems combine several methods of filtration for optimal pollutant removal. Carbon block filtration combined with reverse osmosis units are effective against organic and inorganic pollutants, as are carbon block and distillation combinations.

Where to Find Help

Educating yourself about healthier alternatives is the first step in the move toward an improved diet. The following list provides a variety of information, from where to find a naturopathic physician to sources of organic food.

Locating a Nutritionist or Naturopathic Physician

American Association of Naturopathic Physicians
601 Valley Street, Suite 105
Seattle, Washington 98109
(206) 298-0126
Website: www.naturopathic.org

Contact them for the location of a licensed naturopathic physician in your area.

American College of Nutrition
722 Robert E. Lee Drive
Wilmington, Delaware 28480
(252) 452-1222
Website: www.am-coll-nutr.org

A membership organization that produces a journal and newsletter and also provides lectures on nutrition research.

Metabolic Typing

Metabolic Typing Education Center
(650) 325-1840
Website: www.metabolictyping.com

William L. Wolcott's center provides information on metabolic typing.

Price-Pottenger Nutrition Foundation
P.O. Box 2614
La Mesa, CA 91943-2614
(619) 574-7763

For information on metabolic typing.

Fighting Food Irradiation

Consumers United for Food Safety
P.O. Box 22928
Seattle, Washington 98122
(206) 747-2659

The organization's newsletter, The Food Activist, provides updates on national developments in food irradiation.

Learning More About Organic Foods

The Organic Trade Association
P.O. Box 1078
Greenfield, Massachusetts 01302
(413) 774-7511
Website: www.ota.com

Provides information about organic farming and organic products.

Becoming Vegetarian and Cooking Vegetarian

Vegetarian Resource Group
P.O. Box 1463
Baltimore, Maryland 21203
(410) 366-8343
Website: www.vrg.org

A nonprofit vegetarian resource group whose main goal is to educate the public on health, nutrition, and the environment.

Vegetarian Times
1140 Lake Street, Suite 500
Oak Park, Illinois 60301
(630) 516-4008

A monthly magazine that offers recipes as well as informative articles and the latest news for vegetarians.

Exploring Nutrition and Politics

Community Nutrition Institute
2001 S Street N.W., Suite 530
Washington, D.C. 20009
(202) 462-4700

This organization focuses on consumer protection, food program development, and federal diet and health policies.

Food First/Institute for Food and Development Policy
145 9th Street
San Francisco, California 94103
(415) 864-8555

A nonprofit organization that investigates the root causes of hunger. They survey and study social conditions and develop a profile of society through a "food window."

The Nutrition Action Health Letter
Center for Science in the Public Interest
1875 Connecticut Avenue N.W., Suite 300
Washington, D.C. 20009-5728
(202) 332-9111

A monthly newsletter published to educate the general public, covering all areas of dietary knowledge, studies, and statistics. Excellent reviews of books and recipes included.

Food and Water Ecology

Natural Resources Defense Council
40 West 20th Street
New York, New York 10011
(212) 727-2700
Website: www.nrdc.org

An organization that attempts to steer America away from wasteful and destructive environmental policies. A nonprofit environmental law firm also concerned with public education.

Clean Water Action Project

1320 18th Street N.W., Suite 300
Washington, D.C. 20036
(202) 547-1196

A lobbying group that seeks to protect the environment. They are especially concerned with water, waste, sewage, pollution, and wildlife.

Earth Save

706 Frederick Street
Santa Cruz, California 95062
(408) 423-4069

A nonprofit organization that focuses on helping people realize how their diet affects the planet. Involved in several public education programs.

Greenpeace

702 H Street N.W., Suite 300
Washington, D.C. 20001
(202) 462-1177
Website: www.greenpeaceusa.org

An organization dedicated to monitoring and safeguarding the ecological soundness of the planet.

Sources of Hormone-Free, Nitrite-Free Meat and Poultry

Center for Science in the Public Interest

1875 Connecticut Avenue N.W., Suite 300
Washington, D.C. 20009-5728
(202) 332-9110

You can obtain a list of organic mail-order suppliers or hormone-free beef suppliers, both supermarket chains and mail-order home delivery, from this organization.

Eden Acres Organic Network

12100 Lima Center Road
Clinton, Michigan 49236-9618
(517) 456-4288

Organic Network, a division of Eden Acres, offers an international directory or local statewide directories of suppliers of organic meats, poultry, fruits, and vegetables.

Recommended Reading

All About Vegetarian Cooking (Joy of Cooking). Irma S. Rombauer, Marion Rombauer Becker, and Ethan Becker. New York: Scribner, 2000.

The Body Shaping Diet. Sandra Cabot, M.D. Berkeley, CA: Celestial Arts, 2001.

Diet for a New America. John Robbins. Tiburon, CA: H.J. Kramer, 1998.

Diet for a Poisoned Planet. David Steinman. New York: Ballantine Books, 1990.

Diet for a Small Planet. Frances Moore Lappe. New York: Ballantine Books, 1991.

The Food That Would Last Forever: Understanding the Dangers of Food Irradiation. Gary Gibbs. Garden City Park, NY: Avery Penguin Putnam, 1993.

Macrobiotic Diet. Michio and Aveline Kushi. New York: Japan Publications, 1993.

Metabolic Typing Diet. William L. Wolcott with Trish Fahey. New York: Doubleday, 2000.

Moosewood Cookbook. Mollie Katzen. Berkeley, CA: Ten Speed Press, 1992.

New Laurel's Kitchen. Laurel Robertson, Carol Flinders, and Brian Ruppenthal. Berkeley, CA: Ten Speed Press, 1986.

New McDougall Cookbook. John McDougall, M.D., and Mary McDougall. New York: Plume, 1997.

The New Vegan Cookbook. Lorna Sass. San Francisco: Chronicle Books, 2001.

Staying Healthy with Nutrition. Elson Haas, M.D. Berkeley, CA: Celestial Arts, 1992.

Still Life with Menu Cookbook. Mollie Katzen. Berkeley, CA: Ten Speed Press, 1994.

Transition to Vegetarianism. Rudolph Ballantine, M.D. Honesdale, PA: Himalayan Publishers, 1999.

ENERGY MEDICINE

Energy medicine is a term used to describe both healing bioenergetic therapies and diagnostic screening devices used to measure the electromagnetic frequencies emitted by the body in order to detect imbalances that may be causing present illness or contributing to future disease. These disturbed energy flows can then be returned to their normal, healthy state through the application of bioenergetic techniques or the input of electromagnetic signals that restore a normal energy balance within the body.

IMAGINE THAT YOU are sitting in your doctor's office as he or she takes a small, hand-held probe connected to a meter and, with no further questions, gently presses certain points on your hands and feet while noting the figures displayed on the meter. From this, your doctor is able to tell you which parts of your body are functioning correctly and which organs are causing problems. Some small glass vials containing colorless liquids are placed into a container, which is also connected to the device, and the doctor remeasures some of the points. From this, the doctor is able to tell you why there is a problem. Finally, he or she gives you a few drops of a tasteless medicine and before long you begin to feel better. A description from a futuristic fantasy? No, this is precisely what is happening in some medical clinics around the world today with practitioners of energy medicine.

Equally fantastic to most conventional physicians is the idea that a healer can emit healing energies from his or her hands to improve the health of their patients, in many cases without even needing to actually touch them. Yet this healing approach, referred to in some spiritual traditions as the "laying on of hands," is the basis of a variety of bioenergetic therapies that recognize the existence of a subtle energy body, or biofield, surrounding the physical body, a concept that modern science has only in recent decades begun to accept and verify.

What is Energy Medicine?

Energy medicine refers to various therapies that interact with the body's energy field (biofield) and, in the case of energy medicine devices, use an energy field of their own—electrical, magnetic, sonic, acoustic, microwave, infrared—to screen for or treat health conditions by detecting imbalances in the body's energy field and then correcting them. Energy medicine's basic premise is that both physical matter, including the human body, and psychological processes (thoughts, feelings, attitudes) are expressions of energy. Health is based on the unimpeded flow of energy in the body, and illness is due to blockages or imbalances in this flow.

Practitioners of energy medicine employ a variety of methods and instruments to assess the energetic patterns and fluctuations of the human biofield. This detection of energy imbalances in the body is essential for providing an early warning system for potential disruptions in chemical balance that may lead to disease. Balance can then be restored using holistic therapies, or with treatment devices that rebalance the patient's various energy fields, before further chemical or structural disturbances can occur.

The concept of an invisible biofield surrounding the human body is not new. It has been a core element in the medical philosophies of both Ayurveda and traditional Chinese medicine (TCM) for thousands of years and is also part of the belief systems of most of the world's major religions. Throughout history, various Western healers and medical innovators, beginning with the Greek physician Hippocrates, have taught that the biofield exists and directly influences health and disease. Practitioners of energy medicine also teach that the biofield is comprised of various energetic pathways, known as meridians, and other subtle energy centers. Through these meridian pathways and energy centers, invisible life force energy (known as *qi* to practitioners of acupuncture and *prana* to Ayurvedic physicians) flows and is processed, maintaining the health and harmony of the physical body. Yet, despite mounting evidence that seems to corroborate the existence of both the biofield and this life force energy, the bioenergetic perspective of health is for the most part ignored by conventional physicians.

CULTURAL AND HISTORICAL PRECEDENTS FOR ENERGY MEDICINE

The idea of a vital life force that invisibly animates all life has existed worldwide throughout history. The world's two oldest complete systems of medicine, Ayurveda and traditional Chinese medicine, refer to this subtle energy as *prana* and *qi* (CHEE), respectively, and both systems seek to promote optimal health through various methods designed to harmonize the flow of life force energy throughout the human biofield. In ancient Greece, the mystic philosopher and mathematician Pythagoras referred to this same subtle energy as *pneuma*. A century later, Hippocrates, the father of Western medicine, taught that the unimpeded flow of life force energy was essential for good health. Among the Kung San, the indigenous people of Africa's Kalahari desert, the term used to describe subtle energy is *num*, which the Kung San claim can be accumulated and stored in the lower abdomen and used to treat disease. Similarly, the Kahuna people of Hawaii, in their healing tradition known as Huna, call subtle energy *mana*. They teach that it flows through the body and also surrounds it as an invisible biomagnetic field, which can be affected by one's behavior, emotions, and mental attitudes and beliefs.

In the Judeo-Christian tradition, this healing energy is most commonly known as *spirit*, and throughout European history, many healers and scientists, including Galen, Paracelsus, Sir Isaac Newton, Franz Mesmer, and Samuel Hahnemann, the founder of homeopathy, also recognized the existence of an invisible vital energy upon which good health depended. This same concept has long been a part of the healing traditions of the indigenous peoples of the Americas, most notably the Navaho, Hopi, Mayan, and Incan nations. Since the beginning of the 20th century, this view has also been supported by discoveries in the field of quantum physics, which demonstrate that, at the farthest reaches of the subatomic level, particles (solid matter) are not actually composed of any material substance, but rather packets of light energy known as *quanta*.

Mainstream science, by contrast, is now actively engaged in codifying the human biofield, in part due to conventional medicine's inherent shortcomings. "For most of the 20th century, science and medicine have seen health as being dependent upon the balance of body

chemistry and the functioning of physical structures," notes William Tiller, Ph.D., former professor of Stanford University and a leading figure in the field of energy medicine. "However, attempts to treat illnesses and imbalances chemically often lead to unwanted side effects or the body becoming insensitive to the chemicals." This fact has led many researchers and health professionals to look beyond conventional drug-based therapies to the field of energy medicine.

In addition, many of the most sophisticated diagnostic systems used today in conventional medicine, such as the EKG (electrocardiogram), EEG (electroencephalogram), EMG (electromyelogram), and MRI (magnetic resonance imaging), employ the principles of energy medicine. So too does the SQUID (superconducting quantum interference device), a sophisticated instrument capable of calibrating "the biomagnetic field produced by a single heartbeat, muscle twitch, or pattern of neural activity in the brain." SQUID instruments are now in use in universities and research centers worldwide, where they are being used to further map the human biofield.[1]

While many forms of health care, both alternative and conventional, impact the human energy field, energy medicine's unique focus on working directly with the body's energy systems in order to restore and maintain health sets it apart from other medical specialties and leaves it poised to become a primary form of health care in the 21st century.

How Energy Medicine Works

According to practitioners of energy medicine, the human body is surrounded and permeated by various interconnected fields of energy that can be quantifiably measured and which continuously influence, and are in turn affected by, changes in physical and psychological health, and can also be influenced by the energy fields of others. By working with the biofield and the subtle energies that flow through it and support it, energy medicine practitioners seek to harmonize and maintain the proper flow of life force necessary for optimal psychophysiological functioning. This is accomplished through various diagnostic and therapeutic methods, using instrumented (energy devices) and noninstrumented (bioenergetic therapies) means. A variety of other alternative medicine practices also rely on, at least in part, the principles of energy medicine to accomplish their healthcare goals. In addition to acupuncture, TCM, and Ayurveda, these include guided imagery and visualization, homeopathy, mind/body medicine, flower remedies, light therapy, magnetic field therapy, neural therapy, sound therapy, Qigong, yoga, and certain forms of bodywork, such as Therapeutic Touch, polarity therapy, breath work, and reflexology.

 See Acupuncture, Ayurvedic Medicine, Bodywork, Flower Essences, Guided Imagery, Homeopathy, Light Therapy, Magnetic Field Therapy, Mind/Body Medicine, Neural Therapy, Qigong and Tai Chi, Sound Therapy, Yoga.

According to Rima Laibow, M.D., founding Medical Director of the Alexandria Institute of Natural and Integrative Medicine, in Croton-on-Hudson, New York, all forms of medicine are types of energy medicine—in the broadest sense of the term—in that they input energy into patients for the purpose of healing. "In some forms, the energy is transferred via human intentionality alone, in other forms devices are required, or else conventional drugs or surgery," says Dr. Laibow. "Although we don't usually consider them in this light, drugs, for example, are packets of subatomic particles capable of producing a change in the energy profile of particular enzyme systems in the body." What makes energy medicine unique as a specific medical specialty is the fact that the techniques and technologies that comprise it require little or no direct contact between the patient and the healing agent to produce wholesome biological effects.

Dr. Laibow points out that the term *energy* can refer to familiar and easily measurable frequencies of the electromagnetic spectrum, such as light (including color) and sound, or to less familiar influences of living systems for which measurement is currently more difficult. "These intention-based systems of energy medicine focus human or natural forces on the area of disease to exert their impact," she says. Although conventional science is currently often unable to accurately characterize and measure these subtler forms of energy medicine, growing numbers of practitioners and their patients can attest to the significance of such healing systems.

Whether energy medical devices are employed, or our innate human ability to focus and move energy using bioenergetic approaches, the means by which biological effects are produced is similar, according to Dr. Laibow. "Modern physics has taught us that all matter is composed of vibrating packets of energy which appear to us as particles," she explains. "By interacting with each other, these energy packets create fields of information that are awash in new frequencies. These frequencies interact like ripples in a pool to create new patterns that, in turn, interact again." In healthy biological systems, these patterns are harmonious enough to function well, yet disharmonious enough to allow for growth, change, and flexibility of response. Every cell, tissue, and organ in the body has its own healthy frequencies, both measurable and unmeasurable by conventional scientific methods. Healthy energy patterns are free to communicate, or resonate, with each other, thus creating ever more complex patterns of interaction.

"In illness of any kind, however, these harmonious energy relationships are disrupted," says Dr. Laibow. "An illustration of this is the EKG reading of patients who have suffered a heart attack, which shows that their heart's electrical energy is disrupted and not flowing properly." Energy medicine restores the harmonious interaction of energy within the patient and their environment by imparting new information to the damaged energy system.

One of the reasons that energy medicine is able to restore harmony to damaged or malfunctioning areas is due to the piezoelectric (capable of transforming pressure into electricity) nature of the body and its component parts. According to C. Norman Shealy, M.D., Ph.D., founder of the American Holistic Medical Association, who has been researching energy medicine for over two decades, "we are all living piezoelectric generators," meaning that the body's normal bioelectromagnetic energies are responsible for and regulate its chemical and other biophysical processes. When electromagnetic energy is applied from external sources, it "activates the piezoelectric property of tissue to emit photons, sound waves with a wavelength low enough to resonate with cell membranes."[2] Healing electromagnetic frequencies produce a resonance within the cell membranes that results in greater levels of coherence and intracellular communication. Conversely, exposure to harmful electromagnetic frequencies can, over time, produce disruption and ill health.

The intent of energy healers plays a crucial role in the healing process as well. "It is important to note that, since the energies of the healer and the patient are interacting and creating frequency patterns of their own, the intention of the healer is of crucial importance to the outcome of the process," Dr. Laibow states. "All electromagnetic healing systems pay great attention to the ability of the healer to focus energy for healing purposes through a lens of purity of intent. While little attention has been paid to this aspect of energy medicine, it is important to recognize that human intent also plays a role in the reestablishment of biological harmony and bioenergetic integrity."

Dr. Laibow's view is supported by scientific research. Studies show, for instance, that sincere feelings of appreciation, love, or care produce increased coherence in the heart's electromagnetic field and that the heart itself generates an electromagnetic field that affects others when people touch or are in close proximity. Based on such research, it now appears that the heart may be the source of energy exchanged between practitioners of energy medicine and their patients.[3]

The types of energy medicine fall into two general categories, noninstrumented and instrumented. Noninstrumented forms of energy medicine are also known as bioenergetic healing and generally involve intention-based approaches that are often modeled on the model of "laying on of hands." Instrumented forms of energy medicine involve the use of energy devices that detect or treat health conditions via the application of various energy fields. Another class of instruments protects against the growing health threat posed by electromagnetic fields (EMFs).

Bioenergetic Healing Methods

Bioenergetic healing approaches have been a part of religious and indigenous healing traditions worldwide for millennia and in recent decades a number of modern techniques based on these ancient methods have been developed. All such "laying on of hands" methods of energy medicine involve a process of transferring healing energies from one individual to another. According to Elaine R. Ferguson, M.D., Medical Director of Alternative Medicine, Inc., in Highland Park, Illinois, variants of bioenergetic healing, each adapted to meet the particular needs of their respective cultures, are used throughout the world. Among the most popular modern approaches are Therapeutic Touch, Healing Touch, and Reiki.

Therapeutic Touch: Therapeutic Touch (TT) was developed in 1971 by Dolores Krieger, Ph.D., R.N., Professor Emeritus of New York University Graduate School of Nursing, and her mentor, the late Dora Kunz, a widely respected healer. Together, they originated a nonreligious, secular form of healing that combined the laying on of hands with a number of other ancient bioenergetic techniques, which was initially taught at N.Y.U. as an extension of professional nursing care.

During a TT session, there is generally no physical contact between patient and practitioner, although touch may be employed when treating fractures and parts of the body affected by physical trauma. TT practitioners begin each session by quieting themselves through a process known as "going on center." This enables them to become aware of and more deeply connected with the specific bioenergetic needs of their patients. A brief assessment period follows in which the practitioner places his or her hands two to six inches away from the patient and, using rhythmic, slow-hand motions, determines where block-

ages in the patient's biofield lie. The practitioner then works to replenish the flow of subtle life force energy where necessary, while releasing any congestion or obstruction that may be present. This is accomplished by smoothing the biofield itself, using hand motions, usually beginning at the crown of the patient's head and moving toward the feet, while the TT practitioner visualizes the biofield's energies becoming more coherent and organized. Sessions typically last 20-30 minutes and patients commonly report a variety of benefits, including noticeable feelings of relaxation, improved energy levels, pain reduction, diminished stress, and general well-being.

John Zimmerman, Ph.D., Assistant Professor of Psychiatry at the University of Colorado, has conducted studies to measure the body's magnetic field during the application of Therapeutic Touch sessions. When a trained TT practitioner attempted to heal various parts of test subjects' bodies, such as the eye, elbow, or knee, Dr. Zimmerman was able to quantify several distinct changes in the subjects' magnetic fields. Signals up to several hundred times larger than background noise appeared while the practitioner worked. Investigations by other researchers have documented additional physiologic changes within the human body and in animals during TT treatments, including changes in brain-wave patterns.[4]

Today, Therapeutic Touch provides the greatest amount of credibility for bioenergetic forms of medicine, due primarily to the research of Dr. Krieger and her students. Currently, an estimated 40,000 doctors, nurses, and other health professionals in the U.S. and throughout the world use Therapeutic Touch as an integral part of their practice. It is also included as a viable technique in a number of nursing textbooks. According to Dr. Krieger, TT is also available in over 200 hospitals and taught in more than 100 fully accredited colleges and universities nationwide, as well as in over 75 other nations.[5] Hundreds of research studies have been conducted in American hospitals and universities as well, documenting the efficacy of Therapeutic Touch for a variety of illnesses, both mental and physical, and it is now included in Lamaze classes nationwide in order to help pregnant women better cope with stress and discomfort.

Healing Touch: A variant of Therapeuic Touch, Healing Touch was developed by Janet Mentgen, R.N., in 1981. Like TT practitioners, practitioners of Healing Touch seek to assess and then rectify bioenergetic blockages and disruptions. Besides employing TT methods, practitioners use a number of other bioenergetic techniques that are mastered over four certified levels of training. Healing Touch is used by a growing body of holistically oriented nurses and has been sanctioned by the American Holistic Nurses Association (which also endorses TT) since 1989, due to its ability to hasten the healing process, relieve pain, reduce anxiety, and improve overall well-being.[6]

Reiki: Meaning "the free passage of universal life energy," Reiki involves a transference of energy between Reiki practitioners and their clients in order to restore harmony to the biofield and bolster the body's inherent healing processes. Reiki practitioners claim that its principles evolved from ancient Tibetan Buddhist healing practices that were transmitted from teacher to disciple. Dr. Mika Usui, a Japanese scholar and Christian minister, is said to have rediscovered these principles in the late 1800s. One of his pupils, Saichi Takata, then introduced Reiki to the U.S. in 1937.

Reiki treatments vary according to individual need and are usually administered with clients lying down as the practitioner places their hands on various areas of the body. Prior to becoming a practitioner, students of Reiki undergo a number of training levels in which they are initiated by a "Reiki master" and attuned to healing symbols that are then focused upon as Reiki practitioners send healing energy to their clients. Although Reiki has not received the same degree of scientific study as Therapeutic Touch and Healing Touch, evidence of its efficacy does exist. In one published study on the adjunctive use of Reiki to manage pain, it was found that when Reiki treatments were administered by a second-degree Reiki therapist to patients who were also receiving conventional pain medication, there was a "highly significant reduction in pain following the Reiki treatment." The study involved 20 volunteers who were experiencing pain for a variety of reasons, including cancer.[7] In the last decade, Reiki has become quite popular as a form of bioenergetic healing, and worldwide there are an estimated 200,000 Reiki practitioners.

Applications of Bioenergetic Healing

Numerous studies, especially regarding Therapeutic Touch, now attest to the efficacy of bioenergetic healing.

Plant and Animal Studies: Olga and Ambrose Worrall were two of the most well-known bioenergetic healers in the U.S. during the 1950s and 1960s. Over the years, they successfully treated thousands with diseases deemed incurable by medical science. As their fame grew, doctors throughout the U.S. referred patients to them and the Worralls were voluntarily subjected to a wide range of scientific studies.

Using Kirlian photography, a photographic technique that records the electromagnetic field surrounding animate and inanimate objects, Dr. Thelma Moss, a medical psychologist at U.C.L.A.'s Neuropsychiatric Institute, photographed a leaf of a plant as it appeared in its natural state. The leaf was severely damaged, removed from the plant, and cut. A photo was taken and clearly exhibited a gap over the damaged area. Olga held her hand over the leaf and administered healing into it. The next photo showed dramatic changes, revealing reorganization within the damaged area as well as increased radiation of light.[8] In another series of experiments, Olga was instructed to hold several objects—damaged enzymes, distilled water, and whole blood serum—to see if her touch had any effect. Kirlian photographs of the specimens taken before and after showed clearly visible changes within their electromagnetic fields.[9]

Biochemist Brad Gill, of McGill University in Montreal, Canada, teamed up with Oskar Estebany, another well-known bioenergetic healer who, like the Worralls, had successfully treated many diseases. In this experiment, they used a strain of mice with an increased incidence of thyroid goiters. This strain was selected because of Estebany's previous success treating humans with this disease. The mice were placed on a diet that made them more likely to develop goiters, due to deficient dietary iodine. They were also given a thyroid hormone that acted as a blocking agent. All of the mice were initially held to distinguish the calm ones from the nervous ones. The control group was placed in cages wrapped with electrothermal tape to simulate the warmth of human hands; nonhealers held another group. The experiment lasted 40 days. Compared to the control animals, the mice receiving the healing touch from Estebany showed a significantly slower rate of goiter development.

In another study of the effects of the laying on of hands for wound healing, an area of skin was surgically removed from 48 mice. The mice were evenly divided into three groups: one group was exposed to laying on of hands, another group was treated with artificial heat, while the control group wasn't touched. After 11 days, the wounds of the group exposed to the laying on of hands were significantly smaller than those in the other two groups.[10]

Human Studies: In a double-blind study involving 106 institutionalized elderly people, Therapeutic Touch was shown to be beneficial for treating anxiety. Before and after the patients received TT, their anxiety levels were measured using the Spielberger State Trait Anxiety Inventory. The patients were then divided into groups, with some receiving back rubs and some receiving Therapeutic Touch. The anxiety level of subjects who received Therapeutic Touch was found to be significantly lower than the anxiety levels of subjects who received a back rub without TT, leading researchers to conclude that Therapeutic Touch may enhance the quality of life for elderly, institutionalized populations.[11]

In another study, six volunteers suffering from tension headaches were randomly divided into treatment and placebo groups, with the treatment group receiving TT while the other group received placebo touch. Each volunteer was evaluated prior to intervention, immediately afterward, and four hours later. Ninety percent experienced sustained reduction in headache pain following their TT session, with 70% still reporting improvement of their pain symptoms four hours later. This was twice the average pain reduction experienced during the placebo touch sessions, leading researchers to conclude that TT has potential beyond the placebo effect in the treatment of tension headaches.[12]

Other studies of Therapeutic Touch have shown that it can reduce pain, boost immune function, trigger the "relaxation response," accelerate wound healing, alleviate headaches, reduce fever and inflammation, and ease problems associated with autonomic nervous system dysfunction.[13]

Energy Medicine Assessment and Treatment Devices

Most energy medicine devices are based on the acupuncture meridian system. Acupuncture works on the principle that there is a network of energy channels, called meridians, throughout the body. Different organs are associated with different energy meridians, and health problems in various organs show up as disturbances of energy in the associated meridians. Acupuncture points, or acupoints, are the points along these meridians where energy flow can be measured and manipulated.

Since the 1940s, research has established that acupuncture points possess electrical conductivity.[14] German doctors, led by Reinhold Voll, M.D., measured changes in electrical conductivity at each of the body's acupuncture points. They discovered that the electrical resistance of the skin decreases dramatically at the acupuncture points when compared to the surrounding skin. They also found that each point appeared to have a standard measurement for anyone who is in good health (when there is a steady flow of bioenergy, or *qi,* in the meridians). This measurement changes when health deteriorates.

These discoveries greatly simplified the task of locating acupoints rapidly and accurately. Based on the work of Dr. Voll and his colleagues, and later by researchers in Japan, new energy medicine instruments have been

EDS probes specific points on the hands to gather information about the health, function, and possible toxicity of organs and body systems.

Lymph (Teeth)
Lymph (Throat)
Lymph (Control)
Lung
Organ
Large intestine
Nervous system
NE Meridian
Circulation
Pituitary
Thyroid
Heart
Small intestine
Adrenal
Endocrine
Allergy 1
Allergy 2

Biosource, Inc., Orem, UT

developed both for assessment and treatment. A third class of energy medicine devices has also developed in recent decades to protect against the growing health threat posed by electromagnetic fields (EMFs).

In the United States, electroacupuncture biofeedback devices have been approved on an experimental basis solely for screening purposes, despite the fact that it is estimated that there are between 85,000 and 100,000 practitioners in this field worldwide.

Electrodermal Screening (EDS): Assessment energy devices primarily fall under the category of electrodermal screening (EDS), also known as electroacupuncture biofeedback, which is based on Dr. Voll's research. Dr. Voll developed a precise measuring instrument known as the Dermatron that allowed him to measure the electrical resistance at acupuncture points. He discovered that higher or lower readings than normal at a particular acupuncture point indicate a problem in the organ that corresponds to that acupoint; higher generally means there is irritation or inflammation in the organ and lower usually indicates fatigue or degeneration.

The acupoints that correspond to specific organs and tissues are known as control measurement points (CMPs), because they provide a general indication of the health of the organ or tissue as a whole. There are also specific points that indicate how the various parts of each organ are functioning. If the CMP for a particular organ gives a poor reading, the points for the various parts of that organ can then be checked. Whichever part of the organ shows an imbalance is the site of the dysfunction.

To date, there are over 2,000 such points that have been established as having specific relationships with internal organs. A skilled physician can, in a relatively short time, discover not only which organs have problems, but which part of the organ is malfunctioning and what other organs, if any, it is affecting. Thus it becomes possible to find the root cause of any problem. This assessment technique became known as Electroacupuncture According to Voll (EAV) and is the basis of all EDS devices in use today.

Dr. Voll later expanded his method not only to be able to learn what area of the body is being impacted, but also to determine the exact source of the problem. He found that if a patient held sample homeopathic dilutions of known disease substances, such as bacteria, viruses, or diseased tissue, when the patient came upon the one directly related to the cause of the problem, the EAV reading would return to normal. The reason for this is that homeopathic dilutions of a disease substance are actually remedies, following the homeopathic law of like cures like. Therefore, the body is actually responding positively to what it perceives as good medicine.

Electrodermal screening has been very successful in screening for a wide variety of conditions. However, in screening for cancer it is advisable to also use traditional blood tests as well as blood analysis with a darkfield microscope.

Today, EDS is a quick method used by many practitioners of alternative medicine to identify most underlying conditions, especially those involving toxic or allergenic substances. A blunt, noninvasive electric probe is placed at specific points on the patient's hands, face, or feet, corresponding to acupuncture points at the beginning or end of energy meridians. Minute electrical discharges from these points serve as information signals about the condition of the body's organs and systems, helping the physician in his or her evaluation and development of a treatment plan, while also avoiding the waiting period of laboratory analysis typical of conventional diagnostic tests. When necessary, however, EDS findings

are cross-referenced with specific blood, urine, and stool analyses to confirm EDS results.

According to James Hoyt Clark, of Orem, Utah, an EDS inventor and educator, EDS is a "data acquisition process" in which the trained EDS practitioner conducts an "interview" with the patient's organs and tissues, gathering information about their functional status and their energy pathways. EDS can indicate the degree of stress that is affecting an organ and can also monitor the progress of subsequent therapy, avoiding trial and error and general guesswork. As such, EDS is investigational, not diagnostic, in nature because it requires the physician's knowledge of acupuncture, physiology, and various therapeutic agents (nutrients, herbs, homeopathic remedies) to interpret the energy imbalances, establish their precise focus, and select the most appropriate therapeutic response.

EDS devices are currently manufactured in Germany, France, Russia, Japan, Korea, England, and the U.S. Types of EDS devices include the Vega, which is similar to Voll's original Dermatron device but much faster, and computerized versions of these instruments, such as the Computron, that can quickly perform multiple screenings and allow the practitioner to build a detailed database of patient files useful for research purposes. More sophisticated EDS devices include the LISTEN system developed by James Hoyt Clark, the Omega Acubase, and the Acupro. These devices contain an inventory of energy signals corresponding to several thousand substances, including most homeopathic remedies, pollens, foods, toxic chemicals, dental materials, molds and bacteria, healthy and diseased organ states, and conventional drugs.

Today, EDS devices are widely used in Europe and, in Japan, a system called *Ryo Do Raku* based on similar principles is used by an estimated 40,000 practitioners.[15] In the United States, however, EDS devices have so far been approved on an experimental basis solely for screening purposes, despite the fact that it is conservatively estimated that there are 85,000 to 100,000 practitioners in this field worldwide.[16]

Energy Medicine Treatment Devices

While EDS devices can be a powerful tool for assessing health conditions, treatment devices help complete the circle, allowing the energy medicine practitioner another viable therapy with which to combat disease and illness, often even before it can manifest, by successfully rebalancing the body's energy flow. The following are some of the more commonly used types of treatment instruments.

The MORA: The MORA was created by Franz Morrel, M.D., a colleague of Dr. Voll. He believed that all biological processes are essentially a matter of electro-

ENERGY MEDICINE AND ALLERGIES

Professor Cyril Smith, of the University of Salford in England, has shown that extremely sensitive people can be affected by very small electrical signals of specific frequency. Working with highly allergic patients, he tuned an ordinary laboratory signal generator to specific frequencies causing the patients to experience symptoms of the allergy when exposed to them. He believes it is possible that these symptoms could be alleviated if a second, neutralizing frequency could be found.[17]

Fuller Royal, M.D., of Las Vegas, Nevada, uses EDS devices in combination with homeopathy to determine the source of a patient's allergies and the proper neutralization dose. He tests the patient's diet—all the foods commonly eaten and the artificial dyes found in them—plus all the major chemicals in their environment, along with mold spores, house dust, and various pollens. They can all be tested within an hour with an EDS device.

"For example, if someone is allergic to ragweed pollen, there will be an abnormal reading at the allergy control acupoint," Dr. Royal says. "We then find a specific dilution of ragweed pollen that brings the reading back to zero when it is in the circuit. That solution, given by injection, will neutralize the patient's reaction to ragweed."

To further ensure accuracy, Dr. Royal performs intradermal skin tests as well. When all the tests are finished, separate serums are prepared for each group of allergens and injected for desensitization. Dr. Royal reports a high rate of success using this protocol.

magnetic signals that can be described by a complex waveform. Health can be considered as a smooth wave, while disease is identified by unwanted variations in this wave, both higher and lower.

Dr. Morrel had the idea of taking the electromagnetic signals directly from the body and manipulating the aberrant waveforms by raising or lowering them to create normal waves. These corrected waves are then fed from the device back into the patient through the corresponding acupoints. The signals can be taken from any area of the body, modified, and then returned to that specific area.

Since the MORA uses only the electromagnetic signals coming directly from the patient, it can be characterized as a truly natural therapy. "The crucial point of

the MORA is that disease is considered to be a question of 'wrong' electromagnetic information," says Anthony Scott-Morley, D.Sc., Ph.D., M.D. (Alt. Med.), of Dorset, England. "The MORA instrument 'reads' the wave information of the patient and corrects it. There is no artificial electrical signal introduced. In this sense, it is an extremely pure form of treatment because it deals only with the wave information of the patient."

The MORA has been used successfully for treatment of skin disease, headaches, migraines, muscular aches and pains, and circulation problems, and can be used in combination with homeopathic remedies. Although used primarily for treatment, it can be used as a diagnostic instrument as well.

The MORA can also be used for color therapy, transforming individual colors into appropriate frequencies and transmitting them into the body. "The MORA color instrument reduces the frequency of each color to a lower harmonic, out of the spectrum of visible light to a lower electromagnetic range," states Dr. Scott-Morley. "This allows for deeper penetration of tissue and shorter treatment times than with the use of visible light color treatment."

TENS: A commonly used device for pain relief is the Transcutaneous Electrical Nerve Stimulator, or TENS. Invented by Dr. Shealy, it is widely used in doctors' offices and physiotherapy clinics and can be used at home. It works by applying an electrical current to affected nerves, causing conduction to be blocked and pain to be relieved. TENS units are believed to stimulate the production of endorphins, the body's natural painkillers.

Judy Zacharski, P.T., Director of the Facial Pain and TMJ Clinic, in Menomonee Falls, Wisconsin, uses TENS instruments to treat temporomandibular joint (TMJ) syndrome, a painful condition of the jaw usually caused by stress or injury. A 25-year-old patient of Zacharski's came to her with TMJ syndrome as a result of both an automobile accident (her head struck the steering wheel) and a sports injury (she was hit in the mouth with a baseball). The patient responded positively after the first two TENS treatments and was given a unit to use at home. After ten days, the patient reported considerable reduction in discomfort.[18]

Electro-Acuscope: Using a much lower electrical current than the TENS unit, the Electro-Acuscope reduces pain by stimulating tissue repair rather than by stimulating the nerves or causing muscle contractions. The current is continually adjusted to match the resistance from the damaged tissue in order to facilitate the repair process. The skill of the practitioner is of considerable importance for its effective use. Because of its prolonged effects on tissue repair, the Electro-Acuscope can be applied to a broad range of clinical conditions such as muscle spasms, migraines, TMJ syndrome, bursitis, arthritis, surgical incisions, sprains and strains, neuralgia, herpes zoster infections (shingles), and bruises.

Steve Center, M.D., of San Diego, California, also uses the Electro-Acuscope to treat local skin infections, chronic fatigue syndrome, and carpal tunnel syndrome, though he says he predominantly uses it for acute and chronic pain, mainly of musculoskeletal origin—automobile accidents, lumbosacral (lower back) sprains, shoulder strains, and sports injuries.[19]

"The most impressive results are found in the severe muscle contraction headaches associated with injuries to the muscles of the upper chest, upper thorax, and neck," says George Godfrey, M.D., founding member of the American Trauma Society of the American College of Surgeons and Medical Director of Atlantic Industrial College of Surgeons, in Atlantic City, New Jersey. "At times the headache is gone within 30 seconds." He also uses Electro-Acuscope treatment for chronic problems produced by strains and sprains, carpal tunnel syndrome, whiplash, trauma, skin ulcerations, arthritis, and the palliative care of ruptured disk patients who are either unable or unwilling to undergo surgery.[20]

Light Beam Generator: The Light Beam Generator (LBG) is about the size of a small suitcase, with one, two, or four hand-held heads attached on cords. It uses extremely low current, cold gas light photons to transfer energy frequency patterns to targeted areas of the lymphatic system, a vital aspect of the immune system. Frequency modulation is accomplished with light, and the LBG is safe for use by lay practitioners. "The Light Beam Generator is a valuable tool for restoring proper functioning of the body and immune defense processes," according to Ilonka Harezi, President of ELF International, the manufacturer. It penetrates deeper than lymphatic massage alone and can be used to increase the effectiveness of manual lymphatic massage.

The LBG works energetically to rebalance the charge of the cells' electromagnetic field. Cells in the lymphatic system can clump together and bond electrically with water to create disease conditions of swelling or abnormal growths. The LBG is able to separate these cells and their accumulated fluids and protein wastes, resulting in the rapid dispersal of swelling, tumor masses, and blockages. By opening sealed and calcified vessels, it stimulates blood circulation, reduces edema, and eliminates waste products from tissues.

"The LBG can be used anywhere on the body where there is a problem," says Robert Jacobs, N.M.D., D.Hom. (Med), of London, England. "Because of its pen-

etration, it can help heal organs deep within the body, as well as skin problems." Dr. Jacobs points out that since healthy cells are in a stable energetic state, there are no adverse effects when the LBG is used in 30-45 minute sessions.

Although ELF International makes no claims about the usefulness of the LBG for treating specific diseases, physicians who use the device (about 1,000) have found it beneficial for edema, pain (especially involving soft tissue and tissue congestion due to injury), sciatica, premenstrual syndrome, dermatological conditions, gastrointestinal inflammation, allergies, arthritis, bursitis, diabetes, lupus, fibromyalgia, respiratory conditions, scarring, cellulite, burns, eczema, fibrocystic disease, breast and prostate cancer, prostate enlargement, headaches, and as an aid in surgical recovery. Improvement is due to the LBG's ability to improve lymph flow, while enhancing delivery of oxygen and nutrients through the bloodstream.

Dr. Jacobs had a patient with a severe case of herpes zoster over his upper chest area. The condition was so painful that the man could not raise one of his arms and had difficulty sleeping. Medical treatments had not been able to help him. Dr. Jacobs gave him one 45-minute treatment with the LBG, after which the man was free of most pain. He could move his arm and the pustules were 60% reduced in size. After one additional treatment with the LBG, he was fully healed.

Rena Davis, M.Sc., of St. Helens, Oregon, uses the LBG in conjunction with a dietary and nutritional program to treat a wide range of conditions. One of her patients was a 60-year-old woman with severe rheumatoid arthritis in all of her joints. Davis treated her with the LBG for 14 months, after which time she was completely healed. Davis also finds the LBG is effective in draining varicose veins and for the fluid retention associated with PMS. Sports clinics use it to reduce the swelling of sports injuries.

In 2002, ELF International introduced the ST-8 device, to be used with the LBG or alone. The ST-8 uses scalar technology coupled with an oxygen-feed and extremely low current, cold gas light photons to transfer energy frequency patterns to cells. This allows cells to correct their electromagnetic charge, which improves lymph flow. Physicians who use the ST-8 report that it is especially useful for conditions where the immune system is compromised.

Bio-Electric Field Enhancement (BEFE): Developed by Terry Skrinjar, of Q-Tech Laboratories, in Toowoomba, Queensland, Australia, the BEFE unit is based upon a new quantum resonance theory called Q-Mechanics that alters an external source of artificial energy into an energy format that is similar in nature and compatibility to that of the body. Though not specifically designed to diagnose or treat disease, the BEFE unit has received official approval from the Therapeutic Goods Administration (Australia's equivalent of the U.S. Food and Drug Administration) to be marketed as a therapeutic spa and medical device in Australia.

The BEFE unit consists of a power unit that produces a 24-volt direct current to a water array consisting of copper and special steel plates. According to Skrinjar, the arrangement and constituency of the plates and the material of the array, combined with proprietary electronics, creates a specific electromagnetic signature and harmonics, which are emitted into the medium of water. Users of the unit immerse part or all of their body in water (foot bath or in the bath tub) and then activate it for 20-35 minutes. "The BEFE unit uses water because up to 80% of our body is water, and water contains the necessary electrical patterns to adapt a conventional electrical charge to a bio-charge," Skrinjar says. "The bio-charge is the organic electricity your body produces in order to operate itself on a daily basis. A low bio-charge means you are low on energy, and thus your whole body becomes sluggish and lethargic in all its functions, possibly leading to the development of various physical symptoms in the form of aches, pains, and disease conditions. By giving the body a bio-charge boost, some of these symptoms can be alleviated by your own body and your system can eventually be restored to its full function." In effect, according to Skrinjar, the BEFE unit rebalances the body's meridians, realigning its bioenergy field, which explains many of the benefits commonly reported by those who use it.

"The BEFE unit generates a complex waveform signature that interacts with the water on such a base level as to be synergistic with the bioelectric state of the person being treated," Skrinjar explains. For this reason, persons should be treated one at a time, using clean water for each session, as everyone has an individual and unique bio-signature. The generation and absorption of this bio-charge has been shown to increase the potential voltage in the body's cell membranes, thereby enhancing immunity and helping to maintain cellular function, while at the same time helping to eliminate bacterial, viral, and fungal infections. The BEFE bath has also been shown to stimulate the release of body toxins and foreign material, often resulting in discoloration of the water as the release occurs.

Because of the BEFE unit's ability to improve the body's bio-charge, health practitioners and their patients who use the device have reported numerous health benefits. These include increased vitality, revitalized blood, detoxification and neutralization of toxins, pain and stress

relief, faster recovery time from illness or injury, reduced inflammation, improved sleep, reduced fluid retention, improved endocrine and metabolic function, elimination of menstrual pain, dermal rejuvenation, and improved kidney and liver function. It is recommended that the BEFE unit be used only every other day and never for more than 35 minutes at a time, due to its powerful bio-recharging effects. It should also be avoided by women who are pregnant, anyone using prescription drugs, and anyone with an organ transplant or battery operated implant, such as a pacemaker.

The Sound Probe: The Sound Probe emits a pulsed tone of three alternating frequencies that can destroy anything that is not in resonance with the body, such as bacteria, viruses, and fungi. The pad connected to the instrument is placed anywhere on the body where there is a problem or pain. The alternation of the frequencies ensures that the body does not adjust to the frequency, so that the treatment remains beneficial over time. It can also be used in sequence with the LBG. The Sound Probe is used first to kill off bacteria, viruses, or other microorganisms, then the LBG is used to clear the debris from the system.

The Diapulse: The Diapulse uses radio waves to produce short, intense electromagnetic pulses that can penetrate deep into the tissues of the body. The heat energy produced reaches into tissues to improve blood flow, reduce pain, and promote healing. The Diapulse has been used successfully to reduce edema and inflammation following surgery and may be helpful in functional recovery from spinal cord injuries, according to Gary Emerson, D.C., of Santa Ana, California.

Cymatic Instruments: In addition to the electroacupuncture biofeedback devices discussed earlier, there are also therapeutic cymatic devices, in which a sound transducer replaces the electrodes of the electroacupuncture biofeedback devices. This allows recording of the emitted sound patterns associated with different body parts. The machines can be used for diagnosis as well as treatment. According to Peter Guy Manners, M.D., D.O., Ph.D., of Bretforton, England, each organ, tissue, and molecule has its own harmonic signal. These signals are encoded into the cymatic device, which can be used to deliver to a particular body part a frequency pattern associated with its healthy state, restoring that particular body part to health.

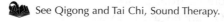 See Qigong and Tai Chi, Sound Therapy.

The **Infratonic QGM:** In the early 1980s, Lu Yan Fang, Ph.D., a senior scientist at the National Electro Acoustics Laboratory, in Beijing, China, discovered that Qigong masters emitted elevated levels of low-frequency acoustical waves, called secondary sounds, from their hands. Although everyone generates secondary sounds, the signals generated by the Qigong masters were 100 times more powerful than the average individual's, and 1,000 times more powerful than those from the elderly or ill.

Using electro-acoustical technology, Dr. Fang constructed an instrument that simulated this infratonic sound (8-14 hertz, 70 decibels). When she directed these massage-like waves into hospitalized patients, she noted numerous improvements, particularly for the management of pain. Other benefits include increased circulatory functioning, migraine suppression, muscular relaxation, and the alleviation of depression. When used on the chest or back, the brain's production of alpha waves is also stimulated.

Today, this machine is medically recognized as an effective pain management tool in China and is also used in Japan, Taiwan, Singapore, France, Spain, Mexico, and Argentina. In the U.S., it is approved by the U.S. Food and Drug Administration as a therapeutic massage device.

Once a physician starts doing energy therapies, that's the point of no return. When you see how dramatically patients respond, you can never practice medicine the same way again.

—MILTON HAMMERLY, M.D.

Devices That Protect Against Electromagnetic Fields

An estimated 80% of people are sensitive to extra low frequency (ELF) electromagnetic fields, which over time can cause organ malfunction and the onset of illness. ELF fields are ubiquitous in most places around the globe, emitted from electrical power lines, computers, televisions, cellular phones, clocks, stereos, household appliances and microwaves, and even water beds. Communication waves and atmospheric disturbances such as electrical storms also generate ELF fields destructive to natural electrical balance in the body.

THE HEALING POWER OF STATIC ELECTRICITY

"Abnormal physiology, such as pain or chronic headache, is associated with abnormal electrical charge, or the abnormal flow of electrons," according to Milton Hammerly, M.D., Medical Director of American Whole Health, in Littleton, Colorado. Dr. Hammerly has found that static electricity, which involves a negative charge, is able to correct such abnormal physical conditions, seemingly on contact. To administer static electricity to his patients, he employs a technique called electrostatic massage (EM). It involves the use of a PVC pipe (Schedule 40, 1 ½ inches in diameter and 12 inches long) that he rubs with a painter's mitt (any fuzzy material can be used) to generate a charge of static electricity. "By sweeping the negatively charged PVC pipe near the body, electrons are pushed to the symptomatic area (in cases of headache, for example, to the head), where they facilitate the normal healing process," Dr. Hammerly explains.

In addition to headaches and pain, EM can also produce benefits in cases of swelling due to water retention, or edema, which often accompanies injury and inflammation. "EM, by moving water accumulated in an area of inflammation, can reduce pressure on the nerves and dissipate the waste products of inflammation," he says. Of 393 patients he treated with EM, 292 (74%) showed a positive response within 15 minutes or less. His patient studies further reveal that EM has a wide application. For cases of muscular pain, 83% responded favorably; for arthritis, 70%; for fibromyalgia, 80%; for rotator cuff tendinitis, 76%; for tension headaches, 84%; and for sinus headaches, 79%.

"After a single office treatment, patients are fully able to continue using EM independently," Dr. Hammerly observes. "While these results are short-term in nature, I see long-term trends in decreased use of medications, fewer office visits, and fewer emergency room visits." Dr. Hammerly adds that "once a physician starts doing energy therapies such as EM, that's the point of no return. When you see how dramatically patients respond, you can never practice medicine the same way again."

Dr. Scott-Morley, along with other researchers, has found that while some people exposed to ELF radiation do not necessarily experience symptoms, most manifest a variety of conditions following ELF exposure, including fatigue, anxiety, emotional highs and lows, depres-

COMMON SOURCES OF ELECTROMAGNETIC FREQUENCIES

Power lines, secondary transformers, electric power meters, electric blankets, hair dryers, electric shavers, TVs, stereo systems, air conditioners, answering machines, portable and cellular phones, refrigerators, blenders, microwave ovens, toasters, vacuum cleaners, washers and dryers, portable heaters, coffee makers, computers, fax machines, copiers, scanners, automobiles, satellite dishes, fluorescent lights.

sion, headaches, migraines, allergies, hormonal imbalances, arthritis, hyperactivity, short attention span, frequent colds, and increased susceptibility to recurring illness and infection. Research strongly suggests that certain types of cancer, as well as greater risk of miscarriage, may be due to prolonged ELF exposure. Unnatural electromagnetic fields (EMFs) produced by televisions and computer screens have also been shown to affect the pineal gland, thereby impacting the normal production of melatonin, a hormone that regulates sleep. Recognizing the growing health risks posed by EMFs, a number of researchers have developed protective devices to neutralize and shield against it.

The Teslar Watch: Named after Nikola Tesla, the inventor of alternating current and 'father' of the scalar non-Hertzian technology it employs, the Teslar Watch produces a scalar wave that has been shown to screen other ELF signals, while radiating its own 8-Hz signal similar to the earth's natural resonance of 7-9 Hz, thus enabling the body to operate within its own natural frequency range. It was developed by researchers at ELF International, who also created the Light Beam Generator.

According to renowned researcher of the human bioenergy field Valerie Hunt, Ph.D., Professor Emeritus at U.C.L.A., scalar energy is created when two identical frequencies meet head on from opposite directions, canceling each other out to leave a stationary energy. "Currently, energy instruments only measure frequencies and wavelengths, not stationary energy," says Dr. Hunt, explaining why scalar energy is not widely discussed by most scientists. "However, studies at the Max Planck Institute showed that the scalar wave, like that created by the Teslar Watch, caused the unclumping of lymph and blood cells. Then the smooth flowing circulatory systems brought nutrients to cells and tissues, and removed chem-

ical and cellular wastes, resulting in improved healing and immune capacity."

The magnetic chip that drives the watch creates the scalar energy, and its active protection is superior to the various stones, metals, and magnets that many people wear today. Dr. Hunt further notes that the 8-Hz cycle wave produced and maintained by the Teslar Watch "constitutes the most important frequency milieu for living tissues to remain functional and to communicate from DNA to genes to tissues, cells, organs, and systems." When worn over the left wrist, the scalar vibrations produced by the Teslar Watch are in direct contact with the acupoints that acupuncturists refer to as the Triple Warmer, where they then spread through the meridian system of the entire body. Dr. Hunt's research has found that the scalar module also creates a protective cocoon, offering maximum protection from absorbing and transmitting destructive EMFs into the body.

Additional research on the Teslar Watch conducted by Dr. Scott-Morley confirms that it eliminates electromagnetic fields from those who wear it. A study of live cell cultures conducted by Glen Rein, Ph.D., at Stanford University Medical Center, showed that the Teslar Watch not only eliminated harmful ELF fields, but actually resulted in a 76%-134% increase in immune response. Additional testing by Dr. Rein also revealed that the Teslar's screening capability created an environment that increased basic biochemical communication between nerve cells, mediated by neurotransmitters. Uptake of the hormone noradrenaline (increases blood pressure) into the nerve cells was inhibited by 19.5%, which may explain the antidepressant effects reported by many wearers of the watch.[21] Other studies now under way indicate that the Teslar Watch is capable of improving athletic performance by as much as 20%, as well as enhancing the circulation of energy throughout the body.

BioElectric Shield: Developed by Charles Brown, D.C., D.A.B.C.N., a chiropractic neurologist, the BioElectric Shield is a pendant that employs a matrix of precision-cut quartz and other crystals to envelop those who wear it in a cocoon of their own bioenergy and to deflect external harmful or incompatible energy. Since 1990, Dr. Brown and his colleagues have tested over 12,000 people using applied kinesiology (AK). Of these test subjects, 98% showed significant muscle weakness simply from holding a cell phone, according to Dr. Brown. But within minutes of wearing the Shield, their strength returned to normal and in many cases even improved. After three weeks of wearing the Shield, Dr. Brown adds, test subjects showed improvements in immune function ranging from 108%-400%, in allergy points, and in liver, kidney, gallbladder, and stomach function, as determined by EDS testing. Strength levels of the test subjects also significantly improved during this period, compared to subjects who wore a placebo device.

In another test, computerized electromyography (used by physical therapists to assess muscle strength) was used with 25 subjects who were instructed to sit before a computer screen after being tested to establish their baseline muscle strength. After five minutes before the screen, the subjects had an average 17% diminishment in muscle strength. They were then given a Shield to wear. Within five minutes, they showed an average gain in muscle strength of over 44%, and 21 of the subjects were actually stronger on their final reading than their initial baseline level. According to Dr. Brown, what makes these studies even more intriguing is that approximately 30% of the test subjects were unaware when their muscle strength weakened or improved, even though the testing devices clearly showed changes occurring.

The Q-Link: The Q-Link is a pendant designed to boost and maintain the body's natural bioenergy, strengthening it against the harmful effects of EMFs. According to its manufacturer, Clarus Products International, when the Q-Link is worn next to the body, its proprietary technology "activates an omnidirectional protective field extending approximately two feet around the body." In 1997, T.M. Srinivasan, Ph.D., an expert in the field of subtle energy research, reviewed independent tests of the Q-Link and the technology used in its manufacture conducted by scientists at the University of California, at Irvine. Among the findings Dr. Srinivasan reported were a 30% or greater reduction in stress responses in organisms exposed to the Clarus field; nullification of EMF radiation generated by computers; reduced problem behaviors among students wearing the Q-Link; and increased heart rate variability (HRV—see Quick Definition) and improved balance in the sympathetic and parasympathetic frequency bands of the HRV, both indicative of improved heart function.[22]

 Heart rate variability (HRV) is the normally occurring beat-to-beat changes in heart rate. Analysis of HRV is an important tool used to assess the function and balance of the autonomic nervous system and is a key indicator of aging and cardiac health.

Applications of Energy Medicine Devices

The level of accuracy of electrodermal screening (EDS) devices is key to their future success and acceptance. In 1989, researchers at the University of Hawaii compared a diabetic population with a control group using electroacupuncture measurements on the spleen-pancreas meridian. The resulting data demonstrated a 95%–97.5% correspondence between EDS assessment and the conventionally confirmed diabetic group.[23] Another study at the University of Hawaii compared EDS assessment of the allergy meridian with six other methods of assessing food allergies. The EDS data gave the highest compatibility with the food-challenge test, the most sensitive of currently available diagnostic techniques for determination of food allergies.[24] Researchers at the University of California, at Los Angeles, and the University of Southern California, were also able to demonstrate an 87% correlation between an EDS diagnosis of lung cancer when compared with standard X-ray diagnosis.[25]

 Electrodermal screening provides a low-cost, highly effective way for screening for physiological and energetic imbalances before they develop into full-blown illnesses. It is an excellent tool for reducing the skyrocketing costs of medical care in this country.

EDS devices can also be used to determine which bacteria, virus, or toxin is specifically responsible for an illness, infection, or disease, and which medications will help a particular health problem. Abram Ber, M.D., of Phoenix, Arizona, reports seeing a patient with Huntington chorea, a hereditary disease of the central nervous system. Characterized by progressive dementia and rapid, jerky motions, there is normally no treatment for this condition. He examined the patient with an EDS device and found evidence of heavy metal toxicity, which he was able to treat with vitamin B_{12} injections and homeopathic remedies. Within a year, the patient's symptoms abated and he is doing well at the present time.

Fuller Royal, M.D., of Las Vegas, Nevada, uses EDS devices exclusively in his practice. He does not treat a specific disease, but rather treats the patient as a whole, looking for the underlying mechanisms that lead to disease. One patient came to him with angina, unable to walk across a room without pain. He had already undergone two bypass surgeries for sclerosis of the coronary artery and was facing a third surgery. Using EDS testing, Dr. Royal discovered the problem to be a wisdom tooth with a mercury amalgam filling. Once this filling was removed, the angina disappeared and the patient recovered completely. In another case, Dr. Royal examined a six-month-old boy who was failing to thrive. The baby had been treated at the Mayo Clinic but still had not improved. Dr. Royal's EDS assessment revealed the presence of a virus contracted from the mother when she had the flu. He treated the problem with homeopathic remedies, and now the child is healthy.

Robert D. Milne, M.D., of Las Vegas, Nevada, also uses EDS devices to screen all his patients, many of whom come to him suffering from chronic fatigue syndrome

VETERINARY ENERGY MEDICINE

Bioenergetic veterinary medicine is identical to that used in humans. The only difference, according to H.C. Gurney, D.V.M., of Conifer, Colorado, is the fact that animals do not have the power to reason whether a treatment is going to work or not; either it will or it won't. Due to an animal's basic impartiality to various treatment modalities, Dr. Gurney views veterinary energy medicine as blazing a trail in energy medicine by offering a workable model with the objective results to back it up.

Today, many veterinary professionals are moving into the field of energy medicine, including Joanne Stefanatos, D.V.M., of Las Vegas, Nevada, President of the American Holistic Veterinary Medicine Association, who devotes her practice almost exclusively to energy medicine. She treats animals ranging from lions, tigers, snakes, and desert tortoises, to birds, domestic cats, and dogs. Using an EDS device to screen for health problems, her treatment therapies include acupuncture, laser acupuncture, electroacupuncture, magnetic field therapy, and homeopathic remedies.

(CFS). Through using EDS, he has found that virtually all female patients have digestive or pelvic problems predating the CFS. Once he treats these problems with diet, food supplements, Chinese herbs, enzymes, and homeopathic remedies, the condition abates. One of Dr. Milne's patients came to him with medically diagnosed intractable thyroiditis (Hashimoto's disease). EDS testing revealed that his body's energy system was congested. Using a combination of acupuncture, herbs, and homeopathic remedies to unblock the energy flow, Dr. Milne was able to resolve the problem to the extent that the patient's antimicrosomal antibody level, an indicator of thyroiditis, returned to normal.

Dr. Scott-Morley also employs energy devices in his practice. One of his patients was a 36-year-old man who came to him with constant pain in the area of his liver. Two extensive medical investigations had found no evidence of anything wrong and a third resulted in the suggestion that the man seek psychiatric treatment. Using an EDS device, Dr. Scott-Morley measured the man's liver acupoints and confirmed chronic inflammation and possible pathological damage. The test further revealed aflatoxin toxicity (frequently caused by a mold found on stale peanuts). Dr. Scott-Morley asked the man if stale

peanuts had any significance for him and was told that he had previously been a truck driver and had transported peanuts from Italy to England, eating several handfuls of them while en route. Upon arrival, the shipment was found to be stale and condemned as unhealthy. Dr. Scott-Morley prescribed a homeopathic nosode (see Quick Definition) of aflatoxin in conjunction with other remedies, and within a few weeks the man fully recovered.

> **QD** A homeopathic **nosode** is a super-diluted remedy made as an energy imprint from a disease product, such as bacteria, tuberculosis, measles, influenza, or approximately 200 other substances. The nosode, which contains no physical trace of the disease, stimulates the body to remove all taints or residues of a particular disease, whether it was inherited or contracted. Only qualified homeopaths may administer a nosode remedy.

Another woman came to Dr. Scott-Morley with pains in her abdomen and digestive disorders. EDS testing indicated liver malfunction along with an impaired right kidney. The toxic agent appeared to be *Bilharzia*, a parasite common in the Nile and irrigation canals of Egypt. But when Dr. Scott-Morley asked the woman when she had last been to Africa, she replied that she had never been outside of England. A second test again showed the presence of *Bilharzia*, leaving both Dr. Scott-Morley and the woman puzzled. Later that same evening, however, the woman phoned to reveal that her mother said she had been born in Egypt and had fallen into an irrigation ditch when she was 18 months old. Dr. Scott-Morley was then able to use a *Bilharzia* nosode to resolve the woman's condition.

Dr. Scott-Morley also uses the MORA device to treat conditions. One of his patients had pain in both of his knees and required crutches in order to walk. After receiving treatment with the MORA device in conjunction with MORA color for 20 minutes, the patient was able to walk free of pain and without the need of crutches and remains pain free three years later.

Energy medicine is also growing in popularity among practitioners of biological dentistry, particularly with regard to electrodermal screening devices. A relationship has been shown to exist between acupoints associated with specific teeth and body organs. Due to this fact, EDS devices are now being used to screen for health problems in the body caused by the related teeth. It can also determine a patient's compatibility with various dental materials and anesthetics before they are used. In this way, dental toxicity can be avoided. EDS devices can detect hidden infections below teeth, which often cause no symptoms and go undiagnosed for years, contributing to degenerative disease elsewhere in the body. In fact, EDS testing is sometimes the only way of detecting these infections.

Philip Jenkins, D.D.S., of Los Gatos, California, uses EDS testing for this purpose. "For years I kept after patients to keep their teeth clean," he says, "but even some patients who followed all the instructions got worse." Now, using EDS testing, Dr. Jenkins can find the infections, identify them, and determine the appropriate homeopathic remedies to treat them.

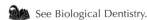 See Biological Dentistry.

The Future of Energy Medicine

The main thrust of conventional chemical-based medicine is crisis intervention rather than prevention. Traditional drug therapies also pose a serious threat of side effects along with an alarming increase in iatrogenic (treatment-induced) diseases and problems. There also appears to be a dramatic rise in the number of chronic degenerative diseases in the Western world for which chemical medicine has no real answer. It is estimated that 60%-70% of the problems presented on a daily basis to primary care physicians defy diagnosis and are usually labeled as neurotic or psychosomatic in origin.[26]

"The medicine of the future will be energy medicine," says Dr. Jacobs, "and chemical medicine will be a subset of medicine as a whole. Probably 80% of medicine will be energy medicine and 20% chemical medicine." According to Dr. Jacobs, Russia is leading the world in the field of energy medicine today. Russian physicians are using microwave energy at acupoints to treat many health problems successfully. At present, it is not known exactly how these different forms of energy work in the body, but there is substantial clinical evidence that they do work.

Just as significant as the treatment applications of energy medicine is electrodermal screening, which can enable a practitioner to screen for the potential for illness before it happens. This makes energy medicine an excellent tool for reducing the costs of medical care in the U.S. By catching diseases early or preventing them from ever occurring, medical costs will be greatly minimized. Research is still needed to prove the value of EDS testing, however. "The problem here is a very practical one," notes Dr. Scott-Morley. "Research costs money and the skilled practitioners of these methods are busy working as doctors, not as researchers. It would take two to three years to train researchers to a high enough level of competency in these methods for the research to be effective. Yet if some enterprising body were to give sym-

pathetic and careful attention to our claims, then I feel we would discover that we have an undreamed of tool available to us, which I'm sure can be further extended and refined."

 Research is needed to prove the value of electrodermal screening. This can easily be verified by comparison of results of competent practitioners with conventional diagnostic methods.

Where to Find Help

For further information about energy medicine therapies and devices, contact:

International Society for the Study of Subtle Energies and Energy Medicine (ISSSEEM)
11005 Ralston Road, Suite 100D
Arvada, Colorado 80004
(303) 425-4625
Website: www.issseem.org

ISSSEEM is an interdisciplinary, nonprofit organization formed for the purpose of improving human health through the advancement of education, practice, training, and research in the emerging field of subtle energies and energy medicine.

Bioenergetic Healing

Nurse Healers–Professional Associates International
3760 South Highland Drive, Suite 429
Salt Lake City, Utah 84106
(801) 273-3399
Website: www.therapeutic-touch.org

Healing Touch International, Inc.
12477 W. Cedar Drive, Suite 202
Lakewood, Colorado 80228
(303) 989-7982
Website: www.healingtouch.net

International Center for Reiki Training
29209 Northwestern Highway, Suite 592
Southfield, Michigan 48034
(800) 332-8112
Website: www.reiki.org

Energy Medicine Devices

Due to various state laws and pending approval by the FDA, we cannot conscientiously offer referrals for energy medicine devices or practitioners who use them. Further information about the energy devices mentioned in this chapter is available by contacting the following organizations.

BioElectric Company
63 Windsong Way
Lavina, Montana 59046
(800) 217-8573
Website: www.bioelectricshield.com

Manufacturers of products (including the BioElectric Shield) proven to reduce stress, fatigue, and overload, while protecting, strengthening, and renewing personal vitality.

Electro Medical, Inc.
1565 Scenic Avenue, Suite D
Costa Mesa, California 92626
(714) 964-6776 or (800) 422-8726

Marketing and education for the Electro-Acuscope and the Myopulse. Referrals to doctors who use this equipment.

ELF Labs
Route. l, Box 21
St. Francisville, Illinois 62460
(618) 948-2394
Websites: www.teslar.com, www.lightbeamgenerator.com

Makers of the Light Beam Generator, Sound Probe, ST-8 and Teslar Watch. Referrals to doctors who use this equipment.

Q-Tech Laboratories
Level 1-453 Ruthven Street
Toowoomba, Queensland, Australia 4350
(011) 61-7-4639-5533
Website: www.q2.com.au

Q—The Experience
10800 E. Cactus Road, Suite 15
Scottsdale, Arizona 85259
(480) 391-8422

Q-Tech Laboratories manufactures the BEFE unit and distributes it internationally, while Q—The Experience distributes the BEFE unit in the United States.

StarTech Health Services, LLC
1219 South 1840 West
Orem, Utah 84058
(888) 229-1114
Website: www.startechhealth.com

For information about the LISTEN System and EDS training seminars. Also provides referrals to practitioners nationwide.

Tools for Wellness
9755 Independence Avenue
Chatsworth, California 91311
(800) 456-9887
Website: www.toolsforwellness.com

Mail-order catalog of nonmedical devices (including the Q-Link), machines, audiotapes, and books.

Recommended Reading

Accepting Your Power to Heal: The Personal Practice of Therapeutic Touch. Dolores Krieger. Santa Fe, NM: Bear & Company, 1993.

The Body Electric: Electromagnetism and the Foundation of Life. Robert O. Becker and Gary Selden. New York: William Morrow, 1987.

Electromagnetic Man: Health and Hazard in the Electrical Environment. Cyril W. Smith and Simon Best. New York: St. Martin's, 1989.

Energy Medicine. Donna Eden with David Feinstein. New York: Tarcher/Putnam, 1998.

Sacred Healing: The Curing Power of Energy and Spirituality. C. Norman Shealy. Boston: Element Books, 1999.

Vibrational Medicine: New Choices for Healing Ourselves. Richard Gerber, M.D. Santa Fe, NM: Bear & Company, 1996.

ENVIRONMENTAL MEDICINE

Environmental medicine explores the role of dietary and environmental allergens in health and illness. Factors such as dust, molds, chemicals, and certain foods may cause allergic reactions that can dramatically influence diseases ranging from asthma and hay fever to headaches and depression. Virtually any chronic physical or mental illness may be improved by the care of a physician competent in this field.

IN THE PAST, CONVENTIONAL medicine has been unwilling to attribute much importance to the complex relationship between individuals and their environment. This attitude has begun to change, however, due to extensive research by environmental specialists over the last 40 years. Today, many physicians cite a link between their patients' illnesses and environmental factors such as diet, pollens, molds, and chemicals.[1]

The field of environmental medicine was pioneered by Theron G. Randolph, M.D., of Chicago, Illinois, a prominent allergy specialist and professor at four medical schools. Since the late 1940s, Dr. Randolph has taught that sensitivity reactions to commonly eaten foods can cause a range of symptoms in susceptible individuals, including headaches, eczema, fatigue, arthritis, depression, and a variety of gastrointestinal disorders.

Further research by Dr. Randolph revealed that chemicals in the environment may have profound negative effects throughout the body. His book *Human Ecology and the Susceptibility to the Chemical Environment*, published in 1962, was the first textbook on the subject. Since then, many other physicians have followed in Dr. Randolph's footsteps, attempting to educate the public that the widespread use of insecticides, herbicides, plastics, food additives, petroleum products, and other chemicals can lead to illness.

"For the past several decades, there has been a rapidly increasing growth in the incidence of more complex and chronic diseases that is directly due to environmental and dietary factors," says Gary R. Oberg, M.D., F.A.A.P., F.A.A.E.M., of Crystal Lake, Illinois, a leading educator in the field of environmental medicine. "Under the current medical model, treatment for these diseases has resulted in rapidly escalating costs, accompanied by a decrease in treatment response rates and

mounting dissatisfaction with the quality of life resulting from such care."[2]

Environmental medicine is a more patient-centered, cause-oriented model that was formed to correct this situation. Environmental medicine has evolved significantly since Dr. Randolph's early discoveries to become one of the most comprehensive forms of holistic medicine. Environmental medicine physicians also recognize the importance of treating the whole person—body, mind, and spirit.

Symptoms of Environmental Sensitivity

Many common illnesses and symptoms can be caused by allergies or environmental sensitivity, according to William Crook, M.D., of Jackson, Tennessee.[3] Traditional allergists routinely treat patients with typical allergy complaints such as asthma, eczema, hives, sneezing, nasal congestion, a runny nose, and itching eyes or throat, as well as other symptoms frequently associated with hay fever. Doctors who specialize in environmental medicine do not limit themselves to these conditions, recognizing that other illnesses, such as headaches, arthritis, chronic fatigue, colitis, and lupus, can also be the result of, or aggravated by, allergies or chemical sensitivity.

Marshall Mandell, M.D., of Norwalk, Connecticut, the father of bioecologic medicine, has discovered that even severe health conditions such as multiple sclerosis, cerebral palsy, and adult post-polio syndrome may be significantly complicated by superimposed allergic reactions and likewise benefited when those allergies are treated.[4] Studies by environmental scientists and physicians indicate that pollutants play a role in the creation of arthritis and autoimmune illnesses.[5]

SUCCESS STORY: AN UNUSUAL TREATMENT FOR MENTAL ILLNESS

In the late 1940s, Theron G. Randolph, M.D., agreed to evaluate Sally, a young woman who had been committed to a mental hospital due to an apparently untreatable psychosis. Dr. Randolph believed that nervous system reactions to certain foods might either be the cause of, or at least a contributing factor to, Sally's psychosis. He thought this could be proved by a test that eliminated those foods from her diet. However, if once the foods were removed she remained as symptomatic as before, then probably they were not the cause.

Sally was hospitalized in an allergy-free environment and started on a spring-water fast. Enemas were given to speed the complete evacuation of her intestinal tract. By the fourth day, her symptoms had cleared and she felt healthy and sane again. In order to ascertain which food or foods affected her physically or mentally and had triggered her psychosis, Dr. Randolph fed her single-food meals. As she reintroduced the foods one at a time into her diet, Sally was monitored for possible reactions.

Sally experienced no problems until she ate beet sugar. Within moments, her face began to contort, she lost contact with her surroundings, and she developed a blank, unknowing stare. She looked and acted as she had during her previous psychotic episodes. By subsequently eliminating beet sugar (fortunately her only food allergy) from her diet, Sally regained her mental health and no longer needed to be hospitalized.

Individuals vary considerably in their specific responses to certain toxins, but in initial stages of toxic exposure, the body defends itself against the toxins through immune and enzymatic responses occurring in the cells. At first, the body allocates available energy to detoxification activities. The duration of this process depends upon the toxicity of the substance and the length of exposure. It also depends upon the body's toxic load—the total number of environmental factors that contribute to a disease. When we undergo prolonged psychological stress without taking measures to alleviate it or expose ourselves involuntarily to pollution, when we eat foods that lack nutritional value on a regular basis or neglect to exercise and resign ourselves to chronic constipation, we essentially invite toxins to gain an upper hand. Once

inside the body, toxins may roam free, creating or worsening conditions that contribute to the development of acute and chronic illnesses.

According to William Rea, M.D., an environmental physician in Dallas, Texas, key detoxification organs, such as the intestines, liver, and the lymphatic system, then become unable to fully detoxify themselves or the body. A pattern of chronic allergies may develop in which the immune system attacks its own unprocessed toxic load. This state of heightened allergic reactivity keeps the immune system on full alert and, eventually, makes it hyperactive.

Toxins place a significant strain on the immune system by diverting energy and resources away from the essential activities of fighting viruses, bacteria, and other microbes. According to Hans Kugler, Ph.D., the immune system of the average person operates at a level that is 50% of what it was 30 years ago and much of that decrease can be attributed to the immunosuppressive effects of environmental toxins.[6] If the campaign against toxins exhausts the cells' stored reserves of nutrients, then cellular function becomes compromised and the body is less able to assimilate key nutrients.

If the body is unable to process toxins due to overload or disease, toxins accumulate in the bloodstream and get stored in fat, brain, and other tissues, which can upset metabolism and damage enzymes (necessary for all life processes). In the case of the central nervous system, pesticides stored in the body over time may cause the nervous system to misfire, causing Parkinson's-like shaking or seizures. Toxins stored in muscles and cartilage may give rise to arthritis. Many toxins are carcinogens, which can cause DNA mutations and impose a higher risk of developing cancer. Toxins also disrupt hormone activity and shift the body's pH, making it unhealthy and too acidic, and produce a higher level of life-shortening and disease-causing free radicals.

 See Allergies, Mental Health.

Richard S. Wilkinson, M.D., of Yakima, Washington, an expert in environmental medicine, points out that the following conditions may be caused by environmental sensitivity or allergies:

- Cardiovascular problems: vasculitis (inflammation of a blood vessel), thrombophlebitis (inflammation of a vein combined with the formation of a blood clot), high blood pressure, angina, arrhythmia, edema (swelling), and fluid retention

- Chronic pediatric disorders: infections, recurrent ear infections, chronic headaches, stomachaches, muscle aches, bed-wetting, and certain types of behavioral and learning disabilities

- Endocrine disorders: autoimmune thyroiditis, hypoglycemia, and premenstrual syndrome (PMS)

- Eye, ear, nose, and throat disorders: hay fever, nasal congestion, sneezing, conjunctivitis, blurring of vision, itchy eyes, tearing, light sensitivity, swelling of the throat, ear infections, dizziness, loss of balance, ringing in the ears, and sinus headaches

- Gastrointestinal problems: canker sores, irritable bowel syndrome, infant colic, gastroenteritis, diarrhea, constipation, gas, bloating, abdominal pains, ulcerative colitis, and Crohn's disease (a chronic inflammatory condition affecting the colon or small intestine)

- Genitourinary illnesses: bed-wetting, recurrent vaginitis, painful intercourse, and chronic cystitis

- Musculoskeletal problems: muscle spasm headaches, lupus (a chronic inflammatory disease with symptoms including arthritis, fatigue, and skin lesions), rheumatoid arthritis, muscle pains, and joint pain

- Nervous system disorders and neurobehavioral manifestations: headaches, epilepsy, sleep disorders, attention deficit hyperactivity disorder, manic-depressive psychosis, sexual dysfunction, eating disorders, schizophrenia, irritability, anxiety, panic, and chronic fatigue syndrome

- Respiratory diseases: asthma and chronic bronchitis

- Skin diseases: eczema, hives, and angioedema (a form of swelling)

Causes of Environmental Sensitivities

Dr. Wilkinson observes that it is not only the specific allergens (substances causing allergic reactions) that need to be identified and treated. Underlying genetic and nutritional factors, as well as exposure to toxic substances, often predispose the person to develop sensitivities to foods, chemicals, airborne allergens, and other materials. Doctors of environmental medicine stress the importance of a thorough environmental and nutrition-oriented history, as well as a careful physical examination,

ALLERGIC ADDICTION SYNDROME

With food allergies, there is a strange paradox: often a person becomes addicted to a food that produces an allergic response—this is called "allergic addiction syndrome." When a person stops eating an allergy-producing food to which their body is "addicted," such as coffee or chocolate, there is a three-day period in which they experience unpleasant withdrawal symptoms, such as fatigue and anxiety. Eating more of this addictive substance can actually improve the situation by suppressing these withdrawal symptoms. This becomes an unhealthy cycle of addiction, craving, and fulfillment that eventually leads to more serious health problems. Allergy experts call this suppression of symptoms by an allergenic food "masking," because it masks or disguises the true allergic symptoms.

in order to uncover possible contributing factors to the patient's illness.

An important question for the environmental physician to answer is: What are the underlying dietary and environmental causes of, and contributing factors to, the patient's physical and mental symptoms? According to the American Academy of Environmental Medicine (AAEM), a network of over 600 physicians, some of the factors that may contribute to an individual's susceptibility include:

An important question for the environmental physician to answer is: What are the underlying dietary and environmental causes of, and contributing factors to, the patient's physical and mental symptoms?

HEREDITY/GENETICS

Sensitivity to dietary and environmental agents appears to be linked to one's heredity. AAEM members recognize that a genetic predisposition to the development of allergies can be passed down through successive generations of a person's bloodline. The number of family members who experienced severe allergies appears to

SICK BUILDING SYNDROME

In the early 1980s, physicians began using the term *sick building syndrome* (SBS) to refer to a host of symptoms produced by low-grade toxic environmental conditions found in living, work, or office spaces. SBS symptoms are numerous: mucous membrane irritation (eyes, nose, and throat), chest tightness, skin complaints (dryness, itching, abnormal redness), headaches, fatigue, lethargy, coughing, asthma, wheezing, chronic nasal stuffiness, temporary weight loss, infections, and emotional irritability. All of these depress the immune system, rendering the individual susceptible to long-term chronic illness.

"Indoor air pollution in residences, offices, schools, and other buildings is widely recognized as a serious environmental risk to human health," explains Michael Hodgson, M.D., M.P.H., of the School of Medicine at the University of Connecticut Health Center, in Farmington. Dr. Hodgson notes that most people in industrialized nations spend more than 90% of their time indoors, that indoor concentrations of pollutants (including toxic chemicals) are often substantially higher than found outdoors, and that small children, the elderly, and the infirm are likely to spend all their time indoors, leading to a permanent chronic exposure to low-grade toxic factors.

In most cases, problems with a building's engineering, construction, and ventilation system are the causes. Studies suggest that symptoms occur 50% more frequently in buildings with mechanical ventilation systems. Among 2,000 office workers in Germany with work-related symptoms, there was a 50% higher than average rate of upper respiratory tract infections that were directly traceable to problems with mechanically ventilated buildings, reports Dr. Hodgson. A U.S. study found that 20% of office workers had job-related SBS symptoms, including a subjective sense of being less productive in their work.

Besides ventilation problems, other sources of indoor toxic pollution include volatile organic compounds released from particleboard desks, furniture, carpets, glues, paints, office machine toners, and perfumes. All contribute to "a complex mixture of very low levels of individual pollutants," states Dr. Hodgson. Bioaerosols are also indoor contaminants and originate as biological agents from mold spores, allergy-producing microbes, mites, or animal dander; then they are distributed through an indoor space by ventilation, heating, or air conditioning systems. Of buildings classified as sources of SBS, one study showed that 70% have an inadequate flow of fresh outside air. It also found that 50% to 70% of such buildings have poor distribution of air within the occupied space, 60% have poor filtration of outdoor pollutants, 60% have standing water that fosters biological growths, and 20% have malfunctioning humidifiers.[7]

---

increase the likelihood of their descendants experiencing allergies as well, and at an earlier age.

POOR NUTRITION

A major cause of chemical sensitivity is poor or inadequate nutrition. A diet of refined, processed foods deficient in vitamins, minerals, enzymes, and other vital nutrients can severely impair the body's ability to function efficiently due to the increased levels of toxins such foods contain. Their ingestion can also result in an increase of free radicals (highly reactive destructive molecules), which can further predispose a person to allergic reactions.

INFECTIONS

Sensitivities to allergens can be developed following severe infections, whether viral, bacterial, parasitic, or fungal (*Candida*). Candidiasis or parasites can cause chronic inflammation or irritation of the lining of the intestinal tract. This inflammation can lead to "leaky gut syndrome," in which bacteria, bacterial toxins, and partially digested foods are able to travel from the intestine into the bloodstream, causing an allergic or immune reaction.

CHEMICAL EXPOSURE

Current research has shown that due to their toxic effects on the body, exposure to pesticides, herbicides, petrochemicals, and other chemicals in the food and water supply, as well as in indoor and outdoor air, can lead to the development of allergic reactions.

STRESS

Increased emotional or physical stress can contribute to allergies in ways that are often both subtle and overlooked.

OTHER FACTORS

- Frequent use of antibiotics, steroids, and other medications

- Hormonal changes due to the menstrual cycle, aging, or surgery

- Glandular disorders such as low thyroid function, thyroiditis, and adrenal insufficiency

- Physical trauma, such as accidents or surgery

- Electromagnetic disturbances of the environment

- Geopathic factors (harmful radiation from the earth)

- Dental amalgam fillings that contain large amounts of mercury or other dental involvement, such as infections under the teeth

 See Candidiasis, Gastrointestinal Disorders, Parasitic Infections, Stress.

Testing for Environmental Illness

An environmental physician may use a number of options for evaluating illnesses to determine if they are caused or exacerbated by allergies. Before embarking upon the often time-consuming and costly regimen of allergy tests, environmental medicine physicians typically begin the diagnostic process by conducting a comprehensive patient interview, which will include a history of prior health problems as well as detailed information on diet, potential exposure to environmental allergens at home or work, and levels of emotional stress. The information disclosed during such discussions can help the doctor assess which tests are indicated in each particular case.

An accompanying physical examination can help assess the level of dysfunction of the organs and systems of the body. Allergy specialist Leo Galland, M.D., of New York City, says that it is important to have more information than simply what allergen causes a person to react. "I want to know why this person is allergic and what factors are aggravating this person's allergy." He specifically looks for individual risk factors, such as parasitic infections and bacterial overgrowth. "Knowing the antecedents of an allergic condition," he explains, "allows me to help the person make more fundamental changes in their life so they are less sensitive to their allergic triggers."

Environmental medicine practitioners use the physical examination and employ various tests to uncover such antecedents. These include tests that screen for toxicity, liver and digestive malfunction, parasitic and bacterial infections, enzyme and nutritional deficiencies, and hormonal imbalances caused by stress. According to Dr.

Wilkinson, "In a thorough evaluation of the chronically ill, the history and physical exam might suggest nutritional problems, the presence of parasites or yeast, thyroid or adrenal disorders, the effect of dental work, psychospiritual issues, and other important considerations."

Laboratory Allergy Testing

Many alternative medicine practitioners consider the ELISA (enzyme-linked immunoserological assay) to be among the most sensitive and useful blood tests in detecting delayed food allergies. The ELISA requires a small blood sample to be taken from the patient, then sent within 72 hours to any of several specialized laboratories that perform this test. At the laboratory, technicians process the sample to collect the IgG antibodies, which are involved in delayed allergic reactions.

RAST (Radio Allergo Sorbent Test) is used by many doctors in diagnosing a patient's allergies. RAST testing can be a means of diagnosing allergies to pollens, molds, dust, and other allergens. RAST testing, however, is not very accurate in testing foods and it can be expensive.

Cytotoxic testing is commonly used by nutritionists to test for allergic reactions to foods and some chemicals. A technician mixes a suspected allergenic substance into a sample of the patient's blood and then examines the blood under a microscope for changes in white cells (lymphocytes, granulocytes, and platelets). Changes in the shape or amount of cells in response to the allergen indicate an allergic reaction.

Elimination-and-Challenge Diet

Often a doctor will suggest an elimination diet to detect food allergies. This involves eliminating the suspected food or foods from one's diet for 10-14 days with the hope that the symptoms disappear. Once the body is cleared of the test foods and the patient's symptoms have disappeared, they are ready to proceed with the "challenge" phase and reintroduce the test foods separately, as single-item meals. If they experience symptoms such as aches, pains, digestive difficulty, fatigue, an inability to think clearly, or any increase in a symptom within a few hours (although it may take up to 72 hours), it may be due to allergy. Ideally, one food is tested each day, and only organic foods are consumed to avoid mistaking a reaction to pesticide residue for a reaction to the food itself.[8] Though these vary from person to person, the foods that most frequently cause a reaction are milk products, wheat, yeast, corn, eggs, coffee, soy, potatoes, tomatoes, beef, pork, chicken, peanuts, oranges, chocolate, and sugar.

Skin Testing

Skin testing is a commonly used and fairly accurate means to test for allergies to pollens and it is about 35% accurate for molds. Unfortunately, it is not an accurate way to identify food allergies.[9] The most commonly used form of skin testing is the scratch test, which is done on the surface of the skin. Many environmental physicians use intradermal testing (an injection into the outer layers of the skin) for dust, molds, and pollens, as well as foods and chemicals. The response to therapy based on the intradermal testing can be more rapid and the testing itself, in the hands of an experienced physician, is a safe procedure.[10]

Provocation/neutralization is used by many environmental physicians for testing foods and determining what may be an effective neutralizing (symptom-relieving) dose. Control of symptoms can be achieved by injecting small amounts of allergenic material intradermally or subcutaneously (just beneath the skin) or by placing a few drops of the allergenic material under the tongue.

In a serial endpoint titration (SET) test, a physician injects a diluted amount of a potential allergen just below the skin. The ratio of dilution is up to the doctor; it may be as high at 1:5 or lower than 1:125. Each person's body will immediately react to the introduction of this foreign substance by forming a wheal of about 4 mm in diameter. Ten minutes after the injection, the wheal is measured again. A 5 mm diameter wheal indicates a non-allergic reaction, while a wheal of 7 mm or higher is a sign of an allergy. Further testing (called progressive whealing) is done with incrementally weaker or stronger amounts of diluted substances to determine the endpoint, or the lowest concentration at which a substance triggers a 2 mm growth in a wheal. In conventional immunotherapy, the endpoint concentration is used as the treatment dose for allergy shots. One advantage of this test is that it shows how strongly the body reacts to varying amounts of the substance; in other words, whether your allergy is mild, moderate, or severe. Allergists generally consider the SET test to be more accurate than the scratch test.

Electrodermal Screening (EDS)

One potentially useful but much less frequently employed method of testing utilizes electrodermal screening to measure minute changes in the electrical conductance of the skin. Changes in energy may be present before any biochemical or physiological change can be measured. Some clinicians claim that this method correlates extremely well with skin testing, is much faster, and avoids the pain and slight risk of an allergic reaction associated with injecting allergens into the skin.

Few clinical studies have tested the effectiveness of EDS as a tool for identifying allergy triggers. A 1997 double-blind, controlled study used EDS with 41 polysymptomatic allergy patients. In the first group of 17 patients, EDS correctly differentiated 82% of the time between house dust mite or histamine (allergens) and saline or water (nonallergens). In the second group of 24 patients, EDS discriminated 96% of the time between allergenic and nonallergenic substances, leading the researchers to state that EDS is a reliable method for detecting allergy triggers.[11]

Although EDS findings are accurate in diagnosis and in identifying food, environmental, and chemical allergy triggers, this information is not adequate for stand-alone diagnosis. The physician should order additional blood, urine, or stool tests to confirm the EDS results in all cases. Investigational device permits have been granted to some practitioners by the U.S. Food and Drug Administration (FDA) in order to review the usefulness of EDS as a diagnostic tool.

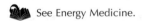 See Energy Medicine.

The Practice of Environmental Medicine

"The practice of environmental medicine is both strategic and comprehensive, rather than a limited treatment modality," says Dr. Oberg.[12] Among the treatment approaches employed by environmental medicine practitioners are the following:

- **Patient Education**—Practitioners of environmental medicine spend a great deal of time in educating patients regarding the causes of their illness and any dietary and lifestyle changes they can make to help regain their health.

- **Therapeutic Diets**—If you suffer from intestinal permeability and constantly eat the same foods over and over again, undigested molecules from these foods will frequently leak into the bloodstream, activating an allergic response. "A repetitive diet can contribute greatly to the development of allergies," says Dr. Mandell. "If someone eats bread every day, for instance, he could easily develop a wheat allergy due to the immune system's continuous exposure to it." A main step in eliminating allergies is to vary your diet. If you are no longer triggering allergic reactions and sending the immune system into chaos, the process of healing a leaky gut and normalizing immune function can begin. The rotation diet is a good way to change repetitive, allergy-inducing eating habits.

- **Detoxification Therapies**—Alternative medicine offers ways to begin "cleaning house" through safe and effective methods of detoxification. Detoxification flushes out toxins circulating in the bloodstream, embedded in soft tissues, and clogging important organs, so that healing and wellness can flourish. Detoxification programs can eliminate accumulated toxins, restore healthy function to key organs, and provide long-term maintenance and support. A detoxification program should be tailored to the individual's specific condition, including disease state, toxic burden, and the functional capacity of their major detoxifying organs (intestines, liver, and lymphatic system). The process must progress at a rate that the body can handle without causing greater injury. Numerous methods of detoxification are available, including fasting on water, juicing, specific diets, colon-cleansing therapies, kidney flushes, and homeopathic remedies. Related therapies for detoxification incorporate bodywork, lymphatic drainage, aromatherapy, antioxidant defense support, and nutrients and herbs to bolster the organs of detoxification. Any program of detoxification must include specific techniques for the mind to foster positive emotions and reduce stress.

  See Detoxification Therapy, Diet, Mind/Body Medicine, NAET, Nutritional Medicine.

- **Nutritional Therapy**—Nutritional supplementation (including vitamins, minerals, herbs, and "superfoods") is also important to correct deficiencies. They can be used in accordance with proper dietary habits to obtain the daily levels of nutrients specific to your needs, to treat diseases or health conditions, or to cope with environmental or lifestyle stresses. It is important to know your individual nutritional needs. The rate at which nutrients should be replaced through diet is dependent upon genetics, gender, exercise level, general health, and stress factors.

- **Immunotherapy**—Immunotherapy, or allergy shots, requires that patients receive injections containing extracts of the allergy-inducing substance. The shots may be given as often as daily in the beginning of the program, decreasing to once or twice a month. With each shot, the allergen is administered in progressively stronger doses until reaching the "maintenance level," the point at which the allergen is "neutralized"—that is, it no longer provokes an allergic reaction. In some cases, sublingual drops of allergen extracts are used instead of subdermal injections.

- **Psychotherapy or Counseling**—Stress is a common part of everyday life, but it can become harmful to the body when it is prolonged or chronic. It affects the body in very real, physical ways by influencing the immune and hormonal systems. For allergy sufferers, this can mean an exacerbation of allergic symptoms; stress can also lead to the onset of allergy and sensitivity. Psychotherapy, counseling, and a number of mind/body therapies can help reprogram negative thought patterns into more healthful ones, deal with stress in a positive way, and incorporate habits for relaxation into your life.

- **Environmental Controls**—Toxins and potential allergens are everywhere in our environment: pesticides in food, mercury in the mouth, industrial wastes in water, carbon monoxide and other chemicals in the air. However, there are many ways to reduce exposure to harmful substances, thereby preventing allergies and sensitivities from developing or helping to alleviate those that already exist. Numerous scientific reports advocate detoxifying the environment to prevent and treat allergies and sensitivities.[13] Many environmental medicine physicians concur with this recommendation, bearing in mind that it's nearly impossible to completely eliminate toxins outside, in the workplace, and in schools. The home is where most people will be able to effectively reduce their exposure to irritants and pollutants. "I try to teach my patients to create a safe haven within their own environment," says Abram Ber, M.D., of Scottsdale, Arizona. "You cannot just purchase things and bring them into the house and hope that everything will be fine. You have to live with consciousness."

- **Drugs**—Pharmaceutical medications are sometimes a necessary first step in allergy treatment by environmental medicine physicians, particularly in cases of acute allergies. However, research shows that antihistamines, cortisone, and other frequently prescribed allergy drugs have many adverse consequences. "The purpose of pharmaceuticals from the model of environmental medicine is to relieve patient symptoms while the underlying causes of their illnesses are being found and corrected," Dr. Oberg says.[14]

SUCCESS STORY: IMMUNOTHERAPY TO ELIMINATE ALLERGIES

Jane, 34, had a distressing list of debilitating allergy-associated symptoms. She had severe eczema on her face, arms, and hands, asthma, multiple chemical sensitivity, herpes, seasonal allergies, sinus infections, and autoimmune symptoms. Prior to seeing Stephen B. Edelson, M.D., of the Edelson Center for Environmental and Preventive Medicine, in Atlanta, Georgia, Jane had been treated by seven physicians (three allergists, two internists, and two dermatologists) but had not improved at all. She was taking prednisone (cortisone), three inhalants, and several antihistamines. "She was given drugs—antihistamines, steroids, and inhalants for her asthma—in other words, Band-Aids for all of her symptoms," comments Dr. Edelson.

Jane had nasal surgery for a deviated septum, hoping it would stop her sinus infections, against which antibiotics were only somewhat helpful. Instead, in the year after surgery, she had eight more infections—and her doctor proposed still more surgery for the problem. More ominous was the fact that the last conventional allergy shot Jane received had produced anaphylaxis, a severe, life-threatening allergic reaction. She ceased the shots after this near-disaster.

Before developing a treatment plan for Jane, Dr. Edelson ran a series of laboratory tests to get more information about her biochemical status. "I consider him somewhat of a detective because he used every means at his disposal to find hidden problems that could be the cause of my medical condition," Jane comments. Over the course of two "intense" days, Jane went through a battery of customized allergy testing. These tests proved that multiple food allergies were at the root of most of her discomfort.

Dr. Edelson also found that Jane had a low level of natural killer cell activity (meaning her immune system was not effective in disposing of disease agents) and she had high levels of two indicators of allergy activity (antibodies IgA and IgG). She was deficient in zinc, magnesium, and selenium, and she also had a positive ANA (antinuclear antibody) reading, indicating an autoimmune disease process.

Dr. Edelson started Jane on a series of enzyme-potentiated desensitization (EPD) injections, spacing them ever farther apart, so that after three years she was getting one injection every six months. In EPD, an allergic patient is given a series of standardized injections of a wide variety of allergens from a single category (such as inhalants), even though some of the items in the category may not be allergens for them. These injections, given over a period of weeks, differ from conventional allergy shots in at least three ways: multiple related allergens are given whereas allergy shots focus on only a few or individual allergens; EPD injects doses that are much weaker than allergy shots; and finally, given along with the allergens is an enzyme called beta-glucuronidase. This last component is important because beta-glucuronidase, injected at a level comparable to that present in the body, acts as a catalyst to make the vaccine more potent—that is, *potentiates* it. The allergens themselves, when given in such low doses, produce an immunity that eventually leads to desensitization.

He also put Jane on a daily nutritional program including vitamin C (12,000 mg) to bolster her immune response and the amino acid lysine (5,000 mg) to reverse her herpes. Within a year, Jane was able to discontinue all her conventional drugs. Today, nearly four years after starting treatment, Jane is "greatly improved," states Dr. Edelson. Of her improvement, Jane notes, "The EPD treatment had a tremendous impact on my quality of life. Although I am still not able to eat some foods and still have slight problems with my asthma when I am overexposed [such as in a smoke-filled room], I feel I am doing at least 90% better."

Conditions Benefited by Environmental Medicine

"Physicians who have been practicing environmental medicine for the past four decades point out that treating illnesses has become more and more complicated over the years due to the increased use of chemicals and medications," says Dr. Wilkinson. Seldom is the solution to a problem as simple as finding a single food that caused all of the patient's symptoms. Effective treatment requires the full participation and cooperation of the patient, who may be asked to make changes in lifestyle, diet, and environment, and perhaps minimize the use of pharmaceutical medications.

Mold and Pollen Allergies

To treat mold and pollen allergies, a person's living environment needs to be as clean as possible. There are also some medications that have minimal side effects and are

ILLNESSES HELPED BY ENVIRONMENTAL MEDICINE

- Allergies
- Angina
- Anxiety and panic
- Arrhythmia
- Asthma and chronic bronchitis
- Autoimmune thyroiditis
- Bed-wetting
- Behavioral and learning disabilities
- Canker sores
- Chronic fatigue syndrome
- Conjunctivitis, blurring of vision, itchy eyes, tearing, light sensitivity
- Dizziness, ringing in the ears, sinus headaches
- Ear infections
- Eating disorders
- Eczema and hives
- Edema (swelling) and fluid retention
- Epilepsy
- Gastroenteritis, diarrhea, constipation, gas, bloating, abdominal pain, ulcerative colitis, Crohn's disease
- Hay fever, nasal congestion, sneezing
- Headaches
- High blood pressure
- Hypoglycemia
- Infant colic
- Irritable bowel syndrome
- Lupus
- Manic-depressive psychosis, schizophrenia
- Muscle aches
- Premenstrual syndrome (PMS)
- Recurrent infections
- Rheumatoid arthritis, joint pain
- Sexual dysfunction
- Sleep disorders
- Sore throat
- Stomachaches
- Vaginitis, chronic cystitis

According to Dr. Mandell, eating the wrong foods during pollen season or peak mold season often makes the symptoms much worse and greatly reduces the effectiveness of therapy.

Food Allergies

Because frequently eaten foods remain constantly present in the system, allergic responses to them are responsible for many forms of chronic physical, mental, and emotional problems that are either misdiagnosed or inappropriately treated, according to Dr. Mandell. One effective and helpful method of treating food allergies is simply for patients to avoid, or at least dramatically decrease, the intake of foods to which they are allergic. This is the most consistent and widely used method of treatment. According to Dr. Mandell, symptoms caused by eating a known food allergen daily or twice weekly may be reduced by eating the same food only once every 7-10 days.

> *Even low-level exposure to a number of different chemicals can cause a wide variety of chronic diseases.*

There are, however, other ways to treat some types of food allergies, such as the provocation/neutralization technique. After skin testing for food allergies, treatments consisting of a mixture of very diluted symptom-relieving solutions of the offending foods can be administered to the patient by either injections or drops given under the tongue. A number of clinicians have found this technique to be an effective treatment for certain patients.[18]

One of Dr. Mandell's most interesting cases was a woman with cerebral palsy who suffered for years from unpredictable attacks of fatigue, painful muscle spasms, and loss of balance. Her neurologist told her that these symptoms were from the cerebral palsy and she should learn to accept them, because "that's the way cerebral palsy is." Dr. Mandell was able to reproduce several episodes of these symptoms in his office by performing symptom-duplicating provocative tests with a tomato extract. These tests were confirmed by having the woman take several single-food (tomato juice and fresh tomatoes) test meals at home at seven-day intervals. If she ate tomato juice and tomatoes once every two weeks, there were no unpredictable flare-ups of her symptoms. However, the attacks could be brought on by eating tomatoes, in any form, less than 12 days apart.

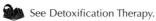 See Detoxification Therapy.

effective for simple hay fever symptoms. These can often be prescribed for short-term, seasonal hay fever. In some cases, it is necessary to test for allergies and then begin specific treatment to increase the body's resistance to those substances. This is best accomplished by using a customized mixture of treatment material prepared from the substances the patient is allergic to and administered in the form of drops taken under the tongue or shots.

ALLERGIES AND CHILDREN

It has been clearly demonstrated that food intolerance is an important cause of hyperactivity in many children.[15] Joseph Egger, M.D., a pediatric neurologist in Germany, has demonstrated an effective treatment for hyperactive children who have their symptoms triggered by food sensitivity. The children avoided the foods to which they were allergic for several months and they were given a very low-dose injection therapy called enzyme-potentiated desensitization (EPD), which is distinguished from conventional methods of desensitization by the fact that a minute amount of a naturally occurring enzyme is added to the antigen solution. The injections were given three times at two-month intervals. Fifteen of 17 patients were cured of their food sensitivities using this method.[16]

Marshall Mandell, M.D., of Norwalk, Connecticut, and Doris Rapp, M.D., past President of the American Academy of Environmental Medicine, have documented the often serious effects that allergies have on the nervous systems of many children with emotional, behavioral, and learning problems, as well as autism and seizures. During feeding tests and tests with sublingual drops prepared from foods and other types of offenders (pollens, molds, food coloring, cigarette smoke), the children suddenly became angry, confused, and hyperactive. Rapid and dramatic improvement was seen in many of these children who avoided or decreased their exposure to the offending substances.

A few years ago, the New York City public school system decided to change the children's school diet. They decreased the amount of sugar, food colorings, synthetic flavorings, and two commonly used preservatives. Over the next four years, there was a dramatic 15.7% increase in academic performance by students in the city's schools. Prior to the dietary changes, academic performance never varied more than 1% up or down in the course of a year.[17]

Chemical Sensitivity and Allergy

Chemical susceptibility was first described by Dr. Randolph. Today, it is commonly accepted that herbicides and pesticides in the food supply and environment pose a hazard to human health. Even low-level exposure to a number of chemicals can cause a wide variety of chronic diseases.[19] In addition, Michael A. Evans, Ph.D., Associate Professor at the University of Illinois College of Medicine, believes 70% to 80% of cancer cases are due to synthetic chemicals that are not themselves completely carcinogenic, but become carcinogenic when they interact with other environmental or genetic factors.[20]

The essential underlying causes of chemical sensitivity and allergies are still debated by medical researchers, even though a National Academy of Sciences workshop estimated that approximately 15% of people in the U.S. are chemically sensitive.[21] Many medical experts believe that at least part of this sensitivity is the result of the post–World War II petrochemical revolution.[22] Today, people are exposed to chemical concentrations far greater than were previous generations. Also, ecological changes in the environment are occurring faster than the body's capacity to adapt to them. There are currently about 55,000 chemical compounds in production: 3,000 chemicals are added to food supplies, over 700 are added to drinking water, and as many as 10,000 are used in the processing and storage of food.[23]

People are constantly exposed to products containing harmful substances that the body cannot properly break down: pesticides, gasoline, paints, industrial waste, household cleaners, smog, food preservatives, and dry-cleaning chemicals. According to the U.S. Environmental Protection Agency (EPA), more than 400 toxic chemicals have been identified in human tissue.[24] Certain pesticides like malathion, diazinon, and dursban accumulate in the nervous system and can cause brain disease, motor dysfunction, and psychological disturbances. Studies have shown that environmental pollutants can cause cancer as well as neurotoxic diseases including depression, apathy, and a diminished capacity to think.[25]

A distinguishing feature of multiple chemical sensitivity (MCS) is its "spreading" effect. After the sensitizing event or chronic low-level exposure to one or more chemicals, an individual becomes sensitive to an increasing number of substances. This may include chemicals that had never triggered reactions before the sensitization, such as glue, perfumes, air fresheners, or gasoline. It may also spread to include food, drugs, alcohol, caffeine, or even airborne allergens. "Switching" is another phenomenon associated with MCS, in which one symptom is replaced by another. For instance, whereas the smell of paint used to make you dizzy, it now gives you headaches.

Chemical sensitivities, like other forms of intolerance, vary in intensity. Some patients note mild irritation or headaches with exposure to certain substances. Others are so sensitive to virtually all chemicals that, to minimize their reactions, they are forced to leave their troubling environment and move to clean housing in unpolluted, rural areas. Frequently the milder forms of chemical sensitivity will improve with adequate intake of antioxidant vitamins and minerals (vitamins C and E, zinc, and selenium) and adjustments in diet, along with treatment for airborne allergens like pollen, mold, and dust mites. The more severe forms of allergies or sensitivity can be extremely complicated to treat. It takes persistence on the part of both the doctor and the patient to produce improvement.

Rheumatoid Arthritis

Rheumatoid arthritis has long confounded physicians. Conventional medicine essentially has nothing to offer the rheumatoid patient except various types of medication (which often cause serious side effects) or surgery to replace damaged joints. Environmental specialists know that adequate treatment of food, inhalant, and chemical allergies is an important factor in decreasing the lingering pain, disabling stiffness, and crippling effects associated with the disease. In a study of 53 patients with rheumatoid arthritis, the elimination of foods to which they were sensitive brought about a remarkable improvement in pain and flexibility.[26]

Dr. Mandell had a patient who was advised by an orthopedic surgeon to have both knees replaced because of severe and painful arthritis. His symptoms were reproduced in Dr. Mandell's office by provocative testing that indicated certain foods were probably the culprits. These foods were definitely confirmed as major offenders by single-food test meals. The arthritis dramatically improved by elimination of these foods. Today, Dr. Mandell's patient is walking comfortably, 12 years after the foods responsible for his severe arthritis were identified. The pain in his knees flares up only when these foods are eaten or after exposure to certain chemical fumes.

Dr. Mandell emphasizes that many people with arthritis may also have migraine headaches, asthma, and colitis that do not occur by coincidence. These symptoms represent bodywide allergies in predisposed individuals who have what Dr. Mandell calls "biological weak spots." He also points out that the condition of the rheumatoid patient is further complicated by fatigue, which he considers a form of brain allergy. He has performed thousands of provocative sublingual tests on patients with arthritis and reports that while one food can cause joint pain and swelling, another can cause headache and fatigue, while a third might bring on all of these symptoms. "Every patient is different," stresses Dr. Mandell. His findings point to the need for a more comprehensive approach to dealing with arthritis.

 See Arthritis.

 With the ever-increasing threat of global pollution, more research is needed to fully understand the impact of environmental factors on health. To support the use of government funds for research in this field, write your elected representatives.

The Future of Environmental Medicine

A thorough understanding of physiology and the interaction of the body with the environment allows specialists in environmental medicine to assist chronically ill patients in their quest for better physical and mental health. "This approach provides powerful insights and tools to improve the quality and cost effectiveness of health care and is effective because it is proactive, cause-oriented, patient-centered, individualized, and preventive," says Dr. Oberg.[27]

Due to advancements in this field, conventional medicine is turning increased attention to the findings of environmental medicine. "It's interesting to observe how conventional medicine is beginning to acknowledge that food and chemicals in the environment can cause a broad spectrum of physical ailments," says Dr. Wilkinson. "When I first became involved in environmental medicine, it was widely ridiculed by the mainstream of my profession."

Though conventional medicine is finally responding to the demands of patients for an environmental medicine perspective, Dr. Wilkinson points out that the realization of a problem does not rapidly translate into effective means of treatment. "Physicians who will continue to lead the way toward effective, physiologic therapy will be those who have spent years listening to their patients and exploring alternatives that offer the hope of helping them," he says.

Where to Find Help

For more information about, and referrals for, environmental medicine, contact the following organizations:

American Academy of Environmental Medicine
7701 East Kellogg Avenue, Suite 625
Wichita, Kansas 67207
(316) 684-5500
Website: www.aaem.com

The academy offers extensive training for physicians interested in learning more about environmental medicine.

American and International Boards of Environmental Medicine (ABEM/IBEM)
65 Wehrle Drive
Buffalo, New York 14255
(716) 837-1380

Provides board certification for medical doctors (M.D.s) and osteopaths (D.O.s) who wish to become certified as experts in environmental medicine.

Environmental Health Center
8345 Walnut Hill Lane, Suite 205
Dallas, Texas 75231
(214) 368–4132
Website: www.ehcd.com

This clinic handles severe cases of malnutrition and chemical exposure. Their therapy also treats heart problems, headaches, and joint pains.

Human Ecology Action League
P.O. Box 29629
Atlanta, Georgia 30359
(404) 248–1898
Website: members.aol.com/HEALNatnl/index.html

Contact HEAL for information on support groups located in many areas of the country that assist patients with environmental illness.

Immuno Labs, Inc.
1620 West Oakland Park Blvd., Suite 300
Fort Lauderdale, Florida 33311
(800) 231–9197
Website: www.immunolabs.com

Specialized allergy and immunology testing for physicians around the world. Provides referrals worldwide to physicians who do allergy testing.

Occupational and Environmental Unit, Tri-Cities Hospital
7525 Scyene Road
Dallas, Texas 75227
(214) 275–1430

Detoxification clinic using dry heat, intravenous supplements, exercise, and massage.

Recommended Reading

Allergy Free: An Alternative Medicine Definitive Guide. Konrad Kail, N.D., and Bobbi Lawrence, with Burton Goldberg. Tiburon, CA: AlternativeMedicine.com Books, 2000.

An Alternative Approach to Allergies. Theron G. Randolph, M.D., and Ralph Moss, Ph.D. New York: HarperCollins, 1990.

Alternative Medicine Guide to Chronic Fatigue, Fibromyalgia, and Environmental Illness. Burton Goldberg and the Editors of Alternative Medicine Digest. Tiburon, CA: Future Medicine Publishing, 1998.

Brain Allergies. William H. Philpott, M.D., and Dwight Kalita, Ph.D. Los Angeles: Keats Publishing, 2000.

Dr. Braly's Food Allergy and Nutrition Revolution. James Braly, M.D. New Canaan, CT: Keats Publishing, 1992.

Dr. Mandell's 5-Day Allergy Relief System. Marshall Mandell, M.D., and L. Scanlon. New York: Harper & Row, 1988.

The Food Allergy Book. William E. Walsh, M.D. New York: John Wiley, 2000.

Help for the Hyperactive Child. William G. Crook, M.D. Jackson, TN: Professional Books, 1991.

Human Ecology and Susceptibility to the Chemical Environment. Theron G. Randolph, M.D. Springfield, IL: Charles C. Thomas Publishing, 1976.

Is This Your Child? Discovering and Treating Unrecognized Allergies in Children and Adults. Doris Rapp, M.D. New York: William Morrow, 1992.

ENZYME THERAPY

Enzyme therapy can be an important first step in restoring health and well-being by helping to remedy digestive problems. Plant enzymes and pancreatic enzymes are used in complementary ways to improve digestion and absorption of essential nutrients. Treatment includes enzyme supplements, coupled with a healthy diet that features whole foods.

FOR EVERY CHEMICAL reaction that occurs in the body, enzymes provide the stimulus. "Enzymes are substances that make life possible," stated Edward Howell, M.D., who pioneered enzyme therapy in the United States. "No mineral, vitamin, or hormone can do any work without enzymes. They are the manual workers that build the body from proteins, carbohydrates, and fats. The body may have the raw building materials, but without the workers, it cannot begin."[1]

Without enzymes, there would be no breathing, no digestion, no growth, no blood coagulation, no sense perception, and no reproduction, states Anthony C. Cichoke, D.C., author of *Enzymes and Enzyme Therapy*. Enzymes are specific biological catalysts, each one stimulating a particular chemical reaction in the body. Thousands of metabolic enzymes are made by the body and are involved in all body processes, including breathing, thinking, talking, moving, and immune function. The body also manufactures digestive enzymes (secreted mainly by the pancreas, but also in the mouth, stomach, and small intestine), which play a vital role in the digestion of food.

Both plant-derived and pancreatic enzymes are employed in enzyme therapy and they can be used independently or in combination. Plant enzymes are prescribed to enhance the body's vitality by strengthening the digestive system, while pancreatic enzymes are beneficial to both the digestive system and immune system. As proper digestive functioning is restored, many acute and chronic conditions may also be remedied.

Enzymes and Digestion

The human body makes approximately 22 digestive enzymes, capable of digesting protein, carbohydrates, sugars, and fats. People digest food in stages: beginning in the mouth, moving to the stomach, and finally through the small intestine. At each step, specific enzymes break down different types of food. An enzyme designed to digest protein, for example, has no effect on starch, and an enzyme active in the mouth will not be active in the stomach. This process is balanced through acidity; each site along the digestive tract has a different degree of acidity that allows certain enzymes to function while inhibiting others.

As enzymes begin digesting food in the mouth and continue their work in the stomach, plant enzymes (derived from food itself or taken as a supplement) also become active. The food then enters the upper portion of the small intestine where the pancreas provides pancreatic enzymes to further break down the food. Final breakdown of remaining small molecules of food occurs in the lower small intestine. Ideally, these enzymes can work together, digesting food and delivering nutrients to cells to maintain their health. Protocols in enzyme therapy are based on this sequence of events.

Plant Enzyme Therapy

As plant enzymes are essential for the proper digestion of food, they can play an important role in promoting good health. This is the basis of treatment in plant enzyme therapy. "The ability to absorb the nutrients in the food we eat is at the foundation of good health," according to enzyme specialist Howard F. Loomis, Jr., D.C., of Madison, Wisconsin. "If we treat digestive disorders, other complaints often clear up as a result." In his practice, Dr. Loomis tests his patients for enzyme deficiency and then replenishes any deficiencies with enzyme supplements. Dr. Loomis adds, "Of course, if a patient is eating a diet of junk food, all the enzymes in the world won't improve basic health. Enzyme therapy needs to be combined with good eating habits. Fresh fruits, vegetables, nuts, and seeds

CAUSES OF ENZYME DEPLETION

- Pesticides and chemicals
- Hybridization and genetic engineering
- Bovine growth hormone (BGH)
- Pasteurization
- Irradiated food
- Excess intake of unsaturated and hydrogenated fats
- Cooking at high temperatures
- Microwaving
- Radiation and electromagnetic fields
- Geopathic stress zones
- Fluoridated water
- Heavy metals
- Mercury amalgam dental fillings
- Root canals

can provide plentiful plant enzymes, and plant enzyme supplements are only meant to supplement those that naturally occur in food."

All four categories of plant enzymes have uses in plant enzyme therapy. Protease digests protein; amylase digests carbohydrates; lipase digests fat; and cellulase digests fiber. Plants are a person's only source of cellulase as the body is unable to produce it. Numerous plant enzyme formulations on the market combine these enzymes.

As plant enzymes are essential for the proper digestion of food, they can play an important role in promoting good health.

Plant enzymes function in the stomach, predigesting the food, and plant enzyme therapy uses this to its advantage. This phenomenon was first proposed by Dr. Howell in the 1920s and the study of this process became his life's work.[2] "If the stomach is performing its proper role and we are eating our foods uncooked, a large portion of the intake will be partially digested before reacting with the stronger digestive juices found there," he stated. "Moreover, fewer of your body's internal digestive enzymes will be called upon to perform the digestive function." It is this easing of the body enzymes' workload that is thought to contribute substantially to the healing effects of enzyme therapy. When the body

receives plentiful supplies of enzymes, according to Dr. Howell, "its internal enzyme supplies are preserved for the important work of maintaining metabolic harmony." As a result, many body systems are strengthened.[3]

This predigestion of food happens during an interim period, before enough hydrochloric acid (HCl) accumulates in the stomach to begin the next stage in digestion, but this is not commonly known. As Lita Lee, Ph.D., of Lowell, Oregon, states, "Many people don't believe this because they are told that gastric HCl excreted by the stomach destroys the enzymes." Actually, it takes 30–60 minutes before enough HCl accumulates in the stomach to initiate the digestion of food. HCl does not destroy but merely deactivates these enzymes by making the environment more acidic. They are reactivated later in the duodenum (upper segment of the small intestine) if the optimum, more alkaline pH is achieved. Enzymes in the stomach can digest 30% to 40% of the starches we eat.[4] And Dr. Lee adds, "By eating raw foods and taking food enzymes, 30% of the protein and 10% of the fat can be digested in the stomach in less than one hour."

Cooking food can destroy these important plant enzymes. They are more heat-sensitive than vitamins and are the first to be destroyed during cooking. They are destroyed by being heated above 118° F,[5] and, as Dr. Lee points out, "are deactivated or destroyed by pasteurizing, canning, and microwaving." However, while raw foods are recommended, a 100% raw foods diet is not necessary. Dr. Loomis points out that some people may have problems digesting uncooked food because of a lack of cellulase. "People who rarely eat raw food can have problems when they finally eat uncooked fruits and vegetables because they don't chew their food thoroughly," says Dr. Loomis. "Chewing liberates the cellulase out of the food, but when they eat the raw food and don't chew properly, the cellulase is never released. Cellulase may also be lacking because of the way the food was handled by the suppliers. Some supermarket vegetables are missing cellulase because they have been sprayed with sulfites, which can destroy these enzymes."

Plant Enzyme Deficiency

In her practice, Dr. Lee has frequently seen the consequences of eating a predominantly cooked-foods diet—inflammation, pancreatic hypertrophy (enlargement), a toxic colon, and allergies. Because of inflammation, conditions such as bronchitis, sinusitis, cystitis, rhinitis, and arthritis may occur, and may be accompanied by fever, redness, swelling, and pain. Pancreatic hypertrophy results when a diet lacking in enzymes puts an extra strain on the enzyme production of the pancreas. If the pancreas falls behind in its work, the organ will enlarge just as a thyroid grows a goiter when it cannot make enough hormones.

Low levels of enzymes can also lead to a toxic colon. Undigested food can remain in the intestine and not be excreted. Here, the molecules are converted into toxins that are transported by the blood to the liver for detoxification. If the liver is overworked, however, it will be unable to properly detoxify the blood. In his practice, Dr. Loomis analyzes the urine and often finds toxins such as phenols (an organic molecule with a structure similar to alcohol) present. Presence of these phenols can lead to a wide range of problems, including allergies, acne, sciatica, and breast pathology.[6]

A meal of predominantly cooked foods can also lead to digestive leukocytosis (an increased white blood count). A rise in white blood cells is a sign that the immune system is being mobilized. It accompanies many pathological conditions, including infections and poisoning, but it can also occur immediately after eating breakfast, lunch, or dinner. "Digestive leukocytosis occurs a mere 30 minutes after eating cooked food," says Dr. Lee. "This does not occur when a person eats raw food because of the presence of plant enzymes in this food." Such a response puts added stress on the immune system. "The concept of the immune system being stimulated every time you eat was first reported in 1897 by Rudolph Virchow, the father of cellular pathology. In other words, your immune system is stimulated, as if you had an infection," confirms Dr. Loomis.

Benefits of Plant Enzyme Therapy

According to Dr. Lee, when a patient's enzyme deficiencies are addressed, many other conditions can resolve, from digestive ailments and common sore throats to hay fever, ulcers, and candidiasis. In one instance, Dr. Lee used plant enzymes to treat a case of chronic digestive disorders. A 57-year-old man had suffered from severe intestinal problems for most of his adult life. A number of medical specialists had provided him with varying diagnoses, including spastic colon, diverticulitis, yeast imbalance, and lactose intolerance, but none of them were able to discover the cause of the condition. He tried several changes of diet without success, and eventually was placed on the drug Lomotil to treat his diarrhea. After meals, he continued to experience painful cramps, diarrhea, headaches, and an overall sense of weakness, and was finally told that there was no cure for this condition. Dr. Lee used a 24-hour urinalysis and blood profile to diagnose the patient's problem as a lipase enzyme deficiency, coupled with fiber intolerance. After four months of

---

HEALTH CONDITIONS AND ENZYME DEFICIENCIES

The following are some of the health conditions commonly associated with shortages of each of the four basic enzymes:

- Protease (digests proteins)—Anxiety; low blood sugar; kidney problems; water retention; depressed immunity; bacterial and viral infections; cancer; appendicitis; bone problems, such as osteoporosis, arthritis, and bone spurs.

- Amylase (digests nonfiber carbohydrates)—Skin problems such as rashes, hives, fungal infections, herpes, and canker sores; lung problems such as asthma, bronchitis, and emphysema; liver or gallbladder disease.

- Lipase (digests fats)—High cholesterol; obesity; diabetes; hardening of the arteries and other cardiovascular problems; chronic fatigue; spastic colon; dizziness.

- Cellulase (digests fiber)—Gas and bloating; acute food allergies; facial pain or paralysis; candidiasis (bowel and vaginal yeast infections).

---

enzyme supplements, the man's condition was completely improved with no recurrence of symptoms.

Plant enzyme therapy can also increase the absorption of nutrients. Dr. Lee recalls a case of myasthenia gravis (a disease characterized by extreme muscle weakness), which is associated with a deficiency in the B vitamins, vitamin E, and manganese. With enzymes, the patient was able to lower the vitamin and mineral dosage since these nutrients were now more easily absorbed. In another case, a young child was diagnosed with severe iron anemia. Given a formulation of iron plus enzymes, the child's condition improved within three days. Dr. Lee points out, "People think that if they simply take vitamins and minerals they will be healthy, but every vitamin and mineral requires an enzyme. You can eat pounds and pounds of vitamins and minerals, but if you don't have the proper enzymes, they won't work."

Many women subject to osteoporosis benefit from taking extra protease and/or lipase enzymes, states Dr. Lee. Protease, the enzyme that digests protein, is required to carry calcium in the blood. Without proper digestion of protein, both protein-bound and ionic calcium levels

HOW TO DIAGNOSE AN ENZYME DEFICIENCY

Along with a patient history and diet survey, many alternative health-care professionals rely on urine analysis to assess a patient's digestive function and enzyme status. The urinalysis provides information on what a person cannot digest, absorb, or assimilate, along with any potential nutritional deficiencies. This test is prognostic rather than diagnostic, except for the identification of substances, such as glucose, not normally found in the urine, which would indicate disease conditions (this is the focus of standard urine tests). In other words, it predicts what lies ahead if you do not clean up your diet and digestion.

Dr. Loomis emphasizes that an individual's total urine output over a 24-hour period must be collected, not just periodic samples. This enables a physician to see how the concentrations of various substances in the urine change over time. The fluctuations are then averaged to give a complete picture of digestive problems. Looking at a 24-hour urinalysis is a way of peeking at the blood, explains Dr. Loomis. The health of the blood takes precedence in the body and cells will sacrifice nutrients in the service of maintaining the blood's relatively narrow pH range of 7.35 to 7.45 as well as its supply of electrolytes, protein, and other nutrients. Thus, the blood takes what it needs from the cells to achieve its necessary balance, or homeostasis.

Another important information-gathering procedure in enzyme therapy is the palpation test. Palpation means to elicit information by touch. Pain and internal organ dysfunction are always accompanied by muscle contraction. The enzyme therapist uses palpation to identify these places of muscle contraction to pinpoint stresses or dysfunction in the body. Dr. Loomis developed a palpation test in which each positive palpation point (meaning there is a muscle contraction) corresponds to a deviation in structure (vertebral subluxation), which, in turn, corresponds to an undernourished organ. Each palpation point also corresponds to one of his enzyme formulations, so palpation serves as both diagnosis and guideline for treatment.

For the test, patients must fast for at least two hours. With the patient lying face-up on a chiropractic table, the practitioner first observes the position of the hips and feet. In most people, one hip is higher or lower than the other, and sometimes one leg is longer or shorter than the other. Then, the practitioner tests palpation points by touch and observes any shift in the position of the hips or leg lengths following palpation. Any observed shift (for example, uneven hips become even) indicates a positive palpation, which means that the person may need the enzyme formulation corresponding to this palpation point. This phase of the test can also reveal nutritional deficiencies and acute conditions such as viral or bacterial infections. Then, the patient eats a meal. After 45 minutes, the palpation test is repeated. Positive palpation points now indicate what the body cannot digest. They also indicate acute and chronic conditions, including inflammation, kidney or urinary tract problems, soft tissue trauma, allergies, and colon problems.

---

in the blood will not be adequate. Lipase is required to carry calcium across the intestinal wall and for the production of female hormones. Thus a deficiency in either of these enzymes could contribute to osteoporosis.

Dr. Lee has also successfully treated patients who have had candidiasis (a *Candida* overgrowth) for years. "They've tried all the popular yeast remedies, including nystatin, probiotics (substances such as acidophilus and *Bifidobacteria* that act to reestablish the intestinal flora), herbals, homeopathics, and fatty acids of many kinds," states Dr. Lee. "Many of them still had the yeast overgrowth plus liver damage due to the nystatin. I used a very potent remedy containing acidophilus, *Bifidobacteria*, and cellulase enzymes. This formula is taken to digest the yeast and reestablish friendly bowel bacteria. Along with this, a protease formula is used to remove the toxic debris. This treatment works very well with homeo-pathics and herbals and I do not hesitate to add these to the enzyme protocol when needed."

It cannot be said that a particular enzyme can help a particular illness. Any treatment is multifaceted, requiring various enzymes plus other modes of care, as well as adherence to a healthy diet with adequate raw foods.

—HOWARD LOOMIS, D.C.

The FDA (Food and Drug Administration) has long approved the use of plant enzymes, but as dietary supplements only. "All we are saying is that by clearing up digestive problems, we've found that many other problems seem to go away and new ailments may be prevented," states Dr. Loomis. "It cannot be said that a particular enzyme can help a particular illness. Any treatment is multifaceted, requiring various enzymes plus other modes of care, as well as adherence to a healthy diet with adequate raw foods."

Pancreatic Enzyme Therapy

The history of pancreatic enzyme therapy predates the work in plant enzyme therapy. In 1902, English embryologist John Beard injected pancreatic extracts directly into tumors of cancer patients with therapeutic success.[7] When others tried this method and failed, mainly due to the impurity of the extract preparations, the therapy fell into disrepute. Later in Germany, Max Wolf, M.D., and Karl Ransberger, Ph.D., used enzymes to successfully treat patients with multiple sclerosis, cancer, and viral infections. The two men provided some of the earliest research on enzymes and co-enzymes.[8]

Hector Solorzano del Rio, M.D., D.Sc., Coordinator of the Program for Studies of Alternative Medicine and Professor of Pharmacology at the University of Guadalajara, in Mexico, is one of the many physicians who uses pancreatic enzyme therapy. He has treated a wide variety of diseases—inflammatory conditions such as rheumatic disorders, soft tissue trauma, viral infections, arthritis, multiple sclerosis, cancer, autoimmune diseases, and AIDS. Dosages are given orally on an empty stomach or by injection and may be combined with plant enzymes.

Pancreatic enzymes are animal enzymes that include protease, amylase, and lipase. Pancreatic enzymes function in the intestine and in the blood. By supplementing the body's own enzymes, pancreatic enzyme therapy, like plant enzyme therapy, promotes health by lessening the demands on the body for supplying enzymes to convert food to usable nutrients and energy. Pancreatic enzymes also play a fascinating role in the immune system, directly assisting the defense mechanisms,[9] and this function has been shown to make a significant contribution to the therapeutic powers of these enzymes.

"Protein molecules that are only partially digested in the small intestine are able to be absorbed into the bloodstream," according to Dr. Loomis. The immune system treats these molecules as invaders. Antibodies couple with these antigens (foreign substances that provoke

VITAMINS, MINERALS, AND ENZYMES

"In enzyme therapy we recommend that patients eat whole, unprocessed foods with plenty of raw foods included," states Lita Lee, Ph.D. "This has many benefits, but not just because these foods provide enzymes. Whole foods also contain vitamins and minerals, embedded in the mother plant, that function as co-enzymes, molecules that also must be present for a chemical reaction to take place."

One of the most important processes in the metabolism of food is the chain of reactions that convert glucose to energy. Several vitamin and mineral co-enzymes are necessary for these reactions and are consumed in the process. Our bodies need a continuing supply. "All the food we eat, which eventually becomes energy, passes through this same set of reactions, whether the food is a hamburger or a raw carrot," says Dr. Lee. "Co-enzymes are always needed, and when the food doesn't provide these, we use the vitamins and minerals stored in our body until these reserves are used up. Only when we eat whole and raw foods can we maintain a good supply of the parts that keep the metabolic machinery going."

an immune reaction) and circulating immune complexes (CICs) are formed. In a healthy person, these CICs may be neutralized in the lymphatic system. But in a sick person, CICs accumulate in the blood where they can initiate an "allergic" reaction. As too many CICs accumulate, the kidneys cannot excrete enough and the CICs begin to accumulate in soft tissues, causing inflammation. This brings unnecessary stress to the immune system. Dr. Loomis comments, "I always wonder why the diets for cancer and AIDS patients include such high amounts of protein when an excess of undigested protein can so obviously lead to demands on the immune system."

It is here that pancreatic enzymes come into play. The pancreatic enzymes are able to break down CICs so that they can pass through the kidneys for excretion. The enzymes are taken between meals so they will not be used for digesting food, but will make their way directly to the bloodstream. Because of their ability to digest foreign proteins, pancreatic enzymes are also able to clear out infecting organisms such as viruses, scar tissue, and the products of inflammation. For this reason, pancreatic enzymes are used in a variety of conditions, including lung infections, tooth infections, bone fractures, and are recommended prior to surgery.

Further research into the benefits of pancreatic enzyme therapy is needed as it has been clinically proven to alleviate a wide range of conditions.

Conditions Benefited by Pancreatic Enzyme Therapy

Pancreatic enzymes have been shown to be beneficial in a variety of disease conditions, including inflammation, viral diseases, heart disease, multiple sclerosis, and cancer.

INFLAMMATION

Inflammation is a response to noxious stimuli and is a way the body rids itself of harmful substances. The classic signs of inflammation are pain, redness, swelling, and heat. Once inflammation takes place, however, healing can begin. With sports injuries, enzymes are used to promote inflammation in order to accelerate healing, and taking them before performing athletics can promote faster healing if injury occurs.

VIRAL DISEASES

Viruses have a protein coat and enzymes are able to initiate reactions that can digest this protective layer so that the viruses can be destroyed. Enzymes help in the removal of CICs that are abundant in viral disease. Research also indicates that enzymes are beneficial in the treatment of herpes zoster (shingles), particularly in patients with immune deficiencies.[10] And enzymes can in part counteract the decreased immune function of HIV (human immunodeficiency virus) infection.[11]

HEART DISEASE

A common precursor of many cardiovascular problems is atherosclerosis, in which the inner arterial walls harden and thicken due to deposits of fatty substances. These substances form a plaque that, with buildup, causes a narrowing of the arteries. High cholesterol is commonly cited as the culprit behind plaque formation. This misguided explanation not only ignores some important facts about cholesterol, including that it is vital to crucial body processes, but dangerously overlooks numerous contributing factors to heart disease.

There is growing evidence that a major culprit responsible for oxidizing cholesterol and producing atherosclerosis is homocysteine, a substance naturally found in the body.[12] Homocysteine is a by-product of protein metabolism (specifically, of the amino acid methionine, found mainly in red meat and milk products). Homocysteine increases free radicals (oxysterol formation), a major factor in damaging blood vessel walls. Enzymes are necessary for converting homocysteine to the harmless amino acid cystathionine.

Vulnerable plaque is another area of recent research in heart disease. It is made up primarily of "soft" cholesterol and is contained in a thin fibrous cap. This cap is weaker than obstructing, hard plaque and more easily ruptured. The body treats vulnerable plaque as an infection and the immune response can break up the cap, releasing powerful coagulants and potentially leading to massive, lethal clotting. The body normally uses enzymes to balance clot formation and dissolution. Fibrinogen (a component of the fibrous cap) levels, clotting activities, and C-reactive protein (an indicator of inflammation) can be reduced using enzyme therapy.[13]

Recent reports also indicate that infections may be a causative factor in many heart attacks. A number of organisms have been implicated, including cytomegalovirus, herpes, and *Chlamydia pneumoniae*.[14] As indicated previously, enzymes are effective at dissolving the protective protein coat of viruses. According to Garry F. Gordon, M.D., enzymes "can be particularly useful in protection against heart attacks and strokes because they can provide safe, long-term management of these various molecular-based risk factors."

MULTIPLE SCLEROSIS

Although the cause of multiple sclerosis (MS) is unknown, it has been shown that demyelination (reduction of the fatty covering of the nerves) occurs. Dr. Solorzano tells of a wheelchair-bound patient diagnosed with MS that no traditional treatment had helped. Trying pancreatic enzyme therapy, the patient gained strength and could dress himself within one month. After three months, he could work (with some difficulty); within six months, his symptoms disappeared and he was able to resume a normal, productive life. One possible explanation for MS is that the demyelination process may be due to CICs accumulating in nerve tissue and causing damage.[15] Enzyme therapy helps stimulate white blood cells to attach to and eliminate the immune complexes and decrease inflammation.

CANCER

Pancreatic enzymes can help in the treatment of cancer in several ways. Enzymes help expose antigens on the surface of cancer cells, so they can be recognized as foreign and destroyed by the immune system. It is now thought that the cancer cell uses a protein called fibrin (or sometimes fats and lipids) to mask its identity, effectively hiding from the immune system. A logical therapeutic strategy would involve degrading the cancer cell's coating, allowing it to be identified by the immune system.[16] Enzymes help destroy CICs produced when cancerous cells shed their antigens into the blood to avoid detection by the immune system. Pancreatic enzymes can stimulate natural killer cells, T cells, and tumor necrosis factor (anticancer agents), all toxic to cancer cells.[17]

According to Dr. Solorzano, by removing the "sticky" coating found on tumor cells, enzymes reduce the risk of tumors adhering to other areas of the body (preventing metastasis).[18] The use of anticoagulants and enzymes can effectively reduce the invasive or metastatic potential of cancer cells.[19] And pancreatic enzymes can enter cancer cells in their reproductive phase, when they are not completely formed and are more susceptible to destruction. Vitamin A increases these effects, as it releases enzymes contained in lysosomes (components of the intercellular digestive system); it is often given in combination with pancreatic enzymes. In Germany, pancreatic enzyme solutions have been injected directly into tumors, causing them to dissolve.[20]

Some European physicians addressing cancer and other illnesses use special enzyme formulations called Wobenzyme® and Wobe-Mugos®, first developed in Germany (available from health practitioners in the United States). These formulas contain pancreatin, papain, bromelain, trypsin, chymotrypsin, lipase, amylase, and rutin (a bioflavonoid), and are administered by injection, tablets, or suppositories. Dr. Wolf started using Wobe-Mugos and other multi-enzyme formulas in 1949. He treated over 1,000 patients using oral doses of 200 mg daily, then raising it to 2-4 g daily. For 107 women who had undergone mastectomies, their five-year survival rate was 84% under Wobenzyme therapy compared to 43% to 48% with conventional therapy, reported Dr. Wolf. Localized application produced better results than systemic use, and long-term use produced the best results in stopping the spread of cancer.

Research reported by the product's manufacturer indicated that pancreatic cancer responded well to this treatment, with 30 patients still alive two years after receiving the enzymes; some of these patients survived 5-9 years. Nicholas Gonzalez, M.D., of New York City, used diet, detoxification, and large doses of enzymes with 11 patients with pancreatic cancer; 81% survived for one year and 45% for two years.[21] This must be seen in contrast to the "standard" survival expectation of seven months for pancreatic cancer. For post-surgical breast cancer patients with Stage I and Stage III cancers, the use of enzymes produced five-year survival rates of 91% and 58%, respectively, compared to 78% and 42% under conventional treatment.[22]

The Future of Enzyme Therapy

There are now over 2,000 enzyme therapists in the U.S. and the field of enzyme therapy is rapidly expanding. "I think enzyme therapy is the wave of the future and will revolutionize the field of nutrition. All preventive therapies will include treatment of enzyme deficiencies and all food supplements will address our need for enzymes," states Dr. Lee.

The use of pancreatic enzyme therapy in the field of medicine has a head start because it already has been the subject of much research in Europe. And Dr. Loomis envisions, "If research funds were currently as available to study all types of enzyme therapy in the United States as they are in Europe, tremendous strides could be taken. The future could be particularly bright for plant enzyme therapy. Depletion of plant enzymes leads to a host of chronic diseases that could in part be avoided if we provided the body with the enzymes it needs. As it is, we are not aware of enzyme deficiencies because they take so long to manifest. When there are signs, the body is already in a state of exhaustion. It is here that the future of plant enzyme therapy lies, in its potentially enormous role in nutrition and the prevention of chronic degenerative disease."

Where to Find Help

For more information on clinics and practitioners using enzyme therapy, contact:

Lita Lee, Ph.D.
P.O. Box 516
Lowell, Oregon 97452
(541) 937-1123

For information on doctors using plant enzyme therapy.

Howard Loomis, D.C.
21st Century Nutrition
6421 Enterprise Lane
Madison, Wisconsin 53719
(800) 662-2630 or (608) 273-8100

For information on doctors using plant enzyme therapy. In the early 1980s, Dr. Loomis formulated his first line of enzymes called NESS (Nutritional Enzyme Support System). Since then, Dr. Loomis's research has led to Thera-zyme, his second generation line of enzymes, available to health practitioners from 21st Century Nutrition. These formulas have a counterpart for consumers called Enzyme Solutions.

Hector E. Solorzano, M.D., D.Sc.
Universidad de Guadalajara
Los Alpes No. 1024 Col. Independencia
44340 Guadalajara, Jalisco, Mexico
(01) 3637-7237, 3651-5476

For further information on clinics and practitioners in Mexico.

Recommended Reading

Complete Book of Enzyme Therapy. Anthony J. Cichoke. Garden City Park, NY: Avery Penguin Putnam, 1998.

The Enzyme Cure. Lita Lee, Ph.D., and Lisa Turner, with Burton Goldberg. Tiburon, CA: Future Medicine Publishing, 1998.

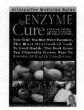

Enzyme Nutrition. Edward Howell, M.D. Wayne, NJ: Avery Publishing Group, 1985.

Enzymes and Enzyme Therapy. Anthony J. Cichoke. Los Angeles: Keats Publishing, 2000.

Food Enzymes for Health and Longevity. Edward Howell, M.D. Twin Lakes, WI: Lotus Press, 1994.

FLOWER ESSENCES

The emotions play a crucial role in the health of the physical body. Flower essences directly address a person's emotional state in order to help facilitate both psychological and physiological well-being. By balancing negative feelings and stress, flower essences can effectively remove the emotional barriers to health and recovery.

BEHIND ALL DISEASE lies our fears, our anxieties, our greed, our likes and dislikes," wrote English physician Edward Bach, M.B., B.S., M.R.C.S., L.R.C.P., D.H.P., in the early 1930s.[1] Dr. Bach based his revolutionary belief upon his personal observations of patients whose physical illnesses seemed to be predisposed by negative psychological or emotional states such as fear, anxiety, insecurity, jealousy, shyness, poor self-image, anger, and resentment. Today, numerous studies conducted at major universities and medical centers have verified Dr. Bach's early conviction, revealing a definite connection between negative emotional and mental states and a reduction of the body's natural resistance to disease.

"True healing involves treating the very base of the cause of the suffering," said Dr. Bach. "Therefore, no effort directed to the body alone can do more than superficially repair damage. Treat people for their emotional unhappiness, allow them to be happy, and they will become well."[2]

In Dr. Bach's day, conventional medicine had no real methodology to address the link between emotional and physical illness, relying instead upon the use of drugs, which often did more harm than good. In an attempt to fill this void, he began to investigate the healing potential of the wildflowers native to the English countryside. After six years of extensive research and testing, he was able to identify 38 flowers of nonpoisonous plants, trees, and shrubs that, when prepared according to a specific homeopathic process he developed, had a profound effect

> *True healing involves treating the very base of the cause of the suffering. No effort directed to the body alone can do more than superficially repair damage. Treat people for their emotional unhappiness, allow them to be happy, and they will become well.*
>
> —DR. EDWARD BACH

on the underlying psychological and emotional states that influence physical illness. These special preparations became known as the Bach® Flower Remedies, renamed the Bach® Flower Essences in America.

Proven effective by licensed health professionals for nearly 70 years, flower essences are a noninvasive therapy sold over-the-counter. They are taken internally by mouth or rubbed topically on pulse points. Because they are nontoxic and nonaddictive, they have no side effects and can be used without professional guidance. "The essences do not interact or interfere with medications or supplements and are totally complementary to all other healing modalities," explains Alicia Sirkin, B.F.R.P., an internationally published Bach Foundation registered practitioner, educator, and expert on the Bach essences. "They even seem to make other modalities work better, a claim made by Dr. Bach himself and later confirmed by therapists in other fields."

According to Sirkin, flower essences are chosen for states of mind, not to relieve physical problems. "Due to the fact that negativity can surround a physical problem, the essences are often an important component in a person's recovery," she says. When emotional distress is eased with the essences, physical problems are often relieved as well. Using this simple therapy, individuals can take control of their healing by first identifying problematic thoughts and feelings, then selecting appropriate flower essences to re-establish harmony and balance. "The result is a more positive outlook, often with feelings of self-

THE ORIGIN OF BACH FLOWER ESSENCES

Dr. Edward Bach was a British physician, bacteriologist, pathologist, immunologist, and researcher. Known for the successful development of conventional vaccines to treat intestinal toxemia, his later research resulted in safer homeopathic versions called Bach Nosodes. Dr. Bach's knowledge and understanding of homeopathic remedy preparation primed him for the groundbreaking work in the discovery and creation of flower remedies, which he called simply "herbs." An early pioneer in the field of mind/body medicine, he dedicated his life to the discovery of a safe and gentle system of self-healing that dealt with the underlying causes of disease. Leaving his lucrative conventional medical practice in London, Dr. Bach spent years searching the countryside of Wales and England for nonpoisonous healing plants. Intuitively, he sensed that dewdrops from certain plants might contain specific healing properties of the plant. Eventually, he hypothesized that the sun's heat could activate and install the plant's healing attributes within the dewdrops themselves.

Bach formulated his 38 essences by experimenting on himself. His senses were so highly developed that by simply holding the petal of a flower in his hand or placing it on his tongue, his body would feel the effect of the flower's qualities. At times, he suffered extreme emotional states that propelled his search for a plant remedy that would effect a cure. His personal trials formed the basis for testing on others, resulting in the applications of the essences as they are used today.

dition of the patient should not be the primary focus of concern. Nora Weeks, Dr. Bach's companion and assistant, summed up his credo in *The Medical Discoveries of Edward Bach, Physician,* "Treat the state of mind or the moods and, with the return to normal, the disease, whatever it might be, would go also." Health practitioners who use Bach flower essences set out to affect physical problems of the body by addressing their emotional and psychological causes. "As the emotions stabilize and general health—especially emotional outlook—improves, the illness begins to dissipate," Dr. Bach wrote. "This seems to be accomplished by the triggering of mechanisms that stimulate the internal healing processes."[3]

Studies from the field of mind/body medicine have confirmed that the psychological and emotional state of a person influences a myriad of bodily processes, for better or worse, by stimulating or suppressing immune activity, adrenal hormones, and neurotransmitters.[4]

 See Mind/Body Medicine, Homeopathy.

Unlike most pharmaceutical drugs, flower essences work subtly, triggering healing mechanisms within the body as they gently resolve underlying emotional stress. Most often, as the essences take effect, one will not even have a sense of having had an emotional problem. Only in retrospect will one be able to determine where attitudes have changed or resolved themselves.[5] Elisabeth Wiley, a psychotherapist and nationally known Bach flower essence practitioner, believes that the essences' bioenergetic frequencies are able to repair imbalances in the human energy field. Research has also shown that Bach flower essences, although clearly different from homeopathy per se, may have a complementary role with homeopathic remedies and share common ground in terms of their respective healing mechanisms.[6] Usually flower remedies prove effective in removing the emotional blocks to recovery in one to 12 weeks. However, in some instances of deeply rooted psychological patterns or beliefs, a longer time period may be required. Once a patient's emotional state has improved, the essences no longer need to be taken. Furthermore, in addition to not creating any physical dependencies, Bach flower essences have a self-diminishing effect.[7] This means that both the need for and the effectiveness of the essences diminish as the patient moves toward a more balanced and healthy emotional level.

According to Sirkin, the essences can be taken any time of day and do not interfere or interact negatively with medications, natural supplements, or any other healing therapy. She cautions, however, that individuals taking the prescription medication Antabuse for alcoholism must not take Bach flower essences due to the small amount of brandy (alcohol) used as a preservative in the liquid.

empowerment," says Sirkin. "By offering relief from the burden of negativity, the essences in effect can work to prevent stress-induced physiological breakdown."

Since the late 1970s, a number of companies have researched and produced additional flower essences derived from flowers native to America and other countries worldwide, but the original 38 remedies discovered by Dr. Bach still remain the core of all flower remedies today.

How Flower Essences Work

"Think of the patient, not the disease; the cause, not the effect," was Dr. Bach's motto concerning health and the use of his flower remedies. He felt that the physical con-

Conditions Benefited by Flower Essences

"All know that the same disease may have different effects on different people; it is the effects that need treatment, because they guide to the real cause," wrote Dr. Bach in *The Twelve Healers and Other Remedies*. Because of this, flower practitioners take little account of a named illness or disease, focusing instead on their patients' emotional states. Flower essences, rather than relating to any specific physical manifestations or symptoms, relate only to specific psychological and emotional states. As there is no universal corresponding psychological equivalent for every physical condition, each patient must be diagnosed individually. "You rarely use the same remedy, or combination of remedies, with any two people," says Abram Ber, M.D., of Phoenix, Arizona, "even if they display similar physical conditions." For example, two patients can suffer from chronic headaches, yet for one fear may be the overriding emotional cause, while for the other it may be loneliness.[8]

"Flower remedies are particularly beneficial in helping to relieve acute trauma associated with accidents, bruises, and injuries, as well as grief following the loss of a loved one," adds Dr. Ber. He also believes that using flower remedies can be a tremendous preventative therapy and that by correcting underlying emotional problems, one can ensure that many physical problems will never recur.

In his writings, Dr. Bach carefully outlined and described the various emotional and psychological states and personality traits for which the remedies are used. Though stated simply, his descriptions coincide with and reveal a more complex assessment of underlying discordant patterns. (For an updated version, see "The 38 Bach Flower Essences and Their Indications for Use" below.)

Alec Forbes, M.D., Medical Director of the Cancer Help Center, in Bristol, England, and a former member of the World Health Organization's Expert Advisory Panel on Traditional Medicine, has used flower remedies for over 30 years. Dr. Forbes states, in addition to personally using flower remedies to help him through many family crises, he has used them in his practice to take hundreds of patients off antidepressants, sedatives, and tranquilizers. "I use flower remedies regularly and find them to be most helpful in alleviating the emotional and psychological stress many of the cancer patients experience," he says.[9]

J. Herbert Fill, M.D., a psychiatrist and former New York City Commissioner of Mental Health, uses flower remedies almost exclusively instead of tranquilizers and psychotropic drugs. He has found flower essences to have

HOW BACH FLOWER ESSENCES ARE PREPARED AND USED

According to Alicia Sirkin, Bach flower essences are prepared from the blooming parts of nontoxic trees, plants, and shrubs in two simple ways, depending upon the plant. In the "sun method," flower petals float on the surface of a glass bowl filled with pure spring water for three hours in direct sunlight in their natural habitat. In the "boiling method," plant parts are boiled in spring water for 30 minutes. Afterward, the flowers are discarded and the remaining liquid is preserved with an equal amount of brandy. Called the "Mother Tincture," this concentrate is used to make a single dilution that is sold to consumers in 10-ml "stock" concentrate bottles.

Sirkin says consumers may then use stock concentrate liquids directly from the bottle according to dosage instructions, or make an additional dilution for daily use in no more than eight ounces of water or other liquid. "This additional dilution conserves the concentrate, since each sip taken from the diluted liquid is as potent as a single dose from the concentrate itself," Sirkin explains. Essences can be taken orally or topically rubbed on pulse points (the inside of the wrists, temples, behind the ears, etc.). For alcohol sensitivities, topical application is preferred. The essences can also be sprayed from an atomizer on or above the body or put in bath water (use 6-10 drops from concentrate). "Since no biological or biochemical plant parts are left in the liquids after preparation, the essences are perfectly safe for anyone to use, without fear of allergic responses or sensitivities," Sirkin notes. To maximize shelf life, the remedies should always be kept tightly sealed and away from sunlight and heat.

a more profound and long-lasting effect on his patients, free from any side effects. "I deal with emotional problems as well as physical ones," Dr. Fill says. "In my observations, these remedies appear to work on a much deeper level, apparently assisting the individual in resolving deep-rooted conflicts, as opposed to simply relieving the symptoms."

John Bolling, a specialist in behavioral and drug abuse problems and former Assistant Professor and Chief Resident in Psychiatry at New York University's Bellevue Medical Center, found significant health improvements in 80% of the patients he treated with flower remedies during a recent clinical study. Although other types of treatment were simultaneously used, such as meditation

RESCUE REMEDY LIQUID AND CREAM

Dr. Bach's only combination formula, Rescue Remedy®, is the world's best known natural stress relief formula. Composed of five flower essences (Cherry Plum, Clematis, Impatiens, Rock Rose, and Star of Bethlehem), Rescue Remedy is designed to help cope with emergencies and crises as well as everyday ups and downs.

The formula has a positive, calming effect in acute emergency situations including bereavement, anxiety, hysteria, a family upset, physical trauma, emotional shock, or accidents. (It should not take the place of emergency medical care, however.) According to Bach flower practitioner Alicia Sirkin, Rescue Remedy can be used to reduce fears before stressful events, such as public speaking, tests, job interviews, airplane travel, quarrels, and dentist or doctor visits, and is also helpful for tension headaches and sleeplessness. Sirkin notes that the cream is effective for healing burns, bruises, small cuts and abrasions, sprains, bug bites and insect stings, rashes, chapped lips, dry skin, and joint pain.

and hypnosis, Dr. Bolling found the most impressive part of the study "was the dramatic improvement shown in the overcoming of blocked emotional patterns by 20% of this group, who prior to the study had been deemed resistant to any form of treatment."

States Dr. Bolling, "Clearly, Dr. Bach's remedies were the primary factor here. In addition to the marked improvement in their emotional state, these patients are now more open and receptive to other treatment modalities which had not been effective before."[10]

Along with medical doctors, many other health professionals have found that flower remedies combine well with their specific treatments. Chiropractors who use flower remedies along with standard chiropractic techniques, for instance, report that using both methods in conjunction has a greater and more permanent health-enhancing effect than using either one alone. "I have used the 38 traditional flower essences over the past number of years with remarkable success," states George Goodheart, D.C., of Detroit, Michigan, the founder of applied kinesiology. "I have found them to alleviate a wide range of emotional problems and emotionally based physical problems. I have seen them dispel worry, anxiety, and negative attitudes, very often in a surprisingly short period of time, instilling a more positive attitude toward recovery."[11]

Harold Whitcomb, M.D., of Aspen, Colorado, uses Bach flower essences in his treatment program for chronic fatigue syndrome. He finds that deep-seated, buried emotions are common in people with chronic fatigue and that the flower remedies help to bring these emotions to the surface and allow them to heal.

 See Acupuncture, Applied Kinesiology, Energy Medicine, Traditional Chinese Medicine.

Flower essences can also be used as an adjunct to acupuncture and traditional Chinese medicine. As acupuncture treatments open blocked energy channels, stored emotional energy is released. Because flower essences work to balance any negative emotional energy, the two therapies work well together, according to Susan Lange, O.M.D., of the Meridian Health Center, in Santa Monica, California, who uses Bach and other flower essences in her practice.

A 40-year-old man suffering from chronic asthma since age 3 came to see Dr. Lange. The man's long treatment history included prednisone (a steroid hormone with the same effects as cortisone) and inhalants. Dr. Lange learned that the initial outbreak of asthma coincided with the onset of his parent's marital difficulties. His parents fought openly in the home and his mother eventually committed suicide. Dr. Lange used acupuncture to open blockages in the man's chest and treated him adjunctively with fuchsia, a flower essence native to America that addresses the repression of deep-seated emotions such as anger and grief. Because the man masked his suffering behind a cheerful facade, Dr. Lange incorporated Bach's traditional flower remedies Elm and Agrimony.

As the energy held in the man's chest released, Dr. Lange treated him for blockage in the solar plexus and administered the flower essence sunflower for issues of self-worth. Finally, he was treated for repressed kidney energy and was given basil and sticky monkey flower essence, and the flower remedy Rock Rose. These remedies addressed his repressed sexual feelings and his fear of intimacy. Within three months, the man was able to discontinue all previous medication and was free of asthma, reports Dr. Lange.

When treating children, Dr. Lange also likes to treat the parents simultaneously. She finds that their problems often interconnect. In one case, a mother was experiencing postnatal depression and couldn't relate to her child. Mariposa lily, a flower essence native to America, was given to both the mother and the child to help them with parent/child bonding. The child was also given pink yarrow essence, which is used to treat those who overly identify with the emotions of others. The health of both the mother and child improved as did their relationship.

Alicia Sirkin has also used flower essences successfully to help her patients cope with a variety of health conditions. "A 55-year-old man came to me with intense back pain," Sirkin recounts. "Full medical testing showed no physiological basis for the problem and repeated visits to his chiropractor were not helping. At the time, he had recently separated from his wife, who wrongly accused him of having an extramarital affair. Now filled with anger, resentment, bitterness, and frustration, he said his wife took his money inappropriately and had been extremely rude. He was very active in his church and the situation was now causing him public difficulties. As a result, he was terribly depressed."

Sirkin addressed only his emotional imbalances, combining four essences into a one-ounce treatment bottle. He agreed that he was feeling great loss, even grief, over the breakup, which pointed to the essence Star of Bethlehem to soothe the heart and for the initial shock of the accusations. Gorse was selected for his depression and feelings of utter hopelessness after having tried many treatments with no hope for recovery, and Holly was used to help him release his anger and hatred. To help him release bitterness and resentment, she also added Willow to his formula. After two weeks, he reported feeling tired physically and mentally, so she added Olive for regeneration.

"Five weeks after his initial visit, he reported that almost all his difficulties were resolved, including his back pain, which only flared up occasionally," says Sirkin. "He recognized that the back pain was a result of his negative emotional state. Now, the anger is completely gone, and he now feels more conciliatory toward his wife."

Among other conditions that Sirkin has seen improved as a result of using Bach flower essences are: insomnia and nightmares, anxiety, boredom, irritability, mental fatigue, fear, lack of trust, impaired motor skills (balance), cuts and bruises, residual physical pain related to emotional trauma, and general lifestyle issues related to stress, overwork, strained relationships, and challenges related to school. She also finds the essences useful for dealing with emotions related to pregnancy, premenstrual syndrome and menopause, and addressing the delayed effects of emotional shock and trauma. "I have observed the essences' beneficial effects in the release of emotional traumas originating as far back as early childhood," she says.

How to Select and Use Flower Essences

Selecting and using flower essences is a simple process. According to Sirkin, the key is to take time to reflect on how you are feeling, noticing what moods, thoughts, and behaviors are bothering you. Then select the essence (or essences) that best describes your state of mind or mood (see "The 38 Bach Flower Essences and Their Indications for Use" below). "When only one of the 38 flower essences seems indicated for your condition, the essence liquid can be taken several different ways with the same result, straight from the concentrate bottle or diluted," Sirkin says.

To take a single flower essence straight from the concentrate bottle, use two drops each time on or under the tongue at least four times a day. To address a passing mood, dilute a single flower essence by putting two drops into a small glass of water; sip frequently, making additional glasses as needed. Do this until you feel better and are satisfied with your improvement. Each sip equals a full dose, just as if you took two drops straight from the concentrate bottle. Minimum daily dose is four sips.

For long-term use, put two drops of a single flower essence into a clean one-ounce, amber-glass dropper bottle. Fill the bottle to the shoulder with spring water. Add one teaspoon of a preservative (brandy, apple vinegar, or vegetable glycerin). Take four drops from this "dilution bottle" on or under the tongue at least four times a day. Each 4-drop dose from the dilution bottle is equal to a 2-drop dose from the original concentrate bottle.

When many unwanted states of mind occur simultaneously, combine up to seven of the essences together in a one-ounce dilution bottle. "Since many of us lead complex lives, using several essences at once can offer a multidimensional healing effect," Sirkin says.

Since each of us is unique and may heal at different rates of speed, there is no definitive answer as to how long it will take before flower essences achieve the results patients are looking for. Generally, a person feels results within several hours to several months, Sirkin notes. "Older or long-standing emotional or mental issues may take even longer to resolve. As patients start to feel better, they may find themselves forgetting to take the essences. This is a cue that the essences have done their job and are no longer needed." However, it's important to be faithful to the dosage until the desired results are obtained. Due to the essences' subtle nature, weeks or months may pass with the feeling that "nothing is happening" until one reflects carefully upon the original condition. Often, family and friends will notice the changes first.

Quite often after taking the essences for a month or more, it will become apparent to the user that other parts of the personality need balancing. "Flower essences seem to peel away immediate difficulties, revealing other layers to be addressed with additional essences," Sirkin says.

"Should this subtle shift occur, hidden or long-standing emotional issues can be positively affected."

Benefits of Consulting with a Bach Flower Registered Practitioner

Although Dr. Bach designed the essences to be self-selecting, a qualified Bach Foundation registered practitioner will take the guesswork out of the selection process. Registered practitioners actively involve the client in the healing process, working with what the conscious mind knows it can handle, Sirkin explains. Practitioners serve as educators and guides to the correct use of the essences, empowering clients toward self-discovery. Other selection methods may reach the core of the issue before an individual can deal with the consequences. As of this writing, there are 49 Bach Foundation registered practitioners in the U.S. and over 800 worldwide. Most practitioners will consult by telephone or e-mail, so it is not necessary to consult with a practitioner in person.

The 38 Bach Flower Essences and Their Indications for Use

Agrimony—Suffering covered by a cheerful or brave facade. Distressed by argument or confrontation, may seek escape from pain or worry with addictive behavior through the use of food, drugs, cigarettes, or alcohol.

Aspen—Vague fears or anxiety of unknown origin. Apprehension, foreboding.

Beech—Critical, intolerant, or easily finding fault. May overreact with annoyance or irritability to the shortcomings of others.

Centaury—Willing servant, overly anxious to please, weak willed, or easily exploited/dominated by others. May neglect own needs to serve others. Avoids confrontation, difficulty saying "no."

Cerato—Lacks confidence in own judgment. Little trust in inner guidance. Constantly seeks advice of others, therefore vulnerable to being misguided.

Cherry Plum—Fear of losing mental or physical control, of doing something desperate or violent. Tantrums, suicidal thoughts, impulse to do something thoughtless or known to be wrong. Fear of letting go. May be near nervous breakdown.

Chestnut Bud—Failure to learn from experience, repeats inappropriate patterns. Difficulty correcting mistakes.

Chicory—Loving, but with expectation of being loved in return. Possessive, emotionally needy, easily hurt or rejected.

Clematis—Lacks concentration, daydreams. Drowsy or "spacey" with a halfhearted interest in present circumstances. Inactive, ungrounded. Trouble materializing dreams.

Crab Apple—Cleansing remedy when feeling toxic, contaminated, or unclean. Ashamed of self-image. Fear of being contaminated. Need for cleanliness. Can be used to assist detoxification, if needed.

Elm—Overwhelmed by responsibilities. Normally capable, now doubts ability to perform tasks. Temporary feelings of inadequacy due to overload. Difficulty prioritizing.

Gentian—Mild despondency or discouragement due to setback, difficulty, or failed expectation. Negativity reverses easily with positive events or successes.

Gorse—Helplessness, hopelessness, sense of futility. Convinced situation will not improve; may not be willing to try remedies.

Heather—Self-centered, self-obsessed, or self-absorbed. Seeks the companionship of anyone who will listen to them. Constant chatterer, poor listener, unhappy if left alone.

Holly—Strongly felt negative feelings: hatred, envy, jealousy, suspicion, revenge, or wrath.

Honeysuckle—Dwelling in the past: old traumas, nostalgia, homesickness, regrets for happier times. Little expectation of future happiness.

Hornbeam—Mental fatigue and tiredness; procrastination. Weary before day or task begins, the "Monday morning" feeling. Difficulty starting.

Impatiens—Impatience, irritability, restlessness, or frustration with slow moving people and events. Quick in thought and action, requires all things to be done without delay. May prefer to work alone.

Larch—Lacks self-confidence despite being capable. Feels inferior. Anticipates failure; may refuse to make effort to succeed.

Mimulus—Everyday fear of known things: heights, public speaking, pain, water, illness, flying, poverty, other people, being alone, etc. For the shy, nervous, or timid personality type.

Mustard—Sudden deep gloom, depression, melancholia, or heavy sadness with no known cause. Condition may come and go.

Oak—Struggling on despite difficulties. Does not give up even if ill or overworked. Strong sense of responsibility and determination. Difficulty resting when exhausted.

Olive—Complete mental and physical exhaustion, sapped energy with no reserve, for example, after a long personal ordeal or illness.

Pine—Guilt or self-reproach, feels unworthy or undeserving. May blame self for another person's mistakes. Not satisfied with own success.

Red Chestnut—Fear for the well-being of others, fearing the worst will happen to loved ones.

Rock Rose—Terror or any great fear (panic, nightmares, etc.).

Rock Water—Self-denial. Strict, perhaps rigid, adherence to a living style or to religious, personal, or social disciplines. Tries to set an example.

Scleranthus—Difficulty in deciding between two choices, seeing value in both. Uncertainty.

Star of Bethlehem—Great unhappiness, grief, loss, trauma, after-effects of shock. Helpful after bereavement.

Sweet Chestnut—Unbearable anguish, has reached the limits of endurance. Dark night of the soul, facing the abyss.

Vervain—Fixed ideas, over-enthusiasm. Attempts to teach, convert, convince, save the world. Champion of justice. Energetic, intense, or driven.

Vine—Overly strong-willed, capable, may become dictatorial or tyrannical. May disregard rights or needs of others. May be power-hungry or merciless.

Walnut—Protection from negative influences or pressures and from the effects of change. Stabilizes emotionally during periods of transition: puberty, adolescence, menopause, aging, job change, new home, relationships, etc. Breaks links to past; facilitates freedom to move forward.

Water Violet—Loners, quiet, aloof, self-reliant. They go their own way and leave others to go theirs. Prefers to bear health or other challenges alone.

White Chestnut—Persistent unwanted thoughts. Mental arguments, worries, or repetitious thoughts that prevent peace of mind and disrupt concentration.

Wild Oat—Career uncertainty, unfulfilled ambition, or boredom with present status and course in life. Although capable and talented, is unclear on which of many paths to take. Frustration or dissatisfaction may result.

Wild Rose—Resigned or apathetic. Indifferent to life's circumstances. Will surrender to health or other problems. Rarely complains. Little effort to improve things or find joy. Emotionally flat or dull.

Willow—Resentful or bitter toward life, blames others. Self-pity over misfortune ("Poor me!"). Sees self as victim.[12]

Where to Find Help

Flower essences, glass dropper bottles, books, audiotapes, and videotapes are sold at health food stores, over the Internet, or at specialty retail stores. For more information regarding flower essences, contact:

Dr. Edward Bach Centre
Mount Vernon, Bakers Lane
Sotwell, Oxon OX10 0PZ, United Kingdom
(44-0)-1491-834678
Website: www.bachcentre.com

The Bach Centre is the official international site for information, education, practitioner educational programs, books, and correspondence courses.

Nelson Bach USA, Ltd.
Wilmington Technology Park
100 Research Drive
Wilmington, Massachusetts 01887-4406
(978) 988-3833 or (800) 319-9151
Website: www.nelsonbach.com

Nelson Bach USA (NBUSA) is America's distribution, sales, and educational division for Bach flower essences.

Flower Essence Society
P.O. Box 459
Nevada City, California 95959
(530) 265-0258 or (800) 548-0075
Website: www.flowersociety.org

FES distributes California flower essences and imports Healing Herbs, made in the United Kingdom, a full line of the 38 flowers discovered by Dr. Bach.

Pegasus Products, Inc.
P.O. Box 228
Boulder, Colorado 80306
(800) 527-6104 or (303) 667-3019

Pegasus manufactures and distributes various flower essences.

Perelandra, Ltd.
P.O. Box 3603
Warrenton, Virginia 20188
(800) 960-8806
Website: www.perelandra-ltd.com

Perelandra sells their own line of flower essences as well as books. Call for a catalog.

Flower Healing
P.O. Box 33-0841
Miami, Florida 33233
(888) 875-6753
Website: www.flowerhealing.com

Directed by Alicia Sirkin, a Bach Foundation registered practitioner. Offers in-person and long-distance consultations, training, and an online self-help newsletter.

Recommended Reading

Bach Flower Essences for the Family. Edward Bach. London, England: Wigmore Publications, 2000.

The Bach Flower Remedies. Edward Bach and F.J. Wheeler. New Canaan, CT: Keats, 1979.

The Bach Remedies: A Self-Help Guide. Leslie J. Kaslof. New Canaan, CT: Keats, 1988.

Bach Flower Remedies for Beginners. David F. Vennells. St. Paul, MN: Llewellyn, 2001.

The Bach Flower Remedies: Illustration and Preparation. Nora Weeks and Victor Bullen. Saffron, Walden, England: C.W. Daniel, 1990.

Bach Flower Therapy. Mechthild Scheffer. Rochester, VT: Inner Traditions, 1987.

Handbook on the Bach Flower Remedies. Phillip M. Chancellor. New Canaan, CT: Keats, 1971.

The Medical Discoveries of Edward Bach, Physician. Nora Weeks. New Canaan, CT: Keats, 1979.

GUIDED IMAGERY

Using the power of the mind to evoke a positive physical response, guided imagery can reduce stress and slow heart rate, stimulate the immune system, and reduce pain. As part of the rapidly emerging field of mind/body medicine, guided imagery is being used in various medical settings and, when properly taught, can also serve as a highly effective form of self-care.

THE IMAGINATION IS probably a person's least utilized health resource," says Martin L. Rossman, M.D., Co-founder of the Academy for Guided Imagery. "It can be used to remember and recreate the past, develop insight into the present, influence physical health, enhance creativity and inspiration, and anticipate possible futures." All of us have to some extent experienced the effects of the imagination on the body. Getting goose bumps while listening to a frightening story, breaking out in chills at the thought of fingernails scratching a chalkboard, or becoming physically aroused from a sexual fantasy are all examples of the body reacting to a sole stimulus—the imagination.

> *If you are a good worrier, and especially if you ever worry yourself sick, you may be a good candidate for learning how to positively affect your health with imagery, as the internal process involved in worrying yourself sick and imagining yourself well are quite similar.*
>
> —MARTIN L. ROSSMAN, M.D.

ing to external events, but to thoughts or images about these events, even though the worrier may not be consciously aware of them. Other thoughts may be verbal, but what all thoughts have in common is that they exist in the mind and the body reacts to them.

"If you are a good worrier," says Dr. Rossman, "and especially if you ever worry yourself sick, you may be an especially good candidate for learning how to positively affect your health with imagery, as the internal process involved in worrying yourself sick and imagining yourself well are quite similar."

David Bresler, Ph.D., L.Ac., Co-director of the Academy for Guided Imagery and former Director of the U.C.L.A. Pain Center, defines imagery as one of the two "higher order" languages of the human nervous system (the other one being the more familiar, educated faculty of thinking in words). Imagery is a natural way the nervous system stores, accesses, and processes information. This makes it especially effective for maintaining the dialogue between mind and body, which is the source of its power in the healing process.

What is Imagery?

Imagery is simply a flow of thoughts that one can see, hear, feel, smell, or taste in one's imagination. As an inner representation of experience as well as fantasy, imagery is a rich, symbolic, and highly personal language. "An image may or may not represent external reality, but it always represents internal reality," says Dr. Rossman. "It is the language of the emotions and the interface between mind and body."

Perhaps the most common human experience of imagery is worrying. Most people worry sometimes and some people worry constantly, even to the point where they experience butterflies in the stomach or tightening in the shoulders. Whatever the case, the body is not react-

The Healing Power of Imagery

Imagery has three main characteristics that lend it great value in medicine and healing:

IMAGERY AND THE BRAIN

According to Martin L. Rossman, M.D., Co-founder of the Academy for Guided Imagery, imagery seems to arise from unconscious processes, body processes, and memories and perceptions from the part of the brain known as the cerebral cortex. Some imagery, however, having to do with smell or feelings, may arise from older, more primitive brain centers. Wherever its origin, imagery is believed to have its effect by sending messages from the higher centers of the brain through to the lower centers that regulate most physiologic functions, such as breathing, heart rate, blood flow and pressure, digestion, immunity, and temperature, as well as waking and sleeping rhythms, hunger, thirst, and sexual function.

Research utilizing advanced methods of brain scanning indicates what parts of the brain are active when a person is performing certain tasks. The scans seem to show that the optic cortex, the same part of the brain activated when a person is seeing, is activated when a person visualizes. Similarly, when people imagine hearing things, the auditory cortex is active, and when they imagine feeling sensations, the sensory cortex is active. It appears that the cortex can create these imaginary realities and, in the absence of conflicting information, the lower centers of the nervous system respond to this information.

This is one reason why health-care professionals use sensory recruitment, an approach that utilizes as many senses in the imagery process as possible. Sensory recruitment increases the subjective reality of the image and probably increases the amount of information sent through the lower brain centers and autonomic nervous system, making it more likely to elicit the desired response.

- It directly affects physiology.

- Through the mental processes of association and synthesis, it provides insight and perspective into health.

- It has an intimate relationship with the emotions, which are often at the root of many common health conditions.

The Physiological Effects of Imagery

Relax for a moment and imagine holding a juicy, yellow lemon. Feel its coolness, its texture, its weight in your hand. Imagine cutting it in half. Notice the cut surfaces— the pale yellow of the pulp, the whiteness of the inner peel, perhaps a seed or two. Carefully cut one of the halves in two and pick up one of the freshly cut lemon quarters. Imagine lifting this lemon wedge to your mouth. Smell its lemony scent. Now imagine biting into the lemon and sucking its sour juice into your mouth. What happened as you imagined doing that? Did you salivate or grimace? Did you have any other kind of physical reaction? Most people do, much more than if you simply asked them to salivate.

This is a simple illustration of the type of physiological response that imagery can induce. If thinking of a lemon makes you salivate, what other more important effects on physiology might certain types of imagery have? For instance, can thinking of pain relief cause endorphins to be secreted?

Research using biofeedback, hypnosis, and meditative states has demonstrated that people possess a remarkable range of self-regulatory capacities. Focused imagery in a relaxed state of mind is a common and central factor in most of these techniques. Imagery of various types has been shown to affect heart rate, blood pressure, respiratory patterns, oxygen consumption, carbon dioxide elimination, brain-wave rhythms, electrical characteristics of the skin, local blood flow and temperature of tissues, gastrointestinal motility and secretions, sexual arousal, levels of hormones and neurotransmitters in the blood, and immune system function.[1]

The healing potentials of imagery go far beyond its remarkable ability to directly affect physiology, however.

Associations and "Getting the Big Picture"

"Recovering from or coping with a serious or chronic illness may demand more than simply imagining getting well," says Dr. Rossman. "It may also require changes in your lifestyle, your attitudes, your relationships, or your emotional state." Imagery can help to develop the insight and self-awareness that it takes to deal with a chronic or life-threatening illness in more positive and constructive ways. This is due to the mental processes of association and synthesis that are central to imagery. "Imagery tends to give us the 'big picture' of a situation and can help us recognize how things are related in ways we might not expect," Dr. Rossman explains. "Becoming aware of these relationships may facilitate a shift in attitude or behavior that can be helpful in relieving, altering, or coping with illness or symptoms."

For example, Dr. Rossman tells of a woman whose chronic arm pain had not responded to medical treatment for two years. She kept seeing an image of her pain as pieces of iron. This made little sense to her until she was asked to describe the qualities of the iron. She described it as hard, cold, and rigid, and then immediately associated these qualities with her grandfather, whom she had been caring for during the past two years, as he displayed these same qualities. This association allowed her to deal with repressed feelings about her role as a caregiver and led to a rapid resolution of her arm pain as well as a great deal of personal growth.

Emotional Connections

Emotions are powerful events in the body. They are physiologically distinct from one another and each affects human physiology in different ways. In fact, Dr. Rossman points out, many physical ailments are direct manifestations of emotions that are locked within the unconscious. "Through imagery, you can access those emotions and consciously alter their effect on your health," he says.

Emotions themselves are a normal, healthy response to life. Failure to acknowledge and express important emotions, however, can be an important factor in illness and is unfortunately all too common. People often suppress those emotions they find to be the most distressing, such as fear, grief, and anger. The natural expression of emotion is often suppressed by family, friends, and society as well. "Yet strong emotion has a way of finding routes of expression," says Dr. Bresler, "and if it is not recognized and dealt with, it can manifest itself indirectly in the form of physical pain and illness, or destructive behaviors like smoking, heavy drinking, and overworking, all of which can in turn lead to serious health problems." In fact, studies in England and the United States have found that 50% to 75% of problems presented to primary care clinics are emotional, social, or familial in origin, though they are expressed by pain or illness.[2]

Studies have found that 50% to 75% of problems presented to primary care clinics are emotional, social, or familial in origin, though they are expressed by pain or illness.

By directly accessing emotions, imagery can help the individual understand the needs that may be represented by an illness and can help develop ways to meet those needs. Imagery is also one of the quickest and most direct ways of becoming aware of emotions and their effects on health, both positive and negative. For instance, one

of Dr. Rossman's patients with inflammatory bowel disease reported that she imagined her bowels being "red, inflamed, and irritated." As this image was explored, she became aware of how her bowels responded to the irritation, frustration, and anger she frequently felt. By learning to recognize what triggered her frustration, and by developing more effective means to express herself when angry, she had progressively less trouble with her bowels. She also learned to use simple relaxation and imagery to imagine her own hands gently soothing her bowels with a cooling, calming balm whenever they became upset. A few minutes of doing this would relieve her abdominal pain and leave her feeling relaxed and at ease.

Imagery in Medicine and Healing

Imagery can be a key factor in dealing with anything from a simple tension headache to a life-threatening disease. It is a proven method for pain relief, for helping people tolerate medical procedures and treatments and reducing side effects, and for stimulating healing responses in the body. Imagery can assist in clarifying attitudes, emotions, behaviors, and lifestyle patterns that may be involved in producing illness. It can also facilitate recovery and be used to help people find meaning in their illnesses, cope more effectively with their health problems, and come to grips with life's limitations.

Learning to relax is fundamental to self-healing, and imagery is a part of almost all relaxation and stress-reduction techniques. For many people, imagery is the easiest way to learn to relax, and its active nature makes it more comfortable than other methods of relaxation.

Treating People Rather Than Symptoms

Beyond simple relaxation, imagery can have specific effects in relieving numerous common symptoms. Dr. Bresler states that because imagery is a way of treating people rather than symptoms or diseases, it can be applied to almost any health-care concern. The following areas of application are some examples of where imagery can be useful, but this list is by no means complete.

Imagery is often used for relief of chronic pain and other symptoms, including headaches, neck and back pain, allergies (including hay fever and asthma), high blood pressure, benign arrhythmia (heartbeat irregularities), stress-related gastrointestinal symptoms (including chronic abdominal pain and spastic colon), functional urinary complaints, and reproductive irregularities including premenstrual syndrome, irregular menstruation, dysmenorrhea (painful menstruation), and excessive uterine

AN IMAGERY RELAXATION EXERCISE

The following exercise is adapted from Dr. Rossman's book, *Guided Imagery for Self-Healing*. This simple technique can be used as a stress reducer either for a few minutes or half an hour. It's best when learning it to have another person read and guide you through the steps until they are familiar. You can also record the exercise yourself and listen to it before going to bed at night.

Get comfortable, either lying down or sitting up. Take a few deep breaths and begin to imagine that with each in-breath, you take in calmness and peacefulness; with each out-breath you release tension, discomfort, and worry. Let your breath find its own natural rate and rhythm and continue to imagine breathing in calmness and peacefulness and breathing out tension and worry.

Invite your body to relax. Imagine breathing calmness into your feet and legs—release any tension on the out-breath. Breathe into your pelvis, hips, and low back, and release on the out-breath; don't struggle or make an effort, just imagine this happening in your own way. Breathe calmness into your abdomen and release tension on the out-breath; breathe into your chest and release tension as you exhale; breathe peacefulness into your neck and shoulders, and release tension as you exhale. Breathe calmness into your arms and hands all the way to the fingertips, and relax as you let go of the breath; breathe into your face and jaws, into your scalp and forehead, into your eyes and release all tension. Allow your whole body to sink into a peaceful, relaxed state.

Now imagine yourself in a place that is particularly peaceful and beautiful, perhaps a place you've actually visited or a place imagined—a special place you'd really like to be. Imagine yourself there now and notice the details—what you see, the colors, shapes, living things. Notice what you hear in this special place, smell any aromas or odors you associate with this place, pay special attention to any feelings of peacefulness and relaxation that you feel and allow yourself to experience them as fully as possible.

Whenever you are ready, simply allow the images to fade and, taking all the time you need, bring yourself back to the outer world, gently opening your eyes and stretching as you return.

bleeding. It can also accelerate healing and minimize discomfort from all kinds of acute injuries, including sprains, strains, and broken bones, as well as from the symptoms of the common cold, flu, and infections. Because imagery can affect immune system function (within limits), there is a great deal of interest among researchers of mind/body medicine for applying it to a broad spectrum of autoimmune diseases, including rheumatoid arthritis, ulcerative colitis, and systemic lupus (a chronic inflammatory disease with symptoms including arthritis, fatigue, and skin lesions).

Imagery has also been utilized by a great number of people with cancer as part of their recovery process. Imagery as a tool in cancer therapy was pioneered by radiation oncologist O. Carl Simonton, M.D. He used imagery as a means of reinforcing traditional medical treatments, suggesting that his patients imagine their cancer cells as "anything soft that can be broken down, like hamburger meat or fish eggs," and their white blood cells as warriors, "aggressive and eager for battle."[3]

Dr. Simonton first employed this technique in 1971 with a 61-year-old patient with throat cancer whose condition had been diagnosed as "hopeless." He was extremely weak, his weight had dropped to 98 pounds, and he was having trouble breathing and swallowing his own saliva. Although he was scheduled to receive radiation treatment, his doctors were concerned that treating him would further deteriorate his condition. Dr. Simonton outlined a program of relaxation and imagery for the man, instructing him to devote five to 15 minutes three times a day. The imagery exercise consisted of imagining the radiation treatment as "bullets of energy" striking his cells, healthy and cancerous alike, with the healthy cells remaining healthy and the cancer cells dying off. The man would then visualize his cancer shrinking in size and his health returning to normal. As a result of this program, the man was able to receive radiation treatment with minimum discomfort. Halfway through his treatment, he began eating again and regaining weight and strength. Within two months, his cancer completely disappeared.[4]

Patricia Norris, Ph.D., a pioneer in the field of imagery, works with people with serious illnesses. Dr. Norris likes to distinguish between two types of imagery: that which uses images preconceived by the therapist as a means of suggesting healing and imagery created by the patient as a way to better understand the meaning of symptoms or to access inner resources. Dr. Norris's most well-known case using the latter type of imagery was that of 9-year-old Garrett Porter, who was diagnosed with an inoperable, terminal brain tumor. By creating an imagery scenario with Garrett (based on his favorite TV show, *Star Trek*), used in combination with biofeedback,

Dr. Norris was able to guide Garrett through a year of intensive therapy, after which the boy's tumor completely disappeared.[5]

Even though cancer patients are not cured through imagery, they report benefits from its use, including relief from anxiety and pain, bolstered self-esteem, and an increased sense of control over their bodies. They also report an increased ability to tolerate chemotherapy or radiation therapy. In addition, by coming to grips with the illness, they are often able to resolve personal and family issues.

Research Confirms the Benefits of Imagery

Since the pioneering work of Drs. Simonton and Norris, a number of studies have verified the positive role imagery can have in treating cancer and coping with its resultant anxiety and pain. In a study of 53 women undergoing radiation therapy for early-stage breast cancer, it was shown that the use of customized guided imagery audiotapes was "an effective intervention for enhancing comfort" and that such tapes were "effective in terms of cost, personnel, and time." This evaluation was made after researchers found that women who used the tapes experienced a significant overall increase in comfort during and after the course of their radiation treatments, compared to women in the control group.[6] Another recent study involved 96 women with newly diagnosed, locally advanced breast cancer. Those who were instructed in the use of guided imagery techniques, in which they visualized their immune cells destroying tumor cells, experienced greater quality of life scores, reduced emotional suppression, and were more relaxed after six cycles of chemotherapy compared to the control group. Although the guided imagery group showed no significant clinical difference in their condition, the researchers concluded that guided imagery should be offered to all patients "wishing to improve quality of life during primary chemotherapy."[7]

Guided imagery has also been shown to significantly decrease pain and reduce the need for pain medication following colorectal surgery, as well as decrease related anxiety levels before and after such operations, according to a study conducted at the Cleveland Clinic Foundation in Ohio. Moreover, among the patients who used guided imagery, the elapsed time to their first bowel movement after surgery was "significantly less" (a median time of 58 hours) compared to the control group (median time of 92 hours).[8] Other recent studies indicate that imagery is useful for a variety of other conditions, including childhood asthma,[9] diabetes,[10] addiction (due to its ability to facilitate a shift in the addictive personality's self-image, thereby increasing the likelihood of

adhering to other treatment protocols),[11] bulimia,[12] and psoriasis.[13]

In addition to being used to explore diseases and symptoms, imagery can be helpful for enhancing tolerance to medical procedures such as MRIs (magnetic resonance imaging) and bone marrow biopsies. Imagery can also help prepare people for surgery and in post-surgical recovery. In fact, imagery can be applied to almost any medical situation where problem solving, decision making, relaxation, or symptom relief is useful. Imagery can be considered as an adjunct treatment to health care no matter how minor the condition.

According to Jeanne Achterberg, Ph.D., past President of the Association for Transpersonal Psychology, establishing healing patterns is far easier when the individual is relatively healthy than when faced with a serious disease. Once someone is diagnosed as being seriously ill, the person often lacks the emotional resources and belief system to employ imagery to its best advantage.[14] In addition, imagery can be an effective tool to help people constructively resolve grief during the anticipation of the loss of loved ones to illness, as well as after their passing.[15]

Interactive Guided Imagery

Beyond these relatively direct applications, "receptive" uses of imagery can have profound effects on health and medical care. These typically involve imaginary dialogues with images representing symptoms or illness, or with an inner store of wisdom or healing that can provide insights into the meaning of body sensations and symptoms. This can lead to better understanding of how lifestyle choices and behavior are affecting health. The following stories demonstrate how imagery can be used to help identify thoughts and fears at the root of physical pain.

Alice, 40, had recently undergone cancer surgery and radiation. However, she continued to have persistent pain in her upper back. Because doctors could not identify the problem, she decided to try guided imagery with Dr. Rossman. First, he asked her to relax and imagine herself at some beautiful place. Alice saw herself on a beach surrounded by cliffs. Next, she was invited to have a dialogue with an imaginary "inner advisor." Alice asked for an image to appear and saw a wise old man tending a fire. He looked like Merlin, the magician of Arthurian legend. When Alice asked him about her pain, he told her that she needed to "ask for help." Alice immediately broke into tears, for throughout her ordeal she had never asked for help from her husband or family. She suddenly realized that she had been afraid to ask for help, thinking she would be too much of a burden on them. Her "inner advisor" then told her how much better her family members would feel if they were included in her healing process. Finally, she imagined asking her husband for help and having him agree to provide it. At the end of session, her pain had substantially decreased and she found the courage to turn to her family for assistance. "In my experience, this receptive use of imagery as an interface language between what we call 'mind' and what we call 'body' often yields the most profound healing response," says Dr. Rossman.

 Natural ability, skills, motivation, practice, and the availability of good instruction are all factors in how effectively you can work with imagery. Some conditions respond better than others, but no matter what the condition, imagery can help you better cope and minimize your suffering.

In a similar case, Dr. Bresler worked with a 52-year-old cardiologist who suffered from excruciating pain in the lower back after receiving successful treatment for rectal cancer. Further surgery was ruled out because the area had been so heavily irradiated and because the man had developed tolerance to his pain medications.

Reviewing the man's medical records, Dr. Bresler read that in a psychiatric evaluation the man had described his pain as "a dog chewing on my spine." Dr. Bresler suggested guided imagery as a way to make contact with the "dog" and invited the man to imagine what it looked like. The patient described "a nasty little terrier" named Skippy. During the following sessions, Skippy began revealing critically important information about the patient, including the fact that he had never wanted to be a doctor but had been pressured into medical school by his mother. As a consequence, the man resented not only his mother, but also his patients and colleagues. Skippy told him that this hostility had contributed to both his cancer and to his subsequent back pain. Finally, Skippy said, "You're a damn good doctor. It may not be the career you wanted, but it's time you recognized how good you are at what you do. When you stop being so resentful and start accepting yourself, I'll stop chewing your spine." Following these insights, the man experienced an immediate alleviation of his pain and, within a few more weeks, it progressively subsided to the point where he felt like a new person.

 Imagery is an adjunctive treatment for illness. Make sure you are aware of all the medical options for your condition and seek proper medical care.

The Future of Imagery

"One of the most appealing aspects of guided imagery is that it lends itself so readily to the process of patient education and self-care," says Dr. Bresler. "It also provides a formal methodology for increasing personal empowerment and self-control. While research studies of its cost-effectiveness are still under way, it appears to offer significant and effective therapeutic benefits after only a few weeks or months of therapy." Dr. Bresler and Dr. Rossman both predict that, in the very near future, training in guided imagery will be an integral part of all psychotherapeutic approaches and that its benefits will become more widely available for medical and psychological problems and as a means of achieving greater personal insight, creativity, and self-actualization.

Where to Find Help

Mastering guided imagery comes with time and training. There are groups and classes that teach imagery around the country. Check local hospitals for wellness programs, patient support groups, or behavioral medical units for referrals. You can also inquire with mental health practitioners, especially those with an interest in health psychology, or with alternative medicine practitioners in your area. For further information, contact:

The Academy for Guided Imagery
P.O. Box 2070
Mill Valley, California 94942
(800) 726-2070
Website: www.interactiveimagery.com

The Academy trains health professionals to use Interactive Guided Imagery, offering a 150-hour certification program. They publish a directory of imagery practitioners and also carry books and tapes for professionals and laypeople, specifically relating to imagery in medicine and healing. Contact for a free catalog.

American Holistic Medical Association (AHMA)
6728 Old McLean Village Drive
McLean, Virginia 22101
(703) 556-9245
Website: www.holisticmedicine.org

Provides a directory of AHMA members (M.D.s and D.O.s) who favor holistic approaches to treating disease and are familiar with and supportive of the use of imagery in healing.

Center for Applied Psychophysiology
Menninger Clinic
P.O. Box 829
Topeka, Kansas 66601-0829
(800) 351-9058
Website: www.menninger.edu

This organization conducts research and provides treatment and workshops in all areas of mind/body medicine, including extensive work with imagery.

Exceptional Cancer Patients (ECaP)
522 Jackson Park Drive
Meadville, Pennsylvania 16335
(814) 337-8192
Website: www.ecap-online.org

This organization, founded by Bernie Siegel, M.D., author of Love, Medicine, and Miracles, *has a referral list of professionals who work with imagery and cancer patients. They also have an extensive catalogue of books and tapes related to healing, with special emphasis on cancer and catastrophic illness.*

Life Sciences Institute of Mind–Body Health
4636 S.W. Wanamaker Road
Topeka, Kansas 66610
(785) 271-8686
Website: www.cjnetworks.com/~lifesci

Offers a variety of mind/body healing approaches, including training in the use of guided imagery and visualization techniques, by a variety of experts in mind/body medicine, including Patricia Norris, Ph.D.

Simonton Cancer Center
P.O. Box 890
Pacific Palisades, California 90272
(800) 459-3424 or (310) 459-4434
Website: www.simontoncenter.com

O. Carl Simonton, M.D., pioneered the use of imagery in people recovering from cancer. His organization has trained professionals around the country in his methods and may be able to refer you to someone in your area.

Recommended Reading

Free Yourself from Pain. David Bresler, Ph.D. Topanga, CA: The Bresler Center, 1992. (Available from The Bresler Center, 115 South Topanga Canyon Blvd., Suite 158, Topanga, California 90290; (310) 455-3634.)

Getting Well Again. O. Carl Simonton, M.D., Stephanie Matthews-Simonton, and James Creighton. Los Angeles: Jeremy P. Tarcher, 1978.

Guided Imagery for Self-Healing. Martin L. Rossman, M.D. Novato, CA: New World Library, 2000.

Imagery in Healing: Shamanism and Modern Medicine. Jeanne Achterberg, Ph.D. New York: Random House, 1985.

Minding the Body, Mending the Mind. Joan Borysenko with Larry Rothstein. New York: Bantam, 1988.

Rituals of Healing: Using Imagery for Health and Wellness. Jeanne Achterberg, Ph.D., Barbara Dossey, R.N., and Leslie Kolkmeier. New York: Bantam Doubleday, 1994.

Staying Well with Guided Imagery. Belleruth Naparstek. New York: Warner Books, 1994.

Why Me? Harnessing the Healing Power of the Human Spirit. Garrett Porter and Patricia Norris, Ph.D. Walpole, NH: Stillpoint International, 1985.

HERBAL MEDICINE

Herbal medicine, also known as botanical medicine or phytotherapy, is the most ancient form of health care known to humankind. Herbs have been used in all cultures throughout history. Extensive scientific documentation now exists concerning their use for major and minor health conditions, including premenstrual syndrome, indigestion, insomnia, liver problems, and heart disease, among others.

HERBS HAVE ALWAYS been integral to the practice of medicine. The word *drug* derives from the old Dutch word *droog* meaning "to dry," as pharmacists, physicians, and ancient healers often dried plants for use as medicines. Today, approximately 25% of all prescription drugs are still derived from trees, shrubs, or herbs.[1] Some are made from plant extracts and others are synthesized to mimic a natural plant compound. The World Health Organization notes that of 119 plant-derived pharmaceutical medicines, about 74% are used in modern medicine in ways that correlate directly with their traditional uses as plant medicines by native cultures.[2]

Yet, for the most part, modern medicine has veered away from the use of pure herbs in its treatment of health disorders. One of the reasons for this is economic. Herbs, by their very nature, cannot be patented. Because of this, drug companies cannot hold the exclusive right to sell a particular herb and they are not motivated to invest in testing or promoting herbs. The collection and preparation of herbal medicines cannot be as easily controlled as the manufacture of synthetic drugs, making profits less dependable. In addition, many of these medicinal plants grow only in the Amazonian rain forest or other politically and economically unstable places, which also affects the supply of the herb.

Before the 1970s, the demand for herbal medicine decreased in the United States because Americans had been conditioned to rely on synthetic, commercial drugs to provide quick relief, regardless of the potential adverse side effects. This viewpoint is changing, however. "The

> *The World Health Organization notes that of 119 plant-derived pharmaceutical medicines, 74% are used in modern medicine in ways that correlate directly with their traditional uses as plant medicines by native cultures.*

revival of interest in herbal medicine is a worldwide phenomenon," says Mark Blumenthal, Founder and Executive Director of the American Botanical Council, the leading nonprofit herbal education organization in the U.S. This renaissance is due to the growing concern of the general public about the side effects of pharmaceutical drugs, the impersonal and often demeaning experience of modern health-care practices, and a renewed recognition of the unique medicinal value of herbs.

"The scope of herbal medicine ranges from mild-acting plant medicines, such as chamomile and peppermint, to very potent ones such as foxglove (from which the drug digoxin is derived). In between these two poles lies a wide spectrum of medicinal plants with significant medical applications," says Donald Brown, N.D., a leading author and researcher on herbal medicine and former Professor of Botanical Medicine at Bastyr University, in Seattle, Washington. "One need only go to the older editions of the *United States Pharmacopoeia* to see the central role that plant medicine has played in American medicine."

What is an Herb?

The word *herb* in herbal medicine refers to a plant or plant part that is used to make medicine, spices, or aromatic oils for soaps and fragrances. An herb can be a leaf, flower, stem, seed, root, fruit, bark, or any other plant part used for its medicinal, food flavoring, or fragrant property.[3]

Herbs have provided humankind with medicine from the earliest beginnings of civilization. Throughout history, various cultures have handed down their accumulated knowledge of the medicinal use of herbs to successive generations. This vast body of information serves as the basis for much of traditional medicine today.

There are an estimated 250,000 to 500,000 plants on the earth today, but only about 5,000 have been extensively studied for their medicinal applications.

There are an estimated 250,000 to 500,000 plants on the earth today, but only about 5,000 have been extensively studied for their medicinal applications. "This illustrates the need for modern medicine and science to turn its attention to the plant world once again to find new medicines that might cure cancer, AIDS, diabetes, and many other diseases and conditions," says Norman R. Farnsworth, Ph.D., Research Professor of Pharmacognosy at the University of Illinois, in Chicago. "Considering that 121 prescription drugs come from only 90 species of plants, and that 74% of these were discovered by following native folklore claims, a logical person would have to say that there may still be more 'jackpots' out there."[4]

How Herbal Medicine Works

In general, herbal medicines work in much the same way as conventional pharmaceutical drugs—via their chemical constituents. Herbs contain a large number of naturally occurring chemicals that have biological activity. Since 1804, chemists and pharmacists have been isolating and purifying the "active" compounds from plants in an attempt to produce reliable drugs. Examples include such drugs as the cardiac stimulant digoxin (from foxglove, *Digitalis purpurea*), blood pressure-lowering reserpine (from Indian snakeroot, *Rauwolfia serpenta*), the anti-inflammatory colchicine (from autumn crocus, *Colchicum autumnale*), the pain-reliever morphine (from the opium poppy, *Papaver somniafera*), and the anti-cancer drug Taxol (from the bark and leaves of the yew tree, *Taxus*).

According to author and integrative medicine proponent Andrew Weil, M.D., because herbs and the dietary supplements made from them use an indirect route to the bloodstream and target organs, their effects are usually slower in onset and less dramatic than those of purified drugs administered by more direct routes. "Doctors and patients accustomed to the rapid, intense effects of synthetic medicines may become impatient with botanicals for this reason," Dr. Weil states.[5]

Herbal medicine often has much to offer when used to facilitate healing in chronic problems. By skillful selection of herbs, a profound transformation in health can be effected with less danger of the side effects inherent in conventional drug-based medicine. However, the common assumption that herbs act slowly and mildly is not always true. Adverse effects can occur if an inadequate dose, a low-quality herb, or the wrong herb is consumed.

The Actions of Herbs

A great deal of pharmaceutical research has gone into analyzing the active ingredients of herbs to find out how and why they work. This is referred to as the herb's pharmacological action, the ways in which the remedy affects human physiology. In some cases, the action is due to a specific chemical present in the herb (as in the antiasthmatic effects of ephedrine and pseudoephedrine in the Chinese herb *ma-huang* or *Ephedra sinica*) or it may be due to a complex synergistic interaction among various constituents of the plant (the sedative action of numerous components in valerian, *Valeriana officinalis,* is an example).

A much older and far more relevant approach is to categorize herbs by looking at what kinds of conditions can be treated with their help. Plants have a direct impact on physiological activity and by knowing what body process one wants to help or heal, the appropriate action can be selected. The actions of herbs that make them beneficial in treating the human body include the following:

- **Adaptogenic:** Adaptogenic herbs increase resistance and resilience to stress, enabling the body to adapt around the problem and avoid the adverse effects of stress, such as fatigue. Some adaptogens are thought to work by supporting the function of the adrenal glands.

- **Alterative:** *Alterative* is a term that is seldom used today, but refers to herbs that gradually restore proper functioning of the body, increasing health and vitality.

- **Anthelmintic:** Herbs that destroy or expel intestinal worms.

- **Anti-inflammatory:** Herbs that soothe inflammation or reduce the inflammatory response of the tissue directly. They work in a number of ways, including inhibiting the formation of various chemicals produced by the body that tend to increase the inflammatory process.

- **Antimicrobial:** Antimicrobials help the body destroy or resist pathogenic (disease-causing) microorganisms. While some herbs contain chemicals that are antiseptic or poisonous to certain organisms, in general they aid the body's own natural immunity.

- **Antispasmodic:** Antispasmodics ease cramps in smooth and skeletal muscles and alleviate muscular tension.

- **Astringent:** Astringents have a binding action on mucous membranes, skin, and other tissues, reducing irritation and inflammation and creating a barrier against infection that is helpful to healing wounds and burns. This may result in the toning and tightening of skin and tissues.

- **Bitter:** Herbs with a bitter taste have a special role in preventative medicine. The taste triggers a sensory response in the central nervous system leading to a range of responses, including stimulating appetite and the flow of digestive juices, aiding the liver's detoxification work, increasing bile flow, and motivating intestinal self-repair mechanisms.

- **Carminative:** Plants that are rich in aromatic volatile oils stimulate the digestive system to work properly and with ease. They soothe the gut wall, reduce any inflammation that might be present, ease griping pains, and help with the removal of gas from the digestive tract.

- **Demulcent:** Demulcent herbs are rich in mucilage and soothe and protect irritated or inflamed tissues. They reduce irritation down the entire length of the bowel, reduce sensitivity to potentially corrosive gastric acids, help prevent diarrhea, and reduce the muscle spasms that cause colic.

- **Diuretic:** Diuretics increase the production and elimination of urine, helping the body eliminate waste and support the whole process of inner cleansing.

- **Emmenagogue:** Emmenagogues stimulate menstrual flow and activity. With most herbs, however, the term is used in the wider sense for a remedy that affects the female reproductive system.

- **Expectorant:** Herbs that stimulate removal of mucus from the lungs. Stimulating expectorants "irritate" the bronchioles (part of the bronchial tubes) causing expulsion of material. Relaxing expectorants soothe bronchial spasms and loosen mucus, which helps dry, irritating coughs.

- **Hepatic:** Hepatics tone and strengthen the liver and, in some cases, increase the flow of bile. In a broad, holistic approach to health, they are of great importance because of the fundamental role of the liver in maintaining health by facilitating digestion and removing toxins from the body.

- **Hypotensive:** Hypotensives are plant remedies that lower abnormally elevated blood pressure.

- **Laxative:** These are plants that promote bowel movements. They are divided into those that work by providing bulk, those that stimulate the production of bile in the liver and its release from the gallbladder, and those that directly stimulate peristalsis (the wavelike contractions of the smooth muscles of the digestive tract).

- **Nervine:** Nervines help the nervous system and can be subdivided into three groups—tonics that strengthen and restore the nervous system, relaxants that ease anxiety and tension by soothing both body and mind, and stimulants that directly stimulate nerve activity.

- **Stimulating:** Stimulants quicken and invigorate the physiological and metabolic activity of the body.

- **Tonic:** Tonics nurture and enliven. They are used frequently in traditional Chinese medicine and Ayurvedic medicine, often as a preventative measure. Tonic herbs like ginseng are thought to build vital energy, or *qi*.

Herbs in Many Forms

Herbs and herbal products come in many forms and are now available not only in natural and gourmet food stores, but also grocery stores, drugstores, and mass market retail stores. Also, a number of mail-order purveyors sell herbal products, as do alternative and conventional health practitioners.

THE POLITICS OF HERBAL MEDICINE

The World Health Organization (WHO) recognizes that nearly 80% of the world population in developing countries is dependent on traditional medicine for primary health care.[6] Herbal medicine constitutes a large part of what is practiced as traditional medicine around the world. WHO has published guidelines for the assessment of herbal medicines in an attempt to help the ministries of health of all governments develop regulations that ensure medicines are labeled properly and that consumers and practitioners are given proper directions for their use.[7]

However, since the early 1970s and through the 1990s, expert panels at the U.S. Food and Drug Administration (FDA) stringently reviewed over-the-counter (OTC) drug ingredients for safety and efficacy and eliminated many herbal ingredients from approved use in nonprescription medicines.[8] This did not come about as a result of finding that herbs were unsafe or ineffective, but because they determined that there was insufficient data upon which to base an evaluation. (The OTC review is a passive system—manufacturers must submit the data to support the safety and efficacy of an ingredient, and members of the herb industry simply did not submit research information on herbs during the 1970s.)

At the same time the FDA was removing the herbal ingredients from OTC drugs, an increasingly large segment of the population began using herbs and other natural medicines. Consequently, the U.S. Congress passed the Dietary Supplement Health and Education Act of 1994 (DSHEA), which created a new legal category called dietary supplements, including vitamins, minerals, amino acids, herbs, and related consumer health products that were ingested as part of the diet. DSHEA allowed herb products to claim limited benefits, so long as these statements were not disease claims (the product did not claim to treat, cure, or prevent a disease). DSHEA also allowed labels to carry warnings of potential adverse side effects, herb-drug interactions, or to proscribe the product's use in people with certain conditions (contraindications).

Herbal medicine is more readily accepted in Europe than in the U.S. The *British Herbal Pharmacopoeia*, though not officially recognized by Parliament, is nevertheless the accepted publication in the field.[9] In 1978, the German Ministry of Health established the respected Commission

E, an expert panel that evaluates the safety and efficacy of herbs sold as nonprescription drugs in German pharmacies. Many of these nonprescription herbal medicines are prescribed by German doctors, who study herbal medicine in medical school and, since 1993, must pass a section on these medicines in their board exams before becoming licensed.[10]

As part of the ongoing unifying efforts among members of the European community, European physicians, health professionals, and researchers have formed ESCOP, the European Scientific Cooperative for Phytotherapy. This organization has published 60 monographs on individual herbs used in clinical medicine as well as for self-medication. These monographs represent the culmination of the scientific and therapeutic information known on each herb.[11]

Additionally, the United States Pharmacopoeia, the organization that has developed official standards for drugs in the U.S. since 1820, is now publishing monographs containing standards for the most popular herbs and other dietary supplements, while the recently established American Herbal Pharmacopoeia is publishing extensive monographs dealing with standards and therapeutic guidelines for the use of many popular herbs. Further, an herb industry consortium called the Institute for Nutraceutical Advancement has begun the process of validating various analytical techniques to ensure that the laboratory methods used by the industry are uniform, replicable, and valid.

There is no licensing body for the practice of herbal medicine in the U.S. The result is that many herbal practitioners are outside of the "system." However, there are numerous qualified practitioners of herbal medicine who utilize approaches based on either the Western biomedical model or on Oriental approaches, such as traditional Chinese medicine and Ayurveda. The American Herbalists Guild is attempting to establish standards for the practice of professional herbal medicine. Within the Western medical community, there are naturopathic physicians who have graduated from four-year accredited schools of natural medicine who employ herbs and nutritional therapies as part of their clinical practice.

HOW TO MAKE AN HERBAL TEA

Loose teas are usually steeped in hot water: three to five minutes for leaves and flowers (this method is called infusion) or 15-20 minutes in a rolling boil for denser materials like roots and barks (called a decoction).

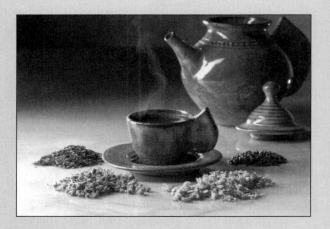

- Infusions are the simplest method of preparing an herb tea and both fresh and dried herbs, such as peppermint, chamomile, and rosehips, may be used. Due to the higher water content of the fresh herb, three parts fresh herb replace one part of the dried herb.

  To make an infusion, put about one teaspoon of the dried herb or herb mixture for each cup of water into a teapot; add boiling water and cover; leave to steep for 5-10 minutes. Infusions may be taken hot, cold, or iced. They may also be sweetened.

  Infusions are most appropriate for plant parts such as leaves, flowers, or green stems where the medicinal properties are easily accessible. To infuse bark, root, seeds, or resin, it is best to powder them first to break down their cell walls before adding them to the water. Seeds like fennel *(Foeniculum vulgare)* and anise should be slightly bruised to release the volatile oils from the cells. Any aromatic herb should be infused in a pot that has a tight-sealing lid to reduce loss of the volatile oil through evaporation.

- For hard and woody herbs, ginger root *(Zingiber officinale)* and cinnamon bark for example, it is best to make a decoction rather than an infusion, to ensure that the soluble contents of the herb actually reach the water. Roots, wood, bark, nuts, and certain seeds are hard and their cell walls are very strong, requiring more heat than in an infusion. These herbs need to be boiled in the water.

To make a decoction, put one teaspoon of dried herb or three teaspoons of fresh material for each cup of water into a pot or saucepan. Dried herbs should be powdered or broken into small pieces, while fresh material should be cut into small pieces. Add the appropriate amount of water to the herbs, bring to a boil, and simmer for 10-15 minutes.

When using a woody herb that contains a lot of volatile oil, it is best to make sure that it is powdered as finely as possible and then used in an infusion, to ensure that the volatile essential oils do not boil away. Decoctions can be consumed in the same way as an infusion.

Whole Herbs: Whole herbs are plants or plant parts that are dried and then either cut or powdered. They can be used as teas or for a variety of products at home.

Teas: Teas come in either loose leaf or teabag form. Because of the obvious convenience, most Americans today prefer to purchase their herbal teas in teabags, which include one or more finely cut herbs. When steeped in boiled water for a few minutes, the fragrant, aromatic flavor and the herb's medicinal properties are released. As a general rule, most teas are consumed for three reasons:

- As alternatives to caffeinated tea or coffee, although some herbal teas do contain caffeine, such as yerba mate *(Ilex paraguariensis)*

- As a component to a meal strictly for the flavor; for example, peppermint *(Mentha x piperita)*, spearmint *(M. spicata)*, rosehips *(Rosa canina)*, lemon grass *(Cymbopogon citratus)*, and anise *(Pimpinella anisatum)*

- For their mild medicinal effects—peppermint and chamomile *(Matricaria recutita)* for upset stomach or to improve digestion; chamomile or hops *(Humulus lupulus)* as a nighttime sleep aid or insomnia remedy; cinnamon *(Cinnamomum zeylanicum)* tea as a home remedy for mild diarrhea.

Capsules and Tablets: One of the fastest growing markets in herbal medicine in the past 15 to 20 years has been capsules and tablets. These offer consumers convenience and, in some cases, the bonus of not having to taste the herbs, many of which have undesirable flavors, from intensely bitter due to the presence of certain alkaloids to highly astringent due to the presence of tannins.

Extracts and Tinctures: These offer the advantage of being quickly assimilated compared to tablets, which take more time to disintegrate and ingest. Extracts and tinctures almost always contain alcohol. The alcohol is used for two reasons: as a solvent to extract the various non-water-soluble compounds from an herb and as a preservative. Properly made extracts and tinctures have virtually an indefinite shelf life. Tinctures usually contain more alcohol than extracts (sometimes up to 70% to 80% alcohol, depending on the particular herb and manufacturer).

Essential Oils: Essential oils are usually distilled from various parts of medicinal and aromatic plants. Some oils, however, like those from lemon, orange, and other citrus fruits, are actually expressed directly from the peels. Essential oils are concentrated, with one or two drops often constituting adequate dosage. Thus, they are to be used carefully and sparingly when employed internally. Because some oils may irritate the skin, they should be diluted in other oils or water before topical application. There are a few exceptions, most notably eucalyptus *(Eucalyptus globulus)* and tea tree *(Melaleuca alternifolia)* oils, which can be applied directly to the skin without concern of irritation.

See Aromatherapy.

Salves, Balms, and Ointments: For thousands of years, humans have used plants to treat skin irritations, wounds, and insect and snake bites. In prehistoric times, herbs were cooked in a vat of goose or bear fat, lard, or some vegetable oils and then cooled in order to make salves, balms, and ointments. Today, a number of such products, made with vegetable oil or petroleum jelly, are sold in the U.S. and Europe to treat a variety of conditions. These products often contain the herbs aloe *(Aloe vera)*, marigold *(Calendula officinalis)*, chamomile, St. John's wort *(Hypericum perforatum)*, comfrey *(Symphytum officinale)*, and gotu kola *(Centella asiatica)*.

Conditions Benefited by Herbal Medicine

Herbal remedies can be used for a wide range of minor ailments that are amenable to self-medication, including stomach upset, colds and flu, minor aches and pains, constipation and diarrhea, coughs, headaches, menstrual cramps, digestive disturbances, sore muscles, skin rashes, sunburn, and insomnia. A growing number of American health consumers use herbal remedies for these conditions, which have been traditionally the domain of nonprescription or over-the-counter drugs. Other conditions that respond to herbal medicine include: digestive disorders such as peptic ulcers, colitis, and irritable bowel syndrome; rheumatic and arthritic conditions; chronic skin problems such as eczema and psoriasis; problems of the menstrual cycle and especially premenstrual syndrome (PMS); anxiety and stress; bronchitis and other respiratory conditions; hypertension; and some allergies.

Herbal medicine can also be used for a number of conditions normally treated by prescription only. One example is milk thistle seed extract for use in cirrhosis and some forms of hepatitis.[12] Another example is the use of hawthorn as a heart tonic.[13] This herb is highly recommended for patients with early stages of congestive heart failure by physicians in Germany (see "The Herbal Medicine Chest" section in this chapter). However, readers are cautioned that they should not self-medicate for suspected cardiac conditions; professional advice is always required.

"When treating chronic illness with herbal medicine, it is extremely important to treat the entire body, as the illness may be simultaneously affecting many systems of the body at various levels," says Mary Bove, N.D., L.M., former head of the Department of Botanical Medicine at Bastyr University, in Seattle, Washington, and now in private practice in Vermont. "The course of the treatment must include nutritional, tonic, and restorative plants in conjunction with herbs that support the body's elimination functions. Alterative and adaptogenic plants can be very effective. Digestive function is also an important consideration in most chronic diseases." The duration of treatment is often longer, with a constant dose of the remedy being given over a longer period of time.

"I had a 38-year-old woman who came in with a ten-year-old case of colitis," Dr. Bove reports. "She had been seen by several M.D.s and N.D.s over the past decade with some improvement. After discussing her long history, I chose to treat her from a different perspective. Primarily, I gave her digestive nervines and tonic herbs like catnip, lemon balm, and tilia flowers. Within three days, she went from 11 stools per day to two per day. I

A DIVERSITY OF HERBAL TRADITIONS

There is a great diversity and richness in the various herbal traditions of the world, some of which still thrive today. Native American cultures contain a cornucopia of healing wisdom as do European traditions, from the Welsh to the Sicilian. There are a number of highly developed medical systems around the world that utilize medicinal plants in their healing work. These include ancient systems such as Ayurveda from India and traditional Chinese medicine. The essential differences between these systems of medicine are their cultural contexts rather than their goals or effects.

Traditional Chinese Medicine: The restoration of harmony is integral to Chinese herbal medicine. Harmonious balance is expressed in terms of the two complementary forces—*yin* and *yang*—and the five elements (fire, earth, metal, water, and wood). The five elements are of particular importance to the Chinese herbalist, because they give rise to the five tastes by which all medicinal plants are evaluated. Fire gives rise to bitterness, earth to sweetness, metal to acridity, water to saltiness, and wood to sourness. Each taste is said to have a particular medicinal action: bitter-tasting herbs drain and dry; sweet herbs tonify and may reduce pain; acrid herbs disperse; salty herbs nourish the kidneys; and sour herbs nourish the *yin* and have an astringent action, preventing unwanted loss of body fluids or vital energy *(qi)*. Herbs that have none of these tastes are described as bland, a quality that indicates that the plant may have a diuretic effect. The taste of a plant can also indicate the organ to which it has a natural affinity. Besides defining particular herbal tastes, the Chinese ascribe different temperature characteristics to herbs: hot, warm, neutral, cool, and cold.

Ayurveda: Ayurvedic medicine, which has ancient roots in the Indian subcontinent, also recognizes five elements: ether, fire, water, air, and earth. These elements manifest themselves in the body to form the *tridosha* or three basic humors: *vata* (the principle of air or movement), *pitta* (the principle of fire), and *kapha* (the principle of water). Ayurvedic medicine sees all universal energies as having their counterparts within the human being. The healing process seeks to achieve in individuals a balance between the elements of air or wind *(vata)*, fire or bile *(pitta)*, and water or phlegm *(kapha)*.

Ayurvedic medicine also holds that the taste of an herb is indicative of its properties. The Sanskrit word for taste, *rasa*,

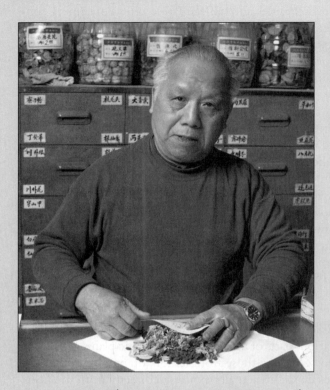

means "essence." There are six essences: sweet, sour, salty, pungent, bitter, and astringent. For example, pungent, sour, and salty-tasting herbs cause heat and so increase *pitta* (fire); sweet, bitter, and astringent herbs have precisely the opposite effect, cooling and decreasing *pitta*. As in Chinese herbal medicine, Ayurvedic texts categorize all plants according to this system, so that their herbalists can prescribe herbs more easily.

Western Medicine: The use of medicinal plants is also fundamental to Western society's pharmacologically based approach to medicine. The majority of medicinal drug groups were discovered or developed from the plant kingdom (or plant *kindom* as some modern evolutionary biologists prefer to call it, acknowledging the kinship and interconnectedness of all living organisms), even if they are now manufactured synthetically. However, most modern health professionals view medicines as biochemical "magic bullets," which should be expected to provide instant results. This approach has been very successful in certain areas, such as the treatment of acute illness, but has major limitations when it comes to chronic or degenerative disease.

 See Ayurvedic Medicine, Traditional Chinese Medicine.

continued with these herbs, adding some others for gut healing. We had excellent results, which were supported by diagnostic imaging."

Herbal medicine has also had great results with arthritic conditions. Consider the case of a 42-year-old woman with rheumatoid arthritis, confined to a wheelchair due to extreme and almost constant pain and swelling. She consulted with David Hoffmann, B.Sc., M.N.I.M.H., past President of the American Herbalists Guild. Her treatment involved herbal medicine and a reevaluation of her diet and lifestyle. Herbs were selected initially to ease the digestive problems (caused by medications she was taking) and to help her sleep. Once such side effects were alleviated, a program was started that enabled her to completely abandon the wheelchair after six months. Though she still had some arthritic pain, she was able to live with it comfortably.

 Additional research into the medical benefits of herbs will speed the integration of herbal medicine into the American health-care system. The National Center for Complementary and Alternative Medicine (NCCAM) at the National Institutes of Health (NIH) is funding millions of dollars worth of well-designed controlled clinical studies on herbs to determine from a valid scientific perspective what benefits they offer.

The Herbal Medicine Chest

ALOE VERA

Aloe is such a widely used ingredient in cosmetics that it is considered a mainstream cosmetic product and many people do not realize it is a medicinal herb. Aloe gel is used externally on the skin primarily for its emollient (skin-softening) property, as well as for its ability to heal wounds and burns. Applied to wounds, aloe gel is a mild anesthetic, relieving itching, swelling, and pain. It is also antibacterial and antifungal, increases blood flow to wounded areas, and stimulates fibroblasts (the skin cells responsible for healing).[14]

Another use for aloe comes from the latex of the inner leaf. Aloe latex is recognized as a safe and effective stimulant laxative ingredient by the U.S. Food and Drug Administration (FDA) as well as by many European countries. Normal precautions regarding laxatives apply to aloe: anthraquinone (a plant-based, organic compound) purgatives like aloe need to be used short-term only and not during pregnancy or lactation. Long-term use or misuse may cause an electrolyte imbalance, resulting in depletion of potassium salts and thus may adversely affect

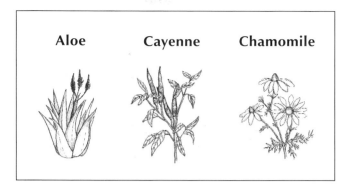

heart function.[15] Keep in mind that these warnings are for aloe latex used as a laxative, not the aloe gel or juice commonly consumed by health enthusiasts for inner cleansing.

BILBERRY (VACCINIUM MYRTYLLUS)

Bilberry is a European blueberry usually sold as a dried concentrate of the blue-purple fruits. These fruits contain compounds known as anthocyanidins that have antioxidant activity. Dried bilberry extracts are used in pill form for various circulatory benefits and to enhance vision, based on the modern legend that Royal Airforce pilots in World War II noticed increased nighttime visual acuity during bombing raids after they had eaten bilberry jam. Several clinical studies have been conducted to test this potential benefit. Bilberry's antioxidant activity and ability to increase microcirculation, especially in the retina, tends to support the ophthalmic benefits. Modern research has supported bilberry as an antioxidant and anti-inflammatory, as well as its ability to stabilize collagen and reduce vascular wall permeability.[16]

CAYENNE PEPPER (CAPSICUM ANNUUM)

Cayenne or red pepper is the most useful of the systemic stimulants, increasing blood flow and strengthening the heartbeat and metabolic rate.[17] As a general tonic, it is helpful specifically for the circulatory and digestive systems and may be used in flatulent dyspepsia (painful indigestion) and colic.[18] If there is insufficient peripheral circulation, leading to cold hands and feet and possibly chilblains (a form of cold injury characterized by redness and blistering), cayenne may be used. It is also useful for debility as well as for warding off colds.[19] Externally, it is used in problems like lumbago (a dull, aching pain in the lumbar region of the back) and rheumatic pains.[20]

CHAMOMILE (MATRICARIA RECUTITA)

Chamomile flower is used in many cultures for its pleasant-tasting tea, often consumed as an after-dinner beverage to help digestion. In Europe, chamomile is noted as a digestive aid, as a mild sedative, and for its anti-inflam-

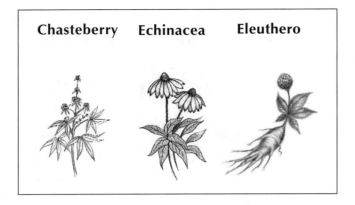

Chasteberry   Echinacea   Eleuthero

matory property, especially in over-the-counter preparations for oral hygiene and in skin creams.[21] In Germany, chamomile is licensed as an OTC drug for intestinal spasms and inflammatory diseases of the gastrointestinal tract. Externally, the extract is approved for skin and mucous membrane inflammation, bacterial skin diseases of the mouth and gums, and as a bath for inflamed conditions of anal and genital regions.[22]

CHASTEBERRY (VITEX AGNUS-CASTUS)

Chasteberry, also called chaste tree or vitex, is becoming widely used as an herb that addresses various hormonal imbalances in women. The clinical results are thought to be due to some regulatory effect upon the pituitary gland.[23] Recent findings confirm that chasteberry helps restore a normal estrogen-to-progesterone balance.[24] It is indicated for irregular or painful menstruation,[25] premenstrual syndrome (PMS),[26] and other disorders related to hormone function. Recent research conducted in Germany supports the use of chasteberry preparations in reducing symptoms associated with PMS.[27] It is especially beneficial during menopausal changes, relieving symptoms such as hot flashes, and may be used to aid the body in regaining a natural balance after the use of birth control pills. Other ailments treatable with chasteberry include fibroid cysts in smooth muscle tissue or body cavities and endometriosis. Several studies suggest that chasteberry can help control acne in teenagers, among both young women and men.[28]

DEVIL'S CLAW (HARPAGOPHYTUM PROCUMBENS)

A native of the deserts of western South Africa and Namibia, where this plant has been used in traditional medicine for centuries, devil's claw is becoming increasingly popular as a safe and effective treatment for rheumatoid arthritis and related inflammation, as well as lower back pain. Clinical studies have strongly suggested its safety and effectiveness.[29] One recent study in France compared devil's claw favorably with a conventional analgesic drug in the treatment of pain in people with

osteoarthritis of the hip.[30] Devil's claw is approved by the German Commission E as an aid to stimulate appetite and for arthritic conditions that affect the arms and legs.[31]

ECHINACEA (ECHINACEA PURPUREA, E. PALLIDA, E. ANGUSTIFOLIA)

Often called purple coneflower, the term echinacea refers to several species of plants that are generally found in the Great Plains region of the U.S. It was the most widely used medicinal plant of the Native Americans of this area, who often exploited echinacea for its external wound-healing and anti-inflammatory properties. Ironically, it was a German researcher, Dr. Gerhard Madaus, who imported echinacea seeds to Europe and initiated the first modern scientific research on the immuno-stimulating properties of this plant.

Echinacea has become one of the most important OTC remedies in Germany, where it is employed for relieving the common cold and flu. Over 180 products are marketed in Germany, including extracts and fresh-squeezed juices from both the roots and leaves of echinacea.[32] The German government has approved echinacea for use in recurrent infections of the respiratory and urinary tracts, progressive systemic disorders such as tuberculosis, leukosis (abnormal growth of white blood cells), connective tissue disease, and multiple sclerosis. When applied topically, echinacea is helpful for wounds with a poor tendency to heal.

Liquid echinacea preparations have immune-stimulating activity when administered both orally and parenterally (any medication route other than the intestine, such as intravenously): increasing the number of leukocytes (white blood cells) and splenocytes (white blood cells of the spleen) and enhancing the activity of granulocytes and phagocytes (cells that have the ability to ingest and destroy substances, such as bacteria, protozoa, and cell debris).[33] While most clinical studies on echinacea tend to support its effectiveness as a treatment for upper respiratory tract infections associated with colds and flu, recent research does not support the use of echinacea as a preventive for such conditions.[34]

ELEUTHERO (ELEUTHEROCOCCUS SENTICOSUS)

Eleuthero, also popularly called Siberian ginseng, is not considered a "true ginseng" but is a member of the same family (Araliaceae) as Asian and American (Panax) ginsengs. Eleuthero is considered an adaptogenic herb, increasing the body's ability to resist and endure stress, and has a very low toxicity.

A wealth of clinical and laboratory research has been conducted on eleuthero in the former Soviet Union. Initial findings from controlled experiments indicate a dramatic reduction of total disease occurrence, especially in diseases related to environmental stress.[35] There is a long list of illnesses that can improve with the use of this herb, including chronic gastritis, diabetes, and atherosclerosis (hardening of the arteries). Results from surgical studies show that eleuthero speeds post-operative recovery and is being used in this way in the treatment of cancer patients, easing the stress response that can aggravate metastasis (the spreading of a tumor to distant sites).[36] Eleuthero has been shown to reduce the cytotoxicity (cell-attacking nature) of cancer-fighting drugs and the narcotic effects of sedatives.[37]

EPHEDRA OR *MA-HUANG (EPHEDRA SINICA)*

Ephedra is a medicinal plant that has been cultivated for over 5,000 years in China, where it was used for asthma and hay fever–like conditions. Also known as *ma-huang*, ephedra's stems contain two primary alkaloids, ephedrine and pseudoephedrine, used in OTC decongestant drugs. Ephedrine has a marked peripheral vasoconstricting action (causing constriction of the blood vessels). Pseudoephedrine is a bronchodilator (able to expand the bronchi in the lungs, necessary for proper breathing), approved for use in asthma and certain allergy medicines. *Ma-huang* and its extracts are found in a number of herbal formulas that are designed to increase energy and reduce appetite.

Due to the relatively large number of adverse reactions (including some deaths) reported to the FDA associated with the use of ephedra-containing dietary supplements, ephedra has become controversial over the last decade. The FDA has tried to limit the amount of the alkaloids in ephedra supplements, their duration of use, and their actual uses; however, another government agency has found the FDA proposal lacking in scientific merit and its adverse event reporting system faulty. At present, the herb and supplement industries have initiated voluntary label warnings and limits on the levels of ephedrine and pseudoephedrine in supplements (usually limited to 25 mg of total alkaloids per dose; a total of 100 mg per day).[38]

Both ephedrine and pseudoephedrine have central nervous system–stimulating properties, with ephedrine being more active. These alkaloids have been characterized as being stronger than caffeine and weaker than methamphetamine. Therefore, this herb should be used with caution or avoided by those with high blood pressure, heart disease, diabetes, glaucoma, prostate conditions, and related conditions where hypertensives are contraindicated.[39] Consumers should check with their physician before taking supplements with ephedra.

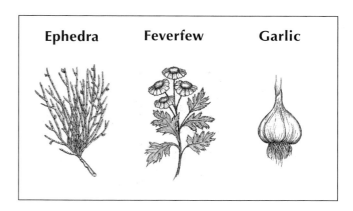

Ephedra   Feverfew   Garlic

FEVERFEW *(TANACETUM PARTHENIUM)*

Feverfew is an herbal remedy that dates back to Greco-Roman times. It was formerly employed as a remedy for difficulties associated with menstrual cycles in young women (the word *parthenium* is derived from the Greek word *parthenos,* meaning "virgin") and was later used in European herbalism to reduce fevers (the name *feverfew* is a corruption of the Latin word *febrifuga,* meaning an agent that lowers fevers).[40]

Interest in this herb has increased in the past 15 years because of several clinical studies published in British medical journals. Research showed that feverfew leaves brought relief in a significant number of migraine patients who had not responded positively to conventional medications and also helped to prevent the onset of additional episodes.[41] The Canadian government's Health Protection Branch (equivalent to the FDA) has approved feverfew leaf extract for migraine prevention, as long as the products contain a minimum of 0.2% parthenolide, a substance in feverfew incorrectly considered to be its primary active component.[42] According to Blumenthal, parthenolide has been shown to be inactive for this use, but can be used as an indicator of the proper plant chemical profile for quality control. Early herbal literature also attributes antirheumatic properties to feverfew, but this has not been confirmed by modern research.[43]

GARLIC *(ALLIUM SATIVUM)*

Garlic is probably the most well-recognized medicinal herb. It is used by traditional medicines all over the world and its applications are as varied as its geographical distribution. The chemistry and pharmacology of garlic is well studied: as of 1998, there were an estimated 1,990 scientific publications on the activities of garlic and chemical compounds from garlic, including chemical, toxicological, pharmacological, clinical, and epidemiological studies.[44]

Garlic is known for its antibiotic, antifungal, and antiviral activities; for helping clear congested lungs; for coughs, bronchitis, and sinus congestion; as a preventive

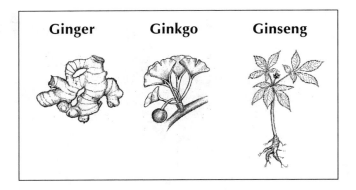

Ginger   Ginkgo   Ginseng

measure for colds and flu; for intestinal worms, dysentery, and certain ulcers; and for gout and rheumatism.[45] Garlic may also help prevent certain cancers. A National Cancer Institute report on a large Chinese population indicated that the consumption of garlic and other members of the *Allium* genus (onions, leeks, shallots) can help lower the incidence of stomach cancer.[46]

Western countries have shown interest in garlic's ability to provide important cardiovascular benefits, including slightly lowering blood pressure, aiding in the thinning of blood, and reducing platelet aggregation (blood coagulation).[47] One four-year study showed that 900 mg per day of a garlic supplement helped reverse arterial plaque buildup, thereby reducing the risk of cardiovascular disease.[48] Garlic has also shown an ability to aid immune function, particularly increasing the activity of natural killer cells.[49]

Studies indicate general benefits from almost any type of garlic—raw, dried, garlic oil, or a prepared commercial product.[50] However, odorless or odor-controlled garlic preparations, such as kyolic, have a high degree of activity and are appropriate for those who do not wish to suffer the problems associated with garlic's characteristic odor, such as bad breath. In Germany, garlic extracts are approved by the Commission E as nonprescription drugs to supplement dietary measures in patients with elevated cholesterol levels and to avert age-associated vascular changes.[51] Although one early meta-analysis (statistical evaluation of many studies) of clinical studies concluded that garlic lowered total cholesterol about 9%–12%, several recent evaluations have found that garlic may only lower cholesterol about 4%–6%.[52]

GINGER *(ZINGIBER OFFICINALIS)*

In addition to its popularity as a food flavoring, ginger is widely used as a medicinal herb in Chinese and Ayurvedic medicine, often added to herbal formulas to increase digestion and the activity of other herbs. In the past 15 years, ginger has become best known for its anti-nausea and anti-motion sickness activity. A number of clinical studies have confirmed ginger's ability to act on the gastrointestinal system and allay nausea.[53] Unlike the leading OTC drug, Dramamine, ginger does not relieve nausea by suppressing central nervous system activity. Rather, the effect is explained by the antiemetic properties of this herb on the digestive tract, which are well documented.[54] A recent study in Thailand on pregnant women has also documented the safety of ginger when used to relieve morning sickness during the first trimester of pregnancy.[55] Ginger is also known to have cardiotonic properties[56] and has been used in traditional medicine for migraine relief.[57] In traditional Chinese medicine, fresh ginger juice is applied topically as a burn remedy.[58]

GINKGO *(GINKGO BILOBA)*

Ginkgo is an excellent example of why protecting plants and animals from extinction can help create new medicines. Ginkgos, the oldest living trees, first appeared about 200 million years ago and, except for a small number in northern China, were almost completely destroyed in the last Ice Age. Ginkgo leaves contain several compounds called ginkgolides and one called bilobalide that have unique chemical structures. The leaves, used as a remedy for lung problems, were mentioned in major Chinese herbal texts as far back as 1436.

A highly concentrated, pharmaceutically prepared standardized extract was developed in the past 30 years in Germany to treat various conditions associated with peripheral circulation.[59] It is currently licensed in Germany for the treatment of cerebral dysfunction (short-term memory problems, dizziness, tinnitus), mainly in older people. A study in the *Journal of the American Medical Association* concluded that ginkgo extract was effective in treating patients in the early stages of dementia associated with Alzheimer's disease.[60]

Ginkgo is also approved in Germany as a supportive treatment for hearing loss due to impaired circulation and for peripheral arterial circulatory disturbances, such as intermittent claudication (a severe pain in the calf muscles resulting from inadequate blood supply).[61] Ginkgo leaf extracts are also used for heart and eye diseases, as well as accidents involving brain trauma. At least three volumes of information on the chemistry, pharmacology, and clinical uses of *Ginkgo biloba* extract have been published.[62]

GINSENG *(PANAX GINSENG,* ORIENTAL GINSENG; *P. QUINQUEFOLIUS,* AMERICAN GINSENG)

Ginseng has an ancient history and has accumulated much folklore about its actions and uses. The genus name *Panax* is derived from the Latin word *panacea* meaning "cure all." Many of the claims that surround ginseng are exaggerated, but it is clearly an important remedy, receiving attention from researchers around the world.[63] Research suggests that it is adaptogenic, aiding the body in coping with stress, primarily through effects upon the functioning of the adrenal glands.[64] Ginseng also has antioxidant, liver-protecting, and hypoglycemic effects.[65] There is a wide range of possible benefits, but the main application is with weak, debilitated, stressed, or elderly people, where these properties can be especially useful.[66]

In addition, ginseng may help to lower blood cholesterol and stimulate a range of immune system and endocrine responses.[67] Several small studies on American ginseng suggest that it can help normalize blood sugar levels in both Type II diabetic adults and normal healthy adults after meals.[68]

GOLDENSEAL *(HYDRASTIS CANADENSIS)*

One of the most widely used Native American herbs, goldenseal root is popularly considered a remedy for colds and upper respiratory tract infections. However, Blumenthal points out that there is a disappointing lack of scientific research to support the potential benefits of this herb. "Many consumers consider goldenseal a tonic remedy that stimulates immune response, although there are no scientific data to support this," he says.

Because of its bitter effects, goldenseal is considered by some to be helpful for digestive problems, from peptic ulcers to colitis.[69] Its bitter stimulation helps in loss of appetite and the alkaloids it contains stimulate production and secretion of digestive juices. Sometimes erroneously called an antibiotic, goldenseal actually has antimicrobial properties, due to the presence of alkaloids, such as berberine.[70] Berberine has a broad spectrum of activity against bacteria, protozoa, and fungi, including *Staphylococcus, Streptococcus, Candida albicans,* and *Gardia lamblia.*[71] For this reason, goldenseal can be useful for helping to treat and prevent traveler's diarrhea. Berberine's action in inhibiting *Candida* prevents the overgrowth of yeast that is a common side effect of antibiotic use. This alkaloid has also been shown to activate macrophages (cells that digest cellular debris and other waste matter in the blood).[72]

Applied externally, it can be helpful in eczema, ringworm, itching, earache, and conjunctivitis.[73] Traditionally, goldenseal has been used during labor to help contractions and, for this reason, it should be avoided during pregnancy.

HAWTHORN *(CRATAEGUS OXYACANTHA)*

Hawthorn has been used in folk medicine in Europe and China for centuries. Hawthorn is one of the primary heart tonics in traditional medicine. Europeans have employed both the edible fruit as well as the extract of the leaves and flowers, primarily for their beneficial effects

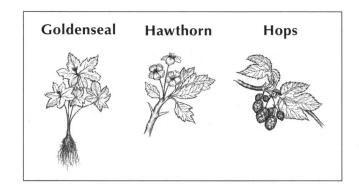

Goldenseal   Hawthorn   Hops

on the cardiovascular system (cardiotonic, sedative, and hypotensive activities).

In Germany, hawthorn extracts are used for a number of heart-related conditions, often in conjunction with digoxin, the primary conventional pharmaceutical drug used for congestive heart failure. Hawthorn has been extensively tested on animals and humans and is known to cause the following actions: decreases blood pressure with exertion, increases the heart muscle's ability to contract, increases blood flow to the coronary muscles, decreases heart rate, and decreases oxygen use by the myocardium (the middle layer of the walls of the heart).[74] Hawthorn extracts are approved by the German Commission E for declining heart performance.[75]

HOPS *(HUMULUS LUPULUS)*

Hops has been used as a bittering and preservative agent in brewing for centuries. In Germany, hops is approved for use in states of unrest and anxiety as well as for sleep disorders, due to its calming and sleep-inducing properties.[76] European researchers have approved the use of hops for such conditions as nervous tension, excitability, restlessness, and sleep disturbances, and as an aid to stimulate appetite. Unlike other types of sedatives, there are neither dependence nor withdrawal symptoms reported with the use of hops, nor are there any reports of adverse side effects.[77] A hops and valerian combination is approved by the German Commission E as a sleep aid, based on scientific research on both herbs; recent research on the combination supports this approval.[78]

HORSE CHESTNUT *(AESCULUS HIPPOCASTANUM)*

Horse chestnut seed extract (HCSE), a standardized extract from the seeds of the horse chestnut tree, is widely used in European phytotherapy to treat "chronic venous insufficiency" (CVI), most commonly poor circulation in the lower legs and the resulting edema (swelling), and nighttime leg cramps. A meta-analysis published in the *Archives of Dermatology* on clinical studies involving 1,100 people concluded that HCSE was safe and effective for conditions associated with CVI. Moreover, adverse effects

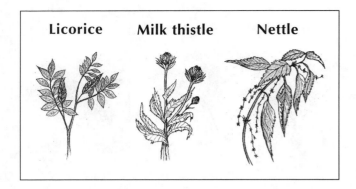

were mild and infrequent.[79] Horse chestnut is also used for varicose veins and hemorrhoids.

KAVA-KAVA (*PIPER METHYSTICUM*)

Kava-kava is the root and rhizome (lateral root) of an herb from the black pepper family from Polynesia, Samoa, Fiji, and Vanuatu. Kava is the most revered herb in Polynesia, being an important part of the culture there. Kava beverages are given to visiting dignitaries as a measure of respect—President Lyndon B. Johnson received kava when he went to U.S. Samoa and Pope John Paul II drank kava in Fiji. Kava is often consumed in a mild, relaxing beverage on a social basis.

European researchers have carried out numerous clinical studies on standardized kava extract to confirm its mild relaxing effects and the herb has been approved by the German Commission E for anxiety.[80] A statistical review of three published clinical trials conducted on a German extract (standardized to 70% kavalactones, the active compounds in kava) showed kava to be safe and effective for treatment of anxiety when compared to placebo.[81]

However, caution is advised when taking kava as recent reports from Europe indicate an association between kava and liver problems. Blumenthal recommends that kava not be used by those with existing liver problems, those taking pharmaceutical drugs that adversely affect the liver, or people who regularly drink alcohol. He also suggests that kava not be taken on a daily basis for more than four weeks and that its use should be discontinued if symptoms of jaundice occur. Anyone with a history of liver problems should consult with their physician before using kava.

LICORICE (*GLYCYRRHIZA GLABRA*)

Licorice is a traditional herbal remedy and modern research has shown it to have effects upon the endocrine system, liver, and other organs. Constituents of this herb, called triterpenes, are metabolized in the body into molecules that have a similar structure to the adrenal hormones, which my be the basis for the anti-inflammatory action of licorice.[82] Glycyrrhizin, a triterpene, inhibits liver cell injury caused by many chemicals and is used in the treatment of chronic hepatitis and cirrhosis, especially in Japan.[83] Glycyrrhizin inhibits the growth of several viruses and inactivates the herpes simplex virus.[84]

Licorice is also used as a treatment for peptic ulcers and gastritis, colic, and bronchial problems such as bronchitis and coughs. There is a small possibility of affecting electrolyte balance with extended use of large doses of licorice. It can cause retention of sodium, thus raising blood pressure. The whole herb has constituents that counter this effect, but it is best to avoid licorice in cases of hypertension, kidney disease, or during pregnancy.

MILK THISTLE (*SILYBUM MARIANUM*)

Historically, this herb has been used in Europe as a liver tonic. Current phytotherapy indicates the use of the standardized extract of its seed (technically, the fruits) for a range of liver and gallbladder conditions, including hepatitis and cirrhosis. A wealth of laboratory and clinical research on this herb reveals its ability to reverse liver damage as well as offer protection from potentially toxic chemical agents.[85] These findings highlight a role for milk thistle in the treatment of toxic/metabolic liver disease (both alcohol- and drug-induced forms), some forms of hepatitis (usually A, sometimes C), cirrhosis of the liver, and fatty degeneration of the liver.[86]

Milk thistle shortens the course of viral hepatitis, minimizes post-hepatitis complications, and protects the liver against problems resulting from liver surgery. It is an excellent remedy for use in the prevention and treatment of many liver disorders. The leading milk thistle extract product from Germany has been termed "undoubtedly the best documented pharmaceutical agent for the treatment of liver diseases."[87]

NETTLE (*URTICA DIOICA*)

Nettle, also known as stinging nettle, is one of the most widely used herbs in the Western world. However, this common plant has received little attention from the medical community. Throughout Europe, nettle is used as a spring tonic and detoxifying remedy. When steamed or boiled, the leaves can be eaten. If used regularly, it can be remarkably successful in cases of rheumatism and arthritis, often when the stinging hairs on the leaves are slapped across a swollen area, producing a counter-irritant effect.[88]

Based upon its traditional uses, it might be inferred that nettle is a safe, immunomodulating tonic. A lectin (plant protein) found in nettle leaf stimulates the proliferation of white blood cells.[89] Traditional use of nettle in the treatment of allergic rhinitis (hay fever) is gaining some limited research support.[90] It is especially indicated for all varieties of childhood eczema. Fresh nettle as a tea has been used as a safe diuretic.[91]

Nettle root has an altogether different use as an aid in treating benign prostatic hyperplasia (BPH), a condition characterized by swelling of the prostate and urinary disturbances. Nettle root extract has anti-inflammatory properties and is approved by the German Commission E for BPH.[92]

PASSIONFLOWER (PASSIFLORA INCARNATA)

Passionflower has enjoyed a tradition of use for its mildly sedative properties. In Germany, passionflower is approved as an over-the-counter drug for states of "nervous unrest."[93] In Europe, passionflower is often added to other calming herbs, usually valerian and hawthorn. Passionflower and hawthorn are used together as antispasmodics for digestive spasms in cases of gastritis and colitis. Pharmacological studies indicate antispasmodic, sedative, anxiety-allaying, and hypotensive activity of passionflower extracts.[94]

PEPPERMINT (MENTHA PIPERITA)

Peppermint has been a popular folk remedy for digestive disorders for over 200 years and is currently one of the most economically significant aromatic food/medicine crops produced in the U.S.[95] In some European countries, peppermint leaf is recognized as a digestive aid due to the gas-preventing and bile-increasing action of the aromatic oil. In Germany, peppermint oil is approved as an OTC drug for upper gastrointestinal cramps and spastic conditions of bile ducts, catarrh (inflammation of mucous membranes) of the upper respiratory area, and inflammation of oral mucous membranes.[96] It is also approved (in enteric-coated capsule form) for irritable bowel syndrome, as the oil exerts a relaxing effect on the smooth muscles of the bowel.[97]

Peppermint oil also has antibacterial properties, as do many essential oils. Peppermint oil and menthol are common ingredients in external analgesic products like balms and liniments. In Germany, this combination is approved for external use for muscle and nerve pain.[98] In addition to the above conditions, peppermint oil is approved by the European Scientific Cooperative in Phytotherapy for gallbladder inflammation and gallstones and skin conditions such as pruritis (severe itching) and urticaria (eruption of wheals with intense itching).[99]

PYGEUM (PRUNUS AFRICANA OR PYGEUM AFRICANUM)

Pygeum bark comes from a hardwood tree in Africa and has become increasingly popular in Europe and the U.S. as a treatment for benign prostatic hyperplasia (BPH). The bark extracts exhibit anti-inflammatory activity and are helpful in reducing the urinary symptoms associated

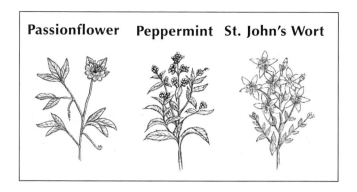

Passionflower   Peppermint   St. John's Wort

with BPH.[100] Numerous clinical studies support its use in modern BPH therapy.[101]

ST. JOHN'S WORT (HYPERICUM PERFORATUM)

A remedy long used as an anti-inflammatory, wound-healing nervine valued for its mild sedative and pain-reducing properties, St. John's wort has recently regained medical attention. Taken internally, it has traditionally been used to treat neuralgia, anxiety, tension, and similar problems. In addition to neuralgic pain, it will ease fibrositis, sciatica, and rheumatic pain.[102] It is especially regarded as an herb to use in the case of menopausal changes triggering irritability and anxiety. Used externally, it is a valuable healing and anti-inflammatory remedy.[103] As a lotion, it will speed the healing of wounds and bruises, varicose veins, and mild burns (especially for healing sunburn).[104]

The primary use of St. John's wort, and the reason for its popularity during the past few years, is its clinically proven benefit for the treatment of mild to moderate depression.[105] It is not effective for cases of more serious or chronic depression, however, and can adversely affect the activity of conventional drugs (antivirals, immunosuppressants, cardiac medications, and possibly others); therefore, people should not use St. John's wort if they are taking conventional medicines, without the consent of their physician.

SAW PALMETTO (SERENOA REPENS)

Saw palmetto is the fruit of an American dwarf palm tree from Florida that has become popular as an herbal remedy for maintaining the health of the male urinary tract. It is most effective in cases of benign prostatic hyperplasia, the noncancerous enlargement of the prostate gland associated with aging.[106] A review of 18 controlled clinical studies on a total of 2,939 men revealed that saw palmetto extract was more effective than a placebo. In three of the studies where the herbal preparation was compared to the leading conventional drug for BPH, finasteride or Proscar®, saw palmetto had about 90% fewer adverse side effects.[107] Another study showed that saw palmetto lowered the levels of the hormone dihy-

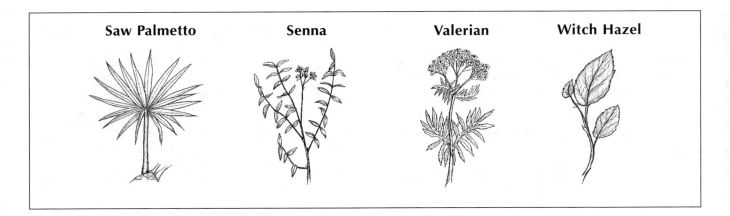

Saw Palmetto Senna Valerian Witch Hazel

drotestosterone (DHT) in prostate tissue. DHT levels are known to increase with age and higher levels are associated with prostate enlargement.[108] An earlier study by the same researchers showed evidence that saw palmetto may help shrink prostate tissue.[109]

SENNA *(CASSIA SENNA)*

Senna is a laxative from the leaves and pods of the senna plant, a member of the pea family, that is derived from ancient Arabic medicine. In Europe and the U.S., extracts from senna are approved in OTC laxatives. The German government has approved senna for all conditions of constipation in which the need for soft stools is indicated. There are no adverse side effects connected with the use of senna, other than those normally associated with the use of stimulant laxatives (long-term use or misuse can result in dependency and electrolyte loss).[110] Like other stimulant laxatives, senna should not be used during pregnancy or lactation unless professionally supervised.

VALERIAN *(VALERIANA OFFICINALIS)*

The odorous root of valerian has been used in European traditional medicine for centuries. In Germany, valerian root and its teas and extracts are approved as over-the-counter medicines for "states of excitation" and "difficulty in falling asleep owing to nervousness."[111] A scientific team representing the European community has reviewed the research on valerian and concluded that it is a safe nighttime sleep aid. These scientists also found that there were no major adverse reactions associated with the use of valerian and, unlike barbiturates and other conventional drugs used for insomnia, valerian does not have a synergy with alcohol.[112] Herbalist and author Christopher Hobbs, L.Ac., notes that other uses for valerian include nervous heart conditions, children's anorexia caused by excitement, trembling, and stomach complaints. He recommends a valerian-hops preparation as a good daytime sedative as it will not interfere with or slow one's reflexive responses.[113] A valerian-hops extract combination has been introduced in the U.S. as a dietary

supplement for aiding sleep, based on clinical studies strongly suggesting the safety and efficacy of this herb combination, as well as the fact that the German Commission E had approved a similar combination based on previous research.[114]

WITCH HAZEL *(HAMAMELIS VIRGINIANA)*

Witch hazel comes from a tree native to North America and is considered a safe astringent for common usage, approved for external use as an OTC medicine. It is found most commonly in the form of a distilled liquid, usually containing about 14% alcohol (which some authors suggest is the actual reason why American witch hazel products possess astringent properties). As with most astringents, this herb may be used wherever there has been bleeding, internally or externally. It is especially useful in easing the pain and swelling of hemorrhoids.[115] Topically, it can be used in the treatment of bruises and swelling and also with varicose veins.[116] Internally, witch hazel teas and extracts have been used to stop diarrhea and aid in the treatment of dysentery. However, commercial witch hazel preparations found in most drugstores are not intended for internal use.

The Future of Herbal Medicine

According to James Duke, Ph.D., an ethnobotanist, former herb specialist with the U.S. Department of Agriculture, and author of numerous books on herbs, one of the reasons that research into the field of herbal medicine has been lacking is the enormous cost of the testing required to prove a new "drug" safe. Dr. Duke has seen that price tag rise from $91 million as of 15 years ago to the present figure of around $500 million. Dr. Duke asks, "What commercial drug maker is going to want to prove that saw palmetto is better than their multimillion dollar drug, when you and I can go to Florida and harvest our own saw palmetto?"

In recent years, however, the research agenda has changed considerably in the U.S. Stimulated by funding from the National Center for Complementary and Alternative Medicine at the National Institutes of Health, millions of dollars have been committed to the development of human clinical trials to test the efficacy of such herbs as St. John's wort, ginkgo, echinacea, black cohosh, and many more. The future looks bright for those who want to explore the benefits of herbal medicine. The demand for natural medicines has grown significantly, to the point that herbal preparations are now available in supermarkets, drugstores, and other large retail outlets. According to a 1999 survey, about 48% of adult Americans had used herbs within the previous year and 24% admit to using herbs regularly.

One of the major problems in the U.S. is the lack of a regulatory system that allows the therapeutic benefits to be put onto the label of herbal products. Without these recognized benefits, consumers will be exposed to media stories that overemphasize the risks and underplay the benefits of these natural remedies.

—MARK BLUMENTHAL, EXECUTIVE DIRECTOR, AMERICAN BOTANICAL COUNCIL

"The use of herbal products requires that people learn about their benefits and their potential risks," says Mark Blumenthal. "People must realize that herbs can have some risks if they are not used properly and responsibly. But one of the major problems in the U.S. is the lack of an effective, rational regulatory system that allows the therapeutic benefits to be put onto the label of herbal products. Without these recognized benefits, consumers will be constantly exposed to media stories that overemphasize the risks and underplay the benefits of these valuable natural remedies."

Where to Find Help

As part of the resurgence in environmental awareness, herbs and herbal remedies are receiving increased attention as a natural, cost-effective alternative to pharmaceutical products. For more information on herbal medicine, or to find a physician who uses herbal remedies, contact:

American Association of Oriental Medicine
433 Front Street
Catasauqua, Pennsylvania 18032
(888) 500-7999
Website: www.aaom.org

The AAOM is a national professional trade organization of acupuncturists who meet acceptable standards of competency. They also can provide names and locations of local members.

American Association of Naturopathic Physicians
8201 Greensboro Drive, Suite 300
McLean, Virginia 22102
(703) 610-9037
Website: www.naturopathic.org

Provides referrals to a nationwide network of accredited or licensed practitioners. Publishes a quarterly newsletter for both professionals and the general public and also offers a series of brochures and pamphlets on a variety of subjects.

American Botanical Council
P.O. Box 144345
Austin, Texas 78714-4345
(512) 926-4900
Website: www.herbalgram.org

The leading nonprofit herbal research and education organization. Publishes HerbalGram, a highly respected peer-reviewed magazine, booklets on herbs, books, reprints of scientific articles, and has an extensive catalog of books, monographs, audio and videotapes, CD-ROMs, and other educational materials for health professionals and consumers. Also provides continuing education for health professionals, plus herbal medicine ecotours of the Amazon and other areas.

American Herbal Pharmacopoeia
P.O. Box 5159
Santa Cruz, California 95063
(831) 461-6318
Website: www.herbal-ahp.org

AHP is a nonprofit educational and research organization that develops national quality control standards for the man-

ufacture of botanical supplements and provides extensive therapeutic information through the publication of comprehensive monographs on herbs.

American Herbal Products Association
8484 Georgia Avenue, Suite 370
Silver Spring, Maryland 20910
(301) 588-1171
Website: www.ahpa.org

AHPA is the major trade association dedicated to ethical and responsible commerce and advancement of the herbal products industry. AHPA's members consist of botanical suppliers, distributors, growers, and marketers who are dedicated to creating products that are used to enhance health through the use of herbs.

American Herbalists Guild
1931 Gaddis Road
Canton, Georgia 30115
(770) 751-6021
Website: www.americanherbalist.com

AHG is a nonprofit membership organization dedicated to meeting the professional needs of herbalists and other practitioners of botanical medicine, offering an academic journal, education guidelines, mentorship opportunities, and national certification standards.

Herb Research Foundation
1007 Pearl Street, Suite 200
Boulder, Colorado 80302
(303) 449-2265
Website: www.herbs.org

Provides research materials for consumers, pharmacists, physicians, scientists, and the industry. Members receive HerbalGram and/or Herbs for Health as benefits.

North American College of Botanical Medicine
1104 Park Avenue S.W.
Albuquerque, New Mexico 87102-2941
(505) 873-8107
Website: www.swcp.com/botanicalmedicine

A leading center for herbal education in the U.S. and a catalyst in the effort to integrate traditional healing practices with contemporary health care. It was founded to meet the growing demands for definitive herbal education and the need for trained professional herbalists.

United Plant Savers
P.O. Box 98
East Barre, Vermont 05649
Website: www.plantsavers.org

An organization committed to the preservation of medicinal plants in North America. Produces conferences, books, and operates a native medicinal plant sanctuary in central Ohio.

Recommended Reading

Magazines and Newsletters

American Herb Association Newsletter. Available from: P.O. Box 1673, Nevada City, California 95959; (530) 265-9552; Website: www.jps.net/ahaherb. This publication covers a wide range of herbal topics: media coverage, research, regulatory issues, quality control, and more.

HerbalGram. Available from: American Botanical Council, P.O. Box 144345, Austin, Texas 78714-4345; (512) 926-4900 or (800) 373-7105; Website: www.herbalgram.org. The quarterly peer-reviewed magazine of the American Botanical Council and the Herb Research Foundation contains scientific updates on herbs, feature articles, updates on legal and regulatory matters, book reviews, and more.

Herb Quarterly. Available from: P.O. Box 689, San Anselmo, California 94979; (800) 371-HERB; Website: www.herbquarterly.com. A magazine dealing with herb gardening and crafting and the medicinal applications of herbs.

Herbs for Health. Available from: 243 E. Fourth Street, Loveland, Colorado 80537; (970) 663-0831; Website: www.discoverherbs.com. The leading consumer magazine on herbs and their potential benefits and uses in self-care.

Medical Herbalism. Available from: Bergner Communications, P.O. Box 20512, Boulder, Colorado 80308; (303) 541-9552; Website: medherb.com. Written primarily for practitioners, this quarterly newsletter deals with the appropriate use of herbs in a clinical setting, including case histories, dosages, contraindications, and toxicity issues.

Robyn's Recommended Reading. Available from: 1627 W. Main, Suite 116, Bozeman, Montana 59715; (406) 585-8006; Website: www.wtp.net/~rrr. Newsletter summarizing some of the latest herbal literature, with reviews reflecting an herbalist's perspective.

Books

101 Medicinal Herbs. Steven Foster. Loveland, CO: Interweave Press, 1998.

The Complete German Commission E Monographs—Therapeutic Guide to Herbal Medicines. Mark Blumenthal, ed.

Austin, TX: American Botanical Council & Integrated Medicine Communications, 1998.

The Encyclopedia of Popular Herbs. Robert McCaleb, Evelyn Leigh, and Krista Morien. Roseville, CA: Prima Publishing, 2000.

Herbal Medicine. V. Fintelmann and R.F. Weiss. New York: Thieme Publishers, 2000.

Herbal Medicine: Expanded Commission E Monographs. M. Blumenthal, A. Goldberg, and J. Brinckmann. Newton, MA: Integrative Medicine Communications, 2000.

Herbal Prescriptions for Health and Healing. Donald J. Brown. Rocklin, CA: Prima Health, 2000.

Herbs of Choice: Therapeutic Use of Phytomedicinals. Varro E. Tyler. Binghampton, NY: Haworth Press, 1999.

Kids, Herbs & Health. Linda B. White and Sunny Mavor. Loveland, CO: Interweave Press, 1998.

Rational Phytotherapy: A Physician's Guide to Herbal Medicine. Volker Schulz, Rudi Hänsel, and Varro E. Tyler. New York: Springer Verlag, 2000.

Women's Herbs, Women's Health. Christopher Hobbs and Kathi Keville. Loveland, CO: Botanica Press, 1998.

All of these books are available from the American Botanical Council at www.herbalgram.org or (800) 373-7105, or from your local bookstore.

HOMEOPATHY

Homeopathy is a low-cost, nontoxic system of medicine used by hundreds of millions of people worldwide. It is particularly effective in treating chronic illnesses that fail to respond to conventional treatment and is also a superb method of self-care for minor conditions such as the common cold and flu.

THE WORD *HOMEOPATHY* derives from the Greek words *homoios*, meaning "similar," and *pathos*, meaning "suffering." Homeopathic remedies are generally dilutions of natural substances from plants, minerals, and animals. Based on the principle of "like cures like," these remedies specifically match different symptom patterns or "profiles" of illness and act to stimulate the body's natural healing response.

Throughout its over 200-year history, homeopathy has proven effective in treating diseases for which conventional medicine has little to offer. However, due to its low cost, which threatens pharmaceutical profits, as well as its divergence from conventional medical theory, homeopathy has been continually attacked by the medical establishment. Nonetheless, homeopathy is practiced around the world, with an estimated 500 million people receiving homeopathic treatment. The World Health Organization has cited homeopathy as one of the systems of traditional medicine that should be integrated worldwide with conventional medicine in order to provide adequate global health care in the 21st century.[1]

In the United States, an estimated 3,000 medical doctors and licensed health-care providers practice homeopathy, and the number continues to rise annually. The U.S. Food and Drug Administration (FDA) recognizes homeopathic remedies as official drugs and regulates their manufacturing, labeling, and dispensing. Homeopathic remedies also have their own official compendium, the *Homeopathic Pharmacopoeia of the United States*, first published in 1897.

> *The World Health Organization has cited homeopathy as one of the systems of traditional medicine that should be integrated worldwide with conventional medicine in order to provide adequate global health care in the 21st century.*

In Europe, homeopathy is far more recognized as a viable medical therapy than it is in America. In Germany, its birthplace, homeopathy is required training for all medical students and used by an estimated 20% of all German physicians. In France, all pharmacies are required to carry homeopathic remedies along with conventional drugs, and they are used by approximately 40% of all physicians. In fact, the homeopathic remedy *Oscillococcinum*™ is the largest selling cold and flu remedy in France. In 1999, the French Medical Association advocated that homeopathy be officially recognized and included as part of French physicians' standard medical training.[2] In Britain, homeopathic hospitals and outpatient clinics are part of the national health system, and homeopathy is recognized as a postgraduate medical specialty by virtue of an act of Parliament. Homeopathy has also enjoyed the patronage of the British royal family for the past six generations.[3] The British Institute of Homeopathy has nearly 9,000 students past and present in 74 countries worldwide. Homeopathy is also widely practiced in India (where over 25,000 doctors use homeopathy), Mexico, Argentina, and Brazil, and in both Europe and the U.S., sales of homeopathic remedies have annually increased by 20% to 30% over the last two decades.[4]

How Homeopathy Works

Homeopathy was founded in the late 18th century by the celebrated German physician Samuel Hahnemann, known for his work in pharmacology, hygiene, public health, industrial toxicology, and psychiatry. Reacting to the barbarous practices of his day, such as bloodletting (the use of leeches) and toxic mercury-based laxatives, Dr. Hahnemann set out to find a more rational and humane approach to medicine.

In Britain, homeopathic hospitals and outpatient clinics are part of the national health system, and homeopathy is recognized as a postgraduate medical specialty by virtue of an act of Parliament. Homeopathy has enjoyed the patronage of the British royal family for the past six generations.

Dr. Hahnemann's breakthrough came during an experiment in which he twice daily ingested cinchona, a Peruvian bark known as a cure for malaria. Soon after Dr. Hahnemann began his experiment, he developed periodic fevers common to malaria. As soon as he stopped taking the cinchona, his symptoms disappeared. Dr. Hahnemann theorized that, if taking a large dose of cinchona created symptoms of malaria in a healthy person, this same substance, taken in a smaller dose by a person suffering from malaria, might stimulate the body to fight the disease. His theory was borne out by years of experiments with hundreds of substances that produced similar results. Based on his work, Dr. Hahnemann formulated the principles of homeopathy:

- Like cures like (Law of Similars)

- The more a remedy is diluted, the greater its potency (Law of the Infinitesimal Dose)

- An illness is specific to the individual (a holistic medical model)

Like Cures Like

According to Dr. Hahnemann, "Each individual case of disease is most surely, radically, rapidly, and permanently annihilated and removed only by a medicine capable of producing (in the human system) the most similar and complete manner of the totality of the symptoms."[5] In other words, the same substance that in large doses produces the symptoms of an illness, in very minute doses cures it.

HOMEOPATHIC POTENCIES

Potency levels of homeopathic remedies are designated with "X", "C", and "M". The "X" means that the remedy has been serially diluted on a 1:10 scale (one part substance to nine parts water), "C" means the remedy has been diluted on a 1:100 scale (one part substance to 99 parts water), and "M" means a 1:1000 dilution. A number value is placed before the scale designator to identify how many dilutions the remedy has undergone. A remedy designated "6X" has undergone six dilutions at one part substance to nine parts water; a remedy that is designated "12X" has undergone 12 dilutions and is stronger than the 6X remedy. Common potencies are 6X, 12X, 30X, 6C, 12C, and 30C.

Dr. Hahnemann referred to this phenomenon as the Law of Similars, a principle first recognized in the fourth century B.C.E. by Hippocrates, who was studying the effects of herbs upon disease. The Law of Similars was also the theoretical basis for the vaccines of physicians Edward Jenner, Jonas Salk, and Louis Pasteur. They would "immunize" the body with trace amounts of a disease component, often a virus, to strengthen its immune response to the actual disease. Allergies are treated in a similar fashion by introducing minute quantities of the suspected allergen into the body to bolster natural tolerance levels.

The More Dilute the Remedy, The Greater Its Potency

Most people believe that the higher the dose of a medicine, the greater the effect. But the opposite holds true in homeopathy, where the more a substance is diluted, the higher its potency. Dr. Hahnemann discovered this Law of the Infinitesimal Dose by experimenting with higher and higher dilutions of substances to avoid toxic side effects.

Today, homeopathic remedies are usually prepared through a process of diluting with pure water or alcohol and succussing (vigorous shaking). Homeopathic solutions can be diluted to such an extent that literally no molecules of the original substance remain in the remedy. Yet, the more dilute it gets, the more potent it becomes. This phenomenon has been the source of great fascination among practitioners and researchers in the field of homeopathic medicine, as from the point of view of conventional chemistry, diluted homeopathic remedies contain no trace of the original substance. In fact, any homeopathic remedy over 24X potency (24 suc-

THE COMPATIBILITY OF HOMEOPATHY WITH CONVENTIONAL MEDICINE

Critics of homeopathy often reject its viability due to its principle of "like cures like" and the fact that many homeopathic remedies are so dilute that they no longer contain molecules of their original substance, supposedly making them incapable of exerting any effect on patients. But according to Daniel Eskinazi, M.D., of the Columbia University College of Physicians and Surgeons, in New York City, neither aspect of homeopathy is in conflict with conventional medicine's biomedical model.

With regard to the principle of "like cures like," Dr. Eskinazi states that a number of pharmaceutical drugs, including aspirin, can produce opposite effects, depending on whether they are administered in low or high doses. Moreover, they can also produce one effect in patients who are ill and another in people who are healthy, very much in accordance to Samuel Hahnemann's first tenet of homeopathy.

As for the issue of dilution, Dr. Eskinazi observes that many pharmaceutical substances used by conventional physicians also remain active in high dilutions. For many homeopathic remedies, the concentration of the original substance after dilution is often less than one part per 100,000. According to Dr. Eskinazi, however, a variety of conventional agents are known to remain active at even greater dilutions, such as certain pheromones, which in some cases are able to produce noticeable physiological effects even at just one molecule. Based on his research of homeopathy, Dr. Eskinazi has concluded that its principles are in fact not incompatible with accepted conventional medical theory.[10]

tion, the explanation of the therapeutic action of the highly dilute homeopathic remedies appears to lie in the domain of quantum physics and the emerging field of energy medicine. A study using nuclear magnetic resonance (NMR) imaging, conducted at Harvard University, demonstrated distinctive readings of subatomic activity in 23 homeopathic remedies. This potency was not demonstrated in placebos (substances having no pharmacological effect).[6] Some researchers believe that the specific electromagnetic frequency of the original substance is imprinted in the homeopathic remedy through the process of successive dilution and succussion, according to Dr. Cook.

See Energy Medicine.

The distinguished Italian physicist Emilio del Giudici has set forth a theory that helps explain homeopathy's mode of therapeutic action. Del Giudici proposes that water molecules form structures capable of storing minute electromagnetic signals.[7] This proposition is given added weight by the findings of Wolfgang Ludwig, Sc.D., Ph.D., a German biophysicist, who has demonstrated in preliminary research that homeopathic substances give off measurable electromagnetic signals. These signals show that specific frequencies are dominant in each homeopathic substance.[8]

If del Giudici's model is accurate, a homeopathic remedy may convey an electromagnetic "message" to the body that matches the specific electromagnetic frequency or pattern of an illness in order to stimulate the body's natural healing response. What Dr. Hahnemann may have been doing in his empirical research was unwittingly "matching the frequencies of the plant extract with the frequency of the [patient's] illness."[9]

Illness is Specific to the Individual

A session with a homeopathic practitioner is a unique experience for someone accustomed to conventional medicine. For instance, you may suffer from chronic headaches, perhaps migraines. While the conventional medical treatment for this condition is the same for most everyone (some form of analgesic or anti-inflammatory drug), homeopathy recognizes over 200 symptom patterns associated with headaches and has corresponding remedies for each.

Your headache may be in the front of your head. It may get worse with a cold sensation and improve with heat. It may be better while you are lying down or while you are sitting up. You may be a person who is thin and easily excited, or the docile, sedentary sort. The first task of the homeopathic practitioner is a process called "profiling," or recording all of the qualities—physical, men-

cessive dilutions and succussions) will have no chemical trace of the original substance remaining.

A report that aired on NBC's *DateLine* in December, 1992, which offered a one-sided argument against homeopathy, contended that a homeopathic remedy received from a prominent homeopathic physician was chemically tested in a laboratory and the results showed that it was "only" water and alcohol. According to homeopathic experts, however, this is exactly the case. After successive dilutions, no molecules of the original substance remain in the remedy.

According to Trevor Cook, Ph.D., D.I.Hom., past President of the British Homeopathic Medical Associa-

tal, and emotional—that will determine the patient's remedy or combination of remedies.

Practitioners of classical homeopathy consult vast compendiums called repertories and *materia medicas* to determine the remedy that most closely matches the total picture of the patient's symptoms. These compendiums catalog the detailed findings of thousands of tests, compiled for over 200 years, which record how healthy individuals reacted to different substances. The homeopathic practitioner's task is to match them exactly to the patient's profile.

The Healing Crisis and Hering's Laws of Cure

In homeopathy, the process of healing begins by eliminating the immediate symptoms, then progressing to the "older," underlying symptoms. Many of these "layers" are residues of fevers, trauma, or chronic disease that were unsuccessfully treated or suppressed by conventional medicine. As the stages of homeopathic healing progress, the patient may get worse before getting better. This is often referred to as the "healing crisis."

In the mid-19th century, Dr. Constantine Hering, the father of American homeopathy, stated that healing progresses from the deepest part of the body to the extremities; from the emotional and mental aspects to the physical; and from the upper part of the body (head, neck, ears, throat) to the lower parts of the body (fingers, abdomen, legs, feet). Hering's Laws of Cure also state that healing progresses in reverse chronological order, from the most recent maladies to the oldest. By Hering's laws, homeopaths are able to track the progress of their treatment and restore a patient's health, layer by layer.

An excellent example of homeopathic treatment is the case of a woman who suffered from lupus, a disease in which the immune system attacks its own tissue. After years of unsuccessful conventional treatment, she was told that she could only expect a life of continued pain and drug dependency. In desperation, she turned to a homeopathic physician.

The highest ideal of cure is the speedy, gentle, and enduring restoration of health by the most trustworthy and least harmful way.

—Samuel Hahnemann,
founder of Homeopathy

First, she was treated for drug dependency and the condition it was to relieve, pericarditis, an intensely painful inflammation of the outer lining of the heart. She was prescribed the remedy *Cactus grandiflorus,* a substance that, in healthy people, produces heart palpitations and depression. The homeopathic dose of *Cactus grandiflorus* reduced the inflammation and a new set of symptoms emerged—anger, bitterness, and stress—powerful emotions she'd experienced prior to the emergence of her pericarditis.

Nux vomica (poison nut) was administered, a substance that produces hyperirritability and nervous cramping in healthy individuals which helped her overcome her emotional problems and progress to the next layer of healing. A recurrence of an old back pain and her phobia of cars emerged, the result of a serious accident and injury. As these conditions were treated, the woman was able to return fully to her life, healthy and free of pain.[11]

Conditions Benefited by Homeopathy

Homeopathy is a complete system of natural medicine that can have a therapeutic effect on almost any disease or health condition. "Homeopathy has been of tremendous value in reversing diseases such as diabetes, arthritis, asthma, epilepsy, skin eruptions, allergic conditions, mental or emotional disorders, especially if applied at the onset of the disease," states George Vithoulkas, Director of the Athenian School of Homeopathic Medicine, in Athens, Greece. "The long-term benefit of homeopathy to the patient is that it not only alleviates the symptoms but it reestablishes internal order at the deepest levels and thereby provides a lasting cure."[13]

Robert D. Milne, M.D., of Las Vegas, Nevada, reports excellent results in the prevention and treatment of acute cold and flu-like symptoms using homeopathic remedies. "The quick use of remedies, such as *Aconite, Bryonia,* and/or *Belladonna,* have been a great help in alleviating the acute symptoms of colds," says Dr. Milne. He also has had success treating conditions such as headaches and women's health problems, including fatigue, irritability, premenstrual problems, neck stiffness, low back pain, and bloating, with homeopathic remedies.

Increasingly, clinical studies are supporting the effectiveness of homeopathic remedies. In a 1991 article published in the *British Medical Journal,* 107 controlled clinical studies (performed between 1966 and 1990) were reviewed. Eighty-one of these studies showed that homeopathic medicines were beneficial in treating headaches, respiratory infections, diseases of the digestive system,

NOT A PLACEBO: HOMEOPATHY IN VETERINARY CARE

Homeopathy has taken on an increasingly important role in alternative veterinary medicine. Carvel Tiekert, D.V.M., of Bel Air, Maryland, Executive Director of the American Holistic Veterinary Medical Association, believes that the reason for this lies in homeopathy's ability to integrate with all other modalities of treatment, thus allowing animals to heal naturally from the inside out. "At least 75% of all animals examined by alternative veterinarians now receive some form of homeopathic treatment," states Dr. Tiekert.

A case history of Christopher Day, M.A., Vet.M.B., M.R.C.V.S., Vet.F.F.Hom, who runs an alternative animal clinic in England, presents a stark contrast between the procedures of conventional medicine and those of homeopathy. "An 18-month-old West Highland white terrier came in with 'dry eye' in one eye," he explains. "Four months previously, the other eye had been affected, treated conventionally for one month, and then been surgically treated. This had relieved the condition, but the initial damage to the cornea remained.

"When the second eye became infected, it was around Easter and no surgery time was immediately available. The dog was then brought to me in order to stabilize her condition until the surgery could be scheduled. I started her on homeopathic injections twice daily, plus artificial tears as necessary. It soon became obvious that the artificial tears were needed less and less often until eventually the impending operation was canceled and the artificial tears were stopped altogether. There

was no damage to the eye and it is still completely healthy without treatment to date."[12]

Other veterinarians, like Richard Pitcairn, D.V.M., Ph.D., of Eugene, Oregon, use homeopathic remedies for the treatment of chronic diseases because they find allopathic methods to be frustrating and ineffective. "My change to holistic medicine has revitalized my practice," says Dr. Pitcairn. "Success with homeopathy, especially with chronic disease, is very personally rewarding. I have used homeopathy as my primary means of therapy since 1978, emphasizing good nutrition and vitamin and mineral supplements. The reason for my switching to homeopathy is simple: it is much more effective than any other system of medicine I have used before."

The reason for this effectiveness and the consistency of the results can be explained very simply, according to H.C. Gurney, D.V.M., of Conifer, Colorado. "Animals do not have the power to reason whether a treatment is going to work or not. It either will or it won't. A drug placebo [a substance having no pharmaceutical effect] will not have the same psychological effect on an animal as it might on a human, and likewise an animal will not be skeptical of an alternative medical approach, as a person might." Homeopathy's efficacy in successfully treating animals goes a long way to debunking claims by critics of homeopathy, who say that its positive effects are due simply to the placebo effect.

---

ankle sprains, postoperative infections and symptoms, and other health-related disorders.[14]

> See Part Three for listings of homeopathic remedies for specific health conditions.

> Official acceptance of homeopathy and its integration into the American health-care system could have an enormous impact on lowering the cost of national health-care due to the low cost, safety, and effectiveness of homeopathic remedies.

Studies attesting to the effectiveness of homeopathic treatment for rheumatoid arthritis have appeared in both *The Lancet* and the *British Journal of Clinical Pharmacology*.[15] In a double-blind study on the effects of homeopathic remedies on influenza, 478 people exhibiting flu symptoms were split into two groups and given either *Oscillococcinum* or a placebo. After a 48-hour period, 17.1%

of those who received *Oscillococcinum* had fully recovered, compared to only 10.3% of the placebo group. Patients in the placebo group also used more drugs to relieve pain and coughing and to reduce fever. In addition, significantly more patients in the *Oscillococcinum* group reported being pleased with the treatment than did those in the placebo group.[16]

Homeopathy can also be useful as an aid in childbirth. In a double-blind study of 93 pregnant women, patients received either a placebo or a 5C combination homeopathic remedy consisting of *Caulophyllum*, *Actea*, *Raemosa*, *Arnica*, *Pulsatilla*, and *Pelsenium*. The women who received the homeopathic remedy were in labor for an average of 5.1 hours, compared to the women in the placebo group, whose labor period averaged 8.1 hours. Additionally, among the homeopathic group, abnormal labors occurred only 11.3% of the time compared to 40% within the placebo group.[17]

Another study was conducted on 69 people with sprained ankles. The group was randomly placed into two groups, one received a homeopathic remedy, while the second group received a placebo. Ten days into the treatment, the patients' pain was evaluated—28 of the 33 people in the homeopathy group were pain free compared to only 13 of the 36 people in the placebo group.[18]

Homeopathy shows indications that it is effective in the treatment of fibromyalgia as well. In 1989, the *British Medical Journal* published a double-blind study which showed that the homeopathic remedy *Rhus toxicodendron* resulted in a 25% reduction in fibromyalgia-related pain compared to a placebo group.[19] Homeopathy may play a significant role in the treatment of fibromyalgia, while conventional methods have proven ineffective in the treatment of the disease.

More recently, a randomized, double-blind, and placebo-controlled study involved 50 patients with perennial allergic rhinitis (chronic inflammation of the mucous membrane due to allergens). All patients were tested to determine the specific allergens causing their symptoms, after which a 30C homeopathic dilution of the offending substance was administered to half of the patients; the other half received a placebo. Patients in both groups received a single dose of their respective remedy and then measured their nasal inspiratory peak flow every morning and evening for one month. At the end of the study, 21% of the patients who received the homeopathic remedy exhibited significant improvement of their symptoms, compared to only 2% in the placebo group. The researchers concluded that homeopathy "provoked a clear, significant, and clinically relevant improvement in nasal inspiratory peak flow, similar to that found with steroids." Of equal importance, the researchers who conducted the study began it intending to prove that homeopathy was a hoax. Based on their results, however, they now admit that it is as effective as conventional medical approaches for treating allergic rhinitis.[20]

Other research shows that homeopathy offers benefit for insomnia and corresponding anxiety,[21] otitis media,[22] and hay fever,[23] as well as dental neuralgic pain following tooth extraction,[24] Parkinson's disease, bronchitis, sinusitis, migraines,[25] and motion sickness.[26]

Combination Remedies

Today, many homeopathic practitioners use combination formulas that contain several remedies to cover a broad range of symptoms for an acute condition. For example, people with a cold experience runny noses, watery eyes, sneezing, fever, and headaches. A combination cold remedy contains remedies for each of these symptoms. The appropriate remedies in a formula will have a therapeutic effect, while the unnecessary remedies will have no effect at all. Combination homeopathic remedies have a unique effect on the body—the body assimilates what it needs and throws off what it doesn't, making homeopathy a completely safe, nontoxic form of medicine. According to Dr. Cook, although this polypharmacy approach is frowned upon by classical homeopaths, it provides a simple source of homeopathic treatments for laypeople as an introduction to this safe, effective, nonaddictive therapy without side effects.

 The government should provide funds for research into homeopathy due to its 200-plus years of clinical success. The results of recent European research also indicate that it deserves to become an integral part of America's health-care system. Write your congressional representatives and demand that research be carried out in this important field of health care.

The Future of Homeopathy

The official acceptance of homeopathy and its integration into the American health-care system could prove to have an enormous impact on lowering the cost of national health-care, due to its low cost and tremendous health benefits. Although controlled clinical studies might prove costly, homeopathy's history of clinical success and the results of studies being carried out in Europe indicate that this is an area where the U.S. government should provide funds for research. Because homeopathic remedies are derived from natural substances and, as such, are unpatentable, no pharmaceutical company will provide the necessary funds for research to gain FDA approval. The low cost of homeopathic remedies also guarantees that it would be impossible for a company to recoup its research investment. Clearly, homeopathy, like other forms of natural medicine, including herbal medicine and nutritional supplementation, is caught in an economic Catch-22. But as part of the growing tide of national awareness of alternative medicine, homeopathy should soon receive the attention it deserves from the U.S. government and become part of the solution to America's national health-care crisis.

HOMEOPATHY IN THE UNITED STATES

Homeopathy has a long and distinguished history in the United States and was popular from the mid-19th to the early-20th century. Dr. Constantine Hering, a student of German physician Samuel Hahnemann, and father of homeopathy in the U.S., established the first homeopathic medical school in the U.S. in 1835 in Allentown, Pennsylvania. By 1844, there were so many physicians claiming to be homeopathic practitioners that the homeopathic medical profession formed the American Institute of Homeopathy, the first national medical association in the U.S. The American Medical Association (AMA) was formed three years later and denounced homeopathy as a delusion. AMA members were forbidden to associate with homeopathic physicians either professionally or socially, and physicians practicing homeopathy were expelled or blocked from becoming members.[27]

Still, homeopathy continued to gain attention in America due in part to its great success in treating acute and epidemic diseases, notably cholera and yellow fever. During an 1849 cholera epidemic in Cincinnati, Ohio, only 3% of those patients treated homeopathically died compared to a 40% to 70% death rate among those treated with conventional medicine.[28] In the 1879 epidemic of yellow fever, homeopaths in New Orleans treated 1,945 cases with a mortality rate of 5.6%, while the mortality rate with standard medical treatment was 16%.[29] At this time, some of homeopathy's more illustrious supporters included John D. Rockefeller, Thomas Edison, and Mark Twain.

By 1900, there were 22 homeopathic medical schools and nearly 100 homeopathic hospitals in the U.S. In fact, 15% of all American physicians practiced homeopathy at the turn of the century, according to Trevor Cook, Ph.D., D.I.Hom., President of the British Homeopathic Medical Association.[30] However, by the same time, the bond between the AMA and the pharmaceutical companies was firmly established. Paid advertisements from pharmaceutical companies in the AMA's journal were the AMA's main source of revenue (as it is today). Prominent physicians were paid to endorse proprietary drugs and doctors were deluged with free samples of pharmaceutical drugs. Through a series of maneuvers including a new rating system for medical schools aimed at eliminating homeopathic colleges, the practice of homeopathy had nearly disappeared as a force in American medicine by 1930.[31]

However, homeopathy is again becoming recognized as a viable alternative medicine, and statistics now show that the American public is returning to this form of treatment in dramatic numbers, with annual sales of homeopathic medicines in the U.S. now reaching $150 million.[32]

Where to Find Help

For more information on homeopathy, contact:

British Institute of Homeopathy and Complementary Medicine
520 Washington Blvd., Suite 423
Marina Del Rey, California 90292
(310) 577-2235
Website: www.britinsthom.com

The largest and one of the most respected centers of learning in homeopathy and complementary medicine in the world, with over 8,000 students in 74 countries. A wide range of courses are available in homeopathy from introductory to postgraduate level. Also offers courses in nutrition, herbal medicine, Bach flower essences, and human sciences.

Homeopathic Educational Services
2124 Kittredge Street
Berkeley, California 94704
(510) 649-0294 or (800) 359-9051
Website: www.homeopathic.com

Offers access to homeopathic books, tapes, and software.

National Center for Homeopathy
801 North Fairfax, Suite 306
Alexandria, Virginia 22314
(703) 548-7790
Website: www.homeopathic.org

Provides a referral list of practicing homeopaths and other information. Gives courses for laypeople and professionals and organizes study groups around the country.

Recommended Reading

Discovering Homeopathy: Your Introduction to the Science and Art of Homeopathic Medicine. Dana Ullman, M.P.H. Berkeley, CA: North Atlantic Books, 1991.

Divided Legacy: A History of the Schism in Medical Thought, Vol. 3: Science and Ethics in American Medicine, 1800-1914. Harris L. Coulter. Berkeley, CA: North Atlantic Books, 1973.

Everybody's Guide to Homeopathic Medicines. Stephen Cummings, M.D., and Dana Ullman, M.P.H. Los Angeles: Jeremy P. Tarcher, 1991.

The Family Guide to Homeopathy: Symptoms and Natural Solutions. Andrew Lockie. New York: Prentice Hall, 1993.

Family Homeopathy: A Practical Handbook for Home Treatment. Paul Callinan. New Canaan, CT: Keats Publishing, 1995.

Homeopathic Medicine for Children and Infants. Dana Ullman, M.P.H. Los Angeles: Jeremy P. Tarcher, 1992.

Homeopathic Medicine Today: A Study. Trevor Cook. Ph.D., D.I.Hom. New Canaan, CT: Keats Publishing, 1989.

Homeopathic Medicines at Home: Natural Remedies for Everyday Ailments and Minor Injuries. Maesimund B. Panos, M.D., and Jane Heimlich. Los Angeles: Jeremy P. Tarcher, 1981.

The Homeopathic Workshop. Trevor Cook, Ph.D., D.I.Hom. London: Crow Wood Press, 2000.

Homeopathy, Healing, and You. Vinton McCabe. New York: St. Martin's Griffin, 1997.

Practical Homeopathy. Vinton McCabe. New York: St. Martin's Griffin, 2000.

HYDROTHERAPY

Hydrotherapy is the use of water, ice, steam, and hot and cold temperatures to maintain and restore health. Treatments include full body immersion, steam baths, saunas, sitz baths, colonic irrigation, and the application of hot and/or cold compresses. Hydrotherapy is effective for treating a wide range of conditions and can easily be used in the home as part of a self-care program.

THE THERAPEUTIC USE of water in all its forms dates back to the beginning of civilization. Hydrotherapy has been used to treat disease and injury by many cultures, including the Egyptian, Babylonian, Persian, Greek, Hebrew, Hindu, Chinese, and Native American. Today, many alternative practitioners prescribe baths, jacuzzis and steam saunas, mineral baths, wraps, rubs, flushes, fasts, enemas and colonic irrigations, douches, sitz baths, and compresses to remedy a great variety of health conditions. Hot or cold water administered externally or internally can be effective in treating conditions ranging from stress and pain to the many toxins, bacteria, and viruses that can cause disease.

How Hydrotherapy Works

External hydrotherapy falls into three categories—hot water, cold water, and contrast applications. "Heat relaxes while cold stimulates," explains Douglas Lewis, N.D., former Chairperson of Physical Medicine at Bastyr University's Natural Health Clinic, in Seattle, Washington. "Hot water produces a response that stimulates the immune system and causes white blood cells to migrate out of the blood vessels and into the tissue where they clean up toxins and assist the body in eliminating wastes." Therapeutically, hot water soothes and relaxes the body and, through the reflex action of the nerves, it can affect nearly every organ and system of the body.

"Cold water discourages inflammation by vasoconstriction (constricting the blood vessels) and through reducing inflammatory agents by making the blood vessels less permeable," says Dr. Lewis. "Cold water also tones muscular weakness and may be useful in cases of incontinence." Dr. Lewis cautions that, contrary to the popular belief, short cold-water treatment may actually increase fever and only extended cold-water treatment pulls heat from the body for fever reduction.

Contrast therapies are those that alternate between hot and cold water in the same treatment. They can stimulate the adrenal and endocrine glands, reduce congestion, alleviate inflammation, and activate organ function. According to Leon Chaitow, N.D., D.O., of London, England, certain contrast therapies are designed to improve circulation in the digestive areas and the pelvis and to stimulate the detoxifying capability of the liver.[1]

See AIDS, Chronic Fatigue Syndrome, Detoxification Therapy, Hyperthermia.

Clinical Application of Hydrotherapy

Many forms of hydrotherapy are used by naturopathic physicians, alternative practitioners, and physical therapists at clinics, hospitals, and health spas to treat a wide range of conditions. Most therapies can also be performed at home; however, the following—hyperthermia, whirlpool baths, and neutral baths—are only available in a clinical setting.

Hyperthermia (fever-induction therapy) deliberately induces fever in the patient who is unable to mount a natural fever response to pathogens (disease-causing organisms and toxins). Fever is often regarded as an undesirable symptom of illness, but holistic practitioners see it as the body's defense against invading organisms. Fever stimulates the immune system by increasing the production of antibodies and interferons (a group of proteins released by white blood cells to combat viruses).[2]

Laboratory research has proven that HIV (human immunodeficiency virus) is temperature sensitive and suffers greater inactivation at progressively higher temperatures above the normal body temperature of 98.6° F.[3] Dr. Lewis believes that a hot immersion bath, if done without raising body temperature and heart rate too quickly, can be used as an adjunctive treatment for "a diverse number of diseases, from upper respiratory infections to sexually transmitted diseases, from cancer to AIDS."

In the treatment of chronic fatigue syndrome, Bruce Milliman, N.D., Associate Professor at Bastyr University, in Kenmore, Washington, reports a 70% success rate using hyperthermia. Hyperthermia can also be used to remove fat-stored chemicals, such as pesticides, PCBs, and drug residues, from the body.

> **CAUTION** Hyperthermia can be hazardous for certain people and conditions and should only be performed under the supervision of a qualified physician.

Whirlpool Baths can rehabilitate injured muscles and joints and alleviate the stresses and strains of everyday life. Whirlpools are also effective in healing skin sores, infected wounds, edema (swelling), and minor frostbite pain. Physical therapists use them to soothe burn patients and improve the circulation of paraplegics and those with polio.

Neutral Baths are a full-immersion therapy that submerges the body up to the neck in water from 92° F to 98° F. The soothing nature of the neutral bath calms the nervous system and is effective for treating emotional and mental disturbances and insomnia. According to Dr. Chaitow, clinical studies reveal that two hours in a neutral bath is effective in reducing excessive fluid retention in patients suffering from mild heart conditions and cirrhosis of the liver.[4] It is also beneficial to the swollen joints of rheumatoid patients. Neutral baths help promote detoxification from alcohol and drug abuse as the neutral bath helps the body rid itself of large amounts of toxin-laden fluids.

> **CAUTION** Those who suffer from eczema and other skin conditions, or acute heart disease, should avoid neutral bathing.

Hydrotherapy at Home

Many of the hydrotherapy techniques used in spas and therapy centers around the world can be performed in the comfort and privacy of your own home. The following section describes these methods. Experiment to find which ones work best for you. Dr. Chaitow suggests that you vary the treatments from day to day, or week to week, to increase the efficiency of your body's response.

> **IMPORTANT** The following methods are recommended for people who are in good health. If you have any health problems or illnesses, consult your doctor before beginning a hydrotherapy program.

> ## NATURAL HEALING WATERS
>
> There are many natural healing waters that spring from the Earth. The balance of minerals in seawater is similar to that of human blood. The water from natural springs carries concentrated levels of sodium, calcium, magnesium, bicarbonate, and sulfur. Bicarbonate spring water can aid in healing cuts, burns, hardening of the skin, digestive problems, and allergies. Sulfur has been known to help arthritis, rheumatism, chronic poisoning, diabetes, skin disease, and urinary problems.

Ice and Contrast are effective therapies for trauma relief. Any injury, like sprains and strains, or acute inflammation like tendinitis, calls for an immediate application of cold. Apply ice as often as 20 minutes every hour for the first 24 to 36 hours post-trauma. Trauma or chronic conditions also respond well to contrast therapy. Alternating hot and cold increases circulation to bring vital nutrients to the area and move waste products out. Simply apply alternating hot and cold packs to the affected area beginning with hot for three minutes, then cold for 30-60 seconds. Repeat three times in one sitting, always finishing with cold, one to three times per day, depending on the severity of the condition.

Baths and Showers are soothing, both mentally and physically. Not only do they relieve general aches and pains, they can also ease internal congestion and digestive ills. Again, water temperature should vary according to individual needs. Hot baths and showers are relaxing and stimulating to the immune system. By inducing perspiration, they facilitate the detoxification process. Cold baths and showers can tonify muscles, reduce inflammation, and act as a bracer against fatigue. Long cold baths are useful for reducing fevers but are not recommended for home use and should only be used under the direction of your physician. Cold showers also can increase the nerve force, stimulate the glandular system, and have a positive effect on the central nervous system.[5] Alternating hot and cold showers can be an excellent way to increase circulation and stimulate organ function. Remember, though, always start with hot and end with cold.

Sitz Baths are a traditional European folk remedy in which the pelvis is immersed in hot or cold water. A hot sitz bath is particularly helpful for problems involving the pelvic region, including uterine cramps, painful ovaries or testicles, and hemorrhoids. A cold sitz bath, taken for two minutes or less, can be used for inflammation, constipation, vaginal discharge, and impotence, but

---

SALT RUBS

A salt rub is excellent for stimulating circulation. Take a small handful of slightly damp sea salts or Epsom salts and vigorously massage them into your already wet skin until it turns slightly pink. One to two pounds of salt is needed for the whole body. Follow with a warm (not hot) shower or bath. Again, vigorously rub your skin while rinsing and drying. The salt rub may make you perspire and help you sleep more soundly. Do a salt rub at least once a month, or weekly as part of your detoxification program. It is not recommended for people with skin rashes or lesions.

---

should not be used for urinary tract infections. (For instructions on how to prepare sitz baths, see "Hydrotherapy Procedures.")

Foot and Hand Baths are excellent for drawing blood away from inflamed parts of the body or drawing congestion away from an organ. They can help relieve insomnia, sore throats, colds, menstrual cramps, foot and leg cramps, and pain from gout, neuralgia, and headaches. A hot foot bath is also an effective remedy for shivering, cold hands or feet, nausea, dizziness, or faintness.[6] To relieve a sore throat or avert a cold, add a tablespoon of mustard powder per quart of hot water to a foot bath container.

Alternating hot and cold foot baths has a profound effect on the nerve and reflex points of the feet. These baths also help relieve toothaches, neuralgia, headaches (when used in conjunction with a cold compress on the head), ankle swelling, foot infections, blood poisoning, and abdominal congestion. Fill two tubs, one with hot water and the other with cold water. Place your feet and ankles in the hot water for three minutes, then plunge your feet into the cold water for 20–30 seconds. Repeat three times, ending with cold water, then thoroughly dry your feet. You may do this several times per day, as needed.

Hands also contain many reflex points that affect the entire body. A cold hand bath can stop a nosebleed and relieve sunstroke. A hot hand bath can relieve cramps in the hands from overuse in athletics, writing, or sewing, and even alleviate asthma attacks.

CAUTION Hot foot baths are contraindicated for those with arteriosclerosis, Buerger's disease, or diabetes.

Cold-Water Treading is another useful preventive water treatment.[7] After a shower or bath, immerse your feet in cold water and march in place for five seconds to five minutes. (For safety, you may need the support of a wall or handle.) Afterward, rub your feet vigorously with a towel, especially the soles. By building tolerance to cold, it is possible to develop resistance to infectious disease, which is why many alternative medicine practitioners recommend this practice as part of a daily self-care routine for their patients, young and old alike.

CAUTION Cold-water treading should not be used if you have rheumatism of the toes or ankles, sciatica, pelvic inflammation, or problems with the bladder or digestive tract.

Steam is an excellent cleanser and deep moisture treatment for the skin. It also helps break up congestion from the common cold and flu. To create a simple home vaporizer, boil water in a clean kettle or pot. Add a few drops of eucalyptus or wintergreen oil, or one to two tablespoons of mint leaves, to the water. Lean over the steaming pot, holding a towel or sheet over your head like a tent, but be careful not to get too close to the boiling water. Breathe slowly and deeply, inhaling the vapors to warm and soothe the respiratory tract.

Compresses and Packs are particularly effective for applying heat or cold to specific parts of the body, as well as for stimulating the immune system and increasing the white blood cell count. One can treat sciatica, for example, by applying hot compresses to the lower back and legs for 30 minutes or longer. For gallstones, intestinal colic, or painful menstrual periods, hot moist compresses can be applied every 30 minutes around the torso, between the shoulders and the navel. (For instructions on how to prepare compresses and packs, see "Hydrotherapy Procedures.")

Hydrotherapy Procedures

The following hydrotherapy procedures, described by Dr. Lewis, are intended to be general and applicable in a variety of situations. According to Dr. Lewis, most of these are best used in conjunction with other treatments to enhance recovery, while some may be used alone. The procedures described in this section correspond to suggestions for hydrotherapy procedures in Part Three: Health Conditions. Please use discretion and consult your physician if you have questions about your condition or the appropriateness of these treatments for you.

Cold Compresses

Description: An application that is applied cold and restored as it warms. It is generally applied as a cold cloth wrung from ice water (not usually as cold as an ice pack).

HEALING BATHS: HERBS, ESSENTIAL OILS, AND HOME REMEDIES

A number of herbs, oils, and minerals may be added to a bath to enhance its therapeutic effects. Here are a few of the more common herbs used in hydrotherapy, available at most natural food stores:

Chamomile: Soothes skin, opens pores, eliminates blackheads, aids digestive problems, and promotes sleep.

Ginger: Relaxes sore muscles, improves circulation, and tones the skin.

Oat straw: Relieves sore feet, ingrown toenails, and blisters.

Sage: Stimulates the sweat glands.

A few drops of various essential oils may also be added to the bath or rubbed directly onto the skin after a shower. The following are a few of the dozens of essential oils available at health stores and body shops:

Cedarwood: Promotes elimination through mucous membranes and acts as an antiseptic and sedative.

Lemon: Increases urine flow and acts as an antiseptic.

Rose: Stimulates liver and stomach functions and acts as an antidepressant.

Tea tree: Enhances skin function and can be used as an antifungal and antibiotic.[8]

Also try adding the following common household ingredients to your bath:

Apple cider vinegar: Detoxifies, combats fatigue, relieves poison ivy, and restores the skin's natural acid covering. Add one cup to your bath.

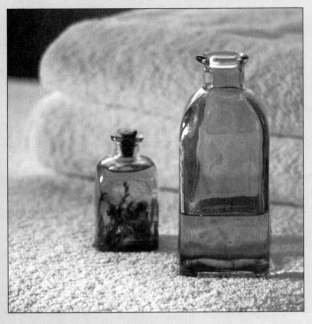

Baking soda: Relieves skin irritation and itching and acts as a mild antiseptic. Add up to one pound to your bath.

Epsom salts: Induces perspiration, aborts illness, relaxes muscles, and relieves swollen and irritated joints. Dissolve ½ pound to one pound in a hot bath.

Cornstarch: Helps reduce itchiness from poison ivy, poison oak, and eczema. Cornstarch can also be an effective cooling agent. Add one cup to one pound of cornstarch to the bath (can be added in conjunction with other substances such as oatmeal).

Oatmeal: Coats, soothes, and restores the skin, and is especially good for itchiness, hives, sunburn, and chafing. Put one cup of uncooked oatmeal in a blender, finely blend it, and add it to a warm or mild bath. (This is also good for soothing diaper rash.)

Purpose: Cold compresses are commonly used where it is beneficial to force blood from an area or to prevent its accumulation. (Such an accumulation might cause congestion, leading to pain or discomfort.) They may also be applied to relieve heat in an affected part.

Uses: To reduce a minor inflammatory reaction, to relieve or prevent headache accompanying fever, following a hot application to stimulate blood flow.

Materials: A cloth of appropriate size to cover the area to be treated and a basin of ice water.

Procedure: Wring a cloth of appropriate size of ice water and apply to the area to be treated. Restore as necessary to keep the cloth cold or for the comfort of the person treated.

Cold Friction Rub

Description: A cold application with friction.

Purpose: The cold friction rub stimulates and increases the function of the various organs.

Uses: Immune stimulation (useful in chronic fatigue syndrome, upper respiratory infections, pneumonia, etc.); to stimulate blood flow into an area to enhance healing.

Materials: Ice water bath and terry cloth towel or mitten.

Procedure: The patient is prepared with a heating process (see the Hot Packs, Immersion Baths, Steam/Sauna, Hot Blanket Packs, and Sprays/Showers sections of this chapter). Briskly rub the area to be treated with the cold, wet cloth until the skin turns pink. Wrap up and keep warm.

Variations: This treatment may be applied to the trunk (front and back) when treating general conditions or it may be applied to a small area or extremity when treating specific conditions.

Precautions/Special Considerations: Adequate pre-heating will produce a better reaction in most people.

Constitutional Hydrotherapy

Description: An application of hot followed by cold to the trunk, front, and back.

Purpose: The treatment is useful to balance body functions, strengthen the immune system, and promote healing.

Uses: Constitutional hydrotherapy is useful as a primary or adjunct treatment of any condition. It is perhaps most useful in the treatment of acute conditions such as upper respiratory infections, bronchitis, asthma, and stomach flu, and in chronic conditions such as irritable bowel, ulcerative colitis, premenstrual syndrome, and arthritis. (When in doubt, try constitutional hydrotherapy.)

Materials: A bed or treatment table, one double sheet folded end to end (or two twin sheets), two wool (or acrylic) blankets, three bath towels (a small bath towel is best, one that when folded in half reaches side to side across the person and from shoulders to hips), one hand towel, and a source of hot and cold water.

Procedure: This is a version of the constitutional hydrotherapy treatment used by naturopathic physicians. It has been simplified for use at home.

- Have the person undress to the waist and lie face up between the sheets, under one blanket. Place two hot, folded bath towels (four layers) on the trunk, shoulders to hips, side to side. Cover with sheet and one blanket, and leave on five minutes.

- Return with one hot bath towel and one cold hand towel. Place the new hot towel on top of two old towels and flip all three towels. Remove the two old hot towels leaving the new hot towel in place. Place the cold towel on top of the new hot towel and flip again. Remove the hot towel, leaving the cold in place.

- Cover the person and add an extra layer of blanket. Leave on for ten minutes or until the cold towel is well warmed.

- Remove the towel. Have the person roll over (face down). Repeat steps applying the towels to the person's back.

Variations: The contrast may be narrowed (not as hot or cold) for the very ill or weak person or may be pushed to the hot for sedation or to cold to tonify and strengthen.

Precautions/Special Considerations: If using the person's bed, take care not to get it wet. Hot water from the tap is usually hot enough. The hot towel should be hot enough that it is just possible to wring it out. The cold towel should be quite cold (use ice water), but wring it out thoroughly and use only one layer. If the person has trouble warming the cold towel, massage the back (through the blankets and towel) and feet. Those with asthma often react negatively to cold applications on the chest. For these persons, begin with a smaller cold towel applied to the abdomen only. With later treatments, gradually increase the size of the cold towel until it covers the entire chest and abdomen without any negative reaction.

Contrast Applications

Description: An application of alternating hot and cold generally applied as three to four minutes of hot followed by 30-60 seconds of cold, repeated three to five times. It may be applied with hot and cold compresses or with immersion.

Purpose: Contrast applications are the most effective for increasing blood flow through an area. This aids in removing wastes that accumulate in areas of inflammation and helps bring nutrients and oxygen into those areas. It is also known to increase the functional activity of the organs that are in reflex relationship to the areas of skin being treated (for example, contrast applied to the skin over the liver will increase the functional activity of the liver itself). Whole-body contrast treatments have been shown effective in stimulating immune function.

Uses: Contrast hydrotherapy is the appropriate treatment to follow ice in acute injuries. Once the acute phase is over (usually 24-36 hours), ice should be discontinued and contrast begun. Contrast is useful in post-acute, sub-acute, and chronic cases of tendinitis, bursitis, and arthritis, as well as local infections such as otitis media, mastitis, urethritis, or even many infected wounds.

Materials: Hot and cold compresses (terry cloth hand, face, or bath towel) or basin of hot and cold water for immersion.

Procedure: Apply hot compress to (or immerse) the affected part in hot water (approximately 110° F) for three to four minutes. Follow with ice water for 30-60 seconds, but not longer—the effects of short cold are desirable here. Repeat three to five times; always end with cold.

Variations: Chemical hot packs and gel cold packs may be used if desired, but wet hot and cold applications are more effective and more readily available. Hand towels and face cloths may be adequately heated from hot tap water and cooled from a basin of ice water.

Precautions/Special Considerations: The same precautions apply as with hot and cold applications alone.

See also the Immersion Baths, Sitz Baths, and Sprays/Showers sections of this chapter.

Enema

Description: An irrigation of the colon using a small amount of water or solution.

Purpose: To aid and encourage elimination from the bowel.

Uses: Used in detoxification from chemical exposure or abuse and to relieve constipation.

Materials: Enema bag (fountain syringe) available at most pharmacies, sea salt, baking soda, and lubricant (hand lotion, surgical lubricant, vegetable oil).

Procedure: Prepare enema solution of one tablespoon of sea salt and one tablespoon of baking soda per quart of water, at about 98° F. Place solution in enema bag and place bag about three feet above the patient. Lubricate the anus and the enema tubing. Insert the tubing just past the inner sphincter (about 1 ½ to 2 inches) and hold in place. Release the valve to allow the solution to enter the colon. Introduce the solution slowly and do not try to take too much (about one pint is usually adequate). Hold the solution for a few minutes before releasing into the toilet. Repeat the procedure several times during each enema.

Variations: It is possible to take the enema while lying on the floor or sitting on the toilet. Choose which is most comfortable for you.

- Often it is useful to stand and walk or massage the abdomen after taking a small amount of solution and before releasing it into the toilet.

- If there is spasm and tension in the bowel, warmer water (about 102° F) will often help relax the bowel.

- If the bowel is weak and flaccid, colder water may help to strengthen it (use water at about 75°-80° F).

- The use of large amounts of solution introduced at once into the bowel during frequent enemas may cause the bowel to become stretched. To avoid this, remember to introduce the smallest amount of solution necessary to produce results.

- It is possible to use water without salt and baking soda. It is also possible to use other solutions for other effects.

Precautions/Special Considerations: Do not use hot water or very cold water. Do not give an enema if there is bleeding from the rectum. Consult your physician before giving enemas to children, the elderly, the very ill, persons with hypertension or bowel disease, or pregnant women. If constipation persists after giving an enema, check with your physician.

Heating Compresses

Description: A heating compress is a cold application that is left in place for a long period of time. It is heated by the body and so becomes a hot application.

Purpose: The heating compress requires an active response from the body and therefore stimulates increased metabolic and healing activity in its vicinity.

Uses: Because it encourages blood flow into an area, it can be used to reduce congestion in another area. (Wet socks may be used to reduce congestion headaches, sinus congestion, and lung congestion.) Its tendency to bring blood into an area makes it useful for chronic joint pain or chronic bronchitis. It may be used in acute and chronic sore throats, tonsillitis, and ear infections. A whole-body treatment may be achieved by the use of the wet sheet pack.

Materials: One pair of light cotton socks and one pair of heavy wool or acrylic socks, or a light-weight cotton fabric cut in width and length to wrap around the area to be treated (joint, neck). You will also need a wool cloth, cotton tee shirt, or wool sweater to cover the body.

Procedure: The wet sock treatment is especially useful in treating children with upper respiratory infections. Before bedtime, wring a pair of cotton socks in ice water, pull over feet, and cover with wool socks; leave in place overnight. By morning, the socks should be warm and dry.

Variations: Knees, ankles, elbows, and wrists may easily be treated by wrapping the area with a cotton cloth wrung from cold water (one or two layers are adequate). Then cover with wool and leave in place several hours until quite warm (overnight is easiest). Throat conditions may be treated in the same way. Shoulders and hips may also be treated this way, but will require more creative wrapping techniques.

You can also use a chest pack. By far the easiest way to make one is to use a cotton tee shirt. Wring the shirt in ice water, pull it on, and cover yourself with a wool sweater. Leave in place overnight.

See also the Wet Sheet Pack section of this chapter.

Hot Blanket Packs

Description: A hot blanket pack with a hot water bottle or electric heating pad.

Purpose: To produce a mild increase in body temperature.

Uses: The hot blanket pack may be used to produce hyperthermia for immune stimulation or detoxification. It may also be used to prepare for cold applications (see also the Wet Sheet Packs, Cold Friction Rub, and Sprays/Showers sections of this chapter).

Materials: A dry sheet, two wool or acrylic blankets, two hot water bottles (or an electric heating pad), and a cold compress.

Procedure: Spread out two blankets with a dry sheet covering them. Have the person undress and wrap in the sheet. Place one hot water bottle on the abdomen and one at the feet (or place the electric heating pad on the abdomen). Mop the face with the cold compress as needed. Leave the person in the pack for 20-60 minutes, depending on the amount of heating desired.

Variations: A hot half-pack may be used where it is desirable to heat only the lower half of the body. In this case, wrap only from the waist to the feet with a hot water bottle or heating pad between the legs. This treatment is milder than the hot foot bath and may be used with people who have peripheral vascular diseases or loss of peripheral sensations. Consult your physician.

Precautions/Special Considerations: Take care not to overheat the person with the hot water bottles or heating pad. Always follow the hot blanket pack with a cool rinse.

Hot Packs

Description: A hot application used to warm a local area.

Purpose: To relieve muscle spasms, produce local hyperthermia, encourage local blood flow, or relieve pain.

Uses: To relieve muscle spasms, to treat local infections, or to prepare for cold applications.

Materials: Commercially available chemical hot packs or towels soaked in hot water from the tap (or heated in the microwave).

See also the Immersion Baths and Hyperthermia sections of this chapter.

Procedure: Prepare hot packs to about 120° F. Place two to three layers of towels over the area to be treated. Place the hot pack on the towels and cover. If the pack gets too hot for comfort, add additional layers of towels as needed. Leave the pack in place 5-20 minutes, depending on the time needed to obtain the desired effect. Packs may need to be restored if they cool too much. Follow with a short (30 seconds) cold application when done. Local redness and perspiration will occur.

Variations: Towels may be wrung from tap water at a temperature that will allow them to be placed directly on the skin. If the desired effect requires that they stay in place for more than five minutes, they should be renewed frequently so that they stay warm.

Precautions/Special Considerations: Hot packs should be used with caution when treating children or persons with decreased sensation. Burns are possible if care is not taken to protect the skin from hot packs. Never apply toweling that has been heated in a microwave directly to the skin. Microwave heating often creates hot and cold spots, so you may not be aware of an area that is too hot. In general, hot packs wrung from hot tap water are the safest. If you can wring them out with your hands, they are not likely to be hot enough to cause burns.

Hyperthermia

Description: A local or whole-body treatment intended to raise the temperature of the tissues (also called artificial fever).

Purpose: To destroy heat sensitive organisms (viruses, bacteria, etc., that are sensitive to increases in body temperature), to enhance immune function, and to encourage elimination of toxic material from the body.

Uses: Hyperthermia may be useful in the adjunct treatment of infectious diseases, ranging from upper respiratory infections to pneumonia, from influenza to AIDS. It is also useful in helping to eliminate toxic material from the body by encouraging sweating. In addition, it has been used in the treatment of many types of cancer.

Materials: A hot tub or deep hot bath, a hot blanket pack, or steam/sauna bath; a basin of ice water and terry cloth towel; and drinking water.

Procedure: Hyperthermia treatments may safely be done by immersing the body in hot water (103°-104° F) for up to 60 minutes at a time. Maintain the bath temperature for the entire time. To prevent a headache, apply cold to the head during treatment. Liberal use of cold water is advised. Begin early in the treatment and a headache can be prevented. (It is much more difficult to get rid of a headache than to prevent one.) Check oral temperature every 10-15 minutes. If temperature exceeds 104° F, cool the bath and apply more cold to the head. Following the treatment, rinse in a cool shower, then wrap up and stay warm.

Variations: If a bath or hot tub is not available, it is possible to heat the body in a sauna or steam bath. The hot blanket pack may also be used to raise body temperature.

Local hyperthermia may be achieved by the use of hot packs or through the inhalation of steam. When inhaling steam for upper respiratory illness, avoid inhaling the steam deeply into the lungs.

Precautions/Special Considerations: Hotter water can generally be tolerated for short periods, but it may cause an increase in body temperature that occurs too quickly. This may cause the treatment to be ended soon and leave the person feeling uncomfortable. Consult your physician before doing this treatment if you have any of the following: high or low blood pressure, serious illness, diabetes, or multiple sclerosis. Do not use this treatment if you are or may be pregnant. Watch for signs of hyperventilation, including numbness and tingling in the lips, hands, or feet. If hyperventilation occurs, reduce the bath temperature; breathe from the abdomen, not the chest; or breathe into a paper bag until the tingling passes. Stand slowly after finishing the treatment and be careful in the shower for the cool rinse. Having an attendant near may be a good idea for the first few treatments.

See also the Immersion Baths, Steam/Sauna, and Hot Blanket Packs sections of this chapter.

Ice Packs

Description: A very cold application using ice or gel packs.

Purpose: To reduce swelling, inflammation, pain, or congestion.

Uses: To relieve swelling and inflammation from acute injuries and conditions such as a sprained ankle, bruises, crushing injuries, tendinitis, and bursitis.

Materials: Commercially available cold pack, crushed ice in a bag, bag of frozen vegetables, ice cubes, frozen paper cup of water, or ice water bath.

Procedure: Apply a cold pack to the affected area for 20 minutes out of every hour for the first 24-36 hours after acute injury, depending on the severity.

Variations: An immersion bath may be used if more convenient (for example, an ankle sprain). Add ice to a basin of water and immerse the affected part as above. (The disadvantage with immersion is that it is difficult to elevate a part that is immersed in a water bath.) In the case of acute tendinitis or muscle spasm, it may be useful to rub the area with an ice cube or cup of ice. Rub vigorously over the painful area until a burning feeling occurs and the area begins to feel numb (usually about 10-12 minutes). This may be repeated hourly in acute cases.

Precautions/Special Considerations: Do not apply cold to suspected frostbite or to areas where there is a loss of sensation. For this reason, it may be inappropriate to apply cold to the extremities of a person with diabetes or peripheral neuropathy.

Immersion Baths

Description: A bath in which all or part of the body is immersed in water. It may be used for contrast or for the effects of hot or cold alone.

Purpose: Immersion may be the easiest way to apply hydrotherapy to the body, either because of the irregularity of a part like a hand or foot or if a large area is to be covered. It may be useful in cases of edema to provide pressure to force fluid back into circulation. Water is also a powerful solvent and may dissolve and remove toxins from the body through the skin.

Uses: Extremities may be treated in the immersion bath for any of the various effects of hot, cold, or contrast. Chemicals may be added for various effects, such as Epsom salts for anti-inflammatory and "drawing" effects. Full immersion baths may be given to produce hyperthermia response (artificial fever), for the relaxing and sedative effects of a neutral bath, to relieve sore muscles, to detoxify, or for the stimulation of a cold plunge.

Materials: A basin (or two for contrast) large enough to accommodate the part to be immersed, filled with hot or cold water (or one of each); plastic wastebaskets are often the best for a foot, leg, or arm. A double-bowl kitchen sink may also serve. A hot tub, whirlpool bath, or bathtub may serve for full immersion when needed.

Procedure: For a local application, cover the part entirely. The hot bath may be approximately 110° F; the cold should be ice water. Most conditions respond best to contrast, unless within the first 24-36 hours of an acute inflammatory condition (see also the Contrast Applications section of this chapter). Epsom salts (generally ¼ pound to ½ pound per gallon) may be added to the hot bath, if desired, for anti-inflammatory action.

Variations: A full immersion bath may be useful in promoting a fever (see also the Hyperthermia section of this chapter), for the relief of aching muscles, or to aid in detoxification. For the latter two conditions, soak in a tub (102°-104° F) for 15 to 20 minutes and follow with a short cold plunge or shower. (Epsom salts may be added, ¼ pound to ½ pound per gallon.) In cases of insomnia, anxiety, or nervousness, a neutral bath (97° F) may be taken for anywhere from 30 minutes to several hours. Do not follow with cold. A cold plunge may be useful after exercise or after any whole-body hot application.

Precautions/Special Considerations: The same precautions apply as with any hot or cold application. Both the hot bath and cold plunge may be contraindicated for persons with cardiovascular disease or during pregnancy. It is also contraindicated for those with peripheral vascular diseases or who have a loss of sensation in the hands or feet. Consult your physician.

Sitz Baths

Description: A bath in which the pelvis is immersed in hot or cold water.

Purpose: To provide the benefits of hot, cold, or contrast to the pelvic organs.

Uses: May be used in infections of the bladder, prostate, or vagina; hemorrhoids; menstrual problems; or bowel problems such as anal fissures, colitis, diverticulitis, or other inflammatory bowel diseases. Cold sitz baths may be used to tonify the pelvic musculature in cases of bladder or bowel incontinence or prolapse.

Materials: One (or two) basins adequate to sit in so that water will cover up to the level of the navel, or a bathtub of water filled to reach the level of the navel, along with a basin of ice water and a bath towel, if needed for contrast treatment.

Procedure: Warm soaks alone may be useful for the treatment of local anal or vaginal irritation. Hemorrhoids and anal fissures may be treated by soaking in a warm bath for 10 to 15 minutes. Other conditions will respond better to contrast. Use one tub of hot water (about 110° F) and one tub of ice water. Follow directions as for contrast applications; three to four minutes hot, 30-60 seconds cold, repeated three to five times. Always end with cold.

Variations: If two tubs are not available, the following is very effective. Sit for three to four minutes in a hot half-bath (water up to the level of the navel in a bath tub), then stand in the hot water and pull a cold towel between the legs and over the pelvis in the front and back. Hold in place 30-60 seconds, then sit back into the hot bath. Repeat (as with contrast) three to five times and end with cold.

Precautions/Special Considerations: When sitting and standing around water, be careful that your footing is secure so you do not slip and fall. Also, when sitting in hot water, it is possible that you may become light-headed and dizzy when standing up. It is best to have an assistant present when doing contrast sitz baths.

Sprays/Showers

Description: A hot or cold spray of water from a hose or shower.

Purpose: Hot—to prepare for cold; cold—to stimulate and increase function.

Uses: Contrast showers—to improve immune function; cold sprays—to increase organ function or stimulate the nervous system.

Materials: A household shower and a hose attached to a faucet or bathtub filler spout.

Procedure: For general immune stimulation, follow a hot cleansing shower with a two-minute cold rinse.

Variations: Following a hot shower (or other heating application), a cold spray on each side of the spine is very stimulating and invigorating. A gentle cold spray over mild varicose veins (without preheating) may help to tone the veins.

Precautions/Special Considerations: Do not use a strong spray over varicose veins. Cold showers and sprays may be approached gradually, starting with cool and working gradually to all cold.

Steam/Sauna

Description: A full-body application of heat in a humid environment.

Purpose: To increase body temperature and/or promote sweating.

Uses: May be used to prepare for cold applications (see also the Contrast Applications, Wet Sheet Packs, and Sprays/Showers sections of this chapter), to produce an artificial fever, or to encourage the breakdown and elimination of toxins.

Materials: Steam room, steam cabinet, sauna.

Procedure: No more than 15-20 minutes should be spent in a steam room or sauna where it is necessary to breathe hot air or steam. This is due to the fact that hot air, moist or dry, reduces the ability of the lungs to exchange oxygen and carbon dioxide. It may be preferable to work your way up to the longer times. Begin with three to four minutes in the hot environment, then exit and do a cool rinse. Gradually increase your time in the heat and increase the degree of cold water for the rinse. It may be useful to take a basin of ice water and a cloth into the steam room to apply cold to the head and face. This may reduce the tendency to headache that can occur with whole-body heating.

Variations: Where available, a Russian steam room or steam cabinet, which allows the head to be outside the hot environment, is preferable. This allows the patient to breathe room temperature air and an attendant may easily apply cold compresses to the face and head. It is possible for a person to remain in this environment for a much longer period of time. Treatment times of up to 60 minutes may be achieved depending on the tolerance and response of the person.

Precautions/Special Considerations: Women who are or may be pregnant should limit applications of heat to ten minutes or less. Persons with cardiovascular disease should consult their physician before doing any treatment involving very hot or very cold temperatures. Persons with multiple sclerosis may not tolerate hot applications well.

Prolonged applications of heat may encourage hyperventilation. If there is tingling in the lips, fingers, or toes, treatment should be discontinued and a cold rinse applied. A headache is a common side effect of prolonged heating, which may occur immediately or some time following the treatment. Most headaches can be avoided by applying cold to the head and face during treatment. It is probably not possible to overdo the use of cold in this way.

Wet Sheet Packs

Description: A full-body wrap in a cold wet sheet. The treatment progresses in three phases: cold or cooling, neutral, and heating.

Purpose: To stimulate, relax, or detoxify depending on the phase.

Uses: The treatment is stimulating and tonifying if it is stopped before the sheet is warmed (first phase). There are easier ways to achieve this stimulation and therefore it is rarely used this way. However, the cold application is useful to control a fever that is rising too rapidly or is too high. The neutral phase is useful to relax and sedate. The final phase of heating is commonly used to aid in cleansing through the skin. It promotes sweating and elimination and is therefore useful in detoxifying from environmental or chemical exposure or from drug, alcohol, or tobacco use.

Materials: A bed or treatment table, wool blankets (one to three may be needed), pillows (one for the head, one for under the knees), a cotton (polyester/cotton) sheet soaked in ice water, a terry cloth bath towel, and a terry cloth hand towel.

Procedure: Spread out one blanket with a pillow for the head and one to support the knees. The blanket should be high enough to fold over the shoulders of the person. Thoroughly wring the sheet from ice water and place it out over the blanket. Have the person undress and lie down on the center of the wet sheet and pull the far half over themselves. Return and arrange the sheet by pulling the far half under the arms and around the far leg. Have the person place the arms in a comfortable position across the abdomen. (If the person is claustrophobic, one arm may be left out.) Wrap the near half of the sheet over the shoulders, arms, and around the near leg. Next, bring the blanket across the person, draping it over the shoulders. Any extra length of wet sheet should be folded up over the blanket. Add extra layers of blanket to hold in heat produced by the body to warm the sheet. (If the treatment is used to reduce fever, extra blankets are not needed.)

If general detoxification is desired, leave the person in the wet sheet until profuse sweating has occurred and as long as he or she tolerates. This may require two to four hours or more. The heating/detoxifying stage will be reached sooner if the person has undergone some sort of heating before getting into the wet sheet pack (exercise, hot shower, hot tub).

Variations: If the relaxing effects of the neutral phase are desired, the person should be removed from the pack before he or she begins to perspire. A warm (not hot) shower following is acceptable. If the tonifying, fever-reducing effects are sought, remove the person as soon as he or she begins to heat the sheet. It may be appropriate and necessary to restore the cold wet sheet one or more times to reach the desired effect of the cold.

Precautions/Special Considerations: Hot drinks such as hot ginger tea will promote sweating. However, do not burn the person (test the temperature of the drinks first) and do not give too much fluid. The need to urinate

could end the treatment too soon if high amounts of fluids are given. Water to drink may be necessary during the elimination phase. The bath towel may be used to cover the person's head and eyes to enhance the heating phase and shade the eyes. The hand towel may be used as a cold compress and to mop the face once perspiration begins in the elimination phase.

The Future of Hydrotherapy

"In Europe, hydrotherapy is commonly found in health clinics, both as a primary and an adjunctive treatment modality," says Dr. Lewis. "In the United States, there is also a definite resurgence of interest in hydrotherapy, which I feel is due to the growing dissatisfaction people have with the overuse of medications. People are looking for other alternatives." Dr. Lewis points out that hydrotherapy has numerous clinical applications and provides a number of safe, natural, and effective adjunct treatments for conditions that include digestive problems, women's health conditions, chronic fatigue syndrome, cancer, and AIDS. The most important application of hydrotherapy, however, may be in the home, where it can be used as a simple and inexpensive means of both preventing and treating the common cold, flu, and many other health conditions. Because of this, hydrotherapy has great potential to play an important role in medicine in the coming years.

Where to Find Help

To find a hydrotherapy facility in your area, look under "Physical Therapy" or "Health Spas" in the Yellow Pages or make inquiries at your local hospital. To find a referral to a naturopathic physician in your area who practices hydrotherapy, contact:

American Association of Naturopathic Physicians
8210 Greensboro Drive, Suite 300
McLean, Virginia 22101
(703) 610-9037
Website: www.naturopathic.org

Provides referrals to a nationwide network of accredited or licensed naturopathic physicians. It hosts an annual convention, and works to move legislature and licensure in various states.

Recommended Reading

Back to Eden. Jethro Kloss. Twin Lakes, WI: Lotus Press, 1989.

Home Remedies. Agatha Thrash, M.D., and Calvin Thrash, M.D. Seale, AL: New Lifestyle Books, 1981.

How to Get Well. Paavo Airola. Sherwood, OR: Health Plus Publishers, 1984.

Hydrotherapy: Water Therapy for Health and Beauty. Leon Chaitow. Boston: Element Books, 1999.

HYPERTHERMIA

Fever is one of the body's most powerful defenses against disease. Hyperthermia artificially induces fever in patients who are unable to mount a natural fever response to infection, inflammation, or other health challenges. It is used locally or over the entire body to treat diseases ranging from viral infections to cancer and is an effective self-help treatment for the common cold and flu, as well as detoxification.

THE BODY PROTECTS itself from viruses, bacteria, and other harmful substances through the use of numerous defense systems. One of these is fever. Fever raises the body's temperature above normal in an attempt to destroy invading organisms and sweat impurities out of the system. Fever is a highly effective and natural process of curing disease and restoring health and has been recognized as such for thousands of years. Hyperthermia deliberately creates fever in the patient in order to utilize this natural healing response.

Hyperthermia takes advantage of the fact that many invading organisms tolerate a narrower temperature range than body tissues and are therefore more susceptible to increases in temperature.

How Hyperthermia Works

A state of hyperthermia exists when body temperature rises above its normal level of 98.6° F. An increase in body temperature causes many physiological responses to occur in the body. Hyperthermia takes advantage of the fact that many invading organisms tolerate a narrower temperature range than body tissues and are therefore more susceptible to increases in temperature (they may die from overheating before harm is done to human tissue). Examples are viruses such as rhinovirus[1] (responsible for half of all respiratory infections), HIV (human immunodeficiency virus),[2] and the microorganisms and bacteria that cause syphilis and gonorrhea.[3]

Hyperthermia treatments may not be able to kill every invading organism, but they can reduce their numbers to a level the immune system can handle. Hyperthermia stimulates the immune system by increasing the production of antibodies and interferon (a protein substance that prevents reproduction of the virus). Hyperthermia is also a useful technique in detoxification therapy because it releases toxins stored in fat cells.

Methods of Inducing Hyperthermia

Body temperature can be swiftly increased by the external application of heat. This approach causes blood vessels to swell and the body to perspire in an attempt to prevent an increase in temperature. An increase in body temperature may be accomplished by such low-tech methods as immersing the body in hot water, sitting in a sauna or steam bath, or wrapping oneself in blankets with a hot water bottle. Other high-tech approaches, more commonly found in hospital and medical centers rather than in alternative medical settings, include the use of short-wave or microwave diathermy, ultrasound, radiant heating, and extracorporeal heating.

- **Diathermy** is the application of radio frequency electromagnetic energy to the body to cause a temperature rise.

- **Ultrasound** is the application of high energy sound waves to cause an increase in body temperature as a result of friction produced at the molecular level that is created as the sound waves strike different body tissues. For whole-body or large area treatments, multiple ultrasound applicators may be used.

- **Radiant heating** devices produce infrared heat that is applied to the body.

- **Extracorporeal heating** is accomplished by removing blood from the body, heating it, and returning it to the body at a higher temperature.

A more recent form of hyperthermia in the United States employs far-infrared energy to treat a variety of disease conditions, including cancer, and to speed detoxification and recovery from muscle sprains and other injuries. Far-infrared (FIR) wavelengths occur just below ("infra") visible red light in the electromagnetic spectrum (see Quick Definition). At the molecular level, FIR exerts strong rotational and vibrational effects that are biologically benign and, in certain processes, biologically beneficial. This is in stark contrast to the health-damaging effects of short wavelengths, such as X rays and gamma rays.

> **QD** The **electromagnetic spectrum** is the entire range of radiant energies, measured as waves of frequencies. *Electromagnetic* refers to the ability to exist as both particle (matter) and wave (energy). The spectrum is usually divided into seven sections, from the longest to the shortest wavelengths: radio, microwave, infrared, visible, ultraviolet, X ray, and gamma-ray radiation. Infrared (IR) wavelengths are further divided into three wavelength segments: near (NIR), middle (MIR), and far (FIR), and are usually measured in microns or micrometers. FIR wavelengths range from 5.6 microns to 1,000 microns.

Although the wavelengths of FIR are too long for our eyes to perceive, we can experience its energy as gentle, radiant heat, which can penetrate up to 1 ½ inches beneath the skin. Among FIR's healing benefits is its ability to stimulate inflammation, which is necessary for a period of time in order to heal injuries such as a pulled muscle. FIR also appears capable of enhancing white blood cell function, thereby increasing immune response and the elimination of foreign pathogens and cellular waste products. Additional benefits include the ability to stimulate the hypothalamus, which controls the production of neurochemicals involved in such biological processes as sleep, mood, and blood pressure; enhancing the delivery of oxygen and nutrients to the body's soft tissue areas; and the removing accumulated toxins by improving lymph circulation.

After more than a decade of use in Europe and Asia, products and devices based on FIR technologies are now increasingly being used by alternative health practitioners in the U.S. and Canada. These include FIR saunas, body wraps, caps and socks, quilts, mats and mattresses, hair dryers, quick-cooking ovens, and shower filters.

Hyperthermia, however it is induced, can be produced either locally or over the whole body. Locally

HISTORY OF HYPERTHERMIA

The beneficial effects of hyperthermia in the form of hot packs, baths, and saunas have been recognized for thousands of years. In 500 B.C.E., the Greek physician Parmenides stated that if only he had the means to create fever, he could cure all illness. The early Romans built elaborate baths, which included saunas, cold plunge baths, and swimming areas. The sauna has long been a part of Finnish tradition and the Russians use steam baths regularly. Native American cultures use sweat lodges in their cleansing practices. Over the last few centuries, physicians have observed that people suffering from certain illnesses, such as cancer, gonorrhea, and syphilis, often become free of these illnesses following a high fever from another infection. This has led to research into the production of fever by various methods (injection of foreign substances, hot packs, hot baths) to treat a wide variety of health problems, from the common cold to AIDS and cancer.

applied hyperthermia is most often employed to treat infections, such as upper respiratory infections (with inhalation of steam or a local application of diathermy) or for infected wounds in a hand or foot (generally produced with immersion in a hot-water bath). Whole-body hyperthermia, on the other hand, is used when there is a general infection, when a local application is impractical, or when a general whole-body response is desirable.

For whole-body hyperthermia, practitioners normally utilize the methods of full-immersion baths, saunas, steam, and blanket packs. In conventional medical settings, whole-body treatment usually involves the more high-tech approaches of diathermy, ultrasound, radiant, and extracorporeal heating; for localized treatments, diathermy and ultrasound are used.

Hyperthermia in all of its forms is often employed in the treatment of bronchitis, pneumonia, sinusitis, and other conditions of the lungs and body cavities, and is used as a modality for physical therapy.

Conditions Benefited by Hyperthermia

Hyperthermia can be used in the treatment of upper and lower respiratory tract infections, bladder problems, and urinary tract infections such as cystitis. For these problems, hot baths are the most common method used to induce hyperthermia. Professional applications of hyper-

HYPERTHERMIA AT HOME

Hot baths are the simplest method of inducing a fever at home and can be used to treat upper respiratory tract infections (colds, flu) and even lower respiratory tract conditions, such as bronchitis and pneumonia. To treat viral infections, hot baths can be combined with hot drinks and blanket-wrapping to stimulate the immune system. After the bath, wrap yourself in dry blankets. You may also want to put a hot water bottle over your abdomen. Allow yourself to perspire heavily for as long as you can tolerate it. This may take several hours. Follow with a cool shower.

It is also possible to produce a mild fever at home by simply wrapping up in a dry blanket pack. Again, you can allow yourself to perspire heavily for several hours and follow with a cool shower.

A wet sheet pack may be used to produce a therapeutic fever as well. Wrap yourself in a very cold wet sheet and several blankets. Like the dry pack, you will need several hours to produce a fever. The cold sheet produces reactions in the body that encourage the production of heat. It is often useful to precede the wet sheet with some kind of heating such as exercise or a hot bath or shower.

Local hyperthermia can also be useful at times. One study shows that the inhalation of steam is useful in the treatment of head colds.[6] Hot soaks or hot packs may also be used to treat local conditions. An infection in a hand or foot might benefit from immersion in hot water. If immersion would be uncomfortable, as in the case of an infected wound, hot packs may be applied to the area instead.

treatment aggravates the situation, but conditions improve considerably after a short time.

It is also useful in treating the common cold and flu, as well as chronic fatigue syndrome. Bruce Milliman, N.D., of Seattle, Washington, reports a 70% success rate using hyperthermia to treat chronic fatigue syndrome. Dr. Lewis has also had good results treating chronic fatigue with hyperthermia. For certain cases, Dr. Lewis prescribes hyperthermia as a form of self-care. In one instance, he suggested a patient take hot-tub treatments at home three to four times weekly. "During the following year, her condition improved wonderfully," reports Dr. Lewis. "While not fully recovered, her energy level is substantially higher and she credits this to her hot-tub routine."

Over the centuries, physicians have observed that people suffering from illnesses such as cancer, gonorrhea, and syphilis often become free of these illnesses following a high fever from another infection. This has led to research into the production of fever to treat a variety of health problems from the common cold to AIDS and cancer.

Acute viral infection is another condition Dr. Lewis treats with hyperthermia. In one case, a patient came to him suffering from a combination of pneumonia and bronchitis. His infection had initially been treated with natural remedies and then antibiotics, both of which produced only minor results. Dr. Lewis prescribed two treatments of hyperthermia, 48 hours apart, with an additional treatment given at home one week later. The patient began to improve with the first treatment and was significantly better by the time of the final treatment. "In treating acute conditions, sometimes the patient will have more difficulty tolerating higher temperatures than those who are suffering from chronic conditions," says Dr. Lewis. "As the fever response is stimulated, however, usually a higher tolerance follows."

thermia are now also commonly being used to treat benign prostatic hyperplasia (BPH), chronic prostatitis, and prostate cancer.

Viral Diseases

Douglas Lewis, N.D., past Chair of Physical Medicine at the Bastyr University Natural Health Clinic, in Seattle, Washington, states that a hot immersion bath, if done without raising body temperature and heart rate too quickly or too high, can be used as an adjunct treatment for a "diverse number of diseases—from upper respiratory infections and sexually transmitted diseases to cancer and AIDS." Hyperthermia in the form of hot baths has also proved useful in the treatment of herpes simplex and herpes zoster (shingles) viral infections. At first, the

HIV Infection

At the Bastyr University Natural Health Clinic, hyperthermia is commonly used in the treatment of HIV. In 1988 and 1989, the Natural Health Clinic conducted a "Healing AIDS Research Project" (HARP). Hyperthermia treatment was included in the treatment protocol developed for the study because of its immune-stimulating, detoxifying, and disinfecting properties. According to Leanna Standish, N.D., Ph.D., director of HARP, participants reported that hyperthermia was the facet of their treatment that had the greatest impact. They found a decrease in night sweats and in the frequency of secondary infection. Also, many participants reported having a greater sense of well-being after hyperthermia treatments.[4]

Laboratory research has proven that HIV is temperature-sensitive and suffers greater inactivation at progressively higher temperatures above 98.6° F. For example, after 30 minutes of heating in a water bath at 107.6° F, 40% inactivation of HIV has been reported, and at 132.8° F, 100% inactivation.[5] "I don't believe that hyperthermia is the answer for all HIV patients," says Dr. Lewis, "but I do think it is an appropriate adjunct treatment for all but a few very sick patients."

CAUTION If you practice hyperthermia at home, you should consult your physician. Be careful to monitor your temperature and not let it rise above 102° F, measured orally.

Cancer

Current medical literature is filled with references to the use of hyperthermia in conventional medical settings as an adjunct cancer treatment. Studies have shown that hyperthermia treatment modifies cell membranes in such a way as to protect healthy cells and make tumor cells more susceptible to chemotherapy and radiation.[7] This makes hyperthermia a useful adjunct in cancer therapy, as its application enables the use of lower doses of chemotherapy and radiation.

Other studies have shown that hyperthermia treatments play a role in stimulating the immune system. White cell counts appear to drop immediately following treatment, but rise within a few hours. Not only do the number of white cells increase, but their ability to destroy target cells appears to increase as well.[8] A recent study has shown an increase in the production of interleukin-1 (a compound produced by the body in response to infection, inflammation, or other immune challenges) with whole-body hyperthermia.[9] These studies indicate that increased body temperature plays a positive role in the healing process of the body. According to Arthur C. Guyton, M.D., an authority in the field of medical physiology, the metabolic rate would be increased 100% for every 10° C rise in temperature.[10] This increased metabolic rate no doubt accounts for some of the increased immune activity.

Among the types of cancer for which hyperthermia has been shown to have benefit are head and neck cancer, breast cancer, lymphoma, lung cancer, soft tissue sarcoma, prostate cancer, pancreatic cancer, rectal cancer, uterine cancer, liver carcinoma, and Bowen's disease (a form of squamous cell carcinoma in situ).[11]

Detoxification

Zane Gard, M.D., and Erma Brown, B.S.N., P.H.N., incorporate hyperthermia as part of their detoxification program known as the BioToxic Reduction (BTR) Program. "The human body stores a mix of toxins in the fat found in cells and cell membranes, as well as in actual fat cells," says Dr. Gard. "These toxins include pesticides, herbicides, and solvents, as well as prescription and recreational drugs." According to Dr. Gard, hyperthermia is an excellent way to stimulate the release of toxins from the cells and allow their elimination, first through the skin and later through the bowels and kidneys.[12]

See Detoxification Therapy, Hydrotherapy.

The program developed by Dr. Gard is comprehensive and requires careful medical supervision. The treatment consists of a daily schedule of exercise and sauna sessions, supplementation (with vitamins, minerals, niacin, trace elements, oils, and amino acids), pre- and post-program blood chemistry analysis, and personality and perception testing. The daily treatments must last for at least two weeks to be effective. Patients are monitored closely after exiting the sauna. Large amounts of toxins are sometimes released into the blood by the hyperthermia treatment and may cause a medical emergency (difficulty breathing, heart problems, and, in the case of recreational drug toxins, flashbacks and hallucinations).

"Traditional wisdom has suggested that saunas work by promoting detoxification through the sweat," says John C. Cline, M.D., B.Sc., C.C.F.P., A.B.C.T., Medical Director of the Cline Medical Centre and Oceanside Medicine Research Institute, on Vancouver Island, British Columbia, Canada. "Saunas also stimulate cells to release toxins, which can then be eliminated by the liver and bowels. Several published studies have now shown that hyperthermic therapy can bring about the rapid removal of a wide range of toxic substances from the body."

Dr. Lewis describes a patient who was being treated at the Natural Health Clinic using hyperthermia produced with a steam cabinet. The patient had a long history of oral and intravenous drug abuse. After a short period of heating, the old accumulation of drug residues was released and he got "high" from the drugs rushing through the bloodstream. Several times during his first few treatments he became incoherent and babbled away about nothing in particular. Gradually, over several sessions, this reaction diminished to almost nothing.

A number of health practitioners also employ far-infrared saunas to improve their patients' ability to detoxify. The FIR energy emitted in such saunas can induce two to three times the sweat volume of conventional saunas, yet they operate at a much cooler air temperature range (100°-130° F compared to 180°-235° F in a conventional sauna). As a result, many patients who cannot tolerate conventional saunas or steam rooms can benefit from using FIR saunas. Moreover, their lower heat range makes them safer for patients with cardiovascular risk factors or fragile health, because lower temperatures don't dramatically elevate heart rate and blood pressure.

Risks Associated with Hyperthermia

When used knowledgeably and with care, hyperthermia is a safe and effective treatment for many conditions. Ill-effects of hyperthermia usually appear only when body temperature exceeds 106° F. However, certain individuals are sensitive to the effects of heat, such as those with anemia, heart disease, diabetes, seizure disorders, tuberculosis, and women who are or may be pregnant.[13] People with these conditions should should use hyperthermia with great care and consult their physicians prior to doing so.

Other reported risks of hyperthermia include herpes outbreaks[14] (including herpes zoster), liver toxicity,[15] and nervous system injury. Some substances used to induce hyperthermia are not recommended. These include blood products, vaccines, pollens, and benign forms of malaria,[16] as secondary infection from the injection of blood products and these other substances is extremely dangerous. Hyperthermia for detoxification should only be performed under medical supervision for the reasons described in the previous section. Additional notes of caution:

- Patients with temperature regulatory problems, especially the old and the very young, should not use hyperthermia.

- Microwave diathermy can burn the tissue around the eyes and should never be used by people with pacemakers.

- People with peripheral vascular disease or loss of sensation should not use hyperthermia due to the risk of burns.

- Caution is advised with patients who have cardiovascular disease, in particular arrhythmia (abnormal or irregular heartbeat) and tachycardia (abnormally rapid heart rate), and severe hypertension or hypotension.

The Future of Hyperthermia

As is true with many treatments that offer little or no potential profit from their development, hyperthermia has seen limited research. Also, to be effective, it is labor intensive and requires the supervision of a qualified medical professional who is able to deal with a crisis situation that can arise as the body eliminates toxins. Because of these factors, Dr. Lewis realizes that many health professionals do not use hyperthermia as a means of treatment.

 At a time when medical treatment consists primarily of high-tech drugs and surgical intervention, it would be useful for some of America's tax dollars to be spent researching low-cost alternative therapies such as hyperthermia.

However, Dr. Lewis foresees the situation changing. "As we begin to recognize the degree to which we have poisoned our environment and ourselves, we will begin to look for effective ways to detoxify," Dr. Lewis says. "And hyperthermia is certainly an important way of doing so, both as a primary and adjunct method. Likewise, as it becomes evident that our immune functions are suffering, we will begin to explore ways to support immune function, and hyperthermia can be a useful tool in that quest." At a time when medical treatment consists primarily of high-tech drugs and surgical intervention, it would be useful for some of America's tax dollars to be spent researching low-cost alternatives such as hyperthermia.

Where to Find Help

For additional help and information concerning hyperthermia, contact:

International Clinical Hyperthermia Society (ICHS)
1502 East Country Line Road South
Indianapolis, Indiana 46227
(317) 887-7651
Website: www.hyperthermia-ichs.org

The ICHS provides a forum for researchers and physicians to discuss their ideas on the use of hyperthermia and to share their clinical findings. Active members include surgeons, medical and radiation oncologists, medical physicists (including basic scientists), nurses, and administrators.

Bastyr University Natural Health Clinic
1307 North 45th Street, Suite 200
Seattle, Washington 98103
(206) 632-0354
Website: www.bastyr.edu

The physical medicine department of the Natural Health Clinic of Bastyr University uses hyperthermia treatment for detoxification and in conditions ranging from upper respiratory infection to chronic fatigue syndrome and HIV.

National College of Naturopathic Medicine
049 S.W. Porter
Portland, Oregon 97201
(503) 499-4343
Website: www.ncnm.edu

NCNM's teaching clinic uses hyperthermia for a wide variety of conditions.

Uchee Pines Institute
30 Uchee Pines Road
Seale, Alabama 36875
(334) 855-4781
Website: ucheepines.org

Uchee Pines Institute is a healing center that provides many health-care alternatives, including hyperthermia treatment.

Far-Infrared (FIR) Products and Devices

High Tech Health, Inc.
2695 Linden Drive
Boulder, Colorado 80304
(800) 794-5355
Website: www.hightechhealth.com

Green Energy Solutions
258 Vega Road
Watsonville, California 95076
(877) 973-7000
Website: www.greenenergysolutions.com

PLH Products
16000 Phoenix Drive
City of Industry, California 91745
(800) 946-6001
Website: www.healthmatesauna.com

Meditherm, Inc.
15824 S.W. Upper Boones Ferry Road
Lake Oswego, Oregon 97035
(503) 639-8496 or (61) 7-5-474-2702 (Australia)
Website: www.meditherm.com

Recommended Reading

Home Remedies. Agatha Thrash, M.D., and Calvin Thrash, M.D. Seale, AL: New Lifestyle Books, 1981.

Lectures in Naturopathic Hydrotherapy. Wade Boyle, N.D., and Andre Saine, N.D. East Palestine, OH: Buckeye Naturopathic Press, 1991.

HYPNOTHERAPY

Hypnotherapy is used to manage numerous medical and psychological problems. Hypnotic techniques can help a person stop smoking, overcome alcohol and substance abuse, and reduce overeating. Hypnotherapy is also effective in treating stress, sleep disorders, and mental health problems such as anxiety, fear, phobias, and depression.

FOR THOUSANDS OF YEARS, the power of suggestion has played a major role in healing in cultures as varied as ancient Greece, Persia, and India. Hypnotherapy uses both the power of suggestion and trancelike states to access the deepest levels of the mind to effect positive changes in a person's behavior and to treat a range of health conditions, including migraines, ulcers, respiratory conditions, tension headaches, and even warts.

In 1955, the British Medical Association approved the use of hypnotherapy as a valid medical treatment. The American Medical Association (AMA) followed suit in 1958, and its Council on Scientific Affairs continues to encourage more research on the subject of hypnotherapy. In the same year, hypnotherapy was also accepted as a valid psychotherapeutic procedure by the American Psychological Association (APA). Hypnotherapy's credibility was further bolstered in 1995, when the National Institutes of Health (NIH) acknowledged its effectiveness for treating chronic pain and recommended that insurance companies reimburse patients who use it for this purpose.[1] In addition, the American Society of Clinical Hypnosis, a professional association of physicians, psychologists, and dentists, has grown from 20 members in 1957 to over 4,300, and attendance at hypnotism courses by physicians and other medical specialists is steadily increasing. Approximately 15,000 doctors now combine hypnotherapy with traditional treatments and recent studies show that 94% of patients benefit from hypnotherapy, even if the only benefit is relaxation.[2]

> *There can be no hypnosis unless the client is willing to participate in the process. The client enters hypnosis in a natural way, of his or her own accord, simply by following the suggestions of the hypnotherapist.*
>
> —A.M. KRASNER, PH.D.,

How Hypnotherapy Works

"Although the exact mechanisms by which hypnotherapy performs its therapeutic work has yet to be elucidated, there is a growing consensus about the reality of its manifested effects," says Gerard V. Sunnen, M.D., Associate Clinical Professor of Psychiatry at the New York University Bellevue Hospital Center, in New York City. "Hypnosis may be conceptualized as a special condition of self-awareness that permits enhanced communication between conscious and unconscious processes, including the workings of the autonomic nervous system. Therapeutic imagery stimulated in hypnosis can be utilized to influence most organ systems in the body in order to boost their performance and heighten their reserve potential. The cardiovascular system, for example, may be given therapeutic affirmations to relax blood pressure, strengthen its basic rhythm, and bring it into harmony with other organ systems."

According to A.M. Krasner, Ph.D., Founder of the American Board of Hypnotherapy, in Santa Ana, California, "All hypnosis is self-hypnosis. The hypnotherapist is a facilitator. There can be no hypnosis unless the client is willing to participate in the process. The client always enters hypnosis in a natural way, of his or her own accord, simply by following the suggestions of the hypnotherapist."

Generally speaking, hypnosis is an artificially induced state characterized by a heightened receptivity to suggestion. The state is attained by first relaxing the body, then shifting attention away from the external environment toward a narrow range of objects or ideas as suggested by the hypnotherapist or by oneself (self-hypnosis).

In the superficial hypnotic state, the patient accepts suggestions but does not necessarily carry them out. Patients who reach the deep, or somnambulistic, state benefit most from hypnotherapy. It is in this state that posthypnotic suggestions (suggestions that take effect after the patient awakens from the trance) to relieve pain are most successful. According to the World Health Organization (WHO), 90% of the general population can be hypnotized, with 20% to 30% having a high enough susceptibility to enter the somnambulistic state, making them highly receptive to treatment.[3]

See Mind/Body Medicine.

Research has demonstrated that a person's body chemistry actually changes during a hypnotic trance. In one experiment, a young girl was unable to hold her hand in a bucket of ice water for more than 30 seconds. Testing showed that the blood levels of cortisol in her body were high, indicating she was undergoing severe stress. Under hypnosis, she was able to keep the same hand in ice water for 30 minutes while there was no rise in cortisol levels.[4]

Research has demonstrated that a person's body chemistry actually changes during a hypnotic trance.

There are many ways of inducing hypnosis. Regardless of what procedure is used, the main concern during hypnosis is to quiet the patient's conscious mind and to make the unconscious mind more accessible. Because the unconscious mind is basically noncritical, suggestions have a better chance of being effective than they would if given during a normal waking state.

People who benefit most from hypnotherapy are those who understand that hypnosis is not a surrender of control; it is only an advanced form of relaxation. Three conditions are essential to successful hypnotherapy:

1. Rapport between hypnotist and subject

2. A comfortable environment, free of distraction

3. A willingness and desire by the subject to be hypnotized

For hypnotherapy to be successful, the late Maurice Tinterow, M.D., Ph.D., an anesthesiologist at the Center for the Improvement of Human Functioning, in Wichita,

HISTORY OF HYPNOSIS

Franz Anton Mesmer, a German physician, introduced hypnosis to the medical community in the late 18th century under the name Mesmerism. Mesmer theorized that a universal fluid, present in all objects, produced disease when it was out of balance in the human body. But Mesmer soon fell out of favor and was banned from France after a committee headed by American statesman Benjamin Franklin and Joseph de Guillotin, a French physician, could not verify his findings. James Braid, an English ophthalmologist, later changed the name to hypnosis based on *Hypnos*, the Greek god of sleep. Although hypnosis is not sleep, the word became entrenched in the English vocabulary.

In the mid-1800s, James Esdaile, an English surgeon stationed in India, performed a variety of operations using only hypnotic anesthesia. Some of the surgical procedures he performed while administering hypnosis included amputations of the arm, breast, and penis, as well as the removal of tumors.

One of the more well-known proponents of hypnosis was Sigmund Freud, the 19th-century father of modern psychiatry. Freud delivered two papers on the subject, and included it in his own practice. "There was something positively seductive in working with hypnosis," he wrote. "For the first time, there was a sense of having overcome one's helplessness; and it was highly flattering to enjoy the reputation of being a miracle worker."

By the early 1890s, however, Freud rejected hypnosis in favor of his own theories of analysis and, shortly afterward, the practice became the focus of dispute, disagreement, and argument. It wasn't until the middle of this century that the British and American Medical Societies recognized its use as an adjunct to treating pain.

Kansas, believed that "the client must be led to accept his or her physician-hypnotist's words as valid descriptions of reality. The therapist must manipulate words and situations in such a way as to lead the subject to believe that the suggestions are literally true statements. These suggestions should be accepted without criticism or analysis."

One of Dr. Tinterow's earliest and most dramatic cases involved a 15-year-old girl who required open-heart surgery in 1960. Because the girl proved allergic to all anesthetic agents, Dr. Tinterow used hypnosis over a period of eight weeks, and by the final session before surgery the girl was able to relax quite easily. She was hypnotized before the operation and remained conscious throughout the four-hour procedure.

Dr. Tinterow had the girl on whom he performed open-heart surgery concentrate on her favorite sport—water skiing. "It was just a matter of having her take deep breaths, close her eyes, and feel herself relaxing from the top of her head to the tips of her toes," he recalled. "You start with the feet and legs and then just have it go all the way to the top of the head." Eventually Dr. Tinterow distracted the girl from the surgical procedure by shifting her attention to what she liked to do best. "I told her to picture herself going to the lake and waterskiing. She was listening to music with her headset on, and we just kept talking to her." Dr. Tinterow even had the girl perform simple arithmetic problems during the surgery to make sure her mind was functioning properly. So successful was his work with her that after the operation the girl didn't even take an aspirin.

What to Expect During a Hypnotherapy Session

During an initial visit to a hypnotherapist, it is common for the therapist to address any concerns that you may have and then perhaps illustrate how suggestion works in everyday life, as well as point out what you can expect while in a trance state. Possible effects, according to Dr. Krasner, include physical relaxation, distraction of the conscious mind, a narrowed focus of attention, increased sensory awareness, reduced awareness of physical surroundings, and increased attention to internal sensations. Following this, you might then be tested for suggestibility based on a variety of methods at the hypnotherapist's disposal.

You may also be asked about your specific condition. The value of this, according to Anne H. Spencer, Ph.D., C.Ht., Founder of the International Medical and Dental Hypnotherapy Association, is that it provides the hypnotherapist with insights into any pattern associated with the condition, as well as an idea of what the client's goals are in terms of wellness. "What I look for in this discussion," says Dr. Spencer, "are clues as to how my client deals with life, as well as indications of any beliefs which may be contributing to his or her condition. These clues very often can provide me with the most effective approach to use in the actual hypnotherapy session."

A hypnotherapy session will usually last 60-90 minutes. The number of sessions required to produce results varies according to each individual. According to Dr. Spencer, six to 12 sessions, one per week, is about the average.

Is Hypnotherapy Safe for Everyone?

Although hypnosis is a very safe practice in the hands of a qualified practitioner, it is a very powerful tool that should be used only with utmost caution. WHO cautions that hypnosis should not be performed on patients with psychosis, organic psychiatric conditions, or antisocial personality disorders. Hypnotherapy is not a cure-all and few doctors are willing to invest the time to master its techniques. Many patients, because of the severity of their conditions, do not make good subjects and are unable to reach the proper depth for posthypnotic suggestions to be effective.

Therapeutic Applications of Hypnotherapy

Hypnotherapy has therapeutic applications for both psychological and physical disorders. A skilled hypnotherapist can facilitate profound changes in respiration and relaxation on the part of the client to create positive shifts in behavior and an enhanced sense of well-being. A physiological shift can be observed in a hypnotic state, as can greater control of autonomic nervous system functions normally considered to be beyond one's ability to control. Stress reduction is a common occurrence, as is a lowering of blood pressure.

Recently, hypnotherapy has witnessed a renaissance in its clinical applications. "Because hypnosis is the most powerful non-pharmacological relaxing agent known to science, in the last few years it has received increasing attention in the medical community," Dr. Sunnen says. "Due to its capacity to induce deep, multilevel relaxation, to quell anticipatory anxiety, to increase awareness of bodily functions, to increase tolerance to adverse stimuli, and to intensify affirmative imagery, it can be adapted to amplify the mind's contribution to healing, both in and out of the hospital."

Dr. Sunnen regularly makes use of hypnotherapy in the hospital setting to prepare patients for surgical procedures and operations. "You can imagine the state of mind of an individual who has never been in a hospital before and who is awaiting quadruple cardiac bypass surgery the next day," he says. "You would be surprised to see such a patient, in spite of all sorts of surrounding noise produced by monitors and intruding personnel, being guided into a hypnotic state so that all such anxiety-producing distractions are pushed back and feelings of peacefulness and tranquility are invited. Add to that positive imagery about the procedure, recruiting all the potential adaptive and healing powers the organism is capable of generating, and you have a patient who is primed to optimally flow through the operative challenge and come out all the better for it."

Dr. Sunnen's view is substantiated by recent studies, which found that hypnotherapy has the potential not only to reduce anxiety due to surgery and other medical procedures, but also to decrease pain resulting from such procedures, improve recovery time, and reduce the need for medication.[5]

Dr. Tinterow employed hypnotherapy to treat a variety of medical conditions and to control pain for conditions such as headaches, facial neuralgia, sciatica, osteoarthritis, rheumatoid arthritis, whiplash, menstrual pain, and tennis elbow.[6] Dr. Tinterow also used hypnotherapy in place of anesthesia in a variety of surgical operations, including hysterectomies, hernias, breast biopsies, hemorrhoidectomies, cesarean sections, and for the treatment of second and third degree burns.[7]

Dentistry is another field where hypnotherapy has been used with excellent results. Kay Thompson, D.D.S., of Pittsburgh, Pennsylvania, regularly uses hypnotherapy in her practice. She describes how hypnotherapy was used for a molar extraction in a patient who was allergic to all procaine-type drugs. To prepare the patient for the extraction, Dr. Thompson taught her how to go into a trance using hypnotic induction techniques. After one session with the patient, Dr. Thompson was able to perform the extraction using only hypnosis. Because the molar was so badly decayed, the operation lasted 45 minutes, yet the patient had no swelling or discomfort afterward and even ate dinner that night. Meanwhile, a co-worker who underwent a similar procedure without hypnosis needed two days off from work because of a swollen jaw, according to Dr. Thompson.

"Most people are not aware that they can control their own healing and even influence their circulation," says Dr. Thompson, who believes that her patient's ability to control her circulatory system through hypnosis enhanced the healing process. Dr. Thompson and her colleagues have also used hypnotherapy to help treat hemophiliacs and have been able to perform surgery on these patients without them having any postoperative bleeding.

According to Dr. Sunnen, while only a small percentage of patients can undergo major surgery using the hypnotic trance as the sole anesthetic, a far greater percentage can benefit from the more subtle therapeutic influence of hypnosis applied in an integrated fashion. "Hypnotic intervention can begin in the preoperative period, be continued during the operation itself, and then be maintained through the postoperative stage to assist the patient through all phases of psychological and physical adjustment," Dr. Sunnen says. In addition, he points out, even when hypnotherapy is unable to totally block pain sensations, it is often able to reduce the dosage of medication and anesthetics used in a variety of medical procedures.

Hypnotherapy is today increasingly being used by a growing number of psychotherapists as well. "In psychotherapy, hypnosis can be seen as a gateway to the unconscious mind," Dr. Sunnen explains. "As such, it can bring insights into consciousness in order to bring about better self-understanding. Equally important, it has the capacity to transform insight into action and execution, a process called 'working through'." In the case of smoking cessation, for example, the mind realizes that smoking is detrimental to health, yet impulses continue to demand the ingestion of smoke. Hypnosis is able to get through to the emotional mind to finally convince it of the futility of smoking.

Gary Lalonde, C.Ht., of Wales, Michigan, uses hypnotherapy to treat various health conditions. One of his clients suffered from reflex sympathetic dystrophy (RSD), a chronic condition where pain does not subside and muscle function begins to deteriorate. "This man had pierced one of his feet with a three-and-a-half-inch nail after stepping on a piece of wood at a construction site," Lalonde relates. "He was treated for the injury, but the pain persisted and grew so bad that he could not return to work. For two years, his condition grew worse. Finally, a thermograph showed that the foot's temperature was 11° F colder than the rest of his body. When his doctors told him it might have to be amputated, he came to see me."

Lalonde worked with this client for seven months, using hypnotherapy not only for pain relief, but also to explore any link between the man's condition and his unconscious beliefs. It was discovered that, within his unconscious, he doubted his ability to provide for his family and that his condition took care of that need by enabling him to collect worker's compensation pay. Lalonde worked with the man to change his belief. As he gained confidence in himself, his pain began to diminish. At the end of 12 sessions, the man was free of all pain and the temperature of his foot returned to normal, something his doctors had told him would not be possible.

The long-term benefits of hypnotherapy are beginning to be borne out. One comprehensive study of hypnotherapy with 178 patients suffering from chronic pain reported that 78% remained pain-free after six months; 47% after one year; 44% after two years; and 36.5% after three years.[8] Another study showed the efficacy of hypnotherapy as compared to psychoanalysis and behavior therapy. After 600 sessions of psychoanalysis, 38% of the patients reported recovery from their conditions; those receiving behavior therapy improved in 72% of all cases

HYPNOTHERAPY DURING PREGNANCY AND CHILDBIRTH

Due to its proven ability to reduce stress and relieve pain, hypnotherapy is increasingly being used in the field of obstetrics (pregnancy and childbirth). The use of hypnotherapy to assist in childbirth dates back to the 19th century, according to Gerard V. Sunnen, M.D. "After falling into disfavor due to competition from chemical anesthesia, the practice of hypnotically assisted deliveries has seen a revival in the last few decades," he says. "One important reason for this comeback is the realization that hypnosis can be useful not only in obstetric analgesia or anesthesia, but in all phases of giving birth, from pregnancy to postpartum recovery."

Dr. Sunnen cites the following advantages for using hypnotherapy in obstetrics:

- Unlike the use of chemical anesthetics, which always carries some risk to both the mother and her infant, hypnotherapy has never been shown to cause injury to either person.

- Hypnosis can make the delivery process more humane and enhance the expectant mother's self-esteem and trust in her own natural resources.

- Should chemical anesthetics still be required, they can be easily and promptly administered and usually in lesser amounts than normal.

- Hypnosis, unlike chemical anesthesia, does not interfere with the normal emotional responses to the birth process and the immediate bonding between mother and child.

- Hypnosis abets both preparation for delivery and the recovery process by minimizing anticipatory anxiety and optimizing the return to normal functioning, unlike chemical anesthetics, which can cause a "hangover" effect lasting up to two days.[10]

ease (for managing the psychological factors that can exacerbate its symptoms); menstrual and menopausal syndromes and various gynecological procedures; glaucoma and cataract removal; tinnitus; and hysterical aphonia (inability to produce speech due to hysteria). Hypnotherapy can serve as an effective adjunct therapy for medical procedures such as chemotherapy, orthopedics, vasectomy, and cytoscopy.[11]

Hypnotherapy can also be helpful for gastrointestinal disorders (peptic ulcer and ulcerative colitis), anorexia nervosa, cardiovascular conditions, skin conditions (acne, eczema, contact dermatitis, psoriasis, warts),[12] asthma,[13] fibromyalgia,[14] irritable bowel syndrome (IBS),[15] cancer pain management,[16] fractures,[17] periodontal disease,[18] insomnia, obesity, phobias, nausea, vomiting,[19] and diabetes (as an adjunctive treatment).[20]

The Future of Hypnotherapy

Since its formal sanction by the AMA in 1958, more and more physicians have come to accept hypnotherapy's value and are making use of its techniques. While hypnosis is still far from being fully understood, it is scientifically respected and has achieved almost unanimous professional acceptance. Experiments to determine how hypnosis works and to quantify its effects are ongoing. And new breakthroughs on how hypnotherapy may be applied to medical and psychological problems are constantly being reported.

In hospitals today, it is not uncommon to find on staff an anesthesiologist, surgeon, nurse, or therapist who is also a trained hypnotherapist. As George Pratt, Ph.D., a clinical psychologist and hypnotherapist in La Jolla, California, notes, "With its focus on the whole person, hypnosis holds the great promise of becoming a humanizing force for the field of medicine as a whole. Realizing that even unconscious patients hear and remember information that pertains to them, physicians, surgeons, nurses, and anesthesiologists will communicate more effectively with comatose, critically ill, and anesthetized patients, thus replacing fear and isolation with encouragement and positive expectations."[21]

after 22 sessions; while hypnotherapy produced a 93% success rate after only six sessions.[9]

According to Dr. Sunnen, hypnotherapy has been shown to provide benefit for the following conditions: burns; multiple sclerosis (as an aid to managing accompanying anxiety, depression, and stress); Parkinson's dis-

Where to Find Help

In choosing a hypnotherapist, it is important that you be assured that he or she has been competently trained and certified. The following organizations can refer you to legitimate practitioners in your area:

The American Society of Clinical Hypnosis
130 E. Elm Street, Suite 201
Roselle, Illinois 60172-2000
(630) 980-4740
Website: www.asch.net

Membership is comprised of M.D.s and dentists trained in the use of hypnosis for treating health conditions. Send a stamped, self-addressed envelope for referrals to practitioners in your area.

American Association of Professional Hypnotherapists
4149-A El Camino Way
Palo Alto, California 94306
(650) 323-3224
Website: www.aaph.org

The AAPH is a worldwide organization that promotes communication between professionals for the promotion and development of ethical methods, techniques, and standards in the field of hypnotherapy. Also publishes a journal and provides an online nationwide directory of AAPH member hypnotherapists.

The National Guild of Hypnotists
P.O. Box 308
Merrimack, New Hampshire 03054
(603) 429-9438
Website: www.ngh.net

The oldest certifying guild in the United States. Offers basic certification programs and trainer programs, and supplies a complete range of books and tapes on hypnotherapy.

American Psychotherapy and Medical Hypnosis Association
280 Island Avenue, Suite 404
Reno, Nevada 89501
(775) 786-5650
Website: www.apmha.com

The APMHA was formed in 1992 to provide a multidisciplinary forum for the ethical use of hypnosis and hypnotherapy. Provides training and offers referrals nationwide.

The American Board of Hypnotherapy/American Institute of Hypnotherapy
2002 E. McFadden, Suite 100
Santa Ana, California 92705
(714) 245-9340 or (800) 872-9996
Website: www.aih.cc

Both the ABH and AIH, founded by Dr. A.M. Krasner, train and certify hypnotherapists in a wide range of hypnotherapy applications.

International Medical and Dental Hypnotherapy Association
4110 Edgeland, Suite 800
Royal Oak, Michigan 48073
(248) 549-5594 or (800) 257-5467
Website: www.infinityinst.com

Trains and certifies M.D.s, dentists, and hypnotherapists in the therapeutic use of hypnotherapy for treating health challenges, with members located throughout the United States, Canada, Europe, Japan, Mexico, and the Virgin Islands. Provides a referral list of certified practitioners throughout the U.S. and Canada, available by sending a stamped, self-addressed envelope.

Recommended Reading

A Primer of Clinical Hypnosis. Gerard Sunnen and Barbara DeBetz. Boston: PSG Publishing, 1985. (Dr. Sunnen's writings on the clinical use of hypnotherapy are also available on the Internet: www.triroc.com/sunnen.)

Hypnosis, Acupuncture and Pain. Maurice M. Tinterow, M.D. Wichita, KS: Bio-Communication Press, 1989.

Hypnotherapy. Dave Elman. Glendale, CA: Westwood Publishing, 1984.

The Wizard Within: The Krasner Method of Clinical Hypnotherapy. A.M. Krasner, Ph.D. Santa Ana, CA: American Board of Hypnotherapy Press, 1990.

LIGHT THERAPY

Light and color have been valued throughout history as sources of healing. Today, the therapeutic applications of light and color are being investigated in major hospitals and research centers worldwide. Results indicate that full-spectrum, ultraviolet, colored, and laser light can have therapeutic value for a range of conditions, from chronic pain and depression to immune disorders and cancer.

MANY HEALTH DISORDERS can be traced to problems with the circadian rhythm, the body's inner clock, and how it governs the timing of sleep, hormone production, body temperature, and other biological functions. Disturbances in this rhythm can lead to health problems such as depression and sleep disorders. Natural sunlight and various forms of light therapy can help reestablish the body's natural rhythm and are becoming an integral treatment for many related health conditions.

More recently, the ability of light to activate certain biochemical substances in the body has become the basis of treatment for skin disorders such as psoriasis and for certain forms of cancer. Exposure to ultraviolet light under controlled conditions has also proved beneficial for certain conditions, particularly when combined with light-sensitive medications.

How Light Therapy Works

When light enters the eye, millions of light- and color-sensitive cells called photoreceptors convert the light into electrical impulses. These impulses travel along the optic nerve to the brain, where they trigger the hypothalamus gland to send chemical messengers called neurotransmitters to regulate the autonomic (automatic) functions of the body. The hypothalamus is part of the endocrine system whose secretions govern most bodily functions—blood pressure, body temperature, breathing, digestion, sexual function, moods, the immune system, the aging process, and the circadian rhythm. Full-spectrum light (containing all wavelengths) sparks the delicate impulses that regulate these functions and maintain health.

After 25 years of clinical research, John Downing, O.D., Ph.D., Director of the Light Therapy Institute, in Santa Rosa, California, has expanded the theory regarding the action of visually perceived light to encompass its effects on other areas of the brain: the cerebral cortex, where it stimulates motivation, learning, thinking, creativity, memory, and even body movements; the limbic system, where visually perceived light brings in the emotional impressions of the world; and the brain stem, where light helps to provide coordination and balance.

The Importance of Natural Sunlight

Poor light poses a serious threat to health, according to the numerous published studies of the late photobiologist John Nash Ott, D.Sc. (Hon.).[1] He firmly believed that the kind of light adequate for maintaining health must contain the full wavelength spectrum found in natural sunlight. Most artificial lighting, both incandescent and fluorescent, lacks the complete balanced spectrum of sunlight and, as Dr. Ott discovered, interferes with the body's optimal absorption of nutrients, a condition he called "malillumination" analogous to malnutrition. Windows, windshields, eyeglasses, smog, and sunscreen lotions all filter out parts of the light spectrum and contribute to this problem. Sunscreens may not block out the most harmful part of the ultraviolet spectrum (UV-C) while inhibiting the uptake of vitamin D. They can also contain toxic chemicals that are absorbed by the skin.

Research reveals that if certain wavelengths aren't present in light, the body can't fully absorb some nutrients.[2] Malillumination contributes to fatigue, tooth decay, depression, hostility, suppressed immune function, strokes, hair loss, skin damage, alcoholism, drug abuse, Alzheimer's disease, and cancer.[3] It has also been linked, in a study at the Clinical Pathology Department of the National Institutes of Health, to a loss of muscle tone and strength.[4]

According to John Zimmerman, Ph.D, founder of the Bio-Electro-Magnetics Institute, in Reno, Nevada, most offices, even those with uncovered windows and

LIGHT AND THE INTERNAL CLOCK

Circadian rhythms are regularly recurring, biological changes in our mental and physical behaviors over the course of the day. As indicated by the term *circadian* (Latin for "around a day"), these rhythms repeat approximately every 24 hours and are primarily controlled by the body's biological "clock." Circadian rhythms are most commonly linked to sleep/wake patterns and account for the fluctuations of alertness and drowsiness throughout the day. Circadian rhythms occur in other physiological processes as well, including blood pressure, body temperature, hormone levels, and the immune system.

The circadian system is regulated by the hypothalamus via the pineal gland. This gland is controlled by the presence or absence of external light and serves to synchronize and coordinate the biological events of the body. "There are neurochemical channels from the retina to the pineal and pituitary glands, the master glands of the whole endocrine system," according to the late photobiologist John Nash Ott, D.Sc. (Hon.). "This regulates your body chemistry and its growth, all organs of your body, including your brain, and how they function."[10]

Melatonin, the chief hormone of the pineal gland, is produced only during darkness (its production is actually inhibited by light). Melatonin has sedative qualities and helps reduce anxiety, panic disorders, and migraines as well as inducing sleep. It is also thought to be a primary regulator of the immune system. Researchers have found that when a person ignores the 24-hour dark-light cycle and keeps irregular hours of work and rest, the body's internal rhythms go awry. The number of hours one sleeps is less important than when one sleeps with respect to daylight.

Studies have shown that being exposed to even a fairly dim light at night can significantly reduce the synthesis of melatonin.[11] People who work in rotating shifts or at night have been shown to experience a higher incidence of heart disease, back pain, respiratory problems, ulcers, and sleep disorders. These people also have a higher rate of error and accidents and often experience a significant loss of alertness and ability to make decisions. However, researchers are using carefully timed, high-intensity bright lighting (5-10 times brighter than ordinary levels), as well as the administration of melatonin, to help shift workers adjust to their schedules.[12]

One of the most prevalent consequences of disrupted circadian rhythms is an illness called seasonal affective disorder (SAD). Travel between time zones often results in jet lag, a less serious but often debilitating and disorienting condition caused by the upset of the body's internal clock. Melatonin, full-spectrum, and bright light therapies are being explored as useful antidotes. Some airports are now considering the installation of full-spectrum lights in their first-class lounges to help passengers adjust to their destination time zones.

---

the lights on, have a light level of only 500 lux (the international unit of illumination, one lumen per square meter) as compared to outdoor light, which has about 50,000 lux, or approximately 100 times more. Night shift workers are usually exposed to a light level of only 50 lux. "By spending 90% of our lives indoors, under inadequate lighting conditions, we cause or worsen a wide range of health problems, including depression, heart disease, hyperactivity in children, osteoporosis in the elderly, and lowered resistance to infection," according to Dr. Downing.[5] In order to maintain health, it is important to be exposed to light containing the full spectrum of sunlight.

Studies indicate that fluorescent light, not exposure to natural sunlight, promotes the development of skin cancer (melanoma).[6] A study carried out by the U.S. Navy compared the risk of melanoma (a malignant skin mole or tumor) for different naval occupations. It was discovered that personnel holding indoor occupations had the highest rates of melanoma, while workers in jobs that required spending time both indoors and outdoors had the lowest rate. In addition, a higher rate of melanoma occurred on the trunk of the body as opposed to the head and arms, which are commonly exposed to sunlight. The authors of the study theorized that the anatomical site of melanoma suggests a "protective role for brief, regular exposure to sunlight."[7] Another study of 900 women who worked indoors under fluorescent lights found that they had twice the normal risk of developing melanoma.[8]

This is consistent with studies that show vitamin D (whose production is stimulated by ultraviolet light) suppresses the growth of malignant melanoma cells. These new findings also call into question the belief that indoor occupations can provide safety for fair-skinned, freckled individuals who are at high risk for skin cancers. This and other studies indicate that an occupational deprivation of sunlight can lead to a vitamin D deficiency, which in turn could favor the development of melanoma.[9]

Forms of Light Therapy

The oldest form of light therapy is natural sunlight. The sun is the ultimate source of full-spectrum light, which means it contains all possible wavelengths of light, from infrared to ultraviolet (UV). Numerous forms of light therapy are now available, including full-spectrum light therapy, bright light therapy, various forms of UV light therapy, syntonic optometry, cold laser therapy, and colored light therapy. Electromagnetic devices such as the Light Beam Generator and the MORA™ also use specific light frequencies in treatment.

 See Energy Medicine.

Full-Spectrum Light Therapy

Light therapy often involves using light boxes, specially designed devices consisting of full-spectrum fluorescent lights that simulate early-morning sunlight. Light boxes typically cost $300-$1,000 and are widely available in a various sizes and styles (wall units, desk lamps, light visors). They usually come in values of 2,500 lux and 10,000 lux. Most standard therapy protocols recommend two hours of exposure to 2,500 lux daily; some doctors recommend using 10,000-lux boxes for only 30 minutes daily. You can perform the light therapy first thing in the morning, sitting before the light box with your eyes open but not staring directly into the light, either at work (assuming you work at a desk or in some manner of stationary pursuit) or at home. (Research has found that external light is sensed by other organs than the eyes— one study, in fact, found that light exposure to the back of the knee suppressed melatonin production. The therapeutic applications of these findings are not assessed at this time.) Generally, it takes about 14 days of light therapy to see benefits.

> **CAUTION** Individuals should never stare into the light during therapy and should be careful to choose light sources that screen out ultraviolet rays. People with eye problems such as diabetic retinopathy or macular degeneration should not employ light therapy without their doctor's consent.

Sunlight and full-spectrum light can be applied to the skin in order to relieve hypertension, depression, insomnia, premenstrual syndrome, migraines, and carbohydrate cravings associated with metabolic imbalances.[13] In a study undertaken by Dr. Ott and his associates, the effect of full-spectrum lighting in the class-room was tested on first grade students in Sarasota, Florida. Using four classrooms, two as a control with standard fluorescent lighting and two outfitted with full-spectrum lights, the researchers tracked the behavior levels of the students for a full semester, using hidden cameras. Their results demonstrated conclusively that the students exposed to the full-spectrum lighting had a marked diminishment of hyperactivity, whereas those in the control classrooms actually became more hyperactive. Similar studies in Canada and elsewhere clearly showed that students in classrooms with full-spectrum light had less absenteeism and a higher academic achievement record when compared with classes conducted under ordinary fluorescent lighting.[14]

> *Most artificial lighting, both incandescent and fluorescent, lacks the complete balanced spectrum of sunlight and interferes with the body's optimal absorption of nutrients, a condition known as malillumination. In order to maintain health, it is important to be exposed to light containing the full spectrum of sunlight.*

Cancer: A ten-year epidemiological study conducted at Johns Hopkins University Medical School, in Baltimore, Maryland, showed that exposure to full-spectrum light (including the ultraviolet frequency) is positively related to the prevention of breast, colon, and rectal cancers.[15] Another report found that exposure to full-spectrum sunlight reduced the risk of developing breast cancer.[16] In Russia, a full-spectrum lighting system was installed in factories where colds and sore throats had become commonplace among workers. This lowered the bacterial contamination of the air by 40%-70%. Workers who did not receive the full-spectrum light were absent twice as many days as those who did.[17]

SAD: Full-spectrum light and bright white light (often preferred because the UV light found in full-spectrum light is not necessary to achieve the antidepressant effect and can be harmful with protracted direct exposure to the eyes) are effective treatments for seasonal affective disorder (SAD), also known as the "winter blues." The symptoms of SAD are depression, excess sleeping and eating, a withdrawn feeling, and lowered sex drive. It is currently being investigated by Charmane Eastman, Ph.D., Director of the Biological Rhythms Research Laboratory at Rush Presbyterian St. Luke's Medical Center, in Chicago, Illinois. Melatonin levels are found to be very high in patients with SAD. Daily exposure to sunlight or to full-spectrum light has been known to eliminate SAD symptoms.[18] In one study, SAD patients who took morning walks and received a minimum of one hour of sunlight showed positive results.[19] Light boxes are used in the majority of SAD cases. Most studies find that early morning sessions, ranging from 30 minutes to two hours using varying intensities of light, bring improvement within a week.[20]

Jaundice: Light therapy is used to treat jaundice in newborn babies. In 1956, Sister Ward of Rochford General Hospital, in England, discovered the treatment by accident. On warm summer days, she would wheel the premature infants into the courtyard. One day a doctor came into the ward and noticed that an unclothed infant was pale yellow except for a bright yellow (heavily jaundiced) triangle across the abdomen. A few days later, laboratory tests on a blood specimen left on a windowsill showed a lower bilirubin (the pigment responsible for jaundice) level than when previously tested. These two events led to the discovery that sunlight was an effective therapy against jaundice. Today, newborns with jaundice are placed near a brightly lit window or, in extreme cases, under intense lights to correct the condition. Often an intense blue light is used, since it has a higher luminosity than full-spectrum light.

Bright Light Therapy

"Bright light therapy involves the use of bright white light ranging in intensity from 2,000 lux to 5,000 lux," says Dr. Zimmerman. While the intensity of this light therapy isn't near that of sunlight (50,000 lux), it is significantly higher than the average workspace (50-500 lux). "Brighter lights in the workplace have been shown to reduce mistakes and drowsiness on the job, especially among night shift workers," adds Dr. Zimmerman. Bright light therapy is also used to treat SAD and other conditions.

Bulimia: Because of the involvement of serotonin (a neurotransmitter) in appetite regulation, bright light therapy has proven helpful in cases of bulimia (bingeing on large amounts of food, followed by self-induced purging). "During two weeks of bright light therapy, 17 women, 20-45 years old, experienced a 50% reduction in the number of binges and purges, as well as in their feelings of depression," says Raymond W. Lam, M.D.,

SUCCESS STORY: SAD NO MORE WITH LIGHT THERAPY

Twenty years ago, Sherrie Baxter left sunny Oklahoma, her native state, for Vancouver, Washington, in the Pacific Northwest. As the years went by, Sherrie became tired and depressed and found herself craving carbohydrates as soon as autumn, with its characteristic overcast skies and dark mornings, would arrive. She'd also stay up late and had trouble getting up in the morning. The depression and fatigue mysteriously lifted by April or May. "One of things I remember was during Christmas: I was walking through the stores and they were playing the holiday music, and I just started crying for no reason. I had no problems like that in spring or summer," she recalls.

In 1985, both Sherrie, 28, and her mother, who had the same symptoms, signed up as research subjects for a study on seasonal affective disorder (SAD) at Oregon Health Sciences University, in Portland. For three weeks, the two women lived in special quarters where the amount of light was strictly controlled. Technicians took regular blood samples day and night to monitor their levels of melatonin. The researchers were testing whether the lack of light in the morning allowed melatonin to be produced later in the day, causing the women's SAD symptoms.

The first week of the study, Sherrie and her mother were kept mostly in near-darkness except for one dim light bulb. The only break was at 2 p.m., when they were told to stay in front of 4-by-6-foot, 2,500-lux light boxes for about two hours. In the second week, the technicians began setting up the light boxes progressively earlier. The third week, the researchers woke the women at 6 a.m. to use the light boxes immediately upon awakening. By the fourth day of that regimen, Sherrie and her mother were no longer depressed and were full of energy. When they got the blood test results, they realized that the positive changes were occurring because the morning light had normalized their melatonin production cycle.

"I tend to be skeptical of things until I see proof," says Sherrie, now 43. "But we were able to see this was a physical thing happening and that was useful to me." After the study, Sherrie starting making light boxes herself and, several years later, started her own business to sell them.

ULTRAVIOLET LIGHT AND THE SUN

Ultraviolet light from the sun can be divided into three types of rays: UV-A, UV-B, and UV-C, depending upon the wavelength. Although there is some difference of opinion concerning the three types, generally UV-C is thought to be most harmful, but because very little of it penetrates the ozone layer, it is not considered dangerous. UV-A penetrates the skin (responsible for slow tanning), but because it has the longest wavelength, it is considered the least harmful.

According to most sources, it is UV-B that poses the greatest danger to humans. UV-B easily penetrates the skin, is responsible for sunburn, and can damage the eyes. Similarly, UV-B reflected from snow can burn the cornea, causing snow blindness. UV-B reflected from the sand and water is responsible for burning the skin more than the direct UV-B rays from the sun. Too much exposure of the eyes to UV-B can lead to cataracts, a clouding of the lens of the eye, so the eyes should always be protected in strong sunlight. Chronic exposure of the eyes to UV-B is also responsible for retinal damage, pterygium (abnormal growths on the cornea), and activation of ocular herpes.[21]

Assistant Professor of Psychiatry at the University of British Columbia, in Vancouver, Canada.

Delayed Sleep Phase Syndrome: Delayed sleep phase syndrome (falling asleep late, around 2:30–3:00 a.m.) may also be treated with bright light. "People who have delayed sleep phase syndrome have seen it disappear for the first time in their lives using light therapy," says Michael Terman, Ph.D., of the New York State Psychiatric Institute at Columbia Presbyterian Medical Center, in New York City. By getting a dose of bright light in the morning, the day starts earlier and patients fall asleep earlier at night. Bright light early at night works similarly for those who fall asleep early and wake early, allowing them to sleep later.

Irregular Menstrual Cycles: Two decades ago, researchers reported that a 100-watt bedside light could shorten and regulate the menstrual cycles among women with long and irregular cycles. "More recently, we repeated this experiment and achieved the same result," according to Daniel F. Kripke, M.D., Professor of Psychiatry at the University of California, San Diego. "This

needs more research, but it offers intriguing implications for treating infertility and improving contraception."

 See Sleep Disorders, Women's Health.

Ultraviolet Light Therapy

In the 1890s, Danish physician Niels Finsen observed that tubercular lesions occurred commonly during the winter but were very rare in the summer. He suspected a lack of sunlight to be the cause of the lesions and successfully treated skin tuberculosis with ultraviolet light. Known as the "father of photobiology," Dr. Finsen won the Nobel Prize in 1903 for his work. Today, ultraviolet light therapies are used to treat diseases ranging from high cholesterol to premenstrual syndrome to cancer.

UVA-1: According to Hugh McGrath, M.D., of Louisiana State University Medical Center, in Shreveport, UVA-1 therapy isolates part of the UV-A wavelength and is being used in patients with systemic lupus, a serious autoimmune disease known to damage the kidneys, skin, blood vessels, nervous system, and heart. Dr. McGrath points out that patients in one study "had decreased joint pain, headaches, rashes, sleeplessness, and need for medication with the chief benefit being a decline in fatigue."

Hemoirradiation: Also known as photophoresis, this therapy involves the removal of up to a pint of blood from the body, irradiating it with ultraviolet light, and reinjecting it. The absorbed light energy activates oxidation of the blood. (The process of hemooxidation therapy involves hemoirradiation of blood to which oxygen has been added.)

In his practice, William C. Douglass, M.D., of Clayton, Georgia, uses an instrument called the Photolume to irradiate blood with UV light. According to Dr. Douglass, UV light can have the following physiological effects: calcium metabolism improves, body toxins become inert, bacteria are killed either directly or indirectly (by increased systemic resistance), chemical balances are restored, and oxygen absorption is increased. He has successfully used ultraviolet light therapy to treat infections, cancer, rheumatoid arthritis, asthma, and symptoms of AIDS. His method has also been used to improve peripheral blood circulation in the treatment of blood poisoning.[22]

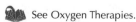 See Oxygen Therapies.

PUVA Light Therapy: In PUVA (psoralen UV-A) light therapy, patients are first given the light sensitive drug psoralen and then, one to two hours later, are exposed

COLORED LIGHT THERAPY

There is mounting evidence that different colors of light have different effects on the body. In 1942, the Russian scientist S.V. Krakov demonstrated that red light stimulates the sympathetic nervous system (which expends body energy and is associated with arousal and stress), while white and blue light stimulate the parasympathetic nervous system (which conserves body energy, slows heart rate, and increases intestinal and most gland activity). Earlier experiments revealed that certain colors stimulate hormone production, while other colors inhibit it.[23] Specific colors can also have an effect on specific diseases. In the early 20th century, it was noted that symptoms of acute eruptive diseases, such as smallpox and measles, were relieved when patients were put in a room with red windows. Melancholiacs also recovered after a few hours in such rooms.

C. Norman Shealy, M.D., Ph.D., of Springfield, Missouri, uses flashing bright lights and colored lights to treat pain and depression. According to Dr. Shealy, these treatments have been shown to alter neurochemical production in the brain and this may account for their positive effects. Dr. Shealy believes the brain has specific responses to different frequencies of flashing light and the frequencies of various colors. "Sleep problems can often be cured in one day by this method," he says, "but mood alteration usually takes 1-2 weeks of treatment." Dr. Shealy believes that it is the relaxation induced by these methods that is responsible for the effects seen in patients suffering from pain. "I believe tension is a primary factor in pain," he says, "and once you relax the tension, the pain eases."

Dr. Shealy has found that photo-stimulation with flashing opaque white or violet lights induces relaxation, reducing stress and chronic pain. "Photo-stimulation, or brain wave synchronization, has been used as a tool to assist relaxation and the induction of hypnosis since 1948," he says. "It has been used with the EEG (electroencephalogram) as an adjunct to the diagnosis of epilepsy."

Another method of colored light therapy known as monochromatic red light therapy is used to treat a range of problems, including pain, endocrine problems, dysmenorrhea, diabetes, gastrointestinal problems, depression, impotence, and frigidity. Gerald Hall, D.C., of El Paso, Texas, uses monochromatic red light therapy to treat the acupoints of the ear as well as points elsewhere on the body.

Ray Fisch, Ph.D., C.H., of Los Angeles, uses therapy involving monochromatic red light (a light-emitting diode or LED) for headaches, arthritis, allergies, sore throat, sinus problems, stress reduction, and wound healing. Preliminary studies have shown that LEDs are helpful for jaundice and ulcers.[24] The red light is applied to acupressure points or to sites of localized pain. For localized pain such as tendinitis, two 5-minute applications directly to the painful area are followed by 10-15 seconds to the surrounding area. This is followed by a gentle massage of the area. Treatment is repeated two to three times a day for a week, then twice a day for a week, followed by once a day for another week. "There are virtually no side effects to this treatment and it can be done at home," says Dr. Fisch.

to full-body UV light. This approach is used to treat vitiligo, a depigmentation problem, and works by stimulating pigment-producing cells to migrate to the skin surface.

Psoriasis, a chronic skin disease, also responds to PUVA light therapy. The ultraviolet light used in treatment helps stop the diseased cells from dividing and can often result in dramatic cures, according to Meyrick Peak, Ph.D., Senior Scientist at the Center of Mechanistic Biology and Biotechnology at Argonne National Laboratory, in Argonne, Illinois. "In study settings, 90% to 95% of [psoriasis] patients respond favorably," adds Warwick L. Morrison, M.D., Associate Professor of Dermatology at Johns Hopkins University, "with the treatment usually involving 30 PUVA sessions spanning ten weeks."

Photodynamic Therapy

"The very thing that can lead to skin cancer can also be used to cure it," says Dr. Peak. In photodynamic therapy (PDT), dyes or medications that absorb light are absorbed by tumors, then exposed to specific types of light. "Light photons are absorbed by the pigment of the dye, which becomes chemically reactive and causes the cancer cells to die," says Dr. Peak. "This therapy has been used in China for over 20 years and has been successful in eliminating some types of tumors." Photodynamic therapy is currently being tested for basal and squamous cell cancers (skin cancers), according to Nicholas J. Lowe, M.D., Clinical Professor of Dermatology at the School of Medicine, University of California, Los Angeles. "However, the concern with some of these treatments is unwanted phytotoxicity—some treatments are likely to make the patient sensitive to sunlight."

DOWNING TECHNIQUE OF COLORED LIGHT THERAPY

When light rays strike the retina of the eye, they are converted into nerve current, sometimes termed *photocurrent*. By measuring the amount of light-generated photocurrent traveling from the retina to the higher brain centers and then comparing them to symptoms of patients, John Downing, O.D., Ph.D., has found many people to have a decreased level of photocurrent transmission. This condition—photocurrent deficit—can cause diminished brain function and can lead to numerous symptoms:

- Learning disabilities
- Poor concentration and memory
- Mental fogginess
- Poor physical coordination and performance
- Sleeping problems
- Lack of self-esteem
- Mood swings
- Seasonal affective disorder (SAD) or depression
- Fear and anxiety
- Hyperactivity
- Fatigue
- Headaches
- Light sensitivity
- Poor peripheral vision and night blindness

Dr. Downing has found that stimulation by way of the eyes with the appropriate colored light can increase the ability of the neurovisual pathways to transmit photocurrent to the brain and thus significantly reduce or eliminate photocurrent deficiency. Dr. Downing developed this modern, comprehensive system of treatment by combining earlier research in the field of light therapy with his own discoveries from hundreds of clinical cases in his optometric vision therapy practice over the last 25 years.

In one case, a 35-year-old woman who was involved in an auto accident suffered pains in the face and head, was mentally sluggish and confused, and severely fatigued. Dr. Downing treated her with 40 sessions of indigo and violet light. The pains disappeared, the mental sluggishness and confusion cleared, and her energy returned to the point where she needed only five hours of sleep a night instead of ten, reports Dr. Downing.

Warren Grundfest, M.D., of Cedars-Sinai Medical Center, in Los Angeles, is using a type of photodynamic therapy called light-activated chemotherapy to treat patients with lung and bladder cancer. "What we're doing is using light to cause a chemical change in the drug," says Dr. Grundfest. "Because it is located only, or predominantly, in the cancer tissue, it causes only the cancer cells to die." Dr. Grundfest reports that after 18 months of treatment, bladder tumors showed an 85% successful response. PDT has been demonstrated effective as a cure for early-stage cancers of the lung, esophagus, stomach, and cervix,[25] resulting in complete remission in 90% of patients.[26]

Syntonic Optometry

Syntonic therapy applies colored light directly into the eyes to augment the control centers of the brain that regulate various body functions. In the 1930s, it was shown by Harry Riley Spitler, M.D., D.O.S., M.S., Ph.D., founder of the College of Syntonic Optometry, in Augusta, Maine, that focusing blue light into the eyes reduces inflammation and pain.

Solomon Slobins, O.D., Director of the College of Syntonic Optometry, uses an instrument called the Lumatron Light Stimulator® for visual evaluation, increasing the visual fields (peripheral vision), relieving headaches, and treating traumatic brain injuries. Developed by Dr. Downing, the Lumatron emits 11 pure wave bands of biologically active light, ranging through the spectrum from ruby to violet. This light is focused into the eyes where it travels to the brain and activates the autonomic nervous system to regulate disruptions in the system, thereby triggering the healing process. Patients sit in a darkened room in front of the Lumatron for approximately 25 minutes while it bathes their eyes with the appropriate colored light, emitted at a rate of two to 16 flashes per second. This exposure is normally found to be immediately soothing, with a lessening of symptoms within a few days.

Cold Laser Therapy

According to Marvin Prescott, D.M.D., of Los Angeles, cold laser therapy, sometimes referred to as soft or low-level laser therapy, utilizes a beam of low-intensity laser light to initiate a series of enzymatic reactions and bioelectric events that stimulate the natural healing process at the cellular level. "Cold laser therapy has been successfully applied to pain control, orthopedic myofascial syndrome (inflammation of the muscles and their surrounding membranes), neurology, trauma, dermatology, and dentistry," says Dr. Prescott, who adds that "the effects on microcirculation, increased synthesis of collagen in the skin, production of neurotransmitters, and pain relief have all been documented."

Cold laser therapy is often used in patients who do not like the needles used in traditional acupuncture. W. John Diamond, M.D., of Reno, Nevada, uses cold laser therapy to treat pain, particularly in children, who are often afraid of acupuncture. He finds it useful for back pain, bursitis, and tendinitis, and uses it in conjunction with homeopathy, herbs, and nutrients to treat chronic problems.

Dennis Tucker, Ph.D., L.Ac., of Nevada City, California, uses cold laser therapy to stimulate acupuncture points as an aid to healing wounds, to reduce inflammation, and to balance the energy flow in the acupuncture meridians. Dr. Tucker also finds cold laser therapy effective in treating infections under teeth. Cold laser therapy is applicable with little prior knowledge, either by a health provider or by self-application, with no demonstrable side effects when used properly. Pen-sized, low-level laser instruments are now available.

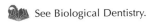 See Biological Dentistry.

The Future of Light Therapy

"Light is the medicine of the future," says Jacob Liberman, O.D., Ph.D., past President of the College of Syntonic Optometry, adding that those working in the field today are discovering new applications for improving one's physical health and psychological well-being. Additionally, many of the new light therapies can be used at home, providing a pain-free and inexpensive alternative to surgery and drugs.[27]

"I remember when people didn't know that smoking was dangerous and people didn't pay much attention to their diets," adds Dr. Eastman. "One of the next steps will be for people to realize that the amount of natural light they receive, as well as when they receive it, is another important component to health. People will watch when they get light just as they now watch their diets and the amount of exercise they get. In the future, it will become commonplace for people to take natural light exposure into account."

Where to Find Help

Though light therapy is a growing field, information may be difficult to find. Below are some organizations that can answer questions and provide you with further information.

College of Syntonic Optometry
15 Western Avenue
Augusta, Maine 04330
(717) 387-0900
Website: www.syntonicphototherapy.com

An organization of optometrists who incorporate optometric phototherapy into their treatments. The college will provide a reference to one of their members who practices in your area.

Dinshah Health Society
P.O. Box 707
Malaga, New Jersey 08328
(856) 692-4676

The Dinshah Health Society, in existence since 1975, advocates the value of color therapy. Through publishing books such as Let There Be Light, *they seek to help people treat themselves with color therapies. Not a referral service.*

Environmental Health & Light Research Institute
16057 Tampa Palms Blvd., Suite 227
Tampa, Florida 33647
(800) 544-4878

The Institute continues the work of light pioneer Dr. John Ott and can provide information on full-spectrum lighting.

Light Therapy Institute
1055 W. College Avenue #107
Santa Rosa, California 95401
(707) 525-4747

Provides colored light therapy using the Downing Technique, conducts training in light therapy, and offers referrals for practitioners.

Society for Light Treatment and Biological Rhythms, Inc.
P.O. Box 591687
174 Cook Street
San Francisco, California 94159
(415) 876-0716
Website: www.sltbr.org

For information on treatment of seasonal affective disorder.

Universal Light Technology
P.O. Box 520
Carbondale, Colorado 81623
(970) 927-0100
Website: www.ulight.com

A company associated with Jacob Liberman, O.D., Ph.D., that presents educational seminars on light therapy for the public and professional communities.

Sources of Full Spectrum Lighting and Light Boxes

Seventh Generation
One Mill Street, Box A-26
Burlington, Vermont 05401-1530
(800) 456-1191 or (802) 658-3773

Verilux, Inc.
9 Viaduct Road
Stamford, Connecticut 06907
(800) 786-6850 or (203) 921-2430
Website: www.ergolight.com

Ott-Lite Systems Inc.
28 Parker Way
Santa Barbara, California 93101
(800) 234-3724 or (805) 564-3467

Recommended Reading

Color Therapy: Healing with Color. Reuben Amber. Santa Fe, NM: Aurora Press, 1983.

Health & Light: The Effects of Natural and Artificial Light on Man and Other Living Things. John N. Ott, D.Sc. Columbus, OH: Ariel, 2000.

Let There Be Light. Darius Dinshah. Malaga, NJ: Dinshah Health Society, 2001.

Light: Medicine of the Future. Jacob Liberman. Santa Fe, NM: Bear & Co., 1992.

Light Years Ahead. Brian J. Breiling, Psy.D. Berkeley, CA: Celestial Arts, 1996.

LONGEVITY MEDICINE

Life expectancy has tripled over the course of human history. While topping the theoretical maximum life span of 120 years remains elusive, it is clear that given the remarkable breakthroughs in longevity medicine, the rate at which we age can be modified. It's entirely possible to live a longer life, with greatly reduced risk of developing age-related illnesses—if you know the primary age-accelerators and how they can be neutralized. Longevity medicine uses the latest findings in genetics as well as proven alternative therapies to detect and prevent age-related illness and extend life span.

AGING—the progressive deterioration with time that makes our bodies less responsive, less viable, and more vulnerable to disease—is part of the human condition. As a result, throughout history, human beings have often pondered: "Why is it that we age? Is it inevitable or is there something we can do to slow the process?" The field of longevity medicine is uncovering the reasons why people age. Factors most commonly cited include defective genes, chronic stress, lower levels of hormone production, increase in free radicals, an accumulation of bodily toxins, progressive clogging of the arteries and lymph vessels of the body, and a tired or overactive immune system.

Whatever the primary forces at play that cause a person to age, what's indisputable is this: as we get older, not only is our physical appearance altered, but other changes take place inside our skins which, like a clock winding down, gradually leave our cells, tissues, organs, and systems less vital with greatly diminished functional capacity. It is this loss of function that tips the scale of balance that normally exists between the processes of building up and tearing down, between youth and age. "Utilizing longevity medicine techniques may add years to your life," says W. Lee Cowden, M.D., of Fort Worth, Texas. "but, more importantly, it should add life to your years."

The Aging Process

In essence, aging is a general process of deterioration that produces a constellation of changes in the body. "Many

> *Utilizing longevity medicine techniques may add years to your life, but, more importantly, it should add life to your years.*
>
> —W. LEE COWDEN, M.D.

subtle and gross changes in the cardiovascular and respiratory systems lead to poor delivery of oxygen and nutrients to the tissues," says Elson Haas, M.D., Director of the Preventive Medical Center of Marin, in San Rafael, California. It is the diminishing levels of oxygen in the body along with nutrient deficiencies that lie behind most of the problems of aging. "Changes occur in the heart and circulation prior to the diminished nutrient supply," he says. "A reduction in heart pumping action with decreased lung capacity reduces oxygen delivery and increases carbon dioxide buildup." At the same time, aging individuals have blood vessels that get increasingly stiff, which leads to high blood pressure, poor circulation, and the risk of heart disease. Other organs also go into a tailspin, especially the lungs and kidneys, which seem to deteriorate faster than the others.

The immune system falters and "cell repair and elimination of defective cells may lessen, leading to an increased incidence of cancer," says Dr. Haas. The musculoskeletal system and the gastrointestinal, sexual, and endocrine organs also register deficits. Good colon function and elimination are important to prevent constipation and diverticular disease, says Dr. Haas, adding that these are two common problems with aging. Kidney function may also diminish with aging, inhibiting clearance of excess nutrients, chemicals, and toxins.

Muscle mass and strength is lost and, as a consequence, so is coordination. Spinal disks shrink, while cartilage and ligaments begin a process of degeneration and diminishing elasticity that leaves an individual less flexible. "With aging there is a loss of height and an increase

A HEALTHY LIFESTYLE EQUALS A LONGER LIFE

The *New England Journal of Medicine* featured a study conducted by James Fries, Ph.D., at Stanford University in California. The study of 1,741 University of Pennsylvania alumni found that middle-aged people who adopted a healthy lifestyle, who watched their weight, didn't smoke, and who exercised, lived longer than those who did not. Furthermore, they experienced fewer years of ill health and remained free of even minor disabilities for up to seven years longer than those who had unhealthy lifestyles. Individuals who had the worst lifestyles were 50% more likely to die by age 75 and twice as likely to be disabled.[1]

in bone fractures," says Dr. Haas. "Arthritis becomes more common with the years and leads to greater joint wear and tear."

As we age, the nervous system can also be affected. Nerve conductance diminishes, our brains decrease in volume, our reflexes slow, and there is a measurable decline in learning capacity and memory. "Senility may result from the diminishing nervous system function along with the effects of reduced brain circulation," says Dr. Haas. In addition, we become prone to age-related illnesses such as Alzheimer's and Parkinson's.

With age, the metabolic rate and thyroid hormone function may diminish, decreasing overall energy level. "Weakened sugar tolerance can lead to diabetes," says Dr. Haas. "Body fat percentages usually increase with age, even with the same dietary intake." Men may find that their sex drive has been dampened because levels of sex hormones have declined. Women may suffer from osteoporosis due to lack of progesterone and estrogen. Both sexes may develop arthritis, cancer, heart disease, or stroke.

Is this grim litany of deterioration inevitable? Many have bought into the belief that frailty and senility are the consequences of aging, over which we have little control. Yet, mounting scientific evidence suggests this is false. The Baltimore Longitudinal Study on Aging (BLSA), begun in 1958, is the oldest and most famous investigation into the process of aging. Since that time, over 600 patient evaluations have been conducted on 1,200 men and women, ranging in age from their 20s to 90s, to assess the metabolic, hormonal, immune system, and mental changes that occur with age. The BLSA has shown that healthy older individuals can have cardiovascular systems and memories as functional as those of

much younger people. Four decades of BLSA research has led to three general conclusions:

1. Disease is not an inevitable by-product of the natural aging process.
2. The human aging process varies greatly from one individual to another. And even in the same person, different organs and bodily systems can age at varying rates.
3. Genetic, lifestyle, and disease processes together affect the rate at which a person ages.

What is Longevity Medicine?

During the period from 1900 to 1990, average life expectancy increased in the U.S. from 47 years to 76 years, a gain attributed largely to improved sanitation and the use of antibiotics. There are currently about two dozen people around the world who are more than 110 years old. Meanwhile, a more recent focus on disease prevention and healthier lifestyles has produced reduced rates of heart disease and other illnesses. Longevity medicine, with its focus on "upstream" diagnosing of imbalances before the onset of age-related diseases, plus tailored methods of enhancing the function of the cardiovascular, immune, detoxification, and endocrine systems, can increase average life expectancy further still.

A recent study in *Science* looked at the average maximum age in Sweden, based on data compiled over the last 140 years. Researchers found that prior to 1970, maximum age increased by 0.44 years per decade; since 1970, it has been increasing by 1.11 years per decade. The increased rate is due to declining death rates from heart disease and cancer, among other factors. Researcher John R. Wilmoth, Ph.D., Associate Professor in the Department of Demography at the University of California, at Berkeley, expects this trend to continue. "Based on available demographic evidence, the human life span shows no sign of approaching a fixed limit imposed by biology or other factors."[2]

Longevity medicine is concerned with: (1) slowing the rate at which an individual ages and thereby extending life expectancy, the number of years a person can expect to live; (2) increasing an individual's "health span," the length of time they are free of age-related diseases such as heart disease, cancer, and diabetes; (3) improving the quality of life through greater vitality, mental acuity, and an overall zest for life.

"Whether a person lives a long life or not, if they are symptom-free and able to live as healthy in their fifties and sixties as they were in their twenties and thirties, that's significant," says Paul Yanick, Jr., Ph.D., a holistic health scientist from Woodbridge, New Jersey. "Claims that people can live to 120, 140, or 150 give the whole field a bad reputation. To gain credibility as a new field, we have to be cautious about what we say in terms of extending life." Dr. Yanick instead talks about "optimal aging" and "optimal health span," rather than "anti-aging." The word *anti-aging* is a misnomer, he says, since nobody can stop the aging process, just slow it down a bit.

Whether a person lives a long life or not, if they are symptom-free and able to live as healthy in their fifties and sixties as they were in their twenties and thirties, that's significant.

—Paul Yanick, Jr., Ph.D.

The roots of longevity medicine—a recognized subspecialty of conventional medicine—trace back to the 1950s when Denham Harman of the University of Nebraska first announced his "free-radical theory of aging," but the formal investigation of the aging process began in 1958 with the inauguration of the Baltimore Longitudinal Study on Aging by Nathan W. Shock, M.D. The BLSA helped establish the field of "biogerontology" and is the oldest and most famous investigation into the changes that accompany the aging process. It was during this same period that Bernard Strehler, Ph.D., of the University of California, helped launch the National Institute on Aging (NIA). Meanwhile, a scientific landmark occurred when Leonard Hayflick, Ph.D., found that human cells possessed a barrier equivalent to the four-minute mile, which for so long daunted runners. Dr. Hayflick found that cells in the human body—with the exception of renegade cancer cells—could multiply up to, but no more than, 100 times. He theorized that this finding was behind the inability of the body to regenerate itself and placed a ceiling on how long a person could live.

Unlike conventional medicine, which focuses on treating disease by way of costly surgery and drugs, longevity medicine is built upon methods of diagnosis and treatment that meet the unique needs and objectives of each person and are inexpensive, noninvasive, and have a low risk of adverse side effects. While longevity medicine has solid roots in preventative medicine (which

focuses on reducing risk factors associated with illness) and environmental medicine (which focuses on reducing toxic exposures and detoxification protocols), it encompasses yet stretches beyond both.

Longevity practitioners are especially interested in distinguishing those factors that play a direct role in causing accelerated aging from those that are merely consequences of aging. Hormones, for example, play a very important role in the aging process, since they affect nearly every aspect of physiological functioning. Body functions influenced by the endocrine system include: fluid volumes inside and outside the cell, the body's pH balance, immune system function, the ability to withstand stress, digestion and nutrient assimilation, and much more. Yet, concluding that aging is simply the consequence of depleted hormone levels is misleading. Decrease of hormones is a consequence of aging but—once decreased—becomes a cause in accelerated aging. There may be an even more fundamental process occurring that causes not only hormone levels to decline, but also other organs and systems of the body to degenerate over time. To achieve optimal results, you need to identify and address root causes, rather than treat symptoms.

Longevity medicine is distinct from conventional medicine, because its approach is based on the following elements:

- Recognizes the deep web of relationship of all parts and levels of the human constitution—immune system to brain to endocrine system to detoxification systems to circulatory system—and how activities on the subtle energetic level cascade down to the physical level, affecting organs and cells.

- Understands biochemical individuality. By virtue of our individual genetics and lifestyle, each of us has different nutritional requirements. Though a central aging theme is emerging at the molecular level common to everyone, accelerated aging involves a different set of factors impacting people in a variety of ways. For this reason, no single longevity method or strategy will work for all people at all times.

- Identifies and seeks to optimize key cellular, organ, and system processes that are known to play an important role in how a person ages. By measuring the capacity of the body's organs and systems, functional status can be determined. This helps guide and fine-tune whatever modalities of treatment are employed, such as nutrients, detoxification strategies, hormone enhancement, and others, so that total body function may be significantly enhanced.[3]

- Makes use of alternative methods of diagnosis and treatment, such as electrodermal screening and homeopathy, that work at the level of the human energy field. Balance and optimal configuration of this field is commensurate with good health and long life.

- Recognizes and actively works in partnership with the inherent intelligence of the body and spirit, which is always working towards health and well-being.

- Focuses upon results and makes use of sensitive, early indicators to provide feedback.

- Includes both a "hard" technology-based side and a "soft" psychospiritually based side. High-tech approaches include special diagnostics, laboratory testing, and nutraceuticals. The "high-touch" psychospiritual aspects involve identifying and eliminating limiting beliefs, reframing negative perceptions, and clearing core emotional issues.

Looking at the Causes of Aging

Compared to their counterparts in the U.S. who live an average of 76 years, residents of Okinawa live an exceptionally long life, typically past 100 years, with a low incidence of chronic and disabling disease. Hoping to find the secret to their longevity, researchers have pointed to their low-fat diet of rice and fish, the simple, stress-free environment that comes with living in an agricultural town, the sense of community and belonging the people have, and the fact that the elderly remain active and engaged, working in the fields even into their nineties.

But what precisely is responsible for their long lives? Is it diet, environment, lifestyle? Or is it simply the good fortune of good genes? According to molecular biologist Ward Dean, M.D., Medical Director of the Center for BioGerontology, in Pensacola, Florida, every human has a potential maximum life span of 120 years. In fact all forms of life have a species-specific life span: a dog's maximum life span is 20 years, a bristlecone pine is 5,000 years, and a tortoise is 150 years. Life expectancy, however, is another matter altogether. It is the additional number of years a person can expect to live at any given age. The "wear-and-tear" on the body caused by environmental factors, toxic exposure, lifestyle choices, diet, stress, and lack of exercise is closely associated with the onset of life-shortening diseases and the obvious discrepancy between actual life span and potential maximum life span.

How Genes Influence Life Span

It is known that activities at the genetic and biochemical level induce changes in cell functioning, changes that ultimately tip the scale from repair and health to degeneration and disease. Aging proceeds according to a genetically determined, biological timetable. Current scientific research seeks to determine what is happening biochemically in the cells to cause degeneration and to find specific genes that govern this process.

Various theories have been developed to explain how genes might place a limit on life span. The telomere theory suggests that the answer can be found in a cell's genetic material (chromosomes), which function as an aging clock. At the ends of each cell's chromosomes are telomeres, spirals of DNA that protect the cell when it divides. Telomeres get shorter and shorter each time a cell divides. After a certain number of divisions have taken place, the telomeres get so short that no more divisions can occur and the cell degenerates dramatically and dies. When large numbers of cells undergo this fate, the specific organ suffers, leading to the eventual deterioration and death of the organism. The more cellular divisions possible, the longer the life span, since the differentiated cells in our body (which number 10 million million) are genetically "hard-wired" to replicate only a certain number of times.[4]

A single gene that affects the production of an enzyme known as helicase has been identified as a possible factor in aging. Helicase plays a role in the metabolism and repair of DNA, making it an important player in the body's ability to repair itself from ongoing damage.[5] An animal's ability to repair certain types of DNA damage is directly related to the life span of its species. Humans repair DNA, for example, more quickly and efficiently than mice or other animals with shorter life spans. This suggests that DNA damage and repair are part of the aging puzzle.

In addition, researchers have found defects in DNA repair in people with a familial susceptibility to cancer. If DNA repair processes decline with age while damage accumulates, as scientists hypothesize, it could help explain why cancer is so much more common among older people. Even within a single organism, repair rates can vary among cells, with the most efficient repair going on in sperm and egg cells. Moreover, certain genes are repaired more quickly than others, including those that regulate cell growth.[6]

Researchers also theorize that the body may possess certain "suicide genes" that, when activated at a specific time, cause cells and tissues to waste away. It is theorized that a master gene may cause cells to overwork and then self-destruct. The master gene forces the others to produce abnormal amounts of protein, which slows down replication and other vital cellular activities. These factors eventually cause organ degeneration and aging. The process becomes apparent in a comparison of old and young skin cells—although both types contain the same array of genes, in older cells the genes work overtime under the direction of a master gene.

Despite the identification of single genes that influence biological activity, many researchers feel that a group of genes, rather than a single aberrant gene, contribute to the aging process. However, no one knows for sure exactly how many. Out of the body's total number of genes, those which influence the aging process may be as few as 100. The completion of the Human Genome Project, which mapped every gene in the human body, should accelerate the process of identifying the genetic causes of aging.

While identifying the genes responsible for aging is a daunting task, so is the other half of the equation—knowing how to turn on certain genes and other genes off. "Theoretically, it's a solvable problem," says Dr. Dean. "Genes are like a computer switch—it's either on or off. The idea is to identify the genes that are associated with the aging process and figure out a way to flip that switch." While theoretically straightforward, the practical implications are not and, at the present time, the answers may be years in the future.

WHAT GENES CAN TEACH US ABOUT LIVING LONGER

Overwhelming scientific evidence suggests that the weak parts in our genetic armor can be compensated for through interventions involving diet, exercise, lifestyle modification, and stress management. Genetics and constitutional factors will make some people more disposed to problems in the cardiovascular system, skin, or memory. Yet, lifestyle factors can be controlled to varying degrees to compensate for genetic weak links.

"Research shows that genetics accounts for only a third of physical and half of mental aging," according to John Rowe, M.D., President of Mount Sinai Hospital in New York, who headed the MacArthur Foundation Research Network on Successful Aging. "The other two-thirds [of aging] relate to lifestyle, our engagement with life, what we eat, the way we manage stress, our social connections, and sense of personal power. It's not all in our genes."

Genes influence health patterns when a person is young. After the age of 50, genetic expression, and thus life expectancy, is more influenced by lifestyle, environment, and nutritional factors. When a person is in their 70s and 80s, there is not much genetic influence left, since a lifetime of environmental influences and personal choices have placed them upon a certain trajectory.[7]

We have far more control over the aging process than we previously thought. We know that certain genes are associated with a greater risk for lung cancer. Yet, as smoking rates have fallen, so too has the incidence of this life-shortening disease. Heart disease incidence in the U.S. has dropped by 45% since the 1950s. This wasn't primarily accomplished through high-tech medicine (heart bypass surgery or drugs), but through improved lifestyles, lower smoking rates among men, and improved diets—all factors that modified biochemical processes governed by our genes. "The genes did not undergo change throughout this period, but their expression was modified as a consequence of environmental factors, resulting in an increase of disease-free years in older age," says biochemist and author Jeffrey Bland, Ph.D., of Gig Harbor, Washington.[8]

Biochemistry of Aging

The characteristics we refer to as aging happen when the body's ability to maintain health declines. The body becomes less able to bring itself back into a state of balance when it is overwhelmed by stressors (physical, chemical, structural, emotional). Not only is there a loss of function as we age, but a loss in organ reserve, a kind of healing "savings account" to draw upon in times of need. These reserves are vital to good health, since they are called upon whenever we experience infection, radiation, physical injury, toxic exposure, or psychological stress, allowing us to bounce back from illness.

A number of factors, including nutritional deficiencies, excessive production of stress hormones such as cortisol, imbalances of life-enhancing hormones, toxins, dental poisons, and immune dysfunction, accelerate the aging process at the cellular level. As we age, these stressors combine to produce changes in a cell's membrane, DNA, and other structural components. The most basic elements of cellular function become less efficient and this eventually culminates in disease as the body deteriorates.[9] Together, these age-accelerators influence activities important to the viability of a cell: the amount of nourishment a cell receives, the cell's ability to rid itself of wastes, the degree of DNA mutation, and the ability of the cell to repair damage.[10]

FREE RADICALS AND ACCELERATED AGING

While it remains unclear if it's the most fundamental process involved in aging, excessive free-radical production is increasingly being regarded as a hallmark of aging. A free radical is an unstable, toxic molecule of oxygen with an unpaired electron that steals an electron from another molecule and produces harmful effects. Free radicals damage cells, which causes the body's organs and systems to lose functional capacity. Free-radical damage also impairs protein synthesis, which is vital to tissue regeneration and repair. Although the body naturally produces certain free radical–neutralizing enzymes, such as superoxide dismutase (SOD) and glutathione peroxidase, it may be unable to prevent all free-radical damage and this gradually causes organs to degenerate.

By lowering oxygen levels and creating acidic conditions in the body, free radicals produce a self-perpetuating cycle, since high acidity increases free-radical production. Perhaps 80% of chronically ill U.S. adults have too much acid in their tissues and about 20% are severely acidic. People with acidosis are more prone to develop chronic, degenerative diseases, such as heart disease, stroke, and arthritis. Excessive free-radical production has also been associated with loss of collagen in the body. Collagen is an essential component of the body's skin and musculoskeletal system; its loss results in tissues that are old and withered.[11]

Free radicals damage the cell's membrane, interfering with its ability to send and receive messages from other cells and to absorb necessary nutrients while eliminating waste products. Free radicals also damage a cell's nucleic acid, DNA, and mitochondria. Mitochondria are the cell's power plant, furnishing the energy needed by cells and tissues to properly function.[12] Deficits of energy cause greater fatigue and pain, and cause organs to function at a reduced capacity.

Free-radical damage is most pronounced in oxygen-rich organs (eyes, brain, liver, heart, lungs, kidneys, and blood) and has been implicated in the following diseases: kidney disease, diabetes, pancreatitis, liver damage, inflammation of the gastrointestinal tract, lung diseases, eye diseases (macular degeneration, cataracts), nervous system disorders (Parkinson's, Alzheimer's, multiple sclerosis), diseases affecting red blood cells (sickle cell anemia, pernicious anemia), iron overload, autoimmune diseases (rheumatoid arthritis, lupus), and most infections (tuberculosis, malaria, AIDS).

AGES AGE US

Another biochemical process that has been found to accelerate aging occurs when excess circulating glucose (sugar) molecules attach themselves to proteins in the blood. This process is known as protein glycation and results in the production of glue-like substances called "advanced glycosylation endproducts" or AGEs. AGEs accumulate in the blood and stick to organs and tissues while accelerating free-radical production. As a result, these organs and tissues stiffen, like leather that is cured. In the skin, AGEs cause wrinkling; in the brain, AGEs play a role in the development of Alzheimer's and other forms of mental impairment.

Diabetes has been regarded as a model of accelerated aging since glycosylation leaves diabetics—who typically have high glucose levels—more vulnerable to certain disorders, such as neurological degeneration, kidney problems, and heart disease, which typically occur in most non-diabetics much later in life. Furthermore, AGEs play a role in heart disease, by directly binding to LDL cholesterol and by stimulating the production of free radicals, which oxidize LDL cholesterol in the bloodstream. This initiates the formation of artery-clogging plaque deposits, leading to hardening of arteries and contributing to high blood pressure.[13] In general, AGEs and free-radical production cause tissue damage, reduce organ capacity, and accelerate biological aging. AGEs have been found to play a role in kidney and pancreatic dysfunction, gastrointestinal inflammation, diabetes, arthritis, and cancer.[14]

HORMONES AND AGING

Hormones are important modulators of cellular activity. Insulin, a hormone manufactured by the pancreas, has profound effects on aging. Some foods that are digested enter the bloodstream as the simple sugar glucose, which the body uses as an energy source. Under the direction of insulin, glucose is able to pass from the bloodstream, through the cell membrane, and into the cell, where it is burned as fuel.

Poor regulation of glucose in the bloodstream can result from insufficient insulin secretion by the pancreas or through the cells' inability to properly utilize insulin, which causes high levels of glucose to remain in the blood. The body then triggers the pancreas to produce more insulin.[15] "Elevated insulin sets off a cascade of disturbances at the cellular level and increases the rate of biological aging," says Dr. Bland. Insulin is a hormone with global actions and can cause high blood pressure, blood fat abnormalities, abnormal immune system function, and accelerated biological aging.

In women, says Dr. Bland, high insulin levels cause the body to shift hormone production away from estrogen—which has a protective effect against osteoporosis, heart disease, and Alzheimer's—and toward production of the male hormone testosterone. Low estrogen and high insulin also alters body composition and shape, causing unhealthy weight gain and increased deposits of abdominal fat. Obesity is a risk factor for high blood pressure, heart disease, and hormone imbalances.

 See Alzheimer's Disease and Senile Dementia, Arthritis, Diabetes, Heart Disease, Obesity and Weight Loss, Osteoporosis.

Underlying Factors That Accelerate Aging

Longevity practitioners strive to address root causes and not merely treat the many degenerative symptoms of aging. It is becoming increasingly clear that to arrive at an adequate understanding of the aging process, we must acknowledge the intricate web of relations that exists within the body. Hormone production, nutrition, stress, toxic load, immune system competence, and brain function influence one another and modify genetic and cellular activities associated with life expectancy.

IMPROPER INTAKE AND ASSIMILATION OF NUTRIENTS

Nutrients, such as vitamins, enzymes, minerals, essential fatty acids, and amino acids, provide the raw materials for optimal cell, tissue, and system function. While Americans are overfed, we're undernourished—and it's killing us. Scientific research has disclosed the many links between what we eat—or don't eat—and how we age. These studies are lending increasing credibility to the important role that nutrition can play in warding off the so-called diseases of aging, such as heart disease, cancer, and diabetes.

Many of us eat too much of the wrong kinds of foods, such as those that cause allergies or processed foods high in sugar and "bad" fats. At the same time, only 9% of Americans obtain the minimum amounts of vitamins and minerals from their regular diet. And there are many reasons to believe that the Recommended Dietary Allowances (RDAs) are arbitrary, set too low in many cases, and do not begin to address unique nutritional needs due to genetics, age, lifestyle, stress levels, and other factors.

What we eat plays a central role in determining our risk of developing diabetes and insulin resistance, impairing the energy-producing capacity of the cell. As we have seen at the biochemical level, insulin resistance, which is characterized by high levels of both insulin and glucose in the blood, leads to increased production of damaging free radicals and AGEs, and to the oxidation of fats in the blood (a contributing factor for heart disease), alterations in a cell's membranes, and hormonal disturbances. High insulin levels lead to diabetes, stroke, and heart disease, and hasten the aging process itself.

Diet affects the acid-alkaline balance of the cells, which plays a role in our level of health and well-being. Hazel Parcells, N.D., who was 105 years old when she died, observed that all decay and disease occurs in highly acidic states. The body of a person who is chronically tired and sleepy is usually acidic, she says, and will age quickly. But when the cells in a body are more alkaline, the person ages less quickly and has more pep and drive.

An individual can alter this chemical balance to favor a more balanced pH by changing how and what they eat (in accordance with their metabolic type).

THE EFFECTS OF STRESS

The field of psychoneuroimmunology (PNI) has provided us with startling insights into how our central nervous system and brain, immune system, and endocrine systems are all linked by way of nerves and chemical messengers called neurotransmitters. As a result of this mind-body connection, there is an interplay between what we think and feel (consciously and subconsciously) and the condition of our bodies.

In our response to stress, free-radical production is increased dramatically; at the same time, our adrenal glands secrete cortisol, adrenaline, and other hormones. This flood of stress hormones has a cascading adverse effect on other hormones related to longevity, such as DHEA, growth hormone, and insulin. This affects the body's ability to repair cells, tissues, and organs. It is in this way that negative mental and emotional states dampen immune system function and deplete organ reserve, predisposing us toward age-related illnesses.

 See Detoxification Therapy, Diet, Stress

TOXIC OVERLOAD

We live in a toxic age, in which high concentrations of toxins from the food we eat, the air we breathe, and the water we drink cause our bodies to accumulate toxins faster than they can be eliminated. "Aging is a slow poisoning, a lifetime accumulation of toxins in the body," suggests Marika von Viczay, N.D., Ph.D., of Asheville, North Carolina. These toxins have lowered our resistance to disease and altered our body's metabolism, causing enzyme dysfunction, nutritional deficiencies, and hormonal imbalances. Toxins can accumulate within a cell, rendering it less able to function properly. Dr. Haas notes that when waste accumulates within a cell, that cell becomes starved for oxygen and other nutrients. This impairs the ability of the cell to heal itself and resume normal function.

In addition, optimal health and longevity is not possible if the gastrointestinal tract is disrupted and an individual is unable to properly digest food, absorb needed nutrients, and excrete waste material and toxins from the body. When unprocessed proteins, bacteria, and microorganisms found in the bowel begin to leak into the bloodstream as a consequence of abnormal intestinal permeability, the result is "leaky gut syndrome." Leaky gut syndrome can lead to a host of problems as toxins overburden the immune system, liver, and kidneys. Cancer and a variety of autoimmune diseases may result.

There is increasing evidence that problems that arise in the mouth can have far-reaching effects throughout the body. Mercury and other toxic heavy metals from dental fillings can leach into the bloodstream and accumulate in tissues and organs, leading to degenerative illnesses. Old dental extraction sites and root canal teeth can become "toxic waste dumps" as resident bacteria migrate to other areas of the body, including the heart (a risk factor for heart disease).

IMPAIRED IMMUNE SYSTEM

The immune system plays a central role in protecting us against infections and diseases caused by ever-present viruses, fungi, and bacteria. The immune system is also responsible for ongoing maintenance and repair work needed to assure the viability of the body's tissues. As a result of environmental insults, chronic stress, improper diet, food allergies, toxins, and other factors, the immune system can be thrown off balance, becoming either overactive or underactive. A dysfunctional immune system can leave us vulnerable to illnesses such as allergies, lupus, multiple sclerosis, and rheumatoid arthritis. Cancer results when the immune system malfunctions and no longer recognizes and destroys cancer cells.

IMBALANCED HORMONES

As people age, the body's glands—gonads, adrenal, thymus, thyroid, pituitary, and pineal—may begin to shrink in size. As they do, hormone production often declines in all these glands. (Some hormone production may increase in an attempt to stimulate failing glands.) This affects the activity of a multitude of processes throughout the body. The pineal gland, for example, produces melatonin, a free radical-fighting antioxidant that affects sleep, body rhythms, and emotional well-being. Melatonin levels decline with age. So does DHEA, produced by the adrenal glands. At age 70, an individual produces just 10% of the DHEA produced at age 25. Reduced levels of DHEA have been linked to heart disease, lupus, skin cancer, and diabetes. Women are well aware of the effects of shifting hormone levels as they age, particularly the symptoms of menopause. But hormone imbalances can also contribute to a number of other health problems, including weight gain, yeast infections, fibroids, and breast cancer. And in males, lower levels of testosterone lead to diminished sex drive, impotence, and loss of bone tissue and muscle mass.

CLOGGED ARTERIES AND LYMPH VESSELS

Arteries and lymph vessels often clog as we age, mostly as a result of some of the other causes of aging—nutritional deficiencies, excess free radicals, eating toxic foods, excess stress, and imbalanced hormones. But once the vessels clog, they become a cause for further accelerating the aging process and producing age-related diseases such as heart attacks, strokes, and some cancers. As arteries clog, blood flow is reduced and nutrient and oxygen supply to the body's tissues is impaired, resulting in greater free-radical formation and less effective tissue repair.

BRAIN SLUGGISHNESS

As a person ages, some brain cells die while others become damaged. Loss of brain weight, reduced reflexes, and a decrease in memory and learning capacity may result. Impaired mental function can be caused by many factors, including reduced blood flow to the brain, food allergy reactions, toxin accumulation, and insufficient nutrients. According to Dr. Haas, changes in brain function and the regulation of balance in the hormonal and nervous systems may be at the core of the aging process.

Dopamine and serotonin are two primary brain messengers (neurotransmitters) that play a central role in many bodily functions. Due to genetic flaws, improper diet, toxins from the environment, microorganisms, stress, and other factors, the levels of serotonin and dopamine may be sub-optimal or out of proportion with each other. This can exert profound effects on other bodily systems, since these chemicals control the region of the brain known as the hypothalamus and thus influence appetite, emotions, the endocrine system, and much more.

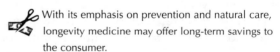 With its emphasis on prevention and natural care, longevity medicine may offer long-term savings to the consumer.

Benefits of Longevity Medicine

The goal of longevity medicine is to modify these aging factors, increasing life span as well as overall health in old age. It brings together a number of modalities for the early diagnosis and treatment of age-related conditions, incorporating techniques from allopathic disciplines, naturopathic medicine, traditional Chinese medicine, nutrition, exercise, and breakthroughs in biotechnology. With its emphasis on early detection of illness, preventative strategies, and lifestyle changes to enhance health, longevity medicine shares many of the same goals as alternative medicine in general. Longevity can be enhanced through improving the diet, reducing stress, detoxifying the body, boosting the immune system, correcting hormone imbalances, improving cardiovascular function, and rebuilding brainpower.

Improving the Diet

Eating a healthy diet is essential to any longevity program. Patricia Huijbregts, Ph.D., of the National Institute of Public Health and the Environment, in Bilthoven, the Netherlands, conducted a 20-year study of 3,045 middle-aged and elderly men in Finland, the Netherlands, and Italy. When the study began, they estimated the dietary intake of their subjects over a 6-12 month period. Each man was given one point for meeting each of the following dietary guidelines: less than 10% of their caloric intake was from saturated fat; 3%-7% was from polyunsaturated fat; 10%-15% was from complex carbohydrates, such as potatoes, beans, and rice. The researchers also made note of whether the subjects ate 400 g of fruits and vegetables, 27-40 g of fiber, more than 30 g of nuts and seeds, and less than 300 mg of cholesterol per day. After accounting for age and lifestyle habits such as smoking and drinking, those men who stuck with the longevity diet lived 13% longer. Researchers found that it was the food groups eaten, not specific foods, that were most important. "The dietary pattern as a whole is more important than specific dietary components with respect to survival among older people," concluded Dr. Huijbregts.[16]

A whole-foods diet is generously filled with a wide variety of different colored vegetables, fruits, and grains (variations in color are due to various minerals, vitamins, and other nutrients important to health); raw seeds and nuts and their butters; beans; fermented milk products such as yogurt and kefir; and fish, poultry, and bean products like tofu. It should also be lower in animal meats, fats, and cheeses as opposed to low-fat milk products. Eating a rich assortment of fruits and vegetables promotes health and longevity especially when these foods are used in the diet in place of simple carbohydrates found in sugar and processed foods. Eating vegetables and fruits also increases the consumption of fiber and other beneficial nutrients, particularly the numerous free-radical fighting antioxidants and other cell-protective phytochemicals (*phyto* means plant).

A whole-foods diet that is predominantly vegetable-based is typically much lower in fat, which reduces the risk of heart disease, cancer, and diabetes, while enhancing immune system function. Men who lower their fat intake to less than 30% of total daily calories have a significant increase in natural killer cell activity, a measure of immune system function.[17] Research also points to the benefits of moving in the direction of a vegetarian-based diet. The British Medical Association reported the findings of a 12-year research program involving 5,000 meat-eaters and 6,100 vegetarians—vegetarians had a 28% lower risk of dying from heart disease and a 39% reduced chance of dying from cancer.[18] The American

EVALUATING BIOLOGICAL AGE

To develop an effective and personalized longevity program, it is important to gather data on health status. Laboratory testing is a part of medicine familiar to us all. Most of us have had fingers pricked for blood samples or been asked to provide a urine sample for analysis. These traditional tests are often useful but, from the vantage of longevity medicine, they are limited in scope. They may be able to provide basic information on cholesterol levels or determine if white blood cell count is abnormally high or they may indicate whether an organ is seriously diseased. They are of limited value since organs and glands have a reserve capacity that masks dysfunction. In other words, abnormal function begins long before conventional medicine reveals the problem. Most traditional tests are not sensitive enough to signal impending problems. So, while routine laboratory tests are useful for the diagnosis of certain illnesses, most are of little value in evaluating biological age and the establishment of benchmarks to gauge the effectiveness of a longevity program.

Longevity-related tests make it possible to assess the health status of your immune, endocrine, and cardiovascular systems, so that imbalances are detected earlier, before a disease fully manifests. "Health status is not to be determined on the basis of any single longevity test," says Jeffrey Bland, Ph.D. Rather, longevity potential and health is better determined through the evaluation of patterns of test results. These "provide a window into the complexity of a person's physiological functioning," according to Dr. Bland.

There are different types of tests to help you develop a personalized longevity program. Electrodermal screening and darkfield blood analysis can help provide a picture of overall health status. Digestive function can be assessed using a stool or urine analysis (these tests are also valuable for getting information on general health). Specific tests are available to assess how well individual body systems are working, including the immune system (T and B Cell Panel, Sedimentation Rate), the endocrine glands (TRH Stimulation Test), and the brain (Brain Electrical Activity Map). Other tests look for possible nutritional deficiencies (Pantox Antioxidant Profile, Functional Intracellular Analysis, Nutricheck USA, Cell Membrane Lipid Profile) or excesses of toxins (hair analysis, ToxMet Screen, DMSA Challenge Test, Functional Liver Detoxification Profile) and stress (Aeron LifeCycles Saliva Assay Report, Adrenal Stress Index) in the body, which can accelerate aging.

NUTRIENTS AND HERBS FOR BRAINPOWER AND LONGEVITY

To Reduce Free-Radical Damage—The following antioxidant nutrients are helpful: vitamins A, C, and E; beta carotene and other carotenoids; bioflavonoids such as pycnogenol, cysteine, NADH (coenzyme of vitamin B3), alpha-lipoic acid, and selenium; zinc, copper, and manganese, important in the formation of superoxide dismutase (SOD); and the enzymes catalase, and glutathione peroxidase. Coenzyme Q10 is a potent antioxidant nutrient found in every cell of the body. It assists the cells with energy production and is beneficial for treating cardiovascular disease. Coenzyme Q10 has no side effects if used properly.[20]

To Improve Brainpower—Phosphatidyl-choline, found in lecithin, is the precursor to acetylcholine, an important brain chemical involved in memory and thought. DMAE (dimethylamino-ethanol) has been shown to increase memory.[21] Phosphatidyl-serine supports and revitalizes nerve cells and has been shown to slow cognitive losses attributed to aging. Vinpocetine (periwinkle extract) enhances memory and concentration.

The amino acids (building-blocks of protein) responsible for nervous system functions include arginine, glutamine, methionine, phenylalanine, and tryptophan. It is recommended, unless under the supervision of a qualified nutritionist or doctor, that people take free-form, formulas containing balanced ratios of amino acids.[22]

Ginkgo biloba helps to improve the circulation to the brain. Standardized extracts of ginkgo have been shown to greatly improve the supply of blood and oxygen to the brain and increase brain function in cases of cerebral dysfunction (dementia related to depression or insufficient blood supply).[23]

Panax ginseng is a potent adaptogenic herb that has the ability to improve mental function and stamina as well as physical endurance. Siberian ginseng is most often recommended to improve mental function.[24]

Proanthocyanidin, a bioflavonoid extract derived from grape seeds or pine bark, provides antioxidant protection to the brain and central nervous system. It strengthens blood vessel walls and improves circulation. Increased blood flow helps prevent ischemia in brain tissue and reduce mental deterioration.[25]

To Reduce the Effects of Aging—Deficiency of the B vitamins can result in numerous conditions related to the brain and nervous system, including memory loss or impairment, disorientation or confusion, irritability or mood swings, fatigue, or depression.[26]

It is estimated that at least 30% of elderly Americans who have been institutionalized are deficient in niacin (vitamin B3).[27] Niacin helps support the healthy functioning of the nervous system, lowers cholesterol levels, and improves circulation throughout the body.[28] Numerous studies have found insufficient levels of vitamin B6 (pyridoxine) in many elderly Americans. Pyridoxine supports the digestive, immune, and nervous systems, and normal brain function.

Vitamin B12 (cyanocobalamin) supports the formation and maintenance of the covering of the nerves (myelin sheath). It is involved in the formation of the neurotransmitter acetylcholine. Folic acid is important during the aging process because it provides nourishment for the brain. Folic acid supports the production of energy and the production of blood cells. Supplementing with folic acid may help in the treatment of depression.

Essential fatty acids (EFAs) are the "healthy" fats required for the maintenance of numerous body systems. Our bodies cannot make essential fatty acids; they can only be obtained through dietary sources or nutritional supplements.

There are two main types of EFAs: omega-3, which is found in fresh, deepwater fish and in some vegetable oils such as walnut or flaxseed; and omega-6, which is found in beans (legumes), nuts, seeds, and unsaturated vegetable oils such as borage and evening primrose. Over 60 health conditions can be helped by supplementing with essential fatty acids.[29]

Ionic minerals (in liquid form) are easily absorbed into the blood through the small intestine. Each ionic mineral (there can be up to 70 in a formula) has either a negative or positive charge and participates as a biochemical co-factor in cellular communication, nerve transmission, and the transport of nutrients. Ionic minerals protect the body from the effects of other, toxic minerals which may be absorbed or ingested.[30]

Dietetic Association has published research showing that a vegetarian lifestyle reduces the risk of heart disease, diabetes, colon cancer, hypertension, obesity, osteoporosis, and diverticular disease.[19]

 See Detoxification Therapy, Diet, Enzyme Therapy, Herbal Medicine, Mind/Body Medicine, Natural Hormone Replacement Therapy, Nutritional Medicine.

Reducing Stress

Although the concept of stress may be commonly discussed today, its role as a contributing factor in many diseases is underappreciated. Estimates suggest that as much as 70% to 80% of all visits to physicians' offices are for stress-related problems.[31] Chronic stress directly affects the immune system and, if not effectively dealt with, can seriously compromise health.

Long before longevity medicine was recognized as a legitimate subspecialty of medicine, Hans Selye, M.D., a pioneering stress researcher, had devoted a considerable amount of thought to stress and its effects on the aging process. Each period of stress, he said, especially if it results from frustrating, unsuccessful struggles, leaves irreversible chemical scars, which accumulate to constitute the signs of tissue aging. "The wear-and-tear of aging—the deposits of DNA-altering proteins in cells, the calcification of organs and blood vessels, the loss of elasticity in the joints, the build-up of arterial plaques associated with heart disease, the narrowing of the arteries, and the cumulative effects of continuously losing brain and heart tissue (that is replaced by scar tissue)—is caused by a lifetime of negative stress or distress," said Dr. Selye.[32]

Stress can deregulate all of the systems of the body, leading to every age-related disease of our time. According to the National Stress Institute, research has increasingly confirmed the important role of stress in heart, gastrointestinal, skin, neurological, and emotional disorders. Stress is also associated with a host of disorders linked to immune system disturbances, ranging from the common cold and herpes to arthritis, cancer, and AIDS. The insidious thing about stress is that it stimulates degeneration of the systems of the body, causing them to lose their resilience; this degeneration, in turn, begets illness, which increases stress, setting up a self-perpetuating cycle of accelerated aging.[33]

Longevity medicine looks for ways to better cope with stress to avoid these deleterious effects. Mind/body treatments, such as guided imagery, Neuro-Linguistic Programming, and biofeedback, can "reprogram" the negative psychological factors that may exacerbate stress, helping you gain greater control over your emotional responses. Other therapies, including meditation, acupuncture, flower essences, and aromatherapy, can be used to mitigate the effects of stress.

Detoxifying the Body

Detoxification is the body's natural process of eliminating toxins and is accomplished by various systems and organs, including the liver, the kidneys, intestines, and skin. If the body's detoxification system becomes overwhelmed, the excessive build-up of poisons can accelerate the aging process, impair the function of our immune and endocrine systems, and leave us more vulnerable to age-related diseases.

"The current level of chemicals in the food and water supply and the indoor and outdoor environment has lowered our threshold of resistance to disease and has altered our body's metabolism, causing enyzme deficiencies, nutritional deficiencies, and hormonal imbalances," says Marshall Mandell, M.D., a pioneer of environmental medicine based in Norwalk, Connecticut. Heart disease, arthritis, multiple sclerosis, Alzheimer's, Parkinson's, fungal infestation, diabetes, lupus, chronic fatigue, allergies, obesity, and many skin problems can be attributed to toxic overload. Symptoms such as headache, fatigue, pain, coughing, and gastrointestinal problems can also be related to toxicity.

Longevity medicine offers ways to begin "cleaning house" through safe and effective methods of detoxification. Detoxification flushes out toxins circulating in the bloodstream, embedded in soft tissues, and clogging important organs, so that healing and wellness can flourish. Specifically, a detoxification program provides the means by which excessive toxins, wastes, fats, mucus, parasites, and bacteria can be filtered and cleared from the body. This will help reduce the toxic load weighing down the immune system, stop the excessive proliferation of age-accelerating free radicals, lessen damage to key enzymes and the loss of other essential nutrients, and prevent the accumulation of heavy metals and other toxins.

Boosting Immune Function

The immune system plays a key role in the repair and maintenance of body tissues, important for regeneration, optimal organ function, and long life. The immune system is the body's primary defense against cancer and a wide variety of bacterial, viral, and fungal infections. With advanced age, immune system function generally declines, raising your vulnerability to many age-related diseases. Another unfortunate effect of the aging process is a propensity of certain parts of the immune system to become overactive, leading to a dramatic increase in inflammatory and autoimmune diseases such as rheumatoid arthritis. The aging immune system is one that is out of balance—most parts underfunctioning, but some parts overactive. Yet this impairment may have more to do with immune suppressive agents, such as stress, environmental toxins, and food allergies, than the aging process itself.

All aspects of the immune defense system can become impaired, less able to detect and protect, as a person ages. Viruses and bacteria previously destroyed and eliminated are ignored and allowed to flourish and multiply due to immune cells that are in improper proportion to one another, too low in numbers, or acting sluggishly. On the other hand, the immune system may also over-react, producing a chronic state of inflammation to common substances (allergic response to dust, pollen, foods) or even attacking the body's own tissues.

"Failure of immune function is what tends to kill you as you get older," says Elmer Cranton, M.D. "If you live to be 120, it will be largely because your immune system demonstrates a superb capacity to deal with the insults of daily living." Immune function and longevity are closely linked. Not only does a robust immune system lessen the likelihood of developing chronic diseases, infections, and other immune-related disorders, but it also enhances DNA replication, insulin sensitivity, and normal thyroid hormone levels, all of which are factors influencing life expectancy. While immune balancing may not allow us to routinely live past our predicted maximum life span of 120 years, it is certain to add years of healthy life we would otherwise not enjoy.

Can the immune system be rejuvenated to function at a higher, more optimal and balanced level (neither underfunctioning or overactive)? The good news is that the answer is yes. Having been in an overactive and dysfunctional state for a prolonged period, often years, the immune system may need intensive support to return it to an optimal level of functioning and enable it to ward off current and future infection. Immunomodulators like beta glucan and arabinogalactan are substances that target and adjust specific weaknesses in the immune system. Enzymes, specific herbs, and certain hormones like DHEA are other natural options for modulating immune function.

Balancing Hormones

Women going through menopause may experience a host of symptoms, including hot flashes, fatigue, night sweats, mood swings, and weight gain. Men are not immune to these problems, either. In their 50s, men sometimes experience "male menopause": a condition characterized by fatigue, less muscle strength and endurance, decreased libido, short-term memory loss, and weight gain around the midriff. What is happening to produce these symptoms? The answer is in your hormones.

Hormones related to aging include the "male" sex hormone testosterone, the "female" sex hormones estrogen and progesterone, as well as hormones found in both men and women including melatonin, growth hormone, cortisol, and DHEA. These chemical messengers regulate metabolism, the body's response to stress, kidney function, blood sugar balance, menstruation, and sexual function. When the hormone levels are imbalanced—from stress, medications, or other causes—there can be system-wide problems. They are critical to the maintenance of normal life processes and are known to be capable of accelerating some aging processes and slowing others.

Since hormones affect virtually every bodily process and act upon organs and systems associated with the rate at which an individual ages, they are regarded as a fundamental factor in the aging puzzle. Together, low levels of certain longevity hormones and impaired communication within the endocrine system create havoc with all the other systems of the body—immune, cardiovascular, detoxification, gastrointestinal, and central nervous system. The net effect is predictable: accelerated aging and an increased vulnerability to the "age-related" diseases that prematurely claim the lives of so many individuals.

If your hormones are imbalanced, one of your priorities should be to detoxify your body systems. Both the liver and gastrointestinal system are involved in the normal processing of hormones. When these organs are not functioning properly, your hormones may become imbalanced. Holistic practitioners generally recommend tending to these systems first through detoxification in order to normalize the body's functions. Alternative medicine also offers a number of therapies to balance your hormones, including dietary and nutritional support, hormone replacement, herbal medicine, homeopathy, and exercise.

Improving Cardiovascular Function

"The average American lifestyle, combining too little exercise, too much stress, and a diet of highly processed foods often deficient in essential nutrients, has rendered this nation's population especially vulnerable to the ravages of heart ailments," says Dr. Cowden. Heart problems can be caused by other aging factors and can also lead to accelerated aging because of a decreased flow of oxygen and nutrients to the body's tissues.

Longevity medicine physicians help to reduce a patient's risk factors for heart disease by considering preventive measures such as stress reduction, exercise, dietary improvement, weight control, and the elimination of smoking. They also work to correct the nutritional and biochemical imbalances that can affect the functioning of the heart and deposition of plaque in the arteries. For example, raising levels of nutrients like vitamin B_6 and

THE FUTURE ROLE OF STEM CELLS FOR LONGEVITY

Stem cells are the "mother cells" of all the cells in our body. They have the capacity to repair any tissue damage in the body, which is why longevity medicine experts are excited about their potential to extend life span and retain the healthy nature of organs in the body. There are three types of stem cells—fetal, umbilical, and adult.

After a very few cycles of replication after fertilization of the egg by a sperm, a structure called a "blastocyst" is formed. The center of this structure is filled with thousands of "pluripotent" stem cells, or cells that can differentiate into or repair any tissue in the body. The number of pluripotent stem cells expands throughout the early development of the fetus, while simultaneously differentiating into the organs that make up the body. Eventually, the number of stem cells peaks, and finally begins to decline as the developing embryo reaches the second trimester.

There are intermediate cells between pluripotent stem cells and final specialized cells such as red blood cells or heart cells, called "multipotent" stem cells. Preliminary research indicates that these cells may have the potential capacity to repair organs composed of a large number of cell types such as the liver and brain. Multipotent stem cells secrete substances that enable them to identify damaged or deficient cells and repair or augment them. This approach is particularly exciting for conditions that involve cells that do not repair or regenerate well, such as the brain and heart, offering new hope for persons suffering from extensive damage in those organs, as well as offering a supply of cells to replace those lost through the aging process.

Although the number of stem cells declines with age, they are found in children and adults. Obviously, the use of fetal stem cells for human therapy is fraught with ethical and moral issues. Therefore, work with umbilical cord–derived stem cells has begun, as well as studies with adult stem cells. However, 12-week-old fetal stem cells are 27 times more potent than adult cells, and nine times more potent than umbilical cells for tissue repair. Furthermore, umbilical and adult stem cells may develop self-antigens, which may result in immune system rejection issues when used therapeutically. Stem cells harvested from a particular individual and then frozen until later use have shown promising results.

Stem cells may play an important role in the future of longevity medicine. These cells, manipulated to develop into specialized cells, offer the possibility of providing the capacity to continually repair damaged tissues or prolong the life span of important organ systems, like the brain and immune system, by supplying a renewable source of new cells.[37]

---

magnesium, as well as antioxidants such as vitamins C and E, coenzyme Q10, and selenium, has been shown to have a positive impact on heart disease.[34] Chelation therapy, acupuncture, and herbal remedies such as hawthorn berries, *Ginkgo biloba,* garlic, and cayenne[35] may also be effective in the treatment of heart disease.

Rebuilding Brainpower

As a person ages, a number of changes typically occur that can impair many aspects of mental function, such as perceptual speed, reaction time, visual-spatial abilities, fluency with words, certain memory functions, and some types of attention. A certain amount of "shrinkage" takes place as neurons whither and die, causing the brain to get smaller; important, say researchers, since brain size and IQ are positively related.

According to endocrinologist Thierry Hertoghe, M.D., of the Academy of General Medicine, in Brussels, Belgium, the aging brain also experiences a loss of density of the tentacle-like dendrites that are part of each brain cell, through which electrical impulses are relayed.

Losing control of your mental faculties as you age isn't inevitable and can be reversed.

—Dharma Singh Khalsa, M.D.

A progressive accrual of a brown-colored slime, known as lipofuscin, accumulates within each neuron and also encrusts it, hampering the transmission of electrochemical messages to other parts of the brain. Over time, suggests Dr. Hertoghe, memory declines and senility and dementia begin. With advancing age, certain biochemical changes also occur, such as deficiencies in important enzymes and neurotransmitters. According to Eric Braverman, M.D., of the New York University Medical Center in New York City, these structural and biochemical modifications of the aging brain reduce its energy (electrical voltage and frequency or speed), causing it to slow down. When this occurs, there are significant impairments in memory, learning, and processing speed, leading to senility, dementia, and other age-related problems.

While growing older is something we must all embrace, unless brain cells have withered and died, the diminishment of our mental abilities is not inevitable. The various causes of mental decline can be reversed and the progression of degenerative changes to the brain's neurons can be slowed. "Losing control of your mental faculties as you age isn't inevitable and can be reversed," says brain longevity expert Dharma Singh Khalsa, M.D., author of *Brain Longevity*.[36] Even in the late stages, Alzheimer's disease can be halted or at least slowed down; catch it early enough and it can be reversed. And if you deal with the possibility of brain decline at mid-life, your chances of preventing it altogether are high.

Dr. Khalsa further states that people 40 to 60 years old "can retain not only an almost perfect memory, but can also have 'youthful minds,' characterized by the dynamic brainpower, learning ability, creativity, and emotional zest usually found only in young people." A comprehensive brain longevity program consists of detoxification, stress reduction, hormone balancing, nutritional support, and exercise (both physical and mental).

The Future of Longevity Medicine

As the world population continues to grow older, longevity medicine will become an increasingly important part of the health-care picture. "This trend is being driven by the lay public seeking higher vitality in to advanced years," says Dr. Cowden. "But I predict that governmental and insurance agencies will join the movement, because proof is accumulating that preventative, longevity wellness care is much more cost-efficient than the crisis-intervention illness care presently being reimbursed by insurance."

With the completion of the Human Genome Project, there may soon be new ways of early detection and treatment of illness. Gene therapies will be able to correct DNA mutations before they manifest as illness. Scientific research continues to validate the use of nutraceuticals for prevention and treatment of age-related illnesses, such as cancer, heart disease, and diabetes. Supplementing with antioxidants, coenzyme Q10, melatonin, growth hormones, "smart drugs" for memory enhancement, natural hormone therapies, phytochemicals, vitamins, and minerals will continue to grow in popularity.

Today, science and medicine have the technology and understanding necessary to appreciate many aspects of longevity medicine. It is becoming increasingly common for the conventional medical establishment to embrace longevity techniques such as nutritional supplementation, lifestyle modification, stress reduction, exercise, and dietary changes.

Where to Find Help

For further information on longevity medicine, contact:

American Academy of Anti-Aging Medicine (A4M)
2415 North Greenview
Chicago, Illinois 60614
(773) 528-4333
Website: www.worldhealth.net

A4M is a membership society of physicians and researchers exploring the process of aging and how it can be slowed or reversed through medical intervention. A4M provides continuing education programs, public forums for disseminating anti-aging research, and legislative advocacy.

International College of Advanced Longevity Medicine (ICALM)
1407-B N. Wells Street
Chicago Illinois 60610
(888) 855-5050
Website: www.healthy.net/icalm

ICALM is a nonprofit, membership organization that provides educational programs and certification in anti-aging/ longevity medicine.

Recommended Reading

Age-Proof Your Body. Elizabeth Somer, M.A., R.D. New York: Quill/William Morrow, 1998.

Age Right. Karlis Ullis, M.D., with Greg Ptacek. New York: Simon & Schuster, 1999.

A Fresh Start. Susan Smith Jones, Ph.D. Berkeley, CA: Celestial Arts, 2001.

Longevity: An Alternative Medicine Definitive Guide. W. Lee Cowden, M.D., Ferre Akbarpour, M.D., and Russ DiCarlo, with Burton Goldberg. Tiburon, CA: AlternativeMedicine.com Books, 2001.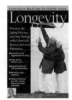

RealAge: Are You as Young as You Can Be? Michael Roizen with Elizabeth Anne Stephenson. New York: Cliff Street Books, 1999.

Stopping the Clock. Ronald Klatz, D.O., and Robert Goldman, D.O., Ph.D. New Canaan, CT: Keats Publishing, 1996.

The Supplement Shopper. Gregory Pouls, D.C., and Maile Pouls, Ph.D., with Burton Goldberg. Tiburon, CA: Future Medicine Publishing, 1999.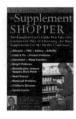

MAGNETIC FIELD THERAPY

Electromagnetic energy and the human body have a valid and important interrelationship. Magnetic field therapy can be used in both diagnosing and treating physical and emotional disorders. This process has been recognized to relieve symptoms and may, in some cases, retard the cycle of new disease. Magnets and electromagnetic therapy devices are now being used to eliminate pain, facilitate the healing of broken bones, and counter the effects of stress.

THE WORLD IS surrounded by magnetic fields: some are generated by the earth's magnetism, while others are caused by solar storms and changes in the weather. Magnetic fields are also created by everyday electrical devices: motors, televisions, office equipment, computers, electric blankets, microwave ovens, the electrical wiring in homes, and the power lines that supply them. Even the human body produces subtle magnetic fields that are generated by the chemical reactions within the cells and the ionic currents of the nervous system.[1] Recently, scientists have discovered that external magnetic fields can affect the body's functioning in both positive and negative ways, and this observation has led to the development of magnetic field therapy.

> *The use of magnets and electrical devices to generate controlled magnetic fields has many medical applications and has proven to be one of the most effective means for diagnosing illness.*

What is Magnetic Field Therapy?

The use of magnets and electrical devices to generate controlled magnetic fields has many medical applications and has proven to be one of the most effective means for diagnosing illness. For example, MRI (magnetic resonance imaging) is replacing X-ray diagnosis because it is safer and more accurate, and magnetoencephalography is now replacing electroencephalography as the preferred technique for recording the brain's electrical activity.

In 1974, researcher Albert Roy Davis, Ph.D., noted that positive and negative magnetic polarities have different effects upon the biological systems of animals and humans. He found that magnets could arrest and kill cancer cells in animals and could also be used in the treatment of arthritis, glaucoma, infertility, and diseases related to aging.[2] He concluded that negative magnetic fields have a beneficial effect on living organisms, whereas positive magnetic fields have a stressful effect.

"Scientifically designed, double-blind, placebo-controlled studies, however, have not been done to substantiate the claims of there being different effects between positive and negative magnetic poles," says John Zimmerman, Ph.D., President of the Bio-Electro-Magnetics Institute, in Reno, Nevada. "But numerous anecdotal, clinical observations suggest that such differences are real and do exist. Clearly, scientific research is needed to substantiate these claims."

Humans need both internal and external sources of magnetic fields for survival. Robert O. Becker, M.D., an orthopedic surgeon and author of numerous scientific articles and books, found that weak electric currents promote the healing of broken bones. Dr. Becker also brought national attention to the fact that electromagnetic interference from power lines and home appliances can pose a serious hazard to human health. "The scientific evidence," writes Dr. Becker, "leads to only one conclusion: the exposure of living organisms to abnormal electromagnetic fields results in significant abnormalities in physiology and function."[3]

Dr. Becker demonstrated that the body concentrates negative electromagnetic energy at the site of an injury for healing.[4] If the body succeeds in sending enough negative magnetic energy to the injury, such as a cancerous growth, then it will heal this lesion. However, in many cases, the body simply does not supply and maintain

ELECTROMAGNETIC FIELDS CAN POSE A SERIOUS HEALTH HAZARD

According to Robert Becker, M.D., John Zimmerman, Ph.D., and many other scientists and researchers, we live in an environment that is filled with stress-producing, electromagnetic fields generated by the electrical wiring in homes and offices, as well as from televisions, computers, microwaves, overhead lights, electrical wiring, and motors that can generate higher than naturally occurring gauss strengths.

The frequency at which a magnetic field is pulsed determines whether or not it is harmful. For example, the voltage of the electrical current used in homes in the United States is 60 cycles per second. In contrast, normal frequencies of the human brain during waking hours range from eight to 22 cycles per second, while in sleep the frequencies may drop to as low as two cycles per second. The higher frequencies present in artificial electrical currents may disturb the brain's natural resonant frequencies and in time lead to cellular fatigue, according to Dr. Zimmerman.

In 1979, Nancy Wertheimer, Ph.D., an epidemiologist at the University of Colorado, found that there was a statistically significant increase in childhood cancers among those who were exposed to the AC (alternating current) electromagnetic fields (EMFs) emanating from the power lines that run along many of the nation's city streets.[7] In 1987, a large-scale study conducted by the New York State Department of Health confirmed Dr. Wertheimer's findings and added that EMFs also affected the neurohormones of the brain.[8] A study at the University of Texas Medical Branch found that workers exposed to EMFs showed a 13-fold increase in brain tumors compared to the unexposed group.[9] Studies of human populations have consistently found associations between residential EMF exposure and cancer, particularly in the case of childhood leukemia.[10] Other studies have shown increases in suicides,[11] depression,[12] chromosomal abnormalities,[13] and learning difficulties.[14]

In another study by Dr. Wertheimer, it was observed that users of electric blankets had a higher incidence of miscarriages.[15] Add to this the possible perils from fluorescent lighting, microwaves, hair dryers, electric shavers, and heaters, and one can see why more research is urgently needed. "Only a few farsighted individuals, such as Dr. Becker, have given much thought to the fact that the new electromagnetic environment created by 20th-century technology may be exerting subtle, yet very important effects upon biology," states Dr. Zimmerman. "This may include alterations in gene expression, immune function, viral pathogenesis, and future genetic tendencies."

Researchers suggest that magnetic therapy can be used to counter the effects caused by the electromagnetic pollution in the environment.

enough negative magnetic energy at the injury to facilitate healing. This is because the human body has some limitations—based on its own energy capacity—on how much negative magnetic energy it can generate. Adding a negative magnetic field from a source outside the body can provide anti-stressful energy of sufficient strength for healing to occur, supplementing the body's effort to heal. The body is then not required to be the sole provider of magnetic energy to its injured area.

"Magnetic field therapy is a method that penetrates the whole body and can treat every organ without chemical side effects," according to Wolfgang Ludwig, Sc.D., Ph.D., Director of the Institute for Biophysics, in Horb, Germany. Magnetic field therapy has been used effectively in the treatment of:

- Cancer
- Rheumatoid disease
- Infections and inflammation
- Headaches and migraines
- Insomnia and other sleep disorders
- Circulatory problems
- Fractures and pain
- Environmental stress

Dr. Ludwig adds that magnetic changes in the environment can affect the electromagnetic balance of the human organism and contribute to disease. Physiologists agree that humans receive approximately 30% of their energy from external sources.[5] Kyoichi Nakagawa, M.D.,

Director of the Isuzu Hospital, in Tokyo, Japan, believes that the time people spend in buildings and cars reduces their exposure to the natural geomagnetic fields of the earth and may also interfere with health. He calls this condition "magnetic field deficiency syndrome," which can cause headaches, dizziness, muscle stiffness, chest pain, insomnia, constipation, and general fatigue.[6] The long-term biological consequences of magnetic deficiency include the development of acute symptoms and chronic degenerative diseases, the loss of normal healing ability, and the unsuccessful defense against infectious microorganisms and environmental toxins.

How Magnetic Field Therapy Works

"The healing potential of magnets is possible because the body's nervous system is governed, in part, by varying patterns of ionic currents and electromagnetic fields," reports Dr. Zimmerman. There are numerous forms of magnetic field therapy, including static magnetic fields produced by natural or artificial magnets and pulsating magnetic fields generated by electrical devices. The magnetic fields produced by magnets or electromagnetic generating devices are able to penetrate the human body and can affect the functioning of the nervous system, organs, and cells. According to William H. Philpott, M.D., of Choctaw, Oklahoma, co-author of *Magnet Therapy: An Alternative Medicine Definitive Guide,* magnetic fields can stimulate metabolism and increase the amount of oxygen available to cells. When used properly, magnetic field therapy has no known harmful side effects.

Almost anything can be magnetized—it's not just a property of iron and other metals. Magnetism happens on an atomic level, where tiny charged particles called electrons orbit around the atom like planets around the sun. These electrons also spin, like the earth on its axis, creating miniature magnetic fields with north and south poles. If you can get all of these electrons spinning in the same direction, you get magnetism.[16] Magnetic fields provide two types of energy response: the negative field spins electrons counterclockwise and the positive field spins electrons clockwise. The spinning of electrons in negative and positive fields is opposite and the biological responses to these magnetic fields are also opposite.[17]

All magnets have two poles: one is called positive and the other negative. However, as there are conflicting methods of naming the poles of a magnet, a magnetometer should be used as a standard method of determination (if one is using a compass to locate the poles, the arrowhead of the needle marked "N" or "North" will point to the magnet's negative pole). Dr. Philpott and other researchers claim that the negative pole generally has a calming effect and helps to normalize metabolic functioning. In contrast, the positive pole has a stressful effect and, with prolonged exposure, interferes with metabolic functioning, produces acidity, reduces cellular oxygen, and encourages the growth of microorganisms.

> **CAUTION** The positive pole has a stressful effect and, with prolonged exposure, interferes with metabolic functioning. In contrast, the negative pole generally has a calming effect and helps to normalize function.

> **IMPORTANT** Industrial magnets often have different positive and negative pole identifications than the magnets used in medicine and therapy. Use a magnetometer or compass to confirm proper identification.

The negative pole calms neurons and encourages rest, relaxation, and sleep. When sufficiently high in strength, it can even produce general anesthesia. And because it is neuron calming, it has been successfully used in the control of neurosis, psychosis, seizures, addictive withdrawal, and movement disorders. A negative magnetic field consistently produces a predictable, long-term healing response, because only this field can ultimately relieve stress or injury. The body itself always responds with negative magnetic field energy to counter any stressor. The negative magnetic field counteracts stress by the following mechanisms: normalizes pH, corrects cellular edema, eliminates free radicals, stimulates hormone production, and releases molecular oxygen.

> *Magnetic field therapy is a method that penetrates the whole body and can treat every organ without chemical side effects.*
> — WOLFGANG LUDWIG, SC.D., PH.D.

Magnetic therapy can be applied in many ways, and devices range from small, simple magnets to large machines capable of generating high magnitudes of field strength. Magnetic blankets and beds have also been manufactured for the purposes of promoting sleep and reducing stress. Specially designed ceramic, plastiform, and neodymium (a rare earth chemical element) magnets can be placed either individually or in clusters above the various organs of the body, on lymph nodes, or on various points of the head. In Japan, small tai-ki magnets have

THE PHYSIOLOGICAL EFFECTS OF POSITIVE AND NEGATIVE MAGNETIC FIELDS

According to many researchers, negative magnetic fields seem to affect all the metabolic processes involved in growth, healing, immune defense, and detoxification. The following chart was prepared by Dr. Philpott and is based on his clinical observations of the effects that positive and negative magnetic fields have upon living organisms.

Negative Magnetic Fields	Positive Magnetic Fields
pH normalizing	Acid producing
Oxygenating	Oxygen deficit producing
Resolves cellular edema	Evokes cellular edema
Usually reduces symptoms	Often exacerbates existing symptoms
Inhibits microorganism replication; slows down infections	Accelerates microorganism replication; speeds up infections
Biologically normalizing	Biologically disorganizing
Reduces pain and inflammation	Increases pain and inflammation
Governs rest, relaxation, and sleep	Governs wakefulness and action
Evokes anabolic hormone production—melatonin and growth hormone	Evokes catabolic hormone production
Clears metabolically produced toxins out of the body	Produces toxic end-products of metabolism
Eliminates free radicals	Produces free radicals
Slows down electrical activity of the brain	Speeds up electrical activity of the brain

been designed to stimulate acupuncture points, but no clinical studies have yet explored this procedure. Magnetic devices are quite popular in Germany, where the use of certain devices is covered by medical insurance. After simple instruction is given to the patient, these devices can be used at home.

The strength of a magnet is measured in gauss units (one gauss is equivalent to about twice the average strength of the earth's magnetic field). The Tesla is another common magnetic measurement: one Tesla equals 10,000 gauss. Every magnetic device has a manufacturer's gauss rating; however, the actual strength of the magnet at the skin surface is often much less than this number. For example, a 4,000-gauss magnet transmits about 1,200 gauss to the patient. Magnets placed in pillow or bed pads will render even lower amounts of field strength at the skin surface, because a magnet's strength quickly decreases with the distance from the subject. The strength of the magnet also depends on its size and thickness. Therapeutic magnets use from 200 gauss to 1,500 gauss (only a fraction of what an MRI machine emits), while a common refrigerator magnet emits just 10 gauss.[18]

 Research into the therapeutic benefits of magnetic field therapy is needed. This type of therapy could provide a safe and effective way to curb rising health-care costs.

Conditions Benefited by Magnetic Field Therapy

Treatments can last from just a few minutes to overnight and, depending upon the situation and severity, may be applied several times a day or for days or weeks at a time. Dr. Philpott has used magnets to help relieve toothaches, eliminate periodontal disease, and eradicate fungal infections like candidiasis. Kidney stones and calcium deposits in inflamed tissues have also been known to dissolve. Magnetic therapy has been shown to be particularly effective in reducing swelling (edema). Studies continue to demonstrate the value of magnetic field therapy for a wide range of conditions, including stress, heart disease, infections, injuries, nervous disorders, cancer, and sleep disorders, among others.

Stress

A negative magnetic field applied to the top of the head has a calming and sleep-inducing effect on brain and body functions, by stimulating production of the hormone melatonin, according to Dr. Philpott. Melatonin has been shown to be antistressful, anti-aging, anti-infectious, anticancerous, and to exert control over respiration and the production of free radicals.[19] A free radical is a highly destructive molecule that is missing an electron and readily reacts with other molecules. This can lead to the aging of cells, hardening of muscle tissue, skin wrinkling, and a decreased efficiency of protein synthesis. As there are literally hundreds of diseases that are related to stress, infections, and aging, magnetic field therapy could be considered an important adjunct in their treatment and researchers are currently studying its contributions.

 See Chronic Pain, Stress.

Heart Disease

A common precursor of heart disease is atherosclerosis, or thickening of the arterial walls. In atherosclerosis, the inner arterial walls harden and thicken due to deposits of fatty substances that form a plaque, which builds up and causes a narrowing of the arteries. Over time, plaque can block the arteries and interrupt blood flow to the organs they supply, including the heart and brain. Atherosclerosis of the coronary arteries (the arteries supplying the muscle of the heart), known as coronary heart disease, is one of the most common forms of heart disease in the U.S. today.

A negative magnetic field oxygenates and alkalinizes body tissues and cells. These two actions oppose the acidity required for the creation of insoluble amino acid and calcium deposits in existing plaques. Since a negative magnetic field has a local effect, magnets must be applied directly over the plaques in order to achieve therapeutic results. According to Dr. Philpott, "Symptoms of cardiac atherosclerosis have been observed to disappear after six to eight weeks of nightly exposure to a negative static magnetic field."

In a case described by Dr. Philpott, a 70-year-old man who had undergone coronary bypass surgery continued to suffer from heart pain. His walk was reduced to a shuffle, his speech was slurred, and he lived in a state of chronic depression. He decided to try magnetic therapy and a plastiform magnet was placed over his heart. Within ten minutes, the pain disappeared. Magnets were applied to the crown of his head while he slept and, within a month, his depression was gone, his speech was clear, and his walking returned to normal.

Sometimes, though, the results of magnetic therapy can be quite dramatic, as in a case cited by Dr. Ludwig. A 46-year-old man had suffered for years from severe heart flutter, diarrhea, and nausea. No treatment seemed to help, but when a magnetic applicator with less than one gauss of energy was placed upon his solar plexus for only three minutes, his symptoms immediately ceased. Two years later, he had experienced no relapse.

Infections

"A negative magnetic field can function like an antibiotic in helping to destroy bacterial, fungal, and viral infections by promoting oxygenation and lowering the body's acidity," says Dr. Philpott. Both these factors are beneficial to normal bodily functions but harmful to pathogenic (disease-causing) microorganisms, which do not survive in a well-oxygenated, alkaline environment. Dr. Philpott theorizes that the biological value of oxygen is increased by the influence of a negative magnetic field and that the field causes negatively charged DNA (deoxyribonucleic acid) to "pull" oxygen out of the bloodstream and into the cell. The negative electromagnetic field keeps the cellular buffer system (pH or acid-base balance) intact so that the cells remain alkaline. The low acid balance also helps maintain the presence of oxygen in the body.

One of Dr. Philpott's patients, Mary, had candidiasis of the vagina and colon, which required constant antibiotic treatment. She also had frequent bladder infections, again requiring antibiotics. Frustrated by her unsatisfactory results, she then exposed her pelvic area to a negative magnetic field and both the candidiasis and urinary infections disappeared permanently.

During a flu epidemic, Susan developed characteristic flu symptoms with profuse mucus drainage from the sinuses, coughing, and general malaise. Her lungs, sinuses, and head were treated 24 hours a day with ceramic magnets. By the third day, she had no symptoms and the magnets were removed. After this, her symptoms still did not return. At the same time, a large number of people in the same community had a severe three-week siege of influenza; those patients who used magnetic therapy like Susan achieved the same results.

Pain and Injuries

A negative magnetic field normalizes the disturbed metabolic functions that cause painful conditions such as cellular edema (swelling of the cells), cellular acidosis (excessive acidity of the cells), lack of oxygen to the cells, and infection. A negative magnetic field is needed to govern all components of the healing process: reducing pain, inflammation, and edema; normalizing the local pH; and activating oxidoreductase enzymes, which neutralize free radicals and release molecular oxygen. As a result, the negative magnetic field inhibits infectious microorganisms, eliminates toxins, relieves inflammation and edema, and facilitates cellular repair.[20] It floods the injured areas with oxygen and stimulates the production of melatonin and growth hormone. In order to supplement the body's own negative field of energy, a negative magnetic field from a static field magnet can be used over any fracture, skin cut, bruise, or injury site.[21]

Dr. Philpott cites the case of a woman in her seventies who had experienced pain and weakness in her left leg for 33 years, stemming from a blood clot in the groin area, and could not climb stairs without stopping several times due to pain. After 12 months of sleeping on a negative magnetic pad, the woman found that she could walk a long flight of stairs without any pain or weakness in her leg.

Jane, a woman in her fifties, had an inoperable, ruptured lumbar disc. She was experiencing chronic pain and was unable to lift any appreciable weight. After sleeping on a negative magnetic bed pad for eight months, her pain was gone. X rays showed complete healing of the ruptured disc.

Central Nervous System Disorders

"When a negative magnetic field is placed directly over an area of electrical activity in the brain, the electrical excitement can be reduced," says Dr. Philpott. It can stop such symptoms as hallucinations, delusions, seizures, or panic without disrupting the patient's mental alertness and orientation. Small disc magnets (made from ceramic neodymium or iron oxide) can be placed around the head to alleviate these kinds of symptoms. Dr. Philpott has pioneered the use of magnetic therapy for numerous psychiatric disorders and he believes that, in the future, subtle uses of magnets will be used to control a variety of symptoms and central nervous system disturbances. Magnet therapy has proven effective in helping those with Alzheimer's[22] and Parkinson's[23] as well.

Cancer

Cancer only develops under certain conditions within the human body, no matter what genetically damaging carcinogens may be involved in the initiation of the disease. The two most important conditions that must exist for the development of cancer are acidity and the lack of oxygen; that is, the pH of the cellular environment must be acid and there must also be a deficiency of oxygen in the cells where cancer is growing.

Magnetic therapy can help alkalinize and oxygenate tissues, thus removing the conditions necessary for cancer cells to survive. This oxygen-rich and highly alkaline environment inhibits the energy-making functions of cancer cells. Because of this fact, a negative magnetic field of sufficient strength and duration can cause the death of cancer cells. Studies are beginning to demonstrate the effectiveness of magnetic fields as a complementary cancer therapy.[24]

Thomas was diagnosed as having prostate cancer with bone metastases (cancer that has spread to the bone). He was treated by Dr. Philpott by placing a ceramic magnet on his lower abdominal area and another on the pubic area, both with the negative magnetic field facing the body. He did this whenever sitting down, about 3-4 hours a day. Furthermore, for 24

SCIENCE DEMONSTRATES THE POWER OF MAGNETIC THERAPY

The French Academy of Sciences published a report in March 1965 on the magnetic treatment of mice with cancer (lymphosarcoma). Every mouse in the untreated, control group died within 18 days. In three other groups, mice began magnetic treatment at different points in time, but with the same strength and duration of magnetic treatment: 620 gauss for two hours a day. The first group received magnetic treatment within five days of starting the test and recovered quickly; all tumors and metastases disappeared. The second group began treatment on day seven and showed the same recovery as the first group; a third group of mice was treated from the tenth day on, but did not recover. These mice all died in 19 to 22 days, just after the untreated mice had died.[25]

These findings were compelling enough to encourage the French Academy of Sciences to conduct another experiment, this time testing the effect of the daily dosage given. In the first group, the mice were treated from the fifth day, with 620 gauss one hour a day; in the second group, the mice were treated with 620 gauss two hours a day, also from the fifth day. Once again, the results were striking. As expected, all the mice in the untreated (control) group died within 15 days; all the mice in the first test group died after 19 days. Meanwhile, the mice in the second test group—they received twice the magnetic treatment per day as the first group—all survived and showed no signs of cancer.[26]

---

hours a day, he wore a flexible magnet, with a ceramic magnet placed on top, across his lower abdomen. He also fastened a flexible magnet across his sacral area (near the tailbone). Three months later, X rays revealed no evidence of bone cancer, and the PSA (prostate specific antigen, a marker for prostate cancer) had dropped from an initial 28 to 2, which is within the normal limits.

Sleep Disorders

The negative magnetic field can influence many biochemical processes within the body that directly relate to maintaining proper sleep patterns. For example, the negative magnetic field is one factor that directly influences the body's acid-alkaline (pH) balance. Oxygen levels are compromised when maladaptive reactions change the cellular and tissue pH in the body to acid. Once oxygen levels are reduced, the painful discomforts of swollen cells may disturb proper sleep patterns. In order to reverse these conditions to the more favorable alkaline and oxygenated conditions necessary for sound sleep, it is important to treat any area of local edema, as well as the entire system, with a negative magnetic field.

A recent study used electromagnetic field therapy to treat 106 insomnia patients. The low-energy magnetic field was administered for 20 minutes, three afternoons per week, for a total of 12 treatments. This protocol produced a significant increase in total sleep time and a decrease in sleep latency. It also improved sleep quality by increasing the number of sleep cycles during the night (more closely resembling normal sleep patterns). The researchers concluded that electromagnetic therapy was "an attractive alternative therapy for chronic insomnia."[27]

Magnetic field therapy is quite effective in treating and preventing all types of sleep disorders. Sleep on a magnetic bed pad composed of mini-block magnets placed sufficiently close together to provide a full negative magnetic field. Exposure to this magnetic bed serves to increase melatonin production.

> **CAUTION** The body's subtle electromagnetic fields can be affected by even the weakest of magnets. Since even minor alterations in the field can cause mild to serious symptoms, magnetic therapy should only be practiced under the supervision of a qualified professional. For some patients, magnetic field therapy can cause pain, while others may have symptomatic reactions to various medications they are taking. Toxins may also be released into the body, causing severe reactions. Dr. Philpott adds the following precautions:
>
> - Don't use magnets on the abdomen during pregnancy.
>
> - Don't use a magnetic bed for more than 8-10 hours.
>
> - Wait 60-90 minutes after meals before applying magnetic therapy to the abdomen to prevent interference with peristalsis (wave-like contractions of the smooth muscles of the digestive tract).
>
> - Do not apply the positive magnetic pole unless under medical supervision. It can produce seizures, hallucinations, insomnia, hyperactivity, stimulate the growth of tumors and microorganisms, and promote addictive behavior.

The Future of Magnetic Field Therapy

With the rising popularity of magnetic field diagnostic techniques such as MRI (magnetic resonance imaging), magnets and electrical devices are beginning to gain mainstream medical acceptance as human diagnostic and treatment tools. According to Dr. Philpott, the application of magnets provides the most predictable results of any treatment he has observed. "It is not only valuable as a medically supervised technique, but for many self-help problems such as insomnia, chronic pain, and tension." Because magnets do not introduce any foreign substance to the body, this makes them safer over the long-term than aspirin or other over-the-counter medications.

As our understanding of magnetic energy improves, says Dr. Philpott, we will see that the negative magnetic field produces the most effective relief of pain caused by infections, local edema, acidosis, and toxicity. Magnets will also prove central to the healing process, particularly with broken bones, bruises, burns, acute environmental allergies, and chronic degenerative diseases such as arteriosclerosis (hardening of the arteries) and Alzheimer's. Negative magnetic exposure can be used to control major mental disorders (delusions, obsessive-compulsiveness, psychotic depression), all types of neuroses, and learning and behavioral disorders (dyslexia, attention deficit disorder, hyperactivity).[28] Finally, negative magnetic field therapy may be the most effective antibiotic treatment for infections (bacteria, viruses, fungi, and parasites).

Where to Find Help

The following organizations offer referrals and information on professional and self-care treatment with magnetic field therapy.

Bio-Electro-Magnetics Institute
2490 West Moana Lane
Reno, Nevada 89509-3936
(702) 827-9099

A private, nonprofit organization established to provide research, education, support, and technical assistance in matters relating to bioelectromagnetics. A national clearinghouse for information relating to both health risks from power line magnetic fields and the health benefits from magnetic therapy.

Enviro-Tech Products
17171 Southeast 29th Street
Choctaw, Oklahoma 73020
(405) 390-3499 or (800) 445-1962

Enviro-Tech provides self-help information, information for physicians, and guidance for research projects under the Institutional Review Board of the Bio-Electro-Magnetics Institute of Reno, Nevada.

MagnetiCo Inc.
5421 11th Street N.E., #109
Calgary, Alberta T2E 6M4 Canada
(800) 265-1119
Website: www.magneticosleep.com

Manufactures and markets a SleepPad™, engineered to produce a negative magnetic field to restore energy while you sleep, as well as other magnetic products.

Norso Biomagnetics
8724-B Glenwood
Raleigh, North Carolina 27612
(800) 480-8601

Offers a full line of biomagnetic wraps, sleep systems, and seating.

Recommended Reading

Cross Currents. Robert O. Becker, M.D. Los Angeles: Jeremy P. Tarcher, 1990.

Healing Magnets. Sherry Kahn, M.P.H. New York: Three Rivers Press, 2000.

Healing with Magnets. Gary Null. New York: Carroll & Graf, 1998.

Magnet Therapy: An Alternative Medicine Definitive Guide. William H. Philpott, M.D., and Dwight K. Kalita, Ph.D., with Burton Goldberg. Tiburon, CA: AlternativeMedicine.com Books, 2000.

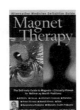

Magnet Therapy: Balancing Your Body's Energy Flow for Self-Healing. Holger Hannemann. New York: Sterling Publishing, 1990.

Magnet Therapy: The Pain Cure Alternative. Ron Lawrence, M.D., Ph.D., and Paul J. Rosch, M.D., F.A.C.P. Rocklin, CA: Prima Health, 1998.

The Magnetic Effect. Albert Davis and Walter Rawls. Kansas City, MO: Acres U.S.A., 1993.

Pain-Free with Magnet Therapy. Lara Owen. Roseville, CA: Prima Publishing, 2000.

The Pain Relief Breakthrough. Julian Whitaker, M.D., and Brenda Adderly, M.H.A. Boston: Little, Brown, 1998.

MIND/BODY MEDICINE

Mind/body medicine is revolutionizing modern health care. Recognizing the profound interconnection of mind and body, the body's innate healing capabilities, and the role of self-responsibility in the healing process, mind/body medicine utilizes a wide range of modalities to help patients most effectively marshall all of their psychophysiological resources to achieve and maintain optimal health.

FOR THE LAST 300 years, Western civilization has been shaped by a rational, scientific, mechanistic worldview that has helped to bring about enormous technological and material advances. The practice of Western medicine reflects this mind-set and relies upon the technology it has produced, according to James S. Gordon, M.D., Director of the Center for Mind/Body Studies and Clinical Professor in the departments of Psychiatry and Community and Family Medicine at the Georgetown University School of Medicine. "Since the philosopher Descartes separated a transcendent and non-material mind from the material and mechanical operations of the body, science has been concerned with ever more accurately resolving the body into its component parts," says Dr. Gordon. "This approach has produced extraordinary achievements in the treatment of infectious diseases, in the synthesis of such desperately needed substances as insulin, and in the creation of exquisitely sophisticated and life-saving surgical procedures."

Unfortunately, the power and real achievements of this biomedical model have tended to narrow human perspective over time. People have come to view all illness as primarily a malfunction of mechanical parts and to regard physicians as technicians responsible for their repair. People have lost sight of the importance of the psychological, social, economic, and environmental influences on health and illness and of the extraordinary power of the mind to affect the body.

The Mind/Body Connection

In the last 30 years, scientists have begun to explore the complex interconnections between mind and body. "Psychological, sociological, and anthropological studies have confirmed what was clinically obvious—that people who are beset with poverty, job dissatisfaction, prejudice, cultural dislocation, long-term loneliness, or the loss of a loved one are far more vulnerable to illness and death than those who are fulfilled in their social and interpersonal world," states Dr. Gordon.

Mood, attitude, and belief can affect virtually every chronic illness. Fear, cynicism, as well as a sense of hopelessness and helplessness, can have a detrimental effect on health, whereas courage, good humor, a sense of control, and hopefulness can all be beneficial. Optimistic people are less likely to become ill and, when they do become ill, tend to live longer and suffer less. Studies at Yale and Rutgers Universities by Ellen Idler, Ph.D., Professor of Sociology at Rutgers, and Stanislav Kasl, Ph.D., Professor of Epidemiology at Yale, indicate that the opinion of one's health status—how well one thinks one is—may be the best predictor of well-being and future health.[1]

 See Biofeedback Training and Neurotherapy, Bodywork, Energy Medicine, Guided Imagery, Flower Essences, Hypnotherapy, Qigong and Tai Chi, Yoga.

The scientific underpinnings for these clinical studies and anecdotal reports may be found in the new and rapidly expanding field of psychoneuroimmunology. The fruits of this approach are already being harvested in comprehensive programs of mind/body medicine at Harvard University, the University of Massachusetts, Stanford University, the University of Miami, and the University of California at San Francisco. Here, people with such life-threatening and debilitating illnesses as cancer, AIDS, heart disease, and chronic pain are learning to change their habits and attitudes, what they eat, when they exercise, and how they think. A number of landmark studies have shown that these men and women are functioning

MIND/BODY MEDICINE AND THE HUMAN ENERGY FIELD

According to Janet Hranicky, Ph.D., Founder and President of the American Health Institute, in Los Angeles, California, our thoughts and emotions have a direct impact on our energy level and on the bioenergy field that surrounds our physical bodies. "In traditional psychiatry and psychology, we are still in a disease model where our focus is on alleviating symptoms," Dr. Hranicky says. "In mind/body medicine, however, if we have patients focus on their problems, dissatisfactions, fears, etc., we tend to see at an energetic level that their energy goes down as they focus on what's not right in their lives. The focus in mind/body medicine, therefore, must be to strengthen the conditioning of the mind to pick a 'better' thought that feels good, rather than to spend extensive time on childhood problems, for example. This doesn't mean that there are not appropriate times to address problem resolutions. However, in mind/body medicine, energy is paramount. It takes energy for the body to heal. Excitement and passion produce high energy states, whereas hopelessness and pain create low energy levels, and fear and anxiety tend to create chaotic energy patterns."

Dr. Hranicky points out that in the conventional model of medicine, patients are usually referred to psychiatry if they display emotional distress. "Their psychological consultation is viewed as a separate issue and is not taken as an essential component of their diagnostic work-up," she says. "In mind/body medicine, emotions are viewed as indicators of the person's state of consciousness, which has everything to do with the bioenergy field. Disturbances in the bioenergy field reflect disturbances in one's consciousness and these disturbances precede the development of illness. We know, for example, that disturbances in the bioenergy field occur weeks, months, and often years before disturbances occur in cells and tissues. In the same manner, changes in consciousness shift the bioenergy field, which then alters the course of disease. Spontaneous remission, for instance, has to do with disturbances in physical matter such as tumors disappearing, often quite quickly, when healthy shifts occur in the strength, coherency, and flow in the bioenergy field."

Research by Dr. Hranicky and others in the field of mind/body medicine indicates that although there are numerous therapies that can be used to address physical or mental/emotional health conditions, if the patient's consciousness doesn't change during the course of treatment, the results achieved usually don't hold. Mind/body medicine, therefore, is ideally suited to facilitate such changes in consciousness and, correspondingly, the bioenergy field, due to its ability to positively shift habitual patterns of limiting negative mental/emotional behavior.

---

far more effectively, feeling better, and, in some particularly striking instances, living longer.[2]

Psychoneuroimmunology

In the 1970s, great advances in the study of the immune system helped to clarify the relationship between body and mind, which gave rise to the field of psychoneuroimmunology (PNI). Researchers found that naturally occurring substances known as peptides or neuropeptides (messenger molecules made up of amino acids) could cause alterations of mood, pain, and pleasure.[3] Among the first of these substances identified were endorphins, which is shorthand for endogenous morphines, or the brain's own morphine. When endorphins are released, they produce pleasurable responses similar to those associated with opiates.

"We theorize that these neuropeptides and their receptors are the biochemical correlates of emotions," says Candace Pert, Ph.D., visiting Professor at the Center for Molecular and Behavioral Neuroscience, at Rutgers University, in New Jersey, and former Chief of the Section on Brain Biochemistry of the Clinical Neuroscience Branch at the National Institute of Mental Health. "It took us 15 years of research before we dared make that connection," Dr. Pert adds, "but we know that these neuropeptides are released during different emotional states.

"But the astounding revelation is that these endorphins and other chemicals like them are found not just in the brain, but in the immune system, the endocrine system, and throughout the body. When people discovered that there were endorphins in the brain that caused euphoria and pain relief, everyone could handle that. However, when they discovered they were in the immune system as well, it just didn't fit, so these findings were denied for years. The original scientists had to repeat their studies many times to be believed."

Emotions, previously thought to be purely psychological, could now be linked to specific chemical processes taking place throughout the body, not just in the brain. Likewise, these peptides were seen to affect the functioning of all the systems of the body, including the immune system. "Viruses use the same receptors [as a neuropeptide] to enter a cell," explains Dr. Pert, "and depending on how much of the natural peptide for that receptor is around, the virus will have an easier or harder time getting into the cell. So our emotional state will affect whether we'll get sick from the same dose of a virus."

> *The immune system, like the central nervous system, has a memory and the capacity to learn. Thus, it could be said that intelligence is located in every cell of the body and that the traditional separation of mind and body no longer applies.*

Statistics have always borne out this relationship between the emotional state of an individual and his or her health, adds Dr. Pert. "You know the data about how people have more heart attacks on Monday mornings, and how death peaks in Christians the day after Christmas and in Chinese people the day after the Chinese New Year," but now science has been able to confirm that emotional fluctuations and emotional status directly influence the probability that a person will get sick or be well.

Researchers also discovered that the immune system, like the central nervous system, has a memory and the capacity to learn. Thus, it could be said that intelligence is located in every cell of the body and that the traditional separation of mind and body no longer applies. Robert Ader, Ph.D., Director of the Division of Behavior and Psychosocial Medicine at the University of Rochester School of Medicine, in New York, considered by many to be the father of PNI, conducted several studies that confirmed this belief. In one study, rats were given an immune-suppressing drug flavored with saccharin. Eventually, they were conditioned to suppress their immune systems in response to the taste of saccharin alone.[4] Another study showed that their immune systems could be similarly enhanced through conditioning. Dr. Ader suggests that people "can learn to influence the balance that maintains health in relation to the outside world."[5]

"Conditioning is a powerful bridge between mind and body," states Joan Borysenko, Ph.D., for "the body cannot tell the difference between events that are actual threats to survival and events that are present in thought alone."[6] The implications of this work for human learning are vast, for they strongly suggest that internal and external stimuli (memories, thoughts, emotions, body movements, sounds, smells, tastes, situations, settings) can affect a variety of previously conditioned immune responses.

 See Stress.

The Effect of Consciousness on the Body

The extent by which consciousness can affect control over the body is remarkable. Biofeedback research, for example, has shown that individuals can learn to control brain-wave activity, affect cardiovascular and respiratory functioning, reduce skin temperature, and voluntarily modify many other autonomic processes of the body. John Basmajian, M.D., Professor Emeritus, Department of Medicine, at McMaster University, in Canada, who is a pioneer in biofeedback research, demonstrated that people could learn to consciously control individual neurons and muscle cells.[7] Single cell control through consciousness offers the possibility that, knowing how this process works, one can affect any part of one's body.

> *This extension of conscious control over involuntary systems has far-reaching implications for psychology and medicine. It suggests that human beings are not biological robots controlled entirely by genes and the conditioning of life experiences.*
> —ELMER GREEN, PH.D., AND ALYCE GREEN

Numerous other studies have demonstrated that consciousness can be used to relieve tension headaches, hypertension, incontinence, temporomandibular joint syndrome, involuntary muscle spasms (dyskinesia), and muscle paralysis caused by cerebrovascular accidents. Consciousness can also be directed toward lowering blood pressure, reducing certain malfunctions of the heart, and modifying gastrointestinal secretions that cause ulcers, stomach acidity, and irritable bowel syndrome.[8]

FIGHT-OR-FLIGHT AND "PLEASURE-FREEZE" RESPONSES TO STRESS

Virtually everyone has experienced the "fight-or-flight" response to some degree. This response is the body's natural, unconscious reaction to threats, either real or imagined. It is often characterized by an adrenaline rush, dilated pupils, and a racing heart, all conditions that equip the body to deal with whatever danger is perceived, be it from an animal, another person, a vehicle, or an imaginary threat, such as a bad dream. The body's physiological processes adapt to the emotional reaction to danger. According to Joan Borysenko, Ph.D., "It's what allows a small woman whose child has been run over to lift a two-ton truck off of that child."

Originally it was thought that the immune system played no part in the fight-or-flight mechanism, but new evidence has pointed to a different conclusion. In one study done immediately after the 1987 Los Angeles earthquake, blood was taken from 19 people 2-4 hours after the event and then again several times over the next year. What the study found was an increase in immune cells (such as antibodies) in the bloodstream just after the earthquake. The distress the individuals were experiencing, coupled with the fear that the "big one" might be coming next, correlated directly with the increase in immune cells.[10] While the alarm response mobilizes the body's ability to fight or get away from a threat, the immune system activation may be seen as the body preparing itself to deal with the results of such a response, such as cuts and bruises sustained while fleeing or injuries from a hostile encounter.

This response is healthy and normal in situations of extreme stress or danger. However, when it manifests too often as a reaction to everyday stresses, the cumulative result can strain the various systems of the body, including the immune system. The body can become conditioned to react in this way, sometimes with little or no impetus, particularly among people who tend to internalize their emotions. This suggests a link between the body's emotional state and its overall health. Relaxation and the "venting" of pent-up emotions, negative or otherwise, have shown positive results counteracting this overactive fight-or-flight response.[11]

While the fight-or-flight response is well-known to most medical practitioners, another type of response to stress is often ignored, according to Janet Hranicky, Ph.D., Founder and President of the American Health Institute, in Los Angeles, California. "Not only can one fight or flee in response stress, one can also detach as a way of neutralizing danger," she says. Such detachment involves repressing or freezing of emotion, according to Dr. Hranicky, and in the long-term can result in what she terms the "pleasure-freeze" response.

"We naturally move towards pleasure (comfort) emotionally and physically unless we have learned to 'hold back' because of previous pain," Dr. Hranicky explains. "Detachment is a defense response to neutralize emotional pain, anger, and fear so as not to feel discomfort. When we use detachment on a regular basis, we get good at numbing ourselves and, emotionally, we lose our normal feedback mechanisms that would ordinarily signal us to make some changes behaviorally. Long-term freezing of, or holding back from, emotions prohibits them from being fluid. When any of our emotions become frozen, the energy they contain is not discharged from the body, which can lead to serious health consequences."

"This extension of conscious control over involuntary systems has far-reaching implications for psychology and medicine," add pioneering researchers Elmer Green, Ph.D., and Alyce Green, Founders of the Voluntary Controls Program at the Menninger Clinic, in Topeka, Kansas. "It suggests that human beings are not biological robots controlled entirely by genes and the conditioning of life experiences."[9]

Steven Fahrion, Ph.D., Co-founder of Life Sciences Institute of Mind–Body Health, in Topeka, Kansas, recalls a 43-year-old middle management executive who came to him for treatment of elevated blood pressure. Dr. Fahrion noted that the man talked rapidly, was over-scheduled, and felt he never had enough time. The patient was given biofeedback exercises so that he could learn to relax by consciously controlling the temperature of his hands and feet. He also learned to meditate and use visualization techniques in order to slow down his racing mind. As the man was able to sit quietly, he also began to have insights into his feelings and the way he managed his life, which he discussed with Dr. Fahrion. After 3 ½ months, the man's blood pressure returned to normal.

MULTIPLE PERSONALITIES

The phenomenon of the multiple personality patient may offer evidence of how mental states directly affect physiology. Often a person with multiple personalities will switch medical conditions when another personality takes over. By changing personalities, they can switch physiological states, going from drunk to sober, sedated to alert, or left- to right-handed.[17]

John Sward, Ph.D., of the Center for the Improvement of Human Functioning, in Wichita, Kansas, witnessed this several years ago when a patient manifested allergies while in a different personality state. Working with an allergist who would first test the woman for a certain allergy, Dr. Sward would then hypnotize her into a different personality state and the reaction would cease. Additionally, Dr. Sward found that the allergist could send the person into a different personality merely by placing different antigens on her skin.

The ability of a multiple personality patient to substitute personalities when in pain is an example of how mind/body states can affect the healing process.

Principles of Mind/Body Medicine

Mind/body medicine extends beyond the parameters of psychoneuroimmunology to include the fields of psychology and physics in a new "science of consciousness," a view that sees energy as the underlying pattern of the universe. This view bears similarities to many Asian philosophies that see human beings as part of an interconnected, universal energy field. These Eastern traditions (Ayurvedic medicine, traditional Chinese medicine) have for centuries believed that consciousness plays an essential role in governing physical and psychological health.[12]

 See Ayurvedic Medicine, Traditional Chinese Medicine.

Mind/body medicine encompasses the following basic principles, which are often ignored or unrecognized by contemporary Western medicine.

Each Person is Unique

No two people are alike, so even if they have the same disease, the paths to recovery may be different. Conversely, the same disease can be the result of different factors with different people. Although these principles have been long recognized in traditional Chinese medicine and Ayurvedic medicine, it is a relatively new concept in Western medicine. One person, for example, may contract pneumonia as a result of a serious infection or cold, while someone else may come down with the same disease as a result of psychological stress. Yet a third person could become susceptible due to a nutritional or biochemical imbalance. Roger Williams, Ph.D., a pioneer in biochemistry, called this phenomenon "biochemical individuality," for he recognized that each of us is genetically unique, requiring slight variations in nutrient intake in order to function optimally.[13]

Chronic Stress

A basic premise in mind/body medicine is that chronic stress and lack of balance contribute to illness. Likewise, relaxation, positive methods of coping with stress, and restoration of balance lead to health. More important than the stressors themselves is the person's ability to cope. When stressors are met as a challenge and the individual feels competent to cope effectively, health may be enhanced. On the other hand, stress can cause people to turn to desperate measures to try to cope, as in the case of substance abuse.

In the general adaptation syndrome model, developed by Hans Selye, M.D., a pioneering stress researcher, chronic activation of the fight-or-flight response leads to strain on an organ system over time and interferes with its ability to adapt. Ultimately, the system breaks down and illness can set in.[14]

British cardiologist Peter Nixon explains that increased stress and arousal causes numerous changes in body functioning that eventually interfere with immune function, protein synthesis, and heart function. Repetitive stress also uses up the body's reserves, leading to increased stress on other physiological functions. This can result in heart disease, cancer, or depression.[15]

If stress contributes to illness, then stress reduction should promote healing. This is the basis of numerous healing modalities such as progressive relaxation, guided imagery, and biofeedback. One such stress reduction method, the relaxation response technique, developed by Herbert Benson, M.D., of Harvard University, is a distillation of basic meditative practice and has been shown to decrease heart rate and blood pressure, enhance health, and reduce the incidence of illness.[16] These basic stress reduction practices can be learned and used by anyone.

Taking Self-Responsibility for Healing

Mind/body medicine supports the view that the patient is an active partner in all stages of treatment, rather than a passive recipient of medical intervention. Lawrence LeShan, Ph.D., a pioneer in mind/body medicine for the treatment of cancer, has documented that cancer patients who took charge of their life direction were more likely to recover than those who passively accepted their diagnosis.[18]

Taking action also decreases the fear and depression that so often accompanies life-threatening illness. By becoming actively involved in self-healing, one shifts from feelings of helplessness and hopelessness, which have been shown to increase depression and the risk of death, to a sense of control.[19]

By becoming actively involved in self-healing, one shifts from feelings of helplessness and hopelessness, which have been shown to increase depression and the risk of death, to a sense of control.

Immune functions are also affected by the experiences of helplessness or control. In one study, animals that were conditioned to experience helplessness were more likely to develop cancer from injected tumor cells and die than other animals. Animals trained to have a sense of control were best able to reject the tumor cells.[20]

The Body's Innate Healing Capabilities

The body has a natural, biological tendency to move toward health and balance, a phenomenon that can be observed in the simple healing of a cut in which the body automatically closes the wound and repairs the damage. The well-known "placebo effect" (in which a neutral substance is found to effectively cure an ailment) also demonstrates the body's capacity to heal itself. Erik Peper, Ph.D., Associate Director of the Institute for Holistic Healing Studies at San Francisco State University, suggests that "the placebo effect can decrease or remove the constraints that are interfering with the body's intrinsic drive toward wholeness." These constraints can include feelings of helplessness and hopelessness, negative beliefs about the illness, and negative self-images.

HOW HEALTHY ARE YOUR THOUGHTS AND BELIEFS?

"It is important to identify if one's thoughts and beliefs and their resultant feelings are healthy or unhealthy," states Janet Hranicky, Ph.D., of Los Angeles, California. To help make this determination, she developed the following questionnaire:

- Are your thoughts based on fact?

- Do your thoughts/beliefs help to protect your life and health?

- Do your thoughts/beliefs help you reach your short- and long-term goals?

- Do your thoughts/beliefs help you avoid your most undesirable conflicts?

- Do your thoughts/beliefs make you feel the way you want to feel?

"If a person answers 'no' to any three of these questions, the belief or thought is considered unhealthy and needs to be changed," Dr. Hranicky says.

Jeanne Achterberg, Ph.D., past President of the Association for Transpersonal Psychology, adds that the effectiveness of the placebo varies "depending upon how much the patient expects to benefit." In other words, those who think they will get better have a significantly greater recovery rate than those who think they will not get better or think they will get worse.[21]

The Importance of the Client-Provider Relationship

The relationship between the client and the physician can strongly influence the healing process. For example, when a physician is perceived as powerful and trustworthy, the client gets better faster, and one study has even shown that physician reassurance and support raises the threshold of pain tolerance in patients.[22]

Mind/body medicine recognizes that the practitioner is constantly communicating (consciously and unconsciously) with the client. Just as the placebo is seen as a way of promoting healing through the patient's belief system, the positive attitude of the doctor can influence the outcome of a given treatment, while discouraging statements or prejudices can evoke what some call a "nocebo" effect by undermining the patient's confidence and hindering the healing process.

Unfortunately, this dimension of the healing process is rarely noticed or addressed. Thus, a doctor who thinks of a patient as hopeless will convey this to the patient even if the thought is unspoken. In the ideal client/provider relationship, the healing process is viewed as a working partnership in which both parties respect the knowledge and intuition of the other. In this respect, the health-care provider seeks to convey the potential for wholeness in each client.

A Systems Approach

Mind/body medicine is based upon a systems perspective that recognizes that human lives are influenced by many interrelated factors, including genetics, family and socioeconomic background, diet, exercise, social support, risk-taking behaviors, attitudes, and spiritual practices. An illness may be a manifestation of imbalance on the physical level, but the imbalance may also originate in other aspects of the self, such as the mental or emotional state.

Any movement toward health mobilizes the other healing potentials of the body. As a person makes a change in one area, other areas tend to change as well. For example, if a person begins to exercise, they may feel more socially confident and might spontaneously change eating habits, thus improving overall physical and emotional health. While any disease may be a problem in but a small part of the total person, the factors that influence its manifestation and subsequent healing can be extraordinarily complex.

The Energy Field Perspective

Each of us has various fields of energy that can be measured with an EKG (electrocardiograph), EEG (electroencephalograph), or electrodermal screening (EDS—a method of testing based on measurement of the electrical properties of acupuncture points). These energy fields are continuously affected by changes in physical or psychological health and can even be influenced by the energy fields of others.

Robert Becker, M.D., a pioneer in the study of the effects of electromagnetism on health, found that small electric currents can stimulate cells to regenerate, fractures to heal faster, and tissue to repair itself.[23] Research in neuropsychiatry over the past few decades has shown that small electric currents between specific points in the brain give rise to the same behavioral changes that are observed with the injection of certain brain-stimulating chemicals.[24]

The energy field perspective can even be applied to hospital settings. Dolores Krieger, Ph.D., R.N., Professor Emeritus of Nursing at New York University, developed a technique known as Therapeutic Touch, which has been proven effective in treating a variety of medical conditions. According to Dr. Krieger, Therapeutic Touch is a "contemporary interpretation of several ancient healing practices in which the practitioner consciously directs or sensitively modulates human energies."[25] The proper use of Therapeutic Touch can increase hemoglobin (enhancing oxygen levels) and decrease anxiety,[26] reduce pain, accelerate the healing of surgical wounds, and help correct dysfunctions of the autonomic nervous system.[27] This technique has been taught to more than 37,000 nurses, doctors, and health practitioners.[28]

In mind/body medicine, one looks beyond the immediate problem to include a larger dimension of one's life. A heart attack may be a signal for a person to become less defensive and hostile, less competitive at work, and to give more attention to relaxation, hobbies, family, and the enjoyment of life.

The importance of human touch is greatly emphasized in mind/body medicine, especially for children. "In a child, absence of touch can cause the pituitary gland to not secrete enough growth hormone," says Dr. Borysenko. "The child will dwarf, developing what is called 'failure to thrive' syndrome. The child can't assimilate nutrients and may actually sicken and die." Handling and physical affection have been shown to increase the survival rate of infants, improve psychological skills and functioning, promote physical growth and immune function, and, most importantly, enable a person to respond effectively to stress.[29] Also, autopsies on animals that were given extra handling and care showed much less damage to their cardiovascular and intestinal systems than those who were not handled.[30]

Illness as Message, Not Enemy

In many ways, conventional medicine conveys the notion of all-out war against disease, in which illness is seen as an enemy and death as a failure. From a mind/body perspective, illness is seen as a communication from the body, a warning signal that something needs attention. People can use this "message" to review the entire mind/body system and see how it is functioning as a whole. If a person experiences back pain, he or she might ask, "Am I carrying too much emotional weight? Am I under too much stress? Am I using my body properly or exercising it well?"

In mind/body medicine, one looks beyond the immediate problem to include a larger dimension of one's life. For example, a heart attack may be a signal for a person to become less defensive and hostile, less competitive at work, and to give more attention to relaxation, hobbies, family, and the enjoyment of life. In this process, a person's heart will heal both literally and symbolically. The highly successful program for healing heart disease conducted by Dean Ornish, M.D., Assistant Clinical Professor of Medicine at the University of California at San Francisco, utilizes these components.[31]

How Healing Occurs from a Mind/Body Perspective

Ultimately, we do not know how healing occurs. The best we can do is to support and encourage the body's intrinsic healing mechanisms. Mind/body medicine often begins by promoting physical and mental relaxation and developing better ways of coping with stress. Various techniques and lifestyle changes may be employed in this holistic approach to health, based on each person's specific needs and preferences.

By taking time to relax, one becomes more mindful of one's condition, grows more aware of the body's subtle signals, and responds to stress long before its destructive effects can take hold. By incorporating short relaxation practices throughout the day and conditioning oneself to relax instead of tensing when encountering a source of stress, the depleted energy reserves can be rebuilt. How a person frames or perceives experiences may also have a direct impact on the immune system. Symbolic threats produce real physiological consequences, as every good worrier knows. Perception of meaning, and the language used, may also be an essential element of healing.

Health Requires Emotional Balance

Grief, bereavement, depression, fear, and panic have been shown to suppress the immune response, while laughter, play, love, faith, hope, and self-acceptance help to stimulate and balance immune function. Part of healing, then, involves the recognition and release of negative emotions such as resentment, guilt, anger, and self-hatred, and fostering of feelings of well-being, adequacy, and self-con-

---

PSYCHOLOGICAL FACTORS ENHANCE HEALTH AND HEALING

In the journal *Science,* 62 studies were cited showing that supportive social relationships—friends, extended family, marital ties, and group membership—had a positive effect upon surgical recovery, recovery from chronic and infectious disease, and improvements of cardiovascular activity and immune function. A lack of these supportive relationships significantly increased the incidence of death.[37] Jeanne Achterberg, Ph.D., cites numerous additional studies demonstrating that:

- Feelings of helplessness and hopelessness increase cancer growth and digestive problems.

- Anxiety and stress increase the production of adrenal corticosteroids, which interfere with healing, compromise the immune system, and encourage cardiovascular disease.

- Fear and anxiety inhibit the cells' repair mechanisms.

- Feelings of security, coupled with the ability to cope, counter the deleterious effects of negative emotions.

- Joy and relaxation increase circulation to painful or wounded areas and improve tissue repair.[38]

---

trol. Studies have shown that having a sense of control, commitment, and connectedness—along with viewing change as a challenge rather than a threat—promotes the maintenance of good health even when under stress.[32]

Sharing and Support

Satisfaction in relationships and work are essential to happiness and health. Healthy relationships are characterized by a mutual flow of giving and receiving, mutual support and respect, and the ability to work out conflicts and difficulties. To be able to share feelings and pain with one another is an essential component to healing, for it shows us that people are not alone and that they have something to offer. This can be accomplished in therapy, in social groups, and through the development of friends or close family relationships. In one study, women with breast cancer who participated in a weekly support group lived twice as long as those who did not.[33]

"There is overwhelming evidence that people who have few social contacts are more likely to get sick and less likely to recover from an illness," says Dr. Peper. One long-term study found that people with the lowest number of social ties were two to three times more likely to die of all causes than those with the most social connectedness.[34] "Isolation and loneliness have been shown to result in immune problems in bereaved individuals who have recently lost their loved ones," adds Dr. Fahrion.

Therapies of Mind/Body Medicine

The goal of mind/body medicine is to provide patients with a better understanding of their thoughts, emotions, beliefs and attitudes, in a manner that enables them to more effectively cope with stress and harness their innate abilities to heal illness and maintain optimal wellness. To achieve these goals, a variety of therapeutic approaches might be employed. These include biofeedback training and neurotherapy, certain forms of bodywork, energy medicine, flower essences, guided imagery and visualization, and hypnotherapy, each of which is covered more extensively in separate chapters. Other approaches include autogenic training, breathwork, "energy psychology," Eye Movement Desensitization and Reprocessing (EMDR), meditation, Neuro-Emotional Technique (NET), and Neuro-Linguistic Programming (NLP).

Guided Imagery

Guided imagery is an important tool for healing. Dr. Achterberg suggests that every image a person has in the mind can affect immune function, blood flow, and heart rate.[35] Other studies have shown that guided imagery can decrease chronic nightmares,[36] reduce substance abuse, and alleviate many other psychological and physiological problems.

Autogenic Training

Based on the research of German neurologist Johannes Schultz, M.D., in the 1930s, autogenic training involves the use of autosuggestions that are intended to induce a reverie, or autogenic state of deep relaxation. Dr. Schultz discovered that regular experience of this deeply relaxed state not only resulted in increased energy and decreased bodily tension, but over time also enabled patients to gain greater control of the autonomic nervous system (ANS) and the various processes of the ANS that are considered involuntary. In that regard, autogenic training has much in common with biofeedback training.

According to Dr. Schultz, the benefits of autogenic training can be achieved by the use of six basic suggestions. People who practice the technique do so by closing their eyes while sitting or lying down. They then tell themselves: "My arms and legs are heavy. My arms and legs are warm. My heartbeat is calm and regular. It breathes me. My abdomen is warm. My forehead is cool." Initially, this exercise is practiced for 5-15 minutes, two to three times a day, under the guidance of a trained professional, until patients become able to easily induce the relaxing effects on their own, simply by repeating the six suggestions to themselves (usually within six months or less of regular practice).

Autogenic training has been found useful for cardiovascular conditions, gallbladder dysfunction, gastrointestinal disorders, headaches, muscle tension and spasm, nausea, respiratory conditions, sexual dysfunction, and vomiting.[39]

Breathwork

Regulation of breathing plays an important role in mind/body medicine, because it is capable of bringing about a state of relaxation. Shallow chest breathing and hyperventilation, for example, are part of the body's response to stress. These dysfunctional breathing patterns can cause increased heart rate, blood vessel constriction, and muscle tension, as well as negative thoughts.

A person who suppresses unpleasant feelings and thoughts may also unknowingly restrict their breathing. Thus, it is important to express and release these emotions in order to maintain proper breathing. Likewise, proper breathing can help facilitate an emotional release. Many psychologically oriented therapies such as Reichian therapy emphasize emotional release through deliberate alteration of breathing patterns.

Slow, conscious, diaphragmatic breathing is a powerful tool for promoting relaxation and awareness. It is an essential component of many therapeutic approaches to the body and the mind and is utilized in most forms of meditation as well as in yoga and Qigong. When heart patients, who are usually shallow chest breathers, learn slow diaphragmatic breathing, there is a 50% drop in recurrence of coronary events.[40] It can also be used to reduce panic attacks, headaches, chest pain, and other symptoms.

In a study at San Francisco State University, Dr. Peper and his student Vicci Tibbets worked with a group of asthmatics to help them learn self-regulation approaches. Participants met in a group for 16 weeks, utilizing the power of group support. They were given diaphragmatic breathing and biofeedback training for calming the upper body muscles. Once breathing techniques were mastered, the participants learned to use them in increasingly stressful situations. As they began to feel in control, their fears decreased and a sense of hope emerged. Those participants who took charge of their lives and continued with their training were found to be in better shape at the 15-month follow-up, showing that self-responsibility contributed to the enhancement of their health.[41]

Energy Psychology

Energy psychology, a term coined by Fred P. Gallo, Ph.D., a leading practitioner in the field, is an outgrowth of the pioneering research of Roger Callahan, Ph.D., developer of Callahan Thought Field Therapy™ (TFT). Dr. Callahan first began to discover the principles of TFT in 1980, while working as a clinical psychotherapist. At that time, one of his clients was a woman who suffered from a fear of water. Dr. Callahan had worked with her for approximately 18 months using conventional psychotherapeutic approaches, but her phobia remained basically unchanged. One day, during a therapy session, the woman remarked that in addition to her fear of water, she was now experiencing stomach symptoms. Familiar with acupuncture's concept of energetic meridian pathways, Dr. Callahan was aware that the meridian that passes along the stomach begins at an acupoint located just below the eye. On a hunch, he lightly tapped this point on the woman's face with his fingertips. To their mutual surprise, her water phobia completely disappeared.[42] Based on this experience, Dr. Callahan developed the specific tapping sequences of TFT, which can be used to treat a variety of psychological conditions.

TFT has been shown to be remarkably effective for providing quick, effective, and lasting relief of most psychological problems, including anxiety and depression, addiction, alcoholism, irrational fears and phobias, limited and self-sabotaging beliefs, panic attacks, post-traumatic stress disorder, sexual dysfunctions, stress, and trauma related to rape and child abuse. More recent research has also found that TFT can provide relief for a number of physical conditions as well, including allergies (food and environmental), attention deficit hyperactivity disorder (ADHD), chronic pain, fibromyalgia, hypertension, seasonal affective disorder (SAD), and sinus problems.[43]

In the past decade, a number of practitioners, including some initially trained by Dr. Callahan, have developed other meridian-based tapping methods, resulting in the emergence of the energy psychology field. Other energy psychology approaches include Emotional Freedom Techniques (EFT), developed by Gary Craig; Energy Diagnostic and Treatment Methods, developed by Dr. Gallo; Emotional Self-Management, developed by Peter Lambrou, Ph.D., and George Pratt, Ph.D.; and Quantum Emotional Clearing, developed by Lee Beymer, Dipl. Ac.

"Energy psychology studies the effects of the body's own energy systems as they relate to emotions, behavior, and psychological health," Dr. Gallo says. "These energy systems include electrical activity of the nervous system, acupuncture meridians, chakras, biofields, and morphogenesis [energetic developmental processes which establish the form of the body and its organs]. While our psychological functioning involves cognitive, hormonal, neurochemical, and environmental causes, energy psychology holds that at a fundamental level, bioenergy significantly accounts for behavior."[44]

In addition to conventional therapy approaches, energy psychology employs various methods that specifically diagnose and address the underlying energetic aspects of a patient's problems. These include muscle testing (kinesiology), sequential tapping or holding of specific acupuncture meridians, body postures, breathwork, and affirmations, and can also focus on the exploration of the relationship among bioenergy, consciousness, thought, intentionality, and spirituality.[45]

"Dr. Callahan's original work discovered that residual energies in the body can cause a repetitive pattern of negative emotions," Beymer adds. "The basic understanding behind the energy psychology phenomena is that negative energy, when it becomes embedded in one's energy matrix, grows and festers, causing repetitive negative emotional and behavioral patterns at various times throughout life. The degree of resultant 'stuckness' relates directly to the intensity of the original trauma, as well as how one internalized it. Serious traumas are frequently repressed and can often be denied completely from memory, but the negativity can continue to affect a person's life for years afterward."

The various methods that comprise the energy psychology field are said to release embedded negative energies from a patient's biofield, or energy matrix, in a way that permanently banishes them and prevents them from causing further interference. Unlike traditional psychotherapy, the techniques are completely noninvasive and do not require patients to "relive" the original traumatic events that led to their problems. Moreover, energy psychology diagnostic methods make it easier to quickly detect, diagnose, and heal problems of which neither the patient nor the practitioner are initially conscious, a process that might take years using conventional psychology procedures.

Eye Movement Desensitization and Reprocessing (EMDR)

Eye Movement Desensitization and Reprocessing (EMDR) was developed in the late 1980s by Francine Shapiro, Ph.D., Senior Research Fellow at the Mental Research Institute, in Palo Alto, California. Since then,

A SIMPLE MEDITATION EXERCISE

The first step to practicing meditation is learning to breathe in a manner that facilitates a state of calm awareness. The following exercise is recommended as an effective method for achieving calmness by Jon Kabat-Zinn, Ph.D., Founder and Director of the Stress Reduction Clinic at the University of Massachusetts Medical Center, in Worchester.

- Find a quiet place where you will not be disturbed and assume a comfortable position, lying on your back or sitting. If sitting, keep the spine straight and let your shoulders drop.

- Close your eyes if it feels comfortable.

- Bring your attention to your belly, feeling it rise or expand gently on the in-breath, and fall or recede on the out-breath.

- Keep your focus on your breathing, "being with" each in-breath.

- Every time you notice that your mind has wandered off the breath, notice what it was that took you away and then gently bring your attention back to your belly and the sensation of your breath moving in and out.

- Each time your attention wanders away from your breath, simply bring it back to your breath, no matter what it has become preoccupied with.

Practice this exercise for 15 minutes at a convenient time every day, whether you feel like it or not. After one week, notice how it feels to incorporate a disciplined meditation practice into your life.

sations associated with their behavioral problems. As they do so, keeping attention on the experiences that disturb them, the patient follows specific hand movements performed by EMDR therapists. Other methods may also be used by EMDR therapists, such as tapping alternate sides of the patient's body or the use of shifting sounds from ear to ear. According to Dr. Shapiro, these techniques enable patients to reprocess how they perceive and respond to what happened to them and to then replace the limiting thoughts and emotions linked to their trauma with those of a more positive nature "that are more congruent with the present."

She cautions, however, that the eye movements associated with EMDR, in and of themselves, are not enough to get the results typically achieved by EMDR, and when used inappropriately can even result in psychological harm. Although the mechanisms by which EMDR works have yet to be fully explained, studies have verified that it is effective in achieving "permanent resolution of deep-seated emotional issues related to trauma and stress, often in as few as one to three sessions."[46] As a result, EMDR is one of the fastest-growing therapies in the mind/body field.

Meditation

According to Dr. Borysenko, meditation can be broadly defined as any activity that keeps the attention pleasantly anchored in the present moment. In this state, the mind is calm and focused, not reacting to memories from the past nor preoccupied with future concerns, two major sources of chronic stress that can negatively impact health.

There are numerous approaches to meditation, most of which fall into two categories, concentrative meditation and mindfulness meditation. Concentrative meditation focuses the attention on the breath, an image, or a sound (mantra) in order to still the mind and allow a greater awareness and clarity to emerge. The simplest form of concentrative meditation is to sit quietly and focus the attention on the breath. When a person is anxious, frightened, agitated, or distracted, the breath will tend to be shallow, rapid, and uneven. But when the mind is calm and focused, the breath tends to be slow, deep, and regular. As the mind becomes absorbed in the rhythm of inhalation and exhalation, breathing becomes deeper and the mind becomes more tranquil and aware.

Mindfulness meditation, according to Dr. Borysenko, "involves opening the attention to become aware of the continuously passing parade of sensations, feelings, images, thoughts, sounds, smells, and so forth without becoming involved in thinking about them." The meditator sits quietly and simply witnesses whatever passes through the mind, not reacting or becoming involved in thoughts,

EMDR has experienced rapid growth in the mind/body and psychotherapeutic fields due to its impressive results in dealing with psychological conditions such as anxiety, depression, phobias, and post-traumatic stress disorder. It is well-known by mind/body practitioners that the initial painful emotions and beliefs caused by trauma and which accompany such conditions often go unresolved, making it difficult to fully recover.

During an EMDR session, the patient places the attention on the thoughts, memories, and physical sen-

memories, worries, or images. This helps produce a calm, clear, and non-reactive state of mind.

The psychophysiological health effects of meditation have been studied in the West since the 1960s. As a result of the large body of research attesting to its many benefits, growing numbers of physicians, psychotherapists, and other health-care professionals are recommending meditation to their patients. Studies have shown that meditation can bring about a healthy state of relaxation by causing a generalized reduction in multiple physiological and biochemical markers, such as decreased heart rate, decreased respiration rate, decreased cortisol (a major stress hormone), and an increase in brain waves associated with relaxation.[47]

Research shows that meditation has benefits for addiction, allergies, Alzheimer's disease, anxiety, arthritis, cancer, cardiovascular disease, chronic pain, depression, diabetes, emphysema, endometriosis, hepatitis, hypertension, indigestion, insomnia, memory loss, menopause, obsessive-compulsive disorder, osteoporosis, premenstrual syndrome (PMS), psoriasis and other skin disorders, recovery from surgery, sexual dysfunction, stroke, and ulcers, reports Dharma Singh Khalsa, M.D., author of *Meditation as Medicine*.[48]

Neuro-Emotional Technique (NET)

In the early 1980s, Scott Walker, D.C., a chiropractor since 1965, began seeking an explanation as to why some of his patients' chiropractic adjustments effectively "held" while others did not, resulting in those patients not getting well when it seemed they should have. Drawing upon a variety of healing disciplines and his own clinical experience, Dr. Walker discovered that the solution to the problem lay in addressing unresolved emotional issues and their harmful effects. Eventually, his research led him to develop a mind/body approach known as Neuro-Emotional Technique to normalize physical and emotional imbalances while assisting the body's natural healing process. Based on his successes using NET to treat patients, he began training others in its use in 1988.

According to Dr. Walker, "NET synthesizes the neuro-mechanisms of speech, general semantics, and acupuncture, and helps re-establish balance of mind and body through the use of physical (spinal or acupressure point) correction in a manner that is simple and pleasant to the patient." Research has shown that emotions are physiological events that are found in all areas of the body, involving molecules known as neuropeptides. It is for this reason that NET practitioners believe NET works. "It may also explain why patients report that NET is so agreeable and sometimes immediately life-changing," Dr. Walker adds.

NET practitioners often compare disease and health care to a baseball diamond, with each base directly influencing the other bases. In this model, first base represents emotional factors, second base symbolizes the effects of toxins on the body, third base stands for nutritional needs, and home plate addresses structural problems. NET practitioners correct each "base" of the diamond as it surfaces. They do so using muscle testing, body reflexes, and verbal constructs to produce clues for patients that enable them to recall the specific emotion, or emotions, associated with what is known as a neuro-emotional complex (NEC) in present time, as well as when it first occurred (the "original sensitizing event").

"The patient mentally holds the emotional memory, which allows the body's physiology to momentarily replicate the emotional/physiological pattern formed by the original event," Dr. Walker explains. "The NET practitioner then makes a safe, gentle, and quick physical correction. Once an NEC is eliminated, annoying behavioral and emotional patterns naturally and sometimes immediately resolve, the patient feels a sense of relief or release, and the nervous system functions more harmoniously."

NET has been found beneficial for a wide range of health conditions and is now used by health practitioners in many fields besides chiropractic. Among the most common physical conditions that respond to NET are physical pain of all types, organ dysfunction, neurological, musculoskeletal, and immunological conditions, and allergies. Commonly treated psychological conditions include phobias, depression, anxiety, obsessions and compulsive behaviors, nightmares, flashbacks, mental/emotional blocks, cognitive distortions, relationship issues, unhealthy impulsiveness, nonassertiveness, and erroneous or unhealthy beliefs and assumptions. Currently, there are over 4,000 NET practitioners in over 30 countries, all of whom are licensed health-care providers.

Neuro-Linguistic Programming

Developed by John Grinder, a professor of linguistics, and Richard Bandler, a student of psychology and mathematics, both at the University of California at Santa Cruz, Neuro-Linguistic Programming (NLP) focuses on how people learn, communicate, change, grow, and heal. *Neuro* refers to the way the brain works and how human thinking demonstrates consistent and detectable patterns. *Linguistic* refers to the verbal and nonverbal expressions of the brain's thinking patterns and *programming* refers to how these patterns are recognized and understood by the mind and how they can be altered, allowing a person to make better choices in behavior and health.

People who have difficulty recovering from physical illness have often adopted negative beliefs about their recovery. They may perceive themselves as helpless, hope-

USING NLP TO HEAL UNPLEASANT MEMORIES

The following exercise can help you learn to adjust memories and feelings, reframing them more positively to enhance your well-being.

- Close your eyes and allow yourself to recall an unpleasant memory. Depending on how you code and process your experiences, the memory will appear to you primarily as an image, a sound, or a feeling. Whichever way it happens will be the way that is most appropriate for you.

- As the memory arises, become aware of the emotions you are experiencing because of it. Now notice the memory itself. If it is visual, notice its size, its proximity, and whether or not you are seeing it in color. If your experience is primarily auditory, notice the qualities of the sounds. Are they loud, grating, or harsh? If the memory evokes a kinesthetic sensation, notice how it feels. By adjusting these qualities, you can literally change the experience itself.

- You can adjust them in the same way that you use the controls on a TV. If you are seeing an image, allow it to become blurry and indistinct. If it is in color, allow it to become black and white. Now allow it to recede, becoming smaller and smaller, until it is so small that you can hardly see it anymore. You can do the same thing with sounds and sensations, changing them until they are comfortable for you. Once you accomplish this, notice how your emotions related to the memory have also changed. You may be surprised to discover how relaxed and in control you feel and how the memory is no longer able to provoke an unpleasant reaction.

- This same exercise can be used to reinforce positive memories, thereby creating more powerful, resourceful states for yourself. As you focus on the pleasant memory, allow it to become clearer, closer, and brighter for you, then add whatever other appealing qualities you wish to create your desired state.

By regularly experimenting with this exercise, you will gain greater control over your emotions and the memories that trigger them. This, in turn, will enhance the way you feel.

---

less, or worthless, and make statements such as "I can't get healthy," "There is no hope," and "I'm not worth the effort." The primary goal of NLP practitioners is to move a person from the present state of discomfort to a desired state of health and well-being by helping to reprogram beliefs about healing. They accomplish this by asking questions to discover how a person relates to issues of identity, personal belief, and life goals. By reading autonomic body changes (skin color changes, moisture changes on the lips or eyes) and other physiological changes, NLP practitioners teach people how to tap into their individual ways of healing, based on how they process information and view their health conditions.

According to Janet Konefal, Ph.D., of Miami, Florida, identity can be a major component of the way people deal with their health conditions, particularly those suffering from chronic disease. "Too often, people tend to identify directly with their illness," Dr. Konefal explains. "A person doesn't usually say 'I'm John, who has this condition of diabetes'—he says 'I'm a diabetic.' The disease moves in and actually shifts a person's identity."

One of the first priorities of NLP is to separate a person's negative or false identifications and help them regain their real identity. Practitioners ensure that any changes will ultimately benefit all aspects of the individual, not just the particular problem being addressed. Special care is taken to keep not only family, social, and work relationships in balance, but also the person's internal systems (thoughts, strategies, behaviors, capabilities, values, and beliefs). Known as an ecology check, this is used to ascertain if NLP will be compatible with the person's specific needs and is accomplished through careful questioning before and after each session.

The practitioner will then ask patients to see themselves in a state of health. This establishes an outcome to facilitate the healing process, since the brain's natural response is to duplicate whatever images or beliefs are created about getting better.[49] The brain then triggers the necessary immunological responses to guide the body toward its goal of health and well-being. As patients are asked questions about their life and health conditions, the NLP practitioner observes their language patterns, eye movements, postures, muscle tension, and gestures, all of which relay information and report internal sensations about how patients relate to their present conditions, both consciously and unconsciously. This reveals limiting beliefs, which can then be positively altered using NLP techniques.

By identifying and removing a patient's limiting beliefs about their condition, NLP has been shown to benefit a variety of health conditions and illnesses, including allergies, pain relief and muscle relaxation, traumatic injury, immunological conditions, and a number of mental/emotional conditions (anxiety, phobia, and compulsive behaviors). Dr. Konefal reports success using NLP in conjunction with other therapies, such as acupuncture, Chinese herbs, homeopathy, and nutrition, to treat patients with HIV/AIDS.

David Paul, M.D., Medical Director of Vail Valley Medical Center, in Vail, Colorado, is a physician who frequently uses NLP in his medical practice, including as a drugless technique for placing dislocated shoulders back into their sockets. He and his colleagues have developed a technique that uses language patterns based on NLP to help patients achieve relaxation and disregard the discomfort involved in the physical manipulation. "Ninety-five percent of the time the shoulder can be put back in its socket in one minute or less without the use of morphine, valium, or similar products," Dr. Paul says. Prior to using this technique, his average success rate was between 40% and 50%.

The Future of Mind/Body Medicine

Mind/body practitioners believe that the present Western medical model will become a subset of the holistic mind/body medicine of the future. As patients recover from surgery or illness, they can be taught skills to speed up the body's healing processes, reduce pain, and reflect upon those changes necessary to improve the quality of their lives. The goal will be not to simply remove the symptom but to help the person attain a greater state of wholeness. It is a process that should continue throughout life. Since this new healing philosophy places so much power and responsibility in the hands of the patient, an educational approach is needed. Relaxation, stress reduction, guided imagery, and behavioral change can and should be taught at all levels, from elementary school to college.

There is already a program in holistic healing studies at San Francisco State University that includes traditional Chinese medicine, Western and Eastern perspectives on holistic health, relaxation training, peak performance training for athletes, meditation, and biofeedback. In addition to cognitive study, students practice daily relaxation, imagery, and other healing techniques. They report decreases in chronic headaches, improved sleep, enhanced self-awareness and self-esteem, and much greater ability to cope with stress. Many have adopted improved dietary and exercise patterns or quit smoking and some have even been able to eliminate long-standing health problems.

Throughout the U.S., major hospitals and university medical centers are also beginning to incorporate the principles of mind/body medicine. At Parkland Hospital, in Dallas, Texas, mind/body medicine has been implemented throughout the organizational system, focusing on what practitioners call "patient-centered" care, which includes personalized attention, education, self-health improvement at home, and prevention. Parkland's seven community clinics have cut their average hospital expenses in half by implementing these types of programs.

At Case Western Reserve University, in Cleveland, Ohio, and at the Menninger Clinic, biofeedback, guided imagery, and other stress reduction techniques are used to treat conditions ranging from migraines to cancer to heart disease. At the University of Massachusetts Medical Center, Jon Kabat-Zinn, Ph.D., established the Stress Reduction Clinic, where patients suffering from chronic pain are taught meditation and a new philosophy of health and well-being. "We need to take what's most valuable from the various consciousness traditions, integrate them into Western behavioral science and mainstream medicine, and study them as best we can in terms of the most sophisticated and stringent scientific methodologies," Dr. Kabat-Zinn states. "We need to ask 'What is it about these ancient traditions that tells us something valuable about healing and the mind?'"

Where to Find Help

For further information about mind/body medicine and the specific therapies covered in this chapter, contact the following organizations:

American Health Institute
12381 Wilshire Blvd.
Los Angeles, California 90025
(310) 820-6042
Website: www.ahealth.com

Founded by Dr. Janet Hranicky, the Institute is an organization devoted to education and research in all aspects of mind/body medicine and provides research-based, targeted stress management programs for individuals and corporations. Also provides a self-contained, mind/body educational program for dealing with cancer.

Center for the Improvement of Human Functioning
3100 North Hillside Avenue
Wichita, Kansas 67219-3904
(316) 682-3100
Website: www.brightspot.org

A medical research, educational organization, the Center offers clinical services, diagnostic testing, educational classes, conferences, and seminars, and performs clinical and basic research.

Center for Mind/Body Medicine
5225 Connecticut Avenue N.W., Suite 414
Washington, D.C. 20015
(202) 966-7338
Website: www.cmbm.org

The Center for Mind-Body Medicine offers an educational program for health and mental health professionals and those interested in exploring their own capacities for self-knowledge and self-care. Directed by James S. Gordon, M.D., its work is grounded in an appreciation of the interpenetration of life's biological, psychological, spiritual, and social dimensions.

Life Sciences Institute of Mind–Body Health
4636 S.W. Wanamaker Road
Topeka, Kansas 66610
(785) 271-8686
Website: www.cjnetworks.com/~lifesci

The Institute has research and treatment programs in all phases of mind/body medicine.

Mind–Body Medical Institute
Beth Israel Deaconess Medical Center
185 Francis Street, Suite 1A
Boston, Massachusetts 02215
(617) 632-9530
Website: www.mbmi.org

Overseen by Dr. Herbert Benson, the Institute provides a treatment program at a medical center where the relaxation response can be learned, using yoga, meditation, and stress reduction.

Stress Reduction and Relaxation Program
University of Massachusetts Medical Center
55 Lake Avenue North
Worcester, Massachusetts 01655
(508) 856-2656
Website: www.umassmed.edu/cfm

The Stress Reduction and Relaxation Program is a training program to teach meditative-type awareness, overseen by Dr. Jon Kabat-Zinn.

EMDR

EMDR Institute
P.O. Box 51010
Pacific Grove, California 93950
(408) 372-3900
Website: www.emdr.com

The EMDR Institute has trained over 20,000 clinicians in the methods of EMDR and maintains an international directory of Institute-trained EMDR practitioners.

Energy Psychology
The following organizations provide information about and training in various therapies within the field of energy psychology.

EMOTIONAL FREEDOM TECHNIQUES (EFT)

Gary H. Craig
P.O. Box 398
The Sea Ranch, California 95497
(707) 785-2848
Website: www.emofree.com

Holistic Communications
P.O. Box 41152
Sacramento, California 95841
(800) 644-5437
Website: www.gettingthru.org

EMOTIONAL SELF-MANAGEMENT

Global Emotional Self-Management Systems
Peter Lambrou, Ph.D., and George Pratt, Ph.D.
Scripps Memorial Hospital Campus
9834 Genesee Avenue, Suite 321
La Jolla, California 92037
(858) 457-3900
Website: www.gem-systems.com

ENERGY DIAGNOSTIC & TREATMENT METHODS

Fred P. Gallo, Ph.D.
Psychological Services
40 Snyder Road
Hermitage, Pennsylvania 16148
(724) 346-3838
Website: www.energypsych.com

QUANTUM EMOTIONAL CLEARING

Lee Beymer, Dipl.Ac.
Radiant Health, Inc.
P.O. Box 2002
Aspen, Colorado 81612
(970) 925-9148
Website: www.quantumemotionalclearing.com

THOUGHT FIELD THERAPY (TFT)

Callahan Techniques, Ltd.
78-816 Via Carmel
La Quinta, California 92253
(760) 564-1008
Website: www.tftrx.com

Meditation

Insight Meditation Society
1230 Pleasant Street
Barre, Massachusetts 01500
(978) 355-4378
Website: www.dharma.org

Provides training and information about the practice of meditation.

Washington Center for Meditation Studies
1834 Swann Street N.W.
Washington, D.C. 2009
(202) 234-2866

Provides training and information about the practice of meditation.

Neuro-Emotional Technique (NET)

NET, Inc.
510 Second Street
Encinitas, California 92024
(800) 434-3030 or (760) 944-1030
Website: www.netmindbody.com

NET, Inc., trains NET practitioners throughout the world and assists the general public in locating the most qualified practitioners in their area.

Our NET Effect (ONE) Foundation
1991 Village Park Way, Suite 201-A
Encinitas, California 92024
(800) 638-1411
Website: www.onefoundation.org

The One Foundation's mission is to establish natural healing as the standard care through NET experimental research, general public education, and humanitarian service.

Neuro-Linguistic Programming

Anchor Point Institute, L.L.C.
505 E. 200 South, Suite 250
Salt Lake City, Utah 84102
(801) 534-1022
Website: www.nlpanchorpoint.com

Provides NLP training to individuals, businesses, and government organizations. References are provided for people with health-related issues.

NLP Comprehensive
12567 W. Cedar Drive, Suite 102
Lakewood, Colorado 80228
(800) 233-1NLP
Website: www.nlpco.com

Offers a variety of training seminars and NLP certification.

Recommended Reading

Creating Wholeness: A Self-Healing Workbook Using Dynamic Relaxation, Images and Thoughts. Erik Peper, Ph.D., and Catherine Holt. New York: Plenum, 1993.

Full Catastrophe Living. Jon Kabat-Zinn, Ph.D., New York: Delacorte, 1990.

Head First: The Biology of Hope. Norman Cousins. New York: Thorndike Press, 1991.

Healing and the Mind. Bill Moyers. New York: Doubleday, 1993.

Imagery in Healing Shamanism and Modern Medicine. Jeanne Achterberg, Ph.D. Boston: Shambhala Publications, 1985.

Mind/Body Medicine: How to Use Your Mind for Better Health. D. Goleman and Joel Gurin. New York: Consumer Reports Books, 1993.

Minding the Body/Mending the Mind. Joan Borysenko, Ph.D. New York: Bantam Books, 1988.

Molecules of Emotion: The Science Behind Mind-Body Medicine. Candace Pert, Ph.D. New York: Touchstone, 1997.

Quantum Healing. Deepak Chopra, M.D. New York: Bantam Books, 1989.

The Relaxation Response. Herbert Benson, M.D. Boston: G.K. Hall, 1976.

Sacred Healing. C. Norman Shealy, M.D., Ph.D. Boston: Element Books, 1999.

Timeless Healing: The Power and Biology of Belief. Herbert Benson, M.D. with Marg Stark. New York: Scribner, 1996.

Breathwork

Breaking the Death Habit: The Science of Everlasting Health. Leonard Orr. Berkeley, CA: North Atlantic Books, 1999.

The Art of Breathing. Nancy Zi. New York: Bantam, 1986.

EMDR

EMDR: The Breakthrough "Eye Movement" Therapy for Overcoming Anxiety, Stress and Trauma. Francine Shapiro and Margot Silk Forrest. New York: Basic Books, 1997.

Emotional Healing at Warp Speed: The Power of EMDR. David Grand. New York: Harmony Books, 2001.

Energy Psychology

Energy Tapping. Fred P. Gallo, Ph.D., and Harry Vincenzi. Oakland, CA: New Harbinger Publications, 2000.

Getting Thru to Your Emotions with EFT. Phillip Montrose and Jane Montrose. Sacramento, CA: Holistic Communications, 2000.

Instant Emotional Healing. Peter Lambrou, Ph.D., and George Pratt, Ph.D. New York: Broadway Books, 2000.

Thought Field Therapy and Trauma. Roger Callahan, Ph.D., and Jane Callahan. La Quinta, CA: TFT Training Center, 1996.

Meditation

Meditation as Medicine: Activate the Power of Your Natural Healing Force. Dharma Singh Khalsa, M.D., and Cameron Stauth. New York: Pocket Books, 2001.

Neuro-Emotional Technique

Good News for People Who Hurt. Lou Ann Hall. Austin, TX: Agape Associates, 1999.

Neuro-Linguistic Programming

Beliefs: Pathways to Health and Well Being. Robert Dilts, Tim Hallbom, and Suzi Smith. Portland, OR: Metamorphous Press, 1990.

NAET

Holistic physicians have long recognized the hidden role that allergy can play in a wide range of disease conditions. All too often, however, allergies go undetected, especially by conventional physicians, who usually are not trained to screen for them. Nambudripad's Allergy Elimination Technique (NAET) is an innovative therapy that not only enables health-care practitioners to more effectively uncover allergies, but also completely eliminate patients' allergic reactions.

THERE IS HARDLY any human disease or condition in which allergic factors are not involved," according to Devi S. Nambudripad, D.C., L.Ac., R.N., Ph.D., of Buena Park, California. "Any organ, group of organs, or portion of the body may be involved, and the allergic responses may show great variations." Over 40 million Americans are known to suffer from allergies of some sort, but Dr. Nambudripad estimates that an additional 50 million or more have hidden allergies of which they are unaware. "They may have other symptoms that keep them going from doctor to doctor, trying all sorts of remedies without getting any relief, not realizing that the underlying cause of their condition is an allergic reaction," she says.

When viruses or bacteria enter the body, the immune system goes into action to rid the body of the invader. This produces many of the symptoms we associate with an illness. Continuous contact with an allergenic substance causes similar reactions to occur, according to Dr. Nambudripad. Among the conditions she claims can be due to allergies are gastrointestinal disorders, migraines, hyperactivity, arthritis, asthma, anxiety, depression, backache, and chronic fatigue.

Dr. Nambudripad's comments may initially seem implausible, yet allergies have for many years been viewed by practitioners of holistic medicine as a potentially critical factor in the onset of a wide range of illnesses. Typically, treatments for allergy sufferers include drugs, the avoidance of all allergic triggers, and dietary changes (some of them very rigorous and lasting for months),

NAET not only makes it easier to determine the various allergens that may be playing a hidden role in disease, it also allows patients to continue to use or be exposed to the implicated substances without further suffering.

along with immune-enhancing measures such as nutritional and herbal supplementation, homeopathy, and acupuncture. But even when the treatments prove successful, patients usually have to diligently monitor or avoid their exposure to the known foods or environmental triggers that caused their illness in the first place. Such vigilance often must last a lifetime.

 See Environmental Medicine.

Dr. Nambudripad claims to offer a more effective and permanent answer to this problem through NAET. According to Dr. Nambudripad, NAET not only makes it easier to determine the various allergens that may be playing a hidden role in disease, it also allows patients to continue to use or be exposed to the implicated substances without further suffering. In her book *Say Goodbye to Illness,* Dr. Nambudripad claims that she will "revolutionize the practice of medicine." This may seem exaggerated, but in nearly 15 years of clinical use with thousands of patients, Dr. Nambudripad reports that NAET alone has entirely relieved allergy symptoms or produced satisfactory improvements in 80% to 90% of her patients.

Sandra Denton, M.D., of Anchorage, Alaska, herself a leading allergy specialist, has experienced the effectiveness of NAET firsthand. Dr. Denton relates how NAET cured her of chronic fatigue syndrome and an attack of asthma that left her hospitalized. "As Dr. Nambudripad began testing me, I was shocked to find that I was reacting to many vitamins and minerals and other essential nutrients of my everyday diet," she reports. Dr.

AN ALLERGY PRIMER

The term *allergy* refers to an exaggerated or unusual response by the body to substances that are harmless, and even helpful, to most people. In many cases, allergies are merely nuisances, but for other people, contact with an allergenic substance can produce toxins in the body that result in a host of health conditions, many of them severe. The majority of allergy sufferers tend to be unaware that they are allergic in the first place, or they are unable to identify the substance(s) causing their allergic response.

Allergenic substances generally fall into one of eight basic categories, depending on how they are contacted: inhalants, ingestants, contactants, infectants, physical agents, genetic agents, molds, and fungi. These categories, in turn, occur in two ways—as food allergies or as allergies caused by environmental influences.

The following symptoms are often signs of an allergic reaction: unnatural or persistent fatigue; weight fluctuations during the course of the day; frequent puffiness in the face, ankles, or fingers; hot flashes (apart from menopause) or perspiration for no obvious reason; inexplicable racing or pounding pulse; a history of food intolerance (certain foods that cause flatulence, sneezing, a runny nose, drowsiness, etc.); cravings for certain foods, particularly bread, sugary foods, milk and other dairy products, coffee, tea, or chocolate; frequent headaches and migraines, asthma, eczema, or gastrointestinal problems.

Many allergic symptoms are hidden or misdiagnosed, but the following are often telltale warning signs that allergies are present. In particular, they can be an indication of food allergies, the most common group of undetected allergens.

Physical Symptoms: dark circles, swelling, or wrinkles under the eyes; vascular headaches; faintness or dizziness; sleepiness soon after a meal; insomnia; frequent waking during the night or premature waking followed by an inability to return to sleep; sinusitis, runny or stuffy nose, or post-nasal drip; excessive mucus; watery eyes and/or blurred vision; ringing in the ears; earaches or recurrent ear infections (particularly among children); sore throat, hoarseness, or chronic coughing; gagging; heart palpitations; chest congestion; mucus or undigested food in the stool; nausea or vomiting; diarrhea or constipation; bloating after meals; flatulence; abdominal pains or cramping; extreme thirst; coated tongue; anal or vaginal itch; hives or rashes; dermatitis; brittle nails and hair; dry skin; dandruff; skin pallor; muscle ache; weakness and fatigue; arthritic symptoms or joint pain; symptoms of PMS; frequent or urgent urination; and obesity.

Psychological Symptoms: anxiety or panic attacks; depression; crying jags; aggressive behavior; irritability; mental dullness or lethargy; confusion; excessive daydreaming; restlessness; poor work habits; inability to concentrate; slurred speech; and indifference or lack of enthusiasm for life.

If you suffer from the above symptoms, you may have hidden allergies and it is recommended that you consult a health-care practitioner trained in their treatment.

Nambudripad eliminated Dr. Denton's reactions to the nutrients using NAET and, within nine days, she was restored to health and able to return to work.[1]

How NAET Works

The key to how NAET works lies in its ability to retrain the patient's brain and nervous system to no longer react to the allergenic substances. This is a radically different approach than the more common method of avoiding allergy triggers for a lifetime, once they have been detected.

Part of NAET's success lies in its effect on the body's energy pathways, or meridians, as they are known by practitioners of traditional Chinese medicine. "When you are exposed to a substance you are allergic to, your brain and meridian system interpret the substance, whatever it may be, as being harmful to you," Dr. Nambudripad explains. "For other people, the substance may be harmless, but for your system it's toxic. As a result, your nervous system 'freezes up' in order to defend against it, which creates blockages in the meridians. So long as the allergy remains, over time, the blockages will lead to further imbalances in the way your body functions—the result is disease."

Allergies, according to Dr. Nambudripad, are a response of the immune system to foreign substances (or their energy fields) around you. "This response triggers different reactions at different times. For instance, one day the reaction might manifest as leg pain and the next time as a headache. It depends upon which area of the body is the one where the energy is blocked." Reversing this process and unblocking the body's flow of energy is the goal of NAET.

 See Acupuncture, Applied Kinesiology, Biofeedback Training and Neurotherapy, Chiropractic, Energy Medicine.

Detecting Your Allergies

NAET practitioners detect allergies through the use of applied kinesiology. Applied kinesiology, first developed by George Goodheart, D.C., of Detroit, Michigan, is the study of the relationship between muscle dysfunction (weak muscles) and related organ or gland dysfunction. Applied kinesiology employs a simple strength resistance test on a specific indicator muscle that is related to the organ or part of the body being tested. If the muscle tests strong (maintaining its resistance), it indicates health.

Patients hold the suspected allergenic substance while the practitioner tests the strength of certain muscles. If an allergy exists, the muscles will exhibit weakness that improves once the patient is no longer in contact with the offending substance. Though this diagnostic method is effective, Dr. Nambudripad also uses a computerized system of muscle testing based on electrodermal screening (EDS—see Quick Definition) and biofeedback. She utilizes a device that can measure minute changes in electrical response (indicating dysfunction) through the skin as the patient holds different materials. This computerized method speeds up the process when there is not simply a single suspected allergen.

 Electrodermal screening (EDS) is a form of computerized information gathering based on physics, not chemistry. A blunt, noninvasive electric probe is placed at specific points on the patient's hands, face, or feet, corresponding to acupuncture points at the beginning or end of energy meridians. Minute electrical discharges from these points serve as information signals about the condition of the body's organs and systems, useful for the physician in evaluation and developing a treatment plan. The key idea is that an energetic event transfers its signal through an acupuncture meridian to the nervous system, with the end result being a cellular pathology. EDS is a "data acquisition process" in which the trained practitioner conducts an "interview" with the patient's organs and tissues, gathering information about the basic functional status of those systems and their energy pathways.

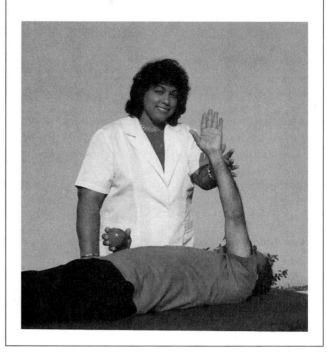

In NAET a practitioner uses applied kinesiology to detect allergies.

According to Dr. Nambudripad, it is possible to use NAET at home to determine whether or not you are suffering from allergies. "To be free of the allergy, you should see a trained NAET practitioner, but if you know what you're allergic to, you can stay away from it until you get the proper treatment." She recommends the following muscle testing procedures:

STANDARD MUSCLE TEST RESPONSE

To do this evaluation, you will need a partner.

1. Lie down on a flat surface and make sure that your fingernails are scrubbed clean and free of any trace of perfume or other substances.

2. Raise your left arm straight up at a 90° angle. Have your partner try to push your arm down toward your toes, applying light pressure. Gently resist as this is done. (Allow five seconds of pushing and resistance.)

3. If your arm goes weak right away, it means your energy is unbalanced. If this is the case, have your partner place his or her right forefinger at a point 1½ inches below your navel, while placing his/her left forefinger at the base of your sternum. Then have your partner gently tap these two meridian points simultaneously for about 20 seconds.

4. Retest the arm by repeating step 2. If the arm now tests strong, proceed to step 5.

5. Using the hand you write with, hold the suspected allergenic substance.

THE ORIGINS OF NAET

Perhaps the most dramatic example of the role allergies can play in compromising health lies with Dr. Devi Nambudripad herself. From early childhood, she suffered from multiple illnesses, including arthritis, bronchitis, sinusitis, migraines, chronic exhaustion, insomnia, and eczema. "I had to live on a special diet that my parents oversaw, and that's how I survived," she says. "Then, when I came to America from India, I started eating health food because my husband was also eating it, due to his own health problems. The result was that I really became crippled, almost bed-ridden. I had almost no energy and was in constant pain."

None of the physicians she consulted were able to help her, until finally she met an acupuncturist, who tested her for allergies. "He helped me understand that my illness was due to allergies, which at first I didn't believe. I thought I had all these other diseases." The acupuncturist told her to eat only white rice and broccoli and that, if she did, her health would improve. "So I tried the diet and within one week I started feeling better. My pain started going away, along with my headaches and arthritis, and that gave me some hope." She lived on that diet for 3 ½ years, during which time she also began her medical training.

Then one day, Dr. Nambudripad ate a carrot, setting the stage for her discovery of NAET. The carrot caused an immediate reaction of faintness. By now trained in acupuncture, she gave herself a treatment to keep herself from going into shock. "When I finished the treatment, I found that I was much better than ever before," she recounts, "even though some of the carrot was still in my hand. Immediately, I associated the electromagnetic field of the carrot being within my body's electromagnetic field and realized that somehow the acupuncture treatment had halted the reaction I was having. I was no longer allergic to carrots—I ate the rest of the carrot and didn't have a reaction."

Because of this experience, Dr. Nambudripad went on to treat herself for most of the other substances she was allergic to, and today they no longer trouble her. "Except for chemicals," she laughs. "They can still get me because there are so many types and, if I haven't treated a particular one, it can still cause a reaction when I'm exposed to it. But now the reactions are very mild and I can instantly treat them."

6. While you hold the substance, again raise your other arm and have your partner try to push it down. You will find that when holding the substances you are allergic to, your arm will be pushed down much more easily, indicating weakness and dysfunction. With substances to which you are not allergic, your muscle strength and resistance will not be weakened. Remove allergenic substances and do not eat or use them until you have seen an NAET practitioner for treatment.

THE "O" RING TEST

With practice, some people can use the following method to muscle test themselves:

1. Make an "O" shape with your hand by bringing the thumb and little finger together. Inserting your index finger of the opposite hand into the "O," apply pressure and attempt to separate your thumb and little finger.

2. If they separate easily, have a partner help you apply step 3 of the standard muscle response test above. If your thumb and little finger remain inseparable and strong, hold the suspected allergen in your other hand and perform step 1 again. If the "O" separates easily, then you are allergic to the substance you are holding; if the "O" remains strong, the substance does not have an adverse effect on you.

Reprogramming the Nervous System with NAET

Once the allergens have been determined, the next step in NAET is to "reprogram" the patient's nervous system to not react to them. Dr. Nambudripad accomplishes this by having the patients hold the substance they are allergic to while she treats them with acupuncture. "Because your energy pathways are unblocked while you are holding the substance during the acupuncture treatment, your body stops reacting to it," Dr. Nambudripad says. "This, in turn, leads your brain to stop viewing it as harmful." Once the treatment is complete, patients are then instructed to avoid exposure to the substance for 25–30 hours, after which time it should no longer cause an allergic reaction.

A recently completed, double-blind study, jointly conducted under the auspices of Dr. Nambudripad's Allergy Research Foundation and the California Acupuncture Association, further attests to NAET's effectiveness. The study, involving 36 volunteers known to be allergic to milk and milk products, was overseen by 21 doctors from different medical fields, including allopathic, chiropractic, applied kinesiology, and oriental medicine.

Participants were randomly assigned to one of three groups: the placebo group received pseudo treatment, the control group received no treatment, and the experimental group received NAET treatment. The study was conducted over a six-week period, with the actual duration of testing lasting one month, then the subjects were tested again after one year and three years. Each subject was tested for milk allergies using a variety of measures, including intradermal milk injections, blood tests, immunoglobulin levels in the blood, kinesiology, electrodermal screening, and other measures, including change in pulse rate and each subject's history and self-assessment of symptoms. Those who received NAET treatment during the initial six-week period showed a "remarkable" decrease in all diagnostic scales used to measure each subject's allergies to milk, according to Dr. Nambudripad. Three years later, the experimental subjects remained without any adverse symptoms from milk consumption.

Conditions Benefited by NAET

Among the conditions Dr. Nambudripad has successfully treated using NAET are: anxiety, addictions, autism, attention deficit disorder (ADD), severe and chronic indigestion, back pain, chronic fatigue syndrome, asthma, genital yeast infections, hypoglycemia, chronic headaches, kidney infection, impaired urination, nausea, and chest pain. The range of potential allergens is quite vast, Dr. Nambudripad explains. "Almost anything can cause an allergic reaction. In my everyday practice, I see patients who are allergic to foods, beverages, water (especially tap water), clothing, plants, chemicals, vitamins, vaccines, furniture, the cars they drive, plastics, metals, cosmetics such as fingernail polish, even wedding rings. In each case, as soon as the offending substance was identified and NAET applied, the accompanying symptoms began to resolve themselves."

Eleanor Chin, D.C., of Mill Valley and San Francisco, both in California, employs NAET as part of her practice and illustrates how potent a therapy it can be. One of Dr. Chin's former chiropractic patients came to her after suffering from excruciating low-back pain for six weeks. "The reason she didn't seek my help right away was because the pain felt like what she had experienced years earlier when she had kidney stones," Dr. Chin explains. "At first, she went to an M.D. and he concurred that the pain was most likely kidney related. So she went to the hospital and they did a number of procedures and nothing helped. Finally, they decided that she should come back for exploratory surgery. That's when she came

CONDITIONS HELPED BY NAET

- Anxiety
- Addictions
- Autism
- Attention deficit disorder (ADD)
- Severe and chronic indigestion
- Back pain
- Chronic fatigue syndrome
- Asthma
- Genital yeast infections
- Hypoglycemia
- Chronic headaches
- Kidney infection and impaired urination
- Nausea
- Chest pain

to see me." Dr. Chin treated her with chiropractic, but it didn't help her condition. Then she asked the woman what she might have done six weeks earlier before the pain occurred. "She told me that she'd undergone cosmetic eyelid surgery," Dr. Chin says. "This led me to suspect a possible allergic reaction to the Novocain™ that was used as her anesthesia." Using muscle testing while having the woman hold an ampule of Novocain, Dr. Chin determined that there was indeed a connection. "I used NAET to treat her for the allergic reaction and later that night much of her pain had subsided. She came back in two days and, after the second treatment, all her pain was gone," Dr. Chin reports.[2]

Not all NAET treatments bring such swift relief, however. For food allergies, Dr. Nambudripad estimates that most allergic responses will cease after 15-20 treatments, usually received once a week. "After that, most patients can eat a wide variety of food without reactions," she says. "If they want to go into more detail to treat other substances they are allergic to, it may take longer. I've had many patients who only needed ten to 12 visits and then I never see them again because they are doing fine. It depends on what they are allergic to, the condition of their immune system, and their lifestyle."

Susan, 19, came to Dr. Nambudripad complaining of low-back pain. She had been experiencing the pain for five days. A urine test suggested a kidney infection, and aspirin and an antibiotic were prescribed. These helped with the symptoms, but later Susan drank a cup of fenugreek herbal tea and experienced a severe reaction of chills, muscular stiffness, and high fever. Dr. Nambudripad then tested her for an allergy to the tea and

CASES FROM DR. NAMBUDRIPAD'S PRACTICE

Here are other successful cases from Dr. Nambudripad's practice that illustrate the wide range of potential allergens as well as NAET's effectiveness for both detecting offending allergens and eliminating their symptoms.

GENDER/AGE	SYMPTOMS	ALLERGENIC SUBSTANCE
Woman, 22	Severe abdominal cramps, indigestion	Sanitary napkins
Man, 62	Lower abdominal pain, frequent urination	Leather belt
Woman, 52	Genital yeast infection, 12 years	Cotton underpants
Man, 32	Severe headaches, nausea, vomiting, belching, sour stomach, 12 years	Raw red onions
Woman, 38	Diarrhea, sweaty palms, anxiety before meetings	Adrenaline
Woman, 34	Itching, burning on thighs	All dietary fibers
Woman, 42	Sore throat, coughing, throat secretions, postnasal drip, breathing difficulties	Smoked rainbow trout
Woman, 32	Dull constant thigh pain, 5 years	Gold
Woman, 44	Severe pain, left leg, 15 months	Diamond ring
Woman, 30	Severe joint pain, both hands, 9 months	Crude pig-iron knife for chopping vegetables
Woman, 30	Chronic fatigue syndrome	Sewing needles, stainless steel, iron, wood
Girl, 3	Coma, 9 days	Pineapple
Man, 37	Leg cramps, muscle spasms	Abalone
Boy, 6	Low-grade fever, 4 weeks	Nutmeg
Girl, 9	Coma, 9 weeks	Peanuts
Woman, 37	Severe chest pain, enlarged spleen	Carob
Woman, 56	Asthma, 7 years	Tap water
Man, 79	Metastasized cancer	Wasp sting
Man, 59	Skin rash, itching on arms	Wheat flour
Man, 44	Chronic athlete's foot, knee pain	Cotton socks
Man, 46	Severe arm pain, 7 months	Artichoke

found that Susan's kidney meridian got blocked by the fenugreek tea and kept generating the allergic symptoms. "The sudden blocking of the meridians is one of the quickest defense mechanisms of the brain to stop the allergen from entering deeper into the body." Dr. Nambudripad used acupressure to treat Susan's kidney meridian and organ imbalance at the same time that Susan held the fenugreek tea in her hand. After the NAET session, Susan was able to resume drinking fenugreek tea without a relapse of symptoms.

Another of Dr. Nambudripad's patients was Thomas, a 28-year-old computer programmer, who came to her complaining of extreme fatigue. His job performance was being negatively affected and it became difficult for him to walk without help. He was then diagnosed with chronic fatigue syndrome. He took a leave from work

and, over time, began to feel better. When he returned to work, however, the symptoms also returned. This cycle continued for four years until Thomas consulted Dr. Nambudripad. She tested him for allergies and discovered that he was allergic to the radiation from his computer screen and the plastic in his keyboard. After NAET treatment, Thomas was able to return to work without his symptoms recurring.

The Future of NAET

It's important to stress that the positive responses attributed to NAET have until recently been entirely anecdotal. That is changing, however. In addition to the recently completed milk allergy study cited above, further double-blind studies exploring NAET's efficacy in treating allergies are now under way. These are needed in order to better understand and validate the efficacy of NAET treatments on foods, drugs, and other allergens.

In the meantime, a growing number of physicians are heralding NAET's merits and incorporating it into their practice, making it one of the fastest-growing new therapies in the field of alternative medicine. Dr. Nambudripad has trained over 4,500 doctors in the U.S., Canada, Europe, Australia, and Israel in the use of NAET and continues to offer monthly seminars to health professionals interested in learning her methods. Many who take her training practice NAET full time, while others combine it with their regular practice. About half of the practitioners are medical doctors, conventional medical allergists, and environmental specialists, with chiropractors and acupuncturists also showing interest.

Where to Find Help

For further information about NAET, and for referrals, contact:

Devi S. Nambudripad Pain Clinic
6714 Beach Blvd.
Buena Park, California 90621
(714) 523-8900
Website: www.naet.com

For information on NAET, training seminars, and referrals to practitioners trained in its use.

Recommended Reading

Living Pain Free with Acupressure: Acupressure Self-Help. Devi S. Nambudripad, D.C., L.Ac. Buena Park, CA: Delta Publishing, 1997.

NAET Guidebook. Devi S. Nambudripad, D.C., L.Ac. Buena Park, CA: Delta Publishing, 2001.

Say Goodbye to Children's Allergies. Devi S. Nambudripad, D.C., L.Ac. Buena Park, CA: Delta Publishing, 2000.

Say Goodbye to Illness. Devi S. Nambudripad, D.C., L.Ac. Buena Park, CA: Delta Publishing, 1999.

NATURAL HORMONE REPLACEMENT THERAPY

Researchers have long known that one of the mechanisms involved in the aging process is the decline in naturally occurring hormones in the body, first occurring after development ceases and then accelerating as we enter our fifties, sixties, and beyond. Chronic illness is also frequently associated with the body's decline in hormone production. Recent research suggests that proper replacement of natural hormones holds great promise in slowing the aging process and as a treatment for age-related diseases.

THE WORD *HORMONE* is derived from the Greek word *hormao,* meaning "to arouse or excite." Hormones are chemical messengers that are usually secreted from the endocrine glands into the bloodstream. Once secreted, hormones then bind with appropriate receptor sites present on the cell membranes of their target organs. "Hormones and receptor sites work like a key and a door," explains Michael Galitzer, M.D., Co-founder of the American Health Institute, in Los Angeles, California. "In order to get into the cell and instruct the DNA to make cell proteins, a hormone must first bind to its receptor. This unlocks the door and delivers a message to the cell."

Hormones play many important roles in the health and maintenance of the body, including influencing the metabolism of carbohydrates, proteins, fats, minerals, and water. They also regulate DNA and RNA production and the subsequent synthesis of cell proteins, are involved in the production of enzymes, and influence the energy production of mitochondria (microscopic structures present in every cell, responsible for converting proteins, carbohydrates, and fats into energy or ATP). In addition, hormones regulate the body's response to stress, kidney function, blood sugar balance, menstruation, and sexual function.

As we age, however, hormone production in the body declines (see "The Decline in Hormones Due to

> *A loss of hormonal balance, as occurs with aging, plays a predominant role in mental and emotional symptoms and in all illness. Restoration of this balance is ideally achieved through natural hormone replacement therapy.*
>
> —MICHAEL GALITZER, M.D.

Aging"). Since hormones affect virtually every bodily process, low levels of certain hormones and impaired communication within the endocrine system creates havoc with all other body systems, including the immune, cardiovascular, detoxification, gastrointestinal, and nervous systems. "A loss of hormonal balance, as occurs with aging, plays a predominant role in mental and emotional symptoms and in all illness," Dr. Galitzer says. "Restoration of this balance is ideally achieved through natural hormone replacement therapy (NHRT)."

Nutritional deficiencies, lack of exercise, and exposure to toxins, can all result in changes in hormone production that can ultimately lead to diminished biological functioning. Stress can also seriously impact hormone production. "Chronic stress among individuals in their prime results in the same blood hormone levels as those of a 70-year-old," Dr. Galitzer says. "This is one of the reasons that we age prematurely with chronic stress." Other factors that can contribute to hormonal imbalances include endocrine disorders, malnutrition, sleep disorders, exposure to electromagnetic fields (EMFs), lack of sunlight, hypothyroidism, insulin resistance, and the use of over-the-counter and prescription medications (pain relievers, heart medications, anti-anxiety drugs, sleeping pills, and nonsteroidal, anti-inflammatory drugs such as aspirin, ibuprofen, and indomethacin).

The Endocrine Glands

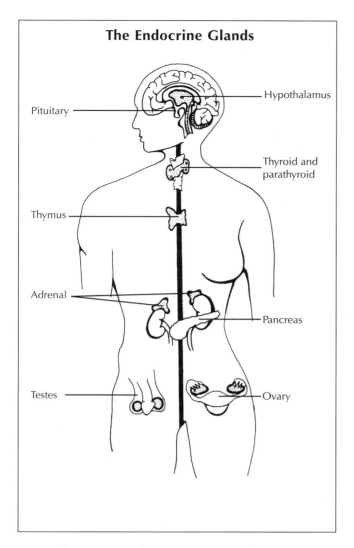

The Endocrine Glands

Pituitary — Hypothalamus

Thyroid and parathyroid

Thymus

Adrenal — Pancreas

Testes — Ovary

THE DECLINE IN HORMONES DUE TO AGING

The levels of various hormones decline as we chronologically age:

- Growth hormone, testosterone, DHEA—50% decline from age 25 to 50, followed by a further 50% decline by age 75.

- Melatonin—sharp, continual decline after age 40.

- Estrogen—30% decline from age 25 to 50, then a slow decline thereafter.

- Progesterone—75% decline from age 35 to 50, then a continual slow decline thereafter.

Research by Michael Borkin, N.M.D., of the National Institute of Endocrine Research, in Las Vegas, Nevada, indicates that the decline in hormone production is also a direct result of physical and emotional stress (for example, youthful hormone levels can be found in seniors over the age of 70, while suboptimal levels are commonly found in teens.)

The endocrine glands are central to the regulation and normalization of all the body's complex, interconnected systems, beginning with the nervous system. The main link between the nervous system and the endocrine system is the hypothalamus, a small gland in the lower brain that acts as the hormone control center. Messages from the brain are sent to the hypothalamus, which in turn releases hormonal messages to the pituitary gland, located just below the hypothalamus. The pituitary gland then produces hormones that stimulate target glands to secrete other hormones.

The pituitary produces follicle-stimulating hormone (FSH) and luteinizing hormone (LH), both of which control menstruation, and hormones that stimulate the production of androgens (male hormones, such as testosterone). The pituitary also controls the thyroid gland by releasing thyroid-stimulating hormone (TSH), activates the adrenal glands through adrenocorticotropic hormone (ACTH), and stimulates overall growth in children by releasing human growth hormone (HGH).

The thyroid gland, located just below the larynx in the throat, acts as the body's metabolic thermostat, controlling body temperature, energy use, and, in children, the body's growth rate. It also regulates the rate of organ function, the speed with which the body uses food, and affects the operation of all body processes and organs. The main hormones synthesized and released by the thyroid are tri-iodothyronine (T3) and thyroxine (T4).

The adrenal glands, located atop the kidneys, help regulate the response to stress by producing the hormones adrenaline and noradrenaline, both of which increase heart rate and blood sugar levels. The adrenals also produce steroid (made from cholesterol) hormones, including progesterone, testosterone, cortisol, pregnenolone, aldosterone, and DHEA (dehydroepiandrosterone). "All steroids are synthesized from cholesterol, the building material used to form stress and sex hormones," explains Michael Borkin, N.M.D., Research Director of the National Institute of Endocrine Research, in Las Vegas, Nevada. "Because of this similarity in structure, these hormones become interchangeable, depending on need."

The pancreas, located behind the stomach, is both a digestive organ that manufactures enzymes and an endocrine gland that produces the hormones glucagon and insulin, which regulate blood sugar levels and help metabolize fats and proteins in the body.

The gonads, or sex organs (ovaries in women, testes in men), are involved in sexual development and reproductive functions. The ovaries produce the primary female sex hormones estrogen and progesterone. The testes also produce progesterone, as well as the male sex hormones (androgens), particularly testosterone.

When endocrine function becomes impaired, over time a variety of physiological functions are impaired as well, including cardiovascular function, organ regeneration, sexual health, cellular immunity, brain function and memory, and protein synthesis. Other conditions associated with endocrine deficiency include decreased lean body mass, decreased glucose tolerance, increased obesity, increased levels of triglycerides and LDLs (low-density lipoproteins, the "bad" cholesterol), decreased high-density lipoproteins (HDLs, the "good" cholesterol), and diminished aerobic capacity.

How Natural Hormone Replacement Therapy Works

According to Dr. Galitzer, natural hormone replacement therapy involves "replacing what is deficient with natural, nontoxic hormones so as to maintain hormones at the levels of one's thirties." If your hormones are imbalanced, one of your priorities should be to detoxify your body systems. Both the liver and gastrointestinal tract are involved in the normal processing of excess levels of hormones. When these organs are not functioning properly, hormones may become imbalanced. Holistic practitioners generally recommend tending to these systems first in order to normalize the body's functions. The hormones most commonly used in NHRT are estrogen, progesterone, testosterone, thyroid hormones, adrenal hormones, melatonin, DHEA, pregnenolone, and human growth hormone.

However, hormones should only be used under the supervision of physicians trained in their use, and not before receiving a proper laboratory and clinical evaluation. Hormones should usually not be given to pregnant women or to people under the age of 35. When taken blindly at excessive doses, serious adverse effects can occur. In addition, relying solely on symptoms and blood tests as the basis for diagnosis without proper accompanying data can easily make the situation worse.

Only within the last few years have tests, such as the hormonal saliva assay report, been perfected. Because these tests are relatively new, many health practitioners are unfamiliar with them and thus they are rarely used. Physicians who have not been trained to interpret the results from saliva are unaware of the value of such testing.

 See Detoxification Therapy, Longevity Medicine.

Testing Hormone Levels

The most responsible way of accurately assessing hormone levels is to perform hormonal circadian testing, also known as "timed hormone capture." This involves looking at hormonal changes that occur during a 24-hour cycle. (With women, this can be extended through an entire menstrual cycle, with collections made every few days.) Testing in this manner provides a comprehensive representation of hormonal activity and the dynamic changes that can occur.

The easiest and most efficient way to perform hormonal circadian testing is the saliva assay report, a simple saliva test that can help determine if you have hormonal imbalances. It can be ordered by both laypeople and physicians and measures up to eight hormones, with the results plotted on graphs for easy interpretation. Testing is performed by taking saliva samples at specific times during a 24-hour period. This is necessary because hormonal fluctuations throughout the day, and especially during sleep, are extremely important. Changing levels can also be plotted over time on the same graph for further testing, or if hormone replacement therapy is begun.

Although hormones are present in saliva only in fractional amounts compared to the blood, saliva testing provides a highly accurate means for determining whether or not hormone levels fall within the normal range for a person's age group. The saliva assay has several advantages over traditional blood testing for hormones, according to Dr. Galitzer. In addition to being painless and noninvasive and easily performed anywhere at anytime, saliva samples are considered to represent the biologically active (or "free") hormones to which cells are subjected. Furthermore, the assay remains stable at room temperature for five days and samples can be mailed to the laboratory. As hormone levels normally are highest in the morning, it is far more convenient to test them at home than to travel to a physician's office later in the day, when hormone levels will typically have fallen off.

The saliva assay is also less expensive than blood testing and can be done frequently, if necessary, to monitor changes brought on by various interventions (diet, exercise, herbs, stress reduction) and to adjust dosages of hormones used in NHRT. In addition, multiple saliva samples collected at different times allow evaluation of hormonal stress responses and circadian rhythm. Overall, it is best to first establish a baseline level of saliva hormones, then test a second time after therapy has begun to measure any changes.

Estrogen

Estrogen refers to a group of female "sex" hormones, produced primarily in the ovaries (and to a lesser extent in the body's fat cells). It is important for adolescent sexual development and for regulating the menstrual cycle—estrogen prepares the uterus for receiving the fertilized egg by stimulating the uterine lining to grow. For the first 10-14 days in a woman's cycle, the uterus is mainly under the influence of estrogen, which begins to climb right before menstruation (from about days seven to 14) and peaks at ovulation. Estrogen also acts as an anti-aging agent; helps to slow down bone loss, thus helping to prevent osteoporosis; improves skin tone; reduces vaginal dryness; and helps reduce heart attack risk (cardiovascular diseases are the major cause of death in menopausal women).

"There are three main types of estrogen that a woman makes during her menstrual years," Dr. Galitzer says. "Estradiol (E1), which accounts for 80% of her estrogen, estriol (E2), and estrone (E3). E2 and E3 each account for approximately 10% of the remaining estrogen." Estradiol is produced directly in the ovaries, estrone is produced from estradiol, and estriol is produced in large amounts during pregnancy and, according to Dr. Galitzer, helps prevent breast cancer. Of the three, estradiol is the most potent form of estrogen.

It is common knowledge that levels of all three types of estrogen decline after menopause. The decline can also occur much earlier, however. "Between the ages of 40 to 44, almost all women are deficient in one of the estrogen hormones," Dr. Galitzer says. Estrogen levels are also linked to progesterone, DHEA, and thyroid hormone levels, and deficiencies can occur due to excess cortisol as well (acute stress raises cortisol levels in the body). Birth control pills can affect estrogen levels, as can diets high in sugars and refined starches; soy products are also estrogenic. Mercury, plastics, and carcinogenic pesticides, herbicides, and insecticides (collectively referred to as xenoestrogens) can contribute to estrogen imbalance as well, as can liver damage from toxins such as alcohol, which elevate estrogen by interfering with its metabolism and excretion.

Signs of estrogen excess include: salt and fluid retention; estrogen synergizes with insulin to promote hypoglycemia and fat synthesis; estrogen promotes histamine release, blood clotting, aging of collagen, and development of fibroids, tumors, and endometriosis. Signs of

---

NHRT AND PATIENT INDIVIDUALITY

Research is causing a change in the way physicians are approaching natural hormone replacement therapy. "The key to natural hormone replacement or enhancement lies in determining the proper priority of treatment," states Michael Borkin, N.M.D. "To accomplish this, the patient has to be approached as an individual. Everyone has a unique sequence of hormones that is the result of their own lifestyle. Once the dynamics of these hormones are analyzed, a treatment plan tailored to each patient's specific needs can be developed to reestablish a healthy hormonal balance. Proper determination is made by using saliva samples taken at least every four hours throughout a 24-hour period."

---

estrogen deficiency include: hot flashes, night sweats, dry eyes, vaginal dryness, sagging breasts and loss of breast fullness, mental fogginess, depression, changes in mood, and decreased sense of sensuality and sexuality.

"Estrogen levels are best kept balanced by eating enough protein and estrogenic foods, keeping thyroid function relatively high, and by always using natural progesterone," Dr. Galitzer says. Estrogenic foods include animal products, apples, barley, brown rice, carrots, cherries, coconut, nightshades, olives, peanuts, plums, wheat, and yams. "These foods can be increased in quantity in women who are perimenopausal and whose estrogen levels are unstable and low, with resulting hot flashes," Dr. Galitzer says. "Such foods should be avoided in women who have symptoms of excess estrogen, however." According to Dr. Galitzer, the herbs black cohosh and licorice root can both be used to increase estrogen levels in women who are estrogen-deficient. However, licorice root should be avoided by people with a history of hypertension.

Eating soybeans and soybean-derived products, particularly fermented soybean foods such as tempeh and miso, can help counteract the negative effects of excess estrogen. These foods contain high levels of genistein, a substance that has a chemical structure similar to estrogen and can be used by the body as a mild estrogen surrogate. Substances like genistein are known as phytoestrogens, which are plant compounds that block estrogens from attaching to cell receptor sites—the places where estrogens exert their effect on the body. Phytoestrogens tend to balance estrogen in the body.[1] Other than soy, foods that are high in phytoestrogens

FACTORS THAT CAN CAUSE WOMEN'S HORMONES TO BECOME IMBALANCED

Estrogen dominance can occur as a result of an excess of estrogen and a deficiency of progesterone. Too much estrogen may be caused by:

- Foods that have hormones added to them, such as commercially produced meat, eggs, and dairy products, and/or a diet high in estrogenic foods

- Herbs that have an estrogenic effect in the body, such as licorice, black cohosh, and damiana

- Birth control pills and other hormone replacement therapy that have high levels of estrogen

- Xenoestrogens (environmental toxins that mimic the action of estrogen); the largest source of xenoestrogens is pesticides

- Exposure to radiation, which increases estrogen levels in the blood

- Chronic constipation, which interferes with the body's ability to eliminate estrogen properly; estrogen then builds up in the colon and can be reabsorbed by the body

- Liver toxicity preventing metabolism of estrogens

Too little progesterone may be caused by:

- An underactive thyroid gland (hypothyroidism)

- Chronic stress

- Ovarian dysfunction such as frequent menstruation without ovulation

- An underactive pituitary gland

- The aging process (after age 35 in women)

include flaxseeds, apples, whole grains, nuts, celery, and alfalfa.[2]

When natural hormone replacement therapy is deemed advisable, it typically combines E1, E2, and E3 in either pill, gel, sublingual (under the tongue), or trans-

dermal (through the skin) forms. When all three estrogens are used, this is known as a Tri-est formula. Some NHRT practitioners advocate against the use of estrone (E3), however, preferring a Bi-est formula that is made up of 92% estriol and 8% estradiol. "Oral estrogens and, to some extent, sublingual estrogens will increase sex hormone binding globulin (SHBG) and thyroid binding globulin (TBG), causing free levels of thyroid hormones and androgens (male hormones such as testosterone and androtestosterone) to fall," Dr. Galitzer points out. "Transdermal estrogen will not increase SHBG and TBG, and this is the preferred route. Transdermal estradiol provides the additional benefit of increasing growth hormone levels."

 See Constipation, Women's Health.

Progesterone

Progesterone is another female "sex" hormone, produced in the ovaries, that prepares the uterus for a fertilized egg; its sudden withdrawal causes the uterus to shed its lining if pregnancy does not occur. When estrogen is high (days 7-14 of the menstrual cycle), progesterone is at its lowest level. Its levels climb to a peak between days 14 and 24, and then dramatically drop off again just before the start of menstruation. In a sense, menstruation is a form of progesterone withdrawal.

Ideally, women should have five to ten times more progesterone than estrogen in the blood, and 50 to 100 times more in saliva. The lower the ratio of progesterone to estrogen, the higher the risk of health problems, especially during menses when there is a surge of estrogen. Lower ratios of progesterone to estrogen result in estrogen dominance, a condition that affects women usually starting at age 35, when progesterone production begins to decline in most women, but it can occur in teens as well.

Progesterone has the unique ability to change its structural form to become other hormones, allowing it to be converted and utilized by the body to the point of depletion. "One of progesterone's major capabilities is to convert to the adrenal stress hormone cortisol," Dr. Borkin says. "This means that all physical and emotional stress can affect progesterone levels." Progesterone helps prevent estrogen from interfering with thyroid function—when estrogen levels become excessive, it can prevent thyroxin from being utilized by the target tissue. In addition, progesterone acts as a precursor to most steroid functions (except those of estrogen and testosterone), which help regulate blood sugar elevation and proper nerve conduction. Balanced progesterone levels are also essential for a healthy libido.

To restore progesterone levels in the body, John R. Lee, M.D., of Sebastopol, California, a leading expert in the use of NHRT, recommends taking a progesterone supplement, which can help turn fat into energy and reduce water retention. While progesterone supplements are available in sublingual drops and capsules, Drs. Lee and Galitzer both prefer the use of a progesterone skin cream or oil, since applying progesterone to the skin allows it to be absorbed into fat layers under the skin, where it can be taken up by the blood as needed. By contrast, if taken in a capsule form, it is more difficult for the body to regulate the amount of progesterone entering the blood. "Progesterone prefers fat and does not dissolve in water," Dr. Galitzer says. "It rides on the membranes of red blood cells and is therefore well absorbed through the skin."

According to Dr. Galitzer, taking progesterone at night can promote restful sleep and restore normal sleep patterns. It also acts as a natural diuretic (increases the flow of urine), helps use fat for energy, is a natural antidepressant, normalizes blood clotting, enhances thyroid hormone activity, normalizes zinc and copper levels (estrogen raises copper levels, lowering zinc, which contributes to PMS), normalizes cell oxygen levels, stimulates new bone formation, restores estrogen receptor activity, and promotes healthy skin through its moisturizing effect. In addition, progesterone helps prevent fibrocystic breast disease and protects against cancer of the breasts, ovaries, and uterus.

Although natural progesterone can be manufactured from a substance called diosgenin, which is found in wild yams and soybeans, the body cannot manufacture progesterone from the raw diosgenin found in these foods. Dr. Lee therefore recommends using products that have been preconverted in the laboratory into progesterone rather than try to obtain it from dietary sources.

Dr. Borkin adds that the primary problem with progesterone supplementation is not dosage but metabolic clearance—the time necessary for inactivation and elimination of the metabolite once it has performed its task. "This can be affected by many factors, depending on the method used to introduce progesterone," he says. "For this reason, I always recommend the use of a transdermal cream because of its high absorption rate and metabolic clearance. Transdermal cream delivers progesterone in a fashion similar to the body's own delivery system. This avoids the problems sometimes associated with other forms of supplementation. Poorly formulated topical progesterone, for example, can build up in the fat cells and cause abnormally high levels of progesterone. This interferes with normal progesterone-estrogen ratios and can cause additional problems, such as constipation, depression, headache, hypoglycemia, and vertigo."

The recommended application of progesterone cream is ⅛ tsp to 1 tsp, 10-80 mg, or 3-10 drops of the oil per day. Premenopausal women with average menstrual cycles (28 days) should apply the cream during days 12 to 26 of their cycle. Those with longer cycles should apply it from days ten to 28. For menopausal women, Dr. Lee indicates that there can be more flexibility in applying the cream. He recommends using it over a 14-21 day period and then discontinuing use until the following month. The cream can be applied to the palms of the hands, the face and neck, the upper chest and breasts, the insides of the arms, and behind the knees. Alternating applications among these sites will increase absorption. Dr. Borkin cautions against using supplements over areas of high fat concentration, however.

When purchasing a natural progesterone cream or oil, there are two points to keep in mind. First, make sure it contains natural progesterone, not just wild yam *(Dioscorea villosa)*. Don't be misled by claims that wild yam creams are the same as progesterone creams. As an herbal supplement, wild yam can have a mild hormone-balancing effect, but it does not provide natural progesterone. Second, make sure you use a brand of cream that has enough natural progesterone in it to make a difference. Dr. Lee advises using only creams or oils that have at least 400 mg of progesterone per ounce, while other NHRT practitioners prefer to use only products that have more than 1,000 mg of progesterone per ounce. Dr. Borkin emphasizes that more is not always better. A high-quality transdermal cream will deliver 95% or more to the bloodstream, compared to oral progesterone that only delivers 5% of what is taken. It is equally important to use a product with a metabolic clearance time of less than four days.

Testosterone

Testosterone is an anti-aging hormone that is responsible for much more than defining sexual characteristics in men or influencing sex drive. Known as an anabolic steroid, testosterone is essential for life, since it helps to regulate basic metabolism, stimulate red blood cell production, and hinder the excessive production of free radicals. Testosterone also facilitates protein synthesis and the building of body tissues. Unlike other hormones that remain on the periphery, testosterone exerts its effects by quickly passing through the membrane of a cell and binding to a specific activation site on the gene. In this way, the protein-manufacturing capability of the DNA shifts into overdrive, enabling the body to repair and rebuild itself.

Testosterone is produced by small groups of specialized cells within the testicles and is also secreted, to a lesser extent, by the ovaries and adrenal glands. The pro-

NATURAL VS. SYNTHETIC HORMONE THERAPY

Synthetic hormones are patented products manufactured by pharmaceutical companies and, according to Michael Galitzer, M.D., of Los Angeles, California, account for the greatest number of prescriptions by physicians. "The number one selling drug for the past several years has been Premarin," he points out. Synthetic hormones are produced by altering the natural structure of the hormone in order to obtain a patent. This changes not only its structure, but also its effect on the body. Many synthetic hormones are derived from animal sources, such as horses, pigs, and sheep. Premarin, for example, is extracted from the urine of pregnant mares, hence its name (*Pregnant mare urine*). It is not the same estrogen as that which naturally exists in the body. "It's a chemical, not natural, with a certain level of toxicity that is indigenous to all chemicals," Dr. Galitzer says. Dr. Borkin adds that Premarin contains 50 different forms of estrogen, among which only three are known to naturally occur in humans.

In the human body, synthetic hormones are foreign and do not have all of the necessary co-factors for them to function properly. In some cases, they do not respond to the enzymes that render them inactive after they complete their goal and continue to function even when unwanted. This can lead to more complicated problems related to estrogen dominance. "In contrast, natural hormones are the exact replicas of those that exist in your body," Dr. Galitzer says. "They are far safer, with far fewer side effects than their synthetic counterparts." Additionally, all the body's necessary enzymes and co-factors make natural hormones work safely and efficiently.

Studies have revealed that the use of synthetic estrogens increase the likelihood of developing breast cancer.[3] Currently, synthetic estrogen remains the primary hormone used to treat PMS and menopausal complaints, yet these conditions can actually be exacerbated by this approach. In addition, depression, blood sugar problems, edema, weight gain, headache, loss of libido, fibroids, osteoporosis, and gastrointestinal problems are all known side effects of synthetic estrogen replacement. One attempt to counter such side effects has been the use of progestins, synthetic hormones similar to progesterone. But progestins can also cause numerous side effects, including water retention, breast tenderness, skin problems, insomnia, liver problems, and increased risk of birth defects.

duction of testosterone is triggered by luteinizing hormone (LH), produced in the pituitary gland. As is the case with other hormones, blood levels of testosterone are monitored by the hypothalamus, which issues a command to the pituitary, causing it to stop secreting LH after levels of testosterone reach a certain level. In the absence of LH, testosterone production ceases.

High levels of testosterone have been associated with balding and overly aggressive behavior. Many elderly men have cancerous cells in the prostate and excess testosterone has been shown to fuel their proliferation. Furthermore, too much testosterone can cause the blood to thicken, as red blood cells clump together; this can place a man at greater risk of stroke.

With age, blood levels of testosterone slowly decrease. Research conducted by the U.S. National Institutes of Health has shown a 1% to 2% reduction per year from age 30 to age 70. Deficiencies vary according to the individual and may produce menopause-like symptoms in some men. Half of men around the age of 80 have testosterone levels that are abnormally low. Men who are testosterone deficient experience a greatly diminished sex drive and have difficulty maintaining erections. They become lethargic and withdrawn and may lose strength and physical endurance. Body composition changes— lean muscle is replaced with fat, since testosterone helps in protein synthesis necessary for building muscles.[4]

Dietary factors can also influence a man's hormone levels. The typical Western diet, with its high levels of fat and low levels of fiber, may have a direct influence on testosterone production, according to clinical studies.[5] Other foods that have been found detrimental to hormone balance include saturated fats (commonly found in fast foods, processed foods, and red meats), hydrogenated oils, preservatives, and products containing refined sugar. The minerals zinc, copper, and selenium are necessary for normal hormone production in men.[6] Selenium, in addition to being required for testosterone production, helps protect the male sex glands against free radicals and heavy metals.[7] If these minerals are lacking in the diet, hormone imbalances may occur.

Men's hormones may be thrown out of balance by xenoestrogens, which are present primarily in pesticides (DDT, PCBs, and dioxin) and industrial by-products. According to some researchers, xenoestrogens may contribute to testicular cancer, urinary tract disorders, and low sperm count. In men, a high level of estrogen slows down the production of testosterone.[8] Many prescription drugs can contribute to sexual dysfunction in men. Exposure to lead, mercury, cadmium, and other heavy metals inhibits testosterone production.[9]

Men's hormone levels can also be adversely affected by certain lifestyle choices. Smoking, in particular, may be a factor in reduced production of testosterone.[10] Excessive consumption of alcohol decreases levels of testosterone and increases estrogen levels in men. However, modest alcohol intake has not been shown to affect hormone levels.[11] In addition, physical or mental/emotional stress can inhibit hormone production. "High levels of stress maintained over an extended period of time can cause testosterone to be converted to the stress hormone DHEA and, in some cases, be abnormally converted to estrogen," Dr. Borkin says.

Since part of the blood supply to the testicles comes from the vas deferens, the duct that transports sperm to the ejaculatory duct of the penis, vasectomy can result in testosterone deficiency. In addition, according to Dr. Galitzer, men lose one testosterone-producing cell (Leydig cell) every four seconds. "With increasing age, the Leydig cells are less sensitive to stimulation by luteinizing hormone, which is why 65% of men between the ages of 70 and 79 are impotent," he says. Dr. Galitzer also suspects that levels of testosterone production may be declining compared to the past. "We are all aware that sperm counts today are 50% less than they were 50 years ago. Might we also deduce that testosterone production is likewise similarly decreased?"

According to Dr. Galitzer, a man's sex hormone profile is determined by his levels of testosterone, estrogen, progesterone, and sex hormone binding globulin (SHBG). "SHBG has two important functions," Dr. Galitzer says. "It binds to cell receptors, so that both testosterone and estrogen can enter the cell. Secondly, SHBG binds excess testosterone, so when SHBG levels are excessive, an imbalance of a man's estrogen/testosterone ratio also develops. The end result is that less testosterone is available to the cells of the body. Ideally, NHRT for a male involves raising his total testosterone and lowering his estrogen and SHBG levels."

Testosterone replacement can heighten sex drive, increase bone density, and improve mood, among other effects. When considering testosterone replacement, the first step is a blood or saliva test to assess levels of the hormone, according to Julian Whitaker, M.D., a nationally recognized alternative medicine educator and editor of *Health and Healing*. If levels are low or even average for your age, testosterone therapy can help alleviate deficiency symptoms and improve overall health, he explains.

CAUTION Men who supplement with testosterone should closely monitor their prostate specific antigen (PSA) levels, as excess testosterone has been linked to prostate cancer. Other possible side effects include testicular atrophy, male pattern baldness, elevated red blood cell counts, elevated blood pressure, and gynecomastia (abnormally large mammary glands in men).

Dr. Borkin recommends the use of transdermal DHEA and androstenedione, since these hormones can convert to testosterone with less likelihood of causing side effects.

The goal of testosterone therapy is to restore blood testosterone levels to those of a healthy man, 25–30 years old. For this, Dr. Whitaker recommends weekly injections of testosterone cypionate (100 mg) or biweekly injections of testosterone enanthate (200 mg). These long-acting versions of the hormone are considered the safest and most effective preparations for use in testosterone replacement. As injection guarantees consistent absorption, Dr. Whitaker considers this to be the preferred method of testosterone supplementation. Skin patches and oral lozenges can also be effective, he reports, however, he advises against oral testosterone in pill form. "With oral testosterone, there is a potential for liver dysfunction and a decrease in protective HDL or 'good' cholesterol levels," he cautions. Further positive effects of testosterone replacement include increased lean muscle mass and protection for the heart, as certain forms of testosterone can improve the ratio between HDL and LDL ("bad") cholesterol and lower cholesterol levels overall.

As an accompaniment to testosterone therapy, Dr. Whitaker generally suggests taking the herb saw palmetto (120–360 mg daily), which has been shown to reduce the conversion of testosterone into dihydrotestosterone (DHT), a stronger version of the hormone. Too much DHT has been linked to various health problems, including prostate cancer.

Nutritional medicine can also help men cope with the natural decline of testosterone. Noted alternative health expert W. Lee Cowden, M.D., of Fort Worth, Texas, recommends the following nutritional supplements be used:

- Vitamin C (2000–3000 mg)
- Vitamin E (500 IU)
- Vitamin B complex (one tablet)
- Zinc (50 mg)
- Manganese (5 mg)
- Magnesium (500 mg)
- Selenium (50 mcg)
- Copper (2–3 mg)
- Evening primrose oil (3000 mg)
- Ginseng (2000–4000 mg)
- Royal Jelly (2000–4000 mg)

Another option employed by Dr. Borkin to maintain adequate testosterone levels is to stop the misappropriation of testosterone while also supplying the necessary building blocks for the production of testosterone. This can be achieved by using transdermal testosterone cream applied to the skin, while also supporting the endocrine system. The typical daily dosage is ⅛ to ½ teaspoon, depending on weight and age, applied to areas of soft skin, preferably upon rising in the morning.

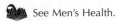 See Men's Health.

Thyroid Hormones

The thyroid gland has four principal hormones: T1, T2, T3, and T4. Thyroid hormones are stored in the thyroid and released to the body as needed. In addition to the marked effect they have on metabolism and the body's ability to oxygenate cells and oxidize toxins, thyroid hormones increase the body's energy and heat production, regulate blood circulation, enhance immune function, and increase heart contractility.

T1 (mono-iodothyronine) and T2 (di-iodothyronine) are not considered especially active. T4 (thyroxine) contains iodine, is produced exclusively in the thyroid gland, and accounts for almost 93% of the thyroid's hormones active in all of the body's processes; its chief function is to increase the speed of cell metabolism or energy conversion. Iodine and the amino acid tyrosine are essential to forming normal amounts of T4. When the body requires more T3 (tri-iodothyronine), T4 can give up its iodine to form T3. While representing only about 7% of the thyroid hormone complement, T3 has a greater biological activity by a factor of three to four times. When T4-to-T3 conversion runs smoothly, normal body temperature and metabolic rates are maintained. If the thyroid is functioning poorly, however, T4 breaks down to form reverse tri-iodothyronine (rT3, a different chemical version of T3). Stress, fasting, illness, or elevated cortisol can contribute to the occurrence of this faulty conversion. As rT3 levels increase, metabolism and body temperature decrease and various enzymes fail to function properly.

The formation and secretion of T3 and T4 are regulated by thyroid-stimulating hormone (TSH or thyrotropin), secreted by the pituitary gland in the brain. TSH, in turn, is directed by another hormone called thyrotropin-releasing hormone (TRH), which is secreted by the hypothalamus gland. When TSH reaches the thyroid gland, it signals it to secrete more hormones (both T4 and T3). The hormones released by the thyroid send a feedback message to the brain, telling it to stop secreting TSH and TRH. TSH blood levels are conventionally taken as the best index for thyroid dysfunction.

Thyroid imbalances, especially hypothyroidism (insufficient thyroid activity), often go undiagnosed. One reason for this is that physicians often confuse the symptoms of hypothyroidism with those of other conditions. According to the American Association of Clinical Endocrinologists (AACE), at least six million Americans suffer from hypothyroidism, yet only half of them have been properly diagnosed. "Thyroid hormone blood tests are frequently in the normal range, even though patients clinically appear to be suffering from hypothyroidism," Dr. Galitzer says. "Identifying these patients and instituting proper thyroid treatment can have great benefit to their overall health."

Subclinical hypothyroidism, the early stage of the disease, is particularly difficult to diagnose because of the action of TSH. During this stage, the pituitary gland recognizes that the thyroid isn't producing enough hormones, so it releases more TSH. The extra TSH causes the thyroid to work overtime to secrete more T4 and T3. A weak thyroid is thus often propped up by high levels of TSH and this masks the symptoms of the condition. Without adequate treatment, the thyroid will continue to deteriorate. To most effectively screen for hypothyroidism and other thyroid imbalances, Dr. Galitzer recommends that doctors request blood tests for thyroid antibodies for all of their patients; 24-hour urine specimens that analyze thyroid hormone metabolites can also be useful.

Thyroid imbalances can be caused by a variety of factors, including environmental pollutants, exposure to radiation, dietary excesses or insufficiencies, certain medications, stress, and yeast infections (candidiasis).

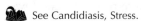 See Candidiasis, Stress.

- **Toxic Environment:** Thyroid problems have been on the rise due to the increasingly toxic environment in which we live. Exposure to radiation, fluoride (in water and toothpaste), mercury from silver amalgam dental fillings, pollutants (thyocyanide) in cigarette smoke, and chlorinated compounds (found in wood and leather preservatives) are just a few of the many causes of thyroid problems.[12]

- **Diet:** Dietary factors include synthetic and genetically engineered hormones in meat, dairy products, poultry, and eggs, which block the release of thyroid hormones. Another dietary factor is excess iodine, which is a powerful thyroid inhibitor. Lack of iodine can also result in thyroid imbalances as well. Raw cruciferous vegetables (cabbage, broccoli, or cauliflower) contain thyroid inhibitors; lightly steaming them eliminates these substances. Liver, while a nourishing food, contains thyroid inhibitors and there is some evidence that soy affects thyroid function.[13] Other dietary influences include vitamin deficiencies (particularly vitamins A and B), mineral deficiencies (zinc, copper, iron, and selenium), and excess intake of polyunsaturated fats (such as those found in soybean, safflower, and corn oils).

- **Medications:** In cases where the thyroid is already impaired, prednisone (an anti-inflammatory drug) can aggravate the condition.[14] Sulfa drugs, commonly used to treat infections, and oral anti-diabetic agents also impair thyroid function. Birth control pills and estrogen replacement therapy (ERT) can lead to estrogen dominance (an excess of the hormone estrogen in relation to progesterone), which inhibits the thyroid. The heart drug Cordarone® and interferon-alpha for hepatitis can cause either an overactive or underactive thyroid.[15]

- **Stress:** The action of thyroid hormones in the body is also uniquely affected by stress. The hormones released by stress, adrenaline and cortisol, interfere with the body's ability to convert T4 into T3. As T3 levels decrease, the body produces even more adrenaline and cortisol to try to speed up metabolism, which further inhibits the conversion.[16] The problem of impaired T4-to-T3 conversion is referred to as Wilson's Syndrome.

Conventional doctors typically treat thyroid conditions with Synthroid®, one of the most commonly prescribed drugs in the U.S. Synthroid can be ineffective since it only contains T4. "Some people can't effectively convert T4 to T3, and thus would benefit more from a preparation that contains both hormones, rather than Synthroid," says Dr. Galitzer, who finds it best to treat with a T4-T3 combination. He prefers Armour Thyroid, a desiccated thyroid formula that contains 80% T4 and 20% T3, or Westhroid, which has an even higher ratio of T3 to T4. "Start with ½ grain and increase the dose every two weeks," Dr. Galitzer advises. "If coffee makes the patient agitated, start with a lower dose and increase it slowly." Taking too high a dose of a thyroid formula can result in a variety of side effects, including anger, nervousness, rapid heart rate, headache, and insomnia, Dr. Galitzer warns.

Diet, nutritional supplementation, and herbal medicine can also help restore a weakened thyroid. Foods known as thyrotrophs stimulate thyroid hormone production and increase the conversion of T4 to T3. Exam-

ples of such foods are seaweed, garlic, radishes, watercress, seafood, egg yolks, raw milk products (kefir, yogurt, cottage cheese), wheat germ, brewer's yeast, mushrooms, organic beef or poultry, amaranth, quinoa, seeds, sprouted beans, watermelon, tropical fruits and fruit juices, and coconut oil.

Nutrients that help enhance thyroid function include vitamins E (800-1,200 IU), A (10,000-20,000 IU, necessary because hypothyroid patients do not effectively convert beta carotene into vitamin A), C (3,000-5,000 mg), and B complex (100-150 mg); the minerals zinc (25 mg), copper (3 mg), selenium (200 mcg), and iron (100 mcg); and the amino acid tyrosine (250-750 mg per day, taken between meals). *Gugulipid*, an Ayurvedic herb that has been used in India for over 2,500 years, is helpful for supporting thyroid function, as is *Coleus forskohlii*, a member of the mint family.

Melatonin

Melatonin, secreted by the pineal gland, regulates the body's internal clock, or circadian rhythm, which determines the 24-hour sleep/wake cycle. The pineal gland receives light-activated information from the eyes by way of the hypothalamus and sends information regarding seasonal and nocturnal changes to the body, which makes adjustments based on whether or not it is day or night, or whether the days are growing longer or shorter. Over 100 body functions fluctuate over a 24-hour period and are dependent on sunlight and darkness as cues.

Melatonin exerts a major influence on the body's biological rhythms, affecting appetite, body temperature, and both sleep patterns and immune system function. It also regulates reproductive activities, growth, blood pressure, motor activity, mood, and tumor growth, and is considered by many scientists to be the "regulator of regulators," according to Walter Pierpaoli, M.D., Ph.D., co-author of *The Melatonin Miracle*. It also plays an important role in human longevity.[17] Melatonin acts as a potent antioxidant that protects the brain and central nervous system from free-radical damage. "Normally present in high concentrations in the nervous system, melatonin appears to play a pivotal part in preventing oxidative damage to the nerves and brain," according to Joseph Pizzorno, N.D., founder of Bastyr University, in Kenmore, Washington. Aged animals and humans are melatonin-deficient and more sensitive to oxidative stress.

Although changes in body size as a person moves from childhood to adulthood may be responsible for fluctuating melatonin levels, the shrinking or calcification of the pineal gland and the resultant drop in melatonin production can also occur due to poor diet, environmental toxins, poor sleeping habits, or the aging process itself.

MELATONIN LEVELS THROUGHOUT LIFE

The pineal gland is roused into action in childhood. Newborn babies don't produce melatonin, since the pineal gland has not matured at the time of birth. At six months, melatonin levels start to rise and three-year-olds have the highest levels. Between the ages of 11 and 35, melatonin production decreases gradually. From 35 to 50, melatonin levels actually increase, after which time levels plummet sharply. The elderly produce half as much melatonin as children. Low levels have been linked to impaired immune activity, increased risk of breast cancer, obesity, heart disease, irritability, low libido, and depression.

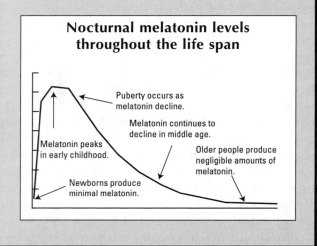

Nocturnal melatonin levels throughout the life span

Puberty occurs as melatonin decline.

Melatonin continues to decline in middle age.

Melatonin peaks in early childhood.

Older people produce negligible amounts of melatonin.

Newborns produce minimal melatonin.

Research suggests that the pineal gland may be sensitive to electromagnetic fields (EMFs)—chronic exposure to extremely low frequency EMFs suppresses nighttime melatonin secretions.[18] Other factors that can interfere with normal levels of melatonin secretion include:

- **Not enough light:** The lack of exposure to bright sunlight, or at least high-intensity artificial (full spectrum) lights, is associated with diminished nocturnal melatonin production. This may be due to the reduced daytime levels of serotonin (needed for the production of melatonin).[19]

- **Improper night lighting:** If you wake up in the middle of the night and are exposed to bright lights, melatonin production shuts off. In one study, six men exposed to bright artificial light (greater than 3,000 lux) from sunset to 2 a.m. on one night experienced inhibition of melatonin urine excretion (indicative of delayed pineal secretion) during the light expo-

sure.[20] Irregular sleep habits can also deplete melatonin supplies.

- **Stress:** As with melatonin, cortisol release is regulated by circadian rhythms, with levels the highest in the dawn hours, the same time that melatonin levels begin to dramatically decline. "There is a balance between cortisol levels and melatonin," Dr. Galitzer says. "You should have high cortisol in the morning and low cortisol at night. Likewise, you should have low melatonin in the morning and high melatonin at night." When large amounts of cortisol are released at night—as a result of physical exercise or emotional upsets—people will likely experience difficulty falling or staying asleep. In one study, nighttime physical stress and the associated high cortisol levels produced a one- to two-hour delay of melatonin release.[21]

- **Drugs:** Several commonly used medications can suppress melatonin production. Short-term use of over-the-counter (OTC) pain relievers, heart medications, anti-anxiety drugs, even sleeping pills, has been shown to interfere with the nocturnal secretion of melatonin. Nonsteroidal, anti-inflammatory drugs (NSAIDs), which include the widely used painkillers ibuprofen, aspirin, and indomethacin, greatly reduce melatonin secretion at night and disturb the amount of restorative deep sleep.[22]

- **Poor Diet:** Caffeine and alcohol have both been shown to impair melatonin production.[23] Deficiencies of magnesium and vitamins B_1, B_6, and B_{12} may also reduce melatonin levels.[24]

Melatonin supplements can be purchased in health food stores and some drug stores. According to Ray Sahelian, M.D., author of *Melatonin: Nature's Sleeping Pill*, melatonin lozenges, as opposed to tablets, seem to be more consistently effective, since they are absorbed directly from the mouth into the bloodstream. While some authorities suggest taking melatonin at the same time every evening to help regulate the pineal gland's production, others suggest it is best used only intermittently.

Richard Wurtman, Ph.D., of the Massachusetts Institute of Technology, reports that a mere 0.1 mg to 0.3 mg is sufficient for inducing sleep. This appears to be a good benchmark for starting supplementation; the dose can be increased until the desired effect is produced without side effects. Since most melatonin tablets contain up to 30 times this amount (3 mg), breaking the tablets into smaller pieces is advised. This practice could help avert some of the side effects that have been observed in melatonin supplement users, such as sluggishness, fatigue, or even nausea. If you take melatonin tablets that also contain vitamin B6, you may find yourself more "hyper" than sleepy at night. This is because B6 tends to raise metabolism in certain individuals. Also, people with altered circadian cycles may require special timing of melatonin supplements. If you have been taking melatonin for an extended period of time, it is best to taper off incrementally over a period of one to two weeks to avoid withdrawal symptoms.

> **CAUTION** Taking too high a dose of melatonin may cause morning grogginess, low body temperature, suppressed sex drive, hangover, or a worsening of symptoms in depressed patients. Individuals with autoimmune disorders, leukemia, or lymphoma should consult their physician prior to use, since immune-suppressing drugs such as prednisone and cyclosporine may react adversely with melatonin. People who are diabetic, depressed, or hormonally imbalanced should also take caution. Pregnant or nursing women should refrain from taking melatonin.

Modification of various lifestyle factors can also boost melatonin levels. Factors known to lower the pineal gland's melatonin production include high-protein diets, overeating, chronic stress, alcohol, caffeine, medications (NSAIDs and beta-blockers), tobacco, lack of natural light exposure during the day, sleep deprivation (or sleeping during the day and not at night), geopathic fields, and sleeping in a room that is not completely dark.

Psychological factors may also depress melatonin production. Individuals who are depressed, have seasonal effective disorder (SAD), panic attacks, and dementia have been found to have suppressed melatonin levels. Studies have found that exposure to electromagnetic fields can suppress the evening production of melatonin. The fields necessary to precipitate a decline in melatonin were about equal to what would be generated by an electric blanket.

Turning lights down earlier in the evening increases the daily supply of melatonin. Going to bed before midnight and getting up at dawn is the healthiest pattern for optimal melatonin production; meditation has also been found to raise melatonin levels. The use of magnets may also help—a negative magnetic field applied to the top of the head stimulates the pineal gland to secrete melatonin, according to William H. Philpott, M.D., of Choctaw, Oklahoma.

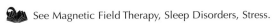 See Magnetic Field Therapy, Sleep Disorders, Stress.

Adrenal Hormones

The adrenal glands are composed of two types of tissue, the adrenal medulla and the adrenal cortex. The adrenal medulla, comprising 10%-20% of the gland, is responsible for the production of the hormones epinephrine (adrenaline) and norepinephrine (noradrenaline). These hormones are released in direct response to the sympathetic nervous system, which is responsible for the fight-or-flight response to stress or physical threats. The adrenal cortex, the outer layer, accounts for 80%-90% of the gland. It is responsible for the production of corticosteroids (also called adrenal steroids). More than 30 steroids have been isolated from the adrenal cortex.

The primary adrenal hormones are aldosterone (essential to maintaining proper fluid levels in kidney cells by regulating amounts of cellular sodium and potassium), androgen (testosterone) and estrogen, cortisol (promotes protein breakdown, regulates insulin and glycogen synthesis, and helps produce prostaglandins), DHEA, pregnenolone, and adrenaline and noradrenaline (also known as catecholamines, they affect heart rate, blood vessels, gastrointestinal tract, kidneys, lungs, bladder, skin, fat cells, liver, pancreas, and eyes). Additionally, the adrenal glands play a central role in maintaining the body's energy levels.

Malfunctioning adrenal glands may result from disease (Addison's, AIDS, cancer, fungal infections, tuberculosis), a defect in the hypothalamus or pituitary gland, or an inadequate amount of the pituitary hormone ACTH, which stimulates adrenal secretion. When the adrenal cortex produces too low a volume of its life-sustaining hormones, a life-threatening crisis will result. Initially, sustained stress causes the over-production of adrenal hormones. Cortisol helps mobilize the body's resources for defense and injury repair. However, in chronic stress, the continuous production of cortisol adversely affects the body by increasing the production of cell-damaging free radicals.

"Many hormonal imbalances are the direct result of adrenal insufficiency," Dr. Borkin says. "When the adrenal glands become exhausted due to overwork, adequate levels of cortisol and DHEA cannot be produced. This, in turn, plays a major role in the usage of all the steroid hormones. Long-term stress can have a serious impact on the adrenal glands and cause them to shrink and reduce production. This causes cellular damage, which sets off a chain reaction that affects all other parts of the body, as well as accelerating the aging process."

Based on his research, Dr. Borkin states, "The adrenal glands hold the key to the hierarchy of hormones. To cause a positive overall hormonal change, it is essential to normalize adrenal activity first, since it is the mainspring in the body's hormonal mechanisms. When the adrenals exhibit dysfunction, all other associated systems will as well." Symptoms of adrenal dysfunction are diverse and can involve the digestive, circulatory, respiratory, and nervous systems, as well as the brain. In addition, poor adrenal function can negatively impact the growth and repair of bones, muscles, hair, and nails.

A simple, noninvasive saliva test known as the Adrenal Stress Index (ASI) can determine whether an imbalance in the adrenal glands exists. The ASI test also evaluates how well the adrenal glands function by tracking their 24-hour circadian rhythm. Four saliva samples taken at intervals throughout the day are used to reconstruct the adrenal rhythm in the laboratory and determine whether the three main stress hormones (cortisol, adrenaline, and DHEA) are being secreted in proper proportion to each other and at the right times. Based on the results, practitioners of NHRT can prescribe the appropriate treatment to restore the balance of hormones.

Dr. Galitzer recommends the following lifestyle changes to enhance adrenal function: exercise, eating regular meals, regular periods of relaxation (including lying down during work breaks), going to bed early (sleep in on weekends when possible), and regular laughter. He also recommends the following supplements: vitamin C (2000-4000 mg per day; the highest concentration of vitamin C in the body is in the adrenal glands), vitamin B5 (pantothenic acid, 500 mg twice daily), magnesium (500 mg per day), and a licorice tincture (ten drops sublingually three times a day) or licorice tea. For severe cases of adrenal exhaustion, adrenal cortical extract (administered intramuscularly, subcutaneously, or sublingually) and Isocort, an adrenal cortex glandular formulation (2-3 times daily), can also be used.

Dr. Borkin adds that it is always necessary to treat the digestive system and the liver at the same time that the adrenals are treated, since dysfunction in either can cause serious chronic stress levels. Dr. Borkin employs a combination of custom compounded transdermal hormone creams and nutritional co-factors to balance the endocrine system and normalize adrenal activity. "This allows for several hormones to be combined with the nutritional co-factors that allow the hormones to function properly," he explains. In addition, he employs a regimen of probiotics, digestive enzymes, and liver detoxification, as well as B-complex vitamin (especially B5 and B6) and vitamin C with bioflavonoids.

"It normally takes four to six months to fully restore adrenal balance," Dr. Borkin says. "Once this is accomplished, focus can then shift to restoring healthy ratios of the steroid sex hormones estrogen, progesterone, and testosterone. It is necessary to affect the hormones in this sequence because, when the body is in the stress mode for an extended period of time, sex hormones are converted to the adrenal hormones DHEA and cortisol. This misappropriation due to stress is the primary cause of abnormal sex hormone levels and ratios. Thus, if adrenal dysfunction is not corrected first, any sex hormone, including progesterone or estrogen, that is supplemented can be converted to a stress hormone. You can do all of the right things, but if you do them out of order you will not get the desired results."

DHEA

DHEA (dehydroepiandrosterone) is the most abundant hormone found in the bloodstream and is sometimes referred to as the "mother of all hormones," because it is used as a building block for many other essential hormones. When the adrenal glands are chronically stressed, production of DHEA can be greatly reduced. DHEA is an important regulator of the thyroid and pituitary glands and DHEA supplementation has also been found to enhance thymus gland function. Many of the positive health benefits derived from DHEA can be traced to its ability to stimulate the production of human growth hormone.

Though the adrenal glands produce most of the body's supply of DHEA, the gonads (ovaries, testes) can also manufacture DHEA when the adrenals are overworked. DHEA exerts powerful effects throughout the body as most cells possess DHEA receptors. As an antioxidant, hormone regulator, and the building block from which estrogen and testosterone are produced, DHEA is vital to health. DHEA also regulates many other hormones, decreases cholesterol, boosts immunity by stimulating natural killer cell activity, increases the sensitivity of cells to insulin, and assists in returning to a balanced state after the stress reaction. DHEA is a good stress barometer, because when stress levels go up, DHEA levels go down.

Generally, DHEA levels tend to decrease with age. DHEA peaks at age 25 and declines at a rate of about 2% per year. It is not until the mid-forties that we begin to feel the effects of lower DHEA levels. By 80, the level of our DHEA is about 15% of what it was when we were in our twenties. By 90, we are down to 5%.[25] Aside from stress and disease, other factors that tend to decrease DHEA levels include sugar, nicotine, caffeine, and alcohol. A vegetarian diet low in cholesterol and healthy fats appears to drain DHEA from the body.[26] While nutritional imbalances in general lower DHEA levels, calorie restriction that does not result in a malnourished state boosts production. Vitamin C has been found to enhance DHEA levels, as does methylsulfonylmethane (MSM), an organic sulfur compound. DHEA levels may also be influenced by pregnenolone, the parent hormone for DHEA. Usually starting at age 45, pregnenolone production slows down and, by age 75, the body produces 60% less pregnenolone than in one's youth.

According to Dr. Galitzer, symptoms of DHEA deficiency include poor memory, poor resistance to noise, anxiety, decreased libido (especially in women), decreased axillary (armpit) and pubic hair, and dry skin, eyes, or hair. To determine whether a DHEA deficiency exists, Dr. Galitzer recommends a 24-hour saliva test as well as a DHEA-sulfate blood test.

Since 1994, DHEA has been classified as a dietary supplement and requires no prescription. Nevertheless, it is best to consult a qualified health-care professional when taking DHEA. C. Norman Shealy, M.D., Ph.D., of Springfield, Missouri, founding President of the American Holistic Medical Association, recommends blood testing to determine your exact DHEA dosage. A typical dosage is 25 mg daily for women and 50 mg daily for men, but since DHEA levels fluctuate significantly (even among people within the same age group), it is important to accurately identify your optimum dose. Some experts also argue that, rather than taking DHEA directly, it is better to take the substance your body uses to make DHEA, namely the hormone pregnenolone. A typical recommended dose of pregnenolone is 50 mg daily, best taken in the morning.

> **CAUTION** Although no serious side effects have been reported in over 5,000 scientific studies on DHEA, some high-dose DHEA users may experience acne, oily skin, facial hair growth (in women), irritability, insomnia, fatigue, and breast enlargement (in men). These symptoms will usually resolve with a lower dose, skipping days, or ending treatment. In addition, since DHEA can convert to estrogen and/or testosterone, monitoring these hormones is also important. Long-term effects of DHEA supplementation are not known. DHEA replacement is not suggested for pregnant or nursing women, individuals under 30 years of age (unless indicated by blood testing), and people at risk for breast, uterine, or prostate cancer.

DHEA can be administered orally (tablet or capsule), sublingually, by injection, or by topical cream. Using DHEA cream or taking it sublingually bypasses the liver, which is important for individuals suffering from liver disease. Raymond Peat, Ph.D., of Eugene, Oregon, advises a dosage of no more than 2-3 mg of DHEA for anyone other than an elderly, sick person, who can take up to 12-15 mg daily (but even then, not without pregnenolone, progesterone, and thyroid glandular). Since pregnenolone converts to both progesterone and DHEA, supplemental pregnenolone is a safer therapy, says Dr. Peat.

COMPOUNDING PHARMACISTS

According to Dr. Galitzer, all natural hormones, with the exception of human growth hormone (HGH) and thyroid hormones, should be ordered from a compounding pharmacist. "Compounding pharmacists make medications from scratch, using raw chemicals, powders, and devices," Dr. Galitzer says. "This allows physicians to prescribe custom-tailored medications for their patients that are not available commercially." Compounding is also necessary to allow pharmacists to prepare small quantities of prescriptions more frequently to ensure stability of the product. In addition, compounding pharmacists can prepare forms free of dyes and preservatives, a significant benefit to the many patients who are allergic to such chemicals commonly found in commercial products.

In the 1930s and 1940s, 60% of all medications in the U.S. were compounded, Dr. Galitzer reports, but compounding decreased due to the advent of manufacturing. "Pharmacists were thankful for the opportunity to fill prescriptions that were pre-made from the manufacturers and, in effect, became dispensers," Dr. Galitzer says. "But since manufacturers must be assured that there will be a return on their investment with a product, there are limited chemical forms, dosage forms, strengths, flavors, and packaging for physicians to prescribe and pharmacists to dispense."

"When supplementing with DHEA, you must distinguish between the pharmacologic doses given to a patient with disease conditions, such as multiple sclerosis, versus the physiologic doses which restore one to the youthful range," Dr. Galitzer cautions. "In addition, it is best to take it in the morning in order to mimic the body's natural circadian rhythm." Supplementing DHEA at levels in excess overwhelms the adrenal glands and creates a variety of problems, such as excess production of estrogen, testosterone, and other hormones. Since DHEA speeds metabolic processes in the body, it is advisable to take antioxidants, such as vitamins C and E, beta carotene, selenium, coenzyme Q10, and grape seed extract, to protect the liver and other organs from excessive free radicals.

A number of dietary and lifestyle changes can also help boost DHEA levels. These include reducing caloric intake; eating a diet rich in essential fatty acids; supplementing with vitamin C (4,000 mg or more), magnesium (400 mg), and chromium (200-400 mcg) daily; reducing stress; and avoiding drugs that artificially inhibit cholesterol formation (required by the body to synthesize pregnenolone, from which DHEA is derived). Stopping smoking is recommended, since nicotine inhibits the enzymatic process necessary for producing DHEA.[27] Siberian ginseng (2-16 ml fluid extract or 100-200 mg standardized extract) can also be beneficial, since ginseng strengthens the adrenal glands, relieves anxiety, and moderates the body's stress response.

Pregnenolone

While DHEA is the parent hormone to testosterone and estrogen, it is derived from pregnenolone. Pregnenolone is made by the adrenal glands and in brain cells. Enzymes convert pregnenolone into either progesterone or DHEA, depending on the tissue and the demands of the body. Pregnenolone also acts as a brainpower hormone in that it enhances memory and concentration, reduces mental fatigue, and generally keeps the brain functioning at peak capacity.

The need for supplemental pregnenolone increases with age. In fact, the older you are, the more likely you are to feel an effect from taking pregnenolone. In a healthy person, the conversion of cholesterol to pregnenolone occurs inside the mitochondria (cellular energy factories). Unlike other hormones, pregnenolone stimulates its own synthesis, so if you take it as a supplement, the body's ability to synthesize it is not suppressed.

Pregnenolone can be purchased in chewing gum form, as sublingual liquids and capsules, and as topical creams. It is typically sold in dosages of 10 mg, 25 mg, and 50 mg. The liquid or capsules (absorbed under the tongue) and the cream (rubbed on the thighs, chest, arms, or stomach) are quickly absorbed into the bloodstream. The usual dose of pregnenolone is about 50-150 mg daily. As with all hormones, more is not necessarily better. Start off with the lower dosages each morning and work up from there until you achieve a noticeable effect. If taking more than 50 mg, do so in divided doses.

> **CAUTION** Since pregnenolone is a precursor to DHEA and other steroid hormones, taking pregnenolone may require a significant reduction in DHEA supplementation. Also, women taking pregnenolone may experience increased levels of progesterone, which may similarly require reduced supplementation. To determine the precise pathway by which the pregnenolone is being converted by the body, blood testing is required.

Human Growth Hormone (HGH)

HGH is a small protein-like hormone (similar to insulin) released by the pituitary gland under the direction of the hypothalamus. Most HGH is released during deep stages of sleep each night, while lesser quantities are released during daytime hours. Though it remains in circulation for only a few minutes, the effects of HGH are profound, delaying many of the manifestations of the aging process. With age, most people lose muscle mass, fat accumulates around the stomach, thighs, and elsewhere, hair turns gray, wrinkles appear, and organs such as the heart diminish in capacity. All of this is influenced by the lack of adequate levels of HGH.

During adolescence, when growth is most rapid, production of HGH is high. After age 20, HGH production decreases at an average rate of about 14% per decade. By age 60, it is not uncommon to measure a growth hormone loss of 75% or more. With even more advanced age, HGH levels become barely detectable.

HGH does not act on tissues directly. Rather, it travels to the liver, which then produces a chemical known as insulin-like growth factor or IGF-1. As the name implies, this substance acts in global ways that are similar to insulin. It is IGF-1 that is directly responsible for HGH's rejuvenatory effects on muscle, bone, cartilage, kidney, and skin tissues. HGH affects protein, glucose, fat, and carbohydrate metabolism; thus, the consequences of low HGH levels range from increased body fat, increased dehydration, wrinkles, impaired vision, and poor memory, to dampened immune function, insulin resistance, low libido, loss of lean muscle mass, atrophy of heart tissue, and the occurrence of chronic, degenerative diseases.

When HGH levels decline below normal, the person's "muscle and bone strength and energy levels most likely will decrease, and tissue repair, cell growth, healing capacity, upkeep of vital organs, brain and memory function, enzyme production, and revitalization of hair and skin will also diminish," according to Edward Lichten, M.D., of Southfield, Michigan. Body fat increases by 7% to 25%, while lean body mass (muscle) decreases to a similar degree. Bones become thinner. Cholesterol and triglyceride levels are increased, and the heart wall becomes thicker, pumping less blood with each beat. Psychological problems also ensue, such as a feeling of social isolation, impaired sense of well-being, depression, inability to concentrate, and fatigue, according to Dr. Lichten.

Researchers have found a strong connection between HGH and insulin/glucose metabolism. It has also been found that supplementing human growth hormone in deficient adults may help avert the onset of some forms of diabetes. Since the pituitary is the master gland (responsible for producing chemicals that trigger the release of other hormones), when other glands run excessively (the adrenals due to stress or the pancreas due to insulin resistance) or underperform (hypothyroidism), this can lead to reduced HGH levels as the pituitary becomes exhausted. Damage or decreased function of the pancreas and liver can also affect HGH levels, since both organs play a role in the synthesis of IGF-1.

It is possible to elevate HGH by reducing or eliminating factors that inhibit HGH production—manage chronic stress, lose weight, eat healthy foods, limit fats to no more than 30% of total calories, avoid sugar and simple carbohydrates (especially near bedtime), refrain from alcohol use, and reverse insulin resistance and diabetes. Sugar in its many forms, found abundantly in processed foods, provokes the pancreas to release insulin. Insulin and HGH are antagonists, meaning that when insulin levels rise, HGH levels fall. Individuals who are obese are often insulin resistant, meaning their blood levels of insulin are high, but the cells are unable to make use of it. This is one reason why obese individuals are often HGH deficient.

Eating less without foregoing the necessary nutrients has been found to elevate HGH levels, as does short-term fasting. Exercise can help stimulate the pituitary gland to produce more human growth hormone; so can a good night's sleep.

Certain nutrients are also vital for the production of HGH. The neurotransmitter acetylcholine regulates HGH secretion, while blood pH (acidity) plays an important role in the body's ability to make use of HGH. The minerals potassium and magnesium influence the release of HGH. Calcium also exerts a strong influence—a rise in calcium will produce an increased release of HGH, while any fall in calcium will result in diminished release. Zinc plays a vital role in HGH release, and the symptoms of zinc deficiency (impaired wound healing, reduced protein synthesis, immunosuppression, reduced sex hormone levels) are directly attributed to the action of HGH.

According to Ron Klatz. D.O., President of the American Academy of Anti-Aging Medicine, in Chicago, Illinois, certain amino acids also help stimulate significant increases of HGH. Dr. Klatz recommends taking the following amino-acid cocktail on an empty stomach: arginine (2-5 g one hour before exercising and before sleeping), ornithine (2-5 g at bedtime), lysine (1 g one hour before exercising and before sleeping), glycine (250-6,750 mg), glutamine (2 g at bedtime), and tryptophan

HOMEOPATHIC REGENERATION OF HORMONES

Many practitioners of NHRT prefer to use homeopathic formulas to regenerate hormone levels, especially when dealing with human growth hormone (HGH) deficiencies. The reason for this has to do with the biophysics of the regenerative process, according to Dr. Galitzer. "Each organ system in the body, while connected to the individual's essential life force, or *qi*, is also a unique bioenergy system, vibrating at a certain resonant frequency," Dr. Galitzer says. "An imbalance in the organ's bioenergy impedes the process of renewing itself. In order to stimulate regeneration, cells and organs need a specific input of energy, certain wave-forms that correlate to the weakened organ. In other words, they need the right amount of energy coupled with the right message."

According to Dr. Galitzer, the best way to stimulate this process is through the use of homeopathy since, unlike nutrients, herbs, and other forms of hormonal therapies, homeopathic remedies do not need to be broken down before they can be converted for use in the body. "This conversion process requires expenditures of energy, which in sick patients may further deplete them, thus impeding regeneration," Dr. Galitzer says. "With homeopathy, this problem does not exist." Dr. Galitzer finds that homeopathic regeneration formulas work well in conjunction with NHRT. "Such formulas provide the proper information, frequencies, and energies to the glands in order to keep them more physiologically active while using natural hormone replacement therapy," he says. "They also enhance receptivity of cell hormone receptor sites to NHRT."

Dr. Galitzer recommends RegenRx formulas to his patients interested in using homeopathic remedies. "The RegenRx formulas contain homeopathic adenosine triphosphate (ATP) 5X, which was found to be the essential energy frequency to assist regeneration in all tissues and organs," he says. Many of the RegenRx formulas have multiple potencies (both X and C dilutions), making them more effective, according to Dr. Galitzer. "When it comes to regeneration, energy by itself is not enough," he says. "There also needs to be a message that tells the cell to move into the regenerative mode. It is the combination of the X and C potencies that acts as the vehicle for delivering this message. In other words, the body is free to choose which of the potencies it needs at any one time."

(500–2,000 mg at bedtime). Dr. Klatz also recommends taking 200–1,000 mg of vitamin B₃ (niacin), a powerful releaser of HGH. Best results are experienced when cycling these hormone-releasing nutrients—use for 4–6 weeks, then cycle off for two weeks.

In addition to the above measures for boosting HGH levels, practitioners of NHRT may also recommend HGH replacement therapy. HGH is typically self-injected four times per week, usually in the evening within one hour of sleep to mimic the body's natural cycle of production. HGH cannot be administered orally, since it will be rendered ineffective by the digestive processes. Getting the correct dose is important, since a dose greater than what the body normally produces can result in adverse side effects. Dr. Lichten suggests that a minimal dose of 0.03 mg/kg of body weight per week will typically produce a positive effect, while minimizing side effects.

As effective as HGH therapy is for some patients, it is clearly not for everyone. Synthetic HGH has to be injected and is expensive. Also, HGH has some side effects and its effectiveness diminishes over time. Finally, injecting HGH does nothing to enhance the functional ability of the pituitary gland to manufacture HGH on its own. The short-term side effects that have been reported—joint pain, carpal tunnel syndrome, fluid retention, high blood pressure, and hypoglycemia—are usually alleviated when the dose is reduced. Some bio-engineered forms of growth hormone have been found to significantly lower insulin levels and, while insulin tends to cause HGH levels to decrease, it is absolutely vital for HGH to be effective.

Monitoring HGH levels prior to treatment and as therapy proceeds is of paramount importance. In this way, HGH levels can be kept within an optimal and safe range. Excessive release of HGH may result in coarse skin; joint enlargement is possible if growth hormone stimulation continues for an excessive amount of time. For this reason, NHRT practitioners typically recommend using HGH for several months, followed by several months of abstinence. They also advise increasing antioxidant levels to counter free radicals. Because of the potential side effects of HGH replacement therapy, many NHRT practitioners, including Dr. Galitzer, prefer to stimulate HGH levels through homeopathic regeneration (see "Homeopathic Regeneration of Hormones"). Dr. Borkin has tested sublingual recombinant HGH with much success. He recommends administering 6–10 sprays (600–1,000 mg/ml) of HGH sublingually at bedtime, for at least six months. He also strongly recommends monitoring sex and adrenal hormones to determine if HGH therapy is having a positive effect on these hormones as well; if not, further

hormonal balancing (adrenal therapy) may be necessary before HGH therapy proves beneficial.

> ⚠ **CAUTION** Reported short-term side effects of HGH replacement in some individuals include nausea, vomiting, increased diabetes risk, night sweats, hyperglycemia, allergic reactions, carpal tunnel syndrome, acute pancreatitis, headaches, visual changes, and neuropathy, among others. The long-term risks of recombinant HGH replacement therapy, IGF-1 injections, and other methods of stimulating HGH secretion are unknown. Though elevated levels of IGF-1 have been shown to increase the risk of prostate cancer, experts debate the findings. Consult a qualified specialist before undertaking a program to stimulate higher HGH levels. It is also important to closely monitor thyroid hormone levels, as elevated levels of HGH tend to boost the body's metabolic rate. This can lead to an increased consumption of thyroid hormone, potentially causing hypothyroidism.

Conditions Benefited by Natural Hormone Replacement Therapy

Research has shown that the use of natural hormones can provide benefit for numerous disease conditions.

ESTROGEN AND PROGESTERONE

According to Dr. Lee, estrogen dominance is a primary cause of almost all female health problems, including fibrocystic breast disease, PMS, mood swings, excessive bleeding, endometriosis, fibroids, infertility, and ovarian cysts. Perimenopause is the time when hormone levels begin to shift in preparation for menopause. It is not so much the decrease in hormones that produces the uncomfortable symptoms associated with perimenopause, but rather the changing ratio between estrogen and progesterone. Chronic or episodic depression, severe mood swings, and anxiety are frequent manifestations of these midlife fluctuations.

Biochemist Phyllis Bronson, Ph.D., and Harold Whitcomb, M.D., of the Aspen Clinic for Preventative and Environmental Medicine, in Colorado, report that almost all of the perimenopausal women they see are suffering from either depression or anxiety caused by hormonal imbalance. "Only a very small percentage feel great naturally," says Dr. Bronson. Anxiety is the result in those who have too much estrogen in relationship to other hormones (estrogen dominance) and depression occurs when the woman has too little estrogen in the hormonal equation (estrogen deficiency).

Other consequences of estrogen dominance can include increased fat storage, tissue damage, bruising, and aging of the skin. It can also damage the pituitary gland and put stress on liver function, reports Dr. Lee. The liver is required to detoxify estrogen and to convert thyroid hormone to its active form. If the liver is not working properly, it will perpetuate the estrogen excess cycle.

Women with estrogen dominance are more prone to the accelerated aging effects of thrombosis (blood clot), embolism (blood vessel blockage), stroke, migraines, hypoglycemia (low blood sugar), edema (fluid retention), and heart attack. Women in this category are much more likely to be vulnerable to migraines and seizures as well. Many menopausal symptoms—hot flashes, profuse perspiration, headache, dizziness, heart palpitations, tinnitus, nervousness/irritability, sleep disturbances, depressive moods—are also due to estrogen imbalances. Osteoporosis is viewed primarily as a disease of postmenopausal women due to decreases in estrogen and progesterone levels that occur at this time, which can contribute to bone loss.

By monitoring and properly adjusting estrogen and progesterone ratios, NHRT practitioners are having great success treating the above conditions. Estrogen may also help prevent Alzheimer's disease, reduce the risk of colon cancer, and prevent tooth loss, while progesterone can act as a protective agent against cancer, serve as a natural tranquilizer, and shows potential benefit for nerve disease.[28]

TESTOSTERONE

Signs of testosterone deficiency, according to Dr. Galitzer, include constant fatigue, decreased ability to concentrate, depression, gynecomastia (breast enlargement in men), hot flashes, loss of confidence, loss of muscle tone, memory problems, nervousness, pale skin, and reduced libido, all of which have been shown to respond to testosterone hormone therapy. Testosterone also lowers cholesterol, protects against heart disease, and prevents osteoporosis, and may play a preventive role against Alzheimer's disease.[29]

THYROID HORMONES

Thyroid imbalances can manifest as either physical or mental/emotional symptoms. Physical symptoms include weight fluctuations, edema, hypoglycemia, skin problems, chronic infections, chronic fatigue syndrome, weakness, low body temperature and cold extremities, slow pulse, hair loss or thinning hair, headaches, infertility, increased liver size, rheumatic pain, muscle aches and weakness, anemia, labored breathing, brittle nails, poor

vision, hearing impairment, menstrual disorders, slow speech, and constipation. Mental/emotional symptoms include apathy, depression, poor memory and concentration difficulties, mood swings, dual personality, paranoia, irritability, inappropriate crying, excessive worry, insomnia, slow reaction time and mental sluggishness, and attention deficit hyperactivity disorder (ADHD).

Other conditions related to insufficient thyroid activity include mitral valve collapse (also known as floppy valve syndrome), joint pain, headache, and increased cholesterol levels. Thyroid conditions can also contribute to heart disease, cancer, hypertension, and multiple sclerosis. All of these conditions, if due to an imbalance of thyroid hormones, may respond to thyroid hormone treatment.

MELATONIN

In experiments, melatonin has reduced the neuronal damage associated with Alzheimer's disease and Parkinson's disease.[30] It has been shown to prevent cataracts (caused by free-radical damage in the eye lens), as well as counteract the free-radical effects of toxins.[31] Further studies have shown that prolonged periods of sleep deprivation—that is, prolonged periods without elevated production of melatonin—cause neuron damage.[32] Low blood levels of melatonin have been implicated in patients with manic depression and schizophrenia; in these cases, restoring patients to normal nighttime levels of melatonin reversed their disorders.[33] Melatonin also helps reduce anxiety, panic disorders, and migraines, as well as inducing sleep.

Research has found that T-helper cells contain receptors specifically designed to fit melatonin molecules. During sleep, melatonin attaches to these receptors and stimulates the production of a factor that stimulates the activation of natural killer (NK) cells, phagocytes, cytotoxic cells, as well as immune cells found in the bone marrow.[34] One study found that increasing nighttime melatonin levels led to a 240% increase in production of NK cells.[35] Researchers have also found melatonin to significantly reduce levels of LDL ("bad") cholesterol and to lower high blood pressure.[36]

ADRENAL HORMONES

The adrenal glands, like the thyroid, help regulate the body's metabolic rate. But whereas the thyroid regulates the chemical reactions occurring in nearly every cell of the body, the adrenal gland regulates the metabolism of proteins, fats, and carbohydrates. In addition, the adrenals constantly monitor nerve energy, physical energy, glandular activity, and the oxidation process. Adrenal hormones aid in blood clotting, enhance bodily strength, and affect circulation, blood pressure, uterine tone, and involuntary muscle contractions. Adrenaline, noradrenaline, and cortisol are stress hormones that regulate and stabilize immune system function by influencing the proliferation of white blood cells. Adrenal hormone therapy is useful for treating allergies and chronic fatigue, muscle weakness, depression, and a magnification of arthritic symptoms resulting from adrenal exhaustion.

Other conditions that can benefit from restoring adrenal balance include age spots, constipation, dark circles under the eyes (shiners), dizziness, edema, hypoglycemia, mood swings, impaired respiration, and poor concentration.

DHEA

A landmark study of 242 men, 50-79 years old, based on 12 years of research, stated that a small supplementation of DHEA (100 mcg/ml) corresponded to a 48% reduction in death from heart disease and a 36% reduction in death from any cause (other than accidents).[37] A Temple University medical researcher reported that DHEA can help a person lose weight by blocking an enzyme known to produce fat tissue. In one study, DHEA supplementation enabled men to lose 31% of mean body fat with no change in body weight in 28 days. Another study, involving 16 middle-aged to elderly men, showed that taking DHEA for one year led to a 75% increase in their sense of well-being—they coped better with stress, felt more physically mobile, and slept better.[38]

DHEA has also been shown to provide a number of life-enhancing benefits, such as improved concentration and memory, increased vitality, enhanced immune system function, increased muscular strength, greater ability to handle stress and depression, and reduced joint pain. DHEA can also have beneficial effects on libido. In men who have decreased testosterone production resulting in lowered libido, DHEA (which can convert to testosterone) can boost libido almost as well as testosterone. DHEA also decreases cholesterol, increases the sensitivity of cells to insulin, and assists in returning the body to a balanced state after stress reactions.[39]

PREGNENOLONE

Pregnenolone has been shown to be effective in ameliorating the adverse effects of stress and enhancing brain function. Both pregnenolone and DHEA have been found to synchronize brain activity and preserve neuronal function. In addition, pregnenolone modulates chemical reactions, calcium-protein binding, gene activation, and enzymatic reactions involved in the storage and retrieval of memory. Pregnenolone also shows promise for treating cases of depression, arthritis, and spinal cord injuries.[40]

HUMAN GROWTH HORMONE (HGH)

HGH replacement therapy has been shown to reverse many of the problems associated with the aging process, such as weight gain, insulin resistance, muscle wasting, dry skin, neurological impairment, low sex drive, and lack of energy. Daniel Rudman, M.D., of the Medical College of Wisconsin, pioneered the use of HGH therapy. In a 1990 study reported in the *New England Journal of Medicine,* involving 21 men, 61-81 years old, Dr. Rudman found that after a six-month period of HGH injections, lean body mass and fat tissue changes were equivalent in magnitude to the changes incurred during 10-20 years of aging. In other words, the test subjects demonstrated a reversal in the aging process, appearing younger, sleeker, and stronger, and benefiting from an increase in muscle mass and a loss in body fat. Lung capacity and heart, immune, and kidney function all improved with HGH.

Human growth hormone supports the production of other hormones, such as testosterone, estrogen, and thyroid hormones. Adults who have an underactive thyroid gland appear to be deficient in growth hormone. When such patients are given adequate HGH, they show gains in energy, muscle strength and mass, mental abilities, and psychological attitude. Scientific studies show that many of the benefits of estrogen (to protect against bone loss), testosterone (in building muscles), and DHEA and pregnenolone (to elevate mood) are due to the stimulation of HGH by these hormones.[41]

Other reported benefits from HGH include revitalization of liver, spleen, and brain functions, increased exercise capacity, increased volume of the thymus gland and enhanced immune function, improved kidney blood flow and efficiency, improved body heat function, a reduced risk for cardiovascular problems, and a general enhancement in the sense of well-being.

The Future of Natural Hormone Replacement Therapy

The popularity of natural hormone replacement therapy has surged in the last decade, and today half of all hormones sold in the U.S. are available over-the-counter in pharmacies and health food stores, by mail order, and over the Internet. At the same time, increasing numbers of physicians, both alternative and conventional, are now exploring the potential benefits of NHRT for their patients. As a result, interest in NHRT is likely to continue to increase in the years ahead.

"We will continue to focus on ideal ways of administering natural hormones, along with nutrients, botanicals, and homeopathic remedies, to maximize glandular function, increase hormonal effects, and improve brain/body longevity," Dr. Galitzer says. "Combining natural hormone replacement therapy with homeopathic regeneration formulas may prove to be the optimal therapy in the future."

Where to Find Help

To learn more about natural hormone replacement therapy, contact:

American Academy of Anti-Aging Medicine
1510 West Montana
Chicago, Illinois 60614
(773) 528-4333
Website: www.worldhealth.net

Dedicated to the advancement of all therapeutic approaches in anti-aging medicine, including NHRT.

American College for Advancement in Medicine (ACAM)
23121 Verdugo Drive, Suite 204
Laguna Hills, California 92653
(800) 532-3688
Website: www.acam.org

ACAM is dedicated to establishing certification and standards of practice for preventive medicine and the ACAM protocol.

American Health Institute
12381 Wilshire Blvd.
Los Angeles, California 90025
(800) 392-2623
Website: www.ahealth.com

A pioneering research organization in the field of longevity medicine and the use of natural hormone replacement therapy.

National Institute of Endocrine Research
1817 S. Eastern Avenue
Las Vegas, Nevada 89104
(805) 496-0275
Website: www.endocrineresearch.com
Provides education and certification for national board specialty in Natural Hormonal Sciences.

Testing Hormone Levels

Aeron LifeCycles
1933 Davis Street, Suite 310
San Leandro, California 94577
(800) 631-7900
Website: www.aeron.com

Sabre Sciences, Inc.
910 Hampshire Road, Suite P
Westlake Village, California 91361
(888) 490-7300
Website: www.sabresciences.com

Compounding Pharmacies

International Academy of Compounding Pharmacists
P.O. Box 1365
Sugar Land, Texas 77487
(800) 927-4227
Website: www.iacprx.org

Apothecure, Inc.
13720 Midway Road, Suite 109
Dallas, Texas 75244
(800) 969-6601

Health Pharmacies
2809 Fish Hatchery Road, Suite 103
Madison, Wisconsin 51713
(800) 373-6704

Medical Center Pharmacy
3675 S. Rainbow Blvd.
Las Vegas, Nevada 89103
(800) 723-7455

Steven's Pharmacy
1525 Mesa Verde Drive E.
Costa Mesa, California 92626
(800) 352-3786

Women's International Pharmacy
13925 W. Meeker Blvd., Suite 13
Sun City West, Arizona 85375
(800) 279-5708

For Libidex Creme (available to health-care practitioners only), contact:

Market Resource International
310 26th Street
Santa Monica, California 90402
(888) 674-9556

For transdermal hormone creams, available to practitioners as well as the public, contact:

Sabre Sciences, Inc.
910 Hampshire Road, Suite P
Westlake Village, California 91361
(888) 490-7300
Website: www.sabresciences.com

For RegenRx products, contact:

Apex Energetics
1701 E. Edinger Avenue, Suite A-4
Santa Ana, California 92705
(800) 736-4381
Website: www.apexenergetics.com

Recommended Reading

Hormonal Health. Michael Colgan. Vancouver, BC, Canada: Apple Publishing, 1996.

Natural Hormone Balance for Women. Uzzi Reiss, M.D., with Martin Zucker. New York: Pocket Books, 2001.

The Second Brain. Michael D. Gershon, M.D. New York: HarperCollins, 1998.

The Superhormone Promise: Nature's Antidote to Aging. William Regelson, M.D., with Carol Colman. New York: Simon & Schuster, 1996.

The Testosterone Syndrome. Eugene Shippen, M.D., and William Fryer. New York: M. Evans, 1998.

Tired of Being Tired. Jesse Hanley, M.D. New York: Putnam, 2001.

The Trouble with Testosterone. Robert M. Sapolsky. New York: Scribner, 1997.

What Your Doctor May Not Tell You About Menopause. John R. Lee, M.D., with Virginia Hopkins. New York: Warner Books, 1996.

What Your Doctor May Not Tell You About Premenopause. John R. Lee, M.D., with Jesse Hanley, M.D., and Virginia Hopkins. New York: Warner Books, 1999.

What's Your Menopause Type? Joseph Collins, N.D. Roseville, CA: Prima Health, 2000.

NATUROPATHIC MEDICINE

Naturopathic medicine treats disease by utilizing the body's inherent ability to heal. Naturopathic physicians aid the healing process by incorporating a variety of treatment options based on the patient's individual needs. Diet, lifestyle, work, and personal history are all considered when determining a treatment regimen.

THE SPIRIT OF naturopathic medicine is reflected in the definition of health advocated by the World Health Organization (WHO)—"a state of complete physical, mental, and social well-being, not merely the absence of infirmity."[1] In fact, WHO, in a report on traditional medicine, has recommended the integration of naturopathic medicine into conventional health care systems.[2]

Naturopathic medicine is not a single modality of healing, but a comprehensive array of healing practices, including diet and clinical nutrition, homeopathy, acupuncture, herbal medicine, hydrotherapy, therapeutic exercise, spinal and soft-tissue manipulation, physical therapies involving electric currents, ultrasound, and light therapy, therapeutic counseling, and pharmacology.

> *In naturopathic medicine, signs and symptoms of disease are seen as the manifestations of the body's attempt to naturally heal itself.*

Principles of Naturopathic Medicine

Although the term *naturopathic medicine* (sometimes known as naturopathy) was not used until the late 19th century, its philosophical roots date back thousands of years. Drawing from the healing traditions of many cultures, including Indian (Ayurvedic), Chinese (traditional Chinese medicine), Native American, and Greek (Hippocratic), naturopathic medicine is a system of medicine based on six time-tested principles:

- The healing power of nature: The body has considerable power to heal itself, and the role of the naturopathic physician is to facilitate this process with the aid of natural, nontoxic therapies.

- Treat the cause rather than the effect: Naturopathic doctors (N.D.s) seek the underlying cause of a disease rather than simply suppressing the symptoms. They avoid suppression of the natural healing wisdom of the body, such as fever and inflammation. Symptoms are viewed as expressions of the body's natural attempt to heal itself, while the causes can spring from the physical, mental/emotional, and spiritual levels.

- First, do no harm: By employing safe and effective natural therapies, naturopathic physicians are committed to the principle of causing no harm to the patient.

- Treat the whole person: The individual is viewed as a whole, composed of a complex interaction of physical, mental/emotional, spiritual, social, and other factors. This multifactorial paradigm results in a therapeutic approach in which no disease is automatically seen as incurable.

- The physician is a teacher: Naturopathic physicians are first and foremost teachers who educate, empower, and motivate patients to assume more personal responsibility for their health by adopting a healthy attitude, lifestyle, and diet.

- Prevention is the best cure: Naturopathic physicians are preventive medicine specialists. Prevention of disease is accomplished through education and a lifestyle that supports health.

How Naturopathic Medicine Works

In the naturopathic system of medicine, signs and symptoms of disease are seen as the manifestations of the body's attempt to naturally heal itself. For example, fever and inflammation are viewed as the body's way of dealing with an imbalance that is undermining the healthy functioning of the body. However, if the cause of the imbalance is not removed, the inflammatory responses will continue, either at a lower level of intensity or intermittently. This can be the origin of chronic disease. Healing a chronic disease requires removal of the underlying cause. This usually culminates in a return of an acute episode, called a "healing crisis" or reaction, a keynote of naturopathic medical theory. Following this, the condition improves.

After identifying which conditions in the patient manifest in disease, the naturopathic physician advises the patient on building better conditions for the return to health.

Although naturopathic physicians emphasize therapeutic choices based on individual interest and experience, as well as the legal parameters of the state in which he or she practices, they maintain a consistent philosophy. All N.D.s have been trained in the basic tools of natural therapeutics and most work with diet and nutrition while specializing in one or more other therapeutic methods.

After identifying which conditions in the patient manifest in illness, the naturopathic physician advises the patient on the methods most appropriate for creating a return to health. In order to become free of illness, it is often necessary for the patient to make both dietary and lifestyle changes. Homeopathy or acupuncture are often used to stimulate recovery. Herbal medicines may be used as tonics and nutritive agents to support and strengthen weakened systems, while specific nutritional agents such as vitamin and mineral supplements and glandular tissue extracts might also be utilized. Hydrotherapy and various types of physical therapy may be required. Additionally, it is important that major emotional stresses be eased to allow the gastrointestinal system to function in the relaxed environment required for proper digestion.

Finally, underlying many illnesses is a spiritual disharmony. This may be experienced as a feeling of deep unease or insufficient strength of will necessary to sustain the healing process. For lasting good health to be established, this disharmony must be overcome. Naturopathic physicians can play an important role in guiding patients to discover the course of action most appropriate.

 With its emphasis on prevention and natural care, naturopathic medicine may offer long-term savings to the consumer.

Conditions Benefited by Naturopathic Medicine

Naturopathic medicine can be applied in any health-care situation, but its strongest area is in the treatment of chronic and degenerative disease. N.D.s are, for the most part, licensed primary care/general practice family physicians. For severe, acute traumas such as a serious automobile accident, emergencies of childbirth, or orthopedic problems requiring corrective surgery, naturopathic medicine is not recommended, although it can contribute to such cases, especially in the recovery phase.

In other acute cases, such as ear infections and common illnesses with fever, the naturopathic physician addresses the associated pain, infection, and fever of the condition, as well as any related concerns of the patient. How this acute condition might relate to underlying causes, such as diet, life stresses, and occupational hazards, is also addressed. The physician will then usually prescribe a variety of means to deal with the immediate problem.

In chronic cases, the procedure is different. Typically, a thorough case exploration will detail the history and nature of the patient's symptoms and complaints, complete health history, and the patient's lifestyle. Finally, a physical examination and appropriate laboratory tests are performed. For naturopathic physicians, understanding the patient as an individual is essential when searching for causative factors, particularly in the areas of the physical, mental/emotional, and spiritual.

After determining causative factors, the physician will discuss the findings with the patient and an attempt will be made to tie together and interpret the symptoms. Symptoms usually relate to a central problem that has many manifestations. As an example, many symptoms can be tied to the effects of toxemia on the different systems of the body, such as the immune system, nervous system, and circulatory system. Others may be due to emotional factors, such as a chronic urinary tract infection when there is a history of sexual abuse.

Finally, dietary factors are determined and appropriate changes are recommended. Any other perceived causes are addressed with counseling, exercise, or other methods of treatment.

 See Acupuncture, Diet, Herbal Medicine, Homeopathy, Hydrotherapy, Nutritional Medicine.

Healing the Person, Not the Disease

Naturopathic medicine does not focus on disease symptoms, but rather the underlying causes. For example, the body has four major organs that assist in elimination: the lungs, kidneys, bowels, and skin. Most skin diseases are viewed by naturopathic physicians to be the result of excessive metabolic toxicity, forcing the skin to be used as an extra route of elimination. The skin excretes both water-soluble and oil-soluble wastes through the sweat and oil glands. Because the elimination of toxins is irritating to the skin, the result is often various forms of skin-related disorders such as dermatitis and acne.

Naturopathic medicine does not focus on disease symptons, but rather the underlying causes.

A woman suffering from dermatitis, an itchy and often inflamed skin rash, sought the help of Jared Zeff, N.D., L.Ac., of Portland, Oregon. She was also partially blind from an incurable condition known as retinitis pigmentosa, a progressive form of retinal degeneration that results in blindness. After assessing her condition, Dr. Zeff viewed the dermatitis as a result of the elimination of toxins through the skin generated by maldigestion. He prescribed a specific diet to help improve her digestion and recommended a series of hydrotherapy treatments, also to improve digestion and to stimulate other mechanisms of elimination. Dr. Zeff also prescribed a botanical digestive tonic and later a homeopathic remedy.

As a result of Dr. Zeff's diagnosis and subsequent treatment, not only did the woman's dermatitis begin to clear, but she reported to Dr. Zeff that instead of seeing him as a blurry shape, she was able to make out the specific features of his face. Her eyesight improved to the point where she could read large-print books. Dr. Zeff had not specifically sought to improve her retinal degeneration, assuming it was not possible for her destroyed tissue to be regenerated. Her story is just one example of the body's amazing capacity to recuperate.

Another patient of Dr. Zeff's was an older gentleman afflicted with bladder cancer. Although this form of

WHAT TO EXPECT WHEN YOU VISIT A NATUROPATHIC PHYSICIAN

A typical office visit with a naturopathic physician takes one hour. One of your naturopathic physician's primary goals is teaching you how to live healthfully, so the time devoted to discussing and explaining principles of health maintenance, as well as your medical condition, is one of the factors that sets naturopaths apart from conventional physicians, who often seem to be rushing from patient to patient.

The relationship begins with a thorough medical history and interview process designed to view all aspects of your lifestyle. If needed, the physician will perform standard diagnostic procedures, including a physical exam and blood and urine analyses. Once a good understanding of your health and disease status is established (diagnosing an illness is only one part of this process), you and your doctor work together to establish a treatment and health-promoting program.

cancer has a high rate of success from conventional treatment, his case had not responded to chemotherapy. When Dr. Zeff applied pressure to specific reflex points of the patient's body, he was told they did not hurt, even though he could see pain expressed in the man's face. When questioned more deeply, it was discovered that the patient's only child had committed suicide five years previously. The man had been unable to grieve and had apparently shut off his feelings, which resulted in a physical manifestation of feeling cut-off from his body.

Dr. Zeff prescribed a diet and a series of hydrotherapy treatments. He also instructed the patient's wife on how to treat her husband at home. She assisted with the hydrotherapy sessions and administered a therapeutic touch technique taught by Dr. Zeff that involved placing her hands over and under her husband's bladder and sacrum for ten minutes each session. Because she was also not well, suffering from chronic bronchitis, Dr. Zeff outlined a specific diet for her as well as a dose of *Ignatia,* a homeopathic remedy to relieve the effects of suppressed grief. Dr. Zeff also instructed the couple to walk together for half an hour each day.

In both husband and wife, the cause of their illnesses—the grief and the inability to release it—was the same, yet on the physical level the unexpressed grief manifested differently. Their illnesses were addressed by informal discussion, a referral to a counselor, and a home-

ORIGINS AND DEVELOPMENT OF NATUROPATHIC MEDICINE

Naturopathic medicine grew out of the alternative healing movement of the 18th and 19th centuries. The European tradition of "taking the cure" at natural springs and spas had gained a foothold in North America by the middle of the 19th century, and this atmosphere helped make the U.S. especially receptive to the principles of naturopathy.

The early naturopaths attached great importance to a natural, healthy diet, as did many of their contemporaries. John Kellogg, a physician and vegetarian, ran the Battle Creek Sanitarium, in Michigan, which utilized natural therapies such as hydrotherapy, while his brother Will built and ran a factory in Battle Creek to produce health foods like shredded wheat and granola biscuits. The Kellogg brothers, along with a former employee, C.W. Post, helped popularize naturopathic ideas about food and at the same time founded the cereal companies that today bear their names.

Naturopathic medicine flourished in the U.S. until the mid-1930s, at which point the medical profession started to conglomerate into the single-view, omnipotent establishment it is today. Naturopathic medicine, and nearly every other natural healing modality, were effectively wiped out. Yet, naturopathic medicine has experienced a tremendous resurgence in the last three decades. This is largely due to increased public awareness of the role of diet and lifestyle in the cause of chronic disease, as well as the failure of modern medicine to deal effectively with these disorders.

opathic remedy, as well as mutual treatments between husband and wife. In ten weeks, the patient was rechecked for cancer. Not only had it disappeared, but his wife's chronic bronchitis had also cleared up.

What is a Naturopathic Physician Trained to Do?

Modern naturopathic doctors provide complete diagnostic and therapeutic services. As family doctors, many practice natural childbirth (usually in the home setting),

pediatrics, gynecology, and geriatrics. Naturopathic physicians make recommendations on lifestyle, diet, and exercise, and utilize a variety of natural and noninvasive healing techniques. The current scope of treatments in which N.D.s are trained include: clinical nutrition; botanical or herbal medicine; homeopathy; acupuncture; hydrotherapy; hyperthermia; physical medicine, including massage and therapeutic manipulation; counseling and other forms of psychotherapy; minor surgery; and natural childbirth and midwifery.

Clinical nutrition: The use of diet as a therapy serves as the foundation of naturopathic medicine. There is an ever-increasing body of knowledge that supports the use of whole foods and nutritional supplements in the maintenance of health and treatment of disease.

Herbal medicine: Plants have been used as medicines since antiquity. Naturopathic physicians are professionally trained herbalists and know both the historical and medicinal uses of plants.

Homeopathy: The term *homeopathy* is derived from the Greek word *homoios*, meaning "similar," and *pathos*, meaning "suffering." Homeopathy is a system of medicine that treats a disease with dilute, potentized remedies that will produce the same symptoms as the disease when given to a healthy individual. The fundamental principle operating here is that like cures like. Homeopathic medicines are derived from a variety of plant, mineral, and chemical substances.

Acupuncture: Acupuncture is an ancient Chinese system of medicine involving the stimulation of certain specific points on the body to enhance the flow of vital life energy know as *qi* (CHEE) along pathways called meridians. Acupuncture points are stimulated by the insertion and withdrawal of needles, the application of heat (moxibustion), acupressure (deep finger pressure), lasers, electrical means, or a combination of these methods.

Hydrotherapy: Hydrotherapy uses water in all its temperatures (hot to cold), forms (ice, steam), and methods of application (sitz baths, douches, spas, whirlpools, saunas, showers, immersion baths, packs, poultices, foot baths, fomentations, wraps, colonic irrigations) in the maintenance of health or treatment of disease. It is one of the most ancient methods of treatment. Hydrotherapy has been used to treat disease and injury by many different cultures, including the Egyptians, Assyrians, Persians, Greeks, Hebrews, Hindus, Chinese, and Native Americans.

Hyperthermia: Hyperthermia is a form of hydrotherapy that deliberately induces fever in the patient who is unable to mount a natural fever response to pathogens (disease-causing organisms and toxins). Fever is often regarded as an undesirable symptom of illness, but N.D.s see it as the body's defense against invading organisms.

Fever stimulates the immune system by increasing the production of antibodies and interferon (proteins released by white blood cells that combat a virus). Hyperthermia can also be used to remove fat-stored chemicals such as pesticides, PCBs, and drug residues from the body.

Physical medicine: Physical medicine refers to the use of physical measures in the treatment of disease. These include: therapeutic exercise, massage, joint mobilization (manipulation) and immobilization techniques, and hydrotherapy. Physical medicine also includes physiotherapy equipment such as ultrasound (high-frequency sound waves that act as a micro-massage to tissues, stimulating or restoring function or blood circulation), diathermy (high-frequency currents used to generate heat within the body), electric currents used in the body to stimulate function or relieve pain, and light therapy (applications of light that are used to stimulate healing responses in the body, such as endocrine function or increased circulation).

Counseling and lifestyle modification: Counseling and lifestyle modification techniques are essential to naturopathic medicine. A naturopathic physician is formally trained in the following counseling areas: (1) interviewing and responding skills, active listening, body language assessment, and other contact skills necessary for the therapeutic relationship; (2) recognition and understanding of prevalent psychological issues including developmental problems, sexual dysfunction, abnormal behavior, addictions, and stress; and (3) various treatment measures including hypnosis and guided imagery, counseling techniques, correction of underlying organic factors, and family therapy.

Minor surgery: Current accreditation and state licensing statutes require all N.D.s to be trained in a variety of minor surgical techniques. These include laceration repair (sutures), skin biopsies, skin lesion removal, sclerotherapy for spider veins and varicose veins, noninvasive hemorrhoid surgery, abscess incising and draining, circumcision, and the setting of fractures.

Natural childbirth and midwifery: The training naturopathic physicians receive enables them to provide pre-, peri-, and post-natal care in the states where they are licensed. As a result, increasing numbers of N.D.s now offer natural childbirth in both home and clinical settings. In doing so, they typically screen both mother and child throughout the pregnancy to minimize the risk of complications. This includes assessing diet and nutritional status and providing counseling to the expectant mother when appropriate. Many N.D.s also work in conjunction with medical midwives.

The Future of Naturopathic Medicine

"To the uninformed, naturopathic medicine, as well as the entire concept of natural medicine, appears to be a fad that will soon pass away," says Michael Murray, N.D., of Issaquah, Washington, a leading naturopathic physician and educator. "To the informed, however, it is quite clear that naturopathic medicine is at the forefront of the future."

 Licensing is currently available for naturopathic physicians in only 11 states. It is important to encourage your state government to license naturopathic medicine in your state.

One of the great fallacies promoted by the United States medical establishment is that there is not firm scientific evidence for the use of many natural therapies. "This assumption is simply not true," says Dr. Murray. "In fact, during the last 20 years, there has been a literal explosion of information in the scientific literature supporting the use of natural medicine."

Today, science and medicine have the technology and understanding necessary to appreciate many aspects of natural medicine. It is becoming increasingly common for medical organizations that in the past have spoken out strongly against naturopathic medicine to embrace it, endorsing naturopathic techniques such as lifestyle modification, stress reduction, exercise, and a high-fiber diet.

"This illustrates the paradigm shift that is occurring in medicine," says Dr. Murray. "What was once scoffed at is now becoming generally accepted as an effective alternative. In fact, in most instances, the naturopathic alternative offers significant benefit over standard medical practices. Undoubtedly, in the future, many of the concepts, philosophies, and practices of naturopathy will be vindicated. Certainly the future looks very bright for naturopathic medicine."

Where to Find Help

Licensing for naturopathic physicians in the United States is currently available in 11 states (Alaska, Arizona, Connecticut, Hawaii, Maine, Montana, New Hampshire, Oregon, Utah, Vermont, and Washington), as well as in five Canadian provinces (Alberta, British Columbia, Manitoba, Ontario, and Saskatchewan). However, the profession is expanding and additional licensing efforts are under way in other states, due to the efforts of the American Association of Naturopathic Physicians (AANP), the leading naturopathic advocacy group in the U.S. There are currently five accredited colleges in the U.S. and one in Canada. These colleges offer four-year degrees in naturopathic medicine and other health-related sciences and are endorsed by the AANP. For further information about naturopathic medicine, contact:

American Association of Naturopathic Physicians
8201 Greensboro Drive, Suite 300
McLean, Virginia 22101
(703) 610-9037
Website: www.naturopathic.org

The leading advocacy group for naturopathic medicine in the United States. Provides a directory of naturopathic physicians and offers referrals to a nationwide network of accredited or licensed practitioners. Also publishes a quarterly newsletter for both professionals and the general public and offers a series of brochures and pamphlets on a variety of subjects.

Bastyr University
14500 Juanita Drive
Kenmore, Washington 98028
(425) 602-3000
Website: www.bastyr.edu

Bastyr University is an accredited educational institution that offers degree programs in the natural health sciences. These include programs in naturopathic medicine, herbal sciences, homeopathy, midwifery, acupuncture, nutrition, Chinese herbal medicine, exercise and wellness, marriage and family counseling, spirituality in health and medicine, and applied behavioral sciences.

National College of Naturopathic Medicine
49 S.W. Porter
Portland, Oregon 97201
(503) 255-4860
Website: www.ncnm.edu

Provides a listing of naturopathic doctors in the United States and offers degree programs in naturopathic medicine and traditional Chinese medicine.

Southwest College of Naturopathic Medicine and Health Sciences
2140 East Broadway Road
Tempe, Arizona 85282
(480) 858-9100
Website: www.scnm.edu

Offers a degree program in naturopathic medicine.

**University of Bridgeport,
College of Naturopathic Medicine**
126 Park Avenue
Bridgeport, Connecticut 06604
(203) 576-4109
Website: www.bridgeport.edu

A comprehensive university offering more than 30 undergraduate and 14 graduate degree programs.

Canadian College of Naturopathic Medicine
1255 Sheppard Avenue East
Toronto, Ontario M2K 1E2, Canada
(416) 498-1255
Website: www.ccnm.edu

Offers a diploma in naturopathic medicine, the Canadian equivalent of a degree in the United States.

Recommended Reading

Divided Legacy: A History of the Schism in Medical Thought, Vol. 3. Harris L. Coulter. Washington, D.C.: Wehawken Book Company, 1973.

Encyclopedia of Natural Medicine. Michael Murray, N.D., and Joseph Pizzorno, N.D. Rocklin, CA: Prima Publishing, 1998.

Lectures in Naturopathic Hydrotherapy. Wade Boyle, N.D., and Andre Saine, N.D. East Palestine, OH: Buckeye Naturopathic Press, 1988.

Textbook of Natural Medicine, Volumes 1 & 2. Michael Murray, N.D., and Joseph Pizzorno, N.D. London, England: Churchill-Livingston, 1999.

Nature Doctors: Pioneers in Naturopathic Medicine. Friedhelm Kirchfeld and Wade Boyle, N.D. East Palestine, OH: Buckeye Naturopathic Press, 1994.

NEURAL THERAPY

Neural therapy uses injections of anesthetics to remove short circuits in the body's electrical network. This process frees up the flow of energy and normalizes cellular function, making neural therapy an effective treatment for a variety of disease conditions, especially chronic pain.

NEURAL THERAPY treats pain and illness and resolves trauma in the body by working to reverse the cumulative effects of injury," says William Faber, D.O., of Milwaukee, Wisconsin. "The structural integrity of the body can be disturbed by injury, causing the energy flow to be blocked."

Neural therapy corrects these blockages in the body through the use of anesthetics injected into the nerve sites of the autonomic nervous system, acupuncture points, scars, glands, and other tissues. The most commonly used anesthetics are procaine and lidocaine. "These are very easily metabolized by the body," explains Marvin Penwell, D.O., of Linden, Michigan, "meaning that the body is able to break down their molecules into other chemical forms that can be readily eliminated. This safeguards against side effects."

By using the pathways of the autonomic nervous system, neural therapy delivers energy to cells short-circuited by disease or injury and helps to regulate biological energy. Although a series of injections is usually required, a single injection can relieve pain instantly and, in many cases, restore complete health, even if the disease has lingered for years.

How Neural Therapy Works

To grasp how neural therapy works, it is necessary to understand a basic premise of biological energy. Everything alive is charged with electricity and every living cell has its own specific frequency range. As long as

Illness begins when energy flow is disrupted, creating what is known as an interference field in the 'ground system' of the body.

energy flow throughout the body is within its normal frequency range, the tissues will remain healthy.

Most chronic illnesses are caused by changes in the electrical conductivity of autonomic nerves and cells. These changes disrupt the flow of biological energy. Illness begins when energy flow is disrupted, creating what is known as an interference field in the "ground system" of the body. The ground system lies between the cell membranes, arteries, veins, lymph vessels, and nerve endings, and is composed of connective tissue—fibroblasts (cells that are the precursors of bone, collagen, and other connective tissue cells), collagen (the protein of the connective tissue), elastin (extracellular protein that makes the tissue elastic), water, and glycoproteins (proteins combined with sugars). When normal electrical impulses travel unimpeded, there is communication among the various systems of the body, fostering vibrant health. If this delicate balance breaks down, however, disruptions in the normal function of cells occur, and eventually chronic disorders develop.[1]

Any part of the body that has been traumatized can create an interference field and can cause disturbances not only at a specific trauma site, but elsewhere in the body. For instance, extracting a wisdom tooth produces an interference field that can frequently cause heart problems.[2] Scars are another form of trauma that can create an interference field.

Neural therapy works not only by restoring dysfunctional nerve balance, but also on a structural basis to restore normal tissue tension. "Scars and injuries can cause a physical tightening of tissues by adhesion," Dr. Faber explains. "This can sometimes be noted by pain and loss

NEURAL THERAPY AND THE NERVOUS SYSTEM

Standard anatomy describes two components to the nervous system. The central nervous system (CNS) comprises the spinal cord (containing millions of nerve fibers) and the brain, while the peripheral nervous system (PNS) is the network of nerves estimated to extend 93,000 miles inside the body. The PNS is the sensory motor branch that pertains to the five senses and how sensory information from the outside world gets translated into muscle movements.

The **autonomic nervous system** (ANS), involving elements of both the CNS and PNS, is controlled by the brain's hypothalamus gland and pertains to the automatic regulation of all body processes, such as breathing, digestion, and heart rate. It can be likened to the body's automatic pilot, keeping you alive without your being aware of it or participating in its activities. Neural therapy focuses its injections of anesthetics into body structures whose nerve supply is linked with the autonomic nervous system.

Within the ANS, there are two branches, the parasympathetic and sympathetic, which are believed to counterbalance each other. The parasympathetic nervous system slows heart rate, inhibits activity, conserves energy, and calms the body, but stimulates gastric secretion and intestinal activity. The sympathetic nervous system involves the expenditure of energy and is associated with arousal and stress. It prepares us physically when we perceive a threat or challenge by increasing our heart rate, blood pressure, and muscle tension. The sympathetic portion links all the cells of the body together; it regulates the contraction and expansion of blood vessels, the activity of connective tissue necessary for regenerating body systems, and the voltage (membrane potential) across the cell membrane in every body cell. Neural therapy primarily addresses this system.

A **ganglion** is a bundle, knot, or plexus of nerve cell bodies with many interconnections that acts like a sorting and relay station for nerve impulses. There are several dozen ganglia throughout the body.

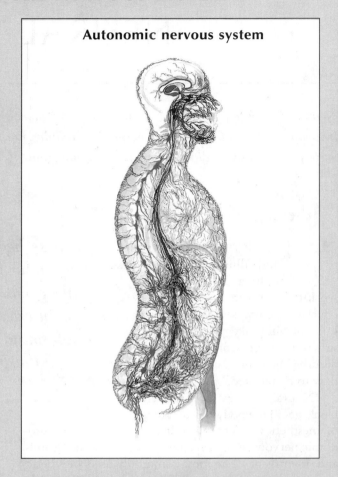

Autonomic nervous system

Membrane potential refers to differing electrical charges, which constantly change around a certain baseline, measured in millivolts, inside and outside of a cell. This, in turn, influences how easily substances (nutrients or toxins) can pass into and out of a cell. Sodium ions are pumped out of the cell (to create the normal resting potential of -80 mV) and potassium ions are pumped in. The three means by which substances are transported across the cell membrane are called ion pumping, ionic channel transport, and carrier protein transport. These mechanisms are voltage dependent and resemble the ebb and flow of tidal water, with nutrients "washing in" and toxins "washing out" with each pulse of the electrical current every 2-5 milliseconds.

of range of motion in areas remote from the actual scars." The following case of Dr. Faber's illustrates this well. Barry, 50, had two gallbladder surgeries one year apart. He fully recovered, but six months later complained of severe knee pain and stiffness. On examination, his knees seemed normal. The gallbladder scars were injected with neural therapy formula. He had immediate improvement of his pain and stiffness, and six weekly follow-up treatments of injections into the abdomen abolished any remnants of his pain and stiffness. That was eight years ago and he remains pain free today.

The task of the neural therapist is to locate the source of the abnormal activity and eliminate the disturbance. Once the cells regain their normal electrical activity, they can eliminate toxic wastes that have built up as a result of this disturbance and begin to function normally again.

All cells in the body can be regarded as organisms, according to Dietrich Klinghardt, M.D., Ph.D., of Seattle, Washington, President of the American Academy of Neural Therapy. "Each cell needs to eat, drink, and detoxify itself, to have the cellular equivalent of a urination and bowel movement," Dr. Klinghardt says. "It does this across the cell membrane, taking in nutrients and eliminating waste products. The rate at which substances are exchanged across the membrane determines how efficiently the cell is working—the more rapid the transport, the more vital the body."

This rapid transport is dependent on the status of the membrane potential, which is a difference in electrical charge on both sides of the cell membrane. "Whenever a cell has lost its normal membrane potential, the ion pumps and ionic channels in the membrane stop working," says Dr. Klinghardt. "In effect, the cell becomes electrically paralyzed and cannot eliminate the waste products of its own cellular processes. This means that abnormal minerals and toxic substances accumulate inside the cell, leading to an inability of the cell to heal itself and resume normal function."

This is where the scar and interference fields enter the picture. Scar tissue can actually produce a measurable electrical charge of up to 1.5 volts. The typical cell's electrical charge is only 80 millivolts. This means the interference field functions like a battery inappropriately implanted in the body, according to Dr. Klinghardt. The interference field generates abnormal electrical signals, which disrupt the autonomic nervous system and membrane potential of nerve ganglia and nerve fibers. The result can be electrical chaos in the spinal cord and brain, and a cascade of nerve disturbances throughout the body that manifest as chronic pain or dysfunction.

"Neural therapy attempts to break this cycle by identifying the 'primary lesion,' or interference field—the structure [scar or focus] that gave the original abnormal

signal in the autonomic nervous system," Dr. Klinghardt says. The local anesthetic, as it infiltrates throughout the cell membrane, temporarily restores the natural membrane potential in the nerve cell at the site of physical trauma. During this respite, which on average lasts 30-120 minutes, the cell eliminates a sufficient amount of the toxic waste to regain normal function, often permanently.

In one case, Dr. Klinghardt treated a man who had been diagnosed with severe arthritis of the hip joints and lower back, which began after a serious bout of prostate gland inflammation. Within seconds after infusing a local anesthetic into the autonomic nerve ganglia surrounding the prostate, the man was pain free, and the pain did not return afterward.

Dr. Klinghardt notes that in many cases involving women with lower back pain, pain relief and lasting cures can be achieved by injecting the Frankenhauser ganglia, which regulates the sexual organs and functions and surrounds the vagina and uterus. Stress from childbirth or prior pelvic infections often create disturbances in the pelvic ganglia that, in turn, generate the pain. "We have consistently observed that with neural therapy, women's premenstrual symptoms and pain during menstruation disappear along with the back pain," Dr. Klinghardt reports.

Interestingly, the people who are the hardest to treat with any other modality are the easiest to treat with neural therapy.

—Dietrich Klinghardt, M.D., Ph.D.

Interference fields often lie dormant until activated by further trauma or by general illness such as malnutrition, emotional stress, or food sensitivity. Interference fields can also be activated by weight gain, as excess weight can stretch scar tissue. Congestion in the lymph system can be especially debilitating. Lymphatic vessels in a chronic state of imbalance can severely disrupt the flow of lymph fluid. Neural therapy can increase the flow of lymph and help clear the tissues of wastes and restore them to normal function.[3]

Indicators of an underlying interference field include failure to respond to other therapies; a condition that worsens after other therapies; a situation where all symptoms are located on only one side of the body; or a sequence of illnesses continually developing one after another. To effect a long-term cure, it is necessary to identify and clear interference fields from the body.

Conditions Benefited by Neural Therapy

German research claims that 40% of all illness and chronic pain may be due to interference fields in the body. Neural therapy has become one of the most widely used treatments for chronic pain in Germany.[4] One study, compiled in Germany in the 1970s, collected statistics from 25 doctors who used neural therapy with procaine to treat 639 cases of trigeminal neuralgia. The results were: 34% cured, 37% substantial improvement, 14% some improvement, and 15% no improvement.

In 267 (42%) of these cases, an interference field was held to be either the cause or a mitigating factor of the disease. This report also stated that those who experienced the least result from neural therapy were those who had previously undergone surgery.[5]

 See Chronic Pain.

There are hundreds of conditions that respond to neural therapy. "About the only conditions that do not respond to neural therapy are metabolic disorders and cancer," says Dr. Klinghardt. "Interestingly, the people who are the hardest to treat with any other modality are the easiest to treat with neural therapy. Those who come to us haven't responded to conventional medicine, chiropractic, acupuncture, nerve blocks, physical therapy, or surgery. This is the very group that is most likely to respond rapidly to neural therapy." Conditions that normally respond to neural therapy include:

- Allergies and asthma
- Arthritis
- Back pain and whiplash
- Bladder dysfunction
- Chronic pain
- Colitis and ulcers
- Depression
- Dizziness
- Ear problems
- Emphysema
- Headaches and migraine
- Heart disease and circulatory disorders
- Hemorrhoids
- Hormonal imbalance
- Glaucoma and inflammatory eye disease
- Kidney and gallbladder disease

- Liver disease
- Menstrual cramps
- Muscle and sports injuries
- Post-operative recovery
- Prostate disorders
- Sinusitis
- Skin diseases
- Thyroid dysfunction

Neural therapy has also been shown effective for treating multiple sclerosis. At the Glasgow Homeopathic Hospital, in Glasgow, Scotland, researchers conducted both a pilot study and a double-blind, placebo-controlled study on the effects of neural therapy on MS patients. Sixty-one participants with MS were selected for the study, each with a Disability Status Score (DSS) or Expanded Disability Status Score (EDSS) grade of 1-7. Each patient received neural therapy injections into trigger points in their ankles and around the circumference of their skulls. The results were impressive: 65% of the patients in the pilot study and 76% of the patients in the double-blind study showed improvement as determined by DSS or EDSS assessments, and follow-up evaluations conducted up to over three years later found that more than 50% of the patients still showed improved ratings. None of the patients experienced any side effects from the treatment and in some cases improvements were rapid. Therapists concluded that neural therapy is an effective, nontoxic, and inexpensive treatment for multiple sclerosis, offering both immediate and long-term benefits.[6]

> *German research claims that 40% of all illness and chronic pain is due to interference fields in the body.*

In Dr. Klinghardt's experience, between one and six treatments, given twice weekly, are usually all that are needed for neural therapy to achieve results. "Often, we can get a person well with one treatment, although it sometimes takes a bit of sleuthing and listening for the body's response to target the source of the problem," he says.

One of Dr. Klinghardt's patients suffered from chronic fatigue syndrome for the better part of a decade. At first, he suspected an appendectomy scar was causing the interference in her body's electrical field, so he injected it with procaine. When this did not bring about the expected result, he used applied kinesiology and found weakness in a strong indicator muscle when she touched her pelvic area. Immediately after injecting the Frankenhauser ganglion, she started coughing. The cough indicated the presence of an interference field in the chest. When Dr. Klinghardt injected her chest, the chronic fatigue syndrome cleared within hours.

In retrospect, the woman remembered coming down with the flu and developing a cough immediately before the chronic fatigue syndrome had set in. Her body's attempt to fight the virus created chest congestion, and this affected the autonomic nerve endings in her lungs and created an obstruction of electrical impulses within her body's ground system. The injection of procaine into her chest reestablished the normal electrical potential of the cells and eliminated the interference field in her lungs so that her energy could circulate freely.

Dr. Penwell, now retired, used neural therapy as a significant part of his practice. He recounts one particular case, an 80-year-old woman who came to him with degenerative arthritis in her knee. She was experiencing a great deal of pain, which extended down her leg and up through her hip joint. This condition had crippled her to such an extent she was forced to depend on a walker and posed a very poor surgical risk. Following his examination, Dr. Penwell gave her several injections in her leg, including her knee joint. When the patient very reluctantly got up off the table to bear weight on the knee joint, she was amazed. Asked to move around, the patient took several steps and smiled broadly. In answer to the doctor's question about how she felt, the woman reached for her walker, folded it up, put it under her arm, and walked out the door and down the hallway. She was given follow-up injections at weekly intervals for four weeks and, as the pain did not return, she concluded the therapy.

Eduardo Guerrero, M.D., P.A., a neural therapist from Houston, Texas, reports that his best results occur when he combines homeopathic remedies with anesthetics to clear interference fields. Dr. Guerrero once treated a man whose two operations failed to relieve his back pain. "He was getting so bad, he couldn't function as a foreman anymore, so he changed to a janitorial job," relates Dr. Guerrero. "One day, while sweeping, the man reinjured his back and couldn't walk. When I administered nerve blocks to the sacral area, he felt pain in the lumbar area. Since the lumbar area corresponds to the urogenital system, I asked him if he'd ever had problems there. He said he'd had gonorrhea while in the army. Within a week of treating him for that complaint, his back pain disappeared."

The most important contribution neural therapy has brought to modern medicine is the understanding of interference fields, states Dr. Guerrero. "As long as you

HISTORY OF NEURAL THERAPY

Neural therapy was developed in Germany by two brothers, Ferdinand and Walter Huneke, both medical doctors. The idea first took shape in 1925, when they published a paper showing how the injection of a local anesthetic affected other parts of the body. Years later, Ferdinand found, to his amazement, that injecting a woman in her leg for pain caused her chronic shoulder pain to immediately disappear. This gave rise to the concept of *ster-felder*, or fields of interference.

In Germany and South America, neural therapy is the most commonly used treatment for chronic pain. Today the "ground system theory," the foundation of neural therapy, is widely accepted in Europe. This theory states that it is actually the connective tissues between cells that control health, and that disease results from disturbances in this tissue. In the U.S., Dietrich Klinghardt, M.D., Ph.D., has trained hundreds of practitioners through his American Academy of Neural Therapy, and there are other practicing neural therapists who have trained outside the U.S..

have a short circuit in the body's electrical network, you cannot recharge your biological energy."

According to Dr. Faber, the head is the most important area for neural therapy. "Doing neural therapy on the head can resolve chronic pain and disability in remote areas of the body," Dr. Faber says. "This is particularly so in the case of jaws and teeth. The head, of course, houses special functions of vision, hearing, smell, taste, voice, balance, emotion, and thought. Neural therapy can be valuable to patients and physicians in the correction of these precious abilities." In one case, a 70-year-old man came to Dr. Faber complaining about his shoulder, which responded well to prolotherapy. But upon further examination, Dr. Faber found the man's head to have irritated nerves. He administered neural therapy to the head to reset the irritated nerves and loosen the tissues. On his next visit, the man stated, "For 70 years, I've had severe problems with anger, frustration, and depression, and that treatment lifted it all off me."

Neural therapy can also be used to treat brain disorders, including poor memory, hyperactivity, dyslexia, autism, cranial nerve dysfunction, epilepsy, and amyotrophic lateral sclerosis (Lou Gehrig's disease), according to Dr. Klinghardt. He points out that no two cases of a particular illness are treated in the exact same fash-

TYPES OF NEURAL THERAPY

Direct technique: The direct or "local" technique in neural therapy treats pain or illness with an injection of anesthetics specifically at the site of the interference field causing the problem. The injections can be made by infiltrating scar tissue, into nerve junctions, or into the area surrounding the spinal cord.

Indirect technique: If the neural therapist cannot pinpoint the exact location of the interference field, the source of pain can be tracked down by injecting related interference fields until the original blockage is found. In other cases, an indirect approach is needed when the problem area is too delicate to receive a direct injection.

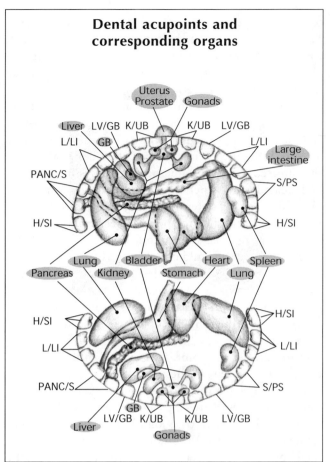

Dental acupoints and corresponding organs

©1983 Ralph Alan Dale

ion and that multiple factors—patient history (including past emotional traumas), physical exam, nutrient status, vaccinations, dental factors and dental amalgam fillings, heavy metal poisoning, allergies, viral infections, current medications, and scars—must all be considered in order to devise the most effective treatment protocol. Each patient's psychological factors should always be treated first, according to Dr. Klinghardt, followed by the appropriate neural therapy interventions, often in conjunction with specific brain detoxification nutrients.[7]

By definition, neural therapy can influence disturbances only if they are due to autonomic causes or if neural or humoral (body fluid) factors are part of the original cause.[8] Neural therapy cannot reverse any major structural changes and therefore does not take the place of orthodox diagnostic or therapeutic measures. Neural therapy is ineffective in genetic disease and nutritional deficiencies, and not beneficial in psychiatric disorders (except depression) or end-stage chronic diseases.

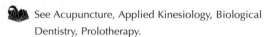 See Acupuncture, Applied Kinesiology, Biological Dentistry, Prolotherapy.

Neural Therapy in Dentistry

In the 1950s, Reinhold Voll, M.D., discovered that each tooth in the mouth relates to a specific acupuncture meridian. He observed that if the organ related to that meridian is not functioning normally, the tooth related to the same meridian may be symptomatic (i.e., painful, decayed). When the meridian is under stress, the acupuncture points are sensitive to local pressure, and this phenomenon can be used for diagnosis and treatment. For example, if the patient suffers a gallbladder attack (intense abdominal pain), the acupuncture point close to his or her right canine tooth will be tender when probed. If neural therapy is used to inject this acupuncture point with a local anesthetic, the abdominal pain will subside. Toothaches, tooth sensitivity, jaw pain, gingivitis, and other local problems respond well when the corresponding oral acupuncture point is treated with neural therapy.

The acupuncture points in the retromolar area (the space behind the last molar of the lower jaw) are indispensable for treating neck pain, low back pain, and temporomandibular joint pain with neural therapy. Acupuncture points in the upper jaw are sensitive to pressure in cases of sinus infections, tension headaches, and indigestion. Sensitivity adjacent to the wisdom teeth indicates heart problems, intestinal disorder, arm/elbow/shoulder problems, vertigo, migraines, and lymphatic problems. Sensitivity in the lower jaw is associated with lumbago, spinal problems, sciatica, indigestion, and hormonal malfunctions. Lingual sensitivities accompany vertigo, cervical syndromes, migraines, hearing difficulties, and kidney/bladder disorders.

Neural therapy has also been shown to be effective as a treatment for symptoms following replacement of dental amalgam fillings. In a recent survey, a questionnaire was mailed to patients who had undergone replacement of dental amalgam fillings and then received mercury detoxification and neural therapy. Forty-two patients responded to the survey, which studied their most distressing symptoms and asked for a personal evaluation following detoxification and neural therapy treatment. Common complaints among the patients included problems with memory and concentration; muscle or joint pain; anxiety and insomnia; stomach, bowel, and bladder complaints; depression; food or chemical sensitivities; numbness or tingling; and eye problems. The most distressing symptoms were headache and backache, fatigue, and memory/concentration problems. Following treatment, 78% of the patients reported they were "satisfied or very satisfied" with the results, compared to only 9.5% who reported dissatisfaction.[9]

CAUTION Neural therapy is contraindicated for several conditions. It should not be used for cancer patients, since the stimulation of the lymphatic system may lead to the spread of cancer cells throughout the body. It is contraindicated in diabetes because it may cause instability of the disease.

Patients allergic to local anesthetics should definitely not receive neural therapy. It should not be used for patients with renal failure or myasthenia gravis (a disease characterized by extreme muscle weakness), or for patients treated with morphine or anti-arrhythmic medications similar in chemical structure to local anesthetics. It is also contraindicated for patients with coagulation disorders (such as hemophilia) or for those receiving anticoagulant therapy.

The Future of Neural Therapy

Currently, chronic pain is the single largest cause of disability in the U.S. Employers and insurance companies have begun researching the far-reaching benefits of neural therapy in efforts to reduce the high cost of health care. According to Dr. Faber, individuals treated with neural therapy for chronic pain are able to resume being productive earlier and with no side effects.

Because neural therapy can remedy a broad range of pain and illness by improving the patient's range of motion, it is gaining respect from health-care professionals who are moving away from drug-based treatments for pain. "These results will hopefully move practitioners into employing neural therapy, realizing that the body has the ability to heal itself, rather than viewing the body as being deficient in some pharmaceutical," says Dr. Faber.

HOW INTERFERENCE FIELDS ARE DIAGNOSED

Locating interference fields begins with a patient history outlining past illness, surgery, or trauma. There are certain empirical relationships between interference fields and illness. Some of these are: tonsils/knee joints; abdominal scars/large joints and low back; leg scars/sciatica; tonsils and teeth/migraine headaches; prostate, stomach, and sinuses/neck; gallbladder scar/shoulder; pelvic scars/premenstrual syndrome; and depression/arthritis, according to Peter Dosch, M.D., of Austria.[10] A scar that crosses an acupuncture meridian is likely to cause disturbances in the corresponding body part. Scars may also be responsible for problems in nearby joints. According to Dr. Faber, scars that do not fade within two years or seem excessively hard or tight across the skin can signal an interference field. Also, the relationship between specific teeth and organs, such as the upper and lower front four teeth to the urogenital system, can be responsible for pelvic pain, chronic kidney disease, and even pelvic malignancies.

Neural therapists listen to the patient to ascertain clues to past problems that the patient may believe to be insignificant. After the initial treatment, patients are asked to keep a record of any changes that occur in the body over the next 48 hours, as these can guide the practitioner in further treatments.

Where to Find Help

For information about neural therapy and referrals, contact:

American Academy of Neural Therapy
1200 112th Avenue N.E.
Bellevue, Washington 98004
(425) 688-8818
Website: www.neuraltherapy.com

Directed by Dr. Klinghardt, the Academy offers introductory and advanced courses in neural therapy and pain management techniques to doctors and provides referrals for neural therapists nationwide. Also offers a variety of training videos and other products related to neural therapy.

Milwaukee Pain Clinic
6529 W. Fond du Lac Avenue
Milwaukee, Wisconsin 53225
(414) 464-7680
Website: www.milwaukeepainclinic.com

Send a self-addressed, stamped legal-size envelope for a list of physicians trained by Dr. Faber in the use of neural therapy. Also offers the videos Neural-Fascial Therapy, an introductory lecture on neural therapy, and Instant Pain Relief, a discussion of neural therapy with Dr. Faber and his patients.

Recommended Reading

Facts About Neural Therapy According to Huneke. Peter Dosch, M.D. Heidelberg, Germany: Karl Haug Publishers, 1985. Available from: Medicina Biologica, 2937 N.E. Flanders, Portland, OR 97232; (503) 287-6775.

Manual of Neural Therapy According to Huneke. Peter Dosch, M.D. Heidelberg, Germany: Karl Haug Publishers, 1985. Available from: Medicina Biologica, 2937 N.E. Flanders, Portland, OR 97232; (503) 287-6775.

Matrix and Matrix Regulation Basis for a Holistic Theory in Medicine. Alfred Pischinger, M.D. Heidelberg, Germany: Karl Haug International, 1991. Available from: Medicina Biologica, 2937 N.E. Flanders, Portland, OR 97232; (503) 287-6775.

NUTRITIONAL MEDICINE

Recent research has demonstrated that diet alone may not be sufficient to supply the nutrients necessary for over-all good health. While most experts agree that nutritional supplements are vital for a variety of illnesses, injuries, and age-related problems, vitamin and mineral supplements can also help to maintain optimal physical and psychological health, and promote longevity and chronic disease prevention.

EVER SINCE THE term *vitamin* was coined almost 100 years ago to describe the discovery of the essential life substances in foods, scientists have debated the issue of nutritional adequacy. Medical science has long held that healthy adults do not need supplementation if they consume a healthful, varied diet. Until recently, it was widely believed that supplements were only considered necessary if a person had an outright or "severe" nutrient deficiency, usually manifested by overt illness.

Today, research indicates that people can have "mild" or "moderate" nutrient deficiencies and that nutritional supplements are necessary to maintain health, according to nutritionist D. Lindsey Berkson, M.A., D.C., of Santa Fe, New Mexico. These mild deficiencies may not cause tangible health disorders, making them difficult to diagnose, but can result in a variety of symptoms along with a general decrease in wellness. Unaddressed, these deficiencies can often put the body at risk for future health problems. Therefore, it is important for individuals to be sure they are receiving the proper amounts of nutrients for overall emotional and physical well-being. Apparently the message is getting through—it is estimated that 80% of adults now take vitamin and mineral supplements, spending $16 billion per year.

The Modern Diet and a New Understanding of Nutrition

"Nutrient density is the hallmark of good food," says Paul McTaggart, a nutrition researcher from Ventura, California. Nutrient density is defined as the relative ratio of nutrients to calories. Foods low in nutrient density are often termed "empty-calorie" or "junk" foods. The leading nutritional problem in the United States today is "overconsumptive undernutrition," or the eating of too many of these empty-calorie foods, says Jeffrey Bland, Ph.D., a biochemist and nutrition expert from Gig Harbor, Washington. Although people in the U.S. consume plenty of food, it is not the right kind of food.

Statistically, studies have concluded that almost two-thirds of an average American's diet is made up of fats and refined sugars having low or no nutrient density. This contributes to nutrient deficiencies that can rob the body of its natural resistance to disease and contribute to aging, while weakening its overall physiological and psychological performance. Consequently, the remaining third of the average diet, which may or may not be from nutrient-dense food, is counted on for the essential nutrients needed to maintain health.

The U.S. Department of Agriculture (USDA) has found that a significant percentage of the U.S. population receives well under 70% of the U.S. Recommended Dietary Allowance (RDA) for vitamin A, vitamin C, B-complex vitamins, and the essential minerals calcium, magnesium, and iron.[1] A separate study found that most typical diets contained less than 80% of the RDA for calcium, magnesium, iron, zinc, copper, and manganese, and that the people most at risk were young children and women (adolescent to elderly).[2] The chart later in this chapter indicates the adult RDA standards for vitamins and minerals, as well as adult maintenance and therapeutic ranges recommended by many nutritional experts.

📖 See Diet, Orthomolecular Medicine.

The standard American diet has been continually cited by numerous studies conducted since the 1960s as a contributing, causative factor in a variety of diseases, including heart disease, atherosclerosis, strokes, high blood

RECOMMENDED DIETARY ALLOWANCE (RDA)

The generally accepted reference standard for nutritional adequacy in the United States is the Recommended Dietary Allowance (RDA). Developed by a group of government-sponsored scientists, its function is to provide levels of essential nutrients that prevent classic deficiency diseases (rickets, scurvy, or beriberi) and set marginal daily guidelines for average population groups. Since the scientists disagreed on exact RDAs, they built within the guidelines instructions to keep reviewing and updating the RDAs (now referred to as Dietary Reference Intake or DRI) every four years as new information is discovered.

The RDAs have since been adjusted to include higher levels of essential nutrients, but a growing number of scientists have begun to dispute the validity of these nutritional guidelines. They maintain that the standards may not be appropriate to prevent mild deficiency reactions such as nervousness, insomnia, mental exhaustion, improper immune function, or proneness to injury. New evidence about the wide variance of nutritional needs for each individual further highlights the inaccuracies of the standards. The nutritional needs of growing children, for instance, do not match those of menopausal women, athletes, or the elderly; then, too, it is important to consider the unique individual needs within a specific age group. Another frequent criticism of the RDAs is that they do not take into account nutrient-deficient food, modern food handling, and environmental factors.[5]

Some scientists support additional revisions of the RDAs to include larger doses of nutrients for the purposes of preventing illness and reducing the effects of environmental pollutants. To accommodate each individual's nutritional needs, these scientists suggest that nutritional screening tests be used to determine specific and unique deficiencies that might deviate from the revised guidelines.

pressure, diabetes, arthritis, and colitis. According to Dr. Berkson, there may also be increased risk of women's health problems associated with diets high in processed fats (trans-fatty acids) and increased consumption of refined sugar and caffeine. Additionally, other contributing factors such as environmental pollution and stressful life patterns are creating even greater nutrient requirements. As the typical American diet is resulting in dangerous deficiencies, people are constantly requiring more

nutrients to maintain good health, even though they may appear to be adequately fed.

Symptoms of Nutritional Deficiency

Historically, doctors and nutritional scientists only recognized nutritional deficiencies if they actually manifested as diseases such as beriberi, pellagra, or rickets. If patients had no overt symptoms or disease, they were regarded as healthy and adequately nourished. Today, doctors are beginning to recognize mild and moderate nutritional deficiencies, the symptoms of which may often be subtle, overlapping, and varied, according to Dr. Berkson. Many times these symptoms are taken for granted as being part of the aging process. Nutritional scientists are learning, however, that these symptoms are actually deficiency signs that can be responsive to nutrient supplementation and dietary improvement. Greater understanding and better testing methods are leading to the diagnosis of more and more subtle nutrient imbalances.

For example, the first signs of B-vitamin deficiency may include subtle changes in behavior: insomnia, mood swings, and an inability to concentrate. These early warning signs, according to Myron Brin, Ph.D., demonstrate that social function may be adversely affected by chronic vitamin deficiency.[3] Other symptoms of nutritional deficiencies can include fatigue, nervousness, mental exhaustion, confusion, anemia, and muscle weakness. It has been reported that marginal deficiencies of vitamins A, C, E, and B_6 may also reduce immunocompetence, impairing the body's ability to ward off disease and repair tissues.[4]

While these can all be signs of deficiencies, they can also have a root in other, separate health problems. Therefore, one needs to always have any deficiencies properly assessed by a qualified health-care provider trained in this field.

Biochemical Individuality

Scientists have increasingly begun to examine whether the standardized RDA guidelines are sufficient for individual nutritional needs. One of the first to question the guidelines was Roger Williams, Ph.D., a pioneering biochemist who discovered vitamin B_5 (pantothenic acid) in the 1930s. In his book *Nutrition Against Disease,* Dr. Williams expressed his belief that each person is genetically unique and therefore requires slight variations in nutrient intake to function optimally. He called this principle "biochemical individuality." Dr. Williams also believed that all living creatures are greatly affected by the overall quality, balance, and quantity of food ingested.

The concept of biochemical individuality has brought about many changes, including the emergence of new preventive diagnostic procedures such as nutrition assessment and risk factor analysis. These utilize physiological data, personal and family health history, dietary analysis, and advanced biochemical screening to help nutritional practitioners determine individual biochemistry and nutritional status.

Essential Nutrients

"Essential nutrients are those nutrients derived from food that the body is unable to manufacture on its own," says Dr. Bland. These are absolutely necessary for human life and include eight amino acids, at least 13 vitamins, and at least 15 minerals, plus certain fatty acids.

Amino acids are the building blocks of protein. The essential amino acids are isoleucine (aids in energy production and hemoglobin formation), leucine (helps heal injured or weakened muscles, fractured or weakened bones, and skin conditions), valine (used by the body to produce energy), methionine (a potent antioxidant), threonine (stimulates the immune system and thymus gland activity), phenylalanine (precursor of the neurotransmitters dopamine and norepinephrine), and tryptophan (precursor of the neurotransmitters serotonin and melatonin).

Essential vitamins are divided into two groups, fat-soluble and water-soluble. The essential vitamins classified as fat-soluble include A, D, E and K. The water-soluble essential vitamins are C (ascorbic acid), B_1 (thiamin), B_2 (riboflavin), B_3 (niacin), B_5 (pantothenic acid), B_6 (pyridoxine), B_{12}, folic acid, and biotin.

The essential minerals include calcium, magnesium, phosphorus, iron, zinc, copper, manganese, iodine, chromium, potassium, sodium, and a number of trace elements. They make up part of the necessary elements of body tissues, fluids, and other nutrients and play an active role in the body's regulatory functions. Low levels of these nutrients have been linked to such conditions as heart disease, high blood pressure, cancer, osteoporosis, depression, schizophrenia, and problems relating to menopause.

Essential fatty acids (EFAs) are unsaturated fats required in the diet. Omega-3 and omega-6 oils are the two principal types. The primary omega-3 oil is alpha-linolenic acid (ALA), found in flaxseed and canola oils, as well as pumpkin seeds, soybeans, and walnuts. Fish oils, such as salmon, cod, and mackerel, contain the other important omega-3 oils, DHA (docosahexaenoic acid) and EPA (eicosapentaenoic acid). Linoleic acid is the main omega-6 oil and is found in most vegetable oils, including safflower, corn, peanut, and sesame. The most therapeutic form of omega-6 oil is gamma-linolenic acid (GLA), found in black currant, borage, and evening primrose oils. EFAs are converted in the body to prostaglandins, hormone-like substances that regulate many metabolic functions, particularly inflammatory

processes. These also play an important role in reducing heart disease and in the treating of conditions such as eczema[6] and premenstrual stress.[7]

Accessory Nutrients

There are also many nonessential nutrients, called accessory nutrients or cofactors, that work in harmony with the essential nutrients to aid in the breakdown and conversion of food into cellular energy and also help support all of the body's physical and mental functions. According to Dr. Bland, some of the accessory nutrients that help support metabolism include B-complex cofactors choline and inositol, as well as coenzyme Q10 (a close relative of the B vitamins) and lipoic acid.

Other accessory nutrients that have demonstrated preventative functions include PABA (para-aminobenzoic acid) and substance P (bioflavonoids), which work with vitamin C. Certain amino acids are also considered nonessential because they can be synthesized by the body from the essential amino acids. These include alanine, carnitine, cysteine, glutamine, taurine, and tyrosine.

Enzymes are specialized living proteins fundamental to all living processes in the body, necessary for every chemical reaction and the normal activity of our organs, tissues, fluids, and cells. Metabolic enzymes are essential for the production of energy required to run cellular functions and also assist in clearing the body of toxins. Enzymes involved in digestion include salivary enzymes, which are responsible for predigestion in the mouth and stomach, and pancreatic enzymes, which carry on digestion in the intestines. The primary digestive enzymes include protease (digests proteins), amylase (digests carbohydrates), lipase (digests fats), cellulase (digests fiber), and disaccharidase (digests sugars).

In addition, the body contains an estimated several trillion beneficial bacteria comprising over 400 species, all necessary for health. Many of these "friendly" bacteria, also called probiotics, reside in the intestines, where they are essential for proper nutrient assimilation. Among the more well-known of these are *Lactobacillus acidophilus* and *Bifidobacteria*.[8] Prior to 1945 and the introduction of mass-market processed foods and industrial agriculture, Americans normally obtained adequate amounts of probiotics from fresh vegetables. Now, supplements may be necessary if you do not consume a diet filled with vegetables and fruits.

How Nutrients Work Together

Vitamins and minerals help regulate the conversion of food into energy in the body, according to Dr. Bland, and can be separated into two general categories: energy nutrients, which are principally involved in the conver-

VITAMIN AND MINERAL SUPPLEMENT RANGES

FAT-SOLUBLE VITAMINS	POSSIBLE SIDE EFFECTS	U.S. ADULT RDA/DRI	ADULT DAILY SUPPLEMENT RANGE
Beta carotene: Converted by the body to vitamin A as needed; primary antioxidant that helps protect the lungs and other tissues.	*Prolonged ingestion of relatively high doses may cause a harmless yellowing of the skin, especially palms and soles. Avoid beta carotene supplements while taking the prescription drug Accutane (isotretinoin), especially during pregnancy.*	Not established	10,000-50,000 IU
Vitamin A (retinol): Essential for growth and development and maintenance of healthy skin, hair, and eyes; prevents night-blindness and supports optical tissues; supports immune system and protects the body from colds, flu, and infections; important for the formation of bones, teeth, and sperm; involved in wound healing.	*Prolonged ingestion of excess vitamin A (over 50,000 IU daily) may be toxic. Avoid vitamin A supplements while taking the prescription drug Accutane (isotretinoin), especially during pregnancy.*	4,000-5,000 IU	5,000-10,000 IU
Vitamin D (cholecalciferol): Essential for calcium and phosphorus metabolism; required for strong bones and teeth; important for the health of the developing heart and nervous system, for proper thyroid gland function, and for normal blood clotting; useful for the prevention and treatment of diminished immunity, calcium deficiencies, osteoporosis, and conditions involving the eyes, including conjunctivitis and glaucoma.	*Prolonged ingestion of excess vitamin D (over 1,000 IU daily) may be toxic and cause hypercalcemia (excess calcium in blood).*	400 IU	200-400 IU
Vitamin E (alpha tocopherol): Primary antioxidant that protects red blood cells and is essential in cellular respiration; important for healthy hair and skin, reducing scarring, and preventing cancer, blood clots, and heart disease;[9] useful for reducing blood pressure, improving athletic performance, preventing muscle cramps, and in treating anemia, autoimmune diseases, cataracts, diabetes, fibrocystic breast conditions, herpes virus (shingles), impotence, PMS, menstrual pain, osteoarthritis, ulcers, and viruses.	*Prolonged ingestion of vitamin E may produce adverse skin reactions and upset stomach.*	12-15 IU	200-800 IU
Vitamin K (phylloquinone): Integrally involved in blood clotting; promotes healthy liver function and the conversion of glucose into glycogen in the liver for storage; useful for liver cirrhosis, jaundice, osteoporosis, heavy menstrual flow, painful menstruation, and nausea and vomiting during pregnancy.	*Unlike the other fat-soluble vitamins, vitamin K is not stored in significant quantity in the liver. Synthetic vitamin K (menadione) is toxic in excess dosages.*	12-15 IU	200-800 IU

WATER-SOLUBLE VITAMINS	POSSIBLE SIDE EFFECTS	U.S. ADULT RDA/DRI	ADULT DAILY SUPPLEMENT RANGE
Vitamin C (ascorbic acid): Primary antioxidant, essential for tissue growth, wound healing, absorption of calcium and iron, and utilization of folic acid. Involved in neurotransmitter biosynthesis, cholesterol regulation, and formation of collagen; useful for preventing constipation, easing arthritis and rheumatism, and preventing blood clots, bruising, and atherosclerosis.	*Essentially nontoxic in oral doses. However, excessive ingestion may cause abdominal bloating, gas, flatulence, and diarrhea. Acid-sensitive individuals should take the buffered ascorbate form of vitamin C supplement.*	60 mg	300-3,000 mg
Vitamin B₁ (thiamin): Essential for food metabolism and release of energy for cellular functions; supports the nervous system and brain function; improves circulation, blood formation, and digestion (stomach acid formation); antioxidant.	*Essentially nontoxic in oral doses.*	1.1-1.5 mg	5-100 mg

VITAMIN AND MINERAL SUPPLEMENT RANGES

WATER-SOLUBLE VITAMINS	POSSIBLE SIDE EFFECTS	U.S. ADULT RDA/DRI	ADULT DAILY SUPPLEMENT RANGE
Vitamin B2 (riboflavin): Essential for food metabolism and release of energy for cellular functions; important in the formation of red blood cells and activation of other B vitamins; promotes healthy hair, nails, and skin; benefits vision, prevents and treats cataracts, and is important for pregnancy.	*Essentially nontoxic in oral doses. Moderate to high doses of vitamin B2 may cause harmless bright yellow coloration of urine.*	1.3-1.7 mg	5-100 mg
Vitamin B3 (niacin): Essential for food metabolism and release of cellular energy; vital for oxygen transport in the blood and fatty acid and nucleic acid formation; a major constituent of several important coenzymes; increases circulation, aids in the metabolism of carbohydrates, fats, and proteins, and in the formation of sex hormones; supports the intestines and nervous system, benefits skin conditions such as acne, helps with high cholesterol levels, various intestinal disorders, headaches, poor memory, mental illness, and vertigo.	*Essentially nontoxic in normal oral doses. High doses (over 100 mg daily) may cause transient flushing and tingling in the upper body area, as well as stomach upset. Prolonged ingestion of excess vitamin B3 (more than 1,000-2,000 mg per day) may elevate liver enzymes and cause liver damage.*	15-19 mg	20-100 mg
Vitamin B5 (pantothenic acid): Involved in food metabolism and release of energy for cellular functions; vital for biosynthesis of hormones and support of the adrenal glands; used for conditions involving stress and fatigue, allergies, arthritis, asthma, headaches, insomnia, psoriasis, post-operative shock, anemia, depression, and anxiety.	*Essentially nontoxic in oral doses. Extremely high doses (over 10,000 mg) will produce diarrhea.*	4-7 mg	10-1,000 mg
Vitamin B6 (pyridoxine): Involved in food metabolism and release of energy; essential for amino acid metabolism and formation of blood proteins and antibodies; helps regulate electrolyte balance; important for nervous system and brain function, formation of RNA and DNA, and antibody production; balances hormones and water levels (B6 is a mild diuretic) in women; useful for premenstrual syndrome (PMS), painful periods, fatigue, and morning sickness in women, as well as allergies, arthritis, asthma, autism, neuritis, epilepsy and convulsions, Parkinson's, schizophrenia, learning disabilities, and carpal tunnel syndrome.	*Prolonged high doses (over 500 mg daily) may be toxic and cause neurological damage. Prescription oral contraceptives may cause a deficiency of vitamin B6.*	1.6-2.0 mg	5-200 mg
Vitamin B12 (cobalamin): Essential for normal formation of red blood cells; involved in food metabolism, release of energy, and maintenance of epithelial cells (found in the skin's outer layer and the surface layer of mucous membranes); important for the nervous system and known to relieve fatigue and increase energy levels.	*Essentially nontoxic in oral doses.*	2 mcg	10-500 mcg
Folate (folic acid, folacin): Essential for blood formation, both red blood cells and white blood cells; involved in the biosynthesis of nucleic acids including RNA and DNA; useful for acne, anemia, atherosclerosis, canker sores, cervical cancer, cervical dysplasia, dermatitis, diarrhea, fatigue, gingivitis, gout, immune weakness, infection, osteoporosis, periodontal disease, pregnancy, restless legs syndrome, and skin ulcers.	*Essentially nontoxic in oral doses. An excess intake of folate can mask a vitamin B12 deficiency*	180-200 mcg	200-800 mcg
B vitamins should also be taken in a B-complex form because of their close interrelationship in metabolic processes.			

VITAMIN AND MINERAL SUPPLEMENT RANGES

WATER-SOLUBLE VITAMINS	POSSIBLE SIDE EFFECTS	U.S. ADULT RDA/DRI	ADULT DAILY SUPPLEMENT RANGE
Biotin: Essential for food metabolism and release of energy; assists in the biosynthesis of amino acids, nucleic acids, and fatty acids; needed for the utilization of other B vitamins; supports the bones, glands, and nerves, and enhances the utilization of insulin (helpful for diabetics); strengthens hair and nails, and prevents baldness and the graying of hair (if a biotin deficiency exists); used to treat skin conditions such as dermatitis, dandruff, eczema, psoriasis (especially in children), and seborrhea.	*Essentially nontoxic in oral doses.*	150-300 mcg	300-600 mcg

MINERALS	POSSIBLE SIDE EFFECTS	U.S. ADULT RDA/DRI	ADULT DAILY SUPPLEMENT RANGE
The functions of minerals are highly interrelated to each other and to vitamins, hormones, and enzymes. No individual mineral can function in the body without affecting the others.			
Calcium: The most abundant mineral in the body; essential for healthy bones and teeth, and for preventing osteoporosis, high blood pressure, insomnia, PMS, and panic attacks; serves as a vital cofactor in cellular energy production and nerve and heart function. The most absorbable forms of calcium are calcium ascorbate, calcium citrate, calcium malate, calcium glycinate, and calcium derived from crystalline hydroxyapatite.	*Prolonged ingestion of excess calcium, along with excess vitamin D, may cause hypercalcemia (excessive calcium in the blood) and calcification in soft tissue (such as joints and kidneys) and may also cause a mineral imbalance.*	1,000 mg	200-1,200 mg
Magnesium: Essential catalyst for food metabolism and energy release; cofactor in the formation of RNA/DNA, enzyme activation, and nerve function; prevents headaches, change in heart rhythm and electrical activity, nerve/muscle problems, and arteriosclerosis.	*Extremely high doses (over 30,000 mg) may be toxic in certain individuals with kidney problems. Doses of more than 400 mg may cause diarrhea.*	310-400 mg	150-600 mg
Potassium: A primary electrolyte, important in regulating pH (acid/base) balance and water balance; plays a role in nerve function and cellular integrity. *A typical healthy diet contains adequate potassium; very active individuals may require additional electrolytes.	*Extremely high doses (over 25,000 mg daily) of potassium chloride may be toxic in instances of kidney failure.*	Not established	1,875-5,625 mg*
Sodium: A primary electrolyte, important in regulating pH (acid/base) balance and water balance; plays a role in nerve function and cellular integrity.	*Prolonged ingestion of excess sodium has been linked to high blood pressure and increased incidence of migraine headaches. Extremely high intake of sodium can result in swelling of tissues (edema).*	Not established	Limit daily intake to 1,500 mg
Phosphorus: The second most prevalent mineral in the body, involved in virtually every metabolic function; constituent of the molecule phosphate, which plays a major role in energy production and activation of the B vitamins; component of RNA/DNA, bones, and teeth.	*Although essentially nontoxic, a disproportionately large amount of phosphorus relative to calcium intake may cause a deficiency in calcium and mineral imbalance.*	700 mg	300-600 mg
Zinc: Cofactor in numerous enzymatic processes and reactions; structural constituent of nucleic acids and insulin; involved in wound healing and digestion; activates metal-containing enzymes; used for protein synthesis; supports immune function.	*Extremely high doses (more than 2,000 mg daily) can be toxic. Excess zinc intake (over 50 mg per day) may cause copper deficiency and mineral imbalance.*	12-15 mg	15-30 mg

VITAMIN AND MINERAL SUPPLEMENT RANGES

MINERALS	POSSIBLE SIDE EFFECTS	U.S. ADULT RDA/DRI	ADULT DAILY SUPPLEMENT RANGE
Iron: Combines with other nutrients to produce blood proteins that are essential components of hemoglobin; involved in food metabolism; cofactor and activator for enzymes.	*Prolonged ingestion of excess iron can be toxic, affecting the liver, pancreas, and heart, and increasing susceptibility to infection. Poorly utilized forms of iron (iron sulfate or iron gluconate) may cause constipation and/or stomach upset. Iron supplements should be taken with food and supplemental vitamin C.*	10-15 mg	10-30 mg
Copper: Essential for production of red blood cells; involved in the maintenance of skeletal and cardiovascular systems; works with vitamin C in the biosynthesis of collagen and elastin (elastic fibers in blood vessels, skin, and vertebral discs).	*Prolonged ingestion of excess copper may be toxic, especially with Wilson's disease, a rare metabolic disorder resulting in an excess accumulation of copper in the liver, red blood cells, and the brain.*	2-3 mg	2-3 mg
Iodine: Essential component of thyroid hormones, which regulate growth and the rate of metabolism; prevents hypothyroidism (underproduction of thyroid hormones).	*Prolonged ingestion of excess iodine may cause "iodine goiter," an enlargement of the thyroid gland. May also induce acne-like skin lesions or aggravate preexisting acne conditions.*	150 mcg	50-300 mcg
Chromium: Vital as cofactor of GTF (glucose tolerance factor), which regulates the function of insulin; involved in food metabolism, enzyme activation, and regulation of cholesterol.	*Essentially nontoxic in oral doses.*	150 mcg	50-300 mcg
Selenium: Important constituent of the antioxidant enzyme glutathione peroxidase, which is contained in white blood cells and blood platelets; synergistic nutritional partner of vitamin E; prevents age/liver spots as well as various heart, liver, immune, and muscle conditions.	*Prolonged ingestion of excess selenium may be toxic.*	55-70 mcg	100-200 mcg

sion of food to energy, and protector nutrients, which help defend against damaging toxins derived from drugs, alcohol, radiation, environmental pollutants, or the body's own enzyme processes.

"The B-complex vitamins and magnesium are examples of energy nutrients," says Dr. Bland. "They activate specific metabolic facilitators called enzymes, which control digestion and the absorption and use of proteins, fats, and carbohydrates. These nutrients often work as a team, their mutual presence enhancing the other's function." In the process of converting food to energy, free radicals are produced that can damage the body and set the stage for degenerative diseases, including arthritis, heart disease, and certain forms of cancer, as well as premature aging. Protector nutrients such as vitamin E, beta carotene, vitamin C, and the minerals zinc, copper, manganese, and selenium play a critical role in preventing or delaying these degenerative processes. Vitamins A, C, and E work together as a team, protecting against breakdown and helping each other maintain adequate tissue levels.

Dr. Berkson notes that vitamins and minerals are what make the chemical and electrical circuitry of the body work and that the body's functioning is therefore profoundly affected by how nutrients either work together or against each other. Nutrients can help each other or inhibit each other when taken simultaneously. For example, iron is best absorbed when taken separately from pancreatic enzymes and should also not be taken with vitamin E, says Dr. Berkson. There are also certain nutrients that can help "potentiate" the other nutrients; for example, vitamin C taken with iron provides the maximum absorption of the iron.

Benefits of Nutritional Supplementation

One of the primary uses of nutritional supplements is to compensate for the inadequacies of the modern diet. While improving the diet should be the necessary first

HOW TO READ A DIETARY SUPPLEMENT LABEL

A product that is ingested orally and contains vitamins, minerals, herbs, amino acids, or other nutrients from food qualifies as a dietary supplement, according to the 1994 Dietary Supplement Health and Education Act. Supplements are not considered drugs under this act and do not need to be reviewed by the U.S. Food and Drug Administration (FDA) before entering the market. The FDA, however, regulates the information a manufacturer can provide about a product. Manufacturers cannot claim that a product will treat or diagnose a disease; for example, claiming that a product treats osteoporosis is illegal. But they can claim that calcium lowers the risk of osteoporosis when scientific studies (reviewed by the FDA) support the link between the nutrient and the health condition. They can also make structure-function claims, which describe the role or function of a nutrient in the body. For instance, a product label can state "Calcium builds strong bones." Every structure-function claim must be followed by a disclaimer: "This statement has not been evaluated by the Food and Drug Administration. This product is not intended to diagnose, treat, cure, or prevent any disease."

Label Front

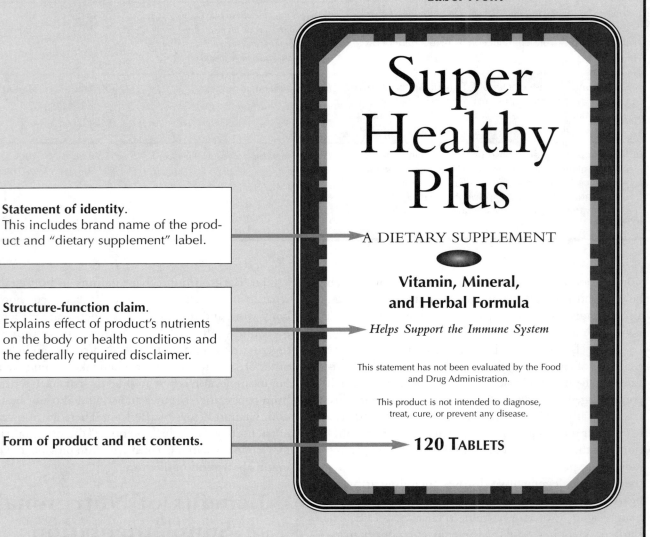

Statement of identity.
This includes brand name of the product and "dietary supplement" label.

Structure-function claim.
Explains effect of product's nutrients on the body or health conditions and the federally required disclaimer.

Form of product and net contents.

Super Healthy Plus

A DIETARY SUPPLEMENT

Vitamin, Mineral, and Herbal Formula

Helps Support the Immune System

This statement has not been evaluated by the Food and Drug Administration.

This product is not intended to diagnose, treat, cure, or prevent any disease.

120 TABLETS

Source: Council for Responsible Nutrition, Washington, D.C., and U.S. Food and Drug Administration's Center for Food Safety and Applied Nutrition.

HOW TO READ A DIETARY SUPPLEMENT LABEL, continued

Label Back

Directions for use: Take one capsule daily.

SUPPLEMENT FACTS

Serving Size: one capsule

	Amount Per Serving	% Daily Value
Vitamin A (as beta carotene)	5000 IU	100%
Vitamin C (from ascorbic acid)	60 mg	100%
Vitamin E (as d-alpha tocopherol)	30 IU	100%
Zinc (zinc citrate)	23 mg	
Echinacea (powdered root)	200 mg	*
Goldenseal (powdered root)	80 mg	*

* Daily value not established

Other ingredients: gelatin, water, binders, and coatings

Manufacturer's
or distributor's name,
address, and zip code

Directions.
Recommended by manufacturer. It is not advised to exceed this amount without recommendations from a health-care professional.

Supplement facts panel.
Lists serving size, amount contained in each tablet or capsule (if the serving size is one tablet), and active ingredients. Also includes "Daily Value," which is percentage of the recommended daily intake for each nutrient. An asterisk indicates that a Daily Value is not established for that nutrient.

Other ingredients.
A complete list of all ingredients used to formulate the supplement. Ingredients are listed in descending order of predominance and by common name or proprietary blend.

Name and address of manufacturer.

step, many studies support the use of nutritional supplements to achieve adequate levels of nutrients. Research by Raymond Shamberger, Ph.D., and Derrick Lonsdale, M.D., of Cleveland, Ohio, found that while consumption of empty-calorie diets can lead to such problems as fatigue, mood swings, insomnia, and a variety of health complaints without other related medical diagnosis, when patients were given supplementary nutrients over a period of 6-12 weeks, many of their symptoms improved. A study at the University of Wales found that the administration of multivitamin supplements to children suffering from marginal nutrient insufficiency brought about significant improvement in their academic performance.[10] A similar observation was made in studying the mental capacity of elderly individuals.[11]

Thousands of studies also support the use of nutritional supplements for the treatment of various health conditions. (While these are too numerous to adequately cover here, you will find additional information on nutrients in each health condition chapter.) For instance, current studies lend strong support to the importance of vitamin C in slowing the development of cataracts, heart disease, and cancer. A study conducted by James E. Enstrom, M.D., an epidemiologist at the University of California at Los Angeles, suggests that men who consume vitamin C every day, at levels five to six times the U.S. RDA, live about six years longer.[12] Robert Cathcart III, M.D., of Los Altos, California, has also documented the effective use of vitamin C in treating various infectious diseases, including the common cold, flu, pneumonia, hepatitis, mononucleosis, and several childhood diseases.[13]

Clinical studies have shown a relationship between low intake of beta carotene and vitamins C and E and a higher incidence of cancer.[14] Research done at Johns Hopkins University, in Baltimore, Maryland, found that there were approximately 50% fewer heart disease cases in a group of people with the highest levels of beta carotene compared to the group with the lowest levels.[15] A similar study at Harvard University found that of two groups with prior evidence of heart disease, the group given a beta carotene supplement had 40% fewer heart attacks than the group given a placebo.[16]

Research has also found that vitamin B3 (niacin) can help combat heart disease, while vitamin B6 can help prevent atherosclerosis.[17] Other studies have shown similar results with vitamin E and heart disease.[18] Large doses of vitamin E have also been found to strengthen immune function and reduce the severity of age-related conditions such as Parkinson's disease.[19]

A 19-year prospective study found that calcium deficiency was associated with a higher risk of colorectal cancer.[20] Calcium supplementation may also decrease

total cholesterol and inhibit platelet aggregation (abnormal blood clotting), both helpful for preventing heart disease.[21] Several studies have also linked chromium deficiency to heart disease.[22] In addition, it has been found that individuals who die suddenly of heart attacks have far lower levels of magnesium and potassium.[23]

Manganese helps maintain the structural integrity of heart and kidney cell membranes and promotes tissue oxygen uptake, food absorption, neurotransmitter synthesis, fertility, insulin synthesis, fat and carbohydrate metabolism, and homeostatic blood-clotting mechanisms.[24] Rheumatoid arthritis sufferers are usually significantly deficient in manganese and supplementation is recommended.

Boron helps to reduce the excretion of calcium and magnesium, important minerals in bone structure and muscle function.[25] Studies in Germany have found that boron can improve joint pain in osteoarthritis as well as decrease bone loss.[26]

A positive relationship has been found between low blood selenium levels and heart disease, possibly related to selenium's antioxidant effects.[27] Selenium supplementation also reduces platelet aggregation,[28] and selenium is a cofactor for glutathione peroxidase, an important antioxidant enzyme. Zinc supplementation has been found to improve progressive hearing loss and other related ear problems.[29]

According to Eric Braverman, M.D., of the New York University Medical Center, in New York City, amino acid supplementation has been used to treat heart disease, as well as herpes, alcoholism, and a variety of psychiatric disorders.[30] Supplementation with the amino acid L-carnitine immediately after an acute heart attack can help damaged heart muscle expand again. In one study, L-carnitine, when given orally at the rate of 2 g daily for 28 days, improved the condition of 51 patients who had experienced heart attacks.[31]

Accessory nutrients can also be taken as supplements for specific purposes. For example, bioflavonoids (plant pigments that act as antioxidants) can help to increase the antiviral activity of vitamin C in treating herpes simplex.[32] Coenzyme Q10 helps to improve heart function.[33] Evidence suggests that gamma-linolenic acid, an essential fatty acid, may help to regulate the cardiovascular, nervous, and immune systems.[34]

 Due to current FDA labeling regulations for nutritional supplements and herbs, health food stores and/or pharmacies are not allowed to present information regarding dosage or treatment of health conditions, regardless of scientific support.

In addition to disease control, nutritional supplements can help people cope with specific lifestyle, environmental, and emotional/psychological factors. For example, smokers require more vitamin E, vitamin C, and beta carotene than nonsmokers, and persons who consume a significant amount of alcohol require more vitamin B_1 and magnesium than the average person.[35] Individuals engaged in heavy exercise programs need to make sure they are getting adequate nutrients to meet their increased caloric demands. Dieters also need supplemental vitamins and minerals to make up for deficiencies that result from reduced calorie intake, according to Dr. Berkson.

Women taking oral contraceptives may need to increase their intake of zinc, folic acid, and vitamin B_6, while pregnant women may require more folic acid for proper fetal development. Lactating women also need additional magnesium and protein, and postmenopausal women require increased calcium and vitamin D to maintain strong bones.

When recovering from surgery, a person may need higher levels of zinc,[36] and individuals who are exposed to smog or other pollutants require higher levels of the protector nutrients such as selenium, vitamin E, and vitamin C.[37] Also, anyone who is under heavy emotional or physical stress will need a higher intake of all the B vitamins.[38]

Using Nutritional Supplements

Today, an estimated 80% of adult Americans take nutritional supplements, many on a daily basis.[39] It is no longer just a fad, but part of a growing trend as people start to take a proactive approach to their own health. Although researchers are learning more every day about the connection between nutrients and health, there is still no definitive scientific "how-to guide" for this very complex issue, especially since each individual's needs are different.

While it is always recommended that a person try to obtain as many nutrients as possible through the consumption of a variety of nutrient-dense foods, this can be unrealistic for many, due to the following reasons: reduced calorie intake; the dislike of certain foods; loss of nutrients in cooking; the variable quality of food supply; lack of knowledge, motivation, or time to plan and prepare balanced meals; and nutrient depletion caused by stress, lifestyle, and certain medications. This is where nutritional supplements can play an important role in filling any nutrient gaps.

Nutritional supplements are not a panacea, however, and it is important to be aware of some potential risks. Prolonged intake of excessive doses of vitamins A, B_6, and D, for example, may produce toxic effects. Other

ANTIOXIDANTS FOR HEALTH

An antioxidant (meaning "against oxidation") is a natural biochemical substance that protects cells against damage from harmful free radicals. Antioxidants work to neutralize free radicals, which, if left uncontrolled, can lead to cellular aging, degeneration, arthritis, heart disease, cancer, and other illnesses. Environmental pollution and stressful lifestyles make daily supplementation with antioxidants a necessity. Extra supplementation may be required if you smoke cigarettes or are exposed to secondary smoke, chemical pollutants, or to high doses of UV (ultraviolet) rays from the sun. When antioxidants are taken in combination, the effect is stronger than when they are used individually. Antioxidants come in a variety of types:

- Amino acids: cysteine, glutathione, methionine, taurine

- Bioflavonoids: anthocyanin bioflavonoids (in grapes, cranberries, and bilberries), citrus bioflavonoids (in grapefruit, lemons, and oranges), proanthocyanidins in maritime pine bark or grape seed extract, stabilized rice bran

- Carotenoids: alpha and beta carotene (in red, yellow, and orange fruits and vegetables and dark green leafy vegetables), lycopene (in red fruits and vegetables, such as red grapefruit and tomatoes)

- Dietary sources: cayenne pepper, garlic, turmeric

- Herbs: astragalus, bilberry, ginkgo, green tea, milk thistle, sage

- Minerals: copper, manganese, zinc (all components of the antioxidant enzyme superoxide dismutase), selenium

- Vitamins: A, B_2, C, and E, coenzyme Q10, NADH (nicotinamide adenine dinucleotide)

- Enzymes: catalase, glutathione peroxidase, superoxide dismutase (SOD)

- Hormone: melatonin

vitamins, minerals, and accessory nutrients can also sometimes cause side effects when they interact with medications, or due to health conditions or simply a person's biochemical individuality. However, alternative practitioners may sometimes recommend dosages higher than those currently considered safe by conventional medicine. The scientific literature and numerous clinical tri-

HOW TO TAKE NUTRITIONAL SUPPLEMENTS

Before taking any nutritional supplement, you should ask what scientific data supports its safety and what are the safe intake levels for the nutrients you are considering. Jeffrey Bland, Ph.D., of Gig Harbor, Washington, and D. Lindsey Berkson, M.A., D.C., of Santa Fe, New Mexico, make the following recommendations:

- Nutritional supplements should be taken with meals to promote increased absorption. Fat-soluble nutrients (such as vitamins A and E, beta carotene, and the essential fatty acids linoleic acid and alpha-linolenic acid) should be taken with the meal that contains the most fat.

- Amino acid supplements should be taken on an empty stomach at least an hour before or after a meal, and taken with fruit juice to help promote absorption. Whenever taking an increased dosage of an isolated amino acid, be sure to supplement with an amino acid blend.

- If you become nauseated when you take tablet supplements, consider taking a liquid form, diluted in a beverage.

- If you become nauseated or ill within an hour after taking nutritional supplements, consider the need for a bowel cleanse or rejuvenation program prior to continuing with supplementation.

- If taking high doses, do not take the supplements all at once, but divide them into smaller doses taken throughout the day.

- Take digestive enzymes with meals to assist digestion. If you are taking pancreatic enzymes for other therapeutic reasons, be sure to take them on an empty stomach between meals.

- Take mineral supplements separately from the highest fiber meal of the day, as fiber can decrease mineral absorption.

- Whenever taking an increased dosage of an isolated B vitamin, be sure to supplement with a B complex supplement.

- A new approach to taking nutrients is using plant-grown vitamins, cultured in a yeast base. According to researcher C. Joe Bentley, of LifeStar Millennium, this makes them a whole food form, enchancing bioavailability.

als support these elevated dosages for short periods of time and only under medical supervision.

Nutritional supplements should also never take the place of appropriate medical care when warranted. If someone is currently under medical care, is taking any medications, or has a history of specific problems, it is important to always consult with a physician before making any changes in diet or lifestyle, including the use of supplements.

It can take years of personal research and experimentation to put together a good dietary and supplement program. To eliminate a lot of guesswork and frustration, consult a qualified health professional trained in the intricacies of nutritional biochemistry, in order to help assess personal needs and develop an effective dietary and nutritional supplement program tailored to biochemical individuality.

High-quality supplements can often be obtained through these professionals or from a source recommended by them. When making a decision to purchase supplements without the advice of an expert, do so as an informed consumer. It is worthwhile to read some of the many books and magazines published about good dietary habits and nutritional supplements. Reputable health food stores are a good source of quality supplements and are usually staffed by people who have a knowledgeable understanding of nutrition and supplementation. Some pharmacies specialize in nutritional and natural remedies as well; there are also mail-order and direct outlets.

The Future of Nutritional Medicine

The current challenge for medicine and nutritional science is to look beyond statistical guidelines in order to gain a greater understanding of the role and proper level of nutrients that will help every individual achieve and maintain a high level of wellness. Through education and involvement, a person can develop an understanding of the proper diet and nutritional needs specifically suited to the body and should make this knowledge an integral part of living well.

Since nutritional supplements cannot be patented, there is little financial incentive for pharmaceutical companies to invest the millions of dollars needed to meet the government's stringent research requirements in order to receive FDA approval for treatment of specific conditions. Alternative sources of funding must be found in order to make nutritional supplements an accepted part of mainstream medicine.

Where to Find Help

To obtain referrals to physicians trained in nutritional medicine, contact:

American Association of Naturopathic Physicians
8201 Greensboro Drive, Suite 300
McLean, Virginia 22101
(703) 610-9037
Website: www.naturopathic.org

Provides a directory of naturopathic physicians and offers referrals to a nationwide network of accredited or licensed practitioners. Also publishes a quarterly newsletter for both professionals and the general public, and offers a series of brochures and pamphlets on a variety of subjects.

American College of Advancement in Medicine
P.O. Box 3427
Laguna Hills, California 92654
(714) 583-7666

ACAM provides a directory of physicians worldwide who have been trained in nutritional and preventative medicine. The directory also provides an extensive list of books and articles on nutritional supplementation.

International Society for Orthomolecular Medicine (ISOM)
16 Florence Avenue
Toronto, Ontario, Canada M2N 1E9
(416) 733-2117
Website: www.orthomed.org

ISOM seeks to further the advancement of orthomolecular medicine throughout the world and to raise awareness of this rapidly growing and cost-effective practice of health care, through publications, conferences, and seminars.

The Society for Orthomolecular Health Medicine
2698 Pacific Avenue
San Francisco, California 94115
(415) 922-6462
Website: www.orthomed.org

This resource serves as a clearinghouse of information and as a referral service for physicians practicing orthomolecular medicine.

Recommended Reading

Encyclopedia of Nutritional Supplements. Michael T. Murray, N.D. Rocklin, CA: Prima Publishing, 2001.

The Nutrition Desk Reference. Robert H. Garrison, Jr., M.A.R., Ph.D., and Elizabeth Somer, M.A., R.D. New Canaan, CT: Keats Publishing, 1997.

Nutritional Influences on Illness. Melvyn A. Werbach, M.D. Tarzana, CA: Third Line Press, 1996.

Prescription for Nutritional Healing. Phyllis A. Balch, C.N.C., and James F. Balch, M.D. New York: Avery Penguin Putnam, 2000.

Staying Healthy with Nutrition. Elson M. Haas, M.D. Berkeley, CA: Celestial Arts, 1992.

The Supplement Shopper. Gregory Pouls, D.C., and Maile Pouls, Ph.D., with Burton Goldberg. Tiburon, CA: Future Medicine Publishing, 1999.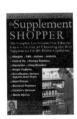

ORTHOMOLECULAR MEDICINE

Employing vitamins, minerals, and amino acids to create optimum nutritional content and balance in the body, orthomolecular medicine targets a wide range of conditions, including depression, hypertension, schizophrenia, cancer, and other mental and physiological disorders.

IN 1968, TWO-TIME Nobel laureate Linus Pauling, Ph.D., originated the term *orthomolecular* to describe an approach to medicine that uses naturally occurring substances normally present in the body. *Ortho* means correct or normal, and orthomolecular physicians recognize that, in many cases of physiological and psychological disorders, health can be reestablished by properly correcting or normalizing the balance of vitamins, minerals, amino acids, and other similar substances within the body.

"Dr. Pauling invented the word *orthomolecular* as a means of confronting the scientific establishment with the importance of medical nutrition," explains Richard A. Kunin, M.D., of San Francisco, California, a leading orthomolecular physician. "For nearly half a century, from the 1930s to the 1980s, nutrition had little credibility among conventional physicians and was likened to quackery. Dr. Pauling's endorsement helped to correct that situation and his phrase has stuck for two reasons. It underscores the scientific validity of physiological factors such as nutrients in healing and it memorializes Dr. Pauling's historic contributions to science and medicine." To acknowledge this physiological approach to medicine, the Orthomolecular Medical Society, which Dr. Pauling supported during his lifetime, recently renamed itself the Society for Orthomolecular Health Medicine and is guided by its motto: "Putting nutrition first in health and medicine."

The premise behind orthomolecular medicine extends back to the 1920s, when vitamins and minerals were first used to treat illnesses unrelated to nutrient deficiency. During that time, it was discovered that vitamin A could pre-

> *Of course, germs are an important consideration in the disease process, but susceptibility is more dependent on nutrition than on exposure to the ubiquitous pathogens that pass our way every day.*
>
> —RICHARD A. KUNIN, M.D.

vent childhood deaths from infectious illness and that heart arrhythmia (irregular heartbeat) could be stopped by dosages of magnesium. Scientific evidence supporting nutritional therapy did not fully emerge, however, until the 1950s, when Abram Hoffer, M.D., and Humphrey Osmond, M.D., began treating schizophrenics with high doses of vitamin B3 (niacin). Their studies showed that niacin, in combination with standard medical therapy, doubled the number of recoveries in a one-year period.[1]

As research continued, it was found that malnutrition and improper nutrition could place a person at risk, directly causing or contributing to the development of disease and psychiatric disorders. Furthermore, it was noted that health can be impaired due, in part, to the consumption of refined, empty-calorie foods such as white bread, pastries, and sugar. Decreased intakes of dietary fiber, bran, minerals, and complex carbohydrates were also found in patients with certain forms of mental illness, along with a loss of vitamins and an increase in dietary fat. At the time, the notion that diet and food choices could improve health or contribute to disease was a new and controversial idea.

Historically, however, the relationship between diet and health has been espoused at least since the time of Hippocrates, 2,500 years ago. "As the great Spanish physician Maimonedes said in the 12th century, 'Anything that can be cured by nutrition should not be treated by any other means'," Dr. Kunin says. "What was obvious then should be no less obvious now: nutrition should come before drugs. Pneumonia, for instance, is not caused by penicillin deficiency, but it is definitely caused by deficiency of vitamins A and C, iodine, zinc, and other vital nutrients. Of course, germs are an important consideration in the disease process, but susceptibility is more dependent on nutrition than on exposure to the ubiquitous pathogens that pass our way every day."

Nutrition is an integral part of body chemistry and physiology. It replenishes the essential molecules that maintain the systems that are the infrastructure of our physical life. Drug therapy can be lifesaving, but nutrition is health-giving. In Dr. Kunin's view, orthomolecular medicine is the foundation of modern scientific medical practice. "Nutrition, pollution, and adaptation are the major categories in this approach," he explains. "Nutrition and pollution are the environmental factors, positive and negative, that affect our health, and adaptation is our response to the environment itself. When adaptation fails, we get sick or perish."

The orthomolecular approach safeguards against such failure by identifying the nutrient imbalances and correcting them. "Nothing is more scientific than that," says Dr. Kunin. "Identifying toxic and infectious agents is equally important and that is equally basic to effective medical practice. The comprehensive manner in which orthomolecular medicine works to accomplish this makes it a true medical advance and a better way to diagnose, treat, and help you understand your individual needs and balance the ever-changing forces in your life."

The Basic Principles of Orthomolecular Medicine

Even today, many physicians disregard the value of proper nutrition in relation to health. The prevalent notion is that a balanced diet will provide all the nutrition one needs. What is overlooked is the fact that the majority of the U.S. food supply is processed and grown in nutritionally depleted soil. Orthomolecular physicians recognize these factors, as well as the fact that biochemical individuality can also play a crucial role in health.

The concept of biochemical individuality is based on the work of Roger J. Williams, Ph.D. In treating his patients, Dr. Williams realized that each individual is unique. Although the Recommended Dietary Allowances (RDAs) for nutrients may prevent severe deficiency diseases, orthomolecular physicians say that these levels do not provide for optimal health and individuals may need many more times the RDA levels. For example, studies of guinea pigs show a twenty-fold variation in their requirement for vitamin C. Similar studies have been done with humans: children have been shown to have varying needs for vitamin B6 and Canadian soldiers and Japanese prisoners of war who suffered from starvation

---

DIAGNOSTIC TESTS USED BY ORTHOMOLECULAR PHYSICIANS

Orthomolecular physicians employ a wide range of diagnostic tests not commonly used by conventional physicians. Richard A. Kunin, M.D., of San Francisco, California, divides such tests into two categories: those that can save your life and those that can improve your health.

Diagnostic tests that can potentially safe your life due to their ability to detect hidden, life-threatening biological imbalances include: erythrocyte sedimentation rate, C-reactive protein, low-density lipoprotein by gel electrophoresis, homocysteine, lipoprotein (a), fibrinogen, soluble fibrin monomers, plasminogen activator inhibitor, protein-S, protein-C, ferritin, complete blood count (CBC), blood chemistry panel, urinalysis, free thyroxine T4/free T3 (tri-iodothyronine), and hemoglobin A1C.

Tests that can improve your health include: vitamin panel, mineral panel (hair, urine, red blood cell), organic acids (urine), amino acids (blood), essential fatty acids (RBC), allergy (IgE, IgG4, ELISA-ACT), and a comprehensive stool analysis.

---

were shown to require a much greater intake of vitamins than usual.

Dr. Kunin summarizes the principles of orthomolecular medicine:[2]

- Nutrition comes first in medical diagnosis and treatment, and nutrient-related disorders are usually curable once nutritional balance is achieved.

- Biochemical individuality is the norm in medical practice; therefore, RDA values are unreliable nutrient guides. Many people require an intake of certain nutrients far beyond the RDA suggested range (often called a megadose), due to their genetic disposition or the environment in which they live.

- Drug treatment is used only for specific indications and always mindful of the potential dangers and adverse effects.

- Environmental pollution and food adulteration are an inescapable fact of modern life and are a medical priority.

DETERMINING THE PROPER DOSE OF VITAMIN C

Robert Cathcart III, M.D., has found that taking vitamin C to bowel tolerance (the amount of vitamin C that can be tolerated by the body before diarrhea occurs) can effectively treat diseases that may involve free-radical damage.[9] These include the common cold, infections, allergies, autoimmune diseases, burns, and viral pneumonia. Free radicals are molecules in the body that contain an unpaired electron; as free radicals seek to replace their missing electrons, they injure body tissues. Free radicals are neutralized by electrons called reducing equivalents that are carried by high doses of vitamin C.

Powdered ascorbic acid (vitamin C) is mixed with water and taken several times in a 24-hour period. The amount taken is increased until diarrhea develops and is slightly adjusted until the diarrhea stops. The more severe the problem, the more vitamin C that can be taken before diarrhea occurs.

Dr. Cathcart suggests the following amounts of vitamin C be taken for certain problems. In many conditions, symptoms are greatly reduced but will return rapidly if the dose levels are not maintained. In serious problems, doses may have to be taken every half hour and delays may prolong the illness.

	Grams/24 hours	Doses/24 hours
Hay fever, asthma	5-20	4-8
Mild colds	30-60	6-10
Influenza	100-150	8-15
Viral pneumonia	50-200+	12-18

CAUTION Before beginning this type of program, it is advisable to seek out the guidance of your physician. People suffering from hypertension or kidney problems should also ascertain that the form of vitamin C they use does not contain sodium ascorbate, a form of salt that can result in heart and kidney complications.

- Blood tests do not necessarily reflect tissue levels of nutrients.

- Hope is the indispensable ally of the physician and the absolute right of the patient.

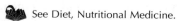 See Diet, Nutritional Medicine.

How Orthomolecular Medicine Works

The basis of orthomolecular medicine lies in creating a healthier diet. Junk foods, refined sugar, and food additives are eliminated. Every effort is made to eat nutritious, whole foods, high in fiber and low in unhealthy trans-fats. Depending on the condition to be treated, various vitamins, minerals, and other nutrients are supplemented. The types and amounts of the nutrients are determined by blood tests, urine analysis, and tests for nutrient levels. Frequently, supplementation is based not only on a patient's symptoms, but also on results reported in medical journals and, quite commonly, the clinical experience of the doctor. Prescribed doses of vitamins are sometimes injected to speed the initial response and follow-up treatment usually consists of vitamin pills several times a day until adequate dosage is achieved. This dosage has often been called a "megadose" because amounts of nutrients taken are often far greater than the levels needed to prevent deficiency. As a result, orthomolecular medicine has also been called megavitamin therapy.

The number of fatalities from overdoses of major pharmaceutical drugs over an eight-year period was 2,556, whereas the total number of fatalities resulting from high doses of vitamin supplements during the same period was zero.

One of the arguments against megavitamin treatment is that high doses of certain vitamins are toxic and may cause certain reactions. A major study, however, indicates that the number of fatalities from overdoses of major pharmaceutical drugs over an eight-year period was 2,556, whereas the total number of fatalities resulting from high doses of vitamin supplements during the same period was zero.[3] A more recent and comprehensive study found that adverse drug reactions were responsible for over 100,000 deaths per year in the U.S. "There is no question that megavitamin therapies are harmless in comparison," Dr. Kunin notes.

Nevertheless, orthomolecular physicians are aware of the problems associated with megavitamin therapy and, if symptoms arise, the dosage of the offending vitamin is reduced. In some cases, these reactions are carefully observed as an indication that the body has been saturated with the vitamin. When this occurs, the dose is lowered until the symptoms disappear and the body is supplied with optimal levels of the nutrient.

Conditions Benefited by Orthomolecular Medicine

Orthomolecular medicine is beneficial for any condition for which nutritional imbalances play a causative role. Since the mid-1950s, for example, niacin has been used as a treatment for schizophrenia. More recently, niacin has been shown to be an effective agent for treating hyperlipidemia (an excess of lipids or fats in the blood). In this capacity, it has been shown to reduce death rates from heart disease and nonfatal myocardial infarction, as well as reducing total cholesterol, low-density lipoproteins (LDLs), and triglycerides, while increasing healthy high-density lipoproteins (HDLs).[4] Orthomolecular physicians recognize, however, that niacin use that is not properly monitored can lead to unpleasant side effects, such as flushing and palpitations and, in excessive dosages, can be toxic for patients suffering from diabetes, gout, hepatitis, and peptic ulcer.

Other orthomolecular discoveries include:

- Studies have shown that higher levels of beta carotene (a precursor of vitamin A) are associated with lower rates of certain cancers.[5]

- Folic acid (a B vitamin) has been used by a number of mainstream physicians to prevent neural tube defects, a condition that causes improper brain and spinal cord development in fetuses.[6] It is now a recommended preventive measure given to pregnant women. Folic acid is also used in the treatment of cervical dysplasia, a pre-cancerous condition of the uterus, and for this reason is also given to women who take birth control pills or who are pregnant.[7]

- Intravenous magnesium sulphate (a mineral compound) is given in some hospitals to heart attack victims to speed recovery time.[8] Injections of vitamin C, magnesium sulphate, vitamin B6, and zinc sulphate are also used by some orthomolecular physicians to help prevent high blood pressure during surgery and post-surgical complications.

- Chromium (a trace mineral) is given to help regulate the body's response to sugar and insulin. It may help those with diabetes[10] and hypoglycemia.[11] It can also aid in lowering cholesterol.

- Essential fatty acids (unsaturated fats that the body cannot make for itself and must obtain from food sources), including omega-3s and omega-6s, are now linked to a decrease in risk factors for heart disease[12] and a lessening of symptoms of other afflictions, including psoriasis[13] and rheumatoid arthritis.[14]

In many of these examples, the doses of nutrients are far greater than the RDAs, but there is general agreement among orthomolecular physicians concerning dosage and usage.

Numerous case histories illustrate the effectiveness of orthomolecular medicine—in many cases, even after other approaches to healing had failed. A dramatic example concerns a patient of Alan R. Gaby, M.D., of Seattle, Washington, former President of the American Holistic Medical Association. The patient, a 36-year-old woman, had a six-year history of muscle pain and spasm, which began after an auto accident. The condition had caused severe and incapacitating symptoms, which had resulted in 11 hospitalizations for persistent pain. She had spent an estimated $100,000 on various treatments over the six years. Numerous prescription medications had been tried with only mild to moderate relief. At the time of her initial visit, she was taking five medications for muscle pain, spasm, and fatigue. Physical examination revealed severe tenderness to light touch at numerous areas of her body.

Dr. Gaby began her treatment with intravenous nutrients consisting of magnesium chloride hexahydrate, calcium glycerophosphate, ascorbic acid (vitamin C), and B vitamins (B6, B5, B1, B12, and B complex). There was no change after the first two injections. After the third injection, however, she reported a 90% improvement in fatigue and muscle complaints. After three days, she discontinued all five of her conventional medications. During the ensuing two months, she received one injection approximately every two weeks. She has reported continued improvement, but the effects of the vitamins begin to wear off after two weeks if she does not maintain her injection schedule.

Jonathan Wright, M.D., of Kent, Washington, reports success in cases of childhood asthma treated with orthomolecular medicine. One of his patients was a 4-year-old boy described by his parents as "being allergic since birth." The boy suffered from chronic nasal congestion and was admitted to emergency rooms numerous times for acute wheezing. When the boy was first brought to Dr. Wright, he was on long-term antihistamine medication.

TREATING ISCHEMIA WITH ORTHOMOLECULAR MEDICINE

"It is no surprise that ischemia, or low blood flow, can cause disease," says Richard A. Kunin, M.D. "Heart attack is the number one killer disease in the U.S. after all, and stroke is not far behind. But the research and media hype have for so long focused on cholesterol and arterial plaque that there has been little attention to the physiology of blood flow itself. We now know, though, that the condition of the blood platelets, the endothelial cells lining the blood vessels, and the blood itself are the major factors in regulating blood flow in microcirculation. And these factors are regulated by nutrients. That is big news, for it transforms our concept of orthomolecular medicine from a focus on chemistry of metabolism to physiology, especially relative to the effects of ischemia."

According to Dr. Kunin, the effects of ischemia are apparent within seconds: cells initially become over-irritable, then reduce activity as free radicals and lactic acid accumulate, ultimately leading to apoptosis (programmed cell death). Apoptosis is a silent or hidden process, because the cell membranes are dissolved by enzymes, says Dr. Kunin. This process is unlike other forms of cell death—caused by trauma, poison, or suffocation—which release undigested debris that, in turn, must be processed by white blood cells and results in pain and inflammation.

Although apoptosis often occurs undetected, the aging symptoms associated with it can be readily apparent. Such symptoms can occur anywhere in the body, especially the skin, muscles, endocrine glands, heart, brain, and pancreas—all organs that weaken and shrink with age and are

susceptible to low blood flow and apoptosis. Aging symptoms linked to the location of apoptosis include:

Brain—stroke, schizophrenia, depression, impaired neurodevelopment

Heart—angina, myocardial infarction, congestive heart failure, arrhythmia

Pancreas—belching, flatulence, malabsorption, abdominal pain

Intestinal tract—duodenitis, irritable bowel syndrome, Crohn's disease, ulcerative colitis

Lungs—asthma, pulmonary fibrosis

Bones—osteonecrosis (hips, knees, jaw)

Muscle—cramps, claudication

Skin—wrinkling, atrophy

Dr. Kunin points out that apoptosis is not confined to aging, but plays a significant role in all diseases. "Orthomolecular medicine can prevent or minimize the damage caused by apoptosis by preserving and enhancing blood flow and by protecting against free radicals that trigger clotting and cause cell damage," he says. What follows is a list of anticoagulant nutrients used by orthomolecular physicians in this regard, along with their mechanism of action and typical dosage range.

CAUTION These nutrients should not be used in this dosage range without proper supervision from a physician competent in the practice of orthomolecular medicine.

NUTRIENT	ACTION	DOSE/DAY
Vitamin C	Antioxidant, lowers Lp(a)	1-4 g
Vitamin A	Anti-prothrombin	5,000-100,000 IU
Niacin (B₃)	Lowers Lp(a), raises HDLs	1,500-3,000 mg
Vitamin B₃ & Statin	Lowers LDL3	1,500-3,000 mg
Pyridoxine (B₆)	Lowers homocysteine	50-100 mg
Vitamin B₁₂	Lowers homocysteine	0.5-1.0 mg
Folic acid	Lowers homocysteine	1-5 mg
Vitamin E	Antioxidant, raises PGI-2	0.5-2 g
Omega-3s	Lowers triglycerides-LDL	2 g EPA
Omega-6s	Lowers triglycerides	0.24-0.48 g
Arginine	Increases nitric oxide	1-3 g
Lysine	Lowers homocysteine	1-3 g

Dr. Wright's examination revealed that the boy had "allergic shiners" under his eyes and showed a maldigestion/malabsorption pattern. Dr. Wright taught the parents how to inject the boy intramuscularly with vitamin B_{12} shots. His parents reported that their son stopped wheezing within the first week of treatment and has slowly been able to reduce medications without ill effects. With additional supplementation of glutamic acid hydrochloride capsules as a digestive aid, a low-dose multimineral complex, and magnesium (50 mg twice daily), combined with B_{12} shots given once every two weeks, he has experienced no further wheezing episodes. When Dr. Wright saw him two years later, the boy was still healthy and his digestive and absorption abilities had also improved significantly. Dr. Wright has also successfully treated numerous other conditions using orthomolecular medicine, including acne, chronic anemia, angina, high blood pressure, cholesterol imbalance, cystic mastitis, headaches, herpes simplex, infertility, and prostate enlargement.[15]

Orthomolecular physicians integrate nutrition and detoxification therapies in a scientific way. They support patients' psychological and hormonal needs, enabling them to better cope with stress in their lives. This is an updated model for the practice of medicine, one that goes far beyond drug therapy and beyond nutrition alone.

—RICHARD A. KUNIN, M.D.

Orthomolecular medicine has also proven beneficial as a treatment for autism. Bernard Rimland, M.D., Founder of the Autism Research Institute, in San Diego, California, was the first to champion a biological cause for this condition in his book *Infantile Autism,* published in 1963. In association with Enoch Calaway, Ph.D., of the University of California, at San Francisco, Dr. Rimland proved the efficacy of orthomolecular factors, specifically vitamin B_6 and magnesium, for treating autistic children. More recently, he has stimulated research that has promoted the benefits of secretin, a little-known neurotransmitter, as an autism treatment.

Dr. Kunin has also researched the biological factors involved in autism, especially the possible link between homocysteine (a sulfur-containing metabolite) and impairment of blood flow. His efforts have led to a new awareness of how vulnerable infants are to low blood flow (ischemia) and the resultant selective damage it can cause. "Infants are small and have smaller arteries," he explains, "but blood clots caused by homocysteine are adult-sized. During the first weeks of life, babies are protected against such clots by delayed production of vitamin K, a principal nutrient involved in coagulation. Research now confirms that there is a strong pro-coagulant trend among children with autism, as well as others in their families." Based on such findings, orthomolecular medicine, due to its judicious use of nutrients to restore proper blood flow, is likely to increasingly become a primary treatment for autism and other conditions caused by impaired circulation.

Commenting on such results, Dr. Kunin adds, "It is obvious that physiology is at the core of health and disease. Orthomolecular physicians integrate nutrition and detoxification therapies in a scientific way. They also support their patients' psychological and hormonal needs, enabling them to better adapt to and cope with the stress in their lives. This is an updated model for the practice of medicine, one that goes far beyond drug therapy and also beyond nutrition alone."

Mood and behavior are other factors that can be improved by orthomolecular medicine. According to Phyllis J. Bronson, Ph.D., a nutritional-biochemical consultant in Aspen, Colorado, amino acid levels in the brain play a significant role. "Chemical impulses in the brain are relayed via nerve transmitters—some of which affect emotions, others affect muscle function," Dr. Bronson states. "Almost all of these neurotransmitters are composed of amino acids. By using supplements of the amino acids that make up specific neurotransmitters, you can actually change the nature and intensity of the brain messages they carry."

Dr. Bronson focuses the large part of her practice on treating people for depression and anxiety disorders. "The traditional treatment for most types of anxiety disorders is the use of Xanex and Valium, which seem to work by stimulating the production of GABA (gammaaminobutyric acid) in the brain," she says. Such drugs have a myriad of side effects, Dr. Bronson points out, and they can also have toxic effects on kidney and liver function. Dr. Bronson prefers to use GABA itself. "GABA is the brain's natural opiate and is related to the endorphins, which are the brain's natural painkillers. It can quiet anxiety, reduce muscle tension, and induce sleep." Dr. Bronson notes that for many people suffering from depression or anxiety disorders, there is a long history of deficient

GABA reserves. "Once they begin taking GABA supplements, their improvement can be quite dramatic," she says. But she cautions against using GABA without the supervision of a competent physician or nutritionist. An individually prescribed supplementation program takes into account the Krebs cycle, which is the final step in the metabolism of fats, carbohydrates, and proteins. Therefore, says Dr. Bronson, to attempt supplementation on one's own is not advisable.

The Future of Orthomolecular Medicine

Unfortunately, there is still some prejudice against nutritional therapy and most medical schools have limited programs in nutrition education. As a result, most graduating doctors have little knowledge of the power of nutrition against disease. Also, since conventional medicine has a history of rejecting nutritional intervention, most doctors are not trained to think along these lines and consequently do not use nutrition in their practices.

Dr. Hoffer foresees a change. "It takes approximately 40 years for innovative thought to be incorporated into mainstream thought," he says. "I expect and hope that orthomolecular medicine, within the next 5-10 years, will cease to be a specialty in medicine and that all physicians will be using nutrition as an essential tool in treating disease."

Richard P. Huemer, M.D., of Vancouver, Washington, a former colleague of Dr. Linus Pauling, and himself a pioneer in the field of orthomolecular medicine, agrees. "We need a paradigm shift and I think it's beginning to occur," he says. "Nutrition needs to be looked at, not as a means of preventing specific deficiency diseases, but as a means of contributing to the overall health of the person and his or her resistance to chronic diseases. We have to start looking for the levels of nutrients necessary for optimum health instead of the minimum amount needed to prevent diseases. This is going to produce a big upsurge in human health in the next 20 years."

Where to Find Help

For more information about nutritional therapy, or to locate an orthomolecular physician, contact:

Society for Orthomolecular Health Medicine
2698 Pacific Avenue
San Francisco, California 94115
(415) 922-6462
Website: www.orthomed.org

This resource serves as a clearinghouse of information and as a referral service for physicians practicing orthomolecular medicine.

Recommended Reading

Dr. Wright's Guide to Healing with Nutrition. Jonathan Wright, M.D. New Canaan, CT: Keats Publishing, 1990.

Nutrition and Mental Illness. Carl C. Pfeiffer. Rochester, NY: Inner Traditions, 1988.

Nutritional Influences on Illness. Melvyn Werbach, M.D. Tarzana, CA: Third Line Press, 1992.

Orthomolecular Nutrition. Abram Hoffer, M.D., and Morton Walker. New Canaan, CT: Keats Publishing, 1978.

Orthomolecular Treatment for Schizophrenia. Abram Hoffer, M.D. New York: McGraw Hill/NTC, 1999.

Putting It All Together: The New Orthomolecular Nutrition. Abram Hoffer, M.D. New Canaan, CT: Keats Publishing, 1996.

The Real Vitamin and Mineral Book. Shari Lieberman and Nancy P. Bruning. Garden City Park, NY: Avery Publishing Group, 1998.

The Roots of Molecular Medicine: A Tribute to Linus Pauling. Richard P. Huemer, M.D., ed. New York: W.H. Freeman, 1986.

OSTEOPATHIC MEDICINE

Osteopathic medicine is a form of physical medicine that helps restore the structural balance of the musculoskeletal system. Combining joint manipulation, physical therapy, and postural reeducation, it is effective in treating spinal and joint difficulties, arthritis, digestive disorders, menstrual problems, and chronic pain.

OSTEOPATHIC MEDICINE, also known as osteopathy, considers and treats the patient as a whole rather than narrowly focusing on a specific ailment. Developed by Andrew Taylor Still (1828-1917) in 1874 as an alternative to the medical practices of his time, osteopathic medicine is the oldest complete system of health care to originate in the United States.

According to Leon Chaitow, N.D., D.O., of London, England, diagnosis of structural problems within the musculoskeletal system and corresponding manipulative treatment are the most fundamental aspects of osteopathic medicine. Doctors of osteopathic medicine (D.O.s, also known as osteopaths) believe that the structure of the body is intimately related to its function and that both structure and function are subject to a wide range of disorders. In treating patients, osteopaths utilize various forms of physical manipulation, which allow the body's innate self-healing mechanisms to operate more efficiently.

Although osteopathic medicine is very effective in treating pain and chronic illness, it typically looks for the deeper causes underlying serious health conditions. One example is heart disease. Osteopathic medicine views this disease as having a musculoskeletal component and, with the appropriate manipulation, substantial benefits can result.

How Osteopathic Medicine Works

"At its simplest, we can say that, when the mechanical structure of the body is normalized or improved, it will

> *The musculoskeletal system is the body's largest energy user. Tension or restriction in this system wastes energy and can cause any number of health problems.*

improve in function," says Dr. Chaitow. To illustrate, Dr. Chaitow points out the implications of one structural problem, a restriction of movement in the upper spinal or rib area that also involves the muscles of that region. The causes of this problem are numerous and can include occupational or sports-related injuries (including overuse through repetitive activities), emotional tension, and internal diseases. "A person with these restrictions may have a breathing problem, such as asthma, bronchitis, and emphysema, or problems relating to a heart condition. Osteopathic treatment can bring more suppleness and mobility to this area, which will ultimately benefit breathing function and help prevent future problems."

Any mechanical restriction in the physical body can influence entire systems and organs. Restriction of any area of the spine can directly affect the organs and systems related to that area. "This is why osteopathic care has been able to, if not cure, allow the patient mobility enough to move in the direction of a cure," says Dr. Chaitow, "especially concerning digestive ailments (including liver and pancreatic dysfunction), bowel disorders, bladder and menstrual problems, prostate congestion, and a multitude of joint and muscle-related problems."

Effects of Musculoskeletal Restriction

The musculoskeletal system is the body's largest energy user. Tension or restriction in this system wastes energy and can cause any number of health problems. "With chronic fatigue syndrome, for instance," says Dr. Chaitow, "it has been found that the person affected has a tendency toward hyperventilation (overbreathing), which is always associated with shortened muscles in the upper chest/neck area and with some restriction of mobility of ribs and the spinal joints." Osteopathic attention to the ribs and spine combined with physical therapy to retrain the area is probably the most effective method for normalizing a problem like hyperventilation, with all of its consequences (phobias, panic attacks, anxiety, fatigue). "This has clearly been demonstrated in the cardiovascular unit of London's Charing Cross Hospital, where hundreds of people have been dramatically helped in this way," concludes Dr. Chaitow

"Chronic muscular tensions in the upper spine are a prime cause of hypoglycemia or low blood sugar," observes psychiatrist Michael Lesser, M.D., "since these tissues are burning fuel at an amazing rate, creating a constant requirement for glucose, which the person may try to meet through sugar-rich snacks and stimulants."[1]

Conditions Benefited by Osteopathic Medicine

Research has confirmed what has already been observed through practical application—that there are few health concerns that cannot benefit from osteopathic care. "Osteopathic medicine can help or resolve many problems that previously have failed to respond to medicine and surgery," states William Faber, D.O., of the Milwaukee Pain Clinic, in Wisconsin.

Osteopathic medicine can help or resolve many problems that previously have failed to respond to medicine and surgery.

—WILLIAM FABER, D.O.

More specifically, osteopathic medicine has provided aid for patients with spinal and joint conditions, arthritis, allergies, heart disease, breathing dysfunction, chronic fatigue syndrome, hiatal hernia, high blood pressure, headaches, sciatica, and various other neuritic (inflammation of the nerves) disorders.[2] Among all alternative therapies, osteopathic medicine, along with chiropractic, has been scientifically verified to be most effective for treating acute low-back pain without complications.[3]

Research into the effects of osteopathic medicine on children has produced marked benefits in terms of quicker recovery rates and fewer negative effects from measles[4] and respiratory infections.[5] For these conditions,

manipulation is used to improve blood circulation, boost immune function, and maintain nerve supply to affected organs and tissues at optimum levels. According to Dr. Chaitow, without a good supply of blood, nutrients cannot be used normally and the defenses of the body are retarded.

Other conditions for which osteopathic medicine has been found to have benefit include neck pain, carpal tunnel syndrome, fibromyalgia, immune deficiency, otitis media (chronic middle ear infection), hamstring injuries, Parkinson's disease, shoulder pain, and impaired neurological development.[6]

The effectiveness of osteopathic treatment depends on a number of factors:

- The level of organic disease
- The level of musculoskeletal involvement
- The patient's nutritional status
- The effectiveness of the body's healing mechanisms

Dr. Faber reports the story of how his plumber suffered from locking in his left knee due to a cartilage tear. An MRI (magnetic resonance imaging) scan confirmed the tear and Dr. Faber referred the man to an orthopedic specialist who treated the condition with physical therapy and a cortisone injection. Two months of treatment failed to correct the problem and the plumber returned to Dr. Faber for help. "I did a myofascial release (a manipulative treatment) of the muscles and connective tissue around the knee," Dr. Faber says. "The results were immediate, with the locking and pain relieved. After a second treatment, the problem was completely resolved."

Just before the 1980 Moscow Olympics, Sebastian Coe, the world record holder for the 1,500 meters, consulted Terry Moule, D.O., a British osteopath, for a recurrent low-back and hip problem that posed a threat to his career. "He had been through the entire medical process without success, including conventional orthopedic treatment," relates Dr. Chaitow. "Within weeks of commencing osteopathic care from Dr. Moule, Coe was pain free and running faster than ever. He went on a few weeks later to win two gold medals in Moscow." The treatment primarily utilized the "neuromuscular technique," an osteopathic soft-tissue treatment now widely taught in the United States.

It is not uncommon for patients with internal organ disease to cite musculoskeletal pain as their primary complaint. For example, an osteopathic physician who treats a patient for pain in the right shoulder would, because of the relationship between the internal organs and the musculoskeletal system, look for reflex pain patterns in the upper thoracic (pertaining to the chest or thorax), lower cervical, and rib regions. In doing so, the physician may find a pain pattern relative to gallbladder disease that would lead to palpating the abdomen and discovering a tender and swollen gallbladder. The osteopathic physician would then treat both the musculoskeletal component of the pain and the gallbladder disease.

What to Expect During an Osteopathic Examination

Osteopathic treatment addresses the cause of mechanical problems within the body. Diagnostic methods include screening and evaluation of:

- Posture and gait—how a person holds their body while standing and sitting, and during activities such as walking.

- Motion—testing evaluates all moving parts for restrictions. For example, a patient may be asked to complete various body movements such as bending, side-bending, extension, or rotation for both specific and general areas of the body.

- Symmetry—to notice one-sided use of any part of the body and subsequent stress. Physicians also look for increased or decreased curve to the normal spinal pattern.

- The soft tissues—using inspection and palpation to look for skin changes, hardening of muscles, temperature changes, tenderness, reflex activity, and excessive fluid retention.

In conjunction with evaluation, X rays, blood tests, and MRI scans are used if there is a suspicion of deeper pathology.[7]

Types of Therapy Used

Different manipulative approaches are available to the osteopathic physician, including:

Gentle mobilization: Moving a joint slowly through its range of motion, gradually increasing the motion to free the joint from restrictions.

Articulation: When motion is severely limited, a quick thrust (similar to chiropractic) may be used.

Functional and positional release methods: Placing the patient in a specific position to allow the body to relax and release muscular spasms that may have been caused by strain or injury.

Muscle energy technique: Gently tensing and releasing specific muscles to produce relaxation.

Myofascial release: This technique is a form of bodywork that releases tension in the fascia (the elastic semifluid membrane that envelops every muscle, bone, blood vessel, nerve, and organ), thereby improving muscle function and restoring balance to the musculoskeletal system.

Other soft tissue techniques: Techniques to relax and release restrictions in the soft tissues of the body.

Cranial manipulation: Very gentle and subtle cranial techniques used to treat conditions such as headaches, stroke, spinal cord injury, and temporomandibular joint (TMJ) syndrome. Cranial osteopathy can be of particular benefit for young children who suffer from hyperactivity, mood disorders, dizziness, or dyslexia. Cranial osteopathy can also be used to provide optimal function and wellness when no illness is present.

 See Bodywork, Chiropractic, Craniosacral Therapy.

Patient Reeducation: Keeping Your Body Healthy

Reeducation is the important final step of osteopathic treatment. Patients who learn how to keep their bodies functioning in a relaxed and healthy state have less anxiety and tension and are better able to cope with stress.

Relaxation techniques may be used to reduce the levels of excessive tension often present in the muscles of people with joint and back problems. These methods, combined with specifically designed exercises and stretches, help the patient to restore functional integrity and balance, coordinate muscular activity, and reduce stress on the joints, making any manipulative treatment easier and more effective.

Improved breathing methods may be taught when necessary, in order to reduce the excessive stress endured by certain muscles in the back and neck when breathing patterns are dysfunctional. This helps restore normal diaphragmatic breathing, allowing for improved lung capacity, while lessening the wear and tear on joints that

ORIGINS OF OSTEOPATHIC MEDICINE

Osteopathic medicine originated in the United States in the last quarter of the 19th century as a result of the work of Andrew Taylor Still, a physician who founded the first school of osteopathic medicine in Kirksville, Missouri, in 1892. Dr. Still continually sought better methods of medical treatment for his patients, especially for those faced with the epidemic diseases of the time and the terrible side effects of the drugs used for their problems.[8]

By the time of Still's death, there were over 5,000 licensed osteopaths in the U.S., and the first school had been established in the United Kingdom. Today, there are 19 osteopathic medical colleges in the U.S., many associated with major universities.

Osteopathic training blends conventional medical, surgical, and obstetrical practices with osteopathic manipulative treatments, providing a comprehensive system of health care. American D.O.s (doctors of osteopathic medicine, of which there are over 44,000) carry the same license and scope of practice as M.D.s. However, some osteopaths focus on the conventional medical approach while others give priority to the manipulative therapies.

There are also many thousands of registered osteopaths in Europe, with schools in France and Belgium. Practitioners trained in the United Kingdom and other English-speaking countries, such as Australia, New Zealand, and Canada, where osteopathic medicine focuses on manipulative treatment, are considered an integral part of alternative and complementary health care.

---

be used as well as the known links between specific nutrients and the tissues of the system.

Health concerns, from heart and breathing dysfunction to fatigue and hyperventilation, can be helped by therapeutic correction of the underlying mechanical disorder. A complete osteopathic treatment to normalize the musculoskeletal system will keep the body working smoothly and efficiently, which is synonymous with health.

The Future of Osteopathic Medicine

Osteopathic medicine is a uniquely American system that has spread worldwide, helping to pioneer the creation of a bridge between conventional and alternative health care. On July 1, 1993, Britain's Queen Elizabeth signed into law the Osteopath's Bill, making osteopathic medicine the first alternative health-care system to achieve legal statutory recognition in Europe, clearing the way for others to follow.

A truly holistic system, osteopathic medicine takes into account all of a patient's needs, with a particular emphasis on a person's structural and functional integrity. In the U.S., however, many D.O.s focus on conventional medicine in place of manipulative therapies, so it is important for patients seeking holistic, alternative care to ask if such therapies are offered before beginning osteopathic care. "If you consider that the musculoskeletal system makes up the largest body system, using far and away the greatest amount of energy," says Dr. Chaitow, "and if you reflect on the fact that it is through the musculoskeletal system that you live your life, you will begin to appreciate osteopathic medicine's importance."

 When seeking an osteopathic physician, ask whether he or she practices manipulative therapies, since many D.O.s focus on conventional medicine.

---

were previously restricted by the excessive contraction of muscles inappropriately overworking.

Postural correction teaches patients how to use their bodies in less stressful, more efficient and economical ways (in terms of energy output), reducing damage and tension affecting the joints and soft tissues, as well as decreasing levels of fatigue. These methods draw on systems such as Feldenkrais Method, the Trager Approach, and Alexander Technique, along with osteopathic innovations, and are particularly useful in relation to patterns of overuse and misuse found commonly in activities related to work and sports.

Individualized nutritional guidance, taking into account the particular requirements of the patient, may

Where to Find Help

For further information on the use of osteopathic techniques in the treatment of health problems, or to locate a doctor of osteopathic medicine, contact:

American Academy of Osteopathy
3500 DePauw Blvd., Suite 1080
Indianapolis, Indiana 46268
(317) 879-1881
Website: www.academyofosteopathy.org

The American Academy of Osteopathy (a practice affiliate of the American Osteopathic Association) represents D.O.s who provide skilled osteopathic manipulative treatments as part of their practices. The Academy publishes a variety of books on osteopathic medicine; contact the Academy for a current catalog of titles.

American Osteopathic Association
142 East Ontario Street
Chicago, Illinois 60611
(312) 202-8200 or (800) 621-1773

All D.O.s are trained in the use of osteopathic manipulative treatments. Some specialize in osteopathic manipulative treatments while others focus less on manipulation and more on other medical specialties. There are many skilled osteopaths in the United States. The American Osteopathic Association is the national organization that represents all D.O.s.

Recommended Reading

Andrew Taylor Still, 1828-1917. Carol Trowbridge. Kirksville, MO: Thomas Jefferson University Press, 1991.

Dr. Fulford's Touch of Life. Robert C. Fulford with Gene Stone. New York: Pocket Books, 1996.

Osteopathic Medicine: An American Reformation. George Northup, D.O. Chicago: American Osteopathic Association, 1987.

Osteopathic Self-Treatment. Leon Chaitow, D.O. San Francisco: Thorsons, 1990.

OXYGEN THERAPIES

Oxygen therapies alter the body's chemistry to help overcome disease, promote repair, and improve overall function. These therapies are effective in treating a wide variety of conditions, including infections (viral, fungal, parasitic, bacterial), circulatory problems, chronic fatigue syndrome, arthritis, allergies, cancer, and multiple sclerosis.

OXYGEN THERAPIES have been utilized in Europe for many years for a wide range of conditions, but in the United States they remain controversial and are currently not approved by the U.S. Food and Drug Administration (FDA). The legality of oxygen therapies varies from state to state.

How Oxygen Therapies Work

Oxygen therapies are classified according to the type of chemical process involved: the addition of oxygen to the blood or tissues is called oxygenation, while the reaction of splitting off electrons (electrically charged particles) from any chemical molecule is known as oxidation. Oxidation may or may not involve oxygen (oxidation refers to the chemical reaction and not to oxygen itself).

Oxygenation Therapies

Oxygenation saturates the body with oxygen through the use of gas, sometimes at high pressure (hyperbaric), increasing the total amount of available oxygen in the body. Insufficient oxygenation may promote the growth of pathogens, whereas excessive oxygenation may damage normal tissues. However, oxygenation employed under strictly controlled conditions can have positive therapeutic effects.

Otto Warburg, Director of the Max Planck Institute for Cell Physiology, in Germany, and a two-time Nobel laureate, proposed that a lack of oxygen at the cellular level may be the prime cause of cancer and that oxygen

All cells, tissues, and organs need oxygen to function. Oxygen therapies utilize oxygen in various forms to promote healing and destroy disease-producing microorganisms and toxins in the body.

therapy could be an effective treatment for it.[1] He showed that normal cells in tissue culture, when deprived of oxygen, become cancer cells and that oxygen can kill cancer cells in tissue cultures.

Oxygen therapy may be professionally administered in many ways: orally, rectally, vaginally, intravenously (into a vein), intra-arterially (into an artery), through inhalation, or by absorption or injection through the skin (subcutaneously). High concentrations of oxygen gas can be given orally through masks, tubes, or via oxygen tents. Ionized oxygen, both positively and negatively charged, can also be administered by inhalation or dissolved in drinking or bath water. Another form of oxygenation used to treat medical conditions is hyperbaric oxygen therapy (HBOT), which introduces oxygen into the body in a pressurized hyperbaric (pressure greater than atmospheric) chamber.

Oxidation Therapy

Oxidation refers to a chemical reaction whereby electrons are transferred from one molecule to another. Oxygen molecules are frequently, but not always, involved in these reactions. The molecules that "donate" electrons are said to be oxidized, whereas the molecules that accept electrons are called oxidants. Hydrogen peroxide therapy uses the process of oxidation.

A healthy state of oxidative balance is necessary for optimal function of the body, but when the body is exposed to repeated environmental stresses, its oxidative function is weakened. When oxidation is partially blocked by toxicity in the body or pathological organisms, oxi-

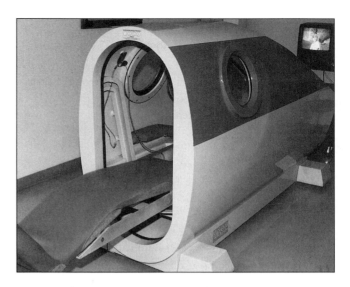

EARLY HISTORY OF OXYGEN THERAPIES

The scientific community has been aware of oxygen and its characteristics for over 200 years. Oxygen was discovered by Englishman Joseph Priestly in 1771. Hydrogen peroxide was discovered by French chemist Louis Jacques Thenard in 1818, and ozone was discovered by Christian Friedrich Schonbein in 1840. The first hyperbaric operating room was created as early as 1879 by a French physician, Dr. J.A. Fontaine.

Doctors and scientists began treating diseases and conditions with oxygen over 100 years ago. Skin conditions were first treated with ultraviolet light (which activates oxidation when absorbed by the blood) in the late 19th century by Niels Finsen, and the use of peroxide appears in the health literature as early as 1884. A.L. Cortelyou, of Marietta, Georgia, successfully treated diphtheria with a peroxide nasal spray in 1898. In the 1919 flu epidemic, Drs. T.H. Oliver and D.U. Murphy administered intravenous hydrogen peroxide, which significantly reduced mortality rates.

Ozone application was used successfully in World War I to combat battlefield infections and, as early as 1924, Frederick Koch, M.D., advocated oral hydrogen peroxide for cancer patients in the United States.

dation therapy may help by "jump-starting" the body's oxidative processes and returning them to normal, according to the late Charles Farr, M.D., Ph.D., Founder of the International Bio-Oxidative Medicine Foundation, in Oklahoma City, Oklahoma.[2]

When properly administered, oxidation therapy selectively destroys disease-producing bacteria, viruses, and other invading microbial organisms and deactivates toxic substances without injury to healthy tissues.[3] For example, if diluted hydrogen peroxide is placed on a wound, the normal cells thrive while the pathogens die. Oxidation therapy must be administered under clinical supervision, since uncontrolled oxidation may be destructive to the body.

Types of Oxygen Therapy

The major types of oxygen therapy used to treat disease are hyperbaric oxygen therapy, ozone therapy, and hydrogen peroxide therapy.

Hyperbaric Oxygen Therapy

Hyperbaric oxygen therapy (HBOT) dates back to the beginning of the 20th century, although its modern use in the U.S. dates only to the formation of the Undersea Medical Society in 1967. HBOT may be administered in individual oxygen chambers that consist of acrylic tubes about seven feet long and 25 inches in diameter. The patient lies on a stretcher, which slides into the tube. The entry is sealed and the tube pressurized at up to two-and-a-half Atmospheres Absolute (over twice the pressure of the Earth's atmosphere at sea level) with pure oxygen for 30-120 minutes. The increased pressure makes it possible to breathe oxygen at a concentration higher than that allowed by any other means. After treatment, the chamber is depressurized slowly with the patient resting inside. Most of the hyperbaric facilities in the U.S. are either part of, or affiliated with, hospitals or the military.

Multiplace chambers, which accommodate many patients at once, and in which oxygen is delivered by mask, are now used at the University of Maryland, Duke University, the University of Texas, Scripps Institute, and the Hyperbaric Oxygen Institute, in San Bernardino, California. These chambers allow nurses and technical personnel to attend to patients during the treatment. An added advantage of multiplace chambers is that a patient can be removed immediately if problems arise, whereas in individual chambers, the patient cannot be removed until the entire chamber is depressurized.

CONDITIONS BENEFITED BY HYPERBARIC OXYGEN THERAPY

The use of oxygen under pressure to treat serious health conditions, including stroke, is medically well-established, but HBOT is not yet widely used in the U.S. compared to other countries. Today in the U.S., HBOT is primarily used for traumas such as crash injuries, burns, wounds, gangrene (death of tissue, usually due to deficient or absent blood supply), carbon monoxide poisoning, decubitus ulcers (bed sores), stasis (the stagnation of the normal flow of fluids), radiation necrosis (death of an area of tissue or bone), and recalcitrant skin grafting. Some microsurgical procedures for the repair and restoration of severed limbs are made possible only by the use of HBOT during the surgery.

According to the late David Hughes, D.Sc., of the Hyperbaric Oxygen Institute, post-surgical HBOT improves early healing in about 60% of cases and guarantees there will be no surgical edema (retention of excessive amounts of fluid by body tissues). "In West Germany, HBOT has been used extensively to treat stroke victims, and government sponsorship of HBOT has reduced aftercare costs for stroke victims by 71%," Dr. Hughes reported. "In France, it is employed for peripheral vascular and arterial problems, and in Russia it is used in drug and alcohol detoxification. In Japan, the medical establishment boasts that no citizen is ever more than half an hour away from a hyperbaric chamber." In Great Britain, more than 25,000 multiple sclerosis (MS) patients have benefited from HBOT.[4]

HBOT's ability to restore the balance of nitrogen and oxygen in the bloodstream via a hyperbaric oxygen chamber was first discovered by researchers who employed the therapy to successfully treat deep-sea divers with the "bends," a sometimes fatal affliction caused by ascending too quickly to the surface. German researchers, recognizing that the loss of extremity function after a stroke is similar to symptoms of the bends, conjectured that HBOT might also have benefit for victims of stroke or heart attack. Their research proved correct and today HBOT may be the single most effective therapy, conventional or alternative, for reversing the damage caused by a stroke.

"Every emergency room in the United States should have a hyperbaric oxygen chamber and every physician should be trained in its use," says David A. Steenblock, M.S., D.O., of Mission Viejo, California, a leading expert in the therapeutic use of HBOT to reduce the effects of stroke and brain injury. According to Dr. Steenblock, "If you can get more oxygen to the brain within the first 24 hours of having a stroke, you can often stop most of the damage and salvage a great deal of brain tissue, eliminating 70% to 80% of the damage. Treating the patient by getting more oxygen to the brain during the first three weeks after the stroke makes it still possible to minimize the damage." In fact, Dr. Steenblock has produced unexpected positive outcomes using HBOT when treating patients as long as 15 years after their stroke.

Since 1971, over 1,000 cases demonstrating a 40% to 100% rate of improvement for stroke victims receiving oxygen under pressure has been reported in scientific journals. Given these positive outcomes, Dr. Steenblock encourages all physicians to consider the merits of HBOT.

 Research is needed on the effects of hyperbaric oxygen therapy for the treatment of early complications of stroke. This type of therapy could prove revolutionary by preventing permanent damage to stroke patients and could also save on health-care costs.

Pulmonary crises such as carbon monoxide poisoning, low blood volume anemia, and cyanosis (a bluish discoloration of the skin due to abnormal amounts of oxygenated hemoglobin in the blood), have also been treated with HBOT. Much work has also been done with HBOT as an adjunct to radiation therapy for cancer and to minimize the side effects of some chemotherapy protocols. "Noncancerous cells are much less sensitive to radiation when the oxygen concentration in their vicinity is increased," Dr. Hughes explained. "HBOT prior to radiation treatment enhances its effectiveness."

According to Dr. Hughes, HBOT has also demonstrated its value as an adjunct to antibiotics in the treatment of anaerobic (able to live without oxygen) infections. He cited the case of an 18-year-old boy involved in a near drowning incident, who was brought to an HBOT clinic after being in a vegetative coma for nine days. After 70 treatment sessions, the boy was able to return to school. He continued with the treatment and made good progress toward a full recovery.

Another of Dr. Hughes's cases involved a 28-year-old woman suffering from viral encephalitis (inflammation of the brain), which left her unable to speak and with right-side hemiplegia (paralysis of only one side of the body). She couldn't walk and had acute optic neuralgia (severe, sharp pain along the optic nerve). After 30 sessions, she had improved enough to walk and talk normally, the optic neuralgia had resolved, and the only persistent symptom was right arm and hand weakness.

HBOT also aided a 70-year-old woman who had been bedridden from MS. After 18 HBOT sessions with Dr. Hughes, she had recovered enough of her motor skills to drive a car and walk without assistance, and within six months she was able to resume her original duties at work.

According to Richard A. Neubauer, M.D., Director of the Ocean Hyperbaric Center, in Lauderdale-by-the-Sea, Florida, MS may be caused by a lack of oxygen in the body's tissues, as evidenced by the fact that providing MS patients with HBOT has been shown to be successful in reducing symptoms of the disease. In his book

HYPERBARIC OXYGEN AND HIV

HBOT has begun to be used experimentally to treat the symptoms of AIDS and HIV (human immunodeficiency virus) infection and their accompanying fatigue. Since 1990, Michelle Reillo, B.S.N., R.N., has been treating AIDS and HIV patients with HBOT at Lifeforce Hyperbaric Oxygen Institute, in Baltimore, Maryland. Reillo and her colleagues concentrate on providing relief and reversing many of the complications associated with AIDS and HIV infection. As Reillo notes in her book *AIDS Under Pressure*, the earlier AIDS and HIV patients can receive HBOT treatments, the better.

"Hyperbaric medicine has well-documented evidence supporting its use in many AIDS-defining complications and infections, regardless of the underlying disorder," Reillo says. "HBOT would be an ideal intervention in the individual recently infected with HIV because it decreases viremia [viruses in the blood], is not toxic to the individual, and decreases the microvascular and neurovascular damage occurring as the initial infection progresses throughout the body." One of Reillo's patients was a 31-year-old man who suffered from debilitating, AIDS-related fatigue and oral yeast infection (candidiasis). After two months of HBOT treatments, administered 2-3 times weekly, his viral load was cut in half. After another two months of treatment, it had dropped to zero. His fatigue resolved, his yeast infection cleared up, he gained ten pounds, and he was again capable of normal physical activity.

Reillo reports that HBOT is also effective for relieving peripheral vascular insufficiency, which results in reduced blood to the hands and feet, leaving them cold and frequently painful. Over a three-year period, 100 AIDS patients with this problem received considerable benefit after receiving only six HBOT treatments over two weeks. First among the symptoms to improve was fatigue, followed by an increase in the ability to exercise and tolerate physical activity, a warming of the extremities, an increase in energy, and less pain in the legs and feet after activity. Moreover, oxygen levels in the patients' tissues climbed from a low 79% to a vigorously healthy 98%. These high levels are not permanent, however, and require continuing HBOT to maintain, Reillo notes, also pointing out that AIDS patients more typically see their oxygen levels climb to the 80%-90% range following HBOT, compared to initial, dangerously low levels in the area of 50%-60%.

Based on her work with AIDS and HIV patients, Reillo also reports that "anti-tubercular medications have been shown to be more effective when used in conjunction with HBOT." In addition, HBOT can provide relief from the severe dermatitis that often accompanies AIDS.

Hyperbaric Oxygen Therapy, Dr. Neubauer states that MS "is a wound or a disease of the blood vessels in the central nervous system." A condition of chronic high blood pressure within the brain and spinal cord damages blood vessels and leads to a lack of oxygen similar to that seen in cases of stroke.

Clinical evidence supports Dr. Neubauer's theory, revealing that 70% of approximately 12,000 MS patients in 14 countries who were treated with HBOT showed improvement in terms of bladder and bowel function and muscular spasticity.[5] Moreover, very few patients who continued with HBOT had relapses or deteriorated any further. In an early study conducted by Dr. Neubauer, involving 250 MS patients, 39% had a "dramatic" improvement, 52% had "minimal to moderate" benefits, and only 9% had no improvement.[6]

Having treated over 1,500 MS patients since 1980, Dr. Neubauer says that MS is "sensitive to the dose of oxygen," but requires long-term therapy. While cautioning that the initial response may be an unreliable guide to the eventual outcome, and acknowledging that HBOT is not a cure for MS, Dr. Neubauer states that it is "the safest, most noninvasive, least expensive [MS] treatment devised to date."

HBOT can also be used to treat a variety of neurological conditions, including emergency situations such as drowning, smoke inhalation, and accidental electrocution, and chronic conditions of decreased blood flow and oxygen to the brain, traumatic brain injury, and cerebral palsy (CP), according to Dr. Neubauer. "As early as 1964, studies published in *The Lancet* demonstrated the positive effects of hyperbaric oxygenation on oxygen-deprived 'blue babies'," he reports. "Thus, using HBOT to treat brain-injured children is not new and it has been more recently acclaimed for its beneficial use in children with cerebral palsy."

In nearly all cases of CP in children, there are areas of the brain that are low in oxygen. HBOT can benefit children with CP due to its ability to increase blood plasma levels by up to 2,000%. Plasma is the solution that holds the red blood cells containing hemoglobin, which transports oxygen throughout the body. "In a 1998 pilot study," Dr. Neubauer reports, "HBOT improved the function in children with paralysis in the legs (spastic diplegia). However, because of the limits of the study (small sample size, no control group, minimal number of treatments), these results must be interpreted with caution and further research is needed to ascertain the true potential of HBOT and its long-term effects for children with CP."

Such studies are already under way or have recently been completed. In one study, conducted at McGill University in Montreal, Canada, the results were highly positive, showing significant improvement in increased motor skills (sitting, walking, and manual dexterity) and decreased spasticity. The results were so encouraging that the Canadian government has authorized a grant of nearly $2 million for further studies. A double-blind study on the use of HBOT and brain injury recently completed at the University of Texas in Galveston showed equally positive results. Furthermore, in Great Britain, 300 children with CP have undergone treatment with HBOT, with results comparable to those of the study at McGill, and evidence of HBOT's usefulness in this regard is now being reported in other countries, including Mexico and Brazil, according to Dr. Neubauer.[7]

Since 1976, HBOT has also been documented to treat radionecrosis, a form of extensive skin damage that can be caused by radiation therapy for cancer, according to Trish Planck, Director of the Hyperbaric Oxygen Clinic, in Reno, Nevada. In one study involving 206 patients afflicted with radionecrosis (after undergoing radiation therapy to treat cancer of the head or neck), 72% had an "excellent" result, 10% a "good" result, 15% a "fair" response, and in only 3% was the therapy ineffective after receiving HBOT to restore dying skin tissue.[8]

Hyperbaric oxygen therapy may cause problems for those with a history of middle ear infections, emphysema, or spontaneous pneumothorax due to the pressure it requires, according to Dr. Hughes. The appropriateness of HBOT for illnesses, including AIDS, heart disease, and detoxification from recreational drug addiction and alcoholism, is still being debated. Yet HBOT is gaining acceptance and is used by both alternative and conventional physicians. Its broad spectrum of applications gives it enormous potential to be used as an adjunct therapy in the future.

> **CAUTION** Hyperbaric oxygen therapy may cause problems for those with a history of middle ear infection, emphysema, or spontaneous pneumothorax due to the pressure it requires.

Ozone Therapy

Ozone, best known for its protective role in the Earth's ecological harmony, has unique biological properties that are currently being investigated for application in various medical fields, according to Gerard Sunnen, M.D., of New York City, author of the first world literature review on the medical uses of ozone.

Approximately 20% of the air we breathe is comprised of two atoms of oxygen (O_2). Ozone (O_3) contains three oxygen atoms and is a less stable form of molecular oxygen. Because of this added molecule, ozone is more reactive than oxygen and readily enters into reactions to oxidize other chemicals. During oxidation in the body, the extra oxygen molecule in ozone breaks away, leaving a normal O_2 molecule. This increases the oxygen content of the blood or tissues. For this reason, ozone therapy is a combination of both oxygenation therapy and oxidation therapy.

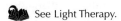 See Light Therapy.

Medical-grade ozone is made from pure oxygen. According to Dr. Sunnen, ozone owes its potent biological action to the large excess of energy contained within its molecule. This accounts for its antiviral, antibacterial, and antifungal actions. "Used externally in topical ozone therapy, ozone/oxygen mixtures readily inactivate a wide spectrum of microorganisms that grow on skin ulcers, such as diabetic leg ulcers, or pressure and decubitus ulcers, poorly healing surgical wounds, and burns," Dr. Sunnen says. "Ozone also increases local tissue temperature, thus enhancing local metabolic processes."

In autohemotherapy, ¼–½ pint of a patient's blood is removed and treated with an ozone/oxygen mixture, then re-infused. This therapy is being investigated for the treatment of viral conditions caused by lipid-enveloped viruses, such as hepatitis B and C, herpes, and HIV. "There is now ample laboratory evidence that ozone readily disrupts the fragile envelope of these viruses through its oxidative action," Dr. Sunnen reports. "Administered for a course of treatments, ozone exerts a culling effect on viral load, thus allowing the immune system to recuperate and regain its competence."

According to Dr. Sunnen, the antiviral action of ozone in autohemotherapy is based on three factors:

1. A direct viral-killing effect. "It should be appreciated that in conditions such as hepatitis C and HIV, up to 10 billion new viral particles are produced daily, thus besieging the beleaguered immune system," Dr. Sunnen notes.

2. The formation of lipid peroxides, which inhibit viral functioning.

3. The ozone-induced formation of cytokines, proteins that activate the immune system.

Laboratory studies have shown that ozone is capable of inactivating HIV *in vitro*.[9] It has also been shown to inhibit the growth of human lung, breast, and uterine cancer cells in tissue culture.[10] According to Dr. Sunnen, some of these effects may be explained by the fact that cancer cells do not possess certain enzymes (glutathione, catalase) that protect normal cells from oxidation. "Cancer cells, exposed to oxidative stress as a result of ozone therapy, are more prone to become disrupted and to disintegrate," he explains, adding that research is needed to determine which types of cancer growth are most susceptible to ozone challenge.

 Because of its potential benefits as a treatment for certain forms of cancer, additional research dollars should be allocated to determining which types of cancer will best respond to ozone therapy.

Ozone can be administered in a variety of ways: topically, intravenously, intra-arterially, intramuscularly, intra-articularly, and subcutaneously. It may also be taken orally, rectally, or vaginally in the form of ozonated water. The intra-arterial route is used (cautiously) to increase oxygenation to limbs afflicted with pre-gangrenous or gangrenous conditions, Dr. Sunnen reports. "Ozone, in such cases, in addition to oxygenating tissues, acts as a vasodilator, thus promoting the delivery of immune factors to diseased tissues and accelerating the removal of toxins," he explains.

Like other oxygen therapies, ozone therapy is widely used and practiced in Europe, but still not readily available in the U.S.

CONDITIONS BENEFITED BY OZONE THERAPY

Test doses of ozone have been found to block the division of cancer cells but not normal cells and this positive effect increased as the ozone doses did, until all cancer-cell activity was virtually halted at high doses.[11] In addition, ozone therapy has been shown to enhance the tumor-fighting ability of standard cancer drugs.[12] German surgeon Joachim Varro, M.D., has worked with hundreds of cancer patients, most of whom had received chemotherapy and radiation. Dr. Varro found that ozone therapy greatly reduced pain among cancer patients, while increasing their energy levels and appetite. Based on his work, Dr. Varro notes the following:

• Patients who received ozone therapy were free of metastases and recurrences for remarkably long periods of time.

• Their survival time could also be prolonged, far exceeding the prognoses of conventional medicine.

• Most patients who underwent ozone therapy shortly after surgery and radiation were able to return to full-time work.[13]

Jonathan Wright, M.D., of Kent, Washington, successfully treated a cancer patient with ozone therapy. The patient had a goose egg–sized tumor on her right ear. Her doctor said it could not be treated and gave her six months to live. Dr. Wright treated the tumor with topical ozone (applied externally to the site of the tumor) and injected ozone directly into the tumor. The tumor regressed in size and, although a small lump remained, the patient recovered.

Dr. Wright also finds ozone therapy effective against any sort of chronic infection, including viruses and candidiasis. He also treats hepatitis B with ozonation of the blood along with an herbal remedy—*Phyllanthus*—and high doses of intravenous ascorbate (a salt of the ascorbic acid vitamin C). He points out that antioxidants such as vitamin C should be given along with any oxidative therapy, since they prevent uncontrolled oxidation, which is detrimental to the body.

 Due to its wide application for a number of health conditions, oxygen therapy can save money in long-term health costs.

Jeff Harris, N.D., of Seattle, Washington, successfully treated a patient suffering from MS with ozone therapy administered by rectal insufflation. When the patient came to see Dr. Harris, she had been unable to work effectively for seven years due to the deteriorating effects of MS, which included numbness in her right leg as well as incontinence, and had spent the last three months on unemployment. Dr. Harris also used vitamin and mineral supplementation, vegetarian diet, dental amalgam removal, counseling, and craniosacral therapy as part of the treatment protocol. She received vitamin B_{12} and folic acid injections daily for two to three weeks and then ozone therapy was started. After the first ozone treatment, she said she felt full of energy. Dr. Harris taught her how to do the treatments herself, which she does daily, and she has now returned to work and states that she is feeling well and full of energy.

CAUTION Adverse effects associated with intravenous ozone have been reported to include phlebitis (inflammation of a vein), circulatory depression, chest pain, shortness of breath, fainting, coughing, flushing, cardiac arrhythmias, and gas embolus (bubbles). Rectal administration of ozone can lead to inflammation of the lower intestinal tract. Although it is easily tolerated in other tissues, ozone in high concentrations causes inflammation of the lung tissues.

THERAPEUTIC APPLICATIONS OF OZONE

The administration of ozone therapy is as varied as the many conditions it can treat. Below are the most typical methods of treatment:

- Intra-arterial (injected into an artery)—for arterial circulatory disturbances and to dissolve atherosclerotic plaque.

- Intestinal insufflation (blown into the intestines from a gas tank using a catheter)—for irritable bowel syndrome and fistulae (abnormal openings).

- Intramuscular (injected into the muscle)—to treat inflammatory conditions, allergic diseases, and cancer (with autohemotherapy).

- Autohemotherapy (ozonation of blood)—to address arthritis, hepatitis, allergies, and herpes infections.

- Ozonized water (ozonation of water that is taken orally, rectally, or vaginally)—disinfection during surgery and dentistry.

- Intra-articular (injected into a joint)—during surgery and with diseased joints.

- External application (by covering the area with a tent and infusing ozone)—for treating fungal infections, leg ulcers, infected or poorly healing wounds, and burns.

OZONE THERAPY AND AIDS

The late German physician Alexander Preuss, of Stuttgart, used ozone as part of a regimen including vitamins, minerals, and other treatments to enhance the immune system. He achieved remission in a number of patients with AIDS-associated infections.[14] In a similar study, French researchers Bertrand Vallancien and Jean-Marie Winkler reported on a group of patients with HIV, herpes, and hepatitis. After nine weeks of transfused ozone, T4 and T8 cells (cells of the immune system) moved toward normal levels in all cases. The ozone treatments caused no further health problems.[15]

Since the FDA has not approved the practice of ozone therapy in the U.S., it is difficult to get data on its use. Many physicians also have been forced to use ozone therapy without calling attention to themselves, for fear of FDA reprisals. However, numerous patient anecdotes are available. One doctor, for instance, reports of good results with HIV-positive patients. He gave these patients three ozone treatments a week for seven weeks. For each treatment, 250–300 cc of blood was removed, treated with ozone, and injected back into the patient. This helped reduce opportunistic infections. Other treatments were also employed to help strengthen the immune system.[16] Patients who have difficulty tolerating AZT (an AIDS medication) treatments may benefit from ozone therapy.

Hydrogen Peroxide Therapy

Hydrogen peroxide is a liquid comprised of two atoms of hydrogen and two atoms of oxygen (H_2O_2). Because it is less stable than water (H_2O), hydrogen peroxide readily enters into oxidative reactions, ultimately becoming oxygen in water.

Hydrogen peroxide is a natural substance manufactured by normal, healthy human cells to regulate metabolism and attack invading pathogens. It also occurs naturally in rain and snow, in fruits and vegetables, and in mother's milk, with particularly high concentrations found in colostrum.[18] In 1920, *The Lancet* reported the use of intravenous hydrogen peroxide by British Army doctors in India, who used it to treat troops suffering from influenza. Its use reduced their death rate from 90% to 50%. In the 1950s, hydrogen peroxide was approved by the FDA as a food additive and for use by farmers to retard spoilage in animal feed. Following this, some farmers, noting an unexpected health benefit in their livestock, started using hydrogen peroxide themselves as a folk remedy for arthritis and other chronic health problems.

Since that time, a number of physicians have experimented with intravenous hydrogen peroxide as a treatment for a variety of conditions, including poor circulation, heart disease, angina, emphysema, bronchitis, asthma, influenza, Lyme disease, chronic fatigue, candidiasis, parasitic infections, and arthritis.[19] It was Dr. Farr who first characterized, in 1984, the oxidative effects of hydrogen peroxide in humans.[20] Today, the use of hydrogen peroxide for its oxidative effects has spread to 38 countries and remains one of the least expensive, yet effective, oxidation therapies.

Oxidation administered through hydrogen peroxide therapy regulates tissue repair, cellular respiration, growth, immune and energy functions, most hormone systems, and the production of cytokines. Oxidation therapy can also work as a defense system, directly destroying invading bacteria, viruses, yeast, and parasites, according to Dr. Farr.

CONDITIONS BENEFITED BY HYDROGEN PEROXIDE THERAPY

Dr. Farr employed hydrogen peroxide for a variety of health problems, including AIDS, arthritis, cancer, candidiasis, chronic fatigue syndrome, depression, lupus erythematosus (a chronic inflammatory disease with symptoms including arthritis, fatigue, and skin lesions), emphysema, MS, varicose veins, and fractures. According to Dr. Farr, other conditions that may benefit from hydrogen peroxide therapy include arteriosclerosis, vascular headaches (migraines, cluster headaches), gangrene, strokes, allergies, asthma, lung infections, diabetes, herpes simplex, herpes zoster (shingles), infections (fungal, bacterial, viral and parasitic), acne, and wounds.[21] Hydrogen peroxide injections have been used for inflamed, damaged, and injured tissues, inflamed nerves such as in herpes, or trigger points causing pain and muscle spasms.[22]

Dr. Farr also demonstrated rapid recovery from Type A/Shanghai influenza with intravenous hydrogen peroxide treatments. Two-thirds of his patients recovered after only a single injection, while a third returned for a second injection; only 10% required a third injection. Recovery time was half that of a control group treated with conventional methods (antibiotics, decongestants, and analgesics).[23]

Robert Haskell, M.D., of San Rafael, California, treated a 44-year-old man with MS who was confined to a wheelchair. After six treatments of intravenous hydrogen peroxide, he began taking a few steps. By the 18th treatment, he was able to walk for four hours without resting.[24]

When properly administered, oxidation therapy selectively destroys disease-producing bacteria, viruses, and other invading microbial organisms and deactivates toxic substances without injury to healthy tissues.

A number of studies have documented the value of combining hydrogen peroxide with conventional cancer treatments. One study, for instance, found that H_2O_2 improved the outcome of chemotherapy using vinblastine.[25] In another study, H_2O_2 injected into the arteries for ten days, followed by mitomycin C (an antibiotic with antitumor properties), enhanced the effectiveness of anticancer drugs.[26] H_2O_2 has also been shown to cause cancer cells to become more sensitive to the effects of radiation therapy, leading researchers to claim an "increased therapeutic ratio" in malignant tumors subjected to irradiation when oxygen levels of the affected

OZONE THERAPY IN VETERINARY MEDICINE

The value of ozone therapy in veterinary medicine was discovered by accident while animal tests were being conducted to substantiate the hazards of ozone to humans. However, the results proved the positive effects of ozone/oxygen mixtures on the survival rate of animals and researchers concluded that the results from the experiments constituted "a critical item worthy of serious consideration."[17]

Ozone therapy can be used on animals to treat intestinal disorders, arthritis, canine paralysis, skin problems, acute and chronic cystitis, oncological disorders, and helminthiasis (intestinal parasites or worms). Ozone is a disinfectant to bacteria and germs and causes inactivation of viruses and fungi. It is used by colonic insufflation for colitis and improves wound healing.

area are increased with hydrogen peroxide.[27] Recently, some doctors have also proposed that hydrogen peroxide could aid in the treatment of Hodgkin's lymphoma.[28]

There are few side effects with hydrogen peroxide therapy. In rare cases, a problem involving inflammation of veins at the site of injection will occur. Hydrogen peroxide should not be taken orally as it causes nausea and vomiting, and rectal administration can lead to inflammation of the lower intestinal tract. Other observed side effects include temporary faintness, fatigue, headaches, and chest pain. Most problems stem from the use of an inappropriate administration route, administration above patient tolerance, the mixing of oxidative chemicals with other substances, or using oxidative chemicals in too great a concentration, according to Dr. Farr.

CAUTION Oxidation therapy needs to be administered under clinical supervision, since uncontrolled oxidation may be destructive to the body.

The Future of Oxygen Therapies

The main stumbling blocks for all oxygen therapies, Dr. Hughes believed, are the FDA, insurance companies, and the entrenched medical establishment. "The problem is that most of the areas of conventional medicine in this country are driven by the pharmaceutical companies," he pointed out. "The incentive is always to sell pills and you can't sell oxygen pills. This tends to hold it back, especially since a large percentage of the research that is done at universities is funded by pharmaceutical companies."

Despite this fact, oxygen therapies are widely used in other countries, particularly Germany and Russia. In the U.S., indications are that the medical profession is becoming more receptive to the potential benefits of oxygen therapy. For example, three decades ago there were only eight indications (in America) for the use of hyperbaric oxygen. By 1992, there were 28 and that number continues to expand. In addition, as more people are becoming familiar with HBOT, there is increased interest by the medical profession about what other conditions it can help, and the same is true for ozone and hydrogen peroxide therapies.

 Research is needed into the many conditions oxygen therapy can benefit. Because oxygen therapy can help the body repair itself, it is an ideal treatment to integrate into a comprehensive health-care system.

Where to Find Help

The following organizations can provide information and answer questions about the various oxygen therapies:

American College of Hyperbaric Medicine
Ocean Medical Center
4001 Ocean Drive, Suite 105
Lauderdale-by-the-Sea, Florida 33308
(954) 771-4000
Website: www.oceanhbo.com

A group of physicians dedicated to the clinical aspects of hyperbaric medicine. Their purpose is to foster ethical growth and development of the science and practice of hyperbaric oxygen therapy. Promotes research and education.

ECH₂O₂ Newsletter
P.O. Box 126
Delano, Minnesota 55328
Website: www.oxytherapy.com

A public forum for those interested in the use of hydrogen peroxide and ozone. Publishes a quarterly newsletter for the public and professionals, addressing thousands of uses for hydrogen peroxide and ozone in areas including farming and agriculture, waste and water treatment, industry, bathing, and dentistry.

International Bio-Oxidative Medicine Foundation
P.O. Box 891954
Oklahoma City, Oklahoma 73189
(405) 478-IBOM

The foundation publishes and distributes a newsletter, as well as scientific research data. Supports educational programs that highlight current research and the therapeutic use of oxidative therapies. Encourages basic and clinical research.

Medizone International, Inc.
P.O. Box 742
Stinson Beach, California 94970
(415) 868-0300
Website: www.medizoneint.com

Developers of an ozone-based treatment for diseases caused by lipid-enveloped viruses, including AIDS, hepatitis B, and herpes. Medizone is also developing patented technology for the decontamination of blood and blood products. Dr. Sunnen serves as Medizone's medical director.

North Carolina Bio-Oxidative Health Center
4505 Fair Meadow Lane, Suite 111
Raleigh, North Carolina 27607
(800) 473-9812
Website: www.carolinacenter.com

Outpatient facility that focuses on metabolic and intestinal detoxification. Comprehensive and synergistic treatment regimens for each patient are developed utilizing therapies such as colon hydrotherapy, intravenous therapies (including ozone), and external ozone hydrotherapy. Supportive elements such as acupuncture and lymphatic massage, as well as techniques to address the psychological/emotional components of health and illness are also part of the program.

Recommended Reading

AIDS Under Pressure. Michelle Reillo, B.S.N., R.N. Kirkland, WA: Hogrefe & Huber, 1997.

Hydrogen Peroxide Medical Miracle. William C. Douglass. Atlanta, GA: Second Opinion Publishing, 1992. To order, call (800) 728-2288.

Hyperbaric Oxygen Therapy. Richard A. Neubauer, M.D., with Morton Walker. New York: Avery Publishing, 1997.

Oxygen Healing Therapies. Nathaniel Altman. Rochester, VT: Healing Arts Press, 1995.

Oxygen Therapies. Ed McCabe. Morrisville, NY: Energy Publications, 1988.

Underwater Medicine and Related Sciences: A Guide to the Literature, Volumes 1 & 2. Charles Shilling. New York: Plenum Publications, 1973, 1975.

The Use of Ozone in Medicine. Siegfried Rilling and Renate Viebahn. Heidelberg, Germany: Haug Publishers, 1987. Available from: Medicina Biologica, 2937 N.E. Flanders, Portland, OR 97232; (503) 287-6775.

PROLOTHERAPY

Prolotherapy rejuvenates the body by injection of natural substances to stimulate the growth of collagen in order to strengthen weak or damaged joints, tendons, ligaments, or muscles. As a simple, cost-effective alternative to drugs and surgery, prolotherapy is an effective treatment for many pain syndromes, including degenerative arthritis, low back and neck pain, joint pain, carpal tunnel syndrome, migraine headaches, and torn ligaments and cartilage.

JOINT, TENDON, ligament, cartilage, and arthritic problems are among the most common afflictions suffered by Americans today. Many remedies are used to treat these problems, such as rest, medication, traction, exercise, cortisone injections, physical therapy, and surgery, but for many patients, these fail to provide lasting relief. In many cases, prolotherapy (also known as reconstructive therapy, sclerotherapy, or proliferative therapy), a nonsurgical method that stimulates the body's natural healing abilities to repair injured tissues and joints, can provide an answer. The word *prolotherapy* is derived from the root *prolo*, which is short for *proliferation*. Prolotherapy is so named because it causes new collagen (see Quick Definition) to grow, or proliferate, in areas of the body where it has been weakened or injured.

"Ligaments, tendons, cartilage, and bones have poor healing abilities due to the lack of blood supply to these tissues," says William Faber, D.O., Director of the Milwaukee Pain Clinic, in Wisconsin, and a leading authority in the field of prolotherapy. "This is why injuries to these areas are so long lasting. When these tissues become damaged, the joint becomes unstable and, in order to compensate, the body forms bony, arthritic spurs. This causes increased friction, increased pain and weakness, and a loss in joint mobility. Further injury often results."

Prolotherapy can facilitate the healing process for specific injuries. In the case of injured joints, a local anesthetic and a natural irritant (sodium morrhuate, a purified derivative of cod liver oil), dextrose, phenol, minerals, or other natural substances are injected into areas where ligaments (see Quick Definition), tendons, or cartilage are torn or weak. "The injection stimulates the body to produce more connective tissue, which helps to strengthen the weak or damaged areas," says Dr. Faber. "As a result, the patient will often experience less pain and greater strength and endurance." Greater mobility and range of motion are other benefits of prolotherapy treatment. The injections are completely safe and trigger the same natural healing response that normally occurs after an injury.

 Collagen is a component of ligaments, tendons, cartilage, muscle, and the outer covering of muscle called fascia. All the soft tissue the body is composed of collagen.

Ligaments are sheets or bands of connective tissues that provide stability to the joints of the body by connecting two or more bones together. When ligaments become weak or damaged, healing is often slow and the injury may not fully recover, primarily because the blood supply to ligaments is limited. Ligaments also contain many nerve endings that can exacerbate the pain a person feels when ligaments are injured or loosened.

Tendons are fibrous connective tissues made out of collagen, which connect muscles to bones. Like ligaments, when tendons become damaged they can cause pain.

How Prolotherapy Works

"Mild, irritating reconstructive solutions cause dilation of blood vessels and a migration of fibroblasts [healing cells] to the injured areas," according to Dr. Faber. "These healing cells lay down collagen to repair the area." This re-growth has been substantiated by research studies dating back nearly 50 years.

In healthy ligaments or tendons, connective tissue, especially collagen fibers, limit themselves to a certain amount of stretch. When ligaments or tendons are injured, however, these connective fibers are also weakened, causing them to lose their ability to prevent further stretch. As a result, ligaments become "loose" and joints and other ligament-based structures become unstable and, ultimately, very painful. Prolotherapy eliminates or reduces pain by stimulating the body to rebuild ligaments and tendons, in many cases producing ligaments and tendons that are stronger and more stable than they were before injury occurred. While prolotherapy cannot reduce abnormal bone growth that has already occurred, it can eliminate the resulting pain. It is most effective when used in conjunction with proper diet, treatment for bacterial and fungal infections, and proper balancing of omega-3 fatty acids.

In a study conducted in the 1950s by surgeon George Hackett, M.D., 1,600 patients with severe sacroiliac sprain were treated with prolotherapy injections. When the patients were examined by independent physicians two to 12 years later, 82% had remained free of pain or recurrences.[1] Dr. Hackett's experiments were repeated in 1983 and 1985 by the University of Iowa's Department of Orthopedic Research. Both studies found that the patients' tendons became more firmly attached to the bone and increased in strength and structure by 30%-40% above normal.[2]

In 1987, at the Sansum Medical Clinic of Santa Barbara, California, rheumatologist Robert Klein, M.D., and internist Thomas Dorman, M.D., conducted a double-blind study of 81 patients who suffered from continuous low-back pain for more than ten years. They found that 88% of the patients injected with a prolotherapy solution of dextrose, glycerine, and phenol demonstrated moderate to marked improvement.[3] A similar study, reported in the *Journal of Spinal Disorders*, showed an 80% improvement.[4] Both studies support Dr. Hackett's findings.

Studies conducted by Harold Walmer, D.O., of Elizabeth, Pennsylvania, show that prolotherapy increases mechanical strength in ligaments and joints.[5] This may explain why so many patients with advanced degeneration of bones and soft tissues, or those who suffer from a wide range of musculoskeletal problems, have improved so dramatically when given prolotherapy injections.

Two placebo-controlled, blinded clinical trials of prolotherapy conducted in 2000 attest to the therapy's effectiveness for treating osteoarthritic conditions. In the first study, 13 patients suffering from osteoarthritis in their knees showed significant improvement in knee pain, swelling, buckling, and joint flexibility after receiving prolotherapy treatments. Additionally, eight of the patients with loose anterior cruciate ligaments found that they tightened following prolotherapy injection alone.[6] The second study investigated the effectiveness of prolotherapy for treating osteoarthritis in finger and thumb joints. Upon completion of the study, prolotherapy was shown to produce significant improvement of pain and joint flexibility.[7]

A 16-year study conducted by Harold Wilkinson, M.D., former Chair of Neurosurgery at Massachusetts Medical Center, also supports prolotherapy's effectiveness. While patients typically require a series of prolotherapy injections before they experience complete elimination of their pain, Dr. Wilkinson reported that "a sizeable portion of people with unresolved chronic pain had more than a year's pain relief with only one injection."[8]

According to Dr. Faber, when a patient does not improve after receiving prolotherapy, typically it is due to the fact that one or more pre-existing conditions are inhibiting the body's healing process; these include infection or the use of cortisone, which can interfere with prolotherapy's effectiveness. Ross Hauser, M.D., founding Medical Director of Caring Medical and Rehabilitation Services, in Oak Park, Illinois, concurs, after observing that some patients who came to him for prolotherapy needed more than the treatments alone to heal. "It is as if some patients have lost the ability to heal, a condition I call 'connective tissue deficiency'," says Dr. Hauser. He points out that the use of synthetic estrogen by women can also inhibit prolotherapy's effectiveness.

Conditions Benefited by Prolotherapy

Prolotherapy has been practiced in the United States for more than 50 years as a treatment for America's most common afflictions: tendon, ligament, and arthritic problems. To date, over one million patients have been successfully treated with prolotherapy, including the former U.S. Surgeon General, C. Everett Koop, M.D., who suffered from chronic back pain until prolotherapy cured it. Common symptoms and conditions that respond well to prolotherapy include:

- Degenerative arthritis
- Back and neck pain
- Torn ligaments and cartilage
- Degenerated discs
- Bursitis
- Carpal tunnel syndrome
- Achilles tendon tears and heel spurs
- Tennis elbow and rotator cuff tears
- Bunions

- Herniated discs
- Fibromyalgia
- Headaches and migraines
- Hip degeneration
- Knee injuries
- Polio
- Sacroiliac sprain
- Sciatica
- Scoliosis and other spinal defects
- Temporomandibular joint (TMJ) dysfunction
- Whiplash

Prolotherapy is also recommended for weak joints; joints requiring a brace; joints that continually pop, snap, and grind; or joints that cannot maintain alignment (particularly when chiropractic or osteopathic manipulations fail to help). It is also effective as a treatment for a wide range of musculoskeletal problems caused by failed surgery, compression fractures, degenerated discs, and muscular dystrophy.

 Prolotherapy can provide a more cost-effective solution to musculoskeletal and joint problems than traditional surgery.

Examples of Prolotherapy's Effectiveness

One of Dr. Faber's cases, involving physician John Parks Trowbridge of Houston, Texas, illustrates how effective prolotherapy can be. Dr. Trowbridge had been experiencing chronic low-back pain since the age of 14. At the age of 30, he had sprained his neck, worsening his condition, and a cervical laminectomy (surgical excision of the vertebral posterior arch) was performed. However, his back problems persisted and, ten years later, he injured his back once again. Diagnosis showed a herniated lumbar disk and another operation followed, but his back pain persisted. When it became so severe that he could barely move without pain, he sought prolotherapy. The pain was relieved immediately, Dr. Faber reports, with his neck and back steadily strengthening during the days after his first treatment. Further treatments provided more relief. "He told me that prolotherapy was the most valuable of any of the treatments he had received, and it only cost a fraction of the $120,000 he had spent on surgery, medications, and other physical therapies," reports Dr. Faber.

Another of Dr. Faber's cases involved a college football player who had suffered repeated injuries to his left shoulder. He relied upon various medications and therapies until the pain became too great, and then under-

went orthopedic surgery; but his condition worsened. Chiropractic treatments afforded him only temporary relief, and his chiropractor suggested prolotherapy. After receiving the injections, his condition improved dramatically. In fact, in a metered punching test, it was found that he ended up with more strength in the left shoulder than in the right.

A third patient of Dr. Faber's suffered from lumbar spondylolisthesis (a forward slipping of one vertebra on the one below it) for more than two years; he experienced constant pain. After receiving prolotherapy from Dr. Faber, he was pain free. Eight years later, he reported no recurrences. Today, he does landscaping, hunts, and even goes waterskiing.

Dr. Hauser has also had many successful outcomes using prolotherapy. One of his patients was a 41-year-old woman who came to him suffering from severe hip pain. After undergoing numerous X rays and an MRI scan, her doctors told her the pain was most likely due to a fall she had suffered some time before, as well as to hereditary arthritis. Over time, the pain became so great that she was forced to stop all physical activity and was sometimes unable to walk for weeks at a time. Finally, after 18 months of anti-inflammatory medication and pain pills, her doctors informed her that the only remaining option was hip replacement surgery. After examining her, Dr. Hauser administered a series of prolotherapy treatments and she became completely pain free. Three years later, she wrote Dr. Hauser to inform him that she was still free of pain and had traveled to Alaska, where she went mountain climbing and hiked to the top of a glacier field.

Degenerative muscle and joint complaints in particular benefit from prolotherapy. James Carlson, D.O., an orthopedic and sports medicine specialist in Knoxville, Tennessee, and past President of the American Association of Orthopedic Medicine, believes prolotherapy is the most effective treatment for Osgood-Schlatter disease, a tendon-insertion ailment that affects adolescents. "These kids have such severe pain in the knees, they can't participate in exercise, sports, or dance, and conventional medicine just dictates 'don't do anything athletic'," says Dr. Carlson. "Prolotherapy is the best thing I've ever seen." His own son, an aspiring baseball catcher, couldn't squat down or kneel. After therapy, he made the team as a catcher and later became a top school athlete.

Marc Darrow, M.D., Co-director of the Joint Rehabilitation and Sports Medical Center, in Los Angeles, California, trains physicians in the use of prolotherapy at the University of California at Los Angeles Physical Medicine and Rehabilitation Residency Program. He became convinced of its effectiveness after years of gymnastics, skiing, tennis, and golf left his left wrist "basically useless because of exquisite pain." After only one prolotherapy treatment, he reports that his wrist was 50% better and, after further injections, he was completely pain free and able to return to an active sports life.

"I have successfully used prolotherapy to treat almost every part of the musculoskeletal system, from head to toe," says Dr. Darrow, noting that his entire staff has benefited from prolotherapy treatments. "It's a shame that prolotherapy isn't taught in every medical school and residency program as core curriculum. If it was mainstream, many of today's musculoskeletal surgeries could be avoided." Dr. Darrow makes it a habit to carry prolotherapy supplies in his car. "The treatment is so simple, I can help people right at the tennis court," he says.

What to Expect from Prolotherapy

Prolotherapy is estimated to be significantly more cost-effective than surgery or joint replacement. Dr. Carlson notes that any pain or discomfort associated with receiving multiple injections is compensated for by the benefits received from prolotherapy. "Dramatic results should be noted by the patient within the first week of treatment," according to Kent Pomeroy, M.D., an Arizona physical medicine and rehabilitation specialist, and Co-founder and past President of the American Association of Orthopedic Medicine. "But if swelling occurs, improvement may not be noticed until the swelling subsides. If marked improvement is not obtained after the first six treatments, then further examination is recommended to find out why the patient's body is failing to reconstruct tissue."

Prolotherapy is significantly more cost-effective than surgery or joint replacement.

Generally, a patient improves dramatically after the first four to six injections. According to Dr. Darrow, often two to four treatments are all that is necessary to bring joints back to full strength and function. However, the response time of the therapy varies from patient to patient, depending on each person's healing ability, and some patients may require as many as 12–30 treatments. Prior to beginning treatment, it is best to be evaluated by a physician trained in prolotherapy. Once treatment begins, the physician can then gauge your response and

PROLOTHERAPY AND TRIGGER POINT THERAPY

While prolotherapy is little known among conventional medical practitioners, and not covered by most insurance, a treatment known as trigger point therapy is endorsed by many physicians and insurance companies. According to Marc Darrow, M.D., of the Joint Rehabilitation and Sports Medical Center, trigger points are "hyperirritable, painful bundles of muscle fibers." When pressed, they can refer pain to other areas of the body, yet they can often be deactivated by injection of a solution such as lidocaine into the tender area, which is what trigger point therapy involves.

"In reality, when trigger or tender points are injected near tendons, ligaments, bones, or muscle fascia, prolotherapy is also being done at the same time," says Dr. Darrow. "Even without a proliferant solution being injected, there is trauma to tissue and a small amount of bleeding, and blood is one of the most effective proliferants of collagen. What is often found is that pain may be reduced or eliminated by one or two injections. Therefore, prolotherapy and trigger point therapy are often performed at the same time without the specific intention of the doctor." For this reason, Dr. Darrow feels that prolotherapy deserves the same degree of acceptance that trigger point therapy currently enjoys.

give you an accurate estimate of how many treatment sessions will be needed.

The benefits of prolotherapy over other methods of treatment include:

- Eliminating the need for drugs or surgery
- Stimulating the body's natural healing mechanism, causing natural re-growth of structural tissue
- A low risk of side effects, when performed correctly
- Permanent results when full treatment course is completed

 Research into the effectiveness of prolotherapy is needed. This type of therapy could provide a revolution in orthopedic medicine by offering rejuvenation rather than surgery, which actually damages and removes tissue.

The Future of Prolotherapy

Although prolotherapy has been used to treat a wide range of musculoskeletal conditions for over 50 years, its practice has not become widespread in the United States. In recent years, however, according to Dr. Faber, the number of practitioners has been growing and currently approximately 400 physicians practice prolotherapy. "One major reason for the slow growth of prolotherapy may be the fact that the substances used in prolotherapy are not patented and therefore would not provide the huge profits that pharmaceutical therapies receive," suggests Dr. Faber. "Prolotherapy also requires specialized training and a serious commitment on the part of the physician to master the procedure."

Prolotherapy can play an important role in the medicine of the future. It may well be the first nondrug, nonsurgical approach to long-lasting musculoskeletal problems, resulting in a much-needed change from the current medical treatment, which involves orthopedics, surgery, physical medicine, and physical therapy. Besides being less expensive and less risky than surgery, prolotherapy is more effective in the treatment of pain, aids in the prevention of future injuries, and has a lasting effect on energy and endurance.

"The initial turning point will be the discovery of prolotherapy by professional athletes," Dr. Faber believes. "Although prolotherapy is well-documented in science and through the case histories of thousands of successful patients, the recovery of a single famous athlete by prolotherapy is what's needed to bring the therapy into the spotlight it so richly deserves."

Such a discovery is already happening, according to Dr. Darrow, who has healed many notable athletes and entertainers using prolotherapy. Among them is Johnnie Morton, Jr., a wide receiver on the Detroit Lions football team. "Johnnie suffered from both a painful sprain where the gluteus muscle attaches to the pelvis and a badly sprained thumb joint from getting clipped during games," Dr. Darrow says. "After only two prolotherapy sessions on each site, he played his first pain-free season in ten years."

Where to Find Help

Physicians can vary greatly in knowledge, skills, and experience in the performance of the art and science of prolotherapy. For further information, contact the following organizations:

Milwaukee Pain Clinic
6529 West Fond du Lac Avenue
Milwaukee, Wisconsin 53218
(414) 464-7246
Website: www.milwaukeepainclinic.com

Directed by Dr. Faber, the clinic provides prolotherapy and other musculoskeletal therapies; training courses in prolotherapy are also available. For additional information, send a legal size, self-addressed, stamped envelope.

Joint Rehabilitation and Sports Medical Center
11645 Wilshire Blvd., 1st Floor
Los Angeles, California 90025
(310) 231-7000
Website: www.jointrehab.com

Overseen by medical director Marc Darrow, M.D., the center specializes in state-of-the-art treatment for joint and muscle pain, back and neck pain, and sports injuries, and provides prolotherapy, chiropractic, exercise physiology, and sophisticated computerized exercise equipment, among other treatment protocols.

American College of Osteopathic Pain Management and Sclerotherapy
5002 East Woodmill Drive
Wilmington, Delaware 19808
(800) 476-6114

A leading organization for the training and promotion of prolotherapy in the United States.

American Association of Orthopedic Medicine
30897 C.R. 356-3
P.O. Box 4997
Buena Vista, Colorado 81211
(800) 992-2063
Website: www.aaomed.org

The American Association of Orthopedic Medicine is a nonprofit organization that provides information and educational programs on various methods of diagnosing and treating musculoskeletal injuries, including manipulation, prolotherapy, neural therapy, acupuncture, nutrition, and hormonal therapies.

Recommended Reading

The Collagen Revolution: Living Pain Free. Marc Darrow, M.D., J.D. Los Angeles: Joint Rehabilitation and Sports Medical Center, 2002.

Pain, Pain Go Away. William J. Faber, D.O. and Morton Walker. San Jose, CA: Ishi Press International, 1990.

Prolo Your Arthritis Pain Away! Curing Disabling and Disfiguring Arthritis Pain with Prolotherapy. William J. Faber, D.O. and Morton Walker. Oak Park, IL: Beulah Land Press, 2000.

Prolo Your Headaches and Neck Pain Away! Curing Migraines and Chronic Neck Pain with Prolotherapy. Ross A. Hauser, M.D., and Marion A. Hauser, M.S., R.D. Oak Park, IL: Beulah Land Press, 2000.

Prolo Your Pain Away! Curing Chronic Pain with Prolotherapy. Ross A. Hauser, M.D., with Marion A. Hauser, M.S., R.D., and Kurt Pottinger. Oak Park, IL: Beulah Land Press, 1998.

Prolo Your Sports Injuries Away: Curing Sports Injuries and Enhancing Athletic Performance with Prolotherapy. Ross A. Hauser, M.D., and Marion A. Hauser, M.S., R.D. Oak Park, IL: Beulah Land Press, 2000.

QIGONG AND TAI CHI

Qigong and Tai Chi combine movement, meditation, and breath regulation to enhance the flow of vital energy in the body, improve blood circulation, and enhance immune function. Because Qigong and Tai Chi can be used by the healthy as well as the severely ill, they represent two of the most broadly applicable systems of self-care in the world.

Q IGONG (also referred to as chi-kung) is an ancient Chinese system of self-healing that stimulates and balances the flow of *qi*, or vital life energy, along the acupuncture meridians (energy pathways in the body). Tai Chi, also known as Tai Chi Chuan, is one of the best known and most choreographed forms of Qigong. Roughly translated, *Tai Chi Chuan* means "Grand Ultimate Martial Art" and is part martial art, part moving meditation.

Like acupuncture and traditional Chinese medicine, the Qigong and Tai Chi traditions emphasize the importance of teaching the patient how to remain well. In China, the various styles of Qigong form the nucleus of a national self-care system of health maintenance and personal development. Both Qigong and Tai Chi cultivate inner strength, calm the mind, and restore the body to its natural state of health by maintaining the optimum functioning of the body's self-regulating systems.

 See Acupuncture, Energy Medicine, Traditional Chinese Medicine.

Recent medical studies in both China and the U.S. show that Qigong and Tai Chi can reduce stress, increase circulation, and provide resistance to disease. Today, most hospitals in China include Qigong as part of their healthcare programs, with certain hospitals devoted solely to its study and practice. Thousands of Qigong institutes also provide Qigong instruction, while major centers in Beijing, Shanghai, and Guangzho train Qigong teachers and carry out government-supported research.

Tai Chi is also quite popular in China and, in the last decade, its popularity has also grown significantly in the U.S. Many Tai Chi practitioners are unaware of or do not

In China, the various styles of Qigong form the nucleus of a national self-care system of health maintenance and personal development.

focus on its martial origins and applications, choosing to focus instead on its many health benefits—improving balance and body awareness, stimulating immune function, increasing flexibility, and improving circulation. According to Roger Jahnke, O.M.D., of Santa Barbara, California, Chairperson of the National Qigong Association, there are multiple styles of Tai Chi, including the long form, which consists of up to 108 movements. "Individuals with serious health issues may not have the stamina to learn the long form of Tai Chi," Dr. Jahnke cautions. "However, some of the shorter forms may be suitable for these patients. Tai Chi is often modified to work with special diagnoses. Individual movements extracted from the longer forms are called Tai Chi Qigong and are easier to learn and practice."

How Qigong and Tai Chi Work

Qigong and Tai Chi practice can range from simple calisthenic-type movements with breath coordination to more complex methods where brain-wave frequency, heart rate, and other organ functions are altered intentionally by the practitioner. When practiced regularly, the combination of movement, deep relaxation, and breathing—common to both forms of exercise—can improve strength and flexibility, reverse damage caused by prior injuries and disease, and promote relaxation, awareness, and healing.

Traditional Chinese medicine holds that Qigong and Tai Chi stimulate and nourish the internal organs by circulating *qi* (see Quick Definition). Regular practice can break down energy blocks and facilitate the free flow of energy throughout the body, promoting blood and lymph flow and the even flow of nerve impulses necessary for proper health maintenance. "The overall benefit of Qigong and Tai Chi is to mobilize and harmonize *qi*, the body's naturally occurring healing resource," Dr. Jahnke says.

> **QD** **Qi** (pronounced CHEE) is a Chinese word variously translated to mean "vital energy," "essence of life," and "living force." In Chinese medicine, the proper flow of *qi* along energy channels (meridians) within the body is crucial to a person's health and vitality. There are many types of *qi*, classified according to source, location, and function (such as activation, warming, defense, transformation, and containment). Within the body, *qi* and blood are closely linked, as each is considered to flow along with the other. The manipulation and readjustment of *qi* to treat disease and ensure maximum health benefit is the basic principle of acupuncture, although other remedies and therapies can be used to influence *qi*.

Like acupuncture, Qigong and Tai Chi activate the electrical currents that flow along the meridian pathways of the body. According to Dr. Jahnke, both health practices stimulate human bioelectrical conductibility. "The human body has the ability to conduct an electrical charge," he explains. This affects the entire body, and it is responsible for maintaining the function of the organs and tissues. For example, one Qigong exercise involves breathing regulation and deep relaxation while lifting the arms and rising upward on the toes. According to Dr. Jahnke, this exercise can help prevent tension headaches, constipation, insomnia, and other disorders by improving circulation of the cardiovascular and lymphatic systems, as well as modulating brain chemistry.

Of the two forms, Qigong has the broadest healthcare applications because it is easier for most people to learn and practice. In the U.S., it is now being taught by qualified instructors in innovative hospital programs, at adult education centers, and in community fitness programs. Applicable to young and old alike, and for people in any state of health, Qigong is unique among fitness programs as it can be performed standing, walking, sitting, or lying down. Qigong exercises can even be performed by those confined to a bed or wheelchair.

In a comprehensive overview of applied physiology and Qigong research, Dr. Jahnke cites a number of current studies in which the following physiological mechanisms are enhanced by regular Qigong practice:

- Initiates the "relaxation response"—triggered by any form of mental focus that frees the mind from its many distractions—which decreases the sympathetic function of the autonomic nervous system. This decreases heart rate and blood pressure, dilates the blood capillaries, and optimizes the delivery of oxygen to the tissues.

- Alters the neurochemistry profile (the balance of neurotransmitters, brain chemicals that bond with receptor sites on tissue, enzyme, immune, and other cells to excite or inhibit their function), moderating pain, depression, and addictive cravings, as well as optimizing immune capability.

- Enhances the efficiency of the immune system through increased rate and flow of the lymphatic fluid and activation of immune cells.

- Improves resistance to disease and infection by accelerating the elimination of toxic by-products from the interstitial spaces in the tissues, organs, and glands through the lymphatic system.

- Increases the efficiency of cell metabolism and tissue regeneration through increased circulation of oxygen and nutrient-rich blood to the brain, organs, and tissues.

- Coordinates right/left brain hemisphere dominance, promoting deeper sleep, reduced anxiety, and mental clarity.

- Induces alpha and, in some cases, theta brain waves, which reduce heart rate and blood pressure, facilitating relaxation, mental focus, and even paranormal skills; this optimizes the body's self-regulative mechanisms by decreasing the activity of the sympathetic nervous system.

- Moderates the function of the hypothalamus, pituitary, and pineal glands, as well as the cerebrospinal fluid system of the brain and spinal cord, which mediates pain and mood and accelerates immune function.

Conditions Benefited by Qigong and Tai Chi

Qigong has been shown to be effective in helping resolve digestive problems, asthma, arthritis, insomnia, pain, depression, and anxiety, as well as helping cancer, heart

TYPES OF QIGONG

Over its long history, Qigong has developed into a number of branches. Personal self-healing and health maintenance practice is called internal Qigong. Internal Qigong performed with little or no movement is known as quiescent Qigong. When internal practice includes movement, it is called dynamic Qigong. According to Roger Jahnke, O.M.D., internal, self-applied Qigong practice may include prone, sitting, standing, or walking forms. Meditation is an example of quiescent Qigong, while Tai Chi is an example of a mildly dynamic Qigong.

One of the most provocative aspects of Qigong is known as external Qigong. In external Qigong, a Qigong master or doctor projects or emits their own *qi* to serve or heal another. When patients are severely ill and their own level of *qi* is very low or stagnant, receiving *qi* from a Qigong master can prove to be a powerful stimulant toward healing. Generally, however, people who receive external Qigong simultaneously do their own internal practice.

"External projection," states Dr. Jahnke, "while seeming to be a fantastic aspect of Qigong, is not unlike what Western cultures call magnetic healing or psychic healing, which both operate through the same natural laws of physics as the phenomena of *qi* emission." In a study conducted by Feng Li-da, M.D., from the Beijing Institute of Traditional Chinese Medicine, a Qigong master practicing external Qigong was able to project her *qi* to both kill and promote the growth of bacteria in test tubes.[1]

nificant improvement. In another study, Qigong eye exercises significantly reduced farsightedness and nearsightedness in a group of Chinese schoolchildren. Sinus allergies, hemorrhoids, and prostate problems have also been effectively treated.[3]

Today in China, many hospitals combine Qigong and Tai Chi with conventional medicine in order to treat cancer, bone marrow disease, and diseases of old age. At the Kuangan Men's Hospital, in Beijing, China, 93 cases of advanced malignant cancer were treated with a combination of drugs and Qigong exercises, while a control group of 30 patients were treated by drugs alone. Eighty-one percent of the Qigong group gained strength, 63% had improved appetite, and 33% were free from diarrhea, compared to control group improvements of 10%, 10%, and 6%, respectively.[4]

Today in China, many hospitals combine Qigong and Tai Chi with conventional medicine in order to treat cancer, bone marrow disease, and diseases of old age.

Qigong is often found to be more effective than chemotherapy, surgery, and even acupuncture for the prevention and treatment of disease. According to Liu Guo Long, M.D., Ph.D., of the Beijing College of Traditional Chinese Medicine, *qi* energy directed to the site of an injury "facilitates the signals to the brain stem." As a result of increased blood and lymph flow, and a greater supply of nutrients regenerating the cells, the area of injury can heal more effectively.

As Director of the Health Action Clinic and Chair of the Qigong and Tai Chi Department of the Santa Barbara College of Oriental Medicine, Dr. Jahnke draws from a broad experience with Qigong. "In classes and at numerous hospitals, we have seen a variety of health benefits of Qigong and Tai Chi. In a study at a senior center, after only two weeks of practice, six people out of a group of 30 had specific improvement—three experienced increased breath volume and relief of constricted breathing, one person found relief from constipation, one person had improved sleep, and one had a lessening of headaches; 25 of the participants reported a heightened sense of well-being in this very brief period of practice. One of our patients had set an appointment for glaucoma surgery before joining a weekly Qigong class. After six weeks in the class, she went to the laboratory for preoperative testing. The results of the tests showed that the

disease, and cases of HIV/AIDS. According to Wong Chong-xing, M.D., Director of Research at the Rei Jin Hospital, in Shanghai, China, several thousand hypertensive patients experienced dramatic improvement after they had been instructed in basic Qigong exercises. His studies suggest that daily Qigong practice lowers blood pressure, pulse rates, metabolic rates, and oxygen demand. David Eisenberg, M.D., a clinical research fellow at Harvard Medical School, says these studies also indicate that Qigong triggers the body's relaxation response by reducing the level of dopamine, a neurotransmitter that controls neurological activity.[2]

Stephen Chang, M.D., a doctor of traditional Chinese medicine, cites numerous scientific studies documenting the effects of Qigong. In one study, 2,873 terminal cancer patients practiced Qigong for six months: 12% of the patients were cured, while 47% showed sig-

glaucoma problem had resolved itself and surgery was no longer necessary."

Dr. Jahnke also cites a group of arthritis patients who have been regular participants in Qigong classes. "After approximately six months, several patients remarked that the stiffness and pain in their hands had diminished and in several cases the deformed knuckles characteristic of arthritis had begun to return to normal," he says. "The most incredible thing about Qigong practice is that people actually can feel the activity of the internal physiological mechanisms of healing in their body. The increase of blood and lymph flow and the shift in neurotransmitters creates an actual sensation that is clearly perceptible to the individual. The Chinese call this '*qi* sensation'."

With Qigong, individuals learn to heal themselves and maintain their health—a profoundly cost-effective feature.

—ROGER JAHNKE, O.M.D.

Tai Chi has been proven to enhance balance control, flexibility, and cardiorespiratory fitness among older patients. In one study, 28 men (average age of 67.5 years) who had practiced Tai Chi for an average of 13 years were compared to a sedentary control group of 30 men (average age of 66.2 years). Measurements of the men's resting heart rate, left and right single leg stance with eyes closed, total body rotation, modified total sit and reach tests, and 3-minute step tests found that the Tai Chi practitioners had significantly better scores than those in the control group.[6]

Often older patients who start an exercise program are not willing to continue that practice. A study of 130 subjects at the Department of Rehabilitation Medicine, School of Medicine, at Emory University, showed that patients who practiced Tai Chi were more likely to continue the practice than a control group because of mental, as well as physical, benefits. Those who practiced Tai Chi reported that the practice affected their everyday life, increased their confidence and balance, and that their practice not only continued, but actually improved over time.[7]

Another study, conducted at the Department of Physical Medicine and Rehabilitation at the National Taiwan University Hospital gauged the overall health benefits of Tai Chi on older individuals. Thirty-eight patients, 58-70 years old, participated in the study. A group of nine men and nine women were in the Tai Chi

A MACHINE THAT PRODUCES *QI* ENERGY

In the early 1980s, Lu Yan Fang, Ph.D., a senior scientist at the National Electro Acoustics Laboratory, in Beijing, China, discovered that the hands of Qigong masters emitted high levels of low-frequency acoustical waves called secondary sound. Although everyone generates secondary sounds, the signals generated by the Qigong masters were 100 times more powerful than the average individual and 1,000 times more powerful than those who were elderly or ill. Using electroacoustical technology, Dr. Fang constructed an instrument that simulated this infratonic sound (8-14 hertz, 70 decibels). By directing these massage-like, secondary sounds into hospitalized patients, Dr. Fang noted numerous improvements, particularly for the management of pain.

Over 1,100 patients were studied and treated. When used on the chest or back, the brain's production of alpha waves is stimulated. Therapeutic benefits include pain reduction (including migraines), increased circulatory functioning, muscular relaxation, and the alleviation of depression.[5]

Dr. Fang's device, the Infratonic QGM, has received awards of recognition from the China Ministry of Health, the China Central Technological Committee, and the National Committee for Traditional Chinese Medicine. It is used as an effective pain management tool in China as well as in Japan, Taiwan, Singapore, France, Spain, Mexico, and Argentina. In the U.S., it is approved for sale by the Food and Drug Administration as a therapeutic massage device. Dr. Jahnke cautions, however, "These machines mimic human *qi*. Remember, it is always preferable to develop one's personal practice to enhance the *qi* instead of just relying on a machine."

group, while the control group was composed of nine men and eleven women. Each session consisted of a 20-minute warm up, 24 minutes of Tai Chi, and ten minutes of cool down. The male Tai Chi group showed a 16.1% increase in maximum oxygen volume, increase in thoracic/lumbar flexibility, and 18.1% increase in the muscular strength of knee extension. The female group showed a 21.3% increase in maximum oxygen volume, increased flexibility, and 20.3% increase in the muscle strength of knee extensor plus 15.9% in knee flexor. In comparison, neither the male or female members of the control group showed any appreciable change in these variables. The study concluded that a 12-month program of Tai Chi is effective in improving the overall health of the elderly.[8]

A study was conducted at the National Taiwan University Hospital on 20 patients who had undergone coronary artery bypass surgery. The study showed that patients who practiced Tai Chi for a year as part of a postoperative outpatient rehabilitation program significantly enhanced their cardiovascular function, compared to patients whose rehabilitation program involved home-based, conventional exercise.[9]

The Pain Management Center of Newark, New Jersey, conducted a study of 26 patients, 18 to 65 years old, to assess the effects of Qigong. The patients, who suffered from late-stage complex regional pain syndrome, were all treatment resistant. The first group received *qi* emission and Qigong instructions from a Qigong master, while the control group received a similar set of instructions from a sham master. Eighty-two percent of the Qigong group reported less pain by the end of the first session, compared to only 45% of the control group. At the end of the last training session, three weeks later, 91% of the Qigong patients reported pain relief, compared to only 36% of the control group. While anxiety decreased in both groups, its reduction was also greater in the Qigong group.[10]

Additional research has shown that Qigong, when regularly practiced, can benefit patients suffering from hypertension, due to its ability to elevate blood levels of HDL ("good") cholesterol while lowering LDL ("bad") cholesterol and triglyceride levels. This was clearly shown by a study involving 100 hypertensive patients, whose mean levels of LDL cholesterol and triglycerides were significantly greater than nonhypertensive patients, and whose HDL levels were significantly lower. The hypertensive patients were divided into two groups—the first group received anti-hypertensive medication and training in Qigong, while the control group received only the medication. After a year, those who practiced Qigong in addition to receiving medication had significant improvements in all areas of measurement, whereas the control group showed no improvement at all.[11]

Qigong has also been found to regulate stress hormone activity, thus helping maintain homeostasis during times of stress. In the study, blood was drawn from patients before, during, and after training to determine the blood levels of stress hormones. Levels of ACTH (adrenocorticotropic hormone) were found to decrease during the training, while cortisol and DHEA levels did not significantly change. Typically, during times of stress, levels of these hormones elevate and, left unchecked, can be harmful to health. By contrast, levels of beta-endorphin, a hormone associated with pleasure, relaxation, and

improved mental functioning, significantly increased during the training period.[12]

Qigong can also benefit patients suffering from bronchial asthma, as shown by a German study involving 30 asthma patients who were taught Qigong techniques. After receiving instruction in Qigong, the patients were asked to practice independently on a daily basis and to keep a diary of their symptoms. One year later, a significant number in the Qigong group, compared to a control group that did not practice Qigong, showed a decrease of at least 10% in peak-flow variability (amount of air they can expire—an indication of airway obstruction). There were also decreased hospitalization rates, less sick leave, reduced antibiotic use, and fewer emergency consultations, resulting in less treatment costs.[13]

Finally, researchers at the International Association of Relaxation Therapy, in Kyoto, Japan, conducted a study of Qigong's benefits for patients with diabetes. In the study, patients were taught Qigong walking, an easy, slow method of walking that involves all of the body's muscles. Ten patients with diabetes and associated symptoms were studied on three separate days. They each practiced Qigong walking or took a 30-40 minute walk half an hour after lunch on one of the three study days. Blood sugar (glucose) levels and pulse rates were measured 30 minutes before they ate and 90 minutes later, then compared to measurements obtained on a day of lunch followed by no exercise. Both regular and Qigong walking were found to decrease glucose levels compared to days of no exercise, but Qigong walking had the additional benefit of not inducing a large increase in pulse rate, which occurred after normal walking.[14]

Qigong Practices

Following is a series of Qigong practices compiled by Dr. Jahnke. They are designed for maximum result along with maximum ease and can be performed by almost anyone, regardless of health, age, or physical condition. To make the practice of Qigong more beneficial and accessible to the person just starting out, Dr. Jahnke suggests:

- Take it easy and don't rush. Excess effort and trying too hard go against the natural benefits of Qigong. Remember, Qigong is intended to help you heal.

- Although Qigong may seem too easy to be beneficial, a dedication to these practices can mobilize one's inherent healing forces.

- Results come over time, so don't overdo it or expect too much too soon.

Practice 1

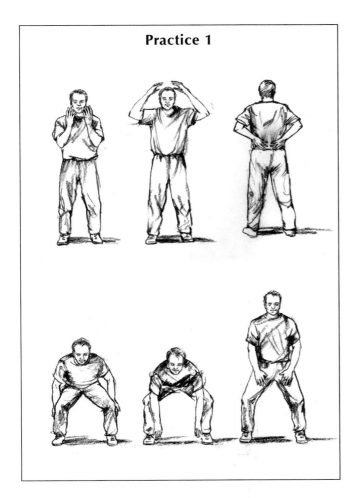

Practice 2

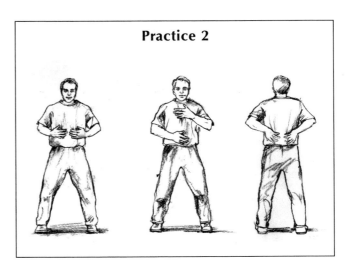

- If performed correctly, Qigong is safe to practice as often as you like.

- Feel free to make up your own routine and to change the practices to suit your needs, likes, and limitations. Modify the methods for seated practice if necessary.

- Always approach each practice with an intention to relax; direct the mind toward quiet indifference.

- Regulate the breath so that both the inhalation and exhalation are slow and deep, but not urgent or exaggerated.

The Practices

1. TRACING ACUPUNCTURE MERIDIANS TO CIRCULATE THE VITAL LIFE ENERGY

The goal of this practice is to move the *qi* along the meridians. Rub your hands together to build up heat—the Chinese say this increases *qi*. Your hands will become warmer if you are relaxed and the environment is comfortable. As if washing your face, stroke the palms upward across the cheeks, eyes, and forehead. Continue over the top and side of the head, down the back of the neck, and

along the shoulders to the shoulder joint. Continue under the arm and down the sides to the rib cage. At the lower edge of the rib cage, move the palms around to the back, across the buttocks, down the back and sides of the legs, and out the sides of the feet. Trace up inside the feet and the inner surface of the legs, up the front side of the torso and onto the face again, beginning the second round. You may rub the palms together before each round.

2. DIRECTING VITAL LIFE ENERGY TO INTERNAL ORGANS

Rub your hands together to build up heat. Apply the right hand to the area over the liver at the lower right edge of the rib cage. Visualize the liver (the largest, most complex organ in the body) receiving the *qi* and benefiting. Apply the left hand to the area over the spleen and pancreas at the lower left side of the ribs. The spleen, an immense lymph organ, is the producer of white blood cells and the pancreas is a critical link in energy metabolism and digestion. Move the hands circularly continuing to create heat, breathe full breaths, and relax. Feel the heat, or *qi*, passing in through the surface of the skin and penetrating to the organs as the entire metabolic process becomes more efficient. Holding the hands still over the organs, continue to feel the heat penetrate. On exhalation, visualize the *qi* circulating from the center of the body out the arms, into the hands, and penetrating from the hands into the organs.

Now, move the palms to cover the navel and breastbone. The navel is the human original connection to life and nourishment, and the Chinese feel that in adulthood it still connects to the whole body. The breastbone protects several vital organs, particularly the heart and the thymus gland. The heart pumps the blood, of course, but the Chinese believe it is the seat of one's emotional and spiritual self. The thymus is the source of T cells, some of the most powerful immune agents. Visualize them benefiting from the warmth, the *qi*, pouring into the navel,

Practice 3

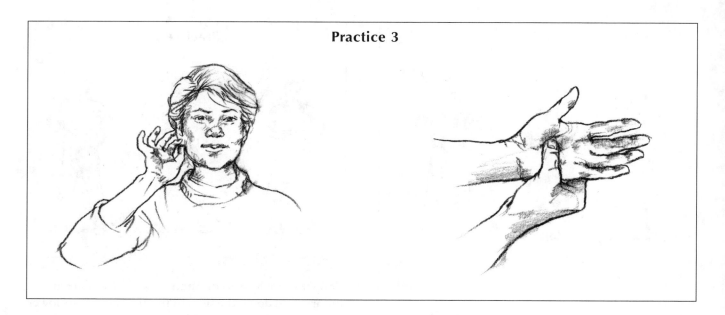

heart, and thymus, enhancing their ability to perform their essential functions.

Move the palms around to cover the lower back. In traditional Chinese medicine, this area is thought to be directly connected to the kidneys, which not only remove toxins from the blood, but also store vital life energies. The adrenal glands rest on top of the kidneys and control much of what the Chinese associate with the regulation of those energies. Rub these areas, penetrating the *qi* deep into the body to improve the ability of the kidneys and adrenals to do their work. Visualize the kidneys and adrenals receiving the *qi* and being empowered to more efficiently help eliminate waste products, produce energy, and activate healing throughout the whole body.

3. MASSAGING THE ACUPUNCTURE MICROSYSTEMS

In modern Chinese medical terminology, the hands, feet, and ears are called reflex microsystems. Pressure applied to these areas, usually with the thumbs, stimulates *qi* throughout the body. With your thumbs, vigorously press all areas of the palms and the soles of the feet. Find sore points and concentrate pressure on them several times.

Practice 4

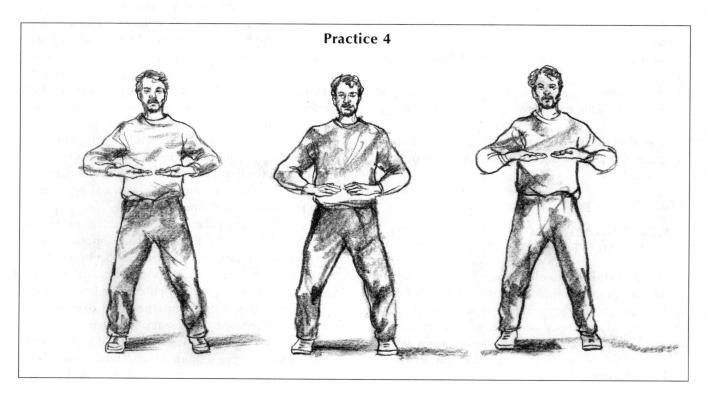

Practice 5

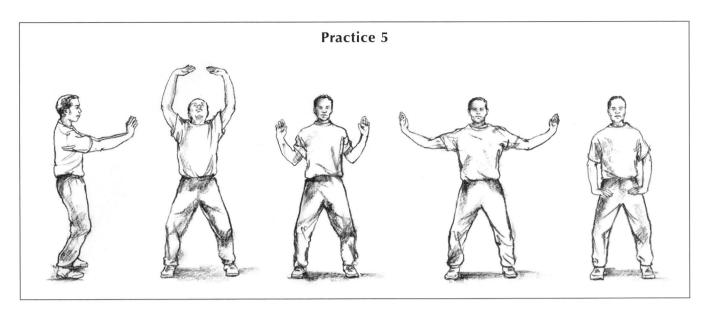

Press out along each segment of the fingers and toes. At the tips of the fingers and toes, press on the lateral sides of the base of the fingernails or toenails (feel for an indentation). Continuing to press, roll the receiving finger or toe under the pressure of the thumb and forefinger of the working hand. Return to give additional pressure to those points that were particularly tender. Now using the thumbs and forefingers, massage the ears simultaneously. Begin with moderate pressure and work over the entire ear on both sides, until the ears begin to feel hot. Notice any areas of discomfort and rub the uncomfortable areas vigorously.

4. BUILDING UP VITAL LIFE ENERGY WITH BREATHING

Sit or stand, keeping your eyes lightly closed or just slightly open, attention focused inward. Shoulders are relaxed and the head rests directly on top of the shoulders and spine. Hands are held palm facing upward, fingertips pointing toward each other two inches below the navel. Slowly inhaling, bring the hands upward to the lower edge of the breastbone. Then, take in three additional short puffs of breath to maximally fill the lungs, raising the hands a bit with each puff to the level of the armpits. Hold for a moment. Turn the palms face down and exhale slowly, lowering the hands slowly to the navel. Exhale three additional puffs of breath to maximally empty the lungs. Lower the hands a bit to the beginning level. Hold for a moment. Repeat.

On the exhalations, you may feel a warm or tingling sensation spreading outward from the center of your body toward your hands. On inhaling, visualize the *qi* accumulating deep inside the pelvic and abdominal cavities (known as the sea of energy). Continue visualizing with exhalation.

5. CONTRACTING AND RELAXING WITH BREATHING

In this exercise, the whole body musculature contracts on exhalation and deeply relaxes on each inhalation. The breath and the contraction together help to cleanse the tissues of the body. While sitting or standing, bring the hands in front of the heart/breastbone, inhale, and relax. Begin to exhale, pressing the hands forward as if pushing something heavy. Contract as many of the body's muscles as possible. Grip the floor or ground with the toes and, while the hands slowly push forward, contract the perineal muscles (located on the pelvic floor between the genital and anal area). When the hands are extended, all muscles are contracted and breath is completely exhaled. Then relax—release tension from all muscles and float the hands back toward the heart with a deep inhalation. Release the toes, the perineum, and the abdomen.

Repeat the same cycle, pressing the hands upward as high as possible, as if lifting a great weight off of yourself, exhaling and contracting. Then relax completely, inhale slowly, and return the hands to the position before the heart. Next, repeat pushing out to the sides, then pressing downward. Continue forward, then up, then to the sides, and finally downward. Contraction and release of muscles pump large volumes of lymphatic fluid away from the tissues, carrying away metabolic wastes through the bloodstream.

6. TWISTING THE WAIST

Standing, with your feet at shoulder width, rotate your torso. This can also be done seated. Upper body movement should come from moving the waist. Shoulders follow the waist and the arms follow the shoulders, they just dangle and swing. Turn the head completely, as far

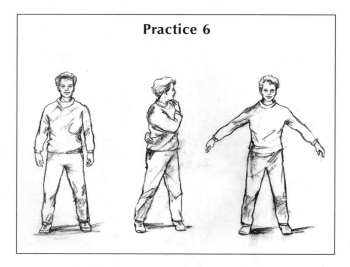

Practice 6

as it will comfortably go, to look behind you. Breathe fully and note a dynamic relationship between action and relaxation. Bring as much relaxation to the movement as possible. Notice that the arms and hands hit the body. This hitting or thumping can become purposeful when aimed at the reflexes of the kidneys, spleen, and liver around the lower torso.

7. SPONTANEOUS MOVEMENT

Spontaneous movement Qigong is very common in China. Instead of following a prescribed set of instructions, each individual is guided to move about or not move at all by an internal sense of the body's needs, a sense of the *qi*. Some people seem to be doing nothing or almost nothing, others may be sitting and moving their arms about in coordination with the breath. Still others may be dancing about in a deeply energized state. Standing with feet at shoulder width or sitting in an armless chair, begin to wiggle the fingers and shake or rock the body; deepen the breath. Increase the body's activity and allow hands and arms to shake. Add shaking of the head and shoulders. Relax the jaw, allowing some sound to be generated on the exhalation, like a giant sigh of relief. This is one of the best exercises to bring about an immediate sensation of the energy or *qi*. Exaggerate the movement, prolong it; shift weight from foot to foot; make sounds; find your own best way to use this exercise.

8. QIGONG MEDITATION

This practice can be done standing, sitting, or lying down. In the severely ill, it can mobilize important healing resources. If the person is healthy, it can help maintain health and coordinate body, mind, and spirit. In this practice, natural forces accelerate through breath, relaxation, intention, and visualization. On inhalation, visualize a concentration of *qi* in the abdominal area. On exhalation, visualize these resources circulating out from the center to all the parts of the body: extremities, organs,

tissues, and glands. Continue, through thought and visualization, to circulate healing energy with deep breathing and deep relaxation.

 With its proven ability to enhance health and prevent disease, Qigong can serve as an effective system of self-care, saving thousands of dollars in health-care costs.

Qigong in America

Qigong and Tai Chi have been widely practiced in the U.S. for many years. Now the health-care and medical community have become interested in gentle self-healing methods that complement both conventional and holistic medicine. "One factor makes Qigong an inevitable innovation in Western culture," says Dr. Jahnke, "the staggering cost of post-symptomatic medical intervention. With Qigong, individuals learn to heal themselves and maintain their health for free—a profoundly cost-effective feature." Dr. Jahnke adds that ancient, low-impact self-healing traditions like Qigong, Tai Chi, and yoga are being referred to as "self-applied health enhancement methods" (SAHEM) in the international medical literature. SAHEM combines gentle body movement, self-massage, relaxation exercises, breathing, meditation, and visualization to create self-healing and health enhancement programs that are now gaining popularity in hospitals, schools, YMCAs, corporate wellness programs, social agencies, churches, and communities at large throughout the U.S.[15]

Evidence of the robust growth of Qigong and Tai Chi is reflected in the fact that the National Qigong Association has grown 1,000% in just six years. In addition, Qigong, Tai Chi, and other aspects of SAHEM are now being studied through the research efforts of the National Center for Complementary and Alternative Medicine (NCCAM) at the National Institutes of Health. "A kind of revolution in self-healing is occurring," Dr. Jahnke concludes. "The Chinese realized thousands of years ago that the most profound medicine is produced within the human body for free. Qigong is a power tool that is easy to learn and use for activating this inner medicine. Tai Chi and Qigong will play a central role in the emerging new health-care system of our country."

Where to Find Help

Though there are many books on Qigong and Tai Chi, classes should be taken with a qualified teacher. Consult your telephone book for a Qigong or Tai Chi center near you, or ask an acupuncturist or doctor of traditional Chinese medicine for a referral.

National Qigong Association (NQA)
P.O. Box 540
Ely, Minnesota 55731
(218) 365-6330
Website: www.nqa.org

A nonprofit organization focused on the integration of Qigong into all facets of our culture, the NQA is a professional organization as well as a community of Qigong enthusiasts with all levels of experience.

International Integral Qigong and Tai Chi Training Institute
Health Action
243 Pebble Beach
Santa Barbara, California 93117
(805) 682-3230
Websites: www.qigong-chikung.com and www.healerwithin.com

Overseen by Dr. Roger Jahnke, this organization offers comprehensive training in Qigong and Tai Chi, publishes books and videos, and presents Qigong training throughout the U.S., Europe, and Asia.

American Qigong Association and East-West Academy of the Healing Arts
P.O. Box 31211
San Francisco, California 94131
(415) 788-2227
Website: www.eastwestqi.com

A chapter of the World Qigong Federation. Brings together scientists, professionals, institutions, and laypeople to promote research and education in Qigong.

The Qigong Institute
561 Berkeley Avenue
Menlo Park, California 94025
Website: www.qigonginstitute.org

A nonprofit organization working to promote Qigong through research and education. The Institute maintains a compilation of extensive clinical and experimental research on the medical applications of Qigong.

Santa Barbara College of Oriental Medicine
Qigong and Tai Chi Training Program
1919 State Street
Santa Barbara, California 93101
(805) 898-1180
Website: www.sbcom.edu

Offers training in all aspects of traditional Chinese medicine, including Qigong and Tai Chi, acupuncture, and Chinese herbalism.

Recommended Reading

Chi Kung: The Ancient Chinese Way to Health. Paul Dong and Aristide H. Esser, M.D. New York: Paragon House, 1990.

The Complete System of Self-Healing: Internal Exercises. Stephen T. Chang. San Francisco: Tao Publishing, 1986.

The Healer Within. Roger Jahnke, O.M.D. San Francisco: HarperSanFrancisco, 1999.

The Healing Promise of Qi. Roger Jahnke, O.M.D. New York: Contemporary Books, 2001.

The Most Profound Medicine. Roger Jahnke, O.M.D. Santa Barbara, CA: Health Action Books, 1990. To order, call (805) 682-3230.

Opening the Energy Gates of the Body. B.K. Frantzis. Berkeley, CA: North Atlantic Books, 1993.

Qigong: Miracle Healing from China. Charles McGee with Effie Pow Yew Chow. Coeur d'Alene, ID: Medipress, 1994.

Qigong: The Secret of Youth. Jwing-Ming Yang. Boston: YMAA Publication Center, 2000.

The Way of Qigong: The Art and Science of Chinese Energy Healing. Kenneth S. Cohen and Bonnie J. Curnock. New York: Random House, 1999.

SOUND THERAPY

Sound and music can have a very powerful effect on one's health. Sound therapy is used in hospitals, schools, corporate offices, and psychological treatment programs as an effective treatment to reduce stress, lower blood pressure, alleviate pain, overcome learning disabilities, improve movement and balance, and promote endurance and strength.

THE ABILITY OF sound and music to heal has been recognized for thousands of years. The writings of Pythagoras and Plato in ancient Greece, the soothing harp music of young David in the Bible, and the chanted hymns of the Vedas in India, all recognize the healing power of sound. In modern times the therapeutic power of sound was medically noted as early as 1896, when doctors discovered that a young boy's brain, partially exposed due to an accident, responded differently when various types of music were played. Certain music increased cerebral and peripheral circulation, while other music stimulated mental lucidity.[1]

Because the ear is not only the primary organ of hearing, but also has powerful influences on eye movement, the rhythms of the physical body, pre-birth brain growth, and general regulation of stress levels in the body, greater emphasis is now placed on the therapeutic union of sound and healing.

Recently, much attention has been placed on the negative aspects of sound, either from music played too loudly or from exposure to the hard noise of industrial machinery. "Calling noise a nuisance is like calling smog an inconvenience," states William H. Stewart, former U.S. Surgeon General, who suggests that "noise must be considered a hazard to the health of people everywhere."[2] Accordingly, one study found that more than 60% of incoming college freshmen have impaired hearing in high frequency ranges due to prolonged exposure to high auditory levels.[3]

How Sound Therapy Works

Sound therapists recognize that certain sounds can slow the breathing rate and create a feeling of overall well-being, while others can slow a racing heart, even soothe a restless baby. Sound can also alter skin temperature, reduce blood pressure and muscle tension, and influence brain-wave frequencies. Although some sounds (like ultrasonic waves) are beyond the range of the human ear, they can have a profound effect on health.

Defined as "oscillating energy waves within the audible range," sound originates and travels from one source to another as waves, each sound with its own velocity and intensity, and each with its own frequency, pitch, and wavelength. (Music is essentially a pleasurable sequence of sound waves.) The intensity of the vibration, or the loudness of sound, is measured in units called decibels. Although volume is a factor, it is not necessary that one be consciously aware of a sound for it to have an effect, because sound creates a response in the entire body, not just the ear.

People respond to sound vibrations in two main ways: via rhythm entrainment and resonance. "Rhythm entrainment describes the phenomenon whereby, in the presence of any external rhythmic stimulus, the natural rhythm of the heartbeat will be overridden and caused to pulse in sync with the sound source," according to Steven Halpern, Ph.D., of San Anselmo, California. This may be the rhythm of drums, or the rhythmic pulse of the music, or it may just be your refrigerator's motor. "Resonance refers to the physical phenomenon in which different frequencies of sound (different pitches) stimulate the body to vibrate in different areas. Typically, low sound resonates in the lower parts of the body and high sound resonates in the higher parts of the body."

Sound is linked to the physical body by the eighth and tenth cranial nerves. These carry sound impulses through the ear and skull to the brain. Motor and sensory impulses are then sent along the vagus nerve (which

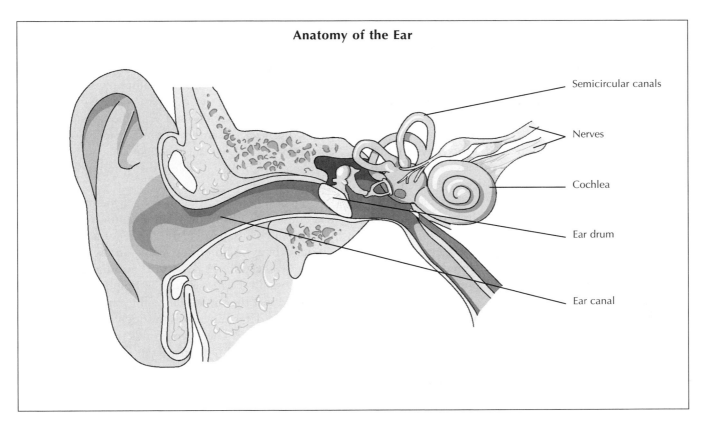

Anatomy of the Ear

Semicircular canals

Nerves

Cochlea

Ear drum

Ear canal

helps regulate breathing, speech, and heart rate) to the throat, larynx, heart, and diaphragm. According to Don G. Campbell, B.M.Ed., author of *The Mozart Effect*, "The vagus nerve and the emotional responses to the limbic system (specific areas of the brain responsible for emotion and motivation) are the link between the ear, the brain, and the autonomic nervous system that may account for the effectiveness of sound therapy in treating physical and emotional disorders."

> *The body has its own rhythmic patterns, and there is growing evidence that the rhythms of the heart, brain, and other organs enjoy a special synchronicity. Illness can arise when these inner rhythms are disturbed.*

Various elements of sound influence separate parts of the brain. Rhythm, for example, engages the hindbrain, while its tempo can alter the sense of time. The human body also has its own rhythmic patterns, and there is growing evidence that the rhythms of the heart, brain, and other organs enjoy a special synchronicity. Ill-

ness can arise when these inner rhythms are disturbed.[4] Tone engages the limbic midbrain, which governs emotion. According to Campbell, "The real power of sound is in the way the tonal or harmonic aspects influence our emotions and midbrain functions."

Sound can also be used to help the body regulate its corticosteroid hormone levels, helping to control the severity of spastic muscle tremors, reduce cancer-related pain, and reduce stress in heart patients.[5]

Auditory Integration Training

Alfred A. Tomatis, M.D., a French researcher and otolaryngologist, was one of the first to notice a strong interrelationship between hearing, the voice, and psychophysiological development. His early work explored the relationship between sounds in the womb and the development of the brain with regard to memory, language, and learning. Dr. Tomatis discovered a direct connection between hearing impairment and vocal range, and a direct connection between hearing impairment and overall health and well-being. The Tomatis Method is now practiced in approximately 250 listening centers in Europe and North America.

Dr. Tomatis discovered that sound acts as a form of brain nourishment and that the ears are designed to energize the brain. While the ear can hear over a wide frequency range, certain sounds can either stimulate or drain the brain of energy. The brain needs the ear to deliver it energy in the form of sounds. "What is important to remember is that the brain doesn't produce the energy," Dr. Tomatis said. "It captures it." He estimated that 80% of the energy that the brain needs is processed through the inner ear. High-frequency sounds energize the brain and charge us up, according to Dr. Tomatis, while low-frequency sounds drain energy away from it and wear us out.

In the early 1950s, Dr. Tomatis designed a system that duplicated how a mother's voice sounds to her unborn child. He then played this filtered voice to children with learning disabilities. In one case, a 14-year-old autistic boy who had not spoken since age four began to babble like a ten-month-old baby. From these experiments, Dr. Tomatis and his colleagues developed the Electronic Ear, a machine that simulates the stages of listening development, used to re-pattern the hearing range and the attention span.

The Electronic Ear is designed to exercise the muscles of the middle ear and improve the ear's response to all frequency ranges. Special headphones equipped with a bone-conduction transducer (to sense vibrations through the bone) deliver sound to the patient via a sophisticated stereo system linked to tuning and filtering components. As lower frequencies are filtered out, the proper auditory preference is introduced. Dr. Tomatis claims to be able to retrain the ear to stop blocking these frequency ranges of sound. Using the Electronic Ear, sound therapists have been able to teach those with dyslexia, autism, learning dysfunction, and attention deficit disorder how to focus and listen more effectively. The Tomatis Method also achieves excellent results with problems seemingly unrelated to the ear, such as post-traumatic stress disorder (PTSD), depression, chronic fatigue, head trauma, motor skill problems, and anxiety disorders. Others have improved their creative skills, musical ability, foreign language learning ability, and organizational skills using the Tomatis Method.

Billie M. Thompson, Ph.D., Director of the Sound, Listening, and Learning Center, in Phoenix, Arizona, used the Electronic Ear as part of her treatment for a hypersensitive six-year-old autistic girl who did not speak and who wore a ski cap 24 hours a day to limit outside stimulation. After three days using the device, the girl discarded her cap and went out to a restaurant with her family for the first time. She also went to church and heard an organ without having to leave in pain. Although she still does not speak more than a few words, she is more social now, participating in many of the family's activities, and no longer retreating into the corner in fear of sound.

While the Electronic Ear is currently being used in treatment centers throughout North America, it is only one aspect of the Tomatis method of treatment, according to Dr. Thompson. "As the ear opens, the individual becomes more receptive and responsive to sound and more motivated to communicate," she says. "By retraining the ear, people of all ages profoundly improve how they learn and relate to others, as we are creatures of movement, rhythm, and sound. With the ear as a key integrator, organizer, and analyzer of information, sound therapy can profoundly enhance thought and communication skills and can make possible a vastly enhanced level of listening."

According to Dr. Tomatis, longer mental and physical endurance can result from listening to Mozart or Gregorian chants, particularly the recordings from the French Abbey of Solesmes. Using an oscilloscope, he measured the Abbey's dawn and midnight masses for Christmas and the masses for the Epiphany and Easter. He found that the sounds fell within the bandwidth he had already determined was uniquely suited for energizing purposes. "There are sounds that are as good as two cups of coffee," Dr. Tomatis says. "If I have a long job to do, I always put on Gregorian chants, because it enables me to remain charged without difficulty."[6]

There are sounds that are as good as two cups of coffee.
—ALFRED TOMATIS, M.D.

Audiotapes based on Dr. Tomatis's work contain enhanced high-frequency sounds that support and enliven the upper register sound of the listener.

Guy Berard, M.D., a French physician, developed a method of retraining, similar to that of Dr. Tomatis, that concentrates on patients who are hypersensitive to high-frequency sounds or who suffer from loss of normal frequency hearing. Often this hypersensitivity can result in behavioral and cognitive problems when certain frequencies are perceived in a distorted manner.

Dr. Berard uses a device called the Ears Education and Retraining System (EERS), which reduces hypersensitivity by optimally allowing all frequencies to be heard with the same comfort and clarity. This device takes music from a sound source (audiotape or compact disc) and filters out the frequencies to which the patient has shown hypersensitivity. The EERS then electronically modulates these frequencies and returns them via headphones to the ears. Dr. Berard has found that after about ten hours of listening to these processed sounds, the listener makes significant progress toward accepting that frequency.

USING MUSIC TO HEAL: SEPARATING FACT FROM MYTH

"The body heals itself most effectively in a state of deep relaxation and using music is one of the simplest and most effective ways to evoke the 'relaxation response'," says Steven Halpern, Ph.D., a pioneering researcher and composer in the sound therapy field. "Studies have shown that music can reduce stress, enhance immune function, balance brain-wave activity, reduce muscle tension, increase endorphin levels, and trigger feelings of inner peace."

However, you must choose the right music to get the right results. Most music is composed for entertainment, dancing, or emotional release, and it excites the nervous system. There is a time and place for this kind of music, but it won't help you reduce stress. According to Dr. Halpern, this has to do with our mental response to music, what he terms our *anticipation response*.

"We have been culturally conditioned to follow melodic, harmonic, and rhythmic patterns in music," he notes. "When we listen to most compositions, we are subconsciously hooked into following the structure and projecting that structure into the future. This projection is the anticipation response." In workshops, Dr. Halpern demonstrates this by singing the first seven notes of a major scale—do, re, me, fa, so, la, ti. "Then I pause to watch people hold their breath or to hear them sing the last note of the scale. They feel the stress that their expectations engender in their minds and bodies and they feel compelled to complete the scale." This dynamic of tension and resolution is the basis for most classical compositions and precisely why such music is generally unsuitable for evoking the relaxation response in most people.

Another factor that can interfere with the listener's ability to relax while listening to music is the intent behind its creation or performance, according to Dr. Halpern. "The state of being of the composer or performer affects the experience of the listener. It's not just the notes, but what comes through, since music is a carrier for consciousness."

Dr. Halpern adds that, when it comes to music, one size does not fit all, which is true even of classical music. "Despite what you might have read, the research does not prove as much as you may have been led to believe. To declare that 'Mozart makes you smarter' or that Mozart's music or Baroque music is the best music for health is a disingenuous position at best and not what the original researchers claimed. The headlines ignore several critical details: Which composition? Recorded by which performer? Making a generic recommendation is basically meaningless. It's like saying vegetables are good for you, without considering if they are fresh or week-old and wilted."

Dr. Halpern cites recent research that found, in deep states of relaxation or meditation, the electromagnetic field surrounding the head "entrains and attunes to the basic electromagnetic field of the Earth itself." This attunement may be the key to understanding how music heals. For inducing relaxation, Dr. Halpern prefers music he describes as "free-flowing soundscapes that invite you to be in the 'hear and now' rather than waiting for the other musical shoe to drop." Ultimately, he recommends that people learn to tune in to their own inner wisdom when selecting music for healing purposes. "Pay attention to your own feelings," he says, "and take responsibility for how you respond to what you listen to."

One of Dr. Berard's patients was an 11-year-old autistic girl who suffered from both a hypo- (low) and hyperacute (high) sense of hearing. Over the course of 20 half-hour sessions using the EERS, Dr. Berard was able to decrease the hyperacute points of the girl's hearing while bringing the deficits up, thus creating a more normal hearing pattern. This also helped correct the girl's dyslexia, attention deficit, and hyperactivity, and today she is a happily married college graduate, working on a research project to help autistic adults.

BioAcoustics

Meaning "life sounds," BioAcoustics™ was developed by Sharry Edwards, M.Ed., Founding Director of the

Sound Health Research Institute, in Athens, Ohio. "Bio Acoustics can most aptly be described as a cross between music therapy and biofeedback," Edwards explains. "It is related to music because specific combinations of sounds are used, but not necessarily sounds that would be considered musical. Biofeedback comes into play as low frequency sounds are presented to elicit specific biological and emotional responses."

 See Biofeedback Training and Neurotherapy.

The principles of BioAcoustics originated with the idea that the brain perceives and generates impulse patterns that can be measured as brain-wave frequencies. These impulses are, in turn, delivered to the body by way

of nerve pathways. Based on her research, Edwards theorizes that these frequency impulses serve as directives that sustain the body's structural and biochemical integrity and maintain emotional equilibrium.

BioAcoustics uses voice spectral analysis to identify and interpret the complex frequency interactions that constantly occur within the body. "The frequencies contained in the vocal patterns provide a holographic representation of the body and its energy patterns," Edwards says. "BioAcoustics seeks to influence the systems within the body that produce, interpret, and use those frequencies in order to create and maintain sound health. My research shows that the body requires a full range of harmonious frequencies working cooperatively in order for health to exist. If even one note is out of tune, as it were, the result is discordant."

Edwards began her research into BioAcoustics as a result of the unusual healing and vocal abilities with which she was born. Audiological tests first conducted over 30 years ago confirmed the fact that Edwards is capable of hearing sounds beyond the normal range of human hearing and can vocally produce sine waves. This testing resulted in Edwards' first project, which revealed her ability to use her voice to control a person's blood pressure levels by as much as 32 points. This, in turn, led her to develop the technology to mechanically reproduce this technique, along with her instructional training program, which is used to certify others in the use of BioAcoustics. Today, approximately 3,000 people have taken her training nationwide, with about 40% of them medical practitioners who use BioAcoustics as a complement to their conventional or alternative therapies.

According to Edwards, BioAcoustics voice spectral analysis can detect hidden or underlying stresses in the body that are expressed as disease. "The vocal print can identify toxins, pathogens, and nutritional supplements that are too high or low, muscles that are weak or strong, and the root cause of disease symptoms," Edwards says. "In addition, it can be used to match the most compatible treatment remedy with each patient." The introduction of low frequency sound to the body, as indicated through vocal analysis, has been shown to control pain, body temperature, heart rhythm, and blood pressure, regenerate body tissues, and alleviate the symptoms of a broad variety of diseases (in some cases, even those that are considered to be incurable).

More recently, microscopic observation has shown that BioAcoustics technology is able to dissolve the ringed protein barrier used by certain pathogens, such as yeast, *Chlamydia pneumoniae,* and the Epstein Barr virus, to avoid detection by the immune system. Once this protective barrier is dissolved, the immune system's white blood cells quickly become activated to attack

and consume the pathogens. Based on such results, Edwards foresees BioAcoustics being used to deal with the rise of such microorganisms and the conditions associated with them. "It has potential in the eradication of such diseases as chronic fatigue, influenza, and HIV," she says, "and it can also help in the fight against antibiotic-resistant pathogens."

BioAcoustics has also been shown to be effective as a predictive diagnostic tool even when patients appear to be symptom-free. As an example of this, Edwards recalls the case of a man who came to her out of curiosity, wondering what BioAcoustics could reveal about his physical condition. "After I gave him a tour of our facility, I analyzed his voice," Edwards recounts. "His vocal print revealed that he might have a serious thyroid problem even though he had no medical history or evidence of that condition. Just to be sure, I suggested that he visit his physician, which he did. The laboratory results taken a few days later indicated nothing abnormal, so both he and his physician dismissed BioAcoustics as having inherent shortcomings. Nine days later, he collapsed with a set of mysterious symptoms that stumped his doctors. His heartbeat was erratic, he was sweating profusely, and was anxious and disoriented. Only after he remembered his vocal test and requested further testing of his thyroid did his physicians find that he indeed had a serious thyroid condition, which was causing his symptoms. BioAcoustics revealed that his thyroid was in stress nine days prior to any physical symptoms or lab results."

The sounds used in BioAcoustics are created by frequency generating and filtering equipment, which patients listen to either in a sound room or through headphones. Depending on the symptoms, treatment can be either short- or long-term, Edwards says. In most cases, reassessment, monitoring, and program adjustment is essential for continued improvement.

Among the conditions for which BioAcoustics has shown benefit are chronic illnesses, such as arthritis, heart disease, diabetes, emphysema, gout, and hypertension; musculoskeletal disorders, including physical trauma, muscle sprains and strains, osteoporosis, sports injuries, and temporomandibular joint (TMJ) syndrome; neurological conditions, including cerebral palsy, multiple sclerosis, Parkinson's disease, and senility; and psychological disorders, such as anxiety, psychosis, attention deficit disorder (ADD), and learning disorders. Edwards is in the process of developing computerized techniques to further improve the BioAcoustics technology, in the hopes that this procedure will become a routine part of preventative and diagnostic health care just like blood work or pulse taking.

Toning

For nine years, the Institute for Music, Health, and Education, in Boulder, Colorado, founded by Don Campbell, has researched and trained students to use toning (making elongated vowel sounds and allowing them to resonate through the body) as a simple way to release stress, balance the mind and body, improve the ear's ability to listen, and improve the speaking and singing voice.

"Toning is the art of making elongated vowel sounds and sensing where they internally vibrate," Campbell explains. Toning causes the brain waves to synchronize and balance within three to five minutes, and this greatly influences the sense of physical and emotional well-being. "Specific areas of the brain are tuned to specific tone frequencies," Campbell adds. "The pitch of the vowel sound determines where it will resonate in the brain."

According to Campbell, toning brings more benefit than singing or speaking, because singing and speaking move the vibratory epicenters so quickly there is no time for the body to balance itself with the sound. To sound the voice through toning is to massage ourselves internally. There is no other way to localize oxygenation, energy flow, and pulsation noninvasively within such a short period of time.

A voice with good timbre and rich overtones will recharge the individual each time it is used, according to Dr. Tomatis. For example, in the 1970s, when he was asked to investigate why monks in a certain French Benedictine monastery had become depressed, tired, and physically uneasy, Dr. Tomatis learned they had abandoned their former habit of chanting in Latin nine times a day. He recommended they resume their chanting. When they did, their energy increased and their depression and fatigue disappeared.

Therapeutic Uses of Sound Therapy

Today, sound has been incorporated into many types of therapeutic settings, including hospital surgery, recovery, and birthing wards, as well as for a variety of physical and psychological conditions.

In the Hospital

Music in hospitals is increasingly being employed due to its ability to reduce pain in surgical, dental, obstetrical, and gynecological procedures. When music therapy is introduced, patients view their hospitalization more positively, report reduced physical discomfort, and experience improvement in mood. Ralph Spintge, M.D., Executive Director of the International Society for Music in Medicine, in Germany, has completed a study of nearly 90,000 patients in the peri- and post-operative phases of surgery. Ninety-seven percent of the patients said music during their recovery helped them relax. Other patients found that music enabled them to get by with less anesthesia. Soft, tonal music was found to be especially effective. Patients who listened to slow Baroque or classical music a few days before surgery, then had it filtering through the recovery room, found that the music minimized postoperative disorientation.[7] Researchers at the Bethesda Naval Medical Center have found that listening to music reduced anxiety in men undergoing sigmoidoscopy compared to control subjects who underwent the same procedure, which involves the passage of a tube through the rectum and into the colon in order to detect cancer and other colorectal disorders.[8]

Abuse

Music therapists who work with victims of domestic violence have found that music can be used to restore the victim's often lost sense of self that can follow such abuse. One survey of 80 therapists who worked with abuse victims found that when their clients (battered women and children) were encouraged to sing songs, chant, and play musical instruments (especially woodwinds, which can enhance respiratory function), they experienced a general sense of improved well-being and greater levels of self-esteem. What made their findings more remarkable is that 75% of the women and 50% of the children suffered from drug problems prior to beginning music therapy.[9]

Attention Deficit Hyperactivity Disorder

Researchers studied 19 children, seven to 19 years old, who were diagnosed with attention deficit disorder (ADD) or attention deficit hyperactivity disorder (ADHD), as they listened to Mozart recordings three times a week during neurofeedback sessions. The researchers reported that the students reduced their theta brain waves in rhythm to the beat of the music and exhibited better focus, mood control, and social skills. Among the children who benefited from this form of music therapy, 70% were found to have maintained their improvement when seen for a follow-up exam six months later.[10]

The Tomatis Method is effective in treating ADHD, according to Pierre Sollier, M.F.C.C., who uses it in his practice as a licensed marriage, family, and child counselor in Lafayette, California. One of Sollier's cases involved an 8-year-old boy who came to him exhibiting all the classical signs of ADHD. During their first session together, the boy fidgeted in his chair, constantly interrupted the conversation with irrelevant questions, and was unable to focus on what he was asked to do. According to his parents, the boy was also "terribly behind" in school, was frequently forgetful, became quickly upset whenever he was frustrated, and showed signs of becoming a bully.

Sollier started the boy on a 15-day program of Tomatis instruction, advising his parents to look for "windows of attention" that might be longer than usual, rather than expecting an overnight miracle. By the end of the initial training, the boy's parents reported that they believed he was paying better attention. He was also acting more obediently and was more punctual in turning in his homework assignments. After a three-week break, the boy returned to Sollier to begin another Tomatis session that lasted eight days. Prior to beginning it, his parents stated that his attention span had continued to improve, he was now doing his homework without supervision, and for the first time in his life he seemed able and eager to express his feelings to them.

Following the second training session, the boy's listening and comprehension skills further improved, as did his sensory integration, which was demonstrated by his performance on the baseball field. In addition, he was now able to recount his daily activities to his parents when they sat down for dinner. According to his mother, it was as if he had awakened from being lost in a world of his own to finally being present with his family.

One month later, the boy began his final eight-day instruction in the Tomatis Method. Upon its completion, his self-image and confidence were noticeably improved. "He could focus his attention, perceive sounds, and reproduce them clearly," Sollier says, "and he made rapid progress in reading and writing. His school teacher noticed his improvement too, referring to him academically as a different child who had almost caught up with his peers."

Cancer

Music therapy along with guided imagery has been shown to reduce nausea and vomiting caused by chemotherapy. Music therapy has also proven useful in the rehabilitation of cancer patients recovering from surgery, resulting in improved motor skills and greater patient self-esteem.[11] In a study at the Ireland Cancer Center, 19 children with cancer who participated in one 30-minute session of music therapy exhibited improved immune function, as evidenced by an increase in immunoglobulin A (IgA) levels, while in a control group of 17 children, IgA levels decreased.[12]

Cerebral Palsy

In a study conducted in 1982, six adult patients with cerebral palsy received 25-minute sound therapy sessions three times a week over a five-week period. During each session, relaxing music was played in conjunction with biofeedback training. When biofeedback training was used alone, the patients exhibited an average 32.5% decrease in muscle tension. But when it was combined with music therapy, average muscle relaxation rates doubled to 65%.[13]

Childhood Learning and Socialization

The Tomatis Method has emerged as a highly successful means of helping schoolchildren eliminate the obstacles to learning. Recently, the Toronto Listening Center, a major Tomatis Method facility in Canada, analyzed the benefits of the Tomatis Method for 400 children following a six-month treatment program. The results, based on answers from both children and parents, showed that 95% of the children benefited. Specifically, attitudes toward school and motivation to learn improved by 87%; achievements in school were up by 90%; reading skills and comprehension increased by 83%, as did relationships with family members and peers; and attention span improved by 86%. In addition, after six months, 83% of the children maintained the gains or continued to make further improvements.

In a study of how music affects the socialization process, 12 handicapped children, three to five years old, were engaged in a music program alongside 15 four-year-old preschoolers without disabilities. The children interacted once a week for eight months, during which time they listened to music as they went about their other activities. By the end of the study, interaction between all of the children had increased from 69% to 93%. More significantly, the handicapped children who chose partners from the other group increased from 7% to 46%, indicating that music makes it easier for students with disabilities to interact with other children.[14]

In Psychotherapy

As early as the 1950s, medical research showed that music can evoke a range of emotions from sadness to joy and can be used to moderate feelings of anger or depression.[15] When music is enhanced by imagery, one's moods and physical sensations can alter rapidly. Recent experiments by Stanislav Grof, M.D., Jean Houston, Ph.D., and Helen Bonny, Ph.D., all show how music helps to deepen many aspects of the therapeutic process. A combination of music, imagery, and breathing can not only bring about a strong emotional release, but can tap into realms of the unconscious that only the most powerful of drugs have been able to access.

Dr. Bonny, former Director of Music Therapy at the Catholic University of America, in Washington, D.C., had used music to facilitate psychotherapy, but began using music to heal herself when she developed heart disease. From her work, Dr. Bonny developed a technique called Guided Imagery and Music (GIM). GIM involves listening in a relaxed state to selected music, a programmed tape, or live music in order to elicit mental imagery, symbols, and deep feelings arising from the deeper conscious self, she says. GIM is used in conjunction with psychotherapy for neurotic patients and as a way to lessen pain and anxiety and explore consciousness in mentally healthy people.

Dr. Berard has found that music therapy can be extremely effective in treating depression, including cases involving suicidal tendencies. One of Dr. Berard's patients was a 16-year-old who was chronically depressed, had exhibited suicidal tendencies since she was five, and had twice tried to kill herself. Neither medical specialists nor strong psychiatric medication had been able to help her. Taking her audiogram (electronic hearing profile) using the EERS device, Dr. Berard found that she was hypersensitive to sounds at 2,000 hertz and 8,000 hertz in her left ear. According to Dr. Berard, such a 2-8 curve is characteristic of suicidal patients, and the deeper the curve is, the more self-destructive the patient is likely to be. Moreover, the absence of strength in the 3,000-7,000 hertz range is often indicative of depression. At the end of 14 listening sessions using the EERS, the girl displayed a drastic change in temperament, becoming more communicative and taking an interest in her appearance. Two years later, a subsequent audiogram showed that her listening and emotional state had returned to normal.

In his book *Hearing Equals Behavior,* Dr. Berard writes that he has treated 233 depressed patients with suicidal tendencies using sound therapy. The results are impressive: 217 (93%) patients were cured after a single course of treatment; 11 patients were cured after two to three treatments, and only five patients showed no improvement.[16]

Headaches

Music therapy can be useful in treating headaches and migraines. Psychologist Janet Lapp, of California State University, trained migraine sufferers to use music imagery and relaxation during two 30-minute, twice-weekly sessions over a five-week period. At the end of the training, they experienced 83% fewer headaches over the next year (and when they did have headaches, they were less severe and not as long lasting). Lapp's trainees also discovered that music could prevent the start of severe headaches. In a Polish study of 408 patients who suffered from intense headaches and neurological disorders, subjects who listened to concert music for six months needed less medication, including painkillers, compared to subjects in a control group.[17]

Hypertension and Stroke

In a study conducted by the University of South Carolina involving 20 coronary patients, it was found that listening to relaxing music helped lower blood pressure levels. Among the patients, music therapy reduced systolic blood pressure levels (from a mean of 124.3 to 118.6), diastolic pressure (78.8 to 75.7), heart rate (from 91.2 to 89.6), and mean arterial pressure (from 94.3 to 75.7). The patients experienced a decrease in anxiety and pain as well. Moreover, their positive shift in physical and emotional states outlasted the therapy itself.[18]

Researchers in Colorado found that, by using rhythmic auditory stimulation for 30 minutes a day for three weeks, they were able to improve cadence, stride, and foot placement among patients who had suffered a stroke. The therapy employed the use of metronome pulses embedded in music of the patient's choice, which was recorded onto audiotapes and listened to with headphones. After the study was completed, the health benefits continued, suggesting that the entrainment effect of the embedded pulses, combined with the music itself, helped strengthen the normal mechanisms in the brain that are typically damaged by stroke.[19]

In Dentistry

For more than 50 years, the healing properties of music have been implemented in dentistry and oral surgery. Wallace Gardner, D.M.D., of Boston, Massachusetts, asserts that loud, stimulating music effectively alleviated pain in 65% of his patients, and a study found that sound stimulation was the only analgesic agent required in 90% of the 5,000 dental operations performed.[20] Additional research shows that due to the release of endorphins (the body's own natural painkillers), audio analgesia with dental patients is comparable in effectiveness to morphine.[21]

Insomnia

The University of Louisville School of Medicine conducted a survey of 25 elderly patients who suffered from sleeping difficulties. After they listened to New Age and Baroque music, all but one of the patients reported more restful sleep and some of the patients were able to discontinue the use of medication for insomnia.[22]

Pregnancy, Labor, and Birthing

The therapeutic application of music can be beneficial for the expectant mother who may be in a state of confusion during labor. Listening to music during the birth process often enhances feelings of comfort and security, and heightens self-esteem, socialization, and sense of personal control over the situation.[23]

The Tomatis Method has proven particularly useful to pregnant women. Researchers at the Vesoul Hospital, in France, found that pregnant women who underwent a month of training in the Tomatis Method spent less time in the hospital and experienced fewer complications during the births of their children. The study divided 50 women into three groups: the first group was given conventional prepartum preparation, the second group received no preparation at all, while the third group were trained in the Tomatis Method in the eighth month of their pregnancy. The Tomatis group experienced only a two-hour labor on average, in contrast to 3 ½ hours for the first group and four hours for the second group. There was also a marked difference in the need for cesarean sections. Only 4% of the Tomatis group required a cesarean, compared to 13% of the prepared group and 15% of the unprepared group. The Tomatis group also required less medication and reported less anxiety about childbirth.[24] In response to this and similar studies, many hospitals now make music therapy available as part of prenatal care.

Music therapy has also been shown to be effective for improving the survival rates of babies born prematurely. Birth weight is extremely important in the survival of such babies. In a study of 153 babies born prematurely, those who listened to Brahms' *Lullaby* six times a day were able to go home an average of one week earlier than babies who did not receive music therapy. The music was shown to relax the babies and reduce crying and unnecessary movement, helping them to better utilize the energy they needed to survive.[25]

Alzheimer's Disease and Senile Dementia

Music therapy can be particularly helpful for patients suffering from Alzheimer's disease or senile dementia. Patients who cannot communicate verbally and are unable to initiate purposeful movement have an increased need for sensory and environmental stimulation that can tap into remote memory. Music and speech patterns (tone and rhythm) are very effective and are utilized not only to provide psychological comfort, but also to enhance communication in an older individual who may be withdrawn, depressed, or institutionalized.

Family members can be trained to improve communication with loved ones using a variety of methods to increase attentiveness, especially for those in the early phase of the disease. These include tapping the hand in rhythm with speech, reading poetry to music, and playing music that has language-based phrasing, such as the slow movement of a Baroque concerto. Music as a time-ordered art form can make music therapy sessions beneficial by helping to reorient patients who become distracted by the symptoms of Alzheimer's. For individuals in the final stages of the disease, music therapy frequently takes a palliative form and can be utilized to provide psychological comfort.

One study of elderly men and women hospitalized with senile dementia and probable Alzheimer's disease found that patients could remember material in songs that were sung dramatically more clearly than spoken material. Each session of the study lasted 20 minutes, and the patients recalled approximately 62% of the sung material compared to only 37% of words that were spoken. When patients were encouraged to sing, hum, or keep time with music, their retention rates increased to 75%. Though memory retention was short-lived, researchers concluded that singing can be an effective way to engage patients in meaningful communication.[26]

For the Dying

Therese Schroeder-Sheker is an academic musicologist who founded the field of music thanatology. Using voice and harp in a 20-year clinical practice, she reconstructed the medieval infirmary music once used within monastic medicine to comfort the dying. Her work has been successfully applied in numerous home, hospital, and hospice settings for the treatment of cancer, respiratory illnesses, and AIDS. This "musical-sacramental-midwifery," as Schroeder-Sheker calls it, is being used at St. Patrick Hospital and at the Mountain West Hospice, both in Missoula, Montana, as well as in other programs in the U.S. and Europe. This can be of great benefit to the person who is making the transition, as well as to their friends and relatives.

Other Conditions

According to Don Campbell, other conditions for which sound therapy has shown benefit include acute pain, aggressive and antisocial behavior, AIDS, allergies, autism, back pain, breathing difficulties (asthma), burns, chronic fatigue syndrome, colds, developmental delays, diabetes, Down syndrome, epilepsy, menopause, neuromuscular and skeletal disorders, obesity, paranoia, Parkinson's disease, rheumatoid arthritis, schizophrenia, substance abuse, tinnitus, toilet training, tooth problems, and trauma.

Instruments in Sound Therapy

An emerging field in sound therapy is the use of devices that utilize specific sound frequencies to achieve therapeutic benefits such as pain reduction or relaxation. Treatments with devices such as the Infratonic QGM and cymatic instruments are currently being used worldwide.

The Infratonic QGM: The Machine That Produces *Qi* Energy

Lu Yan Fang, Ph.D., a senior scientist at the National Electro Acoustics Laboratory, in Beijing, China, discovered that Qigong masters emitted from their hands high levels of waves called secondary sound. She constructed a machine that simulated this infratonic sound and tested it on over 1,100 hospitalized patients. Numerous therapeutic benefits were noted, including pain reduction, headache relief, increased circulatory functioning, muscular relaxation, alleviation of depression, and increased brain production of alpha waves.[27]

Her instrument, the Infratonic QGM, received awards of recognition from the China Ministry of Health and the National Committee for Traditional Chinese Medicine. In China, it is medically recognized as an effective pain management tool. In the U.S., it is approved by the Food and Drug Administration for use as a therapeutic massage device.

Cymatic Therapy

The word *cymatics* is derived from the Greek word *kyma*, which means "great wave," and was coined by the Swiss scientist Hans Jenny, a pioneering 20th-century researcher of the healing properties of sound. According to Peter Guy Manners, M.D., D.O., Ph.D., of Worcestershire, England, inventor of the Cymatic Applicator, cymatic therapy (unlike other sound therapies) is not applied through auditory channels, but directly through the skin, by using sound waves within the audible range to stimulate natural regulatory and immunological systems and to produce a near-optimum metabolic state for a particular cell or organ.[28]

"Every object, whether inanimate or alive, possesses a unique electromagnetic field that exhibits antagonistic, complementary (resonant), or neutral reactions when it interacts with other electromagnetic fields," explains Dr. Manners. Dr. Manners has been researching the relationship between resonate sound frequencies and health for over 30 years. He and other sound researchers have discovered that each cell and group of cells within the body's various organs and tissues possess their own individual sound frequency pattern and emit a vibration specific to this pattern. In addition, the body as a whole also contains an overall, composite sound frequency pattern that is as distinct as a person's fingerprints. When we are healthy, this resonate pattern is steady and constant (resonance may be defined as the frequency at which an object most naturally vibrates), whereas when illness occurs, a state of disequilibrium distorts this harmonic

pattern. Cymatic therapists use the Cymatic Applicator or other cymatic instruments to reestablish equilibrium in the body by transmitting resonant frequencies of sound into the body. These signals pass through healthy tissues, but reestablish healthy resonance in unhealthy tissues.

Dr. Manners has researched the signals given out by healthy tissues. By intercepting electrical messages transmitted via the central nervous system to individual cells, this research has allowed the coding of cymatic signals that cells understand. Each tissue has been given a harmonic factor (H-factor) according to the signal emitted. The Cymatic Applicator adjusts sound frequencies in order to induce beneficial stimulation, activation, and circulation when applied to the body, by direct contact with affected areas or by way of acupuncture meridians. Currently, over 800 sound frequencies are capable of being emitted by the Cymatic Applicator, making it useful for a wide range of disease conditions, including tumors, bruising (both internal and external), calcification, fracture, and bacterial and viral infections.

Cymatic therapy by itself does not heal. Rather, it stimulates the body's inherent ability to heal itself, without pain, surgery, or drugs. According to Dr. Manners, in the future, cymatic therapy will likely concentrate on the skin, peripheral nerves, and bones, since these are the areas capable of regeneration. It may also be useful in organ transplantation, balancing the resonance of the transplanted organ with that of the recipient.

Cymatic instruments have been used by nurses, chiropractors, osteopaths, and acupuncturists in the U.S. and worldwide for over three decades. Training is required to become a cymatic practitioner. Cymatic instruments produce no side effects and their only contraindication is for patients with pacemakers.

The Future of Sound Therapy

The emerging field of sound therapy recognizes that, through sound, people can help tune themselves to a more fundamentally healthy state of mind, body, and spirit. Sound instruments and systems, such as sound tables, auditory floors, brain-wave headsets, and numerous audiotapes and compact discs designed to manipulate brain waves, have also become more widely available during the past decade. "Instruments such as the Electronic Ear have already made great strides in treating patients, such as autistics, whose options were limited with other treatment methods," says Dr. Thompson.

At the same time, sound therapists who realize that the "listening" components (auditory and psychological) are unique for each individual are beginning to test the use of their voices as instruments for physical adjustments integrated with massage, guided imagery, and physical movement. Accordingly, many practitioners believe that sound waves will be elemental in the healing process of the future. Sound will not only be used for treatment, but perhaps also for the diagnosis and prescription of certain tones that can bring the patient's health back into balance.

Where to Find Help

For further information on music and sound therapy, contact:

American Music Therapy Association (AMTA)
8455 Colesville Road, Suite 1000
Silver Springs, Maryland 20910
(301) 589-3300
Website: www.musictherapy.org

The AMTA is an association for music therapists that provides publicity for music therapy; publishes a journal, books, and videotapes on music therapy; accredits schools; and sponsors a national annual conference.

The Chalice of Repose Project (CORP)
St. Patrick's Hospital
312 E. Pine Street
Missoula, Montana 59802
(406) 542-0001 ext. 2810
Website: www.saintpatrick.org

CORP is a nonprofit, seven-institution medical and educational cooperative that is housed at St. Patrick's Hospital in Missoula, Montana. Offering three degree programs, it is a palliative medical teaching and clinical organization that conducts research, publishes, holds conferences, certifies music thanatologists, and trains 25 resident music thanatology interns each year.

Georgiana Institute
P.O. Box 10
137 Davenport Road
Roxbury, Connecticut 06783
(860) 355-1545
Website: www.georgianainstitute.org

Provides education, workshops, consulting, and information on the Berard method.

Inner Peace Music
P.O. Box 2644
San Anselmo, California 94979
(800) 909-0707
Website: www.innerpeacemusic.com

Provides information about the healing power of sound and music, as well as the research and musical recordings of Dr. Steven Halpern.

Mid-Atlantic Training Institute
P.O. Box 414
Saverna Park, Maryland 21146
(410) 757-9719

This organization teaches the GIM method. Provides a training program with internship, as well as 15 programs taught internationally. GIM is also taught in three universities and accredited through the American Music Therapy Association.

Mozart Effect Resource Center
3526 Washington Avenue
St. Louis, Missouri 63103
(800) 721-2177
Website: www.mozarteffect.com

This organization continues the research compiled by Don Campbell in his book of the same name.

Sound, Listening and Learning Center
2701 East Camelback, Suite 205
Phoenix, Arizona 85016
(602) 381-0086
Website: www.soundlistening.com

There are over 180 Tomatis Centers in Europe and now over a dozen in North and Central America that provide education, workshops, consulting, therapeutic sessions, and information on the Tomatis Method.

Sound Healers Association (SHA)
P.O. Box 2240
Boulder, Colorado 80302
(303) 443-8181
Website: www.healingsounds.com

SHA is a nonprofit organization dedicated to the research of sound therapy and the uses of sound and music as therapeutic and transformational tools.

Sound Health Research Institute, Inc.
P.O. Box 416
Athens, Ohio 45710
(740) 698-9119
Website: www.soundhealthinc.com

Directed by Sharry Edwards, M.Ed., developer of BioAcoustics, the Institute offers certification training in BioAcoustics, conducts research related to this technology, and provides BioAcoustic sessions to interested parties on an experimental basis.

Recommended Reading

The Conscious Ear. Alfred Tomatis. Tarrytown, NY: Station Hill Books, 1991.

Healing Imagery and Music. Carol Bush. Portland, OR: Rudra Press, 1995. (CD included)

Mind, Music, and Imagery. Stephanie Merritt. New York: Plume, 1990.

The Mozart Effect. Don Campbell. New York: Avon Books, 1997.

Music and Miracles. Don Campbell. Wheaton, IL: Quest Books, 1992.

MusicMedicine. Ralph Spintge, M.D. St. Louis, MO: MMB Music, 1992.

Music: Physician for Times to Come. Don Campbell. Wheaton, IL: Quest Books, 2000.

Sound Health. Steven Halpern, Ph.D. New York: Harper and Row, 1985.

Sound Choices. S. Mazer and D. Smith. Carlsbad, CA: Hay House, 1999. (CD included)

Sounds of Healing. Mitchell L. Gaynor. New York: Broadway Books, 1999.

TRADITIONAL CHINESE MEDICINE

Traditional Chinese medicine is one of the world's oldest complete systems of holistic health care. It combines the use of medicinal herbs, acupuncture, food therapy, massage, and therapeutic exercise, along with the recognition that wellness in mind, body, and emotions depends on the harmonious flow of life force energy known as qi. Traditional Chinese medicine has proven effective for many conditions, including chronic degenerative diseases, cancer, infectious diseases, allergies, childhood ailments, heart disease, and AIDS.

TRADITIONAL CHINESE medicine (TCM) has been practiced for approximately 5,000 years and, at present, a quarter of the world's population makes use of one or more of its therapies, making it one of the most widely accepted forms of medicine. A complete system of medicine, TCM has been selected by the World Health Organization for worldwide propagation to meet the health-care needs of the 21st century.[1]

TCM's approach to health and healing is very different from modern Western medicine. TCM looks for the underlying causes of imbalances and patterns of disharmony in the body, and views each patient as being unique. Western medicine generally provides treatment for a specific illness, whereas traditional Chinese medicine addresses how the illness manifests in a particular patient and treats the patient, not just the disease. As Roger Hirsh, O.M.D., L.Ac., Dipl. NCCA, of Santa Monica, California, explains, "The conventional Western physician focuses predominantly on the pathogenic factor (the disease), rather than the response of the patient to the factor."

Fundamentals of Traditional Chinese Medicine

The philosophy of traditional Chinese medicine is preventive in nature and views the practice of waiting to treat a disease until the symptoms are full-blown as being

> *The philosophy of traditional Chinese medicine is preventive in nature and views the practice of waiting to treat a disease until the symptoms are full-blown as being similar to "digging a well after one has become thirsty."*

similar to "digging a well after one has become thirsty."[2] In line with this, TCM makes a point of educating the patient with regard to lifestyle so that the patient can assist in his or her own therapeutic process. The TCM practitioner educates the patient about diet, exercise, stress management, rest, and relaxation.

As traditional Chinese medicine views the human body as a reflection of the natural world—the part containing the whole—the TCM doctor thinks and speaks in analogies with nature. The flows of energy and fluids in the body are spoken of as channels and rivers, seas and reservoirs. A diagnosis might describe the body in terms of the elements—wind, heat, cold, dryness, dampness. Despite this poetic language, TCM is not a folk medicine but a comprehensive professional discipline, based on an alternative, complete system of thought.

The terms *yin* and *yang* are used by the TCM practitioner to describe the various opposing physical conditions of the body. These terms stem from a basic Chinese concept describing the interdependence and relationship of opposites. Much as hot cannot be understood or defined without first having experienced cold, *yin* cannot exist without its opposite *yang*, and *yang* cannot exist without *yin*. Together, the two complementary poles form a whole.

See Acupuncture, Qigong and Tai Chi.

Roger Jahnke, O.M.D., Chairperson of the National Qigong Association, explains that, when applying these concepts to the human body, "*yin* refers to the tissue of

The *yin/yang* symbol

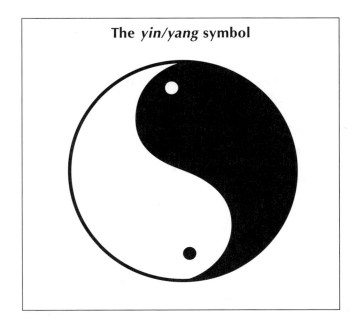

Acupuncture meridians

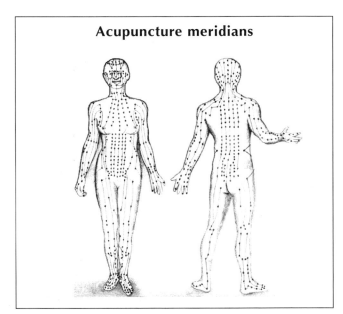

the organ, while *yang* refers to its activity. In *yin* deficiency, the organ does not have enough raw materials to function. In *yang* deficiency, the organ does not react adequately when needed."

These two conditions are forever connected, though, in a system of interdependence and interrelatedness, according to Maoshing Ni, D.O.M., Ph.D., L.Ac., President of Yo San University of Traditional Chinese Medicine, in Marina Del Rey, California. For example, says Dr. Ni, a *yin* deficiency in thyroid hormone levels, the raw material of the thyroid gland, would eventually cause a *yang* deficiency in the thyroid, as its function becomes impaired by the lack of hormones. Likewise, poor thyroid function, a *yang* deficiency, would eventually result in a *yin* deficiency, as the gland's output of hormones decreased.

Traditional Chinese medicine also introduces a major component of the body, *qi* (see Quick Definition), which Western medicine does not even acknowledge. *Qi*, according to Dr. Ni, is difficult to define. "We call it life force and it is all-inclusive of the many types of energy within the body and is essential for life itself," he says. This vital life energy flows through the body following pathways called meridians.

The meridians flow along the surface of the body and through the internal organs, with each meridian being given the name of the organ through which it flows, such as "Liver" or "Large Intestine." Organs can be accessed for treatment through their specific meridians, and illness can occur when there is a blockage of *qi* in these channels. Therefore, it is essential in traditional Chinese medicine to keep the *qi* flowing in order to maintain health. The healthy individual has an abundance of

qi flowing smoothly through the meridians and organs. With this flow, the organs are able to harmoniously support each other's functions.

 Qi (pronounced CHEE) is a Chinese word variously translated to mean "vital energy," "essence of life," and "living force." In Chinese medicine, the proper flow of *qi* along energy channels (meridians) within the body is crucial to a person's health and vitality. There are many types of *qi*, classified according to source, location, and function (such as activation, warming, defense, transformation, and containment). Within the body, *qi* and blood are closely linked, as each is considered to flow along with the other. *Qi* may be stagnant (non-moving), deficient (partially absent), or excessive (inappropriately abundant) from a given organ system. *Qi* has two essential qualities: *yang* (active, fiery, moving, bright, energizing) and *yin* (passive, watery, stationary, dark, calming).

Five Phase Theory

The interrelationship of the organs is another important concept in traditional Chinese medicine. Ten organs are arranged into a system that places each in one of five categories: fire, earth, metal, water, and wood. This system, called the Five Phase Theory, is based on the premise that each organ either nourishes or inhibits the proper functioning of another organ, just as the basic elements also act either adversely or beneficially on each other. "The Chinese have, for thousands of years, watched how things worked around them in order to understand why things happen, why things transform from one thing to

ELEMENT	*YIN* ORGAN	*YANG* ORGAN
Fire	Heart	Small intestine
Earth	Spleen	Stomach
Metal	Lungs	Large intestine
Water	Kidneys	Bladder
Wood	Liver	Gallbladder

another," says Dr. Ni. "They've taken this same conceptual model and applied it to the human body and found it really works well."

For example, as fire melts metal, so does the heart. The heart is associated with fire and controls the lungs, which are associated with metal. Likewise, as metal cuts wood, the lungs control the liver; as wood penetrates the earth, the liver controls the spleen; as the earth dams water, the spleen controls the kidneys; and as water quenches fire, the kidneys control the heart.

The organs are also divided up into two groups of *yin* and *yang* organs. "The heart, spleen, lungs, kidneys, and liver belong to the *yin* group, because they are what we call more substantial organs, more solid," explains Dr. Ni, "whereas the *yang* organs are hollow organs like the small intestine, stomach, large intestine, and bladder, where things just pass through; they're more functional. Remember, *yang* is function and action, and *yin* is more passive, solid, substantial—that's why they're categorized that way."

Dr. Ni adds that there is "a synergistic relationship in all the organs," as in all the elements, so the interactions are a little more complex when deciphering disease symptoms. "A patient came to me with stomach ulcers, for which the prescribed medication gave some relief but had a side effect, constipation. He took a laxative to deal with the constipation, but then he developed a cough and chronic bronchitis. The medication prescribed for the bronchitis also had a side effect, a urinary tract infection. He also developed lower back pain. Additional antibiotics for the urinary tract infection then caused liver problems, a congested feeling and pain. Finally, he became irritable, emotionally unbalanced, and had difficulty sleeping. This was the point at which he came to me.

"Deficiency in earth (stomach) led to deficiency in both metal organs (large intestine and lungs). As the metal organs weakened, it impacted the water organs (kidneys and bladder) and, in turn, affected wood (liver), then fire (heart)—so that all five organs became involved in the Five Phase Theory sequence. The original problem had been caused by excess stomach cold, due to *qi* deficiency. This had been caused by poor digestion of the raw foods diet he had adopted, but the subsequent problems were caused by the medication he had been taking. I took him off the medication and treated him with acupuncture, herbs, and food therapy. After about 2 ½ months, he became healthy."

The Practice of Traditional Chinese Medicine

In treating a patient, a TCM practitioner first looks for patterns in the details of clinical observations of the patient. This allows the practitioner to discover the disharmony in the system of that individual. Familiar with symptoms that are standard to each disease, the doctor also considers what symptoms or behaviors would be especially telling to the individual patient. For example, some people are very active and constantly moving, even red in the face, yet these appearances may not indicate any malady. On the other hand, it is perfectly normal for others to exhibit slowness and inactivity. It is against this individual landscape that the TCM practitioner attempts to correctly assess the pattern of disharmony when an individual becomes ill.

In treating a patient, a TCM practitioner looks for patterns in the details of clinical observations of the patient. This allows the practitioner to discover the disharmony in the system of that individual.

A pattern may be so commonly associated with a certain treatment that the pattern and treatment carry the same name. But often the doctor must develop a strategy by carefully balancing many details. Stomach ulcers, for instance, may originate in very different patterns of disharmony, although the resulting ulcers may appear identical. Because the roots of the disease are diametrically opposed, each type of ulcer may require a very different type of treatment, and the wrong treatment could make things worse. "Yet, in Western medicine, ulcers are generally treated with whatever anti-ulcer medication there may be, without differentiating," says Dr. Ni. "What Chinese medicine does is decipher the response of the patient. How is the patient's body reacting to the illness, to the cause of the illness? It is these patterns that we seek to determine and then treat accordingly." Alternatively, people with different symptoms, but the same pattern of disharmony, can often be treated by the same medicines or therapies.

Methods of Diagnosis

A first-time patient, accustomed to Western medicine, may be surprised that TCM diagnosis does not require procedures such as blood tests, X rays, endoscopy (the inspection of the inside of a body cavity by an endoscope), or exploratory surgery. Instead, the TCM practitioner performs the following, noninvasive methods of investigation:

- Inspection of the complexion, general demeanor, body language, and tongue

- Questioning the patient about symptoms, medical history, diet, lifestyle, history of the present complaint, and any previous or concurrent therapies received

- Listening to the tone and strength of the voice

- Smelling any body excretions, the breath, or body odor

- Palpation (or feeling with the fingers) of the pulse at the radial arteries of both wrists (pulse diagnosis), the abdomen, and the meridians and/or acupuncture points

Through pulse diagnosis, a skilled practitioner can examine the strength or weakness of the *qi* and "blood," which in TCM includes lymph and other bodily fluids, and assess how these affect each of the organs, tissues, and layers of the body. The practitioner will also look at the impact of a wide range of personal and environmental factors. Mood, activity, sex, food, drugs, weather, and seasons of the year can each affect health and the healing process. "All these factors need to be weighed when making a diagnosis," states Dr. Hirsh, "but the presence of one factor doesn't always warrant a disease outcome."

Similarly, one diagnostic method will not always be able to adequately determine a pattern. The TCM practitioner will use these various diagnostic tools to crosscheck and amplify the other methods until the practitioner is certain that the pattern of disharmony is correctly determined.

Dr. Ni explains that what TCM practitioners try to do with all forms of diagnosis is look at illness in the body from the point of view of function. "Too much

---

TRADITIONAL CHINESE MEDICINE TODAY

Today, traditional Chinese medicine (TCM) is a synthesis of the best of China's scholastic and professional medicine, empirically proven and time-tested folk remedies, and modern technology. Since the early part of the 20th century, Chinese doctors began to incorporate elements of modern Western medicine, including modern physiology, pharmaceutical medicines, and treatment and research protocols. In 1949, a special effort to update TCM began when the post-war communist Chinese government began to revise and unify its standards of practice in an effort to improve public health. National committees of the finest TCM doctors of every medical specialty compared the knowledge gained from their own experience. Seeking new ideas, researchers fanned out into the Chinese countryside to interview peasant healers. As a result, many new remedies were added to the repertoire of formally approved TCM treatments.

---

function or too little function—illness can really be simplified in this way," he says. "Either your body is not having enough of a substance or having too much of it in an illness. Or it is functioning too fast or too slowly. If you categorized the body in those simplistic terms, that's what illness is all about. For example, how do you get colds? In Chinese medicine, we recognize that you get colds because your body cannot adjust quickly enough to changes in the environment, such as cold weather. This allows the bacteria or virus, whatever it may be, to invade.

A TCM practitioner looks at the impact of a wide range of personal and environmental factors. Mood, activity, sex, food, drugs, weather, and seasons of the year can each affect the healing process.

"Because of this understanding, TCM treatment, unlike most Western medical practices, will not only treat the inevitable symptoms of the disease—in this case, the actual cold—but will also treat the underlying cause, the body's inability to adapt to change quickly enough to resist the invading microbes."

Treatments in Traditional Chinese Medicine

Historically, a Chinese doctor was known as someone who prescribed herbal medicine, but traditional Chinese medicine today incorporates a wide range of methods of treatment, including herbal medicine, acupuncture, dietary therapy, massage, and energy healing (Qigong).

Herbal Medicine: Herbs are still a primary part of TCM treatment. Chinese herbal prescriptions are generally comprised of a variety of ingredients—perhaps bark, roots, or oyster shell—derived from the vegetable, animal, and mineral kingdoms. The formulas may contain from six to 19 different substances and are assembled with great care. These are prescribed to treat the root of the disease and its manifestation, and the formula must also be balanced within itself. Although the herbs are usually taken internally as decoctions (herbs boiled in water), TCM doctors may also prescribe herbal pills, powders, syrups, tinctures, inhalants, suppositories, enemas, douches, soaks, plasters, poultices, and salves.

Astragalus *(Huang qi),* a popular Chinese herb, is an example of the various benefits the proper herbal remedy can play in TCM. Historically, astragalus has been used by TCM practitioners to strengthen the body's defensive *qi* against external pathogenic factors, thereby enchancing immunity. Modern research has confirmed astragalus is useful in this regard, showing that it increases both specific and nonspecific immunity, such as boosting production of white blood cells. Astragalus also potentiates the anti-tumor effect of chemotherapy drugs, while reversing drug-induced immune suppression.

"Research results with astragalus and many other Chinese herbs provide a scientific understanding of what each herb may do in the body," Dr. Ni says. "What defines mastery in traditional Chinese medicine, though, is the ability of the practitioner to formulate complex combinations of various herbs for a collective purpose. The herbal formulation is often different for every patient due to TCM's personalized objective. That is the beauty of traditional Chinese medicine—to tailor the treatment to each individual patient's needs."

Diet Therapy: The most basic element of TCM is diet therapy, which utilizes the concept of "healing foods." A large body of knowledge on the therapeutic properties of foods has existed for several millennia in China. "For the majority of the Chinese population, folk remedies employing functional foods is the first step to correcting their mind/body imbalances," Dr. Ni says. "Often, a competent practitioner of TCM will recommend a specific diet to the patient based on specific medical needs. In my own clinical practice, I would say most patients expe-

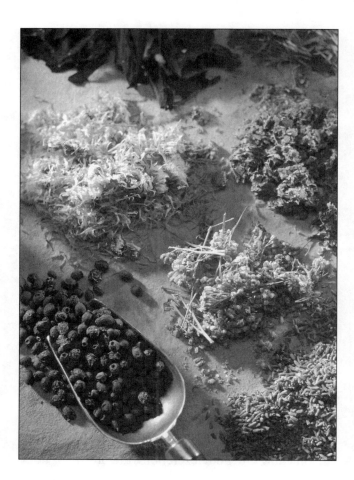

rience up to 50% relief of their medical problems just by making dietary changes alone."

Individual foods may also be part of the protocol. "What we do is learn about the healing properties of each food," says Dr. Ni. "For example, ginger is warming and pungent. It has a healing property of warming the stomach to dispel cold, arresting diarrhea, and settling the stomach from nausea. When you're armed with knowledge like this, then you can begin to apply a whole system, in a very systematic way, for recommending a particular diet to your patients that would assist in their recovery."

Dr. Ni recalls a patient who had been suffering from three weeks of excruciating hemorrhoid pain that his medical doctor felt could only be relieved through surgery. "He couldn't sit, he couldn't sleep, he couldn't walk, every position hurt him so badly," explains Dr. Ni. "In Chinese medicine, this condition is diagnosed as having spleen *qi* deficiency. In other words, his spleen energy was weak and so the rectum was prolapsing, causing hemorrhoids.

"Realistically, with acupuncture, we have to treat continuously every day or every other day for a week or two, but he lived far away and couldn't come in that often. So, I said go home and eat four yams a day. Within a week's time, his hemorrhoids completely disappeared

SUCCESS STORY: ACUPUNCTURE AND CHINESE HERBS STOP MENORRHAGIA

At the age of 45, Claire had an episode of heavy menstrual bleeding so severe that, after six days, she ended up in a hospital. There, after being hooked up to intravenous tubes and given iron supplements, she was told to make an appointment for a D & C (dilatation and curettage, minor surgery to scrape tissue from the uterine lining). However, Claire was terrified of even minor surgery and instead sought help from acupuncturist and herbalist Jason Elias, M.A., L.Ac., of Integral Health Associates, in New Paltz, New York.[4]

After feeling Claire's wrist pulses, which were weak, and looking at Claire's tongue, which was pale and bloated, Dr. Elias determined that Claire was deficient in life force energy or *qi*, particularly in the spleen and kidney organ systems. Claire had been experiencing increased stress in recent years. The stress hindered the smooth flow in the energy channels or meridians throughout her body. In particular, the channels that fed her liver, which circulate through the reproductive organs, were blocked or "stagnated," meaning the energy was not flowing freely. This depleted Claire's liver of energy and prevented it from doing its job of regulating blood flow during menses. The liver was unable to contain the blood and it gushed uncontrollably or, as the Chinese would say, "ran recklessly."

Dr. Elias urged Claire to go ahead with the D & C, just to rule out the possibility that the heavy bleeding could be caused by a serious disorder such as cancer, which a tissue sample from the D & C would reveal.

Through herbs and acupuncture, Dr. Elias would work to correct Claire's *qi* deficiency and "liver *qi* stagnation" and stop the heavy bleeding of her current period. In the first acupuncture session, he used eight acupuncture points, mostly on the legs, feet, and belly, to move energy and strengthen the liver, spleen, and kidney channels.

He also gave Claire a traditional Chinese herbal formula for heavy bleeding, Yunnan Pai Yao (Yunnan White Powder), which contains raw pseudoginseng root, among other ingredients.[5] Dr. Elias also gave Claire an herbal formula of dandelion, nettles, yellowdock, lady's mantle, and agrimony (shepherd's purse)—astringent, blood-coagulating, and iron-rich herbs to nourish the kidneys, liver, and blood. Nettles are particularly rich in nutrients: vitamins A, C, D, and K, calcium, potassium, sulfur, and iron.

Finally, Dr. Elias gave Claire the following lifestyle instructions to assist the herbs and acupuncture in rebalancing her body: avoid caffeine drinks, as caffeine inhibits the absorption of iron; avoid hot showers and baths, which dilate blood vessels and encourage bleeding; eliminate alcohol and aspirin, which thin the blood; and eat iron-rich foods such as spinach, kale, and seaweed. (Dr. Elias would have recommended calf's liver for its iron, B vitamins, and vitamin A content, but Claire was a vegetarian.)

Although dietary changes and the herbal formulas were adequate to correct Claire's nutritional deficiencies, other women with heavy bleeding may wish to use nutritional supplements. For them, Dr. Elias recommends Liquid Floradix Iron (a European herbal formula rich in iron and available at health food stores; follow dosage directions on bottle), beta carotene (25,000 IU daily), and vitamin C (1-5 g daily).

By the next day, Claire's heavy bleeding had stopped. Dr. Elias continued to work with Claire on the deeper underlying imbalances. He also helped her arrive at an understanding of the emotional significance of the bleeding. In her case, it was her blocked creativity trying to break through. Dr. Elias worked with her on taking steps to nourish herself and unblock her creative energy.

and the pain, of course, went away too. When he went back to his proctologist, he was told that hemorrhoids don't just go away, as severe as he had them, and that they wouldn't go away from eating yams. But I know that yams have a healing property for strengthening the spleen *qi* and, therefore, pulling the hemorrhoids back up because that was the cause of his hemorrhoids. I would not recommend yams for every hemorrhoid condition, because, again, in Chinese medicine, hemorrhoids may

have many different causes." This is an example of Chinese diet therapy, where foods are used for their therapeutic properties and not for mere enjoyment.

Acupuncture: Acupuncture is extensively used in traditional Chinese medicine. Using the meridian system and its thousands of corresponding surface points, acupuncture uses special needles placed strategically into these "acupoints" to help correct and rebalance the flow

THE STORY OF MR. HO

Li Shi-zhen, the Chinese doctor revered for reformalizing traditional Chinese medicine in the 17th century, told the story of Mr. Ho: "Mr. Ho was an old woodcutter, bent over with age. He lived alone in the forest, which was a good thing, because he could hardly cut wood anymore and had to forage for food to supplement his tiny income. One day, he came across a large tuber (which looked like a huge potato), scratched it out of the ground, and made a stew of it. This was all he had to eat for several days. But this was very lucky because, to his amazement, he found himself gradually standing up, having more energy and being able to chop more wood. Attributing this to the plant, he consumed it for several months and gained greater energy—so much that he attracted a young woman whom he married and soon they had several children. The tuber he found *(Polygonal multiflorum)* was named 'ho-shou-wu' in honor of Mr. Ho."

In Li Shi-zhen's story, the old woodcutter had kidney weakness, which gave rise to a weak lower back, poor sexual function, and the symptoms of old age. *Ho-shou-wu* helps these conditions and it is a major component of *sho-wu-chih*, a commercially prepared tea taken for health maintenance by millions of Chinese every day.

cises, and the laying on of hands are all incorporated into the overall Chinese medicine approach, as well as an emphasis on spiritual meditation.

"Clinical studies have shown that Qigong can improve the health of people suffering from different chronic medical problems that accelerate the aging process," Dr. Ni reports. Studies also demonstrate that a combination therapy of Qigong and drugs is superior to drug therapy alone, as reported for three medical conditions: hypertension, respiratory disease, and cancer. The results of such studies suggest that practicing Qigong exercises can favorably affect many functions of the body, permit reduction of the dosage of drugs required for health maintenance, and provide greater health benefits than the use of drug therapy alone.

For hypertensive patients, the combination of Qigong and drug therapy resulted in reduced incidence of stroke and mortality, and reduced the need for drugs required for blood pressure maintenance. Among asthma patients, the combination also permitted a reduction in drug dosages, as well as decreasing the need for sick leave, duration of hospitalization, and overall costs of therapy. For cancer patients who practiced Qigong, there was a lowered incidence of side effects commonly associated with conventional cancer care (chemotherapy and radiation).[3]

Conditions Treated by Traditional Chinese Medicine

Traditional Chinese medicine addresses the full range of human illness. While best known for treating chronic illnesses such as asthma, allergies, headaches, high blood pressure, gallbladder disease, lupus, diabetes, and gynecological disorders, TCM also treats acute, infectious illness. Extensive research is continuously being pursued in a wide range of TCM applications and reported in scores of medical journals published around the world.[6]

Research has also shown that TCM can effectively complement modern Western medicine when the two systems are used in concert for acute, chronic, or life-threatening diseases.[7] In China, a combination of TCM and modern Western medicine has been shown to be more effective for treating liver cancer than Western medicine alone.[8] TCM can also minimize the hazardous side effects of some Western medicines while reinforcing their positive therapeutic effects.

In his practice, Dr. Hirsh sees many patients in conjunction with Western doctors for infertility problems and is able to design acupuncture treatments that com-

of energy within the specific meridian, consequently relieving pain and/or restoring health. Moxibustion is also sometimes used, which is the burning of special "moxa" herbs on or above a specific acupoint.

Massage: Massage and manipulation are integral parts of the modern practice of TCM, including professional remedial massage therapies such as osteopathic and chiropractic adjustments. "There are many different massages in Chinese medicine," says Dr. Ni. "We have one massage called *Tui Na*, which is a combination of acupressure, massage, and manipulation." The purpose of massage is not dissimilar to acupuncture, in that the goal is to promote the flow of *qi* and to remove blockages, thereby alleviating any imbalances. Dr. Ni adds that massage is most often used in conjunction with other treatment therapies, such as acupuncture, particularly for musculoskeletal problems such as a sprains.

Energy Healing: Qigong, Tai Chi, and other therapeutic exercises are another aspect of TCM, particularly as a means of stress reduction and preventative therapy. Meditative relaxation, calisthenics, internal energy exer-

plement and support the other medical procedures. He frequently gives acupuncture treatment to women who have just been artificially inseminated, and he works with patients taking Clomid (a fertility drug) to help regulate the woman's fertility cycle. As Dr. Hirsh states, "Traditional Chinese medicine can increase the success rate of Western medicine and at the same time slow down the clock on a woman's aging endocrine system."

East Meets West: A Case History

What is known as hypertension in the West is called "liver fire" in TCM and can be successfully treated according to TCM principles. Dr. Wu, a famous physician in China, was visited by a 42-year-old man who had been diagnosed as having hypertension and the early stages of heart disease. He complained of throbbing temples and soreness at the top of his head. An examination identified the following elements: red (not pink) tongue, deep yellow urine, constipation, poor appetite, painful teeth and eyes, insomnia, pain on the right side of the body, and excessive dreaming. His pulse was "wiry and sinking." The man was diagnosed with "constrained liver *qi* accompanied by liver fire ascending to disturb the head."

The treatment called for harmonizing the liver, cooling the liver fire, and transforming mucus. Twelve herbs were given as a tea for three days and another combination for nine additional days. With this treatment, the patient's blood pressure dropped from 180/130 to 130/90, well within normal range, and soon all his symptoms disappeared. A final herbal prescription was then given, which was taken for a longer period of time to ensure that the patient's blood pressure remained normal.

The Future of Traditional Chinese Medicine

Traditional Chinese medicine is continually evolving. According to Dr. Hirsh, "I believe that diagnostic technology, advanced surgical procedures, electroacupuncture biofeedback testing, and modern homeopathy are aspects of Western tradition that can be integrated with TCM in order to create an 'Integral Chinese Medicine.'

"I see the need for a quantum leap in medical care. With Integral Chinese Medicine, we have a chance to make that leap. Here in America, we have the finest aspects of Western medicine. What we lack is a system of putting this technology together with other diagnostic and treatment techniques, and this is what TCM has to offer. We need to integrate our ability to identify pathogenic [disease-producing] factors with the therapeutic

principles that millions of Chinese practitioners have refined after treating billions of patients.

"The real advantage of Integral Chinese Medicine is that you are integrating this great technology with common sense thinking that has allowed the Chinese to evolve an affordable health-care system for over one billion people."

Where to Find Help

Traditional Chinese medicine is well suited to those looking for safe healing without side effects, answers to medical questions in everyday human terms, and involvement in and responsibility for their own healing. Western patients seeking to avail themselves of the benefits of TCM therapy should contact:

American Association of Oriental Medicine
433 Front Street
Catasauqua, Pennsylvania 18032
(888) 500-7999
Website: www.aaom.org

The AAOM is a national professional trade organization of acupuncturists who meet acceptable standards of competency and can provide you with the names and locations of local members.

American College of Traditional Chinese Medicine
455 Arkansas Street
San Francisco, California 94107
(415) 282-7600
Website: www.actcm.org

The ACTCM seeks to improve the quality of health care by providing graduate education and patient care, enabling students, patients, health-care professionals, and the public to integrate traditional Chinese medicine into their lives.

Recommended Reading

The American Association of Oriental Medicine's Complete Guide to Chinese Herbal Medicine. David Molony and Ming Ming Pan Molony. New York: Berkley Books, 1998.

Between Heaven and Earth: A Guide to Chinese Medicine. Harriet Beinfield, L.Ac., and Efrem Korngold, L.Ac., O.M.D. New York: Ballantine Books, 1992.

Chinese Herbal Medicine. Daniel P. Reid. Boston: Shambhala Publications, 1992.

Chinese Medicine for Maximum Immunity. Jason Elias and Katherine Ketcham. New York: Three Rivers Press, 1999.

The Complete Illustrated Guide to Chinese Medicine. Tom Williams. London: Thorsons Publishing, 1996.

Encounters with Qi. David Eisenberg, with Thomas Lee Wright. New York: W. W. Norton, 1995.

Healing with Chinese Herbs. Lesley G. Tierra. Freedom, CA: Crossing Press, 1997.

Tao of Nutrition. Maoshing Ni, D.O.M., Ph.D., L.Ac., and Cathy McNease. Santa Monica, CA: Seven Star Communications, 1993.

Tao: The Subtle Universal Law and the Integral Way of Life. Hua-Ching Ni. Santa Monica, CA: Seven Star Communications, 1993.

The Web That Has No Weaver: Understanding Chinese Medicine. Ted J. Kaptchuk. Chicago: Contemporary Books, 2000.

The Yellow Emperor's Classic of Medicine. Maoshing Ni. Boston: Shambhala, 1995.

YOGA

Yoga is among the oldest known health practices in the world, and research into yoga has had a strong impact on the fields of stress reduction, mind/body medicine, and energy medicine. The physical postures, breathing exercises, and meditation practices of yoga have been proven to reduce stress, lower blood pressure, regulate heart rate, and even retard the aging process.

YOGA, A SUBSET of Ayurvedic medicine, is a system of psychophysical exercises designed to integrate the physical, mental, and spiritual energies that enhance health and well-being. First systematically set down in writing by Patanjali in the second century B.C.E. in the *Yoga Sutras*, restoring mental and physical health.

Many of the original biofeedback studies at the Menninger Foundation, in Topeka, Kansas, were conducted on yogis (those adept in the practices of yoga). Their union of mind and body gave them control over functions ranging from thyroid output to heart rate. This first alerted medical doctors and scientists to the link between consciousness and physical functioning. Today, yoga is commonly practiced throughout the world and holds a prominent place in the emerging field of mind/body medicine.

See Ayurvedic Medicine, Biofeedback Training and Neurotherapy, Mind/Body Medicine.

The Eightfold Path of Yoga: A Complete System of Health

Classical yoga is organized into eight "limbs" that provide a complete system of physical, mental, and spiritual health, and outline specific lifestyle, hygiene, and detox-

Yoga teaches a basic principle of mind/body unity: if the mind is chronically restless and agitated, the health of the body will be compromised; and if the body is in poor health, mental strength and clarity will be adversely affected. The practices of yoga can counter these ill effects.

ification regimens, as well as physical and psychological practices, that can lead to a more integrated personal development. Yoga helps prepare one for heightened vitality in order to achieve its ultimate goal of spiritual awareness.

The first four limbs of yoga serve to bring the mind and body into harmony through specific postures and breathing exercises. Strong emphasis is also placed upon purification and detoxification of the body and various practices are encouraged, including bowel purification, enemas, nasal cleansing, and cleansing of the eyes. The practices mirror many of the lifestyle changes recommended today by alternative physicians and can be invaluable to maintaining one's health. The remaining four limbs of yoga deal with stages of meditation and advocate service to a "greater good."

Yogic Postures (*Asanas*)

The most widely known yogic practice is *asana*, or Hatha yoga. It includes a variety of physical postures and exercises that create immediate changes in the body. There are two main types of *asana*, meditative and therapeutic.

Meditative *asanas* improve the alignment of the spine and head, promote proper blood flow throughout the body, and instill a state of relaxation and stillness that facilitates increased concentration during meditation. They also help keep the glands, lungs, and heart properly energized.

Therapeutic *asanas*, such as the spinal twist and shoulderstand, are geared toward improving health and

ALTERNATE NOSTRIL BREATHING EXERCISE

The following exercise, known as *nadi shodhana* (purification of the channels), is a simple *pranayama* exercise that purifies the pathways along which *prana* flows through the body, balancing both the flow of breath and the flow of vital energy. *Nadi shodhana* should be practiced at least twice a day, in the morning and evening.

- Sit upright on a cushion or a firm chair with your head, neck, and body aligned. Breathe in a relaxed fashion from your diaphragm for three complete breaths. Inhalation and exhalation should be of equal length and should be slow, controlled, and free from sounds or jerks.

- Close your right nostril with the thumb of your right hand and exhale completely through your left nostril. At the end of the exhalation, close your left nostril with your right index finger and inhale through the right nostril.

- Repeat this cycle of exhalation with the left nostril and inhalation with the right nostril two more times, always making sure to maintain an equal inhalation and exhalation rate.

- At the end of the third inhalation with the right nostril, exhale completely through the same nostril while still keeping the left nostril closed.

- After the exhalation, close the right nostril and inhale through the left nostril. Repeat the cycle of the exhalation through the right nostril and inhalation through the left nostril two more times.

- Place the hands on the knees and exhale and inhale through both nostrils evenly for three complete breaths.

This completes one cycle of *nadi shodhana*. With practice, gradually lengthen the duration of the inhalation and the exhalation.

asana, to provide discipline, awareness, and a relaxed openness. The discipline and awareness help maintain the posture, and the relaxation and openness help stimulate the circulation of *prana* (life energy), allowing the person to fully experience the power and essence of the posture. According to the *Yoga Sutras*, a properly executed *asana* creates balance between movement and stillness—exertion and surrender—which is precisely the state of a healthy body. The practitioner learns to regulate autonomic functions like heartbeat and breath, while physical tensions fade into relaxation.

Breath Control (*Pranayama*)

Pranayama, meaning "regulation of *prana*," focuses on controlling the breath in order to enhance the flow of energy throughout the body. Yoga teaches that *prana* circulates throughout in the body in a system of 72,000 subtle nerves or *nadis*. When the flow of *prana* is interrupted through stress, improper diet, or toxins, one's physical, emotional, and mental health are affected. Chronic blockage of the flow of *prana* can eventually lead to illness. *Pranayama* exercises are designed to help prevent or remove these blockages.

Pranayama can help the practitioner to regulate previously unconscious bodily functions. It has been demonstrated that its practice can aid digestion, heart function, and a variety of physical ailments, and in one study conducted at City Hospital in Nottingham, England, it was found to be particularly effective in reducing the frequency of asthma attacks.[1]

Studies have demonstrated that the practice of pranayama *can aid digestion, heart function, and a variety of physical ailments, and in one study it was found to be particularly effective in reducing the frequency of asthma attacks.*

physical well-being and have been commonly prescribed for patients with back, neck, and joint pain. Originally, therapeutic *asanas* were designed simply to create a condition of ease in the body as a prelude to meditation. Only within the past century have the postures been applied to specific physical disorders, according to Rudolph Ballentine, M.D., Director of the Center for Holistic Medicine, in New York City.

Although yoga postures may involve very little movement, the mind is involved in the performance of every

The connection between the breath and the mind is a basic principle of yoga. If the mind is calm and focused, the breathing will be steady and rhythmic. If the mind is restless and agitated, breathing will be restless and agitated. A fundamental instruction in yogic breathing practices is the elimination of any jerkiness in the breathing motion so as to maintain smoothly flowing breath. This correlates with subsequent smoothness in the flow of thoughts, making yogic breathing exercises useful in calming the restlessness of the mind and creating clarity, focus, and heightened energy. Therefore, *pranayama* is often performed as a preparation for meditation.

Meditation

Meditation is a state of focused concentration that may result in a heightened sense of peace and awareness. Meditation is so thoroughly effective in reducing stress and tension that, in 1984, the National Institutes of Health recommended meditation over prescription drugs as the first treatment for mild hypertension.[2] Meditation has also been shown to have a positive effect on immune function and strengthens the body's defenses against infectious disease.[3] Herbert Benson, M.D., of the Mind-Body Institute at Harvard University, has documented how meditation practice can stimulate certain areas of the hypothalamus, affecting breathing rate, oxygen consumption, brain-wave rhythm, and blood flow.[4]

The final stage of yoga is *samadhi*, or spiritual realization, the culmination of a long, disciplined, and dedicated practice. In *samadhi* one is said to enter a state of awareness separate from, and beyond, the ordinary states of waking, dream, and sleep.

Conditions Benefited by Yoga

The potential benefits of yoga—health, vitality, and peace of mind—are limited only by one's commitment to its practice. Since the early 1970s, there have been more than 1,000 well-designed studies of meditation and yoga, demonstrating their effectiveness in stress and anxiety alleviation, blood pressure and heart rate reduction, improved memory and intelligence, pain relief, improved motor skills, relief from addictions, heightened visual and auditory perceptions, and enhanced metabolic and respiratory functions.[5]

Mary Pullig Schatz, M.D., author of *Back Care Basics,* reports of a 23-year-old diabetic woman who was able to substantially decrease her insulin dependency after beginning the practice of yoga. Studies support this anecdotal data[6] and demonstrate the effectiveness of yoga in the treatment of hypertension, bone marrow depletion, heart arrhythmia, thyroid disorders, menstrual problems, and other physical ailments.[7]

- In several studies, yoga was shown to significantly reduce both blood pressure and the need for drug therapy in adult patients suffering from hypertension. The patients were able to maintain these benefits after the cessation of the yoga therapy with only minimal daily relaxation exercises.[8] And in a study

dealing with the effects of meditation alone on hypertension, subjects were found to have a reduction in systolic blood pressure after meditative techniques had been taught to them and practiced over a period of 20 weeks. The subjects, though, did not show a reduced need for drug therapy as did those in the yoga study, and when they stopped practicing meditation, their blood pressure returned to its original level.[9] Another study involving 42 men with atherosclerosis found that yoga combined with other lifestyle changes (diet, moderate aerobic exercise, and control of risk factors) reduced the episodes of angina, lowered cholesterol, and decreased the size of arterial lesions.[10]

Studies have shown that yoga has a beneficial effect on the respiratory system, from lowered breathing rates and increased lung capacity to a diminishment of asthma attacks.

- Respiratory function has been among the most frequently measured variables in scientific evaluations of yoga. Largely because of the emphasis it puts on the breathing system, especially in *pranayama* practices, studies have shown that yoga has a beneficial effect on the respiratory system, with results ranging from lowered breathing rates and increased lung capacity to a diminishment of asthma attacks.[11] In one study, 17 adult asthmatics, 19-52 years old, were divided into two groups—nine were taught yoga techniques, including *pranayama, asanas,* and mediation; the remaining eight patients served as controls. The test subjects were taught yoga three times a week for 16 weeks. All subjects maintained logs of symptoms and medication use; the researchers also took samples of morning and evening peak flow readings (amount of air they can expire—low levels indicate airway obstruction). Researchers found that the test group reported a significant degree of relaxation and positive attitude compared to the control group. They also tended to use inhalers less than the controls did. Pulmonary function did not vary significantly between groups, but the yoga techniques did prove to prevent exacerbation of asthma attacks.[12]

Another study involving 15 patients with bronchitis found that yoga *asanas* and *pranayama* exercises improved lung function.[13] Other studies have suggested that yoga helps fight allergies by increasing blood levels of histaminase, an enzyme secreted by the adrenal glands that breaks down histamine, a substance involved in allergic reactions.[14]

- Yoga may be helpful for non–insulin-dependent diabetes. In a study of 149 diabetics who participated in yoga therapy for 40 days, 104 patients showed a fair to good response (reduction in hyperglycemia and decrease in the need for drugs to maintain normal blood sugar levels) to yoga.[15]

- There is a preliminary study indicating that yoga *asanas* and relaxation techniques may be useful for carpal tunnel syndrome.[16]

- An aspect of yoga that distinguishes it from other forms of exercise is its attention to the well-being of the endocrine and nervous systems. These systems are toned and stimulated by Hatha yoga practices in at least two ways. First, local increases in circulation are brought about in the endocrine glands and nerve plexuses (the network of nerves) through a variety of *asanas*. For example, during *sarvangasana* (shoulderstand), gravitational effects tend to increase circulation in the thyroid gland, and during *bhujangasana* (cobra position), contraction of the lumbosacral musculature increases circulation to the plexus of that region. A second way is during *pranayama,* when the manipulation of the breathing system has a highly beneficial effect on the nervous system.[17] One study found that yogic techniques were helpful for alleviating anxiety in patients with obsessive-compulsive disorder, allowing some patients to reduce or even discontinue their medication.[18]

- Yoga may be a useful adjunct therapy for certain types of cancer, as indicated in studies of yoga and the control of blood flow. In one study at the Menninger Foundation, a yogi exhibited a high degree of control over his blood flow—it has been recently suggested that if blood flow to the region of a tumor could be restricted, the growth of tumors could be abated.[19]

- Children can benefit from the practice of yoga. A study published in the *Journal of Mental Deficiency Research* reported that, when applied to a group of 90 mentally retarded children, yoga helped produce a "highly significant improvement in IQ and social adaptation."[20]

In the West, more and more physicians are prescribing Hatha yoga classes and "yoga therapy" is a growing field in American health care. The therapeutic results of yoga are starting to make converts of the established medical community, with some insurance companies now covering expenses, thus signaling an acceptance of the economic benefits that yoga can bring to the health-care system as well.

Yoga Therapy

Robin Munro, Ph.D., of Cambridge, England, had a long history of bronchial problems that began with asthma as a child and led to a bronchitis condition as an adult. After a severe bronchial attack at the age of 37, his condition became chronic and could only be controlled through drugs and repeated courses of antibiotics. The condition became so acute that it began to interfere with both his family life and his work.

During the course of exploring alternative therapies for his problem, Dr. Munro met an Indian doctor experienced in yoga therapy. Dr. Munro had already been practicing yoga for over ten years, which, together with deep relaxation, had alleviated his bronchitis but had not cured it.

The new yogic regime prescribed by the Indian doctor consisted of very simple postures and breathing exercises, together with a short session of vigorous exercise. It was first developed at Kaivalyadhama, near Bombay, India, a yoga institute that has been pioneering scientific research on the therapeutic qualities of yoga for 80 years. During the first few months, acupressure was used to overcome acute attacks without medication; after a year, the acupressure became unnecessary as well. Three years after beginning his new program, Dr. Munro's chest was virtually normal and has remained so ever since. "I have not taken a single antibiotic since the day I started," attests Dr. Munro. "That's nearly 30 years ago now."

Personally convinced of the effectiveness of yoga therapy, Dr. Munro founded the Yoga Biomedical Trust in 1983. The Trust's first venture was to carry out a survey of people who practiced yoga. High percentages of people with many different ailments said they considered yoga to have helped them (see "Health Conditions Benefited by Yoga"). Subsequent research has begun to substantiate many of these anecdotal findings.

"The Trust has already carried out successful trials on the benefits of yoga for adult-onset diabetes and rheumatoid arthritis," states Dr. Munro. "And it is currently embarking on a long-term study into the effects of yoga on aging." According to Dr. Munro's research, yoga is particularly valuable in the prevention and management of stress-related chronic health problems. "Yoga

HEALTH CONDITIONS BENEFITED BY YOGA

The 1983-84 Yoga Biomedical Trust survey charted the responses of 3,000 individuals with health ailments who were prescribed yoga as an alternative therapy.

AILMENT	NUMBER OF CASES	% CLAIMING BENEFIT
Back pain	1,142	98
Arthritis/rheumatism	589	90
Anxiety	838	94
Migraine	464	80
Insomnia	542	82
Nerve or muscle disease	112	96
Menstrual problems	317	68
Premenstrual tension	848	77
Menopause disorders	247	83
Hypertension	150	84
Heart disease	50	94
Asthma or bronchitis	226	88
Duodenal ulcers	40	90
Hemorrhoids	391	88
Obesity	240	74
Diabetes	10	80
Cancer	29	90
Tobacco addiction	219	74
Alcoholism	26	100

cannot cure every condition," Dr. Munro says, "but it can substantially help most of them."

A Program of Simple Yoga *Asanas*

While some specific yoga *asanas* can help particular health conditions, the safest and most reliable way to use Hatha yoga therapeutically, says Dr. Ballentine, is to follow a balanced program of postures to achieve an overall normalizing and health-inducing effect. It is best for the beginner to start with a simple program of basic postures. One such beginning yoga program, as suggested by Dr. Ballentine, can be found here and performed in about 30 minutes. An initial structured class or instruction is suggested as a foundation for exercises later practiced on one's own.

Corpse *(Shavasana)*

The first posture, called the corpse, is an excellent posture to start a yoga program. The corpse can also be used between postures, to help relax and prepare the mind for the next posture in the sequence, and at the conclusion of the program to help reduce fatigue.

> *The safest and most reliable way to use yoga therapeutically is to follow a balanced program of postures that will have an overall normalizing and health-inducing effect.*
>
> —RUDOLPH BALLENTINE, M.D.

Lie on your back with your arms spread out about 12-18 inches from your side, palms open and up, and your feet spread about as wide as your shoulders. Place a folded blanket or towel behind your head and neck. Close your eyes and relax, breathing slowly and deeply,

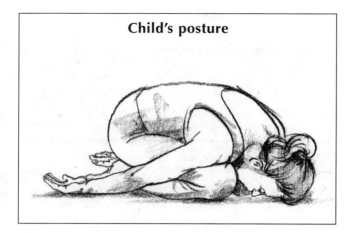

Child's posture

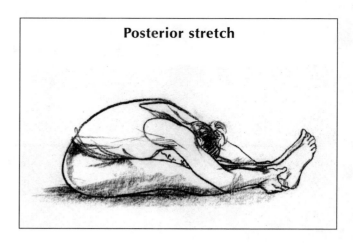

Posterior stretch

allowing the abdomen to expand with each inhalation and contract with each exhalation.

Practice this exercise for five to ten minutes. Its many benefits include:

- Aids circulation and improves the functioning of the nervous system

- Helps relax the skeletal muscles, enabling one to go further into the postures while reducing the likelihood of injuries

- Reduces fatigue

Child's Posture *(Balasana)*

Sit in a kneeling position with the top of your feet on the floor and your buttocks resting on your heels, keeping the head, neck, and trunk straight. Relax the arms and rest the hands on the floor, palms upward and fingers pointing behind you. Exhaling, slowly bend forward from the hips until the stomach and chest rest on the thighs and the forehead touches the floor in front of the knees. As your body bends forward, slide the hands back into a comfortable position.

In the child's posture, the body is completely relaxed and very compact. Do not lift the thighs or buttocks off the legs. Keep the arms close to the body. If you experience discomfort, extend the arms above the head a shoulder's width apart, keeping the arms straight and the palms on the floor.

To release the posture, inhale as you slowly lift the head and trunk and return to a kneeling position. Do not hold this posture for more than five minutes, as it reduces the circulation in the legs. People with excess weight may find this exercise more comfortable if the knees are spread apart.

This exercise provides the following benefits:

- Relaxes the back and promotes healing of back injuries by taking pressure off the intervertebral discs and providing a mild and natural form of traction

- Relieves pain in the lower back that may be caused by other postures; it can be used as a bridge between various *asanas* if lower back pain persists

Posterior Stretch *(Paschimottanasana)*

Sit with your head, neck, and trunk straight and your legs together, extended in front of your body. Inhaling, raise your arms overhead, stretch up and expand the chest. Exhaling, with your back straight and head between the arms, bend forward as far as possible, placing the hands comfortably on the legs. The back of your knees should remain on the floor. Relax, breathe evenly, and hold for 5-10 seconds.

To further the stretch, remain in position, inhale, and stretch forward from the base of the spine to the crown of the head. Exhaling, bring the head further down toward the legs. Relax and breathe evenly.

This exercise provides these benefits:

- Stimulates the peristaltic movement (wave-like contractions) of the digestive tract and prevents constipation

- Stimulates the entire abdominal area: kidneys, liver, stomach, spleen, and pancreas

- Relieves indigestion and poor appetite

- May be therapeutic in the treatment of diabetes

- Stretches the hamstring muscles of the thighs and the muscles and ligaments of the back

- Gently massages the intervertebral discs; develops flexibility of the spinal column

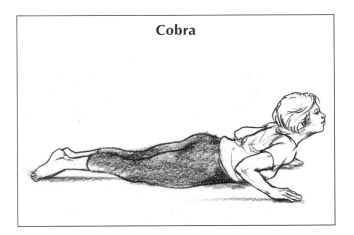

Cobra

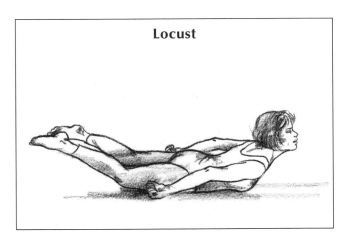

Locust

Cobra *(Bhujangasana)*

Lie on your stomach with your forehead resting on the floor, legs and feet together, with your body fully extended and relaxed. Bend the elbows, keeping them close to the body, and place your hands palm down beside the chest, aligning the fingertips with the nipples.

Inhaling, slowly begin to raise your head, allowing first the nose and then the chin to touch the floor as the head is stretched forward and upward. Without using the strength of the arms or hands, slowly raise the shoulders and chest; look up and bend back as far as possible. Breathe evenly; hold for five seconds. Exhaling, slowly lower the body until the forehead rests on the floor. Relax.

In this posture the navel remains on the floor. Do not use the arms and hands to push your body off the floor, use the muscles of the back only. Keep the feet and legs together and relaxed.

This exercise has many benefits:

- Strengthens the muscles of the shoulders, neck, and back

- Develops flexibility of the cervical vertebrae and corrects deviations of the spine

- Improves circulation to the intervertebral discs

- Expands the chest and develops elasticity of the lungs

- May help low back pain, constipation, stomach pains, and gas pains

Locust *(Shalabhasana)*

Lie on your stomach with your legs together and your arms extended along the sides of your body; place the chin on the floor. Make fists with the hands, placing the thumbs and the forefingers on the floor. Keeping the arms straight, place the fists under the tops of the thighs.

Inhaling, raise both legs as high as possible. Breathe evenly; hold for five seconds. Exhaling, slowly lower the legs and relax.

This exercise has two primary benefits:

- Strengthens the muscles of the lower back

- Reduces lower back pain tendencies

Half Spinal Twist
(Ardha Matsyendrasana)

Sit with your head, neck, and torso straight, with your legs together extended in front of your body. Bend the left leg and place the left foot on the floor at the outside of the right knee. Twist the body toward the left and place the left hand approximately 4-6 inches behind the left hip, fingers pointing away from the body. Bring the right arm over the outside of the left leg and grasp the left foot with the right hand. When bringing your arm over your leg, you may bend slightly forward if necessary; however, do not arch back and then twist your body.

Keeping the back straight, turn to the left, twisting from the lower spine, and look over the left shoulder. Do

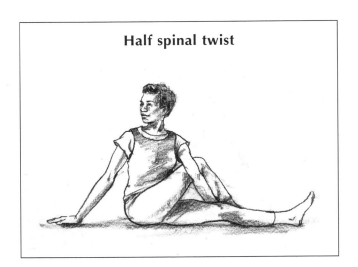

Half spinal twist

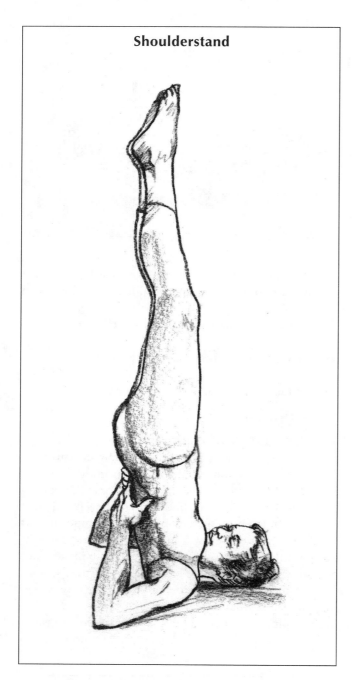

Shoulderstand

- Combats constipation, reduces fat, and improves digestion

Shoulderstand (*Sarvangasana*)

Lie on your back with your legs together, flat on the floor. Bend the elbows and place the hands as close to the shoulders as possible, with fingers pointing toward the small of the back and the elbows firmly on the floor. Raise both legs until they are perpendicular to the floor, lifting the hips toward the ceiling. Press the breastbone against the chin, gently at first and more firmly with experience. Keep the legs straight, relaxed and perpendicular to the floor. Breathe evenly; hold for 20-30 seconds. Slowly increase your capacity until you can hold this posture comfortably for one minute.

As implied in the literal translation of *sarvangasana,* "all member posture" or "entire body posture," this exercise benefits all parts of the body: the shoulders, arms, legs, head, neck, back, and internal organs. Other benefits include:

- Strengthens arms, chest, shoulders, and the back and abdominal muscles

- Places gentle traction on the cervical vertebrae, keeping this important area healthy and flexible

- Venous drainage of the legs occurs quickly and completely, especially benefiting those persons with varicose veins

- Diaphragmatic breathing is easily observed and learned

- Causes higher blood pressure and simple mechanical pressure in the neck, said to rejuvenate the thyroid and parathyroid glands, making them function optimally

- Reduces the occurrence of acute and chronic throat ailments and increases blood supply to all the important structures of the neck

- Called the "queen of *asanas*" and considered a panacea for internal organ ailments, especially those associated with old age; fights indigestion, constipation, degeneration of the endocrine glands, and problems occurring in the liver, gallbladder, kidneys, pancreas, spleen, and digestive system

not use the arms to force your body further into the twist, use them only for balance. Breathe evenly; hold for five seconds. Repeat on the opposite side.

This exercise provides these benefits:

- Provides twist to the spinal column, stretching and lengthening the muscles and ligaments and keeping the spine elastic and healthy

- Alternately compresses each half of the abdominal region, squeezing the internal organs and promoting better circulation through them

Half Fish (*Ardha Matsyasana*)

Sit with your head, neck, and trunk straight, legs together and extended in front of your body. Lean back and place

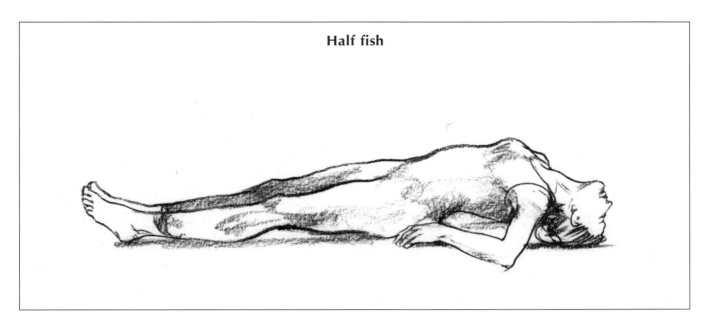

Half fish

the elbows and forearms on the floor in line with the body and legs. Arch the back, expanding the chest, and stretch the neck backward, placing the crown of the head on the floor. Increase the stretch by further arching your back and pulling your head as far as you can toward the back. Be sure to keep the mouth closed to maintain the stretch in the neck. Breathe evenly; hold for 15–20 seconds. Gently lower the body to a prone position. Relax. Once again, conclude with corpse posture to ensure complete relaxation and prevent fatigue.

This exercise provides these benefits:

- Stretches to the cervical vertebrae complementary to that of the shoulderstand; it amplifies the effects of the shoulderstand and eliminates the slight stiffness in the neck and back that results from doing the shoulderstand alone

- Expands the chest, promoting deep inhalation and good ventilation to the top of the lungs and increasing lung capacity

Where to Find Help

There are several forms and schools of yoga available in the West, including Ashtanga, Integral, Iyengar, Kriya, Kundalini, Sivananda, Tantra, and Vini. Each emphasizes a different aspect of the body/mind/spirit relationship. The following organizations may be contacted for further help and assistance.

Himalayan Institute of Yoga, Science, and Philosophy
R.R. I Box 400
Honesdale, Pennsylvania 18431
(800) 822-4547
Website: www.himalayainstitute.org

The Institute offers classes, an extensive catalogue of books, cassettes, and videos, and has centers nationwide.

International Association of Yoga Therapists
P.O. Box 2418
Sebastopol, California 95473
(707) 929-9898
Website: www.yrec.org/iayt.html

This nonprofit organization emphasizes education and research for yoga and yoga therapy, and publishes an annual journal, the Journal of the International Association of Yoga Therapists.

Yoga Research and Education Center
P.O. Box 2418
Sebastopol, California 95473
(707) 928-9898
Website: www.yrec.org

The Center is one of the leading research institutions involved with validating and propagating yoga's many health benefits.

Iyengar Yoga
2404 27th Avenue
San Francisco, California 94116
(415) 753-0909
Website: www.iyiss.org

Offers classes, teacher training, a bookstore, a mail-order catalog, and referrals.

Samata Yoga and Health Institute
4150 Tivoli Avenue
Los Angeles, California 90066
(310) 306-8845
Website: www.samata.com

Samata Yoga and Health Institute specializes in yoga therapy for back pain and stress, and offers group classes and teacher training programs.

Sivananda Yoga
5178 South Lawrence Boulevard
Montreal, Quebec, Canada H2T 1R8
(514) 279-3545
Website: www.sivananda.org

Sivananda centers worldwide, including in the United States, Canada, the Bahamas, India, and Europe.

Yoga Biomedical Trust
Royal Homeopathic Hospital
60 Great Ormond Street
London, England WC1N 3HR
(01) 71-419-7195
Website: freespace.virgin.net/yogabio.med

Founded by Robin Munro, Ph.D., the Trust conducts research into the full range of benefits yoga can provide for both acute and chronic illness.

Recommended Reading

Back Care Basics: A Doctor's Gentle Yoga Program for Back and Neck Pain Relief. Mary P. Schatz, M.D. Berkeley, CA: Rodmell Press, 1992.

Complete Illustrated Book of Yoga. Swami Vishnudevananda. New York: Harmony Books, 1980.

Hatha Yoga: Manual I. Samskrti and Veda. Honesdale, PA: Himalayan International Institute, 1986.

Light on Pranayama. B. Iyengar. New York: Crossroad Publishing, 1992.

Light on Yoga. B. Iyengar. New York: Schocken Books, 1987.

The Yoga Tradition: Its History, Literature, Philosophy and Practice. Georg Feuerstein. San Francisco: Hohm Press, 1998.

Yoga Journal. Available from: 2054 University Avenue, Berkeley, California 94704; (510) 841-9200. Also found at health food stores and health-oriented bookstores.

Part Three

Health Conditions

ADDICTIONS

Addictions afflict millions of people in the United States and result in an annual loss of productivity and health-care costs valued at nearly $250 billion.[1] Alternative physicians believe that conventional methods fail as addiction treatments because they do not recognize the genetic and biochemical imbalances that research has shown to be at the heart of addiction. By focusing on readjusting these imbalances through diet and nutritional supplementation, acupuncture, biofeedback, herbal medicine, and other therapies, alternative physicians are contributing to significant and long-lasting positive change.

ADDICTION CAN BE defined as any physical or psychological dependence that negatively impacts a person's life. Although a person can be addicted to many forms of behavior, such as gambling, over-eating, sex, or reckless behavior, the term *addiction* is most commonly used to refer to dependency on cigarettes, alcohol, and drugs (both legal and illegal). Outward signs of alcohol and other addictions may include depression, frequent accidents, work absences, tremors, anxiety or lethargy (depending on the substance used), hallucinations, mood swings, nausea, and bingeing. In severe cases, addiction can become so obsessive that it may seem to take on a life of its own, and the individual's true identity can take a second place to the personality of the addiction.

According to James Braly, M.D., of Hollywood, Florida, fundamentally all addictions are biochemically the same. He notes that addictive substances become a necessary ingredient of body chemistry, so that withdrawal occurs when the substance is withheld. "Addiction means that the body has made an unhealthy adaptation that must slowly be reversed," Dr. Braly explains. "Until then, nerve impulses are confused and biochemistry scrambled."

When someone with addictive behavior is deprived of, or attempts to abandon, the addiction, the resulting withdrawal symptoms demand a solution. During withdrawal from the addictive substance, something must be done to keep the painful, sometimes unbearable, symptoms at bay. This can lead the person back to the addictive substance or behavior, beginning the destructive cycle anew.

Causes of Addiction

Long perceived as a problem of weak willpower, substance abuse is now considered by most researchers to be a "disease," similar in development to diabetes. In other words, according to Leon Chaitow, N.D., D.O., of London, England, a genetic predisposing condition is usually present that is triggered by familial, environmental, societal, dietary, and other factors. As a result, even when stabilized, an addict must closely monitor the addictive substance throughout his or her lifetime.

Biochemical Imbalances

The body produces its own natural mood enhancers and painkillers, called neurotransmitters, which in healthy individuals work efficiently. Dr. Chaitow cites research into brain function suggesting that the person with addictions or greatest addictive potential may lack these natural stimulants (catecholamines) and relaxants (endorphins). He postulates that the addictive brain may send incorrect or garbled messages to the body through malfunctioning neurotransmitters. "Because of this malfunction, addictive personalities may seek alternatives to natural mood enhancers through the artificial stimulus of addictive substances," he says.

Dr. Chaitow's view, which is shared by growing numbers of researchers in both alternative and conventional medicine, is supported by a recent study that found that some people who become addicted to alcohol or drugs exhibit a flaw in the brain's "decision-making center," impairing their abilities. In the study, conducted at the University of Iowa, in Iowa City, the majority of subjects addicted to drugs or alcohol exhibited the same poor decision-making skills as people with damage to the part of the brain known as the ventromedial prefrontal cortex (VM), which governs decision-making. The study involved 41 substance abusers, 40 healthy controls, and five people with VM damage, all of whom were given a test that simulates real-life decisions. Sixty-one percent of the substance abuse group scored as poorly as the VM patients, compared to only 33% of the control group. The fact that not all people in the substance abuse group scored poorly on the test may help to explain why addiction does not afflict everyone who experiments with drugs or alcohol, while further indicating that the addictive process does impair brain function.[2]

Research also indicates that the brains of those predisposed to alcoholism may not produce enough of the neurotransmitter dopamine, which influences mood and produces feelings of pleasure. Alcohol increases the levels of dopamine in the brain and may stimulate other "feel good" neurotransmitters such as serotonin and glutamate. Chronic heavy drinking can apparently "hardwire" this chemical reward system into the brain's structure, building new neural pathways that insistently demand more and more alcohol to induce the pleasurable feelings. Even those who begin drinking later in life, perhaps in response to high levels of chronic stress, may produce similar changes in brain physiology.[3]

Janice K. Phelps, M.D., author of *The Hidden Addiction—And How to Get Free From It,* believes there is a difference in addictive bodies from birth and that an addictive body may be evident in childhood by the presence of colic, hyperactivity, loss of sleep, irritability, crying, and learning disabilities. Additionally, Dr. Phelps says, "Long before a child can get involved in drugs and alcohol, he's often gotten very addicted to sugar."

Substantiating this line of thought, Dr. Chaitow points to the link between brain chemistry and food addictions. Serotonin is a calming, painkilling substance that is secreted in response to carbohydrate and sugar consumption. Sugar addiction may be an attempt to replenish serotonin in the system. A Massachusetts Institute of Technology study describes groups of people who feel depressed, anxious, and tense—the right conditions for substance abuse—before eating a carbohydrate snack, and who feel peaceful afterward, their bodies satiated with calming serotonin.[4]

Kathleen DesMaisons, Ph.D., of Albuquerque, New Mexico, author of *The Sugar Addict's Total Recovery Program,* believes that many addictive people have a biochemical flaw in the way they process sugar and carbohydrates. This flaw in metabolism causes an addict to respond to sugar as if it were alcohol and to white flour products as if they were sugar. "Genetically, these people have biochemically sensitive bodies which invite chemical imbalance," she explains. "Substances like sugar, by stimulating insulin and rapidly penetrating the cell wall, actually alter the permeability of the cell." In one study, 88% of the alcoholic women had abnormal glucose metabolism.[5]

The normal person, Dr. DesMaisons states, has stronger, more impermeable cells, which prevent the rise and fall of blood sugar and the jagged peaks and valleys of violent emotions that plague addictive personalities. "Sugar is like an opiate drug," Dr. DesMaisons says. "The child who used sugar becomes the adolescent who discovers alcohol, which is the 'perfect' drug because, beyond its high sugar content, it has an anesthetic property. The addictive personality moves naturally into other drugs. The whole syndrome is really about pain management."

Following this line of thought, addiction may be a way of restoring natural body chemicals through artificial, destructive means. Dr. Chaitow says, "We turn to various substances to enhance or replace the body's diminished capacity to produce the chemicals we crave for energy or relaxation."

The Addiction/Allergy Connection

Dr. Braly believes there is a strong correlation between addiction and allergies. "We become addicted to foods as a way of adapting to allergic reactions to them, and we tend to crave foods we're allergic to because we need them to keep withdrawal symptoms at bay," he explains. When we reach this point and need a particular food in order to feel good, or rather in order to not feel bad, we are addicted to it. This topsy-turvy phenomenon is called the allergy/addiction syndrome.

Recent research in the field of addiction suggests that excessive craving for any substance indicates an allergic condition in relation to that substance. "According to this theory," says Dr. Chaitow, "by constantly exposing themselves to an addictive substance, addicts prevent themselves from experiencing the more violent displays of allergic symptoms—the substance 'masks' the allergy."

Furthermore, Dr. Chaitow points out that an addict's withdrawal symptoms are almost identical to the symptoms which occur when an allergenic substance is removed from the diet or environment—ranging from tremors and cramps to sweating, prostration, vomiting, and hallucinations. "Any food or drink which is commonly consumed or craved may in fact be an allergenic substance for an individual if withdrawal from it makes one feel unwell or if consumption produces euphoria," Dr. Chaitow says. Alcohol is the classic substance fitting this description.[6]

Dr. Braly also points out that many of the foods from which alcohol is made—particularly grains, corn deriv-

TRAINING CHILDREN TO BE DRUG ADDICTS

Ritalin, a drug widely prescribed to control hyperactivity and attention deficit hyperactivity disorder (ADHD) in children, is now used by 3%-5% of all U.S. school-children, most of whom are boys. Experts at the International Narcotics Control Board, in Vienna, Austria, which released a report on worldwide Ritalin use, suggest this could pose long-term risks for teenage addiction and compromised well-being. "Our concern is over-prescription," said the U.S. representative to the Board.

A study of 1,000 U.S. pediatricians found that 70% use Ritalin as a diagnostic litmus test to see if children have ADHD, resulting too often in misdiagnosis and inappropriate treatment. The logic is that if the children respond, they must have ADHD. Doctors overuse Ritalin because of time pressures, failure to do a thorough patient workup, and the need to get children treated and out of the office quickly.

It's not only Ritalin that may be making addicts of children. Drug dependency starts in childhood with over-the-counter (OTC) medications, admitted the *Journal of the American Medical Association*.[9] Interviews with 8,145 mothers of 3-year-old children revealed that, in a one-month period, 53% of children had received OTC drugs, most commonly Tylenol and cough/cold medicines. Of these children, 40% received two drugs concurrently, 5% received 3-4 drugs, and 15% received anti-diarrheal medications even though they are not recommended for young children.[10]

atives, sugars, and yeast—are common allergens. He maintains that many alcoholics are also addicted to these foods and thus perpetuate their allergies with excessive drinking. In one study, 73% of the alcoholic women had food allergies, primarily to dairy products and wheat.[7]

Malabsorption of Nutrients

Dr. Chaitow states that the normal population of microorganisms housed in the gut is severely disturbed in alcoholics and may lead to malabsorption of fats, protein, carbohydrates, folic acid, and vitamin B_{12}. This disruption, together with a more permeable or leaky gut, allows foreign and toxic substances to cross the intestinal wall. As a result, allergies may develop and feed alcohol cravings and possible food allergies.[8]

According to nutritionist Inez d'Arcy-Francis, Ph.D., of Kentfield, California, addiction to alcohol, drugs, or foods occurs due to a three-stage process founded on malabsorption of nutrients. The initial factor precipitating addiction is trauma to the body caused by undigested food particles. "It's trauma because the body does not know what to do with these undigested food particles," Dr. d'Arcy-Francis says. "Undigested food molecules are toxins once they pass through the intestinal wall to enter the bloodstream and can cause chaos in the body." Once this occurs, the liver begins to get overwhelmed, the immune system becomes overactive and confused, and chronic allergic reactions are set in motion. In addition, the trauma to the body caused by undigested food particles causes a drop in blood sugar levels and produces food cravings. "This is a physiological reaction to the body trying to protect itself from the now toxic substance," Dr. d'Arcy-Francis explains.

The second stage to this process is known as adaptation, which occurs once the body starts to crave foods it cannot digest. Such foods—typically dairy, wheat, eggs, chocolate, sugar, or alcohol—must then be consumed in increasing amounts so that the body can avoid the pain of withdrawal. A similar adaptation process occurs with regard to other addictive substances, such as nicotine or drugs. The final stage, degeneration, refers to the serious illnesses that can result from addiction, including alcoholism, Crohn's disease, diabetes, and obesity.

Treating Addictions

Substance abuse treatment in the U.S. primarily focuses on Twelve-Step support groups and individual talking therapies, control by medications such as methadone and antidepressants, expensive month-long hospital stays, and, of course, criminal punishment. It is still unknown whether these methods, combined or individually, will be successful in the long run. However, a Rand Corporation study confirmed earlier research, which found that the addictive population studied, once sober or clean, had only a 15%-20% rate of continued abstinence.[11] Compared to such low success rates, the following alternative approaches offer great promise.

Diet

Proper diet is essential in treating addictions, according to Dr. DesMaisons. "My main focus is to reverse symptoms of addiction by changing the person's neurochemistry and nutrient deficiency through dietary intervention," she says. "This principle is called 'biochemical restoration.' If this is accomplished, then the addictive behavior that has previously been unmanaged can be reversed. Ultimately, the goal is to teach people how to recognize and modulate their feelings by paying attention to the foods they eat."

Since Dr. DesMaisons finds that most addictive people have problems processing sugar and carbohydrates, her approach is to immediately place them on a program of three meals a day, with an emphasis on eating proteins at each meal. "Most people in an addictive state are protein deficient," she explains. "Normally, they haven't been eating regularly and they don't have protein when they do eat because their bodies are craving sugar and simple carbohydrates. So by getting them to eat protein foods regularly, which are the most complex foods and take the longest time to break down in the stomach, you start to alter their neurochemistry. They become able to maintain a stable blood sugar level and a consistent supply of serotonin and dopamine to the brain, so that they don't crave the artificial high from alcohol or drugs."

Dr. DesMaisons also instructs people to keep a food journal of what they eat and how they feel afterward so that they have an actual record of how food affects their moods. "We often have people who have been given anti-anxiety medication and no one has bothered to ask them what they eat and drink," says Dr. DesMaisons. "They come in not eating regularly while drinking three pots of coffee a day. That is the source of their anxiety symptoms."

Dr. DesMaisons suggests meal choices based on the person's lifestyle and ethnic background. Typical choices include fish, poultry, meat, cheese, eggs, tofu, and nut butter. In addition, complex carbohydrates are permitted, including beans, grains, and vegetables. "We also encourage a little bit of fat, although not from animal products," Dr. DesMaisons says, "because eating healthy fat leads to the body's production of serotonin, creating a sense of well-being and relaxation. Using olive oil, for instance, is one way to achieve this." Fats in the diet tend to stabilize blood sugar, which in turn stabilizes serotonin production. Those who follow this eating plan will normally notice significant changes in how they feel, often within three to four days, according to Dr. DesMaisons.

Once they begin to experience a positive change, their caffeine and sugar intake is examined and gradually reduced. Dr. DesMaisons also educates people about all of the different sugars found in foods. "Many people are only aware of the overt sugars contained in pies, cakes, cookies, and ice cream," she says. "They have to also be aware of the hidden sugars, particularly the many forms of corn syrup and sugars such as dextrose, maltose, sorbitol, and mannitol. I encourage people to read labels to see what it is they are eating." Because of its high sugar content, fruit is avoided, particularly grapes, cherries, watermelon, and all fruit juices. Citrus fruits, apples, and strawberries, however, can be permitted due to their lower sugar content. "Interestingly, carrot juice is also avoided," says Dr. DesMaisons, "because it's high in sugar."

One of her clients came to her at age 28 after never being sober for more than a month since she was 12. "She'd been in hospitals repeatedly for attempted suicide and had been drinking since she was nine," Dr. DesMaisons says. "One day, she got very upset and went out and drank a gallon of whiskey. She had to be hospitalized, but three days later she walked into my office and said, 'All right, whatever you tell me to do, I'll do.'" She was placed on the food plan and after one month no longer had any cravings for alcohol. After achieving sobriety, she was then able to begin dealing with the emotional issues surrounding her addiction. "Today, she has been sober for four years and her entire life has changed," Dr. DesMaisons relates. "She's in a healthy relationship and has been promoted at her job."

Dr. DesMaisons also incorporates acupuncture, counseling, and guided imagery, with a focus on self-awareness and independence. According to her, 75% of her clients remain sober for two years or more after completing the program.

Nutritional Supplementation

In boosting the body's biochemical defenses against addiction, Dr. Phelps uses nutritional supplements and adrenal support, such as vitamin C, pantothenic acid (vitamin B5), and adrenal extracts, in her treatment regimen. She also stresses that a patient must remove all addictive substances from the diet, including sugar and caffeine.

Megavitamin therapy is commonly cited as one of the most vital tools for replenishing vitamin deficiency, which affects more than 50% of alcoholics, according to Lauri Aesoph, N.D., of Sioux Falls, South Dakota. They are almost always deficient in one or more of the B vitamins, particularly thiamin (B1) and B6. She points out that addicts to narcotics often suffer from a deficiency of essential minerals, especially magnesium, calcium, and potassium. Since alcohol enhances free-radical formation (molecules that damage the body), antioxidants such as selenium, zinc, and vitamins C and E are needed to oppose their effects.[12] Zinc may help the body metabolize and detoxify from alcohol, as does vitamin C.[13] Dr. Aesoph adds that chromium aids in stabilizing the erratic blood sugar seen in alcoholic hypoglycemia, while choline and folic acid are also commonly cited as important supplements to assist in the body's recovery from addiction.

Intravenous withdrawal support for severe cases is often used in Dr. Braly's treatment protocol. He states that those with severe withdrawal problems can benefit from three or four consecutive days of intravenous therapy consisting of vitamin C, calcium gluconate, magnesium sulfate, pantothenic acid, and vitamin B6. "Withdrawal symptoms can often be completely eliminated after one or two days using this approach," Dr. Braly says. Other nutrients that he recommends include evening primrose oil, vitamin B complex, eicosapentaenoic acid (EPA), and glutamine (an amino acid).

"If you had an alcoholic parent, you probably inherited a major deficiency of specific amino acids," according to Billie Jay Sahley, Ph.D., Director of the Pain and Stress Center, in San Antonio, Texas. Roger Williams, at the University of Texas Clayton Foundation for Bio-Medical Research, determined years ago that children of alcoholics have a deficiency of the amino acids GABA (gamma-aminobutyric acid) and glutamine. Glutamine assists in improving mental alertness and memory and also increases levels of GABA. Both GABA and glutamine help stop alcohol and sugar cravings and aid in the absorption of minerals into the tissues. "You can stop the craving for alcohol with 4,000-5,000 mg of glutamine a day," says Dr. Sahley. She also recommends a balanced amino acid complex (in a capsule or powder form) to be taken with the individual amino acids.

The goal is for people to master the keys to their own biochemical and physiological balance. I try to find the key to nourishing the body, so that if there is still any physiological memory of healthy function, the body kicks in again.

—INEZ D'ARCY-FRANCIS, PH.D.

Proper mineral supplementation also offers benefits for people suffering from addiction. Corazon Ilarina, M.D., of the Bio-Medical Health Center, in Reno, Nevada, treated a marijuana addict with an intensive program of mineral supplementation, after a hair analysis showed that he suffered from elevated aluminum, lead, nickel, and beryllium levels. She started a treatment program that included magnesium, chromium, and manganese supplements; thymus and pancreatic extracts; and megadoses of vitamin C to counteract his metal toxicity. Following this program, "there was a dramatic improvement in lowering the toxicity levels of the patient, and his craving for marijuana and alcohol was alleviated," Dr. Ilarina reports.

Dr. d'Arcy-Francis also finds that one of the most effective ways of treating addiction is precise nutritional

supplementation, which she believes helps rekindle the body's "memory" of correct functioning. "I don't make claims to 'cure' anything," she says. "The goal is for people to master the keys to their own biochemical and physiological balance. I try to find the key to nourishing the body, so that if there is still any physiological memory of healthy function, the body kicks in again."

The case of Zoe illustrates this process. When she first consulted with Dr. d'Arcy-Francis, Zoe, 53, stood 5′4″ and was morbidly obese (310 pounds). She was also classified as a "terminal phase drug addict" in recovery, having suffered from alcohol addiction for years. Previously, she had her gallbladder removed, suffered broken ankles and torn cartilage as a result of her obesity, and endured back pain and chronic depression. She also suffered from irregular and painful menstruation, tender breasts, hot flashes, and alternating constipation and diarrhea. "Many of these conditions are directly traceable to insufficient digestion," Dr. d'Arcy-Francis points out.

Zoe's nutritional program began with a tonic consisting of predigested whey powder in a base of unsweetened fruit juice diluted with water (up to 24 oz daily). She also took four teaspoons of vegetable glycerin, which provides the energy of fat molecules without the fat; two teaspoons of dolomite powder daily for easily absorbed calcium and magnesium; 4-8 g of vitamin C ascorbate; and ten drops of liquid dulce, to supply enough iodine to support her thyroid. In addition, Dr. d'Arcy-Francis prescribed a multivitamin/mineral supplement, vitamin B6 (250 mg), gamma-linolenic acid (GLA, an essential fatty acid), chasteberry *(Vitex agnus-castus)* to help stabilize her menstrual cycle (three capsules), and hydrochloric acid (one capsule per meal) along with digestive enzymes to reduce the release of undigested food particles into her bloodstream. The amino acid L-glutamine (1000 mg, five times daily) was also prescribed to help regulate Zoe's blood sugar levels.

Finally, Zoe radically simplified her diet, eliminating sugar, grains, caffeine, dairy products, processed foods, breads, and flours, and replacing them with at least 24 ounces each of cooked root vegetables and other steamed vegetables, plus 3-8 pieces of fruit, 6-8 ounces of protein, and herbal teas.

Within ten months, Zoe no longer had any craving for alcohol or other drugs. In addition, she lost 71 pounds, was no longer depressed, and no longer suffered from food cravings. Her periods became regular and painless as well, and her hot flashes stopped, her breasts were no longer tender, she no longer experienced pain throughout her body, and she was free of diarrhea and constipation.

Traditional Chinese Medicine

Michael Smith, M.D., of Lincoln Hospital, in New York City, has found acupuncture to be the most effective treatment for heroin, cocaine, and crack addictions. Studies have also shown fewer relapses and fewer readmissions to treatment centers for addicts and alcoholics who have had acupuncture.[14] In one study, 118 subjects who had been drinking longer than ten years were given either acupuncture or standard medical detoxification. Those given acupuncture treatments showed a decreased desire for alcohol, fewer depressive symptoms and tremors, and increased participation in psychological counseling programs.[15] Clinical reports indicate that acupuncture is effective in helping people to stop smoking as well.[16]

A more recent study conducted by researchers at Yale University confirmed acupuncture's effectiveness for treating cocaine and heroin addiction. The study involved 82 men and women who were addicted to both drugs. Prior to the study, they were receiving methadone treatment for their heroin addiction, but were still regularly using cocaine. The test subjects were divided into two groups: one received auriculotherapy (ear acupuncture) five times a week, while the control group was given "sham" acupuncture treatments. Eight weeks later, 53.8% of those in the auriculotherapy group tested free of cocaine, compared to only 23.5% in the other group.

Researchers stated that among acupuncture's benefits as a drug treatment were its low cost and lack of side effects, as well as the fact that, unlike pharmaceutical treatments, it can safely be administered to pregnant women. The report cautioned, however, that acupuncture is not a panacea for addiction and should be used in conjunction with other therapies, including psychological counseling.[17]

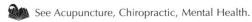 See Acupuncture, Chiropractic, Mental Health.

Jay Holder, M.D., D.C., Ph.D., of Miami, Florida, has developed a specific form of auriculotherapy for addiction treatment and has used it to successfully treat addictions, as well as obsessive behavior related to work, sex, and gambling. In his experience, auriculotherapy has up to an 80% success rate among addicts of nicotine, alcohol, cocaine, heroin, and other drugs.[18] Dr. Holder explains that each type of addiction correlates to specific ear acupoints. "Every drug has a specific receptor site. We meet the needs of that receptor site by supplying and directing endorphins through acupuncture. This allows the body to turn itself back on again. So, the body is helped through the difficult period of withdrawal, until its natural restorative powers return."

Oregon law now requires a series of acupuncture treatments before a heroin addict can qualify for methadone

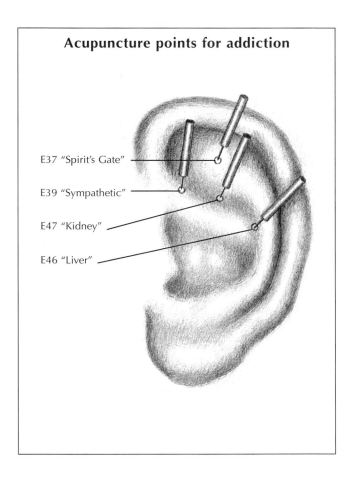

Acupuncture points for addiction

E37 "Spirit's Gate"
E39 "Sympathetic"
E47 "Kidney"
E46 "Liver"

treatment. The state hopes that many people will be able to detoxify with acupuncture alone and not need to start the methadone maintenance program.

William M. Cargile, B.S., D.C., F.I.A.C.A., past Chairman of Research for the American Academy of Oriental Medicine, will often use ginger seeds on ear acupoints rather than needles. The serrated seeds, without penetrating the skin, are placed on the ear with medical tape and are distinctly successful in treating cocaine addiction. Dr. Cargile describes a 46-year-old patient who benefited enormously from ginger seed treatment: "She was a mother of eight children by seven different men and a crack addict. We used whole-body acupuncture in 12 treatments and sent her home with ginger seed on the ears. During the treatment, she had only one relapse. Today, she holds down two jobs and has not had a single relapse."

At Yo San University Clinic, in Marina del Rey, California, Maoshing Ni, D.O.M., Ph.D., L.Ac., practices traditional Chinese medicine, including acupuncture and nutritional guidance. He reports the case of a patient with a 12-year history of drug abuse. He could walk only with difficulty, suffered from shortness of breath, his balance was off, and he had a multitude of physical maladies. "The first acupuncture treatments were applied to the patient's ear points," Dr. Ni relates. "This helped him sleep and

EASE AWAY FROM ADDICTIONS WITH FLOWER ESSENCES

Flower essences, the subtle liquid preparations made from the fresh blossoms of flowers, plants, bushes, even trees, may make it easier to break the cycle of addiction, according to Patricia Kaminski and Richard Katz, co-authors of *Flower Essence Repertory* and founders and directors of the Flower Essence Society, in Nevada City, California.

Flower essence therapy, an approach pioneered by British physician Edward Bach in the 1930s, addresses the emotional, psychological, and spiritual components of health and well-being. In the case of addictions—cigarettes, alcohol, drugs, or emotional codependency such as addictive behavior in personal relationships—flower essences can help overcome the underlying causes of addictive behavior, state Kaminski and Katz. They recommend the following flower remedies to address psychological and emotional causes often associated with addictions:

California Poppy *(Eschscholzia californica)*—This flower encourages inner stability in those with escapist tendencies or a need to experience things from outside themselves. It is particularly helpful for users of hallucinogenic drugs.

Morning Glory *(Ipomoea purpurea)*—This flower is often recommended for thrill-seekers who rely on stimulants to compensate for perceived dullness in everyday life. By encouraging increased awareness of personal surroundings, Morning Glory helps with addiction to stimulants, such as nicotine, cocaine, and amphetamines.

Chrysanthemum *(Chrysanthemum morifolium)*—For those who use drugs or alcohol to avoid confronting painful circumstances, flower essence practitioners often suggest chrysanthemum.

Milkweed *(Asclepias cordifolia)*—Milkweed is commonly prescribed for substance abusers who use alcohol, opiates, or other sedatives to stupefy their consciousness.

Nicotiana *(Nicotiana alata)*—Flowering Tobacco, or Nicotiana, is strongly indicated for those who smoke cigarettes for comfort and relaxation.

Bleeding Heart *(Dicentra formosa)*—Essences of this flower address feelings of pain and loss in personal relationships, especially for people whose emotional connections are motivated by possessiveness or fear. Bleeding Heart is often prescribed for emotional dependency.

Black Cohosh *(Cimicifuga racemosa)*—Useful for people caught in a pattern of abusive or threatening relationships, Black Cohosh helps provide courage to confront abusive situations rather than to retreat from the abuser.

Five Flower Formula—This blend, containing essences of Cherry Plum, Clematis, Impatiens, Rock Rose, and Star of Bethlehem, has a stabilizing effect that is particularly useful as a first step toward healing addiction.

Walnut *(Juglands regia)*—Essence of walnut provides general support in times of change, including the transition between addictive and non-addictive behavior.

Self-Heal *(Prunella vulgaris)*—This flower essence provides healing support and inspires confidence in one's abilities to break an addictive habit.[19]

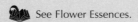 See Flower Essences.

become calmer. We saw immediate relief, and his drug craving was much diminished. I then started him on a program of Chinese herbs to restore the functions of his liver and kidneys since his adrenal glands were depleted. This helped the detoxification and strengthening process. I also put him on a cleansing, very strict, high-fiber, low-fat diet. As a result, his mind began to clear and his appetite returned, and today the patient is recovering well and has suffered no relapses."

Chiropractic

Dr. Holder, working with the University of Miami School of Medicine and the Florida Chiropractic Soci-

ety, conducted the first large-scale human study to prove the effectiveness of chiropractic adjustment in dealing with chemical addictions. Dr. Holder has seen dramatic results from the study, showing that a person receiving chiropractic care is ten times more likely to complete a drug treatment program.

During the 18-month study, patients in a drug-addiction program were divided into three groups. The first group received standard care, including group psychotherapy and medical care. The second group additionally received special chiropractic adjustments. A third group received the standard care and a placebo treatment. Just 56% of the group receiving standard care finished the treatment program, compared to 75% of the placebo group. However, all of those in the chiropractic group completed the program.[20] This 100% retention rate has never been accomplished by any other methodology, Dr. Holder says.

Retention rate, or how long a person stays in a treatment program, is extremely important. "The longer a drug addict is in a treatment center, the better the end results will be and the more likely the person will be successful staying drug-free," Dr. Holder explains. "By removing subluxations that interfere with the normal functioning of the nervous system, a person is more likely to complete their term of stay, because the person now can meet the needs of the other modalities offered as treatment. We have fewer people with drug detoxification or withdrawal symptoms, their physical complaints are almost eliminated, and they can now concentrate on dealing with their addiction."

John, 26, was depressed, displaying psychotic behavior, and strung out on alcohol and cocaine when he came to see Dr. Holder. He'd seen four psychiatrists who had given him different mood-altering drugs, which only worsened his condition. He had started addiction programs twice, but finished neither and attended Alcoholics Anonymous meetings but quit when he found them "boring." He'd go off drugs for a few weeks, sometimes several months, then relapse.

After taking John's case history, Dr. Holder examined him on the treatment table with a system he developed called Torque Release Technique. Dr. Holder was able to tell which vertebrae in John's spinal column were out of alignment (subluxation). "For chiropractors, a subluxation means a separation from wholeness," says Dr. Holder. "It interferes with your body's ability to function in a whole way, which is a form of neurological insult." Dr. Holder maintains that any addicted person will have a spine with one or more vertebrae out of alignment. Using an FDA-approved hand-held spinal adjustment instrument he calls the "Integrator," Dr. Holder makes a few chiropractic adjustments during each visit, painlessly administering a minimum of force and pressure.

What's the connection between a misaligned spine and addictions? It has to do with the interruption of a precise sequence of chemical changes in your brain called the "brain reward cascade." If this cascade is not interrupted, you feel a sense of well-being and pleasure. If the sequence is interrupted, resulting in what is known as "reward deficiency syndrome," you may seek mood-altering substances or activities. The brain chemicals (neurotransmitters) must be released in the right sequence, like falling dominoes, for you to feel good.

In addition to correcting John's misalignments, Dr. Holder started him on a series of four amino acids (precursors or building blocks for proteins) taken daily as oral supplements. They included DL-phenylalanine (750 mg, three times daily), 5-hydroxytryptophan (500 mg, three times daily), L-glutamine (750 mg daily), and L-tyrosine (500 mg, three times daily). John will stay on this amino acid combination for at least a year into recovery.

Although according to Dr. Holder's theory chiropractic adjustment will remove the interference to the natural flow of brain chemicals, it is still necessary to shore up the body's supplies of these substances vital to addiction recovery. The amino acids, especially DL-phenylalanine, will help the brain restore the brain reward cascade. By reducing stress and lifting depression, they will help John make important changes in his behavior and attitude, which are crucial to the success of his treatment program. In addition, John attended Narcotics Anonymous meetings every day and received expert addiction counseling at least once a week. He may also periodically receive the ear acupuncture protocol Dr. Holder has developed as an adjunct to treatment.

The American College of Addictionology and Compulsive Disorders (ACACD), in Miami, Florida, has chosen chiropractic as the profession of choice in training for board certification in addictionology. "The ACACD targeted the chiropractic community because chiropractic is a drugless approach," states Dr. Holder. "People that are chemically dependent must stay away from mood-altering substances their entire lives. What type of primary-care physician is going to be best able to meet the needs of the recovery community? Obviously, someone who isn't going to use mood-altering substances."

Biofeedback Training and Neurofeedback Therapy

Developed by Gene Peniston, Ed.D., A.B.M.P., Chief of Psychology Service at Sam Rayburn Memorial Veterans Center, in Bonham, Texas, and Paul J. Kulkosky, Ph.D., Professor of Psychology at the University of Southern Colorado, in Pueblo, neurofeedback therapy (also know as neurotherapy or brain wave therapy) is a revolutionary treatment for addiction, using biofeedback and visualization techniques to bring about significant behavioral change by altering the addictive personality. "You're changing personal biology, the way someone functions," says Steven Fahrion, Ph.D., founding member of Life Sciences Institute of Mind-Body Health, in Topeka, Kansas, where the treatment is used for a wide range of applications, including alcoholism and drug abuse.

Neurofeedback therapy involves three separate treatment procedures. First, alcoholics and addicts learn how to use biofeedback in association with breathing exercises and relaxation phrases to begin to develop a relaxation response and an orientation to relaxation. According to Dr. Peniston, this allows a patient's alpha brain waves to rise, while also facilitating the ability to descend into a theta state of consciousness (a very deep level of relaxed brain wave activity). This is important, says Dr. Peniston, "because it is only in the theta state that long-lasting physiological or mental change can take place."

The next phase of the program is visualization. This involves the development of alcohol or drug rejection scenarios. Patients visualize themselves standing outside a liquor store or bar, looking in but not going in. They then see themselves walking away and rejecting the purchase of drugs and alcohol. "Before going on to the brain wave training, it is critical that the person be able to visualize himself in situations where he would ordinarily drink or take drugs, and then see himself turning away from that," says Dr. Fahrion.

Brain wave training is the third part of the treatment and is also the most important. In this phase, these new positive images become consolidated and, in effect, stamped on the personality of the patient. Using sophisticated biofeedback equipment, the patient is further induced into an alpha state and then into a theta state. "Alpha is the bridge to theta," says Dr. Peniston. "It only takes being in the deeper theta state of consciousness about 10% of the time during a session for true change to take place. Once a person is in that state, the hippocampus region of the brain is activated. This is where all the experiences a person has had in childhood and adulthood, particularly those that were traumatic and anxiety-provoking, are housed. It's during this state that the hypothalamus system (a region of the forebrain that regulates basic body functions) is reprogrammed."

Dr. Fahrion adds, "Because the brain can't discriminate between created visualizations and actual events, it substitutes the image of the person turning away from the addictive substance for the old behavior. So it really changes the way the person thinks about himself." Dr. Fahrion describes an example of this alteration in thought processes with a patient's account of her visualization: "It's foggy and cold. The air is thick and stuffy, kind of gray. I lean inside my friend's car that smells like cigarette smoke and heavy metal music is playing. They ask me if I want to use and I say, 'No, I don't want to use.' I turn around and start to walk to school. As I walk, the sun starts to come out, the air is lighter and easier to breathe, and everything begins to clear as I walk away. I'm confident in my decisions, feeling lifted up and good about myself."

See Biofeedback Training and Neurotherapy, Hypnotherapy, Mind/Body Medicine.

According to Dr. Peniston, each session lasts about 30 minutes, with the whole treatment program usually requiring at least 30 sessions, depending on the patient's individual needs and disposition going into therapy. In addition to alpha-theta brain wave training, the program also includes instruction in relapse prevention, shame and guilt work, the biology of addiction, spirituality exercises, and self-help groups. "The thing that's so exciting about this is the relapse prevention aspect," adds Dr. Fahrion. "Usually there's a revolving door of relapse, where a person attends a treatment program and, often before he is even out a week or two, he has relapsed again."

"With our first study we had about an 80% success rate," reported Dr. Kulkosky in 1993. "With traditional therapy, such as psychotherapy and anti-craving medication, after 13 months there was only a 20% success rate and, after five years, it had dropped down to zero. We're now five or six years past our first study and we're still seeing about a 70% success rate."

Perhaps the most impressive study involving neurofeedback therapy in addiction was overseen by Dr. Fahrion and his wife, Patricia Norris, Ph.D., also a founding member of Life Sciences Institute and an expert in a wide range of mind/body medical applications. Conducted at the Ellsworth Correctional Facility, in Kansas, over a three-year period in the 1990s, the study involved convicted felons known to suffer from alcohol or drug addiction. Almost all participants had previously tried and failed many other types of addiction treatment.

Each of the participants received a specific protocol developed by Drs. Fahrion and Norris, consisting of neurofeedback therapy, biofeedback training, visualization, and counseling, for three weeks prior to their release. They were then closely followed by their parole officers, which enabled thorough, detailed information to continue to be gathered. Preliminary results after two years of follow-up found that 63% remained drug- and alcohol-free. Success was determined by strict criteria, including no use of drugs or alcohol as determined by frequent urinalysis and no failure of terms of parole. Even more impressive, recidivism for new crimes was only 4%.

The court administrative judge called it "the first good news in 40 years" and stated that neurofeedback therapy could become "the model of addiction treatment for the entire country." Due to the study's success, the Kansas Department of Corrections tripled the number of prisoners at Ellsworth who received neurofeedback therapy and is looking to incorporate it at other prisons. Based on such results, Drs. Fahrion and Norris expect to see "a landslide of desire to start more programs" for addicted prisoners nationwide, once the benefits of neurofeedback therapy become more widely known.[21]

Part of the reason for neurofeedback therapy's high success rate is that if someone does relapse, the body will immediately reject the alcohol or drug, causing a severe flu-like reaction that will usually put the person in bed for several days. "Nobody has an explanation as to why this happens yet, but it's quite consistent all over the country," says Dr. Fahrion. "The other thing that happens is the kick, the high from the addictive substance, disappears. It just doesn't give the person the boost that it did before. Between these two things, it's not something that they like to repeat that much."

Other techniques that are helpful in dealing with addictions include Thought Field Therapy (TFT), developed by Roger Callahan, Ph.D., and Emotional Freedom Technique (EFT), developed by Gary Craig, Ph.D. These techniques incorporate muscle testing to determine the underlying subconscious emotions or decisions that predispose to addiction plus Eye Movement Desensitization and Reprocessing (EMDR) and tapping on key acupressure points while speaking corrective affirmations.

Herbal Medicine

Herbal medicine can play an important role in treating addiction, particularly with regard to the liver, which is one of the body's organs most damaged by substance abuse. As the toxins begin to filter out, cleansing and healing the liver is critical. Dr. Aesoph recommends treating a faltering liver with milk thistle (Silybum marianum), which contains some of the most powerful liver-protective substances known, and not only protects it from damage, but encourages the growth of new cells. Other herbs for supporting liver function include dandelion (Taraxacum officinale) and bupleurum (Radix bupleurum).[22]

Since optimal function of eliminative organs, such as the kidneys and liver, is necessary to battle addiction and sustain recovery, blood-cleansing herbs are also vital. Dr. Aesoph recommends wild oat extract, burdock root, fumitory (Fumaria officinalis), echinacea, and licorice root, which are all useful in this respect.

Like other drugs, the withdrawal symptoms of caffeine, mainly headache, fatigue, and depression, make abstinence difficult. Dr. Aesoph suggests the use of feverfew, lime blossom, and chamomile flowers, which can help break the coffee habit.

Oatstraw (Avena sativa) is one of many herbs useful in addiction treatment, according to Michael Murray, N.D., of Issaquah, Washington. "Oats have long been used in India to treat opium addiction," he explains. "Evidently, they help rebalance the endorphin levels in the brain." Siberian ginseng has been shown to normalize the neurotransmitters in the brain. "This demonstrates that it has some sort of balancing effect. I think that

---

USING HERBS TO STOP SMOKING

According to Michael Murray, N.D., lobelia is the most notable herb used to combat the effects of nicotine withdrawal. "The active ingredient in lobelia, lobeline, has similar actions to nicotine, but it's gentler, has a longer duration of action, and is a suitable alternative to nicotine chewing gum or the nicotine patch," Dr. Murray says. Lobelia has also been shown to have antidepressant action.

"Another herb that's been shown to contain components useful in helping people to quit smoking," adds Dr. Murray, "is ma-huang or Ephedra sinica. Ephedrine, the active constituent in this herb, helps decrease the number of cigarettes smoked. Lobelia is more effective when it's used with a stimulant. So it's possible that by combining lobelia and ephedra (a stimulant), you'll get better results than if you use either alone."

Lobelia, however, is only an interim measure in treating nicotine dependency, warns Dr. Murray. Because the person can become hooked on this herb, it is important to wean the smoker off lobelia over a period of a month. Dr. Murray notes that oat extracts have also induced smokers to decrease the number of cigarettes smoked, even while they claimed to be unaware of the effect.

---

would be very important in someone who needs stimulants or some other addictive substance to function," says Dr. Murray.

Skullcap, valerian, balm (Melissa), kava-kava, and vervain are natural alternatives to pharmaceutical sedatives and tranquilizers used to treat anxiety, inside and outside of addiction treatment. "My first choice," says Dr. Murray, "would be using St. John's wort, due to its antidepressive qualities. Also, it doesn't have strong sedative effects like valerian."

Ayurvedic Medicine

Virender Sodhi, M.D. (Ayurveda), N.D., Director of the Ayurvedic & Naturopathic Medical Clinic, in Bellevue, Washington, practices Ayurvedic medicine, which asserts that each of the three body types has certain weaknesses, which for different reasons can lead to addiction. According to Dr. Sodhi, Ayurvedic medicine holds that an individual develops addictive behavior while attempting to cope with fear and anxiety. Each of the body types—vata, pitta, and kapha—copes with anxiety differently as well. Knowing this, the individual can use these inherent tendencies in an orderly and systematic manner for healing. For example, Dr. Sodhi explains that a *pitta* body type (very driven, overachievers) will not be able to tolerate alcohol. Part of the Ayurvedic diagnostic method outlined by Dr. Sodhi is an examination of the pulse, the tongue, and the eyes, which indicates the condition of inner organs and suggests proper herbs and vitamins needed for treatment. *Ghee* is often used in treatment, as are *ashwagandha* and *calamus*.

Dr. Sodhi relates the case history of a woman addicted for ten years to marijuana. He describes her as "a *kapha* type, slow moving, with a tendency to abuse stimulants for energy," and she was suffering from depression and disorientation. In addition, her adrenal glands were exhausted. Dr. Sodhi administered gotu kola and put her on a vitamin regime, including B_6, B_{12}, and folic acid injections, as well as amino acids to revive the adrenal glands. Dr. Sodhi states, "Within three months, she recovered from the lethargy and depression and soon her glandular functions returned to normal."

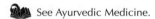 See Ayurvedic Medicine.

Recommendations

- Most addictive people have problems processing sugar and carbohydrates—a program of three meals a day, with an emphasis on eating proteins at each meal, may be helpful.

- Megavitamin therapy is commonly cited as one of the most vital tools for replenishing vitamin deficiency, which affects more than 50% of alcoholics as well as many of those with other addictions.

- Zinc may help the body metabolize and detoxify from alcohol and other drugs, as does vitamin C.

- Chromium aids in stabilizing the erratic blood sugar seen in hypoglycemia of alcoholics and other addicts, while choline and folic acid are important supplements to assist in the body's recovery from addiction.

- Studies have shown fewer relapses and fewer readmissions to treatment centers for alcoholics and other addicts who have had acupuncture therapy, especially auriculotherapy.

- Flower essences may make it easier to break the cycle of addiction.

- A person receiving chiropractic care is more likely to complete a drug treatment program.

- Neurofeedback therapy uses biofeedback and visualization techniques to bring about significant behavioral change by altering the addictive personality.

- Herbs for supporting liver function, important during detoxification, include milk thistle (*Silybum marianum*), dandelion (*Taraxacum officinale*), and bupleurum (*Radix bupleurum*).

- Oatstraw (*Avena sativa*) and Siberian ginseng have proven useful in addiction treatment.

- Ayurvedic medicine asserts that each of the three body types has certain weaknesses that, for different reasons, can lead to addiction. An individual develops addictive behavior while attempting to cope with fear and anxiety. Knowing this, the individual can use these inherent tendencies in an orderly and systematic manner for healing.

Self-Care
The following therapies can be undertaken at home under appropriate professional supervision:

ALCOHOLISM
Acupressure
AROMATHERAPY: Fennel, rose, juniper, rosemary.

FASTING: Detoxifies the body, but only if not malnourished.

HOMEOPATHY: *Berberis, Nux vomica, Sulphur, Lachesis, Lycopodium.*

HYDROTHERAPY: Steam sauna and immersion bath can help rid the body of toxins.

MEDITATION: Alcoholics who practice Transcendental Meditation show a steady decline in alcohol use as well as a 90% sobriety rate after two years.[23]

SMOKING
Meditation / Qigong and Tai Chi / Yoga
HOMEOPATHY: *Daphne ind., Tabacum.*

HYDROTHERAPY: Use immersion bath, wet sheet pack, or steam sauna, one to two times weekly, to produce sweating. Also, consider an enema daily during detoxification.

JUICE THERAPY: A juice fast over 2-3 weeks may be effective for detoxifying the blood from nicotine and to end the craving for cigarettes. Avoid acidifying juices (citrus, tomato).

Professional Care

The following therapies should only be provided by a qualified health professional:

ALCOHOLISM AND DRUG ADDICTION

Acupuncture / Biofeedback Training and Neurotherapy / Chiropractic / Detoxification Therapy / Environmental Medicine / Hydrotherapy / Magnetic Field Therapy / Mind/Body Medicine / Naturopathic Medicine / Ortho-molecular Medicine / Osteopathic Medicine / Oxygen Therapies

SMOKING

Acupuncture / Biofeedback Training and Neurotherapy / Detoxification Therapy / Environmental Medicine / Hypnotherapy / Magnetic Field Therapy / Mind/Body Medicine / Naturopathic Medicine

Where to Find Help

For more information on and referrals for treatment of addictions, contact the following organizations.

American Association of Oriental Medicine (AAOM)

433 Front Street
Catasauqua, Pennsylvania 18032
(888) 500-7999
Website: www.aaom.org

The AAOM is a national professional trade organization of acupuncturists who meet acceptable standards of minimum competency and can provide you with the names and locations of local members.

American College of Addictionology and Compulsive Disorders (ACACD)

975 Arthur Godfrey Road, Suite 500
Miami Beach, Florida 33140
(305) 534-3635

Overseen by Dr. Jay Holder, the college provides instructions to health professionals in Dr. Holder's protocol for treating addictions, as well as offering treatment programs for people suffering from addiction and compulsive disorders.

Ayurvedic & Naturopathic Medical Clinic

2115 112th Avenue N.E.
Bellevue, Washington 98004
(425) 453-8022
Website: www.ayurvedicscience.com

Dr. Virender Sodhi's clinic provides medical training for physicians and health-care practitioners, as well as individual courses for laypeople.

Life Sciences Institute of Mind–Body Health

4636 S.W. Wanamaker Road
Topeka, Kansas 66610
(785) 271-8686
Website: www.cjnetworks.com/~lifesci

The Institute provides research, treatment, and workshops in all areas of mind/body medicine, including extensive work with biofeedback and neurofeedback therapy as a treatment for addiction.

National Acupuncture Detoxification Association (NADA)

P.O. Box 1927
Vancouver, Washington 98668
Website: www.acudetox.com

NADA is a leading organization devoted to researching and furthering the use of acupuncture treatment for addictive behaviors.

National Institute on Alcohol Abuse and Alcoholism (NIAAA)

6000 Executive Blvd., Willco Building
Bethesda, Maryland 20892-7003
Website: www.niaaa.nih.gov

A source of statistics and other information on alcohol abuse. The NIAAA supports research on the causes, consequences, treatment, and prevention of alcoholism and alcohol-related problems.

National Institute on Drug Abuse (NIDA)

6001 Executive Blvd., Room 5213
Bethesda, Maryland 20892
(301) 443-1124
Website: www.nida.nih.gov

A source of statistics and other information on drug addictions.

Sitike Counseling Center

306 Spruce Avenue
South San Francisco, California 94080
(415) 589-9305

One of the premier centers for treating addiction through dietary and nutritional intervention using their Biochemical Restoration Program. Also offers acupuncture and counseling and can provide referrals to similar programs nationwide.

Recommended Reading

Allergy Free: An Alternative Medicine Definitive Guide. Konrad Kail, N.D., and Bobbi Lawrence, with Burton Goldberg. Tiburon, CA: AlternativeMedicine.com Books, 2000.

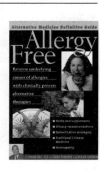

Breaking Your Prescribed Addiction. Billie Jay Sahley, Ph.D., and Katherine M. Birkner, C.R.N.A., Ph.D. San Antonio, TX: Pain and Stress Therapy Center, 1998.

Dr. Braly's Food Allergy and Nutrition Revolution. James Braly, M.D. New Canaan, CT: Keats Publishing, 1992.

Encyclopedia of Natural Medicine. Michael Murray, N.D., and Joseph Pizzorno, N.D. Rocklin, CA: Prima Publishing, 1998.

Food for Recovery: The Complete Nutritional Companion for Overcoming Alcoholism, Drug Addiction, and Eating Disorders. Joseph D. Beasley, M.D., and Susan Knightly. New York: Crown, 1994.

The Hidden Addiction—And How to Get Free. Janice K. Phelps, M.D., and Alan E. Nourse, M.D. Boston: Little, Brown, 1986.

The Sugar Addict's Total Recovery Program. Kathleen DesMaisons, Ph.D. New York: Ballantine, 2000.

AIDS

Worldwide, an estimated 36 million people are HIV-positive or have AIDS and 22 million have died of the disease over the last 20 years. AIDS, more than any other disease, has been surrounded by stigma and mystery ever since it was recognized in the early 1980s. Researchers are still debating its cause and even whether it is, in fact, a new disease. Conventional medicine treats AIDS using drug therapies that, in some cases, can produce toxic side effects that resemble the symptoms of the disease itself. A growing number of alternative physicians are approaching the illness from a different perspective and their work is proving that, contrary to popular belief, AIDS is not a death sentence.

ALL DISEASES, if properly approached and treated in time, are reversible. This includes AIDS (acquired immunodeficiency syndrome), as the following stories illustrate. A man suffering from AIDS for five years came to Joan Priestley, M.D., of Anchorage, Alaska. He'd been diagnosed as terminal and given five months to live. He suffered from severe weight loss and diarrhea, opportunistic infections, and Crohn's disease. After one year of aggressive treatment with Dr. Priestley, the man, despite a continued low T-cell count, which is considered a marker for AIDS and HIV (human immunodeficiency virus) infection, became symptom free, regained 40 pounds, and was able to resume living a productive life.

A patient suffering from night sweats and fever, and diagnosed as HIV-positive (HIV is commonly believed to be the cause of AIDS) was weak and faint all of the time as his T-cell count continued dropping. He sought out Robert Cathcart III, M.D., of Los Altos, California, a pioneer in the use of vitamin C therapy as a treatment for illness. Fifteen months after beginning intravenous vitamin C treatments, the patient's T-cell count had risen from under 300 to 600. He felt healthy and, for the first time in his life, went over a year without having a cold or flu.

In 1984, Jon was diagnosed with Kaposi's sarcoma, a form of skin cancer common to gay men with AIDS. He had also been suffering with hepatitis for a year. After adopting a protocol of nutritional supplementation, herbs,

> *AIDS is defined primarily by what appears to be severe immune deficiency and is distinguished from virtually every other disease in history by the fact that it has no constant, specific symptoms.*

and a healthy diet, under the supervision of Laurence Badgley, M.D., of Foster City, California, his symptoms began to improve. Over nine years later, Jon is healthy and working two full-time jobs.

These are only a few of the many cases of people with AIDS or HIV who have turned their illness around and are now on the road to health. This chapter explains the various methods that they used outside the framework of conventional medicine to keep themselves alive. To understand how and why such treatments work, it is first necessary to examine what AIDS is and what it is not.

What is AIDS?

AIDS is defined primarily by what appears to be severe immune deficiency and is distinguished from virtually every other disease in history by the fact that it has no constant, specific symptoms. Once the immune system begins to malfunction, a broad spectrum of health complications can set in. *AIDS* is an umbrella term for any or all of these 28 previously known diseases and symptoms. When a person has any of these diseases or opportunistic infections, and also tests positive for antibodies to HIV, an AIDS diagnosis is given.

The diseases that mark AIDS differ widely from country to country and even from risk group to risk group. In the United States and Europe, some of the most common diseases associated with AIDS are Kaposi's sar-

HIV/AIDS STATISTICS

- An estimated 36.1 million people worldwide (including 1.4 million children) have HIV/AIDS.

- 47% of those with HIV/AIDS are women.

- In 2000, there were 5.3 million new HIV infections, about 15,000 each day.

- 21.8 million people have died of HIV/AIDS-related diseases through the end of 2000.

- Worldwide, more than 80% of adult HIV infections are the result of heterosexual intercourse.

- Approximately 800,000 to 900,000 people in the U.S. are infected with HIV and a third of them do not know they are infected.

- Of the 40,000 new HIV infections in the U.S. each year, 70% occur in men, 30% in women.

- Among women with HIV in the U.S., 75% were infected through heterosexual intercourse and 25% through injection drug use.

- There have been a total of 438,795 deaths from AIDS in the U.S. through June 30, 2000.

- AIDS is the fifth leading cause of death in the U.S. among those 25-44 years old.

- The number of annual AIDS-related deaths in the U.S. fell 68% from 1995 to 1999.[1]

THE TROUBLE WITH DEFINING AIDS

By January 1, 1993, extreme alterations were being made to the original definition of AIDS. Previously, in order to be diagnosed as having AIDS, it was necessary to have one or more of 25 symptoms listed by the U.S. Centers for Disease Control and Prevention (CDC), as well as being HIV-positive. The CDC added three new conditions—cancer of the cervix, bacterial pneumonia, and tuberculosis—which, when found in combination with the HIV virus, would constitute AIDS. The effect of this decision dramatically and artificially inflated the statistics of people who have AIDS. In the U.S. alone, the figures immediately rose from 250,000 to 400,000, with a huge increase in the number of women with an AIDS diagnosis.

This caused famed British epidemiologist, Gordon Stewart, M.D., to ask the pertinent question: "Will any woman with cervicitis, any man with urethritis, prostatitis, genitourinary cancer or any cancer, or perhaps severe infection, or any other unspecified, wasting, or multiple disease, who happens to be HIV-positive, be diagnosed and registered as having AIDS and treated for HIV disease, because those in the business can expand their domain across any diagnostic code and scruple?"[2]

coma (a form of cancer), pneumocystis pneumonia, candidiasis, and mycobacterial infections such as tuberculosis, toxoplasmosis (a disease caused by protozoa that damages the central nervous system, eyes, and internal organs), cytomegalovirus, and the herpes virus. Other more general conditions not included in the 28 indicator diseases but often associated with the disease include diarrhea, weight loss, night sweats, fevers, rashes, and swollen lymph glands.

There are some striking differences between the various "risk groups" in whom AIDS has remained concentrated. Kaposi's sarcoma, for instance, one of the earliest symptoms by which AIDS was diagnosed, is 20 times more common in gay men with AIDS than in all other American AIDS patients.[3] Tuberculosis, meanwhile, is mainly seen in intravenous drug users. AIDS in Africa, by contrast, lacks the distinction of "risk groups" and occurs evenly among the population and between the sexes. There, AIDS is defined primarily by diarrhea, wasting, fever, and a persistent cough: symptoms that have all been quite common in Africa for decades and are seen in most tropical diseases.

Because of these and other discrepancies, there is much confusion and dissent about what AIDS really is and even if it is accurate to classify it as a disease entity. The common factor that all these disconnected symptoms and diseases revolve around is HIV. If HIV antibodies are detected, these diseases converge as AIDS; if not, then they are diagnosed simply for what they are. In other words, any degree of immune suppression in the presence of HIV is classified as AIDS. But the same degree of immune suppression in the absence of HIV is by definition not AIDS.

This has led to a kind of diagnostic chaos never before seen in medicine. The answer as to who has AIDS and who doesn't may depend on which doctor does the diagnosis. There is also tremendous dispute about whether, in fact, HIV even causes AIDS. This question has been argued in the media, the AIDS community, and in the scientific literature, and still remains unresolved. One camp believes that HIV causes the immune suppression that leads to AIDS, while the other argues that various environmental risk factors such as recreational and pharmaceutical drugs, sexually transmitted diseases, and bacterial infections are the real cause of the immune suppression, and that HIV is simply a by-product of an already suppressed immune system. This also raises questions about how AIDS develops. Does it manifest suddenly or over a period of several years? These questions need to be resolved before the true nature of the relationship between AIDS and HIV can be fully understood.

The HIV Debate

Most AIDS scientists refer freely to HIV as the sole or primary cause of AIDS, yet the body of scientific evidence that supports this notion is ambiguous. Although there is a strong correlation between HIV and AIDS— meaning that most people with AIDS also test positive for HIV—it is not a total correlation, nor is correlation proof of causation. Though at least 200,000 papers have been written on HIV, the evidence that HIV causes AIDS remains tenuous and can best be described as circumstantial: the damage is done, the cells are depleted, and HIV is present at the scene of the crime.[4] So, despite mainstream insistence and billions of dollars and years of research from around the world, the HIV equals AIDS hypothesis still remains in question.

This hypothesis was first announced at a press conference on April 23, 1984, by Robert Gallo, M.D., of the National Cancer Institute. AIDS, he claimed, was a new retrovirus (RNA-containing virus with tumor-causing properties), supposedly isolated in his laboratory, that he called HTLV-III (human T-cell lymphotropic virus type III) and which was later renamed HIV. At the time of the announcement, this hypothesis was based on nothing more than a strong correlation between AIDS cases and HIV. Most, though not all, of the AIDS patients studied showed antibodies to HIV, yet only half of them had detectable live virus. Dr. Gallo's hypothesis soon became accepted as fact. Initial media reports stated that the "probable" cause of AIDS had been found, but very soon the word *probable* was dropped as HIV found its new identity as "the AIDS virus."

Other researchers, reviewing Dr. Gallo's original papers published in *Science,* have concluded that they present no proof that HIV causes AIDS.[5] "Nobody in their right mind would jump into this thing like they did," says Kary Mullis, Ph.D., recipient of the 1993 Nobel Prize in Medicine and inventor of the polymerase chain reaction (PCR), one of the mainstays of AIDS viral technology. "It had nothing to do with any well-considered science. There were some people who had AIDS and some of them had HIV—not even all of them. They had a correlation. So what?"[6]

"There have always been people questioning or disagreeing with the official theory and treatments approach," states Gary Null, Ph.D., an alternative medi-

AIDS WITHOUT HIV?

Growing numbers of cases of severe immune suppression have been reported that appear to be clinically identical to AIDS, but do not test positive for HIV. Peter Duesberg, Ph.D., claims that there may be as many as 5,000 such cases.[9] Because HIV is not present, these cases are not registered as AIDS. The rationale of the U.S. Centers for Disease Control and Prevention (CDC) is simple: AIDS is caused by HIV, therefore, if HIV is not present, the cases cannot be AIDS.

Although several hundred cases of HIV-negative "AIDS" have been documented in the medical literature over the years, it was not until the International AIDS Conference in Amsterdam, in July 1992, that the world media reacted with alarm, writing stories about the "new disease" and criticizing CDC officials for not taking the "handful" of cases more seriously. A single abstract sparked the uproar, written by an American doctor who reported on six cases of AIDS without HIV. Upon hearing the doctor's presentation, several more doctors started to volunteer cases of their own that fit the same description.

Seeking to calm the ensuing chaos, the CDC quickly settled on a new name for the "mysterious new disease," calling it "ICL," which stands for idiopathic CD-4 lymphocytopenia. *Idiopathic* refers to a disease for which the cause is not known.[10]

cine advocate and author of *AIDS: A Second Opinion,* "but they have been silenced. Instead of being urged on in their attempt to help mankind, they were ridiculed and their funding was stopped."[7]

In 1987, molecular biologist Peter Duesberg, Ph.D., Professor of Molecular and Cell Biology at the University of California at Berkeley, launched a frontal attack on the HIV-AIDS hypothesis in the journal *Cancer Research.* Dr. Duesberg, a world-renowned scientist and long-standing member of the National Academy of Sciences, had helped map the genetic structure of retroviruses and is one of the world's foremost experts on retroviruses. After reading every paper on HIV and AIDS published at that time, Dr. Duesberg concluded that the virus was "harmless," pointing out, among other things, that HIV was a latent, inactive virus, which infected very few cells. Dr. Duesberg stated flatly that he "wouldn't mind being injected with it."[8]

Perhaps the most striking point of Dr. Duesberg's critique of the HIV-AIDS hypothesis was that HIV showed very little direct cell-killing activity. In fact, when he viewed HIV under a microscope amidst lymphocytes (cells important in the creation of antibodies), it didn't move at all and the cells remained perfectly intact. According to Dr. Duesberg, this is to be expected. "Retroviruses are not typically cytocidal, that is, they do not kill cells," he explains.[11] But the mainstream AIDS community contends that direct cell killing is not necessary in order to implicate HIV, believing that the virus kills cells by one of several highly complex indirect mechanisms. One of these is known as apoptosis—a mechanism by which HIV is said to program cells to kill themselves in the future. Dr. Duesberg counters that there is no evidence for any of these elaborate mechanisms and that HIV is far too simple genetically to perform these feats. Harvey Bialy, M.D., scientific editor of the journal *BioTechnology*, agrees. "HIV is an ordinary retrovirus," he says. "It only contains a very small piece of genetic information. There's no way it can do all these elaborate things they say it does."[12]

Dr. Duesberg further argues that the HIV-AIDS theory fails to fulfill the standard set of rules used to determine whether or not a particular organism causes a particular disease. These rules, known as Koch's Postulates, were established by German bacteriologist Robert Koch, who determined the causes of tuberculosis, anthrax, and several other infectious diseases using the following rules:

- The suspected organism has to be present in each and every case of the disease and in sufficient quantities to cause disease.

- The agent is not found in other diseases.

- After isolation and propagation, the agent can induce the disease when transmitted to another host.

Dr. Duesberg concedes that there are limitations to Koch's Postulates, especially since most pathogens (disease-causing agents) are pathogenic only when the immune system is already below par. However, he argues, HIV has been shown to fail all three postulates, since it has already been established that the virus is not present in every case of AIDS-like disease; because it is found not in one, but in 28 distinct diseases; and because chimpanzees, when inoculated with HIV, have consistently failed to develop AIDS.[13] In 1993, there were 125 to 150 chimpanzees in captivity around the world that had been injected with HIV, some as long ago as 1983, none of which had developed any symptoms of AIDS.[14]

A British study conducted in 1987 also looked at accidental exposure to HIV by medical personnel (scratched with a needle previously used on infected individuals, for example). The study noted, "One surprising and mildly reassuring fact is that when health workers were examined after needlestick wounds, only one out of 1,500 in the United Kingdom and the U.S. became infected."[15]

A number of researchers have noted that electron micrographs of "HIV" are actually of cell cultures with a variety of particles and cellular debris, which have not gone through the necessary further steps of purification and analysis to isolate a replicating virus. "To identify a virus, a first step is to photograph isolated particles in an electron microscope, and they must look like the viral particles observed in cells, body fluids, or cell cultures to distinguish them from other particles that look like viruses but are not," according to Stefan Lanka, Ph.D., a German virologist. "Proteins making up the viral coat must then be separated from each other and photographed, producing a pattern that is characteristic of the species of virus. A similar procedure must be gone through for the DNA or RNA of the virus. Such evidence has never been produced for HIV."[16] Eleni Papadopulos-Eleopulos, Ph.D., a biophysicist at the Royal Perth Hospital, in Australia, and "dissident" AIDS researcher states, "There is no proof that HIV causes AIDS, because there is no proof that HIV exists."[17]

Another problem with the HIV-AIDS hypothesis are the HIV tests themselves. Since the tests, such as Western Blot and ELISA (enzyme-linked immunoserological assay), measure antibodies to HIV and not the virus itself, they are highly inaccurate, according to Michael Gerber, M.D., H.M.D., of Reno, Nevada. Medical researcher Roberto A. Giraldo, M.D., was surprised to find that the manufacturer of the ELISA test recommended that the blood serum used for the test should be diluted in a 1:400 ratio, a high dilution for such a test. Most ELISA tests use undiluted or only slightly diluted (1:16 or 1:20) serum. An experiment revealed the reason: when he tried the test on undiluted samples, they all tested positive for HIV. "Since there is no scientific evidence that the ELISA test is specific for HIV antibodies, a reactive ELISA test at any concentration of the serum would mean the presence of nonspecific antibodies," concluded Dr. Giraldo. "These antibodies could be present in all blood samples, most likely a result of a stress response, having no relation to any retrovirus, let alone HIV."[18]

The Western Blot test is not standardized, so a positive test in one country would not be considered positive in another country. Antibodies to a variety of viruses, bacteria, and other antigens cross-react with antigens in the tests, potentially leading to false-positive test results.[19] Other conditions that can produce false-positive results are immunizations, herpes, hepatitis, tuberculosis, malaria, parasites, alcoholism and liver disease, pregnancy, and infection with mycobacterium or yeasts (common in AIDS patients).[20] The polymerase chain reaction (PCR) test used to monitor HIV levels is also not specific for the virus, measuring genetic material but not the virus itself.[21]

"In virology as in life, one cannot put the cart before the horse," states Valendar F. Turner, M.D., of the Royal Perth Hospital, in Australia. "What masquerades as proof of the existence of HIV is sets of antibody/antigen reactions between two sets of unknowns (culture proteins and antibodies). For those unlucky enough to possess the cells or antibodies capable of producing similar reactions, the enormous weight of the HIV theory of AIDS becomes their lifelong yoke."[22]

Can a Person Be HIV-Positive and Not Get AIDS?

Though many people do become infected with HIV, a great deal of evidence now points to the possibility that a healthy immune system can keep the virus in check.[23] Australian researchers studied a group of six people who each received contaminated blood products infected by a single common donor. Over ten years later, both the donor and five of the recipients remained symptom free, with no decline of CD4 cells (T-helper cells, involved in immune function and used as a marker for evidence of AIDS) and no sign of the P24 antigen (a specific marker that identifies a cell and causes the production of antibodies to destroy it) in the blood, which are considered signs of worsening AIDS conditions. One of the six recipients died of pneumonia *(Pneumocystis carinii),* but she had received massive immunosuppressive treatment for lupus (an inflammatory disease causing abnormal growth of blood vessels and connective tissue) and cannot be regarded as a typical individual. In only one of the surviving study group members was it possible to even isolate HIV.

The researchers have no clear-cut answer for their findings, stating, "It is not clear whether the benign course of HIV infection was due to host, viral, or other unknown factors."[24] Their belief is that this was possibly a less virulent strain of HIV, but credit for the lack of progression to AIDS could just as easily be due to healthier immune systems, with the exception of the immune-compromised patient with lupus. Even more significantly, the lack of HIV development could be due to the absence of co-factors.

Co-Factors

The AIDS establishment still stands firmly by its conviction that HIV causes AIDS, although they are finally conceding that HIV alone may not lead to AIDS without the help of one or more co-factors. These can include recreational and pharmaceutical drug use, recurrent infections, chronic use of antibiotics, poor nutrition, and pollution, as well as many psychological co-factors, such as stress, fear, and despair.

The AIDS establishment still stands firmly by its conviction that HIV causes AIDS, although they are finally conceding that HIV alone may not lead to AIDS without the help of one or more co-factors.

When AIDS was first recognized, the syndrome was called GRID, for Gay-Related Immune Deficiency, since it was initially only found in gay men. The first few hundred cases were seen in male homosexuals who lived in major cities, particularly New York and San Francisco, who had frequently used both recreational and pharmaceutical drugs and had been exposed to numerous bacterial infections and sexually transmitted diseases. The CDC initially suspected that AIDS was caused by drugs, most specifically amyl nitrates or "poppers," a drug prevalent in gay discos of that era that proved to cause Kaposi's sarcoma in animals. Research now shows that Kaposi's sarcoma is not linked either directly or indirectly to the HIV virus.[25] In 1992, Dr. Duesberg concluded that AIDS was caused by drug consumption and other noncontagious risk factors.[26]

Other groups, though, soon started showing up as targets for the host of opportunistic diseases associated with AIDS. Hemophiliacs, intravenous drug users, and the Third World poor, particularly in Africa, all started coming down with the mysterious disease. As with gay men, these risk groups shared similar symptoms of immune suppression caused by a number of possible co-factors, including drug use, frequent exposure to various bacteria and germs (as from a blood transfusion or a dirty needle), unsafe sexual practices, malnutrition, unsanitary eating and living conditions, or a combination of these factors. Interestingly, in Africa, HIV tests are not required for an AIDS diagnosis.[27] Fever, a 10% weight loss, persistent cough, and diarrhea qualify for a diagnosis of AIDS, even though these symptoms are common to many other illnesses.[28]

Dr. Papadopulos-Eleopulos questions the research behind the assertion that hemophiliacs have been infected with HIV through contaminated blood products. Because the clotting factor (Factor VIII) undergoes rigorous processing, involving freezing, heating, and drying, any HIV present in the serum would not survive, according to Dr. Papadopulos-Eleopulos. "The published data do not prove the hypothesis that such transmission occurs, and therefore HIV cannot account for AIDS in hemophiliacs," she states.[29] It should be noted that while 75% of hemophiliacs have had HIV (according to standard tests) for more than seven years, only 2% develop AIDS-related diseases each year,[30] indicating the importance of co-factors.

In his book *The Virus Within*, Nicholas Regush reviews the AIDS saga and focuses on two medical researchers who have followed the trail of a more virulent virus, HHV-6 (human herpes virus 6). Donald Carrigan, Ph.D., and Konnie Knox, Ph.D., of the Department of Pathology, Medical College of Wisconsin, in Milwaukee, found a damaging presence of HHV-6 in the lymph glands, T4 cells, lungs, livers, kidneys, and spleens of deceased AIDS patients. They note that HHV-6 is commonly found in humans, but is not virulent until the immune system is damaged.

Before HIV was declared to be the single cause of AIDS, many of these various immunosuppressive factors were still being investigated. In 1984, with the discovery of HIV, these other investigations suddenly stopped. Now, there is a vast amount of research on HIV and very little on any of the possible co-factors. "We were all forced into a very dogmatic and simplistic view of what caused AIDS," says Michael Lange, M.D., an infectious disease specialist at St. Luke's Roosevelt Hospital, in New York City. "Today, I think even the greatest proponents of HIV no longer believe that it does all that damage to the immune system by itself. There have to be other factors involved. And because of the HIV hypothesis, there's been little or no research done on what those other factors may be."[31]

 Before HIV was declared to be the single cause of AIDS, many immunosuppressive co-factors were still being investigated. The government should be urged to renew intensive research into these potential co-factors.

Immune System Cells and AIDS

AIDS is often accompanied by a steady decline in CD4 immune cells, which in a healthy person should hover between 900 and 1,600, but in a person with AIDS can decline to as low as zero. In 1989, a CD4 cell count of less than 500 became the cutoff point after which AZT therapy was advised. AZT (zidovudine) is a toxic chemotherapy drug that is believed to stop replication of the HIV virus. Virtually all AIDS therapies, both mainstream and alternative, have used the CD4 count as a marker for immune suppression.

Official doctrine states that HIV also destroys T4 cells, another critical part of the immune system. T4 cells identify invading pathogens and trigger other immune system cells to attack these invaders. With a drastic reduction in T4 cells, the ability to respond against potential disease is reduced. Germs that ordinarily would have no effect on the body become potent enemies. Alternative physicians, even though they have been successful in reviving overall health in persons with AIDS, have struggled with the restoration of full T4 cell counts. It has been observed, however, that high T4 counts do not necessarily correspond with health. Researchers have found people whose T4 counts are almost non-existent (under 10) who show no signs of disease[32] and there is no proof that low T4 counts are sufficient to produce AIDS symptoms.[33] Even conventional AIDS experts are now questioning whether virus-induced killing of immune cells leads to AIDS.[34]

Another phenomenon in people with AIDS is a curious reversal of the ratio between T4 and T8 cells (another cell type vital for proper immune function). While a healthy person has a high T4 cell count and a low count of T8 cells, a person with AIDS has the opposite ratio. The CDC has now applied for permission to say officially that if the absolute ratio of T4 to T8 cells in the body falls below the normal ratio (roughly 1.8 to 1.0), this, along with a positive HIV test, is sufficient for a diagnosis of AIDS.

Prior to AIDS, T-cell counts were rarely performed and scientific understanding of their significance remains unresolved. At the AIDS Conference in Berlin in 1993, researchers stressed that they no longer believed that CD4 counts were a particularly valuable marker for clinical disease progression, because certain drugs had raised CD4s with no improvement in health.

AIDS has thus been simplified by the media, in part to mean nothing more than a deficiency of these immune system cells. While T-cell loss is certainly one of the markers for AIDS, blood tests of a typical patient reveal a far more complicated picture, a kind of immunological chaos that is commonly referred to as "immune collapse." Some scientists feel it is even more complex—that it is a problem of the immune system gone haywire, perhaps even attacking itself in a process known as "autoimmunity."

Dr. Papadopulos-Eleopulos is a prominent critic of the HIV-AIDS theory. Her own research into AIDS, begun in 1981, brought her to the conclusion that excessive and prolonged oxidative stress in the body, caused by multiple co-factors such as drug use, infections, and semen, is what leads to the development of AIDS.[35]

Oxidative stress also reduces the number of T4 cells in the body, one of the primary markers for AIDS.

"It has long been established that the chemistry of the body of most people with AIDS, and those considered to be living at risk, does not look like any typical response to a single viral agent," states Dr. Null. "In terms of chemical interactions, AIDS is far closer to resembling a 'stress response'."[36] The only thing totally clear at present is that the immune systems of people with AIDS are damaged and that the most important thing is to explore what treatments may restore the immune system, thereby restoring health.

AZT and Protease Inhibitors

AZT is a widely used conventional antiretroviral treatment for AIDS, which was originally developed as a chemotherapy treatment for cancer, but then abandoned because it was too toxic.[37] Despite its known toxicity, its use for AIDS is due to the belief that it interferes with the process by which HIV-RNA is converted into DNA, thus neutralizing its effectiveness. This does not happen in all the infected cells, though, leaving a reservoir of infection. Also, if HIV is not the major cause of AIDS, this interference might in itself be of limited value, even if all the infected cells were influenced.

While there may be a short-term (months rather than years) increase in T-cell numbers, this is usually followed by a rapid decline to a point lower than before AZT treatment began. Initially, it was believed that there was a small increased survival rate in those taking AZT, but the results of the Concorde study confirmed in 1993 that the drug neither prolongs life nor staves off symptoms of AIDS in those with HIV but no symptoms. The supposed benefits of AZT also do not take into account its strong negative side effects. When viral DNA synthesis is interrupted by AZT, it stops healthy T cells from being able to synthesize DNA. HIV will also rapidly develop a resistance to the drug, mutating into different strains that are not influenced by it.

In addition, most health experts believe that, even when infection is active, at most one T cell in 500 is infected with HIV. Since one of the main medical theories about HIV is that it does its harm through the destruction of T cells, it becomes clear that AZT is more harmful to the immune system's healthy T cells than HIV. This theory does not even include the damage done by AZT's toxicity, which suppresses the important tasks of bone marrow, causing anemia, neutropenia (abnormally small number of neutrophils in blood, a white blood cell that protects against infection) and leukopenia (abnor-

---

SUCCESS STORY: ESCAPING THE HIV-AIDS TRAP

"I discovered that I was HIV-positive in 1987, while in the process of deciphering non-life-threatening but bothersome health problems that I strongly suspected were not AIDS but the result of other stresses on my immune system," says G. Steven Rose. A gay man, Mr. Rose was trying to go through a process of elimination in order to find out exactly what microbial factors and other stressors were causing his recurring bouts of mononucleosis and depression. He found evidence of several microbes, including cytomegalovirus (CMV), Epstein-Barr virus (EBV), and hepatitis B. "Because I tested positive for HIV, I was put on an AIDS track that seemed to have a mind of its own, winding up in an AZT clinical trial.

"AZT was offered to me as the only hope to deal with HIV infection. I doubted the paradigm from the start, but it took me a while to stand up to it. I finally realized that the AZT was harming me and walked out in disgust. I realized that chasing one killer microbe could not possibly be the way to restore my health, that my health was not as bad as I suspected, and that the only way to heal myself was to not take toxic drugs. I didn't follow any elaborate alternative methods, relying only on diet, rest, and a simple meditation technique. I simply stopped doing the damage and gradually my health returned. Today, as far as I can tell, I'm not dying of AIDS. I've moved away from the medical model and towards living with myself the way I am, and the more I do that, the healthier I become."

---

mal decrease in white blood corpuscles) in up to 50% of people given the drug, with up to half of these requiring transfusions within weeks of commencing use. Other side effects of AZT include muscle wasting, extreme nausea, acute hepatitis, headaches, insomnia, dementia, seizures, and the appearance of cancerous lymphomas (9% of patients), all symptoms identical with AIDS itself.

"I have a large population of people who have chosen not to take any anti-retrovirals," says Donald Abrams, M.D., Director of the AIDS program at San Francisco General Hospital. "They've watched all of their friends go on the antiviral bandwagon and die."[38] Other studies have found that one of the things long-term AIDS survivors have in common is they didn't take antiretroviral drugs.[39]

When comparing AZT treatment studies with the results of the Healing AIDS Research Project (HARP) study conducted by Bastyr University, in Seattle, Washington, which treated HIV-infected patients using alternative therapies (such as nutrition, herbs, psychological counseling, and hyperthermia), it was found that, unlike all the published AZT results involving similar patient groups, none of the HARP patients progressed over a one-year period to AIDS or died;[40] in the AZT studies, the progression rate was between 3% and 7%.[41] This points out that alternative methods, which are much cheaper, produce comparable results over a one-year period as AZT, with no toxicity.

Protease Inhibitors: Since the mid-1990s, the focus of conventional AIDS treatment has turned to the use of protease-inhibiting drugs, which are able to reduce viral loads when taken in very large doses. Protease inhibitors block the enzymes needed for HIV to replicate, thus helping to stop the spread of the virus. However, the body quickly develops resistance to protease inhibitors, so they are typically taken in combination with AZT and other toxic drugs. This combination therapy or "drug cocktail" has proven more effective than AZT alone, particularly in the short-term, but its effectiveness seems to diminish over time. A recent study estimates that 42% of HIV infections will become drug-resistant over the next few years.[42] In addition, protease inhibitors need to be taken in very large doses to enhance absorption and they have some severe side effects, including diarrhea, vomiting, fatigue, headaches, and fever.[43] They also shut down important functions of the immune system. These facts, combined with the high cost of the therapy, have left many AIDS patients looking for safer, more cost-effective alternatives.

Alternative Treatments for AIDS

While the mainstream view of AIDS treatment focuses almost entirely on the elimination of HIV, the alternative view places the emphasis on restoring overall health by first eliminating the co-factors. By concentrating on themselves, rather than on their illness or virus, many long-term AIDS and HIV survivors, working in conjunction with alternative physicians, have succeeded in maintaining good levels of health using a variety of methods that focus on co-factor infections. Prevention of a decline towards AIDS after HIV infection seems to be dramatically helped by using methods that either retard other infections or enhance the natural protective, detoxification, and self-healing roles of the body, including the immune system which, together with the other defensive systems, tries to maintain the body's proper balance for health.[44]

Whether the virus can be held in check seems to depend on a number of factors, namely where the individual who is HIV-infected is starting from—levels of immune function, previous disease or infection, other medical problems, and toxicity from drugs and harmful environmental elements. Other important factors include the person's nutritional status, emotional state, and stress-coping abilities, as well as "lifestyle" choices (including sexual) that may be harming the defense effort. HIV entering a super-efficient immune system may well be overwhelmed and get nowhere. On the other hand, HIV entering a system already compromised by poor nutrition, other illnesses, and drugs, will find its task that much easier.

There are many case histories of people who are HIV-positive and who have developed advanced signs of AIDS (Kaposi's sarcoma) and yet have managed to turn their condition around.[45] Although such stories can be dismissed as "anecdotal," the sheer volume of such anecdotes overwhelms the dismissive arguments of the skeptics. Continuing long-term studies at Bastyr University are also examining the possibility of holding the disease at bay, of keeping people who show early signs of AIDS from degenerating further, and of turning their condition around so that they become active, productive, and self-sufficient once more.[46]

Some of the alternative methods being used today to improve the health and immune function of individuals with AIDS and HIV infection include improving nutritional status, detoxification, mind/body medicine, stress reduction therapies, herbal medicine, homeopathy, and ozone and other oxygen-based treatments.

Diet and Nutrition

"Nutrition is the foundation of natural therapy," Dr. Badgley states. "Broad segments of the American population have been proven to be deficient in specific vitamins and minerals that are critical to immune system function. For example, persons with AIDS are often deficient in folic acid, selenium, zinc, and iron." While there is no universal dietary or nutritional prescription for the treatment of AIDS and HIV, since each person has varying needs in terms of diet and nutrition, there are a few general guidelines a person can follow:

- Eat whole foods with as many essential nutrients and as few additives as possible.
- Fresh, organic vegetables, fruits, and proteins (fish and meat) are suggested whenever possible.
- Avoid processed foods.
- Reduce or eliminate refined carbohydrates (sugars, white flour, pastries) and replace with complex car-

bohydrates (vegetables, whole grains, beans) rich in nutrients.

- Reduce polyunsaturated and saturated fats and oils. Use monounsaturated oils (such as olive oil) with special emphasis on omega-3s (fish oils and certain plant oils).

- Eat smaller portions of food more frequently throughout the day to optimize absorption of nutrients.

- Try to keep a balanced food intake, which ensures that 65% is complex carbohydrates (vegetables, fruits, and grains), 15% protein (fish, yogurt, eggs, and meat), and 20% fat.

- Make sure fruits and vegetables are thoroughly clean and free of parasites and bacteria by steaming lightly before eating.

- Eat a wide variety of foods to help avoid becoming sensitized to specific food families through repeated exposure.

- Eliminate chocolate, caffeine, and alcohol.[47]

Because of a person's biochemical individuality (genetic and environmental differences), each person will have specific nutrient requirements. A qualified healthcare professional should always be consulted in order to receive specific, individual guidelines.

Dr. Badgley reports of a patient who had been HIV-positive for eight years and was diagnosed with AIDS three years later. He eliminated his symptoms through diet and cleansings, beginning with a diet of raw organic fruits and vegetables, emphasizing freshness, moderation, and a variety of foods. He also utilized enemas to rid his system of toxins and to cleanse the colon, where the virus is harbored. He avoided foods that were mucus-forming, like dairy products, eating only cheeses made from sunflower seeds and pumpkin seeds. The patient reported that his T-cell counts rose to normal levels and a liver disease with which he had been diagnosed had gone into remission.

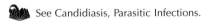 See Candidiasis, Parasitic Infections.

Malnutrition is another common problem associated with people who are HIV-positive and is almost universal in those with AIDS. This is often due to disruptions in the digestive processes caused by the weakening of the immune system. Raw foods, such as vegetables, can be lightly cooked (steamed, stir-fried, added to soups) or juiced to facilitate digestion. Sometimes, though, nutritional supplements taken orally or via injection are the only way to ensure that adequate nutrients get into the body (although with impaired absorption capabilities, the oral route does not always guarantee that what is swallowed arrives where it is needed).

CANDIDIASIS AND AIDS

Candidiasis, or yeast overgrowth in the intestinal tract, is a common feature of anyone who is immune compromised and therefore can be a major problem for people who are HIV-positive or have AIDS. A nutritional strategy that helps discourage yeast overgrowth concentrates on reducing, or cutting out altogether, the intake of simple carbohydrates and sugars, while emphasizing complex carbohydrate intake.[48] In addition, an anti-candidiasis strategy usually employs antifungal foods, such as garlic and olive oil, along with specific substances that kill the yeast, such as caprylic acid (a fatty acid) and aloe vera.

Repopulation of the intestinal tract with friendly bacteria while the yeast is being targeted often involves the use of cultured dairy products such as kefir and live low-fat yogurt, as well as probiotic supplements such as *Lactobacillus acidophilus* and *Bifidobacteria*. *L. bulgaricus* is also sometimes used because of its powerful antifungal and antibiotic potential.[49]

> *Broad segments of the American population have been proven to be deficient in specific vitamins and minerals, that are critical to immune system function. For example, persons with AIDS are often deficient in folic acid, selenium, zinc, and iron.*
>
> —LAURENCE BADGLEY, M.D.

People who are HIV-positive or diagnosed with AIDS are most commonly deficient in the following essential nutrients: vitamin A,[50] vitamin B6,[51] folate, vitamin B12,[52] selenium,[53] and zinc.[54] Nutritional supplementation has been shown in clinical studies to offer great benefits to people already seriously ill with AIDS, and it is seen by many as the cornerstone requirement if there is to be recovery. In a six-month study, vitamins, minerals, amino acids, and essential fatty acids were all supplemented. Among the observed clinical benefits were an improvement in general well-being and a significant decrease in the P24 antigen.[55]

Other nutrients commonly supplemented in HIV-positive and AIDS cases are vitamins A (beta carotene), B complex, and E. In one study, AIDS patients given 60 mg of beta carotene for four weeks showed increased levels of CD4 cells.[56] The B vitamins thiamin (B1), riboflavin (B2), pantothenic acid (B5), pyridoxine (B6), and B12 are essential for improving a weakened immune system.[57] One study found that HIV-infected men with the highest levels of vitamin E in their blood are 34% less likely than others with HIV to progress to AIDS.[58] Vitamin C has also proven to be a powerful antioxidant and inhibitor of viruses and bacteria, as well as having specific and potent immune-enhancing effects.[59] According to Dr. Cathcart, "Preliminary clinical evidence is that massive doses of ascorbate (a vitamin C salt) can suppress the symptoms of disease and markedly reduce the tendency for secondary infections." Working with a group of 102 patients, most taking vitamin C on their own, Dr. Cathcart reports "considerable improvement" in most of the patients' conditions. Some of the improvements included a reduction of diseased lymph glands and the disappearance of Kaposi's sarcoma lesions.[60]

Supplementation of folic acid, biotin, potassium, magnesium,[61] and manganese is also recommended, as well as amino acids and essential fatty acids (particularly omega-3s and omega-6s). Glutathione, a critical amino acid antioxidant, reduces free-radical damage to cells, prevents depletion of other antioxidants, and activates certain immune cells. Counteracting oxidative stress (free-radical damage) may inhibit the progression of AIDS.[62] HIV-infected patients who maintained normal levels of glutathione lived longer than those who were depleted, according to one study.[63] Taking the amino acid N-acetyl-cysteine, lipoic acid, and selenium can help raise glutathione levels. A good multivitamin and mineral supplement can take the place of the individual supplements, but the best advice is to always consult with a qualified health practitioner in order to optimize supplementation.

Dr. Priestley reports good results from placing an HIV-positive patient on a regimen of intravenous nutrition, with supplements taken three times a week. Dr. Priestley also prescribed high doses of oral vitamin C daily and B-complex shots once a week, as well as garlic capsules, Siberian ginseng, beta carotene, zinc, and aloe vera. The patient also began exercising, meditating, and using acupuncture. After beginning treatment, the patient gained 40 pounds and eventually had fewer symptoms, despite having a low T-cell count, according to Dr. Priest-

ley, who continued the patient on a course of nutrients and preventative medicine to guard against infection.

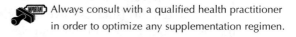 Always consult with a qualified health practitioner in order to optimize any supplementation regimen.

Herbal Medicine

The use of herbal medicines in the treatment of AIDS is widespread today, with additional research ongoing to assess possible further applications and effectiveness. Some of the herbal remedies most often employed include astragalus,[64] Carnivora (Venus' flytrap),[65] echinacea,[66] licorice,[67] and goldenseal.[68] Garlic and isatis root are commonly used because of their broad antibacterial and antiviral qualities,[69] as is ginseng for its tonic effects on the thymus gland in addition to its ability to help resist stress.[70] St. John's wort *(Hypericum perforatum)* is used because of its retrovirus blocking actions,[71] as is hyssop *(Hyssopus officinalis)*.[72]

Aloe vera may also be effective for treating HIV infection. An extract of mannose, one of the sugars in aloe, can inhibit HIV-1. In one study, HIV-1 cells were treated *in vitro* with the mannose extract. Aloe slowed virus reproduction by as much as 30%, reduced viral load, suppressed the spread of the virus from infected cells, and increased the viability (chance of survival) of infected cells. Researchers found that aloe (the mannose extract and perhaps other compounds) stimulates the body's immune system, particularly T4 helper cells (white blood cells that activate the immune response to infection).[73]

Chinese bitter melon, monolaurin (a component of certain fatty acids), and lentinan (extract of shiitake mushrooms) have also shown dramatic anti-HIV effects.[74] According to Subhuti Dharmananda, Ph.D., Director of the Institute for Traditional Medicine, in Portland, Oregon, herbal remedies used in specific combinations can often be much more effective than taking the herbs individually.[75]

Dr. Badgley reports that one of his patients, who suffered with Kaposi's sarcoma, had excellent results with a tea brewed from a mixture of the herbs echinacea, red clover tops, chaparral, dandelion, sarsparilla, and pau d'arco. The patient reports that the tea, in combination with a whole foods diet and nutritional supplements, stimulates his appetite and helps maintain his strength.

CAUTION There are many herbal combinations available, but they should only be administered with the advice of a qualified health practitioner, as all herbal compounds and many individual herbs can be toxic if used incorrectly or in excessive amounts.

 See Diet, Herbal Medicine, Nutritional Medicine, Orthomolecular Medicine.

Acupuncture

Acupuncture has been shown to be an effective and vital tool for the treatment of HIV infection and AIDS, particularly when coupled with other alternative therapies such as herbal remedies. Preliminary studies at the Quan Yin Clinic, in San Francisco, California, have shown acupuncture to increase immune function and T-cell production. It also alleviates many of the symptoms related to HIV infection and AIDS. According to a published report, "Many patients report a reduction in fatigue, abnormal sweating, diarrhea, and acute skin reactions after only 4-6 acupuncture treatments. Many describe an improved sense of well-being, some report weight gain, and are able to return to longer hours of work."[77]

I think that if we had more acupuncture and less AZT and protease inhibitors, we would see a qualitative improvement in these patients' health.

— WILLIAM M. CARGILE, B.S., D.C., F.I.A.C.A.

William M. Cargile, B.S., D.C., F.I.A.C.A., former Chairman of Research for the American Association of Oriental Medicine, has worked with AIDS patients for many years and has been able to increase T-cell counts with acupuncture treatments. "One of these patients had a T-cell count of 30 to 40," he recounts. "We eventually brought it up to 270 and, although this is half the level a person is said to need, he's been doing great for six months." Dr. Cargile adds that the key to understanding acupuncture's influence on cell counts lies partly in its ability to minimize stress and strengthen the body's adaptive mechanisms. "I think that if we had more acupuncture and less AZT and protease inhibitors, we would see a qualitative improvement in these patients' health," he states.

Numerous clinical studies have borne out Dr. Cargile's claims. When 200 patients with AIDS were treated with acupuncture, it was found to reduce levels of secondary opportunistic infections and to be generally beneficial. Also, at Lincoln Memorial Hospital in New York City, out of 27 people with AIDS who received acupuncture treatments, 20 reported that fatigue was reduced and that night sweats and diarrhea improved after 1-3 weeks. Many also gained substantial amounts of weight. Michael Smith, M.D., who oversaw the patients, reports that in some cases T-cell ratios rose dramatically over a 2-3 month period with acupuncture alone.[78] In addition, 15 patients who had acupuncture treatments regularly at Somerville Centre, near Boston, reported improvement in general symptoms and six reported that acupuncture helped reduce side effects of medical treatment for Kaposi's sarcoma.[79]

BITTER MELON

For centuries in Asian cultures, bitter melon has been used as a treatment for a wide variety of ailments. It is believed that eating bitter melon regularly will clean and purify the blood and ward off infections. Since the early 1980s, bitter melon fruits and seeds have been tested as an effective therapy for cancer and HIV. Stanley Rebultan, a Filipino-American man who is HIV-positive, took bitter melon liquid extract for nearly four years as his sole antiviral treatment and saw his T4 cell count increase by 121% (480 to 1,060), his T4-to-T8 ratio improve by 68%, and his CD4 percentage rise by 77%.

At the Amsterdam International Conference on AIDS in 1992, Quingcai Zhang, a Chinese medical doctor and herbalist, presented additional data supporting Rebultan's experience. In Dr. Zhang's study, those who took bitter melon for four months to three years had CD4 counts increase between 33% and 285%. His findings showed that, in most cases, it normalized T4-to-T8 ratios, raised T4 counts over time, and increased energy and sense of well-being. Dr. Zhang also noted that bitter melon blocked HIV-infected macrophages (immune cells that recognize and ingest foreign antigens)—something AZT does not do—as well as infected lymphocytes such as CD4 cells.[76]

Bitter melon extracts or decoctions can be taken orally or rectally. A rectal retention enema is recommended, because the plant is very bitter and unpleasant to drink and may cause nausea. Using an enema also avoids the breakdown of the bitter melon proteins in the stomach acid, allowing them to instead be absorbed directly into the bloodstream through the large intestine.

While bitter melon has shown remarkable results for those who stick with it, many people quit before the therapy can take effect. Rebultan admits that it took him three months before he felt comfortable with the treatment procedure. "It's a long-term therapy," he explains "It takes at least six months to see results, but if I have to do this my entire life to maintain a normal sense of well-being, then I will. Herbal therapy takes a long time. It's not like the overnight miracles of pill popping that American medicine feels so entitled to."

SUCCESS STORY: HOMEOPATHIC GROWTH FACTORS FOR AIDS

Francine, 60, had carried an HIV infection in her system for eight years. She had lost considerable weight (dropping to 104 pounds) and she felt weak and tired much of the time, even though she continued with her job. Barbara Brewitt, M.Div., Ph.D., of Biomed Comm, Inc., in Seattle, Washington, entered her in a clinical study testing the effectiveness of a combination of four homeopathically prepared solutions of human growth factor.

Growth factors are a class of at least 30 different proteins called polypeptides. These regulate cell growth, division, and specialization and also make communication between cells possible. Growth factors are molecules that send signals and set in motion events between cells that can trigger changes in the way the cell uses DNA which, in turn, results in changes in the cell's response to outside events, says Dr. Brewitt. The therapeutic use of growth factors may be a key to reversing the weight loss and immune dysfunction associated with AIDS, suggests Dr. Brewitt. Starting with growth factors prepared by genetic engineering, Dr. Brewitt worked with a homeopath to prepare various homeopathic dilutions of the four substances.

Francine took ten drops of each of the homeopathic formulations four times daily. Each of the medicines was prepared at different strengths, including 30C (low), 200C

(moderate), and 1M (high). Francine also received intravenous nutrients from a naturopathic physician. Her energy began returning and, within seven months, she had gained 17 pounds; during this time, she took no conventional drugs for retroviruses.

In the case of Theodore, 35, he had been diagnosed with HIV infection six years previously. The levels of his CD4 cells had dropped from 560 to 310 cells in 15 months. This was a dangerously rapid loss of immune cells, says Dr. Brewitt. Theodore started AZT and, while his CD4 cells climbed to 600, he suffered from anemia. When Theodore learned of Dr. Brewitt's trials, he quit the AZT and three months later started taking the homeopathic growth factors (ten drops of each preparation three times daily). One year after beginning this treatment, Theodore had gained 22 pounds and felt "very strong." His CD4 cell counts had climbed by 100 and there was no HIV virus detectable in his blood.

In her 12-month clinical trial with 30 AIDS patients using the homeopathic growth factors, Dr. Brewitt observed an average weight gain of almost ten pounds, an absence of opportunistic infections, CD4 cell counts either remaining stable or increasing slightly, and a decrease in the degree of viral infection.[80]

 See Acupuncture, Traditional Chinese Medicine.

Jay Holder, M.D., D.C., Ph.D., of Miami, Florida, has achieved significant results using acupuncture. He describes the case of a man with AIDS, suffering from Kaposi's sarcoma, and given just 22 months to live. Within three weeks of treatment with acupuncture and Chinese herbs, his T-cell count returned to normal and his lesions disappeared.

Most acupuncture treatments for people with HIV or AIDS last approximately 45 minutes and are entirely painless, except for a slight pricking sensation when the needles are inserted. In addition, most acupuncturists today use pre-sterilized, disposable needles to protect both themselves and patients from AIDS, hepatitis, and other infectious diseases.

Hyperthermia

Researchers have proven that HIV is heat-sensitive and will become increasingly inactive as body temperature is raised progressively above normal (98.6° F) for

extended periods of time.[81] Much as a fever is the body's natural defense mechanism against infection and disease, hyperthermia can be used to similar effect by artificially raising the body's temperature. This also stimulates the immune system by increasing the production of antibodies and interferon.

Certain forms of hyperthermia can also be employed as part of a self-care regimen. Hot baths are the simplest method of inducing a fever at home and, for viral infections such as HIV, they can be combined with hot drinks and blanket wrapping to stimulate the immune system. After a hot bath, a person can wrap in dry blankets, with a hot water bottle over the abdomen, in order to perspire heavily for as long as can be tolerated. This may take several hours and should be followed by a cool shower. It is also possible to produce a mild fever with just a hot bath and wrapping in dry blankets after the bath. Again, allow several hours to perspire heavily and follow with a cool shower.

A wet sheet pack may be used to raise body temperature. In this procedure, a person wraps in a very cold, wet sheet, followed by several blankets. Like the dry pack, it will take several hours to produce a fever, the cold sheet causing reactions in the body that encourage the production of heat. It is often useful to precede this procedure with some kind of heating, such as exercise, a hot bath, or a hot shower.

Other more "high-tech" methods are also available, such as shortwave or microwave diathermy (the use of high frequency current to generate heat in a part of the body), ultrasound, radiant heating, and extracorpeal heating (heat administered from a source outside the body), but these are usually administered only in a medical or hospital setting. Infrared saunas are also gaining acceptance for home and spa use. They heat the body from inside out with ambient temperature in the sauna at only 120°-130° F instead of the higher temperatures of a regular sauna. Heating the body to promote sweating helps to detoxify heavy metals, pesticides, and other chemicals and stimulates immune function.

At the Natural Health Clinic at Bastyr University, hyperthermia is commonly used to treat HIV infection. Hyperthermia was also included as part of the HARP study. Participants were given a series of hyperthermia baths (102° F) for 40 minutes. These were administered twice weekly, for three weeks at a time, over the course of a year. According to Leanna Standish, Ph.D., N.D., who oversaw the HARP study, when participants were asked what aspect of the treatment had the greatest impact, the overwhelming response was "hyperthermia." There was a reported decrease in night sweats and in the frequency of secondary infections. Also, many of the participants claimed to have a greater sense of well-being after receiving hyperthermia treatments.[82]

While hyperthermia treatments may not be able to kill every invading virus (with approximately 40% HIV inactivation after 30 minutes in a 107.6° F bath), they reduce their number, making it easier for the immune system to handle the remaining viruses. Hyperthermia is also a useful technique for detoxification, because it releases toxins stored in fat cells.

Precautions: Hyperthermia should only be undertaken with proper supervision, because of the possible damage toxins might cause when released, particularly to the kidneys and liver. Certain individuals are more sensitive to the effects of heat and their condition should be treated with great care. These include people with anemia, heart disease, diabetes, seizure disorders, and tuberculosis. Overall, however, when used knowledgeably, hyperthermia is a safe and effective treatment for HIV, with ill effects appearing usually only when body temperature exceeds 106° F.

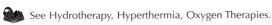 See Hydrotherapy, Hyperthermia, Oxygen Therapies.

Oxygen Therapies

In 1988, Kenneth Wagner, M.D., former head of the Naval Hospital's AIDS unit in Bethesda, Maryland, and Steven Kleinman, M.D., Medical Director of the American Red Cross Blood Services for Los Angeles, along with Michael Carpendale, M.D., of the Veterans Administration Medical Center, in San Francisco, California, and Mark Rarick, M.D., an AIDS researcher at the University of Southern California, all supported the use of oxygen therapy as a primary treatment for AIDS and HIV infection. Their message was direct and simple—oxygen therapy is the safest and most effective method of treating AIDS and its associated infections.[83]

Oxygen therapy uses hyperbaric oxygen, ozone, or hydrogen peroxide to combat HIV in much the same way as the immune system uses self-generated oxygen free radicals (a single oxygen atom) to destroy bacterial and viral infections. The extra oxygen atoms in ozone (O_3) and hydrogen peroxide (H_2O_2) break off and link with the invading molecules, altering their molecular structure, in effect killing the harmful cells and leaving behind only oxygen (O_2) or water (H_2O).

One study found that when HIV-infected blood was removed from the body and treated with ozone, the virus was completely deactivated.[84] Another approach has been to simply inject a diluted form of ozone into the bloodstream. This treatment can be done daily for several weeks at a time. French researchers Bertrand Vallancien and Jean-Marie Winkler studied ozone therapy with a group of patients with HIV, herpes, and hepatitis. After nine weeks of transfused ozone, T4 and T8 cells moved toward normal levels in all cases and the ozone treatments caused no other problems.[85] Ozone has also been found effective for AIDS-related diarrhea.[86] German researchers use bioluminescence (the irradiation of blood with ultraviolet light) in conjunction with ozone therapy to treat viral and other infections.

Hydrogen peroxide, like ozone, can be administered intravenously and can also be taken rectally by enema, vaginally, or transcutaneously (absorption by bathing), according to the late Charles H. Farr, M.D., Ph.D. He advocated the intravenous method of delivery; however, some doctors are using combinations of ozone and hydrogen peroxide and reporting good results as well, because of a synergistic response in the cells. Although hydrogen peroxide can be taken orally, Dr. Farr, who first characterized the effects of hydrogen peroxide in humans, recommended against it, because the enzymes of the stomach are unable to process it properly.

Since 1990, Michelle Reillo, B.S.N., R.N., has been treating AIDS patients with hyperbaric oxygen therapy (HBOT—pure oxygen delivered for 30-60 minutes to patients inside a sealed chamber with high pressure) at

A MULTIMODAL APPROACH SUCCESSFULLY TREATS AIDS

After years of clinical experience with 165 AIDS patients, H.E. Sartori, M.D., and H. Hugh Fudenberg, M.D., conclude that treatment with ozone and a multimodal program can produce a 95% success rate in terms of normalizing laboratory test results and the physical and mental well-being of patients. They call their AIDS treatment approach Life Science Universal (LSU) and it includes a 12-day ozone program (30-35 mg of ozone daily, delivered intravenously), supplementation with vitamins, minerals, and herbs, psychological counseling, "reconditioning" (which involves a 12-step goal-setting program), internal energy exercises, and a mostly vegetarian diet with no dairy products. In addition, they use eight adjunctive therapies, such as homeopathy, Chinese herbs, acupuncture, coffee enemas, heat therapy, thymus glandular extracts, and electrical stimulation (including ear acupuncture using electric currents), when needed.

Of 119 patients for whom post-treatment laboratory results were available, 53 (45%) had their T4 cells return to normal; other key blood factors also normalized. For another 46 patients (39%), T-cell count increased by at least 200. Of 91 HIV-positive patients, 75% saw their conditions change to HIV-negative after completing the program. Most of the patients receiving this treatment "showed a significant improvement of their general well-being and of most of their clinical symptoms," state Drs. Sartori and Fudenberg.[88]

Lifeforce Hyperbaric Oxygen Institute, in Baltimore, Maryland. Reillo and her colleagues concentrate on providing relief and reversing many of the complications associated with HIV infection or AIDS diagnosis. "Hyperbaric medicine has well-documented evidence supporting its use in many AIDS-defining complications and infections, regardless of the underlying disorder," Reillo says. "HBOT would be an ideal intervention in the individual recently infected with HIV, because it decreases viremia [viruses in the blood], is not toxic to the individual, and decreases the microvascular and neurovascular [small blood vessel] damage occurring as the initial infection progresses throughout the body."

HBOT has demonstrated its effectiveness in relieving peripheral vascular insufficiency. This means a reduced supply of blood to the feet and hands, leaving them cold and frequently painful. Reillo reports that, over a three-

year period, 100 AIDS patients with this problem received considerable benefit after receiving only two weeks of HBOT (three treatments per week). First among the symptoms to improve was fatigue, then an increase in the ability to exercise and tolerate activity, followed by a warming of the extremities, an increase in energy, and less pain in the legs and feet following activity. The level of oxygen in the tissues climbed from a low 79% to a healthy 98%, adds Reillo.

HBOT performs well as an adjunct to conventional antibiotic regimens for AIDS patients, Reillo explains. This is especially so in the area of opportunistic infections such as *Mycobacterium avium* complex, a deadly form of tuberculosis that attacks the bone marrow. This complication affects up to 20% of AIDS patients. Getting more oxygen invariably stimulates the appetite and the patients want to eat more, says Reillo. "Oxygen makes you hungry," she says. With appetite improvement, Reillo counsels AIDS patients on the details of a well-balanced, nutritionally rich diet. "The healthier you eat, the less likely you are to lose weight and develop infections," she states.

One of the most serious consequences of AIDS is dangerously low levels of T cells, but here again HBOT is helpful, says Reillo. Over the course of four months of HBOT, Reillo was able to get a woman's T cells to climb from 400 to 800; even better, her CD4 count doubled.[87]

While the oxygen free radicals generated in oxygen therapy are deadly to viruses and bacteria, they can also do damage to healthy tissues if left unchecked. When the body manufactures these oxygen-based defense substances, it follows this immediately by sending protective antioxidant enzymes to quench the process before harm to healthy tissue can take place. Nutritional support is generally recommended with any oxygen therapy, particularly vitamin C supplementation, which acts as a stabilizing antioxidant.

Mind/Body Medicine

There is an absolutely vital relationship between a person's emotional state and their immune system. In cases of AIDS and HIV infection, this relationship has a profound impact on whether the individual maintains or recovers health or slips further down into the disease state.[89] As with cancer, a tremendous negative mental and emotional burden is initially placed on patients diagnosed HIV-positive or with AIDS, because of all the implications that lurk behind these diagnoses. According to Herb Joiner-Bey, N.D., of Bastyr University, without spiritual and mental involvement, people find it difficult to generate the commitment to getting themselves well. This makes the restoration of a positive, realistic outlook that encourages self-reliance a key ingredient in any alternative approach to HIV infection and AIDS.[90]

Emotions such as guilt, hopelessness, suppressed anger, and fear, which are common among many with AIDS, add to the burden of the immune system. Yet, according to Leon Chaitow, N.D., D.O., of London, England, most negative emotions can be resolved with a little effort and attention. "Any stress-coping strategy that reduces these negative influences on the nervous system—relaxation, meditation, visualization, or some form of psychotherapeutic counseling, treatment, or group work—will help immune function," Dr. Chaitow points out.

Jon Kaiser, M.D., of San Francisco, California, specializes in the practice of alternative therapies and the mind/body connection. Nearly 70% of his patients are HIV-positive. One patient's anxiety about being diagnosed HIV-positive has been dismissed by his former doctors. In conjunction with a protocol of diet, nutritional supplements, and herbs, Dr. Kaiser addressed the stress-related symptoms. As a result, the patient regained control over his emotions and his health has improved to the point where he has been asymptomatic for four years. Among the points Dr. Kaiser emphasizes to his patients are the following:

- AIDS is not a death sentence.
- Someone who begins a sound, alternative medicine program early can reasonably consider the possibility of living out a normal life span.
- Maintain a positive attitude.
- Don't panic or give in to the negative messages that the media and the medical establishment promote.
- Follow a balanced, focused treatment program.

Janet Konefal, Ph.D., Associate Professor of Psychiatry at the University of Miami School of Medicine, employs a counseling protocol aimed at "expanding limiting beliefs and altering behaviors among HIV-positive individuals." She places great emphasis on dealing with the distress that permeates AIDS and HIV-associated illnesses. Dr. Konefal's approach is to gradually take the individual—whose negative mental state may carry images of past illness and loss, as well as poor images of future prospects in terms of health, happiness, and survival—toward a position in which positive, hopeful images can start to regularly replace these negative images.

In order to achieve this shift, Dr. Konefal employs techniques that incorporate symbolism, imagery, and goal-setting in a structured and individualized manner. "The result is that the patient's dark, morbid, immunosuppressing thoughts give way to light, life-affirming thoughts that foster the will to live and create an emo-

MASSAGE THERAPY FOR AIDS

Massage can have immense benefits for people with AIDS or HIV. The benefits are both physical (improved circulation and drainage of blood and lymph fluid, relaxation of muscles, and improved joint mobility) and mental and emotional (reduced stress and a greater sense of ease and well-being).[91] According to Robert King, L.M.T., past President of the American Massage Therapy Association, massage provides an environment in which emotions relating to issues such as death, dying, and sadness can emerge, as well as acting as a catalyst that reinforces touching and hugging in daily life. Improvement also takes place in relation to self-image and self-esteem after receipt of a caring massage. A person's sense of isolation and loneliness is also broken down.

The resulting stress reduction derived from massage therapy can have a powerful immune-enhancing effect. Research at the Touch Research Institute, University of Miami School of Medicine, in Miami, Florida, has shown increased natural killer (NK) cell activity and other immune system improvements directly related to massage therapy.[92]

Yet, despite the obvious advantages of massage for AIDS, it is not always readily available. Due to fear, ignorance, and misinformation about how AIDS is contracted, people with AIDS often suffer from the emotional battering of being social outcasts. The result is that touch is one of the first things that leaves their lives once they are diagnosed.

Important: People with AIDS who receive massage often have specific requirements. The massage should not be too fast or too deep, to ensure that the adrenal gland system is not overstimulated, which can challenge the immune system. The person giving the massage should use gentle touch, focusing on relaxation, comfort, and nurturing, rather than on assessing and dealing with postural problems. Massage is always contraindicated for cancer and those with pulmonary problems (pneumonia) require gentle pats rather than rubbing in the affected areas. It is also important for anyone HIV-positive or with AIDS to avail themselves of a licensed massage therapist who has a background in dealing with their condition and emotional state. In many areas, free massage is available for anyone HIV-positive or with AIDS, with many volunteer organizations offering on-site walk-ins.

tionally stronger and more optimistic individual," she says.

 See Bodywork, Guided Imagery, Hypnotherapy, Mind/Body Medicine.

Recommendations

- Eat whole foods with as many essential nutrients and as few additives as possible.

- Fresh, organic vegetables, fruits, and proteins (fish and meat) are suggested whenever possible.

- Avoid processed foods and reduce or eliminate refined carbohydrates (sugars, white flour, pastires) and replace with complex carbohydrates (vegetables, whole grains, beans) rich in nutrients.

- Nutrients commonly supplemented in HIV-positive and AIDS cases are vitamins A (beta carotene), B complex, and E. Vitamin C has also proven to be a powerful antioxidant and inhibitor of viruses and bacteria, as well as having specific and potent immune-enhancing effects. Supplementation of folic acid, biotin, potassium, magnesium, and manganese is also recommended, as well as amino acids and essential fatty acids (particularly omega-3s and omega-6s).

- Herbal remedies most often employed include astragalus, Carnivora (Venus' flytrap), echinacea, licorice, and goldenseal. Garlic and isatis root are commonly used because of their broad antibacterial and antiviral qualities, as is ginseng for its tonic effects on the thymus gland in addition to its ability to help resist stress.

- Acupuncture has been shown to be an effective and vital tool for the treatment of HIV infection and AIDS, particularly when coupled with other alternative therapies such as herbal remedies.

- Researchers have proven that HIV is heat-sensitive and will become increasingly inactive as body temperature is raised progressively above normal (98.6° F) for extended periods of time.

- Oxygen therapy uses hyperbaric oxygen, ozone, or hydrogen peroxide to combat HIV in much the same way as the immune system uses self-generated oxygen free radicals (a single oxygen atom) to destroy bacterial and viral infections.

- Emotions such as guilt, hopelessness, suppressed anger, and fear, which are common among many with AIDS, add to the burden of the immune system. Yet, most negative emotions can be resolved using mind/body therapies.

Self-Care
The following therapies can be undertaken at home under appropriate professional supervision:

Biofeedback Training and Neurotherapy / Guided Imagery / Meditation

AROMATHERAPY: Tea tree oil, garlic.

HOMEOPATHY: *Hypericum.*

Professional Care
The following therapies should only be provided by a qualified health professional:

Enzyme Therapy / Fasting / Orthomolecular Medicine / Magnetic Field Therapy / Traditional Chinese Medicine

Where to Find Help

For information on, or referrals for, treatment of AIDS, contact the following organizations.

AIDS Alternative Health Project
4753 N. Broadway, Suite 1110
Chicago, Illinois 60640
(773) 561-2800
Website: www.danceforlife.org

An organization staffed by professional volunteers who offer chiropractic, acupuncture, bodywork, nutritional and herbal counseling, and massage therapy to HIV-positive individuals.

HEAL
P.O. Box 1103, Old Chelsea Station
New York, New York 10113
(212) 873-0891
Website: www.healaids.com

Offers information to people seeking to strengthen their health and immune systems. Provides information on an alternative approach to health that "precludes toxic, immunosuppressive drugs, but includes physical, emotional, psychological, and spiritual efforts."

Project Inform
205 13th Street, Suite 2001
San Francisco, California 94103
(415) 558-8669
Website: www.projinf.org

A nonprofit organization that provides treatment information, lifestyle strategies, and advocacy for those infected with HIV.

Quan Yin Healing Arts Center
1748 Market Street
San Francisco, California 94102
(415) 861-4964
Website: www.quanyinhealingarts.org

Offers a program for people with AIDS or who are HIV-positive. Services include acupuncture, herbal medicine, yoga, and massage therapy. Also provides a lecture series and discussion groups to provide support and nutritional information.

Acupuncture/Traditional Chinese Medicine

American Association of Oriental Medicine
433 Front Street
Catasauqua, Pennsylvania 18032
(888) 500-7999
Website: www.aaom.org

The AAOM is a national professional organization of acupuncturists who meet acceptable standards of competency and can provide you with the names and locations of local members.

Herbal Medicine

American Association of Naturopathic Physicians
8201 Greensboro Drive, Suite 300
McLean, Virginia 22102
(703) 610-9037
Website: www.naturopathic.org

Provides referrals to a nationwide network of accredited or licensed practitioners. Publishes a quarterly newsletter for both professionals and the general public and also offers a series of brochures and pamphlets on a variety of subjects.

Hyperthermia

Bastyr University Natural Health Clinic
1307 North 45th Street, Suite 200
Seattle, Washington 98103
(206) 632-0354
Website: www.bastyr.edu

The physical medicine department of the Natural Health Clinic of Bastyr University uses hyperthermia treatment for detoxification and in conditions ranging from upper respiratory infection to chronic fatigue syndrome and HIV.

National College of Naturopathic Medicine
049 S.W. Porter
Portland, Oregon 97201
(503) 499-4343
Website: www.ncnm.edu

NCNM's teaching clinic uses hyperthermia for a wide variety of conditions.

Massage

American Massage Therapy Association
820 Davis Street, Suite 100
Evanston, Illinois 60201
(847) 864-0123
Website: www.amtamassage.org

Offers comprehensive information on most areas of massage and bodywork, including an extensive review of scientific research. They also publish the Massage Therapy Journal, *available at many newsstands and health food stores.*

Oxygen Therapy

International Bio-Oxidative Medicine Foundation
P.O. Box 891954
Oklahoma City, Oklahoma 73189
(405) 478-IBOM

The foundation publishes and distributes a newsletter, as well as scientific research data. Supports educational programs that highlight current research and the therapeutic use of oxidative therapies. Encourages basic and clinical research.

Medizone International, Inc.
P.O. Box 742
Stinson Beach, California 94970
(415) 868-0300
Website: www.medizoneint.com

Developers of an ozone-based treatment for diseases caused by lipid-enveloped viruses, including AIDS, hepatitis B, and herpes. Medizone is also developing patented technology for the decontamination of blood and blood products.

North Carolina Bio-Oxidative Health Center
4505 Fair Meadow Lane, Suite 111
Raleigh, North Carolina 27607
(800) 473-9812
Website: www.carolinacenter.com

Outpatient facility that focuses on metabolic and intestinal detoxification. Comprehensive and synergistic treatment regimens for each patient are developed utilizing therapies such as colon hydrotherapy, intravenous therapies (including ozone), and external ozone hydrotherapy. Supportive elements such as acupuncture and lymphatic massage, as well as techniques to address the psychological/emotional components of health and illness are also part of the program.

Recommended Reading

AIDS: A Second Opinion. Gary Null, Ph.D. New York: Seven Stories Press, 2001.

AIDS and Complementary & Alternative Medicine: Current Science and Practice. Leanna J. Standish, N.D., Ph.D., L.Ac., Carlo Calabrese, N.D., M.P.H., and Mary Lou Galantino, P.T., M.S., Ph.D. New York: Churchill Livingstone, 2002

AIDS: The HIV Myth. Jad Adams. New York: St. Martin's Press, 1989.

The AIDS War. John Lauritsen. New York: Asklepios, 1993.

Healing AIDS Naturally. Laurence Badgley, M.D. San Bruno, CA: Healing Energy Press, 1987.

Immune Power: A Comprehensive Treatment Program for HIV. Jon D. Kaiser, M.D. New York: St. Martin's Press, 1993.

Inventing the AIDS Virus. Peter H. Duesberg, Ph.D. Washington, DC: Regnery Publishing, 1996.

Nutrition and HIV. Mary Romeyn, M.D. San Francisco: Jossey-Bass Publishers, 1995.

Poison by Prescription: The AZT Story. John Lauritsen. New York: Asklepios, 1990.

Rethinking AIDS. Robert Root-Bernstein. New York: Free Press, 1993.

Surviving AIDS. Michael Callen. New York: Harper-Collins, 1990.

The Virus Within: A Coming Epidemic. Nicholas Regush. New York: Dutton, 2000.

What If Everything You Thought You Knew About AIDS Was Wrong? Christine Maggiore. Los Angeles: HEAL, 1996.

A World Without AIDS. Leon Chaitow, D.O., N.D., and Simon Martin. Wellingborough, Northamptonshire, England: Thorsons Publishing Group, 1988.

ALLERGIES

Allergies are more widespread than most physicians, including allergists, realize and they can cause far more serious health problems, both physical and mental, than is commonly believed. Allergy sufferers don't need to despair, however. Proper diet and nutrition, combined with other alternative approaches, can relieve and reverse allergies, even after conventional approaches have failed.

AN ALLERGY IS an adverse immune system reaction to a substance that most people find harmless. Allergies can manifest in a variety of ways. Common examples of an allergic response include headaches, fatigue, sneezing, watery eyes, stuffy nose or sinuses, and possibly a skin rash that itches following exposure to dust, pollens, dust mites, animal dander, chemicals, foods, and a variety of other materials. "The allergic reactions themselves can range from mild to severe depending on the person," explains Richard Wilkinson, M.D., who practices environmental medicine in Yakima, Washington. "Many of the conditions are so common that they are almost considered normal by the people who suffer from them." Allergies can cause or contribute to asthma, bronchitis, rheumatoid arthritis, diabetes, ear infections, eczema, hives, migraines or cluster headaches, chronic fatigue syndrome, gastrointestinal disorders, glaucoma, kidney problems, weight gain, seizures, heart palpitations, depression, and even cerebral palsy and multiple sclerosis, among other conditions.

"If you find yourself sneezing and coughing with watery eyes and swollen sinuses each spring, you're probably aware that you have allergies," says Konrad Kail, N.D., of Phoenix, Arizona, author of *Allergy Free: An Alternative Medicine Definitive Guide.* "What might surprise you is that your child's ear infections or your spouse's digestive prob-

> *If you find yourself sneezing and coughing with watery eyes and swollen sinuses each spring, you're aware that you have allergies. What might surprise you is that your child's ear infections or your spouse's digestive problems may stem from allergies, too. Research confirms that allergies manifest as common ailments...and can occur at just about anytime, in just about anybody.*
>
> — KONRAD KAIL, N.D.

lems may stem from allergies, too. Recent research confirms that allergies manifest as various common ailments and disorders—from headaches to autism—and can occur at just about anytime, in just about anybody."

In industrialized nations, the number of people with allergies is rising at an alarming rate and, according to the American Academy of Allergy, Asthma & Immunology, more than 20% of the U.S. population—adults and children—has an allergic condition, making allergies the sixth-leading cause of chronic disease. Of those, more than 15 million have asthma[1] and 40 million experience chronic allergic rhinitis or its seasonal counterpart, hay fever, each year.[2] Allergy expert James Braly, M.D., of Hollywood, Florida, places the figure much higher. "Actually the majority of Americans suffer from allergies," he says. "This is particularly true of food allergy, which is, along with undernutrition, the most commonly undiagnosed condition in the U.S. today."

Conventional medicine currently offers limited treatment options, generally medications, which provide only temporary relief of allergy symptoms. In some cases, the treatment may ultimately lead to new health problems. Alternative medicine practitioners, however, have found that by correcting the underlying causes of allergies, you can eliminate most allergy symptoms for good. Modifying your diet and restoring your normal immune-defense functions may help you breathe, eat, and live allergy-free again.

Types of Allergies

An allergen (a substance provoking an allergy symptom) is a protein that the body judges to be foreign and dangerous. The adverse reaction that follows is called an allergic response. Common symptoms of a typical allergic reaction include breathing congestion, inflamed, bloodshot, or scratchy eyes, tears, sneezing, coughing, itching, nosebleeds, puffy face, flushing of the cheeks, dark circles under the eyes, runny nose, swelling, hives, vomiting, stomachache, and intestinal irritation or swelling. Allergies fall into two categories, those caused by environmental factors and those caused by food.

The typical allergic reactions people have to foods, dust, pollen, and other substances are the body's way of fending off the intrusion of toxins that disrupt the body's equilibrium. Allergens usually enter the body through breathing, absorption through the skin, by eating or drinking foods, or by injection, such as insect bites or vaccinations. Because the body judges the substances to be dangerous to its health, the immune system identifies them as antigens. The mobilized immune system then releases specific antibodies to deactivate the allergenic antigens, setting in motion a complex series of events involving many biochemicals. These chemicals then produce the inflammation or other typical symptoms of an allergy response.

The antibody most commonly involved in the allergic response to pollens and environmental substances is IgE, one of five immunoglobulins, or antibody proteins, involved in the immune system's response. The main types of immunoglobulins are IgG, IgA, IgM, IgD, and IgE. Mast cells, which produce the allergic response and are found throughout the body's tissues, next come into play. When the IgE antibody senses an allergen, it triggers the mast cells to release histamine and at least 28 other chemicals and the allergic response flares into action. An IgE molecule attaches itself, like a key fitting a lock, to the specific allergen; there are different types (shapes and biochemical structures) of the IgE molecules specific for each type of allergen.

The most common allergic reactions occur immediately after exposure to a certain substance (peanuts, pollen, bee stings, or cats). These reactions are typically caused by IgE immunoglobulins, resulting in a runny nose, watery eyes, itching, and skin rashes; more severe reactions include constriction of the bronchial tubes (asthma) and difficulty breathing or even anaphylactic shock. Delayed allergies are another type of allergic reaction, which can manifest symptoms up to 72 hours after exposure to a triggering substance (typically a food). These can commonly appear as seemingly unrelated illnesses or disorders such as lethargy, attention deficit dis-

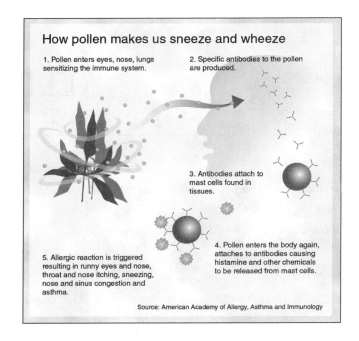

How pollen makes us sneeze and wheeze

1. Pollen enters eyes, nose, lungs sensitizing the immune system.

2. Specific antibodies to the pollen are produced.

3. Antibodies attach to mast cells found in tissues.

4. Pollen enters the body again, attaches to antibodies causing histamine and other chemicals to be released from mast cells.

5. Allergic reaction is triggered resulting in runny eyes and nose, throat and nose itching, sneezing, nose and sinus congestion and asthma.

Source: American Academy of Allergy, Asthma and Immunology

order, fatigue, hyperactivity, acne, itchy skin, mood swings, insomnia, and inflammation in joints or other tissues. Many of these reactions are caused by IgG immunoglobulins. Up to 80 different medical conditions—from arthritis, asthma, and autism to insomnia, psoriasis, and diabetes—have been clinically associated with IgG food allergy reactions.

Conventional medicine has been slow to recognize that both foods and chemicals can trigger adverse responses in the body. Part of the problem is that conventional skin tests do not identify sensitivities before they become full-blown allergies. Additionally, the symptoms may change after each exposure to a sensitizing agent—smelling an offending chemical gives you a headache one time and makes you nauseous the next.

Environmental Allergies

The most common cause of environmental allergies is the pollen of various plants such as trees, weeds, and grass. House dust mites, molds, and tobacco smoke are other causes. Less common, but equally serious, are products often found in the home. "Cosmetics, perfumes, household cleaning agents, the gas we use for heating and cooking, the fabrics in our clothes, and even the metals used by dentists as fillings can trigger allergy attacks in some people," Dr. Wilkinson says.

Chemical sensitivity is a modern phenomenon. It has been directly linked by the work of environmental medicine pioneer Theron Randolph, M.D., to the increasing prevalence of chemicals and toxins in our environment—pesticides in foods, heavy metals in water, vehicle exhaust in the air, and numerous synthetic chemicals in personal hygiene products, cleaning supplies, and building materials. As we now spend up to 90% of our time indoors, often in energy-efficient buildings that re-circulate the same stale air, indoor air irritants are triggering more cases of allergic hay fever than outdoor sources.

In the 1980s, physicians began using the term *sick building syndrome* (SBS) to refer to a host of symptoms produced by sensitivities to low-grade toxic environmental conditions found in living or office spaces. This hazard received national publicity when CBS's *60 Minutes* disclosed that the headquarters of the Environmental Protection Agency in Washington, D.C., was environmentally unsafe for workers. In most cases, problems with a building's engineering, construction, and ventilation system are the causes of SBS. However, evidence is accumulating that the 1,000 new chemicals introduced worldwide each year, even at very low concentrations and exposures, cause allergy and sensitivity.

Food Allergies

The fact that physical and mental disorders can be caused by allergic reactions to food was first discovered during the 1940s by Dr. Randolph. His findings have resulted in a growing number of studies that link food allergies to a wide spectrum of health conditions. Dr. Braly defines food allergies as abnormal or adverse immunological responses to foods that other people eat with impunity. "But food allergies must be distinguished from non-allergic reactions to food, such as enzyme deficiencies or food poisoning," he points out.

Food allergies must also be distinguished from toxic reactions that affect everyone more or less identically, according to Leon Chaitow, N.D., D.O., of London, England, because while a toxic substance such as cyanide will affect anyone who ingests it, any number of people can eat the same food and only those allergic to it will have a reaction. The foods most commonly found to cause allergies include wheat, corn, milk and other dairy products, egg whites, tomatoes, soy, shellfish, peanuts, chocolate, as well as food dyes and additives.

Most adverse reactions to foods are sensitivities, not true allergies. The U.S. Department of Agriculture reports that 15% of the total population suffers from reactions to foods. Of that number, 1.5% experience true, antibody-mediated allergy; the remaining 13.5% suffer from food sensitivities. However, some environmental medicine doctors believe that up to 50% of the U.S. population is sensitive to foods. Symptoms of food sensitivities can be immediate or delayed and often manifest as gastrointestinal problems, such as belching, bloating, gas, and diarrhea; headaches; lack of mental clarity; and fatigue. Additives in foods, such as monosodium glutamate (MSG), tartrazine (FD&C Yellow Dye #5), aspartame (found in NutraSweet™ and Equal™), and sulfites have

---

TOP TRIGGERS OF ALLERGIC REACTIONS

Inhalants
- Plant pollen (ragweed, timothy grass, etc.)
- Animal dander (cat, dog, other pets)
- Cockroach casings
- House dust mite casings
- Mold spores
- Tobacco smoke
- Vehicle exhaust
- Chemical products (paint and cleaning solution fumes, etc.)

Ingestants
- Foods
  —In Children: Milk, egg, peanuts, wheat, soy, tree nuts, corn
  —In Adults: Peanuts, tree nuts, fish, shellfish
- Medications
  —Antibiotics (penicillin, amoxicillin, etc.)
  —Non-steroidal, anti-inflammatory drugs (aspirin, etc.)

Contactants
- Plants (poison ivy, oak, sumac)
- Jewelry (nickel, copper, chromates, etc.)
- Latex gloves
- Beauty products (hair dyes, cosmetics, etc.)

Injectants
- Insect stings/bites
- Some medications

---

been shown to trigger adverse reactions, including headaches and hyperactivity in children.

FOOD ADDICTION

As early as the 1940s, practitioners of environmental medicine, led by Dr. Randolph, found that people with food allergies are often addicted to the very foods they are allergic to. Allergy to addictive foods develops as any other food allergy does—with a leaky gut or improper digestion. According to Dr. Randolph, an allergic reaction to food can last for up to three or more days, making the addiction to the food difficult to discover. This is because the symptoms that a person normally experiences when undergoing withdrawal from an addictive substance can actually improve or be suppressed if the person eats more of the addictive food.

"The relationship between food allergy and food addiction is both extremely close and subtle," Dr. Wilkin-

A FOOD ALLERGY TIMETABLE

Michael Lesser, M.D., of Berkeley, California, has created a timetable, based on patient case histories, that can be used to determine allergenic foods or liquids.[3] When experiencing the symptoms below, notice if they began within the given time frame. If so, they may be due to food allergies.

Symptom	Time after food was eaten
Indigestion or heartburn	30 minutes
Headache	Within 1 hour
Asthma, runny nose	Within 1 hour
Stomach bloat/diarrhea	3-4 hours
Rashes or hives	6-12 hours
Weight gain by fluid retention	12-15 hours
Fits, convulsions, mental disturbance	12-24 hours
Mouth ulcers, joint/muscle pain, backache	48-96 hours

son explains. "If people are allergic to coffee, for instance, they won't usually break into a rash or start sneezing when they drink it. Instead, symptoms such as a headache might occur hours after the coffee is consumed, or they might later experience severe exhaustion if they refrain from having another cup. But most people will tend to drink coffee regularly and thus get relief from their symptoms without realizing that it is the coffee that is causing them."

The suppression of symptoms caused by addictive/allergenic foods when they are eaten has been termed *masking* by Dr. Randolph, as the foods will mask, or camouflage, the actual allergic symptoms. "The likelihood of having an allergic reaction to any given food is directly proportional to how often a person eats it," says Charles Gableman, M.D., a former practitioner of environmental medicine in Lake Forest, California. "This is not true in all cases, but as a rule the foods that we eat the most as a culture tend to be the ones we are most allergic to."

What Causes Allergies?

The underlying causes of allergy and sensitivity are dietary and lifestyle factors that break down your immune system and barrier defenses. Specifically, imbalanced immune function, barrier function default (such as "leaky gut"), and toxic overload are in varying degrees respon-

sible for the development and continuation of allergy and sensitivity.

Imbalanced Immune Function

One of the primary causes of allergies is an imbalanced immune system, which substantially increases the risk of allergic reactions. Dr. Chaitow has found that a number of factors negatively impact the immune function, including increased toxic burden due to pollution in all its forms; disturbance of immune systems through repeated childhood and adult vaccinations and immunizations; and damage to healthy intestinal flora due to over-reliance upon antibiotics and steroids (especially birth control pills).

The immune system may also be weakened by hereditary problems, according to Fuller Royal, M.D., of Las Vegas, Nevada. "Usually this will be reflected in the gastrointestinal tract, so that nutrients are not absorbed and utilized properly. This can then set you up for food allergies." Dr. Royal also agrees that antibiotics can cause allergic reactions and feels that, in many cases, their use is unnecessary. Antibiotics further add to the confusion the immune system is facing, he says, until it is no longer able to tell friend from foe. "When that happens, it starts reacting to all sorts of things that are not foes, which then become treated as allergens. This leads to fatigue and allows viruses, bacteria, and so forth to come in and play havoc."

Other causes of immune dysfunction and food allergies include nutritional deficiencies, a repetitive and monotonous diet, chemicals in the food chain due to pesticides and preservatives, and chronic intestinal yeast overgrowth (candidiasis).[4] "A repetitive diet can contribute greatly to the development of allergies," says Marshall Mandell, M.D., Medical Director of the New England Foundation for Allergies and Environmental Diseases. The diets of allergy patients normally consist of 30 foods or less, which they eat repeatedly. "These 30 foods then become the basis for the most common food intolerances," says Dr. Mandell. "If someone eats wheat bread every day, for instance, he could easily develop a wheat allergy due to the immune system's continuous exposure to it."

 See Addictions, Candidiasis, Children's Health, Gastrointestinal Disorders, Parasitic Infections, Respiratory Conditions.

Barrier Function Default

Barrier function is an important concept in understanding and treating allergy/sensitivity. Barrier functions are those things that keep a person from becoming sensitized (experiencing a negative body response) to sub-

EARLY CHILDHOOD PRACTICES LEAD TO ALLERGY/SENSITIVITY

Research shows that up to 34% of infants born to women who have allergies will develop allergies as well.[5] This is not due to genetic inheritance of allergy, for there is no research supporting the existence of an allergy-causing gene. But the allergic mothers do pass something to their progeny—antigens and their associated antibodies. "One of the immune mechanisms that mediate allergies, an antibody called IgG, transfers through the placenta from the mother's blood into the fetal blood supply," says James Braly, M.D. "This causes the fetus to passively develop allergies to the same foods that the mother is allergic to." Mother's milk, which generally reduces the risk of allergy in children, can also transfer allergens and antibodies to infants.[6]

In one study, a one-month-old breast-fed infant who suffered from chronic allergy-related intestinal problems experienced a full recovery when his mother eliminated cow's milk products, egg, and pork—all commonly allergenic foods—from her diet.[7] Food allergies aren't the only conditions "inherited" *in utero*. Pollen contact *in utero* can sensitize the developing baby to aeroallergens, leading to allergic rhinitis and other allergies upon birth.[8] The transfer of allergen and antibody, however, doesn't fully explain why breast-fed infants become hypersensitive. As it does in all cases of allergy, barrier function default often contributes to infantile allergy development. It's likely that maternal exposure to factors that cause personal barrier function default can also damage the barrier functions of developing fetuses.

According to Dick Thom, N.D., D.D.S., of Beaverton, Oregon, a mother who smokes during her pregnancy can increase the likelihood of her baby developing allergies. The time of year of the birth and weaning are also important factors, Dr. Thom states. "Being born or weaned immediately prior to the peak of pollen season, for instance, can increase the child's risk of becoming allergic to that particular allergen."

Vaccinations Disturb the Immune System—During the past century, vaccinations have become regarded almost as a rite of passage for American children. Beginning as early as a few weeks after birth, the vast majority of children are inoculated against numerous illnesses, including measles, mumps, whooping cough, polio, and tetanus. Most schools actually require immunizations as part of the admissions process. At the same time, childhood cases of allergy and asthma have skyrocketed.

Recent evidence indicates that routine childhood vaccinations contribute to the emergence of chronic allergic problems such as eczema, ear infections, and asthma. While this contention is controversial, a growing number of scientists and physicians maintain that most standard vaccinations permanently disturb the developing immune system, setting the stage for hypersensitive reactions to foods and other common substances. In fact, childhood illnesses such as measles, mumps, and whooping cough may actually reduce the risk of allergy, says Konrad Kail, N.D.

In early 1997, a team of British physicians writing in *Science* made this provocative statement: "Childhood infections may paradoxically protect against asthma." The British physicians noted that the incidence of asthma has doubled in Western countries since 1977 and, in the U.S., it is responsible for 33% of all pediatric emergency-room visits. Yet this growing incidence of asthma seems to be related more to the suppression or absence of respiratory infections than to the commonly cited cause of air pollution. Highly polluted European cities where the use of antibiotics and immunizations is less than in the U.S. have lower asthma rates than comparable U.S. cities. Conversely, in Tucson, Arizona, despite the dry heat and lack of irritants (such as molds, fungi, and dust mites) in the air, the rate of asthma is the same as elsewhere in the country.

This suggests that diseases such as tuberculosis and whooping cough may permanently alter a child's immune system such that they confer a lifetime protection against asthma. Certainly the researchers were not saying that children should have tuberculosis, but they noted that the immune system needs to be tempered by a cell-mediated response, and this best happens during an infectious childhood disease. If this does not happen, the system is left unbridled and subject to overreaction (allergies) to otherwise harmless substances.

ARE YOUR SYMPTOMS DUE TO ALLERGIES?

The following questionnaire, developed by Leon Chaitow, N.D., D.O., of London, England, can help you determine if you have a food allergy. If your answer is "no" or "never" to any question, give yourself a score of zero for that particular question; the other scores are provided with each question.

- Do you suffer from unnatural fatigue? (Score 1 if occasionally, 2 if regularly—three times a week or more.)

- Do you sometimes experience weight fluctuations of four or more pounds in a single day, accompanied by puffiness of the face, ankles, or fingers? (Score 1 if infrequently, 2 if frequently—more than once a month.)

- Do you have hot flashes (apart from menopause) or find yourself sweating for no obvious reason? (Score 1 if infrequently, 2 if several times a week or more.)

- Does your pulse race or your heart pound strongly for no obvious reason? (Score 1 if infrequently, 2 if several times a week or more.)

- Do you have a history of food intolerance, causing any symptoms at all? (Score 2 if your answer is yes.)

- Do you crave bread, sugary foods, milk, chocolate, coffee, or tea? (Score 2 if your answer is yes.)

- Do you suffer from migraine or severe headaches, irritable bowel syndrome, eczema, depression, asthma, or muscle aches? (Score 2 if your answer is yes.)

The most anyone could score on this test would be 14, explains Dr. Chaitow. "If your score is five or higher, there is a strong likelihood that allergies are part of your symptom picture."

to allergies. The second barrier, for inhaled substances (dust, pollens, dander, molds), is the mucus that covers the membranes of the sinuses and respiratory passages. The purpose of the mucus is to trap any irritants and particulates so that they do not come in contact with the membranes and can be removed. The third barrier is the skin; any break in the skin (cut, scrape, burn, rash, or other skin defect) compromises the barrier and sensitization may occur.

- Leaky gut syndrome, or excessive permeability in the digestive tract, can lead to allergies, according to Dr. Braly. "In these cases," he explains, "the immune system reacts to the particles of partially digested foodstuffs (macromolecules) that leak into the bloodstream through the gut as if they were foreign material." Among the causes of leaky gut syndrome, Dr. Braly cites poor digestion, alcohol consumption, the use of steroidal or nonsteroidal anti-inflammatory drugs (NSAIDs), viral, fungal, and bacterial infections, parasites, nutrient deficiencies, excessive stress, antibiotics, and radiation. "These are all factors that one should consider and control as part of an overall approach for treating allergies," he advises.

- Particles that manage to bypass the respiratory defenses are trapped in the mucous membranes, the lining of our respiratory tract, particularly the nose and lungs. Cilia move particles, mixed with mucus, from deep in the respiratory system to the pharynx (part of the upper throat behind the tongue and nasal cavity). From there, the particles are expelled by coughing or they are swallowed, where they are destroyed by stomach acid and digestive enzymes. Lack of humidity and environmental irritants can damage the mucous membranes and allow foreign particles entry into the bloodstream.

- What people sensitize to the most through their skin is what touches damaged skin most frequently. Clothing, fabric chemicals and dyes, laundry products, cosmetics, perfume, aftershave lotions, creams, sunscreens, and even topical medicines can trigger allergic reactions. Perspiration increases the likelihood of sensitization, since perspiration occurs when the skin is hot and the blood vessels to the skin are dilated, which promotes absorption. Deficiencies in water and essential fatty acids, ultraviolet radiation, hormonal irregularities, and stress can impair the skin's repair process, leading the way to allergy and sensitivity.

stances. The barrier function for food sensitivity is digestion. If the person can digest and absorb normally, they do not become sensitized to foods. Inadequate digestion for any reason (infection, inflammation, malabsorption) may result in digestive barrier default, where undigested food particles are absorbed into the bloodstream leading

Toxic Overload

As our food and environment become increasingly saturated with pollutants and chemicals, the body's mechanisms for elimination of toxins cannot keep up with the chemical deluge. All organs involved in detoxification, which include, among others, the allergy barrier systems of the intestines, skin, and respiratory tract, can become overloaded. This overload weakens the barrier functions and can lead to sensitization.

Studies by environmental scientists and physicians indicate that pollutants play a role in the creation of all allergies, as well as arthritis and autoimmune illnesses.[9] According to William Rea, M.D., an environmental physician in Dallas, Texas, when key detoxification organs become unable to fully detoxify themselves or the body, a pattern of chronic allergies may develop in which the immune system attacks its own unprocessed toxic load. The constant circulation of toxins in the body taxes the immune system, which must continually strive to destroy them. An overburdened immune system ultimately becomes hypersensitive and allergies—to food, airborne agents, and chemicals—develop.

Treatment of Allergies

"In order for true healing of allergies to occur, it is necessary to address their cause rather than just treat the outward manifestations or symptoms," says Dr. Wilkinson. "This involves identifying the substances a person is allergic to and eliminating them from the diet and environment. At the same time, the body needs to be purged of toxins and the immune system needs to be stimulated. Since no two people are exactly alike, therapeutic approaches will vary, and usually a combination of therapies is the best course of action." Among the therapies that have proven most effective in treating allergies are diet and nutrition, herbal medicine, desensitization techniques, acupuncture, and homeopathy.

Dietary Recommendations

Foods play a dual role in allergies and sensitivities, as both triggers of and contributors to adverse reactions. The problem with food allergies and sensitivities is that 85% of them involve delayed reactions, manifesting up to 72 hours after consumption of the offending food. You may not realize that the wheat bread you ate two days ago is responsible for your headache today. And the symptoms may shape-shift; that is, change over time and with repeated exposure. "Proper diet is the foundation from which to deal with allergies of all types," says Dr. Thom. "If the body is continually being stressed by the foods that are meant to nourish it, there will be less reserves left over for the immune system to deal with other 'foreign' substances."

ELIMINATION DIET

Once you have identified the foods you are allergic to, the next step is to eliminate them from your diet. Initially, you should completely refrain from eating all allergenic foods for 60-90 days. After this period, you can begin to slowly reintroduce them into your diet. You should also vary the foods that you eat on a daily basis to avoid developing new allergies (see "Rotation Diet" below). In most cases, this diet allows the body to repair intestinal barrier function, enabling patients to reintroduce the reactive foods into their diets. Dr. Braly estimates that only about 5% of delayed food allergies will not subside using the elimination and rotation diets, necessitating the use of other alternative therapies. Remember that eliminating an allergenic food can cause withdrawal reactions. "The majority of people who give up foods they're allergic to go through a mild to moderate withdrawal phase, lasting one to five days, while the body detoxifies itself," says Dr. Braly. Allergic symptoms may get worse during this period and cravings can be intense. Dr. Braly explains that "once the withdrawal phase has passed, the cravings also abate, and the allergy sufferer is free of dependence on that food, free of both the physiological and psychological desire to consume it so frequently and in such great quantities."[10]

ROTATION DIET

One way to ensure that the body is receiving a greater supply of nutrients from food, while at the same time minimizing the risk of exposure to allergenic foods, is to increase the variety of foods eaten and rotate them so that they aren't eaten too frequently. This is known as a rotation diet. According to Dr. Braly, a rotation diet is one of the simplest and most effective measures anyone can take to both prevent and deal with the problems of food allergies. "Normally, I would rotate the foods every four days," he advises. "This means that you are not eating any one food more often than every four days. You might be able to have the same food more than once in a day, but then you wouldn't have it again until four days later. Some people may need to go longer than that, but usually four days is ideal."

Dr. Braly also suggests adopting a diet that includes a wide variety of nonallergenic fresh fruits and vegetables, seeds and nuts, and low-fat, nondairy animal protein. "Grains are important, too," he says. "Although, I make it a general policy to avoid the gluten grains such as wheat, rye, barley, and oats, which many people are not able to tolerate. I would stick to grains like brown rice, millet, and amaranth."

For people with allergies and sensitivities, it is particularly important to keep well hydrated. Most alternative medicine physicians generally recommend eight to twelve 8-oz glasses of water daily, with little or no fluid intake at meals, since it may dilute the stomach's hydrochloric acid, making it difficult to absorb minerals and digest protein. Thirty minutes before or two hours after meals is commonly advised before drinking other than a few sips of water. Additional water is needed if you consume coffee, alcohol, or caffeine products, or eat heavy meats. It's advisable to drink only water that has been reliably purified through reverse osmosis, activated charcoal, de-ionization, or distillation; these filtration methods remove chlorine and fluoride from tap water.

STONE AGE DIET

The "Stone Age" diet is another potentially useful diet plan for allergy sufferers. The theory behind this diet is that our bodies are not genetically adapted to the synthetic, processed foods that constitute much of our modern eating practices. Therefore, we are unable to digest many foods properly, and they become allergenic as our body tries to defend against them.

According to Abram Hoffer, M.D., due to the slow course of evolution, our digestive apparatus has remained the same for 10,000 years. Thus, we are best suited for the foods prevalent during the Paleolithic era—meat, fish, vegetables, fruit, and a few seeds. "You ate different foods in the spring, summer, fall, and winter and never had too much. You also did not load up on any one item," says Dr. Hoffer. Now, we eat an abundance of the same foods, especially grains, every day of the year. "If you overload the gut with one particular item, for instance bread three times a day, then eventually the body breaks down," explains Dr. Hoffer. Malnourishment and a leaky gut are elements of this breakdown.

Dr. Chaitow speculates that the change away from a caveman-type diet over the centuries is associated with the increase in allergies worldwide. Lending weight to this theory is the fact that it is precisely those foods our cave ancestors did not eat—cereal grains, dairy products, and modern processed foods—that most frequently provoke allergic reactions The Stone Age diet requires eating only seasonal produce as well as protein foods, such as meat, fish, and seeds, and very few grains or processed foods. No food chemicals or additives are allowed. Dr. Chaitow reports that patients following the Stone Age diet report impressive results. "In the majority of cases, most allergy problems vanish after a few weeks of eating this way. And with many patients, a gradual reintroduction of the offending foods is possible on a rotating basis."

PROPER FOOD COMBINING

If your food allergies/sensitivities are caused by poor digestion, which allows food molecules to escape the gut barrier, proper food combining may help restore healthy digestion. The general rule, according to Patrick Donovan, N.D., of Seattle, Washington, is that proteins and starchy carbohydrates are never eaten at the same time. Proteins may be eaten with non-starchy vegetables. Carbohydrates (grains, potatoes, and other starchy vegetables) may be eaten with all vegetables as well as legumes. Fruits must be eaten alone, usually as a snack; the same is true with dairy products.

"The rationale for this approach is the difference in digestion time for various food groups," Dr. Donovan explains. "Digestion is optimal if foods eaten together have roughly the same digestion time." Many alternative medicine practitioners have found that food combining helps patients avoid gas, belching, and bloating, which is often caused when sugars from fruits or starchy carbohydrates ferment in the gut because the stomach is busy processing fats. However, some studies have shown that food combining isn't necessarily effective—certain foods may still not be properly absorbed, even if you follow the combining rules. Once again, the efficacy of this diet depends on individual response and how severely digestion is impaired. Supplemental enzymes with food may also help.

Nutritional Supplementation

If digestive disorders are compounding allergies, which is usually the case, they will need to be corrected before any significant improvement can occur. "I find that many people with such complaints suffer from deficiencies in vitamin A, certain B vitamins, zinc, magnesium, and/or essential oils," Dr. Braly says. "Some people, especially as they get older or if their allergies are severe, also require digestive assistance in the form of pancreatic enzymes and/or hydrochloric acid, so supplementing each meal with them can be helpful as well." Alternatively, plant-derived enzymes like bromelain (from pineapple) or papain (from papaya) may be helpful.

Both zinc and vitamin A play an important role in the production of IgA, an antibody secreted from the salivary glands in the mouth and from cells that line the digestive tract. "IgA latches on to what is perceived in the body as allergens or potential allergens in the foods that we eat," Dr. Braly explains. "This results in a protective coat of mucus being formed around these allergens and prevents them from being absorbed into the bloodstream. If you are zinc and vitamin A deficient, you produce less IgA, and therefore your susceptibility to food allergies increases." Zinc also plays a role in the produc-

ALLERGY PREVENTION STRATEGIES FOR CHILDREN

Becoming allergy free can begin as early as infancy and involves what were once common child-rearing strategies: prolonged breast-feeding, later introduction of solid foods, and the avoidance of early immunizations. You can also take steps to protect your children from harmful environmental allergens.

Breast-Feed Your Infant—One of the best ways to decrease the likelihood of developing allergies later in life, according to most alternative medicine practitioners, is to feed an infant on mother's milk. Breast-feeding builds a strong immune system equipped to deal with infection, environmental toxins, and food allergens. Lendon Smith, M.D., a pediatrician in Portland, Oregon, and author of numerous books on children's health, emphasizes that nursing contributes to the child having fewer allergies. He states, "If babies are given anything other than breast milk in the first few months of life, food sensitivities may develop. Their intestines are not meant to digest anything other than breast milk."

Introduce Solid Foods Later—Postponing the introduction of solid foods and prolonging breast-feeding gives an infant's immune system enough time to adequately mature. Studies suggest that a later introduction of solid foods, in particular peanuts, eggs, wheat, and fish, may reduce the incidence of allergies.[11] A study published in the *British Medical Journal* found that children who were started on solid foods before the age of four months were more likely to experience chronic or recurrent episodes of eczema than children of the same age who were not introduced to solid foods.[12] When a child is ready to eat solid foods, usually after six months, parents can give them a healthy start by designing a diet made up of fresh fruits and vegetables, legumes, and low-fat proteins like chicken and fish, with no processed foods, recommends Dr. Smith.

Avoid Early Immunization—Currently in the United States, conventional doctors require that a series of immunization shots be started when an infant is two months old. The first vaccines given are hepatitis B, DPT (diphtheria, tetanus, and pertussis), influenza type B, and polio. In total, an average American child is vaccinated against ten childhood diseases and receives up to 21 shots over a course of the first 15 months of life. It is well documented that certain vaccines can cause immediate allergic reactions in some children; these reactions range from temporary discomfort to death. If you choose not to have your child vaccinated, you should obtain an exemption (medical, religious, or philosophical) since immunization is compulsory in many states in the U.S.

Allergy-Proof Your House—Early exposure to indoor environmental factors, such as house dust mites, molds, smoke, formaldehyde from housing materials, and high levels of radon, can act directly on blocking a person's airways or indirectly by causing sensitivities to allergens. By reducing exposure to air pollutants, the likelihood of developing allergies/sensitivities or suffering chronic allergic reactions can be reduced. Environmental control can be especially helpful in preventing the development of asthma in infants.[13] The following suggestions can reduce exposure to common household allergens by up to 95%.

In the bedroom:
- Wash pillows, blankets, and other bedding monthly in hot water.
- Use washable, organic cotton pillows and enclose mattress and box spring in plastic mite-proof covers.
- Remove stuffed animals from the bed.
- Remove bedroom carpeting or treat carpet with tannic acid, which denatures allergens.
- Eliminate exposure to pets or at least restrict pets' access to the bedroom.

In the house:
- Keep windows closed, especially during "allergy season."
- Avoid tobacco smoke.
- Achieve ideal relative humidity: use air conditioning and dehumidification to help reduce mold production, if your home is too damp; if your home is too dry, use a humidifier.
- Use air filters (electrostatic precipitators and high-efficiency particulate air, or HEPA) and ionizing air purifiers to remove particulate matter and odors from the air. An ozone air purifier can be used in a room where there are no people, animals, or plants while the purifier is running.
- Use low-toxicity mite-specific exterminating chemicals, such as tannic acid.

TESTING FOR ALLERGIES

Currently, a variety of tests are available for identifying allergies. Regardless of which method is used, it is always necessary to demonstrate a cause-and-effect relationship between the exposure to suspected allergen and the outbreak of symptoms if the test is to be relied upon.

Scratch or Prick Skin Test—If you've ever been treated by a conventional allergist, you're probably familiar with scratch or prick skin testing. In each of these tests, the doctor lightly scratches or uses a needle to prick the surface of the skin, usually on the arm or back. Small dilutions of suspected allergens are then introduced on the pricked/scratched skin so that the substances can enter the body. If a wheal, a reddish inflammation resembling a mosquito bite, rises within 20 minutes, an allergy to the substance is confirmed. In conventional immunotherapy, extracts of the allergenic substances are then given as allergy shots in progressively stronger doses until a maintenance level is reached. These tests are limited in that they only measure IgE-mediated allergic responses (asthma, allergic rhinitis, eczema, and hives), which are primarily triggered by inhaled allergens such as pollen, mold, dust, and animal dander. These procedures are only about 15% accurate in spotting food-induced allergic reactions.[15] Thus, delayed food allergies and chemical sensitivities often go undetected by skin testing, according to Konrad Kail, N.D.

IgG ELISA Test—According to James Braly, M.D., testing for food allergies can be far more difficult than determining environmental reactions, because most food allergies are dealt with in the body by IgG antibodies, while most allergy tests only measure the presence of IgE antibodies. Many alternative medicine practitioners consider the ELISA (enzyme-linked immunoserological assay) to be among the most sensitive and useful blood tests in detecting delayed food allergies. The ELISA requires a small blood sample to be taken from the patient, then sent within 72 hours to any one of several specialized laboratories that perform this test. At the lab, technicians process the sample to collect the IgG antibodies, which are involved in delayed allergic reactions. A drop of this serum is placed in each of the tiny holding containers or "wells" in a laboratory testing plate. Each well contains a single potentially allergenic food or a component of highly allergenic foods, such as gluten, which is found in wheat. A computer then analyzes the samples. "We know that one of the fundamental causes behind food allergies is the penetration of undigested or partially digested food from the digestive tract into the bloodstream," Dr. Braly explains. "With the IgG ELISA test, we can measure the actual presence of specific foods and their specific IgG antibodies in the blood to precisely determine which foods a person is allergic to." The test can be done through the mail, as long as samples reach testing labs within 72 hours after the blood is drawn.

Electrodermal Screening (EDS)—This form of testing is widely used in Europe to screen for both food and environmental allergies and to determine what remedy to use to properly neutralize the allergic reaction. A small current of electricity is introduced at specific acupuncture points on the patient. Various allergens are then introduced into the circuitry, enabling the physician to determine any change in the way the patient reacts to the current. As they are found, various treatment doses are also added into the circuit. EDS can accurately test for a full spectrum of allergens, with the entire battery of tests completed in an hour. Few clinical studies have tested the effectiveness of EDS as a tool for identifying allergy triggers. A 1997 double-blind, controlled study used EDS testing with 41 polysymptomatic allergy patients. In the first group of 17 patients, EDS correctly differentiated 82% of the time between house dust mite or histamine (allergens) and saline or water (nonallergens). In the second group of 24 patients, EDS discriminated 96% of the time between allergenic and nonallergenic substances, leading the researchers to state that EDS is a reliable method for detecting allergy triggers.[16]

Applied Kinesiology—Applied kinesiology, first developed by George Goodheart, D.C., of Detroit, Michigan, is the study of the relationship between muscle dysfunction (weakness) and related organ or gland dysfunction. In the case of allergies, when an allergen comes into contact with an allergic person, its energetic properties will block the body's flow of energy, resulting in weakened muscles. To identify an allergen, whether food, chemical, or airborne, the practitioner has a patient hold a glass vial containing a suspected allergen in the less-dominant (non-writing) hand while raising the opposing arm to a 90° angle at the shoulder with the elbow straight. The practitioner then gently pushes on the raised arm down towards the patient's side while the patient resists. A weak muscle response, shown by little resistance to the pressure, indicates an allergy or sensitivity to the substance in the vial.

tion of hydrochloric acid (HCl), which the body needs for proper digestion to occur.

Another group of nutrients that Dr. Braly employs to treat allergies is vitamin P or certain bioflavonoids. "Bioflavonoids are some of the most effective anti-allergy nutrients that I've come across," he says. "Many of my patients who are allergy prone, both to their diet and their environment, over a period of time stop having allergic reactions once these bioflavonoids start taking effect. Quercetin taken orally along with bromelain, vitamin C, and glutamine, has produced wonderful results."

Finally, vitamin C in high doses can have a dramatic effect in improving allergy symptoms, particularly hay fever and asthma, due to its ability to counteract the inflammation responses that are part of such conditions. Robert Cathcart III, M.D., who pioneered the technique of taking vitamin C to bowel tolerance, recommends its use for allergies. In cases of more severe exposure, he advises that the dose of vitamin C be increased as well. Dr. Cathcart bases his recommendations on clinical experience with over 1,000 patients with allergies, the vast majority of whom gained significant relief from this approach.[14]

Herbal Medicine

There are a variety of herbs that offer relief from allergies, according to Dr. Thom. Among those he employs are anticatarrhals, such as goldenseal, red sage, and goldenrod, to help eliminate mucus; and astringents such as yarrow and myrrh (*Commiphora myrrha*) to help contract inflamed tissues and reduce secretions and discharges. To strengthen immune response, Paul Yanick, Jr., Ph.D., of Woodbridge, New Jersey, recommends echinacea, astragalus root, goldenseal root, and *Pfaffia paniculata* (suma or Brazilian ginseng), a Brazilian herb that numerous studies prove is effective and safe for treating weakened immune systems.[17]

One of Dr. Braly's favorite herbs is cayenne pepper. "Its active ingredient is capsaicin, which is a strong anti-inflammatory agent," he says. "This makes cayenne a particularly effective remedy for treating allergies, especially as it is also very inexpensive and readily available." Dr. Braly has reversed allergies, including asthma, simply by instructing his patients to sprinkle liberal amounts of cayenne pepper on their meals. One such case involved a man who had suffered from nightly asthma attacks that were often so bad that his coughs and wheezing would force him to sit up in bed, making sleep extremely difficult. Dr. Braly suggested he use cayenne with his food for a few days and then report back to him. "Four days later, he told me that, after the first day of sprinkling

---

cayenne on his food, he was symptom free for the first time in 13 years," Dr. Braly reports.

Although herbal remedies have shown excellent results in reducing allergy/sensitivity symptoms, using herbs to treat allergies involves an individual approach, according to Dr. Thom. "No one herb will work for all allergy sufferers," he says, although some particularly effective anti-inflammatory herbs are stinging nettle, *Ginkgo biloba,* and licorice. Chinese skullcap, ephedra, and feverfew are others to consider for treating allergy symptoms. Patients whose conditions are severe should consult with a trained herbalist or naturopath.

A major symptom of allergies is gastrointestinal upset, including bloating, gas, abdominal pain, diarrhea, and nausea. Demulcent herbs can alleviate these symptoms (*demulcent* is a term used by herbalists to describe an herb that has a protective effect on the mucous membranes by minimizing irritation). The most commonly used herbs are marshmallow, slippery elm bark, cabbage juice, okra, fenugreek, and aloe vera.

 See Acupuncture, Bodywork, Detoxification Therapy, Herbal Medicine, Homeopathy, NAET.

Desensitization Techniques

Many with allergies and sensitivities will find that they require desensitization treatments to experience complete and possibly permanent remission of their symptoms.

ENZYME-POTENTIATED DESENSITIZATION (EPD)

According to Stephen B. Edelson M.D., Medical Director of the Edelson Center for Environmental and Preventive Medicine, in Atlanta, Georgia, EPD is the most effective therapy for allergies ever developed. First discovered in 1967 by British immunologist Leonard M. McEwen, this applied immunotherapy technique trains the immune system to be nonreactive to substances that usually provoke allergic symptoms. EPD is now used by physicians in at least 12 countries.

In EPD, an allergic patient is given a series of tiny standardized injections of a wide variety of allergens from a single category. EPD injections differ from conventional allergy shots in three important ways: first, EPD injections include multiple related allergens; second, EPD doses are much weaker; and third, EPD injections are given along with an enzyme called beta-glucuronidase. This last component is important because it acts as a catalyst to make the desensitization more potent. According to Dr. McEwen, EPD appears to cause a cloning of certain T cells in the immune system so that they become resistant cells. They then start protecting against the production of T4 cells, which are the ones that lead to allergy symptoms.

EPD has been used successfully to treat about 50 health conditions, mostly of an immune or autoimmune nature. (The latter is when the body attacks its own tissue as if it were an allergen, such as lupus or some forms of arthritis.) It has an overall success rate of between 75% and 80%, with an average 50% decrease in medication use, according to W.A. Schrader, Jr., M.D., of Santa Fe, New Mexico. EPD treatments are generally given once every 2-3 months for six to eight times; 160,000 estimated doses have been given since the late 1960s with no serious side effects reported. Patients take a prescribed list of nutritional supplements in the weeks between shots and follow a specific diet. While EPD significantly reduces one's intolerance to allergenic foods, it does not necessarily eliminate all possibility of reacting to them.

NAMBUDRIPAD'S ALLERGY ELIMINATION TECHNIQUE (NAET)

Nambudripad's Allergy Elimination Technique is a desensitization therapy developed by Devi S. Nambudripad, D.C., O.M.D., Ph.D., of Buena Park, California. It relies on altering energy flow through the body to treat symptoms of allergy and sensitivity. By examining the energy pathways, also called acupuncture meridians, practitioners are able to diagnose allergy/sensitivity triggers. Applied kinesiology, acupressure, acupuncture, and chiropractic are then used to alter the energy flow in an allergic body.

The secret to NAET, according to Dr. Nambudripad, is to retrain your brain and nervous system to no longer react to the offending substance. "We can reprogram our brains to perceive unsuitable energies as suitable ones and use them for our benefit rather than allow them to cause energy blockages and imbalances," she explains.

According to Dr. Nambudripad, your energy system and brain interpret a particular substance as potentially harmful to your body. For other people, this item—a diamond ring, a carob-coated cherry, a peanut—is a harmless, everyday item; but for your system, it's toxic. Your energy pathways freeze up as a way of defending the body against this unsuitable substance. This in turn blocks your energy meridians, and if the condition never changes, the overall functioning of your body suffers. In the past 15 years, Dr. Nambudripad reports that NAET alone has entirely relieved allergy symptoms or produced satisfactory improvements in 80%-90% of her patients.

Acupuncture

Allergies are considered a symptom of immune dysfunction in acupuncture theory, according to William M. Cargile, B.S., D.C., F.I.A.C.A., Chairman of Research for the American Association of Oriental Medicine. In treating allergies, it's vital that we restore the immune system on a systemic level, he says. Acupuncture is ideally suited to accomplish this.

Dr. Cargile treats environmental and food allergies with equal success. One of his patients was a 51-year-old man who came to him with a severe milk allergy. "He had reached a point where he would have immediate diarrhea and other gastrointestinal complaints whenever he had milk, and it had been verified (endoscopically) that he had a stomach ulcer as a result," Dr. Cargile relates. After only two acupuncture treatments given to enhance his immune function, the man was again examined and his ulcer had disappeared. Moreover, he gained immediate relief from his allergies, despite making no change to his diet. "In fact," says Dr. Cargile, "his diet got worse because he began drinking milk again. Instead of experiencing a recurrence of symptoms, he is now able to drink milk without a problem."

Acupuncture has been shown to be particularly effectively in reducing rhinitis symptoms and even desensitizing patients to allergen exposure. In a 1998 study, 24 allergic rhinitis patients were treated with either real acupuncture (using rhinitis-specific acupoints) or placebo acupuncture (nonspecific points) for nine treatments. For two months following treatment, the subjects recorded their symptoms. The real acupuncture group experienced a significant reduction in allergy symptoms compared to the placebo group.[18]

In another study, 102 patients with allergic rhinitis were treated with acupuncture needles containing allergen extracts for two sessions. On the third session, the patients were exposed to the allergen. Allergic reactions were significantly reduced compared to before treatment. The researchers monitored these patients for two years, at which time it was determined that 72% of the patients no longer reacted to the test allergens, while 24% had improved significantly. This outcome was better than that of the control group.[19]

Homeopathy

Homeopathy has widespread applications for the treatment of allergies. In many situations, minute diluted doses of the substance a person is allergic to can be prepared as a homeopathic solution that triggers the body's natural ability to heal itself. "For instance, if someone has a problem with ragweed pollen," says Dr. Royal, "a diluted solution of it, given sublingually or by injection, will often neutralize the person's reaction to it." Dr. Chaitow confirms this, citing the fact that in Europe during hay fever season, hay fever sufferers have been shown to reduce or prevent their reactions by beginning a course of homeopathic pollen supplements a few months before the pollen count rises.

Homeopathic remedies are best prescribed by a competent homeopath. Self-diagnosis is discouraged due to the variety of factors that must be considered before the appropriate treatment is selected. "You have to take an overview of the entire patient and can't afford to overlook anything," Dr. Royal says. He regularly screens his allergy patients for dietary and environmental factors that may be causing their condition, including testing for hydrocarbons, formaldehyde, mold spores, house dust, pollens, monosodium glutamate, and artificial food dyes. From this, he is able to prescribe the most appropriate choice of remedy and reports a high degree of success using this protocol.

Recommendations

- Once you have identified the foods you are allergic to, the next step is to eliminate them from your diet. Initially, you should completely refrain from eating all allergenic foods for 60-90 days. After this period, you can begin to slowly reintroduce them into your diet. You should also vary the foods that you eat on a daily basis to avoid developing new allergies.

- Adopt a diet that includes a wide variety of nonallergenic fresh fruits and vegetables, seeds and nuts, and low-fat, nondairy animal protein.

- For people with allergies and sensitivities, it is particularly important to keep well hydrated. Most alternative medicine physicians generally recommend eight to twelve 8-oz glasses of pure water daily.

- One of the best ways to decrease the likelihood of developing allergies later in life, according to most alternative medicine practitioners, is to feed an infant on mother's milk. Postponing the introduction of solid foods and prolonging breast-feeding gives an infant's immune system enough time to adequately mature.

- Bioflavonoids (such as quercetin taken orally along with bromelain, vitamin C, and glutamine) are effective anti-allergy nutrients.

- Some particularly effective anti-inflammatory herbs are stinging nettle, *Ginkgo biloba,* and licorice. Chinese skullcap, ephedra, and feverfew are others to consider for treating allergy symptoms.

- Many allergy and environmentally sensitive patients will find that they require desensitization treatments, such as enzyme-potentiated desensitization (EPD) and Nambudripad's Allergy Elimination Technique, to experience complete and possibly permanent remission of their symptoms.

- Acupuncture has been shown to be particularly effectively in reducing rhinitis symptoms and even desensitizing patients to allergen exposure.

- With homeopathy, minute diluted doses of the substance a person is allergic to can be prepared as a homeopathic solution that triggers the body's natural ability to heal itself.

Self-Care
The following therapies can be undertaken at home under the guidance of a physician:

Fasting / Guided Imagery / Meditation / Mind/Body Medicine / Qigong and Tai Chi / Yoga

AROMATHERAPY: To calm stress and soothe allergic reactions, use lavender, melissa, and chamomile.

JUICE THERAPY: • Carrot, beet, and cucumber • Carrot and celery

Professional Care

The following therapies should only be provided by a qualified health professional:

Acupuncture / Applied Kinesiology / Ayurvedic Medicine / Biofeedback Training and Neurotherapy / Chelation Therapy / Environmental Medicine / Hypnotherapy / Mind/Body Medicine / NAET / Orthomolecular Medicine / Osteopathic Medicine

BIOLOGICAL DENTISTRY: Hal A. Huggins, D.D.S., reports the improvement or disappearance of food allergies after removing toxic dental mercury amalgams. He believes that food allergies can be caused by the absorption of mercury by food as it is ingested. Sometimes chronic, painless infections in wisdom tooth extraction sites can predispose a person to allergy reactions.

BODYWORK: Reflexology, shiatsu.

CRANIOSACRAL THERAPY: For nasal allergies.

MAGNETIC FIELD THERAPY: Exposure to a negative magnetic field helps to neutralize the acidity of the blood associated with allergies.

OXYGEN THERAPY: Hydrogen peroxide therapy.

Where to Find Help

For more information on, and referrals for, treatment of allergies, contact the following organizations.

American Academy of Environmental Medicine

American Financial Center, Suite 625
7701 East Kellogg Avenue
Wichita, Kansas 67207
(316) 684-5500
Website: www.aaem.com

The academy offers extensive training for physicians interested in learning more about environmental medicine.

American Association of Oriental Medicine (AAOM)

433 Front Street
Catasauqua, Pennsylvania 18032
(888) 500-7999
Web: www.aaom.org

The AAOM is a national professional trade organization of acupuncturists who meet acceptable standards of competency and can provide you with the names and locations of local members.

American Association of Naturopathic Physicians

601 Valley Street, Suite 105
Seattle, Washington 98109
(206) 298-0126
Website: www.naturopathic.org

Provides a directory of naturopathic physicians and offers referrals to a nationwide network of accredited or licensed practitioners. Also publishes a quarterly newsletter, for both professionals and the general public, and offers a series of brochures and pamphlets on a variety of subjects.

Immuno Labs, Inc.

1620 West Oakland Park Blvd., Suite 300
Fort Lauderdale, Florida 33311
(800) 231-9197

Specialized allergy and immunology testing for physicians around the world. Provides referrals worldwide to physicians who do allergy testing.

Nambudripad's Allergy Research Foundation

6714 Beach Blvd.
Buena Park, California 90621
(714) 523-8900
Website: www.naet.com

For a list of NAET practitioners.

National Center for Homeopathy

801 North Fairfax, Suite 306
Alexandria, Virginia 22314
(703) 548-7790
Website: www.homeopathic.org

For information about homeopathy and referrals to homeopathic practitioners.

Recommended Reading

Allergy Free: An Alternative Medicine Definitive Guide. Konrad Kail, N.D., and Bobbi Lawrence, with Burton Goldberg. Tiburon, CA: AlternativeMedicine.com Books, 2000.

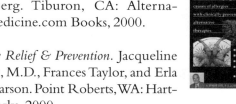

Allergy Relief & Prevention. Jacqueline Krohn, M.D., Frances Taylor, and Erla Mae Larson. Point Roberts, WA: Hartley Marks, 2000

An Alternative Approach to Allergies. Theron Randolph, M.D., and Ralph Moss, Ph.D. New York: HarperCollins, 1990.

Brain Allergies. William H. Philpott, M.D., and Dwight Kalita, Ph.D. Los Angeles: Keats Publishing, 2000.

Dr. Braly's Food Allergy and Nutrition Revolution. James Braly, M.D. New Canaan, CT: Keats Publishing, 1992.

The Food Allergy Book. William E. Walsh, M.D. New York: John Wiley, 2000.

ALZHEIMER'S DISEASE AND SENILE DEMENTIA

A devastating illness with no known single cause or cure, Alzheimer's disease afflicts four million Americans and may affect as many as 22 million people worldwide by 2025.[1] However, some estimates suggest that up to 40% of these patients are misdiagnosed and actually have other forms of senile dementia. Many alternative physicians report success in treating those with Alzheimer's-like dementia by addressing the causes underlying the condition.

ALZHEIMER'S DISEASE is a progressive, degenerative disease that attacks the brain, resulting in impaired memory, decreased intellectual and emotional functioning, and ultimately complete physical breakdown. It is the most common form of senile dementia, afflicting approximately 10% of those over the age of 65 and almost 50% of those over the age of 85.[2] Symptoms vary from depression, fatigue, and occasional forgetfulness to disorientation and aggressive or paranoid behavior. Typically, Alzheimer's disease is characterized by the following:

- Progressive loss of memory (short- and long-term impairment)
- A decline in vocabulary and word understanding
- Repeating the same questions
- Difficulties with numbers
- Problems with spatial and time orientation
- Forgetting simple words and familiar names
- Severe impairment in speaking fluently[3]

This range of symptoms, coupled with the fact that a definite diagnosis can be obtained only in a postmortem examination, causes frequent misdiagnosis. "There are really a number of factors in senile dementia. The best estimates are that 40% of the people diagnosed with Alzheimer's do not, in fact, have Alzheimer's," according to Abram Hoffer, M.D., of Victoria, British Columbia, Canada, a pioneer of orthomolecular and nutritional medicine. "It has come to the point that anyone over the age of 65 with the slightest memory loss

> *The best estimates are that 40% of the people diagnosed with Alzheimer's do not, in fact, have Alzheimer's.*
>
> —ABRAM HOFFER, M.D.

is in danger of being labeled with Alzheimer's. Therefore, we should not let this deter us from developing a treatment approach."

Alzheimer's was first identified in 1907 by German neurologist Alois Alzheimer who, during postmortem examinations, discovered abnormal formations of plaque on nerve endings and tangles of nerve fibers in the brain tissue of individuals who had exhibited symptoms of senile dementia.

The progression of Alzheimer's is characterized by a number of changes that take place in the brain's biochemistry, structure, and function. Dharma Singh Khalsa, M.D., Director of the Alzheimer's Prevention Foundation, in Tucson, Arizona, and author of *Brain Longevity*, says that nerves in the Alzheimer's brain die, severing important links between the two sections of the brain (the forebrain and hippocampus) responsible for thinking and memory. Brain autopsies of Alzheimer's patients show plaques and lesions or clots of dead cellular material, a fact corroborated by Dr. Khalsa and others. "The nerves become encrusted with protein deposits, which turn them into dysfunctional tangled masses of abnormal fibers." These "neurofibrillary tangles" occur most often in the hippocampus, the brain's memory center.

It is the disordered processing of certain proteins in the brain that seems to be the genesis of Alzheimer's. Recent research indicates that the enzymes that normally dispose of defective proteins in the brain may malfunction, thus allowing the plaques of amyloid protein to accumulate.[4] These amyloid plaques fill the spaces between nerve cells and damage the neurons, causing local inflammation and an immune response that may contribute to nerve damage.[5] Innumerable brain cells wither and die as their dendrites (the multiple branching connections between nerve cells) disappear.

There also can be up to a 90% decline in the levels of an important brain chemical (neurotransmitter) called acetylcholine, considered to be the prime molecular carrier of memory. In Alzheimer's patients, the brain is less able to extract oxygen and glucose from which the brain cells derive their necessary energy. At the same time, the enzymes required to synthesize and metabolize acetylcholine are deficient.[6] Eventually, nerve cells swell, then shrink and often die.

Causes of Alzheimer's Disease and Senile Dementia

Currently, the medical establishment spends millions of dollars each year attempting to isolate a single cause of Alzheimer's. Because other forms of senile dementia sometimes mimic the symptoms of Alzheimer's, Dr. Hoffer and other alternative physicians stress the importance of eliminating other possible causes of dementia before arriving at an Alzheimer's diagnosis. "The automatic diagnosis of Alzheimer's can be a real danger," says Dr. Hoffer. "Any type of toxic reaction, even alcoholism, can produce symptoms of dementia."

Joseph Pizzorno, N.D., Emeritus President of Bastyr University, in Kenmore, Washington, explains that two treatable conditions capable of causing senile dementia are often confused with Alzheimer's—pernicious anemia (a blood disease marked by a progressive decrease in red blood cells, muscular weakness, and gastrointestinal and neural disturbances) and cerebral vascular insufficiency (a lack of blood supply to the brain due to constricted arteries). Among the possible causes of senile dementia that can appear as Alzheimer's are multiple strokes, Parkinson's disease (a disease in which the cells that normally produce the neurotransmitter dopamine die off, resulting in a loss of muscle control), Huntington's chorea (a hereditary disease of the central nervous system characterized by progressive dementia and rapid, jerky motions), thyroid disorders, brain tumors, and head injuries. Other causes of senile dementia include drug reactions, environmental toxins and heavy metals, nutritional deficiencies, allergies, candidiasis, depression, alcoholism, and certain infections such as meningitis, syphilis, and AIDS.

Alzheimer's research is beginning to uncover multiple factors that may contribute to the disease. This indicates that the search for a single cause may prove unsuccessful. Possible contributing factors include genetics, impaired blood flow, nutritional deficiencies, environmental influences, and hormone imbalances.

Genetic Tendencies

Researchers have discovered a possible genetic predisposition for Alzheimer's disease—in many families, people in succeeding generations develop Alzheimer's. While genetics is probably not the sole cause, it may be a trigger in a significant number of cases. Scientists think that a genetic mutation may lead to the abnormal production of amyloid proteins or their precursors, which can eventually lead to the formation of plaques in the brain.[7] A specific connection has also been uncovered between Alzheimer's and Down syndrome. Individuals suffering from Down syndrome often exhibit Alzheimer's-like memory problems or dementia in their thirties and forties. Postmortem examinations of the brains of older Down syndrome patients have revealed many of the characteristic abnormalities of Alzheimer's, such as nerve plaques and nerve fiber tangles.[8]

Impaired Blood Flow to the Brain

There may be a relationship between heart disease, reduced blood flow to the brain, and the onset of Alzheimer's. According to Dr. Khalsa, 77% of Alzheimer's patients have cardiovascular disease. More than 85% of people 65 and older who suffer from coronary artery disease also exhibited brain tissue plaques similar to Alzheimer's. What's intriguing is that these Alzheimer's-like plaques seem to clear after coronary artery surgery, suggesting the possibility of a causal relationship, according to Dr. Khalsa, although it has not been conclusively confirmed.[9]

Nutritional Deficiencies

Reduced levels of certain vitamins, minerals, and amino acids have been tentatively linked with Alzheimer's, including folic acid, niacin (vitamin B3), thiamin (vitamin B1), vitamins B6, B12, C, D, and E, magnesium, selenium, zinc, and tryptophan.[10]

The brain functions through the transmission of chemical messenger molecules (neurotransmitters). These neurotransmitters can have far-reaching effects in distant areas of the body. Effective transmission of impulses is dependent upon proper pH (acid–alkaline balance) and the presence of a variety of nutrients (vitamins, minerals, amino acids), hormones, and neurotransmitters. If any nutrients are lacking or present in imbalanced proportions, brain function will be adversely affected and a person will display various symptoms commonly associated with dementia.

DRUGS ASSOCIATED WITH A HIGHER INCIDENCE OF MENTAL CONFUSION

According to the *Physicians' Desk Reference*, the following drugs are associated with side effects of mental confusion (statistics refer to the percentage of individuals affected).[11]

Anestacon Solution (smong most common)

Atrofen tablets (Up to 11%)

Desyrel and Desyrel Dividose (4.9%-5.7%)

Dilantin Infatabs, Kapseals, Parenteral (among most common)

Dilantin-30 Pediatric/Dilantin-125 Suspension (among most common)

Duragesic Transdermal System (10% or more)

Foscavir injection (more than 5%)

Hylorel tablets (14.8%)

IFEX (among most common)

Intron A (up to 12%)

Lioresal tablets (up to 11%)

Marplan tablets (among most common)

Nipent for injection (3%-10%)

Permax tablets (11.1%)

Roferon-A injection (8%)

Stadol injectable, NS Nasal Spray (3%-9%)

Tonocard tablets (2.1%-11.2%)

Wellbutrin tablets (8.4%)

Xanax tablets (9.9%-10.4%)

Xylocaine injections, with Epinephrine injections (among most common)

For example, acetylcholine is the most abundant neurotransmitter in the body. The body's synthesis of acetylcholine is vital because of its role in motor skills and memory; low levels can contribute to lack of concentration and forgetfulness. In order for the body to manufacture sufficient acetylcholine, sufficient choline is necessary (found in seafood, legumes, and lecithin), plus a number of nutrient co-factors, such as vitamins C, B_1, B_5, and B_6, zinc, and calcium.

Environmental Influences

Gary Oberg, M.D., past President of the American Academy of Environmental Medicine, treats patients suffering from environmental illness. "Toxins such as chemicals in food and tap water, carbon monoxide, solvents, aerosol sprays, and industrial chemicals can cause symptoms of brain dysfunction that may lead to an inaccurate diagnosis of Alzheimer's or senile dementia," says Dr. Oberg. Studies have shown that a susceptibility to toxins such as aluminum and mercury is linked to the onset of Alzheimer's and senile dementia.

> *Studies have shown that a susceptibility to toxins such as aluminum and mercury is linked to the onset of Alzheimer's and senile dementia.*

Aluminum: Research indicates that, because of the high levels of aluminum found in the brain cells of Alzheimer's victims, this metal may be a causal factor in the development of the disease.[12] While the source of aluminum toxicity in the body has not yet been proven, aluminum can enter the body through inhalation (by factory workers in certain industries) and by oral ingestion. It has been suggested that aluminum ions may leach into the body from aluminum cooking utensils, cans, and foil, as well as underarm deodorants, antacid pills, and other common products, many of which contain traces of aluminum.[13]

Mercury: Postmortem examination of brain tissue from Alzheimer's victims has also indicated the presence of high levels of mercury.[14] Another study makes a clear connection between the presence of mercury in brain tissue and the presence of "silver" amalgam dental fillings, which contain approximately 50% mercury as well as silver, tin, copper, and zinc.[15] "In a recent test of 7,000 patients, we found 90% to be sensitive to mercury," says Hal A. Huggins, D.D.S., of Colorado Springs, Colorado. "What this means is that while different people will react in different ways to mercury, in 90% of the people with amalgam fillings, the mercury will significantly suppress the immune system." Reactions to high levels of mercury in the body can range from nervousness and depression to suicidal tendencies and severe neurological diseases such as multiple sclerosis, Lou Gehrig's disease (a syndrome marked by muscular weakness and atrophy due to degeneration of motor neurons), and Alzheimer's. "How you react depends on your genetics," says Dr. Huggins. "A person with very strong stock will last a long time before the immune system breaks down. But susceptibility also depends on lifestyle and exposure to other stressors such as poor nutrition and environmental factors."

According to Dr. Huggins, metal fillings also create low levels of constant electrical activity that is conducted directly to the brain, creating aberrant behavior. While the electrical mechanism created by metals in the mouth does not itself directly suppress the immune system, Dr. Huggins cautions that it enables metals to leave the fillings faster and to be absorbed into the blood.

Hormone Imbalances

The hormone melatonin plays a role in the synchronization of brain cells and, as a potent antioxidant, helps protect brain tissue from free-radical damage. Studies show that subjects who have taken melatonin in the evening before bedtime perform better in cognitive tests the next day, possibly as the result of achieving a better night's sleep. According to Ward Dean, M.D., daily concentrations of melatonin appear to decline in those who have Alzheimer's disease. "Many recent studies have found reduced levels of melatonin in the cerebrospinal fluid of patients with Alzheimer's disease," he says.[16]

Stress and the stress hormones, particularly cortisol, play a major role in Alzheimer's as well. "Memory is particularly damaged by cortisol during the aging process," Dr. Khalsa says. Although some cortisol is needed for proper brain function, chronic exposure to toxic levels of cortisol, due to daily stress, injures and even kills brain cells. Clinical studies show that cortisol damages the nerve cells of the hippocampus and blocks their ability to absorb blood sugar (glucose), the brain's sole fuel, causing it to act more sluggishly. Brain scans of Alzheimer's patients show that the temporal (site of the hippocampus) and frontal lobes have a decreased capacity to absorb glucose.[17]

Treating Alzheimer's Disease and Senile Dementia

"When a doctor examines a person who is experiencing symptoms of dementia, the first thing to do is to make an accurate diagnosis and determine what is behind the symptoms. One should not automatically assume it is Alzheimer's," according to Dr. Hoffer. "This should include a survey of all the possible underlying factors. If the doctor is unable to find an explanation, then he can finally assess with greater probability that it is Alzheimer's." Alternative treatments for Alzheimer's and

CAN MERCURY FILLINGS CONTRIBUTE TO ALZHEIMER'S?

New research reported by pioneering dentist Hal A. Huggins, D.D.S., suggests that once even minute amounts of mercury enter the brain, they can seriously damage nerve cells and produce the physical and structural damage of brain tissue now linked to Alzheimer's. The biochemistry is complex, but mercury damages a key enzyme needed for the brain's energy processes called creatine kinase. Autopsies show that the brain of a healthy person contains 2,300% more creatine kinase than the brain of a person with Alzheimer's, according to Dr. Huggins.

The brain needs creatine kinase to make ATP (adenosine triphosphate), which is central to all energy processes in the body. Autopsies also show that a brain impaired by Alzheimer's has reduced ATP levels compared to healthy subjects. ATP, in turn, is needed for the production of tubulin, a protein that gives nerve cells their shape and physical integrity, a kind of molecular scaffolding system. Think of the tubulin structure as a ladder, says Dr. Huggins. In the brain of an Alzheimer's patient, the rungs of the ladder have come undone and the center portion has collapsed into coils. These are the neurofibrillary tangles, as revealed by brain autopsies. "When tubulin, the microstructure of nerve cells, collapses, you have Alzheimer's. The amount of reduction of tubulin activity is directly related to the degree of Alzheimer's," Dr. Huggins says. "No other type of neural degeneration or any other autoimmune disease of the nervous system shows a reduction in tubulin activity."

What does mercury do once it crosses the blood-brain barrier? It destroys tubulin by knocking out the creatine kinase, says Dr. Huggins. According to him, the concentration of a mere six micromoles of mercury in the brain can cause a 60% reduction in tubulin activity; at 11 micromoles, the reduction can be as high as 92%. The result of this process is that you lose brain cells and brain function, says Dr. Huggins. However, the number of mercury fillings does not seem to be related to the severity of Alzheimer's. The real criterion is to what degree the mercury, as a brain toxin, challenges the immune system.

other forms of senile dementia focus on dietary changes, nutritional supplementation, herbs, environmental medicine and detoxification, as well as exercise (mental and physical) and stress reduction.

Diet and Nutritional Supplements

Improving the diet can help Alzheimer's patients and promote brain longevity. In general, maintain a diet that features a balance of proteins, complex carbohydrates (not the simple sugars of the typical fast food diet), and healthy fats. The optimal brain diet steers clear of foods that are processed (monosodium glutamate or MSG and aspartame are two food additives that are proven neurotoxins), genetically engineered, or refined (sugars and flour), while favoring plenty of organic fruits and vegetables and purified water. Alcohol and nicotine are also not recommended, since these substances measurably decrease brainpower.

The amount of protein in the diet is important, since various brain chemical messengers, such as serotonin, dopamine, and endorphins, are manufactured from amino acids and other substances found in the diet such as vitamins and minerals. "The reason that brain cells are dependent upon an optimal intake of amino acids, vitamins, and minerals is the same as for all the other cells in the body—their optimal function cannot occur without these substances providing cell structure, energy, and enzymatic reactions that are essential for such function," says John V. Dommisse, M.D., a nutritional medicine specialist in Tucson, Arizona.[18]

Not only does a whole foods diet provide healthy amounts of fiber, antioxidants, and other nutrients essential for optimal brain function, it also helps to balance pH (an acidic environment inhibits neuron function), normalize blood sugar levels, and prevent insulin resistance. This is important since hypoglycemia (low blood sugar) triggers the body's stress response, causing the brain to be exposed to higher levels of a cortisol.

Nutritional supplementation is an effective approach in treating Alzheimer's. Studies in Japan have shown that daily supplements of coenzyme Q10, vitamin B6, and iron returned some Alzheimer's patients to "normal" mental capacity.[19] In another study, Alzheimer's patients who took a daily regimen of evening primrose oil, zinc, and selenium showed significant improvement in alertness, mood, and mental ability.[20] The following "neuronutrients" are specific vitamins, minerals, fatty acids, and trace elements essential to brain function.

- **Vitamin C:** Vitamin C concentrations are 15 times higher in the brain than in any other body tissue, which means this nutrient is vital for brainpower. Vitamin C extends the life of vitamin E and is needed for the production of several key brain chemicals, including acetylcholine and dopamine. It is important to take vitamin C in staggered doses throughout the day, as the body can fully absorb only 500 mg at a time. Typical dose: 1,000-5,000 mg daily or up to bowel tolerance (just short of producing diarrhea).

- **B-Complex Vitamins:** The B-complex vitamins are important for healthy nerve function. Women using oral contraceptives increase their utilization of the B vitamins and need to supplement their diet with B complex, as should individuals under high stress. Since the B vitamins are water-soluble, they are not stored in the body. These vitamins must be taken when you have food in the stomach; if taken on an empty stomach, pain and nausea may result.

- **Vitamin E:** Vitamin E is an important fat-soluble antioxidant that promotes stable cell membranes and reduces damage to the mitochondria, the cell's energy producer. Vitamin E traps free radicals, interrupting the chain reaction that damages brain cells. Typical dose: 400-800 IU daily.

- **Coenzyme Q10:** CoQ10 is necessary for the generation of energy in all cells and has been found to improve the symptoms of Alzheimer's in some patients.[21] CoQ10 improves cardiovascular fitness and blood circulation to the brain. As a potent antioxidant, it helps to keep the nerve cells free of brainpower-damaging substances. Typical dose: 100 mg daily.

- **Phosphatidyl-Choline:** Phosphatidyl-choline is the major structural and functional component of brain-cell membranes. Without this chemical, brain cells undergo degenerative changes. The brain requires choline to produce acetylcholine, a chemical that plays a vital role in memory. Phosphatidyl-choline is derived from choline and lecithin; natural sources include eggs, soybeans, cabbage, cauliflower, organ meats, spinach, nuts, and wheat germ.[22] Typical dose: one tablespoon of lecithin provides 250 mg of choline or supplement with 1,200 mg of phosphatidyl-choline, 2-3 times daily.

- **Phosphatidyl-Serine (PS):** Phosphatidyl-serine is a large fat molecule found in trace amounts in lecithin and derived from soybeans. Although the brain normally produces PS, if the diet is deficient in essential fatty acids, folic acid, or vitamin B12, PS production may be blocked. PS plays an important role in maintaining the integrity of brain-cell membranes. Perhaps most significant is its ability to lower the level of stress hormones such as cortisol, which damage brain cells and lead to the accumulation of calcified plaques in the brain. Typical dose: 100 mg three times daily.

- **Acetyl-L-Carnitine (ALC):** This amino acid (protein building block) enhances brain energy, helping to improve mood and reduce the effects of age-associated memory impairment. Typical dose: two divided doses of 1,000-2,000 mg each day.

- **Docosahexaenoic Acid (DHA):** DHA is a long-chain fatty acid found in fish, egg yolks, and marine algae, and is the predominant omega-3 fatty acid in brain tissue. As the brain is dependent on dietary fatty acids, reductions in DHA content of the diet may contribute to degenerative changes in the nervous system. Dietary sources include fish (tuna, salmon, sardines), red meats, organ meats, and eggs. Typical dose: 500-1,500 mg daily.

Herbal Medicine

Ginkgo biloba has been shown to improve circulation and increase mental capacity in several clinical trials. In particular, the herb has been effective for treating problems associated with cerebral circulation, neurotransmission (the energetic impulse of nerve cells), neuron membrane lesions caused by free radicals, and neuronal metabolism threatened by lack of oxygen.[23] In a 1995 study, Alzheimer's patients received either 80 mg of *Ginkgo biloba* extract or a placebo. Among the patients taking ginkgo, significant improvement was noticed in cognitive function—memory and attention span increased in the first month of supplementation.[24]

David L. Hoffmann, B.Sc., M.N.I.M.H., of Sebastopol, California, past President of the American Herbalists Guild, reports success using ginkgo with Alzheimer's and senile dementia. "The herb is quite safe, even in doses many times higher than those usually recommended, and clinically it seems to be effective for patients with vascular disorders for all types of dementia and, because of its beneficial effects on mood, for patients suffering from cognitive disorders secondary to depression. For people who are just beginning to experience deterioration in cognitive function, ginkgo might enable them to maintain a normal life."

Environmental Medicine and Detoxification

In addition to taking a comprehensive history, Dr. Oberg screens all his patients for dietary and environmental sen-

sitivities capable of producing Alzheimer's symptoms. Food sensitivities are determined by using an elimination diet. According to Dr. Oberg, if symptoms disappear when a particular food is avoided and then reappear when it is reintroduced into the diet, the person is sensitive to that food and should avoid it (or consider provocative neutralization). Dr. Oberg notes that when toxic substances are removed from the diet, symptoms will often disappear.

For diagnosing environmental sensitivity, he uses a technique called maximum tolerated intradermal dose testing to determine how much of a particular substance is toxic to the patient. The patient can then be desensitized to the substance by being injected with the largest dose of the substance that does not produce a response (such as a skin wheal).

According to William G. Crook, M.D., of Jackson, Tennessee, a pioneer in the field of environmental medicine, overgrowth of the yeast *Candida albicans* in the gastrointestinal tract can contribute to food allergies and poor absorption of nutrients, and it may be related to a number of health and behavioral problems, including depression, hyperactivity, irritability, and "brain fog." Dr. Crook's treatment for patients with *Candida*-related health problems, including Alzheimer's and cerebral dysfunction symptoms, is relatively simple. After performing a thorough physical examination and taking their age into consideration, he puts patients on an elimination diet. Patients whose histories include antibiotics, a high-sugar diet, or birth control pills are treated for yeast overgrowth in the intestines. After the *Candida* is under control, Dr. Crook recommends following a sugar-free diet, including acidophilus (as a supplement or from yogurt) to restore normal intestinal flora.

See Candidiasis, Environmental Medicine.

Garry F. Gordon, M.D., of Payson, Arizona, co-founder of the American College of Advancement in Medicine, reports that chelation therapy can benefit memory in patients with Alzheimer's-like dementia by improving blood flow to the brain. Chelation therapy uses chelating agents (such as EDTA, ethylenediaminetetraacetic acid) administered intravenously to restore proper circulation by removing aluminum, mercury, and other heavy metals from the body. Dr. Gordon cites numerous studies showing an increase in cerebrovascular circulation using EDTA chelation therapy.[25]

The late Charles Farr, M.D., Ph.D., Co-founder of the American Board of Chelation Therapy, successfully used chelation therapy in cases of senile dementia due to either atherosclerosis of the cerebral arteries or toxins in the body. "When a patient is not functioning well, having trouble concentrating and remembering things,

SUCCESS STORY: DETOXIFICATION BEATS ALZHEIMER'S

While physicians throughout the country describe successes with patients afflicted with this "incurable" disease, perhaps the most vivid success story is that of Tom Warren, who wrote a book, *Beating Alzheimer's,* about his recovery from an Alzheimer's-diagnosed illness. Tom was diagnosed with Alzheimer's in June 1983, after undergoing a CAT (computerized axial tomography) scan. "Several doctors read my X rays, but the diagnosis was always the same," he recounts. "I was 50, and I had been experiencing symptoms such as memory loss and fatigue for five years. I was so exhausted there were times when I had to crawl up the stairs. My head ached, my handwriting deteriorated, and conversation became difficult."

Tom began reading everything he could find that might provide a clue to the cause, and a cure. "Sometimes I couldn't remember something I'd read 30 seconds earlier," he says, "but I would somehow know it was important and would mark the passage." When his wife, a pharmacist, came home, she would help interpret his notes and assist Tom with implementing some of the things he discovered.

In his search for a cure, Tom read more than 50 books and sought out a number of medical specialists. Finally, he determined that Alzheimer's and other chronic diseases may be caused by toxic metals and chemicals in the immediate environment. He began a program that included the removal of all his amalgam fillings, testing for food allergies, and a switch to an organic, whole foods diet. Additionally, Tom followed a nutritional supplementation program, a regular exercise regime, and a complete avoidance of household chemical pollutants.

A subsequent CAT scan in 1987 indicated that the disease process had reversed. "Once more, I could appreciate sunsets, remember names, drive a car, converse with friends, think, and plan." He returned to work after an absence of 11 years. "In one way or another," says Tom, "everything I learned pointed to: one, remove poison from the body; two, learn how to live in your environment; three, balance body chemistry; four, avoid junk food as if it were poison; and five, exercise. In time, the body will heal itself."[26]

there is no immediate way of measuring whether it is a circulatory problem, toxicity, or an Alzheimer's-like situation." In cases of senile dementia, Dr. Farr recommended 10-15 chelation treatments, alternating with intravenous hydrogen peroxide, in order to more quickly stimulate the circulatory system. If the patient has atherosclerosis or is suffering from environmental toxins, a turnaround by 10-15 treatments is expected. If not, Dr. Farr assumed it was Alzheimer's.

Biological Dentistry

Dr. Huggins uses a multidisciplinary approach to treat patients with Alzheimer's and senile dementia. He combines the removal of mercury amalgam fillings with numerous other therapies, including dietary supplements and nutritional counseling, acupressure and massage, movement therapy, and psychological support. "What we do is balance chemistry," Dr. Huggins explains. "Our goal is to increase the total efficiency of the chemistry of the body and, to accomplish that, we bring more oxygen into the diseased areas, enabling the body to do the healing."

Removing amalgam fillings is the first step. This process is supported by intravenous vitamin C and other solutions to protect the immune system from stress. Silver fillings are replaced with fillings made of materials that have been tested for biocompatibility. After the fillings are removed, detoxification is performed to remove residues of mercury and other poisons from the body. Mercury poisoning is recognized as a serious risk to the body, but Dr. Huggins stresses that "removing the fillings is only 5% to 10% of the solution. The rest of the picture is extremely complex, but can lead to remarkable recovery. Once you get started, however, the one thing that will destroy your recovery is improper nutrition. Eating just one food to which an individual is allergic can significantly interfere with recovery."

One of Dr. Huggins's patients, a woman who had been diagnosed with advanced Alzheimer's disease, had not spoken for 14 years. "She just sat and glared angrily and looked as if she was ready to beat somebody up," says Dr. Huggins. "We started taking fillings out of her mouth and, on the twelfth day of our 14-day program, she started to mumble something. Her husband said, 'What did you say?' and she snapped at him, 'Nothing!' The patient continued to improve, and recently her husband even called to jokingly request one or two fillings be put back in because she was talking so much."

Dr. Huggins cautions, however, that improvement in Alzheimer's patients is usually slower. "Most of the time, you do not see much progress until perhaps at the end of a month or two; at that point, the patients can tie their shoes, and perhaps a year or two later are out driving a car. That's slow improvement, but it's pretty good when compared to how far they could be going in the other direction."

 See Biofeedback Training and Neurotherapy, Biological Dentistry, Chelation Therapy, Mind/Body Medicine, Oxygen Therapies.

Biofeedback Training

Biofeedback training and neurobiofeedback (NBF) are methods of learning how to consciously regulate normally unconscious bodily functions (such as breathing, heart rate, and blood pressure) through the use of simple electronic devices. NBF devices give immediate "feedback" or information about the biological system of the person being monitored, so that he or she can learn to consciously influence that system. "I have found neurobiofeedback to be an outstanding treatment in many cases of Alzheimer's," says Rima Laibow, M.D., founding Medical Director of the Alexandria Institute of Natural and Integrative Medicine, in Croton-on-Hudson, New York. Dr. Laibow claims that NBF induces the following positive effects in cases of Alzheimer's:

- Reduces excess cortisol levels
- Rebalances the brain's functional capacity
- Along with proper nutrition, NBF enhances new dendritic/neuronal growth
- Where there has been destruction of brain tissue, NBF taps into the holographic nature of the brain, allowing function to be regained

"In the hands of a skilled practitioner, NBF offers the opportunity for effective rehabilitation for many patients," says Dr. Laibow. However, she cautions that NBF should never be used without first undergoing comprehensive testing for toxic allergic and nutritional factors. Biofeedback can be done in the physician's office or a caregiver can be trained to administer the treatments at home in conjunction with frequent consultations with the physician.

Mental and Physical Exercise

Just as exercise physiologists discovered decades ago that the muscles waste away with disuse, so too have neuroscientists found that brain function erodes with idle neglect. K. Warner Shaie, Ph.D., a psychologist at Pennsylvania State University, in State College, believes stimulation is key. "If you don't exercise your muscles, they get flabby. If your brain isn't stimulated, you don't keep growing the new connections that are necessary to maintain optimal mental functioning." People who reach retirement and become inactive and uninvolved in life are most vulnerable to mental decay. "If you don't do

anything, pretty soon you can't do anything," warns Dr. Shaie.

According to Dr. Shaie, the period from ages 60 to 80 is most critical in determining the level of mental degeneration. While most 60-year-olds show little cognitive decline, by age 80 it is rare to find individuals functioning at the same level as they were 20 years earlier. Dr. Shaie suggests that this decline is far from inevitable—continually learning and solving problems stimulates the mind and prevents it from getting "rusty." Mental stimulation that can help maintain brain function includes sharing ideas, discussing news headlines, doing crossword puzzles, playing music, engaging in some artistic endeavor, or even going to movies.

"People who maintain their mental abilities tend to seek out activities that require thinking and decision-making," says Dr. Shaie. "For example, playing bridge is probably a lot better than playing bingo, unless you're playing 25 bingo cards and have to remember them all." Crossword puzzles can help exercise the mind when a person begins to feel information and words are no longer at their fingertips. Jigsaw puzzles help a person's spatial sense. Even square dancing can help, says Dr. Schaie, since it requires a person to figure out how to work through a complex movement.

Physical exercise can also decrease the rate of memory loss. According to Dr. Khalsa, aerobic conditioning has been found to improve mental function by 20%-30%, while increasing blood flow and generating the production of nerve growth factors. While it cannot prevent Alzheimer's, exercise appears to be able to delay it, possibly by reducing other risk factors that lead to the onset of Alzheimer's, such as toxin accumulation, high blood pressure, stroke, and other cardiovascular diseases. It may also prevent the deposition of amyloid plaques around nerve cells in the brain, thought to be a factor in Alzheimer's.

Stress Reduction

In the short term, high stress levels impair a person's ability to pay attention, focus, and easily recall information. However, the long-term effects of stress are more severe, since they accelerate the aging process and cause brain degeneration. According to Dr. Khalsa, meditation provides substantial benefits by inhibiting the release of cortisol and lipid peroxidase (a marker for free-radical activity) and increasing levels of DHEA. Lowered cortisol levels and improved memory function can be documented in subjects who are taught to meditate, according to Dr. Khalsa, who adds that "the use of meditation as a tool for reversing early-stage memory loss is an area ripe for clinical investigation."[27]

While relaxation techniques alone may not be able to reverse Alzheimer's disease, some methods of stress reduction have been found to improve symptoms. Julie Suhr, Ph.D., Assistant Professor of Clinical Psychology at Ohio University, in Athens, studied two groups of mildly to moderately impaired Alzheimer's patients. In a total of five sessions that included at-home practice time, one group was taught progressive muscle relaxation techniques, while the second group simply visualized relaxing scenes. Though both groups experienced less anxiety, only the individuals who were taught to relax experienced an improvement in memory.[28]

Any stress reduction method that effectively disengages the body's fight-or-flight reaction and therefore inhibits excessive cortisol production is useful as a way of ensuring optimal brain longevity. Diaphragmatic breathing, meditation, exercise, guided imagery, and the use of essential oils are just a few examples of the ways available to soothe the body and calm the emotions.

Traditional Chinese Medicine

Maoshing Ni, D.O.M., Ph.D., L.Ac., President of Yo San University of Traditional Chinese Medicine, in Marina del Rey, California, has been treating patients with Alzheimer's and senile dementia for many years. "When we can catch Alzheimer's disease in the first six months to a year, when the symptoms are relatively mild, we seem to be able to stem the progression of the illness," he says. "When it's more progressed—when a person cannot walk well without help, speech is slurring, and memory is going—then degeneration is at a point where we may be able to improve symptoms to a certain degree, but recovery is disappointing."

To halt the advance of the disease in the early stages, Dr. Ni employs a combination of acupuncture, Chinese herbs, nutrition, and an exercise program, the latter of which is critical. "In China, we use a form of therapeutic exercise called Qigong—simple deep-breathing exercise that aids in healing by improving cardiovascular delivery and oxygenating the body." Because it also combines concentration and visualization, Dr. Ni points out that Qigong exercises the brain and balances the body in various ways.

A 72-year-old man who had been diagnosed with Alzheimer's came to see Dr. Ni. He was weak, with slurred speech, and would blank out from time to time, making it difficult for him to remember where he was and why he was there. Over the course of two weeks, Dr. Ni performed four treatments of "scalp acupuncture" to stimulate the energy channels (meridians) in the scalp. Once the needles were placed, Dr. Ni had the man exercise lightly for 20 minutes. This included moving his limbs, walking, stomping his feet, and singing. By the fourth treatment, the patient had regained clarity of speech and claimed to feel better than he had in over a year. Dr. Ni explains that scalp acupuncture can actually clear pathways through the plaque that has accumulated in the brain and therefore alleviate many of the problems associated with Alzheimer's. Other treatments included the herbs ginseng, dong quai, and *ho-shou-wu* to enhance vitality and mobility.

 See Acupuncture, Ayurvedic Medicine, Qigong and Tai Chi, Traditional Chinese Medicine.

Ayurvedic Medicine

Virender Sodhi, M.D. (Ayurveda), N.D., Director of the Ayurvedic & Naturopathic Medical Clinic, in Bellevue, Washington, has had success applying Ayurvedic practices to patients with Alzheimer's disease and senile dementia. Dr. Sodhi combines Ayurvedic therapies with basic homeopathic medicine to help alleviate symptoms. Using a metabolic type analysis, he prescribes a regimen of individualized dietary and herbal remedies and also recommends a cleansing program, noting estimates that as many as 80% of Alzheimer's patients suffer from environmental toxicity.

As part of the program, herbs are used to cleanse the liver. Dr. Sodhi also uses *triphala*, a combination of three herbs, and gotu kola, which he says is good for increasing brain-cell function. For circulation, he prescribes the herbs *Ginkgo biloba* or *macunabrure*. Dr. Sodhi also gives supplements of thiamin (vitamin B_1) and niacin (vitamin B_3), though he cautions that patients with liver damage must be careful not to overload the liver with niacin.

Treatment varies depending on each patient's blood chemistry and individual needs. "My main criterion, however, is to improve digestion and elimination, because if you don't have good digestion and elimination, it does not matter what you put into your body, it all goes down the drain," says Dr. Sodhi.

Recommendations

- Eat a whole foods diet with lots of fruits and vegetables and adequate amounts of protein; they are converted into sugars that fuel the brain. Reduce your consumption of artery-clogging unhealthy fats while ensuring adequate amounts of essential fatty acids such as DHA.

- Helpful nutritional supplements include coenzyme Q10, vitamins B_6, C, and E, evening primrose oil, zinc, and selenium.

- *Ginkgo biloba* has been shown to improve circulation and increase mental capacity.

- Stop smoking (smokers have four times the risk of developing Alzheimer's), avoid products with aluminum, make every effort to purify the living environment of toxins, and avoid foods containing preservatives and artificial colors.

- Detoxification therapies, chelation therapy, and biological dentistry may all be helpful for eliminating toxins and heavy metals (particularly mercury) that may be causative factors in Alzheimer's.

- Physical exercise has many anti-aging benefits. And if it's aerobic, it increases blood flow to the brain, delivering added oxygen to help you think more clearly.

- Think—the old adage "Use it or lose it" applies. Some mind-stimulating activities include balancing a checkbook, reading (out loud, if possible), or anything that requires concentration and focus of attention. Activities such as sketching, drawing, or painting that involve the use of your nondominant hand help enhance communication between the right and left hemispheres of the brain.

- Maintain an interest in people, events, and issues; read books; plan and carry out projects of interest. Education and interesting, meaningful work seem to protect people against the ravages of Alzheimer's.

Self-Care

The following therapies can be undertaken at home under appropriate professional guidance:

Aromatherapy / Guided Imagery / Mind/Body Medicine

HYDROTHERAPY: Constitutional hydrotherapy may be applied two to five times weekly.

Professional Care

The following therapies can be provided by a qualified health professional:

Ayurvedic Medicine / Biofeedback Training and Neurotherapy / Biological Dentistry / Cell Therapy / Chelation Therapy / Herbal Medicine / Magnetic Field Therapy / Naturopathic Medicine / Traditional Chinese Medicine

DETOXIFICATION THERAPY: Depending on the condition of the person.

OXYGEN THERAPIES: • Ozone Therapy—Physicians at the Salvador Allende Hospital, in Havana, Cuba, treated 30 patients diagnosed with senile dementia using ozone

and oxygen therapy for 21 days. Of the patients, 75% showed "marked improvement" in medical status; 83% demonstrated an improved mental condition; 83% were better able to take their own medications; and 80% had greater ease in social interaction and managing daily activities, and had more energy. • Hyperbaric oxygen therapy

Where to Find Help

For more information on, or referrals for, treatment of Alzheimer's disease and senile dementia, contact the following organizations.

American Academy of Biological Dentistry
P.O. Box 856
Carmel Valley, California 93924
(408) 659-5385

The American Academy of Biological Dentistry promotes biological dental medicine, which uses nontoxic diagnostic and therapeutic approaches in the field of clinical dentistry. They publish a quarterly journal and hold regular seminars on biological diagnosis and therapy.

American Academy of Environmental Medicine
American Financial Center, Suite 625
7701 East Kellogg Avenue
Wichita, Kansas 67207
(316) 684-5500
Website: www.aaem.com

The academy offers extensive training for physicians interested in learning more about environmental medicine. For information on physicians practicing environmental medicine, send a self-addressed, stamped envelope stating your request.

American Association of Oriental Medicine (AAOM)
433 Front Street
Catasauqua, Pennsylvania 18032
(888) 500-7999
Website: www.aaom.org

The AAOM is a national professional trade organization of acupuncturists who meet acceptable standards of competency and can provide the names and locations of local members. Referrals by written request only.

American Association of Naturopathic Physicians
601 Valley Street, Suite 105
Seattle, Washington 98109
(206) 298-0126
Website: www.naturopathic.org

Provides a directory of naturopathic physicians and offers referrals to a nationwide network of accredited or licensed practitioners. Publishes a quarterly newsletter for both professionals and the general public. Also offers a series of brochures and pamphlets on a variety of subjects.

American College for Advancement in Medicine (ACAM)

23121 Verdugo Drive, Suite 204
Laguna Hills, California 92653
(800) 532-3688
Website: www.acam.org

This pioneering organization seeks to establish certification and standards of practice for chelation therapy, providing training and education for physicians and scientists. ACAM provides referrals and informational material, including a directory listing of all physicians worldwide who have been trained in preventative medicine as well as in the ACAM protocol for chelation therapy. The organization also provides a copy of the ACAM protocol for chelation to the public.

American Holistic Medical Association

6728 Old McLean Village Drive
McLean, Virginia 22101
(703) 556-9728
Website: www.holisticmedicine.org

A professional organization for holistic practitioners, the AHMA offers information and services for its members and lobbies for holistic issues. It also provides referrals for the public (requests must be in writing).

Ayurvedic & Naturopathic Medical Clinic

2115 112th Avenue N.E.
Bellevue, Washington 98004
(425) 453-8022
Website: www.ayurvedicscience.com

Dr. Virender Sodhi's clinic provides medical training for physicians and health-care practitioners, as well as individual courses for laypeople.

Recommended Reading

An Alternative Approach to Allergies. Theron Randolph, M.D., and Ralph Moss, Ph.D. New York: HarperCollins, 1990.

Beating Alzheimer's. Tom Warren. Garden City Park, NY: Avery Penguin Putnam, 1991.

Brain Allergies. William H. Philpott, M.D., and Dwight Kalita, Ph.D. Los Angeles: Keats Publishing, 2000.

Brain Builders! A Lifelong Guide to Sharper Thinking, Better Memory, and an Ageproof Mind. Richard Leviton. Englewood Cliffs, NJ: Prentice Hall, 1995.

It's All in Your Head. Hal A. Huggins, D.D.S., and Sharon A. Huggins. Garden City Park, NY: Avery Publishing Group, 1993.

Toxic Metal Syndrome. H. Richard Casdorph and Morton Walker. Garden City Park, NY: Avery Penguin Putnam, 1995.

Tracking Down Hidden Food Allergy. William G. Crook, M.D. Jackson, TN: Professional Books, 1980.

The Yeast Connection. William Crook, M.D. New York: Vintage Books, 1986.

ARTHRITIS

Millions of people suffer from some form of arthritis. Because arthritis is commonly believed to be incurable, the standard medical response has been simply to prescribe medication to reduce the symptoms. Substantial evidence, however, now shows that the pain and disability caused by arthritis can be alleviated, and even prevented, through diet, nutritional supplementation, environmental medicine, bodywork, stress reduction, and other alternative therapies.

THE TERM *arthritis* is used loosely as if it encompassed one entity, although over 100 types of arthritis have been identified. Arthritis is an aggregate of illnesses whose common features include an inflammation of the joints, surrounding tendons, ligaments, and cartilage. Among the oldest known afflictions of human beings, it can affect virtually every part of the body: from the feet to the knees, back, shoulders, and fingers. For millions of Americans, arthritis limits everyday movements such as walking, standing, or even holding a pencil. According to the National Institutes of Health (NIH), the effects of arthritis range from slight pain, stiffness, and swelling of the joints, to crippling and disability. Arthritis affects people of all ages. The NIH reports that about 15% of the U.S. population have arthritis or a related disorder and 200,000 children in the U.S. have some form of the disease.[1]

Conventional medicine prescribes a whole "laundry list" of pharmaceutical drugs for arthritis. Many of these drugs block the pain, often very quickly and with little effort on the part of the patients or doctors. While pain relief is important, conventional drugs merely hide the symptoms and ignore the underlying causes of the disease. According to the alternative medicine approach, arthritis is a disease that results from multiple causes, many of them with a less-than-obvious connection to the disease and many causes are not easily detectable. "A number of underlying imbalances, with accompanying physical, mental, and environmental factors, contribute to all forms of arthritis," says Eugene Zampieron, N.D., A.H.G., of Woodbury, Connecticut, co-author of *Arthritis: An Alternative Medicine Definitive Guide*. "When arthritis is viewed through alternative medicine, it becomes a correctable disease that requires adjustments to specific organ systems, diet, and lifestyle."

Types of Arthritis

There are a variety of arthritic conditions, with the three most common forms of the disease being osteoarthritis, rheumatoid arthritis, and gout. Less prevalent types of arthritis include psoriatic arthritis, ankylosing spondylitis, and infectious arthritis.

Osteoarthritis

Osteoarthritis (OA) is by far the most prevalent form of arthritis. The disease affects an estimated 20.7 million Americans. Under the age of 45, more men than women are diagnosed with OA, often due to accidents and injuries. The disease becomes three times more prevalent in women than in men after the age of 45.[2] About a third of adults in the U.S. have X-ray evidence of osteoarthritis in the hand, foot, knee, or hip, and by age 65 as many as 75% of the population have evidence of the disease in at least one of these sites.[3]

Osteoarthritis causes the breakdown of cartilage, the smooth, gelatinous tissue that protects the ends of bones from rubbing against each other. Healthy cartilage shields bones against being worn down by friction, but in OA the cartilage is worn away, allowing bone ends to make direct contact. As the disease progresses, direct contact creates bone spurs and abnormal bone hardening, and leads to inflammation and severe pain as bones continue to rub together without proper cushioning. As a result, bones may become more brittle and subject to fracture.

There are two types of osteoarthritis: primary and secondary. Primary OA is considered "wear and tear" arthritis due to an unhealthy aging process. The onset of primary OA is gradual as the disease usually progresses over the course of many years. Secondary osteoarthritis is the less common of the two types but has a more apparent, direct cause: trauma, injury, previous inflam-

ARTHRITIS: THE BREAKING DOWN OF CARTILAGE

The kinds, symptoms, and causes of arthritis are numerous and almost too varied to be grouped under one term. But the commonality of the various arthritic diseases is the erosion of cartilage (the elastic buffer protecting bones). Under healthy conditions, old or damaged cartilage is replaced by new cartilage constructed by chondrocytes, specialized cells found in cartilage.

Chondrocytes make the primary constituent parts of cartilage called collagen and proteoglycans. The quality or type of cartilage replaced is a function of the raw materials—vitamins, minerals, amino acids, and GAGs (glycosaminoglycans)—available to the chondrocytes and the stresses being placed on the joints. This stress can be physical, toxic, immunological, emotional, or any other type that produces biochemical inflammants and free radicals that attack joints.

Collagen is the structural protein of cartilage and forms the "scaffolding" of the body, which has elastic band-like qualities and is strong and resilient. It is a major part of bone, skin, ligaments, tendons, and all tissues and organs of the body giving us shape and form. When the molecular components of collagen are changed—due to the aging process, increased free-radical production, or poor nutrition—the collagen protein becomes less structured and begins to weaken. The structure of the collagen molecule, which is normally a triple-helix shape, begins to unwind. This is when we begin to wrinkle and become more susceptible to fractures and sprains. As the degeneration of collagen progresses, the molecular bonds that create strong connective tissue begin to weaken and dissolve totally, a process that can contribute to arthritis.

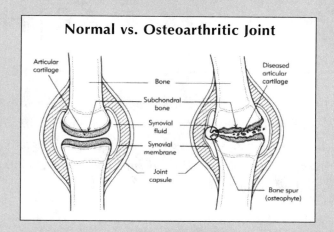

Proteoglycans are attached to and cover the framework of collagen fibers. Proteoglycans have the consistency of gelatin and tend to swell up and absorb water like a sponge, filling in the gaps between collagen molecules. Under a microscope, they look like a long-handled brush used to clean bottles: their long protein core resembles the handle of the bottle brush and the chains of sugar that radiate out from the core resemble the bristles of the brush. Proteoglycans maintain the content and direct the flow of fluids circulating throughout the cartilage as well as in the joints.[7] The sulfur found in proteoglycans has a negative charge—like a magnet, sulfur attracts water molecules to the cartilage, giving the cartilage a cushion to protect the ends of the bones from premature wearing. But the bonds between water and cartilage tend to be weak and easily broken by stress or shock. When these bonds are broken, the water (and cushioning) flows out of the cartilage.

---

mation (even from rheumatoid arthritis), congenital joint misalignment, infection, surgery, or prolonged use of medications.[4]

The symptoms of osteoarthritis include mild early-morning stiffness, stiffness following periods of rest, pain that worsens on joint use, loss of joint function, local tenderness, soft tissue swelling, creaking and cracking of joints on movement, bony swelling, and restricted mobility.

Rheumatoid Arthritis

Rheumatoid arthritis (RA), while less common than osteoarthritis, is a serious and painful joint disease, often resulting in crippling disabilities for young and old alike. Rheumatoid arthritis affects about 2.1 million people in the U.S., most often women.[5] The condition usually starts between the ages of 20 and 50, although it can begin at any age.

Rheumatoid arthritis is an inflammatory disease in which the body's immune system attacks its own healthy tissues. This is called an autoimmune response. The disorder affects many organs throughout the body, but is most noted for its significant disability, deformity, and inflammation of the joints and other structures comprised of connective tissue (which supports and binds together other tissues and forms ligaments and tendons). RA can lead to crippling. It incapacitates the synovial tissue, which is the membrane that lines joints and secretes the lubricant that normally allows bones to move painlessly against other bones. With this condition, joints (most commonly the small joints of the hand) become tender, swollen, even deformed. Over time, the condition can also spread to other parts of the body.

The onset of RA symptoms can be slow with mild discomfort in the joints, morning stiffness, low-grade fever systemically or in the affected joints, and a gradual increase of symptoms. People can also develop rheumatoid arthritis seemingly overnight. Symptoms of rheumatoid arthritis include night sweats, depression, lethargy, fatigue, low-grade fever, weakness, joint stiffness, and vague joint pain. These symptoms can lead to the appearance of painful, swollen joints within several weeks.[6] RA may sometimes affect only one side of the body, but it is common for RA to strike the same joints on both sides of the body simultaneously—in the elbows, for instance. Later in the development of the disease, the affected joints become thicker and deformed.

Gout

Gout is a type of arthritis caused by a buildup in the body of uric acid, which is found in meats and other foods and also produced in the body. When this production is out of balance or there is inadequate elimination of uric acid, gout occurs.[8] When the level of uric acid rises to unhealthy levels in the body, it crystallizes in the joint cartilage and synovial tissue and fluid, causing sharp, needle-like pain in the joints, as well as fever, chills, and loss of mobility.[9] Some of the health problems caused by gout include constipation, indigestion, headaches, depression, eczema, and hives, and those who suffer gout also run a much higher risk of heart and kidney problems.

In 50% of gout cases, the first attack is characterized by intense pain in the first joint of the big toe. If the attack progresses, fever and chills will appear. Initial gout attacks usually strike at night and are preceded by a specific event such as excessive alcohol ingestion, trauma, certain drugs, or surgery. Subsequent attacks are common, with most patients experiencing another attack within one year. However, nearly 7% of gout sufferers never have a second attack. The condition affects approximately three out of every 1,000 adults and is primarily a disease of adult men, 95% of gout sufferers being males over the age of 30.[10]

Less Prevalent Joint Diseases

Ankylosing spondylitis (AS) is an inflammatory disease that bends or fuses spinal vertebrae. Over time, the spine stiffens and causes symptoms that include a severe stooping posture, lower back pain, chest pain when inhaling, weight loss, fatigue, and inflexibility. AS strikes one in 1,000 people under age 40 and is most common in males between the ages of 16 and 35. The disease is found almost exclusively in men who have the HLA-B27 gene;

only 20% of men with that gene, however, actually develop the illness.

Psoriatic arthritis occurs in one out of ten patients who have the skin condition psoriasis. It manifests itself 10-20 years after the onset of psoriasis and includes swelling in many joints, but especially in the end joints of the fingers and toes. There are underlying factors that contribute to the onset of psoriatic arthritis, including improper bowel and liver function as a result of an overgrowth of the yeast *Candida* or infestations of other pathogenic organisms in the microflora of the bowels.

Infectious arthritis, characterized by fever, stiffness, and inflammation, especially in the knee joint, is caused by viral, bacterial, or fungal infections. Researchers have been unable to identify a particular microorganism that causes most types of arthritis; however, they do know that there are two basic types of infectious arthritis. In septic arthritis, microorganisms directly infect the joints. In reactive arthritis, microorganisms found elsewhere in the body indirectly trigger arthritis conditions like rheumatic fever and Reiter's Syndrome. Lyme disease can also cause infectious arthritis. Lyme disease is presumed to be caused by bacteria *(Borrelia burgdorferi)* carried by deer ticks or black-legged ticks. Symptoms may vary, but are usually characterized first by a skin rash, before fatigue, aches, and flu-like symptoms appear. Eventually, these bacteria penetrate the nervous system and attack brain tissue and spinal cells. The incubation period can be lengthy, with initial exposure commonly occurring during the summer and most symptoms developing weeks or months later.

Causes of Arthritis

Arthritis is caused by a variety of factors, including joint instability, injuries, age-related changes, toxins, microbes, altered biochemistry, hormonal factors, and genetic predisposition. Yet other environmental, psychological, dietary, and even dental factors have also been found to bring on the condition. "Five to ten years ago, it would have been heresy to state that allergens could induce arthritis and that, by the elimination of those allergens, arthritis would go into remission," says allergy expert James Braly, M.D., of Hollywood, Florida. "Now it's accepted among most rheumatologists and allergists that some people do have allergy-induced arthritis."

Stress can disrupt the body's hormonal balance as well. When stress interferes with the production of progesterone and thyroid hormones, menopausal difficulties increase. A great many women develop osteoarthritis at this time. Raymond Peat, Ph.D., of Eugene, Oregon, also points out that stress-induced cortisone deficiency can be a factor in some forms of arthritis.[11] When stress

DRUGS ASSOCIATED WITH A HIGHER INCIDENCE OF ARTHRITIS

According to the *Physicians' Desk Reference*, the following drugs are associated with side effects of arthritis (statistics refer to the percentage of individuals affected).[18]

TheraCys BCG Live, Intravesical (1.0%-7.1%)

Tonocard Tablets (4.7%)

Videx Tablets, Powder & Pediatric Powder for Oral Solution (1%-11%)

Wellbutrin Tablets (3.1%)

occurs, body systems release adrenaline and cortisol, a process that weakens the immune system. In this way, bacteria and other detrimental organisms such as *Candida albicans* spread throughout the body.[12]

Five to ten years ago, it would have been heresy to state that allergens could induce arthritis and that, by the elimination of those allergens, arthritis would go into remission. Now it's accepted among most rheumatologists and allergists that some people do have allergy-induced arthritis.

— JAMES BRALY, M.D.

Causes of Osteoarthritis

Osteoarthritis is considered by many to be a natural result of the aging process. To a large degree this is true, with nearly everyone over the age of 60 showing some signs of the disease.[13] Dr. Braly cites age, excess weight, general wear and tear, and a lifetime of inadequate diet and exercise as the chief causes of osteoarthritis. Other research has found additional causes to be skeletal defects, genetic factors, and hormonal deficiencies (as evidenced by the many women who get osteoarthritis after menopause).[14]

The degenerative form of arthritis involves ongoing biochemical processes that negatively alter the structure and regeneration of cartilage and joint tissue. These biochemical processes include free-radical damage, nutritional deficiencies, poor dietary and lifestyle choices, food or environmental allergies, genetic predisposition, and even drug treatments prescribed for pain relief. In various combinations, these factors often cause (or contribute to) changes in the biomechanics of the joints and muscles.

Researchers at Jefferson Medical College, in Philadelphia, Pennsylvania, have identified a possible genetic correlation in osteoarthritis. In some individuals, they have discovered a defect in the gene that instructs cartilage cells to manufacture collagen (the structural protein of the connective tissue), so the collagen is more likely to break down, leading to degeneration of joints.[15]

Patients with osteoarthritis often display insulin resistance or deficiency. Insulin resistance, considered a precursor to adult-onset diabetes, is a blood sugar disorder that occurs when the body fails to "recognize" the effects of insulin in the blood. This makes it more difficult for the body to use sugar (glucose) for energy. The body then begins to break down protein as an alternative energy source, which negatively affects the connective tissue and leads to further destruction within the joints. Diets high in carbohydrates, including sugars and wheat products, tend to increase insulin resistance, disrupting the person's blood sugar levels even more. Excess insulin also stimulates the body to produce more inflammatory prostaglandins, which adversely affect joints.

Biomechanical changes, especially excessive tissue acidity, can contribute to the development of osteoarthritis. When joints lose their full range of motion due to stress, injury, or lack of activity, the "on-loading" and "off-loading" (the exchange of nutrients and waste products) to the cartilage is decreased and breakdown follows. As a result, balanced motion is hindered and the surrounding cartilage starves. The body responds to these biomechanical imbalances by sending calcium to impaired areas to stabilize the weak joint. This results in the formation of hard, inflexible calcium deposits, which cause joint stiffness. Osteoarthritis may also develop from any traumatic injury to cartilage caused by playing sports, accidents, or activity involving repetitive motion.

Yet many people with osteoarthritis never suffer from the aches, pain, and stiffness associated with the disease.[16] Even for sufferers, there is much that can be done to restore arthritis-stricken bodies to functional health, when the underlying, systemic causes of the disease are identified and addressed.[17]

Causes of Rheumatoid Arthritis

Rheumatoid arthritis is classified as an autoimmune disease in which the body attacks its own tissues. In various combinations and severity, food allergies, nutritional deficiencies, toxicity, abnormal intestinal permeability, and microorganisms cause inflammation in the body. For someone who has rheumatoid arthritis, inflammation (the immune system's attack on foreign substances) amplifies and becomes the more destructive autoimmune response.

"A primary cause of most rheumatoid arthritis appears to be delayed food allergy and the often related problem of abnormal permeability of the intestinal wall," says Dr. Braly. This abnormal permeability allows incompletely digested food particles to pass through the walls of the digestive tract and into the bloodstream where, if not cleared, they are eventually deposited in tissues. There they can cause an inflammatory reaction and, because the body is allergic to the deposited food particles, the immune system begins to attack the tissues, especially around the joints. Many scientific studies have documented that there is increased intestinal permeability in over 90% of patients with autoimmune disease and arthritis.[19] The top foods known to trigger rheumatoid symptoms include milk, yeast (both brewer's and baker's), wheat, nightshade vegetables (tomatoes, eggplant, peppers, and potatoes), corn, and eggs.

Other causes of rheumatoid arthritis include genetic susceptibility, lifestyle factors, nutritional factors, toxicity, and microorganisms. There may also be an association between rheumatoid arthritis and abnormal bowel function.[20] These underlying causes work in various combinations to trigger inflammation in the body. In those with rheumatoid arthritis and other types of autoimmune disorders, the immune system never returns to normalcy and remains activated. The immune system resists attempts to suppress itself and begins to produce antibodies that attack the body's own cells, called autoantibodies (meaning "against self").

Causes of Gout

Gout is caused by excessive accumulation of uric acid in the tissues. The underlying cause of uric acid accumulation is unknown, yet research has found that it can basically be attributed to metabolic or kidney problems. Increased production of uric acid may be the result of metabolic enzyme defects, certain types of chronic anemia, or other complex conditions.[21] Dehydration and kidney disease can cause poor clearance of uric acid from the body.

While "high living" may not be the primary cause of gout as it is currently understood, proper diet, nutrition, and metabolic balance all play crucial roles in the prevention and treatment of this disease. In fact, the traditional conception of gout as a condition of affluence has some basis in reality since meats, particularly organ

SYMPTOMATIC DIFFERENCES BETWEEN OSTEOARTHRITIS AND RHEUMATOID ARTHRITIS

OSTEOARTHRITIS	RHEUMATOID ARTHRITIS
Usually affects the elderly	Can affect anyone, even children
Metabolic deficiencies or traumatic injuries are attributable origins	Unproven origin, but infections, particularly bacterial, have been indicated in many cases
Gradual onset of symptoms with mild pain and swelling; mild heat and redness in affected joints	Rapid onset with moderate to extreme pain and swelling; moderate to extreme heat and redness in affected joints
Stiffness from joint damage	Stiffness from swelling
Increased bone density	Loss of bone density

meats, increase production of uric acid, while alcohol inhibits uric acid excretion by the kidneys.[22]

Although most people initiate a gout attack through poor lifestyle choices (obesity, rich foods, alcohol), 10%–15% of gout patients have attacks due to a metabolic problem, such as a deficiency of enzymes (xanthine oxidase) that break down purines or too much purine production by the body. Purines come from certain foods (meat products, especially liver and other organ meats, sausages and other processed meats, anchovies, crab, shrimp, milk, eggs, and many beans, including soy), but are also normally present, in the form of DNA and RNA in the cells. Purines are broken down into uric acid, which is then normally excreted through the urine.

Medications, including aspirin and diuretics, can cause gout by putting extra stress on the kidneys; 25% of new gout cases are caused by these drugs. Kidney stones and other kidney problems are present in 90% of gout sufferers, because urate crystals also accumulate in the kidneys.

Treatment and Prevention of Arthritis

The primary keys for treating and preventing arthritis are proper diet and nutrition, detoxification, and stress reduction. Special care should also be taken to avoid substances that might cause allergic reactions in the body and, when needed, hormonal supplementation and replacement are essential.[23] Vitamins, minerals, herbs, and other natural supplements can provide effective relief without the side effects of conventional drugs.

Detoxification can help arthritis patients reverse the accumulation of toxins in the body caused by bacterial and yeast *(Candida)* infections, parasites, environmental pollutants, and leaky gut syndrome. "Removing toxins from the body has shown to be remarkably therapeutic for arthritis patients," says Dr. Zampieron. Alternative medicine offers a number of safe detoxification strategies.

 See Detoxification Therapy, Environmental Medicine.

Meditation, biofeedback, hypnotherapy, and other mind/body techniques can help reduce stress. Pain management and correction of skeletal/postural problems can also be addressed through a variety of other modalities, including herbal medicine, environmental medicine, bodywork, chiropractic, acupuncture, and Ayurvedic medicine. "With alternative medicine, health is restored to the whole patient, rather than simply providing superficial symptom relief," concludes Dr. Zampieron.

Diet and Nutrition

For decades, medical researchers refused to acknowledge that diet, nutrition, and food allergies could play a role in immune function and arthritis. Today, however, proper diet and nutrition are believed to be key elements in the prevention of all types of disease, including arthritis.

"Dietary practices have a major impact on arthritis. In fact, if you eat the typical American diet, it could be making your arthritis worse," says Ellen Kamhi, Ph.D., R.N., of New York City, co-author of *Arthritis: An Alternative Medicine Definitive Guide.* "Among the offenders are saturated fats (which occur in cooking oils and fried foods), white flour and sugar, red meat, ham, chemical additives, yeast, and milk and dairy products. These foods can increase inflammation, invoke allergies, and interfere with hormone production, cellular integrity, and the function and mobility of the joints." According to Dr. Braly, fatty meats, eggs, margarine, shortening, and dairy products should be dramatically cut down or eliminated from the diet. He also advises the same for caffeine, alcohol, tobacco, and sugars.

Consuming large amounts of soft drinks, which are high in phosphoric acid, can raise the levels of phosphorus in the blood. The normal ratio of calcium to phosphorus in bones is about two to one, although a one-to-one ratio is adequate to maintain skeletal growth.[24] However, in the average American diet, this ratio is extremely skewed, with high amounts of phosphorus relative to calcium. This causes the body to pull calcium from the bones to supplement blood calcium levels,[25] which can exacerbate arthritic conditions.

An important step in treating arthritis lies in achieving normal body weight, as excess weight puts increased stress on weight-bearing joints affected with arthritis.[26] A diet rich in fresh vegetables, fruits, nuts, and whole grains is recommended for maximum nutritional benefit. Whole (unprocessed) foods are rich in the nutrients needed to fight destructive free radicals, promote skin and tissue health, repair bones, muscles, and tendons, and promote bowel regularity.

Dietary fats are an important consideration for anyone with arthritis. The wrong kind of fats can increase inflammation in joints, while the "good" fats will help keep inflammation in check. Hydrogenated fats and trans-fatty acids can directly contribute to inflammation and the destruction of joint tissues. Avoid foods that contain these fats, such as margarine, vegetable shortening, mayonnaise, crackers and chips, cookies, cakes, pastries, packaged breads, candy, and most refined foods. Whole foods are typically high in healthy fats, including the essential fatty acids (see Quick Definition). Cold-water fish are good sources of essential fatty acids, valuable for the prevention of arthritis because of their anti-inflammatory characteristics.[27] Studies have also shown that arthritis patients showed major clinical improvement when supplementing their diets with cod liver oil, which may also reduce the inflammatory process.[28]

QD **Essential fatty acids (EFAs)** are unsaturated fats required in the diet. Omega-3 and omega-6 oils are the two principal types. One important omega-3 oil is alpha-linolenic acid (ALA), found in flaxseed and canola oils, as well as pumpkin seeds, walnuts, and soybeans. Fish oils, such as salmon, cod, and mackerel, contain the other important omega-3 oils, DHA (docosahexaenoic acid) and EPA (eicosapentaenoic acid). Linoleic acid is the main omega-6 oil and is found in most vegetable oils, including safflower, corn, peanut, and sesame. The most therapeutic form of omega-6 oil is gamma-linolenic acid (GLA), found in evening primrose, black currant, and borage oils. Once in the body, omega-3 and omega-6 are converted to prostaglandins, hormone-like substances that regulate many metabolic functions, particularly inflammatory processes. Excess intake of omega-6 oils in relation to omega-3 oils will promote inflammation.

Arthritis sufferers commonly have a high level of acidity (a urine pH that is lower than 6.3), which increases the potential for developing inflammatory conditions. Acidity can be decreased by reducing your intake of acid-forming foods and increasing intake of alkaline-forming foods. The most acid-forming foods for the majority of people are sugar, alcohol, vinegar, coffee, meat, and dairy products. Foods known to increase the alkalinity of the body include all vegetables except tomatoes, aloe vera, and green foods, such as chlorella, barley grass, wheat grass, parsley, and alfalfa.

Dietary treatment for gout sufferers is intended to reduce the production of uric acid to normal levels. Michael Murray, N.D., of Issaquah, Washington, recommends that gout sufferers consume half a pound of fresh or canned cherries per day. Cherries, hawthorn berries, blueberries, and other dark red or blue berries are rich sources of compounds that favorably affect collagen metabolism and reduce inflammation of joints.[29] Bioflavonoids found in black cherries have been used to reduce uric acid levels and decrease tissue destruction associated with gout.[30]

Gout patients should eliminate alcohol intake, which both increases uric acid production and reduces uric acid excretion in the kidneys. Reports indicate that elimination of alcohol is all that is needed to reduce uric acid levels and prevent gout in many individuals.[31] Gout sufferers should also maintain a low-purine diet, which completely omits organ meats, shellfish, yeast (brewer's and baker's), herring, sardines, mackerel, and anchovies. Foods with moderate levels of purines, including dried legumes, spinach, asparagus, fish, poultry, and mushrooms, should also be curtailed. To control gouty arthritic symptoms, refined carbohydrates and saturated fats should be kept to a minimum. Dr. Murray advises weight reduction in obese individuals, using a high-fiber, low-fat diet. Liberal fluid intake should be maintained, because it keeps urine diluted and promotes the excretion of uric acid.

Nutritional Supplements

Many researchers believe a proper balance of vitamins and minerals is essential in the treatment of arthritis. Linus Pauling, Ph.D., of the Linus Pauling Institute for Science and Medicine, in Palo Alto, California, and Robert Cathcart III, M.D., of Los Altos, California, both recommend large quantities of vitamin C.[32] Both an antioxidant and anti-inflammatory, vitamin C helps repair and maintain healthy connective tissue. It is essential for collagen production and the maintenance of the joint lining,[33] helps tissue repair, and reduces the bruising and swelling often associated with arthritis.[34] Vitamins A, B1, B6, E, and niacinamide (a form of vitamin B3) have also proven effective in treating and preventing arthritis.[35] Vitamin D is a fat-soluble nutrient, considered to be both a vitamin and a hormone. It controls the absorption of calcium and phosphorus used in bone formation.[36]

WATER, NOT MEDICATION, TO RELIEVE ARTHRITIC PAIN

The most important life-giving substance in the body, and the one that the body desperately depends on, is water, says Fereydoon Batmanghelidj, M.D., of Falls Church, Virginia, author of *Your Body's Many Cries for Water.* Yet the body has no water storage system to draw on in times of need, according to Dr. Batmanghelidj, who points out that the parts of the body that suffer most from a shortage of water are those without direct vascular circulation, especially the joint cartilage in fingers, knees, and the spinal vertebrae.

Chronic pains are often indicators of chronic dehydration, adds Dr. Batmanghelidj. When any of your joints begin to signal aching pains that come and go, the first thought that should occur to you is that your body is severely short of water. Often, though, when the signs of water deficiency in joint cartilage are not recognized for what they indicate, painkillers are prescribed, frequently resulting in a dependence on addictive medication and possible permanent cartilage damage in the joints.

Rheumatoid joint pain is a direct signal of local water deficiency, explains Dr. Batmanghelidj. If water intake is consciously and regularly adjusted to the needs of each person, in most cases, these pains will gradually disappear. Local swelling of joint surfaces will possibly disappear too. What is more important, the joint structure will begin to repair itself.

Other dietary supplements that have anti-inflammatory and antioxidant effects important for arthritis prevention and treatment include boron, zinc, copper, selenium, manganese, pantothenic acid, and sulfur. Bee pollen, royal jelly (another bee product rich in pantothenic acid), eicosapentaenoic acid (EPA), and evening primrose oil are also beneficial in alleviating arthritis symptoms, especially among rheumatoid arthritics. All these supplements, though, should be taken only under supervision by a qualified health professional.

Cartilage-building supplements provide the raw materials to rebuild damaged cartilage and stop the unnecessary destruction of healthy cells. Julian Whitaker, M.D., of Newport Beach, California, notes that glucosamine sulfate supplementation can be especially effective in helping reverse arthritis. According to Dr. Whitaker, glucosamine plays an integral part in stimu-

CETYL MYRISTOLEATE FIGHTS INFLAMMATION

The existence of a rare anti-arthritis substance (cetyl myristoleate) was stumbled upon in 1962 by Harry W. Diehl, Ph.D., a researcher for the National Institutes of Arthritis, Metabolism, and Digestive Diseases. Assigned to inject an arthritis-inducing agent into laboratory mice for the purposes of testing a new synthetic drug, Dr. Diehl found that the mice were strangely resistant to developing arthritis symptoms. Dr. Diehl eventually identified in the mice an oil called cetyl myristoleate responsible for preventing arthritis.

Cetyl myristoleate occurs in only a few animal species—Swiss albino mice, sperm whales, and the male beaver. To make this useful substance available to the public, Dr. Diehl found that a mixture of myristoleic acid (from fish oils and cow's milk butter) and cetyl alcohol, a molecule found in coconut and palm oils, rendered the same chemical substance found in the mice. Cetyl myristoleate appears to have three modes of therapeutic action that are helpful for both osteoarthritis and rheumatoid arthritis: it acts as a lubricant for smooth motion of joints and muscles, modulates immune system function, and has anti-inflammatory effects.[42]

Typical recommended dose: Cetyl myristoleate is usually given orally for a one-month period at a dose of 10 g to 15 g. It is also available as a topical cream that can be rubbed into sore and painful joint areas. Because cetyl myristoleate is a fatty substance, take it in conjunction with 100 mg of lipase, an enzyme that digests fat.[43]

lating the production of connective tissue and new cartilage growth essential to the repair of arthritis damage. In a study in Milan, Italy, 80 patients with severe osteoarthritis were given a 30-day course of glucosamine sulfate (1.5 g daily). The treated patients experienced reduction in pain, tenderness, and overall symptoms. Examination of cartilage samples from the patients treated with glucosamine sulfate shared many structural aspects of healthy cartilage. The researchers concluded that glucosamine sulfate rebuilt damaged cartilage, thereby reducing pain and other symptoms.[37] Chondroitin sulfate is another supplement, often taken in conjunction with glucosamine, which seems to protect joints from breaking down. While there is debate about the body's ability to absorb chondroitin orally, injectable forms have proven quite effective.

Calcium and magnesium are also vital nutrients in the fight against arthritis. Calcium is essential for bone, joint, muscle, and ligament health, while magnesium is necessary for calcium's proper incorporation into bone, by preventing a buildup of calcium in the soft tissues and joints. Most people, though, consume too much calcium and not enough magnesium. High protein diets, which are common for many Americans, contain a lot of phosphorus, which binds up magnesium and makes it unavailable for the body's use.

Boron helps maintain bone and joint function and activates the metabolism of vitamin D. Low levels of boron in the soil—and thus in foods grown in that soil—have been linked in many countries to increased osteoarthritis levels.[38] Boron supplementation helps to reduce the excretion of calcium and magnesium, important minerals in bone structure and muscle function.[39] Studies in Germany have found that boron can improve joint pain in osteoarthritis as well as decrease bone loss.[40]

Manganese has many functions in the body, including normal growth and metabolism. It helps to activate enzymes, is used for normal bone development, and acts as an anti-inflammatory.[41] Patients with rheumatoid arthritis are usually significantly deficient in manganese and supplementation is recommended.

Sulfur-containing compounds are used by the body to regenerate cartilage cells, maintain cellular functions, and produce the peptide L-glutathione, which is an antioxidant and is used by the liver to process toxins. S-adenosylmethionine (SAMe) is a natural substance produced by the body when the amino acid methionine combines with adenosine triphosphate (ATP), an energy molecule present in all cells.[44] In one double-blind study, SAMe reduced pain in osteoarthritis patients as effectively as the drug ibuprofen and produced fewer side effects.[45] Similar studies have found that SAMe is an anti-inflammatory and pain reliever in arthritis of the hip and knee.[46] Dimethylsulfoxide (DMSO) is also a source of sulfur (derived from wood pulp, garlic oil, or as a by-product of petroleum) and thought to be a free-radical scavenger with anti-inflammatory properties. Methylsulfonylmethane (MSM) is a sister compound of DMSO derived from food sources. MSM is also naturally produced in the body, but levels decrease with age and in degenerative illnesses such as arthritis. Supplementing with MSM can reduce inflammation and scar tissue, relieve pain, and increase blood flow for improved exchange of nutrients.[47] Of special relevance in rheumatoid arthritis, MSM can help normalize the immune system and reduce the autoimmune response.

I. William Lane, Ph.D., author of *Sharks Don't Get Cancer*, reports that shark cartilage in capsule form is now being used to combat the pain of arthritis. Shark cartilage contains large amounts of mucopolysaccharides (carbohydrates that form chemical bonds with water), which stimulate the immune system and reduce the pain and inflammation of arthritis. Additional research shows that shark cartilage stops new blood vessel invasion of cartilage. This eliminates degradation of functioning cartilage. Clinical trials and practical application have shown that shark cartilage orally administered at least 30 minutes before meals is effective in reducing pain for many arthritic patients. In one trial, 80% of osteoarthritis patients at the Comprehensive Medical Clinic in Southern California responded well. The percentage of response for rheumatoid arthritis patients studied in other research was 50% to 60%.[48]

For gout patients, Dr. Murray recommends the following nutritional supplements: eicosapentaenoic acid (1.8 g daily), vitamin E (400-800 IU daily), folic acid (under a doctor's supervision, 10-40 mg daily), and quercetin with bromelain (125-250 mg three times a day between meals).[49]

Herbal Medicine

David Hoffmann, B.Sc., M.N.I.M.H., of Sebastopol, California, past President of the American Herbalists Guild, says that many anti-inflammatory herbs help in alleviating the symptoms of arthritis. Of the many possible combinations, this is a safe mixture that can be taken over a long period of time: combine the tinctures of meadowsweet, willow bark, black cohosh, prickly ash, celery seed, and nettle in equal parts and take one teaspoon of this mixture three times a day. In cases of rheumatoid arthritis, add wild yam and valerian to the mixture.

According to Dr. Murray, yucca and devil's claw may possess anti-inflammatory and analgesic effects for arthritic patients. In clinical trials with gout patients, devil's claw was found to relieve joint pain, as well as reduce blood cholesterol and uric acid levels. For gout sufferers, Dr. Murray recommends 1-2 g of dried powdered devil's claw root three times a day; 4-5 ml of (1:5) tincture three times a day; or 400 mg of dry solid extract (3:1) three times a day. According to the late Robert Bingham, M.D., the use of the yucca plant has proven highly successful as a nonspecific immune stimulator that reduces infection and inflammation. Yucca extract is made from the yucca plant found in deserts in the southwestern U.S. and in Mexico. Yucca extract is safe enough to take for long periods of time to prevent any recurrence of symptoms and can be purchased without a prescription.[54]

ARTHRITIS HELP FROM THE SEA

The green-lipped mussel, an edible shellfish native to New Zealand, is high in a unique kind of fatty acid known to reduce inflammation. ETA (eicosatetraenoic acid) is a previously unidentified type of omega-3 fatty acid with more biological activity than other omega-3s. Green-lipped mussels also contain amino acids, trace minerals, and GAGs (glycosaminoglycans, a component of cartilage). A typical recommended dose is 500 mg, three times per day with food. Precautions: Side effects are rare and mild, but include temporary aggravation of joint pain and tenderness, stomach discomfort, gas, nausea, and fluid retention.[50] People with known shellfish allergies should not use green-lipped mussel.

Sea cucumber (beche-de-mer) is a small marine animal (related to the starfish) traditionally used as an ingredient in Japanese and Chinese soups and stews.[51] Health benefits of sea cucumber include the relief of symptoms of rheumatoid arthritis, osteoarthritis, and ankylosing spondylitis.[52] Sea cucumbers also contain GAGs and chondroitin, which are important components of cartilage tissue.[53] A typical recommended dose is 500 mg twice a day. Precautions: People with seafood or shellfish allergies should not take sea cucumber.

Green tea *(Camellia sinensis)* contains bioflavonoids called catechins, which have anti-inflammatory and antioxidant properties and are helpful in treating rheumatoid arthritis by neutralizing free radicals that act on synovial membranes.[55]

Boswellia serrata, also known as boswella, has been used for centuries by Ayurvedic physicians for arthritic conditions. Its chemical component, boswellic acid, has powerful anti-inflammatory and analgesic activity.[56] Several studies have found that boswellic acid inhibits inflammation-causing agents, prevents interference with GAG (glycosaminoglycan) synthesis, and improves blood and lymphatic circulation to the joints.[57]

Lignum vitae (Guiacum officinale and *Guiacum sanctum)* is a tree native to South Florida, the Caribbean, and South America. The gum of this tree, guaia-gum, contains therapeutic resins and oils used as a pain reliever for arthritis, rheumatism, and gout.[58] Other recommended herbs include licorice and alfalfa. Feverfew has also been found effective in inhibiting the synthesis of pro-inflammatory compounds and decreasing the body's inflammatory response. Herbal remedies that have proven effective for rheumatoid arthritis include turmeric, ginger, skullcap, bupleurum, and ginseng.[59]

Environmental Medicine

"Allergic and allergy-like sensitivities are important factors in a large percentage of arthritis cases," states Marshall Mandell, M.D., Medical Director of the New England Foundation for Allergic and Environmental Diseases. "Allergies may or may not cause arthritis, but they definitely play a role in a majority of cases because they often aggravate and perpetuate the condition. When the substances to which arthritic patients are sensitive are eliminated, avoided, or contacted less frequently, the arthritis is relieved or eliminated."

The link between arthritis and allergic reactions to environmental chemicals and foods was first pointed out by Theron G. Randolph, M.D., the founder of environmental medicine. Dr. Randolph tested over 1,000 arthritis patients with commonly eaten foods as well as chemical substances (ranging from natural gas, auto exhaust, paints, perfume, and hair spray to insecticides, tobacco, and tobacco smoke) to find out which of these substances caused their symptoms.[60] The connection between arthritis and allergies was found to be quite significant.

In his own tests of over 6,000 patients, Dr. Mandell found that foods, chemicals, grasses, pollen, molds, and other airborne substances caused allergic reactions in the joints of nearly 85% of the arthritics he tested. Numerous other studies have shown various foods and food additives, as well as foreign invaders like protozoa, bacteria, yeast, and fungus, can also trigger or aggravate arthritic symptoms.[61]

It usually surprises arthritis patients to learn that both rheumatoid arthritis and the inflammation in osteoarthritis are caused to some degree by a combination of sensitivities to environmental pollutants, food sensitivities, and/or food toxic reactions.[62] There is ample evidence that food antigens (foreign substances) can cross the gastrointestinal membrane, enter the bloodstream, and circulate as injurious immune complexes. High levels of immune complexes have been found in both the blood and the fluid around the joints of arthritis patients.[63]

Although any food can theoretically trigger an allergic reaction in an individual, this list includes the most common food allergens of arthritis patients:

- Dairy products
- Beef
- Wheat
- Yeast (both baker's and brewer's)
- Eggs
- Chocolate
- Oranges
- Sugar
- Nuts (especially peanuts)
- Corn
- Green or yellow wax beans
- Nightshades (eggplants, potatoes, green and red peppers, paprika, tomatoes, tobacco)

All arthritis patients should be tested for food allergies. Once you have identified the foods you are allergic to, the next step is to eliminate them from your diet. Initially, you should completely refrain from eating all allergenic foods for 60-90 days. After this period, you can begin to slowly reintroduce them into your diet. You should also vary the foods that you eat on a daily basis to avoid developing new allergies. "You are likely to find that, as you reintroduce the foods to which you were once sensitive, your old symptoms will not reappear," says Dr. Zampieron. "This is because most food allergies can be cured through abstinence."

Fasting is another method used to reduce allergic reactions and the corresponding arthritic symptoms. During a fast, a patient typically eats only high-nutrient soups, water, and/or vegetable juices. Following this type of diet for several weeks decreases the amount of immune complexes (substances formed when antibodies attach to antigens) circulating in the blood.

Detoxification strategies can help arthritis patients reverse the accumulation of toxins that otherwise promote the destruction of joint tissues and contribute to other degenerative conditions. Several methods of detoxification are currently available, including colon and bowel cleansing therapies, kidney and gallbladder flushes, physical medicine, and homeopathic remedies. Related therapies for detoxification incorporate bodywork, lymphatic drainage, aromatherapy, antioxidant defense support, and nutrient and herbal support to bolster the organs of detoxification.

 See Acupuncture, Ayurvedic Medicine, Biological Dentistry, Bodywork, Chiropractic, Detoxification Therapy, Environmental Medicine, Herbal Medicine.

Bodywork

Osteoarthritis is directly related to skeletal and postural difficulties. Tendons and ligaments can be torn or stretched as a result of injury, exercise, or aging. The fascial tissues (thin sheets of connective tissue that hold muscles, joints, and organs together) tend to thicken and rigidify from overuse. When the body tries to compensate, bony spurs may appear in joints and on bones. Bodywork can alter postural difficulties. Restoration of proper, natural posture through deep massage and movement re-education can enable arthritic sufferers to free themselves from the pain and limitations of the disease.

Massage is one of the most important therapies for the treatment of arthritis. People with arthritis often experience prolonged muscle tension with poor blood circulation in muscle tissues, which can cause nerve and joint pain. Massage helps to break up muscular waste deposits that can cause pain as well as to stimulate circulation in troubled regions in the body, which helps bring more oxygen and other necessary healing nutrients into the tissues and carry toxins away. Dr. Zampieron recommends that arthritis patients pursue a massage program at least two to three times per week in the early stages, then once a week for several months, with a maintenance schedule of twice a month.

Rolfing has been found to help many arthritis sufferers. The procedure was originally devised by Ida P. Rolf, Ph.D., a biochemist who used the technique to treat her own arthritis. She realized that conditions causing arthritic disturbance could be changed by stretching fascial tissues. Rolfing repositions the body in balanced alignment with gravity. "Many diagnoses of 'arthritis' reflect nothing more serious than a shortened or displaced muscle or ligament resulting from a recent or not-so-recent traumatic episode," said Dr. Rolf.[64]

Chiropractic

Chiropractic is an increasingly popular, drug-free treatment for arthritis that has proven highly effective. Certain cases of arthritis, particularly of osteoarthritis, are false diagnoses with the symptoms actually caused by misalignment, or subluxation, of vertebrae and joints. When this is the case, chiropractic adjustments can restore a full range of movement and free the body from pain. William M. Cargile, B.S., D.C., F.I.A.C.A., past Chairman of Research of the American Association of Oriental Medicine, estimates that 95% of osteoarthritic cases have misaligned vertebrae. "If the vertebrae are out of position and there are abnormal stresses, osteoarthritis occurs," Dr. Cargile explains. "Your body begins to grow bones—little stalactites and stalagmites between levels, fusing vertebrae." Hips, knees, ankles, and other joints can also be out of alignment, causing bone spurs to form in these joints.

Manipulation can help arthritis (particularly osteoarthritis in the spine) by restoring proper movement and positioning of the joints. Balanced movement prevents "wear and tear" damage to joints, ligaments, and cartilage. Frequent manipulations help decrease the accumulation of scar tissue after injury, thus preventing later osteoarthritic changes in the joints. Chiropractic adjust-

---

MICROCURRENT TREATMENT FOR ARTHRITIS PAIN

Microcurrent treatment devices generate infinitesimally low levels of electrical current in a form that is compatible with the body's own biocurrents, which occur in healthy tissues. Used to heal muscle-related back injuries or reduce muscle pain, these almost sub-sensory signals are applied to damaged muscle to recharge the cellular "battery," which in turn leads to healing. The pain relief comes from decreases in swelling and spasms and increases in muscle flexibility. Microcurrent is an application within the larger treatment field called electrotherapy, which often uses stronger electrical currents for pain reduction. Nearly all U.S. chiropractic offices, physical therapy clinics, and hospital rehabilitation departments employ some form of electrotherapy for pain control, such as the well-known TENS (Transcutaneous Electrical Nerve Stimulation) unit.

TENS works by applying, for hours or days at a time, a pulsed electrical stimulation to a painful area of the body. By stimulating certain nerves, TENS reduces the neural transmission of pain and produces large amounts of endorphins (natural opiates that block the transmission of pain messages in the brain and body). There are two types of sensory nerve fibers in the body: nerve fibers with a large diameter tend to inhibit pain transmission and prevent pain, while nerve fibers with small diameters tend to facilitate transmission of pain. The application of electrical stimulus to painful areas causes the large-diameter nerves (pain inhibitors) to override the small-diameter nerves (pain transmitters), resulting in reduced sensations of pain.

---

ments, combined with proper nutrition can improve and, in some cases, reverse osteoarthritis.[65]

Acupuncture

According to Dr. Cargile, rheumatoid arthritis is a result of an autoimmune problem that prevents white blood cells from recognizing the joint surface as part of itself. "Acupuncture reduces the aggressiveness of the body against its own tissues and enhances its recognition of the joint tissue," he says. Dr. Cargile uses acupuncture as a whole-body system, utilizing an individual, case-by-case approach to balance the immune system. "We are not just affecting arthritis, we are actually affecting the spleen because of its role in the lymphatic system and its production of white blood cells," he explains.

ARTHRITIS AND DENTAL AMALGAMS

Hal Huggins, D.D.S., of Colorado Springs, Colorado, a leading authority on biological dentistry, has found arthritic symptoms are often associated with mercury dental amalgams. He notes that once the amalgams are removed, the symptoms often disappear, especially if the mercury is then detoxified or chelated from the body.

Dr. Huggins recalls treating a patient, a professional pianist, with arthritis in her hands so pronounced she could no longer perform. She had also suffered from other medical problems for years, including tachycardia, candidiasis, stuttering, and mononucleosis. Dr. Huggins found that she had two mercury fillings and a bridge with a metal base. Both the bridge and mercury amalgams were removed, The patient quickly regained her former energy, and the swelling and pain in her fingers subsided. She was able to play the piano in concert again within two months.

Dr. Cargile cites the use of acupuncture on a 56-year-old woman with a 20-year case of rheumatoid arthritis. She had become almost totally bedridden and her arthritis was being treated with methotrexate, a toxic chemotherapy drug usually used for cancer. The combination of her condition and the drug's extreme toxicity had her near death, but her fear of needles had kept her away from acupuncture. When she finally agreed to try it, she was delighted to discover she felt no pain from the needles. Treatments took place three times a week initially, then two times a week after the second month, and finally, once a week after the third month. She improved dramatically, with a marked decrease in inflammation and an increased range of motion. Her pain decreased as did all the associated symptomatic conditions of her arthritis.

Dr. Cargile has also found much success using a combination of acupuncture with chiropractic for the treatment of arthritis, particularly in cases of osteoarthritis.

Ayurvedic Medicine

According to Virender Sodhi, M.D. (Ayurveda), N.D., Director of Ayurvedic & Naturopathic Medical Clinic, in Bellevue, Washington, Ayurvedic medicine attributes arthritis to problems in the digestion of carbohydrates, proteins, and fats, which create production of intermediate molecules called *ama* and a condition called leaky gut syndrome. This digestive disorder triggers immune and allergic responses and results in the inflammation of the body's joints. Dr. Sodhi describes osteoarthritis as a "complete metabolic dehydration with no fluid left in the joints."

Ayurvedic medicine treats the digestive problems by working with diet and nutrition. Dr. Sodhi recommends that arthritic patients avoid foods that can cause indigestion, like broccoli, cauliflower, and lettuce. He advises patients to take herbs that enhance digestion, such as ginger, cayenne, black pepper, long pepper, and turmeric. Patients are further advised to avoid proteins, especially from animal sources such as beef, chicken, shellfish, and pork (fish protein is acceptable), and to avoid alcohol, coffee, and tea. One liquid he recommends for arthritic patients is pineapple juice with a pinch of turmeric, which helps the body combat leaky gut syndrome.

Dr. Sodhi also tests his arthritic patients for food allergies and for parasites that can cause joint inflammation. Other Ayurvedic herbs are recommended to promote digestion and immune function. In particular, *triphala* helps cleanse the intestines and aids digestion. To increase joint mobility and protect joints from further damage, he recommends flaxseeds, fish oils, and *Boswellia*. Oil massages are beneficial, using sesame or olive oil. For swollen joints, massaging with castor oil helps pull toxins out of the body.

Breathing exercises to relieve the stiffness of the joints and to increase oxygenation are also important, according to Dr. Sodhi. For arthritis patients, he prescribes a regimen of breathing patterns, flexing of the joints of the hands, feet, and elbows, and yoga positions. After exercising, he recommends a soak in hot water enhanced with baking soda or salt, ginger, peppermint, and eucalyptus. He states that Ayurvedic treatment for many patients can turn their condition around in three to four months.

Recommendations

- An important first step in treating arthritis is achieving normal body weight, as excess weight puts increased stress on weight-bearing joints affected with arthritis.

- Whole (unprocessed) foods are rich in the nutrients needed to fight destructive free radicals, enhance tissue health, repair bones, joints, muscles, and tendons, balance the tissue acidity/alkalinity, and promote bowel regularity.

- Dietary fats are an important consideration for anyone with arthritis. The wrong kind of fats (especially hydrogenated oils and saturated fats) can increase inflammation in joints, while the "good" fats (essential fatty acids like EPA) will help keep inflammation in check.

- Vitamin C helps repair and maintain healthy connective tissue. Vitamins A, B₁, B₆, E, and niacinamide (a form of vitamin B₃) have also proven effective in treating and preventing arthritis.

- Calcium is essential for bone, joint, muscle, and ligament health, while magnesium is necessary for calcium's proper incorporation into bone, by preventing a buildup of calcium in the soft tissues and joints.

- Yucca and devil's claw may possess anti-inflammatory and analgesic effects for arthritic patients. *Boswellia serrata,* also known as boswella, has been used for centuries by Ayurvedic physicians for arthritic conditions. Other herbal remedies that have proven effective for rheumatoid arthritis include turmeric, ginger, skullcap, bupleurum, and ginseng.

- Allergies may or may not cause arthritis, but they definitely play a role in a majority of cases because they often aggravate and perpetuate the condition. When the substances to which arthritic patients are sensitive are eliminated, avoided, or contacted much less frequently, the arthritis is relieved or eliminated.

- Restoration of proper, natural posture through deep massage and movement re-education can enable arthritic sufferers to free themselves from the pain and limitations of the disease.

- Chiropractic is an increasingly popular, drug-free treatment for arthritis that has proven highly effective.

Self-Care

The following therapies can be undertaken at home under appropriate professional supervision:

OSTEOARTHRITIS—

Flower Remedies / Guided Imagery / Qigong and Tai Chi

AROMATHERAPY: • Dissolve camphor and mint in vodka or unroasted sesame oil and apply externally. • Lemon oil or marjoram oil (undiluted or mixed with sesame or olive oil) can be rubbed into the affected joints.

JUICE THERAPY: • Celery juice during acute inflammatory stage • Carrot, celery, and cabbage juice • Carrot, beet, and cucumber

EXERCISE AND PHYSICAL THERAPY: Isometric exercises, yoga

RHEUMATOID ARTHRITIS

Guided Imagery / Yoga

AROMATHERAPY: • Detoxify with cypress, fennel, and lemon. • Massage affected joints with rosemary, benzoin, chamomile, camphor, juniper, lavender.

HYDROTHERAPY: • Constitutional hydrotherapy (apply two to five times weekly) or heating compress (apply once daily to affected areas). • Leon Chaitow, N.D., D.O., of London, England, reports that the neutral bath, with the patient immersed in water (35° C) for two hours, has been effective in reducing the swelling of joints in rheumatoid patients.

JUICE THERAPY: • Carrot, celery, and cabbage juice; add a little parsley. • Potato juice • Cherry juice (especially good for gouty arthritis) • Take juice of half a lemon before every meal and before going to bed, then rinse with water afterward. • Carrot, beet, and cucumber • During acute stage, 1-2 pints of celery juice daily. • Radish, garlic • Avoid tomato juice.

Professional Care

The following therapies should only be provided by a qualified health professional:

OSTEOARTHRITIS

Acupressure / Bodywork / Chiropractic / Craniosacral Therapy / Enzyme Therapy / Mind/Body Medicine / Orthomolecular Medicine / Osteopathic Medicine / Prolotherapy / Reflexology

ENERGY MEDICINE: Electrodermal screening (EDS) or applied kinesiology can help detect the underlying causes of arthritis.

RHEUMATOID ARTHRITIS

Enzyme Therapy / Magnetic Field Therapy / Mind/Body Medicine / Naturopathic Medicine / Orthomolecular Medicine / Osteopathic Medicine / Oxygen Therapies / Sound Therapy

ENERGY MEDICINE: Electrodermal screening (EDS) or applied kinesiology can help diagnose and determine the underlying causes of arthritis.

Where to Find Help

For more information on, and referrals for, treatment of arthritis, contact the following organizations.

American Association of Oriental Medicine (AAOM)
433 Front Street
Catasauqua, Pennsylvania 18032
(888) 500-7999
Website: www.aaom.org

The AAOM is a national professional trade organization of acupuncturists who meet acceptable standards of competency and can provide you with the names and locations of local members. Referrals by written request only.

Ayurvedic & Naturopathic Medical Clinic
2115 112th Avenue NE
Bellevue, Washington 98004
(425) 453-8022
Website: www.ayurvedicscience.com

Dr. Virender Sodhi's clinic provides medical training for physicians and health-care practitioners, as well as individual courses for laypeople.

American Massage Therapy Association
820 Davis Street, Suite 100
Evanston, Illinois 60201
(312) 761-2682
Website: www.amtamassage.org

Contact them for the location of a licensed massage therapist in your area.

American Association of Naturopathic Physicians
601 Valley Street, Suite 105
Seattle, Washington 98109
(206) 298-0126
Website: www.naturopathic.org

Contact them for the location of a licensed naturopathic physician in your area.

American Chiropractic Association
1701 Clarendon Blvd.
Arlington, Virginia 22209
(800) 986-4636 or (703) 276-8800
Website: www.amerchiro.org

A major source for information on chiropractic. Monthly publication and newsletter. Provides referrals on request.

The Arthritis Trust of America
7111 Sweetgum Road, Suite A
Fairview, Tennessee 37062-9384

They have a listing of physicians who use one or more of the various recommendations for osteoarthritis, rheumatoid disease, and gout. They are a nonprofit, charitable group, so send a contribution to help defray the cost of services requested.

Recommended Reading

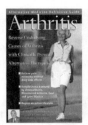

Arthritis: An Alternative Medicine Definitive Guide. Eugene Zampieron, N.D., A.H.G., and Ellen Kamhi, Ph.D., R.N., H.N.C., with Burton Goldberg. Tiburon, CA: AlternativeMedicine.com Books, 1999.

The Arthritis Bible. Leonid Gordin and Craig Weatherby. Rochester, VT: Inner Traditions, 1999.

Arthritis: The Allergy Connection. John Mansfield, M.D. Wellingborough, England: Thorsons Publishers, 1990.

The Arthritis Helpbook. Kale Lorig, R.N., and James Fries, M.D. Cambridge, MA: Perseus Press, 2000.

Arthritis Relief at Your Fingertips. Michael Reed Gach, Ph.D. New York: Warner Books, 1990.

How to Deal with Back Pain and Rheumatoid Joint Pain. Fereydoon Batmanghelidj, M.D. Falls Church, VA: Global Health Solutions, 1992.

Natural Medicine for Arthritis. Glenn S. Rothfeld and Suzanne LeVert. Emmaus, PA: Rodale Press, 1996.

AUTISM

Autism is a severe, sometimes lifelong behavioral disorder with no known single cause or cure. Alternative treatment programs, including diet, nutritional supplementation, environmental medicine, auditory training, craniosacral therapy, and behavior therapy have been helpful in allowing some autistic individuals to participate in society with a greater degree of success, even resulting in cures for a few.

AUTISM IS A MYSTERIOUS illness that has long baffled the medical community. An almost always permanent condition that usually begins shortly after birth, typically before age 2 ½, autism used to occur in approximately four or five out of 10,000 children. Recently, however, there has been an alarming increase in the rate, affecting as many as one in 500 children or perhaps even more.

Autism is characterized by withdrawal and an inability to communicate in a normal manner. In autistic children in whom there is a significant emotional component to their condition, there is a capacity but no willingness to communicate. Autistic individuals often show strong attachments to a particular object rather than to people, display compulsive behaviors such as rocking or arm flapping, and appear to avoid eye contact. While some autistic individuals are mute, others exhibit a bizarre, ritualistic speech pattern. Autistic children may be "mentally retarded," with IQ scores below 70. Studies have shown that many autistic children also have elevated levels of certain brain chemicals, abnormalities in brain-wave patterns, or are prone to epilepsy. They are often institutionalized, particularly if the individual is subject to violent or self-destructive episodes. However, despite severely limited learning capacity, some autistic children show extraordinary talent in a specific area, such as music or mathematics.

Standard Western medicine has no cure or treatment other than drug management of disruptive behavior, usually with antidepressants (Anafranil, Prozac, or Zoloft). Other drugs such as haloperidol, fenfluramine, and naltrexone are used to curb behavioral problems. In the U.S., the annual cost of autism, including special educational programs, is $12 billion. It is estimated that less than 25% of autistic children adjust to adolescence or adulthood, only 5% become self-sufficient as adults, and 40%-70% remain institutionalized for life.

Causes of Autism

"Autism is not a disease with a specific cause, but rather a syndrome with a combination of abnormal behavioral characteristics," according to Bernard Rimland, Ph.D., Director of the Autism Research Institute, in San Diego, California. Although a genetic basis for many cases of autism has long been suspected, only recently have researchers been able to tie specific genes to autism.

"In my clinical experience, all autistic individuals display some form of metabolic disorder," says children's health expert Constantine A. Kotsanis, M.D., of Grapevine, Texas. "However, not all individuals are alike. While it is unclear if the metabolic disorder is a cause or effect of this condition, correction of metabolic issues often yields improved behavior, cognition, and communication." Defects in the breakdown of peptides (simple proteins such as insulin, endorphins, and other neurotransmitters—see Quick Definition) during the digestive process, as indicated by an increased level of urinary peptides, have been found in autistic children.[1]

> **QD** A **neurotransmitter** is a brain chemical with the specific function of enabling communications between brain cells, spinal cord cells, and other nerve cells, all called neurons. Electrical thought impulses cause the release of neurotransmitters at the synapses. Then, these neurotransmitters move a short distance between nerve cells and bind to specific receptor proteins on the adjacent cell, which stimulates an electrical impulse in that cell. Chief among the neurotransmitters identified to date, there are six involved in most mental activities: acetylcholine, gamma-aminobutyric acid (GABA), serotonin, dopamine, L-glutamate, and norepinephrine.

VACCINES, MERCURY, AND AUTISM

The nation is seemingly in the midst of an autism epidemic. The California Department of Developmental Services found a 273% increase of autism between 1987 and 1998.[9] Maryland reported a 513% increase in autism between 1993 and 1998 and several dozen other states have reported similar findings. Hearings in the U.S. House Government Reform Committee were held in August 1999 and April 2000 to investigate the possible causes. Testimony given before the committee included parents of New Jersey's Brick Township, where one in 149 children suffers from autism, a much higher incidence than the national average. These parents contend that their children developed autistic symptoms after receiving childhood vaccinations.

However, there is no conclusive evidence of the connection between autism and vaccines, with studies both supporting and dismissing the hypothesis.[10] It is suspected that autism might be connected to the MMR (measles-mumps-rubella) vaccine. One report by Dr. Vijendra Singh, of the Department of Pharmacology at the University of Michigan, found a higher incidence of MMR antibodies in autistic children.[11]

The National Vaccine Information Center, in Vienna, Virginia, has noted a strong association of the MMR with autistic features. The Encephalitis Support Group, in Sinnington, England, reports that, according to parents who have contacted the organization, children who became autistic after the MMR vaccine started showing early symptoms about 30 days after vaccination. They also report that the DPT vaccine (given at two, four, and six months) has triggered autistic symptoms.

The connection between vaccinations and autism may be mercury poisoning. Thimerosal, a preservative used in many vaccines, contains about 50% mercury. The increases in the occurrence of autism are closely linked to the widespread use of thimerosal-containing vaccines.[12] Mercury is well-documented as a cause of nervous system deterioration, decline in mental function, and learning problems.[13] Certain symptoms of mercury poisoning are similar to autism, particularly defects in coordination and motor skills, visual disturbances, and immune suppression.[14] In addition, many alternative medicine practitioners report significant improvement in autistic children when chelation and other detoxification therapies are employed.[15]

Other possible causes of autism include:

- Fetal alcohol syndrome: In a Canadian study, one in 54 children with fetal alcohol syndrome (a birth defect characterized by deficiencies in growth and mental capabilities) also had autism.[2]

- Brain stem defects: Studies have linked significantly decreased brain stem size to autism.[3]

- Heavy metal poisoning: Elevated blood levels of lead have been found in some autistic children.[4] In an unpublished study done in Dr. Kotsanis's clinic in 1998-1999, all 20 autistic subjects had toxic metals (identified through hair analysis). "It is essential to address this aspect of the metabolic profile in autism, because metal toxicities necessarily affect other metabolic functions," says Dr. Kotsanis. "When toxic metals are identified, a chelation protocol should be considered as part of the overall treatment plan."

- Unusual blood flow patterns in the brain: Total brain blood flow has been found to be significantly decreased in autistic children.[5]

- Viral infections: Rubella (German measles) or cytomegalovirus (related to the herpes virus) during the mother's pregnancy, and severe infections during infancy, may be associated with the onset of autism in children.[6]

- Food allergies: Reports suggest that sensitivities to certain foods, especially wheat, sugar, and cow's milk, may contribute to behavioral symptoms. Because many autistics have food allergies, these allergens need to be identified and eliminated from the diet.[7] Most traditionally trained allergists are not aware that allergies can affect the brain, so a specialist in environmental medicine should be consulted. Dr. Kotsanis has found enzyme-potentiated desensitization (EPD) effective in dealing with allergies in those with autism; however, this therapy is still considered controversial in the U.S.

- Infant vaccinations: Medical historian Harris L. Coulter, Ph.D., of Washington, D.C., believes that autism and many other brain disorders are caused by infant vaccinations, particularly with the pertussis (whooping cough) vaccine.[8] The incidence of autism rose in the 1950s, which coincides with the time vaccinations became popular in the U.S., according to Dr. Coulter.

- A defect in the myelinization process (insulation of nerve fibers): This may account not only for autistic symptoms, but also for the frequent development of epilepsy in older autistic children.[9] What causes this defect is unknown, but one common denominator for both vaccine reactions and mercury is their potential to interrupt myelinization in developing infants.

- Antibiotics: Many children develop autism following antibiotic treatment for repeated ear infections, according to William Crook, M.D., of Jackson, Tennessee.[17] Dr. Crook believes that chronic use of antibiotics destroys the normal bacteria living in the intestinal tract, leading to overgrowth of the yeast *Candida albicans* as well as to "leaky gut syndrome," in which undigested food particles get into the circulation, sparking autoimmune reactions and food allergies, which are common in autistics.

- Digestive deficiencies: Dr. Kotsanis believes that autism has a multifactorial cause and that parasites, yeast infections, food allergies, and a deficiency of digestive enzymes all may play a role. Correction of the digestive environment (returning it to normal flora) is essential in treating autism. Beneficial bacteria (acidophilus, *Bifidobacteria,* and other species) should be supplemented for six months to one year, especially during and after the use of antibiotics.

Treating Autism

The conventional methods of treating autism consist of drugs and behavior modification. Behavioral approaches incorporating a firmly structured, purposeful educational program have proven to be highly beneficial in many cases. In one study, 19 preschool autistic children who received intensive behavioral intervention achieved less restrictive placements in school and had higher IQs than a control group; a follow-up to this study several years later showed that these gains were long-lasting.[18]

Following the work of Nobel Prize–winning ethologist Niko A. Tinbergen, a technique called Holding Therapy seeks to repair the apparently damaged attachment between the autistic child and his or her mother. Using physical contact and emotional connection between mother and child, remarkable results can be obtained in many cases. "Neurological, physical, and biochemical deficits play an undoubted role in the development of autism," says Rima Laibow, M.D., founding Medical Director of the Alexandria Institute of Natural and Integrative Medicine, in Croton-on-Hudson, New York. "But when the mother/child unit is made whole

with Holding Therapy, the enormous capacity for repair that is within us all can be activated." Dr. Laibow has used this technique successfully with dozens of autistic children.

Alternative physicians also claim increasing success using a combination of other therapies, including nutritional supplementation, the elimination of food allergies, environmental medicine, auditory integration training, and craniosacral therapy.

Nutritional Supplements

The causes of the autism are not necessarily the same for every person, but there is usually a strong nutritional factor involved. More precisely, there is often damage to the immune system that will respond to specific nutrients if given according to the child's altered biochemistry. High-dosage (megavitamin) nutritional supplementation is playing an increasingly important role in the treatment of autism. Dr. Rimland states, "Researchers both in the United States and abroad have demonstrated that 30% to 60% of autistic children and adults show significant behavioral and other benefits from the administration of large amounts of vitamin B_6 and magnesium."

Magnesium is employed because the body cannot effectively use vitamin B_6 without adequate magnesium. According to Dr. Rimland, some studies show not only behavioral improvement, but also normalization of brain waves and metabolism. He adds that this approach is far safer, more rational, and more helpful than the use of any drug. A magnesium deficiency has been shown to cause hearing hypersensitivity and hyperirritability, both associated with autism.[19] Dr. Rimland also recommends the supplementation of zinc, as well as the other B vitamins, in his program.

Researchers have demonstrated that 30% to 60% of autistic children and adults show significant behavioral and other benefits from the administration of vitamin B_6 and magnesium.

—BERNARD RIMLAND, PH.D.

Vitamin C has been shown to significantly reduce autistic behavior such as rocking, spinning, and hand flapping.[20] Dimethylglycine (DMG), a nontoxic chemical found in minute amounts in foods, has also proved helpful in treating autism, according to Dr. Rimland. Many

AUTISM AND SECRETIN

Recent autism research has focused on a little-known neurotransmitter called secretin, a chemical messenger involved in digestion. Secretin stimulates the pancreas and stomach to release digestive enzymes and the liver to produce bile. Injections of synthetic secretin in autistic children with gastrointestinal problems have produced some remarkable benefits.

In one study of 20 autistic children experiencing loose stools, 75% had normal bowel movements within 24 hours. In addition, 83% of the parents reported moderate to significant language improvement in the children after secretin treatment, although the therapeutic connection has yet to be determined.[21] It is possible that unrecognized gastrointestinal disorders contribute to the behavioral problems in some autistic patients.[22] Another study found that 76% of 20 autistic children had increased intestinal permeability. After a single injection of secretin, 13 of these children showed a significant decrease in permeability.[23]

Some side effects have been noted with secretin, including hyperactivity and aggressiveness. Further study is warranted to determine safe dosage levels as well as the efficacy of secretin for autism.

parents have reported that within days of starting DMG, their autistic child's behavior improved noticeably and better eye contact was observed, as well as an improvement in the child's speech, adds Dr. Rimland.

 See Diet, Nutritional Medicine, Orthomolecular Medicine.

Diet

Diet is an important factor in treating autism. Dr. Kotsanis recommends that autistic individuals eat a diet of whole, unprocessed, alkalinizing foods such as vegetables, since many autistics have overly acidic blood. "Canned, packaged, and frozen foods contain preservatives and other additives that can have adverse effects on autistics," he adds. "Dairy products should be avoided because of their mucus-producing properties, as should processed sugar, due to the chemicals used in refining. Foods with yellow, red, and green dyes should be completely eliminated from the diet, along with monosodium glutamate (MSG) and aspartame (an artificial sweetener found in NutraSweet®), because at high heat aspartame can potentially break down into formaldehyde."

Another dietary factor to consider when treating autism are allergies to peptides contained in cow's milk and gluten. According to one study, when milk and gluten-derived peptides were removed from the diet, language, social interactions, and behavior all improved. In this particular study, 15 autistic children and adults, 6-22 years old, were treated by restricting or eliminating cow's milk and gluten from their diets. "These patients were socially isolated, were resistant to learning, showed peculiar attachment to certain objects, showed fear of unusual items and situations, and demonstrated both repetitive motor behavior and severe problems with emotional expression," according to the researchers. "Language problems and disturbed attention were also common."

Urine analysis showed that patients had increased levels of cow's milk and gluten-derived peptides. Depending on the specific pattern of peptides in the urine, three types of diets were prescribed to reduce overall peptide levels. Some patients received a gluten-free and milk-reduced diet, others a milk-free and/or gluten-reduced diet, and a third group eliminated milk and gluten from the diet.

After one year, all the study subjects had changed in the direction of the normal spectrum—they were more communicative and showed less bizarre behavior. Other statistically significant changes included improved attention and social integration, improved motor skills, and a decrease in irrational emotional outbursts. Especially noteworthy was the decrease in resistance to learning.[24]

 See Allergies.

Dr. Crook says he has noticeably improved the behavior of autistic children by using an elimination diet. Any food normally consumed more than once a week is removed from their diet. As symptoms improve, each food is added back into the diet one at a time. One of Dr. Crook's patients became more alert, less hyperactive, and more sociable after wheat, sugar, corn, and eggs were removed from his diet.[25]

Environmental Medicine

Environmental medicine explores the role of dietary and environmental allergens in health and illness. According to Stephen B. Edelson, M.D., Medical Director of the Edelson Center for Environmental and Preventive Medicine, in Atlanta, Georgia, autism may be an environmental maladaptation. In his experience with autistic children, 90% showed evidence of toxic chemical exposure and 90% of the mothers had a higher-than-usual exposure to toxic household and industrial chemicals while pregnant. Substances included formaldehyde, toluene, pesticides, and toxins from paints, ceramics, new carpets, and ant and flea sprays. All of the children had allergic sensitivities to foods, inhalants, and chemicals, and exhibited imbalances in key brain chemicals. Further, 40% of the children had nutrient absorption problems, while all had nutrient deficiencies and immune system abnormalities.

On this basis, Dr. Edelson suggests that the origin of autism is both environmental and genetic, that it is a systemic disease involving many organs, and that the liver is unable to clear the body of toxic chemicals. Dr. Edelson institutes an intensive program of nutrient and herbal supplementation, environmental controls, and complete detoxification. Substances administered included amino acids, antioxidants, enzymes, milk thistle (silymarin), gamma globulin, essential fatty acids, and many others, as laboratory tests indicate.

Dr. Edelson's program has resulted in significant improvements in children's behavior and emotions, such as tantrums, disruptiveness, movement, irritability, and relationships. "What needs to be done is to advise the public that until we know more about the effects of chemicals on the developing immature brain, there should be a complete removal from 'chemical environments' of all pregnant women and children during the first few years of life, since we cannot predict who is at risk for autism and the accompanying systemic syndrome," says Dr. Edelson.

 See Detoxification Therapy, Environmental Medicine.

Auditory Integration Training

"Many autistic individuals are highly sensitive and can hear far beyond the normal human range," says Dr. Kotsanis. "To an autistic individual, rain sounds like rocks falling on a roof." This hypersensitivity can result in a number of problems, including blocking out other sounds, fear of noises and people, and an inability to concentrate. Auditory training can bring about a wide range of improvements in speech and behavior in many autistic individuals. The technique is based on the work of two French doctors, Alfred Tomatis, M.D., and Guy Berard, E.N.T. Both the Tomatis and Berard methods provide stimulation to the listener.

Berard training involves listening to ten hours of music (in 20 half-hour sessions) played through Berard's electronic modulating device, known as the Ears Education and Retraining System (EERS). An audiogram is first performed to detect frequencies to which the patient is hypersensitive so that they may be screened out of the music. Then the EERS is used to take music from a sound source, filter out specific frequencies found to cause the individual discomfort, modulate the sound electronically

in an unpredictable manner, and finally send the sounds back to the ears through headphones to exercise the entire hearing apparatus.

The Berard method is based on the idea that behavioral and cognitive problems may arise when people perceive sounds in an unequal manner. Certain frequencies, in other words, may be better comprehended than others, leading to some sounds becoming distorted to the listener, who then may have comprehension and behavior difficulties. Berard claims that the approach can reduce distorted hearing and hypersensitivity to specific frequencies and that, ideally, all frequencies can be perceived equally well.

Favorable results from the Berard method are often achieved within a matter of days. One extremely hyperactive nine-year-old boy overturned furniture and switched equipment on and off on his initial visit to Dr. Kotsanis's office. After two months of auditory training, the patient sat quietly in the reception area, reading while waiting for the doctor. Dr. Kotsanis considers auditory integration training to be the most important factor in his treatment for autistic individuals.

Many autistics have highly sensitive hearing beyond the normal human range. To an autistic individual, rain sounds like rocks falling on a roof. This hypersensitivity can result in a number of problems, including blocking out other sounds, fear of noises and people, and an inability to concentrate.

—CONSTANTINE A. KOTSANIS, M.D.

The Tomatis Method establishes a connection between listening, language, and learning. According to Billie Thompson, Ph.D., Director of the Sound, Listening and Learning Center, in Phoenix, Arizona, the Tomatis Method focuses on listening, which involves more than just hearing. Often in a case of autism, learning disabilities, or attention deficit hyperactivity disorder, the ear is unable to process, organize, and manage the thousands of pieces of sound information coming in from the environment.

Following a listening test, a program to improve auditory processing, audio-vocal control, and desire to communicate is developed. Auditory hypersensitivity is lessened, attention is increased, and the nervous system becomes more balanced, notes Dr. Thompson.

See Biofeedback Training and Neurotherapy, Sound Therapy.

The Tomatis program often, though not always, uses the filtered sounds of the mother's voice as the child would have heard it *in utero*. This is done in order to reintroduce the rhythm and intonation of language and the curiosity and desire to tune in. According to Dr. Tomatis, the mother's voice is not only an "emotional nutrient" for the fetus, but prepares the infant to acquire language and start speaking after birth. A human's first attempt to listen—and the first desire to listen—occurs as a fetus when it hears sounds of its own mother.

Both bone and air conduction are stimulated, and Tomatis's own device, the Electronic Ear, is used to control filtering, balance, timing, and emphasis of different frequencies. The Electronic Ear is designed to exercise the muscles of the middle ear and improve the ear's response to all frequency ranges. Special headphones equipped with a bone-conduction transducer (to sense vibrations through the bone) deliver sound to the patient via a sophisticated stereo system linked to tuning and filtering components. As lower frequencies are filtered out, the proper auditory preference is introduced.

Mozart, Gregorian chants, and children's nursery and folk songs are used in different stages of the program. Dr. Thompson notes that research done by Dr. Tomatis shows that high frequency sounds, achieved through filtering, provide a great deal of stimulation to the cerebral cortex, which helps children and adults access this energy for improved thinking and processing.

When the brain is well-charged with electric potential from high frequency sounds, it enables a person to better focus, concentrate, organize, memorize, learn, and work for long periods of time.

Dr. Tomatis tells about a 14-year-old autistic boy, who had not spoken since age four, who began to babble like a ten-month-old on hearing the sound of his mother's filtered voice. Dr. Thompson describes a hypersensitive 6-year-old autistic girl who did not speak and wore a ski cap 24 hours a day to limit outside stimulation. "After three days, she discarded the cap, went out to a restaurant with her family for the first time, and went to a church and heard organ music without leaving in pain. Though she still does not speak more than a few words, she is more social, does more activities with the family, and does not go to the corner in fear of sound."

> *Auditory training gives autistic children the desire to communicate. It allows them to hear sounds in a different way and can profoundly affect the way they learn and relate to others.*
>
> —BILLIE THOMPSON, PH.D.

To begin, the Tomatis Method is usually given for two hours a day for 15 days. It then continues for at least two additional eight-day intensives. "Auditory training gives autistic children the desire to communicate," says Dr. Thompson. "It allows them to hear sounds in a different way and can profoundly affect the way they learn and relate to others. Our goal is to help the person learn to listen, when possible to speak, and to have more awareness and self-control."

Craniosacral Therapy

Craniosacral therapy manipulates the bones of the skull and the underlying membranes to alleviate pressure and restrictions. The craniosacral system is a body rhythm, somewhat like a semi-closed hydraulic system, involving the flow of cerebrospinal fluid between the cranium (the bones of the skull) and the sacrum (the base of the spine). Disturbances in the craniosacral rhythm can indicate dysfunction in the body.

The Upledger Institute, in Palm Beach Gardens, Florida, uses craniosacral therapy to is treat autism. John Upledger, D.O., reports that in the autistic children treated at the Institute, he found a pattern of cranial restrictions consistent with developmental distortions of the brain, spinal cord, and the bones of the skull. Dr. Upledger has found that the meningeal membranes that line the cranium, especially the dura mater, do not expand normally with the growth of the brain, thereby interrupting normal development. This may be due to biochemical changes in the dura mater brought on by a stressor episode, such as a virus or an adverse reaction to a vaccination.[26]

Craniosacral therapy focuses on releasing restrictions of the cranium and the underlying membranes through gentle hands-on contact with the bones of the craniosacral system, the ribs, and the vertebral column. The therapist monitors the rhythmical movement in the craniosacral system resulting from the increase and decrease in cerebrospinal fluid pressure. When abnormal motion

SUCCESS STORY: UNRAVELING A CHILD'S AUTISM

When he turned 20 months old, Armand, an otherwise healthy and seemingly normal baby, began showing alarming signs of autism. Where once his vocabulary had been large, even precociously so, now it was diminishing into incommunicability. At his best, Armand could mimic a few words, speak in his own peculiar made-up language, or answer in a code picked up from a favorite children's book.

Armand's behavior became erratic and unpredictable. He smacked himself in the face, banged his head against the wall, and barked or screamed in response to questions. He was easily overwhelmed by stimuli and began avoiding eye contact. He couldn't sleep for more than four hours each night and he ate poorly. He was physically uncoordinated, lacking muscle tone in his lower limbs, and was unable to walk on his own.

At 3 ½, when his parents brought him to Zannah Steiner, C.M.P., R.M.T., at the Soma Therapy Centre, in Vancouver, British Columbia, Canada, Armand was still nursing and, for many months, his mother had been unable to leave the house without him. Armand's parents had gone through many doctors, consultations, and diagnoses, and come out nearly bankrupt and almost without hope of a cure. Armand had been diagnosed as having autistic spectrum developmental delay.

There wasn't much in Armand's health history to pinpoint a cause for his autism. Steiner learned that his birth had been difficult and he came out of the womb with his head bent to one side. Shortly after delivery, Armand was given a round of antibiotics for a presumed infection and was kept in intensive care for the first four days of his life.

Once Steiner gave Armand a physical examination, analyzing his craniosacral rhythm, she discovered the source of his problem. It was a mechanical misalignment of the bones and joints of his skull—specifically, of the sagittal suture connecting the left and right parietal bones. One of his cranial bones was overlapping the other rather than lying snugly adjacent, according to Steiner.

This overlap produced a sensation of constant pressure in his head. It had produced a severe compression of his temporal lobes at the base of his skull. Armand's head-banging and nursing (especially the suction and vacuum force created at his palate) were actually his body's strategy for trying to release the pressure in his head, Steiner explains. Armand had restrictions and misalignments in his sacrum as well and these may have cut off much of the nerve stimulation to his legs, thereby accounting for his lack of coordination and poor muscle tone.

Steiner treated Armand three times the first week and up to four times weekly for the next three months. When Steiner released the painful cranial overlap, using craniosacral therapy, Armand immediately stopped hitting himself in the head. She also worked on releasing bones in his palate, as their compression was contributing to the overlap of his cranial bones. When his palate was released, Armand had a markedly reduced need to nurse.

"The results were immediate and dramatic," Steiner relates. After the first week, Armand was able to speak intelligibly again, using sentences. He also responded better to communication from others and he was more reasonable and interactive, including maintaining eye contact. Armand began sleeping normally through the entire night.

The ridge on his skull disappeared after six weeks; the hollows on either side of his forehead filled in and the planes of his face broadened. Over the next two years, Armand enrolled in a special school for children with delayed verbal skills, where he overcame all of his developmental delays and surpassed all his schoolmates in his accomplishments.

---

is detected, the therapist locates the point of restricted movement and brings about a release by gently tractioning and elongating the membranes.

Gentle manipulation seeks to improve motion in the craniosacral system in people with autism and produces improvements in behavior. "As corrections are made, self-abusive behavior such as head banging abates entirely or reduces in severity," says Dr. Upledger. He believes that head banging may be an attempt to relieve the compressive force in the head due to the restrictive dura mater. The effectiveness of craniosacral treatments may be due to alleviating long-standing internal head pain.[27] Dr. Upledger has also seen craniosacral therapy improve socialization skills and increase expressions of love and affection.[28]

"The light touch, hands-on therapy reduces antisocial and self-destructive behavior," according to Bill Stager, D.O., of the Upledger Institute. "It takes two to three treatments for the patient to get familiar with the therapist and begin to respond. After that, progress is quite rapid." Substantial changes are seen within 10-20 sessions, given weekly. A concentrated, two-week program, with sessions lasting for eight hours a day for five days, is available for out-of-town patients. Craniosacral therapy can also be taught to parents to perform on their child at home, along with regular consultations with a skilled therapist. Therapy must be continued until the child is fully grown to maintain the benefits.

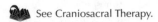 See Craniosacral Therapy.

A Multifactorial Approach to Autism

Dr. Kotsanis has developed a multifactorial approach to treating autism. Although this treatment method has been in use for only a short time, he reports that it has shown dramatic results. Because he has found parasites and yeast infections to be prevalent in autistic individuals, Dr. Kotsanis begins by prescribing a bowel-cleansing program. This consists of Chinese herbs, Biocidin (an antifungal agent made of various herbs), citrus extract, oil of oregano, and antifungal medications. Many autistics are also deficient in digestive enzymes, adds Dr. Kotsanis, and thus must supplement these at every meal.

Furthermore, most of these children have "leaky gut syndrome," permeability in the intestinal walls allowing undigested food particles into the bloodstream. To correct this, he uses butyric acid (a fatty acid derived from butter), L-glutamine (an amino acid), and beta carotene. He believes it is necessary to replenish the normal flora of the digestive system—Dr. Kotsanis recommends acidophilus, aloe vera extract, and garlic extract for this purpose. Vitamins A, B, C, and E, along with calcium, magnesium, zinc, and selenium are also important elements in his treatment protocol, as well as essential fatty acids and antioxidants.

Another key element in Dr. Kotsanis's program is addressing inhalant, food, and chemical allergies and sensitivities. In this phase, offending foods and chemicals are eliminated and the patient is placed on allergy injections for pollen, mold, and animal dander allergies, if these are present. Dr. Kotsanis has found enzyme-potentiated desensitization (EPD) particularly effective in dealing with allergies in those with autism. In EPD, an allergic patient is given a series of standardized injections of a wide variety of allergens from a single category. EPD injections differ from conventional allergy shots in three important ways: EPD injections include multiple related allergens; EPD doses are much weaker; and EPD injec-

tions are given along with an enzyme called beta-glucuronidase. This last component is important because it acts as a catalyst to make the vaccine more potent.

In addition, the patient's surroundings are made as free from irritants (feather pillows, harsh laundry detergents, cigarette smoke, pesticides) as possible. As adverse reactions to vaccinations may be a factor in the onset of autism, Dr. Kotsanis also cautions parents on the use of vaccines for their children. And it is recommended that the patient eat whole, unprocessed, organic foods and drinks purified water.

Next, Dr. Kotsanis utilizes auditory integration therapy twice a day for ten days and, if necessary, repeats it after six months. He considers this an important aspect of the treatment program. At the present time, he is investigating the effect of combining sound and color therapy with voice vibration therapy for the treatment of autism. Dr. Kotsanis also notes that strong psychological support and involvement by the family of the autistic is important for the treatment to be effective.

Dr. Kotsanis has treated several hundred autistic children with this multifaceted approach and reports a high degree of success. The majority of patients had an increase in language and speech capabilities. Additionally, in about three-fourths of patients, treatment resulted in a reduction or complete elimination of hypersensitivity to sound. One nonverbal 11-year-old was so sensitive to light and sound prior to treatment that he spent all day hiding in a closet. After ten days in Dr. Kotsanis's program, he began to speak; within three months, he was playing and engaging in social interactions in a normal manner. According to Dr. Kotsanis, some common remarks made by parents and friends concerning the treated children were that they were calmer, more attentive, exhibited better overall behavior, were more affectionate, and showed a better memory and retention of information.

Dr. Kotsanis stresses that while auditory integration therapy is an extremely important part of the treatment plan, every element mentioned contributes to a positive outcome. He feels that this multidisciplinary approach yields a more optimal result than any single discipline can offer alone.

 See Energy Medicine, Light Therapy, Sound Therapy.

Recommendations

- Behavioral approaches incorporating a firmly structured, purposeful educational program have proven to be highly beneficial in many cases.

- The causes of autism are not necessarily the same for every person, but there is usually a strong nutritional factor involved. Autistic children and adults show significant behavioral and other benefits from the administration of large amounts of vitamin B6 and magnesium.

- Canned, packaged, and frozen foods contain preservatives and other food additives that can have adverse effects on autistics. Dairy products should be avoided because of their mucus-producing properties, as should processed sugar, due to the chemicals used in refining. Foods with yellow, red, and green dyes should be completely eliminated from the diet, along with monosodium glutamate (MSG) and aspartame.

- Another dietary factor to consider when treating autism are allergies to cow's milk and gluten.

- Autism may be an environmental maladaptation. A program of nutrient and herbal supplementation, environmental controls, and complete detoxification may be beneficial.

- Auditory training has been reported to bring about a wide range of improvements in speech and behavior in many autistic individuals.

- Craniosacral therapy manipulates the bones of the skull and the underlying membranes to alleviate pressure and restrictions, which may be a factor in the etiology of autism.

Professional Care

The following therapies can only be provided by a qualified health professional:

Biofeedback Training and Neurotherapy / Craniosacral Therapy / Detoxification Therapy / Environmental Medicine / Enzyme Therapy / Nutritional Medicine / Orthomolecular Medicine / Sound Therapy

Where to Find Help

For additional information on, and referrals for, autism treatment, contact the following organizations:

American CranioSacral Therapy Association
Upledger Institute
11211 Prosperity Farms Road
Palm Beach Gardens, Florida 33410
(407) 622-4706
Website: www.upledger.com

The association promotes increased awareness and acceptance of CranioSacral Therapy among both laypersons and health professionals and oversees the development of certification training for CST practitioners nationwide.

Autism Research Institute
4182 Adams Avenue
San Diego, California 92116
(619) 281-7165
Website: www.autism.com/ari/contents.html

The Autism Research Institute conducts research on the causes, diagnosis, and treatment of autism and publishes a quarterly newsletter that reviews worldwide research. ARI provides referrals to health-care professionals and clinics offering alternative treatment for autism and other childhood behavior disorders. Also maintains a list of auditory training practitioners.

Autism Services Center
Prichard Building, 605 9th Street
P.O. Box 507
Huntington, West Virginia 25710-0507
(304) 525-8014

The Autism Services Center assists families of autistic children and acts as an advocate in designing appropriate therapy. Publishes a quarterly newsletter.

Autism Society of America
7910 Woodmont Avenue, Suite 300
Bethesda, Maryland 20814-3067
(301) 657-0881 or (800) 3-AUTISM
Website: www.autism-society.org

The society has 160 chapters throughout the U.S. and will provide answers to questions on autism. Membership includes a quarterly newsletter with support information and research news. Makes available a wide range of books on autism.

Families for Early Autism Treatment, Inc. (FEAT)
P.O. Box 255722
Sacramento, California 95865-5722
(916) 843-1536
Website: www.feat.org

FEAT is a nonprofit organization dedicated to providing education, advocacy, and support for the autism community.

The Georgiana Organization, Inc.
P.O. Box 2607
Westport, Connecticut 06880
(203) 454-1221

The Georgiana Organization provides education, workshops, consultations, and information on the Berard method.

The Listening Centre, Tomatis Canada
599 Markham Street
Toronto, Ontario, Canada M6G 2L7
(416) 588-4136
Website: www.listening.net

The oldest Tomatis center in North America, The Listening Centre provides therapeutic sessions and information.

Sound, Listening and Learning Center
2701 E. Camelback, Suite 205
Phoenix, Arizona 85016
(602) 381-0086
Website: www.soundlistening.com

Provides education, workshops, consulting, therapeutic sessions, and information on the Tomatis Method.

Recommended Reading

Autistic Adults at Bittersweet Farms. Norman S. Giddan, Ph.D., and Jane J. Giddan, M.A. New York: Haworth Press, 1991.

Brain Allergies. William H. Philpott, M.D., and Dwight K. Kalita, Ph.D. Los Angeles: Keats Publishing, 2000.

Children with Autism: A Parent's Guide. Michael D. Powers, Psy.D., ed. Bethesda, MD: Woodbine House, 2000.

The Conscious Ear. Alfred A. Tomatis, M.D. Barrytown, NY: Station Hill Press, 1991.

Dancing in the Rain: Stories of Exceptional Progress by Parents of Children with Special Needs. Annabel Stehli. Westport, CT: Georgiana Organization, 1995.

Hearing Equals Behavior. Guy Berard, M.D. Los Angeles: Keats Publishing, 2000.

The Mozart Effect. Don G. Campbell. New York: Avon Books, 1997.

Nobody Nowhere. Donna Williams. New York: Times Books, 1992.

The Ultimate Stranger: The Autistic Child. Carl H. Delacato, Ed.D. Novato, CA: Arena Press, 1984.

Vaccination, Social Violence, and Criminality: The Medical Assault on the American Brain. Harris L. Coulter. Berkeley, CA: North Atlantic Books, 1990.

BACK PAIN

Back pain is the leading cause of disability for people under the age of 45, and 80% of all Americans suffer from back pain at some point in their lives. Most people, though, are unaware of the things they habitually do to contribute to this problem. Alternative medicine offers a number of approaches for healing aching backs and preventing future back pain problems.

BACK PAIN IS the second leading cause for doctor visits in the United States, and low back pain is the third most common reason for surgery. The U.S. also has the highest rate of back surgeries of any country in the world, with more than 250,000 operations performed each year. However, according to the Cochrane Collaboration, an international network of health-science researchers that review clinical trials, "the scientific evidence for most [back surgical] procedures is unclear."[1] In addition, new studies have confirmed that whether or not a person undergoes back surgery, four years later the outcome is the same with or without surgery.[2]

"Back pain often appears to have a sudden onset without a known trauma or cause," says Marc Darrow, M.D., a board-certified physiatrist and Medical Director of the Joint Rehabilitation and Sports Medical Center, in Los Angeles, California. "Many patients state that they have never had back pain before and that it doesn't make any sense why they should have it now." The back has many tissues that slowly break down over time, eventually causing instability and pain. However, like a heart attack or stroke, back pain in the majority of cases does not happen unless precipitated by an acute or sudden injury.

"The preamble to back pain is what I refer to as the deconditioning or disuse syndrome," says Dr. Darrow. "As we age, we typically become less active, spending less time in sports and physical activities. This process allows for muscles to atrophy. Also involved is the degeneration of connective tissue made of collagen, such as tendons, ligaments, and joint capsules. Deconditioning and degeneration can be traumatically induced or may continue slowly on its own via the natural aging of the body. This explains why the average age for back surgery is 42. Most

patients around the age of 40 comment that they 'are falling apart.' In a sense, they are."

Back pain can be divided into two basic categories, acute and chronic. Acute pain comes on quickly, either immediately or over a period of several hours. It is often the result of a sudden motion or injury that may come from something as simple as lifting up a heavy object, or from an accident or fall. Chronic back pain, on the other hand, develops slowly and remains for a very long time, sometimes lasting for months or even years, and often flaring up intermittently.

While acute and chronic back pain can manifest in different ways, oftentimes they are interrelated: the acute problem leads to a chronic one or, just as commonly, a chronic condition (which can be hidden for long periods of time) causes the acute symptoms. All too often, according to Doug Lewis, N.D., past Chair of the Physical Medicine Department of Bastyr University, in Kenmore, Washington, the symptoms of back pain are treated without regard for their underlying causes. "The site of the pain is rarely the site of the dysfunction," he explains. "You may make the pain subside, but you're not correcting the dysfunction that caused the pain in the first place. If you leave the pain alone and treat the cause, then you have the pain as a monitor for whether or not your therapy is working."

Causes of Back Pain

When back pain appears, the specific reason or diagnosis of the cause of the pain is often very difficult to ascertain. This is because the back is a complex structure composed not only of bones, but also ligaments, tendons, fascia (covering of muscles and tissues), nerves, muscles, joints, fat, and skin. Other than bones and nerves, these other components, known as soft tissues, are composed of collagen. Ligaments and tendons are basically avascular, meaning they have little or no blood supply to heal them when they are injured, according to Dr. Darrow.

An injury may be acute, which means that it occurred recently, or it can be chronic, which means that the acute phase has passed and the injury did not heal within the first couple of months. If the pain is not resolved during the first few weeks after its onset, it becomes chronic and often remains. For many, this means a lifetime of pain, often from a simple injury like a low-impact car accident or a fall.

According to Dr. Darrow, back pain, with or without accompanying leg pain, can occur due to the following reasons:

- Stretch or tear injuries of muscles, tendons, ligaments, and joint capsules
- Fractures, including spondylolysis (fracture of part of a vertebra that keeps vertebrae aligned) and spondylolisthesis (slipping of a vertebra backwards or forwards on another as a result of spondylolysis)
- Herniated discs or arthritic facet joint (joint between the vertebrae) that may impinge on a spinal nerve that courses down a leg
- Injury, trauma, or arthritis of the joints between the vertebrae
- Degenerative joint or disc disease
- Inflammation of ligament, tendon (tendinitis), or muscle where it attaches to bone
- Vertebral subluxation (abnormal movement of a vertebra from its ideal anatomical position)
- Trigger or tender points (painful point or painful referral patterns from irritated muscle fibers or injured or lax ligaments)
- Tumors
- Pelvic or vertebral instability
- Fibromyalgia
- Local pain syndrome from inflammation of the fascia
- Muscle disease
- Spinal cord injuries
- Spasticity due to increased muscle tone with heightened deep tendon reflexes
- Scoliosis
- Osteoporosis fractures (typically in the thoracic spine, often causing kyphosis, or Dowager's hump)

Other causes include rheumatic diseases, such as psoriatic and rheumatoid arthritis, ankylosing spondylitis, Lyme disease, lupus, and Reiter's syndrome. Psychosomatic causes can also play a role, according to Dr. Darrow, who points out that some people transfer their uncomfortable emotions into physical pain, which is easier for them to deal with.

In order to understand the causes of back pain, says Mary Pullig Schatz, M.D., author of *Back Care Basics*, it is important to understand the anatomy of the spine and its relationship to the rest of the body. "The spine affects and is affected by every movement your body makes," she explains. "The way you stand, the way you sit, the way you move, the way you pick up and carry objects—all these things have the potential to help or hurt your back."[3]

These are some of the physical factors that can be caused, or contributed to, by poor posture and movement, all of which can affect the proper functioning of the spinal column, inevitably leading to back pain, according to Dr. Schatz: foot, ankle, knee, hip, and pelvic alignment; muscle strength in the legs, thighs, buttocks, back, and abdominal wall; abdominal protrusion such as from a beer belly or pregnancy; hip flexibility; the position of the pelvis, especially if it is tilted forward, back, or to either side; the position of the neck in relation to the shoulders; shoulder carriage and the mobility of the arms at the shoulder joints; and the shape and flexibility of the lumbar (lower back), thoracic (upper back), and cervical (neck) spinal curves.[4]

One of the most common postural problems leading to back pain, according to Dr. Lewis, is a twist in the pelvis due to a leg-length discrepancy. This can be anatomical (the legs actually are different lengths) or it can be functional (the legs are different lengths because the pelvis is twisted). This can produce a lateral, or side to side, curvature of the spine (scoliosis), when it becomes pronounced enough. "Anyone who has broken a leg automatically must assume there is a leg-length difference," adds Dr. Lewis. "Also, quite frequently, any injury to a leg during childhood or puberty, before the growth plates have fused, can cause a leg-length discrepancy because it doesn't allow normal growth of the leg."

Muscles in the legs, buttocks, back, and abdomen, when they become too contracted or too tight on one side or the other, can also produce similar pelvis twists and leg-length discrepancies, according to Dr. Lewis, as well as other postural deviations and spinal misalignments that can lead to extreme pain and physical impairment.

Back pain can also be caused by muscle problems that keep the vertebrae in misaligned positions. If muscles in acute cases are not relaxed, back problems can become chronic. Another cause of back pain is stress, both mental and physical, because during stressful situations, the muscles tense and can exaggerate postural strains or musculoskeletal misalignments.

Malocclusion of the teeth—usually as a result of a dentist filling a tooth cavity or putting a crown on a tooth, especially while the back is out of alignment—causes the back to become chronically misaligned, resulting in back pain.

Organic problems may contribute to back pain symptoms. "For example, gallstones, kidney stones, infections, uterine fibroid tumors, and ovarian cysts can all result in severe back pain," says Maoshing Ni, D.O.M., Ph.D., L.Ac., President of Yo San University, in Marina del Rey, California, "because the nerves that go to these organs come from the spine."

Dr. Lewis recounts a patient who came to him with lower back pain. "I treated her for the seeming indications of her pain, and she'd go away and feel great for two or three days, and then by the following week she'd be back in, with exactly the same complaint, exactly the same intensity," says Dr. Lewis. "We did this several times, with the same result, until finally I said to her, 'I think you should see a gynecologist.' She had an exam and discovered a grapefruit-sized cyst on her right ovary, which was removed, and immediately all of her back pain went away."

The reverse situation can also occur, Dr. Lewis notes. "If there's a chronic dysfunction in the musculoskeletal part of the system, it can negatively influence what happens with the organs. Quite often when I have patients with severe or even mild dysmenorrhea (pain associated with menstruation), I will treat the lower back and that will relieve the dysmenorrhea." Dr. Lewis has also found a lot of back pain in smokers, which he believes is related to the destruction of vitamin C in the body as a result of smoking. Vitamin C is necessary for the body to manufacture the collagen that makes up much of the connective tissue of the back. Defective collagen can result in lax ligaments and tendons or degenerative discs.

Because there are so many different factors that contribute to back pain, it is not only important to identify what the problem is, but how the problem arose. This will allow the practitioner to apply the most appropriate form of treatment for a person's ailing back.

Treating Back Pain

"Each medical discipline seems to find the diagnosis of back pain within the standards of what it is taught," Dr. Darrow says. "Often, a patient will be diagnosed with several different causes of pain by different practitioners. This is very confusing to the patient, who doesn't know whom to believe."

Dr. Darrow's view is echoed by David Bresler, Ph.D., of Los Angeles, California, former Director of the U.C.L.A. Pain Center. "When you're dealing with back pain, the type of therapy someone gets often depends on the type of doctor he or she goes to see," he says. "When you see an orthopedist, you'll get physical therapy and cortisone, maybe even surgery. If you see a physiatrist, you'll get exercises and maybe some physical therapy. If you see a chiropractor, you'll get adjusted, and if you see an acupuncturist, you'll get needled. It's a rather arbitrary way to determine what's best for a patient." Dr. Bresler tailors his approach to the specific needs of each patient and, if it seems appropriate, he will refer the person to someone else.

Today, people with back pain can choose from any number of alternative approaches, including all the various physical manipulation techniques and movement awareness therapies, mind/body medicine, energy medicine, acupuncture, and naturopathy. Each of these modalities has been proven effective in some cases, but not in all. Ideally, an alternative practitioner will help the patient explore all the treatment possibilities available and encourage him or her to take an active role in the treatment process.

Dr. Darrow accomplishes this by de-emphasizing diagnostic tests and focusing on his examination findings. "Since we know that half of all people without back pain have positive X-ray and MRI readings, why would we assume that a patient with pain has it because of a positive radiological test?" he says. Many patients visit Dr. Darrow on a whim just prior to a date with the surgeon. Rarely do they end up "under the knife." "About 90% of my back pain patients have nothing more than sprained or lax ligaments, or a strain of a muscle where it attaches to bone," Dr. Darrow says. "Surgery simply cannot help them. My office is filled with patients who come to us after failed surgeries."

Prevention: The Most Effective Solution for Back Pain

Because so many cases of back pain are muscular in origin, the pain usually occurs as a result of the way a person uses, or misuses, his or her body. Faulty habits in the way a person sits, stands, and walks strain the back, pushing and pulling the spine out of alignment and causing weakness, spasms, and sprains in tendons, ligaments, and muscles. The end result is pain, which can be felt either in the back or referred through the nervous system to other parts of the body.

Most back pain can be avoided by taking the simple preventative step of staying in good physical condition. Research has shown that exercise can also be of benefit in the treatment of low back pain and injury. Of particular value are exercise programs that maintain and enhance proper function of the lower back and spine. These include aerobic exercises, stretches, and strength-

STRETCHING FOR RELIEF OF BACK PAIN

Exercise to stretch the rectus femoris muscle

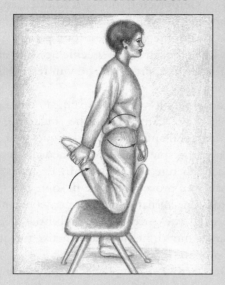

Cat-Cow position

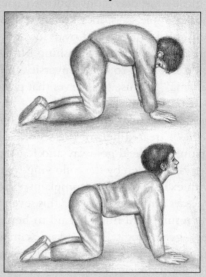

"Without a doubt, stretching is far more important for the relief of back pain than strengthening exercises," says Doug Lewis, N.D., past Chair of the Physical Medicine Department of Bastyr University, in Kenmore, Washington. "We really focus too much on strengthening muscles and I think it's a mistake, until we've done a good job of stretching them." The key is to find what muscles or muscle groups are asymmetrically tight or imbalanced, causing the postural problems and strain leading to back pain. One of the most common muscles associated with this kind of back pain is the rectus femoris, the muscle that runs from above the hip down through the kneecap and into the front of the tibia (the inner, longer bone of the leg between the knee and ankle). "If the muscles in both legs are tight, it can produce an anterior pelvic tilt, where the whole pelvis leans forward. This oftentimes creates a lordosis in the back, which is an excess amount of lumbar curve, commonly referred to as sway back," Dr. Lewis says.

In order to stretch these muscles out to correct the problem, Dr. Lewis instructs patients to stand and put the knee of the leg they want to stretch on the seat of a chair, while holding the back of the chair with the opposite hand for balance. "The idea is to pull the heel of the leg you want to stretch to the buttocks, and push forward with the pubic bone," he says. "This will push the pelvis backward, and you'll feel the stretch all the way from the knee, up the leg, to the front of the thigh."

The "Pelvic Rock" is another stretch to help with low back pain, according to Dr. Lewis, and can be done sitting in a chair. " Sit up straight, back against the chair back so that you have the normal low back curve. Then allow your pelvis to roll back as if you were going to slouch into the chair. Hold that for a few seconds and then come back into the straight position with the normal lumbar curve." Dr. Lewis also advocates the "Cat-Cow" yoga position, "where you're on your hands and knees, and you alternately drop your back into a sway back position, and then arch it like a cat."

One other stretch is frequently quite useful, especially when there is acute back pain, where the person can't move much, as well as for people who are stiff in the morning and have trouble getting out of bed. "While lying flat on the back, perhaps with a pillow under the knees so as not to strain the lower back, alternately push one foot out and then the other," explains Dr. Lewis. "You don't actually have to be pushing against anything. Rather, as you're pushing out with your heel, it's as if you're trying to make your leg longer." This rocks the pelvis back and forth instead of from front to back as in the Pelvic Rock.

"As you do each stretch, hold the stretch, don't bounce. Hold it for 5-10 seconds, then release and relax for 5-10 seconds, then go back into the stretch for 5-10 seconds. Another essential factor to remember is that any muscle you are going to stretch must absolutely be relaxed."

ening exercises such as sit-ups. These both help to stabilize the pelvis and progressively increase the free range of movement of the back.[5]

Proper movement is another key to a strong and healthy back. Often, for example, when walking, one inadvertently overtightens the muscles in the arms, legs, neck, and back with every step taken. This excess strain can eventually lead to chronic pain and illness—both physical and psychological—and can only be corrected when the patient learns how to use their body more efficiently and to maintain new habits and postures through an ongoing process of exercise and self-awareness.[6]

Physical Manipulation Techniques

Physical manipulation techniques aim to move the various parts of the body—muscles, connective tissues, and vertebrae—into proper functional alignment and can often correct serious problems relating to stress and physical pain. Dr. Lewis uses a method known as neuromuscular releasing, a soft-tissue manipulation technique for releasing tissue texture alterations, such as knots, edema (excess fluid in body tissues), fibrosis (abnormal formation of fibrous tissue), and scarring, from various muscle tissue and from the layers between muscles. It involves using thumb pressure on the tissues in order to break up and release any tissue texture alterations that may be inhibiting muscle movement and contributing to back pain.

"Following that, it is essential to relax and stretch these muscles out again, because it is generally my opinion that most dysfunction comes from excessive muscle tension rather than weak muscles," Dr. Lewis says. He also points out that muscles always work in pairs. "When a muscle contracts, the antagonist to that muscle will be held in relaxation," he explains. "For example, in order to lift something with your forearm, the biceps muscle will contract while the triceps on the opposite side of the arm must relax, otherwise we would simply tighten up and not be able to move at all.

"In cases of low back pain, though, one of the most common things is to have a person do sit-ups to strengthen the abdominal muscles. Yet, quite often the abdominal muscles are not weak, but are being held in relaxation because the muscles in the back are in spasm. So if you can get these muscles in the back to relax, they will stop inhibiting the tone of the abdominal muscles."

Other forms of physical manipulation techniques that are used for the treatment of back pain include chiropractic, osteopathic medicine, bodywork, and yoga.

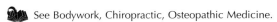 See Bodywork, Chiropractic, Osteopathic Medicine.

CHIROPRACTIC

Chiropractic is the public's number one choice for reducing back and neck pain. In addition to its effectiveness in this regard, it also assists in realigning the body while the other treatment modalities are taking effect. Chiropractors specialize in the manipulation of joints and the vertebrae in the back and neck. Chiropractic theory holds that back pain is often due to subluxations, which are misalignments of the vertebrae. A misaligned vertebra can press on a nerve and produce pain not only in the back but also in areas fed by the affected nerve. Thus, this "referred" pain can be felt in other parts of the body, like the arm or the leg, or can even affect the functioning of organs throughout the body.

Chiropractic treatment has been found to be more beneficial to patients with persistent back and neck complaints than other forms of manipulation.[7] Research in Great Britain found chiropractic to provide "worthwhile, long-term benefits" for patients with low back pain in comparison to hospital outpatient management. This study also found chiropractic benefits to persist for a three-year period, indicating a long-term enhancement of health.[8] For patients with uncomplicated, acute low back pain, chiropractic has also been found to be effective.[9] Finally, a cost comparison study of back-related injuries showed the number of work days lost for patients treated with chiropractic to be nearly ten times less than that of patients treated under conventional medical care.[10]

Chiropractic physicians often use the symptoms of back pain as a diagnostic tool for determining other disorders within the body. Likewise, they believe that by correcting the subluxation causing the back pain, they will also correct the nerve flow, which will in turn lead to the restoration of normal function of any other affected areas or organs. According to Robert Blaich, D.C., of Los Angeles, California, patients with chronic lower back pain who undergo chiropractic for some other problem like headaches or digestive problems often find that, in the course of treatment, the lower back pain goes away as well. Dr. Blaich states that since lower back pain frequently has to do with basic misalignments of the pelvis and spine, chiropractic is a particularly appropriate treatment. As he explains, "Almost all forms of chiropractic involve correcting misalignments, which in turn reduce the stress on joints, help to reduce wear and tear on joints, and help to minimize joint deterioration."

Dr. Blaich contends that chronic lower back pain usually stems from a preexisting weakness. At a minimum, he advises chiropractic treatment every three to six months, although many people benefit from more frequent visits to maintain proper alignment and safeguard against injury to intervertebral disks. The frequency of visits depends on a myriad of predisposing factors,

ALTERNATIVE TREATMENTS FOR SCOLIOSIS

Mainstream approaches to scoliosis, may include many uncomfortable and even dangerous procedures. First, there is little if any preventative aspect available. The protocol calls for monitoring the patient (usually a pre-adolescent or adolescent female) every few months to ascertain if the scoliosis is going to be progressive. If it progresses, then treatments include electrostimulation, exercises, large cumbersome braces, and surgery (everything from spinal fusion to installing rods along the spine to prevent further bending).

Chiropractors consider scoliosis fundamentally a result of misalignments (subluxations) of the spine that cause pressure on the nerves passing between the vertebrae. This in turn causes changes in the muscles along the sides of the spine; that is, it makes them tend to contract more on one side, which pulls the vertebrae to that side, creating the scoliosis.

Within chiropractic, there are many approaches to treating scoliosis, according to Tim Leasenby, D.C., of Aurora, Illinois. "There is a method called Chiropractic Bio Physics (CBP), where we analyze the postural distortions of the spine and correct them with a combined approach of spinal manipulations and exercises to correct the specific distortions found. There is a similar biomechanical method called the Pettibon technique (named after the founder Burl Pettibon), which corrects specific distortions that often include various types of scoliosis." The basic aim of nearly all chiropractic techniques is to reduce the vertebral misalignments, the nerve pressure, and restore normal muscle function in order to return to more optimal spinal architecture. "In many cases of scoliosis, there is an attempt to correct the abnormal curvature of the spine, but often the best outcome is an arrest of the progression of the curve," says Dr. Leasenby. "Even this is preferable to the more invasive mainstream procedures."

Scoliosis may also be treated with acupuncture. Traditional Chinese medicine sees the curvature of the spine as the result of a stagnation or obstruction of the *qi* (the vital energy of the body, which animates the muscles and moves the blood). This creates an imbalance on opposite sides of the spine, again resulting in muscle tightening with pulling of the vertebrae. The application of acupuncture needles (usually to points on each side of the spine) balances the *qi*, allowing the spinal muscles to work more evenly and restoring the spine's alignment. Sometimes electrical current is sent through the needles in order to increase the stimulation and the effect of the treatment.

Biomagnets can also be used as an adjunct to exercise, chiropractic, and acupuncture treatment. Placing the positive pole of the magnets on one side of the curve and the negative pole on the other side has been reported to help balance the muscle tone and relieve or arrest the scoliosis. (This procedure should only be done under the guidance of a qualified practitioner.)

"Whatever treatment is employed, early detection is very important," says Dr. Leasenby. "I have started on patients as young as nine years old with good results. Do not wait to see if a small curve will worsen—take steps to prevent it early and the outcome is much better."

---

including the condition of one's body and lifestyle. As Dr. Blaich puts it, "When you own a car, you wouldn't go 200,000 miles without getting your tires aligned. And if your tires were wearing out prematurely, you would replace the shock absorbers. With alignment, your tires will wear better. That is very similar to what we do in chiropractic as preventive maintenance for the back."

OSTEOPATHIC MEDICINE

By being able to combine methods from both covential and alternative medicine, osteopathic physicians (D.O.s) are in a unique position to help in the treatment of ailing backs. There is also a wide range of osteopathic manipulative approaches for back pain, notes Leon Chaitow, N.D., D.O., of London, England. This allows patients the opportunity to choose among different options in order to find the one most appropriate for their specific needs.

Osteopathic techniques can be used for both chronic and acute back pain, as well as for either joint or soft-tissue problems. The methodology ranges from gentle joint mobilization to specific thrust methods similar to those used in chiropractic. The difference between osteopathic and chiropractic methods lies in variations in basic concepts, as well as in the forms of manipulation most commonly used.

While some osteopaths may manipulate the spine and other joints of the body to relieve back pain and restore alignments, they are also licensed to give injections in order to relieve painful inflammation in the joints. Additionally, they may apply electrical stimulation and various forms of mechanical therapy in order to trigger muscle relaxation, including gentle "muscle energy" techniques, and functional and positional release techniques, all unique to osteopathic medicine.

BODYWORK

Bodywork includes all the various forms of massage, deep tissue techniques, energetic light touch, and movement awareness therapies that can be applied to the treatment of back pain. Because there is such a wide choice of techniques available, the patient is able to select the specific method (or methods) that will best meet their individual needs. Some of the more common forms of bodywork used for back pain and postural problems include Rolfing and Hellerwork. Both of these techniques involve the strenuous manipulation of the muscles, connective tissue, and joints in order to allow the body, muscles, and connective tissue to realign themselves.

Movement awareness therapies such as the Feldenkrais Method and the Alexander Technique have also proved effective for realigning and correcting posture. These methods use light touch as well as visualization and suggestion in order to reprogram the body's ingrained image of itself. By relearning proper posture and movement with these techniques, one is often able to greatly alleviate back pain. There are many other hands-on techniques that effectively treat back pain through energy healing, such as acupressure, *shiatsu*, and reflexology.

YOGA, TAI CHI, AND QIGONG

As well as being an excellent way to keep the body limber and in shape, yoga breathing exercises and postures, Tai Chi, and Qigong also have the potential to reduce much of the tension and stress that can contribute to back pain. A primary focus of these techniques is therapeutic relaxation through gentle exercise, stretching, and meditation. Teachers of these techniques believe that by focusing the mind inward, one is able to profoundly relax and revitalize the body and achieve a greater sense of harmony and well-being.

"When your attention is directed inward, your body receives messages that you are safe and secure and that it is appropriate to relax," explains Dr. Schatz. "So muscles relax, blood pressure drops, nerves are calmed, anxiety is decreased, immunity is heightened, and healing is enhanced."[11] All of these things can greatly improve the ability to deal with both the symptoms and causes of back pain. Likewise, a regular yoga, Tai Chi, or Qigong regimen can help to prevent back pain in the first place.

SELF-AWARENESS, SELF-HELP

The following exercise is a variation on a typical Feldenkrais exercise that can greatly benefit an aching back.

- Lie on your back and take a few deep breaths. Notice how your spine is resting on the floor. Do all the vertebrae touch or are there spaces between your back and the floor? Does one side of your back touch the floor differently than the other? Does one side feel heavier than the other?

- Bend both legs, putting your feet flat on the floor. Gently drop your knees to one side, noticing how far down they go. Bring them back to center and drop them once again to the same side, noticing any differences. Repeat this 25 times and then rest, stretching your legs out. How does your back touch the floor now? Does your breathing seem any different than before?

- Bend your legs and put your feet flat on the floor again and drop your knees toward the other side, noticing how far they go. How does this side compare to the other? Bring your legs back to center and rest. Now imagine doing this movement in the most relaxed and fluent manner. Do this in your mind ten times, and then actually bend your knees to that side. Is the movement easier and more full than before? Do this movement another 20 times, paying attention to how it makes your head move. When your legs drop, does your chin move toward or away from your chest? How does this movement affect your breathing?

- Now stretch your legs back out and rest, noticing how your back touches the floor. What differences do you notice in your breathing, neck, and head? Stand up and walk around slowly, noticing how your body moves and feels. Many people will notice surprising differences in their movement and posture. Indeed, some people find that their backs now lie completely flat on the floor for the first time in their lives, and those with chronic pain may find the problem completely alleviated from this simple five-minute exercise.

A LIFETIME OF PAIN IN THE BACK

Strongly held emotions, if unresolved, can eventually become fixated in the back and prevent the healing of back pain or successful recovery from back surgery. Physicians at the San Francisco Spine Institute, in Daly City, California, interviewed 86 patients (53 men, 33 women, with an average age of 41) who had undergone lower-back surgery. They found that if these patients had experienced three or more serious childhood psychological traumas, they had an 85% chance of not benefiting from back surgery.

Specifically, these traumas or risk factors included physical abuse from a primary caregiver, sexual abuse, alcohol or drug abuse in a parent or primary caregiver, abandonment, or emotional neglect and abuse (such as parents not being available for emotional support, overly criticizing or invalidating the child's emotional needs, or neglecting them). Even the existence of one risk factor reduced the likely success rate by 25%; when a patient had all five factors, the success rate was zero.

The researchers apparently failed to ask the critical question, namely, to what extent did the existence of these unresolved emotional traumas contribute to or create the back problem in the first place? But they urged doctors to assess "the pre-operative psychological status of a patient" before undertaking surgery. Metaphorically, the spine reflects how we hold ourselves in the world—self-image, if you like—and certainly children with serious abuse issues are likely to have a compromised self-image. Expressing this through the spine and back is, metaphorically again, logical.[12]

Prolotherapy

Prolotherapy, also known as regenerative therapy or sclerotherapy, is a technique that can dramatically reduce or eliminate back pain. The technique involves the injection of a proliferant such as dextrose (small quantity of dilute sugar water) with local anesthetic such as lidocaine into the area of pain in order to stimulate the body's natural healing processes via the production of collagen, which strengthens the weakened area and reduces pain.

One of the most prominent proponents of prolotherapy is former U.S. Surgeon General C. Everett Koop, M.D. When he was 40 years old, two separate neurological clinics diagnosed him as having incurable back pain, which radiated down his leg. His pain, however, was completely relieved by prolotherapy, which was basically unknown to modern medicine at the time. Because of his own healing, he used prolotherapy for the remaining 20 years that he practiced medicine.

"Although patients may have had back pain for several years, one to four prolotherapy treatments is often enough to relieve their pain," Dr. Darrow says. "If there is improvement after four treatments, the injections will be continued, usually to a maximum of eight times." One of Dr. Darrow's patients, noted football player Johnnie Morton, Jr., of the Detroit Lions, had back injuries and pain that persisted for ten years. "After only two prolotherapy treatments, he had his first pain-free season," Dr. Darrow reports.

Another of Dr. Darrow's patients was a 61-year-old retired U.C.L.A. emergency room nurse, who came to him with a 15-year history of low back pain. Prior to her first visit, she had spent the previous month in bed taking pain medications prescribed by her doctor, who referred her to Dr. Darrow as a last-resort effort to control her pain. When prolotherapy was explained to her, she said, "The idea that a series of dextrose injections could take away my pain and possibly keep it from reoccurring sounded like a fairy tale to me. To my surprise, I was pain free after the first injections and have remained that way." Prolotherapy is not limited to treating back pain or injuries, but is applicable to all musculoskeletal pain problems including arthritis and headaches, Dr. Darrow points out.

Mind/Body Medicine

According to Dr. Bresler, the connection between mind and body is well established in the rapidly developing field of psychoneuroimmunology (PNI), the study of the interaction among emotions, the nervous system, and the immune system. In applying this perspective to healing, Dr. Bresler uses a combination of guided imagery, relaxation, and biofeedback. In the case of treating back pain, his patients are encouraged to form an image about what's going on in their backs. "They give the pain a voice, asking it, 'What do you want? Why are you here? What do you have to offer?'" says Dr. Bresler. "The pain may indeed have something to offer, like not going to work or not having to make love to one's spouse. When we get an answer, we ask it if there's a way the patient can get what he or she needs without having a painful back. In this way, we honor the body's inner wisdom and intelligence."

Another technique that integrates the body and mind is biofeedback, which teaches how to consciously control heartbeat, respiration, muscle tension, and brain waves. By using this awareness, it is possible to learn how to consciously relax those muscles and improve blood flow to the tissues in the back that are causing one to experience pain.

 See Biofeedback Training and Neurotherapy, Energy Medicine, Mind/Body Medicine, Neural Therapy, Prolotherapy, Qigong and Tai Chi, Yoga.

Melvyn Werbach, M.D., past Director of the Biofeedback Medical Clinic, in Tarzana, California, tells of a mother of two infants who was suffering from chronic back pain. "She had gone through two failed spinal fusions and lifting two babies put her in agony. We used Biofeedback-Assisted Relaxation Training (BART) and it was very successful, far more so than the surgery. Most of the pain disappeared and the rest she was able to control. Several years later, her back pain was still under control." BART seems to affect the immune system and other functions, adds Dr. Werbach, and it can lower the perception of pain. Biofeedback can also affect secondary muscle spasms and thereby reduce muscle tension, which is often the primary cause of pain.

Dr. Darrow teaches his patients that back pain may be a way of handling other uncomfortable issues. "Why is it that, a generation ago, many patients were hospitalized with gastric ulcers and instead, today, we find an epidemic of back pain?" he says. "Back pain may be from subtle or overt emotional, mental, unconscious, or spiritual issues that can rapidly disappear once they are properly dealt with and resolved."

Energy Medicine

Energy medicine techniques such as ultrasound have been used to treat back pain. "Ultrasound helps to break up local edema as well as local fibrosis where there's been inflammation," states Dr. Lewis. "Also, if there has been an injury and some kind of scarring between the muscle layers, the ultrasound can break that up to a certain extent. It will also warm the tissues, which helps to relax the muscles. It can reduce the nerve conduction velocities, which means that the rate at which a pain impulse travels along a nerve pathway to the brain is slowed down, causing a pain-relieving effect."

Energy devices such as the TENS unit (Transcutaneous Electrical Nerve Stimulator) are also used for the relief of back pain. The TENS, which can be used at home, works by applying a small electrical current to the affected nerves in the area of the back pain, causing conduction to be blocked and pain to be relieved. TENS units and other similar energy devices are also believed to stimulate the production of endorphins, the body's own natural painkillers. Microcurrent electrical stimulators such as the Alpha-Stim and Micro-Stim may be

---

HIGH-TECH REJUVENATION OF THE BACK AND NECK

MedX machines are unique, computerized back- and neck-strengthening devices that have been widely studied in the university setting. They were developed by Arthur Jones, the inventor of Nautilus exercise equipment. A three-minute MedX workout twice a week for several weeks can alleviate back pain and prevent back injuries, and a recent study indicates that the MedX might even help avoid back surgery. In the study, 60 patients who were surgical candidates did resistive extension exercise on the MedX; of the 46 participants who completed the program, only three required surgery.[13]

The MedX works by strengthening the musculature of the back and increasing its range of motion, both of which have been found to decrease back pain. While exercising the lower back, the MedX restraints inhibit the use of the pelvis and legs. "This is key, since the major extensors of the back are the buttocks muscles and hamstring muscles," says Marc Darrow, M.D., Los Angeles, California. "The muscles surrounding the vertebrae are usually weak even when the gluteus and hamstring muscles are strong. Once these muscles are strengthened and range of motion is increased with MedX, pain diminishes."

A case history involving tennis pro Jim Pugh illustrates the benefits that MedX can provide. Pugh came to Jason Kelberman, D.C., one of Dr. Darrow's colleagues, suffering from low-back pain that had plagued him for three months, leaving him unable to play or teach tennis. Dr. Kelberman determined that his restricted range of motion and diminished strength were consistent with degenerative disc syndrome. After only three sessions of chiropractic adjustments, Dr. Kelberman was able to significantly reduce Pugh's pain, at which point he had Pugh begin a strengthening program using the MedX. The result was that Pugh's strength quickly improved and he was able to again play tennis at competitive levels.

---

more effective for long-term use than the standard amperage TENS units.

Back pain can be helped by using infrared light or soft (cold) laser devices either on the back or on acupuncture points related to the back. Also, devices like the Light Beam Generator that photomagnetically break up the congestion in the lymph vessels of the back, abdomen, and pelvis can dramatically improve back pain, especially if used in conjunction with manual lymph drainage, dry skin brushing, or rebounding exercise.

Acupuncture and Traditional Chinese Medicine

"Many studies have shown the effectiveness of acupuncture for treating back pain," states Dr. Bresler. "At U.C.L.A., we researched the different styles of acupuncture, comparing Korean, Vietnamese, Japanese, Chinese, and American acupuncturists, and found them equally effective." Dr. Ni adds that traditional Chinese medicine recognizes that psychophysiological problems can also trigger back pain and that "acupuncture works to release the stress that has been internalized into the body."

Back pain that is the result of pinched nerves can be treated through acupuncture, which helps to restore the flow of blood and energy that is needed to bring essential healing nutrients, such as calcium and magnesium, to the injured back. "Acupuncture can also relax muscle spasms or strengthen weak back muscles," states Dr. Ni.

For back pain, Eugene Kozhevnikov, M.D., O.M.D., of St. Petersburg, Russia, uses acupuncture both to relax muscles and to release muscle contractions caused by related damaged organs. Dr. Kozhevnikov claims that 90% of herniated disc cases should be treated with acupuncture first rather than undergoing surgery. His treatment involves electroacupuncture, physical manipulation, and various energy medicine devices.

Naturopathic Medicine

Naturopathic physicians are especially well-equipped to treat back pain, because they are able to provide nutritional support for strengthening and repairing the tissues, herbs, homeopathic remedies, and hydrotherapy for relieving inflammation, as well as soft tissue and joint manipulation for correcting postural dysfunction. Dr. Lewis also counsels his patients on a variety of home therapies for relieving back pain, including slant boards, inversion boots for hanging upside down, and back swings. "All these devices apply some sort of traction to the tissues in the back," Dr. Lewis says, "and that can be very helpful."

Another important tool is shoe lifts for correcting any anatomical leg-length problems. "I tend to be very aggressive about using shoe lifts, especially if the patient is young," says Dr. Lewis, "and I rarely find that they produce any negative response for the patient. They may be sore as their body adapts to the change, but in almost all cases I find it very, very positive." Orthotics, which help to correct flat-footedness plus other inversions and eversions of the foot, are also helpful for back pain, as they correct and balance the foot, which is the foundation of all good posture, according to Dr. Lewis.

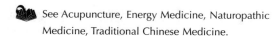 See Acupuncture, Energy Medicine, Naturopathic Medicine, Traditional Chinese Medicine.

NUTRITIONAL SUPPLEMENTS AND HERBS FOR BACK PAIN

Since bone is composed of protein, collagen, and minerals, and muscle fiber is mainly protein with large quantities of minerals comprising the fluid inside muscle, it is logical that nutritional deficiencies in these basic building blocks will compromise the health and function of both bone and muscle. The implications for back pain are obvious. When deficiencies are contributing to your back pain, nutritional supplements are an essential treatment component.

- For acute and chronic back pain: Willow bark, feverfew, rosemary, and the enzyme protease are useful to ease inflammation. For additional support, include a multivitamin, multimineral, amino acid complex, and eicosapentaenoic acid (EPA) from fish oil.

- For degenerated cartilage (osteoarthritis): Glucosamine sulfate and glucosamine HCL are the building blocks of cartilage and connective tissue, which maintain strong and flexible joints.[14] Other useful supplements and herbs include N-acetyl-glucosamine, bovine and shark cartilage, EPA, and antioxidants such as pycnogenol, coenzyme Q10, devil's claw, cat's claw, yucca root, and vitamins C and E. "Vitamin C and bioflavonoids are extremely important for strengthening the connective tissues, especially in smokers who have depleted their vitamin C resources," says Dr. Lewis. He recommends taking 2,000-3,000 mg of each daily, in divided doses throughout the day.

- For acute and chronic muscle spasm: Calcium, magnesium, and potassium supplements, as well as lobelia herb or homeopathic topical creams containing calendula, arnica, and ivy extracts can relieve spasm. "Calcium-magnesium supplements should be taken for muscle relaxation, particularly in instances where there's muscle spasm and twitching," Dr. Lewis adds. He recommends 500 mg of a calcium-magnesium supplement daily, preferably in a citrate form, because it allows for much better absorption.

- For acute and chronic inflammation: Protease enzymes (if no ulcer or gastritis is present), bromelain (enzyme compound from pineapple), mucopolysaccharides (such as bovine and shark cartilage), EPA, evening primrose oil, and the herbs yucca root, *Boswellia serrata,* and wild yam can help ease inflammation.

Recommendations

- Because many cases of back pain are muscular in origin, the pain usually occurs as a result of the way a person uses, or misuses, his or her body. Most back pain can be avoided by taking the simple preventative step of staying in good physical condition.

- Physical manipulation techniques aim to move the various parts of the back—muscles, connective tissues, and vertebrae—into proper functional alignment and can often correct serious problems relating to stress and physical pain. Options include chiropractic, osteopathic medicine, and bodywork therapies.

- As well as being an excellent way to keep the body limber and in shape, yoga breathing exercises and postures, Tai Chi, or Qigong have the potential to reduce much of the tension and stress that can contribute to back pain.

- Prolotherapy, also known as regenerative therapy or sclerotherapy, is a technique that can dramatically reduce or eliminate back pain.

- Mind/body techniques such as guided imagery and biofeedback may be helpful for relieving back pain.

- Energy medicine techniques, such as ultrasound, the TENS unit, microcurrent stimulators, soft lasers, and infrared lights, have been used successfully to treat back pain.

- Many studies have shown the effectiveness of acupuncture or acupressure for treating back pain.

- Naturopathic physicians are especially well-equipped to treat back pain because they are able to provide nutritional support for strengthening and repairing the tissues, herbal and homeopathic remedies and hydrotherapy for relieving inflammation, as well as soft tissue and joint manipulation for correcting postural dysfunction.

Self-Care

The following therapies can be undertaken at home under the guidance of a physician:

Fasting / Guided Imagery / Qigong and Tai Chi / Yoga

ICE: AN IMMEDIATE HOME REMEDY

For years, the standard prescription for any pain was aspirin, a heating pad, and plenty of rest. Although these may have offered minor relief, today most doctors and health practitioners recommend a far more effective home remedy. "Ice is probably the most effective method for treating back pain, particularly acute cases," says David Bresler, Ph.D., L.Ac., of Los Angeles, California. This is especially true when there is swelling, heat, or redness surrounding the painful area. Ice allows the blood to reabsorb the fluids and chemicals that surround the injured area and is particularly effective during the first few days of treatment.

A standard treatment for back pain is to apply ice for ten minutes, then a hot water bottle (not an electric heating pad) for five minutes, then reapply ice, heat, and ice once more for the same amount of time. This can be repeated as often as needed throughout the day. However, if the swelling and pain continues consult a doctor immediately.

ACUPRESSURE: To relieve back pain, briskly rub the backs of your hands over acupoints B23 and B47 (for an illustration of these points, see the acupressure chart in the introduction to the Quick Reference A-Z Section) for one minute. If your back pain is up higher or in deeper, lie down on two tennis balls that are one inch apart wrapped in a towel or sock. Place the balls underneath the tightest parts of your back muscles as you breathe deeply for one minute. Then roll on to another area that is tight or painful and breathe deeply for another minute. Next, put the balls aside and firmly bring your knees into your chest several times with your head on the ground. Immediately afterward, cover yourself while on your back with your legs bent and feet flat on the floor, and deeply relax with your eyes closed for ten minutes. Repeat this two or three times daily to prevent and relieve back pain.

AROMATHERAPY: • For muscular fatigue, use lavender, marjoram, rosemary, clary sage. • For acute pain, use black pepper, ginger, birch.

AYURVEDA: *Kaishore guggulu* (200 mg), generally taken twice a day after lunch and dinner with warm water. *Dashamoola basti:* drink one pint *dashamoola* tea with ½ cup sesame oil three times a week and massage locally with *mahanarayan* oil.

HERBS: The cause of the pain must be identified before appropriate herbs can be prescribed. For example, if related to physical strain or rheumatic problems, drink an infusion of meadowsweet three times a day and rub the area with lobelia and cramp bark. If associated with menstruation, combine equal parts of skullcap and cramp bark tinctures, taking one teaspoon as needed.

HOMEOPATHY: *Arsen alb., Arnica, Actea rac., Rhus tox., Calc fluor., Natrum mur., Ruta grav.* Consult a physician if pain persists.

HYDROTHERAPY: • Hot moist compresses (with water and hot apple cider vinegar) to affected area of back. Follow with alternating hot and cold percussion shower on painful area. • Apply ice to back for ten minutes, followed by five minutes with a hot water bottle; keep alternating ice and heat as needed between hydrotherapy sessions.

LIFESTYLE: In dealing with back pain, it is important to improve posture and to learn proper body use. Regular exercise, especially stretching, can dramatically decrease back discomfort.

Professional Care

The following therapies should only be provided by a qualified health professional:

Applied Kinesiology / Craniosacral Therapy / Environmental Medicine / Hypnotherapy / Neural Therapy

BODYWORK: Acupressure, massage, reflexology, Trager Approach.

DETOXIFICATION THERAPY: Detoxification is indicated, because back pain is often associated with congestive organs, stress, and referred pain. Bowel detoxification with modified juice fasts, herbs, and colonics and lymph detoxification with photomagnetic devices, manual lymphatic drainage, dry skin brushing, and rebounding can be very helpful for chronic back pain.

OXYGEN THERAPY: If pain is caused by injury, hyperbaric oxygen therapy may be helpful.

TRADITIONAL CHINESE MEDICINE: Cupping is an ancient Chinese therapy that helps to regulate the flow of energy and blood. Suction is usually created over the painful area on the body by introducing fire into a cup and placing the cup on the desired point. The amount of suction can be regulated according to the treatment and the age of the patient. Cupping is even more effective when used in conjunction with acupuncture and Chinese herbs.

Where to Find Help

For more information on, or referrals for, treatment of back pain, contact the following organizations:

Acupuncture

American Association of Oriental Medicine
433 Front Street
Catasauqua, Pennsylvania 18032
(888) 500-7999
Website: www.aaom.org

Biofeedback

Association for Applied Psychophysiology and Biofeedback
10200 West 44th Avenue, Suite 304
Wheat Ridge, Colorado 80033
(303) 422-8436
Website: www.aapb.org

Bodywork

North American Society of Teachers of the Alexander Technique
P.O. Box 3992
Champagne, Illinois 61826-3992
(217) 359-3529
Website: www.alexandertech.com

Feldenkrais Guild of North America
3611 S.W. Hood Avenue, Suite 100
Portland, Oregon 97201
(503) 221-6612
Website: www.feldenkrais.com

International Rolf Institute
205 Canyon Road
Boulder, Colorado 80306
(303) 449-5903
Website: www.rolf.org

Chiropractic

American Chiropractic Association
1701 Clarendon Boulevard
Arlington, Virginia 22209
(800) 986-4636
Websites: www.amerchiro.org, www.acatoday.com

International Chiropractors Association
1110 North Glebe Road, Suite 1000
Arlington, Virginia 22201
(703) 528-5000
Website: www.chiropractic.org

MedX

MedX Corporation
1401 Northeast 77th Street
Ocala, Florida 34479
(800) 876-6334
Website: www.medxinc.com

Manufacturer and supplier of MedX machines for the treatment of back pain.

Naturopathic Medicine

American Association of Naturopathic Physicians
8201 Greensboro Drive, Suite 300
McLean, Virginia 22101
(703) 610-9037
Website: www.naturopathic.org

Osteopathic Medicine

American Osteopathic Association
142 East Ontario Street
Chicago, Illinois 60611
(800) 621-1771
Websites: www.aoa-net.org and www.am-osteo-assn.org

Prolotherapy

American Association of Orthopedic Medicine
30897 C.R. 356-3, P.O. Box 4997
Buena Vista, Colorado 81211
(800) 992-2063
Website: www.aaomed.org

Joint Rehabilitation and Sports Medical Center
11645 Wilshire Blvd., 1st Floor
Los Angeles, California 90025
(310) 231-7000
Website: www.jointrehab.com

Marc Darrow, M.D., is the Medical Director of Joint Rehabilitation, which, in addition to prolotherapy, provides chiropractic and MedX computerized exercise equipment to heal back and neck pain.

Yoga

International Association of Yoga Therapists
109 Hillside Avenue
Mill Valley, California 94941
(415) 383-4587

Recommended Reading

The Alexander Technique. Wilfred Barlow. New York: Alfred A. Knopf, 1973.

Awareness Through Movement. Moshe Feldenkrais. New York: Harper and Row, 1972.

Back Care Basics: A Doctor's Gentle Yoga Program for Back and Neck Pain Relief. Mary Pullig Schatz, M.D. Berkeley, CA: Rodmell Press, 1992.

Free Yourself from Pain. David E. Bresler. Ph.D., LAC. Topanga, CA: The Bresler Center, 1992. (Available from: The Bresler Center, 10780 Santa Monica Blvd., Los Angeles, CA 90025; (310) 466-1717.)

Pain Erasure. Bonnie Prudden. New York: M. Evans, 1980.

Rolfing: The Integration of Human Structures. Ida Rolf. New York: Harper and Row, 1977.

Mind Over Back Pain. John Sarno, M.D. New York: Berkley Books, 1986.

Life Without Pain. Richard Linchitz, M.D. Reading, MA: Addison-Wesley, 1987.

CANCER

Despite years of research, with billions of dollars spent per year, the conventional medical establishment's "war on cancer" has been a dismal failure. Today, most people continue to equate cancer with death or, at the very least, an excruciating journey back to health filled with physical debilitation and pain. However, a variety of alternative therapies exist that have proven safer, gentler, and more effective at reversing and preventing cancer than standard conventional techniques.

CANCER IS A DISEASE in which certain cells in the body stop functioning and maturing properly. As the normal cycle of cell creation and death is interrupted, these newly "mutated" cancer cells begin multiplying uncontrollably, no longer operating as an integrated and harmonious part of the body. They also develop their own network of blood vessels to siphon nourishment away from the body's blood supply. This process, if unchecked, will eventually lead to the formation of a cancerous tumor. As the abnormal cells often migrate into and circulate within the bloodstream, the cancer can also spread to other parts of the body. This can cause the formation of more tumors and further sap the body's energy supply, weakening and eventually poisoning the patient with toxic by-products.

Each year, cancer claims the lives of more than half a million Americans, with over one million additional new cases being reported, and one out of every three persons develops cancer within their lifetime.[1] The figures are no less frightening for the rest of the world, as cancer rates continue to climb steadily, particularly among the industrialized nations.[2]

With cancer claiming so many lives each year, the search for a cure has become a global industry. Yet, as enticing as the idea of a "magic bullet" for cancer may seem, because of the multiple factors related to the disease, conventional medicine may never be able to offer the same sort of protection against cancer that it has been able to offer, for example, against polio and tetanus. "Despite some gains, cancer death rates remain unacceptably high, and the disease will kill 554,740 people in the U.S. this year," wrote J. Madeleine Nash in a special edition of *Time* magazine, in 1996 that summarized conventional cancer treatments.[3] Cancer now kills more children between the ages of 3 and 14 than any other illness.[4] Of greater concern is the fact that the numbers of both new cancer cases and

deaths continue to rise. From 1950 to 1980, there was an 8% increase in cancer deaths,[5] but from 1975 to 1989, the number of new cancer cases reported each year increased 13% and the mortality rate rose 7%.[6] Although mortality rates for a few less-common cancers declined, overall rates have continued to rise.[7]

According to John C. Bailar III, Ph.D., Professor of Epidemiology and Biostatistics at McGill University, in Toronto, Canada, conventional medicine is decidedly losing the war on cancer. In 1993, he declared: "In the end, any claim of major success against cancer must be reconciled with this figure," referring to the steady increase in cancer deaths between 1950 and 1990. "I do not think such reconciliation is possible and again conclude [as he had in 1986 when making a similar retrospective review of data] that our decades of war against cancer have been a qualified failure. Whatever we have been doing, it has not dealt with the broadly rising trend in mortality."[8]

Still, there is hope, with much of it coming today from the field of alternative medicine. In order to successfully treat cancer, all insults to the immune system and the rest of the body must be found, then dealt with in a multifactorial, holistic approach. This chapter will examine the most promising alternative therapies for the prevention and treatment of cancer. Because of the stranglehold that conventional medicine has had over the cancer debate, many of these therapies have been suppressed, despite their proven effectiveness. This chapter will also highlight stories of actual cancer survivors—men and women who have beaten the odds and returned to health using a variety of alternative medical methods.

Types of Cancer

In its simplest terms, cancer represents an accelerating process of inappropriate, uncontrolled cell growth—a chaotic process within the order of biology. Cancer cells, when examined under a microscope, are abnormally shaped, inconsistently formed, and disorganized and contain misshapen internal structures—the essence of biological disorder. Cancer, despite its horror for the individual, is a natural phenomenon: it represents the body's response to a continuous attack on its balancing and regulatory mechanisms by numerous factors.

Every cell in the body has the ability to turn cancerous, and many do so on a daily basis. Normally, the immune system is able to protect the body by destroying these cells or reprogramming them back to normal functioning. If the body's defense systems have been damaged, however, this process cannot happen, allowing the cancer to establish itself.[9] If the cancer cells do not spread beyond the tissue or organ where they originated, the cancer is considered localized. If the cancer spreads to other parts of the body, it is then said to have metastasized.

Every cell in the body has the ability to turn cancerous, and many do so on a daily basis.

Among the 150 different types of cancer, five major groups are conventionally recognized.

- Carcinomas form in the epithelial cells that cover the surface of the skin, mouth, nose, throat, lung airways, genitourinary tract, and gastrointestinal tract, or that line glands such as the breast or thyroid. Lung, breast, prostate, skin, stomach, and colon cancers are called carcinomas and are solid tumors.

- Sarcomas form in the bones and soft connective and supportive tissues surrounding organs and tissues, such as cartilage, muscles, tendons, fat, and the outer linings of the lungs, abdomen, heart, central nervous system, and blood vessels. Sarcomas are also solid tumors, but sarcomas are both the most rare of malignant tumors and the most deadly.

- Leukemia forms in the blood and bone marrow and the abnormal white blood cells travel through the bloodstream creating problems in the spleen and other tissues. Leukemias are not solid tumors; they are characterized by an overproduction of abnormal white blood cells.

- Lymphoma is cancer of the lymph glands. Lymph glands act as a filter for the body's impurities and are concentrated mostly in the neck, groin, armpits, spleen, the center of the chest, and around the intestines. Lymphomas are usually made up of abnormal lymphocytes (white blood cells) that congregate in lymph glands to produce solid masses. Hodgkin's disease (cancer growth characterized by progressive enlargement of the lymph nodes, spleen, and liver along with progessive anemia) and non-Hodgkin's lymphoma (lymphatic malignancies without the other Hodgkin's characteristics) are the two most prevalent types of lymphoma in the United States, while Burkitt's lymphoma, rare in the U.S., is common in central Africa.

- Myeloma is a rare tumor that arises in the antibody-producing plasma cells or hemopoietic (blood cell–producing) cells in the bone marrow.

A key characteristic of cancer cells is their greatly prolonged life span compared to that of normal cells. It's ironic, given that cancer can potentially prove fatal to its host and thus to itself as an unwelcome "parasite," that cancer cells are essentially immortal. Cancer cells do not die when they are supposed to and they also fail to develop the specialized functions of their normal counterparts. Masses of cancer cells may become like parasites, developing their own network of blood vessels to siphon nourishment away from the body's main blood supply. It is this process that, unchecked, will eventually lead to the formation of a tumor—a swelling caused by the abnormal growth of cells. If the tumor invades adjacent normal tissue or spreads through the lymphatic system or blood vessels to other normal tissues, this tumor is considered malignant.

The pathological character of such tumors stems from their cells' ability to invade other tissues and travel through the blood and lymphatic vessels to other areas of the body. Most cancer victims die not from the initial multiplication of these abnormal cells, but as a result of this secondary process, metastasis—the spread of cancer in the body. This process represents the cancer cells' tendency to break off from the original tumor, float in the bloodstream, and colonize other tissues.

Cancers that metastasize quickly—even when the total number of cancer cells is still small—are generally considered aggressive, which means more malignant. Aggressive tumors contain cells that are generally less "mature" from a cellular point of view; that is, they are less physically defined and lack some of a cell's standard components. It is often said of these cells that they are less well-developed or well-differentiated.

CANCER SYMPTOMS & STATISTICS

TYPE OF CANCER	POSSIBLE SYMPTOMS	POSSIBLE RISKS	5-YEAR SURVIVAL RATES	ESTIMATED # OF NEW U.S. CASES
	If these occur, see your physician for a physical exam and/or lab tests.		(ALL STAGES) PER CONVENTIONAL TREATMENT	PER YEAR
Bladder cancer	Blood in urine, making it look bright red or rust-colored; pain or burning upon urination; frequent urination; feeling the need to urinate but nothing comes out; urine may appear cloudy because it contains pus.	*Twice as high in whites as in blacks; 2-3 times higher in men as in women; 2-3 times higher in cigarette smokers as in nonsmokers; machinists, truck drivers, and workers exposed to chemicals*	80.7%	52,900
Breast cancer	A lump or thickening of breast; discharge from the nipple; retraction of the nipple; change in skin of breast, such as dimpling or puckering; redness, swelling, feeling of heat; enlarged lymph nodes under arm.	*Increasing age; early menstruation; late menopause; not having a child or having first child after 30; family or personal history; inherited breast cancer gene*	83.2%	185,700
Colorectal cancer	Rectal bleeding (red blood in stools or black stools); abdominal cramps; constipation alternating with diarrhea; weight loss; loss of appetite; weakness; pallid complexion.	*Polyps, ulcerative colitis, or Crohn's disease; family history; residence in urban or industrial area; specific genetic mutations*	61%	133,500
Kidney cancer	Blood in urine; dull ache or pain in back or side; lump in kidney area; sometimes accompanied by high blood pressure or abnormality in red blood cell count.	*Being overweight; twice as high in men as in women; twice as high in cigarette smokers as in nonsmokers; coke-oven and asbestos workers*	57.9%	30,600
Leukemia	Weakness, paleness; fever and flu-like symptoms; bruising and prolonged bleeding; enlarged lymph nodes, spleen, liver; pain in bones and joints; frequent infections; weight loss; night sweats.	*Specific genetic abnormalities (Down and Bloom syndromes); excessive exposure to ionizing radiation and chemicals such as benzene; HIV-1 virus exposure*	68.6%	27,600
Lung cancer	Wheezing "smoker's cough," persisting for months or years; increased, sometimes blood-streaked, sputum; persistent ache in chest; congestion in lungs; enlarged lymph nodes in the neck.	*Cigarette smoking; secondary smoke; asbestos, radiation, radon, or other toxic exposure*	13.4%	177,000
Melanoma	Change in a mole or other bump on the skin including bleeding, or change in size, shape, color, or texture.	*Sun exposure, particularly during childhood; sunburning or freckling easily; 40 times higher in whites than blacks*	86.6%	38,300
Non-Hodgkin's lymphoma	Painless swelling in the lymph nodes of the neck, underarm, or groin; persistent fever; feeling of fatigue; unexplained weight loss of more than 10% in a 6-month period; itchy skin and rashes; small lumps in skin; bone pain; swelling in some part of abdomen; liver and spleen enlargement.	*Lowered immune system function as with the HIV virus; recipients of organ transplants; possibly exposure to herbicides*	51%	52,700
Oral cancer (oral cavity, lip, pharynx)	May often feel a lump in the mouth with the tongue; sometimes a sore spot can be felt while eating or drinking; ulceration of the lips, tongue, or other area inside the mouth that does not heal within two weeks; dentures may no longer fit well; in advanced cases, oral pain, bleeding, foul breath, loose teeth, and changes in speech.	*More prominent in males, with predisposing factors including tobacco and pipe smoking and chewing tobacco; radiation and other toxic exposures*	Not available	28,150
Ovarian cancer	Frequently, few symptoms; abdominal swelling; in rare cases, abnormal vaginal bleeding; women over 40 may experience generalized digestive discomfort.	*Increasing age; never pregnant; residence in industrial country (Japan excluded); family history of breast or ovarian cancer; inherited breast cancer gene*	44.1%	26,700
Pancreatic cancer	Upper abdominal pain and unexplained weight loss; pain near the center of the back; loss of appetite; intolerance of fatty foods; yellowing of the skin (jaundice); abdominal masses; enlargement of liver and spleen.	*Increasing age; cigarette smoking; higher in countries with high-fat diets; higher in blacks than whites*	3.6%	26,300

CANCER SYMPTOMS & STATISTICS

TYPE OF CANCER	POSSIBLE SYMPTOMS	POSSIBLE RISKS	5-YEAR SURVIVAL RATES	ESTIMATED # OF NEW U.S. CASES
	If these occur, see your physician for a physical exam and/or lab tests.		**(ALL STAGES) PER CONVENTIONAL TREATMENT**	**PER YEAR**
Prostate cancer	Urination difficulties due to blockage of the urethra; bladder retains urine, creating frequent feelings of urgency to urinate, especially at night; may have difficulty stopping urination; urine stream may be narrow; bladder doesn't empty completely; burning, painful urination; sometimes bloody urine; tenderness over the bladder and dull ache in the pelvis and back.	*Increasing age; 37% higher in blacks than whites, with twice the mortality rate*	85.8%	317,100
Uterine cancer	Abnormal vaginal bleeding of fresh blood, or a watery bloody discharge in a postmenopausal woman (70%-75% of all cases are postmenopausal); a collection of fluid may also occur in the uterus; painful urination; pain during intercourse; pain in pelvic area.	*Cervical: cigarette smoking; sex before 18; many sexual partners; low socioeconomic status; mortality rate twice as high for blacks as whites* *Endometrial: Early menstruation; late menopause; never pregnant; estrogen exposure, estrogen replacement therapy without progesterone; Tamoxifen; diabetes, gallbladder disease, hypertension, and obesity*	68.3%	49,700

Once metastasis has occurred, cancer is more likely to be fatal, unless checked or reversed by successful multimodal alternative therapies. Metastasis can lead to the formation of more tumors, which further sap the body's energy supply, weakening (and eventually poisoning) the patient with toxins that make one feel fatigued, aching, depressed, and apathetic. Eventually, the unchecked growth overwhelms other body functions. Whatever the immediate cause, the cancer-related death is usually preceded by metastasis and by the establishment of "secondary cancers" that grow as a result of metastasis from the primary tumor site.

Many if not most cancer deaths come as a result of infection by bacteria, viruses, and fungi—microbes that normally would be destroyed by the immune system. In the case of cancer, the immune system becomes severely suppressed, partly because of the systemic weakening brought on by the cancer process and partly because of the negative, toxic effects of conventional cancer treatment—chemotherapy, surgery, and radiation.

Causes of Cancer

As much as science strives to identify single precipitating factors, such as genes or infectious organisms, practitioners of alternative medicine know there is no single cause for cancer, just as there is no single "magic bullet" therapy or substance to end it. Many interdependent factors contribute to the development of cancer. Each type of cancer can be caused by a variety of factors, ranging from air pollution and tobacco smoke, to environmental radiation and industrial chemicals such as asbestos, benzene, and vinyl chloride, to naturally occurring substances such as aflatoxins (toxins produced by fungus commonly found in peanuts, corn, milk, and other foods), as well as the body's own production of free radicals.

Though the causes of cancer are still being debated, science is much closer today to understanding the fundamental factors involved in the process. For some time it has been clear that tumors arise as a result of a series of changes or rearrangements of information coded in the DNA within single cells.[10] Scientists also believe that cancers are generated in two steps, initiation and promotion.

Factors that start the initiation process are called initiators, or triggers. They interact directly with the cellular DNA to start the cell damage process. Initiators can take the form of carcinogens (cancer-causing substances), such as tobacco smoke, environmental pollution, pesticides, heavy metals, and industrial chemicals, as well as specific viruses, radiation, free radicals, and hormones, particularly estrogens.[11]

Initiation of a cancer cell can occur in various ways. For example, low-fiber diets may prolong the residence time of body wastes in the gut, leading to greater exposure of the intestinal lining to cancer-causing agents. A breakdown of metabolic function can also lead to initiation when enzymes, which normally deactivate cancer-

STAGING IN CANCER

In terms of tumor size and severity, oncologists (physicians who specifically treat cancer) distinguish four different phases, which they call stages. Staging refers to an index used by cancer specialists to determine how much cancer exists in the body, its size, location, and containment or metastasis. Stage I, the earliest, most curable stage, shows only local tumor involvement. Stage II has some spreading of cancer to the surrounding tissues and perhaps to nearby lymph nodes. Stage III involves metastasis to distant lymph nodes. Stage IV, the most advanced and least easily cured, refers to cancer that has spread to distant organs.

causing substances, start to function improperly. This causes them to activate the carcinogens instead, allowing the carcinogens to react directly with cellular DNA.[12] In other cases, cellular replication may be so accelerated that cells reproduce too quickly, leaving little or no time for repair. This allows defects in the DNA to become imbedded into the genetic materials passed from one cellular generation to the next as a permanent mutation. DNA repair may also be interrupted by initiators. For example, toxic metals such as lead, mercury, and cadmium can prevent DNA from being repaired.[13]

After the initiation of the cancer process, the disease will often lie undetected for many years, according to the American Institute for Cancer Research.[14] Factors that facilitate the disease process during this latent period are called promoters. While promoters do not directly interact with the cellular DNA, they can further the cellular damage, allowing cancer cells to continue spreading abnormally. Promoters may also hamper the removal of initiated cells by damaging the body's defense systems, particularly the immune system. Lastly, promoters can alter certain tissues of the body in order to make them more favorable for tumor growth. This is usually accomplished by enhancing the conditions for establishing the blood supply necessary for the tumor cells.

The probability is that if a person gets enough exposure to carcinogens, tumors can and will develop even if the immune system is fairly healthy. This is due to the concept of the total body burden—that is, the sum of all factors taxing the immune system including the cancer cells themselves. A tumor or leukemia develops when there is either an increased production of cancer cells because of excess initiators or facilitators (causes) or a decreased removal of cancer cells from the body because of clogged lymphatic drainage or weakened immunity.

The following are among the most common factors associated with the initiation and promotion of cancer.

Sunlight

Solar radiation, particularly ultraviolet-B and ultraviolet-C radiation, is a common carcinogen, accounting for over 400,000 of the overall one million new cases of skin cancer occurring annually in the U.S. Today, even more ultraviolet radiation is present in sunlight because the ozone hole in the upper atmosphere has expanded, weakening the Earth's natural shield against it.

Chronic Electromagnetic Field Exposure

According to an Environmental Protection Agency study, there is growing evidence of a link between exposure to electromagnetic fields (EMFs)—which are generated by electrical currents—and cancer.[15] While EMFs are part of nature and, in fact, are radiated by the human body, the quality and intensity of the energy can either support or destroy health. As a rule, EMFs generated by technological devices or installations tend to be much more harmful than naturally occurring EMFs. We are surrounded by EMFs, produced by electrical wiring in homes and offices, televisions, computers, cell phones, electric blankets, microwave ovens, overhead lights, and electrical power lines. EMFs affect enzymes related to growth regulation, gene expression, and cell division and multiplication—all of which can exert a major influence on tumor growth.[16]

Geopathic Stress

Magnetic radiation from the Earth, presumably connected with geological fractures and subterranean water veins, has been associated with an increased risk of cancer, especially in communities where these geopathic, or pathogenic, influences are more prevalent. According to some experts, the cause of geopathic stress may be localized magnetic anomalies—unusual, sudden changes and magnetic quirks that can upset delicate human physiological balance and thereby create health problems. In 1971, the theory of geopathic stress was supported by research showing that water flowing underground, especially subterranean streams that cross one another, produces measurable increases in magnetic anomalies; these conditions also increase electrical conductivity in the air and soil. While the changes are small, they are still capable of contributing to the development of serious illness, including cancer. One large-scale study by the U.S. government reported that geopathic stress may be a factor in between 40% and 50% of all human cancers and account for between 60% and 90% of all cancers attributed to environmental radiation.[17]

Sick Building Syndrome

In the early 1980s, physicians began using the term *sick building syndrome* (SBS) to refer to a host of symptoms produced by low-grade toxic environmental conditions found in living or office spaces. SBS symptoms are numerous: mucous membrane irritation of the eyes, nose, and throat, chest tightness, skin complaints, headaches, fatigue and lethargy, coughing, asthma, wheezing, chronic nasal stuffiness, temporary weight loss, infections, and emotional irritability. All of these depress the immune system, rendering the individual susceptible to long-term chronic illness and potentially to a cancer process.

"Environmental toxicity is one of the most important areas of cancer causation and cancer prevention and it is yet to receive adequate recognition from the cancer research establishment," states Samuel Epstein, M.D., Professor of Occupational and Environmental Medicine at the University of Illinois School of Public Health. "Neither the National Cancer Institute nor the American Cancer Society has ever given scientific testimony before Congress or any regulatory agency on the importance of avoiding exposure to toxic chemicals." This, despite significant evidence that environmental carcinogens in the home and the workplace are one of the primary causes of cancer. In most cases, problems with a building's engineering, construction, or ventilation system are the causes. Other sources of indoor toxic pollution include volatile organic compounds released by particleboard desks, furniture, carpets, glues, paints, office machine toners, and perfumes. In addition, the carcinogenic effects of certain indoor air pollutants, such as asbestos, environmental tobacco smoke, radon, and formaldehyde, are well described in the clinical literature and are now considered cancer risk factors. The EPA estimates that indoor radon pollution may cause as many as 10,000 cancers a year in the U.S.[18]

Ionizing Radiation

Ionizing radiation consists of high-energy rays that are capable of ripping the electrons from matter, causing genetic mutations that can lead to cancer. This is the type of radiation used in X-ray technology, which may explain why radiologists, who take many X rays each day, have historically had a higher incidence of cancer, as have other workers exposed to low-dose radiation.[19] In fact, medical X rays may cause about 75% of breast cancer.[20] In addition to medical X rays, ionizing radiation also emanates from such common household items as fluorescent lights, computer monitors, and television screens.

Nuclear Radiation

Working or living in the proximity of nuclear power plants presents a cancer risk. Among the hazards are the

---

33 FACTORS THAT CONTRIBUTE TO CANCER

- Sunlight
- Chronic Electromagnetic Field Exposure
- Geopathic Stress
- Sick Building Syndrome
- Ionizing Radiation
- Nuclear Radiation
- Industrial Toxins
- Pesticide/Herbicide Residues
- Polluted Water
- Chlorinated Water
- Fluoridated Water
- Tobacco and Smoking
- Hormone Therapies
- Immune-Suppressive Drugs
- Irradiated Foods
- Food Additives
- Mercury Toxicity
- Dental Factors
- Nerve Interference Fields
- Diet and Nutritional Deficiencies
- Chronic Stress
- Toxic Emotions
- Depressed Thyroid Action
- Intestinal Toxicity and Digestive Impairment
- Parasites
- Viruses
- Free Radicals
- Blocked Detoxification Pathways
- Cellular Oxygen Deficiency
- Cellular Terrain
- Oncogenes
- Genetic Predisposition
- Miasm

---

small amounts of radioactive gases released daily from nuclear reactors. Although these radioactive gas emissions enter the atmosphere at levels deemed "permissible" by the U.S. Department of Energy, evidence suggests that low-level radioactive pollution may pose a significant cancer risk. In England, a higher rate of leukemia has been reported in children living near a nuclear facility. The incidence of childhood thyroid cancer has increased 100 times in those areas of Ukraine, Belarus, and Russia most acutely exposed to the Chernobyl nuclear accident in April 1986, according to a United Nations report. The dangers of nuclear radiation are not limited to those who work in or live close to a reactor, however. Low-level radioactive pollution returns in

NUCLEAR REACTORS AND CANCER

Nuclear reactors directly cause a significant increase in the incidence of cancer, especially childhood cancers, according to data gathered through the efforts of Jay Gould, Ph.D., Ernest Sternglass, Ph.D., and their colleagues at the Radiation and Public Health Project (RPHP), in Miami Beach, Florida, and New York City. Radiation is an extremely potent carcinogen and the more radiation people are exposed to, the greater their likelihood of developing cancer. The effects of radiation exposure are cumulative: a low level of exposure over time does the same—or worse—damage than one large dose. Additionally, nuclear reactors release over 20 radioactive substances into our environment, which are continually reported to the Nuclear Regulatory Commission (NRC).

The incidence of cancer has increased from the beginning of the 20th century, when it struck 3% of the population, to the present day, when 50% of men and 40% of women are expected to develop it. Cancer used to be the tenth leading cause of death in children—it is now second. To conclusively prove that nuclear reactors are contributing to this increase, it is necessary to show that: (1) cancer increased in populations that were most exposed to radiation from reactors and that the increase was proportional to their exposure; and (2) increased amounts of radioactive substances that could only have come from nuclear reactors were found in their bodies.

This is what the scientists at the RPHP were able to demonstrate. First, they gathered data on specific nuclear reactors and how much radioactive contamination was found in the environment. They also compiled the health statistics of the population living in the area, correlated them to the environmental contamination, and compared them to the nation as a whole. They found a unique way to precisely measure the amount of radiation, specifically of strontium-90, within the bodies of affected populations—by collecting thousands of shed baby teeth through the "Tooth Fairy" Project.

Strontium-90 (Sr-90) was chosen because it is produced only through the nuclear fission in the explosion of nuclear weapons and in the operation of nuclear reactors. Sr-90 is an insidious radioactive carcinogen because it binds to calcium in the body and is stored in the bones (and, thus, also in teeth). Sr-90 affects the bone marrow where immune cells are formed, making it an especially high risk factor for all cancers. Although the NRC currently measures the amounts of 20 radioactive substances in the environment, it discontinued the monitoring of Sr-90 in 1982, three years after the Three Mile Island accident.

The RPHP focused on Suffolk County, a 922-square-mile area making up the eastern part of Long Island, in New York, with a population of over 1.3 million. Suffolk County is in proximity to three nuclear power facilities plus a nuclear research facility, the Brookhaven National Laboratory. Highlights of the RPHP report include:

- From 1970-1993, the Indian Point, Millstone, and Oyster Creek reactors released nine times more radioactivity than was released during the Three Mile Island accident.

- From the early 1980s to the mid-1990s, concentrations of radioactive Sr-90 in about 500 Suffolk County baby teeth tested by RPHP rose 40%.

- From the early 1980s to the mid-1990s, cancer incidence in children under age 10 rose 49% in Suffolk County compared to a 12% rise in the U.S.

- In the same period, cancer incidence for young adults in Suffolk County (ages 25 to 44) rose 23% vs. 4% in the U.S.

- An area of northwestern Suffolk County with the highest Sr-90 concentration has a disproportionately large number of rare childhood cancer cases.

These statistics clearly indicate that nuclear reactors are a direct cause of increased childhood cancer. How could the nuclear power industry design, and the government allow to be built, facilities that create such drastic health problems? The answer lies partially in the fact that the effects of low-level radiation were not known in the late 1950s at the beginning of the nuclear power industry. The standard allowable exposure of Sr-90 was set at 1,000 picocuries (per gram of calcium). This was the amount considered "safe" for adults, but it apparently didn't occur to anyone that children were more vulnerable than adults. It is now known that if a newborn infant has an exposure of only 0.8 picocuries of Sr-90, the risk of developing cancer is doubled.

NUCLEAR REACTORS AND CANCER, continued

Can future nuclear power plants be designed to release only 0.001% of the 1957 standards that reactors were designed to meet? There is no foreseeable technology that would bring radioactive contamination anywhere near this level. Current goals are for reactors to limit their discharge of Sr-90 to 3-4 picocuries—still several times the amount proven to cause cancer.

In general, those who live within 50-100 miles of nuclear reactors have the highest levels of exposure and are the most at risk to develop cancer. They inhale it from the air that they breathe and ingest it in the water they drink. But people living hundreds or even thousands of miles away can also be significantly affected. Ninety percent of radiation is spread by precipitation; that is, nuclear plants release radioactivity into the atmosphere and it returns to earth with rainfall. Plus, radioactive toxins get more concentrated as they move up the food chain. Crops absorb radioactive substances from contaminated air, soil, and water, then animals that eat these crops accumulate even higher concentrations. Sr-90 binds to calcium in cows as well as in humans, therefore it gets concentrated in dairy products. Everyone now contains detectable levels of Sr-90 in their bodies.

Laboratory testing can determine the level of exposure and electrodermal screening can ascertain what organs and biological functions are affected. There are a number of modalities that can help eliminate Sr-90 from the body, including oral and intravenous chelation therapy, nutritional supplement regimens that help the body detoxify at the cellular level, and specific protocols targeting the renewal of bones. Certain herbal and homeopathic remedies that assist liver and kidney detoxification can also be used.

rainfall, which then accumulates in the soil to contaminate the food chain. The prime carriers for nuclear fission products are municipal water and air and, to a lesser extent, milk and dairy products.

Pesticide/Herbicide Residues

Clear evidence has linked long-term exposure to pesticides with cancer, leading a consortium of 75 Environmental Protection Agency experts to rank pesticide residues among the top three environmentally derived cancer risks. "Many cancer-causing pesticides and indus-

trial chemicals found in the environment and in our foods tend to accumulate in fatty tissues, whether in fish, cattle, fowl, or people," notes Dr. Epstein. "Although these chemicals for the most part have been banned or strictly regulated, they are very durable and remain in the environment for a long time. Crops grown in soil contaminated with these chemicals will pass on their residue to the animals that are fed them, where they will accumulate in the fatty tissue. If persons choose foods with the highest concentrations of these chemicals, then they too will build up higher and higher concentrations of the same chemicals in their own fatty tissue." This process is known as bioaccumulation and, according to Dr. Epstein, these fat-soluble carcinogens are found in highest concentrations in the body's fattiest tissues, such as the brain, sexual organs, and breasts.

> *Many cancer-causing pesticides and industrial chemicals found in the environment and in our foods tend to accumulate in fatty tissues, whether in fish, cattle, fowl, or people.*
> —SAMUEL EPSTEIN, M.D.

Unfortunately, the use of these poisons is not being curtailed; rather, it has increased tenfold since the introduction of DDT in the 1940s. In the past 50 years, 15,000 chemical compounds and more than 35,000 different formulations have come into use as pesticides and herbicides worldwide. Many of those banned in the U.S. (including DDT) are sold to Third World countries, where they enter food products, such as coffee, fruits, and vegetables, which are then imported into the U.S. In addition to agricultural uses, household and garden pesticides and herbicides represent another major source of toxicity.

Industrial Toxins

A great number of highly toxic chemicals, materials, and heavy metals are released by industrial processes. These toxins later find their way into human tissue, where they have negative health effects, including cancer. By 1980, the Environmental Protection Agency had detected over 400 toxic chemicals in human tissue. Some industrial by-products mimic the activity of estrogen once inside the body, creating havoc in hormonal balance; these estrogen-mimicking chemicals are believed to contribute to breast cancer.

In 1978, Israel banned toxic chemicals such as PCBs, which had been directly linked with breast cancer in a 1976 study.[21] Over the next ten years, the rate of breast cancer deaths in Israel declined sharply, with a 30% drop in mortality for women under 44 years of age and an 8% overall decline, despite an increase in other cancer risks such as dietary factors and alcohol consumption. Meanwhile, worldwide death rates from breast cancer had increased by 4%.[22]

Polluted Water

Polluted water can raise the risk of developing cancer—tap water from municipal sources is increasingly becoming a health hazard in the U.S. One out of every four public water systems has violated federal standards for tap water. It is not only pesticides and agricultural runoff that contaminate public drinking water: according to the Environmental Protection Agency, the tap water of 30 million Americans contains potentially dangerous levels of lead. Tap water can contain many contaminants, including radioactive particles, heavy metals (such as lead and copper), radon, gasoline solvents, industrial wastes, chemical residues, disinfectant by-products, and solid particulates such as asbestos.

 The established link between cancer and toxins in the home, workplace, and environment indicates the need for further research concerning the threat these toxins pose to overall health. To support the use of government funds for research in this field, write your elected representatives.

Chlorinated Water

Disinfecting drinking water with chlorine is standard practice throughout the U.S. While there is little doubt that adding chlorine-type compounds to drinking water protects the public from several kinds of harmful bacteria, chlorine can also form cancer-causing agents when it interacts with other compounds in drinking water. New evidence indicates that chlorinated water increases the risk of cancer for the roughly 200 million Americans who drink it. While the EPA tries to downplay the cancer risk from chlorinating drinking water by asserting that the known risk of water-borne disease in humans, if water is not disinfected, is much greater, a recent study conducted jointly by the Medical College of Wisconsin and Harvard University has found a definite link between chlorine and cancer. The study found that the consumption of chlorinated drinking water accounts for 15% of all rectal cancers and 9% of all bladder cancers in the U.S., or an additional 6,500 cases of rectal cancer and

4,200 cases of bladder cancer each year. Additionally, people drinking chlorinated water over long periods of time have a 38% increase in the chance of contracting rectal cancer and a 21% increase in the risk of contracting bladder cancer.[23]

The dangers from inhaling chlorine can exceed those derived from drinking chlorinated water. The amount of chloroform (the most common trihalomethane in chlorinated water) inhaled or absorbed through the skin during a typical shower may be six times higher than that absorbed from drinking chlorinated water for one day.

Fluoridated Water

Fluoride, a poison second in toxicity only to arsenic, has routinely been added to public drinking water and toothpaste since the 1950s, despite mounting evidence of its multiple health hazards. According to scientific research, fluoride in drinking water can produce cancer, transforming normal human cells into cancerous ones. The National Academy of Sciences has found that fluorine (a component of fluoride) slows DNA repair activity.[24]

 See Detoxification Therapy, Diet.

Tobacco and Smoking

About 30% of cancer deaths in the U.S. can be attributed to tobacco smoke, making it "the single most lethal carcinogen in the U.S.," according to researchers at the Harvard Center for Cancer Prevention, in Cambridge, Massachusetts.[25] Over 2,000 chemical compounds are generated by tobacco smoke and many of them are poisons.[26] Carbon monoxide is released during smoking, reducing the amount of oxygen to the brain, lungs, and heart. Nicotine is not only addictive but also acts as a cancer promoter, making it easier for cancer cells to spread throughout the body.[27] Tar, the leading cancer-causing chemical found in tobacco smoke, contains carcinogenic hydrocarbons and other toxic substances.[28]

 See Respiratory Conditions.

Hormone Therapies

Hormone therapies that increase the levels of estrogen relative to progesterone in women have been linked to some forms of cancer. In particular, prolonged use of oral contraceptives or hormone replacement therapy (HRT) for postmenopausal women have been associated with an increased risk of breast and endometrial cancer. Regarding oral contraceptives, one study indicated that women who took birth control pills for more than four years were twice as likely to develop breast cancer by age 50.[29]

Immune-Suppressive Drugs

The widespread, habitual, and chronic use of a great number of conventional drugs, antibiotics, and even vaccinations can have a seriously suppressive effect on the immune system, acting in concert with all the other factors to prepare the system for a cancer process. Drugs such as aspirin, acetaminophen, and ibuprofen taken for aches and colds, and glucocorticosteroids such as cortisone, decrease antibody production and suppress immune vitality. Antibiotics can directly hinder immune activity and increase the intestinal overgrowth of the yeast *Candida albicans,* which then can suppress the immune system. Research suggests that vaccinations can also suppress immune function.[30] Chemotherapy drugs used to stop cancerous growths have powerful immune-suppressive effects, rendering the individual even more susceptible to new, secondary cancers.

Irradiated Foods

The intent of food irradiation is to kill insects, bacteria, molds, and fungi and thus to extend shelf life, but the results might be dangerous to consumers. The process of irradiation leads to the formation of toxic substances, such as benzene and formaldehyde, and other chemical by-products that have been associated with cancer risk. For example, food irradiation may increase the levels of aflatoxin, a deadly carcinogen;[31] it may allow the botulinum toxin (which causes botulism food poisoning) to remain undetected in irradiated foods;[32] and, over time, it may induce some microorganisms to mutate, giving rise to new, dangerous species. When food additives and food contaminants are irradiated, they are transformed into "unique radiolytic products" of uncertain toxicity. The FDA estimates that 10% of the chemicals in irradiated foods are not found in normal (nonirradiated) foods and are unknown to science.[33]

Food Additives

Of the 3,000 chemical additives introduced into the American food supply each year, only a small fraction have been tested for their effects on humans (most are tested on animals). Among the most common are aspartame, saccharin, and cyclamates, artificial sweeteners that have been linked to a greater incidence of cancer; butylated hydroxytoluene, a food preservative that may contribute to liver cancer; and tannic acid, present in wines and fruits and linked to liver cancer. Other food additives that may increase the risk of certain kinds of cancer include Blue Dye No. 2, propyl gallate, and Red Dye No. 3.[34]

Mercury Toxicity

Mercury, a toxic heavy metal that often comprises up to 55% of "silver" amalgam dental fillings, is a noted carcinogen. Microscopic mercury is released into the body of the person with an amalgam filling every time the person chews. Like other heavy metals, mercury has been shown to cause damage to the lining of arteries and nerve bundles, thereby contributing to cancer. In addition, heavy metals act as free radicals—highly reactive, charged particles that can cause damage to body tissues if inhaled or absorbed. The International Academy of Oral Medicine and Toxicology (IAOMT) cites evidence indicating that dental mercury amalgams are a major contributor to immune dysfunction and free-radical pathologies, including cancer, kidney dysfunction, and cardiovascular disease.[35]

Dental Factors

Alternative medicine health practitioners familiar with the principles of biological dentistry have long noted a link between dental problems and degenerative illness. When a tooth is inflamed or infected or has a root canal in it, it can block the energy flow along one or more of the body's acupuncture meridians, causing the deterioration of a corresponding organ or tissue and, in time, leading to cancer. In effect, a problem in the tooth or tooth extraction socket can focus its energy imbalance elsewhere in the body, a phenomenon known as "dental focus." Dental factors may contribute to as many as 50% of all cancers.

 See Biological Dentistry, Energy Medicine.

Nerve Interference Fields

Dysfunction and imbalances in the autonomic nervous system (ANS—see Quick Definition) can contribute to a cancer process. Most cases of chronic illness involve changes in the ANS, upsets in the electrical activity of ganglia (nerve bundles), according to Dietrich Klinghardt, M.D., Ph.D. The source of this electrical confusion is called an "interference field" or focus. This can be caused by scars from old accidents or surgeries; nerve bundles made toxic from an accumulation of mercury, parasite toxins, solvents, and many other substances; restriction in blood flow to the ANS resulting from strokes or carbon monoxide poisoning; and physical trauma from events such as wounds, surgical injury, or skull fracture.

QD The **autonomic nervous system** (ANS) can be likened to your body's automatic pilot. It keeps you alive through breathing, heart rate, and digestion, without your being aware of it or participating in its activities. The ANS has two divisions: the sympathetic, which expends body energy; and the parasympathetic, which conserves body energy. The sympathetic nervous system is associated with arousal and stress; it prepares us physically when we perceive a threat or challenge by increasing our heart rate, blood pressure, and muscle tension. The parasympathetic nervous system slows heart rate and increases activity of the intestines and glands other than the adrenals.

Diet and Nutritional Deficiencies

Food can make or break our health and, increasingly, factors related to food—its quality, nutritional constituents, even how it is grown and processed—are considered a primary agent for contributing to the initiation and promotion of cancer. According to the National Academy of Sciences, 60% of all cancers in women and 40% of all cancers in men may be due to dietary and nutritional factors.[36]

According to the National Academy of Sciences, 60% of all cancers in women and 40% of all cancers in men may be due to dietary and nutritional factors.

One of the major factors accounting for the steady rise in cancer incidence and mortality rates is nutritional imbalances. The rise of degenerative disease has paralleled the adoption of an overly refined and adulterated, high-protein, high-fat diet over the past 100 years. After World War II, the U.S. population shifted away from regular consumption of whole grains and fresh vegetables and instead increased its consumption of less wholesome, overly refined foods. This so-called affluent diet is high in fat, which can more readily concentrate such chemicals as pesticides, preservatives, and industrial pollutants. The National Research Council's extensive 1982 report, entitled *Diet, Nutrition, and Cancer*, provided strong evidence that much of the rise in cancer rates may be related to typical U.S. dietary practices.

Excessive intake of animal protein: The high intake of animal protein is associated with an increased risk of breast, colon, pancreatic, kidney, prostate, and endome-trial cancers. Excessive protein may produce large amounts of nitrogenous waste in the intestine, some of which can be converted to highly carcinogenic nitrosamines and ammonium salts. Heavy-protein diets may also cause the buildup of metabolic acids in the body and cause large amounts of calcium to be leached from the bones, an obvious problem for women hoping to prevent osteoporosis, but also a serious detriment in the case of bone cancer, when bone-calcium reserves tend to be mobilized and depleted. A causal relationship between red meat consumption and cancer is supported by several large studies conducted in the U.S. Specifically, women with the highest level of meat consumption had double the rate of breast cancer compared to those who consumed small amounts of meat.[37] Men who ate red meat over a 5-year period were nearly three times more likely to contract advanced prostate cancer than men consuming mainly vegetarian fare. High rates of colon cancer have recently been linked to a regular intake of beef, pork, or lamb.[38] In each of these studies, the meat-eating risks are associated with fat intake as well, since American meats are typically high in fat and fat-soluble toxins like pesticides and herbicides.

The link between cancer and meat eaters' exposure to toxic chemicals goes even deeper. All fried and broiled foods contain mutagens, chemicals that can damage or mutate cellular reproductive material, but fried and broiled meats have far more mutagens than similarly prepared plant foods. Additionally, potentially cancer-causing substances are produced when meat, poultry, or fish are fried, broiled, grilled, or barbecued for a long time at high temperatures.[39]

Be wary of contaminated fish: Industrial and agricultural pollution has resulted in chemicals such as mercury, nickel, oil, hydrocyanic acid, and lactronitrile getting absorbed by ocean-borne plankton. These plankton and their toxins travel up the food chain, becoming very concentrated in the tissues of large, fatty predatory fish, like tuna and swordfish. Industrial chemicals such as PCBs (polychlorinated biphenyls) and methyl mercury tend to accumulate in significant amounts in some fish and most shellfish. According to toxicologists, it takes only $\frac{1}{10}$ of a teaspoon of PCBs to make a person severely ill or possibly cause cancer.

Excessive fat intake: Fat intake, especially animal fat, is one of the key factors consistently implicated in higher cancer rates.[40] The cancers most closely associated with high fat intake include breast, colorectal, uterine, prostate, and kidney.[41] Partially hydrogenated vegetable oils, commonly found in margarine and processed foods, are considered a major contributor to the carcinogenic effect of fats.[42] Some evidence suggests that saturated fat consumption may be a factor. The critical factor may not be the quantity of fat in the diet but the quality—many processed fats contain residues of herbicides, pesticides, and other toxins. In breast cancer studies conducted on laboratory mice, tumor growth was enhanced by a high-fat diet only *after* a chemical carcinogen had been introduced.[43] This suggests that fat is probably not an initiator but rather a promoter of cancer. Studies of fat's suppressive effects on the immune system, as well as fat's ability to generate free radicals (lipid peroxidation), support this interpretation.

Eicosanoids: Eicosanoids are hormone-like substances produced from the metabolism of arachidonic acid and other fatty acids. Produced by nearly every cell in the body, eicosanoids are highly potent substances: as little as one billionth of a gram can have measurable biological effects.[44] The human body produces a variety of eicosanoids that, in turn, direct a diverse range of functions, including immune-cell activity, platelet aggregation, inflammation, steroid hormone production, gastrointestinal secretions, blood pressure, and pain sensation. Evidence suggests that one of the eicosanoids, PGE2, promotes the development of various cancers by paralyzing certain key parts of the immune system (specifically, the natural killer cells), stimulating inflammatory processes, and promoting the proliferation of tumor cells. Omega-3 fatty acids appear to reduce PGE2-induced inflammation, inhibit tumor cell proliferation, and enhance immune system function, as demonstrated in a study in which omega-3 fatty acids slowed or delayed the development of metastases in breast cancer patients. Specifically, women who had high fatty tissue content of alpha-linolenic acid (the main omega-3 EFA) were five times less likely to develop metastases than women with a low content.[45]

Excessive intake of refined carbohydrates/sugar: Sugar and white-flour products are believed to have a direct effect on cancer growth, as well as acting to nullify the positive effects of protective foods such as fiber.[46] They can significantly add to the risk of breast cancer, says veteran cancer researcher Wayne Martin, of Fairhope, Alabama. "When someone eats sugar, the body produces insulin, and insulin can promote breast cancer just as estrogen does," he explains. Sugar is remarkably effective at lowering the immune system's ability to work properly. Eating only three ounces (100 g) at one sitting can stunningly reduce the ability of the immune system's white blood cells to engulf and destroy bacteria. The immune-suppressive effect starts within 30 minutes after sugar ingestion and can last for up to five hours. As the average American consumes about five ounces (150 g) of sucrose (granular sugar found in various processed foods) daily, it would seem the immune system of many people is chronically suppressed from dietary factors alone.[47]

Excessive intake of iron: Iron overload refers to an excess of body iron. A Danish study found that iron overload significantly raises the risk of developing cancer.[48] Two other recent reports suggest that even moderately elevated iron accumulations in the body may increase cancer risk.[49] Much of the cancer in the U.S. population today may be related to overconsumption of red meat, a rich source of iron. Citing another recent study showing a relationship between high red meat intake and colon cancer,[50] Neal Barnard, M.D., of the Physicians Committee for Responsible Medicine, states: "Although it is unclear whether the iron in the meat promotes tumor growth any more than the fat does, iron definitely contributes to free radical production, which only increases one's risk of getting cancer." Cooking in iron pots or skillets and the common fortification of bread, rice, pasta products, and multivitamins with iron are further sources of exposure. Iron fortification is largely unnecessary as iron deficiency is uncommon in the U.S., except in menstruating women.

Excessive intake of alcohol: Regular, heavy consumption of alcohol, including beer, is associated with an elevated cancer risk.[51] According to Charles B. Simone, M.D., of Princeton, New Jersey, an alcohol habit can greatly increase the risk for cancers of the breast, mouth, throat (pharynx, larynx, and esophagus), pancreas, liver, and head and neck. Alcohol can accelerate the growth of an existing cancer by suppressing natural killer cells, those immune cells that would otherwise help repel the cancer.[52]

Excessive intake of caffeine: Found in coffee, tea, colas, and chocolate, caffeine is thought to be a factor in the development of cancer of the lower urinary tract, including the bladder. Studies have found the rates for these cancers to be significantly higher in people who drink more than three cups of coffee a day.[53] Caffeine can cause damage to genetic material and impair the normal DNA repair mechanisms, thereby adding to the potential risk for cancer.[54]

Chronic Stress

Numerous studies have linked stress and its related psychological components to susceptibility to cancer.[55] Adults who have recently lost a loved one, or been widowed, divorced, or separated, tend to have the highest

THE TYPE C PERSONALITY

The term *Type C personality* is used in much the same way to describe people at risk for cancer as "Type A personality" is used for people at risk for heart disease. While there is no clear consensus on what exactly makes up a Type C personality, or even if such a thing exists, researchers have found a significant amount of anecdotal and suggestive evidence to support certain psychological features that can greatly increase a person's risk for cancer.

The main psychological aspect associated with cancer is loss, either loss of a loved one or loss of hope. Many cancer patients feel a profound sense of hopelessness and despair, particularly about the meaning of their own existence. Often this feeling has been present as far back as the patient can remember. The other psychological aspect commonly associated with a cancer personality is the suppression or repression of emotions, especially anger. This is seen in people who deny their own needs by holding in their emotions from an early age. These two characteristics often combine into a third feature of the Type C personality—loneliness. This loneliness is usually characterized at an early age by a lack of closeness to one or both parents that carries on into adulthood as a lack of closeness with friends or a fulfilling relationship.

Most people experience one or all of these traits at various times in their lives. This is normal, if it does not become a chronic condition. The people who are most at risk from these psychological factors are those who begin showing these signs at an early age, then carry them into adulthood. Researchers have found that these psychological patterns, along with stress, can greatly add to a person's cancer risk.[58]

cancer rates.[56] In addition, a basic inability to cope with stress has been regarded as a key risk factor in developing breast cancer.[57] Unrelieved, chronic stress increases cancer risk by gradually weakening the immune system. According to Leon Chaitow, N.D., D.O., of London, England, when psychological and emotional changes occur in a person, stress is often produced, resulting in increased adrenaline levels, other hormonal changes, and decreased immune function. "Usually, the body can adapt itself, continuing to function during this temporary condition before returning to normal," Dr. Chaitow says. "But when the stress is too severe or if it becomes

chronic, chemical changes begin to occur in the body, creating an environment that may increase the risk of serious disease, including cancer."

Toxic Emotions

Since the 1970s, research in the field of psychoneuroimmunology (PNI) has documented direct links between emotions and biochemical events in the body. Noted women's health expert Christiane Northrup, M.D., of Yarmouth, Maine, coined the term *toxic emotions* to indicate the powerful, strongly held, and often unconsciously active beliefs and emotions that help generate symptoms to keep illnesses in place. In the view of Dr. Northrup, as well as other alternative practitioners working with cancer patients, beliefs and emotions can be legitimate toxins, contributing to an overall weakening of the immune system.[59]

Depressed Thyroid Action

An underactive or dysfunctional thyroid gland (a key endocrine gland located in the neck) may contribute to a cancer process. Broda O. Barnes, M.D., a doctor who specialized in treating patients with hypothyroidism (underfunctioning thyroid), observed evidence in his clinical practice suggesting a relationship between low thyroid activity and cancer. Research has tended to support Dr. Barnes's clinical observations. In 1954, studies by Dr. J.G.C. Spencer, from Bristol, England, showed that there was a consistently higher incidence of cancer in areas of 15 countries where goiter (enlargement of the thyroid gland) was more prevalent among the population than in the non-goiter areas of the same localities.

Intestinal Toxicity and Digestive Impairment

When the intestines become clogged, toxic, and diseased by what and how we eat and by how poorly we eliminate waste material, the bowel becomes toxic. This creates toxicity for the entire body and results in an inability to absorb the nutrients necessary for health. Around 1900, most people in the U.S. had a brief intestinal transit time, meaning it took only about 15-20 hours from the time food entered the mouth until it was excreted as feces. Today, many people have a seriously delayed transit time of 50-70 hours—more time for the stool to putrefy, for harmful microorganisms to flourish, and for toxins to develop and poison the tissues.

Mucus-producing foods such as dairy products, eggs, and meat contribute to slowing transit time. As a sticky mucoid lining builds up in the intestines as a result of eating these foods along with white flour products, it not only blocks the absorption of essential nutrients into the bloodstream, but also produces a hiding place for bacteria, fungi, yeast, and parasites that are harmful to human health. An overgrowth of these organisms creates a situation called dysbiosis (an imbalance in intestinal microflora), in which the contents of the intestines putrefy and harmful chemicals are generated.

Parasites

The possible presence of parasites in the body, mostly in the intestines, is a little appreciated but major health problem. While people assume they are vulnerable to parasites only if they travel in tropical areas, the fact is that anyone can get them (and many probably already have) from merely staying at home. The damage parasites cause can be extensive: they can destroy cells faster than they can be regenerated; they can release toxins that damage tissues; and, over time, they can depress, even exhaust, the immune system. Of the dozens of specific parasites of concern to human health, the major groupings include microscopic Protozoa, roundworms, pinworms, hookworms (Nematoda), tapeworms (Cestoda), and flukes (Trematoda).[60]

Viruses

According to some researchers, up to 15% of the world's cancer deaths are attributable to the activities of viruses and other microbes. Among the cancer-producing viruses that work through a host's DNA-synthesizing and protein-building mechanisms are human papilloma virus types 16 and 18 (which are sexually transmitted) and associated with cervical cancer, and the hepatitis B virus, associated with liver cancer. Epstein-Barr virus, which produces mononucleosis, is also carcinogenic.[61]

Blocked Detoxification Pathways

In a healthy individual, the body's normal detoxification systems, especially the liver, are generally able to eliminate toxins and thereby prevent illness. To prevent cancer, the liver's detoxification system must be working optimally, says Joseph Pizzorno, N.D., of Seattle, Washington. When the liver is not functioning well, it is unable to process and eliminate the multiplicity of carcinogens entering the body. "High levels of exposure to carcinogens coupled with sluggish detoxification enzymes significantly increase our susceptibility to cancer," says Dr. Pizzorno.[63]

Free-Radical Overload

A free radical is an unstable molecule with an unpaired electron that steals an electron from another molecule, producing harmful effects in the body. Free radicals can be taken in from air, food, and drink or can be generated in the body by energy production and fat metabolism, from the immune response by white blood cells, and by

THE POLIO VACCINE AND CANCER

Did the polio vaccine, given to millions of Americans in the 1950s and 1960s, contain a cancer-causing virus? The answer appears to be yes. Recent scientific studies from researchers worldwide are finding traces of SV40 (a monkey virus that contaminated the polio vaccine in the first few years) in a number of rare tumors in humans. However, U.S. government scientists at the National Cancer Institute (NCI) deny that SV40 has led to any increase in cancer.

Both the polio vaccine of Jonas Salk, M.D., and the later oral vaccine were developed using kidney tissue from monkeys, where the polio virus was grown, then weakened or killed, and used in the vaccine to produce antibodies to polio in humans. The kidney tissue also harbored the SV40 virus. In 1961, researchers found traces of SV40 in the injectable and oral polio vaccines and had evidence that it caused tumors in animals. New procedures were put in place to eradicate SV40 from the vaccine, but there was no recall of tainted virus already distributed—over a year's supply.

Studies in the 1960s and 1970s were inconclusive regarding the cancer-causing potential of SV40. It was not until the late 1980s, with the advent of a new technology called PCR (polymerase chain reaction), which allowed researchers to detect smaller amounts of DNA, that scientists began finding traces of SV40 in human cancers. By 1996, researchers had linked SV40 to a range of brain, lung, and bone cancers. Even more disturbing, there was evidence of SV40 in those who had not been inoculated with contaminated polio vaccine, meaning that the monkey virus might be spread by other means.

In 2000, Michele Carbone, M.D., of Loyola University Medical Center, in Maywood, Illinois, one of the leading researchers of SV40, discovered how SV40 may be contributing to cancer. He found that SV40 binds to immune system cells called tumor-suppressor proteins and disables them, thus weakening the immune response. So, while SV40 may not by itself cause cancer, it suppresses the body's ability to fight it. Even the NCI has finally acknowledged that SV40 "may be associated with human cancer," but it has provided little in the way of research dollars to discover how prevalent it is in the population.[62]

the liver's detoxification process. However, uncontrolled free-radical production plays a major role in the development of at least 100 degenerative conditions, including cancer. What makes the difference between normal functioning of the immune system, which includes the deactivation of free radicals, and the initiation of a potential cancer process is the amount of antioxidants available in the system. An antioxidant (meaning "against oxidation") is a natural biochemical substance that protects living cells against damage from free radicals. Many antioxidants are nutrients like vitamins C and E, while some, like glutathione, are made in the body.

Cellular Oxygen Deficiency

One of the most provocative theories of cancer causation was put forth by two-time Nobel laureate Dr. Otto Warburg. He was a German biochemist who won his first Nobel Prize in 1931 for the discovery that oxygen deficiency and cell fermentation are part of the cancer process.[64] According to Dr. Warburg's theory, when cells are deprived of oxygen, they can revert to their "primitive" state, deriving energy not from oxygen, as normal human and animal cells do, but rather from the fermentation of blood sugar. Blood sugar (glucose) breaks down into lactic acid, which causes an imbalance in the body's acid/base ratio, or pH level (see Quick Definition). As the acidity of the body rises, it becomes even more difficult for the cells to use oxygen normally.[65] "All normal cells have an absolute requirement for oxygen," stated Dr. Warburg, "but cancer cells can live without oxygen—a rule without any exceptions." Humans can become oxygen deficient through several routes, including long-term exposure to air pollution, shallow breathing, clogging of arteries, progressive lung disease, or inadequate exercise.

> **QD** The term **pH**, which means "potential hydrogen," represents a scale for the relative acidity or alkalinity of a solution. Acidity is measured as a pH of 0.1 to 6.9, alkalinity is 7.1 to 14, and neutral pH is 7.0. The numbers refer to how many hydrogen atoms are present compared to an ideal or standard solution. Normally, blood is slightly alkaline, at 7.35 to 7.45; urine pH can range from 4.8 to 8.0, but is usually somewhat acidic, with a normal reading between 5.0 and 6.5.

 The government should examine the wealth of existing studies on oxygen therapy as a treatment for cancer. If approved by the FDA, oxygen therapy could save thousands of lives annually.

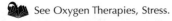 See Oxygen Therapies, Stress.

Cellular Terrain

The term *cellular terrain,* first coined by European practitioners of biological medicine, refers to the general vitality, activity, and biochemical condition of the cells in the body. When the cell becomes imbalanced, conditions are set for infection, illness, and chronic diseases such as cancer. "As we see it," explains Thomas Rau, M.D., Medical Director of the Paracelsus Clinic, in Switzerland, "sickness is not *caused* by bacteria, but the bacteria comes with the sickness. Bacteria, viruses, or fungi can only develop if they have the suitable cellular conditions." Outside influences, such as inadequate nutrition, exposure to carcinogens, chronic organ toxicity, stress, or trauma, provide the impetus to throw the cells out of balance, says Dr. Rau.

Oncogenes

The predominant emphasis in conventional cancer research today is to find individual genes capable of causing, initiating, or triggering cancer growth. First identified in the 1970s, these causal genes are referred to as oncogenes (meaning the gene that starts the *onkos,* or tumor mass). Oncogenes are believed to transform normal cells into cancer cells.[66] Researchers now believe that about 20% of all human cancers are partly brought about by oncogene mutations. In healthy people, the activities of oncogenes are counterbalanced by tumor suppressor genes, also called anti-oncogenes. Under normal conditions, these genes act to prevent uncontrolled cell growth that could lead to tumors.

Genetic Predisposition

The theory of gene causation for cancer inevitably leads researchers into speculations about inherited cancers—genetic configurations or mutations that might predict, if not guarantee, that a given individual will develop a particular form of cancer. The term *family cancer syndrome* is now used to describe the tendency of particular cancers (such as breast, colon, or ovarian) to appear in succeeding generations of the same family. Many scientists now believe that the following inherited cancers may be linked to mutations in certain related tumor suppressor genes: melanoma and pancreatic cancer (MTS1, p16); breast and ovarian cancer (BRCA1); breast cancer (BRCA2); colon and uterine cancer (MSH2, MLH1, PMS1, PMS2); and brain sarcomas (p53).[67]

Miasm

More than 200 years ago, German physician Samuel Hahnemann, the founder of homeopathy, used the term *miasm* to indicate a particular predisposition to chronic disease. Hahnemann's concept of miasms accurately prefigures today's description of oncogenes. A miasm represents an energy residue of an illness from a previous generation, while an oncogene represents a molecular residue of an illness from a previous generation. According to Hahnemann, three miasms underlie all chronic illness and these parallel broad stages in the history of the human experience with primary disease states. The *Psoric* miasm is the foundation of sickness underlying all the diseases experienced by humans—cancer, diabetes, skin disorders, and arthritis as well as serious mental disorders, such as epilepsy and schizophrenia. The *Syphilitic* miasm, which came next in the history of human diseases, derives from syphilis, and is associated with several cancers and dementias. The *Sycotic* miasm, the third layer, arose as a residue of gonorrhea and contributes to arthritis and a few cancers. In recent years, homeopaths have added a *Cancer* miasm, a combination of the effects (or taints) of Hahnemann's original three.

Early Detection

Traditional cancer tests include physical examination, CAT (computerized axial tomography) scans, MRI (magnetic resonance imaging), X rays, and biopsies. Other tests, which are designed to test only one kind of cancer, include mammography for breast cancer, PAP smear for cervical cancer, bone scans for bone cancer, and PSA (prostate specific antigen) blood test for prostate cancer. However, alternative practitioners have other tests at their disposal, which detect cancer located in any area of the body long before it would be apparent through conventional testing. Early detection is imperative for the most effective treatment of cancer. By learning about our bodies and recognizing the telltale signs of cancer, we can do a great deal to ensure that cancer is detected at an early stage. And when it comes to the diagnosis of cancer, the clock is definitely ticking. Consider this— about 35% of those who die from cancer every year would be alive if their cancer had been detected early enough for effective treatment to have been undertaken.[68]

Electrodermal Biofeedback: The prospect of detecting life-threatening diseases such as cancer at the earliest stage has led some alternative medical practitioners to investigate energy medicine, based on the belief that an individual's energy field alters with the onset of disease. This changing energy field can be diagnosed using noninvasive electrodermal biofeedback devices. Electrodermal screening instruments were first popularized in Europe in the early 1970s and have been used in the U.S. since the 1980s. As controversial as they are, their use is becoming increasingly widespread as physicians seek better ways to screen for a wide variety of illnesses and causes before symptoms develop.

Darkfield Microscopy: Darkfield microscopy is a way of studying living whole blood cells under a specially adapted microscope that projects the dynamic image onto a video screen. In this way, the skilled practitioner can detect early stages of illness in the form of known disease-producing microorganisms seen in the blood. Also, the amount of time the blood cell stays viable and alive indicates the overall health of the individual. Darkfield microscopy provides fundamental information on what is happening in the blood. For example, the health of a white blood cell can be determined, whether the cell wall is smooth or ragged, or leaking cytoplasm. It can also tell if a cell has been damaged by free radicals.

AMAS: Until recently, there was no single blood test that could reliably and accurately indicate if cancer was present, either for an initial diagnosis or for monitoring a recurrence. The tests available were sometimes positive when cancer was not present (a false positive) and sometimes negative when it was known that the person had cancer (a false negative). For many years, researchers have been hoping for a cancer marker that could serve as a reliable indicator for a variety of cancers. Possibly the most accurate cancer marker was unveiled in the 1990s, thanks to the efforts of Harvard-trained biochemist and physician Sam Bogoch, M.D., Ph.D., who labored for 20 years before finally uncovering the secret to detecting all forms of cancer in very early stages. Known as AMAS (anti-malignin antibody screen), the test analyzes a sample of blood to reveal whether antibodies to cancer are present. Generally speaking, the test is called an immunoassay, which means it measures the amount present of a specific antibody— in this case, anti-malignin, an antibody that acts against the inner protein layer (malignin) of a cancer cell. Dr. Bogoch found that the anti-malignin antibody serves as a reliable marker for cancers of all kinds. "If there are any cancers that don't respond to the [AMAS] test, we haven't found them yet," says Dr. Bogoch. Although it was approved by the FDA in 1977, it wasn't until late 1994 that the clinical trials with 4,278 patients were completed, validating the test's effectiveness. Now this patented, FDA-approved screen is available to doctors worldwide through Dr. Bogoch's Oncolab. According to Dr. Bogoch, AMAS is 95% accurate on the first test and 99% when repeated; the test can detect cancer up to 19 months before conventional medical tests can find it.

Thermography: A nontoxic, highly accurate, and inexpensive form of diagnostic imaging has been used by progressive physicians in the U.S. and Europe since 1962. Called thermography, it's based on infrared heat emis-

Darkfield view of normal blood

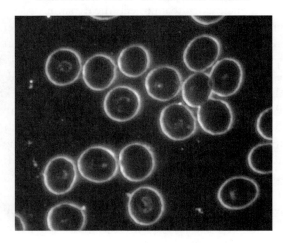

Darkfield view of blood of a person with advanced cancer

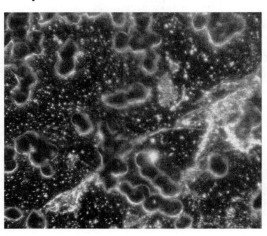

sions from targeted regions of the body. As the body's cells go through their energy conversion processes, called metabolism, they emit heat. Cancerous growths tend to give off more infrared energy and with much less regulation by the autonomic nervous system than normal tissues. Thermography is able to register varying heat emissions, display them on a computer monitor, and thereby provide a diagnostic window into the functional status of a given body area, such as the female breast. For breast cancer, thermography offers a very early warning system, often able to pinpoint a cancer process five years before it would be detectable by mammography. Most breast tumors have been growing slowly for up to 20 years before they are found by typical diagnostic techniques. Thermography can detect cancers when they are at a minute physical stage of development, when it is still relatively easy to halt and reverse the progression of the cancer. Philip Hoekstra, Ph.D., of Thermoscan, in Huntington Woods, Michigan, is a pioneer in the use of thermography. Dr. Hoekstra's clinic has screened more than 50,000 women since 1971. The procedure is simple and noninvasive, says Dr. Hoekstra. The woman stands barechested about ten feet from the device; the imaging takes only a matter of minutes, as results are displayed instantaneously on the monitor; and generally the data can be rapidly interpreted with image-analyzing software. No rays of any kind enter the patient's body; there is no pain or compressing of the breasts as in a mammogram. While mammography tends to lose effectiveness with dense breast tissue, thermography is not dependent upon tissue densities.

Dr. Hoekstra points to the errors, false negatives, and radiation exposure dangers of mammograms. "Mammography is not an acceptable way of screening breasts;

the only reason it's tolerated is that it is a major source of steady income for radiologists," Dr. Hoekstra says. "They have come to covet mammography and want no competition from other approaches." He believes that once women start making demands on their physicians for a different imaging approach, thermography can become the preferred initial screening method. Then mammography will be used only as needed to pinpoint the precise location of breast tumors.

The Hemoccult Test: Colorectal cancer (cancer of either the colon or rectum) is the second most common cancer in the U.S. and surely one of the deadliest. In fact, about one out of every five cancer deaths (20%) in the U.S. is attributed to colorectal cancer and almost half of all colorectal patients will probably die, according to conventional medical statistics. One reason for this heavy death toll may be that the majority of colorectal cancer cases are diagnosed at a late stage of the disease. Detected early, progression of this disease is entirely preventable. Among the more reliable early signs of colorectal cancer is blood on the surface of or mixed in feces. If not visible to the eye, colorectal blood can be detected by chemical tests. In some cases, pain and tenderness are felt in the lower abdomen, but often no symptoms appear until the tumor grows so big that it causes obstruction or rupture of the intestine; at this point, surgery and aggressive forms of treatment become necessary.

For this reason, many doctors now recommend the hemoccult test, in which a sample of feces is applied to a card imprinted with a solution of guaiac, a plant gum. The presence of hemoglobin, hence the name hemoccult (i.e., hidden blood in the feces), is indicated by a

WHAT'S WRONG WITH MAMMOGRAPHY?

Although mammography is the most widely employed screening method for breast cancer, there are a number of compelling arguments for adopting other methods in its place. Current research within conventional medicine provides strong reasons why mammogram screening for detection of breast cancer ought to be reconsidered.

Mammograms Add to Cancer Risk—Mammography exposes the breast to damaging ionizing radiation. John W. Gofman, M.D., Ph.D., an authority on the health effects of ionizing radiation, spent 30 years studying the effects of low-dose radiation on humans. He estimates that 75% of breast cancer could be prevented by avoiding or minimizing exposure to the ionizing radiation from mammography, X rays, and other medical sources. Other research has shown that, since mammographic screening was introduced in 1983, the incidence of a form of breast cancer called ductal carcinoma in situ (DCIS), which represents 12% of all breast cancer cases, has increased by 328%, and 200% of this increase is due to the use of mammography.[69] In addition to exposing a woman to harmful radiation, the mammography procedure may help spread an existing mass of cancer cells. During a mammogram, considerable pressure must be placed on the woman's breast, as the breast is squeezed between two flat plastic surfaces. According to some health practitioners, this compression could cause existing cancer cells to metastasize from the breast tissue.

High Rate of False Positives—Mammography's high rate of false-positive test results wastes money and creates unnecessary emotional trauma. A Swedish study of 60,000 women, aged 40-64, who were screened for breast cancer revealed that of the 726 actually referred to oncologists for treatment, 70% were found to be cancer free. According to *The Lancet*, of the 5% of mammograms that suggest further testing, up to 93% are false positives. *The Lancet* report further noted that because the great majority of positive screenings are false positives, these inaccurate results lead to many unnecessary biopsies and other invasive surgical procedures.[70] In fact, 70% to 80% of all positive mammograms do not, on biopsy, show any presence of cancer.[71] According to some estimates, 90% of these "callbacks" result from unclear readings due to dense overlying breast tissue.[72]

High Rate of False Negatives—Mammography also produces a high rate of false-negative test results. While false positives cause unnecessary distress and intervention, false negatives can be fatal. The breast tissue of women under 40 is generally denser, making it more difficult to detect tumors via mammography. In addition, tumors grow more quickly in women in this age group, so cancer may develop between screenings.[73] As for women aged 40 to 49, even the National Cancer Institute notes that there is a high rate of "missed tumors" in this age category; that is, 40% false-negative test results.[74]

Estrogen Distorts Breast X Rays—Estrogen therapy obscures mammogram results. According to a study of 8,800 postmenopausal women, aged 50 and older, the use of estrogen replacement therapy (ERT) leads to a 71% increased likelihood of receiving a false-positive result on mammogram screening. Mary B. Laya, M.D., M.P.H., study leader at the University of Washington at Seattle, who published the results in the *Journal of the National Cancer Institute* in 1996, also found that women on ERT were more likely to get false-negative readings.

Mammography may also fail to detect advanced tumors measuring less than two centimeters in diameter. Yet a tumor can be felt manually when it reaches about one centimeter (approximately ½ inch) in diameter and, with training in self-examination, women can detect even smaller tumors.[75] In view of this, women should take self-examination more seriously. Many experts believe that early detection through manual examination provides the best results. "It is certainly the safest, least expensive, and least invasive preventive action available to women," says Samuel Epstein, M.D., Professor of Occupational and Environmental Medicine at the University of Illinois School of Public Health. "It also enables women to become familiar with their breast tissue, natural lumps and all, and to report any noticeable changes early."

Mammography is a passing technology, which will soon be replaced by safer testing methods. Two such methods already available include thermography and the Anti-Malignin Antibody Screen (AMAS) test. Thermography uses infrared heat emissions from the body to detect cancer; its advantage is that it does not use radiation. The AMAS test measures serum levels of an antibody found to be elevated in most patients in the early stages of active, nonterminal malignancies.[76]

AN EARLY CANCER DETECTION PRIMER

The message of prevention is that you can beat cancer before it becomes advanced. The key is to detect the presence of cancer early enough so you can treat it with the immune-enhancing, nontoxic treatments of alternative medicine. These methods work best when the body's tumor burden is relatively small—in the *earliest* phases of the cancer's development. Here are signs that may indicate the presence of cancer.

1. A Lump or Thickening in the Breast or Testicles. Self-examination of the breast and testicles offers women and men the best protection against breast and testicular cancer. A lump or thickening in the breast, or any noticeable change in the testicles, are early warning signs. Such signs are grounds for an immediate medical examination.

2. A Change in a Wart or Mole. Changes in warts or moles may be indicative of melanoma or squamous carcinoma. Skin cancers may appear as dry, scaly patches, as pimples that never go away, or as inflamed or ulcerated areas. Warts or moles that grow or bleed should be checked, as should sores in the mouth that persist.

3. A Skin Sore or a Sore Throat That Does Not Heal. Sores that do not heal may also be indicative of skin cancer. A persistent sore throat, hoarseness, a persistent lump in the throat, or difficulty swallowing, may indicate cancer of the pharynx, larynx, or esophagus. These cancers are readily treated when caught early.

4. A Change in Bowel or Bladder Habits. Continuing urinary difficulties, constipation, chronic diarrhea, abdominal pains, rectal or urinary bleeding, or dark tar-like stools should not be ignored; they should be regarded as signals to seek professional help.

5. A Persistent Cough or Coughing Blood. Coughs that become chronic, especially in smokers, should be checked. If there is a cancer in the air passages into the lungs, they may be partially obstructed or irritated or even bleed. Coughing may be a sign of this obstruction or irritation.

6. Constant Indigestion or Trouble Swallowing. Difficulties in swallowing, continued indigestion, nausea, heartburn, bloating, loss of appetite, and abdominal discomfort all may be symptoms of colon cancer or cancer of the stomach or esophagus. Unexplained weight loss is also an indicator.

7. Unusual Vaginal Discharge or Bleeding. The early stages of uterine endometrial cancer and later stages of cervical vaginal cancer exhibit signs of unusual bleeding or vaginal discharge. Prompt attention to these symptoms means a better chance of catching cancer at its most treatable stage. In the case of cervical cancer, Pap tests can detect problems before the later stages cause bleeding.

8. Chronic Fatigue. General feelings of chronic fatigue will often accompany any type of cancer that is rapidly progressing.

If you are experiencing any of these signs and symptoms, contact your physician immediately.

---

color change. The test will sometimes yield false-positive results if the person has recently consumed fresh fruits or vegetables, red meat, iron tablets, aspirin, nonsteroidal anti-inflammatory drugs, or vitamin C supplements. A positive finding with the hemoccult test warrants having a sigmoidoscopy or a colonoscopy, other tests used to detect polyps and tumors in the colon.

T/Tn Antigen Test: The late Georg Springer, M.D., an immunologist who founded the Heather Bligh Cancer Research Laboratories at the Chicago Medical School, uncovered evidence that certain proteins (antigens) on the surface of blood and skin cells can be identified by the immune system (antibodies). Dr. Springer recognized that the T and Tn antigens are specifically associated with cancers of all kinds and that the T and Tn antigens are found in places where cancer has spread, but not in benign tumors. The T and Tn antigens serve as specific markers for the presence of cancer; in the case of breast cancer, the more markers, the more advanced or aggressive the cancer. "What is unique about the T and Tn antibody test is that it enables detection of the majority of cancers before any biopsy can pick up the presence of cancer," said Dr. Springer. "We find that people without any previous cancer, who show positive test results, consistently develop cancer later on."

Prostate Specific Antigen (PSA): The PSA is used for early detection of prostate cancer. Many physicians, both mainstream and alternative, recommend that the

PSA be done annually. However, they also warn of laboratory variability. Physicians should not overreact to an elevated PSA, since many men with prostate cancer do not die from cancer but rather from other unrelated diseases or the complications of conventional treatments.

Prevention

Prevention is the most important and most reliable cancer-fighting tool that exists today, and there is much that an individual can do to prevent cancer. It is especially vital to maintain a strong and healthy immune system. This can be accomplished in a number of ways, including a diet that ensures the optimal intake of immune-enhancing nutrients while decreasing the intake of immunosuppressing foods. Living a life free from continual emotional or mental distress is also important, as well as avoiding carcinogenic toxins in the home and in the environment.

 See Nutritional Medicine, Orthomolecular Medicine.

Diet and Nutrition

With up to 60% of all cancers being related to dietary factors,[77] diet and nutrition are perhaps the most important aspects of any cancer prevention regimen. This is evidenced by the fact that, in 1988, the U.S. Surgeon General called for the reduction of dietary fat as a top priority for the prevention of chronic diseases, including cancer.[78]

Prevention is the most important and most reliable cancer-fighting tool that exists today, and there is much that an individual can do to prevent cancer.

A diet which consists largely of organically grown fresh fruits, vegetables, and whole grains, with little or no fat or meat (particularly grilled, charred, smoked, or cured meats),[79] is highly recommended, especially for women who wish to decrease their risk of breast cancer.[80] The National Cancer Institute (NCI) recommends that Americans reduce their fat intake to no more than 30% of total calories, while increasing their consumption of fresh fruits and vegetables.[81] Additionally, it is essential to avoid highly processed foods, as they can contain partially hydrogenated fats[82] and chemical additives that are potentially

carcinogenic.[83] Cutting down on sugar,[84] caffeine,[85] and alcohol[86] are also highly recommended.

Eating organically grown foods is extremely important, as recent studies have shown that organic foods are not only far more free from carcinogenic pesticide contaminants than conventionally grown foods, they are also richer in the essential nutrients and trace elements necessary for cancer prevention, including beta carotene, vitamin E, and selenium.[87] In a recent five-year study of nearly 30,000 rural Chinese people, researchers from the NCI found that daily doses of these three nutrients reduced cancer deaths by 13%.[88]

Alternative medicine honors individuality, recognizing that each individual has a different biochemistry and different nutritional requirements. Just like fingerprints, each of us has a unique metabolism, that is, how we convert food into energy for running all of the body's processes. In fact, many chronic illnesses like cancer may be symptoms of an underlying disturbance in metabolism. Your body type could be the key to your health. The way to discover this biochemical "fingerprint" is metabolic typing. Metabolic body typing is based on research done by George Watson, Ph.D., William Donald Kelley, D.D.S., Francis Pottenger, M.D., and others. Further refining of metabolic typing has been continued by William L. Wolcott, a researcher and founder of Healthexcel, Inc., in Winthrop, Washington, an organization that performs metabolic typing evaluations.

The following is a list of important cancer-fighting nutrients and foods, along with their sources:

Beta Carotene and Carotenoids—The precursor of vitamin A, beta carotene is found in carrots, sweet potatoes, spinach, and most leafy green vegetables. A diet high in beta carotene and other carotenoids is protective against all cancers, but beta carotene is particularly important for women as a deterrent to cervical cancer.[89] High serum beta carotene (and associated dietary carotenoids) has also been shown to protect the lungs against tobacco smoke and smog, thus inhibiting the development of lung cancer.[90] Ex-smokers who ate green and yellow vegetables high in beta carotene every day decreased their risk of stomach and lung cancer.[91]

Vitamin B6—Found in bananas, leafy green vegetables, carrots, apples, organ meats, and sweet potatoes, vitamin B6 is essential for optimal immune function and helps maintain the health of mucous membranes, which line the respiratory tract and provide a natural barrier to pollution and infection. Vitamin B6 also affords protection against cervical cancer.[92]

Inositol—This natural substance, an unofficial member of the B vitamin family, is found in virtually all cells, where it plays an important role in sending signals between cells and their environment. Inositol is present in high-fiber foods, especially legumes, cereal grains, and citrus fruits. In the body, inositol helps the liver remove excess fat from its tissues; this, in turn, prevents liver stagnation from fat and bile buildup. John Potter, Ph.D., a researcher at the Fred Hutchinson Cancer Research Center, in Seattle, Washington, has identified inositol as one of 15 different classes of phytochemicals that have shown anticancer activity.[93] In fact, it may be one of the key reasons why a high-fiber diet has a protective effect against cancer.[94] One of the best forms of inositol to take supplementally is inositol hexaphosphate or IP-6.

Vitamin C—Found in citrus fruits, cantaloupe, broccoli, green peppers, and many other fruits and vegetables, vitamin C is integrally involved in the maintenance of a healthy immune system as well as protective against a variety of cancers.[95] There is now solid evidence that this vitamin is essential for optimal functioning of the immune system.[96] Among those immune components most actively involved in fighting cancer are the natural killer (NK) cells, which are only active if they contain relatively large amounts of vitamin C.[97] Vitamin C also boosts the body's production of interferon, which has anticancer activity.[98]

Vitamin D—This vitamin, also classified as a hormone, appears to have cancer-killing properties.[99] Though research findings are still preliminary, vitamin D and its metabolites may increase the number of vitamin A receptors on cells ("up-regulating"), inhibit the formation of new tumor blood vessels (angiogenesis), induce the conversion of cancer cells back to normal cells (cell re-differentiation), and induce "cell suicide" (apoptosis) in cancer cells.[100]

Vitamin E (tocopherol)—Found in dark green vegetables, eggs, wheat germ, liver, unrefined vegetable oils, and some herbs, vitamin E is a powerful antioxidant that can directly reduce the damage done by ozone smog. It can also help protect against bowel cancer.[101] Mixed natural tocopherals are much more effective clinically than synthetic vitamin E.

Folic Acid—This substance protects against cervical cancer and is necessary for proper synthesis of RNA and DNA. It is found in beets, cabbage, dark leafy vegetables, eggs, dairy products, citrus fruits, and most fish.[102]

Selenium—An essential trace mineral found in fruits and vegetables, selenium helps the body produce functional glutathione peroxidase, an enzyme essential for detoxification. Low dietary levels of selenium have been correlated with a higher incidence of cancer; accordingly, supplementation of this nutrient acts as a deterrent against cancer in general.[103]

Calcium—This mineral protects against colon cancer and is vital for proper bone formation, blood clotting, and cellular metabolism.[104] It is found in dark green vegetables, most nuts and seeds, milk products, sardines, and salmon.

Iodine—Available in seafood, sea vegetables such as kelp and dulse, and iodized salt, iodine protects against breast cancer and is needed for proper energy metabolism as well as the growth and repair of all tissues.[105]

Magnesium—Found in most nuts, fish, green vegetables, whole grains, and brown rice, magnesium protects against cancer and is necessary in the maintenance of the pH balance of blood and tissues, as well as in the synthesis of RNA and DNA.[106] As a supplement, magnesium malate is one of the most effective forms.

Zinc—This mineral protects against prostate cancer and is necessary for the formation of RNA and DNA and for healthy immune function.[107] It is found in whole grains, most seafood, sunflower seeds, pumpkin seeds, soybeans, and onions. Phytates in grains and beans decrease zinc absorption. If taken as a supplement, zinc oxide and zinc picolinate are the least beneficial forms.

Coenzyme Q10—CoQ10, also known as ubiquinone, is one of a family of brightly colored substances called quinones, which are widely distributed in nature because they are essential for generating energy in living things that use oxygen. The body produces its own coQ10, but usually produces less with aging; therefore dietary sources are important for this coenzyme, especially for older people. It is found in fairly high concentrations in fish (especially sardines), soybean and grapeseed oils, sesame seeds, pistachios, walnuts, and spinach.[108] CoQ10 plays an important part in the body's antioxidant system. When combined with vitamin E, selenium, and beta carotene, coQ10 can significantly reduce free-radical damage in the liver, kidneys, and heart.[109] Another beneficial effect in cancer patients is to increase macrophage activity.[110]

Garlic—Garlic or its components can help lower the risk of tumors in the stomach, colon, lungs and esophagus.[111] Research from China has reported that those who eat a greater quantity of garlic have much lower rates of stomach cancer.[112]

Broccoli—This vegetable has 4.5 g of fiber per cup. One cup, which contains only 45 calories, supplies more than the recommended daily allowance of the antioxidants vitamin C and beta carotene. Broccoli contains a substance called sulforaphane, which research indicates blocks the growth of tumors in mice.[113]

Cruciferous Vegetables—Bok choy, collards, kale, broccoli, cabbage, cauliflower, mustard greens, Brussels sprouts, radishes, and turnips contain a type of flavonoid that activates liver detoxification enzymes. The crucifers are noteworthy due to a wide array of sulfur-containing compounds, but they also contain anticancer and antioxidant vitamins. They regulate white blood cells and cytokines; white blood cells are the scavengers of the immune system and cytokines act as "messengers," coordinating the activities of all immune cells. Since some of the sulfur compounds can inhibit thyroid function, they are best cooked to reduce this tendency.

Tomatoes—Tomatoes contain lycopene (the substance that gives the tomato its deep red color), which belongs to a family of natural pigments (carotenoids) found in plants. According to current research, lycopene is an excellent antioxidant, capable of protecting the body against many degenerative diseases, including prostate, cervical, and gastrointestinal cancers. Men of southern European descent—from regions where tomato-based foods are consumed more frequently as part of the well-publicized "Mediterranean diet"—have a lower incidence of prostate cancer than African-American or Asian-American men who, typically, eat fewer tomato-based items. Even a preexisting family history of prostate cancer did not change lycopene's protective effect, researchers report.[114] One of the fascinating and surprising discoveries is that processed tomatoes (such as pasta sauce) rather than fresh tomatoes produce a greater protective effect.

Mushrooms—A mainstay in Chinese medicine and cuisines, mushrooms help to promote health and longevity. They have an immune-boosting effect, which helps reduce the risk of cancer and enhances heart health. Shiitake mushroom is one of the most studied mushrooms and has been found to enhance immune system function, ward off infection, and neutralize cancerous cells.[115]

Soybeans—Soybeans and other legumes contain diadzein and genistein, naturally occurring "phytoestro-gens" that may block the action of estrogen in the body, thus slowing the growth of hormonally-dependent tumors.[116] Genistein can block the activity of certain oncogenes (chromosomal genes believed to initiate cancer) and has antioxidant, antiestrogenic, and antitumor activity.[117]

Omega-3 Fatty Acids—These fats, essential for the proper functioning of all tissues and cells in the body, may inhibit cancer, especially breast cancer.[118] They're found in fish, such as salmon, mackerel, sardines, haddock, and cod, as well as flaxseed oil.

Fiber—Whole grains, psyllium husks, and other fiber-rich foods are essential to any anticancer diet, as fiber helps facilitate the prompt removal of toxins from the digestive tract. If your metabolic type tolerates grains, it is important to include a variety of whole grains in the diet because the various whole-grain foods contain different kinds of fiber.[119] Consume at least 25-30 g of fiber a day, equivalent to six or more servings of grains (or nuts or seeds) and five or more servings of vegetables (including legumes) and fruits.[120]

Friendly Bacteria—Acidophilus is one of the most common types of *Lactobacilli,* "friendly bacteria" (probiotics) that naturally inhabit the healthy intestine. Among their many health-promoting functions, they: (1) exert direct activity against tumors; (2) prevent cancer by detoxifying or preventing the formation of carcinogenic chemicals; (3) reduce the level of cholesterol, which indirectly aides in cancer resistance; (4) help produce important B vitamins that assist in immunocompetence; and (5) curb or destroy potentially pathogenic bacteria and yeasts.[121] A study of 138 patients with bladder cancer found that those given 1 g of *L. casei* three times a day for 12 months were significantly less likely to develop a recurrence of bladder cancer than those patients receiving a placebo.[122] Other research showed that a derivative of *L. bulgaricus* improved survival among 100 patients with advanced cancer.[123] *Bifidobacteria* are also important friendly bacteria in the colon, due to their suppression of disease-causing microbes.

Spices—Curry powder, turmeric, garlic, ginger, cayenne pepper, sage, thyme, rosemary, and lemon peel are anti-cancer, immune-stimulating, antioxidant, and cholesterol-lowering, and exhibit a multitude of health-enhancing effects.

Water—It is also important to drink only pure, filtered water, in order to avoid any carcinogenic toxins, such as chlorine and lead, which might be lurking in public water systems. Likewise, well water, unless it has been adequately tested, is not to be trusted. Pesticides from farms, as well as industrial toxin runoff, can leach through the soil into underground wells.

Avoid Toxins in Your Environment

It is extremely important to be wary of the carcinogenic chemicals and contaminants found in items many people are exposed to daily, including household and garden products, cosmetics, foods, beverages, medications, and dental filling materials. Such items as furniture polish, car interior cleaners, and even common cleansers contain carcinogens ranging from formaldehyde to crystalline silica. While none of these products alone may present a critical carcinogenic exposure, when multiple exposures are added together, they become cumulative, stressing the body's immune system and damaging cells until, eventually, cancer sets in.[124]

In addition, many chemicals used in cosmetics, pesticides, and other products do not require full safety testing before they are allowed to be marketed and used by millions of consumers. Therefore, it is important to gain as much information as possible about the products to which a person's family will be exposed. For example, among the two leading brands of kitchen cleansers, Ajax contains high amounts of crystalline silica, while its competitor, Comet, does not.[125] "This sort of conscientious buying will enable people to vote with their dollars for an environmental clean-up of all carcinogenic substances used in manufacturing and industry," states Dr. Epstein.

Dr. Epstein also recommends boycotting all consumer products containing carcinogens. "There are a number of substitutes available," he explains. "For example, a combination of plain water mixed with distilled white vinegar and a small amount of baking soda, borax, and lemon juice can clean the home and bathroom as effectively as many higher-priced cleansers." Informed consumerism such as this can bring pressure to bear on the government to require that all products and chemicals be proven safe before they are allowed to be sold to an unsuspecting public.

Reduce Exposure to Electromagnetic Fields (EMFs)

The United States Congress' Office of Technology Assessment recommends a policy of prudent avoidance of EMFs. Prudent avoidance means measuring electromagnetic fields and acting to reduce exposure. To measure electromagnetic radiation, use a gauss meter, a device that measures the amount of gauss, or magnetic flux density, occurring in the home or workspace. It is easy to use and shows which places are safe from chronic exposure and which places are not. Before buying or moving into a new house, apartment, or office, always test for high electromagnetic field levels. Also, avoid living or working in areas with close proximity to power lines and generating stations. Avoid using electric blankets, electric heating pads, waterbed heaters, and similar appliances. Computer shields should always be used as well.

Stress Reduction

In line with the growing body of research regarding stress and its link to serious illnesses, many physicians believe that treating an individual's mental and emotional states is as important as treating any cancerous tumors that may be a result of such conditions. Lifestyle needs to be looked at closely, including examining a person's job, major relationships, living situation, and sexual habits.

"There is overwhelming evidence that people who have few social contacts are more likely to get sick and less likely to recover from an illness," says Erik Peper, Ph.D., Associate Director of the Institute of Holistic Healing Studies at San Francisco State University. One long-term study found that people with the lowest number of social ties were two to three times more likely to die of all causes than those with the most social connectedness.[126] This can be especially true in instances of cancer diagnoses. David Spiegel, M.D., a psychiatrist at Stanford University, demonstrated that women with breast cancer who participated in a weekly support group lived twice as long as those who did not.[127] The letting out of emotions linked to a person's condition, especially for cancer patients, can be very therapeutic.

Alternative Treatments for Cancer

It is important that the cancer patient initially consider the value of both conventional and alternative treatments before making a decision about which approach to follow. Conventional cancer physicians usually view cancer as a tumor that, if not caught quickly enough, will spread its poison throughout the body and eventually cause death.

At present, the three major treatments employed by conventional physicians to treat cancer are chemotherapy, radiation, and surgery. Each of these treatments is risky and can pose severe side effects, and each may actually shorten the cancer patient's life, rather than saving it. For example, the chemicals used in chemotherapy are themselves toxic and carcinogenic and may destroy the immune system, which is why some patients die of chemotherapeutic drugs before they actually succumb to cancer. Alan Levin, M.D., of the University of California Medical School, points out that women with breast cancer are likely to die faster with chemotherapy than without it.[128] And John Cairns, M.D., of the Harvard University School of Public Health, notes that of the approximately half a million people who die each year of cancer, only about 2% to 3% of them actually gain any benefit from chemotherapy.[129]

Surgery to remove cancerous tumors grew out of the premise, since discarded, that localized tumors were isolated manifestations of the disease and that removal of the diseased body part, if caught in time, would prevent the cancer from spreading. Surgery removes as much of the cancer as possible (very often leaving dangerous cancer cells behind), but does not correct the underlying cause of the cancer. Consequently, the tumor often re-occurs. Physicians now know as well that a cancer may already have spread to distant parts of the body long before it becomes detected elsewhere as a lump. This has been borne out by studies that show that mastectomy (the removal of breast tissue, underlying muscle, and all lymph modes in the armpit) presents no advantage, in terms of survival, over a lumpectomy and radiation.[130]

Radiation also poses inherent health hazards. Patients who receive radiation often experience painful sores of the mouth, throat, genitals, and other parts of the body, as well as the onset of ulcers, diarrhea, gastrointestinal disorders, reproductive problems, and birth defects. Ironically, they can also develop further cancer, because patients who undergo radiation therapy face a significantly increased risk of leukemia.[131]

Patients who take chemotherapy for Hodgkin's disease are 14 times more likely to develop leukemia as a result, according to experts from 14 cancer centers who studied 10,000 cases. Use of chemotherapy also increased the risk of bone, joint, and soft-tissue cancer by six times, according to the *Journal of the National Cancer Institute* (May 1995). Radiation therapy increased the risk of developing respiratory cancer by 2.7 times and genital cancers of the uterus and ovaries by 2.4 times.[132] Recent evidence shows that survivors of childhood cancer are six times more likely to get a new malignancy (particularly breast, thyroid, or brain cancer) in early adulthood, almost certainly from the toxic effects of chemotherapy and radiation.[133]

Conventional medicine rarely fully addresses the multiple causes of cancer. Alternative medicine, by contrast, regards cancer as the manifestation of an unhealthy body whose defenses are so imbalanced that they can no longer destroy cells that turn cancerous, as would normally occur in a state of health. Its essential premise is that healthy bodies do not develop cancer and that cancer is a reflection of the dysfunction of the body as a whole, rather than a localized disease. Therefore, alternative therapies seek to strengthen the immune system of the cancer patient and generally shun the use of highly toxic modalities, such as radiation and full-dose chemotherapy. Instead, they prefer to heal the entire body and employ a multifaceted, nontoxic approach, incorporating treatments that rely on biopharmaceutical, immune enhancement, metabolic, nutritional, and herbal, nontoxic methods.

The essential premise of alternative medicine is that healthy bodies do not develop cancer and that cancer is a reflection of the dysfunction of the body as a whole, rather than a localized disease.

Because cancer is a disease with multiple causes, it is important to realize that the best chance of treating it lies in an approach that addresses all of the factors involved. The therapies that follow are among the ones that offer the most promise as cancer treatments. Bear in mind that some of them may work well for certain types of cancers and not for others. Still, they all merit attention.

CAUTION The information presented in this chapter is not to be used in any manner in the nonprofessional treatment of cancer, nor should people with cancer attempt to undertake any of these methods without medical supervision. The material is meant solely as a first step in the education process concerning cancer and the factors involved in its treatment.

Integrating Treatment Methods

One of our primary messages is that there are safe and effective alternatives to conventional, toxic treatments (chemotherapy and radiation) for cancer. Unfortunately, you probably won't hear about them from your conventional doctor. But a closed mind should not stand between you and healing your cancer. Find out about using nutritional substances (vitamins, minerals, and essential oils) to fight cancer, discover the anticancer properties of herbs such as maitake mushroom, and learn the benefits of innovative substances such as shark cartilage, hydrazine sulfate, and antineoplastons. Alternative medicine physicians can guide you on the wide range of natural therapies available as well as the judicious use of conventional treatments.

WILL YOUR CHEMOTHERAPY WORK? A TEST CAN TELL YOU

In the event you decide to include chemotherapy in your cancer treatment program, a new laboratory test can help you determine the most effective chemotherapy drug for your particular cancerous tissues. In addition, the test, called the Ex Vivo Apoptotic Assay, can identify the smallest dosage that will be sufficient to kill your specific cancer. Lower dosages can reduce the severity of chemotherapy's notoriously awful side effects. Without this test, chemotherapy prescription is a process of trial and error as doctors try to determine what kind and dosage of chemotherapy will work best.

The test, developed by Robert A. Nagourney, M.D., involves placing a biopsied piece of your cancer tissue in a test tube with a concentration of one of more than 70 drugs available in chemotherapy regimens. The mixture sits for 72-96 hours to allow the cancer to "grow," after which time the laboratory can determine which drugs caused the most cell death. The test tube simulation provides a reasonable picture of the likely effect of the drug on the body of that individual. Generally, the assay's ability to predict outcomes was scored at 19 out of 21 in a test published in the *Journal of Hematology Blood Transfusion* in 1990.

The process, because it is tailored for each individual, is said to improve the outcome of chemotherapy by about two to three times. Also, the patient doesn't have to endure a battery of different drugs—and their side effects—in the hope that one will work. Let's say your physician tells you that the use of Adriamycin (a chemotherapy drug) induces remissions in 38% of women with breast cancer. How can you tell in advance if you're part of the 38% for whom it works or the 62% for whom it has no effect? "We can now painlessly determine things for a patient in a test tube that they would only be able to find out if they went through the treatments," Dr. Nagourney says. "This is crucial since I've never seen a correctly administered chemotherapy for an 'average' patient."

Robert C. Atkins, M.D., of New York City, says that the key to success in alternative medicine approaches to cancer is to gather as much data as possible on each patient, then to apply the "Hippocratic pecking order." This means using the more benign, nontoxic therapies first and saving the riskier, more invasive therapies for last, if ever. He studies the patient's immune system and the status of its key white blood cells in detail. Dr. Atkins also uses tumor markers (blood tests that detect the presence and extent of tumors) and sonographic or X-ray studies when needed. "The priority is to see whether we are getting a response to our initial treatments," says Dr. Atkins.

Dr. Atkins has observed that, in general, people diagnosed with advanced-stage cancers benefit more from nutrition and other biologic treatments (e.g., enzymes, botanicals, and glandular extracts) than from chemotherapy. For this reason, in most cases he suggests "holding off" on chemotherapy and conventional treatments unless it becomes clear that the safer treatments alone are not getting the job done. By employing nontoxic strategies first, Dr. Atkins is able to support his patients' immune capacity to reverse cancer *before* the system is ravaged by toxic treatments. Those patients who take this approach, says Dr. Atkins, tend to benefit the most from alternative cancer therapies. As one patient told him, "I've gotten to know about two dozen of your patients and the ones who went through chemotherapy before they saw you aren't here or alive anymore."

But the either-or question many patients ask—"Should I go with orthodox treatment or alternative treatment?"—is off the mark. This question is like asking which half of the card deck a person wants to play with, says Dr. Atkins. "As long as both halves are there, let's play with the whole deck. Patients with cancer who seek either orthodox or alternative approaches are entrusting their lives to doctors who are playing with half a deck."[134] In most cases of cancer, Dr. Atkins says that a *complementary* approach is needed, one which emphasizes alternative therapies along with limited and judicious use of conventional methods.

Although Dr. Atkins contends it is a fallacy to think all cancer resides within the boundaries of a tumor, he does find a role for surgery on a case-by-case basis. He finds it rarely necessary in prostate cancer, but in breast cancer, for example, surgery can be appropriate, where possible. "Surgical removal of breast tumors can lead to a complete remission of breast cancer," says Dr. Atkins. "Chemotherapy and radiation are completely unwarranted in this situation and surgery alone, when combined with an integrated immune-enhancement and detoxification program, is almost always sufficient for curing breast cancer."

Dr. Atkins regards chemotherapy as otherwise dangerous and best avoided in treating the majority of cancers. "Only in situations in which chemotherapy is proven to be effective and curative would I recommend it," he says. "In general, this might be testicular cancer, many children's tumors, and extreme cases of Hodgkin's lymphoma. On the other hand, Ukrain (see page 599) can do everything chemotherapy does but without any side effects, so it renders chemotherapy largely unnecessary."

Radiation treatments are typically futile too, says Dr. Atkins. "In some cases, however, we need to shrink tumors if they're encroaching or impinging on more vital parts of the body. In that case, a combination of radiation and hyperthermia [heat treatment delivered by ultrasound or microwave] can be effective." Dr. Atkins was among the first doctors in the U.S. to successfully combine radiation with hyperthermia to help treat prostate cancer.

With so many alternative cancer therapy options, it is literally impossible to do "everything," says Michael B. Schachter, M.D., of Suffern, New York. This is where the *art* of medicine comes in and why it is critical to have a physician well-versed in alternative medicine. To understand patients and their total situation as well as the current available information on alternative therapies, which literally changes every day, the physician must integrate all information and, together with the patient and patient's family, choose the program that will most likely work for that particular person. Then a reasonable trial should be given with careful observation. A willingness to shift gears and either remove or add elements of the program should be maintained in order to increase the chance of a successful result. Many of Dr. Schachter's patients are exposed to conventional therapies before receiving his treatment. He believes that patients receiving conventional cancer therapy while also on an alternative medicine supportive regimen do better than those who undergo conventional therapy without receiving such support.

Biopharmaceutical Therapies

Biopharmaceutical therapies include alkylglycerols, antineoplaston therapy, hydrazine sulfate, shark cartilage, and amygdalin. Each of these therapies has been developed by highly credentialed physicians and medical researchers. What they have in common is the use of nontoxic, naturally derived compounds that rebalance the body's biochemical functioning. Yet, each therapy has been condemned by the orthodox medical establishment.

Alkylglycerols

A group of compounds called alkylglycerols can bolster anticancer defenses and protect the body against the harmful effects of radiation-induced injury.[135] The richest source of these special fats is shark liver oil,[136] but these fats are found to a lesser extent in mother's milk and cow's milk.[137] Animal studies have indicated that alkylglycerols have antitumor activity, probably mediated through macrophages in the form of selective destruction to cancer cells.[138] Cell-culture studies have shown that this "selection" seems to be affected by the cholesterol concentration of the cancer cell; as the cholesterol level drops, the cancer cells die more rapidly.[139]

Extracts of shark liver oil may help people tolerate both chemotherapy and radiation. The administration of alkylglycerols prior to radiation treatment was found to cause advanced tumors to regress toward less advanced stages;[140] alkylglycerols also caused reversal of tumor growth in animal studies.[141] A possible explanation for these findings is that this substance can inhibit a variety of tumor-promoting compounds. One potential area of concern, however, is contamination of shark liver oil by ocean pollutants. No published research, to our knowledge, has addressed this issue nor have the potential toxicities at normal doses been adequately studied.

Antineoplaston Therapy

Stanislaw Burzynski, M.D., Ph.D., based in Houston, Texas, is a graduate of the Lublin Medical Academy in Poland, where he graduated first in his class in 1967. A year later, at the age of 25, he earned a Ph.D. in biochemistry. Dr. Burzynski's treatment is based on the theory that the body has a parallel biochemical defense system (BDS) independent of the immune system. "The mechanism of defense in this system is completely different than in the immune system," Dr. Burzynski explains. "It is a reprogramming of defective cells. It's no longer killing of the cells, but changing the program inside the defective cell, which means that the cell will begin to function normally. In the case of cancer, for instance, if all of the cancer cells will be reprogrammed and function normally, then ultimately we won't have cancer anymore."[142]

Dr. Burzynski has found that the BDS consists of short-chain amino acids known as polypeptides, that are able to inhibit cancer cell growth. He has named these polypeptides antineoplastons (meaning "against new growth"). According to Dr. Burzynski, cancer is largely a disease caused by a malfunction in information processing. "The cell develops according to the program for cellular differentiation," he notes. "Millions of cells are differentiated in the human body every day, bringing up the possibility of errors in the program for differentiation. Taking under consideration such large numbers of cells undergoing differentiation, it is more than likely that a significant number of these cells will develop toward neoplasia [tumor growth]."[143] Antineoplastons, he claims, are able to reprogram cancer cells to restore this process

THE PROACTIVE PATIENT

Perhaps the best illustration of what needs to be done when a person is diagnosed with cancer comes from the experience of Neal Dublinsky. Neal, then 24 years old and recently embarked upon a career as an attorney in Los Angeles, was diagnosed with the most advanced stage (Stage IV) of non-Hodgkin's lymphoma. The bulky tumor had spread to his entire abdomen and there was fluid build-up in his lungs. "I was shocked when I got the diagnosis, and was in extreme physical pain," Neal recalls. "My doctor told me that I had to undergo chemotherapy if I wanted to live. I didn't know better, so I did it."

Neal received chemotherapy for four months. The treatments reduced the tumor, but the reduction was short-lived. They also caused traumatizing side effects, including total hair loss, a feeling of being poisoned, and gastrointestinal distress. "During this time, I was taking an aggressive combination of six different drugs and every three weeks I received more chemotherapy," Neal says. "Afterwards, I was completely incapacitated and each time I returned for another treatment, it got worse."

After the fourth month, Neal underwent radiation therapy for three more weeks. "The radiation only took a minute," Neal notes. "But within an hour, I would be violently ill and retching from my core, and I could no longer eat solid foods." After the daily radiation treatments ended, Neal then underwent a bone marrow transplant using his own bone marrow. "That was the worst time of my life," Neal continues, "but once it was over, it looked like I would be all right." Only four months later, though, a new tumor emerged in his pelvic area that was beginning to compress his right kidney. At this point, all Neal's doctors could offer him was the prospect of another series of even harsher chemotherapy to buy him a little more time, but with no hope of a cure.

By this point, Neal had lost faith in what conventional medicine could do for him. "The physician who performed my bone marrow transplant knew everything about transplants, but almost nothing about other treatment options," he says. "It was that way with each of my doctors. Even though they meant well and were experts in their fields, none of them were able to put it all together and see the big picture." Instead of giving up, Neal contacted alternative cancer associations and also read voraciously, educating himself about every alternative therapy he could find. In addition, he phoned cancer survivors to learn about their experiences with the therapies he was discovering.

Neal was particularly intrigued by the antineoplaston therapy developed by conventionally trained physician Stanislaw Burzynski, M.D., Ph.D., of Houston, Texas. "I spoke with ten of Dr. Burzynski's former patients," he relates. "They had all responded well to his therapy and had suffered from similar kinds of cancer as my own. They spoke of Dr. Burzynski in glowing terms and encouraged me to see him. I decided to follow their advice, but ultimately my decision to go was a leap of faith, because my doctors' attitudes about alternative therapies were dismissive. I figured if I was going to die, I was going to die fighting."

A year after his original cancer diagnosis, Neal began treatment with Dr. Burzynski. The first thing he noticed was that it was not painful. Dr. Burzynski put him on an IV drip of antineoplastons that ran ten hours a day. For ten months, Neal remained on the drip as an outpatient. "Within weeks of beginning the treatment, my biochemical profile improved," he reports. His liver and kidney function progressed, and he started to feel better. His tumor was gradually regressing, showing slow and steady improvement.

After ten months, Neal received four injections of antineoplastons a day, together with oral capsules. Six months later, he achieved complete remission. He stayed with the treatment for another 18 months, taking the capsules for maintenance, then he was taken off the medicine altogether. During this time he also adopted a dairy-less, vegetarian diet, augmented with nutritional and herbal supplements. He underwent a series of localized hyperthermia treatments and colonic irrigations as well, and had his mercury amalgam fillings removed from his mouth. "I began to incorporate elements of many health programs, because I wanted to survive," he says.

He has. Today, Neal continues on in good health. Neal's suggestion to others diagnosed with cancer is simple. "Learn about all the alternative therapies," he says. "You should know more than you will ever use. Read, explore, and research everything, keeping an open mind. Visit the clinics, consult with the doctors. Interview patients, especially those whose histories, type of cancer, stage, and background are most like your own, because different therapies have better track records for different types of cancer. Most importantly, don't become passive. Your treatment is a choice. Don't let others make it for you. Take charge and face this challenge head on."

to normal. They interact with the DNA of the cells, actually becoming part of the DNA and taking the place of carcinogens that would otherwise occupy the same spots on the DNA strand. As this occurs, the antineoplastons redirect the DNA back into normal reproduction.

Antineoplastons can be extracted from blood and urine or manufactured synthetically. Approximately 95% of Dr. Burzynski's patients receive synthetic antineoplastons. Over 2,000 patients have been treated at the Burzynski Research Institute (BRI), most of them diagnosed with advanced or terminal cancer. The majority of them have benefited from antineoplaston therapy, experiencing complete or partial remission, or stabilization of their conditions. In addition, few side effects have been noted. The range of cancers that Dr. Burzynski has treated include lymphoma, breast cancer, leukemia, bone cancer, brain cancer, prostate cancer, lung cancer, colon cancer, and cancer of the bladder.[144]

Dr. Burzynski has successfully used antineoplastons, which he produces himself in an FDA-approved manufacturing facility in his clinic in Houston. As part of a study, he used antineoplastons to treat 20 patients who had advanced astrocytoma, a particularly fast-growing type of brain tumor. Nearly 80% of them responded favorably and a number of them were tumor free four years later.[145] Animal studies in Japan indicate that low doses of an orally administered synthetic antineoplaston help prevent cancers of the breast, lung, and liver.[146]

According to scientific reports presented at the 86th Annual Meeting of the American Association for Cancer Research in March of 1995, Dr. Burzynski's antineoplastons increase the activity of tumor suppressor genes.[147] At this time, there is no other treatment available that is directed to this critical mechanism in the development of cancer. Ironically, instead of being acknowledged for this discovery, Dr. Burzynski has been repeatedly harassed by the FDA and the Texas medical board.

One of Dr. Burzynski's patients, a 10-year-old boy, was diagnosed with an advanced glioblastoma brain tumor. He underwent radiation therapy that proved largely ineffective and in fact damaged the viability of his growth-related pituitary gland. His mental function was also diminished by the therapy, according to his mother. Despite harsh criticism from his physicians, the boy began antineoplaston treatments with Dr. Burzynski. Within one month, the tumor mass began to break down; after six months, he was in complete remission, and he remains cancer free.[148]

714X

This unique compound, developed by biologist Gaston Naessens, consists of nitrogen-rich camphor and organic salts. Jacinte Levesque, O.M.D., of Montreal, Quebec, Canada, a close associate of Naessens, notes that this therapy was developed when Naessens observed that cancer cells required and used up a lot of nitrogen, often stealing it from healthy cells. In order to do this, cancer cells excrete a poisonous compound called co-cancerogenic K factor (CKF), which paralyzes the immune system, allowing the cancer cells to draw the needed nitrogen from the healthy cells. "When 714X is introduced into the system, it acts as an attractor for the cancer cells, because of the high level of nitrogen in the camphor. Now, because the cancer cells are getting their nitrogen from the camphor molecules, they no longer have to excrete CKF to immobilize the healthy cells' defensive systems." While the 714X is engaging the cancer cells, the immune system is able to do its job once again.

In animal studies, 714X was effective against bone cancers and breast cancer. In humans, researchers reported a shrinking of the tumors, weight gain or weight stabilization, reduction or elimination of pain, and extended survival.[149] Dr. Naessens has collected hundreds of case histories in which 714X was effective against melanomas, carcinomas, lymphomas, and other types of cancer.[150]

The usual treatment course involves three consecutive series of injections of 714X directly into the lymph nodes of the groin. The injections are given once daily for periods of 21 consecutive days, followed by a break of two days while the natural defenses of the body are restored. 714X has no harmful side effects, other than burning sensations at or around the site of injection.

Glutathione and N-Acetyl-Cysteine (NAC)

Glutathione is a protein that contains the amino acids cysteine, glycine, and glutamic acid; NAC, a derivative of cysteine, is an amino acid precursor for the body's production of glutathione. Cysteine accounts for glutathione's antioxidant activity and its role in the key antioxidant enzyme, glutathione peroxidase. Blood levels of glutathione peroxidase tend to decrease after the sixth decade of life and are typically lower in patients with malignant cancers.[151] Supplementing regularly with a combination of glutathione and NAC may be especially important for older people who have been exposed to numerous toxins in their diet and environment.

Glutathione reduces free-radical damage to DNA and prevents depletion of other antioxidants. It also helps metabolize various carcinogens, activates certain immune cells, helps synthesize and repair DNA, and may inhibit angiogenesis (a blood vessel-forming process required for tumor growth).[152] Glutathione is also a component of an enzyme that assists in the liver's metabolism of drugs and toxic chemicals. Glutathione and NAC supplements have been found to diminish the toxic side effects of chemotherapy and other conventional treatments.[153] Glutathione is best taken sublingually, rectally, or intravenously.

Hydrazine Sulfate

Often, cancer patients die not from the disease itself but from a process called cachexia, a condition in which the body becomes malnourished and the patient simply wastes away. In 1968, Joseph Gold, M.D., Director of the Syracuse Cancer Research Institute, in Syracuse, New York, discovered that the chemical hydrazine sulfate could reverse cachexia, providing the body with extra strength to fight the disease.

A study of 740 cancer patients (200 with lung cancer, 138 with stomach cancer, 66 with breast cancer, 63 with Hodgkin's disease, 31 with melanoma, and others) reported tumor stabilization or regression in 51% of patients, while 46.6% of the patients reported symptomatic improvements, such as fewer respiratory problems and a decrease in fever.[154] Decreased pain was noted even in cases of metastatic bone cancer, and some patients improved so markedly that they were once again able to walk and care for themselves. In one study, the compound significantly improved the nutritional status and survival of lung cancer patients;[155] it may also aid in treating cancers of the breast and larynx, as well as Hodgkin's disease, desmosarcoma, and neuroblastoma.[156]

Hydrazine sulfate improves appetite, increases a patient's sense of well-being, results in weight gain in those who have lost weight, and may contribute to a shrinkage of tumors. It seems to work by interfering with the liver's ability to produce glucose from lactic acid, a process known as gluconeogenesis. Cancer cells thrive on glucose, which allows the cancer to grow quickly while normal cells in the body break down. This destructive cycle may continue, resulting in a wasting away of the lean mass of the patient. By interfering with gluconeogenesis, hydrazine sulfate inhibits the cancer while allowing normal cells to thrive, thus reversing the vicious cycle. Although the substance is inexpensive and non-patentable, the U.S. Food and Drug Administration has made it illegal for chemical companies to sell hydrazine sulfate to the public.

While hydrazine sulfate can be toxic, the form used in cancer treatment differs from industrial grade versions in that it has been highly purified. Side effects are limited to occasional nausea, dizziness, itching, drowsiness and euphoria. Although there have been occasional reports of patients experiencing numbness in their extremities, this has been alleviated through the use of vitamin B6.

Shark Cartilage

One of the reasons tumors grow is because they develop their own blood supply. Most tissues and organs also do this in a process known as angiogenesis. Cartilage—a tough, elastic, connective tissue found in humans and most animals, including sharks—does not develop a blood supply, because it contains an "anti-angiogenic" substance that stops the blood supply from developing, according to William Lane, Ph.D., of New Jersey, one of the leading proponents of shark cartilage therapy.[161]

The basis for shark cartilage therapy is that if the blood supply to tumors can be interrupted, the tumors will stop growing and eventually die. Research has demonstrated that the anti-angiogenic properties of cartilage can do just that.[162] Robert Langer, Ph.D., of the Massachusetts Institute of Technology, has further demonstrated that shark cartilage contains 1,000 times more of the angiogenesis inhibitor than any other type of cartilage.[163]

In a Cuban study, 14 out of 29 "terminal" cancer patients survived after receiving shark cartilage; of those who died, nine actually died of cancer and six others died of other causes. At 23 months, which was four times the life expectancy, about half (14) of the original group of 29 patients were still alive, doing well, and enjoying completely normal lives. After 33 months of receiving no treatment other than a modest dose of shark cartilage daily, no new deaths had been reported.[164] In a recent pilot study, patients with advanced kidney cancer given an extract of shark cartilage lived twice as long as would be expected without the cartilage.[165]

According to Dr. Lane, ovarian cancer responds the most consistently to shark cartilage, while uterine, cervical, and central nervous system cancers respond positively. Dr. Lane reports that shark cartilage is highly effective against advanced prostate tumors, achieving tumor reduction rates of 15% to 67%. It is also capable of significantly lowering PSA counts in 12-16 weeks. Generally, shark cartilage works best against solid tumors; pancreatic cancers, provided they are not too advanced, also respond well.[166] Shark cartilage is most effective when administered rectally in higher doses than can be tolerated orally.

In 1990, research further confirmed the clinical benefit of shark cartilage by finding a "significant inhibition of angiogenesis."[167] One substance found in sharks, called squalamine, has recently demonstrated the ability to attack tumors via anti-angiogenesis. According to researchers at Johns Hopkins University, animal studies of squalamine suggest a potential therapeutic benefit for patients with brain cancer.[168]

THE ANTICANCER EFFECTS OF CIMETIDINE

According to cancer researcher Wayne Martin, of Fairhope, Alabama, the over-the-counter (OTC) drug cimetidine (nonprescription Tagamet®), which enjoys widespread popularity in the U.S. for the treatment of stomach distress, also holds promise as an anticancer agent, particularly in cases of recurrence of colorectal cancer. To support his claim, Martin cites a number of clinical studies. "The first account of the anticancer effect of cimetidine came from the University of Nebraska in 1979, which reported on two lung cancer patients who had complete remission when they were given cimetidine for stomach distress," says Martin. Since that time, two clinical trials also indicate that the drug may have anticancer properties. In the first trial, patients in Australia who underwent surgery for colorectal cancer, and who also took cimetidine for seven days immediately following their operation, experienced reduced immunosuppressive effects due to surgery, compared with a control group. Follow-up research showed that the three-year survival rate of patients who received cimetidine over the seven days was 93% compared to 59% among those who did not receive the drug.[157]

In 1995, researchers in Japan achieved even better results among colorectal cancer patients who received one year of chemotherapy following surgery. Beginning one week after their operation, half of the patients were placed on cimetidine for the same one-year period, while the remaining patients received chemotherapy alone. At a median follow-up of 3.9 years, 100% of the patients who received the drug were still alive, compared to 53.3% of the patients who only received chemotherapy.[158]

Cimetidine seems to bolster the cancer-fighting activity of natural killer cells[159] and increase the number of helper T lymphocytes.[160] Researchers also believe that cimetidine's effectiveness as an anticancer agent lies in its ability to prevent the normal surge of suppressor T cells that occurs after major surgery. "This is highly immunosuppressive at a time when the surgery for colorectal cancer is sending a flood of cancer cells to all parts of the body," Martin explains. "Cimetidine prevents this surge of suppressor T cells and also inhibits histamine, which is immunosuppressive as well. Additionally, cimetidine also causes cancer cell-killing immunocytes to enter tumors in greater numbers."

Though there have been no trials on cimetidine following any kind of major surgery for cancer other than colorectal surgery, Martin believes that the drug should be just as effective in preventing recurrence of other forms of cancer. "The implication of these two trials is that if every colorectal cancer patient were given cimetidine from one week before surgery until one year after surgery, death from colorectal surgery could be reduced by 80% or more."

Amygdalin/Laetrile

Known technically as amygdalin, or vitamin B17, Laetrile was first synthesized in 1924.[169] Amygdalin is one of many nitrilosides, which are natural cyanide-containing substances found in numerous foods, including the seeds of the prunasin family (apricots, apples, cherries, plums, and peaches), buckwheat, millet, and cassava melons. Much of the experimental work on Laetrile has been conducted by Harold W. Manner, Ph.D., Chairman of the Biology Department at Loyola University, in Chicago, Illinois, whose work is considered to be among the first unbiased studies of the overall value of Laetrile. He reported that Laetrile is virtually nontoxic and that, when used along with vitamin A and certain enzymes, it stimulates the production of antibodies against spontaneous breast tumors in mice; there was complete regression in 76% of the treated mice.[170] The best results using Laetrile are usually obtained when it is used in conjunction with proteolytic enzymes, diet, vitamin A, and other vitamins and minerals.[171]

The noted biochemist Ernest Krebs, Jr., Ph.D., first identified amygdalin as an anticancer agent. Amygdalin has been found to have strong cancer-fighting potential, particularly with regard to secondary cancers, including a 60% reduction in lung metastases.[172] Epidemiologic studies, animal studies, and clinical studies show evidence of amygdalin efficacy. Research indicates that it can extend the lives of both breast and bone cancer patients.[173]

Ukrain

This substance is derived from a combination of a common plant called celandine (*Chelidonium majus*) and thiophosphoric acid (also called thiotepa, one of the original chemotherapeutic agents). The combination appears to neutralize the toxic effects of the alkaloids contained in thiophosphoric acid; by this method, Ukrain has been rendered almost completely nontoxic. Ukrain does not harm the body's healthy tissues and anticancer defenses but actually fortifies them.[174]

Clinical research has shown that Ukrain improves the overall condition and extends the survival of "terminal" cancer patients by giving their immune systems a boost and by blocking tumor growth.[175] In two studies of Ukrain treatment, significant clinical benefits (tumor regression) occurred for both lung cancer and cervical cancer patients.[176] Ukrain helps fortify the immune system in people with a variety of cancers;[177] it consistently increases the number of T helper cells, which coordinate key immune-related activities. At the same time, Ukrain increases the oxygen in both normal and malignant cells. In normal cells, the oxygen then stabilizes; in cancer cells, however, oxygen consumption drops down to zero.[178] Since the cancer cells stop "breathing" at this point, after 15 minutes of Ukrain treatment, they die.

Ukrain also inhibits the synthesis of genetic material and protein in cancer cells, but not in healthy cells.[179] This may account for the findings supporting Ukrain's ability to completely inhibit growth in 57 of 60 human cell lines representing cancers of the lung, colon, kidney, ovary, breast, and brain, as well as melanoma and leukemia.[180] Only two leukemia cell lines and one brain cancer cell line were not inhibited by Ukrain. At high concentrations (100 mcg per ml), however, Ukrain causes "100% growth inhibition" in all 60 human cancer lines. Finally, Ukrain possesses a strong selectivity for cancer cells, and when exposed to ultraviolet light, it glows. For these reasons, it can be used to determine whether a suspicious growth is malignant.[181]

Scientists at the Ukrainian Anticancer Institute, in Vienna, Austria, have carried out clinical studies of Ukrain over a 10-year period on 206 patients with cancers at various stages of development. Total remissions were achieved even in cases of advanced metastatic cancer; the best success rate with Ukrain (93%) was achieved with cancer patients starting treatment at the earliest stage of tumor development (no metastasis). For those starting therapy in Stage II (minimal metastasis), the success rate was 72%, and for those in Stage III (advanced, metastatic cancer), the success rate was 30%.[182]

Immune Enhancement Therapies

Immune enhancement therapies are frequently used by alternative physicians to treat cancer. A strong immune system is one of the keys to the delay and prevention of cancer, but the combination of poor nutrition and exposure to pollutants and natural toxins can cripple immune function, as can the aging of the thymus gland. Immune enhancement therapies seek to restore the immune system to optimum function so that the body can then subdue the cancer. In alternative medicine, this is accomplished without the side effects associated with conventional therapies.

Immunomodulators

An immunomodulator is a substance that can tune, adjust, regulate, or focus—modulate—the activities of the immune system to reverse illnesses.

TRANSFER FACTOR

The first task of our immune system is to recognize what is us and what is not us—what should be in our bodies and what should not—and then to destroy or otherwise neutralize anything harmful. The most well-known immune response is called the humoral response. It involves the production of antibodies, the immune cells that fight off antigens when our bodies recognize their presence. We get sick when our immune systems do not quickly recognize microbial antigens and they're allowed to multiply.

Researchers have suggested that Transfer Factors (TFs) evolved as a way of compensating for the immune system's slow humoral response to foreign substances. Transfer Factors are tiny protein molecules. They are much smaller than antibodies and serve as messengers for the immune system's other major type of response, called the cell-mediated response, which involves other white blood cells (especially T lymphocytes).

A researcher named H.S. Lawrence, using white blood cell extracts, proved in 1949 that an immune response can be transferred via Transfer Factor from a host who tests positive for exposure to a specific antigen to a recipient who tests negative. Early researchers knew that an immune response had been transferred when they saw that persons who received antigen-specific TFs become skin-test positive for that antigen, whereas they had been negative beforehand.

What kind of immunological information is transferred? The TFs can "educate" or modulate a recipient's immune system, teaching it to recognize these specific antigens and communicating the knowledge that they are present. TFs can be procured from either leukocytes filtered from the blood or from milk colostrum. A baby's first exposure to transferred immune response comes from colostrum, the breast milk substance that mothers produce just after giving birth. TFs from colostrum taken as a supplement provide resistance to infection and disease.

IMMUNE NUTRIENTS FROM MILK PROTEIN

One of the most important substances required by the immune system for optimal functioning is an amino acid complex called glutathione. However, supplementation is made difficult by the complexity of the body's system for delivering glutathione to cells. Canadian researchers figured out a way to deliver gluathione effectively in the form of a natural milk protein supplement called Immunocal™, and early research suggests it has benefits for cancer.

Glutathione is a tripeptide, a small protein consisting of three amino acids (glutamic acid, cysteine, and glycine) bound together. The substance functions as a principle antioxidant, scavenging free radicals and toxins such as lipid peroxides that would otherwise damage, even destroy, cells. Further, glutathione regulates the activities and regeneration of other antioxidants such as vitamins A, C, and E. However, when the body is suffering from oxidative stress, supplies of glutathione become depleted. Oxidative stress is a condition in which the body is unable to detoxify itself completely and is overrun by free radicals because antioxidants are depleted.

Glutathione exerts another protective and scavenging role in concert with the liver, the body's primary organ of detoxification and internal cleansing. In the liver, glutathione combines with toxins, carcinogens, and waste products as a way of more effectively securing their elimination from the body. Glutathione has an important role in supporting the activity of white blood cells called lymphocytes (the key players in the body's immune response) as well as antibodies. The tricky fact about glutathione is that you can't simply take more glutathione as a supplement; it must be made inside the cells.

Recognizing this biochemical fact, Canadian researchers developed Immunocal to deliver to the cells the necessary precursors for glutathione. In the course of researching dietary protein sources capable of boosting the immune system, Gustavo Bounous, M.D., of McGill University, in Montreal, Quebec, discovered what became Immunocal. Immunocal is a natural food supplement consisting of concentrated milk protein powder containing unusually high amounts of glutathione precursors. Immunocal concentrates three constituents of the whey portion of milk (albumin, alpha-lactalbumin, and lactoferrin). These contain a large quantity of cystine, an amino acid breakdown product that is a more usable form of cysteine.

Another product, IMUPlus, supplies the three amino acids that make up the tripeptide glutathione: glutamic acid, glycine, and cysteine in the form of cystine. The cystine supplied in IMUPlus can easily be transported to target cells. Mothers' milk supplies cystine in the same alpha-lactalbumin form contained in IMUPlus. IMUPlus also has high levels of the bio-active forms of amino acids leucine, isoleucine, and valine. These amino acids provide a strong source of nitrogen for muscle growth and repair. Another bio-active protein supplied by IMUPlus is lactoferrin, an iron-binding protein that helps block the growth of potentially pathogenic intestinal bacteria. Lactoferrin levels are usually found to be lower in individuals who are very ill. Another immunomodulator made from milk colostrum is Cytolog, which may also prove helpful in boosting the immune system to treat cancer.

Livingston Therapy

In the 1940s, the late Virginia Livingston, M.D., discovered a microbe in human blood that she called *Progenitor cryptocides*. According to Dr. Livingston, this microbe exists in all of us from the moment of conception until the moment of death, and she claimed that it is responsible for cancer. Like other pleomorphic microorganisms, *Progenitor cryptocides* can change size and shape, becoming as small as a virus and as large as a bacterial or fungal microbe. It can be viewed in all of its forms under a darkfield microscope. Dr. Livingston discovered that a certain form of the microbe caused cancer in experimental animal studies, and she found it in virtually all human and animal cancers. Foods can also be contaminated with *Progenitor cryptocides*, including beef, chicken, eggs, and milk, according to Dr. Livingston. This means that eating such foods can provide a basis for the infectious transmission of cancer. Because of this, the Livingston diet emphasizes fresh, raw or lightly cooked plant foods.

The basis of Livingston therapy is restoration of the immune system using a diet of vegetarian raw foods, vaccines, and nutritional supplements. The vaccines are derived from a culture of the patient's own microbe. "It comes from the patient's own tissues, either from the tumor, the urine, the blood, or the pleural [lung] fluid, and it's specific for each person," Dr. Livingston explained. The Bacillus Calmette-Guerin (BCG) vaccine is also used, which is a mild tuberculin vaccine that stimulates the immune system. According to Dr. Livingston, BCG helps stimulate white blood cells to kill cancer cells.

Dr. Livingston also discovered that pleomorphic microbes secrete a hormone that is remarkably similar to human chorionic gonadotropin (HCG). During pregnancy, HCG coats the placenta, safeguarding the fetus from being destroyed by the mother's immune system. Dr. Livingston theorized that when a cancer cell forms, stimulated by *Progenitor cryptocides*, it is protected by a similar hormone. Her research, though initially ridiculed, was proven accurate through the work of researchers at Rockefeller University, Princeton Laboratories, and Allegheny General Hospital, who found that all cancer cells do indeed contain HCG.[183]

Another key to Dr. Livingston's program was her discovery that naturally occurring retinoid abscisic acid (a plant hormone and derivative of vitamin A) neutralizes HCG production. According to Dr. Livingston, abscisic acid is a plant growth regulator that "causes seedlings to go to sleep in the Fall."[184] Similarly, abscisic acid may cause cancer microbes to stop growing. Her research has shown that cancer patients tend to have low levels of this naturally occurring anticancer chemical. Foods rich in abscisic acid include carrots, green leafy vegetables, nuts, seeds, and cereals. Unfortunately, the liver must be functioning optimally in order to convert vitamin A to abscisic acid, plus the acid can be destroyed by cooking. However, the liver function of cancer patients is often subpar. To help counteract this condition, Dr. Livingston recommended drinking carrot juice with liver powder. She also advocated eating a near raw foods diet as a method of preserving their abscisic acid content. No sugar, refined flours, or high-sodium foods are allowed, and few (if any) animal foods, because of their high likelihood of being contaminated.[185]

Dr. Livingston reported success with advanced breast cancer patients, as well as individuals with cancer of the esophagus that had spread to the liver, colon cancer, Hodgkin's disease, and melanoma. Many of these cancers had spread to other parts of the body and the patients were considered terminal. Although she passed away in 1990, Dr. Livingston's work is being carried on by other physicians. Using the Livingston vaccine, they have noted shrinkage or disappearance of tumors, as well as complete remissions in patients with leukemia and malignant lymphoma.[186]

T/Tn Antigen Breast Cancer Vaccine

Cancer cells have proteins, or antigens, on their surfaces that can be recognized by the immune system. The identification of certain cancer-related antigens forms the basis for the approach embraced by the late Georg Springer, M.D. Dr. Springer, an immunologist who founded the Heather Bligh Cancer Research Laboratories at the Chicago Medical School, showed that two antigens called T and Tn play a vital role in the immune system's ability to respond to cancer. The immune system's reaction to T and Tn antigens results in strong cancer cell–killing activity in both animal and human studies.[187]

Using biochemical tests, Dr. Springer detected the T and Tn antigens in over 90% of all cancers. The less aggressive cancers produce a higher proportion of the T antigen, while the Tn antigen predominates in the more aggressive cancers.[188] The overall concentrations of the T and Tn antigens correlate specifically with the aggressiveness of breast cancer.[189]

In 1974, Dr. Springer had his first opportunity to test his experimental vaccine when his wife, Heather Bligh, developed breast cancer and was told she had only a year to live. After receiving the T/Tn vaccine, however, she lived another six years. Encouraged, Dr. Springer began a pilot study with 19 breast cancer patients, all of whom went on to survive at least five years on the T/Tn vaccine; 16 of these women (84%) are still alive, 11 of them after a decade or more of their supposedly terminal diagnosis. In another study, 26 women with advanced breast cancer were given the T/Tn vaccine after undergoing an operation for their primary cancer or after the first recurrence. All survived over five years and only five out of the 26 patients died within 5-10 years; 14 of 18 patients (78%) who were vaccinated over ten years ago are still alive.[190]

Dr. Springer emphasized that nutritional support is also important. He advises his patients to take (once daily) a multivitamin, vitamin C (3-4 g), beta carotene (20,000 IU), and vitamin E (1,600 IU). "The nutritional component is extremely important, because nutrients have been shown to influence both cell-mediated and antibody facets of the immune response," said Dr. Springer. "I recommend that my patients consume a wholesome, high-fiber diet that includes fish and liver to obtain the beneficial nutrients from these foods." In theory, said Dr. Springer, his immune-stimulating vaccine could be used for the treatment of all cancers. However, since the T antigen has not been found in brain tumors or in sarcomas (bone and muscle tumors), the vaccine is unlikely to have any therapeutic impact on these cancers.

Anti-Mycoplasma Auto-Vaccine

Another approach involves the culturing of a patient's blood for a cell wall–deficient bacterium called mycoplasma, found in the blood of all cancer patients. The process produces a vaccine, called the anti-mycoplasma auto-vaccine, for reintroduction into the patient's system. Originally developed in Germany, the anti-mycoplasma auto-vaccine technique is now practiced in North America by Filibert Muñoz, M.D., at the Instituto Medico Biologico (IMB), in Tijuana, Mexico. When this mycoplasma vaccine is given to the patient from whom it was made, the cancer often arrests or regresses. IMB physicians are qualified in the handling of different biological medicine modalities for the nontoxic treatment of chronic degenerative conditions, including cancer. Dr. Muñoz uses the anti-mycoplasma vaccine as part of a multifaceted cancer treatment program that involves ultraviolet photophoresis of the patient's blood, detoxification, dietary change, and nutritional supplementation.

Manuel, 73, was diagnosed with Stage IV prostate cancer with metastases to the spine that were dangerously compressing the spinal cord. Manuel refused chemotherapy, radiation, and surgery, and was willing to try the vaccine protocols used by Dr. Muñoz. First, Dr. Muñoz used a darkfield microscope to study a living sample of Manuel's blood for platelet shape. Platelets are disc-shaped cellular elements in blood that are essential for clotting. Blood platelets can be compromised by bacteria, mycoplasmas, viruses, and parasites such that their shape and ability to clot may be impaired, Dr. Muñoz explains. "The culture allows for the identification of platelet forms typical of many illnesses, particularly of malignant cancers." This test confirmed that there was metastatic prostate cancer and that Manuel had a high amount of toxins in his blood coming from bacterial infections in a root canal tooth and from his dental amalgams.

Next, Dr. Muñoz drew 120 cc of Manuel's blood as the basis for preparing the anti-mycoplasma vaccine. Generally, the results of the platelet test indicate if it is appropriate to prepare an anti-mycoplasma vaccine from the patient's blood, says Dr. Muñoz. Dr. Muñoz explains that a single blood culture from the patient is sufficient to produce enough vaccine to last 4-5 months at the rate of 2-3 injections weekly. Manuel received the vaccine three times weekly for several months, then as his cancer began to reverse itself and he became healthier, the injections were gradually reduced to once monthly. Manuel will need to receive the anti-mycoplasma injection about once every month for the rest of his life as a precaution against any further cancer activity.

During the two months of culturing time for the anti-mycoplasma vaccine, Dr. Muñoz started other treatments. He drew a pint of Manuel's blood each day for the first two weeks and ran it through an ultraviolet photophoresis machine. The process of ultraviolet light therapy killed viruses and bacteria and neutralized toxins in the blood; ozone, a form of oxygen, was also introduced into the blood sample to further purify it, then the blood was reinfused into Manuel. For patients with advanced cancers, Dr. Muñoz does UV blood photophoresis once daily for the first 1-2 weeks.

Therapies also included chelation, sauna, massage, and supplements, including acidophilus, enzymes, glutathione, N-acetyl-cysteine, and both herbal and synthetic antiviral substances, says Dr. Muñoz. These included echinacea, goldenseal, interferon, Pranosine, and Zovirax. In addition, Manuel's diet underwent significant changes, based on a modified macrobiotic approach. He was to eat only fresh fruits and vegetables and fish, and to avoid red meats and minimize his poultry consumption. He also started a regular exercise program to induce sweating and the discharging of toxins through the skin, and he received regular intestinal colonics.

A prime source of Manuel's toxins was his teeth, specifically a toxic substance called di-methylsulphite released from several root canals. Di-methylsulphite is a by-product of the interaction of bacteria and heavy metals placed in the mouth by dental procedures such as amalgam fillings. This substance will depress the immune system and can even weaken the heart. As part of his cancer treatment program, Manuel had his root canal teeth extracted.

Once his cancer was completely controlled and the cancer markers and antigen factors were down to zero, meaning there was no cancer activity, Manuel required spinal surgery for the nerve compression produced by the bony metastases. This operation was necessary to allow Manuel to regain the use of his lumbar nerves and the ability to walk again without pain or fatigue. Two years later, Manuel remained healthy and active, and had taken to traveling all over Mexico.

Coley's Toxins

In the 1920s, New York physician William B. Coley, M.D., found that certain infectious diseases—notably, from bacteria—might stimulate a therapeutic effect against malignancies when introduced into the body in the form of a sterilized vaccine. Dr. Coley found his "toxins" could give the body's anticancer defenses a nonspecific "kick" against the cancer cells by mobilizing them against an easier opponent. Dr. Coley was a surgeon at Memorial Hospital in New York City, one of the leading conventional cancer treatment centers in the U.S., and he refused to believe that cancer was incurable. At the time, surgical methods typically involved amputation of the body parts affected by the cancer; understandably, surgeons who had to perform such operations were more than willing to explore alternatives. Bear in mind that radiation therapy and chemotherapy had not yet been conceived.

Observing that erysipelas, a dangerous skin infection caused by the bacteria *Streptococcus pyogenes,* was followed by a dramatic tumor regression in a cancer patient with advanced sarcoma, Dr. Coley reasoned that certain infectious diseases might stimulate a therapeutic effect on malignancies. Dr. Coley developed a mixture of sterile bacteria, which became known as "mixed bacterial vaccine" or "Coley's Toxins." Specifically, Dr. Coley used *Streptococcus pyogenes* and the bacterium *Serratia marcescens;* the product contained the toxins produced by these heat-killed bacteria and the dead bacteria themselves. His idea was that the bacteria would activate the body's anticancer defenses by mobilizing their forces against the bacteria.

Dr. Coley injected his patients with the bacterial mixture (usually at the site of the tumor or nearby) and claimed success with both partial and complete tumor regression for a number of different types of cancer. For patients receiving the vaccine for sarcoma (cancer of connective tissue and bone), Dr. Coley reported 41% complete cures. He generally recommended a minimum of five months treatment for effective results; treatments lasting only 4-6 weeks often failed. Dr. Coley's death in 1936 coincided with the explosive growth of chemotherapy; as a consequence, his research was buried in the decade that followed. However, during his lifetime, about 50 physicians in the U.S. (including one at the Mayo Clinic) as well as Europe, treated cancer patients with Coley's Toxins.

Five-year survival rates after treatment with Coley's vaccine based on data collected in the 1970s showed the following: 65% for patients with inoperable breast cancer; 69% for patients with inoperable ovarian cancer; and 90% for those with bone cancer.[191] Research conducted at Memorial Sloan-Kettering Cancer Center, in New York City, showed that patients with advanced non-Hodgkin's lymphoma experienced a 93% remission rate versus 29% for those who had only chemotherapy.[192]

Coley's mixed bacterial vaccine can cause some disconcerting side effects, beginning with a shaking chill that lasts 10-15 minutes and typically followed by the development of a fever in the range of 102° F to 105° F. The transient fever is simply the body reacting to the bacterial toxins in the vaccine and has therapeutic benefit to the body.

Pleomorphism and SANUM Remedies

The German researcher Guenther Enderlein, M.D., Ph.D., (1872-1968) opened up a new vista in understanding cancer and devising treatments through his use of darkfield microscopy. In the course of studying live blood under the darkfield microscope, Dr. Enderlein observed protein-based microorganisms, which he called protits, that flourish in the blood cells and plasma, tissues, and body fluids. Protits appear to live in a mutually beneficial (symbiotic) relationship with the body under healthy conditions, but when the body's internal environment—its cellular terrain—changes in terms of pH (acidity/alkalinity ratio), toxic load, or the availability of oxygen and/or nutrients, the protits transform into a disease-causing form. The ability of organisms to undergo sequential shape changes is a theory of bacteriology called pleomorphism.

The microbe that Dr. Enderlein linked with cancer is primarily *Mucor racemosus Fresen*. Under certain conditions, biochemical factors in the body foster develop-ment of the protits into more lethal forms. It has been more specifically identified as the blood parasite *Siphonospora polymorpha*—the most advanced stage of the *Mucor racemosus Fresen,* according to Dr. Enderlein—a major cancer-promoting agent.[193]

Dr. Enderlein noted that a diet rich in animal fats and proteins seemed to promote changes in pH and cause these normally harmless microbes to change into the harmful *Mucor* fungi. Thus, the typical American diet provides the ideal conditions for transforming protits into their harmful forms. This situation is made worse by carcinogenic substances—dietary factors (food additives, pesticides), viruses, alcohol, tobacco, radiation—that can alter the cell's ability to metabolize proteins and fats and to make energy.

The protit, in its altered form, leads to faulty genetic mechanisms that result in incorrect synthesis of proteins such as those used by the immune system.[194] This situation, combined with the "blocking factors" mentioned earlier, may help explain why the immune system often fails to respond appropriately to cancer cells. Dr. Enderlein theorized that disease must be treated at the cellular level and he formulated his remedies accordingly. His formulas, known as SANUM remedies, are dilutions of bacteria and fungi that, once injected into the cancer patient, work according to the principles of homeopathy. By injecting harmless forms of bacteria or fungi exemplifying the microorganism in its benign state, the disease-causing protits revert to their benign form, which promotes normal immune function.

Erik Enby, M.D., of Gothenberg, Sweden, has carried forth the work of Dr. Enderlein and confirmed all his original findings. During Dr. Enby's initial eight-year experience with the darkfield microscope and Enderlein remedies, he successfully treated more than 100 cases of prostate and uterine cancer and effectively stabilized or reversed many cases of breast cancer and leukemia.[195] Dr. Enby notes that Enderlein remedies are most successful when used with an effective program of detoxification.

Dendritic Cell Therapy

Virtually every major cancer center in the U.S. is involved in clinical trials with dendritic cell therapy, a type of cancer vaccine showing remarkable results. But it is already available and proving its worth outside our borders. The new approach seeks to stimulate the immune system to destroy cancer sites and cells. Researchers are attempting to create cancer vaccines through a number of techniques, experimenting with a variety of substances that stimulate different types of immune responses. Presently, the National Cancer Institute alone has 100 active cancer vaccine trials—15 of these are devoted to dendritic cell therapy. Dendritic cells (DCs) are a rare type of white blood cell, generally accounting for less than 0.2% of total blood cells. Dendritic cells were identified only in 1973, by Ralph Steinman, M.D., head of Rockefeller's Laboratory of Immunology and Cellular Physiology, and the late Zanvil Cohn. The critical role dendritic cells play in immunity wasn't appreciated until the early 1990s, when their use in immunotherapy studies first began appearing.

Cancer's causes and the immune system's failure to effectively deal with it are related. Cancer cells have unique and potent defenses against the immune system—they are immuno-suppressive. These defense mechanisms can make the cancer cells undetectable by our immune system and they can also disrupt normal immune responses, weakening or preventing any attack on them. Specifically, they secrete substances called cytokines (some cytokines increase immune response and some suppress it). If we think of the cells of our immune system as an army, dendritic cells are the spies and scouts, alerting the main forces to the number, whereabouts, and vulnerable points of the enemy. The T cells are the main forces. Thus, the actions of cancer cell–produced cytokines have the effect of leaving our immune system's "army" without the knowledge of where the enemy is or how to effectively attack it.

Dendritic cell therapy is designed to overcome these defenses and stimulate the body to mount an effective attack on tumor cells—with no toxic side effects. A crucial discovery was made in 1996, when Drs. Michael Roth and Sylvia Kiertscher of the Jonsson Cancer Center at the University of California, at Los Angeles, reported that dendritic cells could be created outside the body from more common blood cells called monocytes. This made the creation of a vaccine more practical. To create the vaccine, DCs in culture are exposed to all or part of cancer cells from the patient's tumors. The DCs incorporate this material internally, break it down into protein fragments, and present them on their surface as antigens. These antigen-loaded DCs are injected into the patient's body, usually far from the tumor site. This stimulates the T cells to proliferate, each T cell producing many clones containing the same tumor-specific antigen. This creates a new army of T cells able to recognize and effectively attack the patient's cancer.

Dendritic cell therapy is being researched at the University of Heidelberg in Germany, the Institute Curie in France, and hospitals throughout Europe. Practically every major medical center in the U.S. is involved in this work, including Memorial Sloan-Kettering, Cedars-Sinai, Dana Farber/Harvard Medical School, M.D. Anderson, and Johns Hopkins University. They have been conducting clinical trials with dendritic cell therapy for melanoma (skin cancer) and prostate, breast, colon, and other cancers with encouraging outcomes. One private company that has been deeply involved with dendritic cell therapy research is Aidan Incorporated, in Tempe, Arizona. Like other biotechnology firms, Aidan has developed proprietary dendritic cell therapy cancer protocols that are showing remarkable results. And this therapy is available now, not as a clinical trial but as part of an integrated anticancer program, at the BioPulse Clinic, in Tijuana, Mexico. "They have just started using it in combination with their other protocols, but the responses have been very positive," according to Neil Riordan, M.S., P.A.-C., President of Aidan.

Metabolic Therapies

The practitioners of metabolic therapies feel that, because many factors are involved in the onset of cancer, no one therapy will be enough to treat it. Metabolic treatments include an eclectic mix of diet and nutritional supplementation, herbal medicine, detoxification, immune stimulation, and enzyme therapy. The therapeutic goal of such therapies is to rebuild and revitalize the body's life-sustaining functions, thereby eliminating all traces of disease.

Kelley's Nutritional–Metabolic Therapy

Individualized nutrition, detoxification, and the use of pancreatic enzymes make up the therapy advanced by William Donald Kelley, D.D.S. A dentist by training, Dr. Kelley developed his protocol in response to his own metastatic pancreatic cancer, which he reversed in the late 1960s. Dr. Kelley called his program "metabolic ecology" to indicate that the patient's entire way of life must be changed. "The person who has the disease should be treated, not the disease that has the person," he explained.

One of the main points of Dr. Kelley's therapy is that cancer is often caused by the body's inability to effectively metabolize protein; this inability can be linked to improper amounts of proteolytic enzymes. According to Dr. Kelley, these protein-digesting pancreatic enzymes, rather than the immune system, are the body's first defense against tumors. This led him to declare that, fundamentally, cancer is a deficiency of pancreatic enzymes; this deficiency then leads to a disordering of protein metabolism and, from there, to the proliferation of abnormal cells. He believed that excessive protein intake is the most significant cause of pancreatic enzyme deficiency.

His metabolic detoxification therapy calls for coffee enemas, restricting protein intake, and emphasizing a diet of whole grains, fruits, and vegetables supplemented with pancreatic enzymes (taken between meals) and raw juices. Dr. Kelley advised cancer patients to altogether avoid pasteurized milk, peanuts, white flour and sugar, chlorinated water, and all processed foods. He recommended that the diet consist of about 70% raw foods, such as fresh raw salads, to maximize the consumption of living enzymes. Dr. Kelley developed a line of 25 nutritional formulations for hard tumors (solid mass cancers) and 29 for soft tumors (leukemia, lymphoma, melanoma), which the patient takes until they are cancer free for two years. The Kelley protocol is offered by Robert C. Atkins, M.D., of New York City.

Nicholas Gonzalez, M.D., of New York City, a classically trained immunologist, currently employs a cancer treatment that, to a large extent, is based on Kelley's therapy. Dr. Gonzalez' protocol includes six basic concepts first put forward by Dr. Kelley—an appropriate diet for each individual, intensive nutritional support, photomorphogen (raw beef organs and glands) support, digestive aids such as hydrochloric acid, proteolytic enzyme supplementation, and detoxification.[196]

Dr. Gonzalez did not just blindly adopt Dr. Kelley's work though. Rather, his belief that some of Kelley's protocols were valid came as a result of a 500-page, five-year study of Dr. Kelley's cancer patients. The study was conducted under the auspices of Robert Good, M.D., Ph.D., former President of Memorial Sloan-Kettering Cancer Center. Dr. Gonzalez originally tracked 50 of Dr. Kelley's patients, 21-71 years old, all of whom were diagnosed as terminal or with an extremely poor prognosis, encompassing 25 different types of cancer. The results were astonishing, as Dr. Gonzalez discovered the average survival time for the group was ten years and climbing.

To further test Dr. Kelley's results, Dr. Gonzalez decided to track 22 of his patients who had been diagnosed with pancreatic cancer, since this form of cancer had a five-year survival rate with conventional medical therapies of nearly zero percent, as well as a life expectancy of only two to three months. Ten of the patients who only consulted with Dr. Kelley once and then did not follow his treatment program survived only an average of 67 days, or just over two months. Seven who followed his program only partially survived an average of 233 days, or nearly eight months. The five patients who followed his program closely had a median survival rate of nine years; four of the five were still alive and one had died of Alzheimer's disease.[197]

Gerson Therapy

The Gerson therapy was developed by Max Gerson, M.D., a German doctor who immigrated to the U.S. in the 1930s. Shortly after graduating from medical school, Dr. Gerson began to experience severe migraine headaches. He reasoned that he could alleviate his problem by reworking his diet. After succeeding in doing so,

he found that he was able to successfully treat tuberculosis patients with diet alone as well. He then took the next leap, which was to treat cancer patients with his diet. He also treated both Dr. Albert Schweitzer and his wife for various health problems, including diabetes.

Dr. Gerson believed that cancer would not occur in a body with a properly balanced and functioning liver, pancreas, thyroid, and immune system. He found that he could reverse the majority of cancers with his dietary regime, which consisted of a low-salt vegan diet, supplemented ten times a day with freshly crushed fruit (primarily apple) and vegetable (primarily carrot) juices, taken at hourly intervals. This acts to inundate the body with the nutrients from nearly 20 pounds of fresh, organic foods. In addition, patients take 3-4 coffee enemas a day for detoxification and pain relief. There is also supplementation with various substances such as pepsin, potassium, Lugol's solution (a source of supplementary iodine), niacin, pancreatin (a digestive enzyme), and thyroid extracts, which are taken to stimulate organ function, especially the liver and thyroid.

What Dr. Gerson discovered was that cancer patients had an excess of sodium, far outweighing the potassium in their bodies. The sodium acts as a poison in the body, because it is an enzyme inhibitor, whereas potassium is an enzyme activator. The fruits and vegetables in the diet are used to correct this sodium and potassium imbalance. This, in turn, helps revitalize the liver so it can begin to rid the body of malignant cells again. The coffee enemas then aid in the elimination of these dead cancer cells.

Many of Dr. Gerson's cancer patients, whom he treated in the 1940s and 1950s, are documented to have lived in good health for many decades after their treatment period.[198] Although Dr. Gerson passed away in 1959, his work is being carried on by his daughter, Charlotte, and her staff at the Gerson Institute, in Tijuana, Mexico. Gar Hildenbrand, of the Gerson Research Organization, and Shirley Cavin, from the University of California at San Diego's Cancer Prevention and Control Program, compared five-year melanoma survival rates of Gerson therapy patients to rates found in comparable, conventionally treated groups. The study examined 153 cancer patients, 25-72 years old, in various stages of melanoma. Here is a summary of the results:

- Of patients with Stage I and II melanoma (localized), 100% of Gerson therapy patients survived for five years compared with 79% of patients receiving conventional treatment.

- Of patients with Stage IIIa melanoma (regionally metastasized), 82% of Gerson therapy patients were still alive at five years compared with 39% of the conventionally treated patients.

- Of patients with Stage IIIa and IIIb melanoma (regionally metastasized), 70% of Gerson therapy patients were still alive at five years compared with 41% of the conventionally treated patients.

- Of patients with Stage IVa melanoma (a classification proposed by the authors to cover distant metastases), 39% of Gerson therapy patients survived for five years compared with 6% of patients treated by conventional medicine.[199]

Even considering possible weaknesses in the study's design, the substantial differences in survival between the Gerson therapy patients and conventionally treated patients is too great to be dismissed.

Issels' Whole-Body Therapy

The late Josef Issels, M.D., of Germany, came to the conclusion that the only way to attack cancer was not to attack the local manifestation—the tumor—as most conventional therapies do, but rather to strengthen the entire body. "Dr. Issels believes that chronic and especially malignant diseases can only develop if the metabolism and the natural resistance of an organism is negatively changed by various so-called 'causal factors,'" said Wolfgang Woppel, M.D., of Germany, an associate of Dr. Issels. "These include genetic traits, microbes, dental amalgams and infections, abnormal intestinal flora, faulty diet, neural interference, chemical toxins, and radiation."

From this realization, Dr. Issels developed his whole-body therapy, combining many modalities in a single protocol to improve the body's natural defense systems. One of the first things his program recommends is the removal of infected teeth and dental (mercury) amalgams, because these are a tremendous source of toxic stress on the body. A patient's diet is also closely addressed, particularly the removal of tobacco, coffee, tea, alcohol, and other harmful substances from the diet. Organic whole foods are stressed, along with proper digestive support, in the form of the friendly bacteria *L. acidophilus*. Dr. Issels therapy also addresses the patient's emotional state, by having patients unload toxic emotions like stress and anger. This is accomplished through a form of informal psychotherapy.

On top of this framework, Issels' program employs oxygen therapies such as the haemotogenic oxidation therapy. In this therapy, blood is drawn from the patient and oxygen is bubbled through it. Ultraviolet rays are then applied and the blood is left to settle for up to an hour, then returned to the patient by intravenous drip.

This procedure sterilizes and reactivates the blood causing an aggressive immune response. Dr. Issels' therapy also uses hyperthermia to reenergize the immune system. Provoking a fever in the body increases the number of disease-destroying leukocytes (white blood cells). His program employs vaccines for specific types of cancer, using ultrafiltrates of cancer tissues in much the same way as modern vaccines use infectious agents to stimulate antibody production.

In one long-term study, Dr. Issels' protocol was used with 252 terminal patients who had previously undergone conventional surgery and radiation therapy. After five years, 16.6% were still alive and functioning. After 15 years on the program, though, over 92% of the original survivors were still alive and showed no signs of cancer.[202] In another study, 370 cancer patients, with various types and various stages of the disease, followed Dr. Issels' program. After five years, 87% were still alive and showing no signs of the cancer recurring. Further research showed the relapse rate to be only 13% with whole-body therapy.[203] Since Dr. Issels death, there are two doctors continuing his work, Dr. Woppel and Ahmed Elkadi, M.D., of Tampa, Florida.

Insulin Potentiation Therapy

Insulin Potentiation Therapy (IPT) involves the use of a small dose of insulin, which is administered to cancer patients to induce a state of hypoglycemia (low blood sugar). When the patient begins to experience hypoglycemic symptoms, low doses of conventional chemotherapy are administered intravenously. "Insulin can potentiate the effects of many remedies because it has the unique ability to increase a cell's permeability to certain substances," explains Ross Hauser, M.D., Medical Director of Caring Medical and Rehabilitation Services, in Oak Park, Illinois, and one of the few physicians in the U.S. who uses IPT to treat cancer. "Since cancer cells have many more insulin receptors than normal cells, insulin can be used to push anticancer agents into the cancer cells to destroy them."

Insulin also causes certain cancer cells to go into a proliferative growth phase, during which chemotherapy works better. "This is crucial," Dr. Hauser says, "because, in many instances, less than 10% of the cells constituting the tumor mass are actively proliferating by the time the tumor is detected. Thus, the remaining 90% of cancer cells are not susceptible to most chemotherapeutic agents. Most people may not realize that a tumor that has reached the size of clinical detectability has already undergone approximately 30 doublings in size. Only ten further doubling cycles are required to produce a tumor burden of approximately one kilogram (2.2 pounds), which is usually lethal."

CANCER AND HYPERTHERMIA

The body uses its own internally generated heat to protect itself from viruses, bacteria, and other harmful substances. A fever is the body's attempt to destroy invading organisms and to sweat impurities out through the skin. Fever is an effective natural process of curing disease and restoring health—heat therapy, or hyperthermia, represents a way to create fever to call out this natural healing process. A state of natural hyperthermia exists when body temperature rises above its normal level of 98.6° F. An increase in body temperature causes many physiological responses to occur. By increasing the production of antibodies and interferon, it stimulates the immune system. Practitioners of alternative medicine have long recognized hyperthermia as a useful technique in detoxification therapy because it releases from the body toxins stored in fat cells, such as pesticides, PCBs, and drug residues.

The principle behind hyperthermia is simple: heat cancer cells and they can be killed easily. Direct killing of cancer cells begins to occur when the cancerous tissue reaches about 104° F to 105.8° F.[200] "Only a relatively small rise in body temperature can make a huge difference," says Robert C. Atkins, M.D., who includes it in his cancer protocols. Though the principle sounds simple, the technique is far more complicated, thanks to the body's ability to regulate its internal temperature. As any sauna enthusiast will attest, the human body likes heat only to a point. When the body temperature rises, blood flow increases to dissipate the excess heat. One way to circumvent the body's ability to regulate its temperature is to apply the heat locally, targeting a specific tumor. This can be done with the use of microwaves, radio waves, and ultrasound, which can be directed at parts of the body with great precision. Unlike normal tissue, tumors have poor blood flow relative to their metabolic needs and cannot dissipate the heat, so they tend to get hotter than the surrounding area and are more vulnerable to the effects of heat.

At the Duke Hyperthermia Program of the Duke University Medical Center, in Durham, North Carolina, considerable success has been reported in using hyperthermia to treat soft-tissue sarcomas and recurrences of breast cancer. One recent study found that radiation combined with hyperthermia was 30% more effective against breast cancer than radiation treatment alone.[201] Tumors located near the surface of the body generally appear to be more amenable to treatment than deep-tissue tumors.

"I try never to use radiation treatment—which is even more dangerous than most forms of chemotherapy—without also using hyperthermia," says Dr. Atkins. "Thanks to hyperthermia, we can shrink tumors with far less radiation to get the same therapeutic outcome, and our patients' immune systems and overall health are faring much better as a result."

Studies have shown that hyperthermia treatment modifies cell membranes in such a way as to protect healthy cells and make tumor cells more susceptible to chemotherapy and radiation. For this reason, hyperthermia is a useful adjunct in cancer therapy, largely because it enables the use of lower doses of chemotherapy and radiation. Frederich Douwes, M.D., at the Klinik St. Georg, near Munich, Germany, uses infrared-light-induced systemic hyperthermia in conjunction with low-dose chemotherapy, galvanotherapy, and detoxification with excellent results in various metastatic cancers. Hyperthermia treatments play a role in stimulating the immune system, as evidenced by the drop in white blood cell counts immediately following treatment and the rise that occurs within a few hours. Not only do the number of white blood cells increase, but their ability to destroy target cells appears to increase as well. A recent study showed an increase in the production of interleukin-1 (an immune-stimulating compound) with whole-body hyperthermia. Studies indicate that increased body temperature plays a positive role in the healing process of the body. An increase in temperature from 98.6° F to 104° F should increase metabolism by about 30%. This increased metabolic rate accounts for some of the increased immune activity and thus hyperthermia's contribution to cancer reversal.

CAUTION Patients with temperature regulation problems, especially the old and the very young, should not use hyperthermia. Microwave diathermy can burn tissue around the eyes and should never be used by people with pacemakers. People with peripheral vascular disease (poor blood flow to the legs and feet) or loss of sensation should not use hyperthermia because of the risk of burns. Caution is advised with patients who have cardiovascular disease, in particular arrhythmia (irregular heartbeat) and tachycardia (abnormally rapid heart rate), or severe hypertension or hypotension.

IPT was developed in Mexico by the late Donato Perez Garcia, Sr., M.D., in 1930. Today, his work is being carried on by his grandson, Donato Perez Garcia, Jr., M.D. At an IPT training course in February 2001, Dr. Perez Garcia revealed that he's not aware of a single person dying as a result of the therapy. "Because the doses of chemotherapy medications used during IPT are 10% to 25% of the amounts given during conventional cancer care, the risk of side effects is greatly diminished," Dr. Hauser says. "IPT is a great alternative to high-dose chemotherapy with all of its side effects, which can include immunosuppression, hair loss, and injury to the nerves, heart, kidney, and liver. IPT can cause these side effects as well, but they are almost nonexistent because of the low dose of medication used." Dr. Hauser reports that the most common side effect is fatigue on the day of treatment and, in rare cases, nausea.

According to Dr. Hauser, the ideal candidate for IPT is someone newly diagnosed with cancer, with a small tumor load, no metastases, no other medical conditions, and who has not undergone previous cancer treatments. "This doesn't mean that someone who has had previous chemotherapy, has multiple medical conditions, or has a high tumor load can't get IPT," says Dr. Hauser, "but it does signify that the prognosis isn't as good and that the number of treatments and medications used may need to be increased."

Generally, IPT is used until the cancer is arrested or goes into remission, or it is found that IPT is clearly not working. "If, after 6-10 treatments, there has been no tumor regression, the treatment regimen is either stopped or changed," Dr. Hauser says, adding that, although IPT is a pliable treatment, it depends on the particular cancer being sensitive to the chemotherapeutic agent(s) being used. Dr. Hauser reports that IPT has been used successfully and is being studied as a treatment for a variety of cancers, including adenocarcinoma (tumors), lymphoma, squamous cell, multiple myeloma, and others.

A variation on this insulin therapy, called Insulin-induced Hypoglycemic Therapy (IHT), is available at the BioPulse Rejuvenation Center, in Tijuana, Mexico. It involves intravenously introducing insulin to produce a state of profoundly lowered blood sugar. This state lasts for a period of about an hour, with the patient under careful clinical supervision. This hypoglycemic condition changes the environment in the body to one detrimental to cancer cells. Oxygen and glucose are normally metabolized together by healthy human cells. When glucose levels are lowered by insulin, metabolism slows, oxygen accumulates in the blood, and the production of carbon dioxide decreases. This increases the pH of the blood and tissues from an acidic to a more alkaline condition. Cancer cells cannot survive in an oxygenated,

alkaline environment. It has been theorized that the extreme pH of the blood inactivates enzymes responsible for cancer cells' energy and their ability to replicate. Repeated exposure to these conditions does not harm healthy cells, but it kills cancer cells.

Herbal Therapy

Herbs, or botanicals, contain a large number of naturally occurring chemicals that have biological activity. In the past 150 years, chemists and pharmacists have been isolating and purifying active compounds from plants in an attempt to produce safe and effective pharmaceutical drugs. Examples include digoxin (from foxglove, *Digitalis purpurea*), reserpine (from Indian snakeroot, *Rauwolfia serpentina*), colchicine (from autumn crocus, *Colchicum autumnale*), morphine (from the opium poppy, *Papaver somniafera*), and many more.

In China, *Fu Zheng* cancer therapy relies upon ginseng and astragalus, among other herbs. The *Journal of the American Medical Association* reported that life expectancy doubled for patients with rapidly advancing cancers when Chinese herbs were added to their treatment plan. *JAMA* noted that, in general, "patients who received *Fu Zheng* therapy survived longer and tolerated their treatment better than those patients who were treated by Western medicine alone. In addition, the five-year survival rate was twice as high among patients with nasopharyngeal [nasal passage and pharynx] cancer (53% versus 24%)."[204]

Through skillful selection of an herb (or herbs in combination) targeted to the individual patient, major changes in health can be effected with less danger of the side effects inherent in drug-based medicine. However, the common assumption that herbs act slowly and mildly is not necessarily true; adverse effects can occur if an inadequate dose, a low-quality herb, or the wrong herb is prescribed, or if an effective herb causes the body to kill too much cancer too fast and overloads the body's detoxification mechanisms.

In recent years, a great deal of pharmaceutical research has gone into analyzing the active ingredients of herbs to find out how and why they work—an effect referred to as the herb's action. Herbal actions indicate the ways in which the remedy affects human physiology. In some cases, the action is due to a specific chemical present in the herb or it may be due to complex synergistic interactions among various constituents of the plant. In the case of cancer, botanical agents work by:

- Stimulating DNA repair mechanisms (via sulfur-containing compounds)

- Producing antioxidant effects (via the quenching of free radicals by carotenoids and polyphenols)

- Promoting induction of protective enzymes (proteases)

- Inhibiting cancer-activating enzymes (flavonols and tannins)

- Inducing oxygenating effects (via flavonols and rare elements such as germanium)

Among the more recent entries onto the anticancer herbal stage are the following:

Betulinic Acid from Birch Trees—This substance blocked the growth of human melanoma tumors that were transferred to mice, without harming normal cells.[205] Tests in human cancer cell cultures indicated effectiveness against cancers of the lymph, lung, and liver as well.[206] Betulin, a compound that can be converted to betulinic acid, is a major constituent of white-barked birch trees, which are found in abundance throughout the northern hemisphere.

Thuja Tincture—*Thuja occidentalis* (arbor vitae, or tree of life) has served as a successful adjunctive herbal therapy for many cancer cases. An 86-year-old woman had been suffering for 14 years from a large orange-sized tumor in her right breast. It had spread to the lymph nodes and doctors labeled it "inoperable, Stage III breast carcinoma with lymph metastases." The tumor had never been treated. The woman was given tamoxifen, an estrogen blocker, as well as a tincture of thuja herbal extract (20 drops, three times daily), echinacea (one tablet, three times daily), and various vitamins and minerals. She also applied thuja cream locally and later took comfrey, passionflower, sweet violet, cleavers (bedstraw), and chickweed. After one month, the abnormal lymph nodules had disappeared and the tumor was softening; six months later, the tumor had shrunk by 25%; after another six months, no sign of cancer remained.[207]

Bromelain—Bromelain, a mixture of proteases and other enzymes isolated from pineapple stems and fruit, has been used for centuries to treat inflammatory diseases and other health problems. More recently, its anticancer activity has attracted the interest of scientists. Bromelain has been shown to induce differentiation of three leukemia cell lines (in culture) as well as to stimulate the anticancer defenses (monocyte and macrophage cell-killing activity) and to inhibit the growth of cancer cells.[208] The report cites these effects as a possible expla-

nation for the observed tumor-killing potential of bromelain when combined with chemotherapy and notes that such effects are seen even after oral administration. However, rectal administration of bromelain may be preferable for greatest effect.

Phenolic Antioxidants from Mint—Members of the mint family contain special antioxidant compounds that seem to be even more effective than vitamin E (perhaps the premier antioxidant) in helping to prevent recurrences of tumors. One phenolic compound is rosmarinic acid, which is found in high levels in some mints, including wild self-heal *(Prunella vulgaris)*, long deemed by Native Americans and traditional Chinese doctors to be a major herbal medicine.[209]

Centella Extract from Gotu Kola *(Hydrocotyle centella)*—This nutrient-rich herb is said to neutralize and remove toxins, improve mental functioning, and help prevent a nervous breakdown.[210] Scientists at the Amala Cancer Research Center, in Kerala, India, found that gotu kola showed a strong ability to kill cultured cancer cells. They also showed that centella extract more than doubled the life span of mice with tumors and showed a remarkable lack of toxicity even in doses far in excess of those used for therapeutic benefit.[211]

Perillyl Alcohol from Lavender Flowers—The oil of lavender contains a cancer-fighting component called perillyl alcohol. This substance, which is also a derivative of the citrus oil limonene, has been shown in animal studies to inhibit more than 80% of all chemically induced breast cancers. It is thought that the compound blocks tumor growth by inhibiting the gene believed to initiate cancer.[212]

Pollen from Honeybees—Pollen is the male sex cell from a plant; bees pick up this substance when they enter flowers in search of nectar. Research dating back to 1948 found that animals whose diets were supplemented with bee pollen had a significantly lower tumor incidence.[213] A study in *Nature* reported that royal jelly (derived from pollen) protected all mice injected with cancer cells for longer than 12 months, in contrast to those in the control group, injected with the same number of cancer cells, all of which died within 12 days.[214] In studies of women suffering from inoperable uterine cancer, those given bee pollen were found to maintain strong immune systems and to suffer less from nausea, hair loss, and fatigue. Similar results have been reported in studies of cancer patients undergoing radiation treatment.[215]

Other Herbs—Other herbal medicines have been identified as potentially useful adjuncts to cancer treatment, including: pearl barley *(Hordeum vulgare)*; reishi mushroom *(Ganoderma lucidum)*; shiitake mushroom *(Lentinula edodes)*; cauliflower *(Brassica oleracea)*; wax gourd *(Benincasa hispida)*; calendula *(Calendula officinalis)*; chaparral *(Larrea divaricata* and *Larrea tridentata)*; white mulberry *(Morus alba)*; Japanese pepper *(Piper futokadsura)*; thyme *(Thymus serpyllum)*; Chinese cucumber *(Trichosanthes kirilowii)*; and stinging nettle *(Urtica dioica)*.[216]

Rather than consider herbal treatments as alternatives for early or follow-up cancer care, cancer researchers are more likely to investigate the use of herbs as an adjunct conventional treatment. Botanicals have been shown to directly counteract the dangerous effects of chemotherapy and radiation, which are toxic to the body, suppress the immune system, and can cause serious damage to cells. Certain botanicals enhance immunity whereas others stimulate the body's detoxification and antioxidant systems. Still others may block the activity of tumor-stimulating hormones, such as estrogen and prolactin. The use of botanical agents in tandem with conventional treatment may not necessarily be the optimal strategy in every case. Combining these two divergent approaches affords a way for conventional medicine to begin making the transition to a more sensible and ultimately more effective way of treating cancer.

Echinacea

This herb has well-known immune-enhancing abilities. Echinacea was found to increase NK cell activity by 221% in patients with inoperable metastatic esophageal or colorectal cancer.[217] Patients with advanced liver cancer showed a 90% increase in their NK activity when echinacea was combined with a thymus-stimulating agent.[218] In addition, a natural chemical substance in echinacea, arabinogalactan, stimulates the tumor-killing activity of macrophages.[219] Arabinogalactan is also found in larch tree extract (Larix), which has powerful antiviral properties as well. The primary role of echinacea is to provide protection against infection, a common and sometimes deadly complication in advanced-stage cancers.

Essiac

In the 1920s, a Canadian nurse named Rene Caisse introduced a nontoxic herbal tea for treating cancer. The tea was originally named Lasagen by the Ojibway, a Native American tribe based in Ontario, Canada. Caisse obtained the formula for this natural herbal combination from a breast cancer patient who had been healed by an Ojibway medicine man; she renamed it Essiac (which is Caisse spelled backwards) and used it to treat thousands of cancer patients. Although Essiac has never undergone randomized clinical trials, Caisse and her associates recorded many impressive case histories attesting to its efficacy. The recoveries encompass cancers of the pancreas, breast, ovaries, esophagus, bladder, bones, and bile ducts, as well as lymphoma and malignant melanoma.

In 1937, Caisse was introduced to Dr. John Wolfer, then Director of the Cancer Clinic at Northwestern University Medical School. Wolfer arranged for Caisse to treat 30 terminal cancer patients with Essiac under the supervision of five doctors. After 18 months, the doctors concluded that Essiac had relieved pain, shrunk tumors, and improved the survival odds of these patients. Also in 1937, Emma Carson, M.D., spent 24 days inspecting the Bracebridge Clinic, in Ottawa, Canada, where Caisse had done most of her work. Dr. Carson reviewed over 400 cases of cancer patients who had been treated with Essiac and recorded indisputable improvements. She declared: "The vast majority of Caisse's patients are brought to her for treatment after [conventional treatment] has failed and the patients are pronounced incurable. The actual results from Essiac treatments and the rapidity of repair were absolutely marvelous and must be seen to convincingly confirm belief."[220]

According to a recent report, Essiac tea: (1) strengthens the immune system; (2) reduces the toxic side effects of many drugs; (3) increases energy levels; and (4) diminishes inflammatory processes. Studies of some of Essiac's main components—burdock, Indian rhubarb, sheep sorrel, slippery elm—have each demonstrated a significant amount of anticancer activity.[221]

Green Tea

Green tea *(Camellia sinensis)* is a highly popular beverage among the Chinese and Japanese, who consume, on average, 2-10 cups daily. Green tea contains a substance called epigallocatechin gallate, which inhibits the growth of cancers and lowers cholesterol. This is one of a number of chemical compounds known as catechins, which are many times stronger than vitamin E in defending the body against free radicals. The catechins found in green tea support the immune system's responsiveness and have demonstrated powerful anticarcinogenic effects. Studies indicate that green tea consumption can reduce the risk of cancers of the liver and throat.[222] Green tea flavonols (the active bioflavonoids in the tea) may offer substantial cancer protection if consumed on a regular basis.

Hoxsey Therapy

Harry Hoxsey was an herbal folk healer who eventually attracted a devoted following of cancer survivors after he started using an herbal therapy that originated with his great-grandfather. Hoxsey formula comes in a potassium iodide solution and contains the following herbs: red clover (*Trifolium pratense*), buckthorn bark (*Rhamnus purshianus*), burdock root (*Arctium lappa*), Stillingia root (*Stillingia sylvatica*), barberry bark (*Berberis vulgaris*), chaparral (*Larrea tridentata*), licorice root (*Glycyrrhiza glabra*), Cascara amarga (*Picramnia antidesma*), and prickly ash bark (*Zanthoxylum americanum*). The Hoxsey therapy consists of a mix of herbal preparations for internal and external use, and an emphasis on diet, vitamin and mineral supplements, and personal counseling. The external formula (but not the internal one) includes *Sanguinaria canadensis*, also known as bloodroot, which has been used by Lake Superior Native Americans to treat cancer.

Wide-ranging laboratory research has found definite biological activity in the various ingredients of the Hoxsey herbal formula. Studies have shown antitumor effects with components of prickly ash and Stillingia, burdock, and extracts of barberry.[223] In addition, the genistein found in red clover may be responsible for a wide range of anticancer activities, including antioxidant activity, anti-estrogen activity (slowing tumor growth in some cancers), and inhibition of new blood vessel formation (blocks tumor growth).[224] Licorice has a variety of immune-stimulating properties and direct antitumor effects; it also demonstrates the ability to block estrogen's cancer-stimulating effects.[225]

Cancers that have responded favorably to the Hoxsey combination include lymphoma, melanoma, and skin cancer. A five-year preliminary study followed patients with advanced cancer who were treated at three alternative cancer clinics. Six of 16 patients treated at the Hoxsey clinic remained alive and were reported to be disease free after five years. Two of these patients had cancers that are normally considered incurable or "terminal." In contrast, all patients from the other two clinics, where Hoxsey herbs were not used, had died by the end of five years.[226]

CAUTION Individuals taking the Hoxsey tonic are cautioned to avoid tomatoes, alcohol, processed flour, and vinegar because they can negate the tonic's effects.

Iscador (Mistletoe)

Iscador is the trade name for a mistletoe preparation that has been used by European physicians since 1920. Iscador consists of fermented extracts of European mistletoe (*Viscum album*), some forms of which are combined with small amounts of metals to produce anticancer effects.[227] Originally conceived by Rudolf Steiner (1864–1925), Austrian scientist and founder of anthroposophic medicine, the therapeutic success of Iscador has been reported in nearly 5,000 case studies. In animal experiments, Iscador has been found to kill cancer cells, stimulate the immune system, and significantly inhibit tumor formation.[228]

The activity of various immune cells, including NK cells, increases significantly within 24 hours of injecting Iscador.[229] These effects might explain various findings that Iscador selectively inhibits the growth of different types of tumor cells.[230] Two reviews of the clinical research have concluded that treatment with Iscador increases both the length and quality of life, stabilizes the cancer, causes tumors to shrink, and improves the overall condition of the patient.[231]

A study at the Institute for Preventive Medicine, in Heidelberg, Germany, found that Iscador, used as an adjunctive treatment in patients with several types of cancer, extended survival time by 40%. In the study, 396 cancer patients treated with Iscador survived 4.23 years compared to the control group's survival time of 3.05 years. In the subsequent part of the study, mistletoe treatment increased the survival time of 17 breast cancer patients to 4.79 years compared to 2.41 years in the control group.[232]

Iscador's potential as a cancer therapy is strongly supported by the following findings: (1) significantly more breast cancer patients treated with Iscador were alive after ten years compared to patients who received no Iscador; (2) women with cervical cancer who had a combination of surgery, Iscador, and radiotherapy showed an 83% survival rate after five years compared to a 69% survival rate for those who received radiation alone; (3) normally 50% of bladder papillomas become malignant in three years, but with Iscador, only three out of 14 did; (4) among bronchial cancer patients, 75% of those given Iscador were still alive after four years compared to only 35% of those without Iscador; and (5) the survival rate after three years for skin cancer patients on Iscador was 80% compared to 65% for those without it.[233]

Maitake Mushroom (*Grifola*)

According to researchers at the National Cancer Center in Japan, there was complete tumor elimination in about 80% of cancer-induced animals fed extracts from maitake, shiitake, and reishi mushrooms.[234] Compounds in each of these mushrooms increase the tumor-fighting activity of NK cells and improve antibody responses, but maitake seems to have the strongest and most consistent effect. Maitake exhibits potent activity against cancer, inhibiting both carcinogenesis and metastasis, according to researchers. Animal research suggests that maitake supplements increase the body's ability to kill tumors.[235] When maitake was compared to a common form of chemotherapy, maitake demonstrated superior ability to inhibit the growth of tumors (80% versus 45%).[236] Maitake increases immune cells' production of interleukin-1, a protein that aids in defense against cancer and viruses.[237]

Recommendations

- Choose the right doctor. Be sure that your doctor is someone you trust and can communicate with. Think about the following when evaluating your choice of physician: Is the doctor well-qualified to treat you? Are they concerned with your personal needs in treatment? Does your doctor know alternative medicine in cancer treatment? Does your physician realize that your attitude and outlook are just as important as their treatment methods? Will your doctor be completely frank with you about the consequences and risks of every therapy (conventional and alternative), so that you can make the proper decision about your treatment options? Even if you have complete confidence in your doctor, a cancer diagnosis may warrant one or even several second opinions.

- It is a good idea to gather as much information as you can about your type of cancer, its causes, and treatment options. Having this information will not only reduce your anxiety, but also will help you select the best treatments for your recovery. Ultimately, it is your decision as to what treatment program (conventional and/or alternative) you want to pursue and it is best for you to base that decision on sound advice and as much knowledge as you can acquire.

- Contact your conventional physician and inform him about your decision to augment your conventional treatment with natural therapies. No one should self-prescribe or use all of the therapies listed. Certain therapies are contraindicated and cannot be used in combination with other therapies; further, some absolutely require supervision and close monitoring by the physician.

- No one should assume that these therapies offer definitive treatment or a *cure* for cancer. The increased incidence of cancer requires both physicians and the public to carefully scrutinize natural cancer treatment options. Practitioners and patients alike have the opportunity to share information and resources in the challenge to find mixtures of natural therapies that reverse disease when possible and optimize each patient's quality of life.

- The emotional stages that you will typically undergo after a cancer diagnosis are well-documented, but are not any less jarring or painful once you experience them. Rest assured that this is a perfectly normal experience.

- Research suggests that coping style can help prevent the recurrence of cancer. A study of women with recurrent breast cancer found that joy, levity, and happiness are associated with longer periods of being free of symptoms.

- Look at your cancer diagnosis as a wake-up call to examine your life. One of the first steps towards reestablishing health is to take stock and identify what factors in your life have contributed to creating this illness. This "inventory" should include an examination of your personality, lifestyle, relationships, and environmental factors that have created an opportunity for this serious illness to take hold.

- Get support—this is critical to your recovery from cancer. A sense of isolation, of being alone in the cancer process, is the quickest way to deplete your immune system.

Self-Care

Biofeedback Training and Neurotherapy / Guided Imagery / Light Therapy / Mind–Body Medicine

HYDROTHERAPY: Hyperthermia—apply one to two times weekly. • Constitutional hydrotherapy—apply two to five times weekly.

JUICE THERAPY: • Carrot, beet (roots and tops) • Fresh raw cabbage and carrot juice • Grape, black cherry, black currant • Wheatgrass juice • Asparagus juice • Fresh apple juice • Carrot, celery • Carrot, spinach • Carrot, cabbage

Professional Care

Cell Therapy / Chelation Therapy / Enzyme Therapy / Fasting / Magnetic Field Therapy / Traditional Chinese Medicine

OXYGEN THERAPY: • Hydrogen peroxide therapy • Ozone Therapy

Where to Find Help

The following organizations provide information about the alternative therapies discussed in this chapter. They can also provide referrals to patients.

Cancer Control Society
2043 North Berendo Street
Los Angeles, California 90027
(213) 663-7801

Provides listings and information on alternative cancer treatment centers and patients who have recovered from various cancers using alternative therapies (particular emphasis on metabolic therapies). Also sponsors an annual convention showcasing 40-50 alternative practitioners who treat cancer.

Foundation for Advancement in Cancer Therapy
P.O. Box 1242
Old Chelsea Station
New York, New York 10113
(212) 741-2790

A clearinghouse for information regarding alternative cancer therapies, emphasizing nutritional and metabolic approaches.

People Against Cancer
P.O. Box 10
Otho, Iowa 50569
(515) 972-4444

A nonprofit, grassroots membership organization dedicated to cancer prevention and medical freedom of choice. Provides counseling and information on alternative cancer treatments.

World Research Foundation
15300 Ventura Blvd., Suite 405
Sherman Oaks, California 91403
(818) 907-5483

Large research library of alternative medicine, open to the public. Provides a computer search and printout of specific health issues for a nominal fee.

Resources for Specific Therapies and Tests

714X

Cerbe, Inc.
5270 Mills Street
Rock Forest, Quebec, Canada J1N 3B6
(819) 564-7883

AMAS TEST

Oncolab
36 The Fenway
Boston, Massachusetts 02215
(800) 922-8378

ANTI-MYCOPLASMA AUTO-VACCINE

Filiberto Muñoz, M.D.
Circuito Bursátil #9031, Edificio Terra
Zona Rio, Suite 306
C.P. 22320 Tijuana, B.C., Mexico
52-6-683-1398 or 52-6-683-6055

San Diego Clinic
555 Saturn Blvd., Suite B-452
San Diego, California 92154
(619) 778-6828

ANTINEOPLASTON THERAPY

Burzynski Research Institute, Inc.
12000 Richmond Avenue, Suite 260
Houston, Texas 77082
(713) 597-0111

COLEY'S TOXINS

Innovative Therapeutics
2020 Franklin Street, P.O. Box 512
Carlyle, Illinois 62231
(618) 594-8244 or (888) 688-9922

DENDRITIC CELL THERAPY

BioPulse Clinics
10421 So. Jordan Gateway, Suite 500
South Jordan, Utah 84095
(888) 552-2855
Website: www.alternativemedicine.com/healthcenter/biopulse

Aidan Incorporated
621 South 48th Street
Tempe, Arizona 85281
(800) 529-0269 or (480) 446-8181
Website: www.aidan-az.com

ENDERLEIN MEDICINE AND SANUM REMEDIES

Biological Medicine Institute
Avenida de la Paz, No. 16420 Colonia Mineral
Sante Fe, Tijuana, B.C. 22360 Mexico

Enderlein Sales Group
P.O. Box 2352
Santa Rosa, California 95405
(800) 203-3775 or (707) 537-9505

ESSIAC

Flora, Inc. (Flor-Essence®)
805 E. Badger Road
Lynden, Washington 98264
(800) 446-2110

EX VIVO APOPTOTIC ASSAY

Rational Therapeutics Cancer Evaluation
Center
750 East 29th Street
Long Beach, California 90806
(562) 989-6455
Website: www.Rational-T.com

GERSON THERAPY AND ISSELS' WHOLE BODY THERAPY

The Gerson Research Organization
7807 Artesian Road
San Diego, California 92127-2117
(800) 759-2966

Max Gerson Memorial Cancer Center of
CHIPSA
670 Nubes
Playas de Tijuana, B.C., Mexico

The Gerson Institute
P.O. Box 430
Bonita, California 91908-0430
(619) 585-7600

HEAT THERAPY (HYPERTHERMIA)

Friedrich Douwes, M.D.
Klinik St. Georg
Rosenheimer Str. 6-8
83043 Bad Aibling, Germany
49-8061-494-217
Website: www.klinik-st-georg.de

European Society for Hyperthermic Oncology
(ESHO)
Website: www.cv.ruu.nl/radiotherapy/esho

Meditherm, Inc.
15824 S.W. Upper Boones Ferry Road
Lake Oswego, Oregon 97035
(503) 639-8496 or (61) 7-5-474-2702 (Australia)
Website: www.meditherm.com

HOXSEY THERAPY

Bio-Medical Center
P.O. Box 727
615 General Ferreira, Colonia Juarez

Tijuana, B.C., Mexico 22000
011-52-66-84-9011, 011-52-66-84-9081, or 011-52-66-84-9376

HYDRAZINE SULFATE

Syracuse Cancer Research Institute
Presidential Plaza
600 East Genesee Street
Syracuse, New York 13202
(315) 472-6616

BioTech Pharmaca
P.O. Box 1992
Fayetteville, Arkansas 72702
(800) 345-1199 or (501) 443-9148

IMMUNOMODULATORS

Transfer Factor
Chisolm Biological Laboratory
(800) 664-1333 or (803) 663-9777
Website: www.chisolmbio.com

Immunocal™
Immunotec Research Ltd.
292 Adrien Patenaude
Vaudreuil-Dorion, QC, Canada J7V 5V5
(514) 424-9992
Website: www.immunocal.com

IMUPlus and Cytolog
Lifestar Millennium
2175 E. Francisco Blvd., Suite A-2
San Rafael, California 94901
(800) 858-7477 or (415) 457-1400

INSULIN POTENTIATION THERAPY

Caring Medical and Rehabilitation Services
715 Lake Street, Suite 600
Oak Park, Illinois 60301
(708) 848-7789
Website: www.caringmedical.com or www.ipt-cancer.com

ISCADOR

Biological Homeopathic Industries (BHI)
11600 Cochite S.E., P.O. Box 11280
Albuquerque, New Mexico 87123
(505) 293-3843

KELLEY'S NUTRITIONAL-METABOLIC THERAPY

Robert C. Atkins, M.D.
152 East 55th Street
New York, New York 10022
(212) 758-2110

Nicholas Gonzalez, M.D.
737 Park Avenue
New York, New York 10021
(212) 535-3993

LAETRILE AND SHARK CARTILAGE

Oasis Hospital
Paseo Playas de Tijuana, No. 19
Tijuana, B.C., Mexico 22700
52-66-80-1850 or (800) 700-1850

LIVINGSTON THERAPY

Livingston Foundation Medical Center
3232 Duke Street
San Diego, California 92110
(619) 224-3515 or (888) 777-7321

THERMOGRAPHY

Therma-Scan, Inc.
26711 Woodward Avenue, Suite 230
Huntington Woods, Michigan 48070
(248) 544-7500

American Association of Thermology
2740 Chain Bridge Road
Vienna, Virginia 22181
(703) 938-6140

T/TN ANTIGEN TEST

Heather Margaret Bligh Cancer Research
Laboratories Finch University of Health Sciences,
The Chicago Medical School
3333 Green Bay Road
North Chicago, Illinois 60064
(847) 578-3435

Information Resources on the Internet

cancerguide.org

Developed by kidney cancer survivor Steve Dunn, this site reviews the clinical merits and research regarding numerous alternative cancer therapies and substances, such as bovine cartilage, Essiac, and antineoplastons.

www.graylab.ac.uk/cancerweb

This is an England-based multimedia information resource for oncology, providing data on conventional approaches mostly with links to other sites and bibliographic resources.

cancer.med.upenn.edu

Also known as OncoLink, this site provides information on types of cancer, treatment options, clinical trials, and online patient support services; it offers extensive information-searching tools.

www.healthy.net

Sponsored by HealthWorld Online, this site provides information on both conventional and natural health (alternative medicine) through 11 information centers (e.g., health clinics, books, professional association network, library of health and medicine) and 15,000 electronic pages of health data.

www.allabouthealth.com

This site features the latest research findings, events, trends, books, software, products, articles, commentaries, and numerous links to other relevant web sites.

Recommended Reading

Alternative Medicine Definitive Guide to Cancer. W. John Diamond, M.D., and W. Lee Cowden, M.D., with Burton Goldberg. Tiburon, CA: Future Medicine Publishing, 1997.

Alternatives in Cancer Therapy. Ross Pelton, R.Ph., Ph.D., and Lee Overholser, Ph.D. New York: Simon & Schuster, 1994.

Antioxidants Against Cancer. Ralph Moss, Ph.D. New York: Equinox Press, 2000.

Cancer: A Second Opinion. Josef Issels, M.D. Garden City Park, NY: Avery Publishing Group, 1999.

Cancer and Nutrition. Charles B. Simone, M.D. Garden City Park, NY: Avery Publishing Group, 1992.

Cancer Diagnosis: What to Do Next. W. John Diamond, M.D., and W. Lee Cowden, M.D., with Burton Goldberg. Tiburon, CA: AlternativeMedicine.com Books, 2000.

Cancer: Increasing Your Odds for Survival. David Bognar. Alameda, CA: Hunter House, 1998.

The Cancer Industry. Ralph Moss, Ph.D. New York: Equinox Press, 1996.

Cancer Therapy. Ralph Moss, Ph.D. New York: Equinox Press, 1993.

Complementary Cancer Therapies: Combining Traditional and Alternative Approaches for the Best Possible Outcome. Dan Labriola, N.D. Rocklin, CA: Prima Publishing, 2000.

The Journey Through Cancer. Jeremy Geffen, M.D. New York: Crown, 2000.

Life's Delicate Balance: A Guide to Causes and Prevention of Breast Cancer. Janette D. Sherman. New York: Taylor & Francis, 2000.

Options: The Alternative Cancer Therapy Book. Richard Walters. Garden City Park, NY: Avery Publishing Group, 1992.

The Politics of Cancer Revisited. Samuel S. Epstein, M.D. Fremont Center, NY: East Ridge Press, 1998.

Sharks Don't Get Cancer. I. William Lane, Ph.D., and Linda Comac. Garden City Park, NY: Avery Publishing Group, 1992.

Sharks Still Don't Get Cancer. I. William Lane, Ph.D., and Linda Comac. Garden City Park, NY: Avery Publishing Group, 1996.

Third Opinion. John M. Fink. Garden City Park, NY: Avery Publishing Group, 1997.

CANDIDIASIS

Although widespread, candidiasis (yeast overgrowth) is generally overlooked by the conventional medical establishment because its symptoms so closely mimic those of other conditions. Alternative physicians, however, recognize the seriousness of candidiasis and, while conventional medicine has often been ineffective in treating candidiasis, various alternative methods offer safe and effective relief.

EVERYONE HAS *Candida*, a form of yeast *(Candida albicans)* normally confined to the lower bowels, the vagina, and the skin. In healthy individuals with strong, functioning immune systems, it is harmless and kept in check by "good" bacteria, such as *Bifidobacteria* and acidophilus. But if the balance of the intestinal environment is altered by a compromised immune system or other factors, then opportunistic *Candida* proliferates, infecting other body tissues. The *Candida* becomes pathogenic, transforming from a simple yeast into an aggressive fungus that can severely compromise one's health. This potential for mutating from a benign organism to a pathogenic one is why William G. Crook, M.D., author of *The Yeast Connection*, describes *Candida* as a kind of microbiological "Dr. Jekyll and Mr. Hyde." This condition is known as candidiasis.

According to James Braly, M.D., of Hollywood, Florida, the fungal form of *Candida* appears to permeate the gastrointestinal mucosal lining and break down barriers to the bloodstream. "When the fungal form of *Candida* occurs in the body, allergenic substances can penetrate into the blood more easily, where they form immense complexes, and perhaps even promote food allergy reactions," Dr. Braly says. Since their symptoms are often interrelated, he emphasizes that candidiasis should usually be treated together with food allergies.

Candidiasis can affect areas of the body far removed from *Candida* colonizations in the gastrointestinal tract and vagina. One reason for this is that *Candida* produces a number of toxins that can suppress immune function, deplete the body of white blood cells needed to fight infection, and prevent the manufacture of antioxidants such as glutathione.[2] Candidiasis symptoms cover a broad spectrum and the condition can cause a number of

CANDIDA—A STEALTH PATHOGEN?

The concept that *Candida albicans* (or other strains of *Candida*) can pass through the intestines into general blood circulation was first established many years ago, yet in conventional medical circles, the importance of *Candida* involvement in health is still largely undervalued. In 1969, W. Krause, Ph.D., demonstrated that intact *Candida albicans* organisms are capable of escaping the intestinal tract and reaching the blood and urine in humans.

After he was carefully screened for any prior illness or exposure to *Candida*, Dr. Krause ingested a large dose of *Candida albicans* orally. In a surprisingly short time, just a few hours later, he developed numerous symptoms, including headaches and fever. The scientists working with Dr. Krause were able to culture *Candida* organisms from his blood and urine; the colonies were found to be identical to the strain administered.[1] Dr. Krause's bold experiment proved that it is possible for *Candida* to cross the gastrointestinal tract in a viable form and cause systemic illness in healthy patients.

The researchers also concluded that antibiotic use may be a common precursor in cases of systemic candidiasis and increased intestinal permeability. Despite Dr. Krause's experiment, there is still controversy over the idea that *Candida* can systemically translocate to distant sites in the body as a kind of "stealth pathogen" and cause illness.

diseases, ranging from allergies, vaginitis, and thrush (a whitish fungus in the mouth or vagina) to an invasion of the genitourinary tract, eyes, liver, heart, or central nervous system. At its most destructive, candidiasis is involved in autoimmune diseases, such as Addison's disease and AIDS. Other symptoms of candidiasis, according to Dr. Braly, include digestive problems such as bloating, cramping, gas, and diarrhea, respiratory problems, coughing, wheezing, earaches, central nervous system imbalances, generalized fatigue, and loss of libido.

Causes of Candidiasis

Candida infections were rare as recently as a generation ago, but now the illness is relatively commonplace, affecting the health of one in three individuals. "Candidiasis is basically a disease resulting from medical developments like antibiotics, birth control pills, and estrogen replacement therapy," according to Leyardia Black, N.D., of Lopez Island, Washington. "And it can be triggered at a very young age, when children are first being treated with antibiotics."

Leon Chaitow, N.D., D.O., of London, England, agrees. "Fully 35% of women using birth control pills have associated cases of acute vaginal candidiasis," he says, "and there are undoubtedly many others who have less pronounced evidence of yeast overgrowth as immune competence is gradually compromised by the hormonal onslaught."

Since yeast infections enter the body easily through the vagina, and yeast is fostered by estrogen, women of childbearing age are more vulnerable to candidiasis.

 See AIDS, Allergies, Chronic Fatigue Syndrome, Constipation, Gastrointestinal Disorders, Men's Health, Mental Health, Parasitic Infections, Respiratory Conditions, Women's Health.

Murray Susser, M.D., of Santa Monica, California, points out that since yeast infections enter the body easily through the vagina, and yeast is fostered by estrogen, women of childbearing age are more vulnerable to candidiasis. Also, women who have been pregnant are susceptible, since hormonal changes encourage *Candida* overgrowth. When men develop candidiasis, antibiotics,

RECOGNIZING CANDIDIASIS

Candidiasis can cause a wide array of symptoms, including the following:

- Chronic fatigue
- Weight gain
- Depression, anxiety, and irritability
- Hyperactivity, confusion, and loss of memory
- Gastrointestinal problems, such as bloating, gas, cramps, chronic diarrhea, constipation, or heartburn
- Allergies (to both food and airborne allergens)
- Severe premenstrual syndrome (PMS)
- Sexual dysfunction and loss of sexual interest
- Memory loss, severe mood swings, and feeling mentally "disturbed"
- Recurrent fungal infections (such as "jock itch," athlete's foot, or ringworm) or vaginal/urinary infections
- A feeling of being lightheaded or drunk after minimal wine, beer, or certain foods
- Rashes, hives, acne, and scaly skin
- Respiratory problems, including asthma and nasal or lung congestion
- Sinus pressure, hay fever–like attacks, and coughing
- Eye or ear irritation
- Migraines and headaches
- Sleep disturbances
- Heart palpitations

high sugar intake, or immune suppression (from illness, toxins, and stress) are usually the root causes.

Frequently, candidiasis is caused by a combination of factors. As Dr. Chaitow explains, "All too often, more than one influence is operating. Over a few years, a patient may have had several series of antibiotics for a variety of conditions, while using steroids as well, perhaps in the form of the contraceptive pill. If the patient—most commonly a young woman—also happens to be living on a diet that is rich in sugars, then the *Candida* is very likely to have spread beyond its usual borders into new territory."

Dr. Chaitow points out that, when the immune system is completely suppressed (as in AIDS), yeast prolif-

CANDIDIASIS AND PARASITES

Leon Chaitow, N.D., D.O., reports that the presence of parasites in patients can make candidiasis very difficult to treat and that parasite infestation encourages yeast overgrowth. When treatment results for candidiasis are poor, Dr. Chaitow recommends testing for coincidental parasitic infection. Before treatment for candidiasis, all parasites must first be successfully eradicated. Researchers believe that candidiasis can become resistant to treatment because of parasites such as *Giardia lamblia*, amoebas, nematodes, and cestodes.[3] Parasites can be identified by means of blood, urine, and fecal testing, as well as electroacupuncture biofeedback. According to Dr. Chaitow, electroacupuncture biofeedback is also useful for revealing how well the body will tolerate any medications that may be prescribed.

To get rid of parasites, Dr. Chaitow advises pursuing a comprehensive herbal medicine approach rather than medication. "In many cases, anti-parasitic prescription drugs have not proved to be lastingly effective," he points out. "They may diminish symptoms for one or two months, but the symptoms later return with full force." Parasites can be fought with high-dosage probiotics such as *Lactobacillus acidophilus*, *Bifidobacteria*, and *L. bulgaricus*. Treatment may last from eight to 12 weeks. Dr. Chaitow reports an 80% success rate in cases of seriously ill people afflicted with parasites and yeast overgrowth using this method.

---

erates freely and colonizes the body and bloodstream, leading to septicemia (blood poisoning). In less drastic but more prevalent cases, the immune system is temporarily suppressed and helper T cells (lymphocytes that pass into the bloodstream to help fight infection) are destroyed. Such immune suppression can be due to any number of factors, such as poor diet (including ingestion of pesticide residues and preservatives), alcohol use, chemotherapy, radiation, exposure to environmental toxins, antibiotics that injure or destroy the T cells, and stress. Consequently, conditions are created for opportunistic infections—and yeast—to grow.

Antibiotics

According to Dr. Susser, antibiotics—life-saving cures for many diseases—may be the single greatest cause of candidiasis, because antibiotic treatment for infections is nondiscriminatory, killing the "good" intestinal bacteria as well as the "bad" infection-causing bacteria. Both acidophilus and *Bifidobacteria* produce natural antifungal substances (as well as antibacterial materials) as part of their control mechanism over yeast.[4] One of the activities of "good" bacteria is the manufacture of the B vitamin, biotin, which exerts control over yeast. When biotin is lacking, as a result of damage by antibiotics to acidophilus, *Bifidobacteria*, and the normal microflora ecology, yeast has a chance to change into a different organism, an encroaching mycelial (vegetative) fungus.[5]

Antibiotics can cause the altered, imbalanced intestinal environment that *Candida* requires to change into its aggressive form. Dr. Chaitow explains, "*Candida* puts down minute rootlets that penetrate the tissues on which the yeast is growing. When this happens to be the inner wall of the intestines, it breaks down the barrier that exists between the closed world of the bowel and the body. Toxic debris, yeast waste products, and partially digested proteins are allowed into the bloodstream, resulting in allergic and toxic reactions."

If the use of antibiotics is frequent or prolonged (as with a course for acne treatment or an infection), then the spread of *Candida* becomes inevitable. "A vicious cycle may develop as a result," Dr. Chaitow says. "Antibiotics alter the balance of intestinal flora and suppress the immune system. An individual with suppressed immune function is much more susceptible not only to candidiasis but to bacterial infections, which are then treated with antibiotics, which, in turn, increase the growth of *Candida*, and so on."

In addition to medications, we are also exposed to antibiotics and other drugs in the meats and animal products we consume. Antibiotics and steroids are fed to livestock in large quantities to prevent infection and stimulate growth. "If you eat a lot of meat that contains even traces of antibiotics, you may develop a bacteria-yeast imbalance in your intestines," according to Dennis Remington, M.D., and Barbara Higa Swasey, R.D., authors of *Back to Health*.[6]

Antibiotics—life-saving cures for many diseases—may be the single greatest cause of candidiasis.

 See Ayurvedic Medicine, Detoxification Therapy, Diet, Enzyme Therapy, Herbal Medicine, Nutritional Medicine, Oxygen Therapies.

Dietary Factors

Milk and dairy products carry traces of antibiotics, but milk should be avoided for another reason: it contains lactose, a type of sugar that promotes *Candida* growth. Other foods that promote candidiasis are those that contain molds or yeasts, such as breads and pastries, cheeses, dried fruits, and peanuts. However, not all the experts agree that it is necessary to eliminate yeasted foods. They maintain that some foods with yeast—commercially prepared breads and rolls, pastries, and doughnuts—also contain sugar and/or white, processed flour. White flour and sugar are converted into simple sugars (monosaccharides) in the body, the food of choice for yeast. These substances, and not yeast, may be responsible for the *Candida* overgrowth.

The standard American diet now contains higher amounts of refined carbohydrates and sugar than ever before—in breads, pasta, pastries, potato chips, desserts, candy, sodas, and junk foods. High-carbohydrate diets provide plenty of sugars in the body that support the growth of *Candida*.[8] According to Dr. Susser, when sugar is eaten, intestinal fermentation creates a toxin called acetaldehyde, which affects all of the body's physiological functions, including digestion and hormonal processes. Yeast thrives on sugar, therefore a high-sugar diet is one of the predisposing factors for candidiasis.

Alcohol

Candidiasis patients should stay away from all alcohol, since it is composed of fermented and refined sugars. It is also more toxic than sugar and feeds yeast. According to Dr. Susser, alcohol suppresses the immune system, disturbs the whole adrenal hormone axis, and "you can say empirically that it makes anyone with *Candida* worse."

Some candidiasis sufferers will feel, and appear to be, intoxicated. An unusual symptom of certain people with severe candidiasis is the presence of alcohol in the bloodstream even when none has been consumed.[9] First discovered in Japan, and called "drunk disease," this condition is created by strains of *Candida albicans* that turn acetaldehyde (the chemical created by sugar and yeast fermentation) into ethanol. This is a process well understood by distillers of homemade brew. These candidiasis patients whose yeast turns sugar into alcohol are chronically drunk.[10]

Another connection between alcohol and candidiasis has been found in a study of 213 alcoholics at a recovery center in Minneapolis. Test and questionnaire results indicated that candidiasis is a common complication of alcoholism due to the combination of high sugar content in alcohol and the inability of alcoholics to assimilate nutrients. Additionally, female alcoholics with

IT'S NOT JUST IN YOUR HEAD

Individuals who suffer from a *Candida* infection sometimes have a sense that they are not themselves, that something is seriously wrong. Unfortunately, their doctors often cannot find a physical cause and send them home without an adequate diagnosis. Because these patients suffer from depression, anxiety, and moodiness—all symptoms of candidiasis—they are often told that their ailments are psychological in origin. Many doctors will prescribe antidepressant medications and recommend a psychiatrist or therapist.

C. Orian Truss, M.D., of Birmingham, Alabama, a *Candida* expert and author of *The Missing Diagnosis*, says that chronic candidiasis is almost always labeled psychosomatic and treated as a nervous disorder. "Yeast may lead to such a variety of symptoms that the condition is easily confused with illnesses that are psychological in nature," he says. "This has resulted in the heavily disproportionate application of psychiatric methods of treatment in patients whose only psychological problems are those that have been brought on by the failure of the medical profession to correct their long-standing, frustrating illnesses."[7]

candidiasis were significantly sicker than nonalcoholic women with candidiasis.[11]

Many of the symptoms exhibited in alcoholism, such as insomnia, depression, loss of libido, headaches, sinusitis/postnasal drip, and intestinal complaints, overlap with those in *Candida* overgrowth. Obviously, drinking alcohol increases levels of sugar in the system. But other habits of alcoholics are also at fault. Many alcoholics tend to be smokers, for instance, and so are at risk for respiratory infections, which are treated with antibiotics.

Environmental Factors

Damp environments, like musty or moldy basements, may encourage yeast growth. Also, regions with rainy climates tend to have a higher incidence of candidiasis, according to Ann Louise Gittleman, M.S., of Bozeman, Montana, author of *Supernutrition for Women*.[12] Exposure to environmental pollutants, such as pesticide residues, car exhaust, industrial chemicals, and heavy metals (particularly from mercury amalgam fillings), may foster the growth of *Candida* as well.[13]

Diagnosing Candidiasis

Candidiasis causes systemic illnesses that produce a wide variety of symptoms. This makes candidiasis difficult to diagnose accurately, since it shares symptoms with so many other conditions. Dr. Chaitow notes that when symptoms are chronic rather than acute or sudden, he generally suspects a yeast infection. Another clue is if specific symptoms have been previously treated without success, then the diagnosis usually suggests candidiasis.

Some physicians rely on laboratory test results to diagnose the condition. However, while these tests are helpful, it is important not to depend on them exclusively. For example, blood tests can be used to pinpoint *Candida* antibodies. But since most people normally have *Candida* organisms in their systems, the tests may show antibodies even if the patient is not suffering from candidiasis. The truth is there is no single diagnostic test. "The clincher to any diagnosis is not so much what is happening in the laboratory as what is happening in the patient," says Stephen Langer, M.D. The combination of an individual's complete medical history and examination, the patient's response to treatment, and information culled from laboratory tests is the key to a correct diagnosis.[14]

Dr. Chaitow describes the likely candidate for *Candida* overgrowth as someone whose medical history includes steroid hormone medications (cortisone or corticosteroids, often prescribed for skin conditions such as rashes, eczema, or psoriasis), prolonged or repeated use of antibiotics, medications for treating ulcers, or oral contraceptives. Certain illnesses, such as diabetes, cancer, and AIDS, can also increase susceptibility to *Candida* overgrowth.

A qualified practitioner should take your complete medical history to determine if you have a *Candida* infection, but here are a few questions to ask yourself to see if you are at risk (the more questions that you answer affirmatively, the greater your risk):

- Have you recently taken repeated courses of antibiotics or steroids (e.g., cortisone)?

- Have you used birth-control pills?

- Have you had repeated fungal infections ("jock itch," athlete's foot, ringworm)?

- Do you regularly have any of these symptoms—bloating, headaches, depression, fatigue, memory problems, impotence or lack of interest in sex, muscle aches with no apparent cause, brain fogginess?

- Do you experience symptoms of PMS (premenstrual syndrome)?

- Do you have cravings for sweets, products containing white flour, or alcoholic beverages?

- Do you repeatedly experience any of these health difficulties—inappropriate drowsiness, mood swings, rashes, bad breath, dry mouth, post-nasal drip or nasal congestion, heartburn, urinary frequency or urgency?[15]

Additional Tests

Blood Tests—Blood tests can look for *Candida* antibodies in the body. When *Candida* assumes its fungal form, the immune system responds by producing special antibodies to fight off the infection. Consequently, if a large concentration of these antibodies is found in the blood, you may be experiencing a *Candida* outbreak. Dr. Langer notes that "if the yeast antibodies are elevated and the test is positive, the yeast infection is active and threatening."[16] However, as noted earlier, the antibody test may be misleading, because most individuals normally have *Candida* organisms in their bodies.

The blood can also be examined visually using a darkfield microscope to detect the presence of the *Candida* fungus. Darkfield microscopy is a way of studying living whole blood cells under a specially adapted microscope that projects the image (magnified 1,400 times) onto a video screen. The skilled physician can detect early signs of illness in the form of microorganisms in the blood known to produce disease. Specifically, darkfield microscopy reveals distortions of red blood cells (which indicate nutritional status), possible undesirable bacterial or fungal life forms (like *Candida*), and other blood ecology patterns indicative of health or illness.[17]

Stool Analysis—Another test used to diagnose candidiasis is a stool analysis, which can help assess digestive function through laboratory examination of a stool sample. If the stool contains abnormally large amounts of *Candida,* this may indicate candidiasis. The stool analysis can also look at levels of beneficial bacteria in the intestines as well as other digestive markers for determining *Candida* levels.

Electrodermal Screening—Electrodermal screening (EDS) is a form of computerized information gathering that can be used to identify the presence of *Candida.* EDS works by placing a blunt, noninvasive electric probe at specific points on the patient's hands, face, or feet, corresponding to acupuncture points at the beginning or end of energy meridians. Minute electrical discharges from these points serve as information signals about the condition of the body's organs and systems, useful for the physician in diagnostic evaluation and developing a treatment plan. Using EDS, the trained practitioner conducts an "interview" with the patient's organs and tissues, gathering information about the basic functional status of those systems.

Treating Candidiasis

One way that conventional doctors treat candidiasis is to simply prescribe antifungal drugs such as nystatin, ketoconazol, and Diflucan®. However, these drugs should be used as a last resort rather than a first line of defense. Michael Murray, N.D., of Issaquah, Washington, author of *Chronic Candidiasis: The Yeast Syndrome,* says "A comprehensive approach is more effective in treating chronic candidiasis than simply trying to kill the *Candida* with a drug or natural anti-*Candida* agent."[18] Successful treatment of candidiasis first requires the reduction of factors that predispose a patient to *Candida* overgrowth. Secondly, the patient's immune function must be strengthened. Diet, nutritional supplements, herbal medicine, oxygen therapy, Ayurvedic medicine, and acupuncture are some of the choices alternative physicians use to accomplish these ends.

Although self-help is therapeutic for candidiasis, a health regimen should be undertaken with the guidance of a practitioner who understands the condition and is willing to try a variety of treatment options. Recovery from chronic candidiasis seldom takes less than three months and is usually well advanced by six months, but it can take longer to recover completely. Studies show that until bowel *Candida* is under control, local manifestations will continue to appear (such as vaginal thrush). Local treatment alone (for thrush or other symptoms) is not enough.

Diet

Dr. Black says, "In treating *Candida,* my basic dietary taboos are sweets, alcohol, and refined carbohydrates." Sugar must be avoided in all its various forms. These include: sucrose, dextrose, fructose, fruit juices, honey, maple syrup, molasses, milk products (which contain lactose), most fruit (except berries), and potatoes (whose starch converts into sugar).

Many candidiasis sufferers also have allergies and sensitivities to various foods. Although *Candida albicans* yeast is not synonymous to yeast in foods such as bread, a cross-reaction between food yeast and *Candida* frequently occurs. As a result, foods containing or promoting yeast, such as baked goods, alcohol, and vinegar, should be avoided until possible sensitivities are clearly diagnosed. To test patients who are very sensitive to yeast, Dr. Black takes them off all yeast-containing foods for a week. Then

she adds such foods back in the diet, one at a time. If the symptoms reappear, then clearly yeast-containing foods should be avoided.

Similarly, Dr. Braly employs a rotation diet when he suspects food allergies. On this regimen, patients avoid certain suspected allergenic foods and rotate nonallergenic foods every four or more days. They are then later reintroduced into the diet after three to six months to see if symptoms are provoked. Other foods that may have an allergic potential are also rotated, that is, eaten only every four days, in order to avoid further allergic developments. As a result, a greater variety of food is eaten and more nutrients absorbed, while possible allergic reactions are avoided.

Molds are another aspect of *Candida* sensitivity, according to Dr. Susser. These include food molds (found in cheeses, grapes, mushrooms, and fermented foods) and environmental molds (found in wet climates, in damp basements and plants, and outdoors). Molds and yeast can also exchange forms. Therefore, the ingestible molds of cheeses and fermented foods should be avoided. Avoiding food yeast and mold does not attack the *Candida* yeast itself, but is an attempt to ease stress on the immune system caused by substances that can trigger allergies.[19] Even so, food yeast and mold avoidance should be considered case by case for each individual as it may not always be necessary. As Dr. Susser says, "My personal opinion is that most anti-*Candida* diets are too strict. It is unnecessary to take *Candida* patients off of vinegar and mushrooms unless they are allergic to these things."

Dr. Susser also advises patients to avoid yogurt because of its sugar content, despite its high concentration of *Lactobacilli,* which suppress "bad" bacteria and keep other organisms under control. He finds that freeze-dried acidophilus supplements in capsule form are more effective in combating bacteria than even unsweetened raw yogurt.

Candida growth can also be fostered in the diet through consumption of meat, dairy, and poultry products due to the heavy use of antibiotics. Traces of antibiotics given to dairy cows can later show up in milk. Meat eaters should make sure that meat is free of antibiotic contamination. Organic (hormone- and antibiotic-free) meat and poultry should be consumed whenever possible. For candidiasis patients, seafood (free of mercury toxins) and vegetable protein are preferable, since they are not only antibiotic-free, but lower in fat.

Nutritional Supplements

According to Dr. Chaitow, a general nutritional support program is frequently needed to help build immune function and digestive efficiency, which may have become severely depleted or compromised after months

A DIET TO RID YOURSELF OF *CANDIDA*

Acupuncturist and psychologist Jacqueline Young makes the following dietary recommendations to eliminate *Candida*:

Eliminate for at least one month:

- All foods containing yeast, including bread, biscuits, and cakes
- All fermented foods, such as vinegar, soy sauce, and pickled foods
- All forms of sugar and products containing sugar, including sweets and chocolates, honey, maple syrup, sweetened drinks, and sweetened yogurt
- Milk and dairy products and all foods containing trans-fats
- All refined white flour products
- Alcohol, black tea, and coffee
- Foods with artificial sweeteners, colorings, preservatives, and additives

Include these foods:

- Fresh vegetables and salads
- Whole grains—unlike processed white flour, whole grains (such as rye or millet) do not produce much sugar in the intestinal tract; as these grains are digested, they are converted into polysaccharides (long-chain sugar molecules), which do not stimulate the growth of yeast organisms
- Garlic—crushed or finely sliced on salads or vegetables
- Olive oil—extra virgin, cold-pressed olive oil should be the only oil used
- Fresh fruits—only moderate amounts of fruit should be eaten; eliminate completely from the diet for the first week due to high sugar content, then limit to two fruits per day; avoid very sweet varieties and all citrus fruits[20]

tion and increases immune response), and beta carotene (a vitamin A precursor that increases T cells). Antioxidant immune-boosters, such as selenium, calcium, and zinc, are also useful in combating candidiasis. Additional adrenal gland stimulants include chromium, magnesium, and glandular adrenal extract. Essential fatty acids (such as evening primrose oil) may be considered as well.[21]

As routine supplementation, Dr. Braly offers the following regimen:

- Vitamin C (8–10 g daily)
- Vitamin E (400 IU daily)
- Evening primrose oil (6–8 capsules daily)
- Eicosapentaenoic acid (an omega-3 oil, six capsules daily)
- Pantothenic acid (vitamin B5, 250 mg daily)
- Taurine (500–1,000 mg daily)
- Zinc chelate (25–50 mg daily)
- Goldenseal root extract (with no less than 5% hydrastine, 250 mg twice a day)
- *Lactobacillus acidophilus* (one dry teaspoon three times daily; if allergic to milk, use nonlactose acidophilus)

Dr. Braly also recommends supplementation of hydrochloric acid (HCl). He notes that aging, alcohol abuse, food allergies, and nutrient deficiencies create a lack of HCl in the stomach, which prevents food from being digested and permits *Candida* overgrowth. Such supplementation, he says, helps restore the proper balance of intestinal flora. Dr. Braly recommends one capsule of HCl and pepsin at the start of meals, increasing cautiously to two to four capsules with each meal if needed.

Lita Lee, Ph.D., an enzyme therapist based in Lowell, Oregon, uses plant enzyme supplements to treat yeast overgrowth. Many of her candidiasis patients come to her after unsuccessfully trying nystatin, probiotics, homeopathics, fatty acid supplementation, and various herbs. "Certain cellulose enzymes will digest the common kinds of yeast, whereas other yeasts sometimes yield to amylase enzymes," reports Dr. Lee. She uses a probiotic formula and cellulose enzymes to digest yeast and reestablish friendly bowel bacteria.

Every antifungal treatment for candidiasis will reduce the numbers of "friendly" bacteria that inhabit the intestines. In the long run, a healthy growth of these bacteria in the intestines—particularly *L. acidophilus* and *B. bifidum*—is the best defense against yeast infections. Cabbage is one of the best food sources of friendly bacteria; eat it raw or juice it daily. Other foods that can help revitalize the colon and encourage the growth of normal bacteria include rice protein, chicory, onions, garlic, and

or years of chronic candidiasis. Specific nutritional supplementation can be helpful in rebuilding weakened immune function. Recommended supplements include individual B vitamins (increase antibody response and are used in nearly every body activity), vitamin C (stimulates the adrenal glands and is essential to immune processes), vitamin E (the lack of which depresses immune response), vitamin A (builds resistance to infec-

asparagus. *B. bifidum* is also found in yogurt and kefir (a fermented milk drink). Another way to repopulate the intestines with friendly bacteria is to take a probiotic supplement, especially one containing *L. acidophilus* and *B. bifidum*, or is FOS (fructo-oligosaccharide), a sugar that specifically encourages friendly bacteria to multiply. Start with low doses of FOS and increase gradually, as some people get increased bloating from FOS.

In order to overcome candidiasis, sugar must be avoided in all its various forms.

Herbal Medicine

Herbs are often used to kill harmful yeasts and shore up immune function. They are used in teas, dried in capsules or tablets, or taken in suppository form. Herbs that contain berberain (an alkaloid found in the *Berberidis* family) have proven particularly useful as anti-*Candida* agents. These include goldenseal, Oregon grape, and barberry. Berberain fights *Candida* overgrowth, normalizes intestinal flora, helps digestive problems, has antidiarrheal properties, and stimulates the immune system by increasing blood supply to the spleen. Soothing to inflamed mucous membranes, it can be taken as a tea or in other fluid and dry forms.[22]

Dr. Braly's first line of attack on candidiasis is caprylic acid, only after which, if there is no improvement, will he use drugs. In one study, patients taking 3,600 mg of caprylic acid daily for two weeks completely eliminated their *Candida*.[23] Since caprylic acid is readily absorbed into the system, it should be taken in enteric or sustained release forms. Dr. Braly also uses goldenseal root extract, standardized to 5% or more of its active ingredient hydrastine (250 mg twice daily). In a recent study, goldenseal seemed to work better in killing off *Candida* than other common anti-*Candida* therapies, adds Dr. Braly. Other fatty acids derived from olives (oleic acid) and castor beans (undecylenic acid) also are useful.[24]

Garlic, a well-known folk remedy, is a particularly effective antifungal agent. Allicin is the active ingredient in garlic and has been found to be more potent than many other antifungals, especially against *Candida*.[25] A typical recommended dose is 4,000 mcg daily (equal to about one clove of fresh garlic). It is effective against some antibiotic-resistant organisms and can be taken in capsule and deodorized form. In cases of vaginal candidiasis, it can be used as a suppository or douche.

DRUGS AND CANDIDIASIS

The use of drugs to treat candidiasis is the accepted practice in the medical community. These drugs can be exorbitantly expensive and toxic, with dangerous side effects. Virender Sodhi, M.D. (Ayurveda), N.D., of Bellevue, Washington, points out that the most popular of these drugs, nystatin, cannot rid the body of *Candida,* because of *Candida*'s ability to mutate when under attack. Dr. Sodhi formerly used nystatin with patients but found that, even after a year of using it, he was not getting results. According to Dr. Sodhi, nystatin causes *Candida* to mutate into another species of yeast, therefore treatment can continue for long periods and still have little effect. Meanwhile, Dr. Sodhi claims, nystatin lingers in the intestines and kills other potentially helpful organisms.

Pau d'arco bark, obtained from a tropical tree native to Brazil, has long been used to treat infections, intestinal complaints, and genitourinary ailments (cystitis, prostatitis). It is reported to be an analgesic, an antiviral, a diuretic, and a fungicide. However, many products claiming to contain pau d'arco have only trace amounts, or even none, of the herb. These products also may use a part of the tree other than the bark, or may have been damaged in production and shipping.[26] When purchasing products with pau d'arco, be sure that they contain lapachol, an organic compound known for its antibiotic action.

Grapefruit seed extract works as a multipurpose natural antibiotic for bacterial and viral problems in the intestines, against *Candida* infections, and as a vaginal douche.[27] Other antifungal and antibacterial herbs include German chamomile, aloe vera, ginger, cinnamon, rosemary, licorice, oil of oregano, thyme oil, and tea tree oil.[28] Fennel, anise, ginseng, alfalfa, and red clover are also effective.

Oxygen Therapy

Oxygen therapy refers to a wide range of therapies utilizing oxygen in various forms to promote healing and destroy pathogens (disease-producing microorganisms and toxins) in the body. One form of oxygen therapy uses hydrogen peroxide (H_2O_2). Oxidation (a chemical reaction occurring when electrons are transferred from one molecule to another) administered through hydrogen peroxide therapy regulates tissue repair, cellular respiration, immune functions, and the production of cytokines (chemical messengers that are involved in the regulation of almost every system in the body). Hydrogen peroxide therapy can also work as a defense system, directly destroying invading bacteria, viruses, yeast, and parasites, according to the late Charles H. Farr, M.D., Ph.D.

Dr. Farr treated hundreds of patients with chronic systemic *Candida* using intravenous hydrogen peroxide. One patient, Gail, 34, had been suffering with systemic yeast infections for five years and had taken a barrage of antibiotics and practiced rotation and elimination diets, all to no effect. She had a vaginal yeast infection, intermittent diarrhea, headaches, acne, lethargy, joint pain, mental confusion, menstrual irregularities, and had been unable to work for two years. Dr. Farr started her on weekly intravenous infusions of hydrogen peroxide; after only two treatments, Gail reported feeling more alert and able to concentrate better. After the third treatment, her complexion started to improve, all signs of her vaginitis disappeared, and her bowel function became normal. After eight treatments, Gail was free of all the symptoms that had plagued her for five years; and after two more months, she went job hunting.

CAUTION Hydrogen peroxide therapy needs to be administered under clinical supervision, since uncontrolled oxidation may be destructive to the body. Hydrogen peroxide should not be taken orally as it causes nausea and vomiting, and rectal administration can lead to inflammation of the lower intestinal tract. Other side effects include temporary faintness, fatigue, headaches, and chest pain.

Ayurvedic Medicine

According to Virender Sodhi, M.D. (Ayurveda), N.D., Director of the Ayurvedic & Naturopathic Medical Clinic, in Bellevue, Washington, Ayurvedic medicine considers candidiasis to be a condition caused by *ama*, the improper digestion of foods. Dr. Sodhi attributes candidiasis to the widespread use of antibiotics, birth control pills, and hormones, to environmental stresses, as well as to society's addiction to sugar in the diet. "Ayurvedic medicine believes that these stresses on the system cause carbohydrates to be digested improperly," he says. "Furthermore, the immune system in the gut becomes worn down."

From an Ayurvedic perspective, Dr. Sodhi believes that successful treatment of candidiasis depends on strengthening the immune system and improving digestion through stimulation of secretory IgA (an immunoglobulin or antibody). This can be accomplished through a combination of treatments. Grapefruit seed oil and tannic acid are useful in treating *Candida* overgrowth, since they act as antifungals and antibiotics, according to

Dr. Sodhi. He also uses long pepper, *trikatu,* ginger, cayenne, and *neem* before meals to increase immunoglobulins and digestive functions.

Dr. Sodhi begins dosage with ¼ teaspoon of herbs, about 30 minutes before each meal, with dosage increasing gradually to 8-10 teaspoons of herbs a day. Dr. Sodhi also uses acidophilus and recommends that his patients cleanse toxins from their systems using the *pancha karma* program, which involves dietary modification and the use of herbs. Results from Dr. Sodhi's approach usually occur in 4-6 months.

Acupuncture

William M. Cargile, B.S., D.C., F.I.A.C.A., former Chairman of Research for the American Association of Oriental Medicine, has successfully used acupuncture on patients with candidiasis. He advises, "I would start by using meridians that influence genital function, spleen, and stomach. These are *yin* meridians and they correspond to areas of immune system enhancement. You want to normalize the metabolism of the cells in that part of the body." But Dr. Cargile adds that treatment is "a waste of time" if the patient doesn't also pay attention to nutrition, which he calls a significant solution.

Dr. Cargile cites the case of a 41-year-old woman who suffered from severe candidiasis. She was a single mother of three children who had chronic low-grade sore throats and was taking five antibiotic prescriptions. "This had been going on at least three years," Dr. Cargile says. "She was constantly bloated, had colonic distension, and had oral thrush so bad it looked like cotton sticking down her throat. She had clearly destroyed the balance of her intestinal flora." Dr. Cargile gave her a gargle solution of tea tree oil, which reduced the pathogens. He had her change her diet and douche with liquid acidophilus, and he gave her acupuncture treatments through meridians that reached the larynx and throat. "After three treatments over a period of three weeks, she was 90% better," he states. "She had no oral *Candida* like before, and was well on the road to recovery."

Recommendations

- In order to overcome candidiasis, sugar must be avoided in all its various forms.

- Employ a rotation diet to determine if food allergies are a contributing factor. On this regimen, patients avoid certain suspected allergenic foods and rotate nonallergenic foods every four or more days.

- Eliminate all foods containing yeast, including bread, biscuits, and cakes, and all fermented foods, such as vinegar, soy sauce, and pickled foods.

- Avoid alcohol, black tea, and coffee.

- Recommended supplements include individual B vitamins (to increase antibody response), vitamin C (stimulates the adrenal glands and immune processes), vitamin E (the lack of which depresses immune response), vitamin A (builds resistance to infection), and beta carotene (increases numbers of T cells). Antioxidant immune-boosters, such as selenium, calcium, and zinc, are also useful in combating candidiasis.

- Plant enzyme supplements can be used to treat yeast overgrowth.

- To repopulate the intestines with friendly bacteria, take a probiotic supplement, particularly one containing *L. acidophilus* and *B. bifidum*.

- Herbs that contain berberain (an alkaloid found in the *Berberidis* family) have proven particularly useful anti-*Candida* agents. These include goldenseal, Oregon grape, and barberry.

- Antifungal and antibacterial herbs include garlic, German chamomile, aloe vera, ginger, cinnamon, rosemary, licorice, oil of oregano, and tea tree oil.

- Hydrogen peroxide therapy works as a defense system, directly destroying invading bacteria, viruses, yeast, and parasites.

- Ayurvedic medicine and acupuncture may also be helpful for ridding the body of *Candida*.

Self-Care

The following therapies can be undertaken at home under appropriate professional supervision:

AROMATHERAPY: Tea tree oil.

HYDROTHERAPY: Constitutional hydrotherapy (apply two to five times weekly).

Professional Care

The following therapies should only be provided by a qualified health professional:

Detoxification Therapy / Magnetic Field Therapy / Orthomolecular Medicine / Traditional Chinese Medicine

OXYGEN THERAPY: Hydrogen peroxide therapy (IV).

Where to Find Help

For more information on, or referrals for, treatment of candidiasis, contact the following organizations.

American Association of Oriental Medicine (AAOM)

433 Front Street
Catasauqua, Pennsylvania 18032
(888) 500-7999
Website: www.aaom.org

The AAOM is a national professional trade organization of acupuncturists who meet acceptable standards of competency and can provide you with the names and locations of local members.

American Association of Naturopathic Physicians

601 Valley Street, Suite 105
Seattle, Washington 98109
(206) 298-0126
Website: www.naturopathic.org

Contact them for the location of a licensed naturopathic physician in your area.

The College of Maharishi Ayur-Veda Health Center

P.O. Box 282
Fairfield, Iowa 52556
(515) 472-5866

The center provides referrals to health centers that offer methods of prevention and treatment of a broad range of illnesses. They also train practitioners and provide information to the lay public.

Great Smokies Diagnostic Laboratory

63 Zillicoa Street
Asheville, North Carolina 28801
(800) 522-4762 or (704) 253-0621
Website: www.gsdl.com

For information about blood tests and stool analysis for Candida.

Recommended Reading

Candida Albicans: Could Yeast Be Your Problem? Leon Chaitow, N.D., D.O. Rochester, VT: Healing Arts Press, 1998.

Chronic Candidiasis: The Yeast Syndrome. Michael T. Murray, N.D. Rocklin, CA: Prima Publishing, 1997.

Complete Candida Yeast Guidebook: Everything You Need to Know About Prevention, Treatment & Diet. Jeanne Marie Martin, with Zoltan P. Rona. Roseville, CA: Prima Health, 2000.

Dr. Braly's Food Allergy and Nutrition Revolution. James Braly, M.D. New Canaan, CT: Keats Publishing, 1992.

Solving the Puzzle of Chronic Fatigue Syndrome. Michael Rosenbaum, M.D., and Murray Susser, M.D. Tacoma, WA: Life Sciences Press, 1992.

The Yeast Connection. William Crook, M.D. New York: Vintage Books, 1986.

CHILDREN'S HEALTH

Natural and alternative approaches can be very effective in maintaining a child's health, as well as treating common childhood illnesses, with fewer harmful side effects than conventional medicine. Certain standard medical treatments, such as the extensive use of antibiotics and immunizations, are being challenged by researchers, physicians, and government officials with regard to their safety and overall effectiveness. Today, physicians and parents have many options in caring for children, especially in the area of alternative medical care.

CARING FOR CHILDREN is a demanding and sometimes difficult task for parents. When sickness arises, parents may feel frustrated by not being able to identify what is wrong with their child, as well as in determining the severity of the condition. When dealing with a childhood illness, parents need to carefully evaluate their condition and decide what steps to take.

Attention to diet and nutritional supplementation as well as the appropriate use of herbs can have a beneficial effect on a child's health. In addition, homeopathy, traditional Chinese medicine, naturopathic medicine, and Ayurvedic medicine all offer comprehensive approaches to children's health. Though no single approach is meant to replace the advice and supervision of a qualified health-care practitioner, safe alternatives to conventional medical care allow parents to make informed decisions about the types of treatment their children should receive.

Raising a Healthy Child

Concern for the health of a child can begin even before conception. "If you want to give your child the greatest chance for health, consider pre-conception nutrition," Constantine A. Kotsanis, M.D., of Grapevine, Texas, advises parents. "Creation of new life is the single most important event in someone's life. It is the obligation of the mother and father to correct their metabolism and toxicities six months prior to conception." This may include using organic foods, clearing infections from the gastrointestinal and genitourinary tracts, chelation therapy if heavy metals are present, biological dentistry, sauna therapy to clear chemical toxins, ozone therapy for faulty metabolism, and psychological counseling for any unresolved emotional issues.

All parents want their children to be healthy and vibrant. Caring for a child is an all-consuming job for parents, one that practitioners of alternative medicine understand as having several important components. These include a stable and loving environment, a comprehensive understanding of what constitutes proper diet and nutrition, and a thorough knowledge of parental health rights, particularly when choosing a health-care professional, obtaining and retaining medical records, and deciding whether or not to immunize a child.

 See Biological Dentistry, Chelation Therapy, Detoxification Therapy, Diet, Mind/Body Medicine, Oxygen Therapies.

Providing a Loving Environment

According to Lendon Smith, M.D., a pediatrician in Portland, Oregon, and author of numerous books on children's health, the physical, mental, and emotional well-being of a child is dependent upon a sense of security and self-esteem as provided by the parents. As a result, says Dr. Smith, "The foundation for a child's health may well begin with the parents' relationship, even before conception. Following that, the most important thing for the child is to be held, massaged, loved, smiled at, and essentially told that he or she is accepted and worthwhile."

Dr. Smith explains that spending time with children, especially listening to them, is vital. Parents would do well to avoid using too many commands and questions in speaking to their children, points out Dr. Smith. "If children only hear commands and questions that act as challenges to a child's behavior, such as 'What are you doing in there?' or 'Don't get yourself dirty', they tend to develop a low self-image."

ALTERNATIVES TO BREAST-FEEDING

If a mother is unable to breast-feed, for whatever reason, one recommendation by Lendon Smith, M.D., is to see a lactation consultant who can help design a nutritionally balanced substitute to breast milk or discuss ways to encourage lactation.

Dr. Smith has found that goat's milk can be a good replacement for breast-feeding for the first 10-12 months. He suggests diluting it with pure water (three parts goat's milk to one part water). He also cautions parents to be sure to use goat's milk that is supplemented with folic acid, as goat's milk has been associated with a type of anemia related to low folic acid content in the milk. The label on the carton will reveal if the milk contains folate.

Soybean milk is another popular alternative to cow's milk, but because of the popularity of soy it has become a common food allergen, so caution is advised. Other options are amino acid milk, almond milk, and rice milk. However, Eric Jones, N.D., Dean of the Naturopathic Medicine Program at Bastyr University, in Kenmore, Washington, and a naturopathic pediatrician, cautions that these milks by themselves do not provide full nutrition to infants, so you will have to supplement them with nutrients.

Unfortunately, none of these milks are guaranteed to be non-allergenic. Dr. Smith has seen babies who have developed eczema from cow's milk, asthma from soymilk, diarrhea from almond milk, and irritability from goat's milk. Therefore, he suggests rotating them to prevent babies from developing an allergic reaction to any particular one.

Virender Sodhi, M.D. (Ayurveda), N.D., Director of the Ayurvedic & Naturopathic Medical Clinic, in Bellevue, Washington, agrees. "A child's sense of security is very fragile. When parents fight, a child's whole world seems threatened. This creates great stress and the result can be a breakdown in the immune system, followed by recurring illnesses." Dr. Sodhi maintains that growing children should be given a lot of physical affection and verbal encouragement and validation. "This does not spoil the child," he says. "Rather, it helps build good self-esteem."

Growing children should be given a lot of physical affection and verbal encouragement and validation. This does not spoil the child; rather, it helps build good self-esteem.

—VIRENDER SODHI, M.D. (AYURVEDA), N.D.

 See Allergies, Hearing and Ear Disorders, Pregnancy and Childbirth.

Diet and Nutrition

Proper nutrition not only helps create a strong defense against illness, it is crucial to a child's well-being. Dr. Smith notes that a majority of early childhood illnesses and infections are due to food allergies, especially from the early introduction of cow's milk or other allergy-producing foods into a child's diet.

Breast-feeding: Breast-feeding decreases the likelihood of developing allergic sensitivities to certain foods later in life, according to Dr. Sodhi. "Children who are breast-fed not only take in vital nutrients from the mother's milk, but they also receive the antibodies necessary to protect them against childhood illnesses such as ear infections and measles." Human breast milk contains nutrients that are easily digested, contribute to healthy brain development, and provide immunity to infectious agents that the infant will encounter in the environment. It contains anti-inflammatory substances that infants cannot manufacture on their own; stimulates the production of antibodies, which can neutralize a substance foreign to the body before it becomes an allergen; and populates the child's immature intestinal barrier with beneficial microflora.

Dr. Smith emphasizes that nursing for at least 8-10 months contributes to the child having fewer allergies, better jaw formation, good teeth, and a good dental arch. "If babies are given anything other than breast milk in the first few months of life, food sensitivities may develop," says Dr. Smith. "Their intestines are not meant to digest anything other than breast milk. The immature cells lining the intestines will allow foreign food particles to pass through undigested. These particles are antigenic [material that causes immune reactions] and may set up an allergic or antibody response that the child will never outgrow."

Both Drs. Sodhi and Smith recommend that a child breast-feed until he or she no longer wants to nurse, which may take place anywhere from six months to two years of age.

Solid Foods: Dr. Smith notes that when a child is ready to eat solid foods, usually sometime around 4-6 months old, parents can introduce fresh fruits and vegetables, grains and legumes, and low-fat proteins like chicken and fish. Organically grown products are the best choice as they contain fewer environmental toxins, and it is a good idea to avoid foods that are high in processed sugars, fats, or other additives, such as many baby foods, most breakfast cereals, candy, soda, and fast foods.

 Check with your pediatrician to determine the proper order of introducing solid foods into your baby's diet.

Dr. Kotsanis makes the following specific recommendations:

- Avoid wheat products (bread, cereal, cookies, pasta) and dairy products (milk, cheese, ice cream) whenever possible. These are the most common allergenic foods. Breads are available that are wheat-free, gluten-free, and without yeast or sugar. Rice or almond milk can be substituted for cow's milk.

- Avoid fried foods, which are nothing more than rancid and spoiled fats.

- Avoid all food dyes, because they are immunosuppressive. Most processed foods contain dyes, including colas, candy, and chocolate.

However, as children reach school age, it may be more difficult to control their diet, so Dr. Smith recommends keeping the diet at home as healthy and "junk free" as possible in order to offset habits picked up from schoolmates or in other homes. Usually the example of healthy eating set by the parents will win out in the long term, says Dr. Smith.

Maoshing Ni, D.O.M., Ph.D., L.Ac., President of Yo San University of Traditional Chinese Medicine, in Marina del Rey, California, says that the biggest problem today with the eating habits of children is their large intake of sugar. He suggests that parents remove sugar completely from their child's diet. Dr. Ni recommends that a child's diet include a good proportion of beans and legumes, which contain calcium, minerals, and protein. He also recommends soy milk and soy products and discourages using dairy products. (However, one should avoid non-fermented soy products if hypothyroidism is present, because they can exacerbate the condition.) Dr.

PARENTAL HEALTH RIGHTS

Lauri Aesoph, N.D., of Sioux Falls, South Dakota, believes that parents, as health-care consumers, have certain rights when seeking medical treatment for themselves and their children. Here are her suggestions:

Ask questions of your doctor: Ask the physician what he or she finds during an examination and exactly what it means. Ask why tests are ordered and what the results indicate. If you're uncomfortable about the choice of treatment, press for an explanation. If you've read about an alternative therapy you'd like to try, share that information with your doctor. Anytime you feel your doctor has missed something or hasn't asked pertinent questions, say so. Remember, you know your child better than anyone—including your doctor.

Feel free to change doctors: It is a good idea to interview several physicians before choosing one to provide health care for your child. Ideally, parents should join the physician in becoming active members of the health-care team. It is also important to remember that the doctor provides your family with a service and both you and your child should feel comfortable with them.

Obtain copies of medical records and laboratory reports: Ask for copies of your child's medical notes, as well as X rays, blood tests, and other procedures, and maintain an accurate file on the health of your child for future reference. You can save valuable time by collecting medical records and you will be more knowledgeable about your child's medical history.

Learn about your child's condition: Take time to read about your child's current or past illnesses. Educating yourself on the symptoms, as well as the conventional and alternative treatments available, provides you with the tools to ask your doctor relevant questions. This will also place you in a better position to decide if you need to seek a second opinion.

Consider an alternative treatment or practitioner: There is more than one way to view and treat an illness. Even clinicians who practice similar types of medicine may disagree about the appropriate treatment for a particular disease. Your health-care professional need not necessarily be an M.D.—naturopathic physicians, osteopathic doctors, homeopaths, chiropractors, acupuncturists, and other practitioners of alternative medicine use methods that may be effective in treating your child's disorders.

Ni notes that, according to traditional Chinese medicine (TCM), the kidney system is the most important system in the developmental stages of a child. For this reason, Chinese doctors use herbs, such as lycium berries, as well as massage techniques to tone and fortify the kidneys and liver. *Ginkgo biloba* is an herb commonly given to children, often used with alpinia seed (ginger lily).

David L. Hoffmann, B.Sc., M.N.I.M.H., of Sebastopol, California, past President of the American Herbalists Guild, believes that children can greatly benefit from herbs in their diet. Nettle, like spinach, is an excellent fortifier for children. He suggests that parents be creative with salad greens, substituting nettles for lettuce, which he says contains virtually no nutrients. Though Hoffmann understands that it is sometimes difficult to get children to eat raw vegetables, herbs can be incorporated into a child's diet in other ways. Instead of letting children eat jellies that contain large amounts of sugar, Hoffmann recommends that parents experiment with other fruits and herbal berries. Bilberries can be made into a syrup or jam and used to treat children with eyesight problems. Likewise, hawthorn berries are recommended by herbalists to treat children with heart problems or whose family has a history of cardiovascular disease.

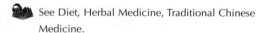 See Diet, Herbal Medicine, Traditional Chinese Medicine.

Factors Influencing Children's Health

Parents concerned about maintaining the health of their children can take measures toward preventing diseases by making sound medical choices. "Conventional medical practices, such as the blanket use of immunizations and antibiotics, have been proven to adversely affect the immune systems of both children and adults," says Dr. Smith. "Allergies to foods and medications have also been shown to impact a child's ability to fight diseases." Alternative treatments, because they work by strengthening the immune system rather than attacking a virus or removing a symptom, may provide better long-term health with fewer potentially dangerous side effects.

Allergies

Researchers and physicians have drawn a link between repeated ear infections and allergic conditions such as hay fever, asthma, eczema, and hives.[1] Allergies to particular foods such as dairy and wheat may encourage ear infections in some children, according to both Drs. Smith and Sodhi. One of the clinical signs that correlate with food allergies is excessive hair and wax in the external ear canals. In such cases, young patients can often be successfully treated by eliminating the offending foods from their diet.[2] When treating an allergic person, the doctor's goal should be to remove as much of the allergenic load (substances the child is allergic to) as possible. In this way, the child's immune system, weakened from fighting the allergens, can recuperate and fend off illnesses more effectively.

Alternative treatments, because they work by strengthening the immune system rather than attacking a virus or removing a symptom, may provide better long-term health with fewer potentially dangerous side effects.

Antibiotics

The conventional treatment for an infection is a course of antibiotics. Antibiotics are usually prescribed for ten days and, once started, the course must be completed, as the bacterial infection can recur and is more difficult to treat the second time around. However, the pediatric literature is full of studies indicating the disappointing results for antibiotic treatment of ear infections.[3] One study from the University of Copenhagen, in Denmark, stated that "88% of patients never need antibiotics and that the frequency of recurrence of otitis media [ear infections] in the untreated group is low compared with those treated with antibiotics." They conclude that if children are treated for an ear infection with an antibiotic within the first day or two of the onset of symptoms, they are much more likely to get another ear infection within a month.[4]

Antibiotics upset the natural balance of the bacteria in the intestines and chronic antibiotic use can lead to yeast infections. "Antibiotics should be used only under life-threatening situations," says Dr. Kotsanis. "If there is pus behind the eardrum or a temporal bone abscess is present, then antibiotic use is a must. However, this is rare and therefore the doctor should use conservative methods first. If the ear is draining, a positive bacterial culture also warrants use of antibiotics for a short time, but this must be followed by probiotics."

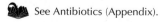 See Antibiotics (Appendix).

Immunizations

Vaccinations are developed to guard children and adults against potentially lethal and previously prevalent childhood diseases such as diphtheria, pertussis (whooping cough), tetanus (lock jaw), polio, measles, mumps, rubella, and influenza. The U.S. government and most conventional physicians pressure parents to start childhood vaccinations as early as two months of age. The first vaccines given are hepatitis B, DPT (diphtheria, pertussis, and tetanus), influenza type B, and polio. In total, an average American child is vaccinated against ten childhood diseases and receives up to 21 shots over the first 15 months of life.

Proponents say that vaccines are the safest and most effective protection against serious childhood illness for both individuals and the community at large. Increased research dollars are spent on developing new vaccines, but little has been done to investigate the possible connection between vaccines and developmental problems (as in the possible connection between the measles-mumps-rubella vaccine and autism). The possible side effects of immunization, including rashes, fever, diarrhea, autism, and even death, have been considered to be minimal when compared to the benefits. Vaccines may even cause serious defects in immune development and function, by bombarding the immune system with "inactivated" antigens suspended in solutions of toxic additives and solvents, including thimerosal (which contains mercury), aluminum, benzoic acid, and formaldehyde.

The potentially devastating side effects associated with immunizations, combined with too many unanswered questions regarding their safety and effectiveness, are causing many health-care experts to now object to blanket immunization.

Supporters maintain that, because parents cannot control their child's activities all the time, immunization is needed to protect the child during exposure to contagious bacteria and viruses. However, the potentially devastating side effects associated with immunizations, combined with the fact that there are too many unanswered questions regarding their safety and effectiveness, are causing many health-care experts to now object to blanket immunization. Today, many parents and physi-

cians are choosing not to automatically pursue a series of immunizations for children. At the same time, many doctors are advising against certain vaccinations they consider unnecessary and, in some cases, potentially dangerous to children.

"In my clinic, more than 50% of parents report normal development of their children until the age of 15-18 months, followed by regression in speech, coordination, and socialization, following vaccinations in the same period," reports Dr. Kotsanis. "Almost all the children that developed problems after vaccination were sick at the time of the vaccinations. They had allergies, chronic infections, were on chronic maintenance with antibiotics, or a combination of these."

Dr. Smith followed the standard pediatric immunization rules for 25 years. "During that period, I insisted that the children who were brought to me received the required immunizations. We [the medical profession] were the experts in preventive care—we knew what we were doing. We were behind the pressure on the legislators to pass a law: 'No shots, no school'. That was medical bigotry at its arrogant best."

Harris Coulter, Ph.D., a medical historian and author of two books on vaccinations, notes that immunization began as an experiment.[5] "Doctors didn't really know what they were doing. It was a tremendous propaganda campaign by the medical profession." Dr. Coulter does not feel all vaccines are necessary and points out that it is important to distinguish between individual vaccines rather than opting for blanket immunization. Of particular concern to many physicians are the diphtheria-pertussis-tetanus (DPT), measles-mumps-rubella (MMR), and polio vaccines.

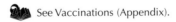 See Vaccinations (Appendix).

DIPHTHERIA-PERTUSSIS-TETANUS

According to Dr. Smith, as a result of the undesirable side effects caused by administering the shot to some infants, DPT has received the most adverse publicity. Most pediatricians see six to eight cases of pertussis (whooping cough) a year. Yet, Dr. Smith points out that some children who have had the complete series of DPT shots and even a booster at 18 months still contract whooping cough. "I began to have mixed feelings about the efficacy of the DPT vaccine," he says, "especially when so many parents reported related fevers and irritability for a day or so after the shots."

Dr. Coulter claims that a mild case of encephalitis (inflammation of the brain) may occur after a DPT shot, followed in some instances by residual damage. "In my opinion, this damage can include epilepsy and seizure disorders, hyperactivity, dyslexia, attention deficit disorder, sudden infant death syndrome, anorexia, and violent behavior."

Dr. Smith suggests that a child be immunized against diphtheria and tetanus, but that parents forego the pertussis vaccine, as it is not as efficient as it should be and is potentially dangerous to health. Dr. Coulter agrees. "Tetanus and diphtheria shots are not as dangerous as pertussis," he says. "However, I don't think the diphtheria shot is really needed because we have few cases of diphtheria in the U.S." He feels that vaccination against tetanus is valuable, but he recommends that the shot be delayed until the child is walking. He points out that tetanus is caused by improperly cleansed wounds and that it is unnecessary to immunize a two-month-old baby, who is unlikely to suffer from a penetrating wound.

Caution: If an unimmunized child catches diphtheria, an antitoxin to the disease must be given the first three days or death is likely, particularly in very young children. If therapy is not instituted immediately, the incidence of nerve damage is high. Tetanus can cause severe brain damage and can also be lethal in young children.

MEASLES-MUMPS-RUBELLA

For parents who choose to vaccinate their children against measles and German measles, Dr. Smith recommends that they follow the protocol to counteract side effects outlined below (see "Taking Precautions During Immunizations"). However, he feels it is better to contract these diseases naturally and be protected by the nutritional protocol he outlines in the treatment section for measles in this chapter.

Caution: Encephalitis occurs approximately once in every 1,000-2,000 cases and is a serious side effect of measles.[6] One child in eight who gets encephalitis will die and half will have central nervous system damage. Bronchopneumonia, otitis media, mastoiditis, brain abscesses, and even meningitis are not rare. Measles can also lead to severe hearing loss in children. Death is also a possibility. Measles can be a serious disease in adults who have not been vaccinated against it as a child; parents may want to take this into consideration when deciding whether or not to vaccinate their children. If a mother plans on having another child, she should be vaccinated before she gets pregnant. This way, if her first child catches rubella, her unborn child will not be affected.

POLIO

Dr. Coulter feels that it is important to vaccinate children against polio. "I had polio myself as a child, a serious case," says Dr. Coulter, whose right leg remains slightly paralyzed. "Polio is a dangerous disease. I have no objections to oral polio vaccinations, although there can be associated side effects."

METHODS OF IMMUNIZATION

The immune system mounts differing defenses to different diseases, depending on the mode of infection. "Because the polio virus enters the system through the alimentary canal," explains Dr. Smith, "it makes sense to give oral polio drops to the child to create an immunity that is as naturally obtained as possible." Dr. Coulter agrees, adding that he believes the oral polio vaccination is also safer than the injectable one.

With measles, mumps, and rubella, the viruses are airborne and enter the body through the nose and throat passages. After being processed through the tonsils, adenoids, and lungs, they move throughout the body to the blood, lymph tissue, spleen, and liver. Because the vaccine for these viruses is shot into the muscle, it induces antibody production but not cellular immunity and this may mean that the vaccination is less effective overall.[7]

TAKING PRECAUTIONS DURING IMMUNIZATIONS

If you choose to have your child vaccinated, the risks associated with immunizations can be reduced through more sophisticated approaches to vaccination. Harold Whitcomb, M.D., of Aspen, Colorado, an internist with more than 45 years of medical experience, achieves this using electrodermal screening (EDS). This is a way of determining in advance whether or not a child is likely to have an allergic reaction to a vaccine and, therefore, whether it is advisable to give the immunization at all. EDS is a form of computerized information gathering that is based on physics, not chemistry. A blunt, noninvasive electric probe is placed at specific points on the patient's hands, face, or feet, corresponding to acupuncture points at the beginning or end of energy meridians. Minute electrical discharges from these points serve as information signals about the condition of the body's organs and systems.

Preparation of the immune system prior to immunizations is important in helping the body counteract the potential side effects of vaccines. Dr. Smith injects his young patients with a mixture of B complex and vitamin C. "Recently," he says, "I have administered the following orally: 1,000 mg of vitamin C, 500 mg of calcium, and 50 mg of vitamin B6 to the child the day before, the day of, and the day after DPT. This mixture needs to be stored up temporarily in the immune system, prior to the inoculation, to the point where the body can process the vaccination in an efficient and safe way. Children following this regimen seem to have no trouble with the shot." Homeopathic remedies may also help reduce the side effects of vaccinations.

Dr. Kotsanis makes the following recommendations regarding vaccinations:

- Parents should understand all the pros and cons of vaccinations, along with the consequences of vaccinating vs. not vaccinating.

- Before vaccinations, give L-glutamine (500 mg), vitamin C (500 mg), and vitamin B6 (50 mg) daily for six weeks. Give probiotics (two times per day) and aloe vera juice (2 oz in divided doses, 2-3 times daily) for three months before and after vaccinations. Make sure the child gets plenty of pure water daily.

- If the child is constipated, take steps to correct the problem. The child should be free of all diseases and immune problems for two weeks prior to vaccination.

- Use pure single vaccines with no preservatives and wait at least 2-3 months between vaccines.

- Wait until the age of 3-4 years before vaccinating, if possible. However, you must keep the child at home during this time to minimize possible contamination from other children.

THE FUTURE OF IMMUNIZATION

As a parent, you have the right to choose whether or not your child will be vaccinated, at what age, and for which diseases. In order to make these decisions, you should be informed of a vaccine's negative effects and weigh those against the vaccine's benefits. It is also highly advised to delay immunization until the child is six months old (rather than two months) and to give only one vaccination at a time. Giving vaccinations to older children allows for greater immune system maturity, while staggering vaccines gives the immune system time to recover and makes it easier to determine which vaccine may be responsible for an adverse reaction.

If you choose not to have your child vaccinated, you must obtain an exemption (medical, religious, or philosophical) since immunization is compulsory in many U.S. states. A medical exemption is obtained from a doctor, usually applies to just one vaccine, and is given following a previous adverse reaction. Religious exemptions are available in 48 states (except Mississippi and West Virginia) and require legal documentation of your decision. Obtaining a philosophical exemption follows the same procedure as obtaining a religious exemption. Your state's health department can provide you with information on the state's immunization regulations and requirements.

"I think immunization should be voluntary," says Dr. Coulter. "Compelling parents to have their children vaccinated will not be tolerated much longer in American society."

> *I think immunization should be voluntary. Compelling parents to have their children vaccinated will not be tolerated much longer in American society.*
>
> —HARRIS COULTER, PH.D.

The U.S. government has finally begun to recognize that vaccinations are not completely safe. Congress has adopted the Vaccine Adverse Effect Reporting System (VAERS) and the National Vaccine Injury Compensation Program (NVICP). The purpose of VAERS, monitored by the Food and Drug Administration and the Centers for Disease Control, is to gather information from physicians regarding adverse reactions to vaccinations. Over 33,000 reactions were reported between 1992 and 1996. Compensation is provided for families with well-founded complaints.[8] The NVICP has paid out over $1.2 billion to parents of children injured or killed by vaccines.

Common Childhood Ailments and Their Treatments

In using alternative therapies for children, caution should be exercised when dispensing any substance, natural or otherwise. Naturopathic pediatrician Eric Jones, N.D., Dean of the Naturopathic Medicine Program at Bastyr University, in Kenmore, Washington, believes that herbs should never be given to a child except under the guidance of a trained practitioner. Likewise, natural therapies such as Ayurvedic medicine, traditional Chinese medicine, or homeopathy should be used only under the supervision of a licensed expert in that field. Lastly, when using vitamins, minerals, or other natural substances, ask a health-care professional what dosage is appropriate for the child being treated.

Colic

Colic refers to spasmodic pains in the abdomen seen in young infants or children and is accompanied by irritability or crying. Colic also refers to conditions of gas or other digestive irritability in infants up to three months old. According to Dr. Smith, colic is often due to an alkaline, high-sodium internal condition, but it can also be caused by overfeeding, swallowing air, or emotional upset.

Though breast milk is recommended for a baby, colicky breast-fed babies may have cramps because of a sensitivity or allergy to some food the mother is eating. A sensitizing food will create a red ring of inflammation on the skin at the anal opening of the baby. The most common offending foods are milk, soy, corn, wheat, and eggs. Garlic, onions, cabbage, and beans commonly produce intestinal gas in both mother and baby. All these foods should be avoided by nursing mothers, according to Dr. Smith.

For babies who are not breast-fed, prepared formulas may contribute to colic. Cow's milk, commonly found in infant formulas, is often the culprit. According to Dr. Smith, up to 50% of infants are sensitive to cow's milk, which can precipitate not only colic but also diarrhea, rashes, ear infections, asthma, and other conditions. Prepared cow's milk formulas may include many additives such as high-fructose corn syrup, which can cause problems for infants.

To treat colic, Dr. Smith recommends giving the baby one tablespoon to one ounce of a mixture of apple cider and water (one teaspoon of apple cider per eight ounces of water). Dr. Smith has found this remedy to be safe and effective.

Up to 50% of infants are sensitive to cow's milk, which can precipitate not only colic but also diarrhea, rashes, ear infections, asthma, and other conditions.

—LENDON SMITH, M.D.

A recent study also found a link between smoking by the mother during pregnancy or immediately after birth and the likelihood that the baby will develop colic. Quitting smoking during this period may help prevent colic.[9]

Ayurvedic Medicine: An Ayurvedic approach, according to Dr. Sodhi, would be to give the child a tea made of fennel (one teaspoon of the herb to one cup of water); a half teaspoon of this infusion taken every hour will relieve colic. A paste made of *asafetida* (⅛ teaspoon of the herb to one teaspoon of water) rubbed on the child's abdomen is another treatment.

Traditional Chinese Medicine: Dr. Ni stresses that, in TCM, the treatment for colic may vary depending on whether the problem arises from a cold, the flu, indigestion, or an allergy. Once the source has been estab-

lished and treatment begins, there are many things a parent can do at home. Dr. Ni recommends applying acupressure to the webbed area between the child's thumb and index finger and massaging that area. Another effective acupressure point is a spot located above the navel at a distance equal to the width of four of the child's fingers. A gentle massaging of that area, and the corresponding area along the child's spine, may bring relief. Also, a tea made of ginger, fennel, a little bit of citrus peel, and some scallions boiled, cooled, and fed to the child, should help to settle the colic, says Dr. Ni.

 See Ayurvedic Medicine, Herbal Medicine, Traditional Chinese Medicine.

Homeopathy: Richard Moskowitz, M.D., a homeopathic physician in Watertown, Massachusetts, suggests that mothers who are breast-feeding stop eating dairy products until the child has outgrown the colic, which usually happens at about three months of age. If the colic persists, he recommends the child be given homeopathic remedies such as *Chamomilla, Colocynthis, Nux vomica,* and *Magnesium phosphorica.*

Herbal Medicine: In Europe and Canada, according to David Hoffmann, parents use a treatment for colic called grippe water, which is simply water infused with dill seed. Though this remedy exists in the *United States Pharmacopeia,* it is rarely used in the U.S. Other herbs believed to help alleviate colic are fennel seed and chamomile. All these herbs contain oils known as carminatives, which reduce inflammation in the bowels and can lessen the production of gas. They are also mildly antimicrobial and antispasmodic (relaxing muscle spasms). These remedies may be effective for older children and even adults with stomach ailments, though they are most effective in younger children.

Stomachache

Even as children grow, stomachaches continue to be a common complaint. Stomach pains stem most commonly from emotional and food-related causes. "For older children," says Dr. Jones, "one of the first things to look at is their emotional state." He estimates that abdominal pains in up to 90% of children are due to functional causes (related to the functioning of the organ and not actual damage) rather than any physical disease process. Occasionally, says Dr. Jones, when a child has an upper respiratory infection, he or she may develop a stomachache from swallowing mucus and phlegm.

Eating habits may contribute to stomachaches. As with adults, when a child eats too fast and on the run, indigestion may result. Consuming foods containing excessive amounts of additives, sugar, salt, and fats can disrupt digestion. Food allergies or intolerances should also be considered.

If the stomach pain is accompanied by other symptoms, such as vomiting, diarrhea, loss of appetite, change in weight, fever, bloody stools, or pain during urination, a visit to the doctor is warranted. It is also important for a parent to remember that a stomachache does not necessarily mean that the problem lies in the stomach—abdominal pain may indicate illness elsewhere.

Ayurvedic Medicine: According to Dr. Sodhi, fennel and anise teas can be drunk in the amount of one tablespoon every hour. The herb *asafetida* can be taken orally by children suffering from stomachaches. An Ayurvedic doctor should be consulted for a prescription.

Traditional Chinese Medicine: A physician practicing TCM will determine if the stomach pain is caused by a specific illness, such as a cold or flu, and then prescribe herbs to treat that illness. According to Dr. Ni, the same remedy used for colic can be applied for any general stomach upset in an older child.

Homeopathy: The homeopathic remedies Dr. Moskowitz uses for colic can also benefit older children suffering from stomach pain. These homeopathics are standard remedies and are adjusted depending on the circumstances of the child's illness, such as whether the symptoms occur at a certain time of the day or whether they are associated with a certain emotional problem.

Herbal Medicine: David Hoffmann states that the older the child is, the less responsive he or she may be to certain herbal remedies. He suggests that parents try the remedies outlined for colic, but if children over the age of five experiencing stomachaches do not respond to those remedies, he recommends using herbs such as chamomile, peppermint, lemon bar, and anise. If these treatments don't work, it may be that the stomachache is due to an infection or diarrhea. Infections should be treated individually. If diarrhea is associated with the stomachache, Hoffmann recommends the herb meadowsweet.

CAUTION If the stomach pain is accompanied by other symptoms, such as vomiting, diarrhea, loss of appetite, change in weight, fever, bloody stools, or pain during urination, a visit to a physician is warranted.

Ear Infections (Otitis Media)

The eustachian tube, a structure that allows for the equalization of air pressure between the middle ear and the back of the throat, provides a pathway through which bacteria can enter the ear. Ear infections usually occur following a cold, when the eustachian tube becomes blocked and infected. The pus buildup formed by the bacterial infection causes extreme pain often accompanied by a high fever. Dysfunctional eustachian tubes may also contribute to the problem.[10] Most children (80%) have at least one ear infection during their first five years. A child suspected of having an ear infection should be examined by a physician. Although antibiotics are usually prescribed by conventional doctors for ear infections, there are many strategies for parents who are interested in a more natural approach to treating infections.

Breast-feeding protects against ear infections. Recent studies show that the longer babies are nursed, the less likely that they will contract otitis media and other infections.[11] Possible reasons for this are that mother's milk contains antibodies that protect against disease and that nursing precludes the use of cow's milk, an irritant to the eustachian tube and a common allergen.[12]

Treatments geared toward boosting the immune system can help children prone to ear infections. "We now know that if a patient is allowed to mobilize the immune system with an approach such as the cold socks treatment, mullein flower oil ear drops, 1,000 mg of vitamin C every hour or two, along with the herbal remedy echinacea and an appropriate homeopathic remedy, he may not get sick for another year," according to Dr. Smith. "These treatment modalities often work faster than antibiotics and are very safe. Once the immune system has been primed and the body learns how to fight off ear infections without antibiotics, repeated infections are rare." Dr. Smith maintains that antibiotics should only be used if the ear infection moves to the mastoid bone, found behind the ear, or the meninges (membranes covering the brain and spinal cord).

CAUTION Any problems that persist or worsen should be referred to a physician or licensed health professional.

Ayurvedic Medicine: Dr. Sodhi suggests an Ayurvedic technique of lymphatic drainage massage for ear infections. He teaches parents how to massage the child's lymphatics (a system of vessels and nodes throughout the body that carry the lymph fluid and help to remove toxins from the body), which will help drain the inner ear tubes. Massaging the child's lymph nodes daily may help keep infections from recurring. Dr. Sodhi also recommends vitamin C and garlic; the latter is best given to children in the form of garlic oil capsules.

Traditional Chinese Medicine: Dr. Ni says that, in the case of a chronic ear infection (usually seen in children who have been given large doses of antibiotics), one must treat the infection while addressing the problem of an immune system weakened by the antibiotics. He prescribes herbs that are powdered and then administered to the child in juice or applesauce. Gentian root, honeysuckle flower, and forsythia are examples of herbs that would be combined in a prescription.

HOMEOPATHICS WORK BETTER THAN ANTIBIOTICS

For cases of otitis media, homeopathic remedies can provide faster pain relief with fewer relapses than standard antibiotics, according to a German study. In the study, 103 children (ages one to 11) received a single homeopathic remedy from among a list that included *Aconitum napellus, Apis mellifica, Belladona, Capsicum, Chamomilla, Kalium bichromicum, Lachesis, Lycopodium, Mercurius solubilis, Okoubaka, Pulsatilla,* and *Silicea*. At the same time, 28 children were given antibiotics, decongestant nose drops, or other conventional drugs.

Those children treated with homeopathic remedies experienced ear pain for only two days, while those on conventional drugs had pain for three days. In other words, the homeopathic remedies produced a 33% pain reduction. Further, the homeopathic remedies were discontinued after 2-4 days, when relief occurred, while the antibiotics were given for 8-10 days. This means the children's bodies also had to cope with the negative side effects of antibiotics, such as the destruction of beneficial intestinal flora, as the price for only moderate relief of symptoms.

After one year, 70.7% of children in the homeopathic group had experienced no recurrences of the ear inflammation, while 29.3% had a maximum of three relapses. In contrast, in the antibiotic group, only 56.5% were free of relapses and 43.6% had a maximum of six recurrences.[13]

Homeopathy: According to Dr. Moskowitz, a critical factor in the long-term treatment of otitis media is the effect of vaccinations on the immune system. He strongly advises parents against vaccinating their children until they are completely over the cycle of ear infections. Many parents don't realize what an added stress a series of vaccinations, such as the DPT booster, poses to the child's weakened immune system, he says.

When treating a child homeopathically for an ear infection, one must consider the child's "constitutional structure," the personality traits of the child. These may include a child's tendency to have certain types of symptoms, such as to become hot or cold, to perspire in a certain way or area, or to sleep in a particular position. With this constitutional profile in mind, it is usually possible to find a remedy that will help the long-term develop-

ment of the child and break the cycle of infection. Along with the homeopathic remedies, Dr. Moskowitz recommends putting 4-5 drops of warm vegetable, sesame, or mullein flower oil in the child's ear and keeping it in place with a cotton ball, which greatly relieves earache pain.

Herbal Medicine: Herbal remedies for ear infections include the internal use of echinacea as well as garlic oil capsules, says David Hoffmann. He also recommends drops of mullein flower oil in the ear, as long as there is no perforation of the eardrum.

Hoffmann tells of a 6-year-old boy who was diagnosed as having neurological deafness (damage to the auditory nerve in both ears). Though the child was not in any pain, he had not been hearing well in school. He and his family all suffered from severe sinus problems. The herbs prescribed to the family members—goldenrod, echinacea, and raw garlic—helped reduce excessive secretion of mucus. Since there are no herbs that can cure neurological deafness, Hoffmann did not expect the child's hearing to improve. However, in treating the whole family for sinus blockage with prescribed herbs and a diet low in mucus-forming foods, the boy's sinus problem cleared up and his hearing did improve. Hoffmann concluded that the child had been misdiagnosed and that 50% of his hearing problem had been due to mucus buildup, resulting from a prolonged infection in the middle ear, and was not related to nerve damage.

 See Homeopathy, Hydrotherapy.

Strep Throat

Often when a child complains of a sore throat, parents worry that it may be strep throat (an infection due to *Streptococcal* bacteria). While this is not true in all cases, there is reason for concern. Most cases of strep throat are short-lived, but a very small number may, if untreated, progress to rheumatic fever or cause heart, kidney, brain, skin, or joint problems. If the infection is not fully cleared, it may return again and again. Therefore, thorough treatment of strep throat is necessary.

Most sore throats are caused by viruses and build slowly over two to three days. Other factors can be environmental, such as a dry atmosphere, cigarette smoking, pollution, or even yelling. Strep throat, on the other hand, occurs suddenly along with a fever, headache, nausea, and general ill feeling. Strep throat is not usually accompanied by cold symptoms, such as a cough and runny nose. Naturopathic physicians are well trained in the diagnosis and treatment of this condition. Some choose to use naturopathic therapies first and monitor the patient's progress. If these treatments are not effective, then the patient may be referred for antibiotics.

"I tend to take a conservative approach with strep because of the potential consequences, particularly in the high-risk group between ages five and 13," says Dr. Jones. After discovering the typical signs and symptoms of strep, he performs a screening test for strep throat on his young patients, a procedure that he says is between 85% and 90% accurate, and a complete blood count. If strep throat is confirmed, Dr. Jones recommends antibiotics. However, he also treats patients with a tincture containing goldenseal, calendula, echinacea, a small amount of oil of bitter orange, and *Galium aparine* (cleavers) if the glands are affected, along with other immune-enhancing remedies. Depending on the child's age, the patient is asked to gargle and then swallow the mixture. Acidophilus is also prescribed to offset the effects of the antibiotics on the intestinal tract. Dr. Jones stresses that it is important to determine whether the illness began because of contact with a carrier or if it is a chronic problem with other underlying causes. The key is early diagnosis and proper treatment.

CAUTION Most cases of strep throat are short-lived, but a very small number may, if untreated, progress to rheumatic fever or cause heart, kidney, brain, skin, or joint problems. If the infection is not fully cleared, it may return again and again. Therefore, thorough treatment is necessary.

Traditional Chinese Medicine: For infections of the throat such as strep, Dr. Ni prescribes a combination of honeysuckle flower and forsythia. Isatis roots and leaves can be very effective as well, he says. He also recommends eating large amounts of watermelon and drinking watermelon juice to cool the "hot" condition associated with strep throat. In his experience, Dr. Ni has been able to treat strep throat without resorting to the use of antibiotics. He stresses that, when beginning treatment with a TCM practitioner, one should stay with that doctor through the entire treatment procedure as natural remedies may take longer in producing results. He has seen parents become impatient with the healing process and hurry to get antibiotics for their children, not realizing that TCM heals by working from the underlying cause out toward the symptoms. This means that symptoms may linger for a short time after the patient has otherwise recovered from the illness.

Homeopathy: When treating bacterial infections, it is important to realize that a new generation of bacteria can evolve in about six hours, genetically selected for those organisms that are resistant to the antibiotic. The *Streptococcus* organism is one that people have been taught to be afraid of unnecessarily, according to Dr. Moskowitz. In fact, like all bacteria, it exists throughout the body and in the environment and may be one of the normal inhab-

---

COLD SOCKS TREATMENT

Randall Bradley, N.D., of Omaha, Nebraska, frequently uses the cold socks treatment, a long-standing naturopathic therapy for stimulating the immune system.[14] Dr. Bradley finds this treatment to be effective in relieving the symptoms of many upper respiratory conditions such as head and chest colds, earaches, the flu, sore throats, and even allergies. With this procedure, he says, relief is often seen within 30 minutes. If not, one can repeat the treatment while the patient remains covered and in bed. After four hours or by morning, the wet socks should be totally dry, the feet warm, and the symptoms gone or improved.

Step 1: Soak the foot part of a pair of 100% cotton socks in very cold water and wring them out thoroughly.

Step 2: Put the child's feet into a basin or bathtub of hot water (as hot as is tolerable without burning). Have the bath deep enough to cover the ankles, have the child sit on a chair or the edge of the bathtub, and keep the rest of the body warm. Soak the feet for 5-8 minutes until they are hot and pink.

Step 3: Remove the feet from the water and pat them dry with a towel.

Step 4: Immediately put on the cold, wet cotton socks and then a pair of dry wool socks over those. The patient should be covered and kept warm.

Step 5: Have the child go directly to bed, keeping the feet covered throughout the night. According to Dr. Bradley, this therapy will fail if the feet are uncovered or if the patient walks around or sits in a chair uncovered.

Dr. Bradley believes that this home remedy works by moving the blood to a specific area of the body—in this case, the feet. When the blood is drawn away from the head to warm the feet, pressure in the head is relieved. As a result, the symptoms of the illness may disappear and children usually fall asleep immediately. People who try this remedy will not only feel better the next day, but the treatment may actually boost the immune system, says Dr. Bradley.

---

itants of a healthy throat. For this reason, Dr. Moskowitz feels it does not make sense to use heavy doses of antibiotics, as this will also kill the natural flora in the child,

THE HOLISTIC APPROACH TO FEVER

Conventional doctors have been taught to treat every symptom that comes to their attention. For instance, medication is often prescribed to reduce childhood fever. Yet fever is the body's mechanism for destroying viruses and bacteria. Alternative practitioners take a different approach—their goal is to bolster and support the child's immune system so that it can learn to recognize and respond quickly to any invading organisms. In fact, according to Richard Moskowitz, M.D., certain childhood infections may be valuable in challenging the child's immune system and consequently strengthening it.

As an alternative to aspirin or acetaminophen, homeopathic remedies for fever and sickness are useful, safe, inexpensive, and have no side effects, says Lendon Smith, M.D. In addition, many herbal preparations such as echinacea not only enhance the immune system, but also act as antimicrobials, killing bacteria and viruses. In most cases, he feels that antibiotics are not required. Consult a physician regarding the instances in which an antibiotic may be indicated.

CAUTION A high fever can cause severe brain damage. Check with your doctor before deciding how best to respond to a fever.

- Homeopathy—According to Dr. Moskowitz, producing a fever is one of the signs of a healthy child. As immune systems develop in children, they respond acutely and vigorously to infections. If parents are worried as to whether or not a fever or infection should be treated by a doctor, Dr. Moskowitz believes that the best thing for them to do is ask: How sick is the child? Is the child vomiting, in pain, not eating, or not responding at all? If the child seems to be coping, says Dr. Moskowitz, the parents may feel confident that the child's immune system will be able to handle the illness with the help of homeopathic remedies. The remedies Dr. Moskowitz recommends do not eliminate fever, but rather help the immune system finish

its job of healing. These remedies might include *Aconite, Belladonna, Ferrum phos., Gelsemium, Pulsatilla,* and *Bryonia.*

- Ayurvedic Medicine—Virender Sodhi, M.D. (Ayurveda), N.D., considers a fever below 102° F to be beneficial in a child, and he does not like to give children medications such as aspirin or Tylenol. He recommends a light, nutritious diet, cold sponging, or homeopathic remedies such as *Belladona, Aconite,* and *Sulfur.* He points out that sometimes a fever can be a reaction of fear or anger and, in these cases, it is helpful for the parent to spend time talking or playing quietly with the child.

- Herbal Medicine—David L. Hoffmann, B.Sc., M.N.I.M.H., believes that a fever may be beneficial in a young child and that a low-grade fever does not need to be reduced. The child should be given a lot of support and comfort along with plenty of fluids. Herbal teas such as peppermint, elder flower, and yarrow will help the body cope with the fever, but will not suppress it. If one wants to reduce the fever, he offers meadowsweet, but he suggests that parents first seek advice from a skilled herbal practitioner.

- Aromatherapy—To cool the system, use peppermint, bergamot, or eucalyptus. To induce sweating, use basil, tea tree, lavender, rosemary, cypress, chamomile, or peppermint.

- Hydrotherapy—To lower a high fever, use a wet sheet pack or immersion bath. A neutral application can also be used to reduce fever to a manageable level.

- Topical Treatment—To lower fever, use a poultice of echinacea root. A cold compress to the forehead and cold pack to the trunk of the body may also be used or rub the body with apple cider vinegar.

lessening resistance to fungi, yeast, and other chronic illnesses. A better solution is to fight the invading organism by strengthening the child's immune system and by helping the child tolerate the symptoms with homeopathic remedies particular to the condition.

Herbal Medicine: According to David Hoffman, one herbal treatment for strep throat that works extremely well is osha root *(Ligusticum porteri).* Holding

this root in the mouth and chewing on it can be beneficial for throat infections. The problem is in getting children to use it, as the taste of the osha root is quite horrible, according to Hoffmann. "Unfortunately, all the things that work well for strep throat taste pretty rotten." He also recommends that children gargle or slowly sip a tea made of sage. Other herbal medications might include echinacea and cleavers, which can be made into a tea or tincture. Teas can be sweetened with honey and tinctures can be added to juice.

Viral and Bacterial Infections

Most viral infections manifest themselves as fever for 72 hours. When the fever dissipates, a watery nose, a strange, croupy cough, or diarrhea appears as the body tries to eliminate the dead virus. The whole disease process lasts about 7-10 days. "If a child gets worse after the first three days or the problem lasts longer than 7-10 days, specific attention and treatment are necessary," says Dr. Smith. "If a fever returns or if previously clear mucus changes to a thick, pus-like green or yellow color, a secondary bacterial infection is likely. If the mucus remains clear and watery, but the symptoms continue, an allergy is usually the cause."

During viral or bacterial infections, the immune system needs support, such as homeopathic and herbal remedies, including echinacea and goldenseal. Vitamin C is a very effective immune booster and probably the safest first line of defense—1,000 mg every hour or two over a 24-hour period (up to bowel tolerance) should produce a favorable result, according to Dr. Smith. Vitamin A and zinc also help the immune system.

Rest and allowing the child to participate in enjoyable, quiet activities can also speed healing. Dr. Smith recommends limiting sugar consumption, including fruit juices, as well as encouraging the drinking of fluids such as diluted vegetable juices and soups. If fruit juice must be given to the child, says Dr. Smith, dilute it with water.

Traditional Chinese Medicine: In the case of infections, before prescribing herbs, Dr. Ni will identify the infection as either a cold type *(yin)* or a hot type *(yang)*. For a *yin* type of infection, he prescribes herbs like cinnamon and ginger, spicier types of herbs that will warm a cool condition. In the case of a *yang* type of illness, which needs to be cooled, herbs like chrysanthemum flowers and peppermint are effective, Dr. Ni says. To reduce a fever naturally, Dr. Ni recommends a tea made of boiled gypsum.

Homeopathy: Dr. Moskowitz reiterates that, in homeopathy, it doesn't matter whether the organism is viral or bacterial—what matters is the way in which the infected individual responds to it and the pattern of that response. A homeopath will analyze the symptoms, asking questions like: Is there a discharge? What does it look like? What does it smell like? Is there an accompanying emotional reaction? Sensitivity to the child on the part of the doctor and the parents helps ascertain the appropriate treatment.

Measles

There are two distinct strains in the measles family: rubeola and rubella. They are viruses and need not cause serious illness if the child's immune system is strong. They can be treated like any other viral infection.

Rubeola, or hard measles, is still around despite vaccinations to protect children against it. It is severe in those with a debilitated immune system, but extra vitamin C can limit it to a minor irritation, says Dr. Smith. The disease begins with a slight fever and dry cough that accelerates over five days, with a rash breaking out at the height of the cough and fever along with red rims around the eyes. The rash begins at the head and reaches the feet within 24 hours. When the fever falls, the rash fades. Ear infections, bronchitis, and bleeding in the skin are possible complications. "Large doses of vitamin A for a short period of time can be protective," says Dr. Smith, "but one must be careful to avoid vitamin A toxicity. Be sure to consult a health-care provider for the correct dosage."

Also called German or three-day measles, rubella is a mild viral infection. It is of serious consequence only to unborn babies whose mothers contract the disease in the first trimester of pregnancy, before all the organs are formed, when it can cause birth defects. Rubella is characterized by a low-grade fever, red cheeks, and a fine rash all over the body. The lymph glands located behind the ears will usually be swollen.

Ayurvedic Medicine: Like other viral infections, the body's response to measles is to get rid of the virus by running a high fever and producing the rashes. Dr. Sodhi recommends that the best thing for parents to do is to ride out the cycle of the virus while making the child as comfortable as possible. To this end, Dr. Sodhi suggests that patients drink plenty of ginger or clove tea to hasten the progress of the disease.

Traditional Chinese Medicine: Dr. Ni also maintains that inducing the eruptions of the skin will quicken the resolution of the disease. To do this, he prescribes herbs such as Bupleurum *(chai-hu)* and peppermint. He also uses a remedy called cicada, which is the ground-up empty shell shed every seven years by the insect of the same name. Dr. Ni says this is a very effective TCM prescription.

Homeopathy: Dr. Moskowitz is opposed to measles vaccinations for children. In fact, he feels that the best way to handle illnesses such as the measles is to expose children to them when they are about five or six years old. At this age, children will come down with the illness and their immune system will be strengthened at an age where the potential side effects are relatively minor. Measles becomes more dangerous in adolescents and young adults and poses the most serious threat to women of childbearing age. If measles are contracted in the first few months of a mother's pregnancy, there is a possible risk of deafness to the baby. Vaccinations given to young children have a ten-year life span and so may not protect children when they reach the age of greatest risk.

He feels that measles is an example of a disease that helps to build a child's immune system for later life. The ability of the body to mount and recover from an illness such as the measles is the prime way the immune system matures in a healthy child, according to Dr. Moskowitz. He feels a disservice is done to the child by not allowing that natural process to happen.

In treating children with a disease like the measles, Dr. Moskowitz will take notes on the totality of the symptoms and the way the individual responds. This response will dictate the homeopathic remedy appropriate for that child. However, a common homeopathic remedy for the measles is *Pulsatilla*.

Herbal Medicine: David Hoffmann says that there are no herbs that specifically fight the measles, though there are many herbs that will control or alleviate the symptoms. One herbal preparation he recommends to help relieve the itching is distilled witch hazel. To ease the discomfort in the eyes, he recommends an eyewash made from a filtered infusion of eyebright.

Ayurvedic Medicine: Dr. Sodhi recalls treating a 14-month-old child who was suffering from a full-blown case of the measles and had a temperature of 106° F. His parents had taken him to a doctor who had prescribed antihistamines and antibiotics, but the child was so sick that he could not swallow this medication and would vomit whenever it was administered. In desperation, they called Dr. Sodhi. Upon examining the child, Dr. Sodhi recommended a concoction containing the herb *khubkalan* (one teaspoon to two cups of water) combined with raisins, boiled and taken every hour. He also told the parents to soak the child in a bath of lukewarm water and ½ cup of baking soda to reduce the itching. Following this regimen immediately produced marked results—within one day, the child's rash had begun to improve, his fever was down, and he was sleeping properly. In addition, the child never developed a secondary infection, which is common with measles.

Chicken pox

Chicken pox, also called varicella (after the varicella-zoster virus), is highly contagious. It is usually a mild illness with a low-grade fever and a blistery rash. Chicken pox is most infectious the day before the rash breaks out. Following that, blisters appear continually for about five days and consequently there will be blisters in different stages of development across the entire body: some just starting, some with heads, some turning milky, and those that are fading and crusty. These blisters are incredibly

itchy. The older the child, the worse the illness. Adults can develop shingles from the same virus if exposed to a child with chicken pox, says Dr. Jones.

Ayurvedic Medicine: During a case of the chicken pox, it is important to watch for a fever over 102° F, which can be kept down with a cool sponge bath, says Dr. Sodhi. Soaking in an alkaline bath containing baking soda will help relieve itching, as will aloe vera gel applied to the rash.

Herbal Medicine: David Hoffmann says swabbing the blisters with witch hazel works best in the case of chicken pox. One can also combine equal parts of dried rosemary leaves and calendula flowers and infuse (boil in water) this mixture. Once the infusion is cooled, it can be applied with a wet cloth by gently dabbing the child's skin where needed.

Traditional Chinese Medicine: Dr. Ni will treat a case of the chicken pox with the same treatment he uses for the measles. A 7-year-old boy in the early stages of chicken pox was brought to Dr. Ni by the boy's mother. The child's pediatrician had told the mother to simply "wait it out," but when the child ran a high fever, suffered from loss of appetite, and experienced severe itching, she wanted to relieve the child's suffering. Dr. Ni's approach was to use herbs to induce the eruptions, which has the effect of speeding the process of the disease and promoting healing. He recommended that the child be given peppermint and Bupleurum as well as a prescription of 12 herbs, some to reduce swelling and others to relieve itching, including an herbal cream. The next day, the mother, very concerned, called to report that the child had broken out in spots everywhere. Dr. Ni assured her that this was the expected pattern and noted that the child's fever was reduced. TCM works by forcing the toxins out of the system, he told her. The mother and child followed Dr. Ni's recommendations and in three days the worst was over. In less than a week, the disease had passed and the child returned to school.

Homeopathy: Dr. Moskowitz feels that chicken pox often need not be treated at all, but notes that common homeopathic treatments to relieve the symptoms and discomfort of chicken pox include *Antimonium tart.*, *Pulsatilla, Sulphur,* and *Rhus tox.*

Mumps

Mumps is characterized by fever and very swollen salivary glands. The glands around the earlobe are those most often affected; however, the sublingual glands (found under the tongue) may also swell.

Herbal Medicine: David Hoffmann feels that the mumps need medical attention as they may become serious. Internally, he recommends the herb cleavers.

Ayurvedic Medicine: Dr. Sodhi explains that with an illness like mumps, it is important that the symptoms not be suppressed but be fully expressed so the disease can "get out" of the body. Swelling is therefore desirable and can be encouraged by drinking "raisin water" made by boiling 20-30 raisins in 1-2 cups of water. According to Dr. Sodhi, taking several cups of this mixture a day helps express the mumps, keeps the virus under control, and aids in nutrition, as many children with this illness find eating difficult. Mustard packs on the glands may be helpful if the disease is not fully expressed. Likewise, a sandalwood pack may reduce swelling if the symptoms are acute and need to be controlled.

Traditional Chinese Medicine: Besides letting a case of the mumps run its course, Dr. Ni prescribes herbs like dandelion, used internally as a tea or externally ground into a powder and made into a poultice with some aloe and applied to the lumps. This will help reduce the swelling.

Homeopathy: Homeopathic remedies for mumps symptoms are *Apis mel.*, *Belladonna, Bryonia,* and *Pulsatilla,* according to Dr. Moskowitz.

Childhood Parasites

The problem of parasites in children can provoke fear and embarrassment in parents, but neither response is necessary, according to Dr. Smith. He refers to parasites as a children's social disease, as children mainly acquire them through their interaction with other children. Parasites can also be acquired from food, contaminated water, and pets.

PINWORMS

Dr. Smith notes that 80% of children 2-10 years of age contract pinworms at some time. Common symptoms include irritability, night wakefulness, teeth grinding, an itchy anal area, and stomachaches. The eggs are carried by children to everything they touch, including the mouth. Eggs are then swallowed and hatch in the lower colon where the worms mate. The pregnant female crawls out at night and lays thousands of eggs around the rim of the anus and the cycle is repeated. The parasites are transmitted from one child to another in social settings.

Dr. Smith recommends that a parent inspect the child's rectal area at night when the child is sleeping for evidence of the parasite. One way to diagnose this problem is to perform a cellophane tape test. To do this, pat the sticky side of the cellophane tape against the area around the child's anal opening first thing in the morning. Fold the tape together with the non-sticky side out and send or bring the tape to your physician to be tested.

To treat childhood parasites, Dr. Smith recommends a garlic enema. Place two cloves of garlic in a quart of water; boil the water for a few minutes, cool the liquid and place the fluid in an enema bag. Bring a chair to the edge of the bathtub and have the child lie face down on the chair, with his or her legs hanging into the tub. Lubricate the anal opening, slide the enema tube in for just an inch or so, and let the fluid run in and then out into the tub.

In treating pinworms, Dr. Moskowitz prescribes the pharmaceutical drug Vermox. He explains that natural remedies for treating pinworms can take a long time to be effective and the process can be very trying for both parent and child. "Vermox is one of my few prescriptions. One dose of it and the pinworms are gone for good."

Herbal Medicine: David Hoffmann suggests peeling a clove of garlic, pricking it with pins so that the oils will leak out, and inserting the clove in the anus of the infected child. This remedy works for adults, but can be irritating for children and they may not be able to tolerate it.

Traditional Chinese Medicine: Dr. Ni approaches the problem of parasites by trying to find out why they are present in the first place. If the immune system is weak, he will work on strengthening it. He sometimes uses pumpkin seeds and watermelon seeds ground into a powder and taken with aloe juice on an empty stomach every morning.

Ayurvedic Medicine: Bitter melon, eaten as a vegetable, is very effective in killing parasites naturally, says Dr. Sodhi. Berberine taken orally also helps, according to Dr. Sodhi, as will tomatoes eaten with ground black pepper.

HEAD LICE

Lice are another common infestation among young children, particularly those of school age, and are usually caused by the child's contact with other children. The most noticeable symptom is a persistent scratching of the scalp. Upon close inspection, parents may find tiny, grey-colored insects crawling among the hairs; these are the adults. The lice eggs (nits) are white and adhere to the hair shafts close to the scalp. The nits have an incubation period of 7-14 days, so patience and strict adherence to recommended treatments are key.

If the child attends school or day-care, a set of treatment guidelines will be required to eliminate all lice and eggs from the child before he or she can return to school. This usually involves washing the child's head with a special shampoo for head lice (either over-the-counter or prescription) and combing out all the nits with a fine-toothed comb. In addition, all clothing, towels, and bed linens used by the infected child must be washed in hot water. Nonwashable items, such as pillows, may be dry-cleaned, set aside in a plastic bag for 5-7 days, or placed in a freezer for 2-3 days. All carpets, upholstery (including car upholstery), and mattresses must be vacuumed and the vacuum bag discarded outside. Any hair-care items or accessories, such as combs, brushes, or barrettes, need to be washed and soaked in medicated shampoo or very hot water. As the condition is extremely contagious, all other members of the household must be examined daily for at least two weeks. Pets, however, do not need to be treated.

Lice shampoos are usually effective instantaneously, since they are essentially insecticides. However, it is recommended that they not be used more than once every seven days. Some parents choose to use natural remedies first. One remedy suggested by Dr. Jones is to use one part essential oil of lavender mixed with three parts olive oil. After scrubbing the child's scalp with the mixture of oils, a vinegar rinse helps to loosen the nits from the hair shaft. Dr. Jones stresses that this must be followed by a thorough combing and removal of the eggs, as well as the usual cleaning procedures.

Hyperactivity/ADHD

Hyperactivity is a complicated and often misunderstood condition. It has been categorized with conditions such as hyperkinetic syndrome, minimal brain dysfunction, and attention deficit hyperactivity disorder (ADHD; also known as attention deficit disorder). A child who is inattentive, overly talkative, impulsive, excessively irritable, and is hyperactive is labeled as ADHD. Dr. Kotsanis does not like putting medically convenient labels such as ADHD on children, because it can stigmatize the child and often obscure the real causes of the heightened or uncontrolled activity. Holistic health practitioners recommend several alternative treatments for this complex condition.

"The first thing I look at," says Dr. Jones, "is if the child has actually been diagnosed as having attention deficit hyperactivity disorder." According to Dr. Jones, at least 50% of ADHD children have been misdiagnosed; he estimates this number actually may be as high as 80% to 85%.

David Hoffmann feels that the diagnosis of ADHD itself is problematic. "I think our culture, especially teachers and harassed parents, have found a new label in hyperactivity to try and control very active, very creative, very alive children," he says. Many parents and physicians are beginning to question the scientific credibility and very existence of the condition. Fred Baughman, M.D., a child neurologist and outspoken critic of the ADHD diagnosis, says that ADHD has never been validated as an objective illness with any proven organic, neurobiologic abnormalities as a cause. The U.S. Department of Edu-

cation, the American Psychiatric Association, and drug manufacturers are among those perpetuating the ADHD designation and the use of drugs such as Ritalin for treatment. "Representing such things as ADHD and learning disabilities as diseases, absent any scientific proof, is to deceive the public," says Dr. Baughman.[15]

The first thing I look at is if the child has actually been diagnosed as having attention deficit disorder. At least 50% of ADHD children have been misdiagnosed.

—ERIC JONES, N.D.

Ritalin, widely prescribed to control hyperactivity and ADHD in children, is now used by at least 5% of all U.S. schoolchildren, mostly boys. There are an estimated 20 million prescriptions for Ritalin. Experts at the International Narcotics Control Board, in Vienna, Austria, which released a report on worldwide Ritalin use, suggest this could pose long-term risks for teenage addiction and compromised well-being. "Our concern is over-prescription," said the U.S. representative to the board. A study of 1,000 U.S. pediatricians found that 70% use Ritalin as a diagnostic litmus test to see if children have ADHD, resulting too often in misdiagnosis and inappropriate treatment. The "logic" is that if the children respond, they must have ADHD. Doctors overuse Ritalin because of time pressures, failure to do a thorough patient workup, and the need to get children treated and out of the office quickly.[16]

Hyperactivity may be caused by other underlying conditions, such as a learning disability, an unstable home life, food allergies, leaky gut syndrome, food additives, excessive sugar ingestion, heavy metal toxicity, or even the need for glasses. Dr. Jones remarks that at least half of his hyperactive patients improved when taken off sweeteners such as sugar and corn syrup. A study performed at Yale University School of Medicine revealed that when ingested by children, sugar releases twice the amount of the stimulant hormone adrenaline into the bloodstream as it does in adults.[17] Several studies have found that hyperactive children tend to be deficient in essential fatty acids (EFAs), unsaturated fats required in the diet.[18]

Caffeine is found in several brands of cola. In a survey involving 800 schoolchildren, those consuming sodas containing caffeine were more likely to be labeled as hyperactive by their teachers than those who drank caffeine-free soda.[19]

Approximately 5,000 additives are used in food products in the U.S.[20] In the 1970s, Benjamin Feingold, M.D., conducted extensive research on the possible link among attention deficit, food additives (flavorings, sweeteners, preservatives), and naturally occurring salicylates (substances in foods such as almonds, apples, berries, coffee, oranges, peppers, and tomatoes). Studies have both supported and dismissed this dietary theory.[21] A 1999 survey by the Center for Science in the Public Interest found that 17 of 23 controlled studies showed some evidence of a link between food additives and other dietary factors and ADHD.[22] In spite of this, many conventional medical experts continue to ignore or deny that diet affects hyperactive children.

 See Diet.

Often, environmental factors can exaggerate a condition such as hyperactivity. Dr. Moskowitz treated a "hyperactive" young girl who was so sensitive to fragrances that, if she smelled a bottle of perfume, she would be "bouncing off the walls for the rest of the day." Through Dr. Moskowitz's long-term treatment, which included various homeopathic remedies, the child's condition improved greatly and she was able to better tolerate these kinds of aggravating stimulants.

Ayurvedic Medicine: Dr. Sodhi recommends that all children, especially those with hyperactive tendencies, be taken off sugar. A nurturing, positive environment, in which they get a lot of attention and very little criticism, can positively affect very active, nervous children. Dr. Sodhi feels that the relationship between the parents can also greatly affect the child's behavior. A calming herb like *Macuna prurens* works very well with hyperactive children, notes Dr. Sodhi. Children, with the help of this herb, may be able to stop taking Ritalin. Another herb he recommends is *ashwagandha*. An Ayurvedic expert should be consulted before using any of these remedies.

Traditional Chinese Medicine: Dr. Ni treats individual cases of hyperactivity according to their manifestations. In TCM, the heart and liver are the two systems that are addressed in cases of hyperactivity. Herbs such as schisandra berries, biota seed, and zizyphus seed are used to calm the system. He also points to a poor diet as a probable cause of hyperactivity and suggests that a nourishing diet be implemented. Dr. Ni recommends parents reduce or eliminate a child's intake of simple sugars and instead provide a diet high in complex carbohydrates, especially beans.

Homeopathy: Dr. Moskowitz also links conditions of hyperactivity with diet, as well as with other chemical stimuli in the environment, such as perfumes, heavy

---

BED-WETTING, ADHD, AND ALLERGIES

Bed-wetting (nocturnal enuresis) is a common occurrence in toddlers and is only recognized as a disorder after the age of five. It is estimated that 3% of youths between the ages of 12 and 18 suffer from chronic sleep enuresis.[23] Some children also experience diurnal enuresis, or daytime incontinence. Less than 1% of nocturnal enuresis cases are attributed to emotional problems.[24] Physiological abnormalities and disorders, including a small bladder, metabolic or hormonal imbalances, urethral stricture, bladder infections, and sleep apnea are associated with the development of this disorder. Food allergies and sensitivities are also implicated.

Research has found that enuresis is significantly more common in children with ADHD than in other children. In fact, 6-year-olds with ADHD are 2.7 times more likely to have nighttime enuresis and 4.5 times more likely to suffer from enuresis than non-ADHD children.[25] Like ADHD, enuresis is often induced by food allergies and can be reversed by eliminating the offending foods. In one study, 21 children who suffered from enuresis as well as ADHD or migraines were placed on an elimination diet. Of those, 12 children were soon able to control their bladders, while another four experienced significant improvements in their enuresis. The hyperactivity and migraines also subsided on the elimination diet. When allergenic foods were reintroduced, symptoms of incontinence, hyperactivity, and migraines recurred.[26]

---

metals, and cigarette smoke. He attributes these ailments to a chronic depression of the immune system, sometimes as a result of vaccinations, congenital problems, or a birth injury. In other cases, it may be caused by an illness such as meningitis. He stresses that a condition such as hyperactivity tends to be a very complicated mixture of things and requires a dedicated relationship with the child on the part of the professional.

Herbal Medicine: For the child experiencing hyperactivity, David Hoffmann notes that there are herbs that may be helpful, provided that psychological factors are being addressed and that dietary irritants are avoided. These herbs include linden flower (especially effective when used in a bath before bed) to relax the child, chamomile for the nervous system, and red clover and milk thistle for liver detoxification. He also recommends

HELPFUL TIPS FOR LEARNING DISABILITIES

Constantine Kotsanis, M.D., of Grapevine, Texas, offers the following general tips for parents of children with learning disabilities and their physicians:

1. Eliminate all allergies by using injections of homeopathic remedies and shark cartilage.

2. Integrate the senses with gross and fine motor control exercises, visual therapy using prism lenses, and sound therapy using auditory enhancement training.

3. Correct all digestive disorders using enzymes, special herbs, antifungals, and "friendly" bacteria supplements (probiotics).

4. Make nutritional changes to avoid "junk" foods, as well as dairy products, food dyes, and sugars. Foods and beverages should be served warm, not hot or cold.

5. Use herbs that support the immune system, such as:

- Ginger: ¼ tsp grated fresh with 1 tsp lemon juice and 1 tsp honey, in a glass of warm water

- Cloves: chew 2-3 cloves daily or add a pinch of clove powder in food, once daily

- Turmeric: add ½ tsp in one cup of warm water or warm rice milk, twice daily

- Garlic: consume 2-3 cloves of fresh garlic daily

that the parents of such children find a way to alleviate their own stress and exhaustion.

Chelation Therapy: "Every hyperactive child that I have examined has had heavy metal toxicity," says Dr. Kotsanis. Once toxicity has been confirmed with hair analysis and urinalysis tests, Dr. Kotsanis may recommend chelation therapy, which refers to a method of binding up ("chelating") toxins, such as heavy metals and metabolic wastes, and removing them from the body. Chelation therapy takes 3-6 months on average and should always be performed under a doctor's supervision.

In one case, Dr. Kotsanis treated a 15-year-old boy with PDD (pervasive developmental disorder) with symptoms of anxiety, low energy, speech delay, and weight gain. First, Dr. Kotsanis corrected the patient's nutrition, healed his leaky gut, and also treated him for yeast infections. Dr. Kotsanis then gave him seven chelation treatments using DMPS (2,3-dimercaptopropane-1-sulfonate) over a period of four months, followed by four months using DMSA (2,3-dimercaptosuccinic acid, an effective agent for heavy metals because it crosses the blood-brain barrier and thus helps remove toxic residues from the

central nervous system). Over the course of treatment, the patient lost weight, improved his speech and eye contact, experienced a decrease in anxiety, and showed improvement in age-appropriate social skills.

Recommendations

- The physical, mental, and emotional well-being of a child is dependent upon a sense of security and self-esteem as provided by the parents.

- Breast-feeding decreases the likelihood of developing of allergic sensitivities to certain foods later in life.

- When a child is ready to eat solid foods, parents can introduce fresh fruits and vegetables, grains and legumes, and low-fat proteins like chicken and fish.

- Maoshing Ni, D.O.M., Ph.D., L.Ac., says that the biggest problem today with the eating habits of children is their large intake of sugar. He suggests that parents remove sugar completely from their child's diet.

- As a parent, you have the right to choose whether or not your child will be vaccinated, at what age, and for which diseases. In order to make these decisions, you should be informed of a vaccine's negative effects and weigh those against the vaccine's benefits. It is also highly advised to delay immunization until the child is six months old (rather than two months) and to give only one vaccination at a time.

Self-Care
The following therapies can be undertaken at home under appropriate professional supervision:

COLIC
AROMATHERAPY: Peppermint, chamomile, fennel
PRACTICAL HINTS: Burping the baby and keeping the abdomen warm by application of a warm water bottle will often bring relief.

EAR INFECTIONS
AROMATHERAPY: Chamomile, lavender, eucalyptus.

VIRAL INFECTIONS
HYDROTHERAPY: Constitutional hydrotherapy (apply two to five times weekly).
HYPERTHERMIA: Apply one to two times weekly.
JUICE THERAPY: Celery, beet, garlic

MEASLES

AROMATHERAPY: Spray or vaporize the room with eucalyptus, tea tree, chamomile, or lavender.

HYDROTHERAPY: • Constitutional hydrotherapy (apply two to five times weekly). • Heating compress, wet sock treatment (several times daily for head or chest congestion, replace socks when dry).

JUICE THERAPY: • Pineapple, pear juice • For the acute stage, try orange, lemon, garlic, and celery.

CHICKEN POX

AROMATHERAPY: Tea tree, bergamot, eucalyptus, chamomile

HYDROTHERAPY: • Constitutional hydrotherapy (apply two to five times weekly). • Heating compress, wet sock treatment (several times daily for head or chest congestion, replace socks when dry).

JUICE THERAPY: Orange, lemon juice

MUMPS

AROMATHERAPY: Lemon, tea tree, lavender

HYDROTHERAPY: • Constitutional hydrotherapy (apply two to five times weekly). • Heating compress, wet sock treatment (several times daily for head or chest congestion, replace socks when dry).

JUICE THERAPY: Orange, lemon

HYPERACTIVITY

HYDROTHERAPY: • Immersion bath or wet sheet pack. • Neutral application as needed for sedation.

Professional Care

The following therapies can only be provided by a qualified health professional:

COLIC

Applied Kinesiology / Chiropractic / Detoxification Therapy / Fasting / Environmental Medicine / Naturopathic Medicine / Osteopathic Medicine / Traditional Chinese Medicine

ORTHOMOLECULAR MEDICINE: Injection of potassium (as little as 1 g of potassium activates the intestinal walls, enhancing digestive abilities).

VIRAL INFECTIONS

Detoxification Therapy / Environmental Medicine / Enzyme Therapy / Fasting / Guided Imagery / Magnetic Field Therapy / Naturopathic Medicine

OXYGEN THERAPIES: • Hydrogen peroxide therapy (IV) • Hyperbaric oxygen therapy • Ozone inactivates lipid-enveloped viruses (mumps, measles).

MEASLES

Naturopathic Medicine / Traditional Chinese Medicine

Oxygen Therapies: • Hydrogen peroxide therapy (IV) • Ozone inactivates lipid-enveloped viruses (mumps, measles).

CHICKEN POX

Craniosacral Therapy / Magnetic Field Therapy / Naturopathic Medicine / Traditional Chinese Medicine

ENVIRONMENTAL MEDICINE: According to Marshall Mandell, M.D., chicken pox is a viral infection in which a small number of cases have been considerably relieved by the use of neutralizing doses of influenza vaccine. It has been reported to relieve itching and shorten the course of the illness.

OSTEOPATHIC MEDICINE: According to Leon Chaitow, N.D., D.O., osteopathic attention to the child includes gentle "spleen pump" techniques, which increase immune activity through enhanced release of white blood cells into the bloodstream, speeding up resolution of the infection.

OXYGEN THERAPIES: Hydrogen peroxide therapy (IV).

MUMPS

Naturopathic Medicine / Osteopathic Medicine / Traditional Chinese Medicine

OXYGEN THERAPIES: Hydrogen peroxide therapy (IV).

HYPERACTIVITY/ADHD

Applied Kinesiology / Craniosacral Therapy / Light Therapy / Traditional Chinese Medicine

BEHAVIORAL OPTOMETRY: Hyperactivity often is tied to sensory dysfunction leading to short attention and loss of context. Behavioral optometry seeks to calm hyperactivity by integrating perception and sensory/motor timing, resulting in sustained focus and emotional stability.

ORTHOMOLECULAR MEDICINE: The common nutrients that are helpful are niacinamide or niacin (1.5-3.0 g per day), the same quantity of vitamin C, and pyridoxine (100-250 mg per day). Zinc may also be required as well, using zinc citrate, if available (15 mg per day).

Where to Find Help

For more information on children's health, or to find a qualified practitioner in your area, contact the following organizations.

American Association of Oriental Medicine
433 Front Street
Catasauqua, Pennsylvania 18032
(888) 500-7999
Website: www.aaom.org

The AAOM is a national professional trade organization of

acupuncturists who meet acceptable standards of competency and can provide you with the names and locations of local members.

American Association of Naturopathic Physicians
8201 Greensboro Drive, Suite 300
McLean, Virginia 22101
(703) 610-9037
Website: www.naturopathic.org

The leading advocacy group for naturopathic medicine in the United States. Provides a directory of naturopathic physicians and offers referrals to a nationwide network of accredited or licensed practitioners. Also publishes a quarterly newsletter, for both professionals and the general public, and offers a series of brochures and pamphlets on a variety of subjects.

Ayurvedic & Naturopathic Medical Clinic
2115 112th Avenue N.E.
Bellevue, Washington 98004
(425) 453-8022
Website: www.ayurvedicscience.com

Dr. Virender Sodhi's clinic provides medical training for physicians and health-care practitioners, as well as individual courses for laypeople.

National Center for Homeopathy
801 North Fairfax, Suite 306
Alexandria, Virginia 22314
(703) 548-7790
Website: www.homeopathic.org

Provides a referral list of practicing homeopaths and other information. Gives courses for laypeople and professionals and organizes study groups around the country.

National Vaccine Information Center
512 W. Maple Avenue, Suite 206
Vienna, Virginia 22180
(800) 909-7468 or (703) 938-3783
Website: www.909shot.com

The National Vaccine Information Center (NVIC), operated by Dissatisfied Parents Together (DPT), is a national, non-profit, educational organization dedicated to preventing vaccine injuries and deaths through public education. NVIC/DPT represents vaccine consumers and health-care providers, including parents whose children suffered illness or died following vaccination. NVIC/DPT supports the right of vaccine consumers to have access to the safest and most effective vaccines as well as the right to make informed, independent vaccination decisions.

Recommended Reading

Beyond Antibiotics: 50 (or So) Ways to Boost Immunity and Avoid Antibiotics. Michael A. Schmidt, D.C., Lendon H. Smith, M.D., and Keith W. Sehnert. Berkeley, CA: North Atlantic Books, 1994.

An Encyclopedia of Natural Healing for Children and Infants. Mary Bove. Chicago: Keats Publishing, 2001.

Healing Childhood Ear Infections: Prevention, Home Care, and Alternative Treatment. Michael A. Schmidt, D.C. Berkeley, CA: North Atlantic Books, 1996.

Help for the Hyperactive Child. William G. Crook, M.D. Jackson, TN: Professional Books, 1991.

The Holistic Pediatrician: A Parent's Comprehensive Guide to Safe and Effective Therapies for the 25 Most Common Childhood Ailments. Kathi J. Kemper. New York: Harper-Perennial, 1996.

How to Raise a Healthy Child...In Spite of Your Doctor. Robert S. Mendelsohn, M.D. New York: Ballantine Books, 1990.

Natural Child Care: A Complete Guide to Safe and Effective Remedies and Holistic Health Strategies for Infants and Children. Maribeth Riggs. New York: Crown Publishing, 1989.

Natural Family Living. Peggy O'Mara with Jane McConnell. New York: Pocket Books, 2000.

New Vegetarian Baby. Sharon K. Yntema and Christine H. Beard. Ithaca, NY: McBooks Press, 2000.

Raising Healthy Kids: A Book of Child Care and Natural Family Health Care. Michio Kushi. Garden City Park, NY: Avery Publishing Group, 1994.

Ritalin-Free Kids. Judyth Reichenberg-Ullman, N.D., M.S.W., and Robert Ullman, N.D. Roseville, CA: Prima Publishing, 2000.

A Shot in the Dark. Harris Coulter, Ph.D., and Barbara Fisher. Garden City Park, NY: Avery Publishing Group, 1991.

Smart Medicine for a Healthier Child. Janet Zand, L.Ac., O.M.D., Rachel Walton, R.N., and Bob Rountree, M.D. Garden City Park, NY: Avery Publishing, 1994.

Vaccination and Immunization: Dangers, Delusions, and Alternatives. Leon Chaitow N.D.,D.O. London: Beekman, 1996.

Vaccines: What Every Parent Should Know. Paul A. Offit, M.D., and Louis M. Bell, M.D. New York: IDG Books, 1999.

Without Ritalin: A Natural Approach to ADD. Samuel A. Berne. Chicago: Keats Publishing, 2001.

CHRONIC FATIGUE SYNDROME

Dismissed for many years as an imaginary ailment, chronic fatigue syndrome (CFS) has only recently been accepted as a medical condition. While conventional medicine has achieved only limited results in treating CFS, alternative physicians are proving that taking a multidisciplinary approach specific to the needs of each individual patient can successfully treat the illness.

WHEN THE FIRST cases of chronic fatigue syndrome were identified in the 1980s among patients in a small Nevada town, the strange disease—marked principally by deep fatigue and muscle aches—was dubbed "Yuppie flu" because it seemed to be concentrated among young, affluent white professionals. Due to this and to the seemingly subjective nature of the symptoms, CFS was the butt of jokes and its sufferers were often not taken seriously by many physicians. Since then, CFS (also known as chronic fatigue and immune dysfunction syndrome, or CFIDS) has become an epidemic and crossed all ethnic and demographic barriers. It is now recognized as a severe, debilitating illness, although the previously dismissive attitude persists in some doctors.

A recent study estimates that 800,000 persons in the U.S. suffer from CFS and that 90% of patients have not been diagnosed and are not receiving proper treatment.[1] Other sources place the numbers much higher. According to Murray R. Susser, M.D., of Los Angeles, California, chronic fatigue syndrome afflicts an estimated three million Americans and possibly 90 million people worldwide. The National Institutes of Health estimates that most CFS sufferers are middle-class and white and at least two-thirds are women.[2] While not defined by the U.S. Centers for Disease Control (CDC) until 1988, and later revised in 1994, CFS has probably been around for centuries, although known under different names. Its symptoms resemble those of "the vapors," common in the 18th

> *A careful medical history, a physical examination, and laboratory tests can pinpoint specific infections, and perhaps the surest way to detect the disease is to inventory the pattern of symptoms.*
>
> —LEON CHAITOW, N.D., D.O.

century, and "soldier's heart," suffered by World War I veterans.[3]

Medical researchers have sought in vain to find a single cause for CFS, at times attempting to link it to the Epstein-Barr virus, candidiasis, and herpes virus. Alternative practitioners such as Dr. Susser believe that CFS is caused by multiple simultaneous infections that must be treated individually, while building up overall immune defenses. Misdiagnosis of CFS is common and creates additional pain and frustration, which could likely be avoided by taking an individualized approach to the patient.

According to Leon Chaitow, N.D., D.O., of London, England, CFS consists of extreme fatigue accompanied by a cluster of symptoms that seem to develop together fairly suddenly, often following an infection. No standard medical tests exist to detect CFS today. "A careful medical history, a physical examination, and laboratory tests can pinpoint specific infections, and perhaps the surest way to detect the disease is to inventory the pattern of symptoms," Dr. Chaitow says.

These symptoms, according to Dr. Susser, can include deep fatigue unrelieved by sleep; muscle and joint pain or weakness; headaches; memory loss; mental confusion and poor concentration; digestive problems; recurring infections; low grade fever (often in the afternoon); swollen lymph glands; food and environmental allergies/sensitivities; severe exhaustion from minor activity; and depression. Other possible symptoms include allergies, autoimmune reactions, dizziness, anxiety attacks, night sweats, rashes, breathing irregularities, hypersensi-

U.S. CENTERS FOR DISEASE CONTROL REQUIRED SYMPTOMS FOR CFS

According to the CDC, in order to be diagnosed with CFS, a person has to be suffering from the following symptoms:

1. New, unexplained, persistent, or relapsing chronic fatigue that is not a consequence of exertion, not resolved by bed rest, and severe enough to significantly reduce previous daily activity

2. Four or more of the symptoms below for at least six months:

- Unexplained or new headaches
- Short-term memory or concentration impairment
- muscle pain
- Pain in multiple joints unaccompanied by redness or swelling
- Unrefreshing sleep
- Post-exertion malaise that lasts for longer than 24 hours
- Sore throat
- Tender lymph nodes in the neck or armpits

OTHER TYPES OF FATIGUE

According to Leon Chaitow N.D., D.O., of London, England, fatigue can result from a variety of conditions other than chronic fatigue syndrome. These include:

- Adrenal insufficiency caused by the overuse of stimulants (tea, coffee, chocolate, cola, alcohol, tobacco, drugs) and/or excessive stress
- Allergies
- Anemia (low levels of iron or vitamin B_{12} in the body can result in anemia)
- Candidiasis, which is often misdiagnosed as CFS in women
- Cardiovascular causes (if breathlessness or chest pain on exertion accompanies fatigue, the heart may be involved)
- Chronic ill health (many chronic diseases have fatigue as a symptom)
- Depression
- Diabetes
- Headaches
- Hypoglycemia (low blood sugar)
- Infections (if fatigue is accompanied by elevated temperature, then an infection is likely to be the cause)
- Nutritional deficiency
- Obesity
- Premenstrual syndrome (the connection will be obvious if it occurs at the same time as the monthly cycle)
- Sleep disturbance or inadequate sleep
- Thyroid gland dysfunction
- Toxicity (increasing amounts of environmentally acquired toxins such as lead, pesticides, and mercury can lead to chronic states of fatigue)

tivity to heat and cold and to light and sound, and irregular heartbeat. The CDC stipulates that a continuance of a number of the above afflictions for six months is a strong indication that CFS is present.[4]

Dr. Susser firmly believes that CFS results from combined infectious conditions. He points out that the principle of the syndrome is that patients suffer from several ongoing, simultaneous infections that weaken the immune system. "The medical establishment talks as if there's only one infection at a time in a person, but there is evidence that more than one can happen," explains Dr. Susser. "In CFS, we often get hidden, concomitant parasite, yeast, and viral infections, which are results of a weakened immune system. One infection puts demand on the immune system, which can't kick it, and another infection may join in, leading from one to another in a domino effect."

According to Dr. Susser, the degree and severity of symptoms often fluctuate, not only over a period of weeks or months, but even from day to day, and a cyclical pattern of illness and reasonable health can emerge. Frequently, after a severe bout of CFS, a patient resumes normal activity and exercise, only to relapse into extreme fatigue after a period of time.

Dr. Susser reports new developments that have made CFS easier to diagnose. For instance, after exercise, brain circulation in CFS patients gets worse, unlike what happens with healthy persons. Therefore, he tests patients after exercise for decreased brain circulation. In addition, he tests the cortisol levels in the blood, which decrease in CFS patients after exercise. Low levels of this hormone (which is vital in dealing with stress) can indicate the likelihood of CFS.[5]

CRIMSON CRESCENTS

One of the primary setbacks to treating chronic fatigue syndrome (CFS) has been the lack of a specific medical marker that would indicate a clinical way to diagnose the syndrome. Burke A. Cunha, M.D., Chief of the Infectious Disease Division of Winthrop-University Hospital, in Mineola, New York, has discovered arch-shaped, bright red, membrane tissue in the back of CFS patients' mouths. Located on both inner sides of the mouth next to the back molars, these "crimson crescents," as Dr. Cunha calls them, intensify in color as the patient's condition worsens and fade as the patient improves.

Dr. Cunha states that the crescents appear in 80% of CFS patients but show up in less than 5% of non-CFS patients with sore throats, and not at all in patients with mononucleosis or strep throat. He states, "If your patient has crimson crescents, you now can say his condition is probably chronic fatigue syndrome."[7] Although Dr. Cunha's findings have not been confirmed by other health practitioners, the existence of such a marker for CFS deserves further investigation.

 See Allergies, Candidiasis, Diabetes, Fibromyalgia, Headaches, Sleep Disorders, Stress, Women's Health.

Causes of Chronic Fatigue Syndrome

According to Dr. Susser, CFS develops as a combined result of nutritional deficiency; acquired toxicity (from the environment, food, and drugs); poor stress–coping abilities; acquired systemic infections (often as a result of excessive use of antibiotics causing candidiasis and parasite overgrowth); and a vicious cycle of lowered immune function, allergy, more infection, and further depleted energy reserves. Individuals with CFS are continually dragged down in a spiral of decreasingly lower levels of energy.

Other factors that can contribute to CFS, according to Dr. Chaitow, include recurrent viral and bacterial infections (such as acne, sinusitis, cystitis); the reaction of the immune system to vaccination and immunization; bowel toxemia and infestation of fungi, protozoa, and parasites; lifestyle factors (inadequate exercise, sleep, and relaxation); hormonal imbalances (particularly thyroid and adrenal); increased muscle tension and breathing pattern changes (hyperventilation); genetic factors; alcohol, drug, and tobacco abuse; and mercury toxicity from dental amalgams. Many experts in the field also believe that a depressed level of immune function lies at the heart of the problem, though whether as cause or result remains a major area of debate.[6]

According to Dr. Chaitow, the conventional medical establishment's search for a single cause of CFS is misguided. He explains, "There has been a search for bacterial, viral, or fungal activity and, in fact, since many of these are commonly found to be present (active or dormant) in people with CFS (ranging from Epstein-Barr virus to herpes simplex and candidiasis), whatever was found was considered to be 'the cause' of the entire syndrome." Dr. Chaitow believes that CFS is a multisymptomatic condition that he describes as being "similar to an onion in which each peeled layer reveals another layer, or another symptomatic factor."

Chronic fatigue syndrome is a multisymptomatic condition 'similar to an onion in which each peeled layer reveals another layer, or another symptomatic factor.'

—Leon Chaitow, N.D., D.O.

"I think that the cause of chronic fatigue is infections, similar to the cause of colds and flu," says Dr. Susser. "There are 2,300 viruses that can cause a cold or flu and if one of those hits you and your body isn't able to get rid of it, then you have a chronic infection. That's really what chronic fatigue behaves like, the flu that never got better. I sometimes call it 'the flu that became always'."

Alternative physicians working with CFS know that removing toxins from the body is an essential phase in restoring patients to health and vitality. Each year, people are exposed to thousands of toxic chemicals and pollutants in the air, water, food, and soil. People living today carry within their bodies a "chemical cocktail" made up of industrial chemicals, pesticides, food additives, heavy metals, and the residues of conventional pharmaceuticals, as well as of legal (alcohol, tobacco, caffeine) and illegal (heroin, cocaine, marijuana) drugs. When combined with multiple infections and nutritional deficiencies, this toxic overload may be the proverbial last straw in the development of CFS.

Viruses and Other Infections

A number of viruses have been implicated in CFS. "The most common infections we find are yeast [*Candida albicans*] and parasites," reports Dr. Susser. "We also find hidden bacterial infections such as Lyme disease [*Borrelia burgdorferi*] and abscesses in the teeth (or jaw) and sometimes chronic prostatitis, chronic sinusitis, and chronic gastritis." Elevated antibody (activated immune protein) levels to certain viruses are frequently found in the blood of CFS patients. These include Epstein-Barr, cytomegalovirus, human herpes virus-6, herpes simplex, rubella, and enteroviruses such as Coxsackie.

The herpes family of viruses (which includes the Epstein-Barr virus and oral and genital herpes viruses) has been a primary focus of interest for the medical profession. The Epstein-Barr virus (EBV), the cause of infectious mononucleosis, has received the most attention since its symptoms are duplicated in CFS sufferers, who also have very high EBV antibody levels. Yet even the National Institutes of Health reports that there is no clear-cut evidence that the Epstein-Barr virus, or any other virus, is the primary cause of CFS.

According to Dr. Susser, CFS has a pattern of illness that includes more than EBV alone. While he concedes that EBV may indeed be a major factor in CFS cases, he rejects it as being the sole cause. He also points out the possibility that EBV might be reactivated due to other weaknesses in immune function.[8] Dr. Susser also reports that recent research has linked CFS to retroviruses, a group of viruses that includes the HIV virus.[9]

"If different virus activity is found in different research efforts, this may mean that it is not the particular virus that matters, but that many viruses seem capable of continued activity if immune function cannot control them," comments Dr. Chaitow. "Therefore, focus on immune function would be more beneficial than focus on the virus, which is simply taking advantage of the situation."

Dental Factors

According to Bill Wesson, D.D.S., of Aspen, Colorado, CFS can be due, at least in part, to amalgam fillings in the teeth, which contain over 50% mercury, a highly toxic substance. He cites the case of a female patient who suffered from CFS for nearly two decades. After undergoing a variety of treatments, which all proved useless, she agreed to undergo the dental work. Dr. Wesson removed silver-mercury amalgam fillings from 14 of her teeth, replacing them with gold and gutta-percha. Afterwards, the patient reported great overall improvement, with her depression, stomach problems, and fatigue particularly alleviated. "Before I removed her fillings, she could hardly walk around the block," says Dr. Wesson. "Now she's rid-

---

LYME DISEASE AND CHRONIC FATIGUE

Lyme disease was first recognized in the U.S. in 1975, after a mysterious outbreak of arthritis near Lyme, Connecticut. It wasn't until 1982 that the spirochete that causes Lyme, *Borrelia burgdorferi,* was identified. Lyme disease is a multisystem inflammatory disease affecting the skin in characteristic rashes (only 50% of patients exhibit these) at first, then spreading to the joints and nervous system later. Many now see the disease not as a simple infection but rather as a complex illness that often consists of other co-infections.

Symptoms are variable, including skin lesions or rashes, flu-like symptoms, sleeping difficulties, muscle pains and weakness, headaches, back pain, fever, chills, nausea or vomiting, facial paralysis, enlargement of the lymph glands or spleen, irregular heartbeat, seizures, blurry vision, moodiness, memory loss, dementia, and joint pains (similar to arthritis). One hallmark of Lyme disease is fatigue unrelieved by rest.

Lyme is sometimes called "the Great Imposter" because it is often misdiagnosed as other diseases, leading a patient (and often the physician) to believe the problem is chronic fatigue syndrome, borderline thyroid gland dysfunction, fibromyalgia, multiple sclerosis, Lou Gehrig's disease, and other debilitating conditions. Joanne Whitaker, M.D., of Palm Harbor, Florida, believes that Lyme is at the base of most chronic fatigue syndrome cases. If you have symptoms associated with CFS or these other illnesses, it is prudent to consider a Lyme disease diagnosis.

---

ing her bike, hiking in the mountains, and cross-country skiing, and her fatigue is completely gone." Dr. Wesson chooses replacement material for fillings according to the strength of a patient's immune system. He tests the compatibility of various elements with the patient's blood to determine the best material to use, and he states that new composite plastic resins are the best options for most patients.

According to Edward Arana, D.D.S., President of the American Academy of Biological Dentistry, in Carmel Valley, California, among the problems caused specifically by mercury amalgam fillings are: chronic fatigue syndrome and lack of energy; tendency toward chronic inflammatory changes, including fibromyalgia, rheumatoid arthritis, and phlebitis; chronic neurological illnesses,

AN IMMUNOLOGICAL TEST FOR CHRONIC FATIGUE

Jay Levy, M.D., of the Division of Hematology and Oncology at the University of California at San Francisco, has developed an immunological test that distinguishes patients with CFS from healthy people and from those with other disorders having similar symptoms, such as lupus, depression, acute viral-like illness, and prolonged fatigue without other CFS criteria.[11] Dr. Levy emphasizes that the test is not yet diagnostic, but is used as a kind of prescreening to identify possible CFS candidates for further study. Dr. Levy and his colleagues have found that the immune systems of people with CFS, unlike those of healthy people, are in a constant overactive state and never return to a normal operating level. This overactivity is what is behind the deep fatigue; paradoxically, this heightened activity overlays a condition of dysfunction and immune incompetency.

In this test, CFS patients with the most severe symptoms (based on a study sample of 147 patients) tend to have increased activation markers on CD8 cells (the proteins on immune system suppressor T cells), with reduced numbers of CD8 suppressor cells. Here is the immune imbalance: one aspect is inappropriately activated, the other exists in insufficient numbers. The test involves monitoring these CD8 cells. "Most noteworthy is the statistical evidence that an individual with two or more of the CD8 cell subset alterations has a high probability (90%) of having active CFS," says Dr. Levy.[12]

especially when numbness is one of the leading symptoms; lowering of the pain threshold; and disturbances of the immune system.

Mercury poisoning can also lead to symptoms such as anxiety, depression, confusion, irritability, and the inability to concentrate, all of which are symptoms of CFS. Such poisoning often goes undetected for years because the symptoms presented do not necessarily suggest mercury as the initiating cause.

The Thyroid and Chronic Fatigue

A major and often overlooked cause of CFS is an underactive thyroid gland. This gland is the largest of the body's seven endocrine glands and its role in all aspects of healthy body functioning is paramount, yet it is also probably the most overlooked factor in a great many health problems, like chronic fatigue. When the thyroid is underactive, every cell and organ in the body generally become

hypoactive as well. The problems occur when clinically severe thyroid conditions go undetected for long periods of time. In those cases, people are erroneously treated for chronic health conditions that are really based on the thyroid and that would respond well and quickly to a small dose of thyroid hormone. Hypothyroidism can be central among the multiple factors involved in creating CFS and therefore to successfully reverse or treat CFS first requires discovering any hidden thyroid imbalance.

This cannot always be done reliably by blood testing only, because some individuals have reverse-T3 syndrome instead of underproduction of thyroid hormone. This condition can be identified by taking the body temperature in the patient's armpit in the morning just before the patient gets out of bed. If the temperature averages less than 97.8° F, then either low thyroid hormone production or reverse-T3 syndrome is present.

Psychological Factors

Some in the traditional medical establishment argue that CFS is a psychogenic or, at least, psychosomatic ailment. Dr. Chaitow acknowledges, "In some instances, mental-emotional factors might lie behind the condition, since there is ample evidence showing that negative emotions and depression lower immune function."

There is no doubt that a positive or negative attitude greatly affects physical health. Nonetheless, the Centers for Disease Control states that depression and anxiety generally develop after the onset of CFS and are secondary reactions to CFS.[10] And Dr. Susser points out that most patients with CFS lead well-adjusted and very active lives prior to the disorder. Furthermore, he reports that many conditions, including heart attacks and cancer, result in depression.

"A reactive depression to the extreme fatigue of CFS should not be surprising," says Dr. Chaitow. "Those with CFS have often been suffering debilitating symptoms for a number of years, barely acknowledged by the medical establishment, and have been offered little appropriate treatment other than a 'chin up' attitude and handfuls of antidepressants."

Treating Chronic Fatigue Syndrome

According to Dr. Susser, CFS is a mixed infection syndrome that will best benefit from a sustained and multipronged approach to healing. Although conventional medical practitioners have had some success using pharmaceutical drugs to treat CFS, they are prohibitively expensive and can have severe side effects and unknown toxic effects on the body.

> *Chronic fatigue syndrome is a mixed infection syndrome that will best benefit from a sustained and multipronged approach to healing.*
>
> —Murray Susser, M.D.

Successfully treating chronic fatigue syndrome draws upon a wide range of alternative medicine therapies. Before designing a treatment plan, extensive testing is required. It is essential to understand the factors that went into creating CFS in each person, because CFS is never caused by one thing alone and no two people have exactly the same causal factors. Most alternative medicine practitioners will use an individualized treatment plan for each patient when treating or reversing the symptoms of CFS.

A number of tests are useful in determining the underlying factors contributing to CFS. Electrodermal screening and darkfield blood analysis can help provide a picture of overall health status. Digestive function can be assessed using a stool or urine analysis (these tests are also valuable for getting information on general health). Specific tests are available to assess how well individual body systems are working, including the immune system (T and B Cell Panel, NK Cell Function, Sedimentation Rate) and the thyroid gland (TRH Stimulation Test). Other tests look for possible nutritional deficiencies (Pantox Antioxidant Profile, Functional Intracellular Analysis, Nutricheck USA, Cell Membrane Lipid Profile) or excesses of toxins (hair analysis, ToxMet Screen, DMSA Challenge Test, Functional Liver Detoxification Profile) and stress (Aeron LifeCycles Saliva Assay Report, Adrenal Stress Index).

 See Life-Saving Tests Your Doctor May Not Know About (Appendix).

In treating CFS, Dr. Susser looks for infections that are the result of toxicity and nutritional deficiency, including yeast and parasites, Lyme disease, abscesses in the teeth and jaw, and sometimes chronic prostatitis, sinusitis, and gastritis. By treating these infections and boosting the patient's nutritional intake with good diet and proper supplementation, Dr. Susser reduces the burden on the immune system.

A major and often overlooked cause of chronic fatigue syndrome is an underactive thyroid gland, a condition known as hypothyroidism. Although, according to conventional medicine, hypothyroidism is a separate illness from CFS and a diagnosis of one precludes a diagnosis of the other, many people with CFS have not been properly tested for thyroid problems. Since thyroid hormones are integral to maintaining optimal body energy levels and are required for proper immune system function as well as nearly all aspects of body function, hypothyroidism can be central among the multiple factors involved in creating CFS. If that is the case, successfully reversing the syndrome will require discovering the hidden thyroid imbalance along with all the other contributing factors.

Detoxifying the body is another important component in promoting the health of the immune system and addressing other factors that may be contributing to chronic fatigue. As our environment and food are increasingly saturated with toxic chemicals, the body's mechanisms for elimination of toxins cannot keep up with the chemical deluge. Given that many people with CFS have chemical allergies as well, it is advisable to take measures to remove these toxins from the body.

Diet and Nutrition

Diet is crucial to reinforcing the immune system and conquering CFS. Enzymes should be one of the first priorities. The poor digestion and intestinal dysfunction that result from enzyme deficiencies deplete the immune system by not providing the body with necessary nutrients and by allowing toxins to leak from the intestines into the bloodstream. Then the body has to expend energy trying to eliminate these toxins. When immunity is already compromised by the presence of multiple viruses or infections, this energy expenditure to remove toxins adds another factor that can tip the balance into creating CFS.

According to Michael T. Murray, N.D., of Issaquah, Washington, a healthy diet avoids "empty" foods low in nutrients and high in sugar and fat. Instead, it concentrates on high-nutrient, high-protein, complex carbohydrate foods—vegetables, grains, beans, fish, and poultry (care should be taken to avoid mercury toxins in fish and antibiotics in poultry). "Your energy level is directly related to the quality of the foods you routinely ingest," says Dr. Murray.[13] He points out the importance of eliminating all allergenic foods and, if one is highly allergic, the rotating of nonallergenic foods. He also advises drinking 8-10 glasses of pure water daily.

For CFS patients suffering from candidiasis, all forms of sugar, including milk products (lactose) and fruit, should be avoided. Caffeine, alcohol, and refined carbohydrates (white flour, white rice) should be completely avoided.

Dr. Murray also advises CFS patients to take a good basic multivitamin/mineral supplement in the most bioavailable and easily absorbable form with adequate

DRUGS ASSOCIATED WITH A HIGHER INCIDENCE OF CHRONIC FATIGUE

According to the *Physicians' Desk Reference,* the following drugs are associated with side effects of chronic fatigue syndrome (statistics refer to the percentage of individuals affected).[25]

Accutane capsules (approximately 5%)
Actimmune (14%)
Anafranil capsules (35%-39%)
Aredia for injection (up to 12%)
Cardura tablets (12%)
Cartrol tablets (7.1%)
Centrax capsules (11.6%)
Cordarone tablets (4%-9%)
Dantrium capsules (among most common)
Depo-Provera contraceptive injection (more than 5%)
Epogen for injection (9%-25%)
Fludara for injection (10%-38%)
Foscavir injection (more than 5%)
Hylorel tablets (25.7%-63.6%)
Hytrin tablets (11.3%)
Intron A (18%-84%)
Lariam tablets (among most common)
Leucovorin calcium for injection (2%-13%)
Lopressor ampules, tablets (10%)
Lozol tablets (5% or more)
Marplan tablets (among most common)
Mesnex injection (33%)

NebuPent for inhalation solution (53%-72%)
Neupogen for injection (11%)
Nipent for injection (29%)
Normodyne injection, tablets (2%-10%)
Norpace capsules (3%-9%)
Parlodel capsules, SnapTabs (up to 7%)
Procardia XL extended release tablets (5.9%)
Procrit for injection (9%-13%)
Proleukin for injection (53%)
Prozac pulvules & liquid, oral solution (4.2%)
Roferon-A injection (89%-95%)
Sectral capsules (11%)
Seldane tablets (2.9%-4.5%)
Supprelin injection (up to 10%)
Tambocor tablets (7.7%)
Tegison capsules (50%-75%)
Tenex tablets (3%-12%)
Tenoretic tablets (0.6%-26%)
Tenormin tablets and I.V. injection (0.6%-26%)
Toprol XL tablets (about 10%)
Trandate injection (up to 10%)
Valrelease capsules (among most common)
Wellbutrin tablets (5%)
Xanax tablets (48.6%)
Zoloft tablets (10.6%)

---

amounts of trace minerals. He particularly recommends the following nutritional supplements for CFS patients: beta carotene (100,000 IU daily), vitamin C (3,000 mg daily), pantothenic acid (150 mg daily, but not at bedtime), zinc (15 mg a day), adrenal extract (1-2 tablets three times a day), and thymus gland extract (1-2 tablets three times a day).

The B vitamins act as a team to help speed up chemical reactions and support overall energy metabolism. Since they are essential for red blood cell formation, B complex deficiency produces anemia (reduced red blood cells), the main symptom of which is fatigue. Fatigue and depression have both been linked to B-vitamin deficiency. A deficiency of any of the B vitamins also interferes with the immune system's ability to fight disease. Additionally, a New Zealand study found that injection of vitamin B12 helped normalize imbalances in red blood cells in CFS patients.[14] Other research has demonstrated that B12 supplementation appears to improve CFS symptoms.[15]

Magnesium deficiency may also be a problem for CFS patients. According to a recent study, in which 20 people with CFS were compared with 20 healthy volunteers, the CFS patients' blood levels of magnesium were lower. In another study, 32 patients with CFS were given intramuscular injections of magnesium; 80% of those receiving the magnesium had reduced symptoms and improved energy, while less than 20% of those on placebo injections reported improvement.[16]

Potassium supports the adrenal glands, which is important for CFS sufferers as these glands are often severely impaired from a protracted period of functioning in a continual state of stress response. Fatigue and muscular weakness are the most common symptoms of potassium deficiency.[17] A review of studies involving a total of nearly 3,000 patients found that 75%-91% of those treated with potassium and magnesium aspartate (1 g of each salt daily) experienced "pronounced relief of fatigue," usually after 4-5 days.[18]

Germanium enhances the availability of oxygen to cells. Between 20% and 50% of CFS patients given germanium experienced substantial to marked relief of their symptoms.[19] Germanium may accomplish this by stimulating the production of interferons (proteins released by white blood cells), which block the spread of viruses and stimulate other immune "workers."[20]

Essential fatty acids (EFAs) are vitamin-like compounds that cannot be made in the body but must be ingested through the foods you eat. Without EFAs, your organs cannot manufacture prostaglandins, substances that are key regulators of immune, digestive, cardiovascular, and reproductive functions. Research suggests a link between CFS and low levels of essential fatty acids.[21] A study of 63 patients with post-viral fatigue syndrome who also had low EFA levels found that three months of supplementation with evening primrose oil and fish oil resulted in normal EFA levels and highly significant improvement in all symptoms, including fatigue, aches and pains, and depression.[22] Evening primrose oil contains GLA (gamma-linolenic acid), a particularly powerful EFA. For CFS patients, Dr. Murray suggests flaxseed oil, one tablespoon per day.[23]

NADH (nicotinamide adenine dinucleotide) is a coenzyme found naturally in a variety of foods and plays a central role in the process by which cells convert food into energy. Recent studies show a role for NADH supplementation in raising energy levels in those with chronic fatigue.[24] Coenzyme Q10 levels are often low in CFS patients and supplementing with coQ10 seems to improve the fatigue levels in these patients.

Supplemental Infusions and Injections

In treating CFS, Dr. Susser also uses infusions of intravenous minerals and vitamins, especially vitamin C, as well as antibiotics, antifungals, antiparasitics, and sometimes even pharmaceutical antivirals (which he says are not generally effective). He states that injections of gamma globulin, the fraction of the blood containing antibodies, and of Kutapressin, a liver extract that is an effective immune system booster, are becoming standard treatment for CFS. Using gamma globulin and Kutapressin together has marked benefit in CFS patients, according to Dr. Susser. Given intravenously, gamma globulin is very expensive and inaccessible to most people, Dr. Susser notes, but given intramuscularly, its cost is moderate. According to Dr. Susser, in most cases, treatment should be weekly for several months.

Herbal Treatment

Matt van Benschoten, O.M.D., M.A., C.A., of Reseda, California, uses herbal medicine to treat the viral infec-

tions and immune suppression found in CFS patients. Prescriptions are individualized for each patient. He primarily uses antiviral herbs combined with herbs that stimulate the immune system. "The initial therapy has to be focused on antiviral measures," he says. "Once that's accomplished and the virus is fairly well eliminated, you can begin to address some of the secondary factors that cause the weakness in the immune system, such as stress-induced weakness, problems in the intestinal tract, heavy metal poisoning (such as dental mercury), and low-level pesticide poisoning."

Using herbal medicines as the primary therapeutic modality, Dr. van Benschoten sees a response in 85% to 90% of his patients. "The time necessary to completely resolve the situation can vary from as short as four to six weeks to as long as 12 to 18 months," says Dr. van Benschoten, "depending upon the duration of the illness and other accompanying health problems."

Dr. Murray recommends herbal regimens for both the acute infectious phase of CFS and the convalescent phase of the syndrome. During the acute phase, he advises using echinacea, goldenseal, and licorice in the following dosages, taken three times a day: as dried root (or tea), 1-2 g; as freeze-dried root, 500-1,000 mg; as tincture (1:5), 4-6 ml (one to 1½ teaspoons); as fluid extract (1:10), 0.5-2.0 ml (¼ to ½ teaspoon); as powdered solid extract (4:1), 250-500 mg. Dr. Murray warns that if licorice is to be used for a long time, it is necessary to increase the intake of potassium-rich foods. During the acute phase of CFS, he also recommends *Phytolacca decandra* or *Phytolacca americana* (dried root, 100-400 mg three times daily) and *Baptisia tinctoria* (dried root, 0.5-1.0 g three times daily).

For the convalescent or chronic phase of CFS, Joseph Pizzorno, N.D., President Emeritus of Bastyr University, in Kenmore, Washington, recommends: goldenseal (in dosages as above); astragalus (dried root), 5-15 g three times daily; licorice (in dosages as above); and Siberian ginseng, as dried root or as tea, 2-4 g three times daily, as fluid extract (1:1), 2-4 ml (½ to one teaspoon) three times daily, or as solid extract (20:1), 100-200 mg three times daily.

In the recovery phase of CFS, Dr. Pizzorno recommends: *Panax ginseng,* as dried root, 1.5-2.0 g three times daily, or as extracts, equivalent to 25-50 mg ginsenosides daily; and Siberian ginseng (dried root), in dosages as above.

Acupuncture and Traditional Chinese Medicine

William M. Cargile B.S., D.C., F.I.A.C.A., former Chairman of Research for the American Academy of Oriental Medicine, has treated CFS patients using acupuncture

HERBS FOR CHRONIC FATIGUE

Immune-Building—aloe vera, astragalus, echinacea, ginger, larch tree extract, maitake mushroom, nettle, noni, *Panax ginseng*

Adrenal Support—ginseng, licorice, wild yam

Antimicrobial—garlic, goldenseal, grapefruit seed extract, licorice, myrrh, olive leaf extract, St. John's wort, yarrow

Fatigue—oatstraw, *Panax ginseng*, Siberian ginseng, suma

Brain Function—ginkgo, *Panax ginseng*, periwinkle

Sleep Disorders—chamomile, hops, kava-kava, passionflower, St. John's wort, skullcap, valerian

Joint and Muscle Pain—cayenne, chamomile, nettle, valerian

Allergies—chamomile, milk thistle

Digestive Disorders—astragalus, cayenne, chamomile, dandelion, ginger, goldenseal, licorice

Anxiety—chamomile, hops, kava-kava, passionflower, valerian

Depression—oatstraw, St. John's wort

alone, concentrating specifically on building the immune system. He says, "If you have an energy depression, it has to do with the immune system, because the immune system is fighting a disease." Dr. Cargile notes that the immune system uses 60% of the body's energy storage compound called ATP (adenosine triphosphate) to manufacture antibodies. As he explains, "You don't have enough energy because your immune system has shifted the use of ATP for the production of antibodies, so there is none left, and that is why you feel so bad."

Dr. Cargile treats CFS using the acupuncture points that relate to autoimmunity and all the meridians (energy channels) in the body. He also strongly advises patients to undergo allergy testing before acupuncture treatment so they can rid their diets of harmful allergens.

Cathie, 54, was diagnosed with idiopathic chronic fatigue, meaning her condition did not have a known cause such as thyroid or endocrine abnormalities. Dr. Cargile states, "She had a 13-year history, with no relief, and a continuous worsening of the condition. She literally did not have the motivation to walk to the kitchen more than once a day." Dr. Cargile used acupuncture to stimulate both her immune system and the production of ATP in her body. After five treatments, Cathie, who

previously had spent up to 20 hours a day in bed, was walking three miles a day, with her energy level restored.

Maoshing Ni, D.O.M., Ph.D., L.Ac., of Marina del Rey, California, also reports successful treatment of CFS. "The people who come to see me have been bounced from one internist to another," he says. "They've been through the mill, rejected by the Western medical establishment." The key to CFS, says Dr. Ni, is improving immunity. "People with CFS have a compromised immune system, which is weak and at the same time hyperactive. My objective is to strengthen and simultaneously desensitize, normalize, and regulate the immune system."

Over a three-month period, Dr. Ni uses a combination of acupuncture, Chinese herbs, and lifestyle changes, including diet, exercise, rest, and meditation. "Herbs are used to support immune function and they are easily assimilated and adapted by the body," he explains. "And I implement a low-stress diet. Up to 40% of the body's energy goes to digestion, so we want to conserve it." Patients reportedly experience a 65% to 80% relief of symptoms after the treatment period and are able to return to a normal life. After a three-month follow-up treatment, Dr. Ni reports that 90% to 95% of his patients have recovered from CFS. According to Dr. Ni, "Acupuncture reprograms the body and the herbs support that reprogramming."

 See Acupuncture, Ayurvedic Medicine, Detoxification Therapy, Diet, Herbal Medicine, Hyperthermia, Nutritional Medicine, Traditional Chinese Medicine.

Ayurvedic Medicine

Using the principles of Ayurvedic medicine, Virender Sodhi, M.D. (Ayurveda), N.D., Director of the Ayurvedic & Naturopathic Medical Clinic, in Bellevue, Washington, treats CFS by improving digestion and eliminating toxins and allergies. Dr. Sodhi puts patients on diet modification and cleansing programs to get rid of toxins and also works on psychosomatic elements to improve sleep patterns. Dr. Sodhi states, "If patients don't sleep well, growth hormones don't get triggered and the body cannot be repaired." Some of the herbs used in Dr. Sodhi's treatment include *ashwagandha, amla, bala, triphala*, and *lomatium*, which are combined according to each patient's particular needs. Acidophilus is also part of the program. According to Dr. Sodhi, *vata* body types are more susceptible to CFS.

A 45-year-old patient of Dr. Sodhi's had been progressively experiencing fatigue for five years, to the point where she could not work at all. After being tested by hospitals and doctors, she was told nothing could be done for her and she was put on antidepressants. The patient refused the medication and came to Dr. Sodhi. He placed her on a diet especially prepared for her specific medical history and body type. The diet consisted of vegetables, fruits, and fish, with no meat or dairy products. "Within three months of starting treatment, she was working and functioning normally," says Dr. Sodhi.

Heat Therapy

Bruce Milliman, N.D., of Seattle, Washington, reports success using hyperthermia as the central element in a treatment program for CFS. Dr. Milliman's treatment involves artificially inducing fever in order to augment the body's ability to fight viral infections. Patients must commit to a three-week course of treatment during which they stay home, get total bed rest, and undergo the fever treatment three times daily. To induce hyperthermia, the patient soaks in a bath (as hot as is tolerable) for a full five minutes, while drinking a 12-ounce glass of tepid water mixed with 2,000 mg of vitamin C.

Emerging from the bath, the patient quickly dries off and gets into a bed prepared with flannel sheets and wool blankets, placing a hot water bottle under the breast (women) or over the liver (men), and remaining under the blankets for 20 minutes. This procedure stimulates a natural fever response and the body will sweat profusely in its attempt to return to a normal temperature.

According to Dr. Milliman, fever is one of the immune system's natural adaptive mechanisms and "turning up the thermostat" enhances immune response. He reports a 70% to 75% success rate with his patients who follow this protocol for the full three weeks. Dr. Milliman reports that most failures in fever therapy occur in individuals unwilling or unable to address simultaneous disorders such as yeast infections, dental amalgam reaction (to mercury), and hypothyroidism.

CAUTION This treatment is intended for extreme cases of CFS in which the patient is virtually incapacitated. This protocol may be contraindicated for certain conditions, such as high blood pressure, diabetes, or endocrine problems. The program must be carried out under the guidance of a qualified physician.

Recommendations

- Diet is crucial to building the immune system and conquering CFS. A healthy diet avoids "empty" foods low in nutrients and high in sugar and fat. Instead, it concentrates on high-nutrient, high-protein, complex carbohydrate foods—vegetables, grains, beans, fish, and poultry (care should be taken to avoid mercury toxins in fish and antibiotics in poultry).

TRANSFER FACTOR FOR CHRONIC FATIGUE

The first task of our immune system is to recognize what is us and what is not us—what should be in our bodies and what should not—and then to destroy or otherwise neutralize anything harmful. The most well-known immune response is called the humoral response. It involves the production of antibodies, the immune cells that identify antigens or foreign substances in our bodies. We get sick when our immune systems do not quickly recognize microbial antigens and the microbes are allowed to multiply. Researchers have suggested that Transfer Factors (TFs) evolved as a way of compensating for the immune system's slow humoral response to foreign substances. Transfer Factors are tiny protein molecules. They are much smaller than antibodies and serve as messengers for the immune system's other major type of response, called the cell-mediated response, which involves other white blood cells (especially T lymphocytes).

A researcher named H.S. Lawrence, using white blood cell extracts, proved in 1949 that an immune response can be transferred via Transfer Factor from a host who tests positive for exposure to a specific antigen to a recipient who tests negative. The TFs can "educate" or modulate a recipient's immune system, teaching it to recognize these specific antigens and communicating the knowledge that they are present. A placebo-controlled pilot study used TFs with 20 chronic fatigue patients—improvement was observed in 12 patients within 3-6 weeks, with an associated increase in the levels of antibodies to Epstein-Barr virus and human herpes virus-6.[26]

TFs can be procured from either leukocytes filtered from the blood or from milk colostrum, the breast milk substance that mothers produce just after giving birth. TFs from colostrum taken as a supplement provide resistance to infection and disease.

- Eliminate all allergenic foods and, if one is highly allergic, rotate nonallergenic foods.

- Dr. Michael Murray advises CFS patients to take a good basic multivitamin/mineral supplement with adequate amounts of trace minerals. He particularly recommends the following nutritional supplements: beta carotene (100,000 IU daily), vitamin C (3,000 mg daily), pantothenic acid (150 mg daily, but not at bedtime), zinc (15 mg a day), adrenal extract (1-2 tablets three times a day), and thymus gland extract (1–2 tablets three times a day).

- Herbs can be useful for treating the viral infections and immune suppression found in CFS. Immune-building herbs include aloe vera, astragalus, echinacea, *Panax ginseng,* larch tree extract, maitake mushroom, noni, and nettle. Antimicrobial herbs include grapefruit seed extract, garlic, lomatium, goldenseal, licorice, myrrh, yarrow, olive leaf extract, and St. John's wort. For fatigue, try *Panax ginseng,* Siberian ginseng, suma, and oatstraw.

- Acupuncture can help to strengthen and simultaneously desensitize, normalize, and regulate the immune system.

- Ayurvedic medicine treats CFS by improving digestion and eliminating toxins and allergies.

- Heat therapy involves artificially inducing fever in order to augment the body's ability to fight viral infections.

Self–Care

The following therapies can be undertaken at home under appropriate professional supervision.

Fasting / Flower Essences

HYDROTHERAPY: • Cold friction rubs (apply two to seven times weekly) • Alternating hot and cold applications.

JUICE THERAPY: Wheatgrass juice

Professional Care

The following therapies should only be provided by a qualified health professional:

Applied Kinesiology / Chelation Therapy / Chiropractic / Detoxification Therapy/ Environmental Medicine / Enzyme Therapy / Magnetic Field Therapy / Nambudripad's Allergy Elimination Technique (NAET)

OXYGEN THERAPY: • Hydrogen peroxide therapy • If the chronic fatigue syndrome is based on Epstein-Barr infection, ozone is reputed to be helpful (applied in autohemotherapy).

BODYWORK: Lymphatic massage, Feldenkrais Method, Therapeutic Touch

TRADITIONAL CHINESE MEDICINE: Acupuncture, moxibustion, herbs, and color therapy

Where to Find Help

The following organizations are good resources for obtaining further information on chronic fatigue syndrome.

CFIDS Association, Inc.
P.O. Box 220398
Charlotte, North Carolina 28222-0398
(800) 442-3437 or (704) 365-2343
Website: www.cfids.org

The largest nonprofit organization dedicated to funding research and disseminating information on chronic fatigue and immune dysfunction syndrome. Publishes a journal, CFIDS Chronicle, *provides a nationwide referral list of physicians and CFIDS associations, and maintains a computer bulletin board with daily updates on CFIDS research.*

CFIDS Buyer's Club
2040 Alameda Padre Serra #101
Santa Barbara, California 93103
(800) 366-6056

Publishes a quarterly newsletter and offers nutritional supplements at substantial discounts. Call for a catalog listing of all products and prices.

American Association of Oriental Medicine
433 Front Street
Catasauqua, Pennsylvania 18032
(888) 500-7999
Website: www.aaom.org

The AAOM is a national professional trade organization of acupuncturists who meet acceptable standards of competency and can provide you with the names and locations of local members.

American Association of Naturopathic Physicians
8201 Greensboro Drive, Suite 300
McLean, Virginia 22101
(703) 610-9037
Website: www.naturopathic.org

Provides a directory of naturopathic physicians and offers referrals to a nationwide network of accredited or licensed practitioners. Also publishes a quarterly newsletter, for both professionals and the general public, and offers a series of brochures and pamphlets on a variety of subjects.

Recommended Reading

Alternative Medicine Guide to Chronic Fatigue, Fibromyalgia, and Environmental Illness. Burton Goldberg and the Editors of *Alternative Medicine Digest.* Tiburon, CA: Future Medicine Publishing, 1998.

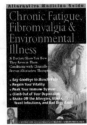

Alternative Treatments for Fibromyalgia and Chronic Fatigue Syndrome. Mari Skelly and Andrea Helm. Alameda, CA: Hunter House, 1999.

Chronic Fatigue Syndrome. Jesse A. Stoff, M.D., and Charles R. Pellegrino, Ph.D. New York: Harper Perennial, 1992.

Chronic Fatigue Syndrome and the Yeast Connection. William Crook, M.D. Jackson, TN: Professional Books, 1992.

Dr. Braly's Food Allergy and Nutrition Revolution. James Braly, M.D. New Canaan, CT: Keats Publishing, 1992.

From Fatigued to Fantastic! Jacob Teitelbaum. New York: Avery Penguin Putnam, 2001.

Recovering from Chronic Fatigue Syndrome. William Collinge, M.P.H., Ph.D. New York: The Body Press/Perigree Books, 1993.

Solving the Puzzle of Chronic Fatigue Syndrome. Michael Rosenbaum, M.D., and Murray Susser, M.D. Tacoma, WA: Life Sciences Press, 1992.

CHRONIC PAIN

Chronic pain has become the most common health disorder in the United States, affecting to some degree 86 million Americans and costing nearly $90 billion a year in medical bills and lost wages.[1] Today, many alternative therapies are available that have proven effective at both reducing chronic pain symptoms and alleviating their causes. Numerous self-help methods can also be utilized, thus reducing the cost of treating chronic pain.

ACCORDING TO David Bresler, Ph.D, L.Ac., former Director of the Pain Control Unit at the School of Medicine, University of California at Los Angeles, pain is divided into chronic and acute pain. "Acute pain refers to any pain from an immediate trauma or condition and usually acts as a warning system for the body to tell a person something is wrong and needs attention," Dr. Bresler explains. "Chronic pain refers to any continual pain that has lasted longer than six months. While acute pain is mostly useful, even vital, in a protective way, chronic pain does not seem to offer any clear purpose. It is very often, and in most senses of the word, useless, having long since served its purpose as a warning."

Pain that lingers long after an injured area has healed is a common example of chronic pain, as well as recurring migraines and headaches, arthritis, recurring back pain, and certain neurological disorders. This type of useless, chronic pain constitutes a major part of the pain problem today, involving enormous costs in terms of medication and therapy, as well as causing a vast degree of misery and disability.

See Allergies, Arthritis, Back Pain, Headaches, Stress.

The Pain Experience

Pain is caused by the stimulation of special sensory nerve endings that respond to bodily irritation, pressure, heat, cold, injury, stress, and certain diseases. However, each person perceives pain differently and that perception can

> *While acute pain is mostly useful, even vital, in a protective way, chronic pain does not seem to offer any clear purpose. It is very often, and in most senses of the word, useless.*
>
> —DAVID BRESLER, PH.D, L.AC.

be influenced by any number of factors, including emotional and mental attitudes, previous experiences, and other health conditions. Social, cultural, and ethnic differences also can affect how one perceives and reacts to pain, as well as early learning and developmental predispositions.[2]

"What we think about pain, how afraid or anxious we are about it, what we believe it represents in health terms, all influence how much pain we report," says Leon Chaitow, N.D., D.O., of London, England. "Aches and pains following exercise can usually be laughed off because we know that they will vanish in a day or so, while the same discomfort caused by a wasting disease or an arthritic condition might be complained of as unbearable."

Dr. Bresler emphasizes this fact, stating that there is not necessarily a direct relationship between the actual sensation of pain and the way people perceive it.[3] "It is important to recognize the complex subjective experience of pain, which involves physical, perceptual, cognitive, emotional, and spiritual factors," says Dr. Bresler. "Pain is an intensely personal experience, and even if no physical explanation for it can be found, all pain is real."

Many people who suffer from chronic pain also feel helpless concerning their condition, an attitude that is very often reinforced by medical doctors who say, "You'll just have to learn to live with it—nothing more can be done." Unfortunately, the ensuing feelings of depression and hopelessness tend to heighten the experience of pain by causing increased heart rate, blood pressure, respiration, sweating, and muscle tension.[4] This can have an ever-increasing spiral effect on people suffering from musculoskeletal pain, as the increased muscle tension augments the sensation of pain, which further increases the anxiety, producing even greater tension and pain.

 Any time pharmacological remedies are used to treat chronic pain, there is a risk of developing a dependency. Over time, this can perpetuate the pain symptoms in order to facilitate and rationalize one's now addictive need for the pain-suppressing drugs.

Coping with Chronic Pain

According to Dr. Chaitow, experts have traditionally been divided on the best approach to understanding and treating chronic pain. Some feel it is best dealt with at the physical, nervous system level, while others tend to emphasize the importance of its emotional and psychological characteristics. "The truth is that both physical and psychological elements are usually intimately combined in most cases of chronic pain, and both require attention when dealing with long-term pain," says Dr. Chaitow. "Central to whatever is done for a person in pain is the need for that person to take some degree of control of the situation, to feel empowered to influence the processes at work, and to not be simply the helpless recipient of other people's efforts." When a person suffering pain understands the causes, nature, mechanisms, and role of that pain, a vital step has been taken in the successful handling of the problem.

Self-help methods therefore become very important in this process, although they should not simply be picked at random. They need to be part of a total therapeutic approach, decided upon mutually by patient and doctor, and designed to meet the needs of the individual's specific problem. Dr. Bresler adds that one of the most important aspects in eliciting a subjective experience such as chronic pain from a patient is the rapport established between patient and doctor.

Change can also be fundamental in the treatment of chronic pain. Often a review of the patient's lifestyle will show certain patterns that contribute to the experience of pain. Sometimes a person can even perpetuate pain in order to receive certain benefits associated with it. For example, a person in pain often attracts positive, caring attention from others that was missing in life before. Or, in the case of Workmen's Compensation benefits, the sufferer may receive financial rewards and, if the person does not care for their job, the continuation of pain can keep them out of an unpleasant work situation. The only way to alleviate these types of chronic pain conditions is to reduce the need that the pain seems able to fill. This kind of change can often only be accomplished through professional counseling.

> *Central to whatever is done for a person in pain is the need for that person to take some degree of control, to feel empowered to influence the processes at work, and to not be simply the helpless recipient of other people's efforts.*
>
> —LEON CHAITOW, N.D., D.O.

In addition, any time pharmacological remedies are used to treat chronic pain, which is the standard tactic of conventional medicine, there is a risk of developing a dependency. This can perpetuate the pain symptoms in order to facilitate and rationalize one's now addictive need for the pain-suppressing drugs. Fortunately, effective nondrug methods of pain relief are available.

Alternative Treatments for Chronic Pain

The body has made a provision for pain to be eased by natural means, such as the production of endorphins, which can produce euphoric and painkilling effects when released. Rather than just suppressing the symptoms of pain, as drug therapy does, doctors and pain therapists using alternative modalities try to utilize and activate these natural healing properties of the body.

Detoxifying the body is an important component in promoting the health of the immune system and addressing other factors that may be contributing to chronic pain. As our environment and food are increasingly saturated with chemicals, the body's mechanisms for elimination of toxins cannot keep up with the chemical deluge. Given that many people with chronic pain have chemical allergies as well, it is advisable to take measures to remove these toxins from the body.

Also, recognizing the complexities of chronic pain, with its physical and psychological components, alternative health practitioners employ a wide variety of treatment methods tailored specifically to the individual. These can include diet and nutrition, hypnotherapy, guided imagery, biofeedback, acupuncture, chiropractic, bodywork, energy medicine, magnetic field therapy, and hydrotherapy. This multidisciplinary approach also includes educating patients about the nature of pain and showing them that they can control their pain.

Diet and Nutrition

According to James Braly, M.D., of Hollywood, Florida, diet and nutrition can both play important roles in the treatment of chronic pain. "I have seen patients who have tried just about everything to relieve their pain, only to finally find relief when they made changes in their diet and added supplements with proven pain-relieving properties," he says. Dr. Braly points out that inflammation, one of the principal mechanisms related to chronic pain, is often caused by an allergic reaction. "Often the reactions are due to food allergies," Dr. Braly notes. "If chronic pain symptoms seem to have no other discernible cause, testing for food allergies is advisable."

Once the allergic foods have been determined, Dr. Braly recommends that they be completely eliminated from the diet for a minimum of three months. After that, they can be reintroduced as part of a rotation diet, with no one food being eaten more than once in any four-day period. Dr. Braly also recommends limiting foods high in saturated fats, including red meats, dairy products, warm-water shellfish, and partially hydrogenated oils, as well as avoiding alcohol and severely limiting caffeine. He suggests a diet high in fiber and nonallergenic complex carbohydrates. "Organic, free-range poultry, cold-water fish, and vegetable protein sources are also good," he says, "while margarine, shortenings, and other sources of partially hydrogenated oils should be omitted. Simple or refined sugars, including fruit juices, sodas, and pastries, are also culprits."

Along with diet, Dr. Braly suggests the following nutritional supplements be taken daily when in pain: vitamin C (a dosage at 90% of bowel tolerance); evening primrose oil and eicosapentaenoic acid (EPA, an omega-3 oil), both of which supply essential fatty acids to reduce inflammation and decrease pain; vitamin E; magnesium; and the amino acid DL-phenylalanine. "DL-phenylalanine is one of the more important nutritional supplements for relieving pain," Dr. Braly says, noting that it has proven effective in increasing blood levels of endorphins and reducing inflammation in about 80% of his patients suffering from chronic pain.

One of Dr. Braly's patients suffered from painful back spasms for years without being able to gain relief. He tested positive for food allergies. The allergenic foods were eliminated, along with alcohol, and he began to follow a rotation diet. "After starting the program, he became pain free for the first time in years," Dr. Braly relates. "He couldn't believe that such dramatic relief could occur without drugs or surgery. But after about 18 months, he strayed from the protocol. Soon thereafter, his back spasms returned. We retested him for allergies, got him back on track, and his pain once more disappeared."

 See Chiropractic, Detoxification Therapy, Diet, Hypnotherapy, Nutritional Medicine.

Hypnotherapy

Hypnotherapy has been approved by the American Medical Association as a clinical adjunct in the management of chronic pain and is currently taught in several medical schools. Although there are numerous ways to induce a hypnotic state, according to Gerald Sunnen, M.D., Associate Clinical Professor of Psychiatry at the New York University Bellevue Hospital Center, in New York City, they all begin by encouraging the patient to enter a deep state of relaxation. The patient may then be given simple suggestions to experience the sensation of pain in a different way, perhaps as a warm or tingly feeling. "This technique is known as symptom substitution and is used to show the patient that it is possible to control the pain," Dr. Sunnen explains. "This can result in a more positive, hopeful attitude toward one's condition."

When chronic pain is the result of an earlier accident or trauma, the hypnotherapist may also use regression to help the patient remember the incident. By re-experiencing the pain and suffering of the past event, the patient can confront and reevaluate the experience. This helps to alleviate anxiety and fear and will often significantly reduce the present experience of pain.

Hypnosis has been used to help alleviate back and joint pain, abdominal pain, pain from burns, and headache and migraine pain.[5] However, Dr. Sunnen notes that hypnosis should always be conducted by a qualified hypnotherapist in order to avoid any potential retraumatization or the triggering of a psychotic reaction.

Guided Imagery

The imagination can be a powerful tool for overcoming pain. In the past ten years, numerous techniques have been devised to harness this power. These techniques, collectively known as guided imagery, encourage more active participation of the patient, which can help the person feel more in control of the problem. Guided imagery can be particularly effective when other pain management approaches have failed.

One common exercise, used by Dr. Bresler, involves visualizing the pain in physical terms, such as a burning fire or a terrible monster gnawing on one's bones. "By mentally extinguishing the flames, or taming the monster, the patient will usually experience an immediate reduction in pain," Dr. Bresler says. "Another very powerful exercise involves the use of an imaginary inner doctor or advisor. First, the patient is taught how to deeply relax and asked to imagine being in some beautiful, restful location. Then, the patient is invited to visualize an advisor, who may appear in any form imaginable—it could be an animal, a religious figure, or an old woman in a cave. Through dialogue with this inner advisor, important information about the pain can emerge and creative solutions for its elimination explored."

Jon Kabat-Zinn, Ph.D., Professor of Medicine at the Stress Reduction Clinic, University of Massachusetts Medical Center, in Worcester, tells his patients to focus on their pain when it comes up and to meditate upon the sensations. "By watching the sensations come and go, very often you will find that they change and that the pain has a life of its own," he says. "When you learn how to work with the pain, to listen to it and to honor it, you discover that it's possible to experience your pain differently. And sometimes, this can result in the sensations actually going away."

 See Biofeedback Training and Neurotherapy, Guided Imagery, Mind/Body Medicine.

Biofeedback Training

Biofeedback training is a technique that uses electronic devices to help a patient learn to regulate various physiological functions, such as brain waves, body temperature, muscle tension, and pulse rate. Through trial and error, the lower centers of the brain learn how to alter these various bodily functions, then later the mind is able to cause the same changes on demand. With proper training, many types of pain can be controlled or eliminated.

George von Hilsheimer, Ph.D., of Maitland, Florida, Diplomate of the American Academy of Pain Management, regularly employs biofeedback when dealing with chronic pain patients. One of his patients was a 42-year-old woman who suffered panic attacks, headaches, and pain in her arm and chest due to an automobile accident three years earlier. "The panic attacks began six weeks after her accident," Dr. von Hilsheimer recounts, "after she was already enduring severe headaches along the left side and top of her head. And this was accompanied by pain down her left arm and hand and behind her left breast."

By the time the woman came to Dr. von Hilsheimer, she was in such a state of panic that she was barely able to leave her home and had to be driven to his office by her mother. Prior to her visit, the woman had seen an orthopedic surgeon and a chiropractor, but neither had been able to help her. Using biofeedback equipment, Dr. von Hilsheimer was able to determine that the nerves and muscles of the woman's left side were overactive,

THE PLACEBO EFFECT

A placebo is defined as a substance that normally has no physiological effect upon the body but, when given to a patient under the pretext of treatment, promotes a healing effect. This phenomenon adds evidence to the notion that a person's beliefs can strongly influence the healing processes of the body. Numerous studies have indicated that placebos provide relief for a variety of pain-related disorders, including arthritis, angina, digestive tract pain, and other chronic pain problems.[6]

In fact, placebos can be nearly as effective as prescription medications. In one study, 82% to 87% of chronic headache sufferers responded to analgesic drugs, whereas 60% responded to a placebo.[7] In another study, 72% of patients suffering from postoperative pain responded to morphine, while 40% responded equally as well to placebo injections.[8] Chronic back pain and cancer pain have responded to placebos as well as, if not better than, conventional pain medications.

One explanation for this phenomenon is that the administration of a placebo produces a reduction of chronic anxiety, which helps to decrease the perception of pain.[9] Placebos can play an important part in the medical intervention of pain and may even help to wean drug-dependent patients from their pain medications.

while being underactive on her right. "Her accident had violently rotated her to the right as her car careened left," explains Dr. von Hilsheimer. "As a consequence, her left-side muscles had been stretched and activated, and her right-side muscles had been compressed and turned off."

Dr. von Hilsheimer had the woman mentally relive her accident, then write about it and discuss her feelings regarding the trauma it had caused her. "She repeated this process until the emotional sting of the accident was relieved," Dr. von Hilsheimer says. "At that point, her panic attacks ended."

Dr. von Hilsheimer then employed biofeedback training to address the woman's pain. "I had her view a screen that vividly portrayed images of her brain-wave activity and she quickly learned how she could speed up the waves," he says. "Then I had her watch the electrical signals from her muscles on a monitor. These signals showed how her posture and defensive movements worsened the imbalance between her muscles to cause pain." Dr. von Hilsheimer taught her exercises and stretches to relieve the pain, and she learned to enhance her performance of them by again watching the monitor. Soon she was able to consciously make her muscles produce more or less electricity, to the point where, after three sessions, she could change the signal simply by deciding to. "As a result," Dr. von Hilsheimer says, "without the use of any invasive procedures or medicines, the woman now enjoys a complete restoration of easy movement and freedom from fear and pain, which she maintains by following a home program of exercise, stretching, and biofeedback."

Acupuncture

Acupuncture has been found to be highly effective in the treatment of chronic pain. "Although the mechanism by which it works is not yet fully understood, it is known to have two pain-relieving functions," Dr. Bresler says. Acupuncture stimulates the release of endorphins and enkephalins (the body's own natural painkillers). At the same time, it can block pain messages from getting through to the brain. The acupuncture needles (or acupressure massage techniques) trigger nerve reactions that travel along thicker and faster nerve channels than the pain sensations do, effectively "shutting the gate" to the brain before the pain messages can even get there.

To date, hundreds of studies worldwide have substantiated acupuncture's effectiveness in treating and managing chronic pain.[10] In 1997, the National Institutes of Health (NIH) released an efficacy statement endorsing acupuncture for a variety of conditions, including postoperative pain, dental pain following surgery, nausea associated with chemotherapy, tennis elbow, and carpal tunnel syndrome.

According to Dr. Bresler, acupuncture was found to be of tremendous benefit, particularly in the treatment of musculoskeletal pain and spasms, arthritis, bursitis, and other similar conditions. Patients treated with acupuncture after oral surgery had less intense pain than those who received a placebo treatment.[11] In one study of over 20,000 patients at the U.C.L.A. Medical Center, acupuncture reduced both the frequency and severity of muscle tension headaches and migraines.[12] Another study, involving 204 patients suffering from chronic painful conditions, resulted in 74% experiencing significant pain relief for over three months after acupuncture treatment.[13] Acupuncture is also helpful in relieving anxiety and depression associated with chronic pain, as well as in helping people reduce their dependence on narcotics and other addictive drugs (and their attendant side effects).[14]

Chiropractic

Chiropractic has been found to be one of the safest and most effective methods in dealing with a wide variety of pain disorders. According to Tim Leasenby, D.C., of Aurora, Illinois, this is because chiropractic adjustments simultaneously affect several pain-causing mechanisms:

- Nerve pressure (pinched nerves)
- Joint compression
- Muscle stretching and/or spasm and trigger points
- Ligament injuries and tissue changes in elasticity and hypersensitivity
- Reflex pain to and from internal organs

"My approach to any person's pain includes all of these as possible components of the pain's origin," says Dr. Leasenby. "Additionally, I consider mental/emotional, metabolic, occupational, and environmental causes." All of the above causes of pain result from the fundamental chiropractic lesion, the subluxation (misalignment in the spine). The subluxation results in nerve pressure and joint derangement, causing muscles to tighten in response to the irritation. The muscle spasm then becomes an additional source of pain. Nerve pressure can result in a distortion of nerve impulses to any internal organ and can subsequently bring about pain and other symptoms related to that organ.

In addition, at some point in life, everyone experiences physical trauma, another common origin for chronic pain. This can be from a single event, like a fall or an automobile accident, or from daily occurrences, like sitting at a computer or holding a phone to your ear with your shoulder. The repetitive wear and tear on the ligaments and joints eventually results in spinal subluxations. This can be greatly alleviated by early and persistent mobilization of the injured joints—another reason chiropractic can be helpful in pain cases.

"When I first see patients with chronic pain, I generally begin by obtaining a history of the pain, a work and family history, a review of all body symptoms, and a chiropractic examination for subluxations and nerve interference," explains Dr. Leasenby. "I most often begin treatment with chiropractic adjustments. A person's complaints will usually begin improving within the first few treatments. Therapy may also include deep muscle massage, traction, exercises, and other treatments that may help the nerves, muscles, and ligaments. Simultaneously, I consider any possibility of pain being referred from an internal illness (for example, blood clots causing leg pain, prostate or kidney problems referring pain to the lower back). If I suspect such a problem, I will run further tests and, when necessary, send the patient to a medical specialist."

Chiropractors may also look at other possible causes of pain, such as the patient's work, hobbies and habits, and relationships with family and friends—these can be a source of mental and physical stressors that feed a chronic pain complex. Also, the person may have nutritional deficiencies, biochemical imbalances, or toxins that contribute to pain. Past or present medications may produce pain as a side effect or from adverse reactions.

One of Dr. Leasenby's patients was a woman in her late thirties with widespread body aches, bouts of extreme fatigue, difficulty concentrating, severe head pain, depression, and uncontrollable emotional swings. She had a condition called environmental illness (see Quick Definition) or multiple chemical sensitivity. She had been suffering with this condition for nine years. "Simply put, it seems like people with this condition are allergic to almost everything—common household items like cleaners, soaps, perfumes, deodorants, and toothpaste," says Dr. Leasenby. She adhered to a very strict diet of organically grown food, because she reacted to the chemicals sprayed on conventionally grown fruits and vegetables and fed to animals. When her husband or child would come in the house, they stopped to clean up with nonallergenic soap and change into clothing made of nondyed or naturally dyed cotton. Her house had no rugs because they trapped molds and other allergens and the walls were lined in foil because of the fumes given off by drywall and paneling. "Even the slightest deviation from this lifestyle would trigger an attack that would last for days," says Dr. Leasenby.

> **QD** **Environmental illness** is a multiple-symptom, debilitating, chronic disorder involving prolonged, heightened, and often incapacitating allergies or sensitivities to numerous common substances found in one's environment. Symptoms may include headaches, fatigue, muscle pain and/or weakness, coughing or wheezing, asthma, weight loss, infections, emotional fluctuations, depression, and irritability. Patients become allergic to and functionally incompatible with many products and substances found in the modern world, such as car exhaust, synthetic carpets, plywood and other building materials, cleaning agents, office machines, and plastics, among others.

When Dr. Leasenby began treating her, she was being helped by a nutritionist who specialized in this sort of disorder. "I used special chiropractic techniques that help alleviate systemic mold, fungal, and yeast infections, and that have a neutralizing effect on allergies. I also used homeopathic, nutritional, and herbal remedies to assist her body in detoxifying and rebuilding normal function." During the 24 months of treatment, her pain subsided and she was gradually able to leave her protective abode for increasingly longer periods—to go to church, see movies, visit friends, go shopping, and even eat at a restaurant occasionally.

NEURAL THERAPY RELIEVES PAIN

Neural therapy, first developed in Germany in 1925 by the physicians Ferdinand and Walter Huneke, demonstrates how the injection of a local anesthetic can favorably influence health problems. Lidocaine or procaine is injected in the body to remove interferences in the body's electrical network and thus relieve chronic pain, reverse injury, and clear energy blockages. The anesthetics are injected into acupuncture points, scars, glands, the nerve bundles in the autonomic nervous system and other tissues. By clearing the local site of interference, neural therapy helps to regulate energy throughout the body. The task of the neural therapist is to locate the source of the abnormal activity and eliminate the disturbance. Once the cells regain their normal electrical activity, they can eliminate toxic wastes that have built up as a result of this disturbance and begin to function normally again.

German research claims that 40% of all illness and chronic pain may be due to interference fields in the body. Neural therapy has become one of the most widely used treatments for chronic pain in Germany.[15] One study, compiled in Germany in the 1970s, collected statistics from 25 doctors who used neural therapy with procaine to treat 639 cases of trigeminal neuralgia. The results were as follows: 34% cured, 37% showed substantial improvement, 14% had some improvement, and 15% showed no improvement. In 267 (42%) of these cases, an interference field was held to be either the cause or a mitigating factor of the pain.[16]

Bodywork

According to Thomas Hudak, L.M.T., of Southbury, Connecticut, massage is one of the most important adjunct therapies for the treatment of chronic pain. Those with pain often experience prolonged muscle tension, which interferes with the elimination of chemical wastes in the muscles and surrounding tissue. Poor circulation in muscle tissues can cause nerve and muscle pain, which can spread to other areas of the body. Pains that seem to emanate from the joints or other areas may actually be coming from "trigger points," focal areas where wastes have accumulated in the muscles.

Massage helps break up muscular waste deposits and stimulates circulation to troubled regions in the body. Deep pressure on trigger points stretches tissues and loosens shortened muscles to restore muscular balance and proper functioning. Most importantly, certain types of pain can be relieved by massage, as the rhythmic motions sedate the nervous system and promote voluntary muscle relaxation. Craniosacral therapy manipulates the bones of the skull and the base of the spine and tailbone in order to treat a range of conditions, from headache and ear infection to stroke, spinal cord injury, and cerebral palsy, and can be helpful in cases of chronic pain.

A typical program of massage would be at least two to three times per week in the early treatment stages, then once a week for several months, with a maintenance schedule of twice a month. Remember that massage therapies should be designed to fit individual profiles.

Energy Medicine

One of the most commonly used energy medicine devices for chronic pain is the TENS (Transcutaneous Electrical Nerve Stimulator), a small device that produces various frequencies and voltages of mild electrical stimulation. By applying electrodes to the affected parts of the body, the TENS electrical current acts upon the nerves, causing nerve conduction to be blocked and pain to be relieved. TENS units are also believed to stimulate the production of endorphins. Patients are often taught how to self-administer this treatment. TENS has been used in the management of post-surgical pain, sports injuries, and other neuromuscular pain disorders. One study, involving 637 patients treated with TENS for chronic post-traumatic pain, showed that 74.2% experienced a reduction in pain, 57.2% needed less medication, and 58.8% had improved sleep patterns.[17]

The Electro-Acuscope™ is another energy device used to reduce pain. It uses a lower electrical current than the TENS unit and works by stimulating tissue repair instead of the nerves. The current is continuously adjusted to match the resistance given off by the damaged tissue in order to facilitate healing. The Electro-Acuscope, because of its prolonged effects on tissue repair, can be applied to a wide range of painful conditions, including arthritis, bursitis, sprains and strains, neuralgia, and bruises. It is also effective in treating acute and chronic pain caused by musculoskeletal disorders, including automobile accidents, lower back sprains, and sports injuries.[18]

The Light Beam Generator (LBG) is about the size of a small suitcase, with hand-held heads attached on cords. It uses extremely low current, cold gas light photons to transfer energy frequency patterns to cells in targeted areas of the lymphatic system, a vital aspect of the immune system. The LBG works energetically to rebalance the charge of the cells' electromagnetic field. The LBG is able to separate these cells and their accumulated fluids and protein wastes, resulting in the rapid dispersal of swelling and other blockages. It also stimulates blood circulation, reduces edema (swelling), and eliminates waste products stored in the tissues. Physicians who use the device have found it beneficial for a wide range of conditions, including pain (especially pain involving soft tissue and tissue congestion due to injury), sciatica, arthritis, bursitis, lupus, fibromyalgia, scarring, and burns.

Another energy medicine device, thermography, is a nontoxic, highly accurate, and inexpensive form of diagnostic imaging that has been used by progressive physicians in the U.S. and Europe since 1962. It's based on infrared heat emissions from targeted regions of the body. As cells go through their energy conversion processes, called metabolism, they emit heat. Pain clusters in the body tend to give off more infrared energy than normal tissues. Thermography is able to register varying heat emissions, display them on a computer monitor, and thereby provide a diagnostic window into the functional status of a given body area.

 See Acupuncture, Aromatherapy, Energy Medicine, Hydrotherapy, Magnetic Field Therapy, Neural Therapy.

Magnetic Field Therapy

According to William H. Philpott, M.D., of Choctaw, Oklahoma, co-author of *Magnet Therapy: An Alternative Medicine Definitive Guide,* magnetic field therapy has many applications for the relief of pain. "The negative magnetic field is ideal for relieving pain symptoms due to its ability to quickly normalize the metabolic functions that create the pain in the first place," Dr. Philpott says. He points out that the negative magnetic field does not act as a painkiller or analgesic, but as a "normalizer of disordered metabolic functions."

Swollen cells caused by toxins, particularly acids resulting from an injury, lead to the most pain. An acid pH and a deficiency of oxygen accompany all injuries and produce these swollen cells. Robert O. Becker, M.D., a researcher in magnetics and author of *The Body Electric,* demonstrated that when an injury occurs, the area of injury initially registers electromagnetic positive and sends a signal of alarm to the brain through the nervous system. A few hours after an injury, the body begins to concentrate a negative magnetic field at the injury site.[19] It is the negative magnetic field that begins the healing process—it floods the injured area with oxygen, stimulates the production of melatonin and growth hormone, and alkalinizes the body's pH. In this way, magnetic therapy can optimize the healing of injuries and reduce pain faster. In order to supplement the body's negative field of energy, a negative magnetic field can be used over any injury site. Studies are now begin-

A MULTI-PRONGED APPROACH TO CHRONIC PAIN

Marc Darrow, M.D., J.D., a physiatrist at Joint Rehabilitation & Sports Medical Center, in Los Angeles, California, treats chronic pain in a substantially different manner than much of the medical community. His first rule is to wean his patients off the drugs that other doctors have placed them on. "I learned early in my residency at the University of California at Los Angeles, that when most patients are off drugs (Neurontin, Prozac, Paxil, vicodin, percocet, and many others), the first thing they experience is a clearing of their consciousness and thinking processes and a start back to self-mastership." After drugs are stopped, the worst complaint they may have is that their pain is the same. "These pain drugs don't do much except to mask the pain and confuse the patient. They certainly do nothing to assist the healing process."

To initiate healing, Dr. Darrow starts his patients on a progressive exercise and rehabilitation program. "My patients joyfully experience the post-exercise soreness of a good workout, which they love, instead of the nagging 'poor me, why should I have this pain for no reason' syndrome. Exercise also stimulates the production of endorphins, reduces pain, and muscular tone returns." Many chronic pain patients have been frightened into inactivity by their doctors, according to Dr. Darrow. This only weakens and atrophies the musculoskeletal system and initiates a progressive road to more pain and depression. Dr. Darrow encourages his patients to exercise as much as they comfortably can.

Dr. Darrow also seeks to rejuvenate areas of the body causing the pain. This is done using prolotherapy to stimulate the growth of collagen in weakened ligaments, tendons, and joints. Prolotherapy (also known as reconstructive therapy) involves injecting small amounts of an irritating solution into areas of pain or dysfunction (strained ligaments or tendons where they join the bone) to produce a healing response. The irritant produces a small focused injury that deactivates the sensitized, painful nerve fibers in the area and causes inflammation; the body then dispatches fibroblasts to the area to produce new collagen to repair the damaged tissues

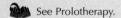 See Prolotherapy.

In addition, Dr. Darrow uses MedX exercise machines (unique, computerized back- and neck-strengthening machines that have been widely studied in the university setting) along with traditional exercise machines and free weights to strengthen the muscles, in conjunction with stretching and chiropractic biomechanics. A diet limiting dairy products, red meat, sugar, bread, and pasta often helps reduce the inflammation of many chronic pain patients. Patients are also prescribed anti-inflammatory supplements such as fish oil, acidophilus and *Bifidobacteria* (to assist digestion), digestive enzymes, and a rice-based anti-inflammatory protein powder.

ning to demonstrate the effectiveness of magnets for pain relief.[20]

One of Dr. Philpott's patients was a woman in her seventies suffering from a clot in her left groin that made climbing stairs painful because it impinged on blood flow to her left leg. Dr. Philpott had her sleep on a negative field magnetic pad with magnets also placed at the crown of her head. After one year of treatment, the woman was climbing stairs freely without pain and it was discovered upon further examination that the clot, which had been present for over 30 years, was healed despite the fact that it had never been treated directly.

Dean Bonlie, D.D.S., of Calgary, Alberta, Canada, a colleague of Dr. Philpott's, also employs magnetic field therapy to treat a variety of chronic pain conditions. One of his patients was a retired member of the Canadian Armed Forces who had been released from the service on medical grounds for being disabled due to low-back injuries. His condition was so severe that he had under-

gone a spinal fusion. He had also tried medications, heat treatments, chiropractic, and physiotherapy, all without long-term results. Dr. Bonlie applied a negative magnet directly on the injured section of the man's back for 25 minutes and he experienced substantial pain reduction. Moreover, upon standing up, he did not experience the flash of burning pain down his right leg that had previously been one of his symptoms. Dr. Bonlie suggested that he begin sleeping on a magnetic sleep pad and the man soon confirmed that, after 25 years, he was finally free of pain.

Hydrotherapy

Hydrotherapy, including compresses and various contrast (hot and cold) techniques, offers a simple and efficient way of treating a variety of factors that contribute to chronic pain. Hydrotherapy can also be used at home. "Cold applications are helpful in reducing the sensitivity of the nerve endings that signal pain sensations,"

HYPERTHERMIA FOR CHRONIC PAIN

Fever is one of the body's most powerful defenses against disease. Hyperthermia (heat therapy) artificially induces fever in patients who are unable to mount a natural fever response to infection, inflammation, or other health challenges, and may be useful for treating chronic pain. A recent form of hyperthermia employs far-infrared (FIR) energy to treat a variety of disease conditions and to speed detoxification and recovery from muscle sprains and other injuries. Far-infrared wavelengths occur just below ("infra") visible red light in the electromagnetic spectrum. At the molecular level, FIR exerts strong rotational and vibrational effects that are biologically beneficial.

Although the wavelengths of FIR are too long for the eyes to perceive, we can experience its energy as gentle, radiant heat, which can penetrate up to 1½ inches beneath the skin. Among FIR's healing benefits is its ability to stimulate inflammation, which is necessary for a period of time in order to heal injuries such as a pulled muscle. FIR also appears capable of enhancing white blood cell function, thereby increasing immune response and the elimination of foreign pathogens and cellular waste products. Additional benefits include the ability to stimulate the hypothalamus, which controls the production of neurochemicals involved in such biological processes as sleep, mood, pain sensations, and blood pressure; enhancing the delivery of oxygen and nutrients to the body's soft tissue areas; and the removing accumulated toxins by improving lymph circulation.

After more than a decade of use in Europe and Asia, products and devices based on FIR technology are now increasingly being used by alternative health practitioners in the U.S. and Canada.

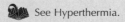 See Hyperthermia.

according to Douglas Lewis, N.D., former Chairperson of Physical Medicine at Bastyr University's Natural Health Clinic, in Seattle, Washington. "Pain generated by inflammation can be eased by use of ice or alternating hot and cold applications. General anxiety, which increases the perception of pain, can also be helped enormously by use of a neutral bath or wet sheet pack."

Blockages in circulation, which can result from inactivity or increased muscle tension and lead to poor oxygenation of tissues and pain, can be alleviated by techniques such as contrast bathing and hot and cold applications, Dr. Lewis notes. "Heating compresses that are applied cold and are then warmed up are also effective. The congestion and swelling caused by a buildup of fluids, as well as muscle stiffness, can be eased with heating compresses and a variety of alternating hot and cold applications or immersions." Generally, cold is more helpful than hot for injuries and inflamed areas, and any hot hydrotherapy methods should almost always end with a short cold application.

Using different substances in water can assist in pain relief, including Epsom salts and a wide range of essential oils. Steam can also be used to reduce the pain of chest and sinus congestion, with or without suitable additions of aromatic herbs and/or oils.

Recommendations

- Central to whatever is done for a person in pain is the need for that person to take some degree of control of the situation, to feel empowered to influence the processes at work and to not be simply the helpless recipient of other people's efforts.

- Detoxifying the body is an important component in promoting the health of the immune system and addressing other factors that may be contributing to chronic pain.

- Inflammation, one of the principal mechanisms related to chronic pain, may be caused by an allergic reaction. Often, significant pain relief can be achieved simply by eliminating allergenic foods from the diet.

- A number of nutritional supplements, taken daily, may help ease pain: vitamin C, evening primrose oil and eicosapentaenoic acid (EPA), vitamin E, magnesium, and the amino acid DL–phenylalanine.

- Hypnosis has been used to help alleviate back and joint pain, abdominal pain, pain from burns, and headache and migraine pain.

- Guided imagery can be particularly effective when other pain management approaches have failed.

- Biofeedback and neurobiofeedback training employs electronic devices to help a patient learn how to use the brain to relax and alter various bodily functions, which can greatly affect chronic pain symptoms.

- Acupuncture stimulates the release of endorphins and enkephalins (the body's own natural painkillers). At the same time, it can block pain messages from getting through to the brain.

- Chiropractic adjustments simultaneously affect several pain-causing mechanisms: nerve pressure (pinched nerves), joint compression, muscle stretching and/or spasm and trigger points, ligament injuries, tissue changes in elasticity and hypersensitivity, and reflex pain to and from internal organs.

- Massage helps break up waste deposits in the muscles and stimulates circulation to troubled regions in the body. Deep pressure on trigger points stretches tissues and loosens shortened muscles to restore proper functioning. The rhythmic motions of massage sedate the nervous system and promote voluntary muscle relaxation.

- The TENS (Transcutaneous Electrical Nerve Stimulator) electrical current acts upon the nerves, causing nerve conduction to be blocked and pain to be relieved. The Light Beam Generator stimulates blood circulation, reduces edema (swelling), and eliminates waste products stored in the tissues; it is beneficial for a wide range of conditions, including pain.

- A negative magnetic field can facilitate the healing process—it floods an injured area with oxygen, stimulates the production of melatonin and growth hormone, and alkalinizes the body's pH. Magnetic therapy can optimize the healing of injuries and reduce pain faster.

- Hydrotherapy, including compresses and various contrast (hot and cold) techniques, offers a simple and efficient way of treating chronic pain.

Self–Care

The following therapies can be undertaken at home under appropriate professional supervision:

Biofeedback Training and Neurotherapy / Exercise / Flower Essences / Guided Imagery / Mind/Body Medicine / Qigong and Tai Chi / Yoga

AROMATHERAPY: • For muscular fatigue, use lavender, marjoram, rosemary, clary sage. • For acute pain, use black pepper, ginger, birch.

Professional Care

The following therapies should only be provided by a qualified health professional:

Applied Kinesiology / Craniosacral Therapy / Environmental Medicine / Hypnotherapy / Neural Therapy

BODYWORK: Acupressure, massage, reflexology, Trager Approach

DETOXIFICATION THERAPY: Detoxification is indicated, because chronic pain is often associated with a build-up of toxins and congestive organs, stress, and referred pain.

OXYGEN THERAPY: If pain is caused by injury, hyperbaric oxygen therapy may be helpful.

TRADITIONAL CHINESE MEDICINE: Cupping is an ancient Chinese therapy that helps to regulate the flow of energy and blood. Suction is created over the painful area on the body by introducing fire into a cup and placing the cup on the desired point. The amount of suction can be regulated according to the treatment and the age of the patient.

Where to Find Help

For additional information on chronic pain, and referrals for treatment, contact the following organizations:

The Academy for Guided Imagery
P.O. Box 2070
Mill Valley, California 94942
(800) 726-2070
Website: www.interactiveimagery.com

The Academy trains health professionals to use Interactive Guided Imagery, offering a 150-hour certification program. They publish a directory of imagery practitioners and also carry books and tapes for professionals and laypeople, specifically relating to imagery in medicine and healing.

American Association of Oriental Medicine
433 Front Street
Catasauqua, Pennsylvania 18032
(888) 500-7999
Website: www.aaom.org

The AAOM is a national professional organization of acupuncturists who meet acceptable standards of competency and can provide you with the names and locations of local members.

American Association of Naturopathic Physicians

8201 Greensboro Drive, Suite 300
McLean, Virginia 22101
(703) 610-9037
Website: www.naturopathic.org

Provides a directory of naturopathic physicians and offers referrals to a nationwide network of accredited or licensed practitioners. Also publishes a quarterly newsletter, for both professionals and the general public, and offers a series of brochures and pamphlets on a variety of subjects.

American Chiropractic Association

1701 Clarendon Boulevard
Arlington, Virginia 22209
(800) 986-4636
Website: www.acatoday.com

A major source for chiropractic information, including a monthly publication and newsletter. Clinical councils with specialization in sports injuries and physical fitness, mental health, neurology, diagnosis and internal disorders, nutrition, orthopedics, physiological therapeutics, diagnostic imaging, and occupational health.

American Society of Clinical Hypnosis

130 E. Elm Court, Suite 201
Roselle, Illinois 60172-2000
(630) 980-4740
Website: www.asch.net

Membership is comprised of M.D.s and dentists trained in the use of hypnosis for treating health conditions. Send a stamped, self-addressed envelope for referrals to practitioners in your area.

Association for Applied Psychophysiology and Biofeedback

10200 West 44th Avenue, Suite 304
Wheat Ridge, Colorado 80033
(303) 422-8436
Website: www.aapb.org

Provides names and phone numbers of chapters in your state (formerly Biofeedback Society of America).

Bio-Electro-Magnetics Institute

2490 West Moana Lane
Reno, Nevada 89509-3936
(702) 827-9099

A private, nonprofit organization established to provide research, education, support, and technical assistance in matters relating to bioelectromagnetics. A national clearinghouse for information relating to both health risks from power line magnetic fields and the health benefits from magnetic therapy.

Recommended Reading

The Chronic Pain Management Sourcebook. David E. Drum. Los Angeles: Lowell House, 1999.

Chronic Pain: Natural Way of Healing. Theresa Digeronimo. New York: Dell, 1995.

Dr. Braly's Food Allergy and Nutrition Revolution. James Braly, M.D. New Canaan, CT: Keats Publishing, 1992.

Free Yourself from Pain. David E. Bresler, Ph.D., L.Ac. Los Angeles: The Bresler Center, 1992. Available from: The Bresler Center, 10780 Santa Monica Blvd., Los Angeles, CA 90025; (310) 466-1717.

Life Without Pain. Richard Linchitz, M.D. Reading, MA: Addison-Wesley, 1987.

Magnet Therapy: An Alternative Medicine Definitive Guide. William H. Philpott, M.D., and Dwight K. Kalita, Ph.D., with Burton Goldberg. Tiburon, CA: AlternativeMedicine.com Books, 2000.

Pain Erasure. Bonnie Prudden. New York: M. Evans, 1980.

Pain Free: A Revolutionary Method for Stopping Chronic Pain. Pete Egoscue. New York: Bantam Doubleday Dell, 1998.

COLDS AND FLU

The common cold and the flu are believed by most physicians to be caused by exposure and susceptibility to a variety of common viruses. Yet not everyone catches a cold or flu when exposed to such pathogens. For this reason, alternative physicians emphasize treating and preventing both colds and flu by strengthening the immune system in order to safeguard it from susceptibility.

ALL OF US HAVE experienced the sore throat, runny nose, aching, and general sense of misery that announce the onset of the common cold. Other familiar signals include a cough, headache, and dry, sore, or sensitive breathing passages. In a given year, nearly half of the United States population will catch a cold and 40% will develop influenza, or the flu.[1]

The symptoms of both the common cold and the flu are often the same, because both are caused by the same family of respiratory viruses. According to John Hibbs, N.D., of Seattle, Washington, the distinction between the two depends on how severe the infection is and the range of symptoms. The flu is usually more severe, develops quickly, and involves more of the body than a cold. A cold also occurs at any time of year, while the flu usually develops in epidemics, normally in late fall and winter.

"Beyond respiratory inflammation, the flu produces a moderate to high fever, aching muscles, and acute fatigue," says Dr. Hibbs. "Vomiting and diarrhea may also develop and, in extreme cases, the flu may lead to pneumonia in particularly susceptible individuals." Other complications of the flu, although rare, include inflammation of the brain (encephalitis) or heart (myocarditis), Reye's syndrome (an illness primarily affecting children, involving abnormal brain and liver function), and croup.

As the body attempts to fight the invading pathogens that can cause colds and flu, white blood cells are rapidly transported to the sites of infection. The chemically mediated inflammatory response of white blood cells causes swelling, which can result in stuffed sinuses and swollen nose or throat. Mucus is also secreted to trap the pathogens. Such reactions are signs of a normally functioning immune system, as are a runny nose, sneezing, and coughing, which serve to expel toxins and infectious organisms in the form of phlegm.

Enhancing the body's ability to remove phlegm is a central feature of the alternative medicine approach to treating colds and flu. In contrast, conventional medicine's approach of suppressing symptoms with drugs can compromise immune function. As a result, though symptom relief may be achieved, the duration of colds and flu can often be prolonged. In addition, the use of antibiotics for secondary infections resulting from colds and flu, such as bronchitis, can disturb bowel function and further weaken the body, making it susceptible to more serious forms of illness.

Other drug side effects can be even more harmful. For example, PPA (phenylpropanolamine), a common ingredient in many popular over-the-counter cold medicines, has caused fatal strokes, according to a warning issued by the U.S. Food and Drug Administration (FDA) in November 2000.

Causes of Colds and Flu

Viruses are commonly thought to be the cause of the cold and flu. However, William M. Cargile, B.S., D.C., F.I.A.C.A., of Lake Park, Georgia, counters this belief. "When everyone in the workplace and at home seems to have a cold or the flu, why do some people not get it?" he asks. "I treat people with the flu all day. Why don't I get it?" Dr. Cargile believes some people can resist viral attacks, while the immune systems in others are weakened and run down to such a degree that they become susceptible to a viral assault. "It comes down to available energy," he says. "The chemicals in the body that regulate stress are deficient and, as a result, the ability to adapt to stress is diminished. These are the kinds of people who are much more susceptible to getting the flu every year."

DRUGS ASSOCIATED WITH A HIGHER INCIDENCE OF THE COLD AND FLU

According to the *Physicians' Desk Reference,* the following drugs are associated with side effects of the cold and flu (statistics refer to the percentage of individuals affected).[5]

Actimmune (most common)
AeroBid inhaler system (10%)
Aerobid-M inhaler system (10%)
Alferon N injection (30%)
Asacol delayed-release tablets (3%)
CHEMET (succimer) capsules (5.2%-15.7%)
Intron A (37%-79%)
Lopressor HCT tablets (10%)
Nipent for injection (3%-10%)
Permax tablets (3.2%)
ProSom tablets (3%)
Rowasa rectal suppositories, rectal suspension enema (5.28%)
Videx tablets, powder for oral solution, and pediatric powder for oral solution (less than 7%)

CAUTION If any complications or severe worsening of either a cold or the flu develop, particularly when the person's immune system is already vulnerable, a physician should be contacted immediately.

The late Emanuel Cheraskin, M.D., D.M.D., of Birmingham, Alabama, agreed. "Three healthy people can breathe the same germs at the same moment," he noted. "One may develop pneumonia, another sniffle his way through a cold, and the third goes unscathed. After all, in most epidemics, those people who succumb represent only a fraction of the number of people exposed."[2] This suggests an ebb and flow in immune levels in each individual, dependant on stress, diet, amount of rest, and other factors. "It is time to put to rest the notion that germs jump into people and cause diseases," Dr. Cheraskin declared. "The evidence is adequate that microbes challenge the internal milieu. The end result depends upon the organism's ability to resist by means of its army of defense systems."[3]

Some physicians go farther, stating that a cold or flu can actually be one of the ways the body detoxifies itself. "Seen from this viewpoint," says Dr. Hibbs, "you can say that the virus causing the cold or flu is an accessory to a natural process." He notes that both the common cold and the flu are primarily caused by improper diet and toxicity and represent the body's attempt to rid itself of toxins through fever, coughing, and the discharge of mucus. "Nature is very homeostatic," he says. "When we run down our immune systems, a cold or flu can arise to detoxify ourselves and bring us back into balance."

It is time to put to rest the notion that germs jump into people and cause diseases. The evidence is adequate that microbes challenge the internal milieu. The end result depends upon the organism's ability to resist by means of its army of defense systems.

—EMANUEL CHERASKIN, M.D., D.M.D.

Poor Diet

Paying attention to the foods you eat can help you avoid creating the nutrient deficiencies or imbalances and toxicity in the body that lead to illness of all sorts, including the common cold and flu, according to Dr. Hibbs. He recommends avoiding all foods that decrease immune function, especially simple sugars, which have been shown to reduce the function of white blood cells.[4] "These are principally the refined sweeteners, cane sugar, corn syrup, and beet sugar," he explains. "But also included are the more natural sources of sugar, such as honey and concentrated fruit sugar found in dried fruit and fruit juice, as well as the sugars in alcohol."

Foods that cause difficulties in digestion or that contain high amounts of toxins, and all junk foods, should also be eliminated. "Meats and animal products in general are notoriously difficult to digest and contain toxins such as bacteria, hormones, pesticides, and antibiotics," Dr. Hibbs points out. "If you do eat meat, make sure your digestion is strong and buy organic, free-range meat products." Food additives, such as synthetic colors, sweeteners, flavorings, and preservatives, as well as hydrogenated oils found in margarine, chips, and many other snack foods, can also toxify the body and stress the mucous membranes and the immune system, Dr. Hibbs notes.

According to William Wolcott in his book *The Metabolic Typing Diet,* eating the wrong foods for one's individual metabolic type causes acid/alkaline imbalances in the tissues, which can make the body more susceptible to colds, flu, and other illnesses. Finally, overeating and improper food combinations can also lead to an accumulation of toxins in the body. "The most common and damaging food combining error people make is consuming foods high in protein, such as meats, milk, eggs, and nuts, with fruit, sugars, and other sweet foods," Dr. Hibbs says.

Allergies

Cow's milk, wheat, and all their derivative foods are often described as "mucus producing." "Whether this mucus production is caused by the alleged high mucus content of food or by an irritation or allergy response that the body has to it is debatable," Dr. Hibbs says. "But the increased congestion of the mucous membranes that these foods can cause correlates with more frequent respiratory infections. Most people who avoid dairy products while recovering from the cold or flu generally have less nasal congestion and throat phlegm. And any food or nonfood (such as monosodium glutamate) to which one is sensitive can cause congestion and susceptibility."

Most people who avoid dairy products while recovering from the cold or flu generally have less nasal congestion and throat phlegm.

—JOHN HIBBS, N.D.

Airborne allergens may also play a role in the cold and flu by decreasing resistance and influencing the respiratory tract. Dust, pollen, molds, and pet dander all aggravate the respiratory tract and increase susceptibility to the cold and flu, just as food allergies can. Inflamed, congested membranes in the nose, sinuses, and throat are more vulnerable to viral attack. Although allergies often share the same symptoms as colds, allergies usually have a seasonal history and are not accompanied by fever or infection as are the cold and flu.

Stress

Stress is another factor that can increase susceptibility to the common cold and flu. During times of stress, hormones are released in the body that cause the thymus gland to shrink, reducing immune activity.[6] The more stress one is under, the greater the chance of viral infection.

PREVENTING COLDS AND FLU

According to Michael T. Murray, N.D., prevention is the best medicine for a cold or flu. "People who suffer from more than two colds a year and whose colds last longer than 4-5 days probably have a weakened immune system," Dr. Murray says. "The immune system can be boosted through proper diet, lifestyle, and supplement strategies, and this will help prevent colds from forming in the first place."

Dr. Murray recommends several steps to enhance the immune system. These include getting adequate rest, since sleep gives the immune system a chance to recover; avoiding sugars, because sugar depresses the immune system; and consuming plenty of water, diluted vegetable juices, soups, and herb teas for proper hydration. He advises taking a daily high potency multivitamin/mineral supplement. Another useful precaution is to frequently wash your hands to avoid spreading infection, especially from hands to eyes, nose, and mouth.

Regular walking can be an effective preventive measure. According to Alice D. Domar, Ph.D., Assistant Professor at Harvard Medical School, a 45-minute walk five times a week serves a preventive function by increasing natural killer (NK) cells that fight infection. Regular walks can also cut sick time in half when a cold or flu does strike. Exercise helps move lymph fluid and white blood cells through the body.

Properly managing stress is another important preventive measure. Taking time out for yourself can be a major step in avoiding infection, as can having support, love, and meaning in your life, all of which help reduce susceptibility to illness.

Should congestion and other symptoms arise, Dr. Murray recommends applying a menthol-based (not petroleum-based) preparation to the upper chest before going to bed. Menthol helps clear the airways and, when applied to the upper chest, may increase the blood supply to the thalamus, one of the main organs controlling the immune system. To help clear mucus from the chest, he recommends a yoga posture known as "the Cobra." To perform this posture, lie on your stomach, then raise yourself up on your forearms, bending at the waist. This will expand the chest and make it easier to cough up phlegm.

This effect was demonstrated in a study that evaluated 420 people for occurrences of stress during the previous year. Job loss, divorce, death, and relocation were among the events included, and fear, sadness, anger, and nervousness were among the emotions monitored. The group was then exposed to one of five cold viruses and tested for antibodies one month later. Of those under the greatest amount of stress, 90% became infected as compared to 74% of those under the least stress.[7] Another study of 100 people showed that those who experienced particularly high degrees of anger and tension were four times more likely to develop a cold or bacterial infection than those who did not experience such emotions.[8]

Stress from lack of sleep can also increase susceptibility to colds and flu, according to David Simon, M.D., Medical Director of the Chopra Center for Well-Being, in La Jolla, California. "About 60% of Americans regularly have trouble sleeping," Dr. Simon points out. "When you don't get enough sleep, natural killer cells that are important in fighting viruses will be less effective."

Treating the Common Cold and Flu

Maintaining a healthy immune system is generally considered to be the key to avoiding the cold and flu. Proper diet, along with nutritional supplements and the avoidance of alcohol, tobacco, and recreational drugs, contribute to enhanced immune function. The cold and flu are always best treated at the onset. Caught early, many natural remedies described below can stop the cold or flu in its tracks.

Diet

"We have between 4,000 and 5,000 microbes of bacteria, viruses, and fungi living in and on every pore and hole in our bodies," says Dr. Cargile. "The real key to health lies in limiting their populations through dietary control and eating the right foods." In addition, Dr. Hibbs notes that getting extra sleep, cutting simple sugar intake, and drinking large amounts of herb tea, water, vegetable juices, and broths for healing a dehydrated respiratory tract will strengthen immune function and enhance detoxification.

"Water flushes the system of toxins," says Dr. Hibbs. He recommends drinking several glasses of pure water a day all year round and eating generously of fruits and vegetables. "Green and orange vegetables are high in beta carotene," he says. "Vegetables highest in beta carotene are leafy greens, carrots, and orange-colored squash. During cold and flu seasons, have at least one of each every day."

According to Jonathan Wright, M.D., of the Tahoma Clinic, in Kent, Washington, "The natural response of the body to illness is to use its energy to fight off the bug, so you may not have much appetite." Since processing food takes a lot of energy, Dr. Wright recommends that people with a cold or flu eat very lightly, or not at all, while forcing fluids to help clear toxins from the body.

 See Diet, Herbal Medicine, Homeopathy, Nutritional Medicine, Yoga.

Nutritional Supplements

Many nutritional supplements can be valuable aids in dealing with a cold or the flu, due to their ability to stimulate immune function and protect the body from the effects of stress. According to Garry F. Gordon, M.D., M.D. (H.), D.O., Director of the Gordon Research Institute, in Payson, Arizona, an effective treatment at the first signs and symptoms of cold or flu is to take high doses of vitamins A and C, plus garlic. He typically recommends a basic regimen over 3-5 days for adults, taking each nutrient in the following dosages every 3-4 hours while awake:

Vitamin C: 2,000-5,000 mg of powdered, mineral ascorbate (this form minimizes excess gas and bowel cramping). The normal daily adult maximum dose is 10,000-20,000 mg. "This dose is continued until all signs of infection have subsided," says Dr. Gordon. "In some cases, though, the dose can go as high as 50,000-100,000 mg daily, depending on the severity of the conditions." The dosage should be reduced, however, if diarrhea occurs.

Numerous studies have shown that people taking large doses of vitamin C (amounts far larger than the U.S. RDAs) report reductions in the incidence, severity, and duration of colds.[9] In several double-blind studies, researchers found that vitamin C supplementation may be useful for lessening the severity of disease as well as reducing transmission of viruses.[10] Beyond its antiviral and antibacterial properties, vitamin C acts as an immunostimulant. It enhances white blood cell production, increases interferon (a group of proteins released by white blood cells to combat a virus), improves antibody responses, and promotes secretion of thymic hormones.[11]

Vitamin A: 100,000 IU of mycelized vitamin A in liquid form. Dr. Gordon stresses the importance of taking high doses of vitamin A at the same time as the vitamin C. "High doses means that as long as a person's weight is over 120 pounds and there is no serious liver condition, you may safely use 100,000 IU of mycelized vitamin A three or four times a day, for a total of

300,000-400,000 IU each day." Dr. Gordon states that no documented evidence exists of serious toxicity due to high doses of vitamin A as long as it is used for only a short period of time. "It is only when these high doses are used for several weeks or months that signs of toxicity develop," he says. "Even then, all reported side effects are completely reversible once supplementation of the vitamin A is discontinued. And certainly vitamin A in high doses is safer than taking larger doses of aspirin or antibiotics, both of which have many possible side effects."

Dr. Gordon emphasizes the importance of taking active vitamin A rather than supplementing with beta carotene, which must be cleaved enzymatically in the liver to form vitamin A. Attempting to enzymatically convert an adequate amount of vitamin A from beta carotene can overtax the liver. (Pregnant women should not take high doses of vitamin A, as it may adversely affect the fetus.)

Garlic *(Allium sativum):* Take in high doses at the same time as the vitamins. Garlic has been shown to protect against flu viruses and to enhance antibody production.[12] The active ingredient in garlic, allicin, which also provides its pungent odor, is rendered inactive by heat. Cooked garlic is not only less odorous, but it has also lost many of its medicinal properties. For this reason, Dr. Gordon recommends 4-6 high-quality deodorized garlic capsules taken 3-4 times a day, which will provide higher, more concentrated doses of allicin than eating garlic cloves, and eliminate the odor problem common to many garlic eaters.

A number of other nutrients have shown promise in treating the common cold and flu:

Zinc: Taking 180 mg of zinc gluconate (in pills containing 23 mg of elemental zinc) every two hours during an episode of cold or flu can speed up recovery time. In a study involving 146 cold sufferers, those taking zinc recovered completely after an average of 3.9 days while those taking a placebo took 10.8 days.[14]

Selenium: According to Earl Mindell, R.Ph., Ph.D., author of *Prescription Alternatives,* taking up to 800 mcg daily of the trace mineral selenium for three days can help your body resist a cold. A normal maintenance dose is 50-200 mcg, Dr. Mindell notes.[15]

N-Acetyl-Cysteine (NAC): This slightly altered form of the amino acid cysteine can reduce the incidence of developing flu. In a six-month study of 262 people (78% were 65 years or older) already susceptible to the Asian

---

NUTRIENT COLD FORMULA

Robert C. Atkins, M.D., Director of the Atkins Center for Complementary Medicine, in New York City, recommends taking this formula every hour or up to ten doses on the first day in which there is a sign of cold or flu. As a general preventive measure, Dr. Atkins suggests taking this blend once or twice daily throughout the year; those who are especially prone to colds or flu, should take it three times daily, he says.[13]

- Beta carotene: 5,000 IU
- Vitamin A: 3,333 IU
- Quercetin: 80 mg
- Zinc gluconate: 25 mg
- Vitamin C: 500 mg
- Calcium pantothenate: 80 mg
- Citrus bioflavonoids: 80 mg
- Selenium (selenite): 30 mcg
- Magnesium (ascorbate): 15 mg
- Garlic (with allicin): 160 mg
- Folic acid: 400 mcg
- Dimethylglycine HCL: 20 mg
- Pyridoxine HCL: 4 mg
- Riboflavin: 2 mg
- Copper (chelate): 1 mg
- Niacinamide: 15 mg

---

influenza virus, 25% of those taking 600 mg of NAC twice daily developed flu symptoms compared to 79% of those taking a placebo.[16]

Herbal Medicine

Herbs have a long history of use as a treatment for colds and flu, due to their ability to stimulate immune function, as well as their antiviral, anti-inflammatory, and anti-catarrhal properties. Some of the herbs that bolster the immune system include echinacea, goldenseal, licorice, elder, St. John's wort, and astragalus (excellent for strengthening the immune system).[17]

If your cold has advanced to the stage in which your throat, sinuses, and lungs are inflamed, the phlegm you cough up is thick, your chest feels tight and sore, and your cold seems to have taken up residence in your lungs, it is still not too late for goldenseal to be of benefit. This herb can help relieve the inflammation of mucous mem-

HAVE A CUP OF BONESET TEA

According to Robert D. Willix, Jr., M.D., a cup of boneset (*Eupatorium perfoliatum*) tea is a frontline treatment in Germany for colds and flu. The herb stimulates the immune system, encouraging white blood cells to destroy viruses and bacteria. Dr. Willix recommends adding 1-2 teaspoons of dry leaves (fresh leaves contain a toxic chemical that dissipates when the leaves are dried) to one cup of boiling water; steep for 10-20 minutes, then drink. Consume two to three cups daily until symptoms disappear.[19]

branes, which under these conditions no longer can protect the body against the influx of bacteria and viruses.[18]

"Lomatium deserves special mention as a flu remedy," says Dr. Hibbs. "It's an antiviral and it stimulates the immune system. I find it to be the most effective flu remedy in the herbal pharmacy." Among patients taking the herb for full-blown flu symptoms, he has observed full recovery on numerous occasions within 24-48 hours. Although not as well-known as other herbs, lomatium is available in most health food stores and herbal outlets.

One of Dr. Hibbs's patients came to him with the flu. "He had nausea but no vomiting and a 102° F fever for two or three days," Dr. Hibbs recounts. "He felt very achy and tired, with moderate coughing and sneezing, and minimal congestion, but it was obviously the flu and not a cold. I simply put him on a lomatium tincture mixed with the herbs ligusticum (*Ligusticum wallichii*) and echinacea. He took it three or four times a day and was told to drink lots of fluids, get plenty of rest, and avoid alcohol and sugar. Within 48 hours, he was 90% better." Dr. Hibbs cautions, however, that lomatium can cause an itchy measles-like rash on the skin of sensitive patients or those who take too large a dose.

Mary Bove, N.D., Chair of Botanical Medicine at Bastyr University, in Kenmore, Washington, recommends the following herbs for general use in the treatment of colds and flu:

- Yarrow, calming to an upset digestive tract, is also an anti-inflammatory and diaphoretic (producing perspiration). These qualities make yarrow particularly useful in influenza and respiratory infections associated with fever, malaise, and decreased appetite.

- Eyebright, an anticatarrhal and anti-inflammatory, is useful in respiratory conditions, specifically, in the nasal pharynx and the sinuses.

- Elecampane (*Inula helenium*) is a soothing, relaxing, yet stimulating expectorant for coughs and bronchial irritations.

- Elder flower, immune-stimulating, anti-inflammatory, anticatarrhal, and diaphoretic, is a good all-purpose herb for the flu and common cold. Dr. Bove notes that these herbs can be easily combined or used singly as teas or tinctures.

Dr. Wright also recommends echinacea (primes the immune system to heightened activity), red clover, myrrh, osha (also known as Porter's lovage, the root has been used traditionally for sore throats and lung congestion), and cayenne pepper during times of cold and flu. These can be taken as a tea (3-5 cups per day), tincture (30 drops, four times daily), or capsules (two capsules, four times daily).

Homeopathy

Alternative physicians are using both traditional and modern methods in homeopathic treatments for the cold and flu. Contemporary methods include injection of homeopathic remedies intramuscularly or intravenously. This approach is employed by Leonard Haimes, M.D., of Boca Raton, Florida, who injects his patients with a homeopathic preparation containing mistletoe *(Viscum album),* a plant that is known for its antiviral and antitumor properties. Along with the preparation, Dr. Haimes gives other herbs, homeopathic formulas, and large doses of vitamin C.

Dr. Hibbs prescribes the following additional homeopathic remedies:

- *Aconitum napellus* for sudden cold or flu symptoms that begin after exposure to cold and in which the patient is chilled but feels better in the open air and worse after midnight. These types of symptoms may include anxiety and extreme thirst.

- *Natrum muriaticum* for the patient with a profuse, thin, watery, nasal discharge. Symptoms include thirst, sneezing, and loss of taste and sense of smell.

- *Allium cepa* for patients whose eyes and nose stream with watery, burning discharge and who sneeze frequently.

- *Nux vomica* for patients who have nasal congestion, especially at night. During the day, the nose can be quite runny and burning, and the person may be impatient and irritable.

- *Eupatorium perfoliatum* for patients who have deep bone ache, are thirsty, cough with chest soreness, and feel worse in cold air.

Other homeopathic treatments Dr. Hibbs prescribes include *Belladonna, Baptisia,* and *Bryonia.* Another popular homeopathic remedy for colds and flu is *Oscillococcinum.* First developed in France in 1919, Oscillo (as it is known in short) has been used successfully as a first-line self-care homeopathic remedy against the flu ever since in over 40 countries. At the onset of symptoms, Dr. Wright recommends taking six pellets, dissolved under the tongue, every six hours. As with all homeopathic remedies, avoid food or beverage for 30 minutes before and after use.

 See Acupuncture, Ayurvedic Medicine, Bodywork, Chiropractic, Hydrotherapy, Hyperthermia, Traditional Chinese Medicine.

Acupuncture and Traditional Chinese Medicine

Dr. Cargile believes that weakened immune systems in people with a cold or flu are a result of depletion of cellular energy stores of ATP (adenosine triphosphate, a substance produced in all cells and responsible for energy) and depletion of cortisol (a stress adaptation hormone produced by the adrenal cortex). To rechannel energy levels in his patients, Dr. Cargile uses acupuncture meridians related to endocrine gland functions, digestion, lungs, and other organs. "When these meridian points are used in conjunction with each other, we have been able to significantly affect the body's immune system and redirect energy in the direction needed," he says. Dr. Cargile says that after treating several patients with acupuncture as a preventative, "people who have had longstanding chronic flu symptoms have not had them now for two years."

Traditional Chinese medicine (TCM) offers another approach to understanding and treating colds and flu. Underlying imbalances and disharmony in the body are described in terminology analogous to the natural world (heat, cold, dryness, or dampness). The concept of balance, or the interrelationship of organs, is central to TCM. According to Marian Small, N.D., L.Ac., of Seattle, Washington, a cold can be caused by six factors: wind, heat, cold, dampness, dryness, and summer heat. "When these factors are strong enough or when a person is in a sus-

ceptible state, then there is an invasion and illness occurs," Dr. Small notes. "Wind usually affects the throat, lungs, and head. Cold weather can create white or clear discharge of body secretions. Heat can manifest as fevers, thirst, dry stools, rashes, and secretions that are yellow and sticky." Dr. Small recommends these Chinese medicine formulas to combat the common cold and flu:

- *Yinqiao,* good in the first stage of a cold or flu, expels wind and heat from the exterior layers of the body. Symptoms can include sore throat, fever with chills, body aches, or headache. It can also be used to help treat certain rashes.

- Natural herb loquat syrup is an expectorant for coughs with phlegm and sinus congestion.

- *Bo ying powder* is for infants and children with a wide range of childhood diseases, including fever, headaches, cough, upset stomach, diarrhea, or vomiting. It can be mixed with food.

- *Bi yan pian* is useful for sneezing, sinus congestion, itchy eyes, or hay fever.

Another herb, Chinese ephedra *(ma-huang),* has been used in China for thousands of years to treat colds, asthma, bronchitis, fever, and other ailments. Ephedra contains ephedrine, which, in a synthesized form, is used in Western medicine in over-the-counter and prescription remedies for conditions such as hay fever and rhinitis. Ephedra roots and branches, taken in a tea, can be very effective in the treatment of cold and flu symptoms.

CAUTION Since ephedra increases blood pressure and heart rate, it should be avoided by those with most heart conditions, high blood pressure, and women who are pregnant.

Chiropractic/Bodywork

Martin Gallagher, D.C., Director of Medical Wellness Associates, in Pittsburgh, Pennsylvania, suggests that many cases of cold and flu may be caused by dysfunction in the nervous system due to mechanical problems in the body, such as spinal misalignments, which adversely affect the immune system. "My main approach to staying well in cold and flu season is improving the function of a person's nervous system, because it integrates all of the systems of the body, including the immune, cardiovascular, and endocrine systems," Dr. Gallagher explains. "We often hear of people getting colds and flu and needing to activate the immune system. But we forget that the nervous system is wired to the immune system, and if you have

HYDROTHERAPY

Hydrotherapy is another method of strengthening and detoxifying the body and immune system. Outbreaks of the common cold and flu often coincide with dramatic changes of temperature, humidity, and season. When done on a regular basis, contrast hydrotherapy, which consists of exposing the body to sudden shifts of hot and cold water temperature, will keep the body and immune system acclimatized. It can be as simple as running the last 30-60 seconds of a morning shower at a colder temperature.

Another hydrotherapy treatment recommended by Jonathan Wright, M.D., is to make a throat or chest compress. Before bed, use a warm washcloth or hot shower on the throat and chest, then dry off and apply a cold cotton wrap or a thin T-shirt, soaked in cold water and wrung out, to the throat or chest. Cover the neck with a wool scarf or the chest with a wool sweater and go to sleep. By morning, the coverings will be dry.

dysfunction in the nervous system, this will affect your health."

Children, in particular, with cranial (head) or cervical (neck) misalignments may have frequent congestion, especially ear infections, because the eustachian tube (which connects the middle ear with the nasopharynx) cannot drain properly, according to Dr. Gallagher. Being misaligned may also interfere with the course of a viral infection and the body's ability to intervene.

Trigger points and drainage techniques can be used to drain the sinuses and relieve congestion, headaches, and post-nasal drip. "There is a point at the center of the eyebrows and points at the side of the nose—you can stimulate these points with finger pressure or with acupuncture needles as well as with light and heat," Dr. Gallagher instructs. "There is another set of points below the collar bone that are neuro-lymphatic reflexes connected to lymph drainage. The lymph system removes toxins and fights infection with T cells and B cells. Stimulating these reflex points in a circular fashion helps lymph drainage in the head and neck."

Another way to support the immune system is by improving the function of the thymus gland. "A chiropractor can check for mechanical misalignments between the shoulder blades, at the first and second thoracic vertebrae," Dr. Gallagher says. "Those are the spinal areas that influence thymus function. Taking thymus glandu-

lar extract, two capsules every two hours, will also activate the thymus gland."

Ayurvedic Medicine

Virender Sodhi, M.D. (Ayurveda), N.D., Director of the Ayurvedic & Naturopathic Medical Clinic, in Bellevue, Washington, employs a number of Ayurvedic approaches to treat patients with a cold or flu. The objective of Ayurvedic medicine, according to Dr. Sodhi, is to rid the body of indigestible toxins, which attract viruses and compromise the immune process. To increase digestion, he uses herbs such as ginger, cayenne, black pepper, long pepper, and holy basil (*Ocimum tenuiflorum*). "I have patients drink lots of warm water and ginger tea throughout the day and use breathing exercises that help them to expectorate mucus," he says. "When people know they have an allergy or the flu, they usually use antihistamines, which dry up the mucus. So you are stuck with a problem—the body wants to expel the mucus, but the use of antihistamines prevents that from happening."

Dr. Sodhi believes it is important to expectorate during a cold or flu in order to clean out nasal passages. He uses a nasal douche for this purpose. "To perform this is very easy," Dr. Sodhi says. "Take a teapot and fill it with sea salt and warm water (one teaspoon of salt per quart of water). Let the water flow from the spout through one nostril and into the other. You should feel the nasal passages clearing within a brief time."

According to Dr. Simon, in Ayuverdic medicine, colds and flu generally fall into a category called *ama,* which represents an accumulation of incompletely digested experiences that the body then stores as toxicity. "A cold can be considered an acute attack of *ama,*" Dr. Simon says. "*Ama* shares many qualities with the Ayurvedic principle of *kapha*—a sluggish metabolic tendency related to the water element, which may prevail during rainy, winter weather. Properties of both *ama* and *kapha* are thick, cold, and stagnant. *Kapha*-reducing herbs and activities can help digest *ama* and move it out of the body."

Like Dr. Sodhi, Dr. Simon recommends the use of ginger or other hot spices to reduce susceptibility to colds. He suggests making a strong tea by grating ginger into a cup of hot water, in order to help mobilize secretions. For a dry cough, he recommends chopped licorice root, which adds a balancing effect to ginger.

Hyperthermia

Hyperthermia can be used to stimulate immune response and detoxification through sweating. "The enhancement of the body's natural tendency to fever during a cold or flu has beneficial effects," says Dr. Hibbs, "including a dramatic stimulation of detoxification through the skin."

Though uncomfortable, fever produces a natural antibiotic effect within the body and additionally appears to shorten the duration of infection.[20] Dr. Hibbs recommends that fever treatments be coupled with a very clean, simplified diet featuring large amounts of water, steamed vegetables, vegetable juice, or broth.

CAUTION People with a heart condition should consult their physician before undertaking hyperthermia.

Dr. Hibbs describes the treatment on a 5-year-old patient. "She had come down with flu symptoms a few hours earlier, including lethargy and fatigue, a fever of 101.5° Fahrenheit, a headache, and a sore throat. She was not hungry and was just encouraged to drink liquids. I gave her a single 90-drop dose of a 50:50 mixture of tinctures of echinacea and lomatium, and she was then given a fever treatment at home. The home treatment consisted of placing her in a hot bath in a very warm bathroom. In the bath, she drank a cup of hot yarrow tea.

"She was attended constantly by an adult and her temperature was taken every two to three minutes orally. When her temperature reached 103°, which took 15 minutes, she was quickly toweled dry and clothed in heavy cotton pajamas. She went immediately to bed, fell into a deep sleep, and woke the next morning feeling completely well and was able to attend school as usual without relapse."

Dr. Hibbs notes, however, that hyperthermia should be used with caution in a patient who already has a fever. "The body temperature should never be permitted to rise above 104° Fahrenheit," he says. "If it does, cool water sponging or medication can be used to reduce it. Medications may also be needed to control fever, particularly in small children. But it should be kept in mind that these drugs interrupt the normal immune response and, while reducing the symptoms, may lengthen infections."

Many people believe that it is necessary to reduce a fever and to take acetaminophen in order to do so. This is actually dangerous medicine, according to Dr. Gallagher, who notes that there are over 70,000 acetaminophen poisonings a year because of adverse effects on the liver. "In the U.S., there are very few harmful fevers (such as yellow fever)," Dr. Gallagher points out. He suggests that patients put on layers of warm clothing. "Wear socks and gloves, even at home, and keep the room warm at 75°-80° Fahrenheit," he says. "Drink warm herbal teas such as echinacea and goldenseal. Get under the covers and sweat. The homeopathic remedy *Belladonna* also potentiates fever. The fever then cooks the poison out of the body. As a result, you will get over an infection more quickly because fever builds the immune system naturally."

Recommendations

- For prevention of colds and flu, get adequate rest and minimize stress. Also, frequently wash your hands to avoid spreading infection and limit social contacts to reduce exposure.

- Eat lightly, emphasizing vegetables high in beta carotene (leafy greens, carrots, squash), garlic, and vegetable broth and fresh-squeezed vegetable juices. Drink plenty of pure spring water or filtered water.

- For 3-5 days, take the following every 3-4 hours while awake: vitamin C in powdered mineral ascorbate form (2,000-4,000 mg); vitamin A in liquid mycelized form (100,000 IU); and garlic capsules (4-6). Other useful nutrients include zinc, colostrum, thymus extract, and beta-1,3-glucan.

- Take homeopathic *Oscillococcinum,* six pellets under the tongue every six hours, at the onset of symptoms. Other useful homeopathic remedies include *Viscum album, Aconitum napellus, Natrum Muriaticum, Allium cepa, Nux vomica,* and *Eupatorium perfoliatum.*

- Exercise, such as 45-minute walks five times a week, helps to significantly boost immune function. For chest congestion, practice the Cobra yoga posture.

- Helpful herbs include echinacea, lomatium, astragalus, cayenne pepper, licorice, goldenseal, elderberry, St. John's wort, eyebright, elecampane, red clover, osha, and yarrow, taken as teas (3-5 cups per day), tinctures (30 drops, four times daily), or capsules (two capsules, four times daily).

Self-Care
The following therapies can be undertaken at home under appropriate professional supervision:

Biofeedback Training and Neurotherapy / Fasting / Guided Imagery / Yoga

AROMATHERAPY: Inhalations and baths with camphor, eucalyptus, lavender, lemon, peppermint, pine, rosemary, tea tree.

FLOWER ESSENCES: For emotional states as appropriate.

JUICE THERAPY: • Lemon, orange, pineapple, black currant, elderberry juice • Carrot, beet, tomato, green pepper, and watercress • Carrot, celery • Carrot, spinach • Carrot, beet, cucumber. Add small doses of ginger, onion, or garlic juice to vegetable juices.

TOPICAL TREATMENT: For a head cold, spray throat and nasal passages with witch hazel.

Professional Care

The following therapies should only be provided by a qualified health professional:

Applied Kinesiology / Chiropractic / Detoxification Therapy / Environmental Medicine / Magnetic Field Therapy / Orthomolecular Medicine / Osteopathic Medicine

BODYWORK: • Acupressure, reflexology, shiatsu • Percussion massage to break up cold congestion

OXYGEN THERAPIES: • Hydrogen peroxide • Ozone

Where to Find Help

For additional information on the treatment of colds and flu, contact:

American Association of Oriental Medicine (AAOM)

433 Front Street
Catasauqua, Pennsylvania 18032
(888) 500-7999
Website: www.aaom.org

The AAOM is a national professional organization of acupuncturists who meet acceptable standards of competency and can provide you with names and locations of local members.

American Association of Naturopathic Physicians

601 Valley Street, Suite 105
Seattle, Washington 98109
(206) 298-0126
Website: www.naturopathic.org

Contact them for the location of a licensed naturopathic physician in your area.

American Herbalists Guild

1931 Gaddis Road
Canton, Georgia 30115
(770) 751-6021
Website: www.healthy.net/herbalists

For information on herbs and for referrals to practitioners.

American Holistic Medical Association

6728 Old McLean Village Drive
McLean, Virginia 22101
(703) 556-9728
Website: www.holisticmedicine.org

Provides referrals, guidelines for nutrition and fitness, and sponsors conferences on holistic medicine for the professional.

Ayurvedic & Naturopathic Medical Clinic

2115 112th Avenue N.E.
Bellevue, Washington 98004
(425) 453-8022
Website: www.ayurvedicscience.com

Dr. Virender Sodhi's clinic provides medical training for physicians and health-care practitioners, as well as individual courses for laypeople.

International Foundation for Homeopathy

P.O. Box 7
Edmonds, Washington 98020
(425) 776-4147

Provides educational courses for professionals and the general public. Offers referrals to homeopathic health professionals.

Recommended Reading

Breathe Free. Daniel Gagnon and Amadea Morningstar. Wilmot, WI: Lotus Press, 1991.

The Common Cold and Common Sense. Dale Alexander. New York: Fireside Books, 1981.

Dr. Gallagher's Guide to 21st Century Medicine. Martin Gallagher. Greensburg, PA: Atlas Publishing, 1997.

Dr. Murray's Total Body Tune-Up. Michael T. Murray, N.D. New York: Bantam, 2000.

Encyclopedia of Natural Medicine. Michael T. Murray, N.D., and Joseph Pizzorno, N.D. Rocklin, CA: Prima Publishing, 1991.

Vitamin C: Who Needs It? Emanuel Cheraskin, M.D. Birmingham, AL: Arlington Press, 1993.

CONSTIPATION

Health begins and ends in the intestines. Unfortunately, constipation is a common problem in the United States, affecting almost 20% of the population, who spend over $700 million annually on laxatives.[1] Despite this fact, conventional medicine gives little attention to this growing national problem, preferring to prescribe drugs that treat symptoms rather than the root causes of the condition. Recognizing that regularity is important to health and that disease starts in the colon, alternative medicine offers a variety of approaches to help cleanse the colon and return it to a natural state of health.

CONSTIPATION REFERS to a difficulty or infrequency in the passage of stools due to sluggish action of the bowels. This can be a serious condition that can result in headaches, fatigue, depression, pain, and other digestive problems. According to James Braly, M.D., of Hollywood, Florida, constipation can undermine the whole body, affecting digestion, the clearing of toxins, energy level, and the absorption of nutrients. Proper elimination is necessary to avoid a buildup of toxins in the body, which can lead to chronic inflammatory and autoimmune diseases, such as rheumatoid arthritis, lupus, ankylosing spondylitis, Crohn's disease, and ulcerative colitis. Improper elimination may even cause a state of toxemia—the longer waste stays in the gastrointestinal tract (longer transit time), the more likely it is that toxins, via osmosis, will pass into the bloodstream and settle into other organ systems. This is called "autointoxication," which brings about a great variety of symptoms and ailments.

There is a wide discrepancy between conventional and alternative health communities concerning what constitutes regular bowel movements. According to the *Physicians' Manual for Patients*, "Daily bowel movements are not essential to health."[2] This view represents the conventional medical outlook. However, alternative practitioners strongly disagree with this idea, feeling that two or three bowel movements per day are ideal for health maintenance.

Still, Leon Chaitow, N.D., D.O., of London, England, points out that different body types have divergent ten-

> *Constipation can undermine the whole body, affecting digestion, the clearing of toxins, energy level, and the absorption of nutrients.*
>
> —JAMES BRALY, M.D.

dencies that require various considerations. For example, he has found that stocky individuals very often have superb bowel function and a rapid transit time. In contrast, Dr. Chaitow has found that lean individuals whose diets are more vegetarian often have a sluggish and slow bowel pattern. He notes that people are different biochemically and emotionally and must be treated on an individualized basis.

Regardless of such individual differences, however, it is now known that irregular bowel movements are directly related to serious health conditions. A study published in *The Lancet* reported that women who have fewer than three bowel movements per week have four times the risk of breast disease than those who have one or more bowel movements per day.[3] Furthermore, colon cancer accounts for over 56,000 deaths each year.[4] Nutritionist Lindsey Duncan, C.N., of Santa Monica, California, says, "I've consulted with 8,000 clients, who come to me with a variety of health problems ranging from fatigue, depression, impaired immune function, and obesity to gas, acne, and lower back pain. The vast majority of these complaints and symptoms are alleviated by cleansing, healing, and supporting the intestinal system."

Causes of Constipation

According to Patrick Donovan, N.D., of Seattle, Washington, constipation can be caused by a number of different factors and conditions, including poor diet and nutrition, dehydration, food allergies, lack of exercise,

TRANSIT TIME

About 100 years ago, most people in the United States had a short intestinal "transit time," meaning it took only about 15-20 hours from the time food entered the mouth until it was excreted as feces. Today, many have a seriously delayed transit time of 50-70 hours. One reason transit times have increased is that our diets now include less fiber from fresh fruits and vegetables. As fiber is indigestible, it helps give stools bulk, while also making them soft and flexible. Another reason is that our modern lifestyle, high in stress, excessive antibiotics, and certain acid-forming foods (such as sugar, eggs, and meat), causes the intestinal tract to accumulate a slimy, sticky substance called mucus.

Increased transit time means there is more opportunity for the stool to putrefy, for harmful microorganisms to flourish, and for toxins to develop and poison the body. Optimal transit time is about 18-20 hours; an acceptable transit time is 24-48 hours. Ideally, everyone should have comfortable, unforced bowel movements about 20 minutes after every meal, just like a baby. A healthy colon produces an easy-to-eliminate stool that is soft but formed, consisting of about 70% water but having enough bulk so that it readily responds to the muscular contractions of the bowel.

microflora," all of which "decreases transit time, reduces colonic pressure, and produces a softer stool."[5]

The relative acidity or alkalinity of food is also important to diet and health. Foods that are too acidic—such as meats, dairy, and sugar—can interfere with the function of the colon, while alkaline foods (like vegetables and fruits) have a natural laxative effect upon the digestive tract. "An acid environment in the body increases transit time while an alkaline one decreases it," says Rima Laibow, M.D., founding Medical Director of the Alexandria Institute of Natural and Integrative Medicine, in Croton-on-Hudson, New York. "Excessively rapid transit time means poor nutrient absorption, while a transit time that is too slow leads to autotoxicity and increases colon cancer risk."

Food sensitivities and allergies can also cause constipation, with dairy products being a common offender. Dr. Braly cites the case of one of his patients, a banker in his mid-forties, who complained of fatigue, lower back pain, dizziness, nausea, weight gain, high blood pressure, headaches, and severe constipation. The patient was dependent on laxatives and also taking two prescription medicines and 6-8 aspirins daily. Dr. Braly changed the patient's diet, eliminating key allergenic foods, and within ten days his chronic constipation disappeared, along with all the other conditions except lower back pain. The patient was able to give up all his medications and lost eight pounds. Dr. Braly states, "No amount of bran or other fiber would have done the trick alone. The elimination of allergies was the crucial factor."

 See Allergies, Diet, Men's Health, Women's Health.

poor posture, emotional upsets and anxiety, imbalances of estrogen and progesterone, imbalances in the autonomic nervous system, drugs and medications, and the misuse of laxatives. Dr. Donovan notes that many older patients' dependence on laxatives and enemas leads to relaxed gut muscles, which make elimination more difficult. Constipation for many patients can also alternate with diarrhea and abdominal cramps in a common condition known as irritable bowel syndrome.

Poor Diet

Dr. Braly points to poor diet as the most significant cause of constipation. Highly processed foods, fast foods, fatty foods, sugars, and salt all contribute to a variety of digestive problems, he notes. Perhaps the single most important cause of constipation is a lack of fiber in a person's diet. The *British Medical Journal* summarized studies on this fact and stated that "fiber increases stool bulk, holds water, and acts as a substrate [catalyst] for colonic

Stress

According to Dr. Braly, anxiety, fear, worry, grief, and frustration have all been known to affect the digestive tract, causing ulcers, diarrhea, or constipation. In some serious cases, peristalsis (the wavelike contractions and dilations of the colon muscles that expel waste matter) becomes extremely weak and the colon becomes severely dysfunctional. When stressed, the nervous system becomes enzyme deficient, saliva flow decreases, and lactic acid accumulates, causing stomach pain and indigestion.

 See Environmental Medicine, Natural Hormone Replacement Therapy, Stress.

Low Thyroid Function

Hypothyroidism (low or underactive thyroid gland function) leads to a sluggish digestive system, often resulting in a number of gastrointestinal problems, including con-

DRUGS ASSOCIATED WITH A
HIGHER INCIDENCE OF CONSTIPATION

According to the *Physicians' Desk Reference,* the following drugs are associated with a side effect of constipation (statistics refer to the percentage of individuals affected).[8]

Anafranil capsules (22%-47%)
Anaprox, anaprox DS tablets (3%-9%)
Aredia for injection (up to 15%)
Asacol delayed-release tablets (5%)
Asendin tablets (12%)
Calan SR caplets, tablets (7.3%)
Clinoril tablets (3%-9%)
Clozaril tablets (5%-14%)
Colestid granules (10%)
Combipres tablets (about 10%)
Cordarone tablets (4%-9%)
DHC Plus capsules (among most frequent)
Daypro caplets (3%-9%)
Desyrel and desyrel dividose (7.0%-7.6%)
Duragesic transdermal system (10% or more)
Empirin with codeine tablets (among most frequent)
Habitrol nicotine transdermal system (3%-9%)
Hivid tablets (less than 6.4%)
Hylorel tablets (21%)
Intron A (up to 10%)
Isoptin oral tablets, sustained release tablets (7.3%)
Limbitrol DS tablets, (among most frequent)
Ludiomil tablets (6%)
Lupron injection (5% or more)
MS Contin tablets (among most frequent)
Marplan Tablets (among most frequent)

Mevacor tablets (2.0%-4.9%)
Nalfon 200 pulvules, Nalfon tablets (7%)
Naprosyn suspension, tablets (3%-9%)
Nicoderm nicotine transdermal system (3%-9%)
Nipent for injection (3%-10%)
Norpace capsules, CR capsules (11%)
Oramorph SR morphine sulfate sustained release tablets
     (among most frequent)
Parlodel capsules, SnapTabs (3%-14%)
Paxil tablets (13.8%)
Permax tablets (10.6%)
Prozac pulvules, liquid, oral solution (4.5%)
Questran light, powder (among most frequent)
Relafen tablets (3%-9%)
Rythmol tablets (2.0%-7.2%)
Sanorex tablets (among most frequent)
Stadol injectable, nasal spray (3%-9%)
Tenex tablets (up to 16%)
Triaminic expectorant DH (among most frequent)
Trilisate liquid, tablets (less than 20%)
Velban vials (among most frequent)
Verelan capsules (7.3%)
Videx tablets, powder for oral solution, pediatric powder
     for oral solution (less than 16%)
Voltaren tablets (3%-9%)
Wellbutrin tablets (26%)
Xanax tablets (10.4%-26.2%)
Zofran injection (11%), tablets (5%-7%)
Zoloft tablets (8.4%)

stipation, gas and bloating, abdominal pain, and decreased absorption of nutrients. Decreased digestive efficiency may lead to a condition called leaky gut syndrome, in which undigested food particles enter the bloodstream causing allergic reactions and depleting the immune system.

Laxatives, Drugs, and Environmental Toxins

The use of some form of over-the-counter laxative is widespread in the U.S. (the Fleet enema is one of the top-selling drugstore products). Yet, according to Dr. Braly, laxatives are only effective as a treatment for occasional constipation. He has found that when laxative use by patients becomes chronic, the laxatives only aggravate the condition. Most over-the-counter laxatives contain ingredients that provide abnormal stimulation of the intestines and slowly paralyze them by damaging intestinal nerves.

Constipation may also result as a side effect from the use of literally hundreds of common medications, including some antibiotics and anti-inflammatory drugs, muscle relaxants, opiates, analgesics, antacids, anticonvulsants, antidepressants, antihypertensives, diuretics, and anesthetics.[6] Physicians prescribe antibiotics to kill the harmful bacteria causing an infection. Unfortunately, these drugs do not distinguish between the unfriendly and friendly microbes that live in our bodies—they cause a massive die-off of friendly bacteria (steroids and birth control pills can have a similar effect). When friendly bacteria are not replaced through diet or supplements, unfriendly bacteria quickly lay claim to the intestines, causing a buildup of toxic materials.

In addition, exposure to some toxic metals (arsenic, lead, and mercury), found in our air and water, are contributing factors to constipation.[7]

Treating Constipation

In treating constipation, Dr. Donovan's aim is to normalize bowel movements, which he believes is absolutely necessary for good health. "The first three things in treating constipation are fluids, fiber, and exercise," he says. "When someone is constipated, it is usually due to an insufficiency of these three things." Alternative medicine offers a variety of methods to help return the colon to a natural state of health, including diet, nutritional supplementation, herbs, stress reduction techniques, and physical therapies, as well as programs from Ayurveda and traditional Chinese medicine.

Diet and Nutrition

Since poor diet is a major cause of constipation, a healthy diet is a key to restoring proper elimination. The general recommendation is to change to a high-fiber diet rich in carbohydrates, vegetables, and fruits, with a proper balance of proteins, vitamins and minerals, roughage, and fluids. Dr. Chaitow recommends a "60/40" diet, where 60% of the total food consumption is fruits and vegetables and the remaining 40% is made up of carbohydrates (20% derived from bread, cereals, and grains), proteins (15%), and fats (5%).

Dr. Donovan emphasizes that increasing dietary fiber increases the frequency and quantity of bowel movements. Major sources of fiber include wheat bran, whole grain products, and beans. The addition of as little as 20 g (0.7 oz) of bran each day can increase fecal weight by 127% and decrease transit time by 40%,[9] two factors that are essential in alleviating constipation and keeping the colon healthy. A study in *The Lancet* showed that an equal quantity of cabbage, carrots, or apples would produce a similar but smaller effect.[10] Sometimes people avoid increasing fiber because they find it less palatable than their usual highly refined diet. Others object to the increase in flatulence and bloating that often results from taking in too much bran too fast. According to Dr. Donovan, this problem can be easily corrected by increasing fiber intake gradually or using more mucilaginous (thick and sticky) forms of bran, such as psyllium or flaxseeds.

The amount of fluids people drink is another important consideration in the treatment of constipation. Dr. Braly recommends a minimum of 6-8 glasses of pure water per day. In order to promote proper digestion, however, high liquid intake should occur away from mealtimes, because consuming excessive liquids with food reduces digestive functions.

According to Steven Bailey, N.D., of Portland, Oregon, juice therapy can be helpful for constipation. One approach involves drinking 16 oz of one of the following juice combinations:

- 8 oz of carrot combined with 8 oz of apple
- 8 oz of carrot, 4 oz of celery, and 4 oz of apple
- 12 oz of carrot combined with 4 oz of spinach

Dr. Donovan recommends combining the intake of fiber and fluids through fruit smoothies. He advises patients to blend a mix of high-pectin fruits like apples, peaches, pears, and berries, with ¼ cup of oat bran and ¼ cup of cracked flaxseed (powder or meal). If there are no dairy allergies, a few tablespoons of yogurt may be added as well.

Donald Brown, N.D., of Seattle, Washington, states that one of the most important nutrients is magnesium, which is naturally found in vegetables and fruits. Although there are a number of effective bulking agents sold in health food stores that help with constipation, Dr. Brown has noted that many people who use them become bloated and still remain constipated. "With these individuals, I usually prescribe a therapeutic dose of magnesium—800 mg daily for adults—and this is often enough to get the plumbing going again. Once this has happened, we can begin work on diet and other bowel conditions," he says.

Dr. Brown also emphasizes the importance of fluid intake and the use of folic acid, particularly with women. Treatment includes a complete medical history, which may show that the problem relates to the use of various drugs and antibiotics. He recommends a stool analysis to check for yeast overgrowth and pays close attention to the function of the liver, which is critical to normal bowel function. Following Dr. Brown's treatment, a patient is usually able to establish healthy, regular bowel movements in three to four weeks, which can then be maintained through improved diet and regular exercise.

Dr. Braly recommends routine nutritional supplementation for constipated patients. He advises using vitamin C (in doses at 90% of bowel tolerance), evening primrose oil (6-8 capsules daily), and increasing dosages of the eicosapentaenoic acid (EPA, a form of essential fatty acid, 3-6 capsules daily).

Probiotics are used to help facilitate the growth of "friendly bacteria" in the colon. Dr. Chaitow recommends daily supplementation with ½ teaspoon of *Lactobacillus acidophilus* in high-potency (over one billion microorganisms per gram) formulations, accompanied by ⅛ teaspoon of *Bifidobacteria bifidum,* taken 20 minutes before meals. He also recommends ½ teaspoon daily of

Lactobacillus bulgaricus, taken with meals to enhance the resident friendly bacteria.

Herbal Medicine

As alternatives to potentially harmful conventional laxatives, a number of natural laxatives are available. Dr. Braly advises every day adding one or two teaspoons of psyllium or ground flaxseed to breakfast cereal or mixed into a beverage. He warns, however, it is possible for some patients to develop severe allergic reactions to psyllium, in which case it should be avoided.

For constipation, Dr. Brown regularly recommends the use of herbs such as aloe, cascara sagrada, senna, and rhubarb. He also advises using dandelion root and silymarin, which help stimulate normal liver functioning and alleviate constipation. Dr. Donovan also uses the medicinal herb blackthorn, which has long been known for its laxative properties; it acts in the large intestine to increase peristalsis.

Stress Reduction

Proper exercise and relaxation play a role in reducing and eliminating constipation, a fact that is recognized by conventional and alternative physicians alike. Exercise tones the abdominal muscles, stimulates the peristaltic action of the colon, decreases emotional stress, and increases breathing and oxygenation of the body, all essential steps in rejuvenating the body and achieving exceptional health. The best exercise, according to Dr. Braly, is a brisk 30-minute walk after a meal, combined with aerobic exercises four to five times weekly. Numerous relaxation therapies, such as meditation, guided imagery, biofeedback, yoga, and Qigong, can also help alleviate stress.

Eating foods slowly, moderately, and in a relaxing environment can also reduce susceptibility to constipation. According to Dr. Laibow, a hormone is released when the stomach is full that triggers the emptying of the colon. Anxiety can override this reflex action.

Dr. Hibbs describes a male patient suffering from many effects of stress, including fatigue and constipation. The patient relied heavily on coffee to keep him going physically and had developed chronic adrenal fatigue. Dr. Hibbs took him off caffeine and sugar, which are both stimulants and were taxing his system. Appropriate exercise and dietary changes were made and he was put on adrenal supportive supplements containing glandular tissue, herbs, and nutrients. His bowel habits normalized quickly and remained that way when he stopped the adrenal supplements several months later.

Physical Therapies

Chiropractic adjustments can help prompt bowel movements. The waves that move material through the colon (peristalsis) occur as a result of nerve excitement that originates at the spinal nerves; adjustments can alleviate spinal subluxations that may be hindering this action.

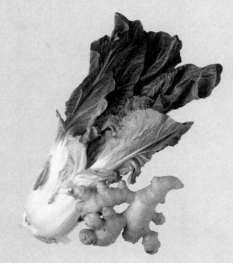

DIETARY GUIDELINES FOR A CLEAN COLON

One way to maintain your intestinal health is to follow these simple dietary guidelines:

- Eliminate or significantly reduce your consumption of white sugar, white flour, white rice, and fried foods
- Make 50% of each meal fresh, raw, unprocessed foods
- Chew each mouthful of food 10-20 times
- Do not eat when emotionally upset
- Each day, eat one serving of protein, at least ½ pound each of two different fruits, six different vegetables (including two ounces of raw fresh sprouts), and at least one serving of whole grains
- Vary foods from meal to meal and from day to day
- Eat your largest meal of the day at noon; do not go to sleep on a full stomach
- Drink a minimum of ½ oz of water per pound of your body weight daily; for example, a 128-pound person needs 64 oz of water; unsweetened fruit and vegetable juices, or herb teas, are also acceptable
- Drink liquids before and after meals, not with them, to avoid diluting digestive fluids
- Eliminate or cut back on stimulants like coffee, black teas, colas, chocolate, and alcohol as well as aspirin and nicotine
- Take a probiotic supplement daily

THE MAYR CURE FOR CONSTIPATION

As an alternative to high liquid intake, Leon Chaitow, N.D., D.O., of London, England, cites a naturopathic cure for digestive problems that involves "reeducating" the digestive system. This diet cure promotes the maximal amount of chewing food: it involves eating dry bread rolls, each morning and before each meal, in order to stimulate salivary flow. During the cure, each mouthful of food is chewed ideally 50 times, until food becomes a paste. This is intended to stimulate the satiety center in the brain and also for marked enzyme mixing with the food, according to Dr. Chaitow.

• Breakfast consists of a stale (three-day-old or dry toasted) roll. Small bites of the dry food should be eaten, with no fluids consumed at all. When the bite of roll has become a paste, place one teaspoon of yogurt (with live cultures) into the mouth. Chew this mixture a few more times (making it a total of 50 chews) and then swallow. Continue following the mouthful of bread paste with teaspoons of yogurt until the roll is consumed. Dr. Chaitow recommends having nothing else for breakfast, but points out that patients will not feel hungry. Thirty minutes after breakfast, Dr. Chaitow advises drinking herbal tea—pau d'arco, lemon verbena, linden blossom, fennel, or sage.

• Lunch consists of another dry roll, consumed as above, followed with lightly cooked vegetables accompanying either a vegetarian, fish, or lean-meat dish. Again, no liquid is consumed with the meal, but herbal tea should follow 30 minutes later.

• The evening meal consists of another dry roll, followed with yogurt, herbal tea, and cooked vegetables.

During the Mayr cure, Dr. Chaitow advises having no fruits, raw vegetables, fatty foods, alcohol, coffee, or sugar. According to Dr. Chaitow, the key to success in this program is the length of time spent chewing food, which is encouraged by the dry roll. If the bowels aren't moving after starting the diet, he recommends taking a teaspoon of Epsom salts in a cup of hot water 30 minutes before breakfast. After 3-5 days, the bowels should start to function efficiently.

Chiropractic adjustments also help normalize the action of the ileocecal valve, the valve that separates the large from the small intestine. If this valve goes into spasms and shuts too tightly, material remains in the small intestine longer than it should, extending transit time. Chiropractic treatment affects the nerve endings connected to the ileocecal valve, which helps to relax it and relieve the spasms.

Massage can help relax the abdominal muscles and encourage normal peristalsis, thus helping to prevent the build-up of fecal material. As stress is also a factor in colon problems, massage acts as a "natural tranquilizer" to restore calm and soothe the digestive tract.[12] Another treatment modality often used by alternative medicine practitioners to treat the colon is reflexology (see Quick Definition). Reflexology therapy stimulates organs of the body through gentle pressure applied to the foot. The reflex areas for the colon are found on the soles of both feet.

> **QD** **Reflexology** is based on the idea that there are reflex areas in the hands and feet that correspond to every part of the body, including the organs and glands. By applying gentle but precise pressure to these reflex points, reflexologists can release blockages that inhibit energy flow and cause pain and disease. Practitioners often focus on breaking up lactic acid and calcium crystals accumulated around any of the 7,200 nerve endings in each foot.

Danish reflexologist Leila Eriksen studied the effectiveness of reflexology treatments among a group of women, 30–60 years old, who had suffered from chronic constipation for an average of 24 years. The average frequency of bowel movements was once every four days. Over a seven-week period, each woman received 15 reflexology treatments lasting 30 minutes each. No other dietary, lifestyle, or treatment programs were used during the study. At the end of the program, the average frequency of bowel motions was once every 1.8 days, or more than twice as frequent as before the study began. In addition, almost half of the women had experienced pain during defecation prior to receiving treatment, but all of the women reported painless bowel movements after treatment. Most were able to reduce their dependency on laxatives as well.[13]

 See Bodywork, Chiropractic, Herbal Medicine, Homeopathy, Osteopathic Medicine.

Ayurvedic Medicine

To treat constipation, Ayurvedic medicine recommends colon detoxification, according to Vasant Lad, M.A.Sc., Director of the Ayurvedic Institute, in Albuquerque, New Mexico. "One method is to use a medicated enema of *dashamoola*, a traditional combination of ten herbs," Dr. Lad explains. He recommends boiling one tablespoon of *dashamoola* powder in one pint of water for ten minutes; strain, cool, and add ½ cup of warm sesame oil. Use this mixture during the *vata* time of day (6-7 a.m. and 6-7 p.m.) until bowel function is improved.

Triphala can also be used, according to Dr. Lad, at a dose of up to one teaspoon of powder in a warm glass of water before bedtime. "Some people may experience a diuretic effect from *triphala*," Dr. Lad says. "In these cases, they can steep the mixture overnight and strain and drink it in the morning. Senna leaves are also used in Ayurvedic tradition to treat constipation, taking ½ teaspoon or less with ginger tea. During pregnancy, however, *triphala* and senna should not be used. Instead, take one cup of hot milk with a teaspoon of ghee (clarified butter) before bedtime. This usually acts as a mild laxative during pregnancy." It is also important to consume some amount of roughage in the diet on a regular basis, such as wheat or oat bran, notes Dr. Lad.

For children with constipation, Virender Sodhi, M.D. (Ayurveda), N.D., Director of the Ayurvedic & Naturopathic Medical Clinic, in Bellevue, Washington, recommends drinking almond oil with a dash of sugar added to increase peristalsis. *Acacia fistula*, a sweet fruit high in vitamin C and fiber, can also be used mixed with sugar, honey, and rose petals.

Traditional Chinese Medicine

Maoshing Ni, D.O.M., Ph.D., L.Ac., President of Yo San University, in Marina del Rey, California, recommends a combination of herbs and exercise, in addition to dietary changes, when treating constipation. "Acupuncture," he states, "can restore the natural peristaltic action of the colon, as can exercise, deep breathing, and massage." Rhubarb root, aloe vera, and senna leaf are often given as a tea by Dr. Ni to alleviate constipation and to help rehydrate the intestines. "But the use of herbs is more complex," Dr. Ni says, "and must be matched to the conditions and constitution of the individual. An elderly or frail person would be given a different herbal compound than someone else, perhaps a mixture of seed lubricants like sesame, apricot kernel, and peach kernel."

In traditional Chinese medicine, diet is also a highly individualized matter, but Dr. Ni generally recommends a high-fiber diet for constipation. "Beets and cabbage have done wonders," he adds, "particularly for people who may find that bran is too harsh."

 See Acupuncture, Ayurvedic Medicine, Traditional Chinese Medicine.

Recommendations

- Increasing dietary fiber increases the frequency and quantity of bowel movements. Major sources of fiber include wheat bran, whole grain products, and beans.

> ### SUCCESS STORY: HOMEOPATHY RELIEVES CONSTIPATION
>
> When his mother brought Robert, 7, to homeopath Sujata Owens, R.S.Hom., of Northfield, Minnesota, he had suffered from severe constipation since birth. In fact, during his first four months of life, Robert had no bowel movements. He had a condition called congenital megacolon or Hirschsprung's disease: a portion of his large intestine lacked the nerve endings necessary to produce peristalsis, the muscular movements leading towards evacuation.
>
> Robert's symptoms included bloating, vomiting, sharp, cramping pains in his abdomen, and frequent, painful urination. On the average, he moved his bowels only once a week and only after great effort. He was always exhausted, looked sad, rarely smiled, and had little interest in anything; he also had difficulties learning, was underweight, sucked his thumb constantly, wet his bed at night, had a poor appetite, and was nervous. "He was a quiet, shy boy with very low energy," says Dr. Owens. He had undergone numerous conventional medical tests and procedures, including ultrasound, surgery, antibiotics, and frequent short-term hospitalizations for pain attacks, but benefited very little from any of it, Robert's mother reported.
>
> Dr. Owens prescribed a single medium-potency dose of *Plumbum Metallicum* 200C, which is homeopathic lead. Two weeks later in a follow-up consultation, Dr. Owens judged the results to be "excellent, with 80% improvement." Robert was a changed boy: he was talkative, energetic, mentally alert, and having 1-3 bowel movements every day. He was free of abdominal pain, vomiting, and bedwetting, his appetite was good, and he urinated without any pain.[11]

- Drink a minimum of 6–8 glasses of pure water per day.

- Probiotics can help facilitate the growth of "friendly bacteria" in the colon.

- Herbs such as aloe vera, cascara sagrada, senna, and rhubarb may be helpful for relieving constipation.

- Exercise tones the abdominal muscles, stimulates the peristaltic action of the colon, decreases emotional

CLEANSE INTERNALLY WITH LIQUID CLAY

Natural clay, especially the form known as bentonite, has been used medicinally for centuries by indigenous peoples around the world. In recent years, bentonite has been increasingly prescribed by practitioners of alternative medicine as a simple but effective internal cleanser to assist in reversing numerous health problems. The name *bentonite* refers to clay first identified in cretaceous rocks in Fort Benton, Wyoming. Although bentonite deposits occur worldwide, many of the largest concentrations are found in the Great Plains area of North America. Bentonite is not a mineral but a commercial name for montmorillonite, the active mineral in many medicinal clays, which comes from weathered volcanic ash.

Liquid clay contains minerals that, once inside the gastrointestinal tract, are able to absorb toxins and deliver mineral nutrients. Liquid clay is inert, which means it passes through the body undigested. Technically, the clay first *adsorbs* toxins (heavy metals, free radicals, pesticides), attracting them to its extensive surface area; then it *absorbs* the toxins, taking them in the way a sponge mops up water. The clay's minerals are negatively charged while toxins tend to be positively charged, hence the clay's attraction works like a magnet.

According to the *Canadian Journal of Microbiology*, bentonite can absorb pathogenic viruses, aflatoxin (the toxic by-product of a mold), and pesticides and herbicides.[14] The clay is eventually eliminated from the body with the toxins bound to its surfaces. Benefits reported by people using liquid clay include: improved intestinal regularity; relief from chronic constipation, diarrhea, indigestion, and ulcers; a surge in energy; enhanced alertness; emotional uplift; improved tissue repair; and increased resistance to infections.

The best way to drink clay is on an empty stomach, at least an hour before or after a meal or immediately before sleeping. Clay is available as a thick, tasteless, gray gel, but it also comes as a powder or encapsulated. Typically, start with one tablespoon daily, mixed with a small amount of juice; observe the results for a week, then gradually increase the dosage to no more than four tablespoons per day, in doses spread throughout the day.

stress, and increases breathing and oxygenation of the body, all essential steps in achieving normal bowel function.

- Eating foods slowly, moderately, and in a relaxing environment can reduce susceptibility to constipation.

- Chiropractic and massage can help relax the abdominal muscles and encourage normal peristalsis.

- Ayurvedic medicine recommends colon detoxification to treat constipation.

- Traditional Chinese medicine uses acupuncture to restore the natural peristaltic action of the colon, along with exercise, deep breathing, and massage.

Self–Care

The following therapies can be undertaken at home under appropriate professional supervision:

Fasting / Qigong and Tai Chi / Yoga

AROMATHERAPY: Massage clockwise around the abdomen with rose, marjoram, camphor, fennel, black pepper, or rosemary.

HOMEOPATHY: *Alumina, Bryonia, Graphites, Natrum mur., Nux vomica, Silicea*

HYDROTHERAPY: • Constitutional hydrotherapy (apply two to five times weekly). • Enema or colon irrigation (apply daily as needed). • For spastic constipation, take a hot sitz bath for more than ten minutes; keep a cold compress on the forehead and drink water. Also, take a hot and cold shower (alternate long hot streams and short cold streams on the abdomen). • For chronic constipation, use a cold compress on the abdomen covered with a large dry towel.

JUICE THERAPY: • Carrot, beet, or celery juice with one teaspoon of garlic or yellow onion juice • For chronic constipation, add garlic, yellow onion, black radish, spinach, watercress, or dandelion to carrot, beet, celery, cabbage, cucumber, tomato • Lemon juice • Apple juice • Carrot, apple • Carrot, celery, apple • Carrot, spinach

LIFESTYLE: Take a brisk walk early in the morning.

Professional Care

The following therapies should only be provided by a qualified health professional:

Biofeedback Training and Neurotherapy / Chiropractic / Craniosacral Therapy / Detoxification Therapy / Environmental Medicine / Hypnotherapy / Magnetic Field Therapy / Mind - Body Medicine / Osteopathic Medicine

BODYWORK: Reflexology, shiatsu, Trager Approach

Where to Find Help

For more information on, or referrals for, treatment of constipation, contact the following organizations.

American Association of Oriental Medicine (AAOM)
433 Front Street
Catasauqua, Pennsylvania 18032
(888) 500-7999
Website: www.aaom.org

The AAOM is a national professional organization of acupuncturists who meet acceptable standards of competency and can provide you with the names and locations of local members.

American Association of Naturopathic Physicians
601 Valley Street, Suite 105
Seattle, Washington 98109
(206) 298-0126
Website: www.naturopathic.org

Contact them for the location of a licensed naturopathic physician in your area.

American Chiropractic Association
1701 Clarendon Boulevard
Arlington, Virginia 22209
(800) 986-4636
Website: www.acatoday.com

A major source for chiropractic information, including a monthly publication and newsletter. Provides referrals on request.

Ayurvedic & Naturopathic Medical Clinic
2115 112th Avenue N.E.
Bellevue, Washington 98004
(425) 453-8022
Website: www.ayurvedicscience.com

Dr. Virender Sodhi's clinic provides medical training for physicians and health-care practitioners, as well as individual courses for laypeople.

Occidental Institute Research Foundation
P.O. Box 100
Penticton, B.C., Canada V2A 6J9
(800) 663-8342 or (250) 497-6020

For information about Mayr therapy.

Recommended Reading

Dr. Braly's Food Allergy and Nutrition Revolution. James Braly, M.D. New Canaan, CT: Keats Publishing, 1992.

Encyclopedia of Natural Medicine. Michael Murray, N.D., and Joseph Pizzorno, N.D. Rocklin, CA: Prima Publishing, 1998.

Healthy Digestion the Natural Way. D. Lindsey Berkson. New York: John Wiley & Sons, 2000.

Herbs for Improved Digestion. C.J. Puotinen. New Canaan, CT: Keats Publishing, 1996.

What Your Doctor Won't Tell You. Jane Heimlich. New York: HarperCollins, 1990.

DIABETES

An estimated 16 million people in the United States suffer from diabetes and about 500,000 new cases are reported each year. Diabetes kills 180,000 Americans annually, which makes it the seventh leading cause of death. Practitioners of alternative medicine combine diet, supplemental nutrients, exercise, and weight loss to help control diabetes and prevent or delay the onset of serious complications.

DIABETES MELLITUS, more commonly referred to simply as diabetes, is a chronic degenerative disease caused by a lack of, or resistance to, the hormone insulin, which is essential for the proper metabolism of blood sugar (glucose). Normally blood sugar rises after a meal as glucose is absorbed into the bloodstream, causing the pancreas to produce enough insulin to return the blood sugar level to its normal range. Diabetic individuals are either unable to produce enough insulin or their cells have become resistant to insulin, and they are unable to move glucose from the bloodstream to the cells, and thus cannot maintain a normal blood glucose level.

Excess glucose in the bloodstream is toxic, according to Peter H. Forsham, M.D., of Evergreen Hospital, in Kirkland, Washington, noting that excess glucose in diabetics can diminish the biological effectiveness of various proteins in the body. For example, when glucose binds to hemoglobin (the iron-containing pigment of the red blood cells), the oxygen-carrying capacity of hemoglobin is reduced.[1]

Diabetes is a leading cause of blindness, kidney failure, limb amputations, and heart disease.[2] The cost of diabetes and its medical complications (resulting from a failure to control the disease) is an estimated $100 billion annually, accounting for about 15% of current health-care spending.[3] "About 95% of diabetes cases can be treated successfully with diet, nutrition, and herbs," says Daniel Dunphy, P.A.-C., of San Francisco, California. "While juvenile diabetes can have a genetic factor, adult-onset diabetes, in most cases, is produced by a combination of factors such as high stress, faulty diet, obesity,

> *Diabetes can lead to heart and kidney disease, atherosclerosis, hypertension, strokes, cataracts, retinal hemorrhages, neuropathy, gangrenous infections, loss of hearing, blindness, and even death.*

impaired digestion, and an overworked pancreas."

Types of Diabetes

There are two major forms of diabetes, insulin-dependent juvenile diabetes (Type I) and non-insulin-dependent adult-onset diabetes (Type II).

In Type I diabetes, the body is unable to produce enough insulin. As a result, glucose builds up in the bloodstream and spills over into the urine, while the body literally "starves" because the cells cannot get the nourishment, which is provided by glucose, to produce energy for the cells' normal functions. Symptoms of Type I diabetes include excessive thirst, hunger, urination, and dehydration, often accompanied by weight loss. Insulin injections are currently the only method in conventional medicine to control Type I diabetes but are not considered a cure. Injections must be administered daily (sometimes several times a day, usually before meals) and must be timed so that the peak action of the insulin will occur when the sugar from the meal elevates the blood glucose to its highest level. Type I diabetes usually begins in childhood, but it may occur later in life if the pancreas is damaged due to injury or disease; 5%–10% of those diagnosed with diabetes are Type I diabetics.[4]

Type II accounts for the majority of diabetes cases and is increasing at epidemic proportions in the U.S., due in large part to poor diet, rising levels of obesity, increasingly sedentary lifestyles, and greater numbers of people living longer. Symptoms are the same as for Type I, with the exception of weight loss. In Type II diabetes, the pancreas still produces insulin, but the cells are resistant to its action and therefore cannot absorb the glucose produced by food intake. The cells of the body may also be unable to properly utilize insulin in the absorption of glucose from the bloodstream. Often Type II diabetes can be remedied by dietary management, exercise, and weight control. Oral medications prescribed to stimulate the body to produce more insulin can also be used until blood sugar levels are brought to normal and stabilized. When the insulin levels in a Type II diabetic are out of control as a result of dietary abuse and lack of exercise, however, insulin injections may be temporarily required to restore balance. Once diet and weight are under control, the insulin shots are usually no longer needed.

Either type of diabetes, when poorly controlled, can lead to heart and kidney disease, atherosclerosis, hypertension, strokes, cataracts, retinal hemorrhages, neuropathy (nerve damage), gastroparesis (loss of peristaltic action in the gastrointestinal tract), gangrenous infections of cuts or sores (with possible amputation of the feet or legs), loss of hearing, blindness, and even death. These complications are easier to avoid in both types of diabetes if blood sugar levels are kept as close to the normal range as possible.

Causes of Diabetes

Although a genetic predisposition appears to govern susceptibility to both types of diabetes, a number of other factors can also be involved. Diet and obesity are key elements in the cause of Type II diabetes. Autoimmune processes, in which antibodies created to fight allergies or certain infections react against the body itself, may also play a role in causing both types of diabetes.

Type I Diabetes

In Type I diabetes the insulin-producing cells of the pancreas are destroyed and become unable to produce insulin. Seventy-five percent of Type I diabetics have antibodies to their own pancreatic cells, as opposed to 0.5% to 2.0% of individuals without diabetes, supporting the theory of an autoimmune cause of the disease.[6]

Microbial infections may be responsible for initiating the autoimmune disease process in Type I diabetes. Microbes that may induce an autoimmune reaction include the pertussis (whooping cough) bacteria, hepatitis virus, rubella virus, Coxsackie virus, Epstein-Barr virus, cytomegalovirus, and herpes virus-6.[7] Also, some people with Type I diabetes have antibodies to the albumin (a simple protein) in cow's milk, which are capable of reacting with the insulin-producing cells in the pancreas.[8]

GESTATIONAL DIABETES

A third type of diabetes, gestational diabetes, is found in pregnant women and is a temporary condition. Characterized by excessive hunger, thirst, and the need to urinate, it is a mild condition and often goes unnoticed, but it is an important condition to treat because elevated blood sugar levels can damage the fetus. Gestational diabetes can usually be controlled with diet but may require insulin. It has been found to respond well, and even to resolve, with a combination of diet and exercise.[5] Jonathan Wright, M.D., Director of the Tahoma Clinic, in Kent, Washington, says he has had success treating, and even curing, gestational diabetes with diet and nutritional supplements, particularly vitamin B6.

Susceptibility to Type I diabetes may also be genetically predetermined. Every individual has a specific "tissue type" (similar to a blood type) that is inherited from the person's parents. Ongoing immunology research shows that many diseases, including Type I diabetes, seem to occur predominantly among persons with specific tissue types.[9]

Type II Diabetes

Diet, obesity, allergies to certain foods, viral infections, and stress are all factors that can contribute to the onset of or aggravate Type II diabetes. An estimated 85% of all Type II diabetics are overweight when diagnosed.[10] After completion of a worldwide study sponsored by the United Nations, Australian scientist Kelly West, M.D., Ph.D., concluded, "The cause of Type II diabetes is usually obesity; the preventative, and often the cure, is leanness."[11] Dr. Ernest Pfeiffer, Professor of Medicine at Ulm University, in Germany, concurs. "It's almost a law that any person 30% overweight for 30 years will become a diabetic."[12]

The main cause of obesity is poor diet, and the key factor is not how much but what is consumed. Largely at fault are processed foods, which are high in calories and stripped of valuable fiber and essential nutrients, according to Jonathan Wright, M.D., Director of the Tahoma Clinic, in Kent, Washington.

A poor diet, in and of itself, is also a major contributing factor for Type II diabetes, as exemplified by what has happened over the years on the Pacific island of Nauru. Until recently, Type II diabetes was unknown in Nauru, where the islanders ate a simple diet consisting mainly of bananas and yams. When phosphates were discovered and mined on the island, the inhabitants

COMPLICATIONS OF DIABETES

Complications with Type I and Type II diabetes can occur when blood sugar levels are not properly controlled. These include ketoacidosis and hyperosmolar coma. When blood sugar levels are not controlled over long periods of time, circulatory problems can occur causing damage to the small blood vessels that supply various tissues, resulting in retinopathy (damage to the retina), neuropathy (nerve damage), nephropathy (kidney disease), strokes, heart attacks, and foot ulcers.

Ketoacidosis: When insulin-dependent (Type I) diabetics do not take sufficient insulin, glucose builds up in the bloodstream. The body must then break down fats for energy, but this process produces ketones, which are toxic to the body and can induce a state of acidosis (excessive acidity in the body). Large doses of insulin are needed to overcome the insulin resistance in this state and hospitalization is often necessary.

Hyperosmolar coma: When severe dehydration occurs (from deficient fluid intake, high blood sugar levels, or physical stress such as infection or surgery), it may result in a condition known as hyperosmolar coma (coma from dehydration). This is a medical emergency requiring hospitalization, as it is fatal in 50% of cases.

Diabetic retinopathy: Damage to the retina in diabetics is one of the leading causes of blindness in the U.S.[17] In poorly controlled diabetes, fragile new blood vessels are formed in the retina in an attempt to bring more oxygen to the eye. However, these vessels often break, hemorrhaging into the eye. Laser treatments help to stop the bleeding, but in doing so destroy much of the retina, which is essential for sight.

Diabetic neuropathy: Damage to the peripheral nervous system is characterized by pain and numbness, most frequently occurring in the feet and legs. It is usually due to severe damage to the small blood vessels supplying the peripheral nervous system.

Diabetic nephropathy: Damage to the kidneys is a leading cause of death in diabetics. It is primarily due to damage to the small blood vessels supplying the kidneys.

Diabetic strokes: Strokes are caused by damage to and clogging in the blood vessels in the brains of diabetics. Large strokes can cause paralysis, speech loss, severe lack of coordination, vision loss, and death. Very small strokes can cause progressive dementia or senility.

Diabetic heart attacks: Heart attacks occur much more commonly in diabetics than non-diabetics.

Diabetic foot ulcers: A lack of oxygen supply and peripheral nerve damage due to diabetic clogging of small blood vessels are the main causes of foot ulcers in diabetics. Without proper treatment, gangrene can form, necessitating amputation. To prevent this, the feet should be kept clean, dry, and warm. Diabetics should never go barefoot, as injuries such as cuts and bruises may not be noticed because of numbness from nerve damage, and ulcers may also occur.

---

attained wealth and settled into a life of leisure, which included adopting a Western diet high in sugar, fat, and carbohydrates. With this change in lifestyle, many began to develop Type II diabetes. Now, according to a study by the World Health Organization (WHO), up to half of the urbanized Nauru population, 30–64 years old, has diabetes, illustrating that adult-onset diabetes may be triggered by poor diet rather than genetic makeup.

The WHO concludes that an apparent epidemic of diabetes has occurred—or is occurring—in adult people throughout the world, a trend that appears to be strongly related to lifestyle and socioeconomic change, and the fact that populations in developed communities in industrialized countries now face the greatest risk.[13] Another telling example of the role of diet in diabetes occurred in England during World War II. When food shortages and rationing removed white flour, sugar, excessive meat protein, and fats from the typical English diet, the death rate from diabetes fell 50%.[14]

Sensitivities to certain foods, as well as viral infections, can result in lower insulin levels in Type II diabetics, causing inflammation and autoimmune damage to the insulin-producing cells of the pancreas.[15] Stress and an individual's ability to manage stress are also important factors affecting the course of diabetes and insulin requirements.[16] Stress can result in the production of adrenaline and cortisol, which increases blood sugar and thus interferes with diabetic control.

 See Obesity and Weight Loss.

Treating Diabetes

The goal for any doctor or patient in treating diabetes is to bring high blood sugar under control and, as much as possible, to stabilize it at a normal level. This can best be achieved by a treatment approach that encourages diabetics to become actively responsible for their own health.

For Type I diabetics, who are usually permanently insulin-dependent, a proper diet and a moderate amount of regular exercise are essential for lowering the overall blood sugar level, which reduces the amount of injected insulin required. Type II diabetics can adequately control their blood sugar levels by experimenting with various foods, frequency and size of meals, and other aspects of their lifestyle such as exercise and stress reduction.[18] They may even be able to forego insulin or oral medicine entirely when blood sugar levels are stabilized by weight reduction, exercise, nutrient supplements, and a sensible food plan. In either case, lowered insulin intake means the likelihood of fewer complications from the disease.[19]

Diet

According to Dr. Wright, a diet emphasizing foods high in complex carbohydrates and fiber, such as whole grains, legumes, and vegetables, reduces the need for insulin by slowing and controlling the release of glucose into the bloodstream. The fiber in plant foods can also be beneficial for diabetics by absorbing water in the body, and forming a natural "sponge" in which food particles are suspended. Dr. Wright suggests that diabetics avoid simple carbohydrates (such as fruit juices) and foods containing refined sugar (such as processed foods, cookies, and pastries), because these foods raise the blood sugar rapidly, thereby requiring a sudden rise in insulin levels, that places stress on the pancreas.

James Anderson, M.D., of the Department of Veterans Affairs at the University of Kentucky, in Lexington, has found that eating a diet high in fiber and complex carbohydrates helps control Type II diabetes and allows the patient to reduce insulin requirements.[21] Dr. Anderson says that patients on oral hypoglycemics (compounds that cause a decrease in blood sugar) and those taking less than 40 units of insulin respond particularly well, as do those who are overweight.

His nutrition plan calls for 55% to 60% of the daily calorie intake to be derived from carbohydrates (two-thirds of these from complex carbohydrates), 14% to 20% from protein (minimum 45 g daily), and 20% to 25% or less from fat (10% or less from saturated fat), with only 200 mg or less of cholesterol daily, plus 40-50 g total dietary fiber daily (10-15 g of this as soluble fiber). According to Dr. Anderson, this plan lowers fats in the

---

WATCH OUT FOR HIDDEN SUGARS

Finding out whether a food product contains sugar requires more sleuthing today than it once did. Only a few manufacturers currently include the word *sugar* in the list of ingredients of their sugar-containing products. Instead, wanting to avoid the sugar stigma that could negatively impact sales, many food producers hide the sugars in their products behind a host of chemical synonyms. Take note that any product listing any of the following ingredients really does contain sugar:

- dextrose
- sucrose
- glucose
- corn sweetener
- fructose
- dextrin
- high-fructose corn syrup
- lactose
- modified cornstarch
- maltodextrin
- maltose
- malt
- fruit juice concentrates
- mannitol
- sorghum
- xylitol
- sorbitol

Although all of these are sugars, fructose does stand apart from the rest. Of all the sugars, fructose (the primary sugar in fruits) has the least severe insulin reaction.[20] However, consuming fructose does increase the rate of cataract formation, especially in diabetics.

---

bloodstream and thus reduces the risk of cardiovascular disease in diabetics. Dr. Anderson points out that since the average American diet contains 11-23 g of fiber daily, some diabetics would need to double or triple their fiber intake. He suggests doing this slowly by adding one high-fiber food per week, particularly whole grains and beans, and increasing fluid intake to help the body adjust to the increased gas production, a common side effect of added fiber.[22]

A vegetarian diet of whole grains and whole fruits and vegetables (rather than juices, which are rapidly absorbed) can be helpful for many diabetics. The American Dietetic Association has published research showing that a vegetarian lifestyle reduces the incidence of diabetes and heart disease.[23] With Type II diabetics, how-

DIETARY GUIDELINES FOR DIABETICS

Jonathan Wright, M.D., of Kent, Washington, recommends the following dietary control measures for all diabetics:

- Totally eliminate refined sugar and sugar products.
- Avoid "junk" foods.
- Eat snacks of protein between meals.
- Eat complex carbohydrates, such as whole grains, fresh fruits, and vegetables, which release their natural sugars more slowly and evenly into the bloodstream.
- Reduce or eliminate the intake of alcohol, tobacco, and caffeine.
- Take off excess weight through exercise and calorie reduction.

ever, Dr. Wright feels that it is necessary to restrict total carbohydrate intake. He recommends moderate amounts of fish and lean meats as sources of protein, along with unsaturated fats and supplementation with vitamins C and E, B-complex vitamins, magnesium, chromium, and zinc. He also suggests small, frequent meals. A daily diet of three small meals, plus mid-morning, mid-afternoon, and bedtime snacks, is the ideal, according to Dr. Wright.

He cites the case of a 47-year-old man who had recently been diagnosed with diabetes. An extensive family history of diabetes included his father, whose condition had led to two cataract surgeries, and two uncles who had suffered heart attacks as a result of diabetes. His doctor had suggested that he reduce his intake of sugar and salt and get more exercise, but said there was little more he could do. Dr. Wright's first recommendation was a change in eating habits, and he used as a model the so-called caveman diet—complex carbohydrate intake combined with moderate amounts of protein and little or no processed foods. To deal specifically with the patient's concern about cataracts, Dr. Wright recommended bioflavonoid supplements to inhibit the enzyme aldose reductase, which has been implicated in the formation of cataracts. In addition, Dr. Wright suggested nutritional supplementation, specifically vitamins C, B_6, and E, as well as cod liver oil, to slow the process of blood platelet clumping, which is associated with various diabetic complications. This, combined with the rest of Dr. Wright's regimen, normalized his blood sugar and blood clotting time, and eventually all symptoms of diabetes were alleviated.

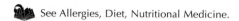 See Allergies, Diet, Nutritional Medicine.

THE GLYCEMIC INDEX

Although pure sugar will cause the greatest insulin response in our bodies, many other foods have a similar insulinogenic (insulin stimulating) effect. To evaluate foods based on their insulin impact, a scientific rating system called the glycemic index was developed by diabetes researchers at the University of Toronto. The index offers a comparison of the insulin effect of different foods, measuring their real-life impact on blood sugar levels. Those foods with a high rating on the glycemic index cause a higher insulin response than those with a low rating.

Richard Podell, M.D., Medical Director of the Overlook Center for Weight Management, in Springfield, New Jersey, indicates that choosing foods with a low glycemic index is "the secret to keeping blood sugar stable and insulin low." Dr. Podell has simplified the index into basic categories, which he presents in his book *The G-Index Diet.*[24] He makes the following general observations:

- Foods with a higher rating, causing a higher insulin response, include white bread, bagels, English muffins, packaged flaked cereals, instant hot cereals, low-fat frozen desserts, raisins and other dried fruits, whole milk and whole-milk cheeses, peanuts and peanut butter, hot dogs, and luncheon meats.

- Foods with a low rating, not causing a high insulin spike, include most fresh vegetables, leafy greens, pitted fruits and melons, coarse 100% whole-grain breads and minimally processed whole-grain cereals, sweet potatoes and yams, skim milk, buttermilk, poultry, lean cuts of beef, pork, and veal, shellfish, white-fleshed fish, most legumes, and most nuts.

- Cooked foods rank higher on the index than raw foods. Similarly, fruits and vegetables that have been juiced or puréed are higher on the index than when eaten whole.

FOOD INTOLERANCES

Dr. Wright recommends that diabetics should be thoroughly tested for food intolerances, which may be contributing to their disease by causing inflammation and autoimmune destruction of the insulin-producing cells of the pancreas. Foods that often are associated with diabetes-related problems include corn, wheat, chocolate, and dairy products.

Research raises the possibility that in some cases of Type I diabetes, the disease may be an autoimmune reaction caused by cow's milk. It is estimated that 75% of Type I diabetics are allergic to their own pancreatic cells and have antibodies to disable them. A recent Australian study showed that children given a cow's milk formula during the first three months of life were 52% more likely to develop Type I diabetes. Conversely, those infants who were exclusively breast-fed during the first three months after birth had a 34% reduced risk of developing diabetes. An Italian study demonstrated an 88% positive correlation between the amount of dairy milk consumed by children and their risk level for Type I diabetes. Apparently, bovine serum albumin, a protein found in cow's milk, closely resembles a molecule found on the surface of certain pancreas cells. This resemblance causes the immune system to react against the pancreatic cells as if they were foreign proteins.[25]

William H. Philpott, M.D., of Choctaw, Oklahoma, has observed the cause of insulin resistance in Type II diabetes to be edema (swelling) of body cells mostly due to reactions to foods and, to a lesser extent, to chemicals and inhalants.[26] The evidence for this was accumulated by examining blood sugar before and after test meals of single foods. When the offending foods were removed, the diabetic reaction vanished. This reversal of the diabetic reaction occurred immediately upon withdrawal of the offending foods, before any weight reduction or nutritional supplementation. Reactions to foods, chemicals, and inhalants as a cause of insulin resistance in Type II diabetes was confirmed by several research studies.[27] Treatment consists of a four-day diversified rotation diet, which leaves out the offending food for three months. This is followed by the gradual re-introduction of these foods back into the diet.

Nutritional Supplements

Abram Ber, M.D., of Scottsdale, Arizona, treats diabetics with diet and nutritional supplementation and feels this is an essential part of therapy. He uses supplements of vitamin B6 and biotin, chromium, magnesium, vanadium, essential fatty acids, and flaxseed oil. He also recommends Jerusalem artichoke (*Helianthus tuberosus*) as part of the diet and uses a mixture of Chinese herbs for his patients. According to Dr. Ber, this treatment can prevent and even reverse the complications of diabetes (such as neuropathy, retinopathy, and nephropathy). He cites the case of a Type I diabetic who had lost most of his eyesight due to diabetic retinopathy and was unable to drive. Over a period of approximately six months on Dr. Ber's supplement program, he regained his vision and is now able to drive and continues to do well.

DIABETES AND STABILIZED RICE BRAN

A study published in the *Journal of Nutritional Biochemistry* (March 2002) found that patients with diabetes (Type I or II) can benefit by eating stabilized rice bran produced by NutraStar, Inc. In the study, participants (20-65 years old) were placed on the National Cholesterol Education Program Step-1 diet, then randomly assigned to the stabilized rice bran regimen or a control group. At the end of the study, those who ate the rice bran (20 g per day for eight weeks) were shown to have significant decreases in fasting glucose (blood sugar) levels compared to the control group, indicating that stabilized rice bran can play a role in managing diabetes symptoms. (For further information, go to www.nutrastar.com.)

There are many nutrients that have proven valuable in treating diabetes.

B Vitamins: Levels of vitamin B6 in the body drop sharply after the age of 50, when Type II diabetes is most likely to occur.[28] Vitamin B6 taken daily can reduce insulin need and improve basic health.[29] Type II diabetics regained normal blood sugar levels with doses of 100 mg daily of vitamin B6 in tests by John Ellis, M.D., who recommends 50 mg daily for maintenance.[30] Symptoms of diabetic neuropathy were reduced or totally eliminated by vitamin B6 supplements in studies at the Thordek Medical Center in Chicago.[31]

Biotin, a component of vitamin B complex, works synergistically with insulin and helps in glucose utilization.[32] Research has shown that biotin is also beneficial for preventing and managing peripheral neuropathy in diabetics.[33] According to Dr. Wright, diabetic neuropathy also responds well to vitamin B12 when it is used in conjunction with topical application of capsicum, a cayenne pepper extract that relieves the pain of neuropathy. Capsicum works by removing substance P, a pain mediator, from the skin. Dr. Wright also finds that niacinamide (vitamin B3) can be beneficial in the early stages of Type I diabetes.

Vitamin C: A high intake of vitamin C has been found to reduce insulin need, maintain eye health, and help prevent cataracts.[34] It is also important in helping to fight infections, to which diabetics are particularly prone. Megadoses of vitamin C have been shown to prevent or delay the vascular complications of diabetes by promoting the production of collagen, which strengthens the blood vessels. However, kidney function should

NUTRIENTS FOR CONTROLLING BLOOD SUGAR

Certain nutrients are required by the body for glucose metabolism, specifically chromium, zinc, B-complex vitamins (particularly pantothenic acid or B5), and vitamin C. The following are dietary sources of these nutrients (foods are listed in descending order of nutrient content):

- Chromium—brewer's yeast, whole wheat and rye breads, beef liver, potatoes, green peppers, eggs, chicken, apples, butter, parsnips, and cornmeal

- Zinc—fresh oysters, ginger root, lamb, pecans, split peas, beef liver, egg yolk, whole wheat, rye, oats, lima beans, almonds, walnuts, sardines, chicken, and buckwheat

- B-complex vitamins—brewer's yeast, beef and chicken liver, mushrooms, split peas, blue cheese, pecans, eggs, lobster, oats, buckwheat, rye, broccoli, turkey and chicken (dark meat), brown rice, whole wheat, red chili peppers, sardines, avocado, and kale

- Vitamin C—acerola cherries, red chili peppers, guava, sweet red peppers, kale, parsley, collard and turnip greens, green peppers, broccoli, Brussels sprouts, mustard greens, cauliflower, red cabbage, strawberries, papayas, spinach, oranges, lemons, grapefruit, turnips, mangoes, asparagus, cantaloupe, Swiss chard, green onions, and tangerines

be tested first because megadoses of vitamin C can be toxic in a diabetic with renal insufficiency. A deficiency of vitamin C has been shown to cause degeneration of the insulin-producing cells of the pancreas.[35]

Vitamin E: According to Evan Shute, M.D., co-founder of Canada's Shute Foundation for Medical Research, vitamin E is essential for the treatment of diabetes.[36] Vitamin E is a powerful antioxidant and has a significant anticlotting effect, which may be a factor in preventing the development of vascular complications, such as damage to the eyes and kidneys, seen frequently in diabetes.[37] Supplementation of vitamin E has freed some Type II diabetics from taking insulin and has also been shown to reduce the rate of blood clotting in Type II diabetes.[38]

Chromium: The body's chromium stores are mobilized immediately when either glucose or insulin enters the bloodstream. According to Dr. Philpott, even the slightest deficiency of chromium upsets the body's tolerance to glucose. The lack of chromium in the modern American diet is acute[39] and is aggravated by consumption of refined sugar, which robs the body of stored chromium.[40]

Chromium supplements are effective in treating hypoglycemia (low blood sugar) and act as a "normalizer" of glucose for insulin-dependent diabetics.[41] Exercise appears to increase the levels of chromium in the tissues and increases the number of insulin receptors on cells in Type I diabetics.[42] Chromium has been shown to restore normal insulin function in Type II diabetics.[43] In a group of Type II diabetics, glucose tolerance was restored to 50% of normal with daily doses of 150 mcg of trivalent chromium (the only type of chromium believed to be biologically active in the human body).[44]

Magnesium and Potassium: Deficiencies of magnesium and potassium create greater glucose intolerance and contribute to damage to organs and the nerves that supply them due to disturbed cell function.[45] Magnesium is essential for the maintenance of a healthy cardiovascular system as well.[46] It reduces fats (lipids) and cholesterol circulating in the blood, is an effective vasodilator (used to widen blood vessels), and helps prevent retinopathy and atherosclerosis. Diabetics who have experienced ketoacidosis are particularly likely to be magnesium deficient. Insulin administration also induces hypokalemia (low blood potassium levels), while potassium supplementation helps improve insulin sensitivity, responsiveness, and secretion.[47]

Vanadium: Vanadium is an essential trace element (found in black pepper, dill seed, unsaturated vegetable oils, and grains) that may mimic insulin to help regulate blood sugar. It is available in supplement form as vanadyl sulfate; typical dosage is 5-20 mg daily.[48]

Zinc: Zinc is essential for the normal production of insulin and the digestion of proteins[49] and has antiviral effects. To confirm a need, ask a doctor for a white blood cell or saliva test, as serum zinc level tests are unreliable, according to Dr. Wright.

Alpha-Lipoic Acid: Alpha-lipoic acid has been prescribed by German physicians for over 30 years to help patients with adult-onset diabetes. Researchers have shown that, when administered intravenously at a dose of 1,000 mg, alpha-lipoic acid can help lower insulin resistance and increase the cellular utilization of glucose by more than 50%. Nevertheless, taking supplements at this dosage is not recommended for everyone and should be done under a doctor's supervision. Dosages up to 100 mg daily generally do not require supervision.

Coenzyme Q10: Also called ubiquinone, coenzyme Q10 occurs naturally in all human cells. Its actions are similar to vitamin E and it also stimulates production of insulin.[50] Taking 80 mg a day for at least three months can help to stabilize blood sugar levels.[51]

Essential Fatty Acids (EFAs): EFAs are unsaturated fats required in the diet. Omega-3 and omega-6 oils are the two principal types. The primary omega-3 oil is alpha-linolenic acid (ALA), found in flaxseed oil as well as pumpkin seeds, walnuts, and soybeans. Fish oils, such as salmon, cod, and mackerel, contain the other important omega-3 oils, DHA (docosahexaenoic acid) and EPA (eicosapentaenoic acid). Omega-3 EFAs have been shown to decrease insulin resistance and vascular complications in diabetics. Linoleic acid is the main omega-6 oil and is found in most vegetable oils, including safflower, corn, peanut, and sesame. The most therapeutic form of omega-6 oil is gamma-linolenic acid (GLA), found in evening primrose, black currant, and borage oils. Omega-6 EFAs can reduce diabetic neuropathy,[52] but should be taken in proper balance with omega-3s.

Amino Acids: Amino acids are the building blocks of the 40,000 proteins in the body, including enzymes, hormones, and neurotransmitters. Supplementing with an amino acid complex assures the body's supply of raw materials for the manufacture of insulin, which is composed of 51 amino acids.[53]

Digestive Enzymes: The use of the digestive enzymes protease, amylase, and lipase is sometimes recommended to aid in the digestion and absorption of nutrients, especially in cases of diabetes, where the pancreas is not functioning optimally.[54] Dr. Wright reports often finding undigested fat and vegetable material in the feces of Type I diabetics, indicating a need for pancreatic enzyme supplementation.

 For older diabetics and diabetics who have problems with absorption of nutrients due to damage to the digestive system, it may be necessary to take minerals and trace elements by intravenous infusion or transdermally, using 30%-40% dimethylsulfoxide (DMSO), a solvent that facilitates the absorption of medicines through the skin.[55] These methods can be very effective for lowering blood sugar levels, insulin requirements, and high blood pressure, but should not be done without first consulting a physician.

Exercise and Stress Reduction

Stress leads to the production of adrenaline and cortisol, hormones that raise the blood sugar level. Relaxation and stress reduction techniques such as yoga, meditation, guided imagery, biofeedback training, and massage are therefore recommended for diabetics.

Research conducted by the National Institutes of Health conclusively proves that exercise in combination with weight loss can reduce the odds of developing diabetes by 58% among people most at risk for the disease, nearly double the rate of risk reduction (31%) achieved by daily use of the diabetes medication metaformin, the only drug known to protect against the disease. Moreover, making this simple lifestyle change poses none of the risks associated with the drug. The study, which involved over 3,000 participants, found that 30 minutes of walking each day, accompanied by an average loss of 15 pounds among participants who were overweight, was all that was necessary to significantly reduce the risk of developing the disease.[56]

Regular exercise should be a priority in any diabetic's lifestyle, as it lowers blood sugar, helps control weight, oxygenates tissues, and stimulates metabolic functions. Although exercise is primarily regarded as a way to burn off fat, it is also effective in stabilizing blood sugar. When you use your muscles vigorously, glucose is absorbed by the cells as an energy fuel without the help of insulin, so the body is less likely to react to sugar intake with surges in insulin.[57] Any program designed to restore healthy blood sugar levels should include daily sessions of light exercise, such as walking, swimming, or cycling.

 Diabetics on insulin should monitor their blood sugar level before exercising and plan on having a snack to prevent hypoglycemia. This is necessary because, once an insulin injection is given, there is no way to neutralize the insulin and it will continue to act to lower the blood sugar level even if the level has naturally dropped below normal as a result of exercise. Also, before beginning any strenuous exercise program, always consult a doctor for a thorough cardiovascular examination.

Herbal Medicine

According to David L. Hoffman, B.Sc., M.N.I.M.H., past President of the American Herbalists Guild, there are many plants with proven hypoglycemic properties that have much to contribute to a comprehensive management program of non–insulin-dependent diabetes. However, herbs will not replace insulin therapy where it is necessary. Some of the herbs traditionally used in the treatment of diabetes include bilberry, goat's rue *(Tephrosia virginiana),* fenugreek, bitter melon, garlic, mulberry leaves, olive leaves, and ginseng.[58]

- Gymnesyl *(Gymnema sylvestre):* Ayurvedic herb used in the treatment of diabetes. It has been shown to reduce the insulin requirement in Type I diabetes, and there is some evidence that it may regenerate or revitalize the cells of the pancreas responsible for producing insulin. Gymnesyl has also shown positive results in Type II diabetes. In fact, some patients were able to discontinue their oral drugs and maintain blood sugar control with gymnesyl alone. In one study of non-insulin-dependent diabetics given gymnesyl along with their oral blood sugar–lowering medication, all patients showed improved blood sugar control, 21 of 22 diabetics were able to reduce their drug dosage considerably, and five subjects were able to maintain blood sugar control with gymnesyl and diet alone.[59] The typical dose of gymnesyl is 400 mg daily in both Type I and Type II diabetes.

- Stevia: herbal sweetener that helps stabilize blood sugar while not requiring insulin for its metabolism.

- Fenugreek seeds *(Trigonella foenum-graecum):* defatted fenugreek seed powder given twice daily (50 g) to Type I diabetics resulted in lowered fasting blood sugar and a 54% decrease in 24-hour urinary glucose excretion. In Type II diabetics, the addition of 15 g of powdered fenugreek seed soaked in water significantly reduced postprandial glucose levels.[60]

- *Huereque*: derived from the root of the *huereque* cactus, which grows in the northwestern Mexican desert. It seems to have a profound effect on lowering blood sugar levels. Daniel Dunphy has used this botanical on 15 insulin-dependent patients with adult-onset diabetes. All 15 are now almost or entirely off insulin. Dunphy reports that the only drawback to *huereque* is that, after about six months, its ability to control blood sugar starts to wear off, as if the body has developed a tolerance to it. However, giving the body a month's rest from *huereque* restores its effectiveness. One option is to switch to *nopal* (another cactus that reduces blood sugar) for a month, then return to *huereque* at a lower dose.

- Bilberry: can aid in the reduction of retinopathy and small blood vessel disease in diabetes.[61]

The appropriate application of hypoglycemic herbs is very important as they can sometimes have a rapid impact on blood sugar levels, and the effect can vary from patient to patient. They can safely be used as part of a comprehensive diabetes management program that is specifically suited for each individual. It is essential that very close observation be kept on blood sugar and urine tests. This necessitates skilled practitioners training the patient. Preventive work to avoid the long-term complications may be undertaken quite safely, even if no attempt is made to deal with insulin levels. Heart and vascular tonics are appropriate to consider for long-term use, especially hawthorn berry and ginkgo.

Chelation Therapy

According to Garry F. Gordon, M.D., D.O., of Payson, Arizona, co-founder of the American College of Advancement in Medicine, chelation therapy is effective in preventing complications of diabetes. Chelation therapy uses chelating agents such as EDTA (ethylenediaminetetraacetic acid), administered intravenously to restore proper circulation. "Over 20 years of clinical experience has shown that people with diabetes who receive intravenous EDTA chelation therapy have fewer amputations, less blindness, less kidney dialysis, and other complications of diabetes than those on conventional treatments," reports Dr. Gordon. Additionally, in a Canadian study involving diabetic patients with unusually high levels of iron, Paul Cutler, M.D., chelated 32 patients with deferoxamine (a chelating agent used to remove iron), resulting in 24 patients no longer needing diabetes medication after 8-13 weeks. Dr. Cutler believes that chelating with deferoxamine could cure a third of adult cases of diabetes.[62]

 See Ayurvedic Medicine, Chelation Therapy, Energy Medicine, Herbal Medicine, Oxygen Therapies, Traditional Chinese Medicine.

Oxygen Therapy

People don't normally think of oxygen as a treatment for diabetes, but according to Frank Shallenberger, M.D., H.M.D., Director of the Nevada Center of Alternative and Anti-Aging Medicine, in Carson City, Nevada, ozone (a less stable, more reactive form of oxygen) can produce remarkable improvements in both the major and secondary symptoms of adult-onset diabetes. The connection between the ozone and diabetes is blood circulation.

Diabetics run the risk of complications, such as loss of vision, heart disease, nerve dysfunction, and gangrenous limbs, because they have considerable circulatory problems such that the actual blood flow to their tissues is diminished, explains Dr. Shallenberger. Patients often have difficulty digesting fats (such as cholesterol and triglycerides) and their arteries tend to thicken and harden. "This is compounded by the fact that what little blood reaches their tissues is less effective than it should be and is unable to deliver oxygen to those tissues," says Dr. Shallenberger. "The tissues become oxygen depleted, which explains why diabetics have problems with gangrene and why they're unable to resist infections."

SUCCESS STORY: REVERSING JUVENILE DIABETES

Perhaps 5% of all cases of diabetes begin suddenly in childhood. When Billy, 5, was brought to Daniel Dunphy, P.A.-C., of San Francisco, California, he had been diagnosed with acute juvenile diabetes. His blood sugar level had been 700 (compared to a normal range of 70-120) and already he had been hospitalized a few times.

His health history revealed the causes of his diabetes. When Billy's mother gave birth to him, she had a yeast infection (candidiasis), which meant Billy was born with a fungal infection. When he drank his mother's breast milk, the candidiasis became seated in his intestines and blood. When he was 6 months old, Billy had a series of ear infections for which he received antibiotics over a four-month period. Since then, he periodically had allergy symptoms, rashes, and sinus and ear problems. When he was 3, Billy started experiencing excessive thirst and frequent urination, which are often early signs of diabetes.

By this time, Billy was drinking 6-7 glasses of fruit juice every day. He craved sugar, and the sugar in these juices fed his yeast infection and made him hyperactive. The antibiotics supported the infection rather than helping to remove it. "The combination of these three factors—candidiasis, ear infections, antibiotics—had exhausted his pancreas and sent him into a diabetic crisis," says Dunphy. Although there was no diabetes in his immediate family, Billy may also have had a genetic predisposition to a weak pancreas.

Billy's insulin doses were so high (he was taking 30 units daily) that he became irritable, developed heart palpitations, and perspired heavily. The high insulin doses nearly sent him into a hypoglycemic (low blood sugar) coma every day. So each day his blood sugar went from very high before his insulin doses to very low after his insulin. His mother was frantic; meanwhile, his doctor was trying his best to manage the sugar swings with insulin.

Dunphy started Billy on an insulin-regulating diet, eliminating all fruits, fruit juices, and dairy products, except for one slice of apple or a cup of berries per day. His diet consisted of proteins, vegetables, and whole grains, thereby replacing sugars with complex carbohydrates. He had frequent small meals instead of large ones.

Then Dunphy put him on vanadyl sulfate (7.5 mg twice daily) and chromium picolinate (200 mcg three times daily). Chromium enhances the cellular activity of insulin and the enzymatic processes necessary for it to function smoothly; chromium is also found in high concentrations in the pancreas and is considered a sugar regulator. Vanadyl, the supplement form of the trace element vanadium, may have activities that mimic insulin. Billy would need to take both supplements for many months. He also gave Billy a homeopathic remedy for the yeast (*Candida*) infection, a nosode of the yeast itself (*Candida* 6C, three times daily for at least two months). In addition, he gave him acidophilus and *Bifidobacteria bifidum* to fortify his intestines with "friendly" bacteria and put him on a bowel- and liver-cleansing program.

"We monitored Billy's blood sugar levels carefully and very slowly reduced his daily insulin," adds Dunphy. "Within three days, his insulin intake was 50% reduced and, within a week, he was taking no insulin. I then instructed his mother not to give him any insulin unless his blood sugar went above 200. This happened only once in the first three months, when Billy had some fruit juice."

Three months into this program, when Billy was stronger and his diabetes under control, Dunphy prescribed a single dose of *Diphtherinum* 200C, a homeopathic remedy that was indicated because Billy's father had suffered from diphtheria and there was still a taint or energy residue of this illness in Billy's system. Over the last three years, Billy has stayed on a program of careful diet plus supplements. His blood sugar only rarely goes above 200, when he resorts to using a small dose of insulin. This case shows that it is possible to significantly help manage and reverse childhood diabetes using diet, homeopathics, and nutritional supplements, but that the disease must be managed with a long-term plan.

A prime reason the red blood cells in the diabetic's blood are unable to release their oxygen is that a key molecule called 2,3-diphosphoglycerate is in reduced supply. Under normal conditions, 2,3-diphosphoglycerate stimulates red blood cells, to deliver oxygen to the tissues, but if there isn't enough of this molecule in the system, the red blood cells can't deliver the oxygen. When you introduce ozone—that is, more oxygen—into the blood, more 2,3-diphosphoglycerate is produced and the oxygen delivery system and the efficiency of blood circulation start to improve. The ozone also appears to enhance the activity of cellular metabolism, the continual conversion of food into energy. Dr. Shallenberger likens the metabolism-heightening effect of ozone to a similar benefit to diabetics obtained through vigorous exercise. It oxygenates the tissues and gets all the body processes running better, he says.

Levels of ATP, an important molecule that stores energy in the cells, are also enhanced through ozonation. Among other functions, ATP helps each cell maintain the integrity of its membrane, thereby enabling it to regulate the passage of materials into and out of the cell, says Dr. Shallenberger. If the cell membrane collapses, the cell dies; if a lot of cells die, you start getting tissue death, and gangrene becomes a possibility.

Dr. Shallenberger often adds another element to the ozonation procedure: chelation. Dr. Shallenberger calls his combined treatment "chezone." Chelation improves blood circulation to the tissues by removing heavy metals, he explains, which means they get more oxygen. This improves their metabolic rate (energy processing efficiency) and enables them to make better use of glucose (blood sugar). When you have higher efficiency in using glucose, you are much closer to controlling diabetes naturally, says Dr. Shallenberger.

Traditional Chinese Medicine (TCM)

Maoshing Ni, D.O.M., Ph.D., L.Ac., President of Yo San University of Traditional Chinese Medicine, in Marina del Rey, California, treats Type I and Type II diabetics with acupuncture and a combination of herbs including astragalus, wild yam, and rehmannia. With Type I diabetes, treatment must begin in the early stages of the disease for TCM to be of any help, but it is quite effective, he says, especially at the beginning and intermediate stages of Type II.

According to Dr. Ni, traditional Chinese medicine can improve circulatory problems and slow down the process of neuropathy. Dr. Ni reports the case of a patient with Type II diabetes who came to his office with painful, swollen legs resulting from neuropathy. After a few treatments, the inflammation, pain, and swelling were resolved and no further symptoms of neuropathy were evident. TCM may also help to stabilize blood sugar levels in Type II diabetics by restoring balance to the endocrine system.

William Cargile, D.C., L.Ac., F.I.A.C.A., past Chairman of Research of the American Association of Oriental Medicine, says he has been successful in treating diabetes with acupuncture. He has found that treatment of the spleen/pancreas point has effects that reduce the autoimmune component of diabetes. He notes that acupuncture is helpful in reversing the neuropathy commonly found in long-term diabetics. In one case, he used acupuncture to treat a 90-year-old patient who had been

bedridden for years and had no feeling in his feet. After the third session, the patient was able to walk again and eventually increased his exercise regimen to three miles a day. His insulin requirements were also lowered by 90% and he regained feeling in his feet.

Dr. Cargile also uses soft laser (or cold laser) acupuncture to treat diabetes and, for Type II diabetics, he uses ear acupuncture to stimulate the autonomic nervous system. Dr. Cargile stresses that acupuncture alone is not sufficient treatment for diabetes and always insists that his patients have concurrent nutritional and conventional medical care.

Ayurvedic Medicine

Virender Sodhi, M.D. (Ayurveda), N.D., Director of the Ayurvedic & Naturopathic Medical Clinic, in Bellevue, Washington, does not differentiate in his treatment of Type I and Type II diabetes. The first thing he addresses is diet modification, eliminating sugar and simple carbohydrates, and emphasizing complex carbohydrates. Protein is limited, since excessive intake can damage the kidneys. Fat is also limited because there is often a deficiency of pancreatic enzymes, making fat digestion difficult. Since many diabetics have autoantibodies (antibodies that are antagonistic to their own bodies), a cleansing program is usually instituted. Dr. Sodhi uses an Ayurvedic method called *pancha karma*, which begins with herbal massages and an herbal steam sauna, followed by fasting to cleanse the body. This is followed by an herbal purge for the liver, pancreas, and spleen. Colon therapy is next, first to cleanse the digestive tract and then to reconstitute the system.

Dr. Sodhi also recommends several herbal preparations for diabetics. "The Indian herb *Gymnema sylvestre* stimulates the pancreas to produce more insulin and also blocks sugar absorption from the gut. Bitter melon and *neem* lower blood sugar, stimulate the pancreas, and also act as liver tonics. A liver tonic is needed, because if the liver is not cleansed, diabetics tend to form gallstones," he says.

Exercise is another key factor, notes Dr. Sodhi, especially for Type II diabetics. He adds that chromium and nutritional supplements are also necessary, as in other forms of diabetic treatment. Dr. Sodhi's program is not a cure for diabetes, though, and the treatment must be continued long-term for the diabetic to remain healthy.

Recommendations

- A diet emphasizing foods high in complex carbohydrates and fiber, such as whole grains, legumes, and vegetables, reduces the need for insulin by controlling the rate of uptake of glucose into the bloodstream.

- Eliminate refined sugar and sugar products and avoid "junk" foods. Eat snacks of protein between meals. Reduce or eliminate the intake of alcohol, tobacco, and caffeine.

- Take off excess weight through exercise and calorie reduction.

- Helpful supplements include B vitamins (especially B6) and biotin, chromium, magnesium, vanadium, essential fatty acids, vitamins C and E, alpha-lipoic acid, and coenzyme Q10.

- Many herbs with proven hypoglycemic properties have much to contribute to a comprehensive management program of non–insulin-dependent diabetes. However, herbs will not replace insulin therapy where it is necessary. Some of the herbs traditionally used in the treatment of diabetes include *Gymnema sylvestre, neem,* goat's rue, fenugreek, *huereque* cactus, bitter melon, garlic, and ginseng.

- Chelation therapy and oxygen (ozone) therapy are effective in preventing complications of diabetes by improving blood circulation.

- Traditional Chinese medicine using acupuncture and herbs can improve circulatory problems and slow down the process of neuropathy.

- Ayurvedic medicine uses diet, detoxification, herbs, and exercise to alleviate problems associated with diabetes.

Self-Care

The following therapies can be undertaken at home under appropriate professional supervision:

Massage / Reflexology / Qigong and Tai Chi / Yoga

AROMATHERAPY: Rub essence of juniper or cedar and olive oil over spleen and pancreas area.

HYDROTHERAPY: Constitutional hydrotherapy, applied two to five times weekly.

JUICE THERAPY: Under a doctor's supervision: • String beans, parsley, cucumber, celery, watercress • Carrot, celery, parsley, spinach • Lettuce, spinach, carrot (add a clove of raw garlic) • Sip one glass three times daily.

TOPICAL TREATMENT: Dry brush massage twice daily to improve circulation.

Professional Care

The following therapies can only be provided by a qualified health professional:

Biofeedback Training and Neurotherapy / Guided Imagery / Herbal Medicine / Mind–Body Therapies / Osteopathic Medicine

ENERGY MEDICINE: Electrodermal screening

MAGNETIC FIELD THERAPY: Sleeping on a magnetic mattress pad can reduce the need for insulin.

OXYGEN THERAPIES: • Ozone Therapy • Hydrogen Peroxide Therapy: The late Charles Farr, M.D., President of the International Bio-Oxidative Medicine Foundation, reported success in treating Type II diabetes using intravenous hydrogen peroxide therapy. Best results are obtained with patients who have never been treated with insulin or any other type of diabetes drug and their diabetic condition can often be reversed.

Where to Find Help

For more information on, or referrals for, the treatment of diabetes, contact the following organizations.

American Association of Oriental Medicine (AAOM)
433 Front Street
Catasauqua, Pennsylvania 18032
(888) 500-7999
Website: www.aaom.org

The AAOM is a national professional organization of acupuncturists who meet acceptable standards of competency and can provide you with the names and locations of local members. Referrals by written request only.

American Association of Naturopathic Physicians
601 Valley Street, Suite 105
Seattle, Washington 98109
(206) 298-0126
Website: www.naturopathic.org

Provides a directory of naturopathic physicians and offers referrals to a nationwide network of accredited or licensed practitioners. Publishes a quarterly newsletter for both professionals and the general public. Also offers a series of brochures and pamphlets on a variety of subjects.

American College for Advancement in Medicine (ACAM)
23121 Verdugo Drive, Suite 204
Laguna Hills, California 92653
(800) 532-3688
Website: www.acam.org

This pioneer organization seeks to establish certification and standards of practice for chelation therapy, providing training and education, and sponsoring semiannual conferences for physicians and scientists. ACAM provides referrals and information, including a directory of physicians worldwide trained in preventative medicine as well as in the ACAM protocol for chelation therapy.

American Holistic Medical Association
6728 Old McLean Village Drive
McLean, Virginia 22101
(703) 556-9728
Website: www.holisticmedicine.org

A professional organization for holistic practitioners, the AHMA offers information and services for its members and lobbies for holistic issues. It also provides referrals for the public.

Ayurvedic & Naturopathic Medical Clinic
2115 112th Avenue N.E.
Bellevue, Washington 98004
(425) 453-8022
Website: www.ayurvedicscience.com

Dr. Virender Sodhi's clinic provides medical training for physicians and health-care practitioners, as well as individual courses for laypeople.

Recommended Reading

Alternative and Complementary Diabetes Care. Diana W. Guthrie and Richard Guthrie, M.D. New York: John Wiley and Sons, 2000.

Controlling Diabetes Naturally with Chinese Medicine. Lynn M. Kuchinski and Bob Flaws. Boulder, CO: Blue Poppy, 1999.

Diabetes and Hypoglycemia. Michael T. Murray, N.D. Rocklin, CA: Prima, 1994.

Diabetes: How to Combine the Best of Traditional and Alternative Therapies. Milton Hammerly, M.D. Holbrook, MA: Adams Media, 2001.

Natural Medicine for Diabetes. Deborah R. Mitchell. New York: Dell, 1997.

Psyching Out Diabetes: A Positive Approach to Your Negative Emotions. Richard R. Rubin, June Biermann, and Barbara Toohey. Los Angeles: Lowell House, 1999.

Reversing Diabetes. Julian M. Whitaker. New York: Warner Books, 2001.

Victory Over Diabetes. William H. Philpott, M.D., and Dwight K. Kalita, Ph.D. New Canaan, CT: Keats Publishing, 1992.

Weight Loss: An Alternative Medicine Definitive Guide. Burton Goldberg and the Editors of *Alternative Medicine.* Tiburon, CA: AlternativeMedicine.com Books, 2000.

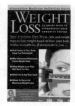

FIBROMYALGIA

Fibromyalgia is a painful muscle disorder that affects millions of people, but it is generally misunderstood. Often people with fibromyalgia syndrome (FMS) get passed around among conventional doctors, sometimes for years, without getting a diagnosis, much less treatment, for their condition. Alternative physicians are proving that the illness can be successfully treated by taking a multidisciplined approach specific to the needs of the individual patient.

FIBROMYALGIA IS a multiple-symptom syndrome primarily involving widespread muscle pain (myalgia), which can be debilitating in its severity. The pain seems to be caused by the tightening and thickening of the myofascia, the thin film or tissue that holds the muscles together. Fibromyalgia, also called fibrositis, shares many of the same symptoms as chronic fatigue syndrome (CFS), including debilitating fatigue, muscle and joint pain, sleep disorders, and digestive problems. Jacob Teitelbaum, M.D., a specialist in the two syndromes, calls CFS the "drop-dead flu" and fibromyalgia the "aching-all-over disease." Given the similarity that these descriptive names embody, Dr. Teitelbaum prefers to put CFS and fibromyalgia in a single category he calls "severe chronic fatigue states."[1]

"Both chronic fatigue and FMS often seem to begin after an infection or a severe trauma," states Leon Chaitow, N.D., D.O., of London, England. "The only obvious difference seems to be that, for some people, the fatigue element is the most dominant while for others the muscular pain symptoms are greatest."[2]

One of the key problems in FMS is the disregulation of the thalamus, the part of the brain responsible for the integration of sensory information, according to Rima Laibow, M.D., founding Medical Director of the Alexandria Institute of Natural and Integrative Medicine, in Croton-on-Hudson, New York. This causes normal feedback from the body to be misinterpreted as pain. Dr. Laibow also considers sleep disorders to be a primary factor in both FMS and chronic fatigue.

An estimated 3-6 million Americans suffer from fibromyalgia, 86% of whom are women, primarily between the ages of 34 and 56. The level of disability caused by fibromyalgia is severe enough that 25% of women and 27% of men affected are unable to work, according to a recent study.[3] Typical tender sites include

SYMPTOMS OF FIBROMYALGIA

- Widespread muscle and joint pains ("hurting all over")
- General fatigue and stiffness
- Allergies
- Headaches
- Sleeping disorders and restless legs
- Irritable bowel syndrome
- Dizziness
- Exercise intolerance
- Anxiety
- Depression
- Irritability and mood swings
- Heightened sensitivity to light, sound, smell, touch
- Dry eyes alternating with watery eyes
- Carpal tunnel syndrome
- Tender skin
- Cold sensitivity
- Numbness or tingling sensations
- Dysmenorrhea (women)

the neck, upper back, rib cage, hips, and knees. Other symptoms include general fatigue and stiffness, insomnia and sleep disorders, anxiety, depression, mood swings, allergies, carpal tunnel syndrome, headaches, irritable bowel syndrome, dizziness, and exercise intolerance. Post-traumatic fibromyalgia is believed to develop after a fall, whiplash, or back strain, whereas primary fibromyalgia has an uncertain origin.

Although fibromyalgia was first described by a physician in 1816 and classified as a distinct disorder (a painful arthritic condition) in 1904, it did not receive recogni-

OFFICIAL DIAGNOSTIC CRITERIA FOR FIBROMYALGIA

In 1990, the American College of Rheumatology (ACR) established the following diagnostic criteria for fibromyalgia. According to the ACR, there must be widespread pain of at least three month's duration in 11 out of 18 tender muscle sites as follows:

- Occiput (on the head): bilateral (on both sides), at the suboccipital muscle insertion
- Lower Cervical: bilateral, at the anterior aspects of the intertransverse spaces of cervical (neck) vertebrae C5-C7
- Trapezius (upper back): bilateral, at the midpoint of the upper border
- Supraspinatus (shoulder blades): bilateral, at origins above the scapula near the medial border
- Second Rib: bilateral, at the second costochondral junctions just lateral to the junctions on the upper surfaces
- Lateral Epicondyle (top of the thigh bone, or femur): bilateral, 2 cm distal to the epicondyle
- Gluteal (buttocks): bilateral, in upper quadrants of the buttocks in anterior fold of muscles
- Knee: bilateral, at the medial fat pad proximal to the joint line.

tion as the debilitating condition it is until fairly recently; in 1987, the American Medical Association cited it as a disabling illness.[4] However, a misconception in the medical community that fibromyalgia is caused by deconditioning—muscles becoming weak and limp as a result of inactivity—has added to the painful burden of those who suffer from the disorder. Furthermore, doctors often misdiagnose this condition as depression and patients have been told "it's all in their head." This blaming of the victim is singularly unhelpful to the patient's state of mind and is also medically inaccurate—most fibromyalgia sufferers were highly active people, overachievers in fact, when the condition struck. Misdiagnosis could likely be avoided by taking an individualized approach to the patient.

 See Allergies, Candidiasis, Chronic Fatigue Syndrome, Sleep Disorders, Stress, Women's Health.

Causes of Fibromyalgia

Many possible triggering events or causes have been implicated in the onset of FMS, including viral and bacterial infections, trauma such as an assault or auto accident, chemical and food sensitivities, chronic stress, hormonal imbalances, mercury toxicity from dental amalgam fillings, breast implants, and irregularities in muscle metabolism. As Dr. Chaitow stated, FMS often seems to begin after an infection or a severe trauma. Researchers have found that those with fibromyalgia have elevated amounts of the neurotransmitters involved in pain responses (Substance P), as well as depressed levels of natural painkillers (such as serotonin) and growth hormone, which helps regenerate muscles. Abnormal sleep patterns, particularly a decrease in slow-wave, Stage 4 sleep, which is most beneficial for the muscles, may also be a factor.

In a study of the possible connection between flu viruses and fibromyalgia, nine out of ten fibromyalgia patients tested positive for antibodies to influenza type A.[5] Influenza A is a viral infection that mainly affects the respiratory and autonomic nervous systems. The sympathetic branch of the autonomic nervous system is associated with arousal and stress, increasing heart rate, blood pressure, and muscle tension. The researchers concluded that influenza A may be implicated in the development of fibromyalgia. Another study found a high prevalence of FMS in patients infected with the hepatitis C virus.[6]

Scientists have found that those with FMS have two to three times the normal levels of Substance P, a neurotransmitter that relays chemical messages about pain, in their spinal fluid.[7] Substance P is a polypeptide (several amino acids bonded together) made naturally in the body. It is released in response to physical injuries to tissues and muscles and is regarded as one of the most potent compounds affecting smooth muscle contraction and inflammation. The overabundance of Substance P may make those with FMS experience pain under circumstances that would not be uncomfortable to others, may suppress levels of serotonin, and can increase sleep disturbances.[8]

At the same time, fibromyalgia patients also have low levels of growth hormone and cortisol. Human growth hormone (HGH), naturally secreted by the pituitary gland in the brain, is a small, protein-like hormone similar to insulin. HGH is secreted in very brief pulses during the early hours of sleep and remains in circulation for only a few minutes. During adolescence, when growth is most rapid, production of HGH is high. After age 20, HGH production declines progressively at an average rate of about 14% per decade. Research indicates that irregularities in HGH secretion may be a factor in fibromyalgia.[9]

Cortisol is a hormone secreted by the adrenal glands, which are located atop the kidneys. Under conditions of chronic stress, high amounts of cortisol are released and then the adrenal glands become exhausted. Imbalances in cortisol secretion are linked with low energy, muscle dysfunction, thyroid dysfunction, immune system depression, sleep disorders, poor skin regeneration, and decreased growth hormone uptake. In other words, people who are short on cortisol because of problems with their adrenal glands experience the same symptoms as fibromyalgia sufferers. Studies have shown that adrenal insufficiency and stress may contribute to many of the neurohormone imbalances and symptoms of FMS.[10]

Fibromyalgia patients show abnormal brain waves during the deepest stage (Stage 4) of sleep. Stage 4 sleep is important for the repair of tissues, the creation of antibodies, and the formation of growth hormone, which is necessary for muscle and bone health. Instead of experiencing the restorative rest that allows muscles to recover from a day of activity, fibromyalgia sufferers wake up during Stage 4 sleep. In fact, this lack of restful sleep is considered a major cause of the symptoms associated with FMS.[11]

Treating Fibromyalgia

The conventional medical solution for fibromyalgia—painkillers—is a prime example of symptom-driven treatment with little understanding of causes and equally slim chances of therapeutic success. The symptoms of FMS are the result of underlying imbalances in the body produced by multiple simultaneous infections and accompanying physical, mental, and environmental factors. Alternative medicine practitioners believe the most effective way of treating fibromyalgia is to combine a variety of approaches.

A number of tests are useful in determining the underlying factors contributing to FMS. Electrodermal screening and darkfield blood analysis can help provide a picture of overall health status. Digestive function can be assessed using a stool or urine analysis (these tests are also valuable for getting information on general health). Specific tests are available to assess how well individual body systems are working, including the immune system (T and B Cell Panel, Sedimentation Rate) and the thyroid gland (TRH Stimulation Test). Other tests look for possible nutritional deficiencies (Pantox Antioxidant Profile, Functional Intracellular Analysis, Nutricheck USA, Cell Membrane Lipid Profile) or excesses of toxins (hair analysis, ToxMet Screen, DMSA Challenge Test, Functional Liver Detoxification Profile) and stress (Aeron LifeCycles Saliva Assay Report, Adrenal Stress Index) in the body.

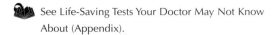 See Life-Saving Tests Your Doctor May Not Know About (Appendix).

"Where a condition has multiple interacting causes, it makes clinical sense to try to reduce the burden of whatever factors are imposing themselves on the immune and repair mechanisms of the body, while at the same time doing all that is possible to enhance those mechanisms," states Dr. Chaitow.[12]

> *Where a condition has multiple interacting causes, it makes clinical sense to try to reduce the burden of whatever factors are imposing themselves on the immune and repair mechanisms of the body, while at the same time doing all that is possible to enhance those mechanisms.*
>
> —LEON CHAITOW, N.D., D.O.

In treating FMS, it is important to look for infections that are the result of toxicity and nutritional deficiency, including yeast and parasites, viruses, abscesses in the teeth, and sometimes chronic gastritis. By treating these infections and boosting nutritional intake with good diet and proper supplementation, a person can reduce the burden on the immune system.

Detoxifying the body is another important component in promoting the health of the immune system and addressing other factors that may be contributing to fibromyalgia. As our environment and food are increasingly saturated with chemicals, the body's mechanisms for elimination of toxins cannot keep up with the chemical deluge. Given that many people with FMS have chemical allergies as well, it is advisable to take measures to remove these toxins from the body.

Diet and Nutritional Medicine

A healthy, balanced diet is essential in treating fibromyalgia. Research has shown that switching to a vegetarian diet improves symptoms of pain, joint stiffness, and sleep disturbances in fibromyalgia patients.[13] According to Michael T. Murray, N.D., of Issaquah, Washington, a healthy diet avoids "empty" foods low in nutrients and high in sugar and fat. Instead, it concentrates on high-nutrient, high-protein, complex carbohydrate foods—

SUCCESS STORY: BODYWORK, VITAMINS, AND EXERCISE HELP REVERSE FIBROMYALGIA

Anika, 54, suffered from chronic low-back pain, muscle soreness, general achiness, fatigue, and depression. She endured years of clinical testing and various drug treatments without getting a diagnosis or relief of her symptoms. Frustrated by her lack of progress with conventional doctors, Anika sought help from Mary Olsen, D.C., a chiropractor based in Huntington, New York. Dr. Olsen identified Anika's condition as fibromyalgia by testing the 18 trigger points associated with FMS—11 of these points must be sore to the touch to qualify as fibromyalgia, according to the conventional medical definition. In Anika's case, 16 of the sites were tender.

Dr. Olsen prescribed a three-part treatment program for Anika. First, she used acupressure on Anika's trigger points, applying pressure in eight-second intervals and repeating the treatment three times at each site. The trigger points in fibromyalgia are actually muscles in spasm and those near the spine often pull it out of alignment. Dr. Olsen administered acupressure to massage the trigger points and chiropractic to realign the spine, then used applied kinesiology to prevent the trigger points from injuring the spine again. Anika saw Dr. Olsen three times a week until her spine began to respond to treatment, and monthly thereafter.

Second, Dr. Olsen prescribed vitamin supplements specifically tailored to fibromyalgia. From her clinical experience, Dr. Olsen has found that fibromyalgia sufferers tend to have low levels of B vitamins and malic acid. The supplement formula she typically uses for this deficiency includes vitamin B1 (25 mg), vitamin B6 (75 mg), manganese (2.5 mg), and malic acid (300 mg). "In most cases, I notice a dramatic improvement within 48 hours of beginning the vitamin therapy," Dr. Olsen says. Anika took this formula two to eight times daily as needed.

Third, Anika began a moderate exercise program, performing a stretching routine (10-15 minutes) five days a week and walking for 20 minutes three times weekly. The exercise would help raise her serotonin levels, which in turn would reduce her fatigue. Dr. Olsen emphasizes that her patients never exercise to the point of pain and this aspect of treatment needs to vary according to the individual. Many people with fibromyalgia are too tired to exercise at all, she says. Dr. Olsen usually waits until the person's condition has improved through vitamin therapy before beginning the exercise program. In Anika's case, she was able to start exercising relatively quickly.

After one year of treatment, Anika reported that her low-back pain was gone, her muscle aches had subsided, and her energy level had increased considerably. As her condition improved, Anika began exercising more, which further boosted her energy level. Her increased energy (and relief from pain) also elevated her mood and Anika no longer suffers from depression.

---

vegetables, grains, beans, fish, and organic poultry (care should be taken to avoid mercury toxins in fish and antibiotics in poultry). "Your energy level is directly related to the quality of the foods you routinely ingest," says Dr. Murray.[14] He points out the importance of eliminating all allergenic foods and, if one is highly allergic, the rotating of nonallergenic foods. He also advises drinking 8-10 glasses of pure water daily.

To further boost energy and build up the nutrient status in fibromyalgia suffers, Meyer's Cocktail may also be effective. The Meyer's Cocktail is an intravenous vitamin and mineral protocol developed in the 1970s by John Meyers, M.D., of Johns Hopkins University, in Baltimore, Maryland. It contains magnesium chloride hexahydrate, calcium gluconate, vitamins B2, B5, and B6, the entire vitamin B complex, and vitamin C. The solution is slowly injected over a 5-15 minute period.

Chanchal Cabrera, M.N.I.M.H, a clinical herbalist practicing in Vancouver, British Columbia, Canada, has found the following to be especially useful for fibromyalgia:

- **Niacinamide**—A form of niacin (vitamin B3), high doses (900–4,000 mg daily in divided doses) of niacinamide are effective in reducing musculoskeletal inflammation, but should only be taken under a physician's supervision.

- **Lipotropic factors (substances that remove and prevent fatty deposits)**—A combination of the lipotropic factors phosphatidyl–choline (lecithin, a neurotransmitter precursor), inositol (component of vitamin B complex), and methionine (an amino acid) can aid in liver function, helping to detoxify the system and correct any excessive fat deposits, which reduce blood circulation and can lead to painful blood clots. Methionine is integral to cartilage so it can improve the strength of joint tissues. The dosage is 1 g of each per day, taken in combination.

- **Vitamin E**—This antioxidant's effective anti-inflammatory action suppresses the breakdown of cartilage while stimulating cartilage growth. A dose of 400-1,200 IU a day is typically recommended.

- **Vitamin C**—This antioxidant nutrient is vital for tissue repair and, when taken in combination with vitamin E, will contribute to the stability of cartilage. The recommended dosage is to bowel tolerance (the point just prior to diarrhea).

- **Eicosapentaenoic acid (EPA)**—An essential fatty acid found in most fish oils, EPA is anti-inflammatory. Essential fatty acids decrease inflammation in the body and supply a source of lubrication for the tissues, which helps decrease pain. An effective dosage is 1.8 g daily.

- **Selenium**—This antioxidant mineral works in combination with vitamin E and inhibits inflammation. Blood levels of selenium tend to be low in fibromyalgia sufferers. The typical recommended dosage is 200 mcg per day.

- **Magnesium malate**—A lack of magnesium can result in aluminum buildup in the brain, which can, in turn, produce fibromyalgia symptoms.[15] Magnesium (1,000-1,500 mg daily) taken in a combination formula with malic acid is an effective supplement.

- **Zinc**—This antioxidant mineral is necessary for tissue repair and may be deficient in people with fibromyalgia. An effective dosage is 25-50 mg daily.[16]

Other nutrients that may be helpful for FMS include:

- **Cetyl myristoleate (CM)**—An oil derived from myristoleic acid (found in fish oils and cow's milk butter) with anti-inflammatory and lubricant properties, which can help alleviate the pain and swelling of joints, muscles, tendons, and other soft tissues in the body. CM also supports the immune system and seems able to stop the depletion of essential fatty acids that typically accompanies chronic inflammation.[17]

- **S-adenosylmethionine (SAMe)**—A natural substance produced by the body when the amino acid methionine combines with adenosine triphosphate (ATP), an energy source present in muscle cells.[18] SAMe is a methyl-donor, meaning that it gives its sulfur molecules to important cellular activity such as rebuilding cell membranes, removing toxins and wastes, and producing mood-elevating brain chemicals (dopamine and serotonin). Studies have found that SAMe is an anti-inflammatory and pain reliever.[19]

Herbal Medicine

According to herbalist Chanchal Cabrera, the following formula treats the symptoms of inflammation and helps ease the pain associated with fibromyalgia, while boosting the immune system. This combination should be taken three times a day, 1 tsp each time. Use equal parts of each: echinacea (immune tonic), black cohosh (*Cimicifuga racemosa*, an anti-inflammatory), devil's claw (*Harpagophytum procumbens,* an anti-inflammatory), licorice (*Glycyrrhiza glabra*, adrenal tonic and anti-inflammatory), dandelion (*Taraxacum officinale,* used to treat liver conditions and aid in toxin removal), and celery (*Apium graveolens*, removes acid wastes from the body). However, before beginning any herbal protocol, people should consult a qualified herbalist, as no single standard formula works for everyone.[20]

Cayenne *(Capsicum annuum)* is an effective systemic stimulant, meaning it invigorates the physiological activities of the body. It is especially helpful for the circulatory and digestive systems, stimulating blood flow and strengthening the heartbeat and metabolic rate.[21] Externally, it is used for muscle and joint pain.[22] The use of cayenne has two benefits for fibromyalgia sufferers: it dissolves the sensation of pain and depletes bodily reserves of Substance P, believed to be overabundant in people with fibromyalgia. The Medical College of Wisconsin, in Milwaukee, treated 45 people suffering from primary fibromyalgia with capsaicin (the active ingredient in cayenne) cream for four weeks. The patients reported less tenderness in the spots treated and a significant increase in their grip strength.[23]

Chamomile (German or wild, *Matricaria recutita*; Roman, *Anthemis nobilis*) produces a calming effect, easing anxiety and reducing tension.[24] It can thus be helpful with overall anxiety, sleep disorders, and muscle tension. Its calming property has a beneficial effect on the gastrointestinal system as well. In Europe, chamomile is recognized as a digestive aid, a mild sedative, and an anti-inflammatory, notably in oral hygiene and skin preparations.[25] Its anti-inflammatory properties also reduce allergic responses.

Prolotherapy and Neural Therapy

Prolotherapy (also known as reconstructive therapy) involves injecting small amounts of an irritating solution into areas of pain or dysfunction (such as strained ligaments or tendons where they join the bone) to produce a healing response. The irritant produces a small focused injury that deactivates the sensitized, painful nerve fibers in the area and causes inflammation; the body then dispatches fibroblasts (bone-building cells) to the area to lay down new collagen (structural protein) to repair the damaged tissues, tendons, cartilage, or ligaments. Prolotherapy evokes the body's natural inflammatory process to heal, stabilize, and strengthen injured tendons and ligaments.

A 16-year study conducted by Harold Wilkinson, M.D., former Chair of Neurosurgery at Massachusetts Medical Center, supports prolotherapy's effectiveness. While patients typically require a series of prolotherapy injections before they experience complete elimination of their pain, Dr. Wilkinson reported that "a sizeable portion of people with unresolved chronic pain had more than a year's pain relief with only one injection."[28] This form of treatment requires a physician and is most often recommended when chronic pain does not respond to physical therapy, anti-inflammatory nutrients, or other alternative approaches.

Neural therapy, first developed in Germany in 1925 by the physicians Ferdinand and Walter Huneke, uses localized injections of anesthetics to favorably influence health problems. Lidocaine or procaine is injected in the body to remove interferences in the body's electrical network and thus relieve chronic pain, reverse injury, and clear energy blockages. The anesthetics are injected into acupuncture points, scars, glands, the nerve bundles in the autonomic nervous system, and other tissues. By clearing the local site of interference, neural therapy helps to regulate energy throughout the body.

Veronica, 42, had suffered from whole-body pain for five years before receiving treatment for fibromyalgia from Ross A. Hauser, M.D., of Oak Park, Illinois. A series of previous diagnoses, physical therapy rounds, and anti-inflammatory medications and antidepressants had brought her no relief. Her neck pain was so intense she had to wear a neck brace; she also had pain in her jaw, arms, legs, and back, and the ligaments in these regions were especially tender. Dr. Hauser treated Veronica with neural therapy, making injections at the tender spots over the ligaments and tendons of Veronica's arms, legs, jaw, back, and neck. Six weeks later, she no longer needed the neck brace and was able to go swimming and walking. Six months later (after a second neural therapy treatment), Veronica experienced pain only with strenuous exercise, but was otherwise "doing great," notes Dr. Hauser. After a third treatment, all her symptoms abated.[29]

 See Acupuncture, Bodywork, Detoxification Therapy, Diet, Energy Medicine, Mind/Body Medicine, Neural Therapy, Osteopathic Medicine, Prolotherapy.

Energy Medicine

Microcurrent treatment devices generate infinitesimally low levels of electrical current in a form that is compatible with the body's own healthy biocurrents. Used to heal muscle-related back injuries or reduce muscle pain, these almost sub-sensory signals are applied to damaged muscle to recharge the cellular "battery," which in turn leads to healing. The pain relief comes from decreases in swelling and spasms and increases in muscle flexibility. Microcurrent is an application within the larger treatment field called electrotherapy, which uses stronger electrical currents for pain reduction. Nearly all U.S. chiropractic offices, physical therapy clinics, and hospital rehabilitation departments employ some form of electrotherapy for pain control, such as ultrasound or the well-known TENS (Transcutaneous Electrical Nerve Stimulation) unit.

TENS works by applying a constant electrical stimulation to a painful area of the body. By stimulating certain nerves, TENS reduces the neural transmission of pain and produces large amounts of endorphins (natural opiates that block the transmission of pain messages at the brain and extremities). There are two types of nerve fibers in the arms, legs, and thorax: nerve fibers with a large diameter tend to inhibit pain transmission and prevent pain, while nerve fibers with small diameters tend to facilitate transmission of pain. The application of electrical stimulus to painful areas causes the large-diameter nerves (pain inhibitors) to override the small-diameter nerves (pain transmitters), resulting in a reduced sensation of pain.

Bodywork

According to Thomas Hudak, L.M.T., of Southbury, Connecticut, massage is one of the most important adjunct therapies for the treatment of fibromyalgia. Fibromyalgia patients often experience prolonged muscle tension, which interferes with the elimination of chemical wastes in the muscles and surrounding tissue. Poor circulation in muscle tissues can cause nerve and muscle pain, which can spread to other areas of the body. A nerve that supplies the muscles also supplies the supporting structures of the joint. Pains that seem to emanate from the joints may actually be coming from "trigger points," focal areas where wastes have accumulated in the muscles.

Massage helps break up muscular waste deposits and stimulates circulation to troubled regions in the body. Deep pressure on trigger points stretches tissues and loosens shortened muscles to restore muscular balance and proper functioning. Most importantly, certain types of pain can be relieved by massage, as the rhythmic motions sedate the nervous system and promote voluntary muscle relaxation. A typical program of massage involves at least two to three sessions per week in the early treatment stages, then once a week for several months, with a maintenance schedule of twice a month. Remember that massage therapies should be designed to fit individual profiles,

In one study, 21 of 26 fibromyalgia patients experienced reduced pain and general improvement after receiving massage therapy. The study discovered a relationship between a fibromyalgia patient's degree of pain and an increase in blood levels of myoglobin (the oxygen-carrying protein of the muscle tissue). The pain may be the outcome of myoglobin leaking from the muscles. Along with the pain reduction after massage, there was a gradual decline in the high levels of myoglobin in the patients' blood.[31]

Osteopathic Medicine

Osteopathic medicine is a treatment method based on the principle that the structure of the body (the musculoskeletal system) is interrelated with the function of its systems and organs, and that disruptions in one can cause problems in the other, making both subject to a wide range of disorders. After a thorough evaluation, an osteopath performs adjustments (manipulations) on the patient, which help the body to correct its structural problems. These manipulations include cranial manipulation, relax and release techniques for the muscles and soft tissues, and articulation (similar to chiropractic adjust-

---

ACUPUNCTURE FOR PAIN RELIEF

Twenty patients with fibromyalgia were treated with acupuncture. Five representative "tender points" were examined before and after therapy. Increased blood flow was registered above all tender points after acupuncture, plus skin temperature had increased in ten of 12 tender points and the number of tender points was reduced from an average of 16.1 to 13.8. Most importantly, pain threshold increased in ten out of 12 tender points. The researchers concluded that "acupuncture is a useful method to treat patients with fibromyalgia; the improvement in circulation above tender points may alleviate pain."[30]

---

ments). Research confirms that osteopathy can provide effective relief of FMS symptoms. In one study of 18 patients who had suffered with FMS for one year or longer, tender point pain was reduced and patients reported an improved daily quality of life. These benefits were achieved after nine treatments spaced one to three weeks apart.[32]

Mind/Body Therapies

Stress is a common part of everyday life, but it can become harmful to the body when it is prolonged or chronic. It affects the body in very real, physical ways by influencing the immune and hormonal systems. For fibromyalgia sufferers, this can mean an increase in pain and inflammation. A basic premise of mind/body medicine is that chronic stress contributes to illness and that relaxation techniques and learning positive ways of coping with stress will improve your health. In a recent review of nontraditional approaches to treating FMS, Brian Berman, M.D., of the University of Maryland School of Medicine, concluded that various mind/body techniques have shown the greatest success so far at improving the symptoms of fibromyalgia.[33] Meditation, biofeedback, guided imagery, and hypnotherapy can help improve pain tolerance and alleviate anxiety and sleep disturbances.

Biofeedback training and neurotherapy (also known as neurobiofeedback or NBF) are methods of learning how to consciously regulate normally unconscious bodily functions (such as breathing, heart rate, and blood pressure) through the use of simple electronic devices. such devices give immediate "feedback" or information about the biological system of the person being monitored, so that he or she can learn to consciously influence that system. Dr. Laibow recommends NBF, along with nutrition, exercise, and lymph detoxification, for the treatment of fibromyalgia. However, she cautions that NBF should never be used without first undergoing comprehensive testing for toxic allergic and nutritional factors. Biofeedback and NBF can be done in the physician's office or a caregiver can be trained to administer the treatments at home in conjunction with frequent consultations with the physician.

Recommendations

- A healthy, balanced diet is essential in treating fibromyalgia. Research has shown that switching to a vegetarian diet improves symptoms of pain, joint stiffness, and sleep disturbances.

- Nutrients such as vitamin B3, antioxidants (vitamins C and E), lipotropic factors (substances that remove and prevent fatty deposits), essential fatty acids, selenium, and zinc may be helpful for fibromyalgia relief.

- Cayenne has two benefits for fibromyalgia sufferers: it dissolves the sensation of pain and depletes bodily reserves of Substance P, believed to be overabundant in people with fibromyalgia.

- Chamomile produces a calming effect, easing anxiety and reducing tension.

- Prolotherapy and neural therapy evoke the body's natural inflammatory process to heal, stabilize, and strengthen injured tendons and ligaments.

- TENS works by applying a constant electrical stimulation to a painful area of the body. By stimulating certain nerves, TENS reduces the neural transmission of pain and produces large amounts of endorphins (natural opiates that block the transmission of pain messages).

- Certain types of pain can be relieved by massage, as the rhythmic motions sedate the nervous system and promote voluntary muscle relaxation.

- Meditation, biofeedback, guided imagery, and hypnotherapy can help improve pain tolerance and alleviate anxiety and sleep disturbances.

Self-Care
The following therapies can be undertaken at home under appropriate professional supervision:

Exercise / Yoga

AROMATHERAPY: • For muscular fatigue, use lavender, marjoram, rosemary, clary sage. • For acute pain, use black pepper, ginger, birch.

Professional Care
The following therapies should only be provided by a qualified health professional:

Acupuncture / Biofeedback Training and Neurotherapy / Chiropractic / Detoxification Therapy / Energy Medicine / Environmental Medicine / Hypnotherapy / Magnetic Field Therapy / Traditional Chinese Medicine
BODYWORK: Feldenkrais Method, myotherapy, Therapeutic Touch

Where to Find Help

The following organizations are good resources for obtaining further information on fibromyalgia.

National Fibromyalgia Awareness Campaign (NFAC)
2415 N. River Trail Road, Suite 200
Orange, California 92865
(714) 921-0150

One of the main organizations devoted to fibromyalgia education. Publishes newsletters and provides pamphlets on FMS.

Fibromyalgia Network
P.O. Box 31750
Tucson, Arizona 85751-1750
(800) 853-2929

Publishes newsletters and other information on FMS.

CFIDS Association, Inc.
P.O. Box 220398
Charlotte, North Carolina 28222-0398
(800) 442-3437 or (704) 365-2343
Website: www.cfids.org

The largest nonprofit organization dedicated to funding research and disseminating information on chronic fatigue and immune dysfunction syndrome. Publishes a journal, CFIDS Chronicle, provides a nationwide referral list of physicians and CFIDS associations, and maintains a computer bulletin board with daily updates on CFIDS research.

American Association of Naturopathic Physicians
8201 Greensboro Drive, Suite 300
McLean, Virginia 22101
(703) 610-9037
Website: www.naturopathic.org

Provides a directory of naturopathic physicians and offers referrals to a nationwide network of accredited or licensed practitioners. Also publishes a quarterly newsletter, for both professionals and the general public, and offers a series of brochures and pamphlets on a variety of subjects.

Milwaukee Pain Clinic
6529 West Fond du Lac Avenue
Milwaukee, Wisconsin 53218
(414) 464-7246
Website: www.milwaukeepainclinic.com

Provides prolotherapy and other musculoskeletal therapies; training courses in prolotherapy are also available. For additional information, send a legal size, self-addressed, stamped envelope.

Recommended Reading

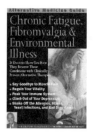

Alternative Medicine Guide to Chronic Fatigue, Fibromyalgia, and Environmental Illness. Burton Goldberg and the Editors of *Alternative Medicine Digest.* Tiburon, CA: Future Medicine Publishing, 1998.

Alternative Treatments for Fibromyalgia and Chronic Fatigue Syndrome. Mari Skelly and Andrea Helm. Alameda, CA: Hunter House, 1999.

Fibromyalgia: A Comprehensive Approach. Miryam Ehrlich Williamson. New York: Walker and Company, 1996.

Fibromyalgia and Chronic Myofascial Pain Syndrome. Devin Starlanyl and Mary Ellen Copeland. New York: MJF Books, 1998.

The Fibromyalgia Handbook. Harris H. McIlwain and Debra Fulghum Bruce. New York: Henry Holt, 1999.

Fibromyalgia: The New Integrative Approach. Milton Hammerly. Holbrook, MA: Adams Media, 2000.

What Your Doctor May Not Tell You About Fibromyalgia. R. Paul St. Amand and Claudia Craig Marek. New York: Warner Books, 1999.

GASTROINTESTINAL DISORDERS

Proper digestion, absorption of nutrients, and elimination of wastes are essential requirements for optimum health. Disorders of the gastrointestinal tract are quite common and can lead to improper digestion, malabsorption, and nutritional deficiencies, all of which may contribute to the development of many other diseases. Alternative medicine treats these disorders with diet, nutritional supplements, herbal remedies, and stress reduction to restore proper digestion and enhance overall health.

A HEALTHY COLON teems with beneficial microorganisms that contribute to the healthy digestion and absorption of food. However, years of poor diet, reliance on medications, stress, and other factors can throw the intestinal ecology severely out of balance, causing a variety of illnesses. Nutritionist Lindsey Duncan, C.N., of Santa Monica, California, says, "I've consulted with 8,000 clients, who come to me with a variety of health problems ranging from fatigue, depression, impaired immune function, and obesity to chronic constipation, gas, acne, and lower back pain. The vast majority of these complaints and symptoms are alleviated by healing and supporting the intestinal system."

Indeed, many illnesses arise from problems in the intestines, including gastritis, colitis, Crohn's disease, irritable bowel syndrome, ulcers, diverticulitis, diarrhea, and hemorrhoids. Most of the digestion and absorption of nutrients that happens in the body occurs along the passageway that comprises the small and large intestines. Keeping this passageway clean and alive with healthy digestive microbes is vital to maintaining overall health.

Causes of Gastrointestinal Disorders

According to Patrick Donovan, N.D., of Seattle, Washington, there are many causes of gastrointestinal (GI) disorders, including dietary and nutritional factors, food allergies, viral and bacterial infections, parasites, and stress.

The typical Western diet of high fat, high carbohydrate, highly processed foods with many additives and preservatives is the root cause of many digestive disorders.

"They can also be secondary to problems with the pancreas, liver, or gallbladder, all of which are involved in the digestive process," Dr. Donovan says. Many of these disorders involve inflammation of part of the digestive tract, which may be secondary to any of the above causes. Disturbance of the digestive system can lead to malabsorption and nutritional deficiencies.

Poor Diet and Nutrition

The typical Western diet of high fat, high carbohydrate, highly processed foods with many additives and preservatives is the root cause of many digestive disorders.[1] Lack of fiber in such a diet makes the digestive system sluggish and leads to improper elimination and constipation. This, in turn, causes a buildup of toxins in the body and may lead to "leaky gut syndrome," in which food particles cross the intestinal wall and enter the bloodstream, inducing an overactive immune response. Nutritional deficiencies can also lead to poor digestion and malabsorption of food, as can deficiencies in digestive enzymes.

Food Allergies

Food allergies lie behind many disease processes and may be a factor in gastrointestinal disorders.[2] Common culprits are milk, dairy products, and wheat. Gluten intolerance can result in celiac disease (intestinal malabsorption). Food allergies may also arise as a result of malabsorption syndrome, which occurs whenever there is injury to the surface layer of the digestive tract, according to Dr. Donovan. With poor digestion, large food particles cross the gut wall and enter the bloodstream, where they can cause food allergies.

Immunologic Factors

Several gastrointestinal disorders involve the immune system. People with deficient immune systems often suffer from malabsorption. If IgA, an antibody normally present in the intestine, is lacking or deficient, the person suffers from an increased amount of gastrointestinal infections. Antibodies in the digestive tract, which normally protect against infection and microbial toxins, help rid the body of parasitic worms and control the absorption of harmful antigens. Evidence suggests that immune mechanisms play a role in colitis (inflammation of the colon) and Crohn's disease (inflammation of the small intestine), since patients with these conditions have antibodies and white blood cells that react with cells that line their GI tract.[3]

Infections

Bacterial, fungal, and viral infections, as well as parasites, can be harmful to the digestive system. Bacteria, fungi, and viruses can cause gastroenteritis, an inflammation of the digestive system often referred to as the stomach flu. They can also release toxins into the system, which result in leaky gut syndrome and cause autoimmune reactions if they enter the circulation. Viruses and bacteria such as Epstein-Barr virus, cytomegalovirus, *Pseudomonas, Chlamydia,* and *Yersinia enterocolitica* have all been associated with Crohn's disease.[4] Parasites also liberate toxins and rob the body of essential nutrients.

An abnormal growth of organisms in the gut is known as dysbiosis. It occurs when pathogenic (disease-causing) organisms in the gut cause the normal flora to be imbalanced. Dysbiosis is a major factor in malabsorption, inflammatory bowel disease, and leaky gut syndrome, according to Dr. Donovan.

High/Low Hydrochloric Acid Levels

Too much or too little hydrochloric acid (HCl) secretion by the stomach is another factor that can lead to digestive problems and malabsorption, according to Virender Sodhi, M.D. (Ayurveda), N.D., Director of the Ayurvedic and Naturopathic Medical Clinic, in Bellevue, Washington. "Too little acid can lead to anemia, as vitamin B12 and folic acid will not be absorbed effectively. And too much acid will give heartburn and gas and may lead to ulcers," Dr. Sodhi explains.

Stress

There is little doubt that psychological stress affects the digestive system, causing excess acid production and poor digestive function. Crohn's disease, ulcerative colitis, and irritable bowel syndrome (irritation of the large intestine) are associated with, and aggravated by, stress, Dr. Donovan points out.

THE GASTROINTESTINAL TRACT

The gastrointestinal (GI) tract is a tube, 25-32 feet in length, which begins at the mouth and ends at the anus. It comprises the mouth, pharynx, esophagus, stomach, small intestine (duodenum, jejunum, and ileum), large intestine (cecum, ascending colon, transverse colon, and descending colon), rectum, and anus. Accessory organs—the liver, pancreas, and gallbladder—all play an important role in digestion.

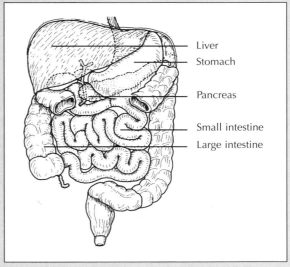

Digestion begins when food mixes with enzymes in saliva. The process is then carried on in the stomach by hydrochloric acid (HCl) and pepsin. Food is liquefied in the stomach and passes into the small intestine, where it is further broken down by digestive enzymes from the pancreas (protease digests proteins, amylase digests carbohydrates, and lipase digests fats). If the pancreas does not produce sufficient enzymes, digestion will be incomplete and absorption of nutrients restricted.

The liver detoxifies toxins, produces proteins and cholesterol, stores the fat-soluble vitamins A, D, E, and K, and produces bile, essential for the absorption of fats and stimulates the small intestine. Any impairment of the liver will thus affect the digestive process. The gallbladder secretes bile to aid absorption of fats and fat-soluble vitamins. Although the gallbladder functions only as a storage vessel for bile, chemical disturbances may result in the formation of gallstones, impeding the flow of bile to the small intestine and the absorption of nutrients.

Most food absorption takes place in the small intestine, while water, electrolytes, and some of the final products of digestion are absorbed in the large intestine.

LEAKY GUT SYNDROME

According to Patrick Donovan, N.D., of Seattle, Washington, the latest research shows that "leaky gut syndrome" has been associated with many disorders and may be the focus from which autoimmune disorders originate. Leaky gut syndrome occurs when the intestinal mucosa is damaged and large food molecules, bacteria, and microorganisms pass across the intestinal wall to circulate through the body. Antibodies are made against these molecules. If the molecules look like normal body components, the antibody cannot distinguish between the two and may attack that body component (autoimmune reaction). This phenomenon can also occur with bacteria and certain drugs. "Bacterial antigens have been associated with rheumatoid arthritis and ankylosing spondylitis," Dr. Donovan reports.

Robert A. Anderson, M.D., founding President of the American Board of Holistic Medicine, has also found that stress can play a significant role in gastrointestinal disorders, as can unresolved emotions. One of his patients, a 58-year-old woman, came to him suffering from chronic diarrhea, for which laboratory tests failed to determine a specific cause. Based on the tests, Dr. Anderson, who knew the woman to be anxious and a perfectionist, suggested that stress might be the cause of her symptoms. She promptly denied this and continued to suffer from diarrhea for four more months, before finally being willing to consider that Dr. Anderson was correct. Eventually, she confided to Dr. Anderson that she was angry with her two sisters, who refused to cooperate by forwarding the information she needed to settle their mother's estate following her death. As the executor of her mother's will, this left the woman both angry and stressful.

Dr. Anderson encouraged her to acknowledge her anger and to write a letter to her sisters in which she expressed all of her resentments towards them. He then instructed her to sign it and give it to her husband to destroy. On the very day that she carried out this suggestion, her diarrhea stopped and she had experienced no further symptoms when Dr. Anderson saw her six months later for a check-up. Moreover, once her resentment had been expressed, the woman wrote her sisters a letter of reconciliation, which served to heal her relationship with them.[5]

Insufficient Exercise

Insufficient exercise leads to a decrease in enzyme and hydrochloric acid secretion needed for digestion, according to Dr. Sodhi. This will lead to malabsorption, nutritional deficiencies, and constipation.

Gastrointestinal Disorders and Their Treatment

Since many gastrointestinal disorders share symptoms such as inflammation, poor absorption, bloating, gas, abdominal cramps, constipation, and diarrhea, the treatments often overlap. The alternative approach to such disorders includes dietary changes, nutritional supplementation, detection and elimination of food allergies, herbal remedies, and stress reduction.

Dr. Donovan recommends a whole foods diet to prevent gastrointestinal problems. "Eliminate all food additives and prefabricated foods and junk foods," he says, "and eat a high–complex carbohydrate, high–fiber, moderate protein, low-fat diet." He recommends staying away from red meat and nuts (unless they are fresh in their shells). Only high-quality, cold-pressed oils should be used, preferably flaxseed or olive oil. "Fats should make up only 10% to 15% of the daily calories," he adds. "I also recommend pasta, beans, vegetables, and protein from fish. If you must have meat, then I recommend organically grown, free-range lamb or poultry."

Dr. Sodhi recommends that black pepper and ginger be sprinkled on foods to aid digestion. Olive oil and lemon may also be useful. In Ayurvedic medicine, treatment depends on body type and different food dressings are recommended for different body types. "Many people have low hydrochloric acid," Dr. Sodhi says. He recommends half a lemon squeezed into ½ cup of water, 10-15 minutes before meals, to stimulate gastric juices. "Ginger tea, or ginger added to the lemon juice, is also effective," he says. "*Trikatu*, a mixture of Indian long pepper, black pepper, and ginger, can be taken as well, an effective dose being ½ teaspoon before meals."

Gastritis

Gastritis is an inflammation of the stomach. "The most common gastrointestinal disorder is viral gastritis," says Dr. Donovan. "You often see it as a combination viral gastroenteritis, which means inflammation of the stomach and intestines—that's the name for the common stomach flu." Bacteria such as *Helicobacter pylori* can cause gastritis, according to Dr. Donovan. "We find a correlation with the presence of *Helicobacter pylori* in about 93% of patients with gastritis and gastric ulcers," he says. Gastritis can also be induced chemically by medications such

RESTORING INTESTINAL VITALITY
WITH FOS AND SOIL-BASED ORGANISMS

An estimated 100 trillion bacteria, both "friendly" and pathogenic, live in the gastrointestinal tract, co-existing within a delicate balance. "Friendly" bacteria, such as *Lactobacillus* and *Bifidobacteria*, support numerous physiological processes in the body, while pathogenic bacteria, such as *E. coli, Staphylococcus*, and *Clostridium*, can harmfully impact, in some cases dangerously, intestinal health. To maintain the balance of the various intestinal flora, practitioners of alternative medicine often recommend using probiotics—the deliberate introduction of live, "friendly" bacteria into the GI tract through food products, such as yogurt, and special supplements.

In recent years, two other approaches have emerged that have been shown to significantly enhance overall gastrointestinal health—prebiotics, which involves the use of nutrients that directly feed the beneficial bacteria that already exist in the large intestine but decline with age; and soil-based organisms (SBOs), which have been shown to bolster overall immune function and normalize and enhance the functions of the GI tract.

Japanese researchers have found that a naturally-occurring form of carbohydrate known as fructo-oligosaccharides (FOS) acts like an intestinal "fertilizer," selectively feeding *Bifidobacteria* in the large intestine so that their numbers increase, thereby discouraging the growth of harmful bacteria. In one study, researchers found that when 23 hospital patients, 50-90 years old, took 8 g (2 tsp) of FOS daily for two weeks, their *Bifidobacteria* levels increased tenfold. FOS is found in foods such as garlic, honey, Jerusalem artichokes, soybeans, asparagus, rye, barley, bananas, tomatoes, and onions. However, Robert Crayhon, M.S., C.N., author of *Health Benefits of FOS*, notes that "there is not enough FOS in foods in the average diet to get an optimal or therapeutically significant dose," which is why the use of FOS supplements is advised.[6]

SBOs are beneficial microbes found in soil, which exhibit the same health-enhancing characteristics of probiotic supplements. Before the advent of modern chemical farming methods, the earth was rich in these organisms, which naturally destroy molds, yeasts, fungi, and viruses in the soil, and perform the same function in the body when present in the food supply. When taken as a supplement, SBOs help detoxify the intestinal tract, improve nutrient absorption, and expel pathogens, including parasites. Research has shown that SBOs facilitate overall cellular health and restore cell function by producing RNA/DNA and metabolizing proteins necessary for cell growth and repair. In addition, SBOs enhance immune function due to their antioxidant properties and their ability to stimulate the production of immune proteins (alpha interferon) and human lactoferrin.[7]

---

as aspirin, ibuprofen, Motrin, Indocin, and steroids, or can be due to an autoimmune reaction destroying the lining of the digestive tract. This often leads to pernicious anemia, an anemia due to interference of vitamin B_{12} absorption.

Alternative treatments for gastritis address the virus to restore balance within the system. These remedies include diet and nutritional supplementation, herbal medicine, and Ayurvedic medicine.

Diet and Nutrition: According to Dr. Donovan, shiitake mushrooms activate the immune system and have a strong antiviral effect. He also recommends vitamin C to just below bowel tolerance (the highest dose that does not cause diarrhea), beta carotene, zinc, and a multivitamin-mineral supplement for the treatment of viral gastroenteritis. "The advantage of vitamin C, zinc, and beta carotene is that they help the lining of the gastrointestinal tract repair and regenerate itself," he adds. He uses

bismuth as an antibiotic and antiprotozoal agent against *H. pylori*, if it is present.

Herbal Medicine: Dr. Donovan recommends the use of herbs that stimulate the immune system while reducing inflammation and encouraging repair of the stomach lining, such as echinacea and goldenseal.

Ayurvedic Medicine: Dr. Sodhi uses meditation, with the type varying with a person's body type. "*Vata* types need chanting or mantras," he states. "*Pitta* types are visually oriented and should meditate with visualization techniques. *Kapha* types are smell and taste oriented and should use incense or flowers."

Colitis and Crohn's Disease

Colitis and Crohn's Disease involve inflammation and possible ulceration of the digestive tract. Symptoms include diarrhea, fever, anorexia, weight loss, gas, and abdominal tenderness. There may be bloody diarrhea if intestinal bleeding occurs. Colitis is confined to the colon,

THE SPECIFIC CARBOHYDRATE DIET

If you suffer from gastrointestinal disorders such as celiac disease, ulcerative colitis, Crohn's disease, severe constipation, chronic diarrhea, diverticulitis, or spastic colon, and think your condition is incurable, you're mistaken, according to Elaine Gottschall, M.Sc. Ever since she watched her own four-year-old daughter recover from ulcerative colitis over 45 years ago, Gottschall has been restoring gastrointestinal health for hundreds of people who thought they were beyond help.

Gottschall calls her approach the Specific Carbohydrate Diet, which is based on the pioneering work of the late Sidney V. Haas, M.D. According to Gottschall, the diet's success rate is excellent, achieving an 80% recovery rate for Crohn's disease and 95% for diverticulitis. Patients following this diet for as little as three weeks will see marked improvement, she says.

According to Dr. Haas's findings, gastrointestinal disorders are due to an imbalanced relationship between carbohydrates and intestinal microbes. When the GI tract becomes unbalanced, bacteria multiply and food absorption declines, producing a vicious cycle that can last for years. The body becomes unable to digest carbohydrates because of microbial overgrowth and toxins. Eventually, numerous illnesses can develop out of this altered intestinal milieu as the system becomes unable to digest most of the foods comprising the standard Western diet.

This trend can be reversed by following Gottschall's Specific Carbohydrate Diet, although she advises that "it is unwise to undertake this regimen unless you are willing to follow it with fanatical adherence." Here are the diet's highlights:

- Proteins to avoid: Processed meats, breaded or canned fish, processed cheeses, smoked or canned meats.

- Proteins allowed: Fresh or frozen meats, poultry, fish, eggs, natural cheeses, homemade yogurt, dry curd cottage cheese.

- Other foods to avoid: All cereal grains in any form, including flour, potatoes, yams, parsnips, chick peas, bean sprouts, soybeans, mung beans, fava beans, and seaweed.

- Vegetables allowed: Most fresh or frozen (but not canned) vegetables and legumes.

- Fruits allowed: Fresh, raw, dried, or cooked fruits, but not canned (except in their own juices).

- Not permitted: Milk or dried milk solids; buttermilk or acidophilus milk; commercially prepared yogurt and sour cream; soymilk; instant tea or coffee, and coffee substitutes; beer; cornstarch, arrowroot, or other starches; chocolate or carob; bouillon cubes or instant soup bases; all products made with refined sugar; agar-agar, carrageenan, or pectin; ketchup; ice cream; molasses, corn or maple syrup; flours made from legumes; baking powder; medications containing sugar; all seeds.

By rigidly following this diet, "many cases of celiac disease, spastic colon, and diverticulitis appear to be cured at the end of a year," Gottschall says.[8]

---

whereas Crohn's disease, though usually affecting the small intestine, can also affect the mouth, esophagus, and stomach. The degeneration of the intestinal mucosa (surface layer of cells) often leads to poor absorption and nutritional deficiencies, says Dr. Donovan. This is a major problem if the distal ileum is involved, since this is where vitamin B12 is absorbed. There may also be an autoimmune component to these diseases. The immune system may react to the cells as they break down or to the food particles or bacteria, which can cross the damaged intestinal walls.

Although colitis and Crohn's disease may result in similar symptoms, the causes are multifactorial and are often the result of autoimmune disorders or food aller-gies. Alternative treatments address these factors through diet, nutritional supplementation, herbal medicine, and Ayurvedic medicine.

Diet and Nutrition: Patients with colitis and Crohn's disease often have decreased food intake and suffer from nutritional deficiencies. Elimination diets are recommended to eliminate food allergies, which may be complicating the problem. According to Dr. Donovan, common allergenic foods are wheat, corn, dairy products, and carrageenan-containing foods (processed foods with stabilizers and suspending agents). Supplements of magnesium, calcium, iron, potassium, and multivitamins are needed to counteract the decreased food intake and decreased absorption from the small intestine.

"One of the best ways to prevent colitis and Crohn's disease is a high-fiber diet," says Dr. Donovan, "but once active colitis is present you cannot use fiber since it is too harsh. As healing occurs, you can use soluble fibers." He suggests a liquid diet in the active phase, consisting of juices from cabbage and green leafy vegetables, because the chlorophyll has healing properties. A good source of chlorophyll is fresh water algae like chlorella. Dr. Donovan also suggests vegetable broths and broths from the seaweeds *wakame, hijiki,* and *kombu,* as well as fish and meat broths for some patients. Vegetables are gradually added back into the diet, then blended fruit juices. This is followed by the introduction of meat and fish broths, then solid fish. When patients are back to normal, they can add animal proteins, grains, and beans.

A patient with a ten-year history of colitis and no relief from conventional therapy came to Dr. Donovan. He fasted the patient for four days and then put him on vegetable juices and lamb bone broth, after having determined which foods he was allergic to. His iron-deficiency anemia was treated with iron-containing herbs and foods such as spinach and kale. His symptoms began to resolve. Over the next ten days, he was put on raw and steamed vegetables and salads and, by the end of a month, he was back on a whole foods vegetarian diet. Within 30 days, he was able to return to work.

Herbal Medicine: Plant flavonoids such as quercetin are helpful in reducing the inflammatory response. According to David L. Hoffmann, B.Sc., M.N.I.M.H., of Sebastopol, California, past President of the American Herbalists Guild, chamomile and peppermint are beneficial for gas, colic, and for associated diarrhea. He recommends astringents such as bayberry, marshmallow root, or plantain and antispasmodics such as wild yam aid the healing process. He suggests a mixture of equal parts bayberry, agrimony, peppermint, wild yam, and valerian for a relaxing effect (one teaspoon taken three times a day). An infusion of chamomile or lemon balm should be taken warm frequently.

Dr. Donovan recommends licorice root tea with marshmallow, slippery elm bark, geranium, yarrow, and goldenseal. He also uses Robert's Formula, which consists of a mixture of marshmallow root (a demulcent, to soften the tissues), wild indigo (for infections), echinacea (an antibacterial that promotes normalization of the immune system), *Geranium maculatum* (to prevent bleeding), goldenseal (to inhibit bacterial growth), poke root (for healing ulceration), comfrey (an anti-inflammatory and promoter of wound healing), and slippery elm (a demulcent).

Dr. Donovan recommends quercetin when food allergies are present. Butyric acid enemas are also part of his treatment. "They have an anti-inflammatory effect

DRUGS ASSOCIATED WITH A HIGHER INCIDENCE OF GASTROINTESTINAL REACTIONS

According to the *Physicians' Desk Reference,* the following drugs are associated with side effects of gastrointestinal reactions (statistics refer to the percentage of individuals affected).[9]

Accutane capsules (approximately 5%)
Alka-Seltzer antacid & pain reliever (4.9% at doses of 1,000 mg daily)
Anturane capsules, tablets (most frequent)
Bayer Aspirin tablets, caplets (4.9% at doses of 1,000 mg)
Bayer Plus Aspirin tablets (4.9%)
Bufferin Analgesic tablets and caplets (4.8%)
Ceptaz (most frequent)
Clinoril tablets (3%-9%)
Cuprimine capsules (17%)
Ecotrin Enteric Coated Aspirin (4.9% at 1,000 mg daily)
Feldene capsules (20%)
Ilosone liquid, oral suspensions, tablets (most frequent)
Lamprene capsules (40%-50%)
Leukine for IV infusion (37%)
Lopid tablets (34.2%)
Marplan tablets (among most frequent)
Meclomen capsules (10%)
Novantrone for injection concentrate (58%-88%)
Paraplatin for injection (17%-21%)
Piroxicam capsules USP (approximately 20%)
Prokine I.V. infusion (37%)
Retrovir capsules, I.V. infusion, syrup (20%)
Rynatuss pediatric suspension, tablets (among most frequent)
Supprelin injection (3%-10%)
Suprax powder for oral suspension, tablets (30%)
Ticlid tablets (30%-40%)
Tolectin (10%)
Toradol IM injection, oral (13%)
Trecator-SC tablets (among most frequent)
Trilisate liquid, tablets (Less than 20%)
Voltaren tablets (20%)

and help the mucosa of the intestine to heal and regenerate," he says. "Butyric acid comes from fiber in the diet and patients with colitis and low butyric acid levels are prone to colon cancer."

Ayurvedic Medicine: "Treatment is mainly focused on relaxing the patient," says Dr. Sodhi. Medi-

NATURAL REMEDIES FOR HEARTBURN

Heartburn, that burning sensation in the upper chest that seems to come in waves about an hour after eating, can be intensely uncomfortable. Many people suffering from heartburn automatically reach for a commercial antacid to neutralize their overly acidic stomach, but there are numerous safe, quick, and effective natural solutions to consider as alternatives.

Exercise Dietary Prudence—First, try to eliminate the probable causes of your heartburn. According to Melvyn R. Werbach, M.D., author of *Nutritional Influences on Illness*, dietary changes known to reduce the incidence of heartburn in those already susceptible include the following: avoid late dinners, fatty meals, alcohol, peppermint and spearmint, chocolate, coffee, milk, orange juice, spicy foods, sugar, tea, and tomato products.[10]

Donald J. Brown, N.D., advises that heartburn symptoms may be eased by taking 600 mg of calcium carbonate (in liquid or chewable tablet form) every 2-3 hours until the discomfort has subsided.[11] According to the late naturopathic physician Hazel Parcells, N.D., Ph.D., D.C., at the first sign of heartburn, sip a glass of warm water into which is mixed one teaspoon of baking soda and heartburn "will go away almost immediately." The baking soda helps to neutralize the overly acidic stomach.

Herbs to Quench the Burning—Taking ½ teaspoon of goldenseal herbal extract (with three tablespoons of water; one dose only per episode) can often relieve burning within 15 minutes. Among its other abilities, goldenseal acts as an astringent and tonic for the mucous membranes lining the gastrointestinal tract. Taken on its own as an encapsulated powder, slippery elm bark exerts a mucilaginous effect on the lining of the esophagus, stomach, and intestines.

For herbal expert James A. Duke, Ph.D., author of *The Green Pharmacy*, a number of common garden herbs are useful in reducing heartburn: "Angelade" (the fresh juice of angelica stalks, carrots, celery, fennel, garlic, parsley, and parsnips); dill (two teaspoons of crushed seeds, steeped

in hot water for a tea; not to be used while pregnant); or gentian (simmer one teaspoon of gentian leaves in 1-2 cups of water for 30 minutes; take 30 minutes before eating).[12]

Homeopathic Remedies—Homeopathy offers a number of first-aid remedies for relief of acute episodes of heartburn, according to type of symptoms, advise naturopathic physicians Robert Ullman, N.D., and Judyth Reichenberg-Ullman, N.D. Among them: *Arsenicum album* (for extreme burning pains in the stomach, anxiety, chills and thirst, abdominal cramping); *Nux vomica* (when heartburn occurs after eating fats or sour foods, accompanied by irritability); and *Sulfur* (when heartburn develops after overeating or eating the "wrong" foods, belching, late morning hunger, early morning diarrhea). They recommend one dose of one remedy (at 30C strength) every four hours until improvement is noticed; then, one dose if symptoms return.[13]

Undoing the Emotional Knots—Chronic heartburn implies an unresolved emotional issue, says Christiane Northrup, M.D. Among the clients she has treated, the underlying emotion is often a kind of addiction to responsibility, compounded by "a feeling of inescapable stress in your life," she comments. One way to gently undo the emotions knotting up your esophagus is with flower essences, taken several times daily for a month or until signs of improvement in your emotional state are noticed, suggest Patricia Kaminski and Richard Katz in *Flower Essence Repertory*. *Elm* is indicated for feeling overwhelmed or overburdened by responsibility and manifesting a perfectionist tendency. *Lavender* is suggested for a feeling of nervous overwhelm, when soothing and calming are needed. *Golden Yarrow* can help with performance anxiety, especially when it registers in the upper abdomen.[14]

CAUTION While a natural approach to heartburn is clearly effective, if heartburn occurs regularly, such as once weekly, it could indicate more complicated problems, such as a hiatal hernia, an enzymatic imbalance or deficiency, or stress or dysfunction in the spleen, adrenal glands, or liver.

tation is recommended. He also believes there is a strong component of food allergies, so these are identified and eliminated. A complete stool analysis is done to see how well food is being digested and if parasites or bacteria are present. Dr. Sodhi uses fish oils and flaxseed oil and the herb *boswellia* to reduce inflammation, along with acidophilus to reconstitute the gut microflora. "Yogurt, cumin, and ginger are also helpful," he says. "But make sure the yogurt does not contain carrageenan, as this can cause bowel cancer."

Irritable Bowel Syndrome

Irritable bowel syndrome (IBS) is a condition in which the large intestine, or colon, fails to operate normally. It is a functional disorder, since there is no evidence of structural damage to the intestine. Symptoms include pain, constipation, diarrhea, gas, nausea, anorexia, and anxiety or depression.[15] The cause is unknown, but food allergies, excess dietary fats, and stress seem to be implicated in IBS. Treatment of IBS aims to reduce the irritation to the digestive system and therefore relies on dietary changes, herbal remedies, and stress reduction.

Diet and Nutrition: The usual treatment for IBS is to increase dietary fiber. To avoid food sensitivities (not allergies, since there does not seem to be an immune component in IBS), fiber from a source other than grains is recommended, such as vegetables, fruits, oat bran, guar gum, psyllium, and legumes (beans and peas). According to James Braly, M.D., of Hollywood, Florida, nuts, seeds, and fruit with small seeds (such as raspberries) should be avoided, as should alcohol, caffeine, and spices. Dr. Braly notes that supplements should include zinc, vitamin A, and evening primrose oil.

Herbal Medicine: Enteric-coated peppermint oil is used in Europe to treat IBS. Without enteric coating, the peppermint oil is absorbed in the upper digestive tract, often causing heartburn and esophageal reflux (stomach acid regurgitating into the esophagus). Ginger also has a long history of use to relieve digestive complaints.[16] Herbs such as chamomile, valerian, rosemary, and balm have antispasmodic effects on the intestines. David Hoffmann recommends a mixture of tinctures of bayberry, gentian, peppermint, and wild yam in equal parts (one teaspoon three times a day) and warm drinks of chamomile or lemon balm.

Stress Reduction: Stress reduction techniques, such as biofeedback and hypnosis, are often helpful in relieving IBS.[17]

 See Stress.

Ulcers

Although traditionally ulcers have been associated with stress, there is evidence that food allergies and nutritional problems may also be responsible, according to Dr. Braly. Excessive dependency on aspirin and other anti-inflammatory medications, including steroids, can also cause ulcers. Symptoms of ulcers include stomach pain or upset, a burning sensation in the stomach, and feelings of acute hunger and pain after eating or lying down. Dr. Donovan has found a high correlation between the presence of *Helicobacter pylori* in the stomach and the occurrence of gastric ulcers. Ulcers are another digestive disorder treated mainly with dietary changes, herbal remedies, and stress reduction.

Diet and Nutrition: Fats, alcohol, and caffeine should be avoided. Avoid aspirin and other anti-inflammatory drugs. Linseed oil on a salad each day is recommended by Dr. Braly, who also suggests drinking three ounces of concentrated aloe vera juice 20 minutes before meals and avoiding foods to which one is allergic. He also advises supplementation with zinc and vitamin A.

Dr. Donovan recommends bismuth for its antibacterial and antiprotozoal effects if *H. pylori* is present and states that bananas and cabbage juice are both effective in treating ulcers in general.

Herbal Medicine: "By using plants that have demulcent, antacid, astringent, and vulnerary [speeding up natural wound healing] actions, it is possible to bring about rapid and complete healing of most ulcers," says David Hoffmann. Some of these plants are marshmallow, calendula, meadowsweet, chamomile, and goldenseal. He suggests drinking an infusion made of one part chamomile and two parts marshmallow root (one teaspoon three times a day). An infusion of chamomile, linden flowers, or valerian may also help. Dr. Donovan recommends licorice root or licorice root tea. It must be deglycyrrhizinated licorice or it will cause high blood pressure over the long term. Cayenne pepper also has a significant healing effect on ulcers, according to Dr. Donovan.

Ayurvedic Medicine: According to Dr. Sodhi, licorice is the best remedy. He recommends taking ½ teaspoon of licorice powder three times a day. He also recommends bananas, coconut (the milk and the fruit), and the herb *ashwagandha*. "A mixture of cinnamon, cardamom, and cloves ground into a powder (¼ teaspoon) can also prove helpful," Dr. Sodhi says. "This reduces acid secretion and relief should be seen immediately." Dr. Sodhi stresses the need to be under the care of a physician when treating GI disorders.

Stress Reduction: Stress reduction techniques such as yoga, meditation, biofeedback, and hypnosis may help

EFFECTS OF HERBS ON THE GASTROINTESTINAL TRACT

Herbs have many properties that can calm, heal, and rejuvenate the gastrointestinal tract.

- Demulcents, such as comfrey, marshmallow, and slippery elm, soothe the lining of the digestive system.

- Anti-inflammatories, such as chamomile, meadowsweet, and marigold, reduce localized tissue inflammation.

- Astringents, such as comfrey and meadowsweet, lessen local bleeding.

- Vulneraries, such as comfrey, chamomile, and goldenseal, speed up local healing.

- Carminatives, such as chamomile, peppermint, and valerian, relieve gas in the lower abdomen.

- Nervines, such as chamomile, valerian, and hops, ease stress.

- Bitters, such as yarrow, wormwood, and gentian, aid in the healing process in the latter stages but are contraindicated in early stages because they stimulate stomach acid and may aggravate the problem.

reduce stress, which is a factor in most digestive system diseases.

Acupuncture: William M. Cargile, B.S., D.C., F.I.A.C.A., former Chairman of Research for the American Association of Oriental Medicine, has had success treating ulcers with acupuncture. He reports on a case of an orthopedic surgeon who was taking Tagamet (a conventional ulcer medication) six times a day, at two to three times the recommended dose, and was getting worse. Dr. Cargile treated the patient with acupuncture, twice on two consecutive days using the Stomach meridian, and he has not needed Tagamet since. In treating ulcer patients, Dr. Cargile uses the acupuncture points associated with stress, anxiety, and stomach/gastrointestinal problems.

Diverticulosis and Diverticulitis

Diverticulosis is a condition in which the walls of the intestines balloon out forming pouches. A small percentage of people go on to develop diverticulitis, an inflammation of these pouches. Problems occur when undigested food particles and small seeds from fruits such as strawberries and raspberries lodge in the pouches. This causes irritation and can lead to inflammation.

"Diverticulosis and diverticulitis are much easier to prevent than to treat," says Dr. Donovan. "They are solely the result of the standard American diet. These diseases do not exist in cultures eating a whole foods, high-fiber diet." Dr. Donovan believes that a major cause of diverticulosis is constipation. "Regular bowel movements, two to three a day, will help prevent diverticulosis," he says.

Diet and Nutrition: A whole foods, high-fiber diet can prevent and relieve the symptoms of diverticulosis and diverticulitis. Dr. Donovan prefers soluble fibers such as ground flax, psyllium, and oat bran, but says a mixture of soluble and insoluble fibers can be used. Flax contains omega-3 fatty acids, which are also beneficial. Foods with small seeds and foods difficult to digest should be avoided.

Patients should be tested for food allergies and any foods to which they are sensitive should be removed from the diet. An ELISA/ACT (enzyme-linked immunosorbent assay/advanced cell test) is the most sensitive way to determine delayed or hidden food allergies and can be used to screen for over 250 types of foods, according to Dr. Donovan.

Fasting: Dr. Donovan recommends a 1-3 day water or vegetable juice fast during acute attacks of diverticulitis. Nutrient-dense broths such as miso or lamb bone broth may also be used until the attack subsides.

Herbal Medicine: Dr. Donovan recommends Robert's Formula, a standard naturopathic remedy, in combination with licorice root tea or deglycyrrhizinated licorice. For daily maintenance, he recommends Robert's Formula with liquid chlorophyll.

Homeopathy: Homeopathic remedies such as *Colocynthis, Bryonia,* and *Belladonna* in low potencies are recommended by Dr. Donovan.

Diarrhea

Diarrhea is a common symptom of many disorders, but should never be taken lightly. Medical attention should be sought if it does not resolve in a few days. Diarrhea results in dehydration, due to loss of fluids, and loss of electrolytes, which can result in death if not replaced. Many people suffer from lactose (milk sugar) intolerance and will suffer from diarrhea if they eat dairy products. A bacterial, viral, or parasitic infection, often from drinking contaminated water, may injure the cells of the small intestine and result in diarrhea. Large amounts of some artificial sweeteners can cause diarrhea, as can megadoses of vitamin C. Diarrhea is often associated with other digestive system disorders such as colitis, Crohn's disease, and IBS.

Diarrhea is usually short-term and self-resolving, but steps can be taken to prevent or treat it. If it becomes chronic, professional advice should be sought.

Diet and Nutrition: According to Dr. Donovan, chronic diarrhea may be due to food allergies, so these need to be identified and eliminated. During the early stages, no food should be eaten. Fluids should be freely consumed and may include fruit and vegetable juices. This should be followed by soups, yogurt, and cooked fruits. Fats and fried foods should be avoided. Vitamin and mineral supplements may be necessary as well, due to excessive nutrient loss.

Dr. Donovan treats children's diarrhea with barley water or rice water. A little sugar can be added to increase the absorption of minerals. Pectin, found in the peel of citrus fruits, apples, carrots, potatoes, sugar beets, and tomatoes, helps relieve diarrhea. *Lactobacillus acidophilus* is needed after diarrhea to reconstitute the bowel flora.

Herbal Medicine: Goldenseal has proved beneficial in bacterial-induced diarrhea.[18] Robert's Formula also has a long history of use in relieving diarrhea, according to Dr. Donovan.

Ayurvedic Medicine: "*Triphala* can be taken as a treatment or a preventive medicine," Dr. Sodhi says. "Also, bael fruit cures many kinds of diarrhea. Bananas are very effective, especially if blended to form a drink. The pectin in the banana absorbs toxins from the body." Goldenseal, Oregon grape, nutmeg, and cumin can also be effective. Care should be taken with cumin, since it can be hallucinogenic, but it can be made into a paste and rubbed on the belly and forehead when treating children.

Hemorrhoids

Hemorrhoids are varicose veins appearing in the anal area. They are not usually evident until the patient is in his or her thirties. Hemorrhoids are caused by a weakness of the veins, excessive venous blood pressure, pregnancy, straining at stool, standing or sitting for long periods, and heavy lifting. While conventional medicine treats hemorrhoids with topical creams or surgery, there are effective natural remedies available.

Diet and Nutrition: Hemorrhoids are rarely seen in parts of the world where high-fiber, unrefined diets are consumed. A high-fiber diet is the most important component in the prevention of hemorrhoids.[19] "A diet rich in vegetables, fruits, legumes, and grains promotes peristalsis and reduces straining during defecation," Dr. Donovan explains. Blackberries, cherries, and blueberries help strengthen the veins, and psyllium and guar gum are good sources of fiber. Dr. Donovan recommends vitamin C and bioflavonoids to strengthen the vascular walls of the colon, rectum, and anus.

Herbal Medicine: Butcher's broom *(Ruscus aculeatus)* and flavonoids are useful in enhancing the integrity of the veins, thus preventing hemorrhoids from developing.[20] David Hoffmann uses equal parts collinsonia,

---

SUCCESS STORY: ENZYME THERAPY FOR CHRONIC DIARRHEA AND SPASTIC COLON

Enzyme therapy can often relieve long-standing gastrointestinal problems, according to Lita Lee, Ph.D., a licensed clinical nutritionist and author of *The Enzyme Cure.* One of Dr. Lee's patients, Frederick, 57, had suffered with chronic diarrhea and a spastic colon for 20 years. "In this condition, you typically have recurrent pain, cramps, or spasms in the abdomen, and diarrhea alternating with constipation," Dr. Lee explains. "Spastic colon is also sometimes associated with irritable bowel syndrome. A lipase deficiency is usually involved."

Frederick would feel sick two hours after eating and experience headaches, weakness, flatulence, and abdominal pain. Laboratory tests had ruled out the possibility of intestinal parasites, and he was taking 4-5 doses of Lomotil every day to cope with his diarrhea. He was also intolerant to milk, so avoided dairy products. But when he first came to Dr. Lee, his diet consisted primarily of refined, processed foods.

Dr. Lee conducted a 24-hour urinalysis, which revealed kidney-lymphatic stress, acidity, severe nutrient deficiencies (vitamin C, calcium, and magnesium), and a toxic colon. It also revealed that Frederick's diet had resulted in excess fat and protein consumption and poor sugar metabolism. "People with spastic colon are usually fiber intolerant and have a tendency to like fats because they produce a feeling of well-being," Dr. Lee says. "They often respond well, even dramatically, to a multiple digestive enzyme formula that is high in the enzyme lipase and contains the enzymes protease, amylase, cellulase, and sugar-digesting enzymes. I used such a formula, which also contained the herbs bilberry, fenugreek and *Ginkgo biloba*, to treat Frederick's spastic colon and diarrhea."

In addition, Dr. Lee prescribed vitamin C and had Frederick take an herbal remedy that helped cleanse his kidneys and decrease stress on his lymph system, which relieved his allergic reactions to dairy products. "In less than one month, Frederick experienced complete improvement," Dr. Lee reports. "He felt great, was off Lomotil, and was able to eat most foods without unpleasant symptoms."

cranesbill, and *Ginkgo biloba* (one teaspoon taken three times a day for relief). For topical application, he recommends a mixture of collinsonia (10 ml) with distilled witch hazel (60 ml), applied after every bowel movement. He also recommends salves made of calendula, St. John's wort, aloe, or plantain. In addition, Dr. Donovan recommends herbal suppositories such as collinsonia and buckeye *(Aesculus),* which tighten the tissues to help get rid of hemorrhoids.

Hydrotherapy: A warm sitz bath (partial immersion of the pelvic region) at a temperature of 100°–105° F is an effective treatment for hemorrhoids.

Exercise: Dr. Donovan has hemorrhoid patients do Kegel exercises, which are classic pelvic wall and rectal exercises. They are done by pulling up the lower pelvic wall and rectum, tightening up, and then relaxing. This increases circulation and pumps the blood away so that it doesn't stagnate in the area.

Recommendations

- Emphasize a whole foods diet, eating plenty of fresh, organic fruits and vegetables and fiber-rich foods. Reduce your intake of high-fat foods and avoid all processed foods, food additives and preservatives, sugar, caffeine, and alcohol.

- Check for food allergies and sensitivities, parasites, and bacterial, fungal, or viral infections, which can contribute to leaky gut syndrome and provoke autoimmune reactions.

- Consider a program of probiotics, the use of soil-based organisms (SBOs), or FOS to restore a healthy balance to the intestinal flora.

- Become aware of and learn how to manage stress and suppressed emotions, which can cause or exacerbate gastrointestinal disorders.

- Enzyme therapy or supplementation of hydrochloric acid (HCl) can often achieve dramatic results for GI disorders due to enzyme deficiencies or low HCl levels.

- Regular exercise helps promote healthy and regular bowel movements.

- For cases of intractable GI conditions, such as celiac disease, colitis, Crohn's disease, diverticulitis, and severe diarrhea or constipation, consider adopting the Specific Carbohydrate Diet.

Self-Care

The following therapies can be undertaken at home under appropriate professional supervision:

COLITIS

Biofeedback Training and Neurotherapy / Fasting / Flower Essences / Guided Imagery / Qigong and Tai Chi / Yoga

HOMEOPATHY: *Merc sol., Aloe, Allium sativa, Belladonna, Colchicum, Nux vomica, Arsen alb., Cantharis.*

HYDROTHERAPY: • Sitz bath (apply contrast daily when acute). • Constitutional hydrotherapy (apply 2-5 times weekly).

JUICE THERAPY: • Cabbage, papaya, carrot juice • Wheatgrass juice • Drink juice of ½ lemon with warm water each morning, followed by carrot and apple or carrot, beet, cucumber. • Aloe juice • Avoid citrus juices.

REFLEXOLOGY: Colon, liver, adrenal, lower spine, diaphragm, gallbladder.

CROHN'S DISEASE

Flower Essences / Mind/Body Medicine / Yoga

AROMATHERAPY: Basil.

HYDROTHERAPY: Constitutional hydrotherapy unless otherwise indicated (apply 2-5 times weekly).

DIARRHEA

Acupressure / Biofeedback Training and Neurotherapy / Fasting

AROMATHERAPY: • For stress-induced diarrhea, use lavender, neroli. • Other antispasmodic oils include eucalyptus and cypress, chamomile.

HOMEOPATHY: *Chamomilla, Colchicum, Sulfur, Arsen alb., Nux vomica, Argent nit., Ipecacuanha, Apis mel., Veratrum alb., Merc sol., Calc carb., Natrum Sulf.*

HYDROTHERAPY: Constitutional hydrotherapy (apply 2-5 times weekly).

JUICE THERAPY: • Carrot, apple juice • Carrot, celery, apple • Carrot, celery, spinach, parsley, garlic • Beets may worsen diarrhea in some cases.

REFLEXOLOGY: Ascending colon, transverse colon, diaphragm, liver, adrenals.

DIVERTICULITIS

Flower Essences

AROMATHERAPY: Rub abdomen with olive oil and essence of cinnamon.

HYDROTHERAPY: Constitutional hydrotherapy unless otherwise indicated (apply 2-5 times weekly).

JUICE THERAPY: • Carrot, celery, beet, cabbage juice • Green juices • Papaya, apple, lemon, pineapple

IRRITABLE BOWEL SYNDROME

Fasting / Guided Imagery / Mind/Body Medicine / Qigong and Tai Chi / Yoga

AROMATHERAPY: Peppermint

HOMEOPATHY: *Merc sol., Aloe, Carbo veg., Nux vomica*

HYDROTHERAPY: Constitutional hydrotherapy unless otherwise indicated (apply 2-5 times weekly).

JUICE THERAPY: Cabbage family, carrot, celery, parsley

ULCERS

Biofeedback Training and Neurotherapy / Guided Imagery / Mind/Body Medicine / Qigong and Tai Chi / Yoga

AROMATHERAPY: Lemon oil, chamomile, geranium

HOMEOPATHY: *Silicea, Arsen alb., Lachesis, Acidum nit., Calendula, Hamamelis, Belladonna*

HYDROTHERAPY: Constitutional hydrotherapy unless otherwise indicated (apply 2-5 times weekly).

JUICE THERAPY: • Drink fresh fruit and vegetable juices. • Wheatgrass juice • For duodenal ulcers, drink raw cabbage juice throughout the day (can be mixed with carrot or celery). • For gastric or stomach ulcers, drink raw potato juice.

REFLEXOLOGY: Diaphragm, stomach, duodenum, reflex pertaining to location of ulcer.

Professional Care

The following therapies should only be provided by a qualified health professional:

COLITIS

Chiropractic / Craniosacral Therapy / Detoxification Therapy / Magnetic Field Therapy / Naturopathic Medicine / Orthomolecular Medicine / Osteopathic Medicine / Traditional Chinese Medicine

BODYWORK: Acupressure, shiatsu, Alexander Technique, Feldenkrais Method, Therapeutic Touch

CROHN'S DISEASE

Acupuncture / Biofeedback Training and Neurotherapy / Chiropractic / Detoxification Therapy / Hypnotherapy / Magnetic Field Therapy / Orthomolecular Medicine / Sound Therapy

TRADITIONAL CHINESE MEDICINE: Barley soup or water

DIARRHEA

Applied Kinesiology / Detoxification Therapy / Environmental Medicine / Enzyme Therapy / Magnetic Field Therapy / Naturopathic Medicine / Neural Therapy / Osteopathic Medicine / Traditional Chinese Medicine

OXYGEN THERAPIES: • Hydrogen peroxide therapy • Hyperbaric oxygen therapy as an adjunctive therapy for nonresponding diarrhea.

DIVERTICULITIS

Acupuncture / Biofeedback Training and Neurotherapy / Chiropractic / Detoxification Therapy / Magnetic Field Therapy / Osteopathic Medicine / Traditional Chinese Medicine

IRRITABLE BOWEL SYNDROME

Acupuncture / Biofeedback Training and Neurotherapy / Chiropractic / Environmental Medicine / Hypnotherapy / Magnetic Field Therapy / Naturopathic Medicine / Neural Therapy / Orthomolecular Medicine / Osteopathic Medicine / Traditional Chinese Medicine

DETOXIFICATION THERAPY: Indicated to assess the effects of diet, unless the person is depleted from diarrhea.

OXYGEN THERAPY: Hyperbaric oxygen therapy can be helpful.

ULCERS

Craniosacral Therapy / Environmental Medicine / Enzyme Therapy / Fasting / Hypnotherapy / Naturopathic Medicine / Neural Therapy / Osteopathic Medicine / Traditional Chinese Medicine

DETOXIFICATION THERAPY: Detoxification is usually helpful.

OXYGEN THERAPY: Ozone therapy

BODYWORK: Acupressure, Feldenkrais Method, Therapeutic Touch

Where to Find Help

For more information on, and referrals for, treatment of gastrointestinal disorders, contact the following organizations.

American Association of Oriental Medicine
433 Front Street
Catasauqua, Pennsylvania 18032
(888) 500-7999
Website: www.aaom.org

The AAOM is a national professional organization of acupuncturists who meet acceptable standards of competency and can provide the names and locations of local members.

Ayurvedic and Naturopathic Medical Clinic
2115 112th Avenue N.E.
Bellevue, Washington 98004
(425) 453-8022
Website: www.ayurvedicscience.com

Dr. Virender Sodhi's clinic provides medical training for physicians and health-care practitioners, as well as individual courses for laypeople.

American Association of Naturopathic Physicians
8201 Greensboro Drive, Suite 300
McLean, Virginia 22102
(703) 610-9037
Website: www.naturopathic.org

The leading advocacy group for naturopathic medicine in the United States. Provides a directory of naturopathic physicians and offers referrals to a nationwide network of accredited or licensed practitioners. Also publishes a quarterly newsletter, for both professionals and the general public, and offers a series of brochures and pamphlets on a variety of subjects.

National Center for Homeopathy
801 North Fairfax, Suite 306
Alexandria, Virginia 22314
(703) 548-7790
Website: www.homeopathic.org

Provides a referral list of practicing homeopaths and other information. Gives courses for laypeople and professionals, and organizes study groups around the country.

Recommended Reading

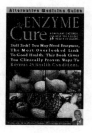

The Enzyme Cure. Lita Lee, Ph.D., and Lisa Turner, with Burton Goldberg. Tiburon, CA: Future Medicine Publishing, 1998.

Breaking the Vicious Cycle: Intestinal Health Through Diet. Elaine Gottschall, M.Sc. Kirkton, Ontario, Canada: Kirkton Press, 1994.

Dr. Braly's Food Allergy and Nutrition Revolution. James Braly, M.D. New Canaan, CT: Keats Publishing, 1992.

Eating for IBS: A Revolutionary Diet for Managing Irritable Bowel Syndrome. Heather van Vorous. New York: Marlowe & Company, 2000.

Eating Right for a Bad Gut. James Scala. New York: Plume Books, 1992.

Food Swings. Barnet Meltzer, M.D. New York: Marlowe & Company, 2001.

Health Benefits of FOS. Robert Crayhon. New Canaan, CT: Keats Publishing, 1995.

Gastrointestinal Health. Steven Perkin, M.D. New York: Harper Perennial, 1992.

Gut Reaction. Gudrun Jonsson. London: Vermilion, 1999.

7 Weeks to a Healthy Stomach. Ronald Hoffman, M.D. New York: Pocket Books, 1990.

HEADACHES

Headaches affect almost everyone. Often, headaches can be a sign of other underlying health conditions. While conventional medicine normally treats headaches by prescribing aspirin and other painkillers to deal with symptoms, alternative physicians treat both the headache and its cause to bring lasting relief from pain.

EADACHES ARE the most common health complaint," states Robert Milne, M.D., of Las Vegas, Nevada. "Whether occasional or acute, headaches are often brought on by other conditions, such as food allergy and environmental sensitivities, hormonal imbalances, trauma, sinus infections, eyestrain, or the flu." Proper treatment of headaches first involves careful diagnosis to locate the disturbance actually causing headache pain. It is then essential to treat the root condition rather than attempting to mask its symptomatic effects with temporary measures such as painkillers or tranquilizers.

Types of Headaches

Current research suggests there are 11 primary headache types, but, as pointed out by Dr. Milne, classifying headaches is far from an exact science. "All headaches, no matter how they are classified, are related, since they are all a response to underlying metabolic, structural, and/or emotional imbalances," explains Dr. Milne. The key to classification is to use the label to get to the underlying systemic disturbance rather than to narrowly define the headache itself.

Tension Headaches

Dr. Milne has found that the most common type of headache is the tension headache, which begins in the back of the neck or head and spreads outward with dull, non-throbbing pain. He estimates that 90% of all headaches involve excessive tension in the muscles of the face, head, and neck. "These headaches often feel like a tight band around the head, and the pain is usually constant," he says.

Dr. Milne attributes the pain to two mechanisms relating to muscle contraction: nerve compression within the muscle caused by poor posture, spinal misalignment,

or physical and emotional stress; and nerve irritation caused by a buildup of metabolic wastes resulting from decreased blood and lymph circulation due to poor diet, constipation, or other digestive problems, and in women, pelvic irritation.

According to physiatrist, Marc Darrow, M.D., of the Joint Rehabilitation & Sports Medical Center, in Los Angeles, California, tension headaches are often caused by lax or injured ligaments in the neck. Many patients with headaches also have neck pain at some time. When the ligaments connecting the vertebrae are loose or injured, surrounding muscles will contract and spasm to stabilize the spinal cord and spinal nerves, and protect them from further injury. The body's intention is to keep the nervous system intact at the expense of all other systems.

Headaches Caused by Vascular Irregularities

Headaches caused by vascular irregularities, including migraines, cluster headaches, and caffeine withdrawal headaches, account for less than 10% of all cases, according to Dr. Milne. With vascular headaches, the alternating constriction and expansion of the arteries of the head exerts pressure on nerves and causes sharp pain.

Migraine Headaches

Migraine headaches are surprisingly common, affecting 15% to 20% of men and 25% to 30% of women.[1] "This is probably because of the hormonal variations that occur due to the menstrual cycle," says Dr. Milne. "Many of my female patients report that they started getting migraines after some kind of hormonal shift, such as at the onset of puberty, while taking or stopping birth control pills, or after a pregnancy. Migraines are also more likely to happen during certain times of a woman's cycle, usually

SUCCESS STORY: ACUPUNCTURE HELPS MIGRAINES

According to Joseph Carter, L.Ac., C.M.T., of Berkeley, California, migraine headaches are linked closely to liver functioning and digestion. One of Dr. Carter's patients, Linda, came to him with debilitating migraines that came up from her neck and along one side of her head, lodging behind her eye.

As he took her history, Dr. Carter discovered that Linda's headaches tended to occur just before the onset of menstruation and that, over the last three years that she had been experiencing headaches, her periods had become progressively heavier, accompanied by more severe head pain. For the previous year, Linda had been unable to go to work during her periods, having to lie in a dark room for two to three days until the headache went away. Linda was also overweight and had long-term problems with her digestion.

Dr. Carter knew immediately that the cause of Linda's headaches was her liver, so after her first acupuncture treatment, he showed her three balancing points on the feet, two corresponding to the liver and one to the gallbladder. Whether or not Linda was experiencing a headache, Dr. Carter instructed her to hold (as often as possible throughout the day) specific acupoints such as Stomach 36 (ST 36) and Spleen 6 (SP 6) to build up her blood, and Liver 3 (LV 3), Liver 4 (LV 4), and Gallbladder 40 (GB 40) to regulate her liver. Each point is actually a pair of points, one on each leg.

In addition, he gave her two blends of Chinese herbs to build up her blood (three tablets, three times a day): Eight Treasures (rehmannia root, angelica, dong quai, condonopsis root, poria fungus, peony root, atractylodes rhizome, ligusticum rhizome, and licorice root), from the end of her period to the middle of her cycle, and Xiao Yao Tong from ovulation to the start of her period. Xiao Yao Tong contains bupleurum root, paeonia root, dong quai, poria fungus, tractylodes rhizome, ginger, licorice root, and mentha leaf. Dr. Carter also gave Linda acupuncture treatments every other week, prescribed a multimineral supplement, and had her drink plenty of water and begin a regular exercise routine. By the time her second menstruation came, Linda reported that her feet had become very hot while he had been stimulating the points, and then her headaches disappeared.

"The fact that her feet were warm meant that blood was staying there, or that her energy had begun traveling more efficiently along the gallbladder meridian, which runs from the head to the feet," explains Dr. Carter. Eventually, after a few more cycles, Linda's headaches stopped altogether.

---

at the beginning or the end of menses, and sometimes during ovulation." This indicates pelvic/ovarian weakness, either inherited or acquired.

"Migraines are very often triggered by food allergies, hormonal changes brought about by stress, and, surprisingly, by chronic dehydration," says Rima Laibow, M.D., founding Medical Director of the Alexandria Institute of Natural and Integrative Medicine, in Croton-on-Hudson, New York.

Migraine symptoms include lightheadedness, throbbing pain on one side of the head, nausea, vomiting, dizziness, blurred vision, hot and cold flashes, and hypersensitivity to light and sound. Migraine sufferers often experience warning symptoms or auras for a few minutes before experiencing pain. These auras consist of blurred vision, muddled thinking, exhaustion, worry, and numbness or tingling on one side of the body.

"Migraine pain is most often severe and localized on one side of the head, usually involving the temple and the eye," Dr. Milne explains. In patients without preceding visual disturbances, there may or may not be any warning signs.

Cluster Headaches

These are the most painful form of headache, with excruciating pain concentrated around the eye. They are often accompanied by tears, facial flushing, and nasal congestion. "Cluster headaches are much rarer than migraines and affect mostly men," says Dr. Milne. As the name suggests, they occur in periodic clusters that can last anywhere from a few weeks to several months. During a cluster attack, sharp, intense pain afflicts the victim for a few hours, then subsides for a few hours more before returning again. "Due to the piercing and vicious nature of the pain involved, the victim can become highly agitated and unable to rest," Dr. Milne explains. "Sometimes a sufferer might even bang their head against the wall just to alter the sensation."

Injured ligaments and muscles in the neck have referral patterns that course up and around the head causing pain, called "trigger points." In addition, nerves from the neck to the head, such as the greater occipital nerve, may be entrapped or inflamed. Dr. Darrow treated a 39-year-old woman with recurring headaches that centered in her left eye—she described the pain as a "hot poker in my eye." He asked if there was any accompanying neck pain, but the patient said no. Nevertheless, the trapezius muscle was palpated and a specific spot was found to significantly increase the eye pain. When the trigger point was injected with a local anesthetic, the eye pain immediately resolved.

More so than for other types of headaches, sufferers of cluster headaches usually fit a certain profile. "The typical victim is normally a male between the ages of 30 and 50," states David Bresler, Ph.D., former Director of the U.C.L.A. Pain Control Unit. "Usually he is also a Type A personality, hard-driving and striving, who often smokes or drinks. A lot of these people commit suicide because of the pain the clusters cause, although often their deaths are attributed to depression instead. But what is depression? It's psychological pain."

Allergy/Sensitivity Headaches

Believed to be a contributing factor in as many as 70% of all headache cases, allergy/sensitivity headaches can take many forms, from migraine, cluster, or sinus-like pain to dull, aching, generalized pain. Attributed to just about any substance that can be eaten, breathed, touched, or worn, these headaches usually occur 4-12 hours after contact with or ingestion of the problematic substance.[2]

According to Dr. Milne, these headaches are among the easiest to treat, since treatment consists of finding the offending substance, eliminating it, and repairing the body through detoxification and nutritional supplements. "However, despite their apparent simplicity, eliminating these headaches often takes patience, since allergies or sensitivities can build up gradually over a period of prolonged exposure, requiring more time for the body to return to normal functioning."

Other allergy headaches can be triggered by poor digestion, yeast overgrowth, dysbiosis, and enzyme deficiencies, according to Dr. Laibow. In this case, foods are improperly broken down and food fragments leak through the gut walls. This can lead to a flood of toxins in the bloodstream, where immune cells attack the food particles causing dangerous cross-reactions in the body. Symptoms such as headaches may result, says Dr. Laibow. However, leaky gut–related headaches can occur 12-96 hours after exposure–making them difficult to pinpoint.

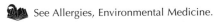 See Allergies, Environmental Medicine.

Trauma Headaches

Also called post-traumatic headaches, trauma headaches are generally attributed to head, neck, and spine injuries, such as those caused by falls and car accidents. Varying widely in intensity, pain from these headaches can be local or generalized and can occur immediately after the injury or, in some cases, develop months later. However, once a trauma headache develops, it usually occurs daily and is fairly resistant to drug-based treatments. "Trauma headaches can be especially confusing, since not only can they mimic the symptoms of migraine and/or tension headaches, but a seemingly insignificant bump on the head can cause debilitating pain," says Dr. Milne.

TMJ/Dental Headaches

Often overlooked by conventional doctors, jaw and dental stress is another underlying cause of headaches, especially when the pain is focused in the mouth or in front of and behind the ear on one or both sides of the jaw. According to Harold E. Ravins, D.D.S., of Los Angeles, California, TMJ/dental headaches are most commonly brought on by jaw misalignments such as temporomandibular joint (TMJ) syndrome or an uneven bite, dental and mouth problems (infected teeth, mercury amalgam poisoning, faulty bridges), or diseases and stressful movement patterns (teeth grinding or jaw clenching). "These headaches are a clear example of how headaches mirror the relationship between the head and the other parts of the body," explains Dr. Ravins, "since when the jaws are not coming together correctly, blood flow is reduced, the brain receives the wrong message, and the entire body is thrown off balance."

Eyestrain Headaches

Often triggered by the strain of long periods of focused visual work, such as working on a computer or reading in poor light, eyestrain headaches are characterized by mild, steady pain felt in and behind the eyes, forehead, and face. Although often accompanied by dry, aching eyes, these headaches aren't attributed to the eyes themselves but to the muscles around the eyes. However, as Dr. Milne points out, digestive disturbances and musculoskeletal misalignments can also contribute to eyestrain headaches, as can chronic stress.

Sinus Headaches

Contrary to popular belief, sinus problems are among the least frequent causes of headaches, affecting less than 2% of all sufferers. "More often than not, so-called sinus headaches are really migraine or tension headaches, since most people with sinus infections rarely get headaches," says Dr. Milne. "However, when they are true sinus headaches, the pain is felt as gnawing painful pressure,

CHILDREN AND HEADACHES

Contrary to popular belief, children can experience serious types of headaches, including migraines. Children of parents who suffer from migraines have an increased risk of developing such headaches. "Sometimes these migraine conditions might take different forms in a child than they would in an adult," according to Robert Milne, M.D., of Las Vegas, Nevada. "For example, headache pain might be vague rather than localized or there may not be head pain at all. Instead, the child might experience spells of nausea, confusion, or dizziness." Children who are prone to motion sickness might also be susceptible to migraines as adults, Dr. Milne notes.

If you suspect your child is suffering from headaches, be sensitive to the situation. "It's important not to focus so much on the problem that you worsen it by increasing your child's tension and fear," says Dr. Milne. "Address the experience in a loving manner and with sympathy, while at the same time gently allowing your child to develop individual coping mechanisms." Parents can help prevent the underlying conditions that can cause their children's headaches in the following ways:

- Keep a record of your child's headaches in a diary. Note what they ate prior to the headache's occurrence. Also, note any activities or stress your child experienced, as well as any exposure to environmental toxins. Such a record will provide clues to what triggers your child's headaches and enable you to eliminate whatever factors are involved.

- By monitoring your child's diet, you will become aware of any food allergies or sensitivities. Once you discover such foods, eliminate them from the diet. Eliminate sugar in all its forms and try not to feed your child too much of the same type of food, such as corn or wheat, as repetition in the diet can trigger headaches and other allergic reactions.

- Ensure that your child adopts regular sleeping and eating patterns.

- Encourage your child to exercise and to spend time outdoors, breathing fresh air. Also help your child develop the ability to relax and enjoy quiet activities, such as reading and drawing.

- Finally, foster your child's ability to express whatever thoughts or emotions they may have, as repressing them can create additional stress and tension.

tenderness and swelling in the sinuses, or in the hollow tunnels in the forehead, nose, and cheekbones." Sinus infections may be caused by an underlying yeast infection, which should be investigated before treatment begins. He adds that sinus headaches are usually accompanied by cold-like symptoms such as a low-grade fever, teary eyes, thick, colored drainage from the nose or back of the throat, sneezing, and loss of the sense of smell.

Rebound Headaches

Headaches related to caffeine and medication withdrawal involve a dull, throbbing pain on both sides of the head and are generally not as intense as migraines or cluster headaches, according to Dr. Milne. Such headaches occur as the body rids itself of the effects of caffeine and other addictive substances caused by consumption of coffee, soft drinks, certain teas, and medications (for weight control, colds and allergies, pain relief, and menstrual aids, among others). "Normally, these headaches strike 12-24 hours after consumption, peaking within 48 hours, and gradually disappearing on their own over five or six days, unless the substance is reintroduced into the body," says Dr. Milne. Such headache sufferers, however, are often unaware that their problem is due to caffeine or medication and so will not avoid it, causing the problem to recur. For frequent users of drugs or caffeine, Dr. Milne recommends a gradual withdrawal over a one-week period. Afterward, several weeks may pass before the headaches caused by these overused substances fully cease.

Exertion Headaches

Usually harmless and short-lived, exertion headaches are brief, throbbing headaches that come on during or immediately after physical exertion (such as lifting, running, or sexual activity) or passive exertion (such as coughing, sneezing, or straining one's bowels). "Although their sudden appearance and extreme disposition make them seem frightening, exertion headaches are rarely the sign of a serious health condition," explains Dr. Milne.

Organic Headaches

Although constituting less than 2% of all headaches, organic headaches are the most serious headache type and should always be ruled out when making a headache diagnosis. Organic disorders such as brain tumors, hemorrhages, glaucoma, swollen and diseased blood vessels, hypertension, and brain infections can all cause severe headache pain. According to Dr. Milne, typical symptoms include headaches that begin suddenly, seizures, projectile vomiting, speech or personality changes, walking difficulty, and increasing pain. A doctor should be consulted immediately if any of these symptoms are present.

What Causes Headaches?

Determining the cause of headaches is a complicated matter, with few established medical facts. "Because there are so many different types of headaches and headache patterns, identifying their underlying causes can be challenging," says Dr. Milne. "But since they are so hard to diagnose, all too often headaches are treated as an isolated problem, separate from the rest of the body. A chronic headache syndrome, however, is a sure sign that there is a systemic disturbance in the body that can be extremely complex and consisting of various conditions that interact and exacerbate one another."

An example of such an interplay of conditions, Dr. Milne notes, is migraine headache caused by hormonal imbalances due to yeast overgrowth (candidiasis). The candidiasis, in turn, can also contribute to food allergies, which many alternative physicians now recognize as one of the primary causes of migraines. "Headaches, therefore, are extremely important and ought not to be ignored because they can direct attention to other health problems that might otherwise have gone undetected and untreated," Dr. Milne says.

While conventional research cites vascular irregularities, genetic predisposition, hormones, sinus problems, and fluctuations in the pain-regulating chemical serotonin as the causes of headaches, alternative practitioners look for the mechanisms beneath these conditions, such as stress, food allergies, chemical and environmental sensitivities, stress, dental factors, structural imbalances, and digestive disturbances.

Stress

According to Dr. Milne, the most common cause of headaches is stress resulting from chemical, emotional, or physical factors. "Many of us carry stress in the muscles of the face, skull, neck, shoulders, and upper back, causing them to contract," he points out. "A person in whom these muscles are persistently contracted is likely to experience chronic tension headaches." Muscles that are constantly contracted can also become fatigued and suffer from a reduced supply of oxygen. In addition, the contractions can cause chemicals such as histamines to accumulate in the body, triggering neurons in the muscles to fire, creating pain. And once the headache occurs, the pain, coupled with the fear of the next headache attack, can result in additional stress and anxiety to perpetuate one of the vicious cycles associated with chronic headache complaints.

Stress can also be due to mental or emotional factors related to the pressures of everyday life, regrets about the past, and worries about the future. Since the mind and body function as a whole, when such concerns are present, the stress that they cause can often result in headache pain.

Leon Chaitow, N.D., D.O., of London, England, points out that another common source of stress that can lead to headaches is eyestrain. "There are many individuals whose chronic headaches disappear when they have their eyes checked," he explains. "If there is a problem that is not corrected, it is common for the head to be held in a tilted manner to try to achieve focus." Dr. Chaitow states that corrective lenses usually eliminate the need to tilt the head and frequently eliminate the headaches as well. In addition, he suggests that eye exercises such as the Bates method may be helpful in curbing eyestrain. Dr. Chaitow also notes that eyestrain and headaches can result from exposure to flickering neon or fluorescent overhead lighting, TVs, and computer screens.

Food Allergies

Based on his own clinical experience, James Braly, M.D., an allergy expert in Hollywood, Florida, states that 90% of all migraine headaches are directly linked to food allergies or to reactions caused by additives, particularly certain preservatives and colorings, caffeine, and chocolate. A study reported in *The Lancet* confirms Dr. Braly's conviction. It cited relief for 93% of the study's migraine sufferers when allergenic foods were eliminated from their diet. Most patients were allergic to more than one food and, not surprisingly, the offending allergens were often among the patient's favorite foods, with the most common offenders being cow's milk, eggs, wheat, cheese, and rye, along with benzoic acid (a preservative) and tartrazine (a popular food dye). A double-blind placebo test also proved that when these foods were reintroduced into the study group's diet, the migraine pain would reoccur.[3] According to Dr. Chaitow, MSG and aspartame (NutraSweet™) have been implicated in many headache cases, as has excessive salt intake.

Dr. Milne warns that food allergies can contribute to headaches other than those specifically classified as migraines. "Food allergies and sensitivities are a much more prevalent factor in headaches than most doctors realize," says Dr. Milne. For example, he cites two common allergens, corn and brewer's yeast, which hide in many recipes and even in some vitamin pills. He recommends that treatment of headaches always start with a careful history of food and chemical intake to discover what role they may play in causing headache pain. If leaky gut is suspected, a history of antibiotic use and testing digestive function is essential.

IS DENTAL STRESS CONTRIBUTING TO YOUR HEADACHES?

Answering "yes" to any of the following questions can be an indication that you are experiencing some form of dental stress, which is most likely contributing to your headaches:

Do you favor one side of your mouth when you chew?

Do you grind your teeth?

Do you have trouble swallowing three or four times in a row?

Do you have a poor sense of balance?

Do you feel tired after eating due to chewing?

Do you have to strain to smile?

Do your gums bleed?

Do you make a clicking sound when you open or close your mouth?

Chemical and Environmental Sensitivities

With over 12,000 substances and pollutants in today's "natural" environment, headaches caused by chemical and environmental sensitivities are a mounting concern for alternative practitioners, especially since they are so difficult to avoid. "Whether you are talking about pollen, mold, cigarette smoke, pesticides, plastics, perfumes, deodorizers, chlorine, hydrocarbons, formaldehyde, radioactive fallout, or carbon monoxide, the substances in the air we breathe and foods and water we consume are creating a crisis in our bodies that mirrors the ecological illness of the planet," says Dr. Milne. "Headaches are the tip of the iceberg."

In addition, exposure to heavy metals (from the combustion of fossil fuels, animal feeds, and water toxicity) has increased several hundred percent over the last century. One particularly insidious form of heavy metal, mercury, lies in the mouths of many unsuspecting headache sufferers. The cumulative build-up of poison caused by silver mercury fillings may be the underlying factor behind many mysterious illnesses, including headaches, depression, allergies, fatigue, and menstrual disorders.[4]

Smoking can cause headaches, according to Dr. Milne. Nicotine constricts the blood vessels while inhaled carbon monoxide overly expands them, thus creating a condition that often triggers migraines and cluster headaches. Dr. Milne also points out that smoking cuts down the effectiveness of pain relievers and may disrupt the nutritional balance of the body.

Blood Clotting

Another common cause of headaches is blood clotting, also known as platelet aggregation.[5] Like the body and mind, blood also responds to stress by tightening, creating little knots—or clots—in the bloodstream. Clotting creates constriction of the arteries, which results in inadequate blood supply to the brain. According to Julian Whitaker, M.D., of Newport Beach, California, the platelets of migraine patients release abnormal amounts of the neurotransmitter serotonin, which enhances constriction of the arteries. Patients on serotonin reuptake inhibitors, like Prozac, should be especially alert to this possibility, according to Dr. Laibow.

Dental Factors

"Teeth that are under continuous stress affect other parts of the body," says Dr. Ravins, who has been treating headaches in his dental practice for over 20 years. He estimates that more than half of his patients come to him because of headaches that they have been unable to cure. Problems such as tooth decay, gum disease, muscle spasm, and low-grade infections from old fillings all cause stress in the lower jaw.

The upper and lower jawbones move together at the temporomandibular joints, located just in front of each earlobe, to produce a pumping action. When the lower jaw hits the upper jaw in harmony, the fluids of the brain can flow through the body properly, explains Dr. Ravins. Dental stress factors can reduce this circulation in the brain area, because when the bones in the skull become more rigid, losing their flexibility and normal motion, they reduce blood flow. This causes the blood vessels to constrict, which can produce a headache.

To rebalance the jaw, Dr. Ravins often has a headache patient use a removable appliance, usually worn at night. This treatment is in addition to healing the gums and teeth and making dietary changes.

Structural Imbalances

A healthy musculoskeletal structure is vital for optimum health, for without a solid foundation, the body becomes susceptible to a wide variety of health problems, including headaches. "External factors such as poor posture, ill fitting shoes, or a traumatic injury, as well as internal ones, such as allergies, digestive problems, or emotional or hormonal imbalances, can all lead to misalignments in the spine and musculature, which affect how the entire body is supplied with blood and energy," says Dr. Milne.

He cites posture as an example of this phenomenon. Poor posture brings about muscle strain, and the result

UNDERLYING FACTORS ASSOCIATED WITH HEADACHES

UNDERLYING FACTORS	POSSIBLE TRIGGERS
Dietary allergy or sensitivity	All dairy products, eggs, wheat, corn, rye, sugar, chocolate, alcohol, pickled or cured meat and fish, shellfish, game (hare, pheasant, venison), fatty and fried foods, pickles, chutneys, some seasonings (bay leaves, cinnamon, chilies, sassafras), some vegetables (onions, broad beans, spinach, tomatoes, eggplant, avocados), some fruits (bananas, seed fruits like peaches, plums, citrus fruits, pineapples, raspberries), nuts, tyramine, MSG, sodium nitrate, aspartame, caffeine, tartrazine, dyes and food colorings, benzoic acid
Environmental allergy or sensitivity	Bright light, noise, high altitude, weather changes, poorly ventilated enclosures causing prolonged exposure to pollutants, cigarette smoke, carbon monoxide, heavy metals, and other pollutants (formaldehyde, phenol, gasoline, plastics, perfumes), pollen, mold, house dust, silver mercury amalgams, contaminated water, pesticides
	Medications: birth control pills, diet pills, blood pressure medications, diuretics, asthma medications, painkillers, antihistamines, estrogen supplements, heart medications
Hormonal imbalance	Low progesterone levels (PMS, irritability, fluid retention, menopause), excess estrogen levels (breast tenderness, fluid retention), hypothyroid (cold extremities), hypoglycemia (low blood sugar, which causes fainting, irritability, dizziness, sugar cravings), Hashimoto's Autoimmune Thyroiditis (HAIT)
Digestive disturbances	Constipation, leaky gut syndrome, candidiasis, hypoglycemia, nutritional deficiencies
Autoimmune disturbances	Abnormal blood clotting, chronic fatigue syndrome
Lifestyle factors	Sleep disturbances (napping, too little or too much sleep), inadequate nutrition, changed meal patterns (hunger, missed or skipped meals, crash diets), over-consumption of sugar and junk food, smoking, fatigue, over-working, uncorrected faulty vision, excessive frowning or squinting and long periods of reading or close-up work (especially in dim light), constant use of computer or TV
Structural disturbances	Musculoskeletal misalignments, head trauma, muscle trauma, coccyx bone trauma, over-exertion, jaw clenching, grimaced face, teeth grinding, poor posture, dental problems, TMJ syndrome
Psychological stress	Stress, anxiety, depression, repressed emotions, anger, boredom

can often be headache pain. However, the classic depiction of bad posture—slouching with round-shoulders and a protruding belly—is only one type of postural distortion, usually caused by poor diet and low energy. Holding oneself rigidly upright in a military-like posture can be just as hard on the body, because maintaining such a stance requires a great deal of muscular tension. In contrast, healthy posture features a spine with slight curvatures and well-toned muscles that maintain these curves.

"Good posture stems from having good energy and standing upright and tall, while still remaining relaxed," explains Dr. Milne. "Shoulders should drop, then be brought back slightly. The pelvis should be tucked in with the knees slightly bent. Shoulder and neck rolls can help relax tight muscles and rebalance posture."

Digestive Disturbances

According to traditional Chinese medicine, the head is seen as a compact representation of the digestive system, meaning that all headaches correspond, in one way or another, to a digestive disorder of some sort. According to Dr. Milne, constipation, nutritional deficiencies, leaky gut syndrome (when damage to the intestinal barrier allows chemicals and partially digested foods into the bloodstream), and hypoglycemia (low blood sugar) are just a few of the underlying digestive problems that may bring about head pain.

Treatment of Headaches

Although aspirin and other painkillers help alleviate headache pain, they usually provide only partial or temporary relief and fail to address the underlying conditions that may cause headaches. Many headache remedies

---

A QUICK FIX FOR MIGRAINE HEADACHES

Robert Milne, M.D., of Las Vegas, Nevada, has found that the following simple procedure can often bring immediate relief for migraine headaches triggered by allergic reactions to food or chemical substances. As soon as migraine symptoms occur, take two tablets of bicarbonate (such as Alka-Seltzer Gold) in a glass of water. Let them dissolve, then drink. "The drink has the effect of creating an alkaline condition in the body," Dr. Milne explains. "This neutralizes the allergic mechanisms and prevents the migraine from fully taking hold."

---

have serious, even potentially life-threatening side effects. Among the nondrug therapies that have proven most effective in treating headaches are diet, nutritional supplements, herbal medicine, prolotherapy and bodywork, relaxation techniques, and hydrotherapy.

CAUTION When headaches are associated with fever, convulsions, head trauma, loss of consciousness, or localized pain in the ear, eye, or elsewhere, rapidly progressing severe pain, dizziness, or blurring of vision, professional help should be sought immediately. Recurring headaches in children and the elderly, or headaches occurring suddenly with no prior history of headache, also require immediate medical attention.

Diet

Because of the link between headaches and food allergies, Dr. Braly recommends that headache sufferers be tested for food allergies. One way to do this is to fast the patient for five days, under medical supervision, during which time only distilled water is consumed. According to Dr. Braly, such a fast is a very effective way of allowing the body to free itself of symptoms as a first step toward determining allergenic foods. He recommends that during the fast the patient be supervised by a competent physician and that the patient avoid smoking and not use toothpaste, mouthwashes, and other personal hygiene products, since they contain chemicals. Once the fast is completed, the patient can then reintroduce individual foods one by one back into the diet. Those that cause a reaction should then be avoided. Keeping a food journal during this time can also be helpful, so that the person can have a record of the offending foods and the symptoms they cause.

After allergenic foods are eliminated, Dr. Braly recommends a maintenance program that incorporates a rotation diet, with no food being eaten more frequently than once every four days. "Such a diet helps prevent the development of further allergies and reactions and also provides a more balanced diet, which supplies a wider range of needed nutrients," Dr. Braly says.

The diet consists of eating foods high in non-allergenic complex carbohydrates and fiber, while avoiding simple and refined sugars (including dried fruit and fruit juices, chocolate, pastries, sodas, and candy), food additives and colorings, preservatives, alcohol, and caffeine. Margarine, shortening, and other sources of partially hydrogenated oils should also be avoided, and saturated fats from red meat, dairy products, eggs, and warm-water fish are limited. These should be replaced with poultry, other types of fish, non-gluten grains, and a variety of vegetables, fresh vegetable juices, and fresh fruit, making sure these foods are hormone-free and organic whenever possible.

Dr. Braly reports that many of his headache patients have experienced substantial relief on this program. One of them was a teenage boy who came to him suffering from two to three migraines a week. He was also 50 pounds overweight, had previously seen a number of headache specialists without success, and was taking several drugs for his pain. He had been diagnosed as being learning impaired and emotionally disabled. By use of the IgG ELISA test, Dr. Braly discovered that the boy was severely allergic to a number of foods, which were then eliminated from his diet. "After he gave up the offending foods and began following the rotation diet, he soon experienced complete relief from his headaches," Dr. Braly says. "He also was quickly able to shed 48 pounds and his learning and emotional difficulties improved. His mother told me I had given her son his life back, but all along the problem had simply been due to the foods he was eating."

Nutritional Supplements

Dr. Braly suggests that as a daily routine for health, the diet should be supplemented with a multivitamin/mineral formula. For headache sufferers, he recommends an increase of vitamin C (2-8 g divided into three doses taken throughout the day), vitamin E (400-800 IU), niacinamide (a form of vitamin B3, 500 mg), and calcium/magnesium (600 mg each). In addition, Dr. Braly has found that evening primrose oil (three to four capsules taken at breakfast and again at dinner), EPA (eicosapentaenoic acid, a form of fish oil), and the amino acid DL-phenylalanine (275 mg taken two to three times daily between meals) should also be included. "Evening primrose oil and EPA are both sources of essential fatty acids that supply the body with anti-inflammatory agents and act to keep the blood vessels from constricting," Dr. Braly explains.

According to Dr. Chaitow, a lack of potassium, which he describes as an excellent nerve tonic, can also contribute to various kinds of headaches. Potassium supplementation in the form of tablets or capsules is undesirable, however, since it can interfere with the functions of other nutrients, according to Dr. Chaitow. Instead, he recommends making a potassium broth. "To make the broth," says Dr. Chaitow, "take an assortment of vegetables, or their skins (potatoes especially), and cover them with cold water. Boil the water and allow the vegetables to simmer for ten minutes. Then strain the liquid from the pot. The broth will be very rich with potassium. Refrigerate and drink several cups of it throughout the day."

Herbal Medicine

There are a variety of herbs that offer relief to headache sufferers. Among them is feverfew, which has been shown to reduce the secretion of serotonin and the production of prostaglandins, an inflammatory agent that contributes to the onset of migraine headaches. In one study, 70% of 270 migraine patients reported that a daily dose of feverfew significantly decreased the frequency and intensity of migraine attacks.[6]

For patients who do not respond to feverfew, Donald Brown, N.D., of Seattle, Washington, recommends *Ginkgo biloba,* which inhibits blood clot formation and increases blood flow to the brain. Garlic also inhibits the formation of blood clots and improves blood circulation and can bring relief when added to the diet. Dr. Brown recommends ginger, which reduces inflammation in the stomach and liver that can contribute to headaches related to digestive disturbances. At the onset of an attack, take 500-600 mg of powdered ginger. The dosage should then be repeated two more times during the day, with four hours between each dose. As an alternative, fresh ginger can be chewed or used in cooking.

Cayenne pepper is another useful herb, especially for cluster headaches. It is an excellent source of magnesium, which has been shown to be a migraine preventative and, according to Dr. Milne, cayenne also reduces the likelihood of a migraine by stimulating digestion, easing muscle pain, and increasing the body's metabolic rate.

Other useful herbs for treating headaches, according to Dr. Chaitow, include chamomile, which is a muscle relaxant and digestive aid; turmeric, a natural anti-inflammatory agent; coriander, which reduces swelling and is an excellent source of potassium; bay leaves, which can be helpful for frontal headaches; skullcap, to soothe headaches due to tension; valerian, a sedative and pain reliever; wild yam, which is an anti-inflammatory useful for correcting hormonal imbalances; and willow bark,

SELF-MASSAGE FOR HEADACHES

The following self-massage can provide effective relief from headache pain: Sit comfortably in a chair, taking care to breathe freely through the diaphragm. Cradle the back of your neck with your hand and squeeze gently, slowly rolling your head in a circle. Release for a few moments, then again squeeze your neck, slightly increasing the pressure. Repeat squeezing and releasing 20 times.

Next, using your fingertips, press into any areas in your neck and shoulders that are sore or tender, moving your arms and shoulders in a gentle, rhythmic motion. Continue this for several minutes, until your headache fades.

Doing these exercises periodically throughout the day will often prevent your headaches from recurring. They can also be performed by a partner. As you seat yourself, have your partner stand behind you and follow the above instructions.

which contains salicylic acid, the ingredient from which aspirin is derived. "Unlike aspirin, however, which is an isolated and concentrated chemical, willow bark acts gently and without aspirin's potential for irritating the stomach," says Dr. Chaitow.

Prolotherapy and Bodywork

Since most headaches have some component of muscular contraction, the question is how to stabilize the vertebrae and calm the irritation. Prolotherapy, an injection technique, can alleviate 80%-90% of headaches over the course of several injections. These findings have been reported in medical journals as early as the work of George Hackett, M.D., in the 1960s. "Why would a patient consider surgical fusion as an answer to neck pain and the accompanying headaches, when a much less invasive process without substantial risk achieves a natural stabilization?" queries Dr. Darrow. Trigger point injections often stop a headache in process and prolotherapy along with the other modalities may provide a permanent resolution of headaches. Chiropractic can be used to align the spine and cervical strengthening can stabilize the weakened neck muscles.

Because of the relationship between headaches and muscle contraction, the field of bodywork has much to offer headache sufferers. "Many headaches occur due to tension spasms in the muscles that run between the base

PROGRESSIVE RELAXATION EXERCISE

The following exercise is a method that headache sufferers can use to learn how to relax and relieve the stress of muscle tension:

Lie down, or lean back in a comfortable chair, in a quiet room with subdued light. Take ten slow, deep breaths, taking a little longer to breathe out than you take to breathe in. The ideal timing is a two-second full inhalation followed by a slow, controlled four- or five-second exhalation. This starts the relaxation process.

Beginning with your feet, clench the muscles and toes tightly for a few seconds, then release. Then tighten the muscles of your leg, and relax. Repeat this process for the rest of your body: buttocks, back, abdomen, hands, arms, shoulders, neck, jaw, eyes, and finally the muscles of the face.

Next, yawn several times, then squeeze your eyes open and shut, taking another ten deep breaths. Now notice how much more relaxed you are. Continue breathing, allowing that relaxation to grow stronger. Then resume your regular activities.

of the skull and along the top of the shoulders," explains William Cargile, B.S., D.C., L.Ac., F.I.A.C.A., former Chairman of Research of the American Association of Oriental Medicine. A variety of bodywork therapies can address this problem by releasing muscle tension and normalizing the neurovascular system. Bodywork methods that are appropriate for treating headaches include Rolfing, Feldenkrais Method™, Alexander Technique, the Trager® Approach, craniosacral massage, and polarity therapy. Such methods require the assistance of a trained professional, however.

For a self-help approach, Dr. Cargile recommends acupressure. "One can achieve a great deal of relief using acupressure self-help techniques," he says. The following acupressure points are useful in treating headaches, according to Michael Reed Gach, Ph.D., Director of the Acupressure Institute, in Berkeley, California:

GB 20: With your thumbs, firmly press underneath the base of your skull into the hollow areas on either side. "These will be located 2-3 inches apart, depending on your head size," Dr. Gach says. "With your eyes closed, slowly tilt your head back and press up from underneath

the skull for one to two minutes. As you do so, take long deep breaths through your diaphragm."

GV 16 with B2: Using your right thumb, press the GV 16 point located in the center hollow of the base of the skull. With your left thumb and index finger, simultaneously press point B2 located in the upper hollows of your eye sockets, near the bridge of your nose. Once again, tilt your head back and breathe deeply for one to two minutes (For illustrations of these acupressure points, see the introduction to the Quick Reference A-Z.)

LI 4: Place your right hand over the top of your left. With your right thumb, press the webbing between the thumb and index finger of your left hand, angling the pressure toward the bone that connects with the index finger. Hold for one minute, then reverse hands and press the point on your opposite hand for an equal length of time. "This point, which is known in acupressure as *hoku*, should not be used by pregnant women," Dr. Gach cautions, "because stimulating it can cause premature contractions of the uterus."

 See Bodywork, Diet, Herbal Medicine, Hydrotherapy, Nutritional Medicine, Prolotherapy.

Relaxation Techniques

Relaxation is crucial to relieve the muscle tension and stress, which cause many headaches. Some sufferers of severe headaches have to make radical lifestyle changes in order to alleviate their condition. A workaholic patient of Dr. Milne, for example, found relief from his throbbing, intensely painful headaches only when he began working fewer hours and spending more time relaxing with his family.

Many techniques for relaxation exist for the headache sufferer. To promote vascular and muscle relaxation, Dr. Braly recommends the regular practice of meditation, deep relaxation, biofeedback, or yoga. He also advises patients to consider undertaking stress and behavior evaluation tests to identify possible emotional and lifestyle factors that might be triggering their headaches.

One of the easiest relaxation techniques suggested by Dr. Milne is slow, deep breathing for approximately five minutes. "Most people do not realize that they usually take short, shallow breaths, and that five minutes of slow, deep breathing will trigger an involuntary relaxation response in muscles all over the body," he explains.

Chronic adrenal fatigue, often a product of ongoing stress, can cause tension in the neck and shoulders and contribute to headaches, says Dr. Laibow. She recommends the following self-help technique:

- Lie on the floor with your head on a pillow and raise your legs so that your calves are resting comfortably on the seat of a chair.

- Close your eyes for 5-10 minutes and let your mind drift. Optional soft music may help you relax during the exercise.

- Afterward, get up slowly. You should feel refreshed and headache free.

Hydrotherapy

Hydrotherapy is another method of treating headaches without the use of drugs. "Hot baths, saunas, heat lamps, and steam baths all reduce tension by increasing blood circulation," says Dr. Chaitow. "This, in turn, removes the metabolic wastes that are often the cause of headaches. A migraine headache, for instance, can sometimes be stopped in its tracks with the combination of a hot shower followed quickly with an ice-cold one." According to Dr. Chaitow, hot water may at first increase the migraine pain by temporarily dilating blood vessels, but this paves the way for fast relief when the vessels are constricted by the cold shower.

This "hot/cold" approach, however, can be too stressful for older people. They can get similar results by placing a piece of cracked ice in the back of the throat at the first sign of pain. "These techniques give the patient a measure of control," says Dr. Chaitow. "They also provide an opportunity to reduce and ultimately omit medication."

For simple headache relief, Dr. Chaitow recommends cold applications of an ice pack to the head along with a simultaneous hot foot or hand bath. For the foot or hand bath, he advises mixing one teaspoon of dry mustard in two gallons of water. "But even a normal bath at body temperature can be therapeutic, especially at the onset of the headache," he notes.

Recommendations

- Because of the link between headaches and allergies, headache sufferers should be tested for food allergies.

- Increase vitamin C (2-8 g divided into three doses taken throughout the day), vitamin E (400-800 IU), niacinamide (a form of vitamin B3, 500 mg), and calcium/magnesium (600 mg each).

- Feverfew has been shown to reduce the secretion of serotonin and the production of prostaglandins, an inflammatory agent that contributes to the onset of migraine headaches.

- *Ginkgo biloba* inhibits blood clotting and increases blood flow to the brain. Garlic also inhibits blood clots and improves blood circulation and can bring relief when added to the diet.

- Bodywork methods that are appropriate for treating headaches include Rolfing, Feldenkrais Method, Alexander Technique, the Trager Approach, and polarity therapy.

- Many techniques for relaxation exist for the headache sufferer. To promote vascular and muscle relaxation, try the regular practice of meditation, deep relaxation, biofeedback, or yoga. Consider undertaking stress and behavior evaluation tests to identify possible emotional and lifestyle factors that might be triggering headaches.

- Hot baths, saunas, heat lamps, and steam baths all reduce tension by increasing blood circulation. This removes the metabolic wastes that are often the cause of headaches.

Self Care
The following therapies can be undertaken at home under appropriate professional supervision:

Fasting / Flower Essenses / Guided Imagery / Mind/Body Medicine / Qigong and Tai Chi / Yoga

AROMATHERAPY: • Lavender, peppermint, rosemary, eucalyptus, chamomile • Rub a drop of lavender oil into temples to relieve pain. • Marjoram

JUICE THERAPY: • Carrot, celery • Carrot, beet, cucumber • Carrot, celery, spinach, parsley

Professional Care
The following therapies should only be provided by a qualified health professional:

Acupuncture / Ayurvedic Medicine / Biofeedback Training and Neurotherapy / Biological Dentistry / Chiropractic / Craniosacral Therapy / Detoxification Therapy / Environmental Medicine / Enzyme Therapy / Homeopathy / Hypnotherapy / Magnetic Field Therapy / Naturopathic Medicine / Osteopathic Medicine / Traditional Chinese Medicine

ENERGY MEDICINE: Electrodermal screening (EDS) can help determine the specific types of headache patients have as well as detect their underlying causes.

OXYGEN THERAPIES: • Hydrogen peroxide • Hyperbaric oxygen therapy

Where to Find Help

For information on headaches, or referrals to a qualified health-care practitioner, contact the following organizations.

American Council for Headache Education
19 Mantua Road
Mt. Royal, New Jersey 08061
(856) 423–0258
Website: www.achenet.org

Provides written information on causes of and treatment approaches to headaches. Also provides referrals to physicians nationwide who specialize in headache treatment, oversees local support groups, and publishes a newsletter.

National Headache Foundation
428 W. St. James Place, 2nd Floor
Chicago, Illinois 60614–2750
(888) NHF-5552
Website: www.headaches.org

Supplies a state-by-state list of physicians who treat headaches, available by written request. Also provides free information on headaches. Membership available for annual fee.

Recommended Reading

Alternative Medicine Definitive Guide to Headaches. Robert Milne, M.D., and Blake More, with Burton Goldberg. Tiburon, CA: Future Medicine Publishing, 1996.

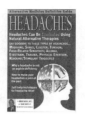

Curing Headaches Naturally with Chinese Medicine. Bob Flaws. Boulder, CO: Blue Poppy Press, 1998.

Dr. Braly's Food Allergy and Nutrition Revolution. James Braly, M.D. New Canaan, CT: Keats Publishing, 1992.

Free Yourself from Headaches: The Natural Drug-Free Program for Prevention and Relief. Jan Stomfeld and Anita Weil. Berkeley, CA: Frog Ltd., 1995.

Freedom from Headaches. Joel R. Saper, M.D., and Kenneth R. Magee, M.D. New York: Simon & Schuster, 1986.

Homeopathy for Headaches. Ursula Stone. New York: Kensington, 1999.

HEARING AND EAR DISORDERS

Disorders of the auditory system affect 28 million Americans. Practitioners of alternative medicine believe that a large percentage of these disorders involve food and environmental allergies, as well as the overuse of antibiotics. Dietary changes, nutritional supplements, herbal therapy, and homeopathic remedies are often highly effective treatments, helping to eliminate the need for antibiotics or surgery.

THE AUDITORY SYSTEM is responsible for the processing of sound and the regulation of balance and is one of the body's most delicate and sensitive systems. When functioning properly, it enables a person to hear the faintest cry or maintain equilibrium in the most extreme circumstances. But the very complexity that allows for such precision also makes the ear susceptible to a wide range of ailments.

Ear disorders can affect people at any age, says Constantine A. Kotsanis, M.D., of Grapevine, Texas, and symptoms may include ear pain and stuffiness, inflammation, tinnitus (ringing in the ears), problems with balance, dizziness, vertigo, nerve damage, and hearing loss. "A slight loss in the ability to hear is not unusual with advancing age," adds Dr. Kotsanis, "but recently more young people are suffering from hearing loss equivalent to someone 40 years their senior." According to studies, more than 60% of incoming college students may have impaired hearing in the high frequency range.[1]

Types of Ear Disorders

There are a wide variety of ear-related disorders, ranging from common ear pain to severe conditions such as chronic otitis media (ear infection), Meniere's disease, tinnitus, and hearing loss.

General Ear Pain

General ear pain is one of the most common complaints. "The usual cause is a buildup of fluid in the middle ear,

> *A slight loss in the ability to hear is not unusual with advancing age, but recently more young people are suffering from hearing loss equivalent to someone 40 years their senior.*
>
> —CONSTANTINE A. KOTSANIS, M.D.

resulting in pressure that swells and closes the eustachian tube," according to Dr. Kotsanis. "When the tube closes, fluid from the middle ear is prevented from flowing and begins to accumulate, and this stagnant fluid can lead to bacterial infection, causing acute pain, fever, and decreased hearing." General ear pain may also be attributed to wax buildup.

Otitis Media

Otitis media is an infection of the ear that is now the most common cause of hearing loss in children. Approximately $2 billion is spent annually on medical and surgical treatment of otitis media in the U.S.[2] Its increased incidence closely parallels the general rise of allergic diseases.[3] There are two basic types of otitis media, acute and chronic.

Acute otitis media is characterized by an infection of the middle ear (usually bacterial) and is often accompanied by an upper respiratory infection or allergy. Earache and irritability are common symptoms, as are fever, chills, and a red, swollen eardrum. Acute otitis media is most common in infants and children, though it may occur at any age. Recurrent acute otitis media is associated with early bottle-feeding, while prolonged breast-feeding (minimum of six months) has a preventative effect due to antibodies contained in mother's milk.[4] It can also occur due to allergies, especially to milk or wheat, or to chronic dehydration.

Chronic otitis media, also known as secretory or serous otitis media, refers to a constant swelling and blockage of the auditory tube and is characterized by a

STRUCTURE OF THE EAR

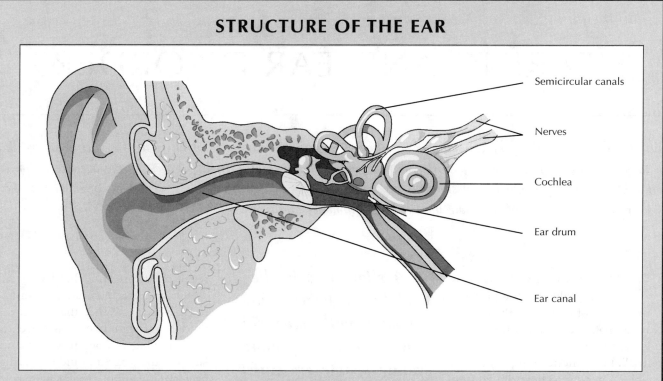

Semicircular canals

Nerves

Cochlea

Ear drum

Ear canal

The ear comprises three distinct sections known as the inner, middle, and outer ear. The inner ear consists of two parts, the cochlea, which is responsible for hearing, and the vestibule and semicircular canals, which are responsible for equilibrium and balance. Lining the inner ear are tiny hair cells that act as sensory receptors to transmit balance and hearing signals to the nerves and the brain.

The middle ear houses the three hearing bones or ossicles (stapes, incus, and malleus) and the auditory (eustachian)

tube, which extends and opens to the back part of the nasal airway. Normally, the middle ear space is filled with air that enters through the nasal opening of the eustachian tube.

The external ear houses the external canal (where wax is produced) and the ear "drumhead." The physical external ear, the external canal, and the eardrum are separated from each other by thin, soft tissue walls.

---

dull, often throbbing pain. It affects 20% to 40% of children under the age of six. "Chronic otitis media is usually accompanied by conductive hearing loss and can be caused by inflammation, swelling, or infection of the middle ear," says Dr. Kotsanis. "Perforation of the membranes of the middle ear is usually present, and there may be a constant drainage from the ear." Dr. Kotsanis warns that any infection of the middle ear left untreated can lead to meningitis (inflammation of the membranes of the spinal cord or brain). Recurrent otitis media has also been linked to hyperactivity in children.[5]

Meniere's Disease

Meniere's disease is a serious dysfunction characterized by a buildup of fluid pressure of the inner ear, which ultimately upsets the balance mechanism and can cause bouts of dizziness, nausea, and vomiting. Three common effects of Meniere's disease are vertigo, tinnitus, and sensory

hearing loss. The sudden, often violent attacks associated with Meniere's disease can last from ten minutes to several hours. Over time, as hearing loss becomes more profound, the number of attacks generally decrease and often cease when hearing loss is total. Conventional treatment consists of diuretics to keep fluid out of the ear canal, regular audiograms to monitor hearing loss, and surgery.

Tinnitus

Tinnitus is characterized by a continuous ringing or hissing in the ear, sometimes accompanied by pain. Causes can include excess earwax, a blocked or impaired eustachian tube, and dysfunction of the auditory nerve. Dr. Kotsanis notes that the onset of tinnitus may also be linked to excessive drug use, aspirin, sustained exposure to loud noise, smoking, trauma, Meniere's disease, and temporomandibular joint (TMJ) syndrome. Tinnitus in the elderly is often due to decreased circulation in and around the ear. People who suffer from tinnitus often complain of vertigo and dizziness, both of which can be symptoms related to problems of the inner ear, the heart, or the brain. These people should see a doctor to rule out anemia, atherosclerosis, labyrinthitis, and hypertension as possible causes of the tinnitus.

Otitis media is now the most common cause of hearing loss in children, with approximately $2 billion spent annually on medical and surgical treatment of it in the U.S.

Hearing Loss

Hearing loss can be sudden or gradual in onset. Problems that develop over a short period of time usually signify a blockage in either the outer or inner ear. Outer ear blockages are most often from wax buildup, while blockages of the inner ear are generally caused by fluid accumulation as a result of infection or allergy. There are two basic types of hearing loss, conductive and sensory.

Conductive hearing loss is associated with problems of either the external ear (wax or infection of the external canal) or the middle ear (eustachian tube dysfunction from infection or allergy, middle ear fluid, or fixation of the bones of the middle ear). Recurrent conductive hearing loss usually results from chronic ear infection or trauma.

Sensory hearing loss in adults is a common occurrence, usually resulting from a deterioration of the cochlea, particularly the loss of hair cells in the inner ear responsible for transmitting sound to the nerves. The most common causes of sensory hearing loss include aging, trauma, injury from high-frequency noise, infection (mainly viral), and metabolic disorders such as diabetes, hypertension, and kidney problems.

Dr. Kotsanis points out that toxins from caffeine, tobacco, aspirin, certain diuretics, and chemotherapy can also cause sensory hearing loss, and adds that, in some cases, vascular damage or benign tumors may be responsible. He recommends that hearing loss secondary to inner ear problems be investigated by an ear specialist. Dr. Kotsanis warns against purchasing a hearing aid without seeing a doctor first as some patients are not candidates for hearing aids even though they have hearing loss and the temporary fix may mask deeper issues.

EXCESSIVE WAX ACCUMULATION

The function of earwax is to clean and moisten the ear canal. A healthy external ear canal produces a constant, small amount of wax, but a buildup can block the ear canal, causing a feeling of fullness in the ear, as well as earaches, deafness, and dizziness. Hearing loss due to wax buildup can be gradual or sudden, depending on whether one is predisposed to excessive wax production. According to Constantine A. Kotsanis, M.D., of Grapevine, Texas, excessive wax in the ears is seen mostly in the elderly and in those with food or mold allergies. He notes that almost all children with excessive wax have an allergy to cow's milk.

It may also be an indication of a deficiency of essential fatty acids (EFAs), according to Rima Laibow, M.D., founding Medical Director of the Alexandria Institute of Natural and Integrative Medicine, in Croton-on-Hudson, New York. She recommends that the ear canals be gently cleansed and nutritional supplementation with EFAs instituted.

For wax buildup, Katie Data, N.D., of Fife, Washington, recommends a washing solution of lukewarm water with a few drops of vinegar or hydrogen peroxide. Virender Sodhi, M.D. (Ayurveda), N.D., of Bellevue, Washington, recommends warm herbal oils such as garlic or mullein mixed in olive oil to remove earwax.

 Individuals who work in a noisy environment should ask their employers for earplugs and muffs. Federal regulations require employers to provide ear protection if the workplace is excessively noisy.

Causes of Ear Disorders

"Many disorders of the ear can be traced to infection, loud noise, and a variety of food and environmental allergies," according to Dr. Kotsanis. Other possible causes include drugs, smoking (as a result of nicotine's negative effects on circulation), trauma, sustained exposure to chlorine (swimmer's ear), and autoimmune and metabolic disorders. Medications such as aspirin, diuretics, and chemotherapy can also cause ear problems.

Infection

Infection and inflammation often follow trauma to the ear. "A common cause is self-injury, usually from the overuse or misuse of cotton swabs and other objects placed in the ear for cleaning purposes," notes Dr. Kotsanis. Infections are also commonly seen after swimming, especially in water that carries a heavy dose of chlorine, bacteria, or fungi. Stubborn and repeated infections are usually fungal and are commonly seen in patients with diabetes, allergies, cancer, candidiasis, and other chronic diseases.

Loud Noise

Twenty-eight million Americans suffer from some form of hearing disorder, of which over a third can be attributed to exposure to loud noise.[6] Depending on one's hearing sensitivity, sustained exposure to any sound over the 80-85 decibel level can cause permanent hearing damage. Potentially damaging sources of noise include airplanes (130 decibels at takeoff), jackhammers (110 decibels), stereos (110 decibels), and rock concerts (over 110 decibels). Sudden intense noise like a gunshot or dynamite blast can damage hearing instantly by tearing the tissue in the delicate inner ear.

Twenty-eight million Americans suffer from some form of hearing disorder, of which over a third can be attributed to exposure to loud noise.

Allergies

Researchers and physicians have drawn a link between repeated ear infections and allergic conditions such as hay fever, asthma, eczema, and hives.[7] Katie Data, N.D., of Fife, Washington, notes that intolerance to particular foods—wheat and dairy products such as cow's milk—may encourage ear infections, inflammation, and hearing loss in some children. She notes that a large percentage of those who come to her with ear infections have problems related to the consumption of these foods. In such cases, young patients can often be successfully treated by eliminating the offending foods from the diet.[8]

According to Dr. Data, other factors to look for when treating infection or inflammation of the ear are environmental allergens such as dust, mold, and animal dander. She pays special attention to environmental allergens where a person sleeps.

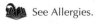 See Allergies.

Antibiotics

Otitis media is the most common reason parents bring their children to the doctor and accounts for 42% of all antibiotics prescribed to children.[9] According to Michael Schmidt, B.S., D.C., C.C.N., of Anoka, Minnesota, while antibiotics are an important means of treating otitis media in some children, research has raised questions about their extensive use. One study from the University of Copenhagen, in Denmark, found that "88% of patients never need antibiotics and that the frequency of recurrence of otitis media in the untreated group is low compared with those treated with antibiotics."[10] The study concluded that if a child is treated for an ear infection with an antibiotic within the first day or two of the onset of symptoms, then the child is much more likely to get another ear infection within a month.

Another study raises doubts about the value of antibiotics in treating children with chronic or long-standing earaches. In this study, children treated with the antibiotics amoxicillin, pediazole, and cefaclor fared no better than those given a placebo and, in fact, suffered recurrent middle ear fluid at a rate two to six times greater.[11] These findings are especially important when one considers that bacteria are only present in 50% to 70% of symptomatic ears; the remainder contain viruses, yeast, or inflammatory material that cannot be treated with antibiotics.[12]

According to William Crook, M.D., of Jackson, Tennessee, antibiotics used to treat ear infections upset the balance of the normal intestinal flora, resulting in an overgrowth of the yeast *Candida albicans*. Dr. Crook points out that this creates a cycle in which the immune system becomes suppressed, leading to recurrent ear infections.

Dr. Schmidt agrees and cites a study in which children treated repeatedly with antibiotics for ear infections developed yeast and fungal infections of the middle ear.[13] Lendon Smith, M.D., a pediatrician in Portland, Oregon, and author of many books on children's health, recommends that antibiotics only be used if the ear infection moves to the mastoid bone (found behind the ear) or the meninges (the membranes covering the brain and spinal cord).

Treating Ear Disorders

Conventional medicine generally treats ear disorders with antibiotics or surgery. Every year, as treatment for otitis media, an estimated one million tympanotomy tubes (tubes inserted through the tympanic membrane) are placed in the ears of American children to facilitate draining. Additionally, an equal number of children are given prophylactic (preventative) antibiotics in an effort to lessen the frequency of ear problems.[14] These approaches,

A NEW APPROACH TO TREATING OTITIS MEDIA

According to Michael Schmidt, B.S., D.C., C.C.N., of Anoka, Minnesota, researchers are beginning to find important dietary, nutritional, and environmental correlations with otitis media. The middle ear fluid of children with repeated ear infections contains highly inflammatory substances that are, in part, related to dietary intake of fats. These inflammatory substances can be reduced by modifying dietary fat intake and by taking antioxidant nutrients and certain trace elements such as zinc, since children who suffer from repeated ear infections are more likely to be zinc-deficient than their healthy counterparts.[18] Children exposed to heavy metals such as lead and mercury during their mothers' pregnancy are more likely to suffer from repeated infections of the ear, nose, and throat as well.[19]

Dr. Schmidt points out that children who suffer viral infections, such as measles and chicken pox, commonly experience decreases in blood levels of vitamin A that may last for six to 12 months. This renders them more susceptible to secondary bacterial infections of the ears, nose, and throat.[20] Also, nutrient deficiencies that affect immune function have been found in various groups of children. For example, U.S. children had the lowest blood levels of vitamin E of any children in the industrialized world—half the level of Japanese children.[21] Again, this may make these children more likely to get ear infections.

A study of 104 children with chronic ear infections investigated the role that food may play. Of these, 81 were found to be allergic to one or more foods. When the offending foods were removed from the diet, 70 children experienced improvement of their middle ear condition. When the offending foods were reintroduced, most of the children experienced a worsening of their condition.[22] Another study found that 19 of 20 children with chronic earaches that had not responded to any other treatment had their condition resolved after food allergy management.[23]

"The questions being raised about the safety and effectiveness of antibiotics and surgery (the placement of tympanotomy tubes), coupled with new discoveries about the role of diet, allergy, nutrition, environment, and other factors, should cause doctors and patients to take a new look at the problem of otitis media in children," says Dr. Schmidt. "At the very least, one should consider the role of food and food allergy. Perhaps we should not be asking 'How can we kill this or that bacteria?' but 'How can we optimize the immune defenses of all children?' Addressing the underlying reasons children become sick, while reserving antibiotics and surgery for those who truly need them, seems to be the sensible solution to the nation's most common pediatric health problem."

however, are often ineffective and can sometimes aggravate a condition. For instance, surgical implantation of ear tubes to promote drainage can lead to recurrent infections. At the same time, children who do not receive antibiotics for ear infections have fewer recurrences than those who do.[15]

When treating ear disorders, practitioners of alternative medicine first seek to identify the cause—diet, intolerance to certain foods or environmental factors, infection, or trauma. Through dietary changes, nutritional supplementation, allergy elimination, herbal remedies, homeopathy, traditional Chinese medicine, Ayurvedic medicine, craniosacral therapy, and auditory integration training, it is possible to alleviate conditions ranging from ear infections to tinnitus to hearing loss.

Dietary Changes

According to John Hibbs, N.D., of Seattle, Washington, making dietary changes such as cutting down on saturated fats and cholesterol, addressing intolerances to certain foods such as wheat and dairy products, and keeping sugar, sweets, and alcohol intake to a minimum (to limit yeast growth, especially if recurrent ear infections have been treated with antibiotics) are smart preventative steps that can have a profound effect on the health and well-being of the auditory system in both children and adults.

One diet-related study reveals a direct correlation between hearing and lipid (fat) levels. Several children with fluctuating sensory hearing loss had their hearing return to near normal when dietary controls were instituted.[16] In another study, over 1,400 patients with inner ear symptoms and increased lipoprotein (proteins that carry fats in the blood) levels were placed on individualized diets. In most patients, dizziness was alleviated, the sensation of pressure in the ears dissipated, hearing improved and stabilized, and tinnitus often lessened in severity and sometimes disappeared.[17]

Nutritional Supplements

Dr. Hibbs points out that a deficiency of protein and iron in a child's diet can lead to ear infections, including otitis media. He recommends that, when necessary, a child's

FOLIC ACID AND VITAMIN B₁₂ FOR HEARING LOSS

Hearing loss is the second most common health complaint (after heart problems) for elderly Americans. But before you buy the latest hearing-aid device, try eating more grains and vegetables high in folic acid (a type of B vitamin) and a B₁₂ supplement. A recent study from the U.S. Centers for Disease Control and Prevention and the University of Georgia found that women (60-71 years old) with hearing loss also had nutritional deficiencies of vitamin B₁₂ and folic acid. The researchers tested 55 women for their hearing abilities and their blood levels of these B vitamins. They found that women with hearing loss had 38% lower levels of B₁₂ and 25% lower levels of folic acid.

Researchers suspect that deficiencies in folic acid and B₁₂ may impair nerve function and blood circulation in and around the ear. Folic acid (found in whole grains, chickpeas, soybeans, spinach, broccoli, and cabbage) is important for red blood cell formation, the breakdown and utilization of proteins, and proper cell division. Vitamin B₁₂ (found in meat, fish, and dairy products) is the only vitamin that contains cobalt, a mineral cofactor and activator of enzymes important for nervous system function and the formation of red blood cells.[29]

diet be supplemented with B vitamins as well as vitamins that contain iron to help prevent anemia, a condition that can lead to frequent ear infections. However, iron should not be given during an infection and should only be given if an iron deficiency has been shown to exist, as excess iron can lower immunity.

When treating chronic otitis media, Dr. Data recommends supplements of beta carotene and vitamin C, along with the amino acid N-acetyl-cysteine to remove the fluid. In cases where otitis media is treated with antibiotics, she stresses the importance of using the "friendly bacteria" acidophilus to reconstitute the normal digestive tract flora. In cases where inflammation puts pressure on the organs of hearing, high-dose pancreatic enzymes have been shown to reduce inflammation and may lead to relief of tinnitus. Nutritional supplementation with vitamins A and C, bioflavonoids, and zinc may also be beneficial.[24] Additionally, thymus extract given orally has been shown to decrease children's food allergies, improve immune function, and may be of particular benefit in chronic otitis media.[25] Vitamins A

and E have proven beneficial in treating hearing loss associated with aging.[26]

MSM (methylsulfonylmethane, an organic form of sulfur) in liquid form used as eardrops can be beneficial for age-related hearing loss. Sulfur is essential to all cells in the body and deficiency results in less permeable cells. MSM produces the effect of easier passage of fluids in and out of cells.[27] In the ears, this results in increased elasticity of the tympanic membrane, which in turn may improve hearing.

Glutamic acid is a neurotransmitter important for brain metabolism. It assists in transporting potassium across the blood-brain barrier and is important for the metabolism of other amino acids, fats, and sugars. Glutamic acid has been shown effective in treating certain forms of tinnitus.[28]

Allergy Elimination

In treating ear disorders, Dr. Hibbs gives high priority to identifying allergies. "I look for related problems such as allergies in the respiratory tract or any indication that other types of allergies might exist, including intolerance to certain foods, as these can create a type of immune weakness that leads not only to mechanical irritation but chronic ear infections as well. When there is an allergy to dairy products or wheat, congestion typically occurs in the middle ear."

When treating infants or children, Dr. Data explains that breast-feeding and the removal from the diet of any food to which the patient is allergic are the recommended preventative measures for otitis media, which occurs most frequently in infants and small children. Human milk provides immunologic protection for the child and avoiding food allergens is important because a child's digestive tract is quite permeable to food antigens.[30] Dr. Data cites the case of a 15-month-old baby suffering from chronic otitis media. The baby had not been breast-fed and had been given a milk-based formula from birth. After examination, she suggested the removal of all dairy and dairy-related products (milk, cheese, and yogurt) from the infant's diet and the use of herbal eardrops. The child's symptoms disappeared almost immediately.

If food elimination and rotation diets do not correct the problem, then allergy treatment using enzyme-potentiated desensitization (EPD) usually gives the best results, according to Dr. Kotsanis. In EPD, an allergic patient is given a series of standardized injections of a wide variety of allergens from a single category. EPD injections differ from conventional allergy shots in three important ways: EPD injections include multiple related allergens; EPD doses are much weaker; and EPD injections are given along with an enzyme called beta-glucuronidase.

This last component is important because it acts as a catalyst to make the vaccine more potent.

Herbal Remedies

Herbal remedies have proven effective in treating a number of ear disorders, according to Dr. Hibbs. To treat ear infections, he uses a combination of goldenseal, mullein, and hypericum (St. John's wort) to reduce ear pain and help draw excess fluid out of the ear. Echinacea and goldenseal can also be used as antibacterials, adds Dr. Hibbs.

Echinacea is an immune-enhancing herb that is an antimicrobial agent, destroying bacteria and viruses found in the body. Echinacea has anti-inflammatory effects and stimulates tissue repair at injury sites. It also increases bacterial and viral resistance.[31] Studies have shown that echinacea fights head colds and related ailments by increasing the number of immune cells in the blood. It also enhances the immune cells' ability to destroy harmful bacteria, inhibits the production of viruses, and controls the duration and intensity of immune responses.[32]

> **CAUTION** Echinacea is not advised for individuals whose immune systems are hyperactive, including autoimmune diseases such as multiple sclerosis, diabetes, lupus, and rheumatoid arthritis. Pregnant women should refrain from using the herb.

Goldenseal *(Hydrastis canadensis)* has been used traditionally to combat bacteria and is also an immune system–enhancer. Berberine, the primary active ingredient in goldenseal, has been shown to be a potent activator of macrophages, the cells responsible for engulfing and destroying bacteria, viruses, and fungi.

For otitis media, David L. Hoffmann, B.Sc., M.N.I.M.H., of Sebastopol, California, past President of the American Herbalists Guild, combines equal parts of echinacea and cleavers tinctures and prescribes one teaspoon three times a day (if this mixture is used for children, he recommends using glycerate forms). Warm mullein flower oil introduced into the ear can be an effective anti-inflammatory, but he warns to avoid this treatment if there is any perforation of the eardrum.

Ginkgo biloba increases circulation in and around the ear and is commonly used to treat tinnitus.[33] Hoffmann recommends combining the tinctures of black cohosh[34] and ginkgo in equal parts and taking one teaspoon of this mixture three times a day. Dr. Kotsanis reports one case of a teenage girl with severe tinnitus whom he successfully treated with ginkgo. Tests revealed an overall hearing level of 20 decibels, meaning the patient had trouble hearing sounds of a lower volume. After six weeks of ginkgo treatments (Dr. Kotsanis's general recommendation is 50-200 mg three times a day for three months), her tinnitus was relieved and her hearing improved to

HOMEOPATHIC REMEDIES OUTPERFORM ANTIBIOTICS FOR EAR INFECTIONS

Parents who may be undecided whether or not to rely exclusively on homeopathic remedies for their children's ear infections (acute otitis media) can take heart from the results of a recent German study. Researcher K.H. Friese, M.D., and his colleagues put 131 young children (average age 5) into two groups. One group of 28 children received conventional remedies such as decongestant nose drops, antibiotics, or secretolytics (12 different drugs in all) when they developed an ear infection. The other group was given one or more of 12 low-potency homeopathic remedies, including *Aconitum napellus, Apis mellifica, Belladonna, Lycopodium,* and *Lachesis,* depending on the exact symptoms reported. In both groups, the children had an average of two previous ear infections.

The results supported the superiority of homeopathic remedies for ear infections. The homeopathically treated group (Group A) had an average of two days of ear pain versus three days for the conventionally treated children (Group B). In Group A, 30% of the children were free of pain within three hours of taking the homeopathic remedy, compared to only 11.5% in Group B. Similarly, Group A required only three days of therapy compared to ten days in Group B. One year later, 70.7% of Group A had no recurrence of ear infections, while the other 29.3% had a maximum of three recurrences. But in Group B, only 56.5% were free of subsequent ear infections after one year and 43.5% experienced a maximum of six recurrences.

"Of the 103 children in Group A," commented Dr. Friese, "five were eventually prescribed antibiotics, but 98 were completely cured by homeopathic treatment." In other words, the homeopathic remedies worked faster, better, and their positive effects lasted longer. Dr. Friese notes that while the conventional approach to treating childhood ear infections is never questioned, it ought to be. "Antibiotics can cause numerous side effects, including allergies, weakening of the immune system, and colonization of the intestines with pathogenic fungi."[35]

the point that she could hear sounds in the 1-5 decibel range.

Tea tree oil drops and diluted grapefruit seed extract drops are helpful for ringing in the ears, clogged ears,

THE INVISIBLE DISABILITY— INFANTS AND HEARING LOSS

According to Katie Data, N.D., of Fife, Washington, although the incidence of pediatric hearing loss is 13 per 1,000 births, the average age of identifying a child with significant hearing loss is 2½ years. This late identification has profound consequences in that it can leave a child unnecessarily handicapped for life. "A child is never too young to be evaluated for hearing loss," says Dr. Data.

Risk factors that can lead to hearing loss include premature birth, low birth weight, newborn jaundice, certain drugs (tobramycin, streptomycin, quinine, gentamicin, furosemide, ethacrynic acid), meningitis, and hereditary disorders such as otosclerosis (scarring of the membranes of the ear). Hearing loss may be present if a child does not respond to a voice or ordinary household sounds. Delayed speech is also a significant sign.

Since the window for language acquisition is birth to four years of age, early identification of hearing loss is essential for normal language development to occur. However, according to Dr. Data, most physicians and health-care providers are not adequately trained to detect hearing loss. Parents whose concerns are hastily dismissed should find a physician who will listen, says Dr. Data, emphasizing that "a child does not outgrow hearing loss" and that "every minute of a child's development is precious." There are many resources available once hearing loss is detected, but early detection (before the first birthday) is critical to minimize the handicap in later years.

diminished hearing, ear pain, itching in the ears, or ear problems caused by yeast infections.

 See Herbal Medicine, Homeopathy.

Homeopathy

Several homeopathic remedies are useful in the treatment of various stages of otitis media. Robert D. Milne, M.D., of Las Vegas, Nevada, recommends *Aconite* and *Ferrum phos.* for the early stages of otitis media. For later stages or recurrent infections, he recommends *Belladonna, Chamomilla, Hepar sulf., Lycopodium, Merc sol., Pulsatilla,*

and *Silicea.* Depending on the symptoms, allergenic food must be eliminated from the diet, according to Dr. Milne.

Dr. Milne points out that many patients who suffer from Meniere's disease have a history of migraines. Depending on the symptoms, he treats Meniere's with specific homeopathic remedies such as *Carboneum sulphuratum* and *Salicylicum acidum*, in addition to the herb ginkgo (to increase circulation), vitamin B_6 (to decrease fluid buildup), and restrictions on sodium, caffeine, and chocolate. The patient should also check for sensitivity to mercury dental amalgams.

Several homeopathic remedies may help in the treatment of tinnitus as well, says Dr. Milne. They include *Salicylicum acidum, Chenopodium,* and *Cinchona officinalis.* The appropriate remedy depends upon the type of noise heard by the patient.

Traditional Chinese Medicine

According to traditional Chinese medicine, ear problems are associated with kidney function. Thus, acupuncture points related to the kidneys, are used to treat a range of ear disorders. Roger Hirsh, O.M.D., of Santa Monica, California, treats ear disorders with a combination of acupuncture and Chinese herbs. He often uses an herbal preparation called *er long zuo gi wan*, a variation of a classical herbal remedy for kidney disturbances.

Dr. Hirsh cites the case of a 35-year-old woman with nerve deafness in her left ear. After obtaining her medical history, acupuncture was recommended—two acupuncture needles were placed in her ankles, two in her knees, two in her hand, and two near the ear. When the knee points were treated with *moxa* (herbs burned on the acupuncture needles), the hearing immediately returned to her left ear. Dr. Hirsh also utilized acupuncture to treat a 65-year-old woman with tinnitus. By increasing the circulation of *qi* (vital life energy) around the ear, the woman reported that, after six sessions, her tinnitus was 80% relieved.

Ayurvedic Medicine

Ayurvedic medicine uses a combination of oils, massage, herbs, and nutritional supplements to treat ear disorders. According to Virender Sodhi, M.D. (Ayurveda), N.D., Director of the Ayurvedic & Naturopathic Medical Clinic, in Bellevue, Washington, the most effective oil for treating ear infections is *neem*, which is both antibacterial and antifungal. Dr. Sodhi combines *neem* with warm *Adardica indica* oil and places it in the ear. Dr. Sodhi also employs lymphatic massage outside the ears to open the eustachian tube and facilitate drainage. In addition, he uses the herb *amla,* which is not only antibacterial and antiviral but a good source of vitamin C. It can be given in raw honey and helps stimulate the immune system.

Dr. Sodhi uses *albad* oil, herbs, and supplements to treat hearing loss. He recommends black pepper and Indian long pepper to improve digestion and elimination and to increase the circulation around the ear. Beneficial herbs include *ashwagandha, bala, and calamus,* all of which are known to increase circulation.

In treating Meniere's disease, Dr. Sodhi uses *albad* oil in the ear to draw out excess fluid. He also gives *albad* oil, sesame oil, and ghee (clarified butter) internally and prescribes rest and lymphatic drainage massage.

For tinnitus, Dr. Sodhi recommends warm *albad* oil in the ear.

 See Ayurvedic Medicine, Craniosacral Therapy, Sound Therapy, Traditional Chinese Medicine.

Craniosacral Therapy

According to John Upledger, D.O., Medical Director of the Upledger Institute, in Palm Beach Gardens, Florida, craniosacral therapy can be beneficial in treating hearing disorders caused by problems associated with the temporal bone (on both sides of the skull at its base, one portion of which encloses the organ of hearing). "When the temporal bone is out of alignment with the rest of the bones of the cranium, hearing can be affected and tinnitus may be the result," says Dr. Upledger. This problem can be solved through craniosacral therapy by adjusting the temporal bone.

Craniosacral therapy manipulates the bones of the skull and the underlying membranes to alleviate pressure and restrictions. The craniosacral system is a body rhythm, involving the flow of cerebrospinal fluid between the cranium (the bones of the skull) and the sacrum (the base of the spine). Disturbances in the craniosacral rhythm can indicate dysfunction in the body.

A child is never too young to be evaluated for hearing loss.

—KATIE DATA, N.D.

"The temporal bone can also be affected if the bite is off and this can interfere with proper hearing," adds Dr. Upledger. "A problem with the bite can also prevent proper drainage of the eustachian tube, leading to a blockage that can result in hearing problems." Craniosacral therapy can successfully address both of these problems. It can also be used to relieve pressure on the temporal lobes of the brain, which may be interfering with the hearing process. "Words may sound scrambled

to the listener, but when the pressure is released, they can hear normally again," says Dr. Upledger.

Auditory Integration Training

Auditory integration training may be effective for patients who are hypersensitive to high-frequency sounds or suffer from loss of hearing in normal frequency ranges. The technique was developed by two French physicians, Alfred Tomatis, M.D., and Guy Berard, E.N.T. Both the Tomatis and the Berard methods provide auditory stimulation to the listener.

Dr. Tomatis theorizes that hearing problems can begin at any time, even *in utero,* due to accident, illness, or physical or emotional trauma. Using a device called the Electronic Ear, Dr. Tomatis established a system of auditory training that emphasizes a connection between listening, language, and learning. Tomatis's method presents different types of sounds to the listener in an attempt to recreate critical periods of listening development.

Specially prepared audiotapes containing music and voice are played into the Electronic Ear, which uses several controls and filters to simulate what Dr. Tomatis believes to be the developmental stages of listening. High- and low-frequency sounds are extracted from the sound source and then played to the listener. Low-frequency sounds are gradually eliminated in part of the program, leaving only the high frequencies that, according to Dr. Tomatis, "energize" the brain. In another part of the program, the person speaks into the Electronic Ear microphone to listen to his or her own voice while repeating words and phrases or reading, in order to establish good audio-vocal control.

A three-year-old girl who had been deaf for the first 18 months of her life was treated with the Tomatis method. When she first began to hear at 18 months, she was not able to process the sounds because they were so foreign to her, according to Billie Thompson, Ph.D., Director of the Sound, Listening, and Learning Center, in Phoenix, Arizona. Over the next year and a half, she was unmanageable, displayed constant tantrums, and continually failed hearing tests. After 60 hours with the Electronic Ear, in conjunction with daily speech therapy, she began to speak, allowing her to enter school, where she is now fully functional.

Similar to the Tomatis method, Dr. Berard's method is based upon the belief that behavioral and cognitive problems can arise when certain frequencies are perceived in a distorted manner and that this altered perception can lead to difficulties in comprehension and behavior. By using a device called the Ears Education and Retraining System (EERS), Dr. Berard claims that distorted hearing and hypersensitivity to specific frequencies are reduced and that, ideally, all frequencies can be perceived equally well.

The device takes music from a sound source (audiotape or compact disc) and filters out the frequencies to which the individual has been found to be hypersensitive. The EERS then electronically modulates these frequencies and returns them via headphones to the ears. Dr. Berard has found that after about ten hours of listening to the processed music (in 20 half-hour sessions), the listener usually makes significant progress toward hearing all frequencies equally well.

One of Dr. Berard's patients was an 11-year-old autistic girl who suffered from both a hypo- and hyper-acute sense of hearing. Over the course of the 20 sessions using the EERS, Dr. Berard was able to decrease the hyper-acute points of the girl's hearing while bringing the deficits up, thus creating a more normal hearing pattern. This also helped correct the girl's dyslexia, attention deficit, and hyperactivity.

Recommendations

- Making dietary changes—cutting down on saturated fats, addressing intolerances to certain foods such as wheat and dairy products, and keeping sugar, sweets, and alcohol intake to a minimum—can have a profound effect on the health and well-being of the auditory system.

- When treating chronic otitis media, supplements of beta carotene and vitamin C may be beneficial, along with the amino acid N-acetyl-cysteine to remove the fluid.

- Vitamins A and E and MSM (methylsulfonyl-methane, an organic form of sulfur) have proven beneficial in treating hearing loss associated with aging.

- For treating infants or children, breast-feeding and the removal from the diet of any food to which the child is allergic are the recommended preventative measures for otitis media.

- *Ginkgo biloba* increases circulation in and around the ear and is commonly used to treat tinnitus. Black cohosh can also help relieve ringing in the ears.

- Tea tree oil drops and diluted grapefruit seed extract drops are helpful for ringing in the ears, diminished hearing, ear pain, or ear problems caused by yeast infections.

- Homeopathic remedies have been shown to work faster, better, and their positive effects lasted longer than antibiotics for otitis media.

- According to traditional Chinese medicine, ear problems are associated with kidney function. Thus, acupuncture points related to the kidneys are used to treat a range of ear disorders.

- Ayurvedic medicine uses a combination of oils, massage, herbs, and nutritional supplements to treat ear disorders.

- Craniosacral therapy can be beneficial in treating hearing disorders caused by problems associated with the temporal bone (on both sides of the skull at its base, one portion of which encloses the organ of hearing).

- Auditory integration training may be effective for patients who are hypersensitive to high-frequency sounds or suffer from loss of hearing in normal frequency ranges.

Professional Care

The following therapies should only be provided by a qualified health professional:

Ayurvedic Medicine / Biofeedback Training and Neurotherapy / Chiropractic / Craniosacral Therapy / Environmental Medicine / Herbal Medicine / Homeopathy / Magnetic Field Therapy / Nutritional Medicine / Sound Therapy / Traditional Chinese Medicine

Where to Find Help

For more information on, or referrals for the treatment of, hearing and ear disorders, contact:

American Association of Oriental Medicine
433 Front Street
Catasauqua, Pennsylvania 18032
(888) 500-7999
Website: www.aaom.org

The AAOM is a national professional organization of acupuncturists who meet acceptable standards of competency and can provide you with the names and locations of local members.

American Academy of Environmental Medicine
7701 East Kellogg Avenue, Suite 625
Wichita, Kansas 67207
(316) 684-5500

Website: www.aaem.com

The academy offers extensive training for physicians interested in learning more about environmental medicine.

American Association of Naturopathic Physicians
8201 Greensboro Drive, Suite 300
McLean, Virginia 22101
(703) 610-9037
Website: www.naturopathic.org

Provides a directory of naturopathic physicians and offers referrals to a nationwide network of accredited or licensed practitioners. Also publishes a quarterly newsletter, for both professionals and the general public, and offers a series of brochures and pamphlets on a variety of subjects.

American CranioSacral Therapy Association
Upledger Institute
11211 Prosperity Farms Road
Palm Beach Gardens, Florida 33410
(407) 622-4706
Website: www.upledger.com

The association promotes increased awareness and acceptance of CranioSacral Therapy among both laypersons and health professionals and oversees the development of certification training for CST practitioners nationwide.

The Georgiana Organization, Inc.
P.O. Box 2607
Westport, Connecticut 06880
(203) 454-1221

The Georgiana Organization provides education, workshops, consultations, and information on the Berard method.

National Center for Homeopathy
801 North Fairfax, Suite 306
Alexandria, Virginia 22314
(703) 548-7790
Website: www.homeopathic.org

Provides a referral list of practicing homeopaths and other information. Gives courses for laypeople and professionals, and organizes study groups around the country.

Sound, Listening, and Learning Center
2701 E. Camelback, Suite 205
Phoenix, Arizona 85016
(602) 381-0086
Website: www.soundlistening.com

Provides education, workshops, consulting, therapeutic sessions, and information on the Tomatis method.

Recommended Reading

The Conscious Ear. Alfred Tomatis. Tarrytown, NY: Station Hill Books, 1991.

Beyond Antibiotics: 50 (or So) Ways to Boost Immunity and Avoid Antibiotics. Michael A. Schmidt, D.C., Lendon H. Smith, M.D., and Keith W. Sehnert. Berkeley, CA: North Atlantic Books, 1994.

Healing Childhood Ear Infections: Prevention, Home Care, and Alternative Treatment. Michael A. Schmidt, D.C. Berkeley, CA: North Atlantic Books, 1996.

Herbal Prescriptions for Health and Healing. Donald J. Brown. Rocklin, CA: Prima Health, 2000.

Music: Physician for Times to Come. Don Campbell. Wheaton, IL: Quest Books, 2000.

HEART DISEASE

Although heart disease causes half of all deaths in the United States,[1] it is one of the most preventable chronic degenerative diseases. It now appears that the primary culprit in heart disease is not high cholesterol levels or even atherosclerosis, but "vulnerable plaque," which is estimated to cause 85% of all heart attacks and strokes. The presence of oxidized cholesterol in the bloodstream is another major risk factor. The risk of heart attacks and strokes can be greatly decreased through dietary changes, exercise, stress reduction, and nutritional supplementation, as well as other alternative therapies.

THE U.S. LEADS the world in death rates from heart disease and over 60 million Americans currently suffer from the disease.[2] Among the conditions included in the category of heart (or cardiovascular) disease are coronary heart disease (decreased blood flow to the heart usually caused by atherosclerosis), congestive heart failure (cardiomyopathy), heart attack (myocardial infarction), stroke, microvascular dementia, chest pain (angina pectoris), high blood pressure (hypertension), arrhythmia, rheumatic heart disease, and hardening of the arteries (arteriosclerosis involving fatty arterial wall deposits, as the most common form).

📖 See Hypertension.

According to the American Heart Association (AHA), every 33 seconds an American dies from some form of heart disease—that's about 954,000 deaths annually or 42% of all mortalities. Every 20 seconds, an American suffers a heart attack, and every 60 seconds somebody dies from one. Among deaths attributed to heart disease, 52.3% are women and 47.7% are men.

"The average American lifestyle, combining too little exercise, too much stress, and a diet of highly processed foods often deficient in essential nutrients, has rendered this nation's population especially vulnerable to the ravages of heart ailments," says W. Lee Cowden, M.D., a cardiologist from Fort Worth, Texas.

> *The average American lifestyle, combining too little exercise, too much stress, and a diet of highly processed foods deficient in essential nutrients, has rendered this nation's population especially vulnerable to the ravages of heart ailments.*
>
> —W. LEE COWDEN, M.D.

Conventional medicine believes that the answer to fighting heart disease lies in treating certain symptoms such as high blood pressure or lowering cholesterol with medication. As a result, the medical cost of cardiovascular disease in the U.S. exceeds $56 billion a year.[3] Expensive coronary bypass surgeries and angioplasties (alteration of blood vessels surgically or with a laser or via balloon dilation) are performed with increasing regularity, while cholesterol-lowering drugs further fuel the skyrocketing costs associated with heart disease. Coronary artery bypass surgery is called an "overprescribed and unnecessary surgery" by many leading authorities.[4]

Some physicians choose to reduce a patient's risk factors for heart disease by considering preventive measures such as stress reduction, exercise, dietary improvement, weight control, and the elimination of smoking. "Although these methods have resulted in some leveling off of the rate of heart disease," says Garry F. Gordon, M.D., of Payson, Arizona, co-founder of the American College of Advancement in Medicine, "the epidemic continues and conventional medicine continues to use drugs and surgery as the primary treatments for heart disease." Equipped to treat heart disease only when it has reached its most serious and life-threatening stages, conventional medicine is largely failing in its battle against the epidemic. Moreover, it is failing to address the primary cause of heart attacks and strokes, vulnerable plaque, which conventional diagnostic procedures such as angiograms do not even usually detect.

Vulnerable Plaque: The Primary Cause of Most Heart Disease

In 1998, the AHA published a monograph, edited by its president, Valentin Fuster, M.D., Ph.D., Director of the Cardiovascular Institute at Mount Sinai School of Medicine, in New York City, which stated that 85% of all heart attacks and strokes were due to vulnerable plaque, a "soft" form of cholesterol, proteins, and blood cells that builds up within the arterial wall.[5] The findings were widely reported in both conventional medical journals and the mainstream media and debunked the accepted conventional wisdom that said heart disease was primarily due to hard arterial plaque that obstructs the artery. Despite the coverage the report received, for the most part practitioners of conventional medicine today still focus on treating and minimizing what many experts now view as the secondary causes of heart disease, often ignoring the issue of vulnerable plaque altogether. While such secondary causes are important, addressing them alone is at best an incomplete approach to treating and preventing heart disease, and at worst can result in needless death and physical impairment.

"Vulnerable plaque has come under scrutiny only very recently," Dr. Gordon says. "Until recently, it had not usually been noticed during traditional cardiovascular diagnostic testing, because it rapidly builds up within the wall of the artery itself, extending outwards very little." It is primarily composed of soft cholesterol and clotting proteins (rather than the more mineralized crystalline form of obstructing plaque common in atherosclerosis), which is contained by a fibrous cap that is thinner and weaker than obstructing plaque, and so is much more easily ruptured.

"The body tends to respond to vulnerable plaque as an infection, sending defensive blood cells that attack and inflame the cap," continues Dr. Gordon. "The tendency to breakage that results from this is what gives vulnerable plaque its name. The interior of the plaque contains powerful coagulants that, if released into the blood, can create massive, lethal clots. This is what makes vulnerable plaque so deadly."

According to Dr. Gordon, the discovery of vulnerable plaque and the primary role it plays in most cases of heart disease explains why there has never been a significant reduction in heart attacks or deaths in surgical patients. "It also lends itself to a kinder, noninvasive, supplement-based protocol that can give immediate protection against heart attacks and strokes," Dr. Gordon says.

The body tends to respond to vulnerable plaque as an infection, sending defensive blood cells that attack and inflame the cap. The tendency to breakage that results from this is what gives vulnerable plaque its name. The interior of the plaque contains powerful coagulants that, if released into the blood, can create massive, lethal clots. This is what makes vulnerable plaque so deadly.

—Garry F. Gordon, M.D.

Seen and Unseen Plaque

Understanding vulnerable plaque explains why some people with little or no blockage due to atherosclerosis have heart attacks, while other people with almost completely blocked arteries may never experience any symptoms of cardiovascular disease. "All arterial plaques are actually thought to be the body's way of repairing damage to the arterial wall," Dr. Gordon explains. "Small tears might be caused by high blood pressure due to stress, the effects of smoking, and a number of other factors." In response to such tears, collagen, clotting proteins, and various other substances are released into the bloodstream and adhere to the injured site, attracting platelets (special cells responsible for clotting). "The core of the plaque contains many fat-laden cells derived from white blood cells known as leukocytes, which contain a large amount of tissue factor, a powerful coagulant," Dr. Gordon says. "This core is separated from the bloodstream by a fibrous cap. It is the integrity of the cap that determines the stability of the plaque."

Because the body tends to treat the buildup of soft cholesterol in vulnerable plaque as an infection, it releases germ-fighting blood cells that inflame the plaque and enzymes called metalloproteinases that eat away at the fibrous cap. "Vulnerable plaque is a lethal combination of powerful clotting substances stored in the artery wall and separated from the bloodstream only by the weak cap that is being attacked by the body's defense mechanism," Dr. Gordon states. Biomechanical studies have shown that no more stress than that caused by a normal heartbeat can rupture these plaques, he adds.

Blood vs. Blood Vessel

"The information about vulnerable plaque strongly suggests that the current surgical approaches to cardiovascular disease are as misguided as removing your lung if you have pneumonia," Dr. Gordon says. "The focus has to be on the blood, not the blood vessel."

The information about vulnerable plaque strongly suggests that the current surgical approaches to cardiovascular disease are as misguided as removing your lung if you have pneumonia. The focus has to be on the blood, not the blood vessel.

—GARRY F. GORDON, M.D.

Dr. Gordon notes that although more than one million angiograms are performed annually in the U.S., they usually do not reveal vulnerable plaque deposits. "But angiograms can be replaced by another test using an ultra-high-speed magnetic resonance imaging (MRI) scanner that often does detect vulnerable plaque," he says. "This new test, necessitating more ultra-high-speed MRI machines, will certainly take the financial sting out of cardiovascular disease testing by resulting in fewer angiograms." Darkfield microscopy, a diagnostic technique that views a patient's live blood through a special microscope as the sample is illuminated with angled halogen light, can also be used to detect clotting, according to James Privitera, M.D., of Covina, California, an expert in its use.

"The pharmaceutical industry also sees tremendous opportunity in developing new, patentable drugs specifically aimed at stopping vulnerable plaque from rupturing," Dr. Gordon says. But while conventional medicine is just beginning to look for new drugs for this purpose, for over 20 years, many alternative physicians have been prescribing natural substances and supplements that balance the blood itself, remove the elements that attack and

rupture vulnerable plaque, repair existing arterial lesions, and prevent their further development.

"What is exciting today is that we finally have the means to analyze the components in the bloodstream and improve the risk factors identified therein," Dr. Gordon says. "Now we can focus upon the sick or unhealthy components of the bloodstream that cause irreparable damage and, rather than cutting out the areas in which they become lodged, we can provide the blood itself with the necessary nutrients and other factors that will restore it to health."

The Role of Infections

It is now recognized by many researchers that infection can trigger the formation of vulnerable plaque, causing heart disease. "The infection aspect of heart disease has been given added validation by a recent report published in the *Journal of the American Medical Association,* showing that up to 55% of heart attacks appear to be prevented by treatment with proper antibiotics," Dr. Gordon says. "In addition, evidence published in *Science* (February 1999) implicates *Chlamydia pneumoniae* (an infectious bacteria that 95% of us are exposed to during our lives). Cytomegalovirus (CMV) and herpes (common retroviruses) as well as *Helicobacter pylori* have been shown to be closely connected with heart attacks."

Analysis by researchers at the National Public Health Institute, in Helsinki, Finland, of blood samples taken from Finnish patients who suffered heart attacks found that 70% tested positive for antibodies associated with *C. pneumoniae,* despite the fact that the rate of heart attacks in Finland "did not follow the six-to-seven-year cycles of acute *C. pneumoniae* outbreaks." This led the researchers to speculate that heart attacks are caused by chronic, not acute, *C. pneumoniae* infections.[6] As Paul W. Ewald, Professor of Biology at Amherst College, points out in his book *Plague Time,* the proposed link between infection and heart disease is not new—in fact, it was first theorized in the 1820s. And the first evidence that *Chlamydia* was involved in arterial disease occurred in the 1940s.[7]

Given the role infection can play in heart disease, Dr. Gordon says, "When vulnerable plaque is actively infected is when the body—trying to prevent the spread of this active infection in one small part of the blood vessel system—causes the blood going through this area to become hyper-coagulable and viscous, and a clot may also form, so that the blood can barely flow through that area." Left untreated, this process can eventually result in the major symptoms of heart disease and possibly death.

COMMON TYPES OF HEART DISEASE

Heart Attack: Atherosclerosis that occurs in the coronary arteries can deprive the heart of oxygen-rich blood until the affected area of the heart literally dies, causing a myocardial infarction (heart attack), sometimes leading to cardiac arrest (stopped heartbeat) that often results in death. Heart attacks are responsible for about 500,000 deaths annually in the U.S., and there are an estimated 1,500,000 new and recurrent cases every year.[8] Often, a diminished blood supply to the heart exhibits few symptoms until the blockage is so great that a heart attack results. But while a heart attack may appear to come on suddenly, it often begins with years of physical neglect, such as a poor diet and lack of exercise. Genetic predisposition can also be a crucial factor.

Coronary Stenosis: In coronary occlusion, arteries that course over the surface of, and penetrate into, the heart muscle become narrowed so that blood flow through them is restricted. The heart muscle stops receiving adequate amounts of oxygen and nutrients and a person develops angina. This means the heart muscle's pumping capacity has been exceeded. Coronary stenosis is commonly caused by atherosclerosis, the buildup of plaque and clogging in the arteries that can lead to heart attacks.

Angina: Angina (discomfort, heaviness, or pressure in the chest or throat) can result when there are lesions in the coronary arteries or valves of the heart. These lesions diminish the supply of oxygenated blood to the heart muscle, causing discomfort to radiate from the throat or chest to the shoulder and down the left arm, in some cases.

"Silent angina" is a form of angina that manifests without discomfort, other than shortness of breath, numbness in the arm, dizziness, or other vague symptoms caused by overexertion or emotional stress. About 50% of all people with coronary stenosis develop silent angina. Often, their first awareness of having heart disease is when they have a sudden heart attack. Overall, however, angina is a warning sign that there are problems with the heart, but is not necessarily a precursor of a heart attack if appropriate treatment is initiated.

Congestive Heart Failure: Congestive heart failure (cardiomyopathy) is failure of the heart muscle. The heart becomes congested with blood and dangerously weakened. Congestive heart failure is most commonly caused by coronary stenosis or occlusion and heart attacks. Repeated heart attacks can damage large sections of the heart muscle, so that there is not enough heart muscle left intact to pump blood out of the heart. Cardiomyopathy can also be caused by viral infections that damage the heart muscle. As the pressure and volume of blood inside the heart's pumping chamber increases, additional pressure is placed on arteries and veins in the lungs, resulting in fluid leaks into the lungs and the start of the cardiomyopathy process. A typical sign of congestive heart failure is shortness of breath, either with minimal exertion or when lying down at night.

Stroke: Twenty-five percent of the blood pumped from the heart goes to the brain and, if the blood flow to a part of the brain is interrupted for any reason, the affected brain cells are deprived of oxygen and die, resulting in a stroke, the third leading cause of death in the U.S.[9] Stroke can lead to loss of speech, physical movement, or eyesight, depending on the area of the brain affected. Of the 500,000 Americans who suffer a stroke every year, nearly two-thirds become handicapped. There are currently over two million people in the U.S. disabled by stroke.[10]

Atherosclerosis of the cerebral arteries can affect blood flow to the brain and increase the risk of stroke. A stroke can also result from a blood clot that has formed in a narrowed cerebral artery or as a result of a clot formed elsewhere in the body, usually in the heart or arteries of the neck, and carried in the bloodstream to the head as a thromboembolus. Other causes include a blood vessel that ruptures or hemorrhages, causing blood to spill into the brain, not only damaging the brain cells directly, but resulting in further damage to brain tissue due to lack of oxygen when the blood supply is interrupted. Strokes have also been associated with inherited disorders, birth defects, and certain rare blood diseases.[11]

How Plaque Forms

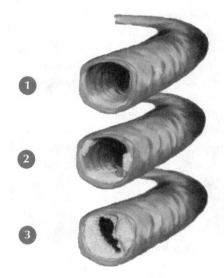

1. A normal, healthy artery.
2. The beginning of cholesterol plaque buildup within the artery.
3. Severely restricted artery with plaque filling the majority of the passage; note further breakdown and ballooning of inner artery wall.

Atherosclerosis and Oxidized Cholesterol

A common precursor of heart disease is atherosclerosis, in which the inner arterial walls harden and thicken due to deposits of fatty and protein substances. These substances form a plaque, which in turn causes a narrowing of the arteries.[12] Over time, plaque can block the arteries and interrupt blood flow to the organs they supply, including the heart and brain. Atherosclerosis of the coronary arteries (the arteries supplying the muscle of the heart), known as coronary heart disease, is one of the most common forms of heart disease in the U.S. today. Coronary heart disease can lead to angina and heart attack, while atherosclerosis of the cerebral arteries (the arteries that supply blood to the brain) can precipitate strokes.

Atherosclerosis may be well under way even at birth. In investigating the deaths of newborn babies in Scandinavia from a variety of causes, it was found that nearly 97% had some degree of arterial thickening, the first step

in heart disease.[13] Plaque formation in arteries usually follows prior damage to the inner lining of the arteries.

According to Dr. Cowden, deficiencies of nutrients such as vitamin C, vitamin E, and magnesium make this inner lining more susceptible to damage and plaque formation. "Small tears can occur in the lining of the arteries after a sudden, very high blood pressure episode of brought on by stress," Dr. Cowden explains. "The vessels cannot always dilate rapidly enough to accommodate the sudden increase in pressure and tearing occurs."

When tearing occurs, collagen (a protein of the connective tissue), clotting proteins, and other chemical substances are released to repair the tear. "Other cells are attracted to the repair site, including white blood cells laden with oxidized cholesterol, which is deposited at the site and initiates soft plaque formation," Dr. Cowden says. "Calcium is then attracted to the site and solid plaques, which are more difficult to remove, are formed."

Cholesterol is Not All Bad

Cholesterol, a steroid that has long been cast as the villain in heart disease, is a waxy, oily substance necessary for the maintenance of the body's cells. Cholesterol also plays a role in the manufacture of key male and female sex hormones and steroidal hormones, including pregnenolone, testosterone, estrogen, progesterone, and cortisol. These are critical for the health of the immune system, the mineral-regulating functions of the kidneys, and the smooth running of the hormonal systems in men and women. "The fact is that cholesterol, unless it is oxidized, is a valuable nutrient that the body has to manufacture every day in order to help build the membranes of new cells that we must continually form to replace dead and dying cells," Dr. Gordon says.

 See Natural Hormone Replacement Therapy.

According to Dr. Cowden, the human liver synthesizes about 3,000 mg of new cholesterol in any 24-hour period, a quantity equivalent to the amount contained in ten eggs. "This new cholesterol is used to repair cells," he says. "In fact, in most people, less than 5% of the cholesterol in the bloodstream gets there through diet."

Cholesterol levels in the body are determined by measuring the blood levels of lipoproteins (proteins that carry fats in the bloodstream), including high-density lipoproteins (HDLs) and low-density lipoproteins (LDLs). Testing cholesterol levels allows physicians to determine how effectively the body is metabolizing cholesterol and how much remains in the bloodstream. LDL cholesterol is often referred to as "bad" cholesterol because it appears to deposit fats on arterial walls and causes the most arterial damage.[14] HDLs are often called "good" cholesterol because high levels are associated with a reduced risk of heart disease. HDLs may also contribute to the removal of "bad" cholesterol from the body.[15]

However, LDL cholesterol becomes harmful only after it has been oxidized (the process of a substance combining with oxygen) from exposure to free-radical substances such as unstable oxygen molecules, homocysteine (an amino acid), or chlorine (from drinking chlorinated water), according to Dr. Cowden. Therefore, oxidized cholesterol should be considered the real culprit in atherosclerosis, as it can work to initiate plaque formation on arterial walls, leading to atherosclerosis and ultimately to heart attacks and strokes.[16] This view is echoed by noted health researcher Richard Passwater, Ph.D., who states, "We've been living on cholesterol phobia for years, but nothing matters unless you prevent the oxidation of cholesterol."

In most people, less than 5% of the cholesterol in the bloodstream gets there through diet.

—W. LEE COWDEN, M.D.

Conventional medicine continues to ignore the distinction between oxidized and nonoxidized cholesterol, focusing instead on simply lowering LDLs. In May 2001, for example, new guidelines were issued by the National Cholesterol Education Program stressing the need for "more aggressive treatment" of people with high cholesterol levels. Included in the guidelines was the suggestion that statins, a new class of cholesterol-lowering drugs, be administered to 36 million Americans (a 300% increase from previous criteria). These recommendations are now being followed by the majority of conventional M.D.s, despite the fact that in August 2001, Baycol (one of the most popular statin drugs) was withdrawn from the marketplace by its manufacturer after findings showed the drug was linked to more than 30 deaths due to rhabdomyolysis, a rare muscle-wasting disease. Statins in general also cause inflammation of the liver and can result in serious adverse reactions when used with other drugs.[17]

How Oxidized Cholesterol is Formed

Oxidized cholesterols (known as oxysterols) enter the bloodstream either from processed foods, from the metabolism of ingested animal products, from environmental pollutants such as chlorine, fluoride, and pesticides (like DDT), or from various stressors such as infection, trauma, and emotional stress.[20] According to

---

DRUGS ASSOCIATED WITH A HIGHER INCIDENCE OF HEART DISEASE

According to the *Physicians' Desk Reference*, the following drugs are associated with side effects of congestive heart failure (statistics refer to the percentage of individuals affected).[18]

Emcyt Capsules (3%)

Ethmozine Tablets (1%-5%)

Lupron Depot 3.75 mg Injection (5% or more)

Novantrone for Injection Concentrate (Up to 5%)

Rythmol tablets (0.8%-3.7%)

Tambocor Tablets (Approximately 5%)

Tonocard Tablets (4%)

Zoladex (5%)

In addition, research has shown that Celebrex and Vioxx, two popular "COX-2 inhibitors" used to treat arthritis, can increase the risk of heart attack, stroke, and other cardiovascular conditions by as much as 200%, compared to the older, generic arthritis drug naproxen.[19]

---

researcher Joseph Hattersley, M.A., of Olympia, Washington, many oxysterols reach people through the air-dried powdered milk and eggs used in processed foods, as well as in fast-food products.[21] Lard that is kept hot and used repeatedly to cook French fries and potato chips is loaded with oxysterols, as are gelatin preparations, says Hattersley.

Another source of oxysterols is methionine, an essential amino acid found in red meat, milk, and milk products. Methionine is converted in the body to homocysteine, which is then normally converted to the harmless amino acid cystathionine. But in individuals deficient in the enzyme necessary to convert homocysteine to cystathionine, homocysteine will be abnormally high. This excess homocysteine is capable of generating free radicals that produce oxysterols.

In 1969, heart researcher Kilmer S. McCully, M.D., proposed that homocysteine could, when allowed to accumulate to toxic levels, degenerate arteries and produce heart disease. Put simply, the homocysteine theory suggests that heart disease is attributed to "abnormal processing of protein in the body because of deficiencies of B vitamins in the diet," stated Dr. McCully. In short, "protein intoxication" starts damaging the cells and tissues of arteries, "setting in motion the many processes that lead to loss of elasticity, hardening and calcification, and for-

C-REACTIVE PROTEIN AND INFLAMMATION

Inflammation plays an important role in the development of heart disease. According to Harvard University Physicians' Health Study, a comparison of 543 men who had suffered heart attacks with the same number who had not found that elevated levels of inflammation throughout the body increased heart attack risk by 300% and stroke risk by 200%.[27]

By doing a blood test for C-reactive protein (CRP), a molecule produced by the liver in response to invading bacteria and chemical toxins (both of which can cause inflammation), physicians can determine the degree of inflammation in the body. Although CRP is almost always present in the body, levels that are consistently in the high-normal range or above accurately indicate chronic infection with a strong likelihood of subsequent heart disease, particularly heart attack, stroke, and angina.[28]

Moreover, high CRP levels are a likely indicator of heart disease in patients otherwise considered to be at low risk. In one study, 64 patients who experienced an initial "uncomplicated" heart attack, received hospitalization treatment and were found to be "without residual ischemia or abnormal left ventricular function." The overall average CRP levels for each patient was 2.04 mg/dL, yet during an average follow-up period of 13 months, patients who subsequently died of a second heart attack had an average CRP level of 5.09 mg/dL, despite being considered at low risk for reinfarction. Additionally, among those who experienced new-onset angina or another nonfatal heart attack, average CRP levels were 3.61 mg/dL compared to an average of 1.48 mg/dL among patients with no further heart disease.[29] Subsequent research confirmed that CRP levels serve as "an exquisitely sensitive objective marker of inflammation" relative to the long-term prognosis in heart disease patients, as well as in patients who are apparently healthy.[30]

Overall, according to Garry F. Gordon, M.D., elevated levels of CRP are associated with as much as an eightfold increased risk for heart attack or stroke. "Fortunately, we have many nutritional and other safe, natural strategies that will improve arterial function and lower CRP levels," Dr. Gordon says, adding that, first, patients and physicians alike must come to understand the importance of measuring CRP.

mation of blood clots within arteries." Men with high homocysteine levels are up to three times more susceptible to heart attacks than men with low levels.[22]

Oxysterols can also be generated internally through exposure to environmental pollutants and pesticides. Chemicals that oxidize cholesterol include chlorine and fluoride, both ingested from tap water.[23] Chlorine has been shown to have an adverse effect on the arteries and fluoride lowers thyroid function, which in turn allows levels of cholesterol and homocysteine to rise.[24] Chlorine in drinking water also forms trihalomethanes (carcinogens formed when chlorine interacts with organic chemicals in water), which, according to Hattersley, also create oxysterols.[25]

 See Biological Dentistry, Environmental Medicine.

Other Risk Factors for Heart Disease

Additional risk factors for heart disease include genetic predisposition, hypertension, diabetes and insulin resistance, hypothyroidism, smoking, mercury poisoning, toxic foci (from gum disease, root canal teeth, extraction sites, chronic tonsillar disease), and nutritional deficiencies (especially coenzyme Q10, magnesium, and selenium).

Genetic Predisposition

A variety of genetic factors can play a role in heart disease. According to Robert A. Anderson, M.D., founding President of the American Board of Holistic Medicine, this is particularly true in rare but serious hereditary patterns involving impaired cholesterol metabolism. In such cases, male family members are prone to heart attacks as early as their twenties, according to Dr. Anderson. Hyperhomocysteinemia, a condition characterized by poor metabolism of the amino acids methionine and cysteine, is a more common, yet less severe genetic risk factor, although some researchers believe that it may account for 20% of heart attacks and strokes. Elevated blood fibrinogen levels, another serious risk factor for heart disease, can also be influenced by heredity.[26]

Hypertension

Hypertension (high blood pressure) can significantly increase the risk of heart disease if left untreated, due to the additional damage it can cause to the arteries' delicate inner lining. Because typically the symptoms of hypertension are not obvious, patients who suspect they may be susceptible to the disease are advised to undergo regular medical screenings. According to Dr. Anderson, the current guidelines for hypertension are as follows:

- High normal pressure: 130-139/85-89
- Stage 1 hypertension: 140-159/90-99
- Stage 2 hypertension: 160-179/100-109
- Stage 3 hypertension: 180-209/110-119

"These levels are based on an average of at least three readings with the patient at rest and free of acute stress," Dr. Anderson says.[31]

Approximately 95% of hypertension is labeled by conventional doctors as "essential" or cause unknown. However, a large percentage of these hypertensive patients have nutritional deficiencies, heavy metal toxicity (especially lead, mercury, nickel, and cadmium), toxicity from pesticides and chemical poisons, or marked autonomic nervous system imbalance. When these issues are corrected, the hypertension usually dramatically improves or resolves.

Diabetes and Insulin Resistance

Diabetes mellitus, particularly Type II (adult-onset) diabetes, has been recognized as a risk factor for heart disease since the 1960s. "The presence of diabetes accelerates premature degeneration of arterial walls, inducing circulatory deficiencies," Dr. Anderson says. Type II diabetes can also cause a number of biochemical changes, including increased levels of corticosteroids, increased biochemical stress, and the production of high levels of free radicals, Dr. Anderson adds.[32]

Insulin resistance (sometimes referred to as syndrome X), which can trigger Type II diabetes, may also play a role in heart disease, especially in families with a history of early heart disease. Research shows that the cluster of biochemical imbalances related to insulin resistance tends to be associated with heart attacks or blood-vessel blockage at an early age (55 for men, 65 for women). Researchers also found that such individuals with heart disease had higher insulin levels in addition to higher triglycerides, higher fibrinogen, and lower HDL cholesterol, compared to their siblings without heart disease.[33] Insulin resistance and Type II diabetes both often have deficiency of organic chromium or presence of environmental toxins as contributors to their development.

Hypothyroidism

Hypothyroidism (underactive thyroid) can contribute to heart disease and the propensity for a heart attack, according to Broda O. Barnes, M.D., a Connecticut physician who specialized in identifying and treating the many unsuspected disease conditions associated with low thyroid activity. Dr. Barnes demonstrated the correlation of hypothyroidism and heart disease in a study of 1,569 patients, grouped according to six categories of age or heart status. As a frame of reference, he used the Framingham Heart Study (begun in 1949), which tracked the health status of thousands of men and women over several decades.

Dr. Barnes found that among women 30-59 years old, while there were 7.6 expected coronary cases according to the Framingham results (where no thyroid treatment was given), among his thyroid-treated patients there were no cases. Similarly, for those women with high risk of heart disease, Framingham results predicted 7.3 cases, but among Dr. Barnes's patients there were none. For women over 60, Framingham predicted 7.8 cases; Dr. Barnes's group had none. For men ages 30-59, the ratio was 12.8 (Framingham) to 1 (Barnes); for high-risk males, it was 18.5 to 2; and for men 60 and over, it was 18 to 1. In summary, out of an equivalent patient population, Framingham results expected 72 coronary cases, but among Dr. Barnes's thyroid-treated patients, there were only four cases.[34]

Smoking

Heart disease specifically related to smoking takes the life of an estimated 191,000 Americans every year. This is 44% more people than are killed by smoking-related lung cancer.[35] In other words, smoking can be worse for your heart than for your lungs. Smoking also endangers the heart health of those around you. An estimated 37,000 to 40,000 people are killed annually by cardiovascular disease caused by secondary smoke, according to the American Heart Association.

Recent research shows that habitual exposure to secondary smoke nearly doubles the risk of heart attack and death in nonsmokers. The level of risk (91% higher), determined in a ten-year study of 32,000 women, is far greater than scientists previously thought. The study also found that even occasional exposure produced a 58% higher risk. "The 4,000 chemicals in tobacco smoke just about do everything that we know that is harmful to the heart," Dr. Ichiro Kawachi of the Harvard School of Public Health said. "They will damage the lining of the arteries, increase the stickiness of your blood, and therefore increase the chances that you will develop clotting and a heart attack."[36]

Mercury Poisoning

Mercury toxicity plays an often hidden role in cardiovascular disease. As a result, growing numbers of alternative physicians are beginning to routinely screen for mercury poisoning (and other heavy metal toxicities) as part of a comprehensive treatment program for heart disease. Mercury poisoning is most commonly caused by dental amalgam fillings, but can also be caused by various vaccines, as well as exposure to mercury in the environment and from certain fish.

Russian research, first reported in 1974, found that when electrocardiograms were prepared from rabbits exposed to mercury vapor, abnormal changes were apparent in the readings, most likely due to an inactivation by mercury of certain heart enzymes necessary for heart muscle contraction. Other research has identified mercury as a contributing factor in arterial disease as well as other problems affecting the heart and arteries. Mercury appears to interfere with the normal processing of nutrients that supply arterial smooth muscle, leading to their becoming rigid.

Mercury toxicity may also interfere with the processing of cholesterol from arterial cell walls and in depositing cholesterol in the liver for removal from the body. Further, because it interferes with certain fat-removing enzymes, "mercury may be contributing to the high total cholesterol" characteristic of those people vulnerable to arterial disease. Because this is so, any time there is an unexplained elevation of cholesterol, the physician should check for mercury toxicity.[37]

Dr. Cowden recommends that patients with coronary disease have all the mercury amalgam fillings removed from their teeth. Aside from the documented effect that mercury can leach from dental fillings and be distributed throughout the body, it can also leak into specific nerve ganglia that regulate heart function, as Dr. Cowden has observed in some heart disease patients. "Because the mercury was poisoning those ganglia, or nerve bundles, the patient's heart started having problems, such as impaired blood supply or disturbed heart rhythm," he says. "When we got the mercury out of their teeth, then used chelating agents to get the mercury out of their body tissues, the heart problems cleared up and they were able to discontinue their heart medications for arrhythmia and angina."

Gum Disease and Other Oral Disease

Research conducted over the last few decades has shown that gum disease (periodontitis) can significantly increase the risk of stroke. In one study, 10,000 adults who participated in a health survey from 1970 to 1992 found that those with gum disease were at increased risk for stroke. According to researchers, the bacteria associated with gum disease enter the bloodstream, damaging the lining of blood vessels and stimulating clotting. Based on their findings, the study's lead researcher advised, "People may need to pay more attention to their oral health, as it may influence their systemic health."[39]

Preventing and Reversing Heart Disease

Through the use of a variety of natural therapies, the risk of heart disease may be greatly reduced. These same approaches may also benefit those already suffering from heart disease. They include dietary changes, nutritional supplementation, herbal medicine, chelation therapy, detoxification, oxygen therapy, exercise and stress reduction, traditional Chinese medicine, and Ayurvedic medicine.

During the teenage and young adult years when bad dietary and exercise habits can most easily be altered, much can be done to protect the body against heart disease. Although initial damage done to the arteries can cause the buildup of plaque, it can be corrected and reversed through diet and nutritional supplements.

Diet

Dietary management can be highly effective in reversing heart disease. Dean Ornish, M.D., Assistant Clinical Professor of Medicine at the University of California at San Francisco, used a vegetarian diet, exercise, and stress-reduction techniques to reverse arterial buildup of plaque.[40] His "reversal diet" is almost entirely free of cholesterol, animal fats, and oils. Dr. Ornish found that the condition of those patients who followed the diet improved, while the condition of those who continued eating a diet high in fat got worse.[41]

According to Dr. Cowden, however, the success of Dr. Ornish's diet is due not primarily to low levels of cholesterol and fats, but to both low levels of methionine (an amino acid found in red meat, milk, and milk products, and a precursor to homocysteine, a free radical capable of oxidizing cholesterol) and to a high intake of vegetables and grains. These foods are rich in those vitamins (B$_6$, C, and E, and beta carotene) that act as co-factors for antioxidants and antiatherogenics (substances preventing atherosclerosis).

To reduce the level of oxidized cholesterol in the bloodstream, Dr. Passwater suggests combining a dietary regime (under 30% of daily calories from fat so as not to raise LDL cholesterol levels) with a personalized nutritional supplementation program. "What needs to be done," says Dr. Passwater, "is to first control the LDL cholesterol through diet, then raise the antioxidant level to prevent oxidized cholesterol from doing damage." Clearly, a healthy diet that limits homocysteine-generating food, such as red meat and fried foods containing oxidized or hydrogenated fats, can keep the body's systems operating more smoothly.

Eating onions and apples and drinking green or black tea can also contribute to heart health. These items contain high concentrations of the bioflavonoid quercetin and are inversely associated with coronary heart disease mortality rates. A bioflavonoid is a pigment in plants and fruits that acts as an antioxidant to protect against damage from free radicals. In the body, bioflavonoids enhance the beneficial activities of vitamin C and therefore help keep the immune system strong.[42] A recent study found that men in the highest third of dietary quercetin levels had a 53% lower risk of coronary heart disease than those in the lowest third.[43]

Apples and green or black tea are also rich in catechins, another bioflavonoid, as is chocolate. In a ten-year study recently completed in the Netherlands, it was found that elderly men who consumed the most catechins per day (an average of 72 mg, which can be obtained from four apples, two cups of tea, or a small piece of chocolate) were 51% less likely to die of ischemic heart disease compared to those who consumed the least amount.[44] Ischemic heart disease is caused by clogged arteries, which reduce the amount of blood and oxygen supply to the heart.

Supplementing the diet with essential fatty acids (EFAs) may help to lower the level of homocysteine.[45] Omega-3 EFAs are useful in reducing high LDL levels and may prevent heart attacks by eliminating clotting and arterial damage. Omega-6 EFAs have been shown to decrease the aggregation or stickiness of platelets, allowing them to pass through the arteries without danger of clotting.[46] Dr. Cowden notes that the best natural sources of omega-3s are flaxseed oil and eicosapentaenoic acid (EPA) from ocean algae or from cold saltwater fish, such as Scandinavian salmon, orange roughy, and halibut. Omega-6s are most abundantly found in borage oil, black currant oil, and evening prim-

rose oil. Grapeseed oil is 76% linoleic acid (an omega-6 oil) and has a high concentration of vitamin E, making it a significant source for this nutrient. These oils should not be rancid and should be cold-pressed so that no fatty acids are lost. Dr. Cowden recommends taking at least equal amounts of omega-3s (especially EPA) whenever taking omega-6s.

While EFAs are beneficial to heart health, elevated levels of "free" fatty acids associated with high dietary intake of saturated fats and trans fats (from hydrogenated oils) can pose serious cardiovascular risks. In a study that tracked the 22-year medical histories of 5,200 healthy men between the ages of 42 and 53, researchers found that those men with elevated blood levels of "free" fatty acids were up to 70% more likely to experience sudden cardiac death than men with lower levels.[47] Free fatty acids enter the bloodstream primarily from fat stored in body tissue.

Both saturated and trans fats are known to increase the risk of heart disease, due to their ability to raise LDL levels. New research indicates that trans fats pose the greater danger. In one study, 29 healthy, nonsmoking adults followed two diets, each for a period of four weeks. The first diet contained 9.2% of total calories from trans fats, while the second contained the same amount of calories from saturated fats. Researchers monitored each participant's blood vessel function by measuring dilation in response to blood flow. It was found that the trans-fat diet reduced blood vessel function by 29% and also reduced healthy HDL levels by 20%, compared to the saturated-fat diet.[48] The primary food sources of trans fats are ready-made baked goods, margarine, vegetable shortening, and fried fast foods.

According to Dr. Cowden, the following dietary guidelines are helpful in preventing heart disease:

- Eat minimally processed foods (avoid additives and preservatives or foods containing powdered eggs or powdered milk).

- Buy organic foods (free of pesticides, herbicides, steroids, and antibiotics) whenever possible, especially when buying meats and dairy products.

- Avoid irradiated foods whenever possible.

- Increase fiber from green leafy vegetables, fresh raw fruits, bran, whole grains, and psyllium.

- Reduce fat intake, especially fried foods, animal fats, and partially hydrogenated oils. Increase complex carbohydrates such as whole grains, beans, seeds, and potatoes.

- Use monounsaturated oils (such as cold-pressed olive oil), omega-3 oils (flaxseed oil or oils from deep ocean fish), and omega-6 oils (borage, black currant oil, or evening primrose oil).

- Reduce meat, sugar, tobacco, and alcohol consumption, which are all sources of free radicals.

Dr. Cowden puts many of his heart patients through a detoxification regimen consisting of a vegetarian diet, vegetable juices mixed with garlic and (in some cases) cayenne, as well as low-temperature saunas. This program helps to cleanse the body of toxins that may be contributing to free-radical damage to the artery walls and the buildup of arterial plaque. He also often uses homeopathic remedies to aid in detoxification.

Nutritional Supplements

Because atherosclerosis and heart disease take many years to develop, a daily regimen of supplements may be helpful as prevention. The amount of supplements needed varies from one individual to another depending on body weight and absorption levels, and it is best to consult with a nutritionally skilled physician or naturopathic physician before embarking on a routine of supplements.

Matthias Rath, M.D., author of *Eradicating Heart Disease,* and former Director of the Linus Pauling Institute of Science and Medicine, in Palo Alto, California, is a leading proponent of nutritional supplements to both prevent and reverse heart disease. "I firmly believe that America's number one killer can be prevented by an optimum intake of essential nutrients," Dr. Rath declares. One of the many successful outcomes Dr. Rath has achieved using his nutritional protocol involved a man in his fifties, who came to him after experiencing sudden cardiac failure, a severe heart muscle weakness that results in decreased pumping function and enlargement of the heart chambers. The man was no longer able to work full-time and had to give up most physical activities. Sometimes he felt so weak he had to hold an object with both hands to keep from dropping it, and he was unable to climb stairs. Dr. Rath put him on a supplement program for heart health. "Soon, he could again fulfill his professional obligations on a regular basis and was able to undertake daily bicycle rides," Dr. Rath says. After two months on the supplement program, his cardiologist found that his heart enlargement had decreased. One month later, he went on an overseas business trip and reported that physical limitations were no longer interfering with his work.

The following nutrients are among those used by Dr. Rath and other alternative physicians to promote heart health:

BETA CAROTENE

Research done at Johns Hopkins University, in Baltimore, Maryland, found that there were approximately 50% fewer heart disease cases among those study participants with the highest levels of beta carotene (a vitamin A precursor) compared to the group with the lowest levels.[49] Dr. Cowden recommends supplementing with mixed carotenoids rather than beta carotene alone.

NIACIN

Niacin (vitamin B3) helps to lower cholesterol levels and lessen the risk of heart disease.[50] It has also been shown to increase the longevity of patients who have suffered one heart attack. In one study, over 8,000 middle-aged men who had experienced one heart attack were given supplements of niacin, estrogen, thyroid hormone, or a placebo. Results showed that only niacin was beneficial in lowering the death rate and increasing longevity.[51] Abram Hoffer, M.D., Ph.D., of Victoria, British Columbia, Canada, saw a patient in 1992 who was a pilot and had not been able to fly since 1985 because of heart problems. Dr. Hoffer put him on niacin (3 g daily) and, after 18 months, he was given a clean bill of health and was able to fly again. Another of Dr. Hoffer's patients came to him 20 years ago with angina pectoris. This patient was also treated with niacin and, according to Dr. Hoffer, has had no signs of angina since.

VITAMIN B6

Researchers have found vitamin B6 (pyridoxine) to be a safe and inexpensive supplement that may be helpful in preventing heart attacks and strokes.[52] Vitamin B6 is needed for the conversion of homocysteine to the harmless chemical cystathionine, thus preventing the homocysteine-induced oxidation of cholesterol.[53] It has also been suggested that vitamin B6 inhibits the platelet aggregation which occurs in atherosclerosis.[54] The typical American diet, however, leaves many people significantly deficient in this vital nutrient.

In 1949, Moses M. Suzman, M.D., a South African neurologist and internist, gathered a group of pre-cardiac patients who showed signs of arterial damage and had them take 100 mg of vitamin B6 per day, while patients who had already had heart attacks or angina were given 200 mg per day (half from a B-complex including choline). In addition, the patients with the most serious conditions were given folic acid (5 mg), vitamin E (100-600 IU), magnesium, and zinc.[55] Over the next 23 years, Dr. Suzman's patients recovered rapidly, as their angina and electrocardiographic irregularities diminished or disappeared. Those who dropped out of the vitamin and diet regimen, however, soon found their cardiac problems returning.[56]

Interest in vitamin B6 deficiency and its relationship to heart disease began when Dr. McCully found that heart patients had nearly 80% less of the vitamin than healthy individuals. From this, he postulated that B6 may help the body resist the arterial damage that precipitates heart disease. He also found that patients who had already suffered a heart attack or angina and were then given 200 mg of B6 daily (half in a B-complex including choline)—combined with a low-fat, mostly vegetarian diet—recovered rapidly.[57]

VITAMIN B12

A deficiency of vitamin B12 is associated with elevated homocysteine levels. When vitamin B12 is supplemented, homocysteine levels decrease.[58] This effect can be increased by also supplementing with choline, folic acid, riboflavin, and B6.[59]

FOLIC ACID

Folic acid is essential for the proper metabolism of homocysteine.[60] Recent studies have shown that vitamins B6, B12, and folic acid can dramatically lower homocysteine, one of the major contributing factors in heart disease.[61]

VITAMIN E

Vitamin E is a fat-soluble antioxidant that can help prevent abnormal blood clot formation. Dr. Passwater believes that any nutrient that prevents the oxidation of cholesterol—vitamin E, beta carotene, and coenzyme Q10—offers a protective factor. Supplementation of vitamin E inhibits platelet aggregation and helps repair the lining cells of blood vessels.[62] Two studies published in the *New England Journal of Medicine* suggest that vitamin E can contribute greatly to the prevention of heart disease in both men and women.[63] The first study, done at Harvard Medical School, involved a group of 87,245 female nurses—it was found that those who took 100 IU of vitamin E daily for more than two years had a 46% lower risk of heart disease.[64] The second study, also at Harvard, involved 39,910 male health professionals who reduced their risk of heart disease by 37% after daily supplementation with 100 IU of vitamin E.[65] In another study funded by the World Health Organization, it was shown that, among 16 European populations, those with low blood levels of vitamin E were at greater risk for heart disease than those with high blood pressure and high cholesterol levels.[66]

 High dosages of vitamin E are not recommended for people with hypertension, rheumatic heart disease, or ischemic heart disease except under close medical supervision. However, in hypertensive or ischemic heart disease patients, if the dose of vitamin E is raised gradually, the blood pressure will usually not rise significantly and there will not be a greater workload placed on the heart, according to W. Lee Cowden, M.D.

VITAMIN C

The use of vitamin C (ascorbic acid) is believed to help prevent the formation of oxysterols.[67] By combining the amino acid lysine with vitamin C, it may be possible to dissolve clots in the bloodstream.[68] In an animal study, it was found that the equivalent of the U.S. Recommended Dietary Allowance (RDA) of vitamin C offered virtually no protection against arterial damage. When the amount of vitamin C was increased to a dose equivalent to 2,800 mg for a 154-pound person, the researchers were able to reverse the damage.[69] Studies also reveal that vitamin C is required for collagen synthesis and is therefore necessary to maintain the integrity of the walls of arteries.[70] Nobel laureate Linus Pauling, Ph.D., believed that a deficiency of vitamin C may precipitate arteriosclerosis because it causes defects in the arterial walls due to reduced collagen synthesis.[71] Dr. Pauling and Matthias Rath, M.D., have shown that vitamin C supplementation can reverse arteriosclerosis.[72]

"Vitamin C reverses oxidation and prevents free-radical formation," according to Dr. Cowden. "In a diet that involves reducing fats, vitamin C is an integral part of helping the body to repair itself." In patients with existing cardiovascular disease, Dr. Cowden recommends that vitamin C be taken to bowel tolerance (the maximum amount a person can take before causing loose stools or diarrhea). He suggests a minimum of 3-4 doses daily, increasing the amount until reaching bowel tolerance. Stay on bowel tolerance until cardiovascular disease is resolved and then go on a maintenance dose of at least 3,000 mg daily. For those who are well but want to prevent cardiovascular disease, 3,000-10,000 mg daily is sufficient. Higher doses of vitamin C should be taken with adequate amounts of water, magnesium, and vitamin B6, Dr. Cowden adds.

 According to W. Lee Cowden, M.D., high amounts of the ascorbic acid form of vitamin C taken over a prolonged period of time can leach calcium and other minerals out of the teeth, bones, and other tissues. He recommends that high amounts of ascorbic acid be balanced by mineral ascorbates containing magnesium, potassium, zinc, and manganese.

COENZYME Q10

Over 40 years ago, Karl Folkers, Ph.D., a biomedical scientist at the University of Texas, in Austin, discovered that coenzyme Q10 helps to strengthen the heart muscles and energize the cardiovascular system in many heart patients. Studies reveal that coQ10 may protect against atherosclerosis and it has been shown to have antioxidant properties that may protect against the formation of oxysterols.[73] Dr. Gordon reports success in helping infants avoid risky surgery using supplements of coQ10, amino acids, and herbs. "In one case," he relates, "I went to see a newborn diagnosed with myocardiopathy, a disease of the heart muscle. With the family's permission, I treated the baby with coenzyme Q10, carnitine [an amino acid], magnesium, vitamin C, a multivitamin/mineral formula, liquid garlic, and hawthorn berry extract. The baby recovered without the heart transplant surgery that was being recommended by the university medical center."

PROANTHOCYANIDIN (PCA)

Pycnogenol, an antioxidant derived from maritime pine bark or a comparable PCA extract from grape seeds, enhances heart health by protecting LDL cholesterol from oxidation and by protecting the integrity of the artery lining. In addition, according to Dr. Passwater, "[PCA] helps keep the blood platelets from becoming stickier and developing a tendency to unnecessarily clump together. This reduces the undesirable formation of the blood clots that cause coronary thrombosis resulting in myocardial infarction."[74] PCA has also been shown to reduce histamine levels, thereby minimizing damage to arterial linings caused by invading mutagens and free-radical scavengers.[75]

SELENIUM

A positive relationship has been found between low blood selenium levels and cardiovascular disease, possibly related to selenium's antioxidant effects.[76] Selenium supplementation also reduces platelet aggregation[77] and selenium is a co-factor for glutathione peroxidase, an important antioxidant enzyme.

 Research is needed into the role of nutritional supplements in preventing and reversing heart disease.

MAGNESIUM

It has been found that individuals who die suddenly of heart attacks have far lower levels of magnesium and potassium than control groups.[78] Magnesium helps to dilate arteries and ease the heart's pumping of blood, thus preventing arrhythmias (irregular heartbeats). Magnesium may also prevent calcification of the blood vessels, lower total cholesterol, raise HDL cholesterol, and inhibit platelet aggregation.[79] But simply taking magnesium supplements may not be sufficient. Dr. Cowden explains: "Most doctors don't use the best form for optimum absorption. It's more effective to use magnesium malate, glycinate, taurate, or aspartate, or even herbal magnesium such as red raspberry, but some patients need intravenous or intramuscular magnesium to quickly raise their magnesium to ideal levels." Magnesium oxide has very poor absorption and therefore should probably not be used.

Alan R. Gaby, M.D., former President of the American Holistic Medical Association, has found that cases of congestive heart failure respond well to an intravenous injection of a "cocktail" composed of magnesium chloride hexahydrate, hydroxocobalamin, pyridoxine hydrochloride, dexpanthenol, B-complex vitamins, and vitamin C. (This is a modification of the nutrient cocktail popularized by John Meyers, M.D.)

CALCIUM

Calcium supplementation may decrease total cholesterol and inhibit platelet aggregation.[80] Dr. Cowden finds herbal forms of calcium to be more effective for heart disease patients.

CHROMIUM

Chromium supplementation has been shown to lower total cholesterol and triglycerides and raise HDL cholesterol.[81] It is even more effective in lowering cholesterol when combined with niacin (vitamin B₃).[82] A chromium deficiency has been linked to coronary heart disease by several studies.[83]

POTASSIUM

Hypertension (high blood pressure) is often present in heart disease. It has been found that supplements of potassium can help reduce a patient's reliance on blood pressure medication or diuretic drugs.[84]

AMINO ACIDS

The amino acid L-arginine, when given intravenously (20 g over a one-hour period), can produce significant increases in stroke volume and cardiac output in patients with congestive heart failure. Arginine therapy can also lower arterial blood pressure.[85] Supplementation with L-carnitine immediately after a heart attack can help damaged heart muscle expand again. In one study, L-carnitine, given orally (2 g daily for 28 days), improved the condition of 51 patients who had undergone heart attacks.[86] Specifically, the amount of damaged heart muscle after 28 days was significantly less, the incidence of angina and arrhythmia was reduced by 50%, and the number of car-

DANGERS OF CONVENTIONAL CARDIOVASCULAR TREATMENT

Cholesterol-Lowering Drugs: Since many people with heart disease also have elevated blood cholesterol levels, physicians have traditionally prescribed cholesterol-lowering drugs as part of their treatment program, even though new research shows that it is not the levels of cholesterol but the levels of oxidized cholesterol that represent high risk for heart disease. However, recent research has called into question the safety and efficacy of cholesterol-lowering drugs. It has been found, for instance, that the drugs used to lower LDL (low-density lipoprotein) cholesterol actually raise it in people who already have the highest levels.[87] In addition, these medications can lead to serious complications. A study conducted in Finland reported that deaths from heart attacks and strokes were 46% higher in those taking cholesterol-lowering drugs.[88] Newer drugs being touted as safer also have harmful side effects. Studies have shown that lovastatin lowers the blood levels of coenzyme Q10, an antioxidant that helps the body resist heart damage.[89]

Aspirin and NSAIDs: Although long-term use of anti-inflammatory drugs help prevent heart attack and strokes, and taking aspirin when one is having a heart attack can increase survival, there is a serious downside to taking aspirin and/or other nonsteroidal, anti-inflammatory drugs (NSAIDs) daily. "These can cause internal bleeding, plus liver and kidney damage, and are linked to 20,000 deaths and over 125,000 hospitalizations annually," Dr. Gordon says. "Fortunately, we do not have to rely on such drugs, nor wait for new drugs to be developed, for there are a number of safe, natural substances that can be used instead, which are documented to have the same health benefits without the side effects."

Angioplasty and Bypass Surgery: In 1992, Nortin Hadler, M.D., Professor of Medicine at the University of North Carolina School of Medicine, wrote that none of the 250,000 balloon angioplasties performed the previous year could be justified and that only 3% to 5% of the 300,000 coronary bypass surgeries done the same year were actually required.[90] His views echoed those made more than a decade earlier at a symposium of the American Heart Association by Henry McIntosh, M.D., who stated that bypass surgery should be limited to patients with crippling angina who do not respond to more conservative treatment.[91]

The inability of most angioplasty and bypass surgery procedures to extend life following a heart attack has also been demonstrated by a 1997 report in the *New England Journal of Medicine*, which found that the death rate of U.S. and Canadian heart attack patients after one year was 34%. Among the U.S. patients, 12% had received angioplasty and 11% had bypass surgery, compared to the Canadian patients, with only 1.5% receiving angioplasty and only 1.4% had bypass surgery. U.S. patients are also five times more likely (34.9% to 6.7%) to have coronary angiography (catheterization of heart arteries) than Canadians, with one-year survival rates between patients in both countries basically remaining equal.[92]

More recent research has found that five years after heart bypass surgery, 42% of patients "show a significant decline on tests of mental ability, probably from brain damage caused by the surgery." The researchers of the study noted that "it highlights an ugly truth that surgeons know but are not eager to discuss with patients."[93] In addition, other research indicates that having bypass surgery soon after a heart attack or angina may actually increase the risk of stroke within months after the procedure is performed.[94]

Heart Catheterization: According to a 1996 study, the conventional diagnostic medical procedure called "right heart catheterization" can significantly increase a patient's risk of death. The test involves inserting a catheter (tube) through the neck to measure blood pressure inside the heart, yet it has never undergone strict scientific trials and should therefore be considered experimental. Nonetheless, it is estimated that over 500,000 patients in the U.S. receive heart catheterization each year.[95] In addition, according to Julian Whitaker, M.D., author of *Reversing Heart Disease*, catheterization "leads to a dramatic increase in the use of bypass surgery and angioplasty because physicians then try to open up observed blockages."[96] Yet, research shows that when catheterization is followed by either of these procedures, the death rate of heart attack survivors increases by 36%.[97]

FISH OIL FOR PREVENTING HEART ATTACKS

In the early 1980s, physicians began prescribing aspirin as a preventative to those patients at risk for heart attacks and strokes. Many cited aspirin's anticoagulant effects, noting that aspirin prevents the blood from clotting in plaque-occluded arteries. Cardiologist W. Lee Cowden, M.D., suggests that this approach may be misguided, since aspirin has been known to cause gastrointestinal bleeding and even perforated ulcers in some cases. Eicosapentaenoic acid (EPA) from fish oils has no such risks and has also been shown to significantly reduce death from coronary heart disease.[102] In addition, EPA (especially when taken in conjunction with adequate antioxidant nutrients like vitamins E and C and beta carotene) works on reducing the stickiness of clotting cells in the blood by affecting prostaglandin ratios (like aspirin does). However, EPA also favorably alters blood lipid ratios and helps to lower blood pressure (which aspirin does not).[103]

diac events of any kind for those on L-carnitine was 15.6% compared to 26% for those taking a placebo.

 See Diet, Herbal Medicine, Nutritional Medicine, Orthomolecular Medicine.

Herbal Medicine

According to David L. Hoffman, B.Sc., M.N.I.M.H., of Sebastopol, California, past President of the American Herbalists Guild, "Some herbs have a potent and direct impact on the heart itself, such as *Digitalis purpurea* (foxglove), and form the basis of drug therapy for heart failure." One of the most promising herbal remedies for the treatment of heart disease is the extract from the hawthorn berry, a commonly found shrub. Hawthorn berry has been found to help improve the circulation of blood to the heart by dilating the blood vessels and relieving spasms of the arterial walls.[98] According to Dr. Gordon, "Hawthorn berry may render unnecessary medications that decrease the rate and force of heart contraction in the treatment of heart disease, as it performs a similar function to these drugs."

Garlic and ginger have many properties that make them valuable in treating heart disease. Garlic contains sulfur compounds, which work as antioxidants and also help dissolve clots.[99] Ginger has been shown to lower cholesterol levels and make the blood platelets less sticky.[100] Evidence is mounting that an extract from olive leaves has extensive therapeutic benefits, including lowering blood pressure and working against free-radical activity. The active component of the olive leaf is oleuropein (the bitter element removed from olives when they are processed). The leaf also contains natural vitamin C helpers or bioflavonoids, such as rutin, luteolin, and hesperidin, which are needed for maintenance of the capillary walls.[101]

While it is best to consult a skilled herbalist before taking herbs, the following is an example of a cardiac tonic that Hoffman recommends: an equal combination of the tinctures of hawthorn berries, *Ginkgo biloba*, and linden flowers (½ teaspoon three times a day). He also suggests the addition of tincture of motherwort to prevent palpitations and garlic to help manage cholesterol.

Chelation Therapy

There is mounting evidence that chelation therapy offers an alternative to the hundreds of thousands of bypass surgeries and angioplasties performed each year. Chelation therapy is traditionally used to treat poisoning from toxic metals by removing them from the body with a chemical agent. Norman Clarke, Sr., M.D., Director of Research at Providence Hospital, in Detroit, Michigan, hypothesized that since chelation with EDTA (ethylenediaminetetraacetic acid) removed calcium from pipes and boilers, it may be useful to remove calcium plaque in patients with arteriosclerosis. His experiments confirmed his theory, and angina patients treated by Dr. Clarke reported dramatic relief from chest pain.[104]

EDTA chelation therapy has since proven to be safe and effective in the treatment and prevention of ailments linked to atherosclerosis, such as heart attacks, stroke, peripheral vascular disease (leading to pain in the legs and ultimately gangrene), as well as arterial blockages. According to current drug safety standards, aspirin is nearly 3½ times more toxic than EDTA.[105] During a chelation therapy session, EDTA is given intravenously to remove plaque and calcium deposits from the arterial walls and then the unwanted material is excreted through the urine. The treatment is usually administered several times per week over a course of two or three months in order to restore complete circulation.

In a 1988 study of 2,870 cases, Efrain Olszewer, M.D., and James Carter, M.D., head of nutrition at the Department of Applied Health Science, School of Public Health and Tropical Medicine, at Tulane University, documented that EDTA chelation therapy brought about significant improvement in 93.9% of patients suffering from coronary artery blockage.[106] Elmer Cranton, M.D., of Troutdale, Virginia, estimates chelation therapy can help avoid bypass surgery in 85% of cases. He points out that during the time that chelation therapy has been

ALTERNATIVE TREATMENTS FOR STROKE

In the same manner that coronary arteries can become blocked by plaque, causing a heart attack, so can arteries supplying the brain become blocked, leading to a stroke. The effects when the oxygen supply to a portion of the brain is blocked include loss of speech, movement, or eyesight. Until now, most stroke victims had little choice but to spend months working with physical therapists, sometimes recovering only minimal function. Researchers, particularly in Germany, have recognized that the loss of functioning of an arm or leg after a stroke was similar to symptoms of the "bends," a sometimes fatal affliction deep-sea divers can get from ascending too quickly. Restoring the balance of nitrogen and oxygen in the blood cured divers of the bends, and physicians suspected that victims of stroke might be helped in a similar manner.

A hyperbaric oxygen chamber, which alters the atmospheric pressure, forces oxygen into the tissues so that it reaches the cells in its most easily utilized state. According to David Hughes, Ph.D., of the Hyperbaric Oxygen Institute, in San Bernardino, California, the treatment has been used quite successfully in Germany. Hyperbaric oxygen therapy increases oxygen to the brain and the increased atmospheric pressure may have therapeutic benefits for swollen tissues.[107] An infusion of highly diluted hydrogen peroxide into the bloodstream may have the same effect, and hydrogen peroxide has been shown to dissolve lipids from the arterial walls.[108]

W. Lee Cowden, M.D., has noticed that if patients can be treated within the first 12 hours after a stroke with a combination of high antioxidant intake, essential fatty acids, and either hyperbaric oxygen therapy or "body-bag" ozone therapy, then a dramatic regression of stroke symptoms can occur. Patients regain sensation, strength, and mental clarity, as well as motor and sensory skills and orientation. In his treatment, Dr. Cowden uses the antioxidants vitamin E, beta carotene, ascorbyl palmitate (a form of vitamin C), and proanthocyanidins (an antioxidant found in maritime pine bark or grape seeds), as well as the essential fatty acids eicosapentaenoic acid (EPA) and docosahexaenoic acid (DHA) to help prevent damage to brain cells.

Harvey Bigelsen, M.D., Medical Director of the Center for Progressive Medicine, in Scottsdale, Arizona, uses biological therapies developed by the late German bacteriologist Gunther Enderlein, M.D., Ph.D., to help alleviate the symptoms of stroke. According to Dr. Bigelsen, Dr. Enderlein theorized that disease must be treated at the cellular level and formulated his remedies accordingly. The remedies are extracts of plants and fungi that, once injected into the patient, work according to the principles of homeopathy. Dr. Enderlein maintained that bacteria can take on both harmless and harmful forms; by injecting harmless forms of bacteria, those harmful entities in the body will revert to their harmless state. Dr. Bigelsen uses these remedies intravenously to bring strokes-in-progress to a halt.[109] One such patient was treated intravenously and within five minutes the crisis of the stroke was broken and the symptoms alleviated. The patient was then treated with cell therapy to stimulate the brain tissue and chelation therapy to help clear out the arteries. He was able to walk out of the hospital with no residual disability and resumed work a few days later.

Margaret A. Naeser, Ph.D., Associate Research Professor of Neurology at Boston University School of Medicine, has conducted research on the use of low-energy lasers (20 milliwatt red to infrared laser light) in the treatment of paralysis in stroke. Five of her six subjects showed improvement and patients with mild-to-moderate paralysis responded better than those with severe paralysis, according to Dr. Naeser. The improvements were observed even when treatments were begun three or four years after the stroke.

David A. Steenblock, M.S., D.O., of Mission Viejo, California, a specialist in alternative treatments (especially hyperbaric oxygen) for stroke, offers the following recommendations for stroke prevention:

- Avoid tobacco smoke and alcohol.
- Don't use amphetamines, cocaine, or other illicit drugs as these can be harmful to the heart.
- After age 50, have your carotid arteries checked every five years for atherosclerosis.
- Monitor your blood pressure.
- Exercise daily.
- Eat fresh, nonprocessed vegetables. Eat a high-fiber diet. Avoid fats, cholesterol, and sugar and keep your weight down to help prevent diabetes, which affects the heart.
- Take magnesium, calcium, vitamins E and C, and bioflavonoids.
- If you are a woman over 35, avoid birth control pills.
- Quickly correct any medical problems that develop.

administered according to established protocol, not one serious side effect has been reported.

Dr. Gordon points out that EDTA chelation can be beneficial for bypass candidates even when the therapy appears unsuccessful in reducing the amount of calcification in coronary arteries. The reason for this, according to Dr. Gordon, has to do with the fact that 85% of heart attacks, strokes, and other types of cardiovascular disease are caused by the rupture of vulnerable, non-calcified arterial plaque and subsequent clot formation.

"It is now widely accepted that the underlying cause of death in heart attacks and strokes is from a blood clot related to this vulnerable, soft or non-calcified, plaque due to an active infection in the arterial wall," Dr. Gordon explains. "Unfortunately, most patients are unaware of this information about vulnerable plaque or that it is readily detected by currently available vascular tests. As a result, patients who choose chelation therapy instead of bypass are usually disappointed should they learn they still have calcified coronary vessels and may then mistakenly opt for surgery, despite the fact that their so-called 'unsuccessful' chelation treatments have enabled them to sustain a far higher level of physical activity than before treatment." Dr. Gordon adds that improved oxygenation of heart tissues usually results from intravenous chelation. "This, in and of itself, is a reasonable goal for patients with cardiovascular conditions," he says.

Because new evidence suggests that most heart attacks and strokes are due to blood clots caused by vulnerable plaque, Dr. Gordon believes that a "carefully and rationally developed" oral chelation formula can be as beneficial as intravenous chelation in helping to prevent such conditions, but in a different manner and without producing the longevity benefits routinely observed with I.V. EDTA. "There appears to be benefits from both therapies," Dr. Gordon says, "but intravenous administration of EDTA cannot permanently reduce inflammation or excessive clotting tendencies. For this reason, most patients believe their I.V. chelation treatments are reversing their arteriosclerosis, yet all too often we are learning that is not the case."

To ensure that his heart patients receive the most comprehensive care, Dr. Gordon developed and employs his own oral chelation protocol. "I have been able to document significant improvements of blood flow to the legs, head, and heart of patients experiencing problems of clot, heart spasm, and arrhythmia with the use of oral chelation, so that fewer than 5% have had to have heart surgery," Dr. Gordon reports. One example of such a patient was a man in his mid-fifties, who came to Dr. Gordon after a series of monthly small, recurring strokes. "An arteriogram revealed that he had bilateral, high-grade obstructions of both carotid arteries," Dr. Gordon

says. "After being told that the surgery being recommended for his condition in itself involved a high risk of stroke, he came to me. Since being placed on oral chelation therapy six years ago, he has had no further incidents of stroke."

Enzyme Therapy

In Germany, the Mucos company has developed an all-natural combination enzyme-bioflavonoid product called Wobenzym-N that is widely available in most countries, including the U.S. Unlike most enzyme products on the market, this enzyme is specially designed not to digest food but to be used in the bloodstream to deal with many factors that can lead to cardiovascular conditions and other serious diseases, according to Dr. Gordon, including elevated fibrinogen and C-reactive protein. "This product provides all the benefits of anti-inflammatory medication without the high incidence of gastrointestinal bleeding and other side effects associated with long-term use of aspirin and NSAID," Dr. Gordon says.

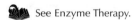 See Enzyme Therapy.

Oxygen Therapy

Studies at Baylor University about 30 years ago found that an intravascular drip of hydrogen peroxide into leg arteries of atherosclerotic patients cleared arterial plaque. In cardiopulmonary resuscitations, hydrogen peroxide infusions often stopped ventricular fibrillation (rapid, ineffective contractions by the ventricles of the heart), the heart's response to insufficient oxygen.[110] The late Charles Farr, M.D., Ph.D., of Oklahoma City, Oklahoma, reported success alternating treatments of I.V. diluted hydrogen peroxide and chelation therapy to bring patients out of high-output heart failure (where the heart fails even though it is pumping a high amount of blood). Ozone therapy can also be used to treat arterial circulatory disturbances and to dissolve atherosclerotic plaque. Typically, injection of ozone into an artery is the method employed for this type of treatment.

Hyperbaric oxygen therapy (HBOT) is a form of oxygen therapy that is particularly effective as a treatment for stroke. "Every emergency room in the United States should have a hyperbaric oxygen chamber and every physician should be trained in its use," says David A. Steenblock, M.S., D.O., of Mission Viejo, California, a leading practitioner of HBOT for stroke. "If you can get more oxygen to the brain within the first 24 hours of having a stroke, you can often salvage a great deal of brain tissue, eliminating 70% to 80% of the damage. Treating the patient by getting more oxygen to the brain during the first three weeks after the stroke makes it still possible to minimize the damage." In fact, Dr. Steenblock has produced unexpected positive outcomes when treating people as long as 15 years after their stroke. The goal is to get as much oxygen into the brain as possible. This helps to revive oxygen-starved brain tissue that was damaged but not entirely destroyed when the stroke occurred. Since 1971, over 1,000 cases demonstrating a 40% to 100% rate of improvement for stroke victims receiving HBOT have been reported in scientific journals.

 See Biofeedback Training and Neurotherapy, Chelation Therapy, Guided Imagery, Oxygen Therapies, Yoga.

Stress Reduction and Exercise

Stress-reduction techniques and exercise have been shown to be highly effective in reversing heart disease. In a study conducted by Dr. Ornish, an experimental group following a routine that combined a low-fat vegetarian diet, stress management, the elimination of smoking, and moderate exercise had a 91% decrease in the frequency of angina, as opposed to a control group that experienced a 165% increase in angina.[111]

An international study, conducted in Canada, the U.S., and Israel, evaluated the effectiveness of an intervention aimed strictly at hostility reduction in patients with coronary artery disease. The study found the heart patients who released at least some of their hostility reduced their blood pressure as well. Participants learned listening skills to help reduce antagonism and techniques to avoid cynicism and anger. Patients who attended the full, eight-session course were observed to be less hostile and healthier than other patients. Patients recovering from a heart attack took a six-hour program consisting of stress management training with mind/body techniques and emotional support, resulting in a 50% reduction in subsequent rates of cardiac death.[112]

Stress reduction can also play an important role in preventing heart disease, in light of research showing that emotions such as anger, depression, and hopelessness can increase its likelihood of developing. People with an angry temperament, who are prone to lose their temper at the slightest provocation, are found to have nearly twice the risk of developing heart disease compared to people who get angry only when they have good cause, such as being unfairly treated or criticized. This is true even of people with angry temperaments who have normal blood pressure levels.[113]

People who are angry and hostile also tend to have higher levels of homocysteine, which increases heart disease risk. In addition, homocysteine levels are higher in men who suppress feelings of anger or hostility compared to angry or hostile men who express such emotions.[114] Patterns of poorly managed feelings of anger can begin to strain the heart as early as age 8, according to a

---

SUCCESS STORY: ELIMINATING THE NEED FOR A HEART TRANSPLANT

While conventional medicine often relies on the high-risk procedure of heart transplant in treating heart disease, this radical method can often be avoided. W. Lee Cowden, M.D., of Fort Worth, Texas, reports the case of a 45-year-old physician who was suffering from pneumonia and an enlarged heart. When given an ejection fraction test (measuring the percentage of the blood contained in the ventricle that is ejected on each heartbeat), his heart was only ejecting 16% of its contents (60% is normal), and his doctor told him his only hope was to receive a heart transplant. When he came into Dr. Cowden's office, he could barely walk across the room without becoming out of breath.

Dr. Cowden immediately put him on a detoxification program that included a vegetarian diet and a three-day vegetable juice fast with garlic. He also had him follow a nutritional supplementation regimen including coenzyme Q10, vitamin C, magnesium, vitamin B complex, trace minerals, omega-3 fatty acids, lauric acid (an essential fatty acid), and carnitine, as well as the antiviral herbs St. John's wort, *Pfaffia paniculata*, and *Lomatium dissectum*. Within three months, Dr. Cowden reports, the patient could jog ten miles a day, and upon repeating the ejection fraction test, his score was up to 30%. Now he works 60 hours a week and continues to jog ten miles daily.

1999 study of 123 healthy children, 8-10 years old, and 78 teenagers, 15-17 years old. The study found that participants in both groups who had two or more cardiac risk factors also rated "significantly higher in hostility" than their peers who had less cardiac risk.[115] Feelings of depression and hopelessness can also increase heart disease risk, especially among men and the elderly.[116]

Dr. Cowden includes stress-reduction exercises as part of his treatment. He believes that deep breathing and imaging techniques aimed at reducing stress should be conducted frequently throughout the day to reduce the output of stress hormones and lower the level of platelet aggregation. He encourages patients to do these techniques before meals and at bedtime, as they not only reduce stress but also can improve digestion. "The nutrients we are giving have to be absorbed out of the gastrointestinal tract. If the gut is in a stressed state, it will

STOPPING A HEART ATTACK WITH YOUR HANDS

According to Glenn King, Director of the King Institute for Better Health, in Dallas, Texas, there are particular locations on your body called "Energy Sphere Points," which, when you press gently on them with your fingers, can stop a heart attack or other serious conditions. King is the foremost U.S. practitioner of a little-known Asian health practice called *Ki-Iki-Jutsu*, which means "breath of life." He describes it as "a finger-delivered form of therapy that allows the body, by its own tremendous power, to heal itself by unconstricting any stagnation or blockage of the natural energy circulatory patterns." Subtle bodily energy, known as *qi* or *ki*, flows along meridian pathways throughout the body, according to traditional Chinese medicine. By pressing certain pairs of points along the meridians, you can energetically, successfully treat seizures (as King experienced personally), heart attack, and other serious health conditions.

If you witness someone having a heart attack, place your right fingertips on the person's fifth thoracic vertebra (midway between the most prominent parts of the shoulder blades on the back) and, with your other hand, hold the little finger of the person's left hand. "This prompt action has consistently stopped heart attacks in progress," King states. On average, this process can shift a person from being on the verge of entering cardiac arrest into a state of no sign of heart arrhythmia, pain, or discoloration within 2-4 minutes, King adds, noting that these results have been confirmed by cardiologists.

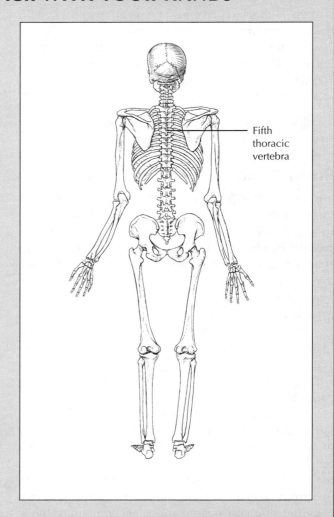

Fifth thoracic vertebra

---

not absorb those nutrients nearly as well as if it is in a relaxed state."

Even ten minutes of extra exercise per day can significantly reduce the risk of heart disease.

—W. LEE COWDEN, M.D.

CAUTION If you are in ill health or over the age of 40, check with your physician before beginning an exercise program.

It is also important for people with heart disease to get plenty of exercise. "Even ten minutes of extra exer-

cise per day can significantly reduce the risk of heart disease," adds Dr. Cowden. However, many people have difficulty building a regular program of exercise into their lives. David Essel, M.S., of Fort Myers Beach, Florida, provides some helpful tips to accomplish this:

1. Move at least a little. Set a goal to walk, swim, skate, jump rope, aerobic dance, run, or ride a bike, three times a week for 20 minutes if possible, but even a ten-minute walk is better than nothing.

2. Exercise can help you control or lose weight. This will likely have a positive effect on your cardiovascular health. Again, the amount of time you exercise is not the most important factor; that you exercise at all is what counts.

3. Increasing lean muscle mass can improve your heart's

health. A twice-weekly strength-training program using calisthenics, free weights, or exercise machines, in which the major muscle groups of the body (chest, back, legs, etc.) are exercised for up to three sets of 8-12 repetitions, can increase lean muscle tissue. This allows the body to burn more calories during the day, thereby assisting in weight loss.

4. Keep to the program because exercise regularity is important. To stick with any program that enhances cardiovascular fitness, consider the following: invite a friend to exercise with you one or several days each week; schedule your exercise session in your daily planner so it has the same or higher priority as any other meeting for that day; or listen to your favorite music, book on tape, or motivational audio to inspire (or entertain) you during your workout.

By following a regular exercise program, you may achieve a reduction in your blood pressure (if it was high), a reduction in the blood levels of triglycerides and LDL cholesterol (which, if elevated, can harm the heart), and an increase in HDL cholesterol (the kind that is beneficial to your system).

Traditional Chinese Medicine

Traditional Chinese medicine (TCM) views heart disease as a problem stemming from poor digestion, which causes the buildup of plaque in the arteries. Harvey Kaltsas, Ac.Phys. (FL), D.Ac. (RI), Dip.Ac. (NCCA), recommends herbs to strengthen digestive functioning. "It has been understood in China for thousands of years that the circulation needs to flow unimpeded," states Dr. Kaltsas. An herbal extract made from a plant known as mao-tung-ching *(Ilex puibeceus)* is often used to dilate the blocked vessels. According to Dr. Kaltsas, a study was conducted in China in which mao-tung-ching was administered daily (four ounces orally, 20 mg intravenously) to 103 patients suffering from coronary heart disease. In 101 of the cases, there was significant improvement.[117]

Maoshing Ni, D.O.M., Ph.D., L.Ac., President of the Yo San University of Traditional Chinese Medicine, in Marina del Rey, California, views heart disease as either a weakness or a block in the body's energy system. For acute problems such as pain or abnormal heart rates, he uses acupuncture, but usually refers acute heart problem patients to a Western physician. He says that TCM is more suited to the treatment of chronic heart problems. For these, Dr. Ni uses a combination of acupuncture and herbs to dissolve plaque, lower cholesterol levels, raise blood flow rates, and relieve angina. One patient came to Dr. Ni after having an angioplasty because of 70%

blockage of the coronary arteries. After the angioplasty, he still had 55% blockage. Dr. Ni treated him with herbs and acupuncture and, within four months, the blockage was reduced to 35%.

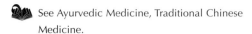 See Ayurvedic Medicine, Traditional Chinese Medicine.

Ayurvedic Medicine

In treating heart disease, Ayurvedic physicians use several methods that result in the reduction of the generation of free radicals, which can contribute to the disease process in the arteries and heart. "Meat, cigarette smoke, alcohol, and environmental pollutants all generate free radicals," explains Hari Sharma, M.D., F.R.C.P.C., Professor Emeritus of Ohio State University's College of Medicine and Public Health. By using specific herbal food supplements and *pancha karma* (detoxification and purification) techniques, says Dr. Sharma, "free radicals and lipid peroxides are reduced." As it is especially important for those with heart disease to lower their level of stress, Dr. Sharma also recommends a program of Transcendental Meditation.

Virender Sodhi, M.D. (Ayurveda), N.D., Director of the Ayurvedic and Naturopathic Medical Clinic, in Bellevue, Washington, reports an interesting case of heart disease involving a 55-year-old Asian male with chest pain so severe that he could not walk more than ten steps before having to sit down. He came to Dr. Sodhi's office after receiving word from the local hospital that he needed immediate bypass surgery. Refusing the surgery, doctors told him, would mean certain death.

Before beginning treatment, the man underwent a battery of tests ordered by Dr. Sodhi. Angiographic studies showed that the patient's coronary arteries were blocked—the left main coronary artery was 90% narrowed, the anterior descending was 80% narrowed, and the right coronary was 30% blocked. Blood tests indicated elevated cholesterol levels at 278 and decreased HDLs at 38. Dr. Sodhi determined his patient's metabolic type and started him on an appropriate cleansing program that included dietary changes and appropriate herbs. (See the Ayurvedic Medicine chapter for discussion of metabolic types.)

After three months, the man's cholesterol levels reportedly dropped more than 30% and his HDLs rose to 48. More importantly, though, his exercise tolerance had dramatically improved. "He was doing the treadmill exercise," Dr. Sodhi reports, "at the speed of five miles per hour for 45 minutes without any angina." More than two years later, the patient was still doing fine, with improved EKG readings and able to jog up and down hills with no symptoms. According to Dr. Sodhi, there is a hospital in Bombay, India, that has treated 3,300 cases of coronary heart disease using this method, with about 99% success.

The Future of Heart Disease Treatment

Conventional treatments for heart disease tend to rely heavily on technological interventions such as bypass surgery, angioplasty, heart transplant, and even the artificial heart. Coronary artery bypass surgery is called an "over-prescribed and unnecessary surgery" by many leading authorities.[118] Complications from such treatments are common and the expense to the health-care system is extraordinarily high. For the most part, medicine is more equipped to treat heart disease only when it has reached its most serious and life-threatening stages.

An announcement in 1993 by the Mutual of Omaha Insurance Company, one of the nation's largest insurers providing coverage for about ten million people, may help point the way for heart disease treatment in the future. The company now offers insurance coverage for individuals participating in pilot programs testing Dr. Ornish's therapy, including a vegetarian diet, exercise, meditation, and support groups. According to Dr. Kenneth McDonough, Mutual of Omaha's Medical Director, "This isn't only a pilot program for coronary artery disease, it's a pilot for medicine in general."[119]

"No longer can we remain secure by following the old, completely inadequate recommendations made by the American Heart Association and other so-called health authorities," says Dr. Gordon. "Their recommendations have led to today's unhealthy, 'one-size-fits-all' fat-restricted diets, which lump beneficial and detrimental fats together, along with using the ill-advised cholesterol-lowering drugs so commonly relied upon. For those who are going to avoid dying of heart disease, it is essential to comprehend the paradigm shift toward understanding and dealing with vulnerable plaque and infection/inflammation inside the arteries, along with the development of newly recognized molecular markers for heart disease, such as C-reactive protein, fibrinogen, and homocysteine. Not only can you avoid virtually every heart attack and stroke if you have these risk factors measured and learn how to adequately control them, but if we base our treatment approaches on these new developments—using those which are most natural and with the least potential for harm—we can actually make death from heart attacks and strokes virtually a thing of the past."

Recommendations

- Eighty-five percent of all heart disease is caused by vulnerable plaque, which cannot usually be detected by conventional cardiovascular diagnostic tests. Moreover, evidence suggests that vulnerable plaque can be triggered by chronic infection, including *Chlamydia, Helicobacter pylori,* cytomegalovirus (CMV), and the herpes family of retroviruses. To effectively screen for vulnerable plaque, ultra-high-speed magnetic resonance imaging (MRI) may be required. Darkfield microscopy can also be useful. People at risk for heart disease should also be screened for infectious agents, as well as oxidized cholesterol, fibrinogen and homocysteine levels, and free-radical damage.

- Emphasize organic foods (free of pesticides, herbicides, steroids, and antibiotics) whenever possible. Increase fiber from green leafy vegetables, complex carbohydrates, fresh raw fruits, bran, whole grains, and psyllium. Use monounsaturated oils (like olive oil), omega-3 oils (fish oils or flaxseed oil), and omega-6 oils (borage oil or evening primrose oil). Avoid processed foods (with additives and preservatives or foods containing powdered eggs or powdered milk) and irradiated foods whenever possible. Reduce intake of harmful fats, especially fried foods, animal fats, and partially hydrogenated oils, and eliminate sugar, tobacco, and alcohol.

- Proper nutritional supplementation can significantly improve cardiovascular conditions, as well as prevent them from occurring in the first place. Useful nutrients include beta carotene; vitamins B_3 (niacin), B_6, B_{12}, C, and E; folic acid; the minerals calcium, chromium, magnesium, potassium, and selenium; the amino acids L-arginine, L-taurine, and L-carnitine; coenzyme Q10; and pycnogenol.

- Useful herbs for heart disease include foxglove *(Digitalis purpurea),* hawthorn berry, garlic, ginger, *Ginkgo biloba,* linden flower, and motherwort. For best results, consult a skilled herbalist.

- Both exercise and stress reduction can help mitigate heart disease risk and improve recovery.

Self-Care

The following therapies can be undertaken at home under appropriate professional supervision:

Fasting / Yoga

AROMATHERAPY: • To strengthen the heart muscle, use garlic, lavender, peppermint, marjoram, rose, rosemary. • For palpitations, try lavender, melissa, neroli, ylang-ylang.

HYDROTHERAPY: Constitutional hydrotherapy (2-5 times weekly).

JUICE THERAPY: • Carrot, celery, cucumber, beet (add a little garlic or hawthorn berries) • Blueberries, blackberries, black currant, red grapes

Professional Care

The following therapies can only be provided by a qualified health professional:

Biofeedback Training and Neurotherapy / Environmental Medicine / Guided Imagery / Hypnotherapy / Magnetic Field Therapy / Mind/Body Medicine / Osteopathic Medicine

BIOLOGICAL DENTISTRY: Hal A. Huggins, D.D.S., reports the improvement or disappearance of many cardiovascular problems including angina, unidentified chest pains, and tachycardia (rapid heartbeat for no apparent reason) after removing toxic dental amalgams.

BODYWORK: Acupressure, Alexander Technique, reflexology, shiatsu, massage

CHIROPRACTIC: To improve mid-back mobility and breathing.

HYDROTHERAPY: Leon Chaitow, N.D., D.O., reports that the neutral bath—patient immersed in water (35° C) for two hours—has been effective in treating mild heart problems that result in fluid retention.

Where to Find Help

For additional information and referrals concerning treatment for heart disease, contact the following organizations.

American Association of Oriental Medicine (AAOM)

433 Front Street
Catasauqua, Pennsylvania 18032
(888) 500-7999
Website: www.aaom.org

The AAOM is a national professional organization of acupuncturists who meet acceptable standards of competency. Provides referrals to members nationwide.

American College of Advancement in Medicine (ACAM)

23121 Verdugo Drive, Suite 204
Laguna Hills, California 92653
(800) 532-3688
Website: www.acam.org

ACAM provides training and education, sponsors conferences for physicians and scientists, and provides referrals to physicians trained in preventative medicine and in the ACAM protocol for chelation therapy.

American Holistic Medical Association (AHMA)

6728 Old McLean Village Drive
McLean, Virginia 22101
(703) 556-9245
Website: www.holisticmedicine.org

A professional organization for holistic practitioners, the AHMA offers information and services for its members and lobbies for holistic issues. It also provides referrals for AHMA physicians (M.D.s and D.O.s) nationwide.

Ayurvedic and Naturopathic Medical Clinic

2115 112th Avenue N.E.
Bellevue, Washington 98004
(425) 453-8022
Website: www.ayurvedicscience.com

Operated by Dr. Virender Sodhi, the Clinic is a leading center for Ayurvedic and naturopathic medicine in the U.S.

Ayurvedic Institute

11311 Menaul Boulevard N.E.
Albuquerque, New Mexico 87112
(505) 291-9698
Website: www.ayurveda.com

The Institute, directed by Dr. Vasant Lad, trains people in most of the aspects of Ayurveda, and provides Ayurvedic treatments for a wide variety of health conditions.

King Institute for Better Health

P.O. Box 118495
Carrollton, Texas 75011
(800) 640-7998 or (214) 731-9795
Website: www.kinginstitute.org

Provides information and training in the art of Ki-Iki-Jutsu.

Gordon Research Institute (GRI)

708 E. Highway 260
Payson, Arizona 85541
(520) 472-4263
Website: www.gordonresearch.com

Directed by Dr. Garry F. Gordon, GRI is a leading research institution in the field of clinical nutrition and chelation therapy (both oral and I.V.) and the repository of over 40 years of Dr. Gordon's clinical research. Also provides protocols for the proper use of chelation therapy and information about Dr. Gordon's proprietary oral chelation and other nutritional supplement formulas.

The Raj/Maharishi Ayur-Veda Health Center

1734 Jasmine Avenue
Fairfield, Iowa 52556
(641) 472-9580
Website: www.theraj.com

Residential treatment center offering Ayurvedic treatments and education.

Recommended Reading

Alternative Medicine Guide to Heart Disease, Stroke & High Blood Pressure. Burton Goldberg and the Editors of *Alternative Medicine.* Tiburon, CA: Future Medicine Publishing, 1998.

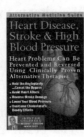

Bypassing Bypass. Elmer Cranton. Charlottesville, VA: Hampton Roads Publishers, 2000.

Coping with Angina. Louise M. Wallace. London: Thorsons, 1990.

Dr. Dean Ornish's Program for Reversing Heart Disease. Dean Ornish, M.D. New York: Ballantine, 1990.

Encyclopedia of Natural Medicine. Michael Murray, N.D., and Joseph Pizzorno, N.D. Rocklin, CA: Prima Publishing, 1998.

Good Cholesterol, Bad Cholesterol. Eli M. Roth, M.D., and Sandra L. Streicher, R.N. Rocklin, CA: Prima Publishing, 1993.

Heart Frauds: Uncovering the Biggest Health Scam in History. Charles T. McGee, M.D. Colorado Springs, CO: Health Wise Publications, 2001.

Heart Myths. Bruce D. Charash, M.D. New York: Viking Penguin, 1992.

The Johns Hopkins Complete Guide for Preventing and Reversing Heart Disease. Peter Kwiterovich, M.D. Rocklin, CA: Prima Publishing, 1998.

The New Supernutrition Book. Richard A. Passwater. New York: Pocket Books, 1991.

Plague Time: How Stealth Infections Cause Cancers, Heart Disease, and Other Deadly Ailments. Paul W. Ewald. New York: Free Press, 2000.

Preventing Silent Heart Disease. Harold L. Karpman, M.D. New York: Henry Holt, 1991.

Reversing Heart Disease. Julian M. Whitaker, M.D. New York: Warner Books, 1995.

HYPERTENSION

Hypertension, or high blood pressure, affects nearly one out of four Americans. Conventional medicine uses drugs to relieve the symptoms of hypertension, but does little to address the underlying causes. Alternative therapies can provide a natural and effective way of preventing or reducing hypertension, resolving the underlying factors without the many side effects associated with high blood pressure medications.

APPROXIMATELY 60 MILLION Americans, two-thirds of whom are under 65 years of age, suffer from hypertension, indicating that this condition is not an inevitable result of aging but rather a condition affected by a number of risk factors, including smoking, obesity, chronic stress, excessive alcohol consumption, and a diet high in fats and salt. "Individuals with diabetes are especially susceptible, as are those with a family history of hypertension," according to W. Lee Cowden, M.D., a cardiologist from Fort Worth, Texas, and author of *Longevity: An Alternative Medicine Definitive Guide.* "Stress and a sedentary lifestyle are other factors to consider when diagnosing and treating this condition."

To understand high blood pressure, you need to know a few facts about the heart. The human heart beats 70 times per minute on average, 100,000 times a day, and 2.5 billion times over the course of an average life. With each heartbeat, about 2.5 ounces of blood are pumped through the heart—that is 1,980 gallons every day. The term *blood pressure* refers to the force of the blood against the walls of arteries, veins, and the chambers of the heart as it is pumped through the body. More than normal force exerted by the blood against the arteries (when high blood pressure is present) begins to damage the cellular walls and makes it easier for harmful substances, such as toxins and oxidized cholesterol, to form dangerous deposits on the arterial walls.

High blood pressure takes two forms: essential hypertension, when conventional doctors have not been able to determine a cause, and secondary hypertension, when damage to the kidneys or endocrine dysfunction cause blood pressure to rise. Of the diagnosed cases of hypertension in the United States, over 90% are labeled by conventional doctors as essential hypertension.[1] The symptoms of hypertension appear throughout the body and may include dizziness, headaches, fatigue, restless-

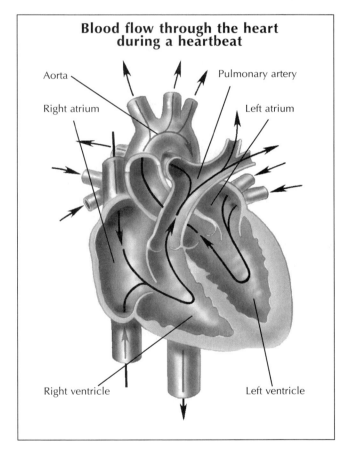

Blood flow through the heart during a heartbeat

Aorta

Pulmonary artery

Right atrium

Left atrium

Right ventricle

Left ventricle

ness, difficulty breathing, insomnia, intestinal complaints, and emotional instability. In advanced stages, the hypertensive person often experiences cardiovascular disease as well as damage to the heart, kidneys, and brain.

Causes of Hypertension

"High blood pressure often occurs due to a strain on the heart, which can arise from a variety of conditions,

773

DIAGNOSING HYPERTENSION

Hypertension is the technical name for high blood pressure. Blood pressure is measured by placing an inflatable cuff around the upper arm. As the cuff is inflated, the arm is squeezed tight. At this point, the pulse cannot be heard through the stethoscope. As the cuff is slowly deflated, the pulse is heard again. This is the high number and measures the systolic pressure, when the heart is contracting to pump blood into the body. As the cuff is deflated even further, the pulse sound through the stethoscope disappears again. That reading is the low number and measures the diastolic pressure, when the heart is relaxing to refill with blood. The ratio of the two numbers represents blood pressure, as in 120/85, an "average" or healthy reading. A patient has hypertension if the high (systolic) reading is above 140 and the low (diastolic) reading is above 90 when tested on two separate occasions at least a few hours apart.

including diet, atherosclerosis [hardening of the arteries], high cholesterol, diabetes, environmental factors, as well as lifestyle choices," according to Dr. Cowden. When these factors combine with a genetic predisposition, hypertension can occur in two out of three individuals.[2]

Dietary Factors

Hypertension is closely associated with the Western diet and is found almost entirely in developed countries.[3] Recent studies of residents in remote areas of China, New Guinea, Panama, Brazil, and Africa show virtually no evidence of hypertension, even with advanced age. But when individuals within these groups moved to more industrialized areas, the incidence of hypertension among them rose. These studies concluded that changes in lifestyle, including dietary changes and increased body mass and fat, significantly contributed to the higher levels of blood pressure.[4] And obesity, regardless of the presence of other factors, increases the risk of hypertension.[5]

Although a combination of genetic and environmental factors such as behavior patterns and stress contribute to hypertension, the main cause appears to be a diet high in animal fat and salt (sodium chloride),[6] especially if high in relation to potassium and magnesium, according to Dr. Cowden. Research concurs that a diet high in sodium chloride and deficient in potassium has been associated with hypertension. Lack of potassium and other nutritional deficiencies play a significant role in the development of hypertension. Magnesium levels have been found to be consistently low in patients with high blood pressure.[7]

Lifestyle Factors

Lifestyle choices, including smoking and consumption of coffee and alcohol, have been shown to cause hypertension. A study conducted in Paris, France, showed higher systolic and diastolic levels in coffee drinkers, and levels rose in direct correlation to the amount of coffee consumed each day.[8] Even moderate amounts of alcohol can produce hypertension in certain individuals, and chronic alcohol intake is one of the strongest predictors of high blood pressure.[9] Restricting alcohol and avoiding caffeine are recommended.

Smoking is a contributing factor to hypertension directly and is due to the fact that smokers are more prone to increased sugar, alcohol, and caffeine consumption.[10] Even smokeless tobacco (chewing tobacco, snuff) causes hypertension through its nicotine and sodium content.[11] In addition, a lifestyle that includes chronic levels of stress raises the risk of developing high blood pressure.[12]

Although a combination of genetic and environmental factors such as behavior patterns and stress contribute to hypertension, the main cause appears to be a diet high in animal fat and salt.

—W. Lee Cowden, M.D.

Environmental Factors

Environmental factors such as lead contamination from drinking water, as well as residues of heavy metals such as cadmium and mercury, have been shown to promote hypertension.[13] Even a low level of lead exposure and accumulation in tissues in adults is now linked to both hypertension and impaired kidney function.[14] In two studies involving over 1,000 men, the exposure to lead was at levels previously considered safe. Those with the highest bone levels of lead were 50% more likely to have hypertension than those with the lowest. Researchers at the Harvard School of Public Health found that high levels of childhood exposure to lead are linked to adult obesity, according to their 1995 study of 79 overweight adults.[15] Adults who had absorbed high lead levels as children gained the most weight between the ages of seven and 20. Both excess weight and high lead concentrations are associated with high blood pressure in adults.

People with hypertension have been shown to have blood cadmium levels three to four times higher than those with normal blood pressure.[16] It is important to rule out lead, cadmium, and mercury toxicity when treating hypertension.

 See Chelation Therapy, Heart Disease.

Treating Hypertension

Conventional medicine uses drugs to treat hypertension by reducing heart output, lowering arterial resistance to blood flow, or reducing fluid retention through the use of diuretics. These medications may relieve the symptoms of hypertension but do little to address the cause. As many of these drugs have unwanted side effects, an alternative approach to reducing blood pressure may be preferable.

A careful evaluation of the factors contributing to the illness may reveal a need for dietary changes, nutritional supplementation, and lifestyle changes such as increased exercise, weight loss, and stress management. Other therapies include various forms of mind/body medicine, herbal medicine, detoxification therapies, Ayurvedic medicine, and traditional Chinese medicine.

Diet and Nutritional Supplements

Cardiologist Stephen T. Sinatra, M.D., of the New England Heart Center, in Manchester, Connecticut, recommends a diet that consists of 30% fats, 20%-25% protein, and 45%-50% carbohydrates. The fats should come from fish such as salmon, mackerel, Greenland halibut, cod, and blue fish (but not tuna because of possible mercury contamination). Large amounts of red meat should be avoided, while fresh fruits and vegetables are emphasized. This is basically the so-called Mediterranean diet. A now classic study conducted in the 1980s, investigating the rate of heart attacks over a ten-year period for individuals in European nations, revealed that the island of Crete reported no heart attacks as a cause of death, even though many of the residents had dangerously high cholesterol levels, a presumed risk factor for heart disease.

According to Dr. Sinatra, "the Mediterranean diet, rich in monounsaturated fat (olive oil) and antioxidants, has proved to be crucial in cardiovascular protection." Dr. Sinatra says this diet is low in saturated fats (such as dairy products and meats), high in fiber and antioxidants (vitamin C, beta carotene, and vitamin E) from fresh fruits and vegetables, and high in essential fatty acids, found in fish, flaxseed oil, and other omega-3 oils. Avocados and

asparagus, commonly eaten in this diet, are rich in L-glutathione, an amino acid that can scavenge for harmful free radicals. And olive oil is "the healthiest of oils, no doubt," says Dr. Sinatra. Also, garlic and other members of the onion family (prominent in this diet) help because they significantly reduce blood pressure.[17]

Making relatively simple changes in diet can lower blood pressure as effectively as conventional hypertension drugs. This was confirmed in a study directed by the Kaiser Permanente Center for Health Research, in Portland, Oregon, in cooperation with researchers at Johns Hopkins, Harvard, and Duke Universities.[18] The study enrolled 459 adults (50% women, 60% African-American) with a starting blood pressure of 160/80-95 (high blood pressure was considered 140/90 or higher). The participants were divided into three groups, each following a different diet. The first group ate a conventional American diet (typically high in fats, sugar, meat, and processed foods); the second group ate the same diet complemented with fruits and vegetables. The third group practiced a diet low in fats, comprising only 31% of the total calories, kept their consumption of cholesterol low, and their consumption of fruits, vegetables, and low-fat dairy products high. Changes in blood pressure were noticeable within two weeks. For those in the third group, blood pressure values dropped by an average of 5.5/3.0, while for those in the second group, the readings declined an average of 2.8/1.1.

Another study compared the effects of omega-3 fatty acids in fish or fish oil supplements in 125 men with moderately high blood pressure consuming high-fat or

---

A BOWL OF OATMEAL FOR YOUR HEART

In recent years, at least 37 clinical studies have affirmed the ability of oatmeal and oat bran to reduce blood cholesterol levels, lower blood pressure, and generally reduce the long-term risk of heart disease. In recognition of these well-established benefits, in 1996 the U.S. Food and Drug Administration (FDA) granted manufacturers/packagers of oatmeal the right to make specific health claims about this food, stating that diets high in oatmeal or oat bran may reduce the risk of heart disease. It was the first such permissible health claim ever accorded to a food by the FDA, an agency that generally has favored drugs over natural substances.

In 1995, researchers at Johns Hopkins University, in Baltimore, Maryland, reported that people who regularly consumed even a modest portion of oatmeal (one ounce cooked, daily) had lower blood pressure and cholesterol readings than those who never ate oatmeal.[20] The study was based on the evaluation of 850 men, 17-77 years old, living in China; their oatmeal consumption was 25-90 g daily.

The researchers stated that "the higher the oats intake, the lower the blood pressure," regardless of other factors such as age and weight, or alcohol, sodium, or potassium intake, which are known to affect blood pressure. According to chief researcher Michael Klag, M.D., it is oatmeal's high content of water-soluble fiber (beta glucan) that produces the heart benefits. A six-year study involving 22,000 middle-aged Finnish males showed that consuming as little as 3 g daily of soluble fiber (from the beta glucan fiber component of oats, barley, or rye) reduced the risk of death from heart disease by 27%.[21]

low-fat diets. The subjects ate fish, took fish oil supplements, or had a combination providing an average total of 3.65 g per day of omega-3 fatty acids. There was a significant reduction in both systolic and diastolic blood pressure in the subjects eating fish and/or taking fish oil supplements, particularly in those on a low-fat diet.[19]

Eric R. Braverman, M.D., Director of Place for Achieving Total Health (PATH), in New York City, treats hypertension with a program centered around diet and nutritional supplementation. Dr. Braverman's diet is low in sodium, low in saturated fat, high in vegetables from the starch group, and high in protein (particularly fish). In addition, the diet features large amounts of fresh salad.

Simple sugars, alcohol, caffeine, nicotine, and refined carbohydrates are reduced dramatically or eliminated altogether. His nutritional supplement program for a typical hypertensive patient includes fish oil, garlic, evening primrose oil, magnesium, potassium, selenium, zinc, vitamin B6, niacin, vitamin C, tryptophan, taurine, cysteine, and coenzyme Q10.

Studies have shown that nutritional supplementation, particularly with potassium, calcium, and magnesium (nonchloride salts), along with antioxidants and zinc, can help reduce hypertension.

Sodium and Potassium: In order to reduce blood pressure, sodium intake must be restricted while potassium intake is increased.[22] Individuals with high blood pressure should be aware of "hidden" salt in processed foods. Although their salt intake is comparable, vegetarians generally have less hypertension and cardiovascular disease than non-vegetarians because their diet contains more potassium, complex carbohydrates, polyunsaturated fat, fiber, calcium, magnesium, and vitamins A and C.[23] According to Dr. Cowden, regular consumption of potassium-rich fruits such as avocados, bananas, cantaloupe, honeydew melon, grapefruit, nectarines, oranges, and vegetables such as asparagus, broccoli, cabbage, cauliflower, green peas, potatoes, and squash can lower high blood pressure. Steaming rather than boiling vegetables helps prevent vital nutrient loss.

Calcium: Calcium has been shown to lower blood pressure in hypertensives.[24] Because many with high blood pressure have a lower daily calcium intake than people with normal blood pressure, calcium-rich foods, including nuts and leafy green vegetables such as watercress and kale, should also supplement the diet.[25] A recent analysis of the research on calcium and hypertension shows that either increasing calcium in the diet or using calcium supplements will usually have a positive effect on systolic blood pressure.[26]

Magnesium: In one study, magnesium supplementation lowered blood pressure in 19 of 20 hypertensives.[27] Dietary magnesium is found in nuts (almonds, cashews, pecans), rice, bananas, potatoes, wheat germ, kidney and lima beans, soy products, and molasses.

Antioxidants and Zinc: Research has found that antioxidants are linked to an increase in nitric oxide activity.[28] Nitric oxide helps open blood vessels, which in turn may help lower blood pressure. Zinc may be helpful because it activates SOD (superoxide dismutase), an antioxidant enzyme. A study of 21 patients with hypertension found that daily supplementation with a combination of antioxidants and zinc (500 mg of vitamin C, 50,000 IU of beta carotene, 600 IU of vitamin E, and 80 mg of zinc) lowered blood pressure from 165/89 to 160/85.5 in eight weeks.[29]

Other beneficial supplements include vitamins A, C, and E, niacin (vitamin B₃), bioflavonoids (particularly rutin), and the amino acid taurine.[30]

 See Diet, Nutritional Medicine, Orthomolecular Medicine.

CAUTION High dosages of vitamin E are not recommended for people with hypertension, rheumatic heart disease, or ischemic heart disease except under close medical supervision, starting at a low dose and building up cautiously.

Lifestyle Changes

Lifestyle plays a major role in the development of hypertension, and any program to reduce blood pressure must take this into consideration. Dr. Cowden notes that any changes that are implemented must be maintained if blood pressure is to be controlled on a long-term basis. Smoking should be moderated, or preferably totally avoided, and alcohol intake should be kept to a minimum. Weight loss reduces blood pressure in those with and without hypertension and should be a primary goal for hypertensives who are obese or moderately overweight. Other factors for reducing and controlling hypertension are increased exercise and stress management.

EXERCISE

Regular exercise reduces stress and blood pressure, so it is highly recommended as an integral part of your life. Consistent aerobic exercise can both prevent and lower hypertension.[31] In a study of 902 people with hypertension, 45 to 69 years old, positive long-term effects on blood pressure and cholesterol levels were achieved with increased exercise along with a lower fat diet.[32] Swimming, which is frequently prescribed as a nonimpact exercise to lower high blood pressure, can produce a significant decrease in resting heart rate (a sign of cardiovascular health) and systolic blood pressure in previously sedentary people with elevated blood pressure.[33]

CAUTION Before undertaking any exercise program, an individual with hypertension should consult a physician.

STRESS MANAGEMENT

Stress-reduction techniques from the various disciplines of mind/body medicine, such as biofeedback, yoga, meditation, Qigong, relaxation exercises, and hypnotherapy, have all proved successful in lowering blood pressure.[34] In fact, meditation is so effective in reducing stress that in 1984 the National Institutes of Health recommended meditation over prescription drugs for mild hypertension.[35]

Biofeedback has proven particularly valuable in working to lower hypertension.[36] Patients in one study were able to sustain lower blood pressure readings after three years of using biofeedback.[37] Combining biofeedback with other stress-reduction techniques can also help patients achieve optimal results. A study of mildly hypertensive men treated with biofeedback, autogenic training, or breathing relaxation training showed a significant reduction in both systolic and diastolic blood pressure. The higher the pretreatment blood pressure level, the greater the effects of these types of relaxation training.[38]

Self-guided relaxation techniques can be a quick and effective way to lower blood pressure, according to researchers at the National Taiwan University, in Taiwan.[39] Hypertension is widespread there, with 27% of men and 13% of women having readings of at least 140/90. Based on a study group of 590 individuals with high blood pressure, researchers found that practicing progressive relaxation techniques (from an audio cassette) coupled with home study of healthful practices led to an average drop of blood pressure to 130/85 after two months. No drugs or other treatments were involved other than the power of self-directed relaxation.

 See Biofeedback Training and Neurotherapy, Guided Imagery, Hypnotherapy, Herbal Medicine, Mind/Body Medicine, Qigong and Tai Chi, Yoga.

Herbal Medicine

Many botanicals and herbs have hypotensive (blood pressure–lowering) properties. These include the garlic family, mistletoe, olive leaves, hawthorn berries, and periwinkle.[40]

Garlic: According to David Hoffmann, B.Sc., M.N.I.M.H., of Sebastopol, California, eating a clove of raw garlic daily will help considerably in preventing or reversing the effects of high blood pressure. While garlic has been used for centuries in traditional cultures throughout the world as a multipurpose medicinal food, in recent decades more than 2,000 clinical studies have validated many of the folk-healing claims for "the stinking rose," as garlic was once called.

Prominent among these substantiated claims is garlic's ability to lower blood pressure, inhibit cholesterol production and reduce triglyceride levels, promote blood circulation, and discourage clot formation. Yu-Yan Yeh, Ph.D., of the Department of Nutrition at Pennsylvania State University, reviewed extensive multi-laboratory studies on garlic's ability to reduce cardiovascular disease and concluded: "Collectively, the results suggest that garlic may lower the risk for this disease by reducing plasma lipids [fats in the blood], lowering blood pressure, and

DRUGS ASSOCIATED WITH A HIGHER INCIDENCE OF HYPERTENSION

According to the *Physicians' Desk Reference*, the following drugs are associated with side effects of hypertension (statistics refer to the percentage of individuals affected).

Alfenta injection (18%)
Aredia for injection (up to 6%)
Dobutrex solution vials (most patients)
Epogen for injection (up to 25%)
Habitrol Nicotine Transdermal System (3%-9%)
Lupron Depot 3.75 mg (among most frequent)
Methergine injection, tablets (most common)
Orthoclone OKT3 sterile solution (8%)
Polygam, Immune Globulin Intravenous, Human (3%-6%)
Procrit for injection (Up to 24%)
Sandimmune I.V. ampules for infusion, oral solution (13%-53%)
Sandimmune soft gelatin capsules (13%-53%)
Tolectin 200-600 mg (3%-9%)
Velban vials (among most common)
Ventolin inhalation aerosol and refill (fewer than 5%)
Wellbutrin tablets (4.3%)

depressing platelet adhesion and aggregation [clotting]." A scientific panel of the European community has endorsed garlic for its cardiovascular benefits.[41]

Olive Leaf Extract: The primary active part of the olive leaf is oleuropein (the bitter component removed from olives when they are cured) and the flavonoids rutin, luteolin, and hesperidin, which are natural compounds needed for maintenance of the capillary walls. Recent analysis of oleuropein at the University of Messina, in Italy, demonstrated that olive leaf extracts have distinct heart benefits. Researchers concluded that oleuropein produced "a strong coronary dilatory effect and a significant decrease in arterial blood pressure;" in other words, increased blood flow to the heart and lowered blood pressure.[42]

Hawthorn *(Crataegus oxyacantha):* Hawthorn has been used in folk medicine in Europe and China for centuries. Europeans have employed the edible fruit as well as the leaves and flowers, primarily for their beneficial effects on the cardiovascular system. Hawthorn is one of the primary heart tonics in traditional herbal medicine. Fruit and leaf extracts are known for their cardiotonic, sedative, and hypotensive activities. Hawthorn has been extensively tested in animals and humans and is known to cause a decrease in blood pressure with exertion, increase in heart muscle contractility (the ability to contract or shorten), increase in blood flow to the heart muscle, decrease in heart rate, and decrease in oxygen use by the myocardium (the contracting middle muscular layer of the walls of the heart).[43] "An infusion of hawthorn berries taken twice daily is a gentle and effective way of helping the body to normalize blood pressure," says Hoffmann. "The infusion can be strengthened by combining linden flowers or by adding chamomile or valerian, if tension or headaches are present."

Maitake Mushroom: Prized for centuries by Japanese herbalists for its ability to strengthen health, maitake mushroom (which means "dancing mushroom") is now being investigated in Japan and America for its healing abilities in a number of diseases, including hypertension. In over 30 cases, maitake gradually decreased high blood pressure to normal levels.[44]

Reishi Mushroom: Chinese herbal medicine physicians regard the reishi mushroom as an "elixir of immortality." Research confirms that reishi is an effective cardiotonic. In a study of 54 people, average age 58.6, whose blood pressure was higher than 140/90 and who were unresponsive to conventional medication, those taking reishi mushroom extract three times a day for four weeks experienced a significant drop in their blood pressure compared to the control group.[45]

Detoxification

Detoxification is the body's natural process of eliminating internal toxins and is accomplished through various systems and organs, including the liver, kidneys, intestines, and skin, with toxins eliminated through urine, feces, and perspiration. Everyone has a specific level of tolerance to toxicity that cannot be exceeded if good health is to be maintained; if the system becomes overwhelmed, various symptoms can occur, including hypertension.

Dr. Cowden puts hypertensive patients through a detoxification regimen consisting of daily saunas, homeopathic remedies, and a vegetarian diet supplemented with cayenne and garlic. "Cayenne (*Capsicum annuum*) mixed with vegetable juices or lemon juice is excellent for lowering blood pressure," says Dr. Cowden. He adds that after a few days of treatment, alternating cayenne/vegetable juice with cayenne/lemon juice, patients are often able to come off medication because this regime helps to cleanse the body of toxins that may be causing the high blood pressure.

Dr. Cowden notes that individuals with hypertension often suffer from a liver insufficiency, in which the liver does not properly clear steroid hormones (sex hormones and hormones of the adrenal glands) as well as toxic substances from the blood. Saunas and a vegetarian diet can help to restore liver function and lower blood pressure. (Patients with more severe hypertension should have their saunas medically supervised.)

A toxic lymphatic system can also contribute to hypertension. Dr. Cowden suggests deep breathing exercises and ten minutes daily of dry brushing of the skin (vigorously brushing the entire body with a dry brush) in the direction of lymph flow, for three weeks. Another way to stimulate lymph flow and to clear the lymph system of toxins is by using a small trampoline or rebounder for 5-10 minutes, 2-3 times a day, says Dr. Cowden.

Dr. Cowden reports the case of a severely hypertensive woman, with a blood pressure of higher than 240/140, who had tried every prescription hypertensive drug and had adverse reactions to all of them. Due to years of poor dietary habits and an unhealthy lifestyle, her system was highly toxic. He put her on a detoxification program that included a vegetarian diet, vegetable juice and lemon juice fasts with garlic and cayenne, supplements of magnesium, saunas, simple stress-reduction techniques, and cranial electrical stimulation (the use of microelectric impulses to stimulate the production of endorphins). Within two weeks, her blood pressure decreased to 140/80, which is ideal, according to Dr. Cowden. She went off her hypertension medications and her blood pressure remained in that range during her follow-up visits over the next six months.

Ayurvedic Medicine

Ayurvedic medicine treats hypertension according to each person's metabolic type. Virender Sodhi, M.D. (Ayurveda), N.D., Director of the Ayurvedic & Naturopathic Medical Clinic, in Bellevue, Washington, says that hypertension is found most often in *pitta* and *kapha* types and is usually due to a combination of genetics and lifestyle. Patients of Dr. Sodhi's are put on a diet low in sodium, cholesterol, and triglycerides (the latter causes the blood to become viscous and therefore raises blood pressure).

Yoga breathing exercises help to relax the body and stimulate the cardiovascular system, effectively reducing hypertension, says Dr. Sodhi. "Breathing first with one nostril, then the other, for 10-15 minutes, two to three times a day, is highly effective in lowering blood pressure. I have patients try this in the office and, after ten minutes, their blood pressure drops considerably."

Herbs also play an important role in treating hypertension. Herbs are usually used in combinations, depending on the patient's individual needs, and are often combined with rose water and minerals such as calcium, magnesium, silicon, and zinc. According to Dr. Sodhi, the following herbs are indicated for hypertension:

- *Sankhapuspi (Convolvulus pluricaulis)* has a calming effect, reduces anxiety and anger, and lowers cholesterol while increasing high-density lipoproteins (this helps to improve circulation and lower blood pressure).

- *Ashwagandha* also has a calming effect and helps to reduce stress and thus blood pressure.

- Coral in rose water is an excellent tonic for the heart, as it contains calcium and magnesium, usually deficient in hypertensives.

- Rauwolfia and its extract, reserpine, are particularly useful in helping to regulate blood pressure. Care must be taken when prescribing rauwolfia and reserpine, however, because they can cause neurological biochemical imbalances and depression and should not be given to patients already suffering from (or with a past history of) depression.

 See Ayurvedic Medicine, Detoxification Therapy, Qigong and Tai Chi, Traditional Chinese Medicine.

Traditional Chinese Medicine

According to traditional Chinese medicine (TCM), essential hypertension is usually due to a problem in the circulation of energy *(qi)* in the body. Poor diet and long-term emotional distress such as chronic nervousness, anger, and depression can lead to this condition. "Treatment is aimed at bringing the energy flow of the body back into balance through a combination of acupuncture and herbs," says Harvey Kaltsas, Ac.Phys. (FL), D.Ac. (RI), Dip.Ac. (NCCA), of Sarasota, Florida. "Secondary hypertension often occurs when the energy reserves become exhausted (called 'kidney *yin* deficiency') and can also be treated with a combination of acupuncture and herbs to build up and restore one's energy."

With early diagnosis and treatment, not only can hypertension be alleviated but also complications (including damage to the heart, brain, kidneys, and liver) can be prevented. Other important elements of treatment include Qigong exercises, meditation, and a diet high in vegetables and low in fat, sugars, and alcohol.

Mark T. Holmes, O.M.D., L.Ac., Director of the Center for Regeneration, in Beverly Hills, California, relates two cases in which TCM successfully controlled hypertension. The first case involved a 46-year-old attorney with essential hypertension, whose blood pressure was 160/90. His additional symptoms included impotence, insomnia, red eyes, nervousness, and a decreased desire to exercise. An inability to relax after work, combined with a nightly habit of drinking two bottles of expensive wine, were determined to be causative factors. Laboratory tests revealed elevated liver enzymes. In TCM, this is referred to as a "flaring up of liver fire." After seven months of daily herbal intake combined with regular acupuncture treatments, the patient's hypertension was reversed. All other symptoms abated except the impotency, which significantly improved.

Dr. Holmes also successfully treated an 80-year-old woman suffering from secondary hypertension with a combination of TCM and Western medication. Normally, her blood pressure remained high, around 210/90. This dropped moderately to 180/90 with the use of her prescribed medication. Using Chinese herbs combined with bimonthly acupuncture and homeopathic remedies, Dr. Holmes was able to stabilize her blood pressure at 130-140/85. A subsequent Western clinical examination revealed a 20% increase of carotid artery circulation.

Recommendations

- Reduce your weight.

- Eliminate salt (avoid salty foods and add no salt to food) and avoid alcohol, caffeine, and smoking.

- Change your diet to include more potassium-rich foods (potato, avocado, cooked lima beans, bananas, flounder), fiber, and complex carbohydrates. Eat more celery, garlic, onions, and vegetable oils high in omega-3 fatty acids, but eat much less animal fat.

- Take supplements, including calcium (500-1,000 mg daily), magnesium (500-1,000 mg daily), vitamin C (1-3 g per day), zinc (15-30 mg per day), and flaxseed oil (1 tbsp per day).

- Take hawthorn herbal extract (100-250 mg, three times daily).

- Take coenzyme Q10 (50-60 mg, three times daily).

- Exercise more and practice stress-reduction techniques (biofeedback, self-hypnosis, yoga, meditation, muscle relaxation).

- A detoxification regimen may be necessary for relief from hypertension.

Self-Care

The following therapies can be undertaken at home under appropriate professional supervision:

Fasting / Yoga

AROMATHERAPY: Ylang ylang, marjoram, lavender

HYDROTHERAPY: Constitutional hydrotherapy (apply two to five times weekly).

JUICE THERAPY: • Celery, beet, and carrot or cucumber, spinach, and parsley. Add a little raw garlic to vegetable juices. • Run a clove of garlic through a juicer, followed by enough carrots to make eight ounces of juice. Drink once per day.

Professional Care

The following therapies should only be provided by a qualified health professional:

Acupuncture / Chelation Therapy / Detoxification Therapy / Environmental Medicine / Hypnotherapy / Orthomolecular Medicine

BODYWORK: Acupressure, reflexology, shiatsu, massage, Rolfing, Feldenkrais Method, Alexander Technique, Therapeutic Touch

ENERGY MEDICINE: W. Lee Cowden, M.D., uses cranial electrical stimulation to treat hypertensive patients, reporting that it can lower blood pressure and alleviate panic attacks within 30-40 minutes.

MAGNETIC FIELD THERAPY: Recent studies from Russia show that magnetic treatments reduce blood pressure in certain patients with hypertension.[46]

Where to Find Help

For additional information and referrals for hypertension treatment, contact the following organizations.

American Academy of Environmental Medicine
American Financial Center, Suite 625
7701 East Kellogg Avenue
Wichita, Kansas 67207
(316) 684-5500
Website: www.aaem.com

Offers training for physicians in environmental medicine. For information on physicians practicing environmental medicine, send a self-addressed, stamped envelope stating your request.

American Association of Oriental Medicine
433 Front Street
Catasauqua, Pennsylvania 18032
(888) 500-7999
Website: www.aaom.org

The AAOM is a national professional organization of acupuncturists who meet acceptable standards of competency and can provide the names and locations of local members.

American Association of Naturopathic Physicians
8201 Greensboro Drive, Suite 300
McLean, Virginia 22101
(703) 610-9037
Website: www.naturopathic.org

Provides a directory of physicians and offers referrals to a nationwide network of accredited or licensed practitioners. Also publishes a quarterly newsletter, and offers a series of brochures and pamphlets on a variety of subjects.

American College for Advancement in Medicine
23121 Verdugo Drive, Suite 204
Laguna Hills, California 92653
(800) 532-3688
Website: www.acam.org

ACAM provides a directory of physicians worldwide trained in nutritional and preventative medicine as well as an extensive list of books and articles on nutritional supplementation.

Ayurvedic & Naturopathic Medical Clinic
2115 112th Avenue N.E.
Bellevue, Washington 98004
(425) 453-8022
Website: www.ayurvedicscience.com

Dr. Virender Sodhi's clinic provides medical training for physicians and health-care practitioners, as well as individual courses for laypeople.

International Society for Orthomolecular Medicine (ISOM)
16 Florence Avenue
Toronto, Ontario, Canada M2N 1E9
(416) 733-2117
Website: www.orthomed.org

The ISOM seeks to further the advancement of and raise awareness about orthomolecular medicine throughout the world, through publications, conferences, and seminars.

Recommended Reading

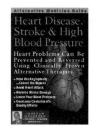

Alternative Medicine Guide to Heart Disease, Stroke & High Blood Pressure. Burton Goldberg and the Editors of *Alternative Medicine.* Tiburon, CA: Future Medicine Publishing, 1998.

Choices for a Healthy Heart. Joseph C. Piscatelli. New York: Workman, 1987.

Control High Blood Pressure Without Drugs. Robert L. Rowan, M.D., with Constance Schrader. New York: Fireside, 2001.

Dr. Dean Ornish's Program for Reversing Heart Disease. Dean Ornish, M.D. New York: Ivy Books, 1996.

High Blood Pressure Solution: Natural Prevention and Cure with the K Factor. Richard Moore, M.D., Ph.D. Rochester, VT: Healing Arts Press, 1993.

Overcoming Hypertension. Kenneth Cooper, M.D., M.P.H. New York: Bantam, 1991.

The Relaxation Response. Herbert Benson, M.D., with Miriam Z. Klipper. New York: Wholecare, 2000.

Reversing Hypertension. Julian Whitaker, M.D. New York: Warner, 2000.

Stress Management. James S. Gordon, M.D. New York: Chelsea House, 2000.

MEN'S HEALTH

Normal function of the male genitourinary tract is essential to the overall health of a man's body. Because this system is susceptible to a number of conditions and disorders, special attention must be paid to its health in order to maintain healthy sexual function, proper elimination, and general vitality.

STATISTICALLY, MEN experience higher rates of heart disease, cancer, chronic lung disorders, liver diseases, and diabetes than women, all of which contribute to an average life expectancy seven years less than women. These conditions, however, are not unique to men. Therefore, when a person thinks of men's health, the focus is primarily on disorders of their genitourinary organs. Because the genitourinary tracts of men and women are distinct, each requires its own specific set of health requirements.

Women's health issues have been well publicized and discussed with relative openness. Men's health issues, on the other hand, are just beginning to be seen as equally important. This is partly due to men in general, who traditionally have been less likely to seek medical attention than women, especially for minor problems, which often serve as warning signs for more serious underlying illness. The result is higher mortality rates resulting from the advanced state of the illness when it is eventually discovered. Social and economic pressures, as well as a lack of understanding of what constitutes normal function, also contribute to men's ambivalence in issues of health.

Types of Men's Health Disorders

The health of the genitourinary organs reflects a man's overall well-being, according to Dana Ullman, M.P.H., Director of Homeopathic Educational Services, in Berkeley, California. Individual sexual habits can also influence

It is estimated that 10-30 million men in the U.S. are experiencing some form of impotence, of which only about 200,000 per year seek medical help.

—TOM KRUZEL, N.D.

a person's state of health, just as the health of the body and the reproductive system can be a determining factor for sexual habits and sexual drive. The most common men's health concerns include impotence, benign prostatic hypertrophy (BPH), prostatitis, and prostate cancer.

Impotence

Impotence is defined as the inability to sustain a satisfactory erection to perform intercourse and ejaculation. "It is estimated that 10-30 million men in the United States are experiencing some form of impotence, of which only about 200,000 per year seek medical help," states Tom Kruzel, N.D., of Scottsdale, Arizona. Although impotence has long been associated with aging, Dr. Kruzel points out that growing older is not necessarily an inevitable cause. "Rather, the amount and force of ejaculation decreases, while the recovery period between ejaculations becomes longer," he says. "This varies from person to person, depending on their overall health and vitality."

There are two forms of impotence, primary and secondary. "Primary impotence is rare and is almost always associated with severe psychopathology," says Dr. Kruzel. "This may include unreasonable fear of engaging in intercourse, fear of intimacy, or extreme feelings of guilt or anxiety about the act of intercourse. Low male sex hormone levels can also be a cause." In cases of primary impotence, men are unable to engage in sexual intercourse.

Secondary impotence is the more common type of impotence and Dr. Kruzel estimates that it is related to psychological causes about 80% of the time. "Men who suffer from secondary impotence are only able to engage in intercourse 25% of the time," he says. "This is most often situational in nature, as the person may have become bored with the relationship or the place and time may be less than optimal. Emotional factors such as low self-esteem, immaturity, performance anxiety, and depression can also play a role."

By age 50, about 30% of men will start to experience difficulties with urination related to enlargement of the prostate gland.

—Tom Kruzel, N.D.

One way of evaluating the cause of impotence is to evaluate whether or not an erection occurs while sleeping, which generally happens during REM (rapid eye movement) sleep. The usual method of doing this is called the "stamp test," which involves placing a ring of paper around the penis prior to bedtime. If the ring has been disrupted in the morning, the man has experienced an erection at some time during the night. This indicates that the cause of impotence is most likely due to psychological factors rather than to physical causes.

Illness, such as diabetes and heart disease, can contribute to impotence, according to Dr. Kruzel, as can certain endocrine disorders such as hypothyroidism and hypopituitarism. Vascular diseases can play a role due to their effects on the vessels of the penis. Neurological disorders from injury or brain disease (Parkinson's disease or multiple sclerosis) have also been found to be causes, as have the various surgeries of the genitalia. Medications (antihypertensives, antidepressants, and psychotropics) may cause impotence, especially in elderly men taking multiple prescription drugs. Other causes of impotence include low levels of testosterone, zinc deficiency, high cholesterol, and alcohol or drug addiction.[1]

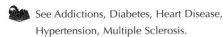 See Addictions, Diabetes, Heart Disease, Hypertension, Multiple Sclerosis.

Benign Prostatic Hypertrophy

According to Dr. Kruzel, by the age of 50, about 30% of men will start to experience difficulties with urination related to enlargement of the prostate gland or benign prostatic hypertrophy (BPH). Increases in the number of times a man has to urinate, along with a frequent sensation of having to urinate (especially at night), are among some of the early signs. In addition, a reduction in the

---

THE PROSTATE GLAND'S RELATIONSHIP TO HEALTH

The prostate gland lies at the base of the bladder, surrounding the urethra, and weighs less than an ounce. The size of a walnut, it is bordered by the rectum, bladder, pubic bone, and pelvic muscles. Its purpose is to secrete substances that protect or enhance the functional properties of sperm cells and to provide a fluid support system for the sperm cells. It does this by secreting a thin, milky alkaline fluid during ejaculation to enhance delivery and fertility of the sperm. In addition, the prostate acts as the genitourinary system's first line of defense against infection and disease.

Prostate fluid consists of zinc (in the male body, the prostate has the highest concentration of this mineral and zinc may be largely responsible for the prostate's ability to defend against infection and disease), citric acid, potassium, fructose, prostaglandins, proteolytic enzymes, prostate specific antigen (PSA), and acid phosphatase. Levels of these last two substances, when elevated, are considered reliable indicators of prostate cancer.

Some of the more common problems associated with the prostate are benign prostatic hypertrophy (BPH), prostatitis, and prostate cancer. All of these conditions are greatly influenced and accelerated by the aging process and therefore need to be monitored regularly, especially as men move through middle age into older age.

---

force and caliber of urination is also characteristic of prostatic enlargement. Instability of the detrusor muscle (the outer muscle layer of the bladder) can even result in urinary incontinence. "This occurs in up to 3% of patients with BPH," Dr. Kruzel says. "These symptoms often lead to an increased sense of frustration and embarrassment, as well as the disruption of normal activities."

Enlargement of the prostate is usually caused by an abnormal overgrowth or swelling of the tissue of the prostate, which then blocks the urethra (opening from the bladder). Problems associated with this condition usually continue to worsen with age, increasing in incidence to about 50% of all men by the age of 60 and up to 80% past age 70.[2] Most physicians consider this to be a normal consequence of aging.

The growth of prostate tissue that results in BPH occurs due to the hormone testosterone, which is produced by the testicles and the adrenal glands, according to Dr. Kruzel. As a person ages, the conversion of testosterone to its more active form of dihydrotestosterone (DHT) becomes greater. "The more active DHT results in a greater growth of tissues in the prostate gland, which ultimately leads to the obstruction of the urethra which passes through it," Dr. Kruzel explains.

The increased uptake of testosterone by the prostate appears to be related to the amount of another hormone called prolactin, secreted by the pituitary gland in the brain. Prolactin also increases the activity of the enzyme responsible for converting testosterone to DHT. Research indicates that both emotional stress and alcohol (especially beer) result in higher prolactin levels. As a result, prolonged periods of emotional stress or ongoing alcohol consumption may play a significant role in BPH.[3]

Chronic constipation has been implicated as a contributing factor to prostatic discomfort when there is an already enlarged gland. A correction of the constipation will bring some symptom relief, since the rectum puts pressure on the prostate gland when it is enlarged. In addition, there is a buildup of waste products in the circulation with chronic constipation, which will indirectly have an effect on the function of the prostate.

"BPH is merely prostate cancer waiting for a place to happen," according to Jeffrey L. Marrongelle, D.C., C.C.N., of Schuylkill Haven, Pennsylvania. "It almost always evolves into cancer, given enough time." The reason for this, Dr. Marrongelle says, is that, immunologically, there is only a quantitative difference between BPH and prostate cancer. "It's a continuum of stress on the prostate gland until the tissue generates into abnormal tissue and cancer begins," he adds.

BPH is merely prostate cancer waiting for a place to happen. It almost always evolves into cancer, given enough time.

—JEFFREY L. MARRONGELLE, D.C., C.C.N.

In Dr. Marrongelle's view, one of the primary factors that drives the prostate gland along the continuum of inflammation to enlargement to cancer is stress, which can occur in many forms—emotional, nutritional, toxic (environmental), lifestyle, and career. Since stress, over time, wears down the immune system, vulnerable organs like the prostate absorb the consequences of an overly stressful life. "When you're always stressed and don't pay

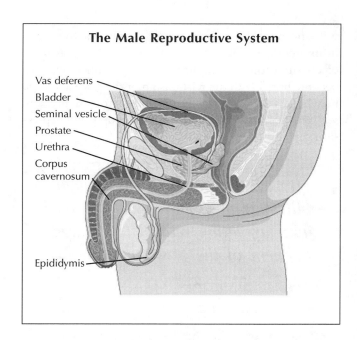

The Male Reproductive System

Vas deferens
Bladder
Seminal vesicle
Prostate
Urethra
Corpus cavernosum
Epididymis

attention to the 'stop signs' and 'red lights' in your life, but keep pushing yourself, you're going to compromise your immune and endocrine systems and stress your adrenal glands, testes, and prostate, setting yourself up for disease," Dr. Marrongelle explains.

Prostatitis

Prostatitis is an inflammation or infection of the prostate gland, most often seen in men between the ages of 20 and 50. It is commonly viewed as being due to an infective agent such as a bacteria or *Chlamydia* (an intracellular parasite transmitted through sexual contact). Bacteria in the urine, which passes through the urethra, can settle in the prostate. Noninfective forms of prostatitis are also recognized and may be associated with autoimmune disorders.[4] Several researchers have suggested that infective agents may not be the cause of the condition but instead are acting opportunistically upon a depleted glandular environment.[5]

Depletion of glandular elements such as zinc, ascorbic acid (vitamin C), and proteolytic enzymes make it easier for an infection to occur, according to Dr. Kruzel. Prostatitis can also follow increased amounts of sexual activity, particularly with multiple partners, which depletes the prostate of enzymes and zinc needed to sterilize the urethra and protect the gland from infection and introduces additional bacteriological factors. (It is advised that all sexual activity, including masturbation, be eliminated during infection in order to allow the prostate to renew itself and to keep the infection from spreading further.) Excess caffeine, alcohol, and spicy foods may contribute to a lack of glandular nutrition, which ultimately adds to depletion of the prostate and lowered immune function.[6]

Symptoms of prostatitis include difficulty, frequency, and urgency during urination, along with a burning sensation or pain, and a discharge from the penis after bowel movements. These symptoms can range from mild to severe, and come and go over time, with the prostate gland being susceptible to both acute and chronic infection or inflammation. According to Dr. Kruzel, an acute condition is often signaled by severe pain and tenderness in the region of the prostate, sometimes extending up into the genitals, pelvis, and back. Fever, chills, and overall fatigue can also follow.

Symptoms of a chronic condition are similar, but milder. Often, these symptoms will be disregarded and treatment will be delayed or foregone completely. If the condition is caused by an infection that is untreated or unrecognized, it may result in the infection of the sex partner as well and can lead to more severe complications, such as a kidney infection, epididymitis (an inflammation of the epididymis, a tube along the backside of the testicles), and orchitis (a painful swelling of the testicles). Bladder obstruction and prostate stones may also occur if chronic prostatitis is allowed to persist untreated.

Prostate Cancer

Cancer of the prostate is responsible for 35,000 deaths every year in the U.S., with an additional 165,000 men developing the disease in the same period.[7] It is the most commonly found cancer in males over 50 and is the second most common cancer afflicting men. The highest incidence is found in African-American males, who are 40% more likely to be stricken with the disease.[8] A study by the American Urological Association showed the incidence of precancerous prostate gland lesions to range from 22% to 41% in men between the ages of 30 and 49.[9] "This suggests that cancer of the prostate is more prevalent than previously thought," Dr. Kruzel says.

Cancer of the prostate is responsible for 35,000 deaths every year in the U.S., with an additional 165,000 men developing the disease in the same period.

About 20% of enlarged prostates are the result of cancer, but 80% of these cancers either do not metastasize or are of the slow-growing variety, often causing little if any problem.[10] The remaining forms spread more rapidly, primarily to the bones of the spine and lymph nodes of the pelvis. "One of the problems with cancer

---

DRUGS ASSOCIATED WITH A HIGHER INCIDENCE OF IMPOTENCE

According to the *Physicians' Desk Reference*, the following drugs are associated with side effects of impotence (statistics refer to the percentage of individuals affected).[15]

Anafranil capsules (up to 20%)

Lupron Depot 3.75 mg (among most frequent)

Lupron injection (5% or more)

Normodyne injection, tablets (up to 4%)

Paxil tablets (1.9%-10.0%)

Proscar tablets (3.7%)

Roferon-A injection (6%)

Wellbutrin tablets (3.4%)

---

of the prostate is that it may be present without any detectable symptoms or with symptoms identical to those found in BPH," Dr. Kruzel explains. "Few of the classic cancer symptoms of weight loss, blood in the urine, urinary retention, pain, or the swelling of tissues (due to the accumulation of lymph) are present early in the disease and may not show up at all until metastasis has occurred. This can lead to its continued growth and subsequent spread throughout the body."

The precise cause of prostate cancer is unknown. Genetic factors seem to play a role—there are more occurrences in some families than in others, with African-American men showing a greater incidence than other ethnic groups. Hormonal factors may also affect the prostate as early as puberty by delaying sexual development and maturity. Persons who enter puberty later seem to have higher incidences of prostate cancer, probably due to that late development, according to Dr. Kruzel. Hormone levels certainly influence the course of cancer once it has become established. According to Dr. Kruzel, higher incidences of cancer found as the male population ages are related to the change in hormone levels, from testosterone to the more active DHT, that is normally part of the aging process.

 See Cancer, Natural Hormone Replacement Therapy.

Several studies indicate that men who undergo a vasectomy have an increased risk of developing prostate and testicular cancers.[11] This may be due to the production of allosperm antibodies, which are formed following the procedure; these antibodies lower immune

THE DANGERS OF VIAGRA

Since receiving approval by the U.S. Food and Drug Administration (FDA) as a treatment for impotence, Viagra® (sildenafil) has become one of the most popular—and publicized—drugs in recent history. In 1998, the first year of its availability, more than 1,000,000 prescriptions for Viagra were written in the U.S.

Viagra is said to work by relaxing the muscles that line the arteries of the penis. This increases the flow of blood into the corpus cavernosum, the spongy tissue that makes up the penile shaft. Estimates are that Viagra works between 60% and 90% of the time and it is most effective as a treatment for milder forms of impotence, or erectile dysfunction, caused either by psychological factors or side effects from other medications.

Despite its benefits for impotence, Viagra is not without its risks. During the first six months following its launch, a number of men died while taking the drug, although Viagra itself was never conclusively found to be the cause of their deaths. Even so, though the FDA continues to approve the sale of Viagra, it was banned in a number of other countries, including Canada, Japan, Australia, and Israel, once the deaths were reported.

Viagra is not appropriate for patients with heart disease who are taking nitroglycerin or other nitrate-based drugs, since the combination of Viagra with such drugs can lead to dangerously low blood pressure levels. In addition, Viagra can cause a number of other side effects, including abnormal vision, diarrhea, indigestion, severe headaches, and urinary tract infections. For these reasons, alternative physicians choose to treat impotence and other men's health conditions using safer, more natural methods.[16]

Treatment and Prevention of Men's Disorders

Conventional Western medicine tends to view all genitourinary disorders as conditions that can be treated solely with medication, surgery, or medical devices. Alternative physicians, by contrast, look at the underlying causes, whether physical or mental, internal or external. This approach can result in a more pronounced and longer lasting improvement in overall health. Some of the alternative modalities most often used in the treatment of men's health issues include diet and nutrition, herbal medicine, homeopathy, natural hormone thereapy, acupuncture, traditional Chinese medicine, and Ayurvedic medicine.

 See Diet, Herbal Medicine, Homeopathy, Nutritional Medicine.

Diet and Nutrition

"Poor nutrition is a primary cause of most conditions of the genitourinary tract," Dr. Kruzel states. "A good diet and nutritional program is a must for normal function. An avoidance of spicy foods, caffeine, alcohol, tobacco, and foods high in fat and carbohydrates is also imperative to the treatment of any disease of the prostate, as these factors can serve as irritants, negating the effects of essential nutrients such as vitamin C, vitamin E, and zinc." Supplementation of these nutrients is crucial for treating any prostate disorders as they are among the more prominent elements found in prostate tissues. These nutrients are also necessary for the formation of seminal fluid.[17]

Vitamin C is a major component of the seminal vesicles and prostate gland and high amounts are found in prostatic secretions. Vitamin E is also present and acts as an antioxidant, stabilizing membranes and lipids. Zinc has long been used in the treatment of prostate disease because of its prominent role in the metabolism of prostate tissue as well as its sterilizing effect, which keeps the gland and urethra free of microorganisms.

A general vitamin and mineral supplementation routine is beneficial, especially one high in B vitamins and magnesium. In numerous studies, magnesium has been shown to be an important nutrient that is deficient in most people. Garlic in its natural clove form can also help supply the body with vitamins and minerals and, most importantly, help to prevent infection.

Essential fatty acids, such as fish oils, olive oil, evening primrose oil, and eicosapentaenoic acid (EPA), are also needed in large amounts by the prostate gland. These become especially important if there is a high level of

response and the body's subsequent ability to destroy cancerous cells.[12]

It has also been noted that there are higher rates of prostate cancer (as well as other cancers) in men who are exposed to chemical toxins. Workers in the petrochemical, rubber, and textile industries have among the highest cancer rates for industrial employees.[13] Urban areas have higher incidences of prostate cancer, which is thought to be due to pollution.[14]

SUCCESS STORY: RESOLVING IMPOTENCE HOLISTICALLY

According to Michael Borkin, D.C., N.M.D., of Westlake Village, California, impotence is generally due to a combination of psychological and physiological factors, all of which must be addressed for the problem to be resolved. Dr. Borkin's holistic treatment approach is illustrated by the following case history.

Rupert, 50, a stomach cancer patient recovering from surgery, chemotherapy, and radiation, complained of loss of libido and erections that were "terribly painful," the few times he was able to achieve them. "Rupert's cancer and cancer treatment had exerted great trauma on every system of his body, including low back pain, digestive malabsorption, and a compromised gastrointestinal tract, in addition to his impotence and erection problems," Dr. Borkin reports.

Dr. Borkin began Rupert's treatment using chiropractic, along with a supplementation program using nutrients, herbs, and natural hormone therapy. He also employed magnetic field therapy to help redirect energy flow through Rupert's pelvic region and homeopathic remedies to stimulate the drainage of toxins caused by the chemotherapy and radiation treatments. Chiropractic adjustments were necessary in Rupert's case because his stomach cancer and resultant surgery had compromised the integrity of his abdominal muscles, causing his back to go out of alignment," Dr. Borkin explains. "My goal was to realign lumbar vertebrae, particularly lumbar-5, which is associated with the nerve supply to the reproductive organs. When nerve transmission is blocked by a misaligned vertebra, this essentially turns off the message from the brain to the penis." Dr. Borkin prescribed several nutrients for Rupert:

- Zinc, to bolster immune response and sexual function
- Manganese, essential for healthy sexual function
- Niacin (vitamin B3), to improve circulation
- Lipoic acid, which acts as an antioxidant
- Trace minerals, to provide foundational support for the other nutrients
- Saw palmetto, which helps oppose the unhealthy influences of estrogen on prostate tissues
- Prostate PMG and Orchex, to supply the genetic blueprint that directs nutrients to the prostate and testes

Within two weeks, Rupert was able to experience painless erections and soon thereafter his libido also began to increase. However, Rupert and his wife had become physically estranged and emotionally aloof. When Rupert explained the problem to his oncologist, he was put on Paxil, an antidepressant. "Using Paxil when you already have a libido problem is counterproductive," Dr. Borkin says. "Rupert didn't know that one of the side effects of Paxil is loss of libido, so taking it only compounded his problem." Dr. Borkin, in consultation with Rupert's oncologist, took him off Paxil, then began phase two of Rupert's treatment. This entailed dietary changes and gastrointestinal refortification, Neuro-Emotional Sensory Training (NEST), natural hormone replacement, exercise, and marriage counseling.

Since chemotherapy had ravaged Rupert's beneficial intestinal flora, allowing pathogenic bacteria to proliferate, Dr. Borkin prescribed acidophilus to recolonize the intestines and improve nutrient absorption and waste elimination. He prescribed a combination of hydrochloric acid and pancreatic enzymes and eliminated all dairy products (except butter) from Rupert's diet after determining he was allergic to them. Using a saliva test, Dr. Borkin determined that Rupert had high levels of cortisol and low levels of DHEA, caused by the cumulative effects of long-term stress. "Chronic stress, in which adrenaline and cortisol are constantly released, begins to affect the endocrine system and reproductive organs," Dr. Borkin says. To help rebalance Rupert's hormones and emotions, he prescribed Libidex Creme, a natural transdermal endocrine cream.

NEST, a combination of chiropractic and emotional release work, was used. "When a strong emotion becomes a physiological event, such as discomfort in the solar plexus, it creates a negative feedback mechanism that can continue indefinitely," Dr. Borkin says. The goal of NEST is to interfere with this unhealthy loop, undo energy blockages in the body, and restore healthy communication between the brain and the rest of the body. The combination of approaches, along with exercise (swimming three times a week) and marriage counseling, resulted in a 95% improvement in Rupert's impotence problems and overall health.

sexual activity, which can deplete the prostate of nutrients needed for normal function. They can also act to reduce blood clotting associated with prostate cancer, thus lowering the potential for the spreading of tumors.[18]

Glandular therapy has proven to be effective in the treatment of disorders of the prostate gland. Extracts of bovine (cattle) or porcine (pig) prostatic tissue taken orally or administered intramuscularly provides essential nutrients and growth factors to the gland. This is often coupled with other nutritional or herbal medicines. Several researchers have also speculated that the prostate gland may be susceptible to autoimmune diseases. Glandular therapy may provide a protective function against circulating autoantibodies due to the similarity of their cellular structures.[19]

In addition, Dr. Marrongelle recommends Wobenzyme, a German enzyme formula that can help reduce inflammation of prostate tissue, and colostrum, which is high in immunoglobulins (specialized immune defense proteins) that protect against infections. Alternative physicians also recommend that men drink pure, filtered water in place of tap water, as the water supply of many municipalities has been shown to contain heavy metals and pesticide residues. Such contaminants tend to settle in the body's fatty tissues, found in high concentrations in the prostate gland.

Herbal Medicine

Herbal medicine can offer many of the same therapeutic benefits for treatment of genitourinary tract disorders as drug therapy, without any of the potentially severe side effects. Herbal medications need to be specific to the individual condition in order for them to be most effective, according to Dr. Kruzel, and should always be taken under the guidance of a trained health practitioner to ensure maximum result.

Impotence: *Corynanthe yohimbe* and *Ginkgo biloba* are often used for the treatment of impotence due to their ability to stimulate vascular flow to the penis. Yohimbe has also been shown to increase libido and decrease the latency period between ejaculations, as well as have a positive effect on impotence problems due to depression.[20] Several studies have confirmed the beneficial action of ginkgo, including one in which a *Ginkgo biloba* extract was found to increase penile blood flow in a group of patients who had not responded to traditional drug therapy; half the group regained potency within six months.[21]

True unicorn root *(Aletris farinosa)* has been reported to be an excellent herb for impotence in men and has been used to promote fertility in both men and women.[22] Also, saw palmetto *(Serenoa repens)* works well for impotence, especially if included with other medicines. *Strych-*

nos nux-vomica is used for the treatment of sexual dysfunction, especially if it is caused by an excess of alcohol, cigarettes, or dietary indiscretions. Since it contains small amounts of strychnine alkaloids, it can be toxic if taken improperly and is only available through physicians trained in its use. It can also be used in a homeopathic dose with equal or better effect.[23]

Additionally, Siberian ginseng *(Eleutherococcus senticosus)* is widely believed to have aphrodisiac properties for which it has been prized over the centuries. Known as an adaptogen, it affects whichever system of the body may be in need of support. Its American counterpart, *Panax quinquefolius,* does not possess quite the stimulating properties, but is safer to use over the long term.[24]

Benign Prostatic Hypertrophy: Saw palmetto berries contain about 15% saturated and unsaturated fatty acids and sterols that have been found to reduce prostate swelling, stimulate immune function, and prevent the conversion of testosterone to its more potent DHT form. When used in clinical trials, saw palmetto has been shown to result in a significant decrease in prostate size and relief of symptoms.[25]

The powdered bark of the *Pygeum africanus* tree has also been used for centuries as a treatment for urinary disorders. Scientists in France who isolated its active compounds concluded that the herbal preparation was antiinflammatory, reduced swelling, and lowered cholesterol. Studies have clearly shown this herb to promote the regression of symptoms associated with BPH with no toxic side effects observed, even at large doses and with prolonged use.[26] Another herb indicated for problems associated with prostatic hypertrophy is true unicorn root *(Aletris farinosa)*.[27]

A 68-year-old man complaining of blood in his urine, difficulty with urination, decreased urinary flow, slight urgency, and a full sensation in his rectum was diagnosed as having an enlarged prostate gland and a bladder stone. The patient was started on saw palmetto extract, glandular extracts of animal prostate, and a combination of herbal medicines, which included *Pygeum africanus,* horsetail, and cornsilk, to reduce the size of the bladder stone. Within ten days, the patient reported a decrease in visible blood with urination, an increase in urinary flow, and a decrease in the sensation in his rectum. Microscopic examination of the urine three months later was normal and the patient was placed on a low dose of saw palmetto to prevent further problems. According to Dr. Kruzel, this case is typical of patient response to treatment for an enlarged prostate gland or bladder or kidney stone.

Prostatitis: *Chimaphila umbellata,* or pipsissewa, is an evergreen plant used in the treatment of urinary tract disorders. It is especially useful for the treatment of chronic prostatitis, as well as kidney and bladder stones. It contains arbutin, the active ingredient in uva ursi, a powerful urinary tract antiseptic that helps provide the urinary tract and prostate with increased blood flow and nutrition.[28] Horsetail is an excellent herbal medicine in the treatment of acute prostate infection. It is also indicated for urinary problems due to inflammation of the bladder or prostate and can be used for the treatment of bladder and kidney stones as well.[29]

Purple coneflower *(Echinacea angustifolia)* is a powerful herbal antimicrobial agent that can be used against any infective process, including prostatitis.[30] The herbs *Delphinia staphysagria,* Oriental thuja *(Thuja occidentalis),* and pulsatilla *(Anemone pulsatilla)* are also indicated for inflammation of the prostate gland. These herbal agents act to decrease pain, bladder irritation, swelling, and impotence associated with prostatitis, according to Dr. Kruzel.

Prostate Cancer: Numerous herbal formulas are available for the treatment of cancer of the prostate. In general, herbal medicines are not specific for the different types of tumors encountered but rather act as an overall immune system stimulant. "Herbal medications perform a variety of functions when attacking cancerous tissue," Dr. Kruzel says. "They act to stimulate production and activation of T and B lymphocytes (white blood cells). Additionally, herbal preparations will adhere to the tumor cell surface, making it easier for the lymphocytes to attach and destroy the cell. Certain components of herbal medicines will also enter the tumor cell to disrupt its function, making it more vulnerable to destruction by the immune system."

CAUTION Consult your physician immediately if you suspect you may have cancer.

Saw palmetto and *Pygeum africanus*—because of their ability to inhibit testosterone conversion, decrease swelling, and provide increased blood flow to the prostate—are essential parts of any herbal medicine program for prostate cancer. Less specific but equally important is the use of medicines such as pokeroot *(Phytolacca decandra),* periwinkle *(Vinca rosea),* mistletoe *(Viscum album),* colchicine *(Colchicum autumnale),* hemlock *(Conium maculatum), Berberis aquifolium, Echinacea angustifolia,* foxglove *(Digitalis purpurea),* and burdock *(Arctium lappa).*[31] These herbs have been found to effectively help treat cancer of the prostate and, when used along with a holistic therapy program, have as good as, or better, survival rates than conventional therapy, Dr. Kruzel states.

For a 69-year-old man diagnosed with prostate cancer, the immediate surgical removal of his testicles and prostate was recommended, as well as a course of chemotherapy. Dr. Kruzel placed him on saw palmetto

extract, Hoxsey formula (an herbal formula, developed by the late Harry Hoxsey, N.D., used to treat cancer), plus mistletoe, pokeroot, and high doses of vitamins C and E. He was also given the homeopathic remedy *Lycopodium* and had already changed to a primarily vegetarian diet.

"Over the next six months, the tumor size was monitored by the prostate specific antigen (PSA) test and rectal ultrasound," Dr. Kruzel recounts. "Within the first 60 days, the PSA dropped from a high reading of 4.5 to 3.0 (a normal reading is 0.5-4.0), but there was no change noted on ultrasound. By the end of the six-month period, the tumor had decreased in size upon ultrasound examination and the PSA level had decreased to 2.6." According to Dr. Kruzel, this patient will be kept on immune-stimulating herbs and saw palmetto extract until the tumor disappears completely. It is his view that the patient has a very good prognosis as long as he continues to follow the dietary, herbal medicine, and vitamin recommendations.

Homeopathy

By itself, homeopathy may work for a wide variety of urological conditions. It is often combined with other treatments, such as herbal medicines and nutrition, to increase the healing action of the remedy and the degree of healing experienced. Homeopathic remedies may work extremely well for problems of impotence, especially if the condition is due to psychological causes. Numerous homeopathic medications are also available for the treatment (both short-term and long-term) of BPH.

According to Dr. Kruzel, severe urethral obstructions that require catheterization respond well to homeopathic treatment. A number of his patients reported a change in the indwelling catheter diameter during the course of homeopathic therapy as the prostate gland reduced in size. "Initial reduction in size occurred within the first week to ten days of therapy," he reports. "Ultimately, the patients were able to urinate without them as normal urinary function returned over the next 6-8 weeks."

Homeopathy has been used to treat all forms of prostatitis and works especially well with chronic prostatitis that has been unresponsive to conventional antibiotic treatment. "The patient may have experienced prolonged discomfort, sometimes lasting for years, because the condition was incompletely treated initially," Dr. Kruzel says.

Dr. Kruzel treated a 38-year-old man with severe pains in his hips, thighs, testicles, and prostate gland. His condition had been diagnosed 12 years earlier as gonococcal urethritis and was treated with antibiotics. Almost immediately after the disappearance of the discharge, the pains began in his hips and thighs. He received several courses of antibiotics over a three-year period, which did nothing to relieve his symptoms. He was later diagnosed by a rheumatologist as having arthritis and placed on nonsteroidal, anti-inflammatory drugs. Dr. Kruzel started him on homeopathic *Berberis* 30C; at his one-month follow-up, the man reported that he was about 60% better. After three months on the homeopathic medication, he was completely pain free and no longer taking the arthritis medicine.

Dr. Marrongelle has had good success treating prostate conditions using combinations of homeopathically prepared substances that encourage the flushing of toxins, including heavy metals, fungi, and yeast, from the body and help relieve the lymphatic system of congested debris.

Natural Hormone Replacement Therapy

Testosterone replacement can heighten sex drive, increase bone density, and improve mood, among other effects. When considering testosterone replacement, the first step is a blood or saliva test to assess levels of the hormone, according to Julian Whitaker, M.D., a nationally recognized alternative medicine educator and editor of *Health and Healing*. If levels are low or even average for your age, testosterone therapy can help alleviate deficiency symptoms and improve overall health, he explains.

The goal of testosterone therapy is to restore blood testosterone levels to those of a healthy man, 25-30 years old. For this, Dr. Whitaker recommends weekly injections of testosterone cypionate (100 mg) or biweekly injections of testosterone enanthate (200 mg). These long-acting versions of the hormone are considered the safest and most effective preparations for use in testosterone replacement. As injection guarantees consistent absorption, Dr. Whitaker considers this to be the preferred method of testosterone supplementation.

Skin patches and oral lozenges can also be effective, he reports; however, he advises against oral testosterone in pill form. "With oral testosterone, there is a potential for liver dysfunction and a decrease in protective 'good' cholesterol levels," he cautions. Further positive effects of testosterone replacement include increased lean muscle mass and protection for the heart, as certain forms of testosterone can lower cholesterol levels.

As an accompaniment to testosterone therapy, Dr. Whitaker generally suggests taking the herb saw palmetto (120-360 mg daily), which has been shown to reduce the conversion of testosterone into dihydrotestosterone (DHT). Too much DHT has been linked to various health problems, including prostate cancer.

 Men who supplement with testosterone should closely monitor their prostate specific antigen (PSA) levels, as excess testosterone has been linked to prostate cancer. Other possible side effects include testicular atrophy, male pattern baldness, elevated red blood cell counts, elevated blood pressure, and gynecomastia (abnormally large mammary glands in men). Dr. Borkin recommends the use of transdermal DHEA and androstenedione, since these hormones can convert to testosterone with less likelihood of causing side effects.

Another option employed by Dr. Borkin to maintain adequate testosterone levels is to stop the misappropriation of testosterone while also supplying the necessary building blocks for the production of testosterone. This can be achieved by using transdermal testosterone cream applied to the skin, while also supporting the endocrine system. The typical daily dosage is ⅛ to ½ teaspoon, depending on weight and age, applied to areas of soft skin, preferably upon rising in the morning.

Traditional Chinese Medicine

Disorders of the genitourinary tract are commonly regarded by practitioners of traditional Chinese medicine (TCM) as a combination of disease symptoms and the effects of the patient's lifestyle. A patient is always evaluated for constitutional state, *qi* (vital life energy), and nutritional status. The causes of the condition are viewed as either internal (psychological causes or internal organ disharmony) or external (physical causes such as spicy foods, alcohol, or drug use). The person is then diagnosed as being either *yin* or *yang,* hot or cold, possessing dampness or moisture, hot or dry.

Prostatitis and urethritis are generally viewed as conditions of damp heat by TCM practitioners. Herbal medicines that promote the removal of dampness and excess water, such as *polyporus, akebia,* or *cephalanoplos,* and *Dianthus* formulas with their potent herbal combinations, may be used to treat these conditions, according to Dr. Kruzel.

"Impotence, along with premature ejaculation, is seen by TCM primarily as a functional disorder, with stress and nutritional indiscretions being the main contributors," Dr. Kruzel says. "Impotence due to low hormone output is considered a deficiency of kidney *yang,* while premature ejaculation is considered a deficiency of the kidney storage vessel."

Herbal medications such as Siberian ginseng *(Eleutherococcus senticosus),* which enhances blood flow, is considered superior by many TCM physicians in the treatment of impotence.[32] This is not to be confused with its counterpart *Panax ginseng,* which has long been prized as an aphrodisiac. "Many herbalists and physicians consider *Panax* too stimulating for long-term use as it tends to burn out the kidney fire," Dr. Kruzel says. "Lycium berries, which are specific for enhancement of kidney and liver *qi*, are used as a *yin* tonic for sexual dysfunction." Herbs such as cascara sagrada and lotus seed have also been found to enhance sexual function and eliminate premature ejaculation.[33]

A number of acupuncture points (along the Conception Vessel channel) can be used with certain Spleen and Bladder points to increase energy or *qi* flow to the sexual organs. Treatments are usually done over a period of weeks and tend to have a cumulative effect, gradually restoring normal function.

Nocturia (frequency of urination at night) is one the most common symptoms seen with BPH and is treated with both acupuncture and herbal medicines. According to Rick Marinelli, N.D., M.Ac.O.M., of Beaverton, Oregon, BPH responds very well to acupuncture and TCM. A person may remain on herbal medication for several months as the gland recovers, but Dr. Marinelli usually sees some improvement within the first 3-6 weeks of treatment, especially if coupled with acupuncture. With chronic BPH, Dr. Marinelli sometimes suspects a low-grade inflammation of the prostate as well, often finding symptoms of burning, urgency, and fullness in the perineal area (the external region between the anus and the genitals). In these cases, he suggests a more aggressive treatment plan until the symptoms have resolved.

Similar to the Western medicine view, cancer of the prostate gland is seen as a silent disease in that it may be present without symptoms long before it is found. Yet, where conventional medicine tends to focus on the prostate tumor, TCM tends to focus on the symptom complex presented by the whole body. A treatment plan is therefore designed to address the deficient immune system, based on the symptom picture provided by the patient. The *Fu Zheng* treatment, which increases the body's energy flow, is used specifically to strengthen immune function.

In China, most hospitals have departments of both Western and traditional Chinese medicine, which combine their efforts in the treatment of cancer. According to both Drs. Kruzel and Marinelli, patients undergoing conventional treatments such as chemotherapy or radiation often tolerate them better if they are combined with TCM.

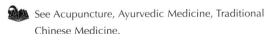 See Acupuncture, Ayurvedic Medicine, Traditional Chinese Medicine.

NATURAL PROGESTERONE AND MEN'S HEALTH CONDITIONS

Topical application of natural progesterone may prove beneficial in the treatment of prostate conditions. One doctor reports working with 12 men, all in their late seventies, who were suffering from osteoporosis. As it has been established that natural progesterone, applied topically, can relieve osteoporosis, the physician suggested that the men systematically massage it into their skin on a daily basis. All of them began to experience relief from their condition and, after three months of daily massage, they were also experiencing an improved urine flow, with less pressure on the prostate gland and a noticeable decrease in nightly urination. Each patient had been suffering from an enlarged prostate, but had not mentioned it in the original exam (simply attributing the condition to old age). Although this report is anecdotal, it suggests an area of research to determine exactly how natural progesterone can work to reverse prostate disorders.

Ayurvedic Medicine

According to Virender Sodhi, M.D. (Ayurveda), N.D., Director of the Ayurvedic and Naturopathic Medical Clinic, in Bellevue, Washington, Ayurvedic medicine can employ a number of herbal treatments to combat prostate problems, including *amla, triphala, neem,* and *shilajit.* Exercises such as the *ashiwin mudra,* which is the squeezing and relaxing of the anal sphincter, are also effective at helping relieve congestion and aiding circulation in the prostate, notes Dr. Sodhi.

Dr. Sodhi recalls treating a 65-year-old man who had been diagnosed with BPH five years before, but had not wanted to undergo surgery, so he sought out alternative therapy. "When he came to me, he was not able to urinate properly. A slow, feeble stream was all that was coming out," says Dr. Sodhi. "I had him practice the *ashiwin mudra* and gave him the herb *yashad bhasam,* as well as a combination of *shilajit* and zinc, plus other herbs such as *amla, triphala, ashwagandha,* and *bala.* We also did prostatic massage. Within three months, he was able to urinate properly and the prostate gland was softer and more gel-like, indicating significant improvement."

For prostatitis, Dr. Sodhi recommends three things:

- Changing sexual behavior if the infection is due to, or exacerbated by, sexual overstimulation.

PROSTATIC MASSAGE

Quite often, a buildup of pressure in the prostate can be due to lack of intercourse and ejaculation, according to Tom Kruzel, N.D., of Scottsdale, Arizona. "When this occurs, ejaculation through intercourse or masturbation is often recommended in order to relieve pressure," he notes. "In addition, prostatic massage is an effective therapy for relieving pressure due to prostate enlargement." The massage is normally administered by a physician, who inserts a gloved finger in the patient's rectum to massage the prostate directly.

Done weekly for the first few weeks until symptoms begin to abate, periodic treatments follow as needed to relieve pressure. Prostatic massage does not affect the cause of the enlargement, but will only relieve symptoms. Excessive pressure during the massage can also result in bleeding and soreness of the gland, Dr. Kruzel points out. "Prostatic massage is contraindicated in cases of prostatitis, as it may cause the spread of the infection to other parts of the body, and in cancer, as it may disrupt the integrity of the tumor, causing the cancer to migrate," he says.

• Increasing diuresis (flow of urine) so that the patient will urinate more frequently, thereby helping to rid the body of infection. This can be accomplished by drinking large amounts of water. The congestion can also be relieved with the help of the *ashiwin mudra* exercise and by soaking the testicles in cold water.

• Taking antibiotic herbs such as *neem* to help stop the infection. *Amla* and *shilajit* can be taken as supportive herbs as well.

When a 33-year-old male who had been treated unsuccessfully with antibiotics for his prostatitis came to see Dr. Sodhi, he immediately had the patient stop all sexual activity. "He was upset because his doctor had said he could have as much sexual activity as possible," Dr. Sodhi says. "I started him on berberine and *neem* as well as on zinc supplements. I also had him soak his testicles and do the *ashiwin mudra* exercises. Within three months, all symptoms of his prostatitis were gone."

Prostate cancer can be more difficult to treat, according to Dr. Sodhi, "because sometimes by the time it is diagnosed, it has already metastasized and spread to the spine or organs of the body." One of Dr. Sodhi's patients, an 80-year-old man, had been told he had only two months to live. "He didn't want to go through a lot of treatment because he felt he had lived a good life and if he only lived another couple months, that was okay," Dr. Sodhi recounts. "I prescribed an *amla* tonic, a preparation of *amla* and extracts of various herbs. I thought this was the best preparation for fighting the cancer and regenerating the immune system."

Dr. Sodhi then lost track of the man until two years later when he was lecturing in Phoenix, Arizona. "A man walked up to me and said, 'Dr. Sodhi, I don't know if you remember me, but I'm your patient who was diagnosed with prostate cancer and I'm still living and it's almost two years.'" The man had been reordering his prescription from Dr. Sodhi's office all this time. "I think the *amla* was very helpful to him," states Dr. Sodhi, "but I believe the man's mental attitude was equally as important, because he wasn't afraid of death or his cancer."

Prevention

Prevention is the best approach to maintaining the health of the male organs. "Considering the far-reaching effects problems of the genitourinary tract can have in terms of discomfort, the side effects of standard treatments, and the enormous costs that are brought to bear, not to mention quality of life, prevention of these disorders should be undertaken by all men, of all ages," says Dr. Kruzel. "Periodic examination coupled with a blood test for levels of prostate specific antigen (PSA) provide the best method of early detection for both BPH and cancer of the prostate. This should be coupled with a complete physical that includes a digital rectal examination."

It is recommended that males over the age of 40 receive yearly examinations for the presence of prostate enlargement and cancer. Reluctance to undergo examination on the part of many men often causes early treatment to be postponed, allowing the condition to become worse. It is only after symptoms become unbearable that many men seek treatment.

Early detection has become much simpler and more refined with the introduction of a few relatively noninvasive diagnostic procedures such as blood tests, digital rectal examination, urinalysis, and ultrasound. Rectal ultrasound for visualization of the tumor is beneficial when used with these other tests. Because the procedure is relatively new, it should be done by a physician experienced in the interpretation of ultrasound imaging.

Along with frequent examinations, there should be changes in dietary habits. Several studies have found that decreasing the consumption of sugar leads to lower levels of prostate cancer, and decreased incidences of cancer in general are found in cultures that have a lower intake of refined sugar.[34] High-fat diets, especially diets

MALE MENOPAUSE

As men enter midlife, levels of their male hormones, known as androgens, decline and can become unbalanced. When this occurs, a variety of symptoms begin to manifest, including fatigue, less endurance and muscle strength, loss of libido, weight gain (especially around the midriff), joint aches, sagging skin, and moments of depression, emotional malaise, insomnia, decreased short-term memory, irritability, mood swings, and even panic attacks. Such symptoms are indications of the andropause complex, also referred to as "male menopause," a diagnosis that is increasingly gaining acceptance among physicians.

According to Gary S. Ross, M.D., of San Francisco, California, the andropause complex of symptoms is usually noticeable by the time a man is in his fifties, although they may appear much earlier. All such symptoms are signs that a man's hormones, both in terms of their levels and their ratios to one another, are in a state of flux, shifting into a new, midlife configuration. "Hormone levels, especially of testosterone, start off high in puberty and peak throughout the teenage years," Dr. Ross says. "Then, as men pass the age of 30, they begin a slow drop, so gradual at first that most men don't notice it. But by the time they are 40, 45, or 50, they start experiencing the male menopause symptoms."

Declining hormone levels, and the resultant symptoms that can accompany them, are not inevitable, and may be slowed or reversed by a number of alternative therapies, including natural hormone replacement therapy and the use of glandular extracts. Other important approaches (often used in conjunction) include proper diet, appropriate nutritional supplementation, detoxification, exercise, herbal medicine, and homeopathy. Among the hormones alternative physicians use to balance and restore proper hormonal levels are testosterone, human growth hormone (HGH), thyroid glandular extract, and DHEA, depending on individual need. When appropriate, Dr. Ross also uses transdermal creams and homeopathic formulas.

"As a person ages, it is crucial to make adjustments in the diet to reflect changing hormonal patterns," Dr. Ross says. He typically recommends a diet that has a sufficient amount of cleansing foods (high-fiber fruits, vegetables, and grains) to balance the high level of congesting foods (breads, pasta, dairy products) commonly consumed by most people. This helps prevent the kidneys, liver, and intestines from getting clogged and working less efficiently, which leads to reduced absorption of nutrients and increased accumulation of toxins.

Dr. Ross also recommends a weekly liquids-only diet based on vegetable broths or fresh juices. "This gives the digestive system a break and enables it to clean itself," he says. "Taking psyllium husk powder, a natural laxative and intestinal cleanser, is also a good idea, as is the use of digestive enzymes to enhance digestion and nutrient absorption." Depending on need, appropriate nutrients or herbal remedies may also be prescribed.

Regular aerobic exercise is also important to help maintain good blood circulation, especially in the reproductive area, and can be augmented with weight training, which can help stimulate the body to release growth hormone.

"Men today are very active and want to stay at their best rather than letting themselves go, getting old and fat," Dr. Ross says. "They want to keep going at the same pace and have a proactive attitude about resolving symptoms of male menopause as they appear." Thanks to the comprehensive treatment approaches employed by Dr. Ross and other alternative physicians, their success in doing so is increasingly possible.

high in animal fats, also contribute to higher rates of prostate cancer. Consumption of large amounts of red meat is associated with high fat intake due to the fattening process cattle go through. Cultures that consume high levels of red meat have higher levels of prostate cancer.[35] A low-fat diet with a balance of proteins is the most beneficial to men over age 30.

Lifestyle changes, especially those associated with sexual habits, are important for prevention of genitourinary problems, as well as for a person's overall health, Dr.

Kruzel notes. "Protected intercourse through the use of condoms not only helps to prevent unwanted pregnancy, but also to avoid contamination of the male urethra by vaginal flora," he says. "Likewise, it is the only defense, short of abstinence, a man can take against sexually transmitted diseases, from herpes to AIDS."

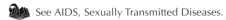 See AIDS, Sexually Transmitted Diseases.

Recommendations

- Emphasize a diet rich in fresh, organic fruits and vegetables, high-fiber grains, and drink lots of pure, filtered water. Avoid milk and dairy products, starchy carbohydrates, spicy foods, caffeine, alcohol, tobacco, and foods high in fats.

- Consider detoxifying the gastrointestinal tract to relieve or prevent constipation, which contributes to prostate dysfunction. Self-care approaches include psyllium husk powder and a weekly liquid-only diet consisting of vegetable broths or fresh-squeezed juices. To enhance digestion and nutrient absorption, take digestive enzymes with each meal or add hydrochloric acid (HCl), if necessary. To replenish intestinal flora, supplement with *Lactobacillus acidophilus*.

- Useful nutritional supplements include vitamins C, E, B₃ (niacin), and B-complex, the minerals manganese and zinc, essential fatty acids (omega-3s and omega-6s), lipoic acid, and trace minerals.

- Helpful herbs include saw palmetto, yohimbe *(Coryanthe yohimbe), Pygeum africanus, Echinacea angstifolia, Panax ginseng, Ginkgo biloba,* and Oriental thuja *(Thuja accidentalis).*

- Depending on need, testosterone, thyroid glandular extracts, human growth hormone (HGH), natural progesterone, DHEA, and pregnenolone, can be extremely useful in preventing and reversing men's health conditions and minimizing male menopause.

- Exercise 20-30 minutes at least three times a week. Swimming, in particular, is a useful exercise for men with prostate problems, as it helps free up pelvic nerve supply.

- Minimize stress, which impairs immune function and weakens the reproductive organs.

Self-Care
The following therapies can be undertaken at home under appropriate professional supervision:

IMPOTENCE
Biofeedback Training and Neurotherapy / Mind/Body Medicine / Yoga
AROMATHERAPY: Sandalwood, jasmine, rose, clary sage, ylang ylang
HYDROTHERAPY: Sitz bath (apply contrast 2-5 times weekly).

JUICE THERAPY: Red cabbage, celery, and lettuce juice, twice daily

PROSTATE DISORDERS
Qigong and Tai Chi / Yoga
AROMATHERAPY: For inflammation, use lavender, cypress, thyme.
JUICE THERAPY: • Pumpkin juice • Carrot and celery with a little horseradish and watercress added • Carrot, cucumber, beet, radish, and garlic.
HYDROTHERAPY: Sitz bath (apply contrast daily). Alternate hot and cold sitz baths—three minutes hot, 30 seconds cold; repeat three times. Hot and cold sitz baths cause a flushing effect on the prostate, increasing blood flow to the gland, which results in increased metabolism as well as elevating the white blood cell population. Additionally, there is an effect upon nerve flow to the pelvic organs allowing for better function.
PRACTICAL HINTS: Walk outdoors an hour daily.
REFLEXOLOGY: Reproductive glands, bladder, lower spine, pituitary, adrenals, prostate area.

Professional Care
The following therapies should only be provided by a qualified health professional:

IMPOTENCE
Chiropractic / Hypnotherapy / Magnetic Field Therapy / Osteopathic Medicine / Traditional Chinese Medicine
BODYWORK: Acupressure, Feldenkrais Method, reflexology, shiatsu.
CHELATION THERAPY: Many people with impotence may also have a diminished blood supply. Chelation therapy may be indicated to improve both conditions.

PROSTATE DISORDERS
Detoxification Therapy / Magnetic Field Therapy / Naturopathic Medicine / Osteopathic Medicine / Traditional Chinese Medicine
BODYWORK: Acupressure, reflexology, shiatsu.

Where to Find Help

For information on men's health, and referrals to a qualified practitioner, contact the following organizations.

American Association of Naturopathic Physicians
8201 Greensboro Drive, Suite 300
McLean, Virginia 22102
(703) 610-9037
Website: www.naturopathic.org

Provides a directory of naturopathic physicians and offers referrals to a nationwide network of accredited or licensed practitioners. Also publishes a quarterly newsletter, for both profes-

sionals and the general public, and offers a series of brochures and pamphlets on a variety of subjects.

American Association of Oriental Medicine
433 Front Street
Catasauqua, Pennsylvania 18032
(888) 500-7999
Website: www.aaom.org

The AAOM is a national professional organization of acupuncturists who meet acceptable standards of competency and can provide you with the names and locations of local members.

Ayurvedic Institute
11311 Menaul N.E., Suite A
Albuquerque, New Mexico 87112
(505) 291-9698
Website: www.ayurveda.com

The institute trains people in most of the aspects of Ayurveda.

National Center for Homeopathy
801 North Fairfax, Suite 306
Alexandria, Virginia 22314
(703) 548-7790
Website: www.homeopathic.org

Provides a referral list of practicing homeopaths along with other information. Gives courses for laypeople and professionals and organizes study groups around the country.

Recommended Reading

Encyclopedia of Natural Medicine. Michael Murray, N.D., and Joseph Pizzorno, N.D. Rocklin, CA: Prima Publishing, 1998.

Maximize Your Vitality and Potency: For Men Over 40. Jonathan Wright, M.D., and Lane Lenard, Ph.D. Petaluma, CA: Smart Publications, 1999.

Thriving: The Complete Mind/Body Guide for Optimal Health and Fitness for Men. Robert Ivker and Edward Zorensky. New York: Crown, 1997. Available from: Thriving Health, Inc., (888) 434-0033 or via online ordering at www.sinussurvival.com.

Prostate Troubles. Leon Chaitow, D.O., N.D. Wellingborough, England: Thorsons Publishers, 1988.

MENTAL HEALTH

Any disturbance in behavior, emotion, or cognition can be considered a form of mental disorder. Recent evidence suggests that depression, anxiety, antisocial behavior, learning disorders, or schizophrenia can be caused by biochemical imbalances, toxins, allergies, food sensitivities, and other environmental factors. Advances in nutritional therapy, orthomolecular medicine, mind/body medicine, environmental medicine, and other alternative therapies now offer many solutions to the treatment of mental disorders.

ACCORDING TO THE National Institute of Mental Health, nearly 30% of Americans suffer from some type of mental disorder severe enough to require psychiatric treatment.[1] Incidences of depression and suicide are also rapidly increasing, especially among children and adolescents.

Types of Mental Disorders

Although there is no clear-cut way of defining mental disorders, they can be divided into several overlapping categories, loosely defined as emotional, personality, and thought disorders.

Emotional Disorders

Two of the most common emotional disorders are depression and anxiety. Depression is characterized by feelings of persistent sadness, fear, unhappiness, pessimism, hopelessness, worthlessness, or despair. Serious depression, if not treated, can even lead to suicidal thoughts and feelings. Physiological symptoms may include a change in appetite (either increased or decreased), constipation, sleepiness, or sleeplessness.

Anxiety disorders, including phobias, affect roughly 10 million people,[2] with symptoms ranging from mild unease to intense fear and panic. These symptoms can often be manifested physically by tightness in the chest, hyperventilation, heart palpitations, or gastrointestinal problems.

Personality Disorders

Personality disorders are characterized by a person's inability to effectively relate socially for a variety of reasons. People suffering from paranoia, for instance, are overly suspicious, narcissistic people who tend to be selfish and self-centered, and antisocial people fail to conform to societal rules and regulations. Other personality disorders can include overdependence, insecurity, obsessiveness, compulsiveness, passiveness, and aggression. Patients with borderline personality disorders often have difficulty maintaining stable relationships and are often socially inappropriate and moody. Addictions to alcohol, drugs, and gambling are also considered forms of personality disorders.

Thought Disorders

Thought disorders include conditions such as behavioral problems, learning difficulties, schizophrenia, dementia (confused thinking), delusions, and brain dysfunction. Manic and depressive behaviors can also be considered forms of thought disorders.

Causes of Mental Disorders

Until recently, most mental disorders were considered either psychological in nature or genetically predisposed. Treatment options were generally limited to psychotherapy or to medication, electroshock treatment, or surgical intervention. Today, however, many psychiatrists, psychologists, and researchers recognize that numerous factors can contribute to the onset of mental disorders, including social and cultural factors, age and gender, nutritional deficits, allergies and food sensitivities, bioenergy imbalances, alcohol and drug addictions, and even prescription drugs, including those prescribed to treat mental illness. Peter Breggin, M.D., a Harvard-trained psychiatrist, points out that drug therapy, while suppressing the symptoms of depression and other mental disorders, can make a person chemically toxic, which will actually deepen the problem.[3]

THE DANGERS OF PSYCHIATRIC DRUGS

Increasingly in the U.S., psychiatric care is administered by physicians, not psychiatrists. Managed care organizations and HMOs are emphasizing psychiatric drugs in place of conventional psychotherapy for the sake of cost-effectiveness.[4] But the use of such drugs can result in serious health risks and even death. These risks are compounded by the fact that psychiatric drugs are increasingly prescribed to adolescents and infants, before the brain has fully developed. According to the U.S. Food and Drug Administration (FDA), in 1994, doctors wrote 3,000 prescriptions for Prozac for children less than one year old, and another 150,000 prescriptions of psychotropic (affecting mental/emotional behavior and function) drugs were written for children between the ages of two and four. What is particularly alarming about medicating children at such early ages is that the use of such drugs has not been approved for children younger than six and no data exist on safety and efficacy for such age groups.[5] The following are some of the health risks associated with such drugs, which include stimulants (Ritalin), antidepressants (particularly tricyclic drugs), and drugs such as clonidine, used to treat insomnia.

Ritalin (methylphenidate), an amphetamine primarily prescribed for attention deficit disorder (ADD), has more potent effects on the brain than cocaine, according to a recent study. "The data show that the notion that Ritalin is a weak stimulant is completely incorrect," stated psychiatrist Nora Volkow.[6] Side effects attributed to Ritalin include brain damage, stunted growth, negative behavioral changes, and suicidal tendencies, as well as the deaths of a number of children.[7] Other side effects include insomnia, loss of appetite, stomachache, headaches, dizziness, and suppression "of the vitality and basic personality of the child."[8] The most recent statistics about Ritalin use reveal that it has been prescribed for approximately 20% of U.S. schoolchildren[9] and that prescriptions in the U.S. account for 90% of Ritalin use worldwide. Moreover, 50% of U.S. children diagnosed with ADD are prescribed Ritalin without first receiving psychological or educational testing.[10]

Compounding this problem is the fact that many researchers and practitioners dispute whether ADD is actually a legitimate medical condition. Renay Tanner, an expert in human rights and psychiatry, states "The important thing to remember is that no child has ever died of ADD, yet a number of children have died from the 'treatment.' One has to ask why children are being targeted for the myth of chemical imbalance when no one can show that an alleged sufferer has a chemical imbalance and no one, certainly not the medical community, even knows what such a chemical imbalance might be."[11]

Prozac and similar antidepressant drugs, such as Paxil and Zoloft, have seen a significant increase in use over the last decade, with approximately 28 million Americans having used the drugs and 70% of the prescriptions for them written by physicians rather than psychiatrists.[12] Joseph Glenmullen, Ph.D., author of *Prozac Backlash*, considers this trend both dangerous and reckless, pointing out that antidepressants can have severe side effects. These include uncontrollable facial and body tics (which can be signs of severe neurological damage), hallucinations, dizziness, nausea, anxiety, withdrawal symptoms, sexual dysfunction, and electric shock–like sensations in the brain. Dr. Glenmullen cautions that a small percentage of people can become homicidal, suicidal, or both as a result of Prozac use.[13] Other research suggests that Prozac and other drugs that work by enhancing serotonin activity in the brain can, over time, cause permanent structural changes in the brain due to their ability to interfere with its metabolism.[14]

The tricyclic antidepressant Norpramin can cause serious side effects and has been implicated as the primary factor responsible for the sudden deaths of a number of children.[15] Research shows that the use of antipsychotic drugs can lead to tardive dyskinesia (movement disorders) in 5% of users and symptoms of the disease in another 12.5%. An additional 34% are likely to develop Parkinsonism. Such risks are high for every age group, with children being particularly susceptible.[16]

Clonidine, a commonly prescribed drug for sleep disorders, ADD/ADHD, and other behavioral problems—despite the fact that it has received FDA approval only for managing hypertension—can cause serious side effects, including a high incidence of overdose, low heart rate, depressed respiration, mood alteration, diminished cognitive and planning skills, and depressed levels of consciousness. It has also been implicated in the deaths of a number of children.[17] In addition, according to the *Physicians' Desk Reference*, certain nonpsychiatric drugs can cause side effects of mental depression, including Depo-Provera Contraceptive Injection and Roferon-A Injection.[18]

Illness can also be a major contributor to mental illness, as well as stress, both physical and emotional, chronic and acute. Exposure to environmental stresses from chemicals, toxins, and electromagnetic fields can play a major role in one's mental health as well.

Diet and Nutritional Factors

Diet and nutrition are probably the most significant determining factors, other than psychological or genetic causes, that predispose one to a mental disorder. Virtually any nutrient deficiency can result in depression. In fact, research shows that deficiencies in vitamins C, B_1 (thiamine), B_3 (niacin), B_6, and B_{12}, and folic acid could be specifically linked to depression and other emotional disorders.[19]

In 1991, researchers found that babies deficient in iron, even though treated, scored lower on IQ and mental function tests than babies with normal iron levels, when checked at age five.[20] As far back as the 1950s, when the late Carl Pfeiffer, Ph.D., M.D., former Director of the BrainBio Center (now the Carl C. Pfeiffer Institute), in Princeton, New Jersey, discovered that trace metal imbalances could contribute to mental disorders, violent, criminal, and delinquent behaviors in both children and adults have been linked to these imbalances.

"We've tested thousands of people in prisons, and many thousands more with behavior disorders, and found that 95% suffer from inborn chemical imbalances that predispose them to bad behavior," says William Walsh, Ph.D., a former research scientist at the Argonne National Laboratories and a colleague of Dr. Pfeiffer. Dr. Walsh discovered that violent individuals often had elevated copper-zinc ratios and extremely low levels of sodium, potassium, and manganese. These people were considered underachievers and had learning difficulties and attention deficit.

People with severe antisocial tendencies (lacking in remorse or conscience) showed a different biochemical pattern. They were low in copper, zinc, sodium, potassium, and manganese, but high in calcium and magnesium, often with toxic levels of lead. Studies in Texas have shown that when levels of the trace element lithium, commonly found in very small amounts in drinking water, are extremely low, the rates of suicide, homicide, and rape are significantly higher. When these levels are corrected by careful supplementation, aggressive behavior drops significantly.[21]

Another trace metal pattern involved people who were delinquent, impulsive, and irritable. Dr. Walsh found them to be low in all trace metals including calcium and magnesium. They also had low levels of most nutrients and amino acids, which may be caused by problems relating to nutritional absorption. "Many of these people have insufficient stomach acid," says Dr. Walsh. "When you correct the stomach acid, the body will often take over and treatment can be stopped."

Dr. Walsh classified a fourth type of individual who, though not violent or delinquent, did poorly in school and work, got irritable after eating sugar, and felt drowsy after meals. The basic problem, Dr. Walsh discovered, was hypoglycemia. Dr. Walsh's findings parallel an experiment conducted by the New York City public school system. Over a period of four years, they decreased the amount of sugar, food colorings, synthetic flavorings, and two commonly used preservatives in foods served at 803 schools. A dramatic 15.7% increase in academic performance was noted, compared to prior years in which no more than a 1% increase or decrease was reported.[22]

According to orthomolecular psychiatrist Harvey Ross, M.D., of Los Angeles, California, many patients who complain of depression have hypoglycemia, which, in some cases, may even be the sole cause of the patient's depression. "Many times, patients can feel depressed without being able to say why," says Dr. Ross. "They may also be experiencing low energy, feel irritable, or be having attacks of anxiety or fear, sometimes even to the point of developing phobias. Diabetes may be part of their family history, but from a medical standpoint nothing seems wrong. Often they will be referred to a psychotherapist, usually without much success, when what they really need is to see a physician who treats hypoglycemia."

Leon Chaitow, N.D., D.O., of London, England, notes that another recently identified cause of depression is the excessive use of aspartame, the artificial sweetener widely used instead of sugar in diet colas and foods. "This is because aspartame is made up of amino acids and, when they are metabolized, they can cause an imbalance in brain chemistry because of their extreme concentration," Dr. Chaitow says. Depression may also be due to a specific food or chemical to which one is sensitive or allergic, Dr. Chaitow points out.

 See Allergies, Children's Health, Diabetes, Diet, Environmental Medicine, Enzyme Therapy, Nutritional Medicine.

According to the late Benjamin Feingold, M.D., nearly half of all hyperactive children are sensitive to artificial food colors, flavors, and preservatives.[24] Although overwhelming evidence from around the world has supported Dr. Feingold's hypothesis, it remains a controversial topic, due in part to several negative studies conducted in the U.S. that were financed in part by such major food manufacturers as Coca Cola and General Foods.[25] Other countries have already restricted the use of artificial additives in foods because of their potential harmful effects.

Children who suffer from behavior problems such as attention deficit disorder (ADD) or attention deficit hyperactivity disorder (ADHD) have been shown to respond particularly well to dietary intervention, such as the Feingold diet, and the elimination of food additives and artificial colorings. In one Australian study, 55 children suspected of having ADHD followed the Feingold diet for six weeks. By the end of this period, 75% exhibited significant improvements in behavior. Moreover, the positive change lasted 3-6 months after the diet was discontinued. In addition, researchers determined that symptoms of 14 children were directly triggered by artificial food coloring.[26] A similar study, involving 78 children with ADHD, found the same percentage of improvement after the children were placed on a food elimination diet. Researchers also were able to show that "exposure to reactive substances was significantly associated with hyperactive behavior and with impaired psychological test performance."[27]

More recently, a scientific review of research published between 1985 and 1995 (primarily double-blind, placebo-controlled studies) found a "definite connection" between diet and behavior and concluded that a wide range of foods and food additives can adversely affect children's behavior.[28] Other studies have shown that food additives alone are sometimes not enough to provoke reactions in children and that other food sensitivities are often involved. These include allergic reactions to milk, soy products, chocolate, grapes, oranges, apples, peanuts, wheat, corn, tomatoes, eggs, refined sugar, fish, and oats.[29] Doris Rapp, M.D., past President of the American Academy of Environmental Medicine, has demonstrated how just a few drops of allergenic substances can suddenly provoke anger, confusion, and hyperactivity in children.

Addiction and Substance Abuse

According to Karl E. Humiston, M.D., of Albany, Oregon, when asked about their very first cigarette, most smokers will readily admit it made them pretty sick. "But after a bit of persistence, one gets used to it, builds up a tolerance for it, and actually comes to like it and is uncomfortable only when going too long without smoking," Dr. Humiston says. "The same can basically be said about regular alcohol and drug users as well."

Orthodox physicians and psychiatrists usually give no thought to this phenomenon, however. "But for the human body to no longer be distressed by something as noxious as cigarette smoke, and perhaps even come to enjoy it, a profound change of some sort has to occur in one's body chemistry," Dr. Humiston points out. "It is not just a psychological adaptation."

HISTAMINE LEVELS AND SCHIZOPHRENIA

In the 1950s, when the late Carl Pfeiffer, Ph.D., M.D., found that trace metal imbalances (copper, zinc, lithium, cobalt) were linked to mental illness, he also found that nearly half of those suffering from schizophrenia had low levels of histamine, a chemical present in cells throughout the body. He called these people histapenics. Histapenics are often classified as paranoid schizophrenics who suffer from severe depression, experience hallucinations, and become suicidal. Laboratory tests show that histapenics also have low levels of basophils (white blood cells that store histamine), deficiencies in zinc and folic acid, along with unusually high levels of copper.[23]

Dr. Pfeiffer also found that nearly a third of the schizophrenics he analyzed had too much histamine in their systems. Histadelics, as Dr. Pfeiffer referred to them, are often obsessive-compulsive and delusional with severe impairment in their thinking and high basophil levels. They are also suicidally depressed and may even become catatonic.

This phenomenon is called a "specific adaptation"—the body has adapted, at the chemical and energy levels, to a specific substance that is actually toxic or to which it is allergic. "This protects the body from instantly getting sick, but at the price of a heavy chronic stress that can grind away at one's immune system," says Dr. Humiston. "For example, most smokers don't get lung cancer, but all become much less healthy. Plus, in order to maintain the adaptive protection, you must maintain the exposure. In other words, you have to keep taking the stuff. If you go too long without it, then you get sick and can only be relieved by taking it again."

This is the physical basis for addiction. It is also the physical basis for many forms of mental and emotional illness. Adaptive/addictive reactions to toxic or allergenic foods and chemicals account for much depression, confusion, irritability, anger, compulsive behaviors, and even psychosis, according to Dr. Humiston, as well as for obvious addictions such as to cigarettes, alcohol, and drugs. "Since symptoms mainly appear when you are not exposed to the substance, or occur in a chronic or erratic pattern, neither the patient nor the physician is likely to think of the connection unless trained in environmental medicine," he notes. "The person whose worst fits of anger occur on the days when he doesn't have toast for breakfast is not likely to think of this as reflecting a wheat allergy. Similarly, the person who knows that coffee works best to relieve his morning headache is not likely to see this headache as a withdrawal symptom from an adaptive addiction to coffee, but that's what it is."

Environmental Factors

In a 1981 study, Stephen Perry, M.D., of Staffordshire, England, reported that people who lived near high-voltage lines had unusually high levels of depression and suicide.[30] A second study showed that apartment-dwelling people who lived closest to the building's main power supplies and electrical cables showed as much as an 82% increase in depression.[31] A third study, conducted by David Dowson, M.D., of Southampton, England, also showed an increase in depression from those who lived near power lines.[32]

 See Addictions, Candidiasis, Light Therapy.

Numerous studies have shown that exposure to heavy metals, solvents, paints, and other toxic substances and fumes can produce many psychological symptoms, including depression and fatigue,[34] as well as contributing to violent behavior. Post office slayer Patrick Sherril had extraordinarily high levels of lead and cadmium (in addition to a severe copper-zinc imbalance), which the University of Oklahoma attributed to his handling of ammunition. James Huberty, who shot 24 people at a McDonald's in San Ysidro, California, had an extremely high level of cadmium, which may have come from his 17 years of work as a welder.[35] Scientific studies have also attributed many childhood learning disorders to high levels of mercury, cadmium, lead, copper, and manganese.[35]

The quality and quantity of light can also affect one's mental state, according to pioneering photobiologist John Nash Ott, Sc.D. (Hon.).[36] Dr. Ott discovered that artificial lighting (incandescent or fluorescent) not only interferes with the body's optimal absorption of nutrients, but also contributes to a variety of mental and physical disturbances, including fatigue, depression, hostility, alcoholism, drug abuse, a shortened life span, Alzheimer's disease, and cancer.[37] John Downing, O.D., Ph.D., Director of the Light Therapy Institute, in Santa Rosa, California, confirmed these findings, stating that "by spending 90% of our lives indoors, in inadequate light conditions, we are causing or worsening a wide range of health problems, including depression, heart disease, hyperactivity in children, osteoporosis in the elderly, and lowered resistance to infection."[38]

Another form of this photobiological sensitivity is called seasonal affective disorder (SAD), a condition resulting from inadequate amounts of sunlight, usually during the winter months. According to Dr. Chaitow, 5% to 10%

of the population suffers from this disorder, which is often characterized by marked depression, extreme fatigue, and increased appetite. Hugh Riordan, M.D., founder of the Center for the Improvement of Human Function, in Wichita, Kansas, adds that seasonal depression can also be triggered by mold and pollen allergies. Dr. Riordan notes that a monthly cycle of depression may point to hormonal imbalances, especially in women.

 See Natural Hormone Replacement Therapy, Women's Health.

According to Dr. Humiston, depression in women is often caused by toxicity from an overgrowth of yeast *(Candida albicans)* in the intestines, especially when the yeast organisms are stimulated by the artificial form of the hormone progesterone, commonly found in birth control pills.

Stress and Lowered Immune Function

While many physical conditions and disorders have been shown to cause psychological stress, studies have also found that psychological stress can likewise contribute to physical illness. The central nervous system, the endocrine system, and the immune system all respond to psychological stress. Depressed immune function is associated with many kinds of stress including bereavement, divorce, job loss, examinations, anxiety, depression, loneliness, and sleep deprivation.[39] Up to 80% of health problems in the U.S. are considered stress-related. In large-scale studies conducted in 1967, those who became seriously ill reported having more stressful life events than those who were well.[40]

Multiple daily stress has been shown to undermine health.[41] British cardiologist Peter Nixon, M.D., suggests that when the body systems are overstimulated by stress, illness is likely to occur and cardiac disease may set in.[42] Jeanne Achterberg, Ph.D., past President of the Association for Transpersonal Psychology, adds that feelings of helplessness and hopelessness increase digestive problems and cancer growth. Fear, anxiety, and stress can also interfere with healing, compromise the immune system, and encourage cardiovascular disease.[43]

According to Carl Simonton, M.D., Director of the Simonton Cancer Center, in Pacific Palisades, California, stress is the greatest single factor in cases of recurring cancer.[44] One study found that depressed men are more likely to develop cancer in the following 20 years and twice as likely to die of it; in another study, women who experienced stress were more likely to get breast cancer.[45] Studies have also shown that psychotherapy helps to improve long-term health and immune function in cancer recovery patients. David Spiegel, M.D., of

Stanford University, demonstrated that women with metastatic breast cancer who participate in a weekly support group live twice as long as those who do not.[46]

Grief and social isolation can lead to weakened immune function, increased risk of cancer, and earlier death. One large nine-year study found that people with the lowest amount of social ties are 2-3 times more likely to die of all causes than those with the most social connectedness.[47]

One experiment showed that the more stress a person is under, the greater the chance of viral infection. In the study, 420 people were evaluated for occurrences of stress during the prior year. These included such events as job loss, death in the family, moving, and divorce; feeling frightened, nervous, sad, angry, or irritated; or feeling unable to cope with current demands. They were then exposed to one of five cold viruses and tested one month later for antibodies. Ninety percent of those who were under the greatest stress became infected, compared to 74% who experienced the least amount of stress.[48] In another study, the results indicated that people who experience stress (particularly tension and anger) are four times more likely to develop a cold or bacterial infection.[49]

Researchers who have reviewed the influence of stress on immunity have concluded that, since the effect is not universal (with some people handling the stress well and showing no decline in immune efficiency), it is not the stress that is to blame but the individual's means of handling it. "This has been called the 'hardiness factor'," says Dr. Chaitow. "It comprises a tendency to see problems as challenges, not threats; having a commitment to involvement in society rather than having a sense of detachment from it; and having a feeling of control over life rather than a sense of being subject to the whims of fate."

According to Dr. Chaitow, these three elements can be learned via appropriate counseling and therefore the absence of one or all of them from a person's personality profile is not necessarily a permanent feature, since "people can learn to cope with stress so that it does not negatively affect them." This is also the basis of numerous healing modalities such as progressive relaxation, guided imagery, and biofeedback, which can be used effectively to treat both psychological and physiological disorders.

Viral Brain Infections

"My clinical experience indicates that there is a common starting point for all organic brain disorders—a viral infection from the herpes family, namely, Epstein-Barr, cytomegalovirus (CMV), and human herpes virus 6," states William H. Philpott, M.D., of Choctaw, Oklahoma. According to Dr. Philpott, these infections occur during the gestation period in which the mother has a flare-up

THE MIND/BODY CONNECTION

Research conducted in the fields of psychoneuroimmunology and mind/body medicine over the past two decades has established a definite and intimate relationship between the physiological and psychological processes of the body. Neurochemical substances known as neuropeptides, discovered by Candace Pert, Ph.D., a leading neuroscientist currently teaching at Rutgers University and a former Section Chief at the National Institute of Mental Health, were found to cause alterations in mood. Even more significant, perhaps, was the discovery that these substances can be found not only in the brain, but in the spinal cord, glands, organs, and other body tissues.[50] Among the most well-known of the neuropeptides are endorphins, which can have a pain-relieving and pleasure-inducing effect when released. Dr. Pert looks at the neuropeptides as the "biochemical units of emotion" and as "the bridge between the mental and the physical."[51]

Neuropeptides are the key to changes in emotion, because they increase or decrease the transmission of messages to and from the brain. Because these neuropeptides are found throughout the body, they can also affect the functioning of all the body's systems, including the immune system. "Viruses use the same receptors as a neuropeptide to enter into a cell," explains Dr. Pert. "Depending on how much of the natural peptide for that receptor is around, the virus will have an easier or harder time getting into the cell. So our emotional state will affect whether or not we'll get sick from the same loading dose of a virus."[52]

of infectious mononucleosis, herpes, or other viral invasions. She then passes the infection on to the fetus. "The infectious invasion into the child's brain can also occur in early childhood," Dr. Philpott says. "As the child progresses through the early years of brain development, these viruses actually infect the neurons of the brain, producing a mild swelling within the brain. When this occurs, perception, judgment, and the ability to concentrate are often severely damaged."

The viruses Dr. Philpott attributes to organic brain disorders are chronic and fluctuating, meaning they remain active in the body and brain, though the severity of symptoms they cause can fluctuate. As they grow in strength due to varying stresses within the child's life, they place additional stress on the immune system, eventually compromising immunity. "This additional stress makes the child much more prone to maladaptively react to specific foods in the diet and to chemicals and inhalants in the environment," Dr. Philpott says.

Schizophrenia is an example of a mental disorder for which viral infection may be implicated. "Schizophrenia is a state of disordered brain function in the areas of perception, mood, thought, and motor function," Dr. Philpott explains. "Acute mental symptoms can be triggered by maladaptive reactions to foods, chemicals, or inhalants to which the subject is allergic, addicted, or otherwise hypersensitive. From studying schizophrenia, I have concluded that its origin is the aforementioned viral infections. After being infected in the brain, the child often experiences learning difficulties or hyperactivity. In adolescence or in their early twenties, the person develops full-blown schizophrenia, manic depressive reactions, or psychotic depression. All suffer from maladaptive reactions caused by the viruses and also have multiple and often severe nutritional deficiencies."

Dr. Philpott's observations were recently given added weight by research conducted at Johns Hopkins University and the University of Heidelberg, in Germany, which discovered that a retrovirus from the HERV-W family (the same class of pathogen as the HIV virus) is present in the DNA of up to 30% of schizophrenia patients.[53]

Treatment of Mental Disorders

A growing number of doctors and health practitioners have found that mental disorders, in many cases, can be successfully treated through means other than the traditional practices of psychotherapy, drug therapy, electroshock treatment, and surgery. These include nutritional and herbal supplements, dietary changes, exercise, mind/body medicine (biofeedback, EMDR, energy psychology, relaxation, flower essences, guided imagery), and magnetic field therapy.

Diet, Nutrition, and Herbal Medicine

According to Richard Kunin, M.D., of San Francisco, California, the most important dietary rules to follow for optimal psychological and physiological health are:

- Variety: Eat a little of a lot of different foods.

- Moderation: Don't overeat or binge.

- Whole foods: Eat natural foods (whole grains and fresh vegetables) rather than processed foods.

- Purity: Eat foods free of pesticides and additives, preferably organic.

- Balance: Eat a diet that is specifically suited to your own individual needs and body.

By following these basic guidelines, a person can do much to prevent mental disorders. However, when certain conditions exist that contribute to the deterioration of one's mental state, more direct nutritional steps are often required.

For treating psychological problems caused or exacerbated by hypoglycemia, Dr. Ross will have his patients begin an individualized program that includes a strict diet and the use of nutritional supplements. He recommends a high-protein, low-carbohydrate diet, and in addition to three meals daily, the patient eats smaller snacks every two hours between meals until bedtime. After the first four months, patients are introduced to a maintenance diet that includes no more than three servings of fruit a day. Ideally, the patient will refrain from processed foods and sugars, but may occasionally have a small amount of sugar. However, in times of increased stress, it may be necessary to return to the stricter dietary program.

Raising serotonin (a biochemical important in sleep and sensory perception) levels in the body can also help reduce depressive symptoms, according to Dr. Riordan, who recommends drinking walnut tea (which is high in serotonin) several times a day. To make this tea, simply steep a broken half of an English walnut in boiling water. Dr. Riordan adds that drinking plenty of water and breathing deeply are also effective ways to reduce depression. Studies conducted by Dr. Riordan showed that a nondepressed person breathes in six times the amount of air than does a person who is depressed.

Numerous herbs and botanicals have antidepressive effects. For example, *Hypericum perforatum,* commonly known as St. John's wort, has been used historically as a mood elevator. One clinical study demonstrated that a standardized extract of hypericum led to significant improvement in symptoms of anxiety, depression, and sleep disorders in 15 women.[54]

One of the earliest and most important breakthroughs in understanding the link between nutrition and mental health was made in 1952, when Abram Hoffer, M.D., Ph.D., President of the Canadian Schizophrenia Foundation, and his colleague, Humphrey Osmond, M.R.C.P., F.R.C.P., of Tuscaloosa, Alabama, found that schizophrenia could be treated with megavitamins. Drs. Hoffer and Osmond demonstrated that vitamin B3 (nicotinic acid or nicotinamide) can double the recovery rate of acute schizophrenics.[55] This discovery challenged some of psychiatry's basic concepts of schizophrenia and paved the way for orthomolecular medicine, which combines nutrition and the use of individualized supplements with other medical treatments.

These early studies, however, did not seem to help chronic patients, but progress was made when vitamin B3 therapy was combined with other treatments. "I examined the treatment outcome of 26 chronic patients who remained under my care for ten years and more," says Dr. Hoffer. "Eleven are working, two are married and looking after their families, two are single mothers caring for their children with no difficulty, and three are managing their own businesses. One patient received his B.Sc., one was awarded her M.A., and another got a certificate from community college. From this group, 18 are well, three are much improved, five are improved, and one has shown no improvement."[56] Compared to research that showed only a 5% significant recovery using traditional psychiatric treatment,[57] orthomolecular treatment of mental disorders, Dr. Hoffer believes, may soon become a standard medical practice.

In treating schizophrenia patients, Dr. Walsh has found that those with low histamine levels are much easier to treat with nutritional therapy than those with elevated histamine levels. To elevate histamine in such patients, his medical staff prescribes folate and nutrients, basophil enhancement, and a specialized treatment that causes their bodies to get rid of excess copper. After several months of treatment, the nervousness, depression, and hallucinations often disappear. Paranoid symptoms, however, may take as long as a year to subside.[58]

With people whose histamine levels are high, treatment may begin with megadoses of calcium (1,000 mg twice daily), which helps to release excess histamine from the body cells. Megadoses of the amino acid methionine (1,000-1,500 mg) hastens the exit of histamine from the body. Patients with elevated histamine levels must also avoid multivitamins that contain histamine-elevating agents such as niacin and folic acid. "Unfortunately," adds Dr. Walsh, "these people may also have to stay away from many kinds of nutritious foods, like green leafy vegetables, or they will get worse." In each case, Dr. Walsh recommends individual nutritional counseling.

Dr. Walsh, along with the late Dr. Pfeiffer, has also treated children effectively with nutritional therapy, noting improvements in learning disability, hyperactivity, and attention deficit disorders. "After our first 1,000 patients, we found we were getting major improvement with 70% of our behavior-disordered kids," says Dr. Walsh. "Twenty-two percent had improvement that was clear but not complete, 8% had little or no improvement. With learning disorders, 53% showed great improvement and 34% were better but still had a learning handicap. Approximately 13% showed no improvement at all."[59]

In one case, Dr. Walsh treated a ten-year-old boy who had explosive bouts of anger and hysteria, hitting people and destroying things. After four months of treatment,

his parents reported that his behavior had significantly improved and he was getting good grades in school. Another case involved a 16-year-old girl who was extremely emotional, with wild and erratic behavior, who lied, was deceitful, and was an underachiever in school. After four months of nutritional treatment, her fighting and emotional upheavals were gone, although she continued to do poorly in school.

In order to treat behavior and learning disorders, careful testing (blood, urine, and hair analysis) must be carried out in order to identify each patient's biochemical individuality. Over 120 different determinations need to be made, including testing for blood levels of histamine, lead, copper, and zinc; thyroid, kidney and liver function; protein levels; and electrolyte levels.

"Many children who don't improve appear to have allergy problems in addition to biochemical imbalances," says Dr. Walsh. "For this particular group, diet is especially important." Some children are particularly sensitive to food dyes, particularly yellow and red, or sugar, while others may have a reaction to taking multivitamins and minerals. "Multivitamins are wonderful for most people, but if you happen to have the wrong biochemistry, it might make you dramatically worse. This is particularly common for those with learning disabilities. One young man I saw had an extraordinary copper/zinc ratio. He was taking multiple vitamins that contained copper and this was like poison to him."

Treatment in such cases is to avoid multiple vitamins and enriched foods containing copper, prescribing instead a supplement that will bring the copper and zinc levels back to normal. "We make sure that they don't drink water that may be copper-bearing and suggest that they stay away from other possible sources of copper," Dr. Walsh says. "Swimming pools, for example, are treated with anti-algae agents that are loaded with copper and patients ought to make sure they shower afterward and not drink any of the water."

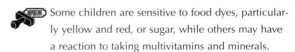 Some children are sensitive to food dyes, particularly yellow and red, or sugar, while others may have a reaction to taking multivitamins and minerals.

A study involving 15 autistic people, 6-22 years old, indicated that autism can also be treated through the use of diet. The patients were socially isolated, resistant to learning, showed peculiar attachments to objects, fear of unusual items and situations, and demonstrated repetitive motor behavior and severe problems with emotional expression. Language problems and disturbed attention were also common. Urine analysis showed that the patients had increased levels of peptides (simple proteins). Depending upon the specific pattern, three types of diets were prescribed to reduce the overall pep-

ORTHOMOLECULAR MEDICINE

The term *orthomolecular* was first used in 1968 by Nobel Prize-winning scientist Linus Pauling, Ph.D., referring to the connection between nutrition and the mind. In 1991, Melvyn Werbach, M.D., published a 370-page volume that summarizes research studies supporting Dr. Pauling's original ideas about this connection. "It is clear that nutrition can powerfully influence cognition, emotion, and behavior," states Dr. Werbach. "It is also clear that the effects of classical nutritional deficiency diseases upon mental function constitute only a small part of a rapidly expanding list of interfaces between nutrition and the mind."[60] He notes that patients in hospitals and nursing homes are often nutritionally deficient, adversely affecting their mental state.

Orthomolecular medicine has come a long way from the original discovery that large doses of B and C vitamins could improve the mental condition of schizophrenic persons. Yet, according to Joseph Beasley, M.D., Director of the Department of Medicine and Nutrition at the Brunswick Hospital Center, in Amityville, New York, conventional medicine has largely ignored the overwhelming extent to which poor nutrition and toxic environments have damaged physical and mental health.[61] As further research is completed, though, it will become increasingly more difficult to ignore this important link between nutrition and mental health.

tide levels—some patients received a gluten-free and milk-reduced diet, others received a milk-free and/or gluten-reduced diet, and a third group received a milk- and gluten-free diet.

Milk reduction was achieved by eliminating milk and cheese, and gluten reduction was achieved by giving only gluten-free bread and cakes. After one year, all the study subjects had changed toward the normal spectrum: they were less psychotic and more communicative and showed less bizarre behavior. Other statistically significant changes include increased attention and social integration, improved motor ability and skills, and a decrease in emotional outbursts. Especially noteworthy is the decrease in resistance to learning demonstrated by all cases.[62]

Mind/Body Medicine

A variety of mind/body approaches can be helpful in treating mental and behavioral disorders.

BIOFEEDBACK AND RELAXATION TECHNIQUES

Several studies have found that children suffering from hyperactivity and attention deficit show improvements in academic performance when trained in biofeedback and relaxation techniques.[63] These findings provide further evidence that mental conditions can be improved through the use of exercises designed to reduce stress and promote physical awareness.

In many cases of extreme anxiety, according to Dr. Chaitow, hyperventilation patterns are pronounced, with breathing rapid and extremely shallow. This is something also seen frequently in people displaying phobic behavior or who are subject to panic attacks. The person affected in this way will often report a sense of oppressive pressure on the chest and an inability to take a full breath. Breathing retraining, coupled with expert bodywork to release the rib structures and breathing muscles, as well as relaxation measures, will usually correct any habitual tendency toward hyperventilation. This nondrug approach is widely used in Europe for the treatment of chronic phobias and anxiety.[64]

 See Biofeedback Training and Neurotherapy, Bodywork, Flower Essences, Mind/Body Medicine, Yoga.

EYE MOVEMENT DESENSITIZATION AND REPROCESSING (EMDR)

Since its development by Francine Shapiro, Ph.D., in 1990, EMDR has become one of the most rapidly growing modalities in the field of mind/body medicine. Today, it is employed by over 20,000 psychotherapists as a treatment for a variety of mental and behavioral disorders, including addiction, anxiety, stress, and post-traumatic stress disorder (PTSD). It is as a treatment for PTSD that EMDR is best known, due to its high level of rapid success. Research has shown that 84% to 90% of people suffering from PTSD due to rape, natural disasters, catastrophic illness, the loss of a child or other loved one, or other traumas, fully recover after only three sessions of EMDR.[68]

ENERGY PSYCHOLOGY

An outgrowth of the pioneering research of Roger Callahan, Ph.D., energy psychology addresses mental and emotional problems by the use of acupressure techniques, kinesiology, and specific affirmations and breathing patterns. Its basic premise is that many mental/emotional problems, such as addiction, anxiety, depression, phobias, PTSD, irrational or uncontrollable feelings of anger, guilt, loneliness, panic disorders, rage, and rejection, are due to blockages or disturbances in a person's bioenergy field.

According to Fred P. Gallo, Ph.D., developer of a form of energy psychology known as Energy Diagnostic and Treatment Methods, such conditions can be resolved by having the patient think about or emotionally reconnect with mental or emotional issues while tapping specific acupuncture meridian points. "Thinking about a trauma you have experienced, typically triggers a painful emotion," Dr. Gallo explains. "The tapping techniques of energy psychology cause such emotions to go away, essentially by balancing out an energy system that is fundamental to the emotion, after which you can think about the event and no longer be bothered by it." Like EMDR, energy psychology is experiencing rapid growth among health professionals due to its effectiveness in rapidly and completely resolving mental/emotional disorders.[69]

BACH FLOWER THERAPY

Based on the work of British bacteriologist and homeopathic physician Edward Bach in the first half of the 20th century, Bach flower therapy is ideally suited for treating various mental/emotional conditions. "The combination of psychotherapy and Bach therapy tends to be very fruitful as a rule," according to Mechthild Scheffer, author of *Bach Flower Therapy*. "Psychotherapy in combination with Bach therapy will be accelerated. The essential point is reached more quickly and side issues threatening to bog things down are resolved more easily. People not suitable for [psychotherapeutic] treatment often become suitable after a period of Bach flower therapy."[70] In certain cases, Bach flower therapy can also be useful as a self-care approach for treating mental/emotional problems.

Magnetic Field Therapy

Dr. Philpott suggests that many psychological disorders are caused by electromagnetic imbalances in the body and that these can be corrected through the application of magnetic therapy, which uses specially designed magnets placed on or above different parts of the body. "Anxieties, phobias, obsessions, compulsions, depression, psychosis, and seizures evoke an abnormal rise in the electrical activity of the central nervous system," he says. Such conditions, according to Dr. Philpott, can be controlled through proper placement of negative magnetic energy devices, thus eliminating or reducing the severity of the mental disorder. Schizophrenics, he notes, have abnormally high electrical discharges deep within the brain and, through properly applied magnetic energy, a calming effect can be produced to alleviate their symptoms.[71]

USING WRITING AND GUIDED IMAGERY TO PREVENT NIGHTMARES

One out of ten people suffer from frequent nightmares. These people often also suffer from depression, hypochondria, and hysteria, and use more alcohol, tobacco, caffeine, and tranquilizers than others.[65] At the University of New Mexico, in Albuquerque, researchers found that two forms of behavior therapy could be used by patients at home to reduce the number of nightmares. The first technique, called desensitization, involves recalling the nightmare in detail while relaxing and then writing it down on paper. The second technique, called rehearsal, is a form of guided imagery in which the person relaxes and then, through visualization, changes the plot and the ending of the nightmare prior to writing it down.

It took only one session to teach a group of 28 people how to do these exercises. After seven months, 23 people reported having fewer nightmares (average reduction from 4.4 to 2.2 per week) using either technique. In four cases, nightmares ceased entirely and one woman was able to eliminate her nightmares after three days of rehearsal practice. Previously, she had been plagued by nightmares four times a week for 30 years.[66]

Additional research has found that the practice of keeping a daily journal can provide significant benefits for people dealing with mental or emotional problems, while simultaneously improving physical symptoms associated with such issues.[67]

Dr. Philpott reports that magnetic field therapy is replacing electro-convulsive therapy (shock treatments) for depression and other major mental disorders. "It is also replacing tranquilizers, antidepressants, and anti-seizure medications for the same conditions," he adds.

One of Dr. Philpott's patients was a professor named Gerald, who suffered from psychotic depression. His condition was so severe that he would neither eat nor drink, and tranquilizers and antidepressants did not improve his symptoms. After six weeks in the hospital, Gerald's wife was told that the only therapy left with potential value was electric shock treatment (EST), which she declined, choosing instead to consult with Dr. Philpott. "I told Gerald's psychiatrist that EST produced a magnetic anesthesia which would be helpful, but that there was also a magnetic treatment without the side effects of EST," Dr. Philpott says. He had Gerald recline on a massage table covered with magnets and placed a stack of eight magnets under Gerald's head. He also administered an intravenous solution for hydration that contained various nutrients (vitamins C and B6, calcium, and magnesium). Within an hour, Gerald's condition was reversed. "It would have taken a dozen or more electric shock treatments to achieve this same goal, and there would more than likely have been at least temporary memory loss associated with EST," Dr. Philpott says.

Recommendations

- Emphasize a whole foods diet, free of processed foods, preservatives, sugars, additives, and pesticides. If possible, eat only organic foods and vary your menu plan, eating meals specifically suited to your biochemical needs.

- The following nutrients are often deficient in people suffering from mental disorders: vitamins C, B1, B3, B6, B12, and folic acid, sodium, potassium, manganese, and zinc. Screen for excess levels of copper, lead, and other metals.

- A number of herbal remedies can be useful for treating mental conditions without the same risk of side effects associated with psychiatric drugs. St. John's wort, for example, is a mood elevator shown to be helpful for anxiety and depression.

- Screen for trace mineral imbalances, food and environmental allergies or sensitivities, excess histamine levels, hypoglycemia, and viral brain infections.

- Use caution when considering the use of psychiatric drugs, including Ritalin, Prozac, and other commonly prescribed drugs for mental and behavioral disorders, due to their high risk of side effects and even sudden death.

Self-Care
The following therapies can be undertaken at home under appropriate professional supervision:

DEPRESSION

Fasting / Flower Essences / Mind/Body Medicine / Reflexology / Yoga

AROMATHERAPY: • Sedative oils including chamomile, clary sage, lavender, ylang ylang, and sandalwood may be helpful. • Neroli, jasmine, bergamot, melissa, rose, and geranium are antidepressants. • Propolis tincture.

HYDROTHERAPY: • Constitutional hydrotherapy, immersion bath, or wet sheet pack (apply two to five times weekly). • Neutral application as needed for sedation.

SCHIZOPHRENIA

HYDROTHERAPY: • Constitutional hydrotherapy, immersion bath, or wet sheet pack (apply two to five times weekly). • Neutral application as needed for sedation.

JUICE THERAPY: • Seasonal fruit and vegetable juices. • Short juice fasts (under medical guidance).

Professional Care
The following therapies should only be provided by a qualified health professional:

DEPRESSION

Acupuncture / Applied Kinesiology / Chiropractic / Craniosacral Therapy / Environmental Medicine / Guided Imagery / Hypnotherapy / Magnetic Field Therapy / Osteopathic Medicine / Sound Therapy

BIOLOGICAL DENTISTRY: Hal A. Huggins, D.D.S., reports the improvement or disappearance of many emotional problems, such as depression, irritability, and suicidal tendencies, after removing toxic dental amalgams. Silver fillings contain approximately 50% mercury and only 20% to 30% silver.

BODYWORK: • Massage, shiatsu, acupressure, Feldenkrais • Rolfing is helpful if used in conjunction with psychotherapy.

SCHIZOPHRENIA

Acupuncture / Magnetic Field Therapy / Naturopathic Medicine / Orthomolecular Medicine / Sound Therapy / Traditional Chinese Medicine

BODYWORK: Rolfing

Where to Find Help

The following organizations can provide information on alternative approaches to treating mental illness, as well as referrals to alternative practitioners.

American Counseling Association
5999 Stevenson Avenue
Alexandria, Virginia 22304-3300
(703) 823-9800
Website: www.counseling.org

The counseling profession grew out of education and therefore is largely based on principles of human development and of activating the power within.

American Holistic Medical Association (AHMA)
6728 Old McLean Village Drive
McLean, Virginia 22101
(703) 556-9245
Website: www.holisticmedicine.org

Leading organization of physicians (M.D.s and D.O.s) who practice holistic medicine and are trained to treat the "whole person"—body, mind, and spirit. Provides referrals to members nationwide.

Center for the Improvement of Human Function International
3100 North Hillside Avenue
Wichita, Kansas 67219
(316) 682-3100
Website: www.brightspot.org

Medical, research, and educational facility specializing in the treatment of chronic illness. It is at the forefront of research in nutritional medicine. Treatments include counseling, stress reduction, biofeedback, acupuncture, hypnosis, pain control, and massage.

Foundation for the Advancement of Innovative Medicine
485 Kinderkarmack Road
Oradell, New Jersey 07649
(877) 634-3246
Website: www.faim.org

Organization of professionals and laypeople advocating holistic and alternative practices, including those geared towards treating mental illness. Provides referrals.

Recommended Reading

Brain Allergies: An Update. William H. Philpott, M.D., and Dwight Kalita, Ph.D. Chicago: NTC/Contemporary Publishing, 2000.

EMDR: The Breakthrough "Eye Movement" Therapy for Overcoming Anxiety, Stress, and Trauma. Francine Shapiro, Ph.D., and Margot Silk Forrest. New York: Basic Books, 1997.

Energy Tapping. Fred P. Gallo, Ph.D., and Harry Vincenzi, Ph.D. Oakland, CA: New Harbinger Publications, 2000.

Magnet Therapy: An Alternative Medicine Definitive Guide. William H. Philpott, M.D., and Dwight K. Kalita, Ph.D., with Burton Goldberg. Tiburon, CA: Alternative Medicine.com Books, 2000.

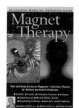

Prozac Backlash. Joseph Glenmullen, Ph.D. New York: Simon & Schuster, 2000.

Solving the Depression Puzzle. Rita Elkins, M.H. Pleasant Grove, UT: Woodland Publishing, 2001.

Talking Back to Prozac: What Doctors Won't Tell You About Today's Most Controversial Drug. Peter R. Breggin, M.D., with Ginger Rose Breggin. New York: St. Martin's Press, 1995.

The Betrayal of Health. Joseph Beasley, M.D. New York: Times Books, 1991.

Toxic Psychiatry. Peter R. Breggin, M.D. New York: St. Martin's Press, 1994.

MULTIPLE SCLEROSIS

Nearly 350,000 Americans are affected by one of medicine's least understood diseases, multiple sclerosis (MS). Although conventional medicine offers no known cure for MS, alternative medicine has recognized a number of contributing factors to its onset and progression. Often, the early detection and identification of underlying causes, combined with strict dietary and lifestyle guidelines, can stabilize or reverse the symptoms and, in some cases, even result in complete remission.

MULTIPLE SCLEROSIS affects the central nervous system and usually occurs in early adult life. The disease, which was first diagnosed in 1849, typically affects people between the ages of 20 and 40, with women at twice the rate of men. Symptoms rarely show up before age 15 or after age 60 and for reasons not clearly understood. MS is five times more prevalent in temperate climates, such as the northern U.S., Canada, and northern Europe.

Normally, nerve fibers are surrounded by a layer of insulation called myelin. MS results when the nerve fibers of the central nervous system develop multiple patches of demyelination (removal of the myelin sheath). "What seems to happen in MS is that the immune system attacks the myelin sheath, following a pattern of inflammation occurring as randomly distributed plaques in the central nervous system," according to Etienne Callebout, M.D., of London, England. "The damage to the myelin sheath impairs nerve transmission, either slowing down or stopping impulses from the brain directing muscles to move." The *multiple* nerve sheaths that have lost their myelin covering become scarred and hardened, called *sclerosis*.

Nerve transmission is disrupted, leading to feelings of pins and needles in the hands and feet, numbness, loss of balance and clumsiness, partial or complete paralysis, sensitivity to heat and cold (for about 60% of MS patients, heat makes symptoms worse), blurred or double vision, pain, and difficulty walking. "In advanced stages of MS, walking becomes more difficult, movements become more spastic, arms and hands may become weak, speech can become slurred, and chronic urinary urgency or incontinence may develop," says Patrick Kingsley, M.D., of Leicestershire, England, a specialist in nutrition

> *Although the stereotype of an MS sufferer is that of a person in a wheelchair, many people are able to walk and continue working.*

and environmental medicine who has treated over 2,000 multiple sclerosis patients. "Fatigue, one of the 'silent' and most disabling symptoms of multiple sclerosis, may render even the smallest tasks difficult." Although the stereotype of an MS sufferer is that of a person in a wheelchair, many people with MS are able to walk and continue working.

Multiple sclerosis is often described as a relapsing/remitting disease, where attacks are followed by remission, leaving the MS sufferer worse off than before the exacerbation. The disease can be benign, with a few minor attacks spread over many decades, or deterioration can be rapid. Most cases fall somewhere between these extremes. Because no two cases of MS are identical, the severity of attacks and the state of health following a remission period differ from patient to patient. Unless steps are taken to slow or halt the disease, patients with chronic symptoms will probably become progressively worse.

Causes of Multiple Sclerosis

By the time multiple sclerosis is actually diagnosed—usually in a person's twenties or thirties—the disease is well established, having taken root in either adolescence or childhood. The medical establishment generally contends that there is "no known cause" for MS, yet billions of dollars have been spent researching potential causes and cures.

Alternative medicine, however, regards MS as a complex, multifactorial disease involving several causes. "It

The Myelin Sheath

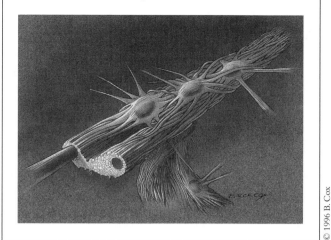

© 1996 B. Cox

has been known that the degree of symptoms in MS is inconsistent with the degree of demyelination. In fact, minor demyelination may be accompanied by major symptoms and vice versa," says Rima Laibow, M.D., founding Medical Director of the Alexandria Institute of Natural and Integrative Medicine, in Croton-on-Hudson, New York. "Therefore, it is more likely that other factors, such as dietary and nutritional depletion, allergies, toxins, stress, and infections, may be causing the progression of MS, while the demyelination is of secondary importance." When these factors are addressed, the symptoms may be alleviated or even reversed.

Dietary and Nutritional Deficiencies

People with multiple sclerosis typically have nutritional deficiencies. Studies show that essential fatty acids, the building blocks of the brain and nervous system, are lacking in many MS patients.[1] Multiple sclerosis is most common in Western countries where people consume large amounts of meat, dairy products, and processed foods—all foods low in essential fatty acids—and is least common in countries where diets are high in unsaturated fats, including seed oils, olive oil, oily fish, fresh fruits, and vegetables—all foods high in essential fatty acids. A predominantly meat versus vegetarian diet seems to be a significant risk factor.[2] The connection with saturated fat intake was first noted in 1950 by Roy Swank, M.D., of Oregon Health Sciences University, in Portland, Oregon, and has been confirmed in more recent studies.[3]

Stephen Davies, B.M., B.Ch., of London, England, has found that, even with a balanced diet, MS patients have difficulty absorbing essential nutrients. Although these differ from person to person, says Dr. Davies, the most common deficiencies are vitamins B_1, B_6, and B_{12}, magnesium, zinc, folic acid, amino acids, manganese, and selenium, as well as essential fatty acids. Deficiencies of

MORE THAN MYELIN

The pioneering research of the late German physician Hans A. Nieper, M.D., who treated 3,500 MS patients over the course of 35 years, has shown that this disease affects not only the brain and spinal cord, but upsets the integrity of cellular membranes potentially anywhere in the body. Dr. Nieper explained that the myelin sheath around the nerve fibers (axons) resembles a large tobacco leaf, with anywhere from five to 30 wrappings. Each layer is structurally identical to a typical cell membrane, he said, and the sheath is multilayers of cell membranes. However, the myelin sheath is more than an insulator for nerves, as is commonly presumed—there seems to be a flow of electrical current between the myelin sheath and the central nerve axon.

Dr. Nieper found that a substance called colamine phosphate (now known as calcium-AEP) is necessary for an appropriate electrical charge on the surface of the myelin sheath and the nerve cell membrane. When it is not present, the MS process begins, as well as other autoimmune diseases manifesting throughout the body. "We have found that in the MS patient, all cell membranes are affected, not just those in the myelin sheath," he said. "Their porosity is defective—even the membranes of red blood cells allow too much stuff to pass through." This porosity impairs the cells' electrical activities and leaves them open to "aggression" from immune cells and toxins. "During MS attacks, the sheath is partially destroyed by so-called killer T cells, leaving patches of scar tissue in the myelin sheath," said Dr. Nieper.

biotin, a member of the B vitamin family that plays a role in the metabolism of fatty acids, causes symptoms similar to MS.[4]

Food Sensitivities and Leaky Gut Syndrome

Intolerances or allergies to certain foods are common in those with multiple sclerosis. Among the most frequent are milk and dairy products, caffeine, tannin, yeast, sugar, wheat, gluten (found in wheat, spelt, kamut, barley, oats, and rye), corn, food additives, and fermented products such as ketchup, vinegar, and wine. In one study, it was found that of 135 MS patients, 65.9% had a history of sinusitis, a classic symptom of intolerance to milk and dairy products.[5]

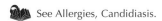 See Allergies, Candidiasis.

HISTAMINE FOR MULTIPLE SCLEROSIS

Histamine is a compound in the body, released during allergic reactions, that causes a number of bodily responses—dilation of blood vessels, contraction of smooth muscles, and stimulation of gastric acid. It is formed from the essential amino acid histidine. Since the 1950s, studies have indicated that histamine may be useful for relief of MS symptoms. Current research using transdermal (absorbed through the skin) histamine with MS patients has shown improvements in extremity strength, bladder control, fatigue, and cognitive function. Several mechanisms of action have been suggested, including improved digestion (from increased gastric acid secretion), increased blood flow in the brain, suppression of autoimmune responses, and stimulation of remyelination of nerves.[8] Further research is needed to uncover the connections among allergies, gastrointestinal dysfunction, and MS.

Candidiasis, an abnormal overgrowth of the intestinal yeast *Candida albicans*, is a major cause of food intolerances and mycotoxin production and, like nutritional deficiencies, can add to the stress on individuals with multiple sclerosis. William G. Crook, M.D., of Jackson, Tennessee, first made the connection between MS and the yeast *Candida albicans*, documenting several cases in which symptoms improved once the candidiasis was treated.[6]

The result of both food intolerances and candidiasis may be a body-wide condition of poisoning as toxins leach out of the intestines into the bloodstream and other tissues (known as "leaky gut"). Food particles and toxins that enter the bloodstream are detected by the immune system, which mounts a defense to protect the body. This places a strain on the immune system and weakens it, allowing other pathogenic viruses and yeasts to multiply—further compounding the load on the immune system.[7] Also, circulating immune complexes (CICs), which result whenever an antibody attaches to a foreign substance such as a toxin or food particle, can become embedded in the tissues of the body. The immune system may then respond by attacking not only the CICs but the body's own cells to which they are attached. Over time, the result can be autoimmune diseases such as rheumatoid arthritis and multiple sclerosis.

Environmental Toxins

Gary Oberg, M.D., past President of the American Academy of Environmental Medicine, notes several ways in which environmental toxins may contribute to multiple sclerosis. "Toxins may cause metabolic poisoning, interrupting the body's normal metabolic pathways and damaging the myelin sheath of nerves, which is the basic defect in MS. Certain substances, while not toxic to everyone, may initiate an autoimmune reaction in susceptible individuals. These individuals make antibodies to the foreign substance that cross-react with myelin, thus damaging the nerves and inducing symptoms characteristic of multiple sclerosis." According to Dr. Oberg, some of the substances that can produce or aggravate MS symptoms include chemicals in food and tap water, carbon monoxide and diesel fumes, fumes from gas water heaters, solvents, aerosol sprays, and chipboard and foam in furniture and carpets.

Toxicity from Mercury Dental Amalgams

Mercury is a highly toxic metal that, when used in dental amalgam fillings, can seep into body tissues, where it accumulates and becomes capable of producing symptoms that are indistinguishable from those of multiple sclerosis.[9] According to Hal Huggins, D.D.S., of Colorado Springs, Colorado, mercury poisoning often remains undetected because patients' symptoms do not necessarily suggest mercury as the initiating cause. But the effects of mercury toxicity are potentially devastating and accumulative.

Mercury was first recognized as a poison in the 16th century, yet mercury amalgams have been used in dentistry since the 1820s. Mercury has been shown to bind to the DNA of cells and to cell membranes, causing cell distortion and inhibited cell function.[10] When this happens, the immune system no longer recognizes the affected cell as part of the body and initiates an autoimmune reaction, destroying myelin in the process. MS patients have been found to have seven times higher levels of mercury in their cerebrospinal fluid (the fluid that surrounds the brain and spinal cord) compared to neurologically healthy patients.[11]

Electromagnetic Fields

Electromagnetic fields (EMFs) are a low-level type of radiation that is generated when electric currents flow through wire coils. Every time you turn on an electric appliance, it produces EMFs. Common household and office appliances emit very low frequency (VLF) or extremely low frequency (ELF) electromagnetic fields. We are surrounded by stress-producing, electromagnetic fields generated by the electrical wiring in homes and offices, televisions, computers and video terminals, microwave ovens, overhead lights (particularly fluorescent), electrical poles, and the hundreds of motors that can generate higher than naturally occurring field strengths.

An electromagnetic field can be likened to an invisible energy web (shaped somewhat like the contour lines on a topographical map) produced by electricity. While EMFs are part of nature and in fact are radiated by the human body and its individual organs, the quality and intensity of the energy can either support or damage health.

Electromagnetic changes in the environment can adversely affect the energy balance of the human organism and contribute to disease. EMFs interact with living systems, affecting enzymes related to growth regulation, pineal gland metabolism, regulation of the hormones melatonin and serotonin, and cell division and multiplication. MS patients typically show calcification of the pineal gland as well as decreased brain levels of melatonin and serotonin, according to Dr. Laibow.

Melatonin is important in MS because it is a potent antioxidant that protects the brain and central nervous system from free-radical damage. "Normally present in high concentrations in the nervous system, melatonin appears to play a pivotal part in preventing oxidative damage to the nerves and brain," according to Joseph Pizzorno, N.D., founder of Bastyr University, in Kenmore, Washington. Numerous studies show that chronic exposure to extremely low frequency EMFs suppresses nighttime melatonin secretions.[12] Not enough daytime light—the lack of exposure to bright sunlight or at least high-intensity artificial (full spectrum) lights—is also associated with diminished nighttime melatonin production.

Trauma and Stress

Dr. Kingsley notes that a first episode of MS often follows a physical trauma or period of emotional stress and that initial symptoms sometimes appear at the site of an injury (for example, numbness in an arm or leg following a trauma in which that limb was injured). In addition, recent research shows that most Parkinson's disease patients have sustained a blunt injury to the top of one foot, which causes dysfunction in the Stomach, Spleen/Pancreas, and Gallbladder meridians, demonstrated by the fact that treating these helps reverse the condition. Several alternative practitioners are finding a similar blunt trauma and meridian disturbance in MS patients.

Viral and Bacterial Infections

Medical researchers have long suspected a viral involvement in MS. Recent research on patients infected with the Epstein-Barr virus (a form of herpes virus believed to be the causative agent in infectious mononucleosis) shows that levels of essential fatty acids are very low after the illness, similar to the low levels found in MS patients.[13] This virus interferes with the body's ability to metabolize essential fatty acids, causing a partial breakdown of the immune system. An acute episode of infection with the Epstein-Barr virus during adolescence could leave the door open to chronic illness such as MS some years later.

Another theory holds that MS may be initiated by stealth pathogens. The term *stealth pathogen* refers to bacteria that have cell walls that are deficient in structure and thus lack rigidity. This feature enables such cell wall deficient (CWD) bacteria to easily move DNA between cells and for groups of CWD bacteria to fuse together and "facilitate genetic experiments," explains microbiologist Lida Holmes Mattman, Ph.D., a leading authority in this field. Such "genetic experiments" can include many of today's more baffling autoimmune diseases such as MS and rheumatoid arthritis.[14]

According to Philip Hoekstra, Ph.D., of Huntington Woods, Michigan, the bacterium that may be the organic cause of MS is *Borrelia mylophora*, so named because its characteristics resemble those of *Borrelia burgdorferi*, the bacteria believed responsible for Lyme disease. In multiple sclerosis, the myelin sheath surrounding nerves gets eaten away by the immune system, explains Dr. Hoekstra. "Most of the destruction of the myelin sheath takes place from actions of the white blood cells and their antibodies. But their primary target is not the myelin sheath at all, it's the *B. mylophora* bacteria in the nervous system." Unfortunately, the myelin sheath sustains a lot of collateral damage as the immune cells attempt to find and destroy the microbe, Dr. Hoekstra says.

There is no question that those MS patients who show the greatest improvement are the ones who start treatment earliest.

—ROY SWANK, M.D.

Genetic Predisposition

Although multiple sclerosis is not a hereditary disease, it is considered familial. First generation relatives of MS patients show a greater risk (by a factor of 30-50 times) of developing the disease than the general population.[15] This familial pattern strongly suggests a transmissible microbe as one of the causative agents in MS.

Treating Multiple Sclerosis

An early diagnosis is an essential first step in treating multiple sclerosis. For the best rate of success, treatment of the disease should begin as soon as possible after diagnosis. Once the disability has gained a hold, it becomes harder to reverse the damage. "There is no question," says Dr. Swank, "at least in the minds of alternative physicians, that those MS patients who show the greatest improvement are the ones who start treatment earliest."

Many health-care professionals believe that, if treatment begins soon enough and is adhered to, it is possible to control multiple sclerosis in many, if not all, patients. "Cure is possible if the cause or causes can be found and then eliminated," says Dr. Kingsley. "If mercury is eliminated from the body, and if the food and environmental sensitivities of the individual are pinpointed and sorted out, in addition to addressing any nutritional deficiencies, then I believe it is perfectly possible to cure people. But they must accept the fact that, if they then return to their former diet and have mercury fillings put back in their teeth, they will probably get MS again because they have a predisposition toward it."

Dr. Callebout and other alternative practitioners recommend thorough testing to get a clear picture of the individual's condition. "First, I would do a 'sweat mineral test' to detect possible heavy metal toxicity and general mineral status," he says. "In many respects, this yields more accurate information than either a hair analysis or blood test. You place a special plaque on the patient's back and produce mild perspiration over the course of an hour; then you analyze the perspiration for minerals." He also assesses the patient's antioxidant capacity to see if the body is equipped with the necessary nutrients and systems to counteract toxins. Other common tests include: an adrenal stress test to indicate how well (or poorly) the adrenal glands are functioning as measured over a 24-hour period; a stool analysis to assess digestive function and nutrient assimilation; a urine analysis to check biochemical status and organ function; a glucose tolerance test to monitor blood sugar levels; and a full standard blood count and biochemistry panel.

Because multiple sclerosis affects each patient differently, treatment programs are individualized. Dietary and nutritional needs are often addressed, as are food allergies and environmental toxins. Recommendations may be made for detoxification therapy, as well as for the removal of mercury amalgam dental fillings. Among practitioners of alternative medicine, there is a degree of consensus—not generally shared by conventional doctors—that MS can be controlled. This type of approach involves fundamental nutritional, environmental, and lifestyle changes. It is important that treatment be followed under the guidance of a qualified practitioner trained in these fields.

Diet

The most well-documented success with multiple sclerosis patients is Dr. Swank's work with a low-fat diet. He found that MS patients who ate the lowest amount of saturated fat realized the greatest improvement, and those who ate saturated fat in amounts larger than the prescribed maximum fared the worst.[16] Dr. Swank recommends that the maximum safe level of saturated fat for anyone with MS not exceed 15 g (about three teaspoons) a day. Patients need to be especially careful of hidden saturated fat found in processed and packaged foods. For best results, he advises the elimination of all saturated fat and a switch to the polyunsaturated type.

Dr. Swank suggests oils such as sunflower, safflower, and olive, which contain either polyunsaturated or monounsaturated fats (a minimum of four teaspoons of unsaturated oils a day, up to ten teaspoons for patients leading an active life). While Dr. Swank's emphasis is on first reducing saturated fat intake, other doctors believe that the priority should be to increase an MS patient's intake of essential fatty acids, found in polyunsaturated and monounsaturated oils. Either way, the result is a low saturated fat and high polyunsaturated fat diet.

Dr. Callebout makes the following general dietary recommendations for MS patients:

- Avoid: solid fats, hydrogenated oils, margarine, red meats, dairy products, cooked eggs, shellfish, alcohol, sugar, chocolate, monosodium glutamate (MSG), yeast, additives, fermented foods, most fast foods and prepared foods, hydrolized vegetable proteins, and (as much as possible) salt.

- Include: tofu, mung bean sprouts, millet, organic oatcakes (unless allergic to gluten), fresh organically raised poultry, some nuts and seeds, tahini, most vegetables, and selected fruits.

Nutritional Supplements

"Replenishing of fats and minerals is absolutely crucial, but which ones and how they are provided becomes the dividing line between success and failure in many cases," comments Dr. Laibow. Important supplements include essential fatty acids, vitamins, minerals, trace elements, and amino acids.

Essential Fatty Acids: The two families of essential fatty acids (EFAs) are omega-3 and omega-6. Omega-3 EFAs in particular have been found deficient in MS patients. Increasing the intake of omega-3 oils reduces the production of pro-inflammatory immune cytokines (chemical messengers of the immune system, such as interleukins, interferons, and eicosanoids).[17] The primary omega-3 fatty acid is alpha-linolenic acid (ALA), which is abundant in flaxseed oil. Other food sources of omega-3 fatty acids include dark-green leafy vegetables; hemp seed, soy, and walnut oils; pumpkin seeds, sesame seeds, walnuts, almonds; and the wild plants chia, cattail, and purslane. Other types of omega-3 fatty acids beneficial to MS patients include eicosapentaenoic acid (EPA) and docosahexaenoic acid (DHA), found in salmon, bluefish, bass, trout, and brown and red algae.

Gamma-linolenic acid (GLA), a member of the omega-6 family, is found in evening primrose oil, black currant oil, borage oil, and spirulina. Known primarily for its anti-inflammatory effect, GLA is necessary for the healthy functioning of the immune system and helps to produce vital regulators of inflammation called prostaglandins (biologically active unsaturated fatty acids) in the body.

Dr. Callebout often recommends a procedure called oil instillation, originally developed by a Swiss physician, which is performed after a chamomile enema. This herbal enema, given before going to bed, relaxes and cleanses the intestines, which tend to spasm in MS. The oil instillation involves inserting, by way of a catheter-tipped syringe, about 50 cc of organic cold-pressed flaxseed oil, walnut oil, or sunflower oil into the colon for quick absorption by the intestines. The enema and instillation are done every night for three weeks; eventually the body requires less oil and the dose can be reduced to around 5-10 cc, three times weekly.

"You couldn't eat or digest enough oil-based products or the oil itself to get the same effect as direct intestinal absorption," says Dr. Callebout. "Yet the typical MS patient needs to absorb a massive amount of essential fatty acids to repair the myelin sheath. The oil is absorbed by the body during the night as you sleep." The clinical strategy is to provide the nutrient precursors for the "good" prostaglandins that slow down or halt the autoimmune process.

See Diet, Nutritional Medicine.

Vitamins, Minerals, Trace Elements, and Amino Acids: Specific vitamins, minerals, trace elements, and amino acids may be recommended to make up for deficiencies as well as to act as co-factors for the efficient metabolism of essential fatty acids and the repair of myelin. These co-factors include vitamins B_1 (thiamine), B_3 (niacin), B_6, B_{12}, and C, zinc, and magnesium. Other supplements frequently recommended are all the other B vitamins, including vitamin B_5, calcium, and selenium.

Women with MS are at an increased risk of developing osteoporosis and should supplement with vitamin D.[18] Dr. Laibow also recommends antioxidants for MS sufferers, including L-glutathione, carotenoids including beta carotene, folic acid, vitamin E, choline, L-carnitine, dimethylsulfoxide (DMSO) or methylsulfonylmethane (MSM), bioflavonoids, methionine, cysteine, and alpha-lipoic acid.

- Vitamin B_{12} is proving highly effective for decreasing symptoms of MS, especially when associated with mercury poisoning. Dr. Kingsley sometimes prescribes doses "as high as 12,000 mcg once a week by intravenous infusion, usually with other essential nutrients. However, intramuscular doses are commonly 4,000-8,000 mcg once a week, and this can continue for many weeks until the person has become mercury negative." He says that, in some cases, he has been able to stop a relapse. "We have been able to completely clear an MS relapse within half an hour of administering a suitably high dose of vitamin B_{12} intravenously," says Dr. Kingsley.

Dr. Kingsley adds that textbooks on the subject of multiple sclerosis do not even mention the value or use of vitamin B_{12}.[19] "Many academics have been arguing that vitamin B_{12} is not necessary because they consider the condition to be a central nervous system disease. Their main reason for not recommending B_{12} to patients has been because the levels of B_{12} in the blood of MS patients are nearly always within the normal range. Now, however, studies are showing that the B_{12} levels in the cerebrospinal fluid of patients with MS are lower than those of control groups."[20]

One woman suffering from MS and experiencing numbness in her arms, legs, and hands, as well as pain in her arms, consulted with Dr. Kingsley. These symptoms had been occurring for approximately two years, and over that time she was eating a great deal of cheese and drinking six cups of tea and two cups of coffee daily. Dr. Kingsley identified milk and dairy products, tannin, caffeine, and yeast as the foods and substances to which she was allergic. At his suggestion, she made dramatic changes in her diet, eating plenty of fish, chicken, salads, fruit, and drinking herbal teas. Like all of Dr. Kingsley's patients, she had her mercury amalgam fillings replaced and began chelation therapy to clear her system of heavy metals. She also received regular injections of vitamin B_{12} in variable doses. "After about seven months, she became symptom free for the first time, but then suffered periodic relapses, each of which cleared with a suitable treatment of vitamin B12. Apart from additional relapses in relation to a developing flu or when under stress, the gap between each infusion of vitamin B12 has become longer and longer as time has gone by."

- Dr. Callebout prescribes oral calcium-AEP (2.5-3.0 g daily). Calcium-AEP is an essential component of cell membranes, but in MS it becomes dangerously deficient; the body may become unable to synthesize adequate amounts of this substance. In 1965, the German Federal Health Authority (the equivalent of the FDA) declared calcium-AEP to be a registered anti-MS medicine. Despite this precedent, the substance is nearly unobtainable in the U.S.

- Magnesium has consistently been found deficient in MS patients.[21] Dr. Davies stresses the importance of magnesium, as spasticity can often be traced to low levels of this mineral. (To accurately determine magnesium levels, use a test that measures magnesium inside the cell; blood tests are useless clinically.) One patient, a man who was diagnosed with MS at age 40, sought Dr. Davies' advice and was tested for nutrient levels and possible allergies. Very low levels of magnesium were found, so the patient was given weekly injections over two to three months. Allergies to wheat and all milk products were identified and it was recommended that the patient remove those foods from his diet. Also recommended were a multivitamin/mineral, evening primrose oil, and cod liver oil. Dr. Davies notes that the patient now has MS under control and is no longer plagued by bouts of double vision. He says that, although the patient still has a limp, he is able to work full time.

- The importance of selenium, which is often deficient in people with MS, is its activity as an antioxidant and anti-inflammatory. Selenium works in conjunction with vitamin E in cell membranes to fight free radicals.[22] Selenium can also protect against the absorption of heavy metals such as aluminum, mercury, and lead.[23] The small amount of selenium needed by the body is often hard to obtain through the diet because foods are now grown in mineral-poor soils.[24] If grown in fertile soil, grains are a good source of selenium, as are liver and fish.

- Coenzyme Q10, also called ubiquinone, occurs naturally in all human cells. It has actions similar to vitamin E, assists in cellular energy production, improves circulation (increasing oxygen delivery to tissues), and supports and stimulates the immune system.[25] CoQ10 is an antioxidant and can help relieve the debilitating fatigue of MS.

- Amino acids are the building blocks of proteins. Amino acid supplementation is important since there seems to be a deficiency in the blood-brain barrier functions with regard to the amino acid precursors of several neurotransmitters, which are present at abnormal levels in the brain and spinal fluid of MS patients, according to Dr. Laibow. Research has found significantly low levels of GABA (gamma-aminobutyric acid), aspartic acid, glutamic acid, and glycine in those with MS.[26]

5-HTP (5-hydroxytryptophan), a precursor for the hormones melatonin and serotonin, is also recommended for MS patients. "Serotonin deficiency contributes to several of the manifestations of the disease, including the high incidence of depression and suicide, sleep disorders, pain syndromes, heat sensitivity, fatigue, cognitive deficits, spasticity, and dysfunction of bladder control," says Dr. Laibow. She notes that extremely large doses may be needed because of underlying metabolic deficits.

A few alternative physicians are finding good clinical response in MS patients by giving daily intravenous L-glutathione (600-2,500 mg), an antioxidant tripeptide often lacking in the chronically ill. This treatment works best in concert with other dietary, nutritional, and detoxification therapies.

Once environmental toxins are removed, it is entirely possible that remission can occur.

—GARY OBERG, M.D.

Environmental Medicine

When treating MS patients, Dr. Oberg initially searches for the environmental or dietary factors that exacerbate multiple sclerosis symptoms. Dietary factors are examined by using an elimination diet—removing a particular food or substance from the diet and observing if the symptoms disappear. If they do, and reappear on reintroduction of the food into the diet, then that food must be avoided.

To diagnose dust, mold, pollen, food, or chemical sensitivities, Dr. Oberg uses a diagnostic technique called maximum tolerated intradermal dose testing. By inject-

MS AND BEE VENOM THERAPY

You may find it difficult to imagine voluntarily getting stung by a honey bee, but patients with MS who use bee venom therapy take about 4,000 stings a year, at the rate of 20-40 live bee stings per sitting, three times a week. Using bee stings for medicinal purposes (called apitherapy) is clearly not for the faint-hearted, but who would rather be sick for life when, after a few pinpricks, you could enjoy dramatic improvement?

While the medicinal uses of bee products are known widely around the world and have been used in China since antiquity, their use in American holistic medicine has started only recently. With more than 1,500 papers on the healing benefits of bee stings published in European and Asian scientific journals, the idea of stinging for health is now gathering momentum in America. The therapeutic use of honey-bee stings is still in its early days: exact dosages and length of treatment are still being investigated. Helping this progression along is the pioneering work of the International Apitherapy Study (IAS), begun in 1983, which is now gathering follow-up data on more than 12,000 patients. According to IAS, the anecdotal reports of remarkable successes are increasing and the number of licensed physicians willing to experiment with bee venom therapy is also growing.

Bee venom can be injected into the skin of the patient either by hypodermic needle or by the direct contact of the honey bee. Here, the practitioner holds a live honey bee in a pair of tweezers, places it in contact with a particular spot on the patient's body, and lets nature do the rest. Dosage is determined by how long you let the stinger remain in the skin: for example, you can remove it instantly or let it remain for five minutes.

Treating MS requires the most prolonged treatment, according to IAS data, which is tracking 4,500 individuals with MS. Yet patients report an easing of symptoms, such as less fatigue and reduced cramps, after only 20-40 stings. The bee therapy field is rich with almost unbelievable stories of crippled, bedridden MS patients walking and leading productive lives again within 6-18 months of beginning bee sting treatment.

Peer-reviewed studies of bee venom published in scientific journals have begun to unravel how this natural substance gets such astonishing results. First, the bee venom works both locally, at the site of injection, and systemically, through stimulating the immune system. Second, bee venom contains substances whose anti-inflammatory effect is 100 times stronger than hydrocortisone (and you don't get unpleasant drug side effects with bee venom). Research also indicates that bee venom is a potent antioxidant.[28]

All these benefits do come with a slight risk. Scientists estimate that about 2% of the population is allergic to honey-bee stings and will experience an allergic or even anaphylactic shock reaction to the venom.

---

ing an extract of the offending substance in the largest dose that does not cause a reaction (such as a skin wheal), the patient can be desensitized. "Once environmental or dietary substances to which the patient is individually sensitive are removed," says Dr. Oberg, "it is entirely possible that remission can occur." Electrodermal screening may also prove beneficial in determining toxins and allergens complicating MS.

 See Biological Dentistry, Chelation Therapy, Detoxification Therapy, Environmental Medicine, Enzyme Therapy, Neural Therapy, Oxygen Therapies.

Biological Dentistry

The removal of mercury-containing dental fillings is an intrinsic part of the treatment of multiple sclerosis. According to Dr. Huggins, mercury vapor escaping from dental fillings can interfere with the action of key enzymes, thus disturbing important enzymatic functions in the body. He adds that mercury vapor is implicated in chronic fatigue, a common MS symptom.[27]

Replacing mercury fillings with other kinds of material, however, is not as straightforward as it seems. Dr. Huggins warns that some plastic materials can contain aluminum and thereby create different problems for the patient. Before any work is begun, patients of Dr. Huggins first receive a "serum bio-compatibility blood test" to determine which alternative material is biologically compatible. Dr. Huggins explains, "The patient's blood is tested against multiple dental materials. Some dental materials cause immune reactions and others immune suppression. Neither are healthy conditions. Since no material is 100% safe, we do immunologic testing on each patient's blood to determine where reactivity is. After identifying the allergen-like and immuno-suppressive reactivity levels, a computer matches available dental materials with reactivity and suggests the safest materials for that particular patient."

Dr. Huggins's treatment is individualized and based on the results of extensive tests. After removal of the mercury fillings, a detoxification program is developed according to the requirements of each patient and can include nutritional support, acupressure, and massage treatments. Chelating agents such as DMSA (2,3-dimercaptosuccinic acid), DMPS (2,3-dimercaptopropane-1-sulfonate), and vitamin C can be used either intravenously or in tablet form to remove mercury residues. As DMPS and DMSA also remove vital minerals from the body, zinc, copper, magnesium, selenium, and manganese should be taken in addition to the other usual supplements. The program also has a psychological component and Dr. Huggins warns that emotional release often occurs during detoxification. The program is then followed up with nutritional supplements to balance body chemistry and boost immune function, as well as individualized dietary and lifestyle guidelines. Recommendations are also made concerning the use of saunas and bodywork to enhance the detoxification process.

Dr. Huggins has seen approximately 400 cases of MS at his center, 85% of which have improved. Positive changes include patients who are able to walk again after having been confined to a wheelchair.

Hyperbaric Oxygen Therapy

In hyperbaric oxygen therapy (HBOT), a patient is placed in an oxygen chamber. Atmospheric pressure is then elevated in order to increase the amount of oxygen entering the body's tissues. The method and its technology were originally developed in the 1930s by the military for diving operations, decompression sickness, and air embolism, but it has been used in hospitals since then for the treatment of burns and wounds and carbon monoxide poisoning. As well as oxygenating the tissues, David Hughes, D.Sc., Director of the Hyperbaric Oxygen Institute, in San Bernadino, California, notes that HBOT may also enhance the immune system, reduce inflammation via its effect on prostaglandins, help in the repair of damaged blood vessels, stimulate the circulation in the small blood vessels, and in a variety of ways assist in the production of myelin. Bladder and bowel dysfunction are two of the symptoms of MS that most improve with HBOT.[29]

Exactly how this procedure works for patients with MS is still a matter of conjecture and debate. One theory is that MS is a "wound or a disease of the blood vessels in the central nervous system," contends Richard A. Neubauer, M.D., of Lauderdale-by-the-Sea, Florida, author of *Hyperbaric Oxygen Therapy*. A condition of chronic high blood pressure within the brain and spinal

cord damages blood vessels and leads to a lack of oxygen similar to that seen in cases of stroke. HBOT reoxygenates these oxygen-deprived tissues, he says.

While some medical literature refutes HBOT's effectiveness, in Britain several thousand people with MS have received HBOT treatments. From 1983 to 1987, 500,000 individual sessions were provided, and nearly half of the 4,000 people involved benefited in one or more ways.[30] HBOT was effective in keeping many people from getting worse, often improving their general condition and reversing many minor symptoms. Dr. Neubauer likens HBOT to insulin for diabetes: "It provides a significant chance for control and stabilization of MS." Documented benefits include a lessening of fatigue and pain, and improvements in balance, bladder control, vision, upper and lower limb mobility, coordination, and speech.

Dr. Neubauer suggests that, on average, 20 HBOT sessions annually (1-2 per month) are enough to prevent a recurrence of MS. For best results, he recommends starting HBOT treatment as early as possible following the initial MS diagnosis.

Enzyme Therapy

According to Hector H. Solorzano del Rio, M.D., D.Sc., Chairman of the Program for Studies of Alternative Medicine at the University of Guadalajara, in Mexico, pancreatic enzymes can help patients with multiple sclerosis. He cites the case of a 40-year-old male patient confined to a wheelchair, who had not benefited from orthodox medical treatments. After a month of enzyme treatments, he had gained sufficient strength to begin taking care of himself. Three months later, he began to walk, and after six months he was leading a productive life.

Why does an MS patient need enzymes? Studies suggest a strong correlation between digestive dysfunction and the worsening of the disease. The problem lies in what are called circulating immune complexes (CICs), undigested food particles surrounded by immune cells that circulate in the blood, never digested or removed from the body. As CIC levels decrease, MS patients have longer periods free from relapse. Enzyme supplementation breaks up CICs, improves digestion and assimilation, and gives the MS patient a respite between the flare-ups of symptoms.

Hundreds of MS patients in Mexico and Germany have sought out enzyme therapy. These patients are also given unsaturated fatty acids and often supplements of selenium. Apparently, response to enzyme therapy is much faster if patients have not previously been given treatment that has suppressed the immune system.

Magnetic Field Therapy

While electromagnetic fields (EMFs) may exacerbate MS symptoms, magnetic field therapy using weak, pulsed EMFs has shown success in alleviating some of those symptoms. Dr. Laibow estimates that 60%-70% of MS patients experience some improvement with pulsed magnetic field therapy. Studies have shown that pulsed EMFs can improve MS symptoms, including alexia (the loss of the ability to understand written language)[31] and partial cataplexy,[32] as well as bladder control, spasticity, and fatigue.[33]

MS patients should also consider using devices to protect themselves from harmful EMFs. Dr. Laibow recommends that her MS patients wear the Teslar Watch (named after Nikola Tesla, the inventor of alternating current and 'father' of the scalar technology the Teslar Watch employs). The Teslar Watch screens harmful signals while radiating its own signal similar to the Earth's resonance of 7-9 Hz. This enables the body to operate within its own natural frequency range.

Attitude and Lifestyle Changes

Dr. Kingsley advises that "taking an active role in treatment should be the first concern of a person diagnosed with multiple sclerosis. This includes positive cooperation with the practitioner, as well as possible fundamental lifestyle changes in work, relationships, and environmental conditions. Changes may be necessary to improve a person's condition; it may be inadvisable, even impossible, to carry on as if nothing has happened."

Dr. Swank finds stress to be the second most important cause of MS after high-fat diets. "Continuing stress, such as from legal actions and family problems, can cause MS," he says. Dr. Swank treats these patients with mild sedatives to help them sleep and be more relaxed during the day. For mild stress, he suggests taking a short rest in the afternoon and, for more severe stress, he advises a rest mid-morning as well. Meditation, biofeedback, guided imagery/visualization,[34] hypnosis,[35] Tai Chi,[36] and other methods can help those with MS by facilitating deep relaxation, which supports the body in its processes of maintenance and repair and replenishes its stress-fighting resources.

MS patients who smoke cigarettes should quit. One recent study found that people with MS who smoked experienced a deterioration of motor function immediately after smoking, probably due to the effects of nicotine on the central nervous system.[37]

"Exercise is very important for MS patients for a wide variety of reasons, ranging from its anti-depressive impact to its immunomodulatory effect," says Dr. Laibow. Many people with MS are more disabled than they need be. Gentle exercise will help keep someone with MS toned, supple, and mobile. Any type of exercise will do, although yoga is particularly suited for helping patients regain lost movement. Aerobic exercise (three 40-minute sessions per week) has been found to improve quality of life, fitness, and emotional/social behavior in MS patients.[38]

CAUTION MS patients should avoid excessive heating of the body. In particular, avoid sedentary hyperthermic exposure (for example, sauna or sunbathing) as opposed to medically sanctioned aerobic exercise. MS patients should consult with a qualified health-care practitioner before beginning an exercise program.

Recommendations

- Early diagnosis is an essential first step in treating multiple sclerosis. For the best chance of success, treatment of the disease should begin as soon as possible after diagnosis. Electrodermal screening can help diagnose MS before standard tests become abnormal or classic symptoms develop.

- Adopt a low-fat diet—MS patients who eat the lowest amount of saturated fat realize the greatest improvement, and those who eat saturated fat in larger amounts fare worse.

- Avoid: solid fats, hydrogenated oils, margarine, red meats, dairy products, cooked eggs, shellfish, alcohol, sugar, chocolate, monosodium glutamate (MSG), wheat products, yeast, additives, fermented foods, most fast foods and prepared foods, hydrolized vegetable proteins, and (as much as possible) salt.

- Include: tofu, mung bean sprouts, millet, organic oatcakes (unless allergic to gluten), fresh organically raised poultry, some nuts and seeds, tahini, most vegetables, and selected fruits.

- You can boost your dietary intake of omega-3 fatty acids by eating more dark-green leafy vegetables; flaxseed, soy, and walnut oils; pumpkin seeds, sesame seeds, walnuts, almonds; and the wild plants chia, cattail, and purslane. Other types of omega-3 fatty acids beneficial for MS include eicosapentaenoic acid (EPA) and docosahexaenoic acid (DHA), found in salmon, bluefish, bass, trout, and brown and red algae.

- Supplements frequently recommended are vitamins B₁, B₃ (niacin), B₆, B₁₂, and C, as well as zinc, magnesium, calcium (especially calcium-AEP), and selenium. Important nutrients for MS sufferers include L-glutathione, mixed carotenoids including beta carotene, pantothenic acid, folic acid, vitamin E, choline, L-carnitine, dimethylsulfoxide (DMSO) or methylsulfonylmethane (MSM), bioflavonoids, methionine, cysteine, and alpha-lipoic acid.

- Search for and eliminate the environmental or dietary factors that may be exacerbating MS symptoms (especially geopathic stress fields, chemical pollutants, and food allergens).

- The proper removal of mercury-containing dental fillings and subsequent mercury detoxification are critically important parts of the treatment of MS.

- Hyperbaric oxygen therapy may enhance the immune system and reduce inflammation.

- While some electromagnetic fields (EMFs) may exacerbate MS symptoms, magnetic field therapy using weak, pulsed EMFs has shown success in alleviating some of those symptoms. It is estimated that 60%–70% of MS patients experience some improvement with magnetic field therapy.

- Meditation, biofeedback, guided imagery/visualization, hypnosis, Tai Chi, and other methods can facilitate deep relaxation.

- Gentle exercise will help keep someone with MS toned, supple, and mobile.

Self–Care
The following therapies can be undertaken at home under appropriate professional supervision:

Detoxification Therapy / Exercise / Mind/Body Medicine / Yoga

AROMATHERAPY: Rub affected part with mixture of 95% olive oil and 5% essence of juniper or rosemary.

AYURVEDA: The herb *ashwagandha* is recommended.

HYDROTHERAPY: Constitutional hydrotherapy should be applied two to five times weekly.

JUICE THERAPY: Short fasts with fruit and vegetable juices.

PRACTICAL HINTS: Avoid the use of electric heating pads, chlorinated water, and fluoride (in water, toothpaste, and mouthwash).

Professional Care
The following therapies should only be provided by a qualified health professional:

Biofeedback Training and Neurotherapy / Cell Therapy / Chelation Therapy / Diet / Guided Imagery / Hypnotherapy / Nutritional Medicine / Traditional Chinese Medicine

BODYWORK: Massage, Feldenkrais Method.

DETOXIFICATION THERAPIES: Unclogging the lymph system is an important part of any detoxification strategy and can help with MS. Techniques that can help unclog the lymph include manual lymph drain massage, light beam therapy, dry skin brushing, exercise, dietary recommendations and herbs, herbal wraps, acupressure, and reflexology.

OSTEOPATHIC MEDICINE: To relieve symptoms.

Where to Find Help

For additional information on, and referrals for, treatment of multiple sclerosis, contact the following organizations.

American Academy of Biological Dentistry
P.O. Box 856
Carmel Valley, California 93924
(408) 659-5385

The purpose of the AABD is to promote biological dental medicine, which uses nontoxic diagnostic and therapeutic approaches in the field of clinical dentistry. The academy publishes a quarterly journal and holds regular seminars on biological diagnosis and therapy.

American Association of Oriental Medicine (AAOM)
433 Front Street
Catasauqua, Pennsylvania 18032
(888) 500-7999
Website: www.aaom.org

The AAOM is a national professional organization of acupuncturists who meet acceptable standards of competency and can provide you with names and locations of local members.

American College of Hyperbaric Medicine
Ocean Medical Center
4001 Ocean Drive, Suite 105
Lauderdale-by-the-Sea, Florida 33308
(954) 771-4000

For information and referrals for hyperbaric oxygen therapy.

Foundation for Toxic Free Dentistry
P.O. Box 608010
Orlando, Florida 32860-8010

A nonprofit group whose main goal is to educate and refer the general public to biological dentists worldwide. Send a self-addressed, stamped envelope (with enough postage for two ounces) and they will send information and referrals.

Huggins Diagnostic Center
P.O. Box 49145
Colorado Springs, Colorado 80919
(719) 522-0566
Website: www.hugnet.com

For information on removal of mercury fillings.

Oregon Health Sciences University
Multiple Sclerosis Center of Oregon
Department of Neurology, UHS 42
3181 S.W. Sam Jackson Park Road
Portland, Oregon 97201
(503) 494-5759

For additional information on the Swank diet and other approaches to MS.

Recommended Reading

It's All in Your Head: The Link Between Mercury Amalgams and Illness. Hal Huggins, D.D.S. New York: Avery Penguin Putnam, 1993.

Multiple Sclerosis—A Self-Help Guide to Its Management. Judy Graham. Rochester, VT: Inner Traditions, 1990.

The Multiple Sclerosis Diet Book. Roy L. Swank, M.D., Ph.D., and Barbara Brewer Duggan. New York: Doubleday, 1987.

Natural Way with Multiple Sclerosis. Richard Thomas. Rockport, MA: Element, 1995.

Reversing Multiple Sclerosis: 9 Effective Steps to Recover Your Health. Celeste Pepe, D.C., N.D. Charlottesville, VA: Hampton Roads, 2001.

OBESITY AND WEIGHT LOSS

Obesity clearly poses a danger to health, having been associated with numerous health problems, including heart disease, high blood pressure, diabetes, and certain types of cancer. However, diets for weight loss have been shown to be ineffective and even damaging to health. A well-balanced diet that avoids the wrong dietary fats, refined sugars, and excess calories (which all contribute to weight gain), regular exercise, drinking adequate amounts of pure water, and stress reduction can help maintain a healthy weight.

WEIGHT LOSS has become a national obsession in America. As many as 40% of women and 24% of men in the U.S. are trying to lose weight at any given time through such diverse methods as diets, special dietary supplements, exercise, behavior modification, and drugs. While this obsession is often fueled by psychological needs (the urge to conform to an artificial standard of beauty fostered by media, fashion, and peer pressure) rather than physical needs, it is estimated that 97 million Americans are overweight.[1] The World Health Organization estimates that over 300 million adults are obese worldwide. Obesity (defined as being 20% or more over average weight) among U.S. adults increased by 50% between 1991 and 1998.[2] Even more troubling, according to Joseph E. Pizzorno, N.D., President Emeritus, of Bastyr University, in Kenmore, Washington, is the fact that the number of severely obese children in the U.S. nearly doubled between 1965 and 1980. This trend, if it continues, will only lead to an even greater frequency of adult obesity as these children grow up.

This is alarming because excess weight has been linked to a number of health problems, including high blood pressure,[3] heart disease, stroke,[4] diabetes,[5] gallbladder disease, respiratory conditions, as well as breast, endometrial, and uterine cancers in women, and cancer of the colon and rectum in men.[6] In fact, 85% of Type II diabetes cases are attributed to obesity, along with 45% of hypertension, 35% of heart disease, and 18% of high cholesterol.[7] Obesity has also been shown to result in a decreased life span for both women and men[8] and may be a contributing factor in as many as 300,000 deaths each year.[9] About $65 billion is spent each year on health complications related to obesity. Add indirect costs, such as disability and lost work productivity, and the total climbs above $100 billion.[10]

The answers to weight gain and weight loss, though, are not always simple and easy. Under controlled settings, most people trying to lose weight are usually able to lose about 10% of their total body weight, but up to two-thirds of that weight is regained within a year. Every year, 80 million Americans go on a diet and up to 95% of them gain back any weight they lose within five years; one-third gain back more weight.[11] "Fad diets can be a very temporary way to get started, but recognize it is not long term," says Gary Ewing, M.D., of the University of South Carolina School of Medicine's Department of Family and Preventive Medicine. "Anything you can do in a few days, you can undo in a few days."[12]

To achieve significant and permanent weight loss, you need to come up with a plan—incorporating healthier eating, exercise, stress reduction, and healing any underlying imbalances—that will last a lifetime.

Causes of Obesity and Weight Gain

Obesity is indicated by an abnormally high proportion of body fat, but, according to Timothy Birdsall, N.D., of Sandpoint, Idaho, "although it is commonly assumed that obesity is due to overeating, there is, in fact, a complex interaction between one's culture, environment, exercise habits, and eating styles, as well as one's genetic makeup, biochemical individuality, and physiological set point." Individual metabolism is inherent and created by lifestyle, diet, and exercise habits. Researchers have found that obesity tends to run in families. This may be partially due to genetics, but could also be influenced by dietary and lifestyle habits learned as a child, including the kinds of food you tend to eat (for example, high-fat or processed foods) and how often you eat.

The set point theory states that one's size and body fat are determined by genetics, eating patterns, and calorie intake at certain key times in life such as early adolescence. These patterns are relatively fixed, says Elson Haas, M.D., Director of the Preventive Medical Center of Marin, in San Rafael, California, and author of *Staying Healthy with Nutrition*. Attempting to arrive at a weight above or below one's set point range causes physiological mechanisms that ultimately force behavioral changes and a return to one's previous weight. A good example of this is the rapid weight gain that can happen after coming off a diet, especially a low-calorie starvation diet. The body reacts to what it perceives as a threat, quickly regaining the weight to once again reach its natural set point.

Perhaps, living in the "consumer culture" of the United States, it is our just reward to be consuming ourselves to death. Not only are we eating more, but also the kinds of foods we consume—fast foods, processed and high in fat—offer the least nutrition and the most potential for adding fat to our hips. And we're eating too much, period: average calorie intake is over 2,000 calories per day compared to 1,800 calories in the 1970s.[13] The food industry is doing its part to keep us "living large"—it spends $36 billion every year on advertising and a typical child sees up to 10,000 food commercials every year.[14]

Perhaps, living in the "consumer culture" of the United States, it is our just reward to be consuming ourselves to death. Not only are we eating more, but also the kinds of foods we consume—fast foods, processed and high in fat—offer the least nutrition and the most potential for adding fat to our hips.

There are also cases where excess weight is gained because of conditions such as food allergies and nutritional deficiencies, which are often treatable. Food allergies cause water retention and weight gain, as well as food cravings and many physical and emotional problems. Recent research suggests that food addictions may be another explanation for obesity—it was found that obese individuals have fewer dopamine receptors in their brains (dopamine is the brain chemical that triggers feelings of satisfaction).[15] Weight gain may also be due to a sluggish

metabolism, chemical toxicity, insulin imbalance, impaired thermogenesis (the mechanism by which fat is burned to produce body heat), excessive dieting, or psychological factors. In some cases, obesity occurs as a signal that a more serious disease is present, such as hypothyroidism or Cushing's syndrome (hypersecretion of adrenal hormones).

Sluggish Metabolism

Thin people have higher metabolic rates and burn calories at a much faster rate than their obese friends, says Majid Ali, M.D., Associate Professor of Pathology at Columbia University, in New York. Metabolic rate can be understood as being the rate by which the body utilizes energy. The basal metabolic rate (BMR), which varies tremendously between individuals, is the minimum amount of energy needed to maintain normal body functions. Age, sex, body size, and fat-to-muscle ratio are all factors that influence how efficiently an individual burns calories. Even when individuals are matched for all of these factors, they can exhibit a 30% difference in BMR.[16] The types of food a person eats may also affect metabolic rate. According to Dr. Birdsall, carbohydrates are most effective in raising the metabolic rate. He points out that while fats can also increase the metabolic rate, they contain more calories per gram than carbohydrates and are therefore relatively less effective.

An inefficient thyroid gland (hypothyroidism) can be the cause of sluggish metabolic rate, says Dr. Birdsall. And while it is possible that laboratory tests will not indicate the existence of hypothyroidism, other tests, such as basal body temperature, and symptoms, such as chronic constipation, fatigue, feeling cold, and a tendency to gain weight, may point to subclinical hypothyroidism. When metabolism slows, the body will store rather than burn calories, causing an accumulation of fat. Insufficient thyroid hormones and the consequent slowing of metabolism affects nearly every function in the body and several of these have a direct connection to weight problems:

- Many people with low thyroid function have puffy, thick skin and retain fluid throughout their bodies. This is because of an accumulation of hyalouronic acid, a sugar that binds with water in the body, causing swelling and an increase in weight.[17]

- Hypothyroidism leads to a sluggish digestive system, often resulting in a number of gastrointestinal problems, including constipation, gas and bloating, abdominal pain, and decreased absorption of nutrients. Decreased digestive efficiency may lead to a condition called leaky gut syndrome, in which undigested food particles enter the bloodstream causing

TRUTHS AND FALLACIES ABOUT OBESITY

According to Gus Prosch, Jr., M.D., of Birmingham, Alabama, an obesity specialist who has treated thousands of overweight patients, there are seven critical fallacies relating to the problem of obesity, as well as seven truths or facts. These fallacies and truths are accurate 99% of the time, says Dr. Prosch. Understanding these before entry into a weight-control program will save an overweight person much time, effort, money, and disappointment.

The seven fallacies about obesity:

1. Fad diets can successfully make you lose weight and keep the weight off.

2. Most physicians can successfully help you lose weight and keep the weight off.

3. Today's many and varied weight-loss programs and clinics can successfully and permanently make you lose weight and keep the weight off.

4. Past experiences show that counting calories is a good way to help you lose weight and keep the weight off.

5. Your weight problem is caused from overeating and/or lack of exercise alone.

6. If you could only lose enough weight to get slim, you could keep your weight off from then on.

7. There is no way that you can lose your weight successfully and keep the weight off.

The seven truths about obesity:

1. If obese, you have a lifetime disease.

2. Your metabolic processes will always tend to be abnormal.

3. You cannot eat what others eat and stay thin.

4. Anyone can lose weight and stay slim provided the causes of weight gain are determined, addressed, and corrected.

5. Understanding insulin metabolism is the key to losing weight intelligently.

6. There is absolutely no physiological requirement for sugar or processed foods in your diet.

7. You cannot lose weight and keep it off successfully by strictly and solely following any special diet, or by taking a weight-loss pill, or by following an exercise program. To succeed, you must address all the contributing factors causing obesity. And you must make exercise and physical activity a lifetime effort.

allergic reactions and depleting the immune system. Weight gain is one of the potential results of these digestive disturbances.[18]

- Hypothyroidism is linked to pancreatitis, a decrease in insulin production by the pancreas due to inflammation. Insulin is the hormone that controls how the body processes sugars. When insulin imbalances occur, blood sugars, rather than being burned off, are turned into fat.[19]

- Decreases in the levels of thyroid hormones reduce the body's thermogenic or fat-burning capacity, leading to increased fat storage.[20]

Impaired Thermogenesis

Stephen Langer, M.D., of Berkeley, California, author of *Solved: The Riddle of Weight Loss*, describes the different ways the body uses calories. "Energy output," he says, "actually breaks down into three parts: basal metabolism (how fast you burn up energy in your cells in a resting state); thermogenesis (energy, in the form of heat, given off above the metabolic resting rate); and, of course, physical exercise."[21] The first two ways of burning calories are unknown to most people. If either basal metabolism or thermogenesis is impaired, your body loses one of its outlets for burning calories. These calories then accumulate in your body as fat, even if you are dieting and exercising.

The body contains two types of fat tissue, white adipose tissue, which stores fat, and brown adipose tissue (BAT), which burns fat to produce heat. Evidence indicates that an impairment of the thermogenesis system in BAT may lead to obesity.[22] If fat from the diet is not burned up by BAT, it is stored as fat in white adipose tissue, thus contributing to excess body weight. Chronic dieting can alter BAT's responsiveness, lowering thermogenesis and causing increased hunger, according to Dr. Birdsall.

"Brown fat may well be the most important discovery to explain why some people can remain thin while eating everything in sight, while others, no matter how restricted their caloric intake, still cannot lose weight," says nutritionist Ann Louise Gittleman, M.S., of Bozeman, Montana, author of *Beyond Pritikin*.[23]

Toxic Load

The liver serves as a filter for the toxins that the body absorbs from food, air, and water. Unhealthy lifestyles, poor diet, and exposure to industrial chemicals and pesticides can overload the liver with poisons, creating toxic conditions in the body that may cause a buildup of fat. Most people do not associate weight gain with exposure to toxic substances, but the truth is that the poisons that accumulate in our bodies can lead to a host of degenerative diseases. However, well before these diseases take hold, our bodies will begin to accumulate fat in response to the increased toxic burden. Toxicity is one of the primary causes of excessive weight, particularly in people who have problems keeping weight off.[24] When the liver becomes overloaded with toxins, it causes certain imbalances that lead to weight gain, including blood sugar imbalance, essential fatty acid deficiency, and slowed metabolism.

Many people who are overweight or obese are, in fact, "lymph fat." Stagnant lymph fluid holds water and toxins so that body bulk accumulates. People with this type of obesity often have hands and feet that appear small compared to their body bulk. Lymphatic detoxification using manual lymph drainage massage, lymphatic exercises such as rebounding, and other therapies can help stimulate the flow of lymph fluid in the body.

Unhealthy or compromised intestinal function can also have a major impact on your weight. Many people with a toxic colon simply may not be able to absorb the nutrients from the foods they're eating and may overeat as a result. "When the bowel fails, the whole body goes into a nutritional crisis. Metabolic shock waves flow to every cell and tissue," says nutritionist Bernard Jensen, D.C., Ph.D., of Escondido, California, who has treated thousands of colon patients during his 60 years of practice.[25] Nutritionist Lindsey Duncan agrees that a clean colon aids in digestion and the ability to metabolize food. "Over 90% of the people I see are metabolizing less than 55% of what they are eating," she says. "They think it's normal to have a bowel movement once every few days. I often startle my clients with the question, 'If we eat three meals daily but only eliminate once a day, or once every other day, where do you think all the rest of that food is hiding?'"

Toxic by-products from the colon can drain the body of energy, lower metabolism, and overburden other detoxifying organs, such as the liver and kidneys. The importance of removing toxic waste from the bowel is to stop damaging by-products from recycling back into the body. Once the colon is clean, metabolism is more likely to work properly and a major obstacle to weight loss is eliminated.

Insulin Imbalance

Many cases of obesity are due to an imbalance of the hormone insulin, says David K. Shefrin, N.D., of Beaverton, Oregon. Insulin allows the body to utilize glucose (sugar) and carbohydrates. Factors such as genetic predisposition, food allergies, eating habits, and stress may interfere with glucose and carbohydrate utilization, result-

ing in a condition known as glucose intolerance. Excessive sugar consumption (refined carbohydrates) may also contribute to glucose intolerance and obesity.[26]

If insulin is not rapidly cleared from the bloodstream after a meal, it will cause an individual to feel hungry, says Dr. Shefrin. Usually insulin will signal the body to stop eating, but if a person has chronically elevated glucose levels due to inefficient insulin, he may eat more. Thus, the more refined carbohydrates a person eats, the hungrier he or she may become. Research also shows that overweight individuals burn sugar less effectively than individuals of normal weight and that dieting only makes this problem worse. The same research concludes that this trait is a part, not a consequence, of obesity.[27]

When an overweight person becomes more obese, the insulin problem becomes worse as well, because the individual becomes more unresponsive to the action of insulin, says Gus Prosch, Jr., M.D., an obesity specialist from Birmingham, Alabama. In such a person, the simple carbohydrates are triggering the release of increasing amounts of insulin, but the body cannot use it efficiently. This is why we see high insulin levels in overweight people. Apparently the insulin receptors on their body cells are blocked from performing their function. This prevents insulin from stimulating the transfer of glucose to the cells to give them energy, which explains why so many overweight people feel tired so often. To make matters worse, since the insulin is not converting the glucose to energy, more glucose is then moved into the fat cells to create more fat.

Ultimately, either the insulin receptors or the pancreas itself wears out or becomes exhausted, in which case diabetes will result, according to Dr. Prosch. This excess insulin in overweight people can lead to other problems and complications, including:

- Increased salt and water retention

- Sleep disorders caused by insulin interference with neurotransmitters

- The production of more LDLs, or bad cholesterol, by the liver due to insulin stimulation

- Interference with the thyroid hormone thyroxine, thereby aggravating low metabolism

- Hypoglycemia, hunger, and a further craving for simple carbohydrates

These factors illustrate why sugars and simple carbohydrates are so detrimental to the health of America, says Dr. Prosch. The number of overweight and obese people in this country is constantly increasing, and the problem will continue to get even worse until our health leaders learn the truth and fulfill their responsibility to inform citizens of these facts. "We are so inundated with bad foods and obesity-generating products—from sodas to cookies to breads and other baked goods—that it is a challenge for every person to eat a healthy diet," says Dr. Haas.

We are so inundated with bad foods and obesity-generating products—from sodas to cookies to breads and other baked goods— that it is a challenge for every person to eat a healthy diet.

—ELSON M. HAAS, M.D.

Lack of Exercise

The amount of exercise you get on a regular basis will strongly affect your weight. Our lives in general are less physically active compared to previous generations and most of us aren't getting enough exercise to make up for it. Children in America now spend an estimated 2½ hours per day watching television.[28] A quarter of the population is completely sedentary, while 55% are "inadequately active," according to the CDC.[29]

Exercise is important for long-term weight management because it speeds metabolism and preserves lean muscle. Muscles burn more calories and, in the absence of exercise, muscle mass can be lost during a restricted calorie diet. While dieters may lose weight, those who incorporate regular moderate exercise are building muscle that increases their metabolism and improves their overall health.

In a recent study, three groups of dieters were assessed on their weight management over the course of two years. The first group was assigned to a restricted-calorie diet, the second group was prescribed diet and exercise, and the third group assigned an exercise program only. A year later, the dieters lost an average of 15 pounds, the dieters who exercised lost 20 pounds, and the exercisers lost six pounds. During the second year, however, dieters regained about a pound, the dieters who exercised regained all of the weight they had lost, and the exercisers regained less than half a pound. "We were shocked," said researcher John Foreyt, Ph.D., of Baylor College, in Waco, Texas. "We'd put our money on the diet-plus-exercise group, but apparently the negative effects of restrictive dieting—feelings of hunger and deprivation—eventually lead to overeating."[30]

Dieting

With thousands of diets and a multimillion-dollar industry dedicated to weight control, shedding a few pounds should be easy. Unfortunately, the weight lost by dieters is almost always regained. As a result, many dieters fall into the yo-yo trap—a repetitive cycle of weight loss and gain. This is primarily because, after losing weight on a diet, people go back to their previous ways of eating, which results in the same body plus a few pounds.

Susan Kano, a national speaker and author on dieting and eating disorders, tells a story about a friend who had not only been trying to lose weight for years, but was also in the dieting business. Initially, she struggled to get from 165 pounds down to 120. After a while, her weight returned to the 165-pound mark. Over the years, as she tried one diet after another, her weight went up and down. Today, she continues to diet and weighs over 200 pounds.

There are several reasons why this happens and why food restriction for the purposes of weight loss should be avoided. We have gotten fatter as a culture over the last few years, says Kano, partly because of dieting. Whenever the body is deprived of food, whether from famine or dieting, it ensures survival by decreasing the metabolic rate in order to compensate for fewer calories. Energy is stored so efficiently in adipose (fat) tissues that someone of normal weight can survive for two months without eating. The desire to binge after food restriction, although disheartening to dieters, is another built-in survival mechanism intended to click on after a famine.[31] Our innocent cellular metabolism has no way to tell the difference between self-imposed starvation and life-threatening famine.

Dieting can be a cause of obesity and not the way to lose weight, adds Dr. Ali. Dieting not only slows down the metabolism, but leads to the emaciation of muscle cells, bloating of fat cells, accumulation of toxic fats in tissues, and fatigue. The more rapid the weight loss, the higher the risk of heart complications from muscle loss as well. An obese person needs to gain muscle mass and increase the amount of fat-burning tissue, continues Dr. Ali. Increased muscle mass will improve metabolism. This usually means a slight initial weight gain, or at least absence of weight loss (because muscle tissue is heavier than fat tissue). Only then can someone hope to increase the rate of burning, and losing, fat, says Dr. Ali.

THE DIET CRAZE

No doubt you've fallen for one or more of the diet-of-the-week schemes over the years, promising quick and painless weight loss. Over the last 30 years, we've seen quite a few diets come and go: the Grapefruit diet, Atkins diet, Pritikin Plan, Fit for Life, Beverly Hills diet, the Rotation diet, Scarsdale diet, Ornish plan, Cabbage Soup diet, the Zone—the list goes on and on. Every time you look, there's another diet book on top of the best-seller lists or the latest diet "guru" promising miracles on the talk shows.

First, you're told to count calories. Then, it's not about calories but about eating low-fat foods. Others told you that the magic formula for weight loss was eating lots of protein and cutting back on carbohydrates. Still others advocated high-carbohydrate diets. What you end up with is a glut of confusing and conflicting messages about weight loss.

A recent survey by the Calorie Control Council found that 27% of adult Americans are on a diet, while another 39% are trying to control their weight but do not consider themselves to be dieting. "Dieting is now perceived as a quick-fix, short-term, on-again, off-again solution to a weight problem," concludes John Foreyt, Ph.D., Director of the Nutrition Research Clinic at Baylor College of Medicine, in Waco, Texas. However, those trying to control their weight see this as "something to be permanently incorporated into their lifestyle, recognizing that to be successful at maintaining a healthy weight, they'll have to develop lifelong habits incorporating diet and exercise." In this same survey, people were asked why they had failed to stay at their desired weight. The number one answer was that they weren't getting enough exercise (56%).

The fad diets, by concentrating on food restrictions, ignore the importance of incorporating physical activity into one's life. Other reasons given for failure: bingeing on favorite foods (41%) and watching only fat intake and not calories (34%). "Counting fat at the exclusion of calories and bingeing are two symptoms of a diet gone awry," says Dr. Foreyt. "The fact that dieters are more prone to these behaviors is further evidence that diets usually fail."[32]

According to a study done by *Consumer Reports* magazine, commercial diet programs don't work either. *Consumer Reports* evaluated programs offered by Diet Center, Jenny Craig, Nutri/System, Physicians Weight Loss Centers, Health Management Resources, Medifast, Optifast, and Weight Watchers. Most of these programs prescribe a low-calorie diet of about 1,000-1,500 calories a day, exercise, and counseling. The *Consumer Reports* study found that "most individuals who go through a commercial diet program typically regain half their lost weight in a year and much of the rest in another year." In general, the researchers concluded, "there is no evidence that commercial weight-loss programs help most people achieve significant, permanent weight loss."[33]

Psychosocial Factors

Psychology may play a significant role in weight gain: many people who overeat do so in response to stress, anger, sadness, boredom, or other emotional factors unrelated to hunger or nutritional needs.[34] Food is an intricate and tightly woven part of social activities, childhood memories, and the psyche. Food is used to help celebrate almost all major holidays and events. In the U.S., birthdays are marked by cakes and ice cream; Halloween is centered around candy and other treats; July Fourth celebrates with picnics; and Thanksgiving, with its traditional feast of turkey, stuffing, and gravy, isn't complete without a thick slab of pumpkin pie and whipped cream. Even romantic dating centers around eating.

Foods affect moods by triggering the release of endorphins, the body's natural painkillers, and the brain chemical serotonin, a mood regulator. Unfortunately, these foods (chocolate, carbohydrates, sweets) not only elevate your mood but also trigger cravings for more.[35]

This kind of "emotional eating" can contribute significantly to weight gain if you lead a stressful life or have unresolved emotional issues. Any attempts at weight loss will prove unsuccessful until these issues are resolved. "People that are overweight can be using food as a tranquilizer or a reward or a substitute for affection," says Douglas Ringrose, M.D., Director of the Ringrose Wellness Institute, in Edmonton, Alberta, Canada, which specializes in the treatment of eating disorders. "Others eat because it's something to do when they're bored or to turn themselves into a fortress against the world."

Everybody has consumed foods for reasons other than that they were hungry. Occasional "emotional eating," to relieve anxiety or make you feel better, is perfectly normal. But when it leads to overeating, significant weight gain, and poor dietary choices, emotional eating can seriously affect your health. Food can also become a substitute for or an escape from addressing the under-

DIET AND SELF IMAGE

As you explore your emotional issues, it is important to keep in mind that your inner desires and feelings regarding body weight are shaped by what you see and hear every day. You need to distinguish between feelings and desires that are your own and those that come from social pressure. "Rapid weight loss at any price, so you can fit into a particular dress or feel comfortable in a swimsuit, is about image," says Jeremy Kaslow, M.D. "Weight management however, is about the pursuit of lifelong health, and the two are very different."

Many individuals try to lose weight in pursuit of a sexier, slimmer image. However, the yearning to "look good" is almost always motivated by a need to conform to someone else's ideal of what you should look like. As you explore what has been driving you to gain weight, ask yourself why you feel the need to reduce. It is important not to confuse the yearnings to satisfy someone else's demands with your own desire to be healthy and live at your peak physical level.

Because of the diet culture and the commercial interests that bombard us with images of ultra-thin models, we learn to hate our own bodies and, in turn, are led to destructive and self-defeating eating behaviors. The reality is that most of us can never attain the cultural ideal, no matter how hard we try, because of our innate body type. "The standard for a beautiful body, the movie-star, magazine-model body, is natural for only a fifth of the population. This has created a whole generation of women who are dieting and exercising compulsively, and often uselessly, at the expense of their health in pursuit of an unrealistic ideal," says psychologist Kathleen Pichola, Ph.D.[38] Freeing yourself from such ideals may be the best thing you can do to restore your health.

These dependency patterns can be established early in life. "Feeding children sweets to comfort, distract, or amuse them encourages both the brain and body to develop chemical and behavioral pathways leaning toward food (especially simple carbohydrates) as support," says Rima Laibow, M.D., founding Medical Director of the Alexandria Institute of Natural and Integrative Medicine, in Croton-on-Hudson, New York. "These patterns can literally be deadly later on in life."

Feeding children sweets to comfort, distract, or amuse them encourages both the brain and body to develop chemical and behavioral pathways leaning toward food as support. These patterns can literally be deadly later on in life.

—RIMA LAIBOW, M.D.

Stress also causes biochemical changes in the brain that induce cravings for sweets. Sarah Leibowitz, Ph.D., of Rockefeller University, says that the production of cortisol, one of the hormones secreted by the adrenals during stress, stimulates the production of a brain chemical called neuropeptide Y. This chemical can set off an alarm within the body for sweet or starchy foods. As we satisfy this desire by eating a candy bar or some other similar food, the neurochemical buzzer quiets down and we usually feel better. If the alarm goes off in the morning, however, it may stay "turned on" all day, causing a relentless craving for sweets.[37]

Are You Overweight?

You probably know if you're overweight—your clothes seem a little tight or your body just feels uncomfortable or bulky to you. A quick look in the mirror may confirm the extra pounds. However, an ideal weight for you should be based on feeling healthy, not on how you or others think you should look. One of the easiest ways to get a general picture of where you are on the weight scale is to use the guidelines issued by the U.S. Department of Health and Human Services. These general guidelines give normal weight ranges based on height and age.

When you've found your correct weight range, keep in mind your frame size (small, medium, or large) and gender when considering where you fall in a given range.

lying psychological problems—these buried feelings can also be detrimental to your health.

"In situations such as boredom and loneliness, eating becomes a way to fill the emotional void," according to Elizabeth Somer, M.A., R.D., author of *Food and Mood*. "While preventing boredom and developing meaningful relationships take time and effort, eating is easy and relatively effortless. Boredom, anxiety, anger, depression, jealousy, and other emotions are a normal part of life, but using food to treat them or to avoid resolving them is not a long-term solution for feeling better."[36]

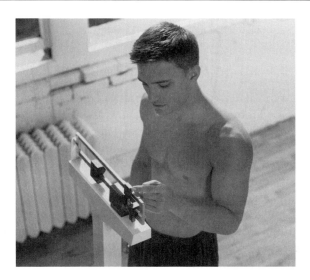

HEIGHT	WEIGHT (IN POUNDS)	
	Ages 19-34	Ages 35 and up
5' 0"	97-128	108-138
5' 1"	101-132	111-143
5' 2"	104-137	115-148
5' 3"	107-141	119-152
5' 4"	111-146	122-157
5' 5"	114-150	126-162
5' 6"	118-155	130-167
5' 7"	121-160	134-172
5' 8"	125-164	138-178
5' 9"	129-169	142-183
5' 10"	132-174	146-188
5' 11"	136-179	152-194
6' 0"	140-184	155-199
6' 1"	144-189	159-205
6' 2"	148-195	164-210
6' 3"	152-200	168-216
6' 4"	156-205	173-222
6' 5"	160-211	177-228
6' 6"	164-216	182-234

Specifically, those with smaller frames should be on the lower end of a given range while those with larger frames will be on the higher end. Men will generally fall on the higher end of each weight range because they tend to have higher muscle and bone mass and women will be on the lower end of the range. Again, these are meant as general guidelines, not as absolute numbers—you need to always bear in mind your unique physiology.

 No single table or measurement should be relied on solely to indicate a weight problem. Use these measurements as a general guide. If they indicate a potential weight problem, it is best to check with your health-care professional for further evaluation.

Body Mass Index (BMI)

Calculating your body mass index is another way to determine if you are overweight, with a little more precision than the height–weight charts. The BMI is the ratio of your weight to your height. The BMI is based on the metric system, so pounds and inches will need to be converted to kilograms and meters.

1. Multiply your weight in pounds by 704. For example, if a person weighs 160 pounds, multiply 160 by 704, which equals 112,640.

2. Convert your height to inches (5′10″ equals 70 inches), then multiply it by itself. In this example, 70 inches multiplied by 70 inches equals 4,900.

3. Divide the answer from step 1 by the answer in step 2: 112,640 divided by 4,900 equals 22.99, which should be rounded to the nearest whole number. This is your BMI. So, our 5′10″ person who weighs 160 pounds has a BMI of 23.

The higher your BMI, the greater your health risk. Physicians generally consider a BMI between 20 and 25 to be acceptable; those with a BMI from 27 up to 30 are considered overweight and at a higher risk for weight-related diseases; those with a BMI of 30 and higher are considered obese.[39]

BMI should not be used by pregnant women, bodybuilders or other competitive athletes, children, or the elderly (particularly those who are sedentary or frail).

Body Fat or Body Lean?

These charts and calculations are intended to help you determine if you have a weight problem. They are relatively easy ways of estimating your body fat based on standards for your height and age. Overall weight is used as an indicator of excess body fat. However, you can also more directly measure your body fat (as opposed to lean body tissue such as muscle and bone).

"Experts are beginning to realize that their best measure of overall health is not weight-to-height-to-sex-to-age ratios, but the ratio of body fat to body lean tissue," states Daniel B. Mowrey, Ph.D., Director of the American Phytotherapy Research Laboratory, in Lehi, Utah. Dr. Mowrey believes that putting aside the old concept of weight management in favor of fat management is more useful.[40]

There are a number of ways of measuring body fat, all of which are generally performed in a physician's office, health club, or weight-loss clinic. One method uses calipers to measure skinfold thickness at various points on the body. Another method is called hydrostatic weighing, where a person is weighed repeatedly both in and out of water; since fat is lighter than water, the proportion of fat to other tissues can be calculated. A third way of determining body fat is through bioelectric impedance, in which a small electric current is passed through the body; because fat tissue is a poor conductor compared to lean body mass, the percentage of fat in the body can be estimated. Cost and convenience may be factors in whether or not you choose to use one of these methods.

How Do You Feel?

One last determinant of whether or not you have a weight problem is how you feel. Your level of health and vitality is the final measure of your ideal weight. So, answer a few questions about your overall state of health:

- Do you have plenty of energy? Or would you like to have more?

- What health problems do you have?

- Does your weight hamper your movements or activities?

- Do you feel comfortable with your size?

- Do you have eating disorders, like compulsive overeating, that leave you debilitated physically and emotionally?

- Would you like to feel better than you do?

Use these questions, along with the other measurements, to assess if weight may be a factor in any health problems you may be experiencing and if you might benefit from a weight-loss program.

Treating Obesity

Dr. Birdsall believes that proper diet and exercise are the most effective ways to lose weight. However, he feels that it is not a matter of how much a person eats, but what the person eats that is important, and that one's diet must be high in complex carbohydrates. Other approaches to treating obesity include detoxification, stimulating thermogenesis, and correcting any underlying condition affecting one's weight, such as insulin imbalance or hypothyroidism. Herbs and nutritional supplements may also prove beneficial in some cases.

 See Detoxification Therapy, Diet, Herbal Medicine, Mind/Body Medicine, Nutritional Medicine.

Diet

The typical American diet includes more refined and processed foods than the diet of any other nation. When food is refined and processed, not only is fiber removed but simple sugars often replace complex carbohydrates. A diet low in fiber and high in simple sugars can be a major contributing factor to excess weight gain. Fiber, on the other hand, can help weight loss as evidenced by the almost complete absence of obesity in cultures that consume a diet high in fiber.[41] Fiber has been shown to not only reduce cholesterol, but also to pull dietary fat from the body into the feces. Other benefits of roughage include increasing chewing time, thus slowing down the eating process and inducing satiety, preventing constipation, and stabilizing blood glucose levels.[42]

A whole foods, whole grain, high-complex carbohydrate, low-fat, high-fiber diet is recommended by Dr. Birdsall. He suggests a maximum of 25% of the daily food intake be in the form of fat and all of this should be healthy vegetable oils from nuts and seeds and olive oil. In general, this amounts to 45-50 grams per day, which represents about 450 calories.

Dr. Haas points out that certain people will do better on different types of diets, with the one consistent factor being that the diets are low in fat. For instance, some people will do better on a low-carbohydrate diet, instead of one that is high in carbohydrates, he says. As long as the fat content of the diet remains low, the overweight person can have success. This was verified by a Cornell University study, which showed that when women were allowed to eat as much as they wanted, with the only restriction being that they had to consume low-fat foods (only 20% to 25% of calories as fat), they lost weight.[43] This is due to the fact that fat contains more than twice as many calories per gram as protein or carbohydrates. A Swiss study also revealed that, unlike carbohydrates, approximately 90% of excess fat consumed during a meal is converted to body fat.[44] Very fatty foods may also encourage overeating because more needs to be consumed in order to maintain the body's storage of glucose.[45] Weight loss should therefore be directed toward a change in eating habits rather than dieting.

Alcohol should also be avoided or minimized, since it has been found to act like a sugar and be converted to fat in the body, affecting the liver with fatty deposits and promoting weight gain. J.P. Flatt, Ph.D., from the University of Massachusetts Medical School, estimates that one ounce of alcohol represents ½ ounce of fat in the diet.[46] Cigarettes, which are used by many people to manage their appetite, also appear to steer extra fat to the abdomen. In addition, both of these substances should be especially avoided by those who are prone to glucose intolerance.

Alternative medicine practitioners recognize that individuals have different nutritional requirements. As Ralph Golan, M.D., author of *Optimal Wellness*, explains, "A successful weight-loss regimen requires a diet tailored to individual needs. Some may lose weight and thrive on a high-protein, low-carbohydrate diet, whereas others get results on a high-complex-carbohydrate, low-protein diet."[47] The key is to match the diet to individual physiological needs.

Nutritional Supplements

- Vitamin A facilitates the efficient absorption of nutrients by strengthening the lining of the digestive tract. Along with vitamins C and E, it bolsters the immune system and thus makes the body more resistant to infection from parasites and yeast overgrowth, two common causes of weight gain. Vitamin A is also necessary for the production of thyroxin, a thyroid hormone, and helps the thyroid to absorb iodine, a key nutrient.[48] The healthy functioning of the thyroid is essential to maintaining metabolism and preventing the accumulation of body fat.

- Vitamin B1 (thiamin) and vitamin B2 (riboflavin) primarily serve in the maintenance of mucous membranes, formation of red blood cells, and metabolism of carbohydrates. Deficiencies of vitamin B1 may lead to blood sugar imbalances.

- Vitamin B3 (niacin) is necessary for oxygen transport in the blood and fatty acid and nucleic acid formation. It is also vital to the actions of more than 150 enzymes in the body—without these enzymatic reactions, our body's energy production would quickly shut down.

- Vitamin B5 (pantothenic acid) is vital for synthesis of hormones and support of the adrenal glands. Pantothenic acid deficiency can cause fatigue, insomnia, and depression.[49] Some researchers claim that vitamin B5 also increases the rate at which fat and carbohydrates are metabolized.

- Vitamin B6 (pyridoxine) strongly influences the immune and nervous systems. It aids in fat and protein metabolism and the conversion of the amino acid tryptophan to the brain neurotransmitter serotonin, which helps to control appetite.[50]

- Choline is a B vitamin that helps the body break down fats and transport them in and out of cells.

- Inositol is a B vitamin important for bone marrow, eyes, and intestines. It assists in metabolizing fats in the blood and liver and lowers cholesterol.

- Chromium is a mineral essential for regulating the production of the hormone insulin, which is responsible for stabilizing blood sugar levels and preventing the conversion of blood sugar into fat. Over the years, research has demonstrated that chromium deficiency impairs glucose tolerance, decreases circulating insulin levels, boosts blood sugar levels, and elevates levels of triglycerides and cholesterol.[51]

- Iodine, along with the minerals copper, zinc, and selenium, is part of the structure of thyroid hormones (especially thyroxin), which regulate how fast the body burns calories.

- Amino acids are the building blocks of proteins, each one having a specific function. Certain specific amino acids are helpful for weight loss, although it is generally recommended that a complex of free-form amino acids be taken instead of individual ones. Isoleucine aids in energy production, hemoglobin (carries oxygen in blood) formation, and in the regulation of energy from blood sugars. Methionine helps prevent excessive accumulation of fats in the liver and vascular system and detoxifies heavy metals and toxins. Alanine promotes immunity and assists the body in metabolizing glucose. L-carnitine helps bring fat molecules to the "furnaces" of the cells, the mitochondria, so they can be burned for energy instead of stored in fat cells.

- Hydroxycitric acid (HCA) is derived from the dried rind of the tamarind fruit (*Garcinia cambogia*). It helps to clear fats from the liver, helps suppress appetite, and slows the rate at which the body converts carbohydrates into fat. Studies show that HCA reduces food consumption by approximately 10%.[52] HCA has been found to be more effective when taken in combination with chromium.

- Fiber helps flush wastes from the body, works to reduce blood sugar levels, and contributes to feelings of fullness.

Detoxification

Obesity is almost always associated with toxicity, as many toxins are stored in fatty tissue, according to Dr. Haas.

SPECIFIC DIETS FOR WEIGHT LOSS AND WEIGHT MANAGEMENT

According to Elson Haas, M.D., Director of the Preventive Medical Center of Marin, in San Rafael, California, and author of *Staying Healthy with Nutrition* and *The False Diet*, the following diets may prove effective for both weight loss and weight management as part of a general health maintenance program.

The Fish-Fowl-Green Vegetable Diet includes fresh ocean fish, tuna, shrimp, and trout, plus organic poultry and green vegetables, both raw and cooked. This is basically a protein-vegetarian, low-carbohydrate diet, which has become more popular in the last decade. These foods can be eaten in any quantity desired, within reason. One piece of fresh fruit and one cooked egg are also suggested daily. Some bran and/or psyllium can be used to support bowel function. Salad dressing should be limited to 1-2 tablespoons of vegetable oil, such as olive or flaxseed, with some fresh lemon juice or vinegar. If no oils are used, an essential fatty acid supplement should be taken. A few raw nuts or seeds could also be used.

Daily fluid intake should be 8-10 glasses (eight ounces each) of good clean water, such as home-purified water or bottled spring water, and/or herbal teas. Two to three glasses should be drunk first thing in the morning and then again 30-60 minutes before each meal. Clear soup broth is also acceptable. A general multivitamin should be taken daily. Several pounds a week can be lost fairly easily with this diet even with only moderate activity, but the diet should be followed no longer than one or two months at the most, says Dr. Haas.

The High-Fiber Starch Diet can be a good weight-loss plan for overweight vegetarians, especially if they avoid excessive sweets, according to Dr. Haas. Complex carbohydrates, such as whole grains, legumes, pasta, potatoes, and starchy vegetables are eaten at the beginning of a meal in order to provide bulk, thus decreasing appetite and giving a feeling of fullness, he explains. These are relatively low-calorie foods if they do not have sauces, gravy, butter, or oil added to them. Vegetables can be consumed as desired, at least several cups daily. Dr. Haas also suggests a couple of pieces of fruit daily. Dairy foods, red meats, and any fried, fatty, or refined foods should be avoided, as should sweets.

Water intake should be maintained at 8-10 glasses daily. A multivitamin can also be taken, along with some extra vitamin B12. Care should be taken that iron and calcium

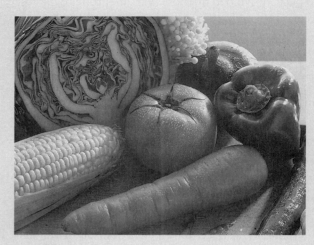

intakes are adequate. These and other minerals might be supplemented, though most should be found in sufficient amounts in this diet.

The Allergy-Rotation Diet is becoming more popular for weight loss as well as for general health, especially when there are food allergies present. Any foods shown to be a possible problem should be eliminated from the diet for one to two months, depending on the degree of sensitivity. If a person seems to be addicted to any foods—craving them and eating them every day, sometimes even at every meal—those foods should be completely removed from the diet for at least several weeks before testing them, although avoiding them even for only four days will allow the body to be sensitive to their true effects, says Dr. Haas. Testing them involves a food challenge, whereby an adequate portion of the food is eaten by itself and then the person is monitored over the next 24 hours or so for reactions. Some reactions can even take 3-4 days to appear. Keep in mind that there are many ways to react to foods, some of which are not allergies. Laboratory tests can also elucidate which foods are problematic.

To desensitize to other possible food allergies, a rotating diet means setting up a four-day rotation plan. Any food eaten on one day must be excluded from the diet for the next three days, Dr. Haas explains. For example, if apples, corn, and peas are eaten on Monday, you would not eat them again until Friday. Eliminating allergenic foods also reduces water retention through reduced immune reactions and secondary inflammation, allowing the person to feel much better while slimming down.

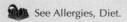 See Allergies, Diet.

SPECIFIC DIETS FOR WEIGHT LOSS AND WEIGHT MANAGEMENT, continued

The Ideal Diet is a well-balanced diet that incorporates aspects of all the previous diets. It is a rotation diet, good for food allergies; it has a high-fiber content from whole grains and vegetables; it is low in fat; and it contains good quality protein. The diet is as follows:

- Early morning: one or two pieces of fruit.

- Breakfast: starch, such as cereal grain or potatoes

- Mid-morning: snack of fruit most days and occasionally nuts or seeds

- Lunch: protein and green and other vegetables

- Mid-afternoon: snack, vegetable or fruit

- Dinner: starch or protein with vegetable

- Evening snack: vegetable or fruit, if needed

Water should be consumed as usual, 8-10 glasses per day, mainly taken about one hour before meals, and a multivitamin/mineral supplement can also be used. Additional water and fiber and more filling low-calorie foods will help in decreasing the appetite, Dr. Haas says. They will also support good colon function, which is helpful to detoxification and reducing food cravings.

Detoxification programs can eliminate accumulated toxins, restore healthy functioning of key organs, and provide long-term maintenance and support. Specifically, a detoxification program provides the means by which excessive toxins, wastes, fats, mucus, parasites, and bacteria can be cleared from the body. This will help reduce the toxic load weighing down the immune system, stop the excessive proliferation of free radicals, lessen damage to key enzymes and the loss of other essential nutrients, and prevent the accumulation of heavy metals.

The benefits of detoxification include increased vitality, reduced blood fats (cholesterol and triglycerides), improved assimilation of vitamins and minerals, and mental clarity. Individuals who have undergone detoxification programs report better sleeping patterns, more efficient metabolism (which often translates into weight loss), and more energy. Several methods of detoxification are available, including fasting on water, juicing, specific diets, colon cleansing, liver and kidney flushes, lymphatic detoxification, and homeopathic remedies. Related therapies for detoxification incorporate bodywork, lymphatic drainage, aromatherapy, antioxidant defense support, and

nutrient and herbal support to bolster the organs of detoxification.

When we lose weight, we reduce our fat and thereby our toxic load. However, during weight loss, we release more toxins and thus need protection through greater intake of water, fiber, and antioxidant nutrients such as vitamins C and E, beta carotene, selenium, and zinc. Dr. Haas adds that L-cysteine can also be used, as it helps liver and intestinal detoxification processes.

Michelle Pouliot, N.D., from Torrington, Connecticut, recalls a woman in her mid-forties who sought help for a weight problem. The woman had had many surgeries and an extensive history of prescription drug use. Dr. Pouliot helped to stabilize the woman's health, then put her on a detoxification program using a whole foods diet, an occasional two-day vegetable juice fast, mild exercise, and meditation. To help the woman release toxins through her skin, Dr. Pouliot instructed her to soak in an Epsom salts bath and do dry brush massages three times per week. Drinking eight glasses of water per day supplemented with cranberry juice extract helped her kidneys flush out poisons. Fiber supplements moved waste out of her colon and milk thistle helped her liver detoxify more effectively. Finally, deep breathing exercised her lungs. After three weeks, she had lost 17 pounds.

CAUTION Many health professionals use fasting for therapeutic reasons other than weight loss, particularly detoxification. While weight is invariably lost during any fast, the results are not usually permanent, unless one uses the fast as a transition into a healthier diet and healthier habits. Juice cleansing is a great catalyst for change. Still, if you are considering a fast for any reason, do so only under the guidance of a trained health-care provider.

Correcting Insulin Imbalance

Rather than being concerned about calories, you should always try to eat foods low on the glycemic index (see below). Here are some other basic dietary rules for blood sugar health:

- Eat whole, fresh, and unprocessed foods as much as possible

- Avoid simple or refined carbohydrates and sugar products and replace them with complex carbohydrates, such as whole grains, beans, and vegetables; complex carbohydrates are easier on the pancreas and promote insulin balance

SUCCESS STORY: THE INDIVIDUAL APPROACH TO WEIGHT LOSS

Amelia, 41, was a retired executive who had fought with her weight her entire life. She was 5'7" and weighed 340 pounds. Her body mass index or BMI was 53 (body mass index is a ratio of your weight to your height; a BMI of 27 or higher is considered overweight). After she turned 40, Amelia began to have more problems with her weight and her physician told her that she had high blood pressure, high cholesterol, and that she was diabetic. Her physician recommended medications for each of these problems, but Amelia wanted another option.

She came to see Frances Gough, M.D., and Teresa Girolami, M.D., of Sound Weight Solutions in Bellevue, Washington. Amelia was put on a comprehensive program of dietary changes, exercise, and counseling. "Our philosophy is that life is a series of decisions and choices and being enabled to make good, confident decisions about diet and exercise leads to success," says Dr. Gough. "Positive changes need to be a priority and worked at every day."

Amelia's diet consisted of large amounts of meat, cheese, and butter. She disliked vegetables of any type and incorporated few of them into her diet. Dr. Gough instructed her to keep a food diary, writing down everything she consumed for a week. "The diet diary helps people understand what they're actually eating," says Dr. Gough. "They're quite surprised when they write it down—they forgot about that cookie they grabbed on their way out the door and little things like that."

Amelia then met with a holistic nutrition specialist for a full assessment of her food intake. The nutritionist used a special computer program to design dietary guidelines specifically for Amelia. She was advised to convert to a whole foods diet, primarily vegetarian with five servings of fruits and vegetables every day, and cut back on meat consumption to once or twice weekly. She discovered that, while she disliked cooked vegetables, she actually enjoyed eating raw ones. Amelia was quite enthusiastic about the vegetarian approach and even bought a rice cooker to start eating more rice and vegetables. One session with the nutritionist involved a trip to the grocery store to help Amelia make healthier choices when shopping for foods as well.

How do you get people to make better food choices? "You take the worst habits and begin to modify them," says Dr. Gough. "Then, that builds and builds until, over a few weeks, they're eating things that are far more healthful and that they feel comfortable with."

Amelia participated in weekly group therapy sessions to help with the emotional issues surrounding weight problems and trying to lose excess weight. The therapy program also focuses on lifestyle changes (in behavior, attitude, and self-esteem) that are helpful in maintaining weight loss. Items that might be discussed in a typical therapy session include: issues of loneliness, depression, and isolation and how they relate to food bingeing; sabotage from others—family members who bring home high-calorie foods, chocolates, cookies, and other snacks; and how to stay on a healthful eating plan while maintaining a hectic schedule. Peer support greatly improves the chances of maintaining weight loss, according to Dr. Gough. "Some type of therapy, particularly in a group, is highly beneficial and helps solidify their motivation and their feelings about what they're going through," she says.

Amelia also began an exercise program with a personal trainer, working out for one hour three times per week. Her program began with a body composition assessment using bioelectric impedence, in which a small electric current is passed through the body to measure levels of body fat. This measurement is more specific than simply stepping on a scale, allowing the person to see how much fat they may be losing and muscle they're gaining from an exercise regimen. Based on this analysis, the trainer then designed an exercise program for Amelia, including both cardiovascular exercises and weight training.

In nine months on this program, Amelia lost 60 pounds. That amounted to a 5% reduction in body fat and a 5% increase in lean body mass. Her BMI dropped from 53 to 42. Her blood pressure dropped from 160/110 to 130/80 and her cholesterol, triglycerides, and blood sugar levels were all within normal ranges. More importantly, Amelia learned to incorporate these healthy changes into her life and continues to lose weight. "You could say that the supplement we use is an educational supplement," explains Dr. Gough. "Education to help people make the choices they need to make to get out of the situation they're in. We help them make good choices nutritionally, good choices behaviorally, and good choices in terms of exercise."

- Eat at least three regular meals per day or, alternatively, eat five or six smaller meals throughout the day; this helps stabilize the release of blood sugar

- Eat adequate amounts of protein (meat, chicken, fish, eggs, dairy, beans, tofu, nuts) at each meal, including breakfast; proteins take longer to break down in the body, thus stabilizing blood sugar levels

- Avoid foods made with hydrogenated oils and incorporate adequate amounts of healthy fats, such as organic, unprocessed olive, sesame, or flax oils; healthy fats extend the release time for sugar into the bloodstream

- Reduce your intake of fruit juices and dried fruits and drink vegetable juices (except carrot and beet) and herbal teas instead; fruit sugars can cause a rapid rise in blood sugar levels

- Reduce your intake of caffeinated beverages, which stimulate blood sugar and insulin, and alcohol

- Avoid artificial sweeteners and products containing them[53]

To evaluate foods based on their insulin impact, a scientific rating system called the glycemic index was developed by diabetes researchers at the University of Toronto. Richard Podell, M.D., Medical Director of the Overlook Center for Weight Management, in Springfield, New Jersey, indicates that choosing foods with a low glycemic index is "the secret to keeping blood sugar stable, insulin low, and hunger in check." Dr. Podell has simplified the index into basic categories, which he presents in his book *The G-Index Diet*.[54] He makes the following general observations:

- Foods with a higher rating, causing a higher insulin response, include white bread, bagels, muffins, packaged flaked cereals, instant hot cereals, low-fat frozen desserts, raisins and other dried fruits, whole milk and whole-milk cheeses, peanuts and peanut butter, hot dogs, and luncheon meats.

- Foods with a low rating, not causing a high insulin spike, include most fresh vegetables, leafy greens, pitted fruits and melons, coarse 100% whole-grain breads and minimally processed whole-grain cereals, sweet potatoes, skim milk, buttermilk, poultry, lean cuts of beef, pork, veal, shellfish, white-fleshed fish, most legumes, and most nuts.

- Cooked foods rank higher on the index than raw foods. Similarly, fruits and vegetables that have been juiced or puréed are higher on the index than when eaten whole.

Vitamins that help to both restore and maintain insulin potency are zinc (20-30 mg daily), manganese (5-10 mg daily), and vitamin C (3,000 mg daily). For maximum benefit, take these supplements once per day. A B-complex vitamin (50 mg, three times daily) is also useful for controlling blood sugar levels; deficiencies of vitamin B_1 tend to mimic and aggravate hypoglycemia, B_5 helps support the adrenal glands, and biotin enhances glucose utilization and reduces sugar cravings.[55] The trace mineral vanadium also helps regulate blood sugar levels. It is present in small amounts in unsaturated vegetable oils and grains and is also available in supplement form as vanadyl sulfate; typical dosage is 10-20 mg daily.[56]

Herbs may also be helpful for controlling blood sugar. *Gymnema sylvestre* is an Ayurvedic herb often used to treat diabetes. *Gymnema sylvestre* inhibits the taste of sugar and also blocks the absorption of sugar by as much as 50%, making this herb useful for blood sugar control. In addition, some evidence suggests that it can enhance the activity of insulin in the body.[57] *Stevia rebaudiana*, a South American herbal sweetener, helps stabilize blood sugar while not requiring insulin for its metabolism. Stevia is over ten times sweeter than sugar and contains only one calorie per ten leaves. Available in powder or liquid forms, stevia can safely be used as a sugar substitute in cooking.[58] Ingredients in green tea *(Camellia sinensis)* may influence the way sugars are absorbed and processed by the body. It is thought that green tea slows the release of carbohydrates, which prevents an insulin surge and stimulates fat burning rather than fat storage.[59]

Exercise

Food fuels the furnace of metabolism; exercise stokes its fire, says Dr. Ali. Yet, almost as important as exercise, is what kind of exercise one does. Exercise that causes sweating and heavy breathing is sugar-burning exercise. Overweight people need fat-burning exercise, which requires slow, sustained activity. Dr. Birdsall recommends 45-60 minutes of vigorous walking or other aerobic activity every day, if possible, or at least five times per week. Stretching daily is also recommended. Exercise such as walking possesses many health benefits, including lowering the set point and increasing the metabolic rate.[60] The key is finding an activity one likes and then changing exercise plans periodically to alleviate boredom.

Boosting Thermogenesis

Gamma-linolenic acid (GLA), an omega-6 essential fatty acid, has been shown to be effective at reactivating brown fat and increasing thermogenesis.[61] Normally, the body can manufacture GLA from dietary sources of linoleic acid, another omega-6 oil; sources of linoleic acid include safflower, sunflower, corn, soybean, and flaxseed oils.

Medium-chain triglycerides (MCTs) are saturated fats that promote weight loss. MCTs are a form of natural fat found in certain seeds that tend to accelerate metabolism while lowering blood levels of cholesterol. Naturopath Michael T. Murray, N.D., says that MCTs, unlike other types of fat, tend to be rapidly burned up rather than stored as fat. In fact, one study found that those who added just 1-2 tablespoons of MCTs to their normal diet burned 5% more calories.[62] Good sources of MCTs are grapeseed and coconut oils, available at most health food stores.

Carnitine is a nutrient primarily found in meats and dairy products that can boost your metabolism by helping your body burn off fat more efficiently. "Carnitine is the forklift that takes fat to the fat incinerators in our cells—the mitochondria," says Robert Crayhon, M.S., author of *The Carnitine Miracle.* "Unless fat makes it into the mitochondria, you can't burn it off no matter what you do or how well you diet." As part of a weight-loss program, Crayhon typically recommends 1,000-4,000 mg of carnitine daily.[63]

Ginseng has an ancient history and as such has accumulated much folklore about its actions and uses. Common varieties are Oriental ginseng *(Panax ginseng),* American ginseng *(Panax quinquefolius),* and Siberian ginseng *(Eleutherococcus senticosus).* In traditional Chinese medicine, ginseng is used as a general tonic to improve stamina during exercise, sharpen mental abilities, and relieve fatigue. Research indicates that ginseng may be able to raise basal metabolic rates as well. Ginseng should not be abused, however, as serious side effects can occur, including headaches, skin problems, and other reactions.[64]

Ephedra, also known as *ma-huang,* has become a popular ingredient in natural weight-reducing formulas. Its effectiveness and ability to enhance the burning of fat, especially when taken with green tea or coffee, is due to the active ingredient ephedrine. Many people, particularly women who have a history of chronic dieting, can benefit from this herb as it helps to stabilize and enhance their metabolic rates. An over-the-counter preparation containing ephedrine can stimulate the brown adipose tissue to burn fat, which produces heat that is dissipated by the body.[65] It also has a mild appetite suppressant action, according to Dr. Birdsall. The effects of ephedrine can be enhanced by caffeine, theophylline (a white, crystalline alkaloid derived from tea), and aspirin.[66] These preparations offer a way to burn excess fat in patients with thermogenic deficiencies.

Many people, however, will experience side effects like irritability, anxiety, insomnia, hyperactivity, rapid heart rate, and increased blood pressure. Used alone, ephedra can lead to rapid weight loss, but the pounds usually return once the herb is discontinued. Although herbs can have adverse side effects, Dr. Birdsall says they are rare and only short-term. In eight years of practice, he has only had three patients who had to discontinue ephedra. He finds herbs to be highly effective, but cautions that they should only be used under professional supervision. For best results, ephedra should be part of a comprehensive program that includes permanent lifestyle changes, including diet and exercise.

> **CAUTION** Ephedra should be used only under medical supervision. Ephedra should not be used by anyone with heart disease, high blood pressure, thyroid disease, diabetes, or benign prostatic hypertrophy. If using antidepressant drugs or medication for hypertension, avoid ephedra. Pregnant women should also avoid taking this herb.

Psychological Counseling

Obviously, one way to prevent the weight-gaining effects of stress is to avoid stressful situations. However, since stress is not always avoidable, it is important to be able to control how you react to a stressful situation. Mind/body treatments, such as guided imagery, Neuro-Linguistic Programming, neurobiofeedback, and hypnotherapy, can "reprogram" the negative psychological factors that may be contributing to weight gain, helping you gain greater control over your emotional responses. These therapies help you "stockpile positive emotions and sweep out negative thoughts," according to Dr. Ringrose. "You're programming your computer, the brain, for the emotions that you want, rather than any that are trying to intrude and sabotage your weight-loss efforts." Other therapies, including meditation, acupuncture, flower essences, and aromatherapy, can also be used to mitigate the effects of stress.

Lauri Aesoph, N.D., from Sioux Falls, South Dakota, recalls a woman in her early forties who decided to investigate weight loss after her husband left her because he thought she was too fat. Over a series of visits, the woman was instructed in how to select foods that were healthy for her and was encouraged to exercise regularly. Midway through her program, it was discovered that she had been sexually molested as a young woman. Eventually the woman came to understand that she might have gained weight to protect herself from sexual intimacy. To help her open the door to her feelings, she was given weekly guidance concerning the physical and emotional changes that were taking place in her life. The homeopathic remedy *Calcarea carbonica,* which fitted her constitutional symptoms, was prescribed. As the remedy began to work, her fears and apprehensions around sex and being thin surfaced, but as she continued to openly discuss her feelings and fears, her weight dropped until she reached her desired goal. At that point, she no longer resisted feeling sexually attractive and, according to Dr. Aesoph, she began to enjoy her new lifestyle and body.

Recommendations

- A whole foods, whole grain, high-complex carbohydrate, low-fat, high-fiber diet is recommended.

- Vitamin B6 (pyridoxine) aids in fat and protein metabolism and the conversion of the amino acid tryptophan to the brain neurotransmitter serotonin, which helps to control appetite.

- Chromium is a mineral essential for regulating the production of the hormone insulin, which is responsible for stabilizing blood sugar levels.

- Fiber helps flush wastes from the body, works to reduce blood sugar levels, and contributes to feelings of fullness.

- Obesity is almost always associated with toxicity, as many toxins are stored in fatty tissue. Detoxification programs can eliminate accumulated toxins, restore healthy functioning of key organs, and provide long-term maintenance and support.

- Rather than being concerned about calories, you should always try to eat foods low on the glycemic index.

- Exercises, such as walking possess many health benefits, including lowering the set point and increasing the metabolic rate.

- Gamma-linolenic acid (GLA), an omega-6 essential fatty acid, has been shown to be effective at reactivating brown fat and increasing thermogenesis.

- Medium-chain triglycerides are saturated fats that have been shown to promote weight loss.

- Carnitine is a nutrient primarily found in meats and dairy products that can boost your metabolism by helping your body burn off fat more efficiently. Typical recommended dose is 1,000-4,000 mg of carnitine daily.

- Psychology may play a significant role in weight gain: many people who overeat do so in response to stress, anger, sadness, boredom, or other emotional factors unrelated to hunger or nutritional needs. Mind/body therapies such as neurobiofeedback can help you explore and gain control over these issues.

Self-Care
The following therapies can be undertaken at home under appropriate professional supervision:

AROMATHERAPY: Fennel, juniper, rosemary.

JUICE THERAPY: • Celery, watercress, parsley • Lemon, grapefruit, pineapple, grape • Carrot, celery • Carrot, spinach • Carrot, beet, cucumber • Cantaloupe, watermelon

Professional Care
The following therapies should only be provided by a qualified health professional:

Acupuncture / Detoxification Therapy / Hypnotherapy / Mind/Body Medicine / Naturopathic Medicine / Orthomolecular Medicine

Where to Find Help

For more information on, and referrals for, treatment of obesity, contact the following organizations.

American Association of Naturopathic Physicians
8201 Greensboro Drive, Suite 300
McLean, Virginia 22101
(703) 610-9037
Website: www.naturopathic.org

Provides a directory of naturopathic physicians and offers referrals to a nationwide network of accredited or licensed practitioners. Also publishes a quarterly newsletter, for both professionals and the general public, and offers a series of brochures and pamphlets on a variety of subjects.

American Society of Bariatric Physicians
5600 S. Quebec Street, Suite 109A
Englewood, Colorado 80111
(303) 779-4833

Provides referrals for bariatric physicians (weight disorders specialists) to the general public and has a dial-a-tape phone line of prerecorded messages on nutrition, eating disorders, and weight loss.

Overeaters Anonymous
6075 Zenith Court N.E.
Rio Rancho, New Mexico 87124
(505) 891-2664
Website: www.overeatersanonymous.org

The aim of OA is to help people stop eating compulsively by offering support groups and a Twelve-Step method of healing. Call for the location of the nearest chapter.

Recommended Reading

The Butterfly and Life Span Nutrition. Majid Ali, M.D. Denville, NJ: Institute of Preventive Medicine, 1994.

A Cookbook for All Seasons. Elson M. Haas, M.D., and Eleonora Manzolini. Berkeley, CA: Celestial Arts, 2000.

Dr. Braly's Food Allergy & Nutrition Revolution. James Braly, M.D. New Canaan, CT: Keats Publishing, 1992.

Eating Well for Optimum Health. Andrew Weil, M.D. New York: Quill, 2001.

The False Fat Diet. Elson M. Haas, M.D., and Cameron Stauth. New York: Ballantine Books, 2000.

Feeding the Hungry Heart. Geneen Roth. New York: Plume, 1993.

The Metabolic Typing Diet. William L. Wolcott with Trish Fahey. New York: Doubleday, 2000.

The Schwarzbein Principle. Diana Schwarzbein and Nancy Deville. Deerfield Beach, FL: Health Communications, 1999.

Staying Healthy with Nutrition. Elson Haas, M.D. Berkeley, CA: Celestial Arts, 1992.

The Supplement Shopper. Gregory Pouls, D.C., and Maile Pouls, Ph.D., with Burton Goldberg. Tiburon, CA: Future Medicine Publishing, 1999.

Weight Loss: An Alternative Medicine Definitive Guide. Burton Goldberg and the Editors of *Alternative Medicine.* Tiburon, CA: AlternativeMedicine.com Books, 2000.

OSTEOPOROSIS

Osteoporosis is a disabling disease affecting an estimated 28 million Americans.[1] Currently, a third of post-menopausal women in the United States have osteoporosis, and the U.S. has the highest rate of osteoporotic fractures in the world.[2] However, the condition can be halted, and even reversed, using alternative treatments such as nutritional supplementation, diet, herbs, and natural hormonal therapy.

OSTEOPOROSIS IS generally regarded as a metabolic bone disorder—the rate of bone loss (resorption) speeds up while the rate of making new bone tissue slows down. Levels of calcium and phosphate salts decline so that the bones become porous, brittle, and susceptible to fracture for lack of new bone tissue to replace old tissue. You end up with literally less bone (or skeletal mass) in the body and the bone you have is more fragile and subject to fracture.

Each year in the U.S., 1.5 million people over 45 years of age experience bone fractures associated with osteoporosis, mainly in the vertebral column, wrist, and hip.[3] While these fractures can be painful, and vertebral fractures can lead to skeletal deformity, hip fractures are even more serious—20% of older people with hip fractures die within a year of the fracture.[4] The resulting immobility of hip fractures becomes debilitating in and of itself and causes a downward spiral with rapid loss of muscle, bone, endurance, strength, and appetite. The estimated health-care costs due to osteoporotic fractures is $10-$15 billion per year.

While people commonly associate easily broken bones with osteoporosis, many may not realize just how serious the disease is. A woman's risk of developing osteoporosis is higher than the combined risks of developing uterine, ovarian, and breast cancers, and osteoporosis is the fourth leading cause of death in American women.[5] According to John R. Lee, M.D., of Sebastopol, California, osteoporosis affects women more than men because women have less bone mass than men and begin to lose bone far earlier. "Up to age 35, men and women have equal bone stability. For women, the most rapid rate of bone loss occurs in the first five years after menopause, beginning around age 45, when body hormone supplies undergo a dramatic change. Virtually all women lose 5% to 10% of bone mass during this period. The rate of bone

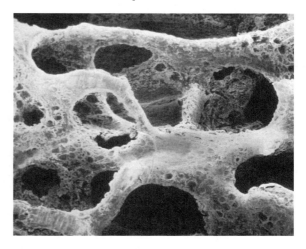

Osteoporotic bone

Osteoporosis is a metabolic bone disorder in which the rate of bone loss speeds up while the rate of making new bone tissue slows down. Levels of calcium and phosphate salts decline so that the bones become porous, brittle, and susceptible to fracture for lack of new bone tissue to replace old tissue.

© 1993 SPL/Custom Medical Stock Photo

loss then drops to about 1% per year." Men don't experience bone loss until after age 70, but once they do contract osteoporosis, the condition can be severe.

Causes of Osteoporosis

Conventional wisdom regards the loss of bone mass as an inevitable part of aging. In actuality, osteoporosis, like heart disease, is "a disease of Western civilization created by our lifestyles," according to Susan E. Brown, Ph.D., Director of the Osteoporosis Education Project, in Syracuse, New York, and author of *Better Bones, Better Body*.

RISK FACTORS OF OSTEOPOROSIS

The following factors are linked to a higher risk of osteoporosis:[9]

- Small bone structure, thin build, and short in height
- High-protein diet and/or high-salt diet
- Low calcium intake (less than 1,200 mg daily)
- Caucasian or Asian heritage (living in the U.S.)
- Fair skin, freckles, blonde or reddish hair
- Cigarette smoking
- Lack of exercise or sunlight
- High caffeine consumption (more than two cups of coffee daily) or high alcohol intake (more than two drinks daily)
- Early menopause (before age 43), either naturally or through surgery such as removal of the ovaries
- Absent or irregular menstrual periods
- Prematurely gray hair (half gray by age 40)
- Use of certain conventional drugs, including glucocorticoids (such as prednisone), anticonvulsants (such as Dilantin), tranquilizers, mood-altering drugs, aluminum-containing antacids
- Frequent indigestion, bloating, and gas
- Family history of osteoporosis
- Never having children
- Thyroid problems, celiac disease (intestinal malabsorption), kidney disease, or liver disease

Early Warning Signs of Osteoporosis

If you have several of the following symptoms, you could be suffering from osteoporosis. Bone screening for the condition may be advisable, especially if a number of the risk factors above are also present in your life.

- Height loss
- Tooth loss and periodontal disease
- Brittle fingernails
- Transparent skin
- Leg cramps at night
- Joint pain
- Insomnia and restless behavior

Some gradual decline in bone mass is a natural fact of aging in all cultures, but in non-Westernized societies it rarely progresses to the point of causing easy fractures. "The highest osteoporosis rates are found in the most prosperous and technologically advanced societies. Conversely, the lowest rates are typically found in poorer, less technologically advanced societies," says Dr. Brown.[6] Nature has designed our bones to last a lifetime, and that includes after menopause, she says.[7]

Osteoporosis is viewed as a disease of postmenopausal women because menopausal drops in estrogen and progesterone levels can contribute to bone loss, and the consequent fractures generally occur later in life. However, osteoporosis can begin in a woman as early as age 35 if her lifestyle includes such factors as chronic stress, cigarette smoking, lack of exercise, and a poor diet. Contrary to popular belief, even if a woman's estrogen levels stay high and she consumes adequate calcium, she can still develop osteoporosis because these lifestyle practices promote the disease.

These bone-depleting lifestyle factors, now attributed to the rise in osteoporosis, have become the focus of alternative care. "Never before have humans been so physically inactive, eaten so much processed food, spent so much time indoors under artificial lighting, taken so many drugs and medications, undergone so many surgical procedures, or exposed themselves to a vast array of chemical, electromagnetic, and informational pollution," states Dr. Brown.[8]

Dietary Factors

When it comes to diet and bone health, it is necessary to maximize the intake of nutrient-dense, bone-building foods and minimize the intake of substances that limit bone health. The standard American diet of processed foods, carbonated soft drinks, caffeine, and high protein, sugar, and salt consumption can promote osteoporosis. According to Dr. Lee, "Processed foods lead directly to calcium loss because these foods are nutrient deficient. This in turn stimulates a need for protein, which, eaten in high amounts, can cause the body to lose calcium."

Researchers have known this relationship between protein intake and calcium loss since 1920, but protein continues to be considered synonymous with being "well-fed."[10] The body cannot store protein, and the excess is metabolized and excreted in urine. Excess protein creates an excess of the waste products that result from the breakdown of protein, including ammonia and acids. Ammonia prevents calcium from being reabsorbed by the kidneys. The acids, which need to be buffered by calcium in the body, also deplete bones of this mineral. This may be why vegetarians seem to have a definite advantage in calcium balance. In one study involving 1,600 women, lacto-ovo vegetarians (vegetarians who eat milk and eggs) of 20 years had only 18% bone loss compared to omnivores (people who eat all types of food), who had lost 35%.[11]

Another source of calcium loss is a high-sodium diet. Women eating 3,900 mg of sodium daily excreted 30% more calcium than those eating 1,600 mg daily.[12] Sugar has been linked to loss of calcium as well and can cause metabolic problems that eventually lead to mineral imbalances.[13]

Soft drinks and caffeine also put bones at risk, according to Dr. Lee. Consuming large amounts of soft drinks high in phosphorus can lead to high levels of phosphorus in the blood. Since the body needs to maintain blood levels of phosphorus and calcium in equal amounts, high phosphorus causes calcium to be drawn from the bones to meet the demand. Caffeine not only increases calcium excretion in the urine, but also allows more calcium to be secreted into the gastrointestinal tract.[14] One study found that individuals who drink more than three cups of coffee a day increase their risk of osteoporosis by 82%.[15]

Research has also linked alcohol consumption and bone loss; specifically, drinking more than a few ounces of alcohol a day inhibits calcium absorption, contributes to calcium loss, and disturbs mineral balance in the body. A study at the Veteran's Affairs Medical Center, in Portland, Oregon, found that alcohol consumption of just one to two drinks daily is "clearly linked with reduced bone mass."[16]

Alan R. Gaby, M.D., of Seattle, Washington, proposes that calcium is receiving more attention than it deserves and that other nutrients may be equally critical to the prevention of osteoporosis. "Vitamin K, silicon, boron, folic acid, magnesium, and manganese all play a role in bone building and need to be consumed through diet or supplements," he says. To prevent osteoporosis, you must get sufficient levels and the proper ratio of these bone nutrients. Unfortunately, they are often deficient in the modern diet, which may be one of the reasons why osteoporosis is a disease of Western civilization. Dr. Gaby notes that our diets have a far lower vitamin and mineral content than those of our ancestors. "Studies indicate that modern farming practices deplete the soil of essential minerals, resulting in lower levels of these minerals in our foods," says Dr. Gaby. Added to this, overconsumption of nutrient-empty foods, such as sugar and white flour, further deprives us of vitamins and minerals.[17]

Hormonal Factors

Conventional medicine views osteoporosis primarily as an estrogen deficiency occurring at menopause. If this were so, then all women around the world would get osteoporosis at menopause, but this is not the case.[18] Further, vegetarian women, who have lower estrogen levels than their meat-eating counterparts, still tend to have more bone mass.[19] "A reduced supply of hormones is the primary cause of menopause-related osteoporosis, a condition that is generally attributed to a lack of estrogen, but the major hormone deficiency of concern in osteo-

porosis is that of progesterone," says Dr. Lee. Progesterone is the hormone that stimulates monthly ovulation, but it also stimulates bone formation by activating osteoblast-mediated mineralization of bone.

Menopause-related osteoporosis is generally attributed to a lack of estrogen, but the major hormone deficiency of concern in osteoporosis is progesterone.
—JOHN R. LEE, M.D.

"Before menopause actually begins, the body starts to decrease its output of progesterone," points out Dr. Lee. "Because of the lack of progesterone, bones slowly begin to lose their mass even prior to menopause." One study of 66 premenopausal women, ages 21 to 41, all of whom were marathon runners, measured hormone levels and bone loss over a year. The researchers found that "while there was no correlation between the rate of bone losses and levels of estrogen, there was a close relationship between progesterone and bone loss."[20] With a combination of low progesterone and poor diet, osteoporosis may already be well under way as women approach menopause. Then, when menstruation ceases, osteoporosis accelerates because estrogen levels fall and the already diminished bone mass is even more rapidly depleted.

Conventional medicine's standard use of estrogen replacement therapy (ERT) on women at menopause is problematic for a number of reasons, not the least of which is that it overlooks the role of progesterone in maintaining bone health. While estrogen can help prevent bone loss, progesterone is needed to build bone.

Environmental Factors

Dr. Gaby says the polluted world is another contributor to the widespread incidence of osteoporosis. Heavy metals such as lead, cadmium, tin (from tin cans), and aluminum are particularly at fault, he says. These heavy metals are found in products to which we are exposed daily and are also delivered to us by acid rain. "Acid rain leaches heavy metals out of the bedrock, moving them into our rivers and lakes, and eventually into the water we drink," says Dr. Gaby. "Acid rain has also caused our drinking water to become more acidic, which challenges our body's buffering capacity, drawing calcium out of

HOW BONES GROW AND CHANGE SHAPE

Bones grow and develop throughout childhood and adolescence, and in a person's twenties bone mass increases by 15%. Every bone has a combination of compact tissue and spongy tissue, with the amount and proportion in constant flux. Some bones are so dense they appear solid, while others are primarily a complex webbing of bone tissue.

Two types of bone cells reshape bones. The osteoclast detects older or slightly damaged bone matter and slowly dissolves it, leaving behind a space. The osteoblast then moves into this space and spins out new bone matter to fill the space. With osteoclast/osteoblast equilibrium, bone mass remains stable. When the equilibrium shifts, bone mass is altered.

Bone, like all living tissue, requires adequate nutrition for proper growth. Bones need sufficient levels of minerals, especially calcium, phosphorous, magnesium, manganese, zinc, copper, and silicon, plus vitamins A, C, and K. Also, vitamin D is necessary to ensure proper intestinal absorption and utilization of calcium. Physical stresses on a bone caused by gravitational pull and the contraction of muscle also stimulate it to increase in size. An arm placed in a cast for a week or two will lose bone mass, as will the bones of astronauts in the gravity-free environment of space flight.

Hormones direct bone-building action. In females, estrogen exerts some control over the osteoclast after puberty, suppressing excessive bone loss, while progesterone stimulates the osteoblast to make new bone. In males, these functions are mediated by testosterone. For both sexes, the thyroid hormone calcitonin helps maintain proper blood levels of calcium while enhancing bone formation.

bones to provide alkalinity for balance. All this can lead to osteoporosis."

Fluoride, once touted as an osteoporosis treatment, is in fact toxic to bone cells, according to Dr. Lee. "When given in treatment doses, fluoride causes an apparent increase in bone mass, but the resulting bone is abnormal and lacks strength." Recent studies have shown that even smaller amounts of fluoride than found in drinking water increase the risk of hip fracture.[21]

Other Osteoporosis Risk Factors

There are a number of other risk factors for osteoporosis, including insufficient calcium absorption, the use of conventional drugs, hysterectomy, excess thyroxin (a hor-

mone secreted by the thyroid gland), low body fat, smoking, and lack of exercise.

Fluoride, once touted as an osteoporosis treatment, is in fact toxic to bone cells.

—JOHN R. LEE, M.D.

Insufficient Calcium Absorption: Calcium is ingested in the form of relatively insoluble salts, whether the source is food or dietary supplements. According to Dr. Lee, for calcium to be absorbed, it requires not only vitamin D but also adequate hydrochloric acid (HCl) in the stomach. With age, the amount of HCl secreted decreases. Since 50% of those 70 or older produce less HCl than is needed for calcium absorption, Dr. Lee recommends taking a supplement of either HCl or calcium citrate (which is better absorbed under these conditions than other calcium compounds) with meals.

Conventional Drugs: Antibiotics used to treat a variety of diseases can often deplete normal intestinal flora that supply the body with vitamin K, which is needed in the building of bone. Yogurt and other unpasteurized cultured milk products or supplements of *Lactobacillus acidophilus* and *Bifidobacteria bifidum* can help replace this flora.

Glucocorticoid medications, such as prednisone, not only impair calcium absorption, but also inhibit bone formation, which can lead to osteoporosis. Research has found that taking more than 7.5 mg of prednisone daily for six months or longer significantly increases your risk of osteoporosis.[22] Progesterone supplements taken with these medications can protect against this dangerous side effect, according to Dr. Lee. Other conventional medications that increase your risk of osteoporosis include anticonvulsants such as Dilantin (for seizures), anticoagulants (blood thinners), aluminum-containing antacids, certain chemotherapy drugs, and lithium, among others.[23]

Hysterectomy: A hysterectomy (removal of the uterus) is another risk factor for early osteoporosis, even if the ovaries are still intact. "This is because anywhere between 16% and 57% of all women who undergo uterus removal suffer from premature loss of ovarian function with its associated rapid bone loss," explains Dr. Brown.[24] Unfortunately, this surgery, a conventional medical solution for uterine fibroids and endometriosis, is all too common among premenopausal women. Every year in the U.S., 750,000 women undergo hysterectomies (many including ovary removal);[25] about 90% of these are unnecessary and many are performed on women in their twenties and thirties who have no children, according to Vicki Hufnagel, M.D., of Beverly Hills, California.[26]

High Levels of Thyroxin: Thyroxin, a hormone secreted by the thyroid gland, stimulates minerals to be drawn out of the bones as part of the natural and ongoing process of bone remodeling. In hyperthyroidism, an excess of thyroxin causes bone depletion. Thyroid medication, which supplies thyroid hormone to the body, functions in the same way. People taking thyroid medication should have routine monitoring of their dose to check if it is in excess of what is needed.[27]

Low Body Fat: Being excessively lean, whether from weight loss or excessive exercise, such as training for marathon running, impairs hormone production and eventually bone synthesis. Low body fat causes reduced progesterone and, if menstruation also ceases, both progesterone and estrogen are lowered. Under these circumstances, the consequences for bone mass are the same as they are from menopause. In fact, studies show that bones stressed by the weight of a large body are healthier than the bones of a small, thin person.[28] After menopause, estrogen levels are also higher in heavier women, as the hormone is synthesized in fat tissue.[29]

Smoking: Studies indicate that cigarette smoking appears to promote osteoporosis by inhibiting estrogen's effect on osteoclast cells[30] and by lowering estrogen concentration in the blood. In addition, hampered breathing because of smoking prevents carbon dioxide from leaving the body as it normally does in an exhaled breath, and this too can affect bones. According to Dr. Lee, carbon dioxide retention leads to higher blood levels of carbonic acid, which the body attempts to neutralize with calcium taken from bones.

Lack of Exercise: Unless bones are stimulated by weight-bearing exercise, they become sluggish and stop building bone mass. The key is weight-bearing exercise, as in running, dancing, or brisk walking versus swimming. The force of impact such exercise delivers to bones is a stimulant to bone building.[31] Lifting weights can also provide bone-building stimulation by exerting weight and pull on bones.[32] In addition to stimulating bone growth, exercise also improves blood circulation to the bones, an important aid in preventing osteoporosis. A four-year study at the University of Vienna showed that regular running significantly reduced bone loss in middle-aged women.[33]

Treatment of Osteoporosis

Alternative treatments for osteoporosis focus on supplementation with natural sources of calcium and other

HOW TO TEST FOR OSTEOPOROSIS

The initial test for osteoporosis, according to Katherine O'Hanlan, M.D., of Stanford University, in Palo Alto, California, is measuring for a loss in height. "With osteoporosis, vertebrae shrink and this leads to height loss, which can be observed," explains Dr. O'Hanlan. "This test, done carefully, should be performed routinely at regular office visits, as this is the earliest symptom of osteoporosis. A loss of a half inch from the height you've been all your life is significant." Once a loss of height is confirmed, bone density should also be measured.

Bone density is best measured by DXA (dual X-ray absorptiometry), which has a 1% error rate, states Dr. O'Hanlan. "DPA (dual photon absorptiometry) is not the way to go, though it will be offered because a lot of people have the equipment, but it has an 8% error rate, so it may not pick up a 1% to 2% change in bone density." Regular X rays can only detect osteoporosis after 25% of the bone mass has been lost. John R. Lee, M.D., of Sebastopol, California, also endorses DEXA (dual energy X-ray absorptiometry), which is 95% to 98% accurate and can detect a bone mass change of 3% to 5%.

In diagnosing osteoporosis, it is more effective to monitor certain bones, according to Dr. Lee. He feels it is best to target a trabecular (spongy) area of bone, such as the spongy bone at the end of a long bone, a vertebra, or the heel bone, rather than a cortical bone (a denser bone of the limbs). The turnover rate of the spongy bone is more rapid and changes will show much earlier. He recommends using the lumbar spine, since four vertebrae can be measured, reducing the chance of an erroneous reading. Lumbar bone mineral density should be monitored at regular intervals as a progress check in treatment.

nutrients, balancing the body's hormone production, as well as exercise and regulating diet. These approaches can be very effective without leading to side effects.

There are numerous steps you can take to prevent the development of the disease or to halt and reverse its progress. Many of these steps can be accomplished relatively easily by making dietary and lifestyle modifications and eliminating as many of the known risk factors present in your life as possible. For example, quitting smoking, keeping alcohol consumption to a moderate level, eliminating your use of aluminum products such as cookware and aluminum-containing antiperspirants and

ANTI-OSTEOPOROSIS SUPPLEMENT PROGRAM

Susan Brown, M.D., recommends the following bone nutrients to help prevent and reverse osteoporosis:[40]

- Calcium: builds healthy bones (1,000-1,500 mg daily)

- Magnesium: helps regulate calcium metabolism (450 mg daily)

- Boron: helps regulate calcium, magnesium, and phosphorus metabolism (no more than 3 mg daily)

- Copper: aids in bone formation (1.5-3.0 mg daily)

- Manganese: needed for cartilage and collagen (3.5-7.0 mg daily)

- Phosphorus: combines with calcium to form essential bone mineral salts (1:1 ratio with calcium)

- Silica: needed for collagen (no established rate, possibly 20-30 mg daily)

- Zinc: necessary for osteoblast and osteoclast formation and helps manufacture collagen matrix that holds bones together (12 mg daily)

- Vitamin A: helps increase osteoblasts, the bone-building cells (4,000-5,000 IU daily)

- Vitamin B$_6$: necessary for hydrochloric acid production, needed for calcium absorption (2 mg daily)

- Vitamin B$_{12}$: required by bone-building cells to maintain optimum function (2-3 mcg daily)

- Folic acid: detoxifies homocysteine, a substance that can cause osteoporosis (400 mcg daily)

- Vitamin C: helps form collagen (250-2,000 mg daily)

- Vitamin D: essential for calcium absorption (200 IU daily)

- Vitamin K: required to manufacture the bone protein matrix (70-140 mcg daily)

- Protein: builds bones and needed to absorb calcium (44 g daily)

- Essential fatty acids: help bone structure and development (omega-3s and omega-6s, dosages vary per individual)

diet, nutritional supplements, hormone balance, exercise, and avoidance of known toxic factors such as fluoride and cigarette smoking," states Dr. Lee.

Diet and Nutritional Supplements

Nancy Appleton, Ph.D., a nutritional consultant in Santa Monica, California, believes that the standard American diet produces metabolic imbalances that reduce absorption and retention of minerals, including calcium. A diet of excess protein, dairy products, sugar, soft drinks, alcohol, caffeine, and fried foods has an acidifying effect on the body, causing calcium to be drawn from the bones to buffer this condition.

Dr. Lee's recommended diet for treating osteoporosis is vegetarian-based, with whole grains, legumes, fruits, vegetables, nuts, and seeds, plus optional small amounts of organic meats and dairy products. Leafy green vegetables, beans, and fish are used as primary calcium sources. If dairy products are used for calcium, yogurt is the preferred source since many older people are lactose intolerant and, in yogurt and other fermented dairy products, the lactose has been consumed by the fermenting culture and converted to lactic acid. Also, make sure to get adequate amounts of essential fatty acids (EFAs). Research has shown that two essential fatty acids in particular contribute to calcium balance and bone calcium content: EPA (eicosapentaenoic acid), an omega–3 EFA found in fish such as salmon, cod, and mackerel; and GLA (gamma–linolenic acid), an omega–6 EFA found in evening primrose, black currant, and borage oils.[34]

Research has found that a diet high in soy foods appears to help prevent osteoporosis. "Soy protein does not cause calcium excretion like animal protein," says fitness and nutrition consultant Linda Ojeda, C.N.C., Ph.D.[35] In addition, tofu, tempeh, and other soy foods contain calcium and plant estrogens, or phytoestrogens. "Recent work suggests that the isoflavones [phytoestrogens] in soybeans also have a direct benefit on bone health, possibly by inhibiting bone resorption," Dr. Ojeda says.[36] Phytoestrogens are so named because they can act like hormonal estrogen in the body, attaching to estrogen receptor sites and serving to restrain bone loss. In preliminary studies, synthetic isoflavones, such as ipriflavone, have also shown effectiveness in slowing bone loss.[37]

Some health practitioners also recommend calcium supplements. Michael T. Murray, N.D., of Issaquah, Washington, recommends the more soluble forms—calcium citrate, calcium lactate, and calcium aspartate. Combinations of calcium and other minerals are also prescribed. Recommended quantities of calcium range from approximately 800 mg to 1,500 mg per day, a significantly wide range that is still debated. Dr. Appleton also cautions

antacids, making sure to get enough exercise and sunshine, and cutting down on excessive protein consumption are all important preventive measures. "A treatment plan for osteoporosis should recreate the conditions under which normal bone building occurs, including proper

about possible side effects associated with calcium supplementation. "Excess calcium can be redistributed in the body and is often deposited in soft tissues, possibly causing arthritis, arteriosclerosis, glaucoma, kidney stones, and other problems," she says. "Excess calcium can also imbalance stores of other minerals in the body."[38] Less calcium is needed if magnesium intake is adequate. Consult your health-care professional in order to determine whether calcium supplementation is appropriate.

Other nutrients, such as the B vitamins, vitamins C and D, phosphorus, magnesium, and zinc, are also important for bone health. Dr. Murray emphasizes the effectiveness of boron. "Boron can potentiate estrogen's role in building bones and it also helps in the conversion of vitamin D to its active form, which is necessary for the absorption of calcium." He adds that though 5 mg of boron per day is the optimum intake, the average American is only consuming 1-3 mg. Whole plant foods (whole grains, nuts, seeds, fruits, and vegetables) are good sources of boron.

Honora Lee Wolfe, Dipl.Ac., of Boulder, Colorado, recommends supplements of natural microcrystalline calcium hydroxyapatite complex (MCHC), a compound of calcium, phosphorus, magnesium, and fluoride, in amounts equal to the normal physiological proportions found in bone. MCHC has been found to not only halt bone loss but also to restore bone mass in cases of osteoporosis.[39]

Natural Hormone Therapy

Natural progesterone, made from sterols (a group of substances related to fat) found in wild yams, is now drawing attention as a likely replacement for synthetic progesterone (progestin), which is used as a treatment for osteoporosis. "It is virtually the same molecule as the progesterone the body makes," explains Dr. Lee. By contrast, synthetic progestin has additional chemical groups that change its shape. The danger is that cells that bind progesterone will receive this molecule, but once in place, the false progesterone cannot function properly, adds Dr. Lee. For example, with natural progesterone, sodium stays outside cells where it belongs. With progestin, sodium moves into the cells and brings water along with it. The result can be water retention and hypertension, and there are many other examples of similar dysfunction.[41]

Natural progesterone in any form does not produce the mood changes and more serious side effects associated with synthetic progesterone. The safety of natural progesterone has been confirmed through extensive testing by Joel Hargrove, M.D., at the Department of Obstetrics and Gynecology, Vanderbilt University, in Nashville, Tennessee.[42] Dr. Hargrove and his associates prescribe natural progesterone for premenstrual syndrome and as

hormone replacement therapy for menopausal and postmenopausal women.

Dr. Lee has used natural progesterone in his clinical practice, with positive results, since 1982. In a clinical trial of 100 patients, 38-83 years old, Dr. Lee reports a treatment program of diet, nutritional supplementation, and natural transdermal (absorbed through the skin) progesterone was virtually 100% successful in building bone mass. "The average increase in bone mass was 15%. The bone status of women with relatively good initial bone mass density (BMD) remained stable, while the BMD of women with the lowest scores gained over 40%," states Dr. Lee. "Women with postmenopausal osteoporosis routinely showed true reversal of their disease, with significant improvement in bone mass and the virtual elimination of osteoporotic fractures."

Dr. Lee's typical recommended dose for natural progesterone is one ounce of 3% cream per month. At bedtime, apply about ¼ teaspoon to soft tissue skin such as on the thighs, stomach, breasts, and inside the upper arms, alternating the sites of application; do this nightly for two to three weeks of your monthly cycle (the two weeks before your period if still menstruating; three weeks if postmenopausal).

 Report any occurrence of unusual vaginal bleeding to your physician, as it may be a sign of hormonal imbalance.

Exercise

Regular exercise that delivers the force of impact to bones (dance versus swimming) builds bones, as does weight-bearing exercise. While simple walking can help maintain bone mass, more rigorous activity is required to build bone. Walkers can use weighted bracelets to add weight-bearing exercise to their aerobic activities. In one study, 30 women increased their spinal bone mass by 0.5% in one year with 50 minutes of vigorous walking four times a week, irrespective of calcium intake, while non-exercisers lost 7% of spinal bone mass.[45]

Simply because you are not an athlete or have not exercised much in your life doesn't mean you should resign yourself to osteoporosis. Research shows that beginning exercise even after menopause can help build bone strength. In other words, it is never too late to begin an exercise program and start reaping the benefits.

Herbal Medicine

Herbalist Susun Weed, of Woodstock, New York, has found that herbal medicine can enhance an osteoporosis prevention and treatment program. Here are some of the more helpful herbs she uses, which are particularly

ARE CONVENTIONAL TREATMENTS EFFECTIVE?

In treating osteoporosis, conventional medical practice relies chiefly upon both hormone replacement (estrogen) and pharmaceutical drugs such as etidronate. Since estrogen has been shown in studies to slow bone resorption, it has become a standard prescription for women at menopause. But estrogen does nothing to maintain new bone formation. With drugs such as etidronate, the bone retained by treatment is made up of a larger percentage of old bone cells, which are inhibited from being absorbed into the blood. At the same time, new bone growth decreases. The resulting bone is more crystalline and brittle and may be more subject to fracture.

Further, since bone loss appears to resume at a pretreatment rate once the drug is stopped,[43] therapies must be continued uninterrupted for 20-plus years until bone loss abates around age 70. Unfortunately, the longer estrogen is taken, the greater the risk of side effects and secondary diseases such as salt and water retention, increased fat, uterine fibroids, gallbladder and liver disease, heart disease, stroke, breast cancer, and endometrial cancer. To offset the cancer risk, manufactured progesterone (progestin) is now added to help balance the estrogen. This seems to slightly improve osteoporotic bones, but progestin may in turn increase the chances for undesirable side effects of its own.[44]

effective when combined with bone-promoting dietary and lifestyle changes.[46]

- Horsetail *(Equisetum arvense)*—restores bone density; take as a daily tea made from dried herb, or use the Bone Brew infusion below.

- Dandelion root tincture—improves absorption of minerals by hydrochloric acid, 10-15 drops before meals.

- Bone Brew—calcium-rich infusion of three dried herbs: nettle *(Urtica dioica)*, 1 tbsp; horsetail 1 tbsp; and sage *(Salvia officianalis)*, 1 tbsp. Put the first two herbs in a quart container, crush, and then add the sage. Fill container with boiled water and close cap tightly. Let sit for a minimum of four hours. When ready, remove herbs and drink tea, hot or cold. One

cup of tea has as much calcium as a cup of milk, according to Weed.

Dr. Ojeda suggests that certain herbs be incorporated into an osteoporosis prevention program because they have hormone-stimulating properties. Unlike synthetic hormone replacement therapy, they do so safely and gently. The herbs can be taken as supplements or teas. Dr. Ojeda cites the following herbs as estrogen-stimulating: black cohosh, alfalfa, hops, sweetbriar, horsetail, buckwheat, sage, rose, and shepherd's purse. Among the herbs she recommends to support progesterone are wild yam, chastetree berry, sarsaparilla, and yarrow.[47]

 See Diet, Herbal Medicine, Natural Hormone Replacement Therapy, Nutritional Medicine, Traditional Chinese Medicine.

Traditional Chinese Medicine

According to traditional Chinese medicine, the health of the bones is directly related to the health of the kidneys. Treatments for osteoporosis therefore focus on increasing the energy of the kidneys. As Wolfe states, "It is common for people in China, once they turn 50, to begin taking low-dose herbal formulas that boost kidney energy and to continue this for years. Traditional Chinese medicine views the aging of the kidneys as the aging of the body, and herbal therapy can slow down this process." According to Wolfe, two Chinese herbal formulas—Two Immortals Decoction or *er xian tang* and Eight Flavor Rehmannia or *shai di huang*—can be effective. However, she cautions, specific recommendations for each person's needs should be prescribed by a professional.

Maoshing Ni, D.O.M., Ph.D., L.Ac., President of Yo San University of Traditional Chinese Medicine, in Marina del Rey, California, provides the following anecdote. "A patient came to see me who was menopausal and complaining of back pain. According to tests, she had lost 30% of her bone density. The woman was Persian and because of certain beliefs did not want to take hormones. We began to treat her condition using acupuncture and herbs, in particular *eucommia, dipsaci,* and *dong quai.* The acupuncture sessions were given twice a week for the first month and then tapered down after that. After six weeks of treatment, she was no longer experiencing the pains associated with the osteoporosis and there was a 50% increase in bone density. Blood tests showed that her estrogen and progesterone levels had come back too. There was not a complete reversal of the condition, but traditional Chinese medicine can indeed contribute to healing."

Recommendations

- Emphasize leafy green vegetables and whole grains. Limit red meat to three or fewer times per week. Avoid excessive protein and all soft drinks. Also, limit alcohol consumption and restrict intake of fat, caffeine, and salt, which are implicated in excessive calcium loss.

- Nutritional supplements: vitamin D (350-400 IU daily); vitamin C (2,000 mg daily in divided doses); beta carotene (15 mg daily, equivalent to 25,000 IU of vitamin A); calcium (goal of 800 mg daily by diet and/or supplement). Vitamins B_6 and K, magnesium, zinc, manganese, strontium, boron, silicon, and copper may be recommended. Add hydrochloric acid (HCl), if needed, to support nutrient absorption.

- Hormonal supplements: Progesterone—One ounce of 3% cream per month; apply approximately ¼ teaspoon at bedtime over a 2-3 week time period each month. Alternate among different smooth skin sites. Estrogen—If needed for hot flashes or vaginal dryness, use 0.3 mg to 0.625 mg daily of conjugated estrogen for three weeks, timed to coincide with progesterone use. Do not use if contraindicated for any reason (check with your physician).

- Exercise: 20 minutes daily or half an hour three times a week.

- Helpful herbs include horsetail (*Equisetum arvense*) and dandelion root tincture.

Self-Care
The following therapies can be undertaken at home under professional guidance:

Fasting / Reflexology

JUICE THERAPY: • Green juice • Beet, carrot, and celery • Lemon, papaya, pineapple

Professional Care
The following therapies can be provided by a qualified health professional:

Acupuncture / Chiropractic / Herbal Medicine / Homeopathy / Magnetic Field Therapy / Osteopathic Medicine / Traditional Chinese Medicine

AYURVEDIC MEDICINE: A traditional Ayurvedic formula for osteoporosis consists of one part sesame seeds (black seeds, if possible), a half part *shatavari* (the main Ayurvedic rejuvenative herb for the female), and a half part ginger, with raw sugar added to taste; eat one ounce daily. The Ayurvedic herb *amla* is also recommended for osteoporosis.

ENVIRONMENTAL MEDICINE: Excessive exposure to lead can cause a negative calcium balance, and cadmium can cause a decrease in the mineral content of bones and contribute to osteoporosis.

Where to Find Help

For more information on, or referrals for, the treatment of osteoporosis, contact the following organizations.

American College for Advancement in Medicine (ACAM)
23121 Verdugo Drive, Suite 204
Laguna Hills, California 92653
(800) 532-3688
Website: www.acam.org

For referrals to a physician knowledgeable about natural hormones.

American Association of Oriental Medicine
433 Front Street
Catasauqua, Pennsylvania 18032
(888) 500-7999
Website: www.aaom.org

The AAOM is a national professional organization of acupuncturists who meet acceptable standards of competency and can provide you with the names and locations of local members.

American Association of Naturopathic Physicians
8201 Greensboro Drive, Suite 300
McLean, Virginia 22101
(703) 610-9037
Website: www.naturopathic.org

Provides a directory of naturopathic physicians and offers referrals to a nationwide network of accredited or licensed practitioners. Also publishes a quarterly newsletter, for both professionals and the general public, and offers a series of brochures and pamphlets on a variety of subjects.

Foundation for the Advancement of Innovative Medicine (FAIM)
P.O. Box 7016
Albany, New York 12225-0016
(877) 634-3246
Website: www.faim.org

FAIM seeks to serve both as a forum for exchange and a constituency for change, to educate both those within the field and the general public as to the benefits of innovative medicine, to secure freedom of choice for patients, and to encourage research and development of promising new approaches.

Professional and Technical Services
333 Northeast Sandy Blvd.
Portland, Oregon 97232
(800) 648-8211 or (503) 231-7244

This organization provides information concerning natural progesterone cream.

Transitions for Health
621 Southwest Alder, Suite 900
Portland, Oregon 97205
(800) 888-6814 or (503) 226-1010

A source for natural progesterone.

Recommended Reading

Alternative Medicine Guide to Women's Health 1 & 2. Burton Goldberg and the Editors of *Alternative Medicine.* Tiburon, CA: Future Medicine Publishing, 1998.

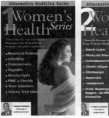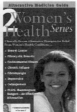

Better Bones, Better Body. Susan E. Brown, Ph.D. Los Angeles: Keats Publishing, 2000.

Everything You Need to Know About Osteoporosis. Sheila Dunn-Merritt and Lyn Patrick. Roseville, CA: Prima Health, 2000.

Food and Our Bones. Annemarie Colbine. New York: Plume, 1998.

Healthy Bones: What You Should Know About Osteoporosis. Nancy Appleton, Ph.D. Garden City Park, NY: Avery Penguin Putnam, 1999.

Hormone Replacement Therapy, Yes or No? Betty Kamen, Ph.D. Novato, CA: Nutrition Encounter, 1996.

Managing Menopause Naturally with Chinese Medicine. Honora Lee Wolfe. Boulder, CO: Blue Poppy Press, 1998.

Menopausal Years. Susun S. Weed. New York: Ash Tree Publishing, 1992.

Dr. Susan Lark's Menopause Self-Help Book. Susan Lark, M.D. Berkeley, CA: Celestial Arts, 1990.

150 Most-Asked Questions About Osteoporosis: What Women Really Want to Know. Ruth S. Jacobowitz. New York: William Morrow, 1996.

Preventing and Reversing Osteoporosis. Alan R. Gaby, M.D. Roseville, CA: Prima Publishing, 1995.

PARASITIC INFECTIONS

Three out of five Americans will be infected by parasites at some point in their lives. Easily spread from person to person and through contaminated food and water, harmful parasites cause our bodies to lose their biological balance by secreting toxins and damaging vital organs. While living off the human body, these tiny organisms can contribute to a variety of acute and chronic illnesses, often going undetected. Proper diagnosis and treatment is essential in order to maintain health and restore normal bodily functions.

ALTHOUGH TECHNICALLY any organism that lives off another organism can be defined as "parasitic," according to Murray Susser, M.D., of Santa Monica, California, the term *parasite* refers specifically to those protozoa (single-cell organisms), arthropods (insects), and worms that invade and feed off host organisms, often causing harm. "Parasites have been co-evolving with humans for millions of years," says Dr. Susser, "and, like viruses and fungi, their presence in the body serves no known purpose."

> *Parasites have been co-evolving with humans for millions of years and, like viruses and fungi, their presence in the body serves no known purpose.*
>
> —MURRAY SUSSER, M.D.

Illness can often result when disease-promoting parasites, which frequently contaminate food and water supplies, are ingested. Parasites also infest the skin, as with scabies and lice, or can enter the bloodstream through insect bites, as with malaria and yellow fever parasites. They can deplete the body of essential nutrients, taxing and overwhelming the immune system, which can lead to serious illness and even death.[1]

A complicating factor of a parasitic infection is that most people who have parasites don't know it. Medical researchers are beginning to recognize that parasitic infections contribute to a variety of major diseases, including Crohn's disease, ulcerative colitis, arthritis and rheumatoid symptoms, chronic fatigue syndrome (CFS), and AIDS. A number of digestive complaints, such as diarrhea and irritable bowel syndrome, are now being linked to past or present parasitic infections.

What are Parasites?

"Americans today are host to more than 130 kinds of parasites," says nutritionist Ann Louise Gittleman, M.S.,

of Bozeman, Montana, author of *Guess What Came to Dinner: Parasites and Your Health.* These parasites can range in size from microscopic single-cell protozoa to tapeworms up to 15 feet long. Although many may regard parasite infections as a problem of developing nations, the truth, according to the U.S. Centers for Disease Control and Prevention (CDC), is that one in six Americans is host to a parasite.[2]

In the U.S., the most common parasites in humans, apart from head lice, are of the microscopic protozoal variety, which can be transmitted by air, food, water, insects, animals, or other people. These tiny parasites include *Giardia lamblia*, a virulent form found in the contaminated waters of lakes, streams, and oceans, and a common cause of traveler's diarrhea; *Entamoeba histolytica*, which can cause dysentery and injure the liver and lungs; *Blastocystis hominis*, which is increasingly linked to acute and chronic illness;[3] and *Dientamoeba fragilis*, which is associated with diarrhea, abdominal pains, anal pruritus (intense itching sensation of the anus), and loose stools.[4] Another parasite, *Cryptosporidium*, poses a significant threat to those with immunologic diseases such as AIDS.[5]

Besides lice, the most common of arthropod parasites are mites, ticks, and fleas. These parasites, in turn, can carry other, smaller infectious organisms, such as *Borrelia burgdorferi*, a coiled spirochete-shaped parasite that is implicated in causes Lyme disease, and *Yersinia pestis*, which causes the dreaded bubonic plague.[6]

The other type of parasite, commonly known as "worms," include pinworms, roundworms, tapeworms, *Trichinella spiralis* (worms usually acquired from eating tainted pork that inhabit the intestines and muscle tissue), hookworms, Guinea worms, and filaria (threadlike worms that inhabit the blood and tissues). Such worms can be contracted by those traveling in remote and underdeveloped regions of the world, as well as from contaminated water or from pets. Roundworms, for example, infect about 25% of the world's population and cause up to one million cases of disease annually.[7] Roundworms are particularly difficult to get rid of due to their high reinfection rate and the ability of their infective eggs to resist treatment.[8] They are particularly prevalent in the Appalachian Mountains and adjacent regions[9] and are the second most common intestinal worm in the U.S. Pinworms, the most common type of intestinal worm, are especially found among children.

Sources of Parasites

Parasites can be transmitted through contaminated food and water, foreign travel (particularly to countries with poor sanitary standards), and household pets or other animals.

FOOD

The U.S. food supply is commonly thought of as the safest in the world. Nevertheless, according to the CDC, up to 80 million illnesses occur in this country every year due to contaminated food supply. Approximately 9,000 of these reported illnesses result in death.[10] The influx into this country of food grown around the world, as well as the popularity of ethnic foods such as sushi and sashimi, which are uncooked or undercooked, contributes to the spread of parasites.[11] Raw or undercooked beef and pork may contain tapeworms or the roundworm *Trichinella*, while raw fish (sushi or smoked salmon, for instance) may also contain tapeworms or anisakid worms.

The influx into this country of food grown around the world, as well as the popularity of ethnic foods such as sushi and sashimi, which are uncooked or undercooked, contributes to the spread of parasites.

Fruits and vegetables, particularly from countries where parasites are prevalent or where human wastes may be used as fertilizer, may pose a risk of parasite contamination if they are not washed thoroughly before eating.

Without adequate safeguards, both farming and processing practices may lead to contamination. Aquatic vegetables, such as watercress and bamboo shoots, may contain parasitic cysts. Poor hygiene in the storage and preparation of food may lead to parasite infestation, in restaurants, nursing homes, daycare centers, or at home. Food handlers can contaminate the food they are preparing as can insects, such as flies or cockroaches.[12]

Sometimes, simply poor digestion is a contributing cause of parasitic infection. "Someone who has a low acid level in the stomach won't digest food properly, so whatever parasites come through in the food won't get sterilized out," says Maoshing Ni, D.O.M., Ph.D., L.Ac., President of Yo San University, in Marina del Rey, California. "That's what the hydrochloric acid does, it sterilizes the food and kills off all the germs. When it's not effective at doing that, they get passed along into the intestines. That's why kids get a lot of parasites, because their digestive system is not yet as sophisticated as an adult's."

WATER

"Don't drink the water" is the advice commonly given to travelers heading abroad. Unfortunately, this adage could readily apply in the U.S.—contaminated water is a common source of parasites in this country as well. Our drinking water comes from rivers, lakes, and reservoirs, all of which are threatened with contamination from agricultural runoff, waste products from farm animals, and human sewage.

Chlorination is no protection either. Two of the most common parasites, *Giardia* and *Cryptosporidium,* can survive in chlorinated water for up to 18 months. "Giardiasis [infestation with the *Giardia* parasite] may be a rampant problem in the U.S. today, since over 50% of our water supply is contaminated with it and, unlike bacteria, it is not killed by chlorination," says Steven Rochlitz, Ph.D., author of *Allergies and Candida*.[13] Water filtration systems may help remove *Giardia* from tap water, but few eliminate *Cryptosporidium*, which is so small that it simply passes through most filters. Many urban water systems have no filtration systems at all. Even springs and mountain streams are increasingly becoming contaminated with parasites from wild animals and human visitors.[14]

FOREIGN TRAVEL

Hermann Bueno, M.D., of New York City, an international authority on parasitic disease, explains that, as international travel has increased, parasite infections have become more common in the U.S. "Parasites recognize no national borders," he says. "The world is getting smaller and parasites, generally associated with tropical diseases and Third World countries, where climate and unsanitary living conditions encourage their growth, are now appearing in the United States." Dr. Bueno is not just talking about a case of traveler's diarrhea: some people return from their journeys carrying unsuspected parasitic infections such as malaria, roundworms, or blood flukes.[15]

PETS

There are 240 diseases that can be transmitted from animals to humans (65 transmitted by dogs and 39 by cats), according to Gittleman. With an estimated 118 million pets in the U.S., it is easy to see how pets may be a major source for parasites. Roundworm, hookworm, and toxoplasmosis may be more common than most people think. "It is estimated that 50% of adult Americans may carry latent taxoplasmosis infections acquired from cats," according to Gittleman. *Giardia* is a highly contagious parasite and can be carried by virtually any species—wild animals, cats, and dogs—as well as people. Parasites are transmitted from animal to human through contact with animal feces, fur containing parasite eggs, or infected fleas.[16]

OTHER SOURCES

Parasites can also be transmitted by insects (mosquitos, flies, cockroaches, and fleas), through sexual contact (common sexually transmitted parasites include *Giardia lamblia, Entamoeba histolytica,* and *Trichomonas vaginalis*), or even inhaled from the air.

Giardiasis is particularly serious among those who live in institutions and overcrowded communities and can be spread by drinking or swimming in feces-contaminated water and from person to person, or animal to person, contact. Day care centers are one of the primary sources for parasitic infections in children.[17] Dennis Juranek, of the CDC Division of Parasitic Infection, in Atlanta, Georgia, reports that the current infection rates due to *Giardia* in day care centers range from 21% to 44% in the U.S.[18] Pediatric and dental clinics are another source for the spread of parasites, according to a study by the University of California at Los Angeles, which found 38% of the attending children infected.[19]

Parasitic Infection and Disease

Large numbers of people throughout the world have parasitic infections compromising their health and contributing to illness, according to Leo Galland, M.D., of New York City, yet most who are infected don't even know it. Many parasites go undetected for years because they don't produce any serious symptoms, or only pro-

duce symptoms at one stage in their lives, which can easily be attributed to another cause. Parasite longevity is another factor in their contribution to chronic diseases. In one recent study of chronic giardiasis, the mean duration was found to be 3.3 years,[21] with infection from *Strongyloides stercoralis*, an intestinal worm, often persisting for 20-30 years.[22]

Martin Lee, Ph.D., a biochemist, microbiologist, and Director of Great Smokies Diagnostic Laboratory, in Asheville, North Carolina, conducted a study on the presence of parasites in chronically and acutely ill people. "In one group of lower-income immigrants who were acutely ill, 70% had parasites, with 20% of these parasites proving to be pathogenic (disease-producing)," Dr. Lee recounts. "In a second group, comprised of a broader and more affluent socioeconomic cross section of chronically ill people, 20% tested positive for the presence of parasites." Dr. Lee's results have subsequently been verified by the CDC.

Many parasites go undetected for years because they don't produce any serious symptoms, or only produce symptoms at one stage of their lives, which can easily be attributed to another cause.

 See AIDS, Allergies, Candidiasis, Chronic Fatigue Syndrome, Constipation, Gastrointestinal Disorders.

Dr. Galland feels that major health problems can be caused by even mild parasitic infection. In his research, he reports that nearly half of the people diagnosed as suffering from irritable bowel syndrome had intestinal parasites and that most were cured of their symptoms when treated for parasitic infection. Eighty-two percent of those who suffered from chronic fatigue syndrome were relieved of these symptoms as well. Dr. Galland's findings indicate that any person with chronic gastrointestinal complaints, such as bloating, diarrhea, abdominal pain, flatulence, chronic constipation, and multiple allergies (especially to food), and patients with unexplained fatigue, should be screened for intestinal parasites.

Candidiasis, the overgrowth of the yeast *Candida albicans* in the intestinal tract, is reaching epidemic proportions in the U.S. and is often found as a complication of giardiasis. Candidiasis is an opportunistic infection (develops when the body is compromised by other infections) and has serious consequences—it increases gut perme-

A PARASITE PRIMER

Parasites are organisms that survive by feeding off another living organism—the host—usually causing damage to the host. Protozoa, Trematodes (flukes), Cestoda (tapeworms), and Nematoda (roundworms and hookworms) are the four main types of parasites.

Protozoa

Protozoa (microscopic, single-celled organisms) are the most common type of parasite found in the U.S. They reproduce rapidly in the intestinal tract and can migrate to other organs (liver, pancreas, heart, and lungs).

- *Giardia*—a common parasite, transmitted via contaminated water and food. *Giardia* infests the small intestine, incubating up to three weeks before causing symptoms. Infection can damage the intestinal lining; symptoms include foul-smelling stools, cramps, bloating, headaches, and fatigue.
- *Cryptosporidium parvum*—the most prevalent waterborne parasite in the U.S.; it can also be spread by contact with feces. Symptoms include diarrhea, nausea, cramps, and fever.
- *Trichomonas vaginalis*—transmitted through sexual contact or from contaminated toilet seats, towels, or bath water. The infection is often symptom-less, but can cause vaginal discharge, yeast infections, and painful urination in women or an enlarged prostate and urinary inflammation in men.
- *Entamoeba histolytica*—spread through water or food; may incubate for up to three months, then spread through the digestive tract or migrate to other organs. Abdominal pain, bloating, and diarrhea are common symptoms.
- *Toxoplasma gondii*—infection generally comes from cats; undercooked meats are another source. It may cause flu-like symptoms (fever, headache, swollen lymph nodes, and fatigue).

Flukes (Trematodes)

Flukes are leaf-shaped flatworms that attach to the host using abdominal suckers. Flukes usually begin their life cycle in snails, then as larvae they infect fish, vegetation, or humans. Flukes can migrate to the lungs, intestines, heart, brain, and liver. Trematode eggs can cause inflammation by releasing toxins that damage tissues.

- **Intestinal Fluke** *(Fasciolopsis buski)*—contamination usually from eating infected water vegetables (water chestnuts, bamboo shoots, or watercress). The worms live in the small intestine, where they cause ulcerations and allergic reactions. Common symptoms are diarrhea, nausea, abdominal pain, and vomiting.
- **Sheep Liver Fluke** *(Fasciola hepatica)*—fresh watercress is the most common source. This worm attaches itself in the gallbladder and bile ducts, causing inflammation and local trauma. Symptoms include jaundice, fever, coughing, vomiting, and abdominal pain.
- **Oriental Lung Fluke** *(Paragonimus westermani)*—found mostly in Asian countries; spread by eating undercooked crabs and crayfish. The worms can penetrate the intestines and migrate to the lungs or brain. Symptoms include coughing fits and blood in the sputum.
- **Blood Flukes** *(Schistosoma japonicum, S. mansoni, S. haematobium)*—transmitted by swimming in contaminated water, blood flukes burrow into the skin and migrate to the heart, lungs, liver, or bladder. They can live in the body for up to 30 years.

Tapeworms (Cestoda)

Tapeworms are flat, segmented, and ribbon-like and are the largest intestinal parasites, growing up to several feet in length. The most common source of infection is eating undercooked meat or fish containing the larvae. The worms develop in the body and attach to the small intestine, surviving by absorbing nutrients from partially digested food. Often tapeworms produce no symptoms.

- **Beef Tapeworm** *(Taenia saginata)*—enters the body in raw or undercooked beef; this tapeworm can live in the intestines for up to 25 years, growing to a length of eight feet. Symptoms include diarrhea, cramps, nausea, and loss of appetite. Long-term infection may lead to vitamin deficiencies.
- **Pork Tapeworm** *(Taenia solium)*—undercooked pork, smoked ham, or sausages are common sources. The adult worms attach in the intestines, causing symptoms similar to those of the beef tapeworm. The larvae can infect the heart, liver, muscles, eyes, brain, and spine.
- **Fish Tapeworm** *(Diphyllobothrium latum)*—infestations caused by eating undercooked or raw fish. It grows up to 15 feet in length and symptoms include vomiting, heartburn, diarrhea, and loss of appetite.

ability to undigested foods and bowel toxins, which then enter the bloodstream and may induce an autoimmune response, promoting intolerances or sensitivities to common foods.

Intestinal parasitic infections are also being linked to chronic fatigue syndrome. In one study, over a third of the CFS patients tested were infected with *Giardia lamblia*. Their complaints included depression, muscular pain and weakness, headache, and flu-like symptoms present for an average of two to three years.[23]

Research has shown a connection between HIV (human immunodeficiency virus) and parasites. According to Leon Chaitow, N.D., D.O., of London, England, parasites are a common problem seen in people with AIDS. He finds AIDS patients often have treatment-resistant candidiasis due to immunosuppressive factors caused by parasites. A study at the University of Virginia reports that a pathogenic species of amoeba *(Entamoeba histolytica)* produces a substance that attacks the immune defense cells that can inactivate the HIV virus. Because of this ability to actually disarm the body's own defense mechanism, amoeba parasites may play a role in the onset of AIDS.[24]

Symptoms of Parasitic Infections

Parasitic infection is usually evident within three to five days of exposure, sometimes beginning with explosive and watery diarrhea. Giardiasis is the leading cause of diarrhea in children and causes a variety of physical, behavioral, mental, and emotional problems.[25] Other symptoms may include intermittent diarrhea and constipation, indigestion, rashes, hives, gas, fatigue, and allergic reactions to food. If left untreated, rheumatoid and arthritic symptoms may emerge. Mucus in the stool, anorexia, cramping, constipation, nausea, vomiting, night sweats, and fever may also occur.

Acute cases can produce compromised immunity; malabsorption and malnutrition; deficiencies of vitamins A, B$_6$, and B$_{12}$, potassium, calcium, and magnesium; electrolyte imbalances; and severe weight loss. The toxicity produced in extreme cases of parasite infestation can also cause blackouts, muscular and skeletal pain, wide swings in blood sugar levels, and menstrual irregularities.

Different parasites often infect different regions of the body as well. While giardiasis affects the functioning of the small intestine, amoebiasis (amoeba infestation) mainly involves the colon, and extreme cases can result in liver and lung abscesses. An amoebic infection can be hard to distinguish from ulcerative colitis (ulcer of the colon lining).

Diagnosing a Parasitic Infection

Symptoms and personal history are the first two things a physician should check when diagnosing a possible parasitic infection. "I always begin with a detailed picture of the symptoms and then gather a complete history that will indicate if exposure to parasites should be factored in," says Dr. Galland. "Red flags are things like a recent trip out of the country, extensive use of antibiotics (which weaken the immune system), or having a child in day care, where it's estimated 30% of staff are infected." Alternative medicine practitioners typically ask patients the following questions to assess the likelihood of a parasite exposure:

- What is your travel history (inside and outside the U.S.)?

- What is the source of your drinking water? Have you ever drunk water from streams or rivers while camping?

- Do you have pets in your household or are you in close contact with animals?

- Do you frequently eat out, particularly at ethnic restaurants, sushi bars, or salad bars?

- Do you like to eat raw fruits and vegetables?

- Do you like raw or undercooked meat or fish?

- Do you work in a hospital, day care center, sanitation department, around animals, or in a garden?

- Do you engage in oral or anal sex?

- Do you have some or all of these symptoms—dark circles under your eyes, distended abdomen, bluish lips, allergies, diarrhea or constipation, anemia, skin eruptions, anal itching, chronic fatigue, loss of appetite, insomnia, depression, or sugar cravings?[26]

After determining whether a parasite infection may exist from a patient's symptoms and history, physicians generally then confirm the diagnosis with various testing procedures. Different parasites require different formulations to kill them, so an accurate diagnosis is an important step in any treatment program. Unfortunately, parasite infections are often overlooked by mainstream physicians, partly because they simply fail to use the right diagnostic test. According to David Casemore, M.D., of the Public Health Laboratories in Great Britain, parasitic infection is "almost certainly underdetected, possibly by a factor of ten or more."[27] If you suspect you may have an intestinal parasite, or just want to be tested as a preventative measure, make sure your physician, hospital, or laboratory follows the guidelines set up by the CDC and the *Manual of Clinical Microbiology*. A number of diagnostic tools can be useful in determining if you have parasites, including a purged stool test and mucus and blood tests.

Stool Analysis—Gittleman recommends using a purged stool test for parasites. This method differs from standard stool analysis: the patient ingests 1½ ounces of a high-

sodium solution on an empty stomach to encourage more frequent and powerful bowel movements. These induced stool samples have higher levels of mucus, which provide greater numbers of organisms. Parasites generally begin to appear after the fourth bowel movement, but sometimes it may take as many as 12 bowel movements to dislodge them. The purged stool test may be more accurate than conventional stool analysis for diagnosing a parasite infection. The problem with a random stool sample is that parasites cling to the wall of the intestines and simply may not be present in the feces.[28] A purged stool test is not recommended for individuals with high blood pressure as the high-sodium solution may exacerbate their problem, according to Gittleman. Pregnant women and those suffering from an intestinal obstruction or appendicitis should not take this test.

Bueno-Parrish Test—Another test procedure recommended by alternative care practitioners is the Bueno-Parrish test. Developed by Dr. Bueno, this test involves the use of a rectal mucus swab to identify parasites. The procedure, technically called an anoscopy, involves taking a sample of mucus from inside the rectum with a cotton swab. A stain that makes even fragments of parasites visible is then applied to the swab material and the sample is examined with a microscope. This procedure has helped identify parasite infections in patients who had previously been misdiagnosed.[29]

Blood Tests—Blood tests may be useful for diagnosing some parasitic infections. Elevated levels of a special white blood cell called an eosinophil may indicate a parasite infection. Blood tests can also measure levels of antibodies to some parasites, including *Entamoeba histolytica*, most types of flukes, malaria, and *Trichinella*. Abnormal blood levels of some nutrients may indicate parasites. For example, low levels of iron, folic acid, and calcium may indicate the presence of *Giardia*.[30]

Some physicians also supplement conventional diagnostic testing for parasites with diagnostic tools such as electrodermal screening to discover the type and degree of dysfunction within a particular organ that may be infested with parasites. Such methods can also be helpful for determining the body's tolerance of medications or remedies that may be prescribed.

Treatment of Parasitic Infections

Although antibiotics and other drugs are often used to treat parasitic infections, such approaches can pose a threat to one's overall health by upsetting the natural balance of the immune system, especially for those who are already immunosuppressed or chronically ill, according to Dr. Galland. Also, due to the toxicity of most of these drugs, they cannot be taken over an extended period of time, which can be a serious impediment in the treatment of *Giardia* and other long-standing, resistant infections. Because of this, the cure rate for these drugs is considerably decreased, with the likelihood of recurrence greatly increased.

Many alternative physicians employ a multifaceted approach to treating parasitic infections. Among the options they make use of are detoxification therapy, diet and nutrition, herbal medicine, traditional Chinese medicine, and Ayurvedic medicine.

CAUTION Before beginning any parasite elimination program, consult a qualified health-care professional. This is especially important if you are pregnant.

Detoxification

Like other toxins, parasites can make it harder for the liver, kidneys, and intestines to detoxify and eliminate wastes from the body. If testing reveals that you have a parasitic infection, you may want to consider a detoxification program, says W. Lee Cowden, M.D., of Fort Worth, Texas, to rid your system of parasites. Parasites tend to embed themselves in the intestinal wall, but over the course of several weeks, you can flush them out by using some of these natural substances (preferably in combination): psyllium husks, agar-agar, citrus pectin, papaya extract, pumpkin seeds, flaxseeds, comfrey root, beet root, and bentonite clay (take bentonite only in combination with another substance, such as psyllium). Extra vitamin C (minimum 2 g daily, but higher amounts up to individual bowel tolerance are more useful) can help flush out the intestines.

Irrigate the colon with 2-16 quarts of water via enema. To the water, you may add black walnut tincture or extract, garlic juice, vinegar (two tablespoons per quart of water), blackstrap molasses (one tablespoon per quart of water), or organically grown coffee. Use filtered or distilled water for the enema; further sterilize it by boiling or ozonating it for 10-15 minutes before use, including before using it to prepare the coffee.

Diet and Nutrition

If you suspect a parasitic infection, eliminate all uncooked foods from the diet and cook all meats until well done. It is also advisable to eliminate coffee, all sugars including fruits and honey, and all milk and dairy products, with the possible exception of raw goat's milk. Raw goat's milk contains secretory IgA and IgG immunoglobulins,

types of antibodies that help strengthen the immune system. According to naturopath Steven Bailey, N.D., of Portland, Oregon, IgA and IgG are helpful in the treatment of parasites.

Gittleman says that the best diet for a parasite infection is one that "supports the host and starves the parasite." Specifically, she recommends against eating any sugar, white flour, or processed foods (such as prepackaged snack foods). Once inside the body, these foods provide ideal conditions for parasites to breed. She has found that a diet composed of 25% fat, 25% protein, and 50% complex carbohydrates (the type of starch found in vegetables and whole grains) is best for people with parasite infections.

Gittleman also advises limiting your intake of raw fruits and vegetables; instead, cook both fruits and vegetables. Sufficient levels of vitamin A are particularly important for preventing parasites, as this vitamin seems to increase resistance to penetration by larvae. Good dietary sources of vitamin A include properly cooked carrots, sweet potatoes, squash, and salad greens. A combination formula of digestive enzymes, taken between meals, may also be helpful for eliminating parasite larvae or eggs in the intestines.

Certain foods are anti-parasitic, according to Gittleman, and you should incorporate more of these foods in the diet. These include pineapple and papaya, either as fresh juice or in supplement form, eaten in combination with pepsin (a stomach enzyme) and betaine hydrochloric acid (a supplement form of stomach acid). Avoid all meats and dairy products for at least one week at the beginning of therapy. Also consider pomegranate juice (four 8-ounce glasses daily), papaya seeds, fresh figs, finely ground pumpkinseeds (¼-½ cup daily), or two cloves of raw garlic daily. Because pomegranate juice can irritate the intestines, do not drink it for more than four to five days at a time. Other anti-parasitic foods include onions, kelp, blackberries, raw cabbage, and ground almonds.[31]

Since an intestinal parasitic infection may be only one element in the much larger issue of immunosuppression, nutritional supplementation is also important for the restoration of normal bowel and immune function. Nutrients should include vitamins A and B12, calcium, magnesium, and a probiotic, which can include *Lactobacillus acidophilus, Bifidobacteria,* and *L. bulgaricus.* Dr. Chaitow recommends that any anti-parasitic protocol include high-dosage probiotics to help rebuild intestinal flora ravaged by the parasitic infestation, as well as by other opportunistic infections, such as candidiasis. Probiotics are also imperative for fighting off any further infestation.

Herbal Medicine

The following herbal remedies have been found to be safe and effective for the treatment of parasitic infections. Any of these remedies can also be used as a preventative for parasitic infection when water or food conditions are questionable. According to Dr. Galland, it is advisable to continue any treatment regimen until at least two parasitological tests, performed one month apart on purged stool specimens, are negative.

Citrus Seed Extract: Citrus seed extract is highly active against viruses, protozoa, bacteria, and yeasts, and has been used extensively in other countries for the treatment of parasitic infections. It is not absorbed into the tissues, is nontoxic and generally hypoallergenic, and can be administered for up to several months, which may be required to eliminate *Giardia* and the candidiasis that often accompanies it. Since citrus seed extract also kills beneficial organisms, supplementing with probiotics is recommended after treatment.

> **CAUTION** Before using any of these herbal remedies, it is important to first consult with a health professional who has been properly trained in their use. *Artemisia annua* should not be used during pregnancy.

> See Detoxification Therapy, Diet, Herbal Medicine, Nutritional Medicine.

Artemisia annua: This is an herbal remedy of Chinese origin. Its antiprotozoal activity is especially effective against *Giardia*, but some caution is advisable. It can initially cause a worsening of symptoms, allergic reactions, and some intestinal irritation. *Artemisia annua* is often prescribed by Dr. Galland, along with citrus seed extract. It may be used with other anti-parasitic herbs and can also be used in conjunction with conventional drug therapy.

Artemisia absinthium: This is one of the oldest European medicinal plants, similar to the *Artemisia annua* of Chinese herbal tradition. Known as "wormwood," it was highly prized by the Greek physician Hippocrates and used to expel worms. *Artemisia absinthium* taken alone can be toxic, though, and therefore should be used in combination with other herbs to nullify its toxicity.

Aloe vera: Known as "the potted physician," the aloe plant is filled with a clear gel that acts as a digestive tonic. Studies have shown that aloe can destroy bacteria, yeasts, and parasites in the intestines.[32]

Garlic *(Allium sativum):* Aside from its use in cooking, garlic is also an effective and well-researched medicinal herb, used in traditional medicines all over the world. Garlic and its preparations are known for their antibiotic, anti-fungal, and antiviral activity. It is effective against roundworms, tapeworms, pinworms, and hookworms.

Goldenseal *(Hydrastis canadensis):* One of the most widely used American herbs, goldenseal is considered to be a tonic remedy that stimulates immune response and is directly antimicrobial itself. Goldenseal's antimicrobial properties are due to berberine, an alkaloid that is effective against bacteria, fungi, and parasites, particularly *Giardia*.[33]

Traditional Chinese Medicine

In traditional Chinese medicine, herbs are the primary treatment for parasites and the type used depends on the location of the parasites in the body, according to Dr. Ni. For intestinal parasites, purgative herbs are usually used. Pumpkin seeds and quisqualis seeds are two common remedies. The pumpkin seeds are eaten raw, while quisqualis seeds are usually roasted. Both are taken every morning on an empty stomach, approximately 10–12 seeds of each, for about two weeks. "Quisqualis and pumpkin seeds are mild and safe enough for adults and children to take daily as a preventative measure as well," says Dr. Ni.

Meliae seeds are much stronger than either pumpkin seeds or quisqualis and should only be taken in more severe cases. The meliae seeds paralyze the parasites for approximately eight hours, allowing the body to eliminate them through the bowels. Betel nut is another typical treatment for intestinal parasites. The nut is chewed raw like chewing tobacco. "It can give a certain sense of euphoria, too, because it is slightly toxic," says Dr. Ni. "This is negligible, but some people might get diarrhea."

Depending on the type of parasite, they may be able to get through the intestinal walls and into the bloodstream. "In situations like this, you have to use some very strong antibiotic-like herbs, such as goldenseal and coptidis, which are anti-parasitic as well," says Dr. Ni. While eliminating the parasites with herbs, Dr. Ni also strengthens the immune system in order to get at the underlying cause of the parasitic infestation. He reports that nutrition and herbs such as ginseng, ligustri berries, and schisandra berries can accomplish this. He has had good success with his three-month treatment program addressing both components.

Dr. Ni recalls treating a woman previously diagnosed with chronic fatigue syndrome, candidiasis, and severe stomach difficulties. "We did a stool test and found that she also had parasites. This woman was tremendously underweight. When she came to see me, she weighed 86 pounds and was 5´4˝ tall. It took about three months for us to work on nourishing her body. Besides using herbs to kill off the parasites, I also used them to boost her immune system and to deal with the yeast problem and her digestive weakness. That's why she got the parasites in the first place. After three months of treatment, her stool tests cleared up and remained clear, all her symptoms went away, and her weight went back up to 108 pounds."

 See Ayurvedic Medicine, Traditional Chinese Medicine.

Ayurvedic Medicine

Ayurvedic medicine, a 5,000-year-old health-care tradition from India, has many natural remedies that address specific parasitic infections. According to Virender Sodhi, M.D. (Ayurveda), N.D., of Bellevue, Washington, the most effective herbs for *Giardia*, amoebas, *Cryptosporidium*, and protozoal intestinal parasites are *bilva*, *neem*, and berberine, which can be taken in combination. He also recommends bitter melon, as well as such nutritional support as psyllium husk, turmeric, and *L. acidophilus* for the enhancement of the intestinal microflora. It may take several months to eliminate intestinal parasites.

Dr. Sodhi had a patient who came to him for a long-standing asthma condition. She had previously been treated with a variety of standard drugs, which had not helped. "She was also having alternating constipation and diarrhea, and her white blood cell count was high," says Dr. Sodhi. "I suggested a stool test, which came back positive for *Giardia*. When we started treating her for *Giardia* with *bilva*, *neem*, and berberine, her asthma cleared up too. It's a well-known fact that whenever there are parasites, the white cell count gets higher and you get more allergy-prone, so there is some link there, although we don't know completely how it occurs."

Although the Ayurvedic remedies mentioned here are safe and easy to self-administer, Dr. Sodhi recommends consultation with a qualified practitioner before beginning any treatment protocol in order to determine which of the various options will be best suited to individual needs.

HOW TO AVOID PARASITES

There are several precautions that will help you avoid parasites:

Food

- Do not eat raw beef—it can contain tapeworms and other parasites.
- Do not eat raw fish or sushi—you are almost certain to get worms if you eat raw fish.
- Wash hands after handling raw meat or fish (including shrimp)—don't put your hands near your mouth without washing them first.
- Use a separate cutting board for meat—spores from meat can seep into a cutting board and contaminate vegetables or anything else you put on the board.
- Wash utensils after cutting meat.
- Wash vegetables and fruit thoroughly—particularly salad items, as they often harbor parasites. Wash in one teaspoon Clorox (or a few drops of grapefruit seed extract) per one gallon of water; soak for 15-20 minutes. Then soak in fresh water for 20 minutes before refrigerating.
- Do not drink from streams and rivers.

Pets

- Do not sleep near your pets—they harbor worms and other parasites.
- De-worm your pets regularly and keep their sleeping areas clean.
- Do not let pets lick your face.
- Do not let pets eat off your dishes.
- Do not walk barefoot around animals.

General

- Always wash your hands after using the toilet.
- Wash your hands after working in the garden—the soil can be contaminated with spores and parasites.

When Traveling

- Don't drink the water.
- Start taking Chinese herbs or other preventive medications two weeks before traveling and continue them while you travel.

Recommendations

- Parasites tend to embed themselves in the intestinal wall, but over the course of several weeks, you can flush them out by using some of these natural substances (preferably in combination): psyllium husks, agar-agar, citrus pectin, papaya extract, pumpkin seeds, flaxseeds, comfrey root, beet root, and bentonite clay.

- Eliminate all uncooked foods from your diet and cook all meats until well done; soak both organic and inorganic vegetables in salted water (one tablespoon per five cups) for a minimum of 30 minutes before cooking. It is also advisable to eliminate coffee, all sugars including fruits and honey, and all milk and dairy products.

- Anti-parasitic foods include pineapple and papaya, onions, kelp, blackberries, raw cabbage, and ground almonds.

- Herbal remedies found to be safe and effective for the treatment of parasitic infections include citrus seed extract, *Artemisia annua*, and *Artemisia absinthium*.

- Traditional Chinese medicine and Ayurvedic medicine both offer detoxification protocols and herbs to eliminate parasites from the body.

- If you have children and/or pets, they must be treated at the same time as the adults in the household to prevent reinfection.

- During treatment, drink more pure water (not from the tap) than usual to help the body flush out the now dead parasites from your system; at least 64 ounces of water per day for a 150-pound adult.

- Sanitize your environment. When you have almost finished treatment, wash all pajamas and bedding before using them again.

- Although alternative medicine anti-parasitic therapies are milder than conventional treatments, no treatment program can successfully remove parasites from the body without causing some stress. This is because parasites create a toxic load in the body as they are killed off. Side effects of any treatment will thus often include intense and uncomfortable reactions, such as abdominal discomfort, joint pain, exhaustion, or other flu-like symptoms. Consequently, an effective anti-parasite treatment program should include measures that will help strengthen the body's natural cleansing and detoxifying systems.

Self–Care
The following therapies can be undertaken at home under appropriate professional supervision:

Fasting / Flower Essences

AROMATHERAPY: • Bergamot, chamomile, camphor, lavender, peppermint, melissa • For ringworm, tea tree or thyme oil

AYURVEDA: • *Neem* may be effective in eliminating parasites. • *Pippali* or Indian long pepper *(Piper longum)* is often used for worms. • As a broad spectrum antibiotic, use an herbal mixture of *vidanga* (300 mg), *trikatu* (300 mg), *chitrak* (200 mg), and *kutki* (200 mg), generally taken twice a day after lunch and dinner. *Triphala* may also be helpful (½ teaspoon with warm water 30 minutes before sleep).

HERBS: Make an infusion of fresh pumpkin seeds—one ounce of crushed seeds to a pint of boiling water. Drink a cup three times a day, six days a week, for three weeks. Eat one ounce of pumpkin seeds a day as well.

Professional Care
The following therapies should only be provided by a qualified health professional:

Acupuncture / Magnetic Field Therapy / Naturopathic Medicine

DETOXIFICATION THERAPY: May be indicated, depending on the condition of the person.

OXYGEN THERAPY: Hyperbaric oxygen therapy

Where to Find Help

When possible, use laboratories of teaching institutions or universities where state-of-the-art equipment and procedures are available. The following laboratories may also be used or contacted for further information.

Center for the Improvement of Human Function International
3100 North Hillside Avenue
Wichita, Kansas 67219
(800) 447-7276
Website: www.brightspot.org

A medical, research, and educational organization with four major divisions: Center for Healing Arts treats people who have not responded to standard medical care; Bio-Center Laboratory provides diagnostic services for physicians and hospitals; Bio-Medical Synergistics Education Institute provides learning opportunities for physicians, nurses, and health-care personnel; and Bio-Communications Research Institute gathers clinical data about the effectiveness of treatment protocols and engages in clinical and basic research.

Great Smokies Diagnostic Laboratory
63 Zillicoa Street
Asheville, North Carolina 28801
(828) 253-0621 or (800) 522-4762
Website: www.gsdl.com

Offers a comprehensive profile that includes the tests recommended in this chapter.

Lexington Professional Center
133 E. 73rd Street
New York, New York 10021
(212) 988-4800
Website: www.lexpro.com

For information on the Bueno-Parrish test.

Parasitic Disease Consultants Laboratory
2177-J Flintstone Drive
Tucker, Georgia 30084
(770) 496-1370
Website: www.parasitic.com

For information on blood tests for parasites.

Uni Key Health Systems
P.O. Box 7168
Bozeman, Montana 59771
(406) 586-9424 or (800) 888-4353
Website: www.unikeyhealth.com

For information on purged stool tests for parasites.

Recommended Reading

Guess What Came to Dinner. Ann Louise Gittleman. New York: Avery Penguin Putnam, 2001.

Solving the Puzzle of Chronic Fatigue Syndrome. Michael Rosenbaum, M.D., and Murray Susser, M.D. Tacoma, WA: Life Sciences Press, 1992.

Superimmunity for Kids. Leo Galland, M.D. New York: Dutton, 1989.

PREGNANCY AND CHILDBIRTH

The decisions a woman and her partner make during preconception, pregnancy, and childbirth will shape the life of their child. As alternative medicine increases in popularity, future parents and caregivers are looking toward natural therapies such as nutritional supplementation, homeopathy, herbal medicine, massage, and aromatherapy in order to give birth to a healthier child.

THERE ARE MANY available choices surrounding pregnancy and childbirth—a hospital birth is no longer seen as the only safe option for delivery. Many couples are opting to have their babies at home or in birth centers that offer the kind of care that is tailored to each couple's needs. Currently, holistic practitioners in the field of childbirth are addressing the need for dietary changes, abstinence from harmful substances, childbirth classes, and emotional support during the birth. Other options range from the modern technology of a hospital birth to water birth in the home; obstetric care to midwifery and doula care; and medical drug intervention to labor-inducing herbs.

> *A preconceptual checkup, including personal and family medical history, present lifestyle, and an assessment of both partner's health is an excellent beginning.*
>
> —HELEN BURST, R.N., M.SC.

health of any child she brings into the world. This would include a complete head-to-toe physical examination and screening for breast and cervical cancer, sexually transmitted diseases, drug, alcohol, or tobacco abuse, as well as any history of sexual, physical, or verbal abuse."

"The preparation for pregnancy begins six months to a year from the time of desired conception," according to Maoshing Ni, D.O.M., Ph.D., L.Ac., President of Yo San University of Traditional Chinese Medicine, in Marina del Rey, California. "This entails having the parents evaluate their diet and take herbs so that the egg and sperm are fortified at the time of conception and the health of their future child is maximized."

Preconception

"The idea of preconceptual preparation dates back to ancient times," according to Molly Linton, N.D., L.M., a naturopathic physician and licensed midwife, from Seattle, Washington. "Many cultures recognized the need to follow a balanced diet, exercise, and take proper relaxation for a period of time prior to conception, in order to cleanse and tonify the body to ensure optimum health for the child."

"A preconceptual checkup, including personal and family medical history, present lifestyle, and an assessment of both partner's health is an excellent beginning," says Helen Burst, R.N., M.Sc., Professor of Nurse Midwifery at Yale University. "Preconceptual care is a marvelous opportunity to screen for a wide range of factors that could be critical to not only the mother's health but the

Diet and Nutritional Influences

According to the late Roger Williams, Ph.D., a pioneer of nutritional science, "Nature is so intent upon the continuance of the race that people will continue to propagate even when nutritional conditions are poor." A woman with very poor dietary habits, Dr. Williams stated, may not become impregnated at all. With a slightly improved, but still poor diet, she may conceive but then miscarry. And perhaps with yet a slightly better, albeit deficient nutritional intake, she may give birth to a baby with physical or mental anomalies.[1] A vivid example of the effect of poor nutrition on the unborn child is the increase in congenital deformities that occurs during times of famine.[2] While studying people from traditional cultures, Weston A. Price, D.D.S., discovered that it only takes one generation of eating a typically Western diet—

one high in fats, salt, sugar, and low in complex carbohydrates—to compromise an offspring's health.[3]

A well-balanced diet is vital to ensure a healthy baby. Inadequate nutrition may also disrupt a woman's and man's reproductive system. Specific nutrients influence the production and maintenance of the egg and sperm and thus affect the conception and subsequent health of the fetus, according to Dr. Linton. For example, studies on women suggest that folic acid and fatty acids play a role in fertility.[4] More specifically, health officials at the U.S. Centers for Disease Control and Prevention (CDC) now recommend that all women of childbearing age take folic acid (0.4 mg daily) to protect their future newborns from developing a neural tube defect, an anomaly of the spinal cord.[5]

Avoiding Drugs and Alcohol

The number one requirement for the good health of babies is the parents' avoidance of harmful substances, such as caffeine, nicotine, recreational and some prescription drugs, and alcohol, according to Dr. Linton.

Caffeine: Studies on the effect of caffeine on the human reproductive cycle are mixed. One investigation indicated that women who consume a lot of caffeinated drinks are less fertile than those who drink caffeine occasionally or not at all.[6]

Nicotine: Approximately a third of men and women in their reproductive years smoke cigarettes. Aside from the many diseases that smoking causes, fertility is also negatively affected. Women who smoke may experience more ectopic pregnancies (in which the fertilized egg attaches to, and grows in, the fallopian tube). These women may also reach menopause earlier than their nonsmoking counterparts. They also risk compromising the health of their eggs, fallopian tubes, and cervix.[7] Male smokers risk damage to their sperm from the carcinogenic substances found in cigarette smoke. Researchers claim that if a mutated sperm successfully fertilizes an egg, it may produce adverse effects in the developing fetus.[8]

Recreational and Prescription Drugs: The avoidance of recreational drugs is vital during preconception. Marijuana, for instance, once viewed as a fairly innocuous substance, carries a dual danger. The deep, extended inhalation that is a typical practice among marijuana smokers allows more tar and carbon monoxide to enter the lungs than regular cigarette smoking. Genetic material can be damaged by marijuana and, in animal studies, it has been linked to an increase in fetal deaths and malformations.[9]

Cocaine may be responsible for decreasing the concentration of sperm in semen. It is also thought to create deformities in the sperm's shape and to reduce the speed at which it swims after ejaculation.[10] Tests have shown that men who use drugs increase their chances of producing abnormally developed offspring and the preconceptual use of cocaine has been linked to cases of neurological damage in children.[11]

In the case of the effect of prescription drugs on fertility and conception, contact your physician for advice.

Alcohol: Alcohol consumption presents several threats to the health of potential parents and their future offspring. Alcohol depresses immune function and has a tremendous impact on the egg and sperm. Researchers studying the effects of alcohol consumption on rodents state that there may be a direct connection between moderate consumption by the parents and genetic damage to their offspring.[12] Miscarriage and mental and physical handicaps were also noted as possible results of alcohol consumption.

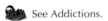 See Addictions.

Adverse Environmental Effects

"Besides the poisons taken voluntarily, there is a myriad of unavoidable environmental hazards that can be detrimental to the health of future parents and, as a result, their offspring: toxins in the workplace, vehicle emissions, water and air pollution, to name but a few," says Dr. Linton. It is important to be aware of these environmental hazards and to minimize exposure to them whenever possible.

In an experimental investigation of two lamp factories, conducted in Italy, researchers tested the reproductive health of the women working in each factory—one group was exposed to mercury vapors on a daily basis while the other was not. The mercury group experienced more menstrual difficulties, increased infertility, and a rise in vaginal bleeding during pregnancy. They also showed more miscarriages, preterm deliveries, and fetal malformations compared to the non-exposed group.[13]

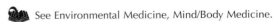 See Environmental Medicine, Mind/Body Medicine.

Emotional Factors

People are continually reminded that stress is detrimental to their health. Emotional and mental stressors have been linked to a host of illnesses ranging from fainting, nausea and weakness, and heart disease to dental cavities and the common cold.[14] "Stress can tear your health down faster than can inadequate nutrition," according to Dr. Linton. Therefore, during preconception, it is impor-

THE DEVELOPMENT OF THE FETUS DURING PREGNANCY

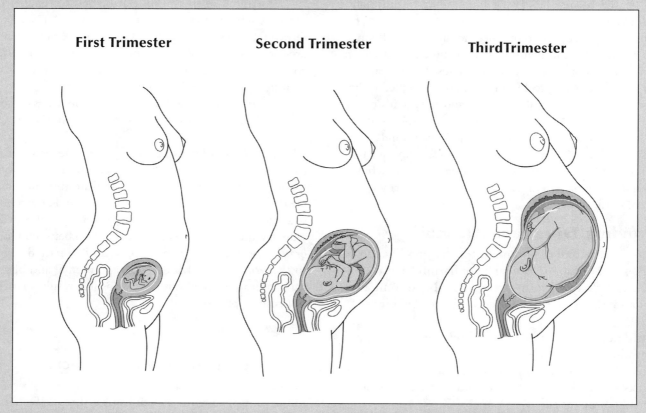

First Trimester   **Second Trimester**   **ThirdTrimester**

The first three months of pregnancy mark a period of intense development for the growing fetus. These early weeks are a critical time, because during this period the various organ systems are being fundamentally elaborated. It is at this stage that they are most sensitive to environmental chemicals, drugs, and viruses, which can cause birth defects.[17] During the second trimester, developmental changes are less rapid and the baby's growth takes over. By the third trimester, the baby's growth slows and the development of the senses as well as the brain and the sex organs is completed.

The First Trimester
The first organs form around the third week, after the formation of a primitive spinal cord. Then the nervous system and the cardiovascular system begin to develop. The first blood cells are produced. Circulation of blood begins and, by day 21, a primitive heart is functioning. Skeletal, nervous, and digestive systems are rapidly developing. Around this time, the mother misses her period.

During the fourth week, small swellings that will eventually develop into arms and legs appear on the upper and lower sides of the body, as well as near the top of the head

where the eyes will form. The liver is formed and the intestines, stomach, gallbladder, pancreas, and lungs begin to form. The fifth week shows an increase in the size of the head and brain. The embryo's nervous system is beginning to function and it will display reflex movements in response to touch.

At week six, arms and legs begin their primitive formations. The upper lip, throat, windpipe, and voice box form. The olfactory lobe, which deals with the sense of smell, and the pituitary gland begin formation in the brain. Around day 40, jaws, teeth, and facial muscles start to develop. The sexual organs are determined during week seven and cartilage and some bone starts to form.

During week eight, the external genitalia are formed—the female clitoris and male scrotum develop around day 50. By the end of this week, the embryo is 1¼ inches long. All of its organ systems are roughly formed, lower limbs have grown, and the embryo looks vaguely like a human infant.

Week nine marks the end of the embryonic stage. In this week, the fetus undergoes a growth spurt and virtually doubles its size. Fingernails, toenails, and hair follicles appear.

DEVELOPMENT OF THE FETUS DURING PREGNANCY, continued

The skin thickens and becomes less transparent and baby teeth begin to form under the gums. In the male fetus, the penis becomes distinguishable.

By week ten, connections between the nervous system and the brain are mature enough to transmit sensory information. Consequently, the skin all over the body is now responsive and the fetus will move in reaction to touch. Fetal blood is now manufactured in the spleen and bone marrow.

During week eleven, the vocal cords are formed. Several digestive organs become functional: the liver secretes bile, the pancreas secretes insulin, and the intestines form into folds lined with villi and glands.[18] As the neural system matures, breathing, sucking, and swallowing motions begin. Week twelve marks the end of the first trimester. The fully formed baby is about 3½ inches from the top of the head to the rump and weighs only one ounce.

The Second Trimester
During the fourth month, the fetus experiences an enormous growth spurt. This takes place largely in the body and limbs, which brings its proportions close to those of a newborn. As fetal movements become more pronounced and varied, the mother may feel them for the first time.

In the fifth month, a fatty tissue called brown fat forms in the areas around the neck, chest, and crotch. This fat helps the fetus maintain its body temperature. Vernix, a fatty substance secreted from glands in the skin, forms a thick coating over the baby's skin to protect it during the long exposure to the amniotic fluid. A fine hair appears all over the body, together with the formation of eyebrows and hair on the head.

During the sixth month, due to a lack of fat under the skin, the fetus appears lean and wrinkled. Its skin is a reddish color, a sign that the capillary system is developing. By the end of the month, the lungs are developed to such an extent that it is now possible, for the first time, that the baby could survive outside the womb. Hearing and visual systems are now functioning primitively. The fetus has grown from eight inches to 12 inches.

The Third Trimester
By the seventh month, the baby's senses are already fully developed. It can hear, see, smell, and taste. White fat forms in the innermost layer of the skin and smoothes out wrinkles. In male babies, the testes descend into the scrotum. The brain increases in size and sophistication. It is just as advanced as that of a newborn; more refined movement and learning is now possible. During the eighth month, the baby's growth slows down and the new appearance of fat makes the body look more full and rounded.

As the fetus begins its ninth month in utero, its growth slows even more, but white fat is still produced and the baby becomes plumper. Most of the fine hair that covered the body has disappeared and the vernix now only covers the back. The baby receives antibodies from the mother's blood to protect and stimulate its immature immune system.

---

tant that both partners try to maintain a positive state of mind. In terms of reproductive health, science provides an abundance of evidence showing that stress harms both men and women. Negative emotions can decrease sperm count and movement, as well as increase a woman's prolactin, the hormone responsible for milk production and breast growth during pregnancy.[15] Most importantly for the future child, a couple must want to become parents—a 22-year Czechoslovakian study found that children born to mothers who were denied abortions grew up with more emotional and psychological scars.[16]

Pregnancy

Fertilization usually takes place in the fallopian tube. Only one of the millions of sperm will pass through the mem-

brane of the ovum (female egg) achieving conception. Once the sperm has fertilized the ovum, enzymes in the egg alter the inner membrane and make it impossible for more sperm to enter. Once introduced, the nuclei of the sperm and the egg, each containing 23 chromosomes, unite to form one fertilized egg with the 46 chromosomes needed for human development. The whole process of intermingling takes 24 hours. The fertilized egg then travels to the womb where it embeds itself like a seed in the lining of the uterus and begins to grow.

Physical Changes in the Mother During Pregnancy
During the first trimester, the uterus, a small, hard, pear-shaped organ becomes a soft, spherical sac through which the baby can be easily felt. By the end of the first

trimester, the uterus has expanded out from the pelvic cavity and touches the abdominal wall. It continues to grow and, at term, the uterus is between 500 and 1,000 times its prepregnant size. The actual growth of muscle fibers, not just the stretching of the uterus, is responsible for most of the increase in size. At the end of the ninth month, the uterus almost touches the mother's liver just under the lower right rib.

The prepregnant cervix is firm and muscular. During pregnancy, from as early as the first trimester, the cervix begins to soften, caused by an increase in the number of blood vessels and mucus glands in the cervical lining. The cervix also becomes spongy in texture and creates a mucous plug that seals the cervical opening soon after fertilization takes place. This plug is released some time around the start of labor.

Soon after conception, the vagina experiences an increase in blood flow and as a result it takes on a violet hue. Throughout pregnancy, the vaginal wall thickens, elongates, and becomes looser and more elastic in order to prepare for the enormous amount of stretching that it will go through during the delivery. The opening to the vagina and the vulva become swollen and vaginal discharge becomes thick, white, and acidic, which helps guard against infection.

Within a couple of weeks of conception, the breasts can feel full, heavy, and sore. These sensations are due to the enlargement of ducts and lobules known as alveoli. During the first trimester, the breasts begin to increase in size. As time progresses, the areola, the pigmented area around the nipples, become wider and darker and the nipples themselves become larger and darker. After the first trimester, some women may notice a slight discharge of colostrum, a highly nutritious, yellowish liquid that the newborn suckles on until the milk comes in, around the third day after birth.

How to Have a Healthy Pregnancy

Although each individual responds to pregnancy differently, and there is no such thing as a perfect pregnancy, there are many ways to contribute to a healthy one. "Probably most important is that the woman realizes the physiological impact carrying a child has on her health and that she listens to her body's needs," says Dr. Linton. "Adequate rest, including naps, 'mental' breaks, and sufficient sleep, is essential. Maintaining a positive outlook and keeping stress to a minimum are beneficial to both mother and baby. Comfortably paced, regular, non-jarring exercise, such as low-impact aerobics, walking, yoga, and swimming, can increase stamina for labor, strengthen muscles used during delivery, and may enhance the ability to cope better with labor."

HARMFUL FACTORS AFFECTING THE FETUS

Maternal exposure to alcohol and cigarettes, recreational drugs (marijuana, cocaine, heroin, and LSD), medications such as lithium (to treat depression) and tetracycline (an antibiotic), pesticides, petroleum products, heavy metals such as lead and mercury,[19] caffeine,[20] and even over-the-counter medicines such as aspirin can harm the fetus and should be limited if not avoided altogether. Recent research also suggests that mothers having high homocysteine levels (an amino acid linked to heart disease), being overweight, or having urinary tract infections can increase the risk of birth defects and later impairment to children, as can the use of the acne drug Accutane.

There are two periods of pregnancy when the maternal consumption of alcohol is particularly threatening to the development of the fetus: from the 12th to the 18th week and from the 24th to the 36th week. Experts at the U.S. National Institute of Alcohol Abuse and Alcoholism claim that three or four beers or glasses of wine a day can cause any one or more of the following defects: mental retardation, hyperactivity, a heart murmur, facial deformity such as a small head, or low-set ears.[21] Consuming even small amounts of alcohol during pregnancy can increase the risk of newborn children developing behavioral problems later in life. In a study of 506 women, researchers found that children born to mothers who drank the equivalent of one cocktail a week during pregnancy were three times as likely to exhibit behavioral problems such as aggression, delinquent behavior, and attention problems by ages 6 to 7 compared to children born of mothers who completely abstained from alcohol from conception to birth. This was true after the researchers took into account other factors that can influence children's behavior.[22]

Cigarette smoking cuts the amount of oxygen available in the maternal blood, which directly affects the growth of fetal tissue. Studies have shown that babies born to mothers who smoke 13 or more high-tar cigarettes a day are smaller and in poor physical condition compared to those of nonsmoking mothers.[23] In addition, more recent research has found that mothers who are heavy smokers (15 or more cigarettes per day) during pregnancy and shortly after birth are twice as likely to have babies who develop infant colic or who are fussier than normal and seemingly inconsolable.[24]

Research also indicates that high levels of homocysteine may be a marker during pregnancy for preeclampsia and umbilical placental vascular disease. Moreover, infants born of mothers with high homocysteine levels tend to be born earlier than normal and to weigh significantly less at birth.[25] Homocysteine has also been shown to cause birth defects.[26]

Babies born of mothers who are overweight or obese prior to conceiving are 36% more likely to be born with a birth defect compared to babies born of women of normal weight, according to a recent study conducted by the CDC. The researchers noted that the study has "important implications for prevention, given the increasing prevalence of obesity."[27]

The CDC recently released a report that some women become pregnant while taking the acne drug Accutane, despite the fact that the drug causes severe birth defects and despite the fact that the drug contains a warning symbol to that effect on its packaging. According to the CDC, many women were unable to determine what the symbol meant. The CDC advises women taking Accutane to use two forms of birth control, be tested for pregnancy each month, and register with a survey that monitors the experiences of women who use the drug.[28]

New research shows that urinary tract infections (UTIs) during the third trimester of pregnancy can increase the risk of mental retardation in infants by 40% and double the likelihood of fetal death, if left untreated. UTIs occur in approximately 5%–7% of all pregnancies. However, the research also showed that women who were treated with antibiotics within the first few days of UTI symptoms (burning sensations during urination and/or a frequent urgency to urinate) had no increased risk of their babies being harmed.[29]

Over-the-counter drugs such as aspirin, when used during the first half of pregnancy, have been linked with lower-than-average IQs in those babies.[30] Research into the effects of valium on chickens revealed an impairment of muscle-cell development in their chicks and suggests a possible risk in human pregnancy.[31]

Environmental factors, such as pesticides, lead, and chemicals brought home from a work environment on a parent's clothing, can harm an unborn child.[32] X-ray exposure to the mother, as well as preconception X-ray exposure to the father, is also harmful.[33] Although most studies have not substantiated the claim that video display terminals (VDTs) adversely affect the fetus, many individuals are not convinced. In 1991, in response to this concern, San Francisco, California, mandated that companies with 15 or more employees protect their workers against potential adverse health effects from VDTs. They were required to provide wrist rests, antiglare shields, adjustable chairs, and regular breaks from sitting in front of a VDT screen. Louis Slesin, publisher of *Microwave News*, claims that the effects of using VDTs during pregnancy are unknown. He points out that studies concluding that VDTs are not harmful to the fetus do not assess the situation accurately. As so many people

are now using VDTs in their workplace, more reliable investigations need to be conducted.

Nutrition During Pregnancy

It is important to the health of both mother and fetus that the mother eats a well-balanced and varied diet. Fresh fruits and vegetables, whole grains, legumes, beans, and fish are essential. Limit refined sugars, processed foods, and saturated fats. Organically grown produce, meats, and poultry are preferable. However, if produce is not organic,

---

REDUCING THE RISK OF PREECLAMPSIA

Preeclampsia, or toxemia during pregnancy, can occur in the late stages of pregnancy and, if left untreated, can pose serious health risks (including death) to both the mother and fetus, due to epileptic seizure. Symptoms of preeclampsia include high blood pressure, fluid retention, and protein in the urine. There are no known markers to screen women for their risk of developing preeclampsia. However, research indicates that the risk is greater among women whose mothers developed the condition or who are impregnated by a man whose mother experienced preeclampsia-related complications during their birth. Women who have never before borne children are also at greater risk for the disease, and poor diet and nutritional deficiencies are other known risk factors.[34]

According to Alan Gaby, M.D., high-protein diets appear to reduce the risk of preeclampsia, as does supplementation with vitamins B6, C, and E, calcium, magnesium, and rutin (a flavonoid antioxidant). Dr. Gaby recommends a diet high in fiber-rich foods that avoids all refined sugars, processed foods, caffeine, and alcohol, as well as medicinal drugs, unless they have been prescribed by your physician. He also cautions against supplementing with high doses of vitamin A.

In cases of severe preeclampsia, pregnant women can be hospitalized and treated with high doses (20 g or more over a 24-hour period) of intravenous magnesium sulfate. "While that treatment is effective to some extent, it is not without risk," Dr. Gaby says. He recommends a safer dosage of 1,000 mg of magnesium sulfate and 300 mg of vitamin B6, which he says provides the same benefits and additionally is more effective in reducing fluid retention.[35]

it should be washed to remove as much of the agricultural chemical residue as possible.

Most physicians recommend eating plenty of dairy products during pregnancy, due to their calcium and protein content. Helen Burst also suggests her patients use milk products. "If a woman is lactose intolerant," says Burst, "obviously you're going to find other ways of getting her the protein. If she's not lactose intolerant, I don't see any problems in using milk and the dairy products."

Other doctors are more wary about suggesting dairy as a mainstay of a pregnant woman's diet. Lendon Smith, M.D., a pediatrician and author of several books on children's nutrition, explains, "Many babies will develop a milk sensitivity before they are born because the mother followed the obstetrician's dictum: 'Drink a quart of milk every day so the baby will get the calcium.' If a mother is already sensitive to dairy products and takes in milk, cheese, and ice cream, she may not be absorbing the calcium from those foods she is ingesting." Foods such as nuts, soybean products such as tofu and soymilk, and goat milk products provide alternative sources of protein. Seaweed, green vegetables, and a mixture of sunflower, sesame, and pumpkin seeds are alternatives for calcium. No one food, including dairy, should be eaten on a daily basis, Dr. Smith advises, as this increases an individual's chance of developing a food sensitivity.

Although a well-chosen vegetarian diet may be healthy for some pregnant woman, vegetarians who consume no animal products at all, including dairy and eggs, should use a vitamin B_{12} supplement. This is especially true in light of a recent study which found that women who are deficient in B_{12} have a greater risk of infertility or repeated miscarriages. One woman in the study had suffered seven miscarriages before her B12 deficiency was discovered, and then went one to have three healthy children in separate pregnancies after supplementing with the vitamin.[36]

"Women who are vegetarians must carefully combine their grains and beans in order to achieve adequate protein intake," cautions Alan Gaby, M.D., past President of the American Holistic Medical Association and a noted nutritional expert. "Even with proper food combining, a protein supplement may be necessary for some vegetarian women. To assure adequate intake of vitamins and minerals, a well-formulated prenatal supplement should be used."[37]

The idea that a pregnant woman needs to eat for two is a myth. A baby is not a parasite that depletes the mother of all her nutrition. Both undereating and overeating have a negative impact, according to Dr. Linton. "The usual obstetric advice of increasing daily intake by 300 calories is not supported by all, and some nutritionists feel that hunger, not calorie counting, is a more reliable guide to eating during pregnancy," she says.

Eating five to six small, nutrient-dense meals a day is a sensible idea. Restricting weight gain, which was very popular 20 years ago, was thought to ease a woman's labor. We now know that this is not necessarily so. Guidelines issued in 1990 by the Institute of Medicine, in Washington, D.C., recommend weight gains for healthy pregnant women. The range of optimal weight gains depends on the weight of the mother early in pregnancy:

- 28-40 pounds for "underweight" women
- 15-25 pounds for "overweight" women
- A minimum of 15 pounds for "obese" women[38]

These guidelines "reflect current interests in preventing low–birth weight babies and thus reduce the incidence of infant mortality and mental and physical retardation."[39] Pregnancy is not the time to diet. Dr. Linton offers a simple formula. "If you are eating a whole foods diet, drinking plenty of water, and getting adequate exercise such as walking or swimming, then the weight you gain in your pregnancy is appropriate."

Opinions vary on the amount of protein that is needed during pregnancy. The U.S. Recommended Dietary Allowance (RDA) indicates that a woman's requirements rise from 46 g to 60 g per day. Some experts advocate consuming even more protein than the RDA. "I think that dietary protein is probably the most common nutrient deficiency in pregnancy," says Timothy Birdsall, N.D. "Pregnant women need 70-100 g of protein daily, which most people will not get with a normal diet." These levels of protein, adds Dr. Birdsall, help feed increasing blood volume and guard against complications during pregnancy, such as preeclampsia.

Helen Burst agrees with Dr. Birdsall's sentiments. "I believe in protein and calorie increases during pregnancy and certainly when breast-feeding, too," she says. "To me, the amounts given in the RDA are too low. You can make a significant difference in the birth weights of babies born to women eating a good balance of protein and calories." Both Dr. Birdsall and Burst point out that a protein increase must be accompanied by more calories or the protein will be used for energy rather than the construction of tissues, such as blood, the placenta, and an expanding uterus.

Salt Intake During Pregnancy: Sodium is needed to maintain fluid balance and blood volume. For this reason, salt restriction is one common nutritional advisement that does not apply during pregnancy. Restricting sodium and using diuretics, once routine treatments to prevent preeclampsia and swelling, are not only unnecessary but also potentially harmful.[40] It is best to use salt to taste.

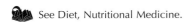 See Diet, Nutritional Medicine.

Nutritional Supplements

If there is any concern that a mother's diet does not provide all the vitamins and minerals needed for a healthy pregnancy, she may want to add a prenatal supplement. Requirements for many nutrients increase during this time and supplementing a poor diet results in a healthier pregnancy.[41] Dr. Linton notes that it is most important for pregnant women to eat well and then use supplements to optimize their health. Supplements of specific vitamins and minerals can also be used as safe treatments to certain problems during pregnancy. For example, vitamin B6 may help alleviate morning sickness[42] and calcium can decrease hypertension.[43]

However, like any substance taken during this time, discretion should be used. "Ideally, we get our nutrients from foods," says Dr. Birdsall. "The unfortunate part is that none of us live in an ideal situation. We're all exposed to varying levels of toxins in our environment and in the food chain. Most of us are have levels of stress in our lives that deplete us of nutrients. Many of the foods we consume are deficient in nutrients compared to what they were 75 or 100 years ago." A prenatal supplement, he explains, acts as an insurance policy, providing it contains reasonable amounts of vitamins and minerals.

Vitamin C is a nutrient that is chronically underdosed, according to Dr. Birdsall. He points out the vital role of vitamin C in the formation of collagen, a protein found in connective tissue, cartilage, and bone. Some doctors are concerned over a condition called rebound scurvy, thought to affect newborns whose mothers have ingested large amounts of vitamin C. In Dr. Birdsall's experience and research, this is a very rare phenomenon. "I have only been able to find two documented cases of rebound scurvy in the medical literature," he explains. If it does develop, he says, the infant recovers with no treatment in a relatively short period of time.

Folic acid, a B vitamin found in green leafy vegetables, nuts, and whole grains, can prevent neural tube defects in fetuses.[44] However, artificial supplementation of folic acid can decrease zinc absorption, a mineral required for proper fetal growth and immunity.[45] In unusually large doses (1,000 mcg), folic acid is associated with maternal infection and abnormally slow fetal heart rate.[46]

Extra iron may be warranted if the mother's hemoglobin tests suggest a deficiency. Yet routine supplementation of iron can block zinc absorption and has been linked with infection, cancer, and other conditions.[47] However, Dr. Birdsall states that iron is the only nutrient that the current dietary guidelines for pregnancy say

should be supplemented and he sees adding this mineral to his pregnant patients' regimen as valuable.

Vitamin D should also be taken judiciously to avoid toxicity. The fetus can drain as much as 300 mg daily of calcium from the mother during the third trimester, in order to facilitate bone development. However, absorption of vitamin D (a nutrient that aids in calcium uptake) and calcium are enhanced during pregnancy. Consequently, some experts are debating whether the current RDA of 1,200 mg of calcium daily during pregnancy is perhaps too high. Excessive levels of this mineral in the body can result in its spillage into the urine. One in every 1,500 pregnant women who consumes high amounts of calcium may develop kidney stones, slightly higher than in nonpregnant women.[48] Dr. Birdsall feels that physicians have tended to over-supplement pregnant women with calcium for two reasons: "We tend to ignore the relationship between calcium and the other minerals, particularly magnesium and zinc. And most of the research done on calcium supplementation is done with relatively inefficient forms of calcium." Calcium citrate or citrate/malate are the most absorbable forms—the more efficiently the mineral is absorbed, the less you need to ingest.

While it is true that milk contains substantial amounts of this mineral, some experts question the availability of dairy's calcium. "There is now some good research to indicate that dairy consumption by the mother can induce an allergic condition in the baby," Dr. Birdsall says. Using alternative calcium foods, such as dark green leafy vegetables, and avoiding calcium-robbing foods, such as coffee, sugar, and salt, will ensure adequate nourishment for a pregnant woman. With regard to salt, pregnancy is not a time to restrict salt intake, but it should be used in moderation as large amounts will decrease available calcium. Calcium supplementation can also help ease leg cramps during pregnancy.[49] Vitamins B6, D, and K, and boron are nutrients that are also involved in bone metabolism.

CONTRAINDICATED VITAMINS, MINERALS, AND HERBS

Pregnant women should use caution in taking vitamins and minerals. One nutrient that should be supplemented with caution during pregnancy is vitamin A, which recent research shows can increase the risk of birth defects, such as heart abnormalities, cleft lip, or cleft palate. Doses of vitamin A as low as 15,000 IU have been associated with microcephaly, a congenital abnormal smallness of the head often seen in mental retardation.[50] (However, no evidence exists linking similar or higher doses of vitamin A obtained through the diet to such birth defects.)[51] "There is no question that very large doses of vitamin A

STRETCH MARK PREVENTION OINTMENT

Most women are concerned about stretch marks during pregnancy. Although many doctors feel stretch marks are hereditary, prevention is a good remedy. The consistent application of a mixture containing a blend of specific oils is your best protection. This should be applied once or twice a day and massaged into the abdomen, breasts, and thighs. The best times to do this are in the morning when you wake up and before bed at night. Start using this prevention routine as soon as your abdomen begins to swell as it is then that the skin begins to stretch.

All of the following ingredients can be found in most health food stores. Sweet almond oil can also be purchased where massage supplies are sold.

- 1 oz vitamin E oil
- 5 tbsp (2½ fluid oz) cocoa butter
- 4½ oz sweet almond oil

Carefully melt the cocoa butter in a double boiler—do not overheat it. Once the cocoa butter has turned to a liquid, add the vitamin E and sweet almond oils. Place the mixture in an eight-ounce plastic container. The ointment will solidify as it cools and may be stored at room temperature.

can cause birth defects," Dr. Gaby says. "What we do not know is the optimal intake of vitamin A for pregnant women, nor do we know the maximum safe level. Everyone agrees that 10,000 IU per day is safe. If there is a medical reason to take larger amounts of vitamin A during pregnancy, the risks should be carefully weighed against the benefits."[52]

Beta carotene, which is converted by the body into vitamin A, is relatively nontoxic and probably safe. However, Dr. Birdsall says, "I err on the side of caution in situations like that and normally would not, at least early in pregnancy, use high doses of beta carotene either." Regarding the use of supplementation during pregnancy, only take what is absolutely necessary.

Although many herbs are useful during pregnancy and childbirth, there are many that are discouraged. According to Dr. Birdsall, herbs such as autumn crocus, barberry, goldenseal, juniper, male fern, mandrake, pennyroyal, poke root, rue, sage, southernwood, tansy, thuja, and wormwood may trigger a miscarriage. Use herbs with discretion and only under the guidance of a professional. "There are some herbs that are absolutely contraindicated in pregnancy," Dr. Birdsall says. His list of

herbs to avoid during this time includes some fairly common plants, such as the laxatives senna and cascara sagrada found in both herbal preparations and over-the-counter drugs. Senna encourages menstruation and may promote miscarriage.

Herbs with high concentrations of the alkaloid berberine, found in goldenseal, barberry, and Oregon grape root, should not be used during pregnancy. "Historically," says Dr. Birdsall, "goldenseal was used to stop postpartum uterine hemorrhage and it does that because it causes strong uterine contractions." Licorice contains estrogen-like substances and is to be avoided during pregnancy. Juniper can harm the fetus and possibly induce a miscarriage.

Preparing the Body for Childbirth

Ease the stress, pain, and anxiety precipitating and accompanying childbirth by taking the proper steps to prepare one's body and mind. Exercises that strengthen the body are easy to do, but equally important are exercises that strengthen the intimacy between the expectant parents.

Kegel Exercises: The muscle that surrounds the vagina is called the pubococcygeal (PC) muscle. It is usually in good tone; however, during pregnancy and childbirth it supports a lot of weight and can become slack. To keep the PC muscle toned, it is important to practice Kegel exercises on a daily basis, both before and after the birth.

To find your PC muscle, sit on the toilet and spread your legs apart. As you start to urinate, see if you can control the flow of urine without moving your legs. The PC muscle is the one you use to turn the flow on and off.

- Slow Kegels: Tighten the PC muscle as if to stop the urine. Hold for a slow count of three and then relax. Repeat ten times.

- Quick Kegels: Tighten and relax the PC muscle, as quickly as you can, five times. Relax and repeat ten times.

- Pull in, Push out: Pull up the entire pelvic floor as though trying to suck water into the vagina. Then push out or bear down as if trying to push the imaginary water out. This exercise uses the stomach and abdominal muscles as well as the PC muscle. Do this 4–5 times in a row. Repeat ten times.

Ideally you should repeat each of these exercises five times a day, beginning at the start of pregnancy. After a few months, you will notice an improvement in your performance and can gradually increase the amount of practice times each week. These exercises can be done anytime and anywhere: practice while driving the car, watching television, washing dishes, or waiting in line. They will enhance vaginal elasticity and improve bladder control. It is also good to practice during sexual intercourse as this can help elevate sexual awareness and pleasure.

Perineal Massage: The perineum is the area between the vagina and anus. During the last six weeks of pregnancy, it should be massaged daily in order to prepare for the stretching it will experience during birth. This technique can also help reduce the need for an episiotomy (a small surgical incision in the perineum made by obstetricians to facilitate the emergence of the baby) and protect against tearing. This technique should be delayed if there are any vaginal problems, such as an active herpes sore or vaginitis. It can be resumed when the vagina has healed. Perineal massage can be performed by you or your partner.

Roy Dittman, O.M.D., of Santa Monica, California, offers these guidelines for a perineal massage:

- Wash your hands. Have a mirror handy, and find a warm, private place to practice.

- Lubricate your perineum and your thumbs with vegetable oil, cocoa butter, KY jelly, or vitamin E oil. You can also use your own body secretions if you wish.

- Placing your thumbs about 1½ inches inside your vagina, press down and to the sides at the same time. Gently and firmly stretch the skin until you feel a slight tingling or burning sensation. Continue to hold this pressure for an additional two minutes until the perineum becomes more numb and the tingling is not as distinct.

- Take 3-4 minutes to massage the oil along the outside of the lower half of the vagina. Avoid moving upward toward the urethra.

- Pulling gently outward or forward, massage the lower part of the vagina with your thumbs. This massage motion helps to stretch the perineal skin, similar to the way your baby's head will stretch it during birth.

Intimacy During Pregnancy

A woman's physical and emotional comfort with her pregnancy determine her sexual attitudes and enjoyment at this time. Her feelings are often influenced by her partner's attitude to her appearance. This issue is complex and it is therefore vital that women and men discuss their feelings, fears, and beliefs about the changes that are shaping their lives and consequently affecting their lovemaking.

During pregnancy, a woman's libido can oscillate from high to low. She may become anorgasmic for a period or the symptoms of pregnancy may dampen her sexual drive. During the latter months, the awkwardness of her shape may inhibit her from lovemaking. Some couples are concerned that intercourse may harm the fetus and it is reassuring for them to learn that the penis rarely touches the cervix. The vagina lengthens during sexual excitement and the mucous plug covering the cervical opening to the uterus also provides protection. Semen is rich in prostaglandins, natural bodily chemicals that can help ripen and soften the cervix, and intercourse may initiate uterine contractions. However, these actions will not induce labor unless a woman is nearing the end of her pregnancy.

Helen Burst feels that sexual activity should depend on how the woman feels. "There are many things in terms of alternatives to actual intercourse itself, if that is a problem," she explains. "The only time that I restrict sex is if she's having signs and symptoms of preterm labor." Other exceptions to sex or orgasm during pregnancy would be cases in which vaginal bleeding occurs, if the woman experiences continuing or painful cramps after intercourse, or if the woman has a new sexual partner with a sexually transmitted disease or AIDS. If there is a history of preterm labor, Burst advises the use of condoms for sexual intercourse.

The father or birth coach should participate in the many decisions and educational opportunities during pregnancy. This includes touring the hospital (if this is the chosen location for birth) and learning about the different stages of labor. The partner should discuss any concerns for the birth with both the pregnant woman and the birth attendant. He or she should feel free to disclose any feelings, positive or negative, surrounding the upcoming event, so that there are no uncertain feelings to hinder the support of the mother during labor.[53]

Childbirth

All the planning, preparation, and events around pregnancy culminate with the birth of the child. Regarding childbirth, expectant parents must make some very important decisions including where the birth will take place, what type of practitioner will deliver the care, and what method will be used.

It is best to prepare for childbirth well in advance, preferably before conception. "It is important that expectant mothers know all of their options in order to make informed decisions," says Heather Allen, a doula and childbirth educator, in Clinton, New York. She recommends that parents-to-be read books on the subject, interview care providers, and tour hospitals and birth centers, even requesting their statistical data regarding birthing interventions, cesarean rates, and so forth.

"I urge pregnant women to enroll in quality prenatal classes and to get professional assistance in developing healthy nutrition and exercise programs," Allen adds. She also suggests considering working with a midwife or doula (labor assistant) and advises women to become aware of their hospital's birthing policies so that they can negotiate, well before labor, if they desire care that is different than the policies normally allow. "One way to do this is to write a birth plan that both you and your physician sign off on," she says. Most importantly, Allen counsels women to "believe in yourself, your body, and the birth process itself."

Medical Intervention

Medical technology has its place in childbirth. However, the routine use of many standard interventions typically used in hospitals, such as pain medication, cesarean sections, and episiotomies, are being reevaluated. According to Susanne Houd, Program Director of the Department of Midwifery at the Michener Institute, in Toronto, Ontario, Canada, criticism of home births is unjustified, especially when it is based on hospital knowledge. "It's like comparing oranges to apples," she says.

A Canadian study discovered that the level of intervention increased when low-risk maternity patients delivered at facilities specializing in high-risk situations.[54] This situation has been referred to as the cascade effect—in an otherwise normal circumstance, one type of medical intervention can lead to complications and then more intervention. For example, a woman hooked up to a fetal heart monitor needs to remain inactive. As a result, her labor slows down due to tension and inactivity. To hasten the labor, the physician may order a rupture of membranes, which then enhances pain. Pain medications or anesthesia may follow, finally culminating in a cesarean section.[55]

Recently, the World Health Organization (WHO) confirmed a view held by many alternative health practitioners: fewer medical visits during pregnancy do not adversely affect birth outcomes. WHO researchers conducted a multicenter, randomized, controlled trial in order to compare current standard prenatal care with a newer model that emphasizes "actions known to be effective in improving maternal or neonatal outcomes" with fewer doctor visits. Over 12,500 women in Argentina, Cuba, Saudi Arabia, and Thailand were assigned to clinics offering the newer model, while 12,000 were provided with care under the standard model. Both groups were screened for problems such as low birth weight, preeclampsia, severe anemia after birth, and urinary tract infections. The average cost of care under both models was also considered.

The study found that women who received care under the newer model averaged only five doctor visits, compared with an average of eight visits under the standard model, and that "women in the new model were no more likely to give birth to a low–birth weight baby, have anemia during pregnancy, or spend longer in the hospital than women who had more prenatal visits." A subsequent review by the WHO researchers of previous trials involving 57,000 women found similar outcomes, with the only noticeable difference being that the newer model often meant reduced costs.[56]

ELECTRONIC FETAL HEART RATE MONITOR (EFM)

EFM is a machine used to determine the heart rate of the fetus and mother's uterine contractions. EFM uses either ultrasound or electrodes attached to the baby and prints out a graph with the results. "I'm glad its there when we need it, because it can save lives," says Helen Burst. "And there are times where there are clear indications for fetal monitoring. To use it as a routine in perfectly normal pregnancy and childbirth, I think is not the way management of care should be done." Risks involved, says Burst, include the fact that neither EFM readings nor their interpretations by practitioners are always totally accurate. When EFM was compared to auscultation (listening to the heartbeat with a stethoscope) in a series of studies at the University of Denver, there was no difference in fetal death and health between the two groups. The most glaring disparity was the 16.5% cesarean rate in the EFM group versus 6.8% in the non-EFM group.[57] Some experts have suggested that EFM has a positive influence on a child's neurological development later on, but there has been no support for this theory.[58]

PAIN MEDICATION

Medications for pain relief are a risk during childbirth, with part of the risk due to the drugs the baby receives through the placenta. When pethidine (a pain medication) is given to women in labor, it sedates newborns to the point of disturbing their early suckling pattern and possibly inhibiting successful breast-feeding.[59] Epidural analgesia, local pain medication injected between the spinal vertebrae, may diminish the bearing down reflex and perineal sensation. This can in turn delay the second stage of labor and lead to early surgical intervention or use of forceps and a vacuum extractor.[60] There is even speculation that drug use during labor may be responsible for drug use among children and teens today.[61]

EPISIOTOMY

The most common surgical procedure in childbirth and medicine overall is the episiotomy, an incision in the muscular wall surrounding the vagina intended to widen the opening and ease delivery. A Canadian study now recommends that routine episiotomies be abandoned. Instead, researchers suggest, this surgery should be reserved for cases of fetal distress or if a woman is unable to deliver her child without help. Episiotomies do not, as previously thought, prevent perineal tears or trauma, enhance later sexuality, or benefit the baby.[62] They are also not mandatory for all forcep or vacuum extraction use.[63] Burst says that when she saw this study it angered her. The results, she says are "what we've been saying for years, but it's not until the M.D.s come out with an article that anybody pays attention to it."

VACUUM EXTRACTION AND FORCEPS

The use of forceps and vacuum extraction has recently been associated with decreased oxygen delivery and intracranial bleeding of the fetus during birth. Such instruments are used to forcibly pull the baby from the vagina and it is suggested that these methods are used more frequently on women who are less educated about childbirth. Forceps may later impair the baby's vision and cause foot problems. Vacuum extraction has resulted in leg problems.[64] One article, entitled "Fatal Forceps," recounts a pathologist's findings that some infant deaths may be due to delivery by forceps.[65] Recent research has also found that mothers whose babies are born via vacuum extraction or forceps delivery are nearly twice as likely to develop fecal incontinence (difficulty controlling bowel movements and gas) than women who give birth without such procedures.[66]

CESAREAN SECTION (C-SECTION)

Approximately 25% of all births in the U.S. are performed by c-section. One researcher claims that the high c-section rate is related in part to its financial compensation for the attending physician and hospital.[67] An English teaching hospital conducted an exercise to assess the need to perform c-sections in a number of birthing situations. Not only did auditors disagree with each other as to whether a c-section was indicated in each case, but also when given identical information at different times, auditors were inconsistent with their own decisions.[68]

"When necessary, a cesarean can be a life-saving technique for the mother and/or the baby," Heather Allen says. "But a cesarean section is a major form of abdominal surgery and, whenever it is contemplated, the physi-

cian must weigh its risks and benefits compared to birthing the child vaginally." According to Allen, there are certain situations when c-sections are safer than vaginal birth. These include fetal distress, fetal malpresentation, placenta previa (a placenta implanted in the lower uterus), and cord prolapse. She notes, however, that c-sections are sometimes performed for other reasons than the well-being of the mother or fetus, such as avoidance of patient pain, convenience factors, and legal concerns of the hospital or physician ("defensive medicine"), and that cesarean rates are also higher for women who have private medical insurance and for women who are private, rather than public, clinic patients.

"Compared with vaginal birth, c-sections tend to cause greater pain and debility, sometimes for months," Allen says. "The surgery itself increases the risk of maternal death, hemorrhage, surgical injury to other organs, infection, blood clots, and rehospitalization for complications caused by the procedure. C-sections, when performed for reasons other than the baby's health, increase the risk of the baby being born in poor condition or having trouble breathing." C-sections also lead to lower rates of breast-feeding and increase by 30 times the need for emergency hysterectomy due to post-operative bleeding.[69]

In the early 1970s, only 3% of births were by c-sections, according to the World Health Organization, which states that the rate should be no higher than 10% in any developed country.[70]

Contrary to popular belief, it is possible for a woman to have a vaginal birth after a cesarean. It is recommended by the American College of Obstetrics and Gynecology that appropriate patients try vaginal birth after previously having had a c-section.[71] Statistically, vaginal births create fewer complications. Although it is estimated that 50% to 80% of VBACs (vaginal birth after cesarean) are successful, uterine rupture, the main concern with VBACs, occurs in less than 0.5% of cases. VBACs are not recommended for women with serious medical problems, such as diabetes, a multiple birth, a small pelvis, or a classical (vertical) c-section incision scar.[72]

There are a number of benefits for babies born vaginally, as well as for their mothers, according to Allen. The advantages for babies include the fact that they are born when they are ready, tend to be better prepared for life outside the womb due to a surge of catecholamines (biochemicals affecting the nervous and cardiovascular systems, metabolic rate, body temperature, and smooth muscles) that occurs as the baby moves through the birth canal, are much more likely to be born with healthy lungs, tend to enjoy more frequent early contact with their mothers, and are much more likely to be breast-fed. Benefits to the mother include decreased risk of infection (2%-4% compared to as high as 35% for c-section births), decreased risk of other surgical hazards, quicker recovery times, decreased risk of postpartum depression, and lower medical costs.

Delivery

Originally, all women gave birth in their home environment. This first began to change in North America at the beginning of the 20th century, when childbirth gradually migrated from a female-assisted experience in the home to a medical procedure based in a hospital. Once the trend away from home birth had begun, the percentage of babies born in hospitals escalated and reached 90% in the 1950s.[73]

HOSPITAL BIRTH

An obstetrician (OB), a medical doctor specializing in the care of women during pregnancy and childbirth, will typically deliver babies in a hospital. A hospital environment is populated with modern technology, routine testing, and conventional medicines.

The rate of medical intervention (invasive medical procedures such as episiotomies, pain medications, and c-sections) is higher in a hospital than in a home environment and, according to Lewis Mehl, of the Waisman Center at the University of Wisconsin, normal variations of childbirth can often be mistaken for complications by hospitals. This may be due to several reasons: the higher levels of tension in the hospital, the availability of consultants, modern tests, and equipment, and the state of mind of hospital staff as they mediate between both high-risk situations and potentially normal births. It is also suggested that some physicians fear that the practice of minimum intervention could be translated by their colleagues as incompetence.[74]

However, the demand for a more natural approach to labor and delivery has motivated many hospitals to construct birth rooms or centers within their facilities. Such birthing rooms offer a more relaxed and personable atmosphere while maintaining contact with all the hospital benefits.

If a woman wants to have her baby in a hospital but still wants to have a natural birth, it is important that she make her wishes clear to the obstetrician beforehand. Many women find it helpful to write a birth plan, illustrating their wishes regarding medical intervention and the choice of birth position. These can be discussed with the woman's OB 6-8 weeks before the due date. Usually a copy is sent to the hospital with the additional paperwork and many women carry an extra copy with them.

FREE-STANDING BIRTH CENTERS

Free-standing birth centers (FSBCs) offer a compromise between a hospital and a home birth. They usually offer a homelike setting and are very casual about friends and relatives attending the birth. They are generally run by midwives, who follow the prenatal care and deliver the baby. Occasionally obstetricians will be called in to deliver the baby.

In the 1970s, there were only 30 such centers in the U.S., but now there are more than 300 nationwide. In the case of an emergency or complication, they all have a written or verbal transfer agreement with a nearby hospital. Although most FSBCs offer technologies such as pain medication and fetal heart monitors, their care offers less intervention, is more personalized, and allows parents more active participation.

Birthing in an FSBC is safe and can often be more economical. FSBC clients are carefully screened to confirm their low-risk status, so they can be assured a more natural childbirth. Some FSBCs also offer the use of warm water tubs for labor and birth. Prenatal education, one-on-one care, and occasionally the use of natural remedies, such as homeopathic remedies and herbs, are part of an FSBC program.[75]

HOME BIRTH

During the 1950s and until fairly recently, it was considered risky to give birth at home. Today, more people are considering home birth a viable option. Although hospital technology is not so readily at hand in home birthing situations, there are many advantages to birthing at home: familiarity and comfort, more control over the actual birth procedure, less chance of intervention, full-time supervision and care, and less expense.[76] Recent investigations have determined that when low-risk women choose a home birth, it is as safe (if not safer) than a hospital birth in terms of interventions, birth injuries, and maternal hemorrhaging.[77] However, it is important that women are adequately screened for risk factors. High-risk factors include hypertension and heart disease, kidney disease, anemia, diabetes, epilepsy, multiple births, women who have had a cesarean section, and first-time mothers over the age of 35. A home birth is generally not advisable if you fall into any of these categories.

BIRTH ATTENDANTS

"It's interesting that midwifery is the exception in the U.S. and not the norm," observes Susanne Houd. Houd, a practicing midwife, former World Health Organization employee, and native of Denmark, offers a worldly view to the past and current state of midwifery. She notes that "sage femmes," Europe's female folk healers who also assisted in childbirth, were once trained by priests but gradually shifted to a medically based education. The Midwives Act, legislation regulating the practice of midwifery, went into effect around 160 years ago in most European countries. This did not happen in North America, she says. Instead the doctors just took over. "It was a new country," she explains. "The tradition may not have been that strong."

Today, the option of using a midwife is available to many women. A midwife (or in some states in the U.S., a naturopathic doctor or N.D.) will usually attend a home birth. Certified nurse midwives (CNMs) are trained nurses with additional midwifery education and state certification. CNMs are permitted to attend hospital births and can also give sole care for women wanting a home birth. A midwife gives more personalized care than an OB, especially during labor and delivery. Most CNMs will have a backup doctor at a hospital that they use on a regular basis, in case of complications.

Midwives are more likely to have some knowledge of natural therapies, such as herbal medicine and homeopathy, and may be able to suggest natural solutions to common health problems during pregnancy. Their philosophies usually support minimal intervention. Services generally include prenatal care, delivery, and postpartum checkups.

It is important for a woman to very carefully choose the professional who will deliver her baby. Prospective birth attendants should be interviewed thoroughly. It is essential that a woman feel completely comfortable and trusting of the person who is going to guide her through one of the most challenging and intimate moments of her life. She should also feel that this person's philosophies surrounding the birth mirror hers as much as possible, whether this person is an obstetrician or a midwife. In order to prepare for the daunting task of choosing a birth attendant, it is helpful to write down any thoughts and questions about the birthing process. Whether considering a midwife or OB, one can present this preliminary birth plan to him or her.

WATER BIRTH

Pioneered by Drs. Michel Odent in France and Igor Tjarkovsky in Russia, birthing in water is increasing in popularity in the U.S. It is a method of natural childbirth that is thought to ease the passing of the child from the dark and watery sanctuary of the womb to the outside world of air and gravity. Dr. Odent used hot tubs in his birth center as a means of relieving stress and pain during labor. He discovered that the allure of water often resulted in women delivering their babies underwater. This experience may lessen the length of labor and the difficulty of pushing during labor.

DOULA CARE

"Doulas are trained labor assistants who provide information and lend physical and emotional support to women and their partners before, during, and after childbirth," says Heather Allen, a doula and childbirth educator, in Clinton, New York. "They are a recent addition to the 'modern maternity team' and are filling a void that has existed for generations in our maternity care system."

In addition to providing high-quality support during the labor process, doulas make prenatal visits to assist expectant parents in becoming better informed about their childbirth options. They may help parents write their birth plan and take part in conversations between parents, their physician, and other birth-care providers. During labor, doulas can provide nonmedical care in the form of massage and guidance with body positions and breathing, as well as offering continuous emotional support. They will usually remain with the mother in the initial hours after birth and then make postpartum visits to help her identify any problems, such as those related to breastfeeding and postpartum depression. "Doulas can also enhance the father's participation before, during, and after childbirth," Allen says. "Most fathers report that they feel assured and relieved by the doula's presence."

Research has shown that the assistance of a doula during labor can significantly improve the health of both the mother and the newborn child. Benefits include:

- Shorter labor duration
- Reduced need for c-sections, painkiller and oxytocin use, and forceps[78]
- Reduced incidence of maternal fever and infection
- Reduced risk of health complications and hospitalizations of the baby[79]
- Reduced risk of vacuum extraction, anxiety, and postpartum depression
- Increased incidence of successful breast-feeding and feelings of a positive birth experience[80]
- Reduced maternal bleeding after birth[81]

Doula care has also been found superior to the Lamaze method, leaving first-time mothers feeling more secure[82] and increasing the chance of spontaneous vaginal birth.[83] Because of such proven benefits, a number of insurance companies now provide coverage for doula care.

Women who have experienced water births report that they felt relaxed during their labor. Some women maintain that their weightless feeling in the water eased their pain. Others felt that being in the water reduced the risk of perineal tearing. Advocates of water birth claim it is the least stressful way to give birth for both mother and baby.

In Europe, some of the more progressive hospitals now offer water birth. In the U.S., however, it is a technique generally confined to free-standing birth centers or to women birthing at home. FSBCs usually provide large tubs rather like oversized baths for the process. A home water birth can be done in a portable inflatable tub—much like a portable spa tub—that can be rented specifically for water birth purposes.

During labor, the midwife or OB will usually allow the mother to enter the pool when her cervix has dilated to 5-8 centimeters. Entering the pool before this can slow down or halt the labor. When it is time for the baby to emerge, the midwife simply guides the infant out into the water where it may float for a second before being lifted out of the water by the midwife to be placed at the mother's breast. As the baby does not draw in breath until air hits its lungs, there is no risk of it drowning or breathing in water. The infant continues to get air through the umbilical cord until it stops pulsating some minutes after birth. Mother and baby remain happily in the water until it is time for the placenta to be delivered, which is usually done outside of the tub.

Preparing for Childbirth with Prenatal Classes

Although most expectant parents tend to participate in some form of prenatal preparation, expert opinions on the subject are divided. Elizabeth Noble, author of *Childbirth with Insight*, maintains that such prepared labor techniques are tiring and sometimes impossible to follow during labor. She explains that birth is of an "uncontrollable nature" and that control is not possible or desirable. Noble recommends that a laboring woman should be supported with common sense and intuition to better serve her needs.[84] For instance, it is important that she feels free to adopt whichever position is comfortable to her at the time and that she is encouraged to move around if she feels the urge to do so. Sometimes a woman will feel the need to vocalize—this is a natural instinct and can help tremendously during labor. Food and drink should be readily available to replenish her supply of energy, adds Dr. Linton.

On the other hand, Penny Simkin, P.T., of Seattle, Washington, who has been intimately involved in childbirth for over 30 years as an educator, labor support person, lecturer, consultant, and author, states, "For most women, this is the greatest physical challenge they will ever meet." She explains that most other physical and mental challenges, such as mountain climbing, meditation, and playing a musical instrument, are prepared for with training that includes specific breathing techniques and, she adds, "I can't see that childbirth should be an exception to that." Simkin maintains that, when a person is in pain, gasping is often the result. There are, of course, exceptions and she explains that if a woman feels loved and cared for and is able to remain calm, she can perhaps rely on her instincts to guide her breathing. Very few women, however, allow themselves to follow their instincts during the birth process.

Most expectant parents take prenatal classes during the third trimester. According to Simkin, the earlier a woman can take a class, the better. The information offered in a prenatal course will help eliminate some of the doubts and fears that surround childbirth, as well as provide practical information such as prenatal nutrition. Classes will vary, so when researching those available, all prospective students should inquire about class size, number of classes in the course, cost, philosophy, subjects covered, background, and training of the instructor. Couples should choose the class that fits comfortably with their own philosophy and needs. Techniques used in prenatal classes are varied, but all work toward preparing the couple for childbirth by teaching them how to reduce pain and anxiety.

Hypnosis: Hypnosis was used as early as 1837 for women giving birth. It was believed that having subjects focus on an idea rather than on the pain of labor would produce a state of anesthesia. These early ideas were taken further in Russia in the 1920s. The Russians believed that hypnosis altered conditioned or learned reflexes, so that a negative reflex perceived as painful could be supplanted by a positive reflex perceived as a 'sensation.' By the 1960s, the Russians had used hypnosis in thousands of births.

Today, in England, self-hypnosis is taught as a method of alleviating pain during labor. Gowri Motha, M.D., is an obstetrician who believes that preparing for birth by learning self-hypnosis techniques and using alternative therapies to clear the body of toxins and unnecessary tension will result in a stress-free and possibly pain-free labor. At her clinic in Northeast London, she has developed a prenatal birth program that encompasses self-hypnosis, reflexology, massage, osteopathic medicine, yoga, and other alternative healing methods so that women may have a more pleasant birth experience. She delivers the majority of her patients' babies in water and many of her women labor for under six hours.

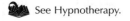 See Hypnotherapy.

The Grantly Dick-Read Method: An English obstetrician, Grantly Dick-Read, M.D., developed a theory that pain is not a necessary part of labor and childbirth. In delivering a baby to a woman who felt no pain during the process, he surmised that pain was essentially due to images of fear that women had learned from their society. He felt that these images could create muscle tension in the uterus, cervix, and abdomen, and cause real pain.

The Grantly Dick-Read method of prenatal classes employs three techniques. First, it teaches women about the physiology and anatomy of childbirth. The classes are structured in a way that attempts to dispel the notion that childbirth must be painful. In fact, the word *pain* is never used as it is thought that this alone would conjure up fear and, moreover, that the sensation felt during childbirth cannot be compared to any other known feeling of pain. Second, mothers are taught relaxation, physical conditioning, and breathing exercises. They are encouraged to relax between contractions. Finally, the method stresses the importance of the relationship between the mother and her birth attendant. The woman must have absolute faith in her attendant to prevent fear, which ultimately creates tension within the body and thus pain.

Psychoprophylaxis: Psychoprophylaxis was developed in Russia in the 1940s and stemmed from the old technique of hypnosis. Doctors believed that pain is a learned reflex and that women can be reeducated not to focus on the pain during the birth process. Like the Grantly Dick-Read method, mothers are taught anatomy in order to illustrate why birth does not have to be painful. They are also taught breathing techniques, relaxation, pushing methods, and positions to use during labor.

Lamaze: Lamaze was developed by a French obstetrician who adopted and changed the Russian method of psychoprophylaxis. He too taught anatomy and physiology, but went into greater detail, adding instruction on how the fetus develops. Dr. Lamaze also showed how a woman, through conditioned reflexes, could learn to replace pain and fear with joyful expectation and redefine contractions as sensations instead of birth pains. To the classes that taught breathing, relaxation, and delivery exercises, he added a pant-blow breathing technique to help with pushing in the second stage of labor. Today, Lamaze is one of the most popular methods of prenatal preparation.

The Bradley Method: This program was developed from a combination of the Lamaze and Grantly Dick-Read methods and incorporates the best elements of both with additional elements of its own. The key characteristic of the Bradley method is the emphasis on the father as the main labor coach.

The Birth

Emotional support during labor and delivery, whether from a partner, midwife, or birth assistant, is one of the most valuable forms of care a woman can receive. Women who feel their needs are being met emotionally have fewer complications, less pain, a shorter labor, and less postpartum depression than those who don't.[85]

Penny Simkin has reinforced this approach through her own research. She wanted to assess women's long-term memory of their birth experience and compared the birth stories of 20 female pupils who took her prenatal classes between 1968 and 1974 with information she gathered from in-depth interviews and questionnaires more than 20 years later. "I found that women don't forget," she relates, "and the amount of detail that they recall is really very impressive." When she asked women to grade the satisfaction they felt during childbirth, a higher satisfaction and positive memories were associated with control and a sense of accomplishment. These birth experiences had enhanced the women's self-esteem. Simkin adds that these women had also "remembered positive words and actions from their doctors and their nurses." Those women that rated their satisfaction as lower felt entirely different—they held negative memories of a lack of control, fear, discomfort with doctors, and pain. The length of labor, however, did not influence satisfaction ratings.

A partner doesn't need to be experienced or trained in the birthing process to be effective. Sharing in the moment, being aware of the woman's needs, and ensuring her physical comfort are sufficient. Any friends or family who are also assisting should complement the father's role without creating additional tension.[86]

Birthing Positions: "It has been found that standing and walking, activities that many women naturally gravitate toward during labor, can actually enhance the dilation of the cervix and aid the baby's descent," says Dr. Linton. "An active labor also reduces the need for medication as many women find it easier to cope with the pain when they can move around. Exclusive bed rest during labor can compress major blood vessels and compromise circulation." These two actions decrease maternal blood pressure, decrease uterine blood flow, and may result in fetal distress. The mother's breathing is also impaired when lying down.

"Some women find it helpful to squat with their partner supporting them," adds Dr. Linton. "It has been found that squatting increases the pelvic opening by 0.5-1.0 centimeter, and when you are talking about a 9.5-centimeter head, that is significant." Others are more comfortable on their knees, supported in the front by a pile of cushions. Many women are also attracted to warm water during labor, such as a bath or jacuzzi. Yelling during labor is a common urge and a natural way of releasing tension and trapped emotions. It is extremely beneficial and ultimately helps relax the muscles in the uterus and vagina.[87]

During the final phase of labor, many women automatically feel an urge to be upright or squatting and grasping something, such as the back of a chair, a partner's hands, or a support bar. This is called the fetus ejection reflex. These instincts, as well as dilated pupils and the need to drink, are due to a rush of adrenaline. An advantage of this physiological process is that it enables a mother to be alert during the first few moments with her newborn.

Herbs: There are several botanicals and homeopathic remedies useful during childbirth. Some commonly used herbs are blue cohosh, bethroot, and homeopathic *Calophyllum*. All are used to help stimulate uterine contractions to either initiate labor or to restart a stalled labor.

- Blue cohosh—3-8 drops of blue cohosh tincture can be taken in a glass of warm water or herbal tea; repeat every half hour until contractions are regular.

- Bethroot—Bethroot tincture, widely used by Native Americans, starts and strengthens contractions; take ¼ to ½ tsp in warm water or tea, every 30 minutes.

- *Calophyllum*—Homeopathic *Calophyllum* 200X can be taken every 30 minutes for two hours.

 It is always advisable to consult an herbalist, homeopath, naturopathic physician, midwife, or other expert before taking herbal or homeopathic preparations during pregnancy.

Essential Oils During Labor: Essential oils are aromatic substances extracted from certain flowers, fruits, and leaves. Due to their high concentration and ability to penetrate the skin, they have enormous healing potential. During labor, certain essential oils can be used to relax and calm the mother. A few drops of an essential oil can be diluted in a base oil and massaged into the back and abdomen by the partner. Oils can also be put into a small amount of water and used in a diffuser or on a cotton ball on a warm radiator. Lavender, geranium, or neroli oils are excellent during labor.

- Lavender is calming and has a slight analgesic effect. It also stimulates circulation, beneficial for both mother and baby, and has anti-inflammatory and antiseptic properties.

- Geranium is one of the best oils to stimulate circulation, which facilitates easy breathing. It has a contractive effect and helps pull together dilated tissues, so it is healing for the uterus and endometrium after the birth. Geranium is also an antidepressant and known for its uplifting effect.

- Neroli targets the nervous system, where it helps make breathing easier. It has a calming effect, increasing blood and oxygen to the brain. Use in low doses for relaxation—1-2 drops in water in a diffuser—as in higher doses it is a stimulant. Neroli is an antiseptic and antidepressant.

After the Birth

Once the baby has been born, it is vital for the mother and her infant to bond. Placing the baby at the mother's breast will usually initiate suckling. This is very important to future breast-feeding. Most infants will imitate crawling motions toward the breast soon after delivery and will be suckling in less than an hour if not drugged or disturbed.[88] Even though the mother's milk has not yet come in, the baby will suckle on the colostrum, a nutritious pre-milk fluid that is naturally present in the mother's breast.

The umbilical cord is often cut and the placenta discarded as soon as possible. Most physicians will wait for the cord to stop pulsating before severing it. However, many European doctors and natural childbirth attendants wait until the placenta is delivered or longer before cutting so the newborn can benefit from the oxygen-rich blood from the cord and placenta.[89] Likewise, Helen Burst adds that the placenta may be wrapped in a blanket and used as a warmer alongside the infant immediately after delivery.

Medications for the Infant: Check with local laws concerning procedures commonly performed on newborns at birth, such as silver nitrate, erythromycin, or tetracycline eye drops and vitamin K shots (given during labor to prevent hemolytic disease, characterized by anemia, jaundice, enlargement of the liver and spleen, and generalized edema) as they are required in most states and provinces.[90] Dr. Linton recommends allowing the baby to nurse before administering eye drops because they blur the vision. She also prefers to check the mother's diet during pregnancy to see if she is deficient in vitamin K rather than automatically giving a shot. "If she is eating enough squash and dark green leafy vegetables such as spinach, chard, and kale, there is no reason to assume that the baby will be vitamin K deficient," she says. "If an expectant mother has not eaten these foods by the end of her pregnancy, we supplement with oral vitamin K during the last month of pregnancy. There is evidence that it crosses the placental barrier." There have been studies linking intramuscular vitamin K shots with childhood cancer, but no such ties were found when vitamin K was administered orally.[91]

Circumcision: This is a routine surgical procedure that is not required. It has been argued that this procedure is medically beneficial to prevent urinary tract infections and penile cancer. Scientific evidence now shows that the advantages of circumcision are insignificant when compared to the surgical risks.[92] "There is no medical reason to perform circumcision," Dr. Linton says. "It is totally a cosmetic decision on the part of the parents. In fact, most insurance companies no longer cover it, because it is considered cosmetic surgery."

Postpartum Care

The care taken around pregnancy should not end with childbirth. After delivery, both the mother and baby will have health concerns that can be addressed through alternative medicine.

Maternal Physical Changes After Birth

During the 6-8 weeks after the birth, the mother's body begins to return to its prepregnant self. Her reproductive organs shrink and she begins to lose her pregnancy weight. Pregnancy demarcations, such as skin pigmentation and enhanced hair growth, fade away. Estrogen and progesterone levels plummet and the vagina regains its original tone.

The uterus gradually begins to involute, or shrink, and returns to its normal size within 5-6 weeks. Nursing and uterine massage assist in this process and, during the first few days, prevent excessive blood loss. It is normal for a bloody vaginal discharge, called lochia, to flow from the uterus for 4-8 weeks after the birth. At first, lochia is heavy and red, but it gradually decreases in volume and changes to pale pink and finally to a white, yellowish, or brown color. Breast-feeding, body position, and activity may increase the flow of the lochia. Afterpains caused by uterine contractions may occur during the first week after birth, especially while nursing or if the mother has given birth previously. Resting and deep breathing will allay some of this discomfort.

The perineal area may be sore, particularly if an episiotomy was performed or if there is a perineal tear. The cervical opening decreases in size, however there remains a somewhat wider aperture than before. The labia shrinks, but remains larger, looser, and darker in color than its prepregnant state.

Besides the delivery of the baby and placenta, and the loss of a cup or more of blood, weight sheds gradually over the next few months to a year. At the beginning, frequent urination and increased perspiration expel up to five pounds of fluid during the first five days. Excess fat slowly recedes with exercise and a sensible diet. Lax abdominal muscles regain tone in about six weeks. There are mixed opinions and experiences on whether nursing aids in weight loss. Stretch marks will fade, but not completely unless precautions have been made during the pregnancy.

Maternal Emotional Changes

The emotional impact of new parenthood is one of the most difficult alterations to come to terms with. Some women experience much anxiety about caring for a new infant, while others experience mood swings from exhilaration to depression. Most mothers, both new and experienced, feel extremely tired. Unless the mother takes adequate and proper rest, chronic fatigue can intensify the physical and emotional challenges of adjusting to a new baby.

Breast-Feeding

Nursing mothers have an increased level of the hormones prolactin, often called the mothering hormone, and oxytocin (a pituitary hormone that stimulates release of milk from the mammary glands). These hormones, together with the baby's instinctive sucking motions, are essential to the cycle of milk production. For the first 3-4 days, the infant will feed on colostrum, an easily digested liquid that is high in protein and antibodies and low in fat and carbohydrates. The mother's milk ducts do not start producing mature milk until around 2-4 days after birth.

Whether a woman nurses or not, the first lot of mature milk will still be produced and her breasts will pass through a stage of engorgement when they are hard, hot, and painful. Dr. Birdsall recommends vitamin B6 and sage as natural remedies used to suppress lactation (the production of milk), if desired. Cabbage leaves are wonderful for taking the heat out of engorged breasts. A couple of leaves can be torn off and placed under the bra. The leaves are removed and discarded when they become warm and replaced with new ones.

If a woman is not nursing, menstruation resumes in one to two months. A breast-feeding mother can expect her period to begin in several months to a year or two after the birth, depending on how long she continues to nurse.

The Father's Participation

The father's response to the newborn will depend on how settled he is, his experience with infant care, medical and financial pressures, and the preconceived expectations he has of himself and the new mother. The

THE BENEFITS OF BREAST-FEEDING

Today, there is more evidence than ever illustrating the positive health effects of nursing for both mother and child.

For the infant, breast-feeding:

- Enhances bonding between the mother and infant.[93]
- Provides optimum nutrition.[94]
- Provides disease-fighting constituents, such as lactoferrin, lysozyme, immunoglobulin A,[95] T and B lymphocytes,[96] and macrophages.[97]
- Encourages appropriate growth and development.[98]
- May increase survival rate for low–birth weight newborns.[99]
- Decreases severity of gastrointestinal infections, such as diarrhea.[100]
- Supplies protection against necrotizing enterocolitis, a serious complication of the intestinal tract that occurs most often among premature or low–birth weight babies.[101] Breast-feeding also protects against ear infections, decreases the risk of colic and food allergies, and may increase a child's intelligence.[102]

For the mother, breast-feeding:

- Stimulates contractions of the uterus and aids in controlling postpartum blood loss.[103]
- Increases mother's confidence in parenting skills.[104]
- Is convenient and economical.[105] It is easier, especially at night, and less time-consuming than bottle-feeding. The milk is ready to serve, always at the perfect temperature, and there is no preparation guesswork involved in the feeding process.
- Can help—if used with little or no supplementation—lengthen and space the birth of children by suppressing ovulation (although breast-feeding should not be relied on for birth control).[106]

it is normal for her partner to feel displaced and perhaps resentful of the new baby. However, with a little bit of planning, he can share in welcoming the new child to the world and enhance bonding time with the baby.

Before the birth, time with the child can be arranged by helping to prepare and freeze meals ahead of time, ensuring extra help during the first week or two after the birth from family, friends, or hired help, and learning about infant care. If possible, the father should consider taking some time off from work after the baby's birth in order to spend precious moments with his new family.

Many fathers are present during their child's birth and even assist in this process. Once the baby is delivered, the father can help in baby care such as changing, dressing, bathing, and bringing the baby to the mother for nursing. When the baby is old enough, the mother may consider pumping her milk so the father can take over one nighttime feeding with a bottle. This will not only give the mother more uninterrupted sleep, but allows the father to more closely bond with the baby. This same strategy can be used when the mother wants to leave the house by herself or return to work.

For fathers who feel left out of the natural mother-child bond during the first few months, it is reassuring to know that this will gradually change as the child gets older and grows more independent. If the father develops a positive attitude toward the baby in the beginning, this will help foster a healthy, happy relationship within the entire family.

Postpartum Changes and Care

Pregnancy, labor, and delivery are taxing on a woman's body. It is important to recognize this. How the mother cares for herself after the baby comes depends on the nature of her delivery, whether the baby was born in the hospital, a birthing center, or at home, and whether or not there were any complications. If a woman is discharged early or her baby is born at home, she will need help with household tasks so she can devote her first postpartum week to bonding with her newborn and recovering from the birth. In fact, comments Helen Burst, "One of the nice things about home birth is that the couple assumes that responsibility (of caring for the baby) right from the beginning."

Women who have no complications can usually get up and move around shortly after birth. Not to do so, explains Burst, is physically and mentally unhealthy. A woman must take care of herself postpartum "and part of taking care of yourself is getting up and around."

It is also important to do postpartum exercises, which should include Kegels to strengthen the pelvic muscles. It is, of course, more difficult to adhere to this plan when

introduction of a new family member, whether a first or additional child, often sets up a love triangle among mother, father, and baby. With the mother focusing her attention on her infant, together with disrupted sleep, a change in sexual patterns, and less freedom as a couple,

other children are present. Women who are having their second or third child may take longer to recover than with their first. The mother should be guided by her own body and activities such as work, sex, housework, and exercise should be resumed only when she feels ready. In Western culture, people have demanding schedules and are used to instant results. It is therefore important for a woman to be aware of the stress her body has endured and the recovery it must make. Lack of sleep, nursing, and child care make extra demands on her body. Pacing oneself and taking slow steps are key in maintaining normal activities and optimum health.

Nutrition while nursing remains as important as during pregnancy. Eating a varied diet with plenty of whole foods and fluids still applies. Aggressive dieting during this time of healing and nurturing is detrimental to the health of both mother and baby.

Care of the Perineum: Correct perineal care is essential in order to prevent infection, particularly if an episiotomy was performed or a tear occurred and stitches were made. Douching and tampons should be avoided during this period. For the first 24 hours, 30 minutes of ice packs placed on the perineum with a cloth in between, followed by 15 minutes of rest, helps reduce swelling. After the first day, heat in the form of a hot water bottle or heating lamp (not ultraviolet or sunlamp) should replace cold treatment. Warm water sitz baths (20 minutes) are also helpful. Witch hazel or essential oil of lavender applied to a sanitary napkin can help with swelling.

Urination during the first week may be difficult and painful. Cleansing the perineum after urination will help. Warm water should be applied using a peri bottle available from the hospital or midwife. Women should always wash and wipe from the front to the back toward the rectum to avoid reinfection. Constipation may occur and/or bowel movements may be painful. To keep stools soft, drink a lot of fluids and eat plenty of fiber such as fresh fruits and vegetables.

Sleeping: Adjusting to a new sleeping schedule is probably the most important habit to acquire. Exhaustion from the delivery and frequent awakenings for night feeding is inevitable. New mothers should nap when the baby is sleeping and go to bed early.

Healing Remedies: In addition to rest and sound eating habits, overall recovery and healing can be enhanced by using Chinese medicines, homeopathic remedies, and nutrient supplementation, according to Dr. Dittman. He adds that acupuncture is effective in balancing hormones and strengthening the *qi* (the body's vital life energy) by retonifying the spleen, liver, kidneys, and uterus. In addition, Dr. Dittman recommends manipulating muscles, tendons, and ligaments using *cheng kua*, an ancient Chinese method. Prenatal vitamins and min-

---

REDUCING THE RISK OF SUDDEN INFANT DEATH SYNDROME

Sudden Infant Death Syndrome (SIDS) kills nearly 5,000 babies in the U.S. each year and refers to the sudden and unexplained death of infants under the age of one. Although its causes have yet to be determined, and there are no means of predicting it, the following recommendations by the National Institute of Child Health and Human Development can help reduce the risk of SIDS.[108]

- Receive early and regular prenatal care, eat a healthy diet, and eliminate smoking, alcohol, and drugs.

- Unless advised otherwise by your physician, place your baby on his or her back at night and during naps. This is important and runs contrary to the advice many mothers have received that the best sleeping position for their babies is on their stomachs. Consult with your physician to determine if your baby has any health conditions that might necessitate a different sleep position, such as birth defects, breathing difficulties, heart or lung problems, or regularly spitting up after eating.

- Make sure your baby sleeps on a firm mattress or other surface. Avoid using fluffy blankets or comforters and keep soft stuffed toys or pillows out of the crib.

- Be aware of the temperature in your baby's room. Babies should be kept warm yet comfortable. Avoid overheating.

- Keep your baby away from all sources of smoke, including cigarettes and cigars.

- Consult with your physician at the first signs that your baby might be ill.

- If at all possible, breast-feed your baby, since breast milk helps keep babies healthy.

---

erals can be continued. Vitamin C, zinc, and beta carotene during the first week will accelerate healing of perineal wounds. The homeopathic remedy *Arnica* is helpful during the first few days immediately following birth and is indicated for injuries, shock, trauma, and bruising.[107]

Sex and Birth Control After the Birth

It is advisable to wait 6-8 weeks before resuming sexual intercourse. Some health professionals believe that it is possible to get a uterine infection from early intercourse. However, a woman must determine for herself when she is ready. Thirty years ago, when Helen Burst graduated from nursing school, episiotomies were a regular procedure and left most women with stitches and a sore perineum. "Most women didn't feel like having sexual intercourse for 4-6 weeks because of the episiotomy," Burst recalls. "I learned many of them were having sex before I saw them at six weeks postpartum." Consequently, Burst decided that family planning discussions were necessary before the scheduled six-week checkup. She maintains that a woman should resume sexual relations when she feels ready.

Engorged breasts may also diminish a woman's sexual desire. Sexual drive, however, varies among new mothers from no or diminished libido to normal or enhanced drive. This is an area where communication between sexual partners is important. Many things can contribute to decreased libido including depression, anxiety, irritability, fatigue, pain, nursing, interruptions, and fear of pregnancy. Planning for intimacy can offset some of the frustrations of lovemaking. As with so many other areas of adjustment, sleep is one of the best aphrodisiacs—it softens the edges of irritability and feeds the libido. Sex for many new parents may get designated to bedtime when both partners are exhausted. A few hours of sleep before lovemaking may help. Hiring a babysitter away from home in the middle of the day when mother and father are more rested can also help partners resume sexual activity and intimacy.

A woman's natural vaginal lubrication may decrease during this time. Using an artificial lubricant, such as vegetable oil or KY jelly, can eliminate painful intercourse. Use sexual positions that don't irritate the healing perineum or press on engorged breasts. Be aware that a slack vagina will tighten with time and the help of Kegel exercises.[109]

Probably the most important thing to feed a healthy sex life is a healthy relationship. Parents are often taught that children come first. But if a marriage or relationship is not attended to, there is no family. Partners should get out by themselves on a regular basis and find ways to attend to each other emotionally and not just sexually. Setting aside 10-15 minutes per day for discussing the events of the day is a pleasant way for partners to connect.

While breast-feeding appears to suppress ovulation somewhat and help in the spacing of children, it is not a guaranteed form of birth control. The baby's frequent sucking while nursing initiates the release of hormones that appear to suspend menstruation and ovulation.[110] However, it is possible to ovulate and become fertile before menstruation returns. There are several effective

and safe forms of birth control that can be used, such as natural family planning, which involves the daily charting of fertility signs (basal body temperature, consistency of the cervical mucus, and positioning and width of opening of the cervix), and condoms and other barrier methods such as a diaphragm used with spermicidals. Do not use oral contraceptives while nursing.

Recommendations

- A healthy pregnancy begins with proper planning. Prior to conception, both parents should receive a full medical check-up to screen for any potential risk factors. Both parents should also educate themselves about diet, nutrition, lifestyle choices, birthing options, what to expect during the course of pregnancy, the delivery itself, and postpartum care.

- Emphasize fresh, organic fruits and vegetables, whole grains, organically raised meats and poultry, and fish. Wash nonorganic produce prior to eating to remove agricultural chemicals. Avoid all processed foods, refined sugars, saturated fats, caffeine, alcohol, cigarettes, and recreational drugs. If using conventional medical drugs, consult with your physician to assess potential health risks.

- Useful nutrients include vitamins B_6, B_{12}, C, D, K, and folic acid, and boron, calcium, and zinc. Extra iron may also be warranted if deficiencies are present in mother's hemoglobin. Avoid excess vitamin A (above 10,000 IU per day) to reduce the risk of birth defects.

- Avoid the use of herbal medicines without proper consultation with a medical herbalist.

- Educate yourself about healthy lifestyle choices (including exercise, such as breathing techniques and Kegel exercises) and become informed about the many medical options available to you during pregnancy, labor, and the birth itself. Once your baby is born, consider breast-feeding, which has been shown to increase young babies' health and can deepen the emotional bond between mother and child.

- In addition to your physician, consider working with a midwife and/or doula to further increase the likelihood of a healthy pregnancy and delivery.

Professional Care

The following therapies should only be provided by a qualified health professional:

Acupuncture / Environmental Medicine / Herbal Medicine / Hypnotherapy / Traditional Chinese Medicine

Where to Find Help

For more information and referrals to a qualified professional, contact the following organizations.

American College of Nurse Midwives
818 Connecticut Avenue N.W., Suite 900
Washington, D.C. 20006
(202) 728-9860
Website: www.acnm.org

Maintains a list of accredited nurse midwife programs. Will make referrals to midwives in your area.

Doulas of North America (DONA)
13513 North Grove Drive
Alpine, Utah 84004
(801) 756-7331
Website: www.dona.org

An international association of over 3,000 doulas trained to provide the highest quality support to birthing women. Provides certification and referrals to doulas nationwide.

Global Maternal/Child Health Association
Waterbirth International
P.O. Box 1400
Wilsonville, Oregon 97070
(503) 673-0026
Website: www.waterbirth.org

GMCHA is working to alter the current technological dependency, excessive drug use, and rising cesarean rate, which are predominant in the U.S., by educating medical professionals and the public on the benefits of family-centered, natural childbirth, midwifery as the model for maternity care, and the use of warm-water immersion during labor and birth.

Hypnobirthing Institute
146 Sheep Davis Road
Pembroke, New Hampshire 03275
(603) 225-3441
Website: www.hypnobirthing.com

Provides instruction in relaxation techniques to enable expectant mothers to eliminate fear, tension, and pain in order to give birth in an alert and relaxed state of body and mind. Also provides referrals to certified hypnobirthers nationwide.

Informed Birth and Parenting
P.O. Box 3675
Ann Arbor, Michigan 48106
(313) 662-6857

This program certifies childbirth educators and birth assistants. Books and videos on pregnancy, childbirth, and parenting are available for sale. Referral service for midwives throughout the U.S. and Canada.

International Association of Parents and Professionals for Safe Alternatives in Childbirth
Route 1, Box 646
Marble Hill, Missouri 63764
(314) 238-2010

Educational organization that encourages natural childbirth in hospitals. Working to establish guidelines for safe home births. Provides parental education.

International Cesarean Awareness Network
1304 Kingsdale Avenue
Redondo Beach, California 90278
(310) 542-6400
Website: www.ican-online.org

A nonprofit organization dedicated to lowering the rate of unnecessary cesareans, supporting vaginal birth after cesarean (VBAC), and encouraging positive birthing through education and advocacy.

International Childbirth Education Association (ICEA)
P.O. Box 20048
Minneapolis, Minnesota 55420
(612) 854-8660
Website: www.icea.org

ICEA unites people who support family-center maternity care and believe in freedom of choice based on knowledge of alternative medicine. They offer teaching certificates, seminars, continuing education workshops, and a mail-order book center.

National Association of Childbearing Centers (NACC)
3123 Gottschall Road
Perkiomenville, Pennsylvania 18074
(215) 234-8068
Website: www.birthcenters.org

Provides an extensive range of resources for expectant mothers, including referrals to birthing centers nationwide.

Read Natural Childbirth Foundation
P.O. Box 150956
San Rafael, California 94915
(415) 456-8462

A nonprofit educational program preparing expectant parents for childbirth. Using the principles of Grantly Dick-Read, M.D., and the exercises developed by Mabel Lum Fitzhugh, R.P.T., the foundation certifies birthing teachers.

Sudden Infant Death Syndrome Alliance
1314 Bedford Avenue, Suite 210
Baltimore, Maryland 21208
(800) 221-7437
Website: www.sidsalliance.org

The SIDS Alliance provides training for professionals through national and local conferences and, through its 50 local affiliates, assists families and others dealing with the death of an infant.

Recommended Reading

A Child is Born. L. Nilsson. New York: Dell Publishing, 1990.

Birth Without Violence. F. Leboyer. New York: Alfred A. Knopf, 1990.

Evolution's End. Joseph Chilton Pearce. New York: Harper Collins, 1992.

Heart and Hands: A Midwife's Guide to Pregnancy and Birth. Elizabeth Davis. Berkeley, CA: Celestial Arts, 1997.

Making a Baby. Debra Fulghum Bruce and Samuel Thatcher. New York: Ballantine, 2000.

Nutrition in Pregnancy and Lactation. B.S. Worthington-Roberts, J. Vermeersch, and S.R. Williams. St. Louis, MO: Times/Mirror Mosby College Publishing, 1985.

Pregnancy, Childbirth and the Newborn. Penny Simkin, Janet Whalley, and Ann Keppler. New York: Simon & Schuster, 2001.

The Secret Life of the Unborn Child. Thomas Verny, M.D., with John Kelly. New York: Delacorte Publishing, 1981.

Water Babies. Eric Sidenbladh. New York: St. Martin's Press, 1982.

RESPIRATORY CONDITIONS

For the millions of people with respiratory difficulties, the simple act of breathing can be a constant struggle. Alternative medicine has much to offer such people, for many respiratory problems that have defied conventional medical treatment can be effectively alleviated through such methods as diet, nutritional supplements, herbal medicine, hydrotherapy, acupuncture, and traditional Chinese medicine.

BREATHING IS ALMOST taken for granted. Yet, as John A. Sherman, N.D., of Seattle, Washington, states, "This constant motion has a profound effect on our overall health. The lungs relentlessly pump oxygen, which helps rejuvenate blood vessels, digest food, stimulate the heart, and maximize brain function. The lungs also act as a major eliminative organ, where gaseous exchange can be accomplished."

The respiratory system is a complex and sensitive network of organs that provides an immediate link with changes in the atmosphere. There are miles of air passages in the lungs, but by the time air reaches them, it has already been warmed and moistened by the nose, filtered through nose hairs and in the lungs, and then constantly refiltered through millions of tiny cilia (hair-like cell projections) to remove any particles that could damage the lungs.[1]

"We can fast, we can even restrict our fluids for long periods, but without a proper source of oxygen, we're gone in about six minutes," says Dr. Sherman. "This is why breathing properly is so important." Proper breathing is associated with regulation of the autonomic nervous system, brain-wave and immune function, stress reduction, pain control, and digestion.

"Ninety-two million Americans—more than one out of three—suffer from one of the four most common chronic respiratory illnesses: sinusitis, allergic rhinitis (hay fever), asthma, and bronchitis," states Robert S. Ivker, D.O., past President of the American Holistic Medical Association and author of *Sinus Survival* and *Asthma Survival*. "According to a survey from the Centers for Disease Control and Prevention, chronic sinusitis is now our

> *Chronic sinusitis, when combined with allergic rhinitis, asthma, and chronic bronchitis, make respiratory disease our first environmental health epidemic.*
> —Robert S. Ivker, D.O.

nation's number one chronic ailment, allergy is number four, asthma is number eight, and chronic bronchitis is number nine. By comparison, in the 1960s, not one of these four conditions was listed in the top ten."

According to Dr. Ivker, chronic sinusitis was the primary reason for nearly 12 million office visits to physicians in 1995 and for more than 200,000 sinus surgeries in 1998. "Chronic sinusitis, when combined with allergic rhinitis, asthma, and chronic bronchitis, make respiratory disease our first environmental health epidemic," he says. "The modern-day plague of air pollution is insidiously destroying our respiratory tracts and, according to the Environmental Protection Agency (EPA), 60% of all Americans live in areas where the air quality makes breathing a health risk. Pollutant-laden air acts as a chronic irritant that can cause respiratory mucous membranes to become hypersensitive, hyper-reactive, and inflamed. The longer you breathe unhealthy air, the more likely it is that you'll develop sinus or other respiratory conditions."

Respiratory problems can begin as increased mucus secretion, congestion, or coughing, and develop into allergic rhinitis or obstruction of the ostia (the openings of the sinus drainage ducts), resulting in sinus infections, bronchial spasms, wheezing, and other increasingly debilitating symptoms. Airborne pollutants can also be fatal, Dr. Ivker points out, citing a 1993 study performed by the EPA and the Harvard School of Public Health, which found that up to 60,000 deaths occur in the United States each year caused by particulate air pollution.

The Respiratory System

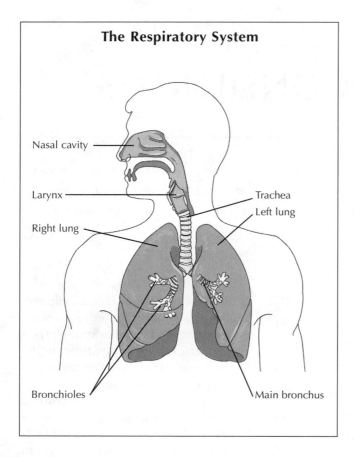

Nasal cavity

Larynx

Right lung

Trachea

Left lung

Bronchioles

Main bronchus

Respiratory Conditions and Their Causes

Respiratory problems can be caused by any number of factors, including viral and bacterial infections, pollen, environmental pollution, and smoking, as well as by a poor quality diet, food toxins and allergies, a stressful and inactive lifestyle, and the misuse of antibiotics. Respiratory problems manifest in a variety of symptoms related to a number of troublesome conditions, including hay fever, bronchial asthma, bronchitis, pneumonia, sinusitis, and emphysema.

Hay Fever

Allergic rhinitis, or hay fever, affects as many as one out of every ten Americans.[2] It is an inflammation of the nasal mucous membrane that can be seasonal or chronic. Its primary symptoms are nasal mucus discharge (rhinorrhea), itching of the eyes, nose, or throat, nasal congestion or obstruction, and sneezing.

Allergic rhinitis results from an antibody-type immune response following exposure to an allergen. It is most commonly associated with pollen, but, says Dr. Sherman, "people allergic to pollen are only a subgroup of a larger group of sufferers who are sensitive to all kinds of environmental aggravations, including dust, cat and

dog dander, mold spores, foods, medications, insect bites, even perfume. These allergens can affect a person year round and cause a host of symptoms, including hives, eczema, digestive disorders, breathing difficulties, swelling, headaches, and even chronic fatigue syndrome."

According to Dr. Sherman, hay fever is a disorder of the immune system. "Just as the immune system is activated by a virus or bacteria, it also interprets a grain of pollen or dust particle as an intruder," he says. "Thus, whenever a person already has a weakened immune system from dealing with chronic food allergies or a vitamin deficiency, it tends to create a more severe reaction to the pollen."

The immune system can also be weakened by other sources of environmental pollution such as cigarette smoke, auto exhaust, or house dust. "People wondering if their runny noses and itchy eyes are caused by the common cold or by hay fever need to remember an allergic reaction will more often than not produce clear secretions, no fever, and bouts of multiple sneezes," Dr. Sherman adds.

Asthma

Asthma is a chronic and sometimes acute condition in which the smooth muscles that surround the smaller air passages into the lungs (bronchi and bronchioles) go into spasms, narrowing the bronchial passageways and making it difficult for air to flow in and out of the lungs. Asthma is also characterized by excessive mucous membrane secretions that can block the bronchioles.

Asthma is the leading cause of disease and disability in children and teens 2-17 years old. Five million children under the age of 18 suffer from asthma,[3] making it the leading cause of hospitalization and school absenteeism for children.[4] It is also relatively common among all age groups, ranking eighth on the list of chronic disease conditions in the U.S., with 65% of sufferers developing symptoms before the age of five.[5] More than 15 million Americans have asthma, a 33% increase from 1990 and a 66% increase from 1980.[6] Occupational asthma, which develops in adults due to substances they are exposed to at work, accounts for 15.4% of all cases of asthma in U.S.[7] In 1997, 5,400 people died from severe asthma attacks,[8] more than double the asthma death rate in 1980.[9]

Asthma takes a high toll on health-care finances as well, with total related medical costs at an estimated $14.5 billion per year.[10] Asthma patients tend to also suffer from allergic rhinitis. A recent study showed allergic rhinitis occurred in 99% of asthmatic adults and 93% of asthmatic adolescents; the same study reports that severe rhinitis is associated with an exacerbation of asthma.[11]

Asthma generally manifests itself in the form of an asthma attack. Between these attacks, an asthmatic will usually seem perfectly healthy. An attack is characterized by a narrowing of the bronchial passages, along with an excessive excretion of mucus, resulting in impaired breathing, with the severity of the symptoms often accelerating rapidly. "The greater the obstruction, the more difficult breathing will become," notes Dr. Sherman. An attack will usually begin with an unproductive cough, followed by rapidly progressing difficulty in breathing. While the respiratory rate does not increase, expiration becomes prolonged and labored, resulting in wheezing that can often be heard from a distance.[12]

A number of allergic and environmental agents can precipitate asthma attacks, including pollen, dust, mold, animal dander, feathers, textiles such as cotton and flax, detergents, petrochemicals, air pollution, and smoke. According to James Braly, M.D., of Hollywood, Florida, wheat, milk, and eggs are among the most likely foods that will trigger an asthma attack. He adds that chemical additives such as food coloring and preservatives can also be at fault. Sensitivity to aspirin, exposure to cold air, and exercise can also prompt an asthmatic reaction.

 See Allergies, Environmental Medicine.

Dr. Sherman points out that when asthma originates during infancy, it is generally due to food allergies; when it strikes between ages 10 and 30, it is usually due to inhalants; and when it occurs after age 45, it is commonly due to infections. "These factors can exist at any age and in any combination, however," he says.

He also notes that asthma attacks that occur only in the summer are normally caused by pollens or mold spores, while those that occur only in winter are usually due to infections. And attacks that occur at night tend to be emotionally related and may be due to suppressed anger. In addition, up to 90% of asthmatics are or were mouth breathers (versus breathing through the nose), making it much easier for dust, pollution, organisms, and cold air to enter the lungs. Breath retraining can be of immense help in alleviating this additional cause of asthma.[13]

Bronchitis

Bronchitis refers to chronic or acute inflammation of the bronchial tubes, with symptoms ranging from chills, fever, and coughing, to difficulty breathing and pain in the chest. Acute bronchitis is a mild, short attack, sometimes accompanied by a secondary bacterial infection, while chronic bronchitis is characterized by constant inflammation, often accompanied by irritation of the bronchi, but without any infectious component. Other symptoms of chronic bronchitis include cough, hypersecretion of

ASTHMA AND STRESS

A growing body of research indicates that asthma attacks can be triggered by stress. In a 1999 study, for example, 30 adolescents with asthma and 20 controls were subjected to a stressful situation—a frustrating computer task. Heart rate, blood pressure, respiratory rate, deep inhalations, and sighs were measured, as were asthma-specific processes such as lung function, wheezing, coughing, and breathlessness. The subjects also recorded their emotions during the task. All measurements indicated that the subjects were undergoing high levels of negative emotions and stress. None of the asthmatic participants experienced airway obstruction, wheezing, significant periods of coughing, or reduction in lung function. However, all of them suffered from breathlessness, many of them severely. Moreover, the breathlessness experienced was higher than the breathlessness provoked by irritating substances before the test. The researchers confirmed that while stress may not trigger a full-blown asthma attack, it may induce breathlessness in patients with asthma.[14]

In another study, 130 adults with asthma documented their stressors, frequency of asthma symptoms, peak flow readings (a measure of how much air the lungs can expel), and use of beta-agonist bronchodilators. Stress was positively correlated with lowered breathing ability as measured by peak flow rates and increased symptoms of asthma and use of bronchodilators.[15] Researchers suggested that stress provokes breathing problems because it appears to promote the adhesion of leukocytes (white blood cells) to bronchial ciliary cells, causing accelerated allergic inflammatory reactions and asthma.[16]

The asthma-stress link is compounded by the fact that asthma is itself a major source of stress, especially for children and their parents. Asthmatic children in particular appear to be bound in a vicious cycle, whereby stress contributes to asthma attacks, which causes more stress, leading to more attacks as well as stress-related psychological problems. Studies have shown that in severely asthmatic children, those who are plagued by depression and persistent family conflict are at a greater risk than others for suffering a fatal asthma attack.[17] Moreover, in a study comparing asthmatic children with non-asthmatic controls, the asthma group had significantly more total anxiety disorders, past school problems, past psychiatric illnesses, and family stress.[18]

FINDING THE ROOT CAUSE OF RESPIRATORY INFECTION

Conventional medicine usually considers bacterial or viral infection as the cause of congestion in the lungs. Many alternative physicians, however, consider the opposite to be true: that infection is the result of lung congestion. "Organisms only grow in the body when the 'soil' is right," explains John A. Sherman, N.D., of Seattle, Washington. "In the lungs, this means that congestion provides fruitful soil for the growth of infection. By only removing the infection, we do not solve the underlying problem."

David L. Hoffmann, B.Sc., M.N.I.M.H., past President of the American Herbalists Guild, adds, "One factor most often related to congestion is diet. If the body gets too much mucus-forming food, it increases secretion into the lungs as part of the natural cleansing process. Yet, if we inhibit the production of secretions with antibiotics, we can nurture congestion in the future and perhaps sow the seeds for chronic, degenerative diseases."

Respiratory difficulties that thrive on excessive mucus, such as asthma, require a diet low in mucus-forming foods. Dr. Sherman advises restricting the intake of dairy products (including goat's milk and yogurt), eggs, gluten-rich grains (wheat, oats, rye, and barley), sugar, potatoes, and other starchy root vegetables. Fresh fruits and their juices are good replacements, as long as one is careful about the high fructose content of beets, carrots, and many fruits.

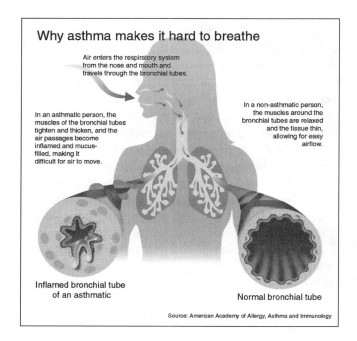

Why asthma makes it hard to breathe

Air enters the respiratory system from the nose and mouth and travels through the bronchial tubes.

In an asthmatic person, the muscles of the bronchial tubes tighten and thicken, and the air passages become inflamed and mucus-filled, making it difficult for air to move.

In a non-asthmatic person, the muscles around the bronchial tubes are relaxed and the tissue thin, allowing for easy airflow.

Inflamed bronchial tube of an asthmatic

Normal bronchial tube

Source: American Academy of Allergy, Asthma and Immunology

mucus, expectoration of sputum, and increased susceptibility to bronchial infection.

Bronchitis can be caused by infection, exposure to cold, or noxious agents. It is seen much more commonly in the winter, as it usually follows some form of upper respiratory infection, such as a cold. In addition, food or chemical allergies can provoke symptoms of bronchitis. Smokers or those exposed to excessive second-hand smoke may also be more vulnerable to chronic bronchitis.

Pneumonia

Pneumonia is defined as a severe inflammation of the lungs. It ranks as the fifth leading cause of death in the U.S., leading all other infectious diseases in mortality.[19] It is particularly threatening for the elderly, according to Dr. Sherman. "Like bronchitis, pneumonia is much more common during the winter months," Dr. Sherman says. "It is also a frequent complication of other serious illnesses and is the most widespread of all fatal hospital-acquired infections." Symptoms include chest pain, coughing, difficulty in breathing, shortness of breath, fever, and single episodes (but not persistent) of shaking chills.

Joseph Pizzorno, N.D., President Emeritus of Bastyr University, in Seattle, Washington, reports that pneumonia is usually seen in immune-compromised persons, including drug and alcohol abusers. People with HIV are especially vulnerable to the disease. Chronic lung diseases and debilitating illnesses can also cause pneumonia, as well as the use of immunosuppressive drugs or respiratory therapy.

Bacteria, fungi, and viruses can also be at fault, notes Dr. Sherman. The typical organisms that cause pneumonia are *Pneumococcus, Staphylococcus, Streptococcus, Klebsiella, E. coli, proteus, Pseudomonas, Hemophilus,* and fungi. "Patients with bacterial pneumonia, though, are much more likely to have complications such as lung abscesses, pleurisy (inflammation of membrane enfolding the lungs), and the spreading of infection through the bloodstream to other organs," Dr. Sherman says. While antibiotics have greatly reduced fatality rates for pneumonia patients, their use has expanded the range of pathogens responsible for the disease, Dr. Sherman adds. This is especially true of hospitalized patients, because the pathogens are more resistant to commonly used antibiotics.[20]

Sinusitis

Sinusitis is an inflammation of the mucous membranes of one or more sinus cavities. It can be acute, as in a sinus infection, or chronic, in which the inflammation persists and may involve a low-grade infection with periodic flare-ups. Chronic sinusitis symptoms usually include constant postnasal drip, head congestion, headaches or facial pain, fatigue, diminished sense of smell, and nasal drainage. Other symptoms of sinusitis include general malaise, fever, and a nasal or hoarse voice. With chronic sinusitis, prolonged or repeated inflammation in the nasal passages can lead to degeneration in the tissues that make up the mucous membrane, hampering the ability of the sinus to drain properly.

According to Dr. Ivker, numerous external and internal factors can trigger sinus inflammation and infection. External factors include tobacco smoke, common cold viruses, extremely dry air, cold air, and air pollutants in home or work environments. "Both colds and smoking can paralyze the cilia, the minute hairs that line the upper airways and protect them against infection," Dr. Ivker adds. "The common cold is also most often the trigger for acute sinusitis. Colds that persist beyond two weeks, accompanied by headache or facial pain, yellow/green nasal and postnasal mucus drainage, and fatigue are the primary symptoms of a sinus infection."

Internal factors include food allergies and sensitivities, gastroesophageal reflux disease (GERD), dental infections, immunodeficiency, structural problems (such as nasal polyps, cysts, or a deviated septum), and emotional stress. "Emotional stress is a major factor in weakening the immune system and allowing infection to occur," Dr. Ivker says, based on the fact that nearly all of his patients with chronic sinusitis also had significant emotional issues, especially anger. "Chronic sinusitis patients tend to be high-achieving perfectionists who are frequently angry with themselves for making mistakes," he notes.

"Another primary cause of sinusitis, and respiratory illness in general, is the overuse of antibiotics," Dr. Ivker points out. "This has created antibiotic-resistant bacteria, as well as an epidemic of *Candida albicans* fungal infection." The use of antibiotics to treat sinusitis is not only inefficient but also pointless, since conventional antibiotics are not effective against fungi. In 1999, a study conducted by the Mayo Clinic reported that an immune system response to fungus, rather than to bacterial infection, is more often the cause of chronic sinusitis, and that the immune response to fungi in patients with the disease is markedly different than in healthy people. This unusual reaction is responsible for the chronic inflammation, pain, and swelling of the mucous membrane that is associated with sinusitis and is now referred to as allergic fungal sinusitis. Although the researchers of the study stated that we must begin looking at chronic sinusitis as a dysfunction of the immune system mediated by a fungus, they failed to speculate on the impact that multiple

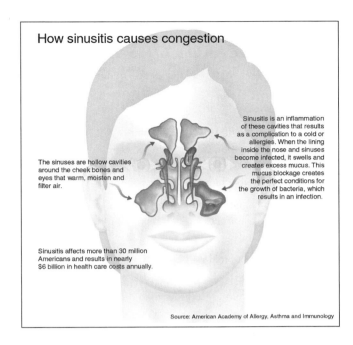

How sinusitis causes congestion

Sinusitis is an inflammation of these cavities that results as a complication to a cold or allergies. When the lining inside the nose and sinuses become infected, it swells and creates excess mucus. This mucus blockage creates the perfect conditions for the growth of bacteria, which results in an infection.

The sinuses are hollow cavities around the cheek bones and eyes that warm, moisten and filter air.

Sinusitis affects more than 30 million Americans and results in nearly $6 billion in health care costs annually.

Source: American Academy of Allergy, Asthma and Immunology

courses of broad-spectrum antibiotics might have had on their patients' unusual immune response.

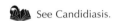 See Candidiasis.

Emphysema

Emphysema is characterized by a permanent enlargement of the air sacs and ducts in the lungs, along with destruction of the walls of these air spaces. In addition, there is a loss of the small blood vessels that supply these spaces, resulting in the lung tissue becoming inflamed and hardened. According to Dr. Sherman, these changes are what produce the "barrel chest" effect common among emphysema sufferers, who are often referred to as "pink-puffers" because of the difficulty they have breathing. Symptoms of emphysema include wheezing, a hard and spasmodic cough, copious sputum production, as well as difficulty in breathing, varying from mild exertion to a marked lack of oxygen even while resting. Even the mere act of conversation by people with emphysema can initiate coughing attacks, Dr. Sherman notes.

The single major cause of emphysema is cigarette smoking, with the risk running higher as the number of packs and years of smoking increase.[21] Certain types of environmental pollutants are linked with an increased incidence of emphysema, including cadmium fumes, which can be found in high concentrations in tobacco smoke as well. Emphysema has also been associated with gastric or duodenal ulcers (ulceration in the first part of the small intestine) caused by increased respiratory acidosis, an acidic condition due to an insufficient supply of oxygen to the lungs that results in the retention of carbon dioxide.[22]

THE HAZARDS OF SMOKING

It is no secret that smoking poses numerous health risks. The following is a brief list of some of the harmful effects associated with smoking.

- Each cigarette steals away eight minutes of life. A pack a day equates to losing a month of life each year and two packs a day means 12-16 years off the life expectancy for lifetime smokers.

- Just one cigarette can increase the heart rate 20-25 beats per minute and can increase blood pressure significantly.

- Cigarettes contain 4,000 known toxic poisons.

- Smoking one pack of cigarettes a day depletes more vitamin C (500 mg) than most people ingest in a day.

- Cigarettes increase carbon monoxide levels in the blood, which compete with oxygen so thoroughly that it takes the circulatory system six hours to return to normal after smoking just one cigarette.

- Smoking is so immunosuppressive that it takes three months to reverse its direct damage to the immune system[23] and many years to reverse its indirect or long-term effects.

- A direct link has been found between lung cancer and flue-dried tobacco, especially that to which sugar has been added, while no significant correlation between traditional sugar-free, air-dried tobacco and cancer has been found.

- Secondary cigarette smoke inhaled by nonsmokers can also pose health hazards. According to the Environmental Protection Agency, it has been linked to 20% of lung cancer cases in the U.S. not directly attributed to smoking. This equates to approximately 3,000 lung cancer deaths each year among nonsmokers. This risk is doubled for nonsmoking spouses married to people who smoke. Secondary smoke also causes 150,000 to 300,000 cases of respiratory illness among infants and young children. And babies are three times more likely to die if their mothers smoked during and after pregnancy.[24]

Treatment of Respiratory Conditions

A variety of alternative treatments exists for respiratory conditions, including diet and nutrition, herbal medi-

cine, hydrotherapy, homeopathy, and acupuncture. "The primary goals of the holistic treatment for respiratory disease are to heal the mucous membranes lining the nose, sinuses, and lungs and to strengthen and restore balance to the immune system," Dr. Ivker says. "If it is suspected or definitively diagnosed that *Candida albicans* is involved in the patient's condition, then its elimination will require a major commitment and will become the third goal."

Hay Fever

An allergic reaction to airborne pollens, animal dander, dust, or to foods, hay fever traditionally has been remedied with antihistamines or other drugs given orally or as nose drops. The following treatments may offer relief for hay fever sufferers with fewer side effects.

Hay Fever "Advance" Prevention: To lessen the effects of environmental allergens on hay fever victims, Dr. Sherman advises maintaining an active advance prevention program. This is done by determining what time of year to expect certain allergens and symptoms. "If you know when to expect allergens, you can start treating yourself for several weeks in advance of exposure," Dr. Sherman says. Dr. Sherman advocates testing for specific allergens in your "off season," while your immune system is at its peak. Blood tests, applied kinesiology, and measuring changes in galvanic skin response are the methods he recommends using.

Leon Chaitow, N.D., D.O., of London, England, also reports that in Europe it is common for hay fever sufferers, sensitive to pollen, to start taking pollen extract supplements a few months before the season in which they are most likely to be troubled. This effectively desensitizes patients and usually reduces their symptoms dramatically, he says.

Diet and Nutrition: A diet of high-fiber, whole foods including fruits (non–citrus), vegetables, grains, nuts, and raw seeds may be helpful in combating hay fever and reducing mucus production in the sinuses. It is also helpful to drink lots of fluids. Raw juices, in particular, are beneficial, particularly celery, cucumber, spinach, and parsley.

Since hay fever is allergy-related, according to Dr. Sherman, it is best to avoid dairy products, wheat, eggs, citrus fruits, chocolate, peanuts, and shellfish, which are common allergens. "Food coloring can also cause hay fever and sinus congestion," notes Dr. Braly. "These should be avoided, as well as all preservatives, especially metasulfites, which are often used to keep food fresh in restaurants. Also, eliminate caffeine, alcohol, tobacco, and refined sugar."

Dr. Braly recommends nutrient supplementation for hay fever sufferers, particularly of vitamins A, C, and E,

CREATING A HEALTHY INDOOR AIR ENVIRONMENT

Robert S. Ivker, D.O., recommends the following steps to prevent and help treat chronic asthma, bronchitis, hay fever, and sinusitis.

"The simplest and most effective way to heal damaged mucous membranes is to stop breathing unhealthy air," Dr. Ivker says. "While in many parts of the country, it will be years before outdoor air quality improves, technology has made it possible for anyone to breathe healthy indoor air." Dr. Ivker defines healthy air as being clean (odor-free and without smog), moist (35%-60% relative humidity), warm (65°-85° F), and rich in negative ions and oxygen (100% saturation). "Negative ions can make a dramatic difference in indoor air quality," he says. "Optimum levels for good health are 3,000-6,000 ions per cubic centimeter, yet the average indoor environment contains only 200 ions per cubic centimeter."

To improve negative ion levels in your home and work environments, Dr. Ivker recommends purchasing a negative ion generator, which has the added benefit of cleansing air of dust, pollen, molds, animal dander, and bacteria, and can also help repair damaged mucosa by stimulating the cilia lining their surface. "Look for a unit that emits a minimum of one trillion ions per second and is self-regulating," Dr. Ivker advises. If you are unable to find an ion generator, another option is an air cleaner with a HEPA filter. "HEPA filters actually remove negative ions from the air," he cautions, "but at least they will clean your air of unhealthy airborne particles."

To keep air moist, Dr. Ivker recommends humidifiers, even if you live in a humid climate. "Humidifiers are particularly important during the winter months, when the windows are typically closed and the heat is on, making indoor air extremely dry," he says. "A warm mist room humidifier is best. For a central humidifier (one that attaches to the furnace), be sure to use a flow-through type without a tray of standing water." Plants can also increase the moisture content of indoor environments, as well as improve oxygen levels. In addition, certain plants, such as chrysanthemums, philodendron, and spider plants, act as effective air filters.

"Ensuring good ventilation is extremely important, to allow for optimal levels of oxygen and fresh air, and to minimize indoor air pollution," Dr. Ivker says. "Air duct cleaning and carpet cleaning, without using toxic chemicals, are other valuable ways of creating healthy indoor air. A good furnace filter on a forced-air heating and air-conditioning system can also be quite helpful." Be sure to change your filters regularly. Also, avoid synthetic or plastic furnishings and building materials, especially in your home, as these tend to emit toxic gases. To minimize the effects of dust, remove rugs and stuffed toys from bedrooms and damp dust twice a week.

As part of his overall treatment protocol for respiratory conditions, Dr. Ivker recommends that his patients drink good quality water throughout the day. "Not only is water essential for optimal health, it also benefits the mucosa of the respiratory tract," he explains. "The wetter the mucous membrane, the thinner the mucus and the more easily it can flow and drain." Based on his clinical experience, Dr. Ivker recommends that adult patients drink 1/2-2/3 ounce of water per pound of body weight each day. "This means that a healthy, sedentary adult weighing 160 pounds needs to drink about 80 ounces of water each day, while a more active person in the same weight category should drink 104-112 ounces," he says.

To further ensure the health of the mucous membranes, Dr. Ivker recommends a regular practice of breathing steam and nasal irrigation. "Breathing steam is an excellent way to care for your entire respiratory tract," he explains. The easiest way to breathe steam is to cover your head with a towel and bend over a pot of boiling water. For added benefits, you can add a few drops of eucalyptus oil to the water. Sitting in a steam room or sauna will also work. Nasal irrigation has been a part of the Ayurvedic and yoga traditions for centuries. It involves pouring salt water through each nostril to cleanse the membranes of the nose and sinuses and flush out mucus. Dr. Ivker recommends the use of a Neti pot or a device called the SinuCleanse. "To make an irrigation solution, mix 1/3 teaspoon of noniodized salt into an eight-ounce glass of nonchlorinated or filtered water and add a pinch of baking soda," he says. The most convenient method of both moistening and irrigating is to use a saline nasal mist spray.

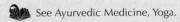 See Ayurvedic Medicine, Yoga.

SUCCESS STORY: CHIROPRACTIC FOR CHILDHOOD ASTHMA

Spinal misalignment and other types of physical trauma can sometimes precipitate cases of childhood asthma, according to Norman Allan, Ph.D., D.C., of Toronto, Ontario, Canada. When such structural misalignment contributes to asthma, chiropractic can help relieve it, as illustrated by the following case history involving one of Dr. Allan's patients.

Larry, 10, was brought to Dr. Allan with symptoms of bronchial asthma and allergies that had persisted since he was six years old. In order to adequately breathe, he required an inhaler throughout the day, was dependent on steroids during times of crisis, and had once needed to be rushed to the emergency room for relief of a severe asthma attack.

In reviewing Larry's medical history, Dr. Allan learned that he had fallen out of a tree one week before experiencing his first asthma flare-up. Larry's mother had mentioned this fact to the numerous conventional physicians she had previously consulted, but all of them had dismissed it as a potential contributing factor. Dr. Allan found that Larry's fifth thoracic vertebra was out of alignment at about the level of the sternum. Misaligned vertebrae in the upper chest can impair the function of nerves serving the lungs and thus lead to respiratory problems.

Dr. Allan gave Larry the appropriate chiropractic adjustments. The next day, Larry's mother reported that he was about 80% better. Over the next three months, Dr. Allan adjusted Larry weekly, at which time Larry's asthma was "well-controlled." He no longer required his inhaler every day and, over the next two years of follow-up care, his asthma symptoms returned in mild form only under conditions of high stress, usually of an emotional nature, or if he over-exercised.

Dr. Allan reports that, of the children with asthma with whom he's worked, about one-third respond dramatically to chiropractic intervention, especially when there is a strong emotional component and some degree of a physical, structural problem, while another third respond on a more limited basis.

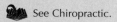 See Chiropractic.

essential fatty acids, and vitamins B_5 (pantothenic acid) and B_6 (pyridoxine). He has used coenzyme Q10, raw thymus glandular extract, bee pollen, royal jelly, geranium, and zinc to good effect as well. Multivitamin/mineral tablets are used as a simple supplement for children.

Dr. Ivker reports that proanthocyanidin, or grape seed extract, is also effective in treating hay fever. He notes that in, France, it has become the most commonly recommended natural remedy for allergies. He also recommends the bioflavonoid quercetin to all his patients with hay fever.

Herbal Medicine: Dr. Sherman reports that nettle *(Urtica dioica)* has the ability to clear the sinuses and can greatly reduce the symptoms of hay fever. Tincture of licorice is also often recommended (½ to one teaspoon should be taken in warm water twice daily, five days a week). This regimen is believed to be most effective if it is initiated a month before the season when symptoms usually appear.

A combination of black cohosh, skullcap, pleurisy root, catnip, and red pepper has also proven effective for hay fever sufferers, according to Dr. Sherman. He also suggests a teaspoon of horseradish diluted in water and taken slowly over several hours to drain and help dry out the sinuses. Comfrey tea and fenugreek tea taken daily can be beneficial as well, as can the fresh juice of coriander. Other herbs found to be effective include ginger root, angelica, astragalus, dandelion root, eyebright, goldenseal, ephedra, and mullein.

⚠️ CAUTION Comfrey can be toxic and should only be used under competent supervision.

Hydrotherapy: Dr. Chaitow recommends a variety of hydrotherapy methods that are useful in helping to decongest the sinuses. These include nasal irrigation, alternating hot and cold compresses, hot footbaths, and steam inhalation.

Asthma

The advantages of using natural methods instead of conventional treatments for asthma are obvious, according to Dr. Sherman. The most common medications used by conventional medicine in the treatment of asthma include prednisone, a cortisone derivative, which can cause severe adverse reactions, including fluid and electrolyte disturbances, muscle weakness, peptic ulcers, impaired wound healing, headaches and dizziness, menstrual irregularities, and glaucoma; prednisone may also help manifest latent diabetes.[25] Approaches such as diet and nutrition, herbal medicine, neurobiofeedback, and hydrotherapy have shown positive results in the treatment of asthma, without the negative side effects associated with drug-based therapies.

Diet and Nutrition: "Strengthening the immune system is of primary concern in the treatment of asthma," states Dr. Braly. This can be accomplished by eliminating allergens in foods, correcting digestive problems, establishing the proper balance of essential fatty acids, such as those found in cold-water fish, and supplying other nutrients important to the immune system. Good dietary management also needs to be maintained in order to resist asthma. According to Dr. Braly, this can be accomplished by rotating the diet and avoiding all artificial colorings (especially FD&C Yellow No. 5) and flavorings. He also advises avoiding caffeine, alcohol, tobacco, sugar, and all preservatives.

In addition to eliminating allergenic foods, Alan Gaby, M.D., past president of the American Holistic Medical Association, suggests supplementing the diet with nutrients such as vitamins B6, B12, niacinamide, and C, essential fatty acids, and the minerals magnesium chloride and calcium glycerophosphate. For acute asthma attacks, he recommends an intravenous injection of these same vitamins and minerals. Other nutrients of direct benefit to asthmatic patients include quercetin (a bioflavonoid), beta carotene, selenium, and manganese. Bee pollen has also proven helpful for some asthmatics affected by airborne allergens.

Dr. Sherman points out that cases of asthma associated with low blood sugar respond well to a hypoglycemic diet. This diet seems to especially help exercise-induced asthma.[26] In addition, if asthma is due to a high-stress lifestyle, Dr. Sherman recommends adding ½ teaspoon each of sea salt and baking soda to juice for immediate relief. Research has also found that many patients are able to reduce their incidence of asthma attacks by taking one tablespoon of olive oil twice daily.[27]

Herbal Medicine: Dr. Sherman recommends several herbal remedies for asthmatics, which can be taken in the form of teas or tinctures. Among these are ephedra (in its natural rather than synthetic form), which he calls a very effective bronchodilator, especially when combined with thyme, an antispasmodic. Mullein tea soothes the mucous membranes and is especially good for night attacks. It can be combined with marshmallow and slippery elm tea for an additional mucus-secreting effect. Dr. Sherman also recommends passionflower tea or tincture for cases of asthma due to tension or nervous conditions.

According to Dr. Pizzorno, licorice root, Indian tobacco, capsaicin (from cayenne pepper), skunk cabbage, gumweed, horse chestnut, jujube plum, green tea, onions, and garlic are valuable aids for those suffering from asthma. Dr. Ivker also recommends lobelia and the Ayurvedic herb *Coleus forskholin* for treating asthma.

A VEGAN DIET FOR RESPIRATORY CONDITIONS

Joseph E. Pizzorno, N.D., President Emeritus of Bastyr University, in Seattle, Washington, has found that a vegan diet (elimination of all animal products, including dairy) can have a long-term positive effect on respiratory conditions, primarily asthma. In one study, Dr. Pizzorno noted significant improvement in 25 patients treated with a vegan diet.

The diet excluded all meat, fish, eggs, and dairy products, and drinking water was limited to spring water. Chlorinated tap water was specifically prohibited, as were coffee, tea, chocolate, sugar, and salt. Herbal spices and 1½ liters of herbal teas a day were allowed. Vegetables used freely included lettuce, carrots, beets, onions, celery, cabbage, cauliflower, broccoli, cucumber, radishes, Jerusalem artichokes, and all beans except soy and green peas. A number of fruits were allowed, including blueberries, strawberries, raspberries, cloudberries, black currants, gooseberries, plums, and pears. Apples and citrus fruits were not allowed. Grains were either eliminated or severely restricted.

Dr. Pizzorno says that 71% of the patients showed favorable results from the diet within just four months and, after one year, a 92% success rate was reached.

Homeopathy: According to Konrad Kail, N.D., of Phoenix, Arizona, the following homeopathic remedies are useful for treating asthma symptoms.

Ammonium carbonicum—Indicated for severe asthma, accompanied by exhausted breathing, shortness of breath with wheezing, bronchial constriction and congestion, difficulty in expectorating, burning in chest, cough with palpitations, slow labored breathing, bubbling sounds, lung swelling, and slimy sputum with specks of blood. Symptoms worsen around 3 a.m., on cold, cloudy days, in the damp open air, during menstruation. Symptoms improve while eating, lying on abdomen, or in dry weather.

Aralia racemosa—Indicated for dry cough with first sleep, asthma on lying down at night, tickling in throat or sensation that something is stuck, strong spasmodic cough, constriction of chest, whistling while breathing, frequent sneezing, hay fever accompanied by excessive nasal discharge, and salty, bitter taste in mouth. Also feel raw burn-

TREATING ASTHMA WITH MAGNESIUM

A co-factor in more than 300 enzymatic reactions involving energy and nerve function, magnesium stimulates adrenal and immune function, relaxes smooth muscles, and serves as a natural bronchodilator and antihistamine. Numerous studies prove that intravenous administration of magnesium can stop acute asthma attacks when convention drugs have failed. In one study, ten children suffering from acute asthma attacks were treated with an intravenous infusion of magnesium, while a control group received a placebo. None of the patients had responded to earlier administration of beta-agonists or corticosteriods. Thirty minutes after treatment, the magnesium group experienced significant improvements in peak expiratory flow and a reduction in asthma symptoms compared to the control group. This improvement persisted for at least 90 minutes following treatment.[28] Inhaled magnesium has proved as effective as conventional drugs in blocking bronchial constriction in severe asthma attacks.[29]

Oral supplementation of magnesium is useful in minimizing asthma symptoms. In a double-blind, controlled study, researchers placed 17 asthmatic subjects on a low-magnesium diet for a week, after which they administered oral magnesium supplements (400 mg daily) to some subjects while treating the rest with placebos. A week later, the researchers provoked all subjects with an asthma-inducing irritant. The magnesium-treated group experienced a significant reduction in asthma symptoms compared to the placebo group.[30]

Conventional asthma drugs, especially glucocorticoids, have been shown to disrupt magnesium absorption, leading to magnesium deficiency in asthmatics.[31] Magnesium deficiency can cause anxiety, muscle tremors, confusion, irritability, and pain. Processed food or foods cooked at high temperatures can be depleted of their magnesium content. Food sources of magnesium include tofu, nuts and seeds, and green leafy vegetables, especially kale, seaweed, and chlorophyll. Magnesium is absorbed well when taken as an oral supplement. Use magnesium glycinate, fumerate, or citrate, which are usually better absorbed with less of a laxative effect. RDA: 400 mg; therapeutic dose: 500–1,000 mg.

CAUTION Very high doses of magnesium (30,000 mg or higher) may be dangerous if kidney disease is present. Doses of 400 mg or higher may produce a laxative effect, causing diarrhea.

ing behind sternum; may become drenched with sweat during sleep. Symptoms worsen between 9 p.m. and 11 p.m., after a nap, or being in a draft. Symptoms improve while lying with head high or sitting up.

Arsenicum album—Indicated for wheezing cough that may be alternately dry and loose, cough worsens during drinking and while lying on back, accompanied by burning in the chest, darting pain in the upper portion of the right lung, bloody sputum, and scanty, frothy expectoration. Feel restless and anxious, chilly, need for warm water but only drinks in sips; also can't lie down due to fear of suffocation or death. Symptoms worsen between 11:30 p.m. and 3 a.m., when consuming cold drinks, or in cold air.

Arsenicum iodatum—Indicated for hay fever–induced asthma, dry, hacking cough with little or difficult expectoration (yellow/green foul-smelling mucus), air hunger (difficulty getting deep breath), short of breath, burning heat in the chest. Feel thirsty and chilly. Symptoms worsen in dry, cold weather or when it is windy and foggy, after indoor exertion, eating apples, or breathing tobacco smoke. Symptoms improve in the open air.

Cuprum metallicum—Indicated for spasmodic asthma alternating with vomiting, cough with gurgling sound, feel like suffocating, painful chest constrictions and spasms, loud rattle in chest; breathing worsens while bending backward. Symptoms worsen around 3 a.m., when angry, in hot weather, or when raising arms. Symptoms improve upon consuming cold drinks.

Ipecac—Indicated for constant constriction in chest, persistent or suffocating cough with every breath that causes nausea, vomiting; may cough until blue in the face; rattle in chest without expectoration; voice may be hoarse (but painless). Feel thirstless and chilly. Symptoms worsen in warm or damp weather, with a moist warm wind, after overeating, or lying down. Symptoms improve in open air.

Kali nit—Indicated for dry, short, hacking cough in the morning accompanied by chest pain and bloody, sour-smelling sputum, constriction in chest and right lung, severe shortness of breath (can't hold breath long enough to drink), heart palpitations. Feel burning internally but cold externally. Symptoms worsen when walking in cold, damp weather, lying with head low, or eating veal. Symptoms improve with gentle motion and drinking sips of water.

SUCCESS STORY: HYPNOTHERAPY STOPS STRESS-INDUCED ASTHMA

Some physicians believe there is often a strong emotional underpinning to asthma, but it isn't always easy to help a patient identify and then clear that emotion. In such cases, hypnotherapy has a role, according to clinical hypnotherapist Joseph Riccioli, C.Ht., NBCDCH, Director of the Hypnosis Healing Center, in Totowa, New Jersey.

Rosie, 28, had lived with asthma for 20 years. She had a history of stress-related problems, including insomnia, and had several times consulted a psychiatrist for relief of her anxiety. Rosie wasn't happy with the outcome of these consultations because she was reluctant to take the powerful conventional drugs these doctors had prescribed. When Rosie told Dr. Riccioli that she had officially been diagnosed as having anxiety disorder, he replied, "In hypnotherapy, we do not diagnose—we directly communicate with and probe the subconscious mind to find a probable cause for a person's unhealthy state, be it physical or emotional."

Hypnotherapy helps patients understand that emotional states are linked to illness. "When an unresolved issue is held onto for a period of time," explains Dr. Riccioli, "it can create a conflict between the subconscious and conscious minds. If it remains unresolved, it may manifest itself emotionally, as depression or anxiety, for example. If this persists, it may eventually internalize and manifest itself physically as symptoms."

Dr. Riccioli's clinical interest was in discovering Rosie's feelings about her condition. "The subconscious mind remembers everything. It is just a question of getting to that information," he says. During regression hypnosis, Rosie's memory took her back to her childhood, when she was eight years old. "This was the first time she experienced feelings of anxiety," says Dr. Riccioli. She remembered that her parents fought continuously; on one occasion, they had a particularly vigorous altercation that so upset Rosie that she began crying. Her parents paid no attention to her distress and made no effort to comfort her. "This experience is what we call the initial synthesizing event," says Dr. Riccioli. "Soon after this argument, Rosie developed asthmatic symptoms. The primary causes of her bronchial constriction and spasm were her nerves acting on her lungs."

During the regression therapy, Rosie appeared to relive this painful experience—she cried, became nervous, and showed signs of breathing difficulty. These were positive signs, as the pall of childhood emotional trauma was about to be lifted from Rosie's lungs. Using a combination of psychological techniques, such as working with the inner child, seeking forgiveness, and reframing, Dr. Riccioli helped Rosie understand and resolve the cause of her anxiety and simultaneously release the cause of her asthma. "After that single session, Rosie was like a new person," says Dr. Riccioli. Shortly thereafter, her asthma improved so much that she was able to finally discontinue all of her conventional asthma drugs after two decades of suffering.

According to Rima Laibow, M.D., founding Medical Director of the Alexandria Institute of Natural and Integrative Medicine, in Croton-on-Hudson, New York, neurobiofeedback (NBF) is another technique that unlocks emotional trauma and disentangles it from asthma symptoms. It is typical for asthmatic patients doing NBF to have original events like Rosie's come to mind—and body—powerfully during a session. If properly handled by a skillful therapist, this is often the patient's last asthma attack. NBF deals with the underlying immune, emotional, and stress management aspects of the condition simultaneously.

Lachesis—Indicated for dry, fitful coughs, sensation of suffocating while lying down, painful larynx; breathing almost stops when falling asleep; feel like must take a deep breath. Feel thirsty and cold. Symptoms worsen upon waking, consuming warm drinks, swallowing, going from cold to warm weather. Symptoms improve in open air, upon consuming cold drinks, and when bathing.

Lobelia—Indicated for asthma attack accompanied by weakness in the stomach and preceded by prickling all over, rattle in chest, difficulty in expectorating, chest constriction causing shortness of breath. Feel sensation of pressure in chest. Symptoms worsen after sleep or smoking. Symptoms improve after rapid walking, in the evening, in warm places, or after eating a little.

Natrum sulpuricum—Indicated for asthma attacks in damp or cold air; cough with thick green mucus, hold chest while coughing, feel pain in left part of lower chest, need to take a deep long breath. Recommended for children.

Pulsatilla—Indicated for asthma marked by dry cough at night that loosens up in the morning, thick yellow/green mucus, shortness of breath, pressure on and soreness in chest, and air hunger. Feel smothered when lying down, thirstless, discouraged, desirous of sympathy, and whiny. Symptoms worsen in warm room or in warm air, in the evening, before menstruation and during pregnancy, and after eating rich foods and fats. Symptoms improve in open air, with erect posture, or upon crying.

Sambucus—Indicated for children that awaken with throat spasm or feeling of suffocation; also mucus obstruction, spasmodic cough, whistling while breathing, difficulty in expectorating, chest pressure accompanied by stomach pressure or nausea. Wake up sweating profusely but feel dry, burning heat while asleep. Not thirsty. Symptoms worsen in dry, cold air, during sleep, after consuming cold drinks or eating fruit, or while head is low. Symptoms improve while sitting up, wrapped up, and in motion.

Spongia tosta—Indicated for dry, barking, deep cough accompanied by severe dryness in airways, including larynx (which is also painful to touch), wheezing, panting, grabbing throat when swallowing. Symptoms worsen during inhalation and before midnight, in a dry, cold wind, upon being awakened, after raising arms, or using voice. Symptoms improve when lying with head low, after eating, and after coughing.

Sulphur—Indicated for difficult and irregular breathing, violent cough with mucus rattling, shortness of breath at night, burning and pressure in chest, pains shoot to back, rapid morning pulse, red/brown spots over chest. Feel thirsty and chilly. Symptoms worsen at night and while standing and bathing. Symptoms improve while sitting up.

Hydrotherapy: For asthma sufferers, Dr. Sherman advises hot fomentations to the chest, especially for those suffering from acute attacks. He recommends combining these with hot footbaths, with the head kept cool using a fan or cool water. The body should be covered up with wool or cotton blankets. Dr. Sherman adds that Russian baths (a sauna with the head left outside the cabinet or steam bath) can also be effective, but it is important the patient not get chilled afterward.

A 20-minute hydrogen peroxide bath can help relieve asthma attacks as well, according to Dr. Sherman. Fill a bathtub with water at 98°-100° F; add 13-16 oz of hydrogen peroxide and soak while the release of oxygen relieves symptoms. Afterward, be sure to rest.

Traditional Chinese Medicine and Acupuncture: Both acupuncture and traditional Chinese medicine (TCM) can be effective in treating asthma and other types of respiratory conditions. Mark Cooper, N.D., L.Ac., of Portland, Oregon, recalls treating a woman suf-

fering from a case of constant, acute asthma attacks. Using a variety of natural therapies, including herbs, homeopathy, and spinal manipulation, he was able to alleviate only about half the symptoms. As a last resort, in a process called moxibustion, a cone of moxa (a Chinese herb) was placed over a specific acupuncture point on the woman's chest, on the lower part of the breast bone. The herb was then burned until the patient could no longer stand the heat. According to TCM, this particular treatment is performed only once, but Dr. Cooper reports that the results in this case were dramatic and long lasting. The woman became free of her dependency on medications and gradually improved to the point where only mild wheezing was present. Dr. Cooper adds that this method can also be used in emergencies to alleviate difficult breathing in asthmatics.

Several studies attest to acupuncture's effectiveness in relieving asthma symptoms. In one study, 17 patients with long-standing histories of asthma were treated with acupuncture. After ten weeks of acupuncture therapy, more than 70% of the patients reported a significant improvement in their asthma symptoms, which continued for six months after treatment.[32] In another study, 94 patients with asthma who were treated with acupuncture experienced a significant reduction in symptoms compared to 49 patients in a control group. Acupuncture reduced bronchial hyper-reactivity, promoted the function of cell beta-adrenergic receptors, and elevated concentrations of T lymphocytes and other important immune cells.[33]

Yoga: Scientists have found that yoga can be therapeutic for people with asthma.[34] In one study, 17 adult asthmatics, 19-52 years old, were divided into two groups—nine were taught yoga techniques, including breathing exercises (*pranayama*), physical positions (*asanas*), and mediation, while the remaining eight patients served as controls. The test subjects were taught yoga three times a week for 16 weeks. During this time, all subjects maintained logs of the symptoms and medication use; the researchers also took samples of morning and evening peak flow readings (amount of air they expired—low levels indicate airway obstruction). Researchers found that the test group reported a significant degree of relaxation and positive attitude compared to the control group and they also tended to use inhalers less than the controls did. Lung function did not vary significantly between the groups, but the yoga techniques did prevent exacerbation of asthma attacks.[35]

Bronchitis

In most cases of bronchitis, it is important for mucus to be cleared from the lungs. Coughing can help this, notes Dr. Sherman, therefore cough suppressants should be

SPECIAL THERAPIES FOR ASTHMA

The following physical therapies—one that must be administered by a trained practitioner, the other you can learn for yourself—are specially suited to help alleviate the respiratory difficulties associated with asthma.

Infraspinatus Respiratory Response (I.R.R.) Therapy: The Infraspinatus Respiratory Response (I.R.R.), sometimes also called the Infrascapula Respiratory Reflex, is a neuromuscular response that has a direct connection to the sympathetic nervous system. A nerve reflex prompts bronchial spasm, making the bronchioles constrict and produce phlegm, causing an asthma attack. The I.R.R. is also implicated in the onset of pneumonia and bronchitis. Manipulating this muscular response can relieve, even reverse, asthma symptoms and other respiratory ailments, according to Harry H. Philibert, M.D., of Metairie, Louisiana.

Dr. Philibert has helped more than 5,000 patients experience immediate remission from respiratory disorders using a special protocol that treats the I.R.R. He developed this I.R.R. therapy after he discovered that palpating the infraspinatus muscle caused pain in patients with asthma and other respiratory diseases but not in others. Recognizing a dysfunction in the neuromuscular reflex, Dr. Philibert developed a type of neural therapy whereby he injects the muscle with lidocaine (an anesthetic). This simple technique has demonstrated remarkable results with medication-dependent chronic asthmatics. While chronic asthma takes at least a few treatments to respond, there is usually an immediate reversal of the acute symptoms. Interestingly, the pain in the muscle also disappears.

During I.R.R. treatments, the patient lies prone with arms hanging over the sides of the exam table. The infraspinatus muscle is palpated and if pain is present, the muscle is injected with lidocaine. A few minutes after administering the lidocaine, the practitioner palpates the muscle again and repeats lidocaine injections if pain persists. This procedure is repeated until the patient is free of pain. Patients with chronic asthma are seen every two weeks until the respiratory symptoms and muscular pain subside.

Dr. Philibert reports that in a study of 25 asthmatics over a six-month period, all but one reported feeling better after I.R.R. treatment. Sixteen experienced dramatic improvements in the peak flow meter readings, while another seven felt that they were completely free of asthma. Approximately half of the subjects voluntarily stopped using their inhalers. Acupressure applied to a point on the chest parallel to the I.R.R. treatment point on the back also provides almost instantaneous relief from respiratory distress.

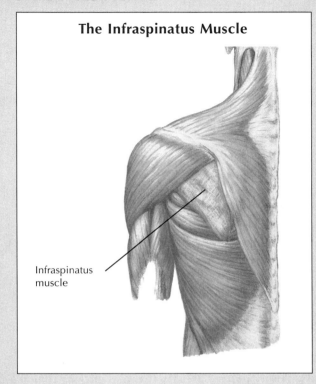

The Infraspinatus Muscle

Infraspinatus muscle

Buteyko Breathing Reconditioning Technique: The Buteyko Breathing Reconditioning Technique is an effective method for helping asthmatics breathe normally again. Designed by Russian-born scientist Konstantin Pavlovich Buteyko, Ph.D., the technique consists of easy-to-learn shallow breathing exercises. Butekyo's theory is that asthmatics tend to hyperventilate, lowering their carbon dioxide levels, which causes blood vessels to spasm and deprives the tissues of oxygen. In moderate amounts, carbon dioxide is a smooth muscle dilator.

Most conventional breathing techniques for asthma work on expanding the lung's capacity to inhale and take in deeper breaths. Yet, despite the seeming contradiction of clinical thinking, the Buteyko method has been validated in research. In one study of 35 asthma sufferers, 27 reported a decrease in symptoms after $4\frac{1}{2}$ months. Seven were able to overcome all attacks and 15 overcame most; 12 totally reduced their use of bronchodilators and 14 reduced their steroid use. Twenty-three of the 35 stated that the technique was superior to conventional asthma treatment.[36]

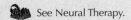 See Neural Therapy.

avoided unless the patient is extremely weak from lack of sleep. Patients who cough once a minute for 20 minutes have shown a 41% clearance of mucus from the lungs in X rays.[37] Deep breathing has also been shown to encourage mucus removal.

Diet and Nutrition: For bronchitis sufferers, Dr. Sherman first advises eating hot, spicy foods, which open the air passages to bring relief. These foods include garlic, onion, chili peppers, horseradish, and mustard. Dairy products, starches, sugars, and eggs should be avoided in order to produce less mucus. In addition, a whole foods diet will strengthen the immune system and drinking lots of fresh fluids is essential. Dr. Sherman reports that vitamins A, C, and E are effective in relieving bronchitis. Zinc, proteolytic enzymes (taken between meals), garlic, thymus gland extract, selenium, and bioflavonoids are other beneficial supplements.

Herbal Medicine: "Dry, irritating bronchitic coughing can be eased with a mixture of equal parts dried mullein, coltsfoot, and anise seed, drunk as a hot infusion several times a day," says David L. Hoffmann, B.Sc., M.N.I.M.H., of Sebastopol, California, past president of the American Herbalists Guild. Elecampane, horehound, goldenseal, echinacea, raw garlic, and ginseng are other medicinal herbs that have proven beneficial. Dr. Sherman recommends a blend of poke root, licorice, echinacea, grindelia, and lobelia taken as a tea or tincture 3-4 times daily. This formula can be obtained from most naturopathic physicians or herbalists.

Hydrotherapy: Doug Lewis, N.D., former Chair of Physical Medicine of Bastyr University, recommends that bronchitis patients receive a cold friction rub or hyperthermia, applied every 48 hours. Walking (treading) in cold water for a few minutes daily to strengthen the body is also useful, as are full, hot baths taken for 20-60 minutes.

Pneumonia

According to Dr. Sherman, generally it takes a patient 2-3 weeks to recover from pneumonia. Fever may come and go before any definitive treatment and recovery is completed.

Diet and Nutrition: For pneumonia, Dr. Sherman first advises patients to remove all known food allergens from the diet and to drink plenty of fluids and fresh juices. "Diluted pear juice is especially effective at loosening up congestion in the lungs," he notes. "The juices of green and yellow vegetables and fruits are also beneficial, including lemon juice. Dairy products and processed food products should be avoided." He adds that fresh garlic, cayenne pepper, and chili peppers have proven effective for pneumonia as well.

Vitamins A and C, beta carotene, zinc, proteolytic enzymes (taken between meals), acidophilus, bioflavonoids, and thymus gland extract are additional nutrients that have been found by Dr. Sherman to be of value in battling pneumonia.

Herbal Medicine: Dr. Sherman lists the following herbal remedies as valuable for easing pneumonia symptoms: lobelia and sanguinaria used as expectorants, hydrastis as an infection fighter, plus the antiviral herbs *Arctostaphylos,* uva ursi, *Cephaelis ipecacuanha,* St. John's wort, juniper *(Juniperus communis),* and *Piper cubeba.*

Hydrotherapy: According to Dr. Sherman, pneumonia can be greatly relieved by using a "pneumonia jacket" applied by a professional. He recommends that the jacket treatment be combined with a hot footbath and a cold compress to the forehead; the feet should not be chilled. Patients with strong vitality should follow the jacket treatment with a cold mitten friction rub, done after the chest is thoroughly reddened (about 20 minutes) and the feet are warmed.

Acupuncture: William M. Cargile, L.Ac., D.C., F.I.A.C.A., past Chair of Research of the American Association of Oriental Medicine, has had dramatic success using acupuncture in the treatment of pneumonia. Dr. Cargile recalls a man who mistakenly took Chinese weight-loss herbs designed for another person who had a completely different constitution. The patient developed pneumonia almost immediately and conventional medical treatment could not cure him, even after three weeks. "His condition was such that he could not lie down and had to sleep sitting in a chair in order to breathe," Dr. Cargile says. "When he came to me, he had so much fluid in his lungs that his respiratory capacity was only about 40%." After only one treatment, the patient was coughing up chunks of red, fleshy sputum and, within two days, had returned to 80% of his normal breathing capacity.

Sinusitis

Based on curing his own the debilitating chronic sinusitis, Dr. Ivker developed a comprehensive "Sinus Survival" program that treats the whole person. In addition to addressing his patients' physical health, Dr. Ivker pays attention to their home and work environments (see "Creating a Healthy Indoor Air Environment"), helps them deal with mental and emotional issues that can contribute to their illness, and encourages them to deepen their spiritual and social connections including healing troubled relationships and improving social communication skills. "After about two months of incorporating the recommendations for physical and environmental health into your daily routine, you can begin the mental/emotional components, followed by the social/spiritual components," he says. After just one month of making a commitment to the program, the majority of chronic sinusitis patients experience significant improvement, he reports. "If the commitment is maintained, within six months patients are usually healthier than they have been in years. Over 90% of my patients have cured their chronic sinusitis in this time period."

Dr. Ivker's program is in stark contrast to conventional medical approaches for treating sinusitis, which employ a variety of antihistamines, decongestants, steroid nasal sprays, and antibiotics, and, if the condition still persists, resort to surgery—cutting away the swollen mucous membrane and attempting to establish artificial drainage pathways. In Dr. Ivker's estimation, such approaches seek to provide "quick fix" solutions that largely fail because they do not address the root causes of sinusitis. "There is no quick fix in the process of curing chronic sinusitis or in experiencing optimal health," he says. He is not opposed to using antibiotics in all cases, however. "If there is no sign of improvement after strictly following my program for two to three weeks, then antibiotics might be appropriate," he says, although in most instances, the lack of response is due to candidiasis. In the majority of such cases, Dr. Ivker usually recommends an aggressive anti-fungal treatment program that includes medication (Diflucan or Sporanox) or an anti-candidiasis homeopathic formula, along with following a strict anti-candidiasis diet and supplementation with probiotics.

Overall, however, Dr. Ivker recommends his Sinus Survival program for patients who have not responded to antibiotics or surgery; those who cannot tolerate drugs or undergo surgery, or who are not candidates for surgery; and anyone who is interested in self-care, preventing and curing sinusitis, and experiencing optimal well-being.

> *There is no quick fix in the process of curing chronic sinusitis or in experiencing optimal health.*
> —ROBERT S. IVKER, D.O.

Diet and Nutrition: "With specific regard to the respiratory tract, the change I most often recommend is to avoid milk and dairy products, since the proteins they contain, especially in cow's milk, can increase and thicken mucus secretions," Dr. Ivker says. He also advises the elimination of sugar, caffeine, and alcohol, and avoidance of red meat, salt, simple or refined carbohydrates (white breads, pastries, commercial pastas), packaged and "junk" foods, food additives (BHA, BHT, sodium nitrite, sulfites), artificial colors and sweeteners (saccharin, aspartame, cyclamates), and unhealthy fats (hydrogenated or trans fats). "I also usually recommend eliminating foods most likely to cause congestion," he adds. "In addition to milk and dairy, these include wheat, corn, chocolate, and soy products. If other foods seem suspicious, I suggest eliminating them from the diet for three weeks, then reintroducing each food individually for three or four days to see if there are any changes in the patient's symptoms."

Foods that Dr. Ivker recommends include fresh, organic fruits and vegetables; whole grains low on the glycemic index (meaning they are absorbed slowly and therefore provide better nutrition), such as brown rice, amaranth, quinoa, barley, kamut, oats, and millet; nuts and seeds; legumes (beans and peas); and lean, organic fish and poultry. In addition, he advises his patients to drink plenty of pure, filtered water ($^1/_2$ to $^2/_3$ oz of water per pound of body weight). For patients whose sinusitis is caused or exacerbated by nasal allergies, Dr. Ivker recommends garlic, onions, citrus fruits, and horseradish, all of which are highly beneficial for strong immune function.

Dr. Ivker also recommends the following regimen of nutritional supplementation for sinusitis. The lower dosages represent preventive levels, while the higher dosages can be used as part of a comprehensive treatment program.

- Vitamin C (polyascorbate or ester C): 1,000-5,000 mg three times per day
- Beta carotene: 25,000 IU 1-3 times per day
- Vitamin B6: 50-200 mg twice daily
- Multivitamin complex: 1-3 times per day
- Vitamin E: 400 IU 1-2 times per day
- Calcium (citrate or hydroxyapatite): 1,000-1,500 mg
- Chromium picolinate: 200 mcg
- Flaxseed oil (or omega-3 fatty acids in fish oil): 2 tbsp daily
- Garlic extract: 1,200-2,000 mg 1-3 times per day
- Magnesium (glycinate, citrate, or aspartate): 500 mg daily
- Proanthocyanidins (grape seed extract): 100 mg 1-3 times per day on an empty stomach
- Selenium: 100-200 mcg daily
- Zinc picolinate: 20-60 mg daily

CAUTION These dosages are for adults only. Women who are pregnant or undergoing menopause and children should first consult with a physician before beginning a nutritional supplementation program.

Herbal Medicine: The primary herb Dr. Ivker employs in his program is echinacea (200 mg or 25 drops, 2-5 times per day). As part of a treatment program, he also recommends goldenseal (200 mg or 20 drops, 3-5 times per day).

According to Richard Barrett, N.D., of Portland, Oregon, other useful herbal remedies include purple coneflower, ephedra, Oregon grape, horseradish, poke root, yarrow, garlic, wild indigo, and elder flowers. A good herbal formula for acute sinusitis, recommended by Dr. Barrett, is made using one part each of tinctures of eyebright, goldenseal, yarrow, horseradish, and ephedra. "Proper dosage is 30 drops every two hours for two days, then four times a day until symptoms are gone," he says.

Dr. Barrett also suggests an herbal formula for sinusitis attacks accompanied by infection: two parts purple coneflower and wild indigo, with one part poke root. Proper dosage is 30 drops every hour until the condition improves, then four times daily. Other herbs Dr. Barrett recommends are stinging nettle, goldenrod (as a tincture), and eyebright compound.

Hydrotherapy: Drs. Ivker and Barrett both recommend nasal irrigation (also known as nasal lavage) using saltwater and steam inhalations to loosen nasal secretions, cleanse the nasal passages, and assist the sinuses in draining. An alternative method, according to Dr. Barrett, is to use one teaspoon of powdered goldenseal mixed in a cup of warm water. He also recommends hot footbaths with a cold compress placed over the affected sinuses. Additionally, a hot compress can be applied over the sinuses for three minutes, followed by a cold compress for 30 seconds; repeat at least three times, being sure to finish with the cold application.

Homeopathy: Sinusitis can also be treated with homeopathy as a form of self-care. "A reasonable approach to home treatment would be to match the remedy with your symptoms and then take two pellets of 30C potency every 3-4 hours, apart from food and other medicines, until symptoms abate," Dr. Barrett explains. "Afterward, repeat less frequently as needed." The following are some of the main homeopathic remedies for acute sinusitis. If none of these remedies seem to match the symptoms, seek out a homeopathic practitioner for treatment.

Arsenicum album—Use if the discharge is thin, watery, and burning; the condition worsens with exposure to the open air; or there is a tendency to feel chilly, a desire for warm drinks, and a sense of restlessness and anxiety.

Kalium bichromium—Use if there is a feeling of pressure at the root of the nose and a foul smell or loss of smell; if the frontal sinuses are chronically stuffed up, with con-

stant postnasal drip and nasal obstruction; or if the symptoms are relieved by warm applications and worsen from exposure to cold damp air.

Nux vomica—Use if passages are stuffed up, especially at night and outdoors; if frontal headaches are experienced, which ease with pressure placed against them; or if patients are chilly, irritable, and cannot bear noises or light.

Mercurius iodatus—Use if nostrils are raw and ulcerated, if patients are worse at night and suffer from extremes of temperature, either hot or cold; if the nasal discharge is yellow/green and tinged with blood; or if they perspire easily, which aggravates the condition.

Silicea—Use if there are dry hard crusts in the nose which bleed easily, as well as pain experienced over the frontal and maxillary sinuses; if the nasal bones are sensitive to touch; if the nose is obstructed, with a loss of smell. *Silicea* types are not particularly resilient and tend to be fair-skinned and very sensitive to the cold.

Research has shown that the nasal spray *Euphorbium compositum*, a preparation of eight homeopathic remedies, is effective as a treatment for chronic sinusitis. In one study, 172 patients were divided into two groups, with each patient receiving either the homeopathic spray or a placebo (two dosages, four times a day, for four months). Those who received the homeopathic spray experienced considerable improvement—reduced headaches, sinus pressure, and breathing difficulties—compared to the placebo group. Another study involving 3,510 patients found that 75% of the patients rated results from *Euphorbium compositum* as "good" to "excellent."[38]

Acupuncture: Dr. Cargile states that he has never had a patient with sinusitis who has not responded to acupuncture treatments. "The irony is that in almost all of my sinusitis cases, I'm the last person the patients came to and everything else they tried, including the pharmaceutical treatments, failed," he says. One of Dr. Cargile's patients was a tennis player who was stricken with sinusitis in the midst of competing in a tournament. "She was trying to reach the finals and was having severe difficulty because of how excruciating her symptoms were and the way her eyes were tearing," he says. She received one acupuncture treatment from Dr. Cargile and gained immediate relief, remaining well throughout the rest of the tournament. After receiving seven additional treatments spaced over three weeks, her sinusitis completely cleared up and did not return.

According to Dr. Cargile, sinusitis is often linked to toxins in the bowel and intestines. "To effectively treat sinusitis, you want to stimulate the body to detoxify, so that it will raise its energy," he explains. "Once this happens, often the sinusitis will be better within minutes. And in some cases, the relief will last for weeks and sometimes months, without the need for further treatments."

Lifestyle: Although patients with sinusitis often may be adverse to physical exercise, Dr. Ivker recommends 20-30 minutes of aerobic exercise, three to five times a week. "With the possible exception of diet, regular exercise can contribute more to optimal health than any other health practice," he says. "Among its many benefits are decreased tension, depression, anxiety, and 'fight-or-flight' response; enhanced aerobic capacity and energy levels; improved metabolism and quality of sleep; and greater self-esteem. However, anyone suffering with chronic sinusitis or asthma should begin a regimen of aerobic exercise very gradually." He also recommends stretching exercises and strength conditioning, as well as getting plenty of sleep.

Mental and Emotional Health: "Improving your mental and emotional health can make a significant difference in how you feel physically," Dr. Ivker says. "What you eat, for instance, is sometimes far less important than what's 'eating' you." Proper stress management is an important factor, both at home and at work. Essential mental/emotional components of his program include: modifying beliefs and attitudes through affirmations and visualizations; developing clarity about personal and professional objectives; undergoing counseling or psychotherapy, if appropriate, or practicing biofeedback; learning to express painful emotions, especially the safe release of anger, grief, and fear; keeping a journal; and finding more humor, optimism, and play in life.

"Many energy medicine modalities, which work on both the physical and mental/emotional levels, can also be beneficial in treating and preventing chronic sinusitis and other respiratory conditions," Dr. Ivker says. Among them are Healing Touch and Therapeutic Touch, Reiki, Qigong and Tai Chi, and the various therapies in the field of energy psychology.

See Biofeedback Training and Neurotherapy, Energy Medicine, Mind/Body Medicine, Qigong and Tai Chi.

Spiritual and Social Health: "Spiritual health encompasses not only a conscious awareness of the Divine, but also an intimate connection to ourselves and to our families, friends, and communities," Dr. Ivker says. "The spiritual practices I find most helpful in this regard are prayer, meditation, gratitude, and spending time in nature." Intimacy with a spouse, partner, or close friend is the essence of optimal social health, according to Dr.

Ivker. It also consists of a strong, positive connection to family members and others in the community. Opportunities for improving social health include practicing forgiveness, developing friendships, performing selfless acts and being altruistic, and participating in support groups.

Emphysema

According to Dr. Sherman, the first and foremost thing that must be done in order to heal emphysema is to immediately stop smoking. Once that is accomplished, the alternative therapies will be much more effective.

Diet and Nutrition: "An increased quantity of raw foods in the diet will prove beneficial, as will hot and spicy foods such as garlic, onions, chili peppers, horseradish, and mustard," says Dr. Sherman. "Cold-pressed olive oil can be taken daily as well, and seaweed may also bring substantial relief." He has found that grapes and raw grape juice provide beneficial aid, as do the raw juices from other fruits, including oranges, lemons, and black currants. "Raw vegetable juices, such as carrot, spinach, celery, and watercress, are strongly recommended and are even more beneficial when a small amount of garlic juice is added to them," he says. In crisis situations, Dr. Sherman suggests a fast of 3-10 days, drinking only vegetable juices. Avoid mucus-forming foods such as dairy products, salt, eggs, meat, processed foods, "junk foods," and white flour products.

Nutritional supplements recommended for emphysema include zinc and vitamin B_6, to chelate cadmium from the body; vitamin E, for decreasing the patient's dependence on oxygen tank therapy;[39] lecithin, to reduce the surface tension of fluids in the lungs, enabling easier elimination;[40] and vitamins A and C, protein, and folic acid, to help reestablish connective tissue elasticity. Chlorophyll, coenzyme Q10, the amino acids L-cysteine, L-methionine, and L-glutathione, and vitamin B_{12} are also beneficial, according to Dr. Sherman.

Herbal Medicine: For emphysema, Dr. Sherman recommends a variety of herbal remedies. Coltsfoot tea and thyme are effective in helping eliminate mucus. Anise oil mixed with honey is beneficial taken before each meal. Ephedra tea quiets bronchospasms and mullein helps prevent infections and aids in excreting fluid from the lungs.[41] Comfrey, fennel seed, fenugreek, licorice root, rosehips, and rosemary are other beneficial herbs.

"Relief from coughing may be expedited with a mixture of equal parts of coltsfoot, mullein, and licorice, taken three times a day," adds David Hoffmann. "The flowers of these herbs, combined into an infusion, are not only effective but taste delicious." A blend of marshmallow, coltsfoot, violet, mullein, and red poppy flowers in equal parts, taken three times a day, is another very

THERAPIES TO HELP STOP SMOKING

John A. Sherman, N.D., suggests the combination of these three therapies to aid smokers in giving up their life-threatening addiction.

Aversion Therapy: Stop smoking except for one hour daily. Smoke constantly during that hour. Take 15 drops of lobelia tincture 30 minutes before the first cigarette and again at 15 minutes before the last cigarette. Take this same quantity of lobelia tincture every 15 minutes during the remainder of the smoking hour. This will produce nausea. Its association with smoking can eliminate the desire for cigarettes in just 5-6 days, according to Dr. Sherman.

Hydrotherapy: A simple Epsom salt bath, using ½ pound of salt per bath, helps pull nicotine and tar from the skin to prevent its introduction into the bloodstream. Shower or bathe normally after the Epsom salt bath to rinse them off. Dry with a white towel. The brownish residue of nicotine excreted by the skin visually enforces the desire and need to stop smoking. Exercise and colonic irrigations may also be useful in helping the body to eliminate toxins from smoking.

Diet: The best withdrawal diet is similar to one used to treat hypoglycemia, which maintains constant blood sugar and avoids developing a flood of food cravings. This diet consists of six meals a day, largely consisting of fresh fruits, vegetables, proteins, and complex carbohydrates (whole grains and pasta). Sugar and baked flour products are to be avoided. This diet will help maintain a fairly even blood sugar level through the day.

"pleasant" medicine. White horehound is also highly effective in battling coughing, but its unpleasant taste needs to be masked by combining it with licorice or anise seed.

Hydrotherapy: According to Dr. Sherman, the pneumonia jacket treatment is also beneficial for emphysema sufferers with excessive or viscous mucus production. Once again, he cautions that it should only be administered under professional supervision. Dr. Sherman also recommends long-term constitutional hydrotherapy. "This form of water treatment utilizes hot and cold water packs placed over the chest and abdomen at specific time intervals," he explains. "Sine-wave electrical pads can also be employed to stimulate both the digestive tract and nervous system, helping to clear the lungs."

Fomentations, or hot compress applications, are also beneficial, states Dr. Sherman. A thick, folded flannel cloth is usually applied a number of times in succession at high temperatures to essentially produce a local vapor bath. "This procedure is employed when it is necessary to reduce swelling, stimulate absorption of fluid, increase local blood supply, and awaken functional activity," Dr. Sherman says. "Full fomentations include a steam pack to the back, a hot footbath, and cold compresses to the face, head, or neck."

Recommendations

- Take steps to improve the indoor air quality of your home and work environments. Consider the use of a negative ion generator or air filter. Change filters in heating systems regularly, vacuum regularly, damp dust twice a week, and remove rugs and stuffed toys from bedrooms. Avoid secondhand smoke and if you smoke, stop.

- Avoid the use of household furnishings and other products that are synthetic or made from plastic.

- Emphasize a diet of fresh, organic fruits and vegetables, whole grains, fish, and organic poultry. Eliminate milk and dairy products, sugar, caffeine, and alcohol, and minimize your salt intake. Also consider an elimination diet, in which you abstain from eating foods to which you may be sensitive or allergic. Garlic and onion boost immune response and help nourish the respiratory tract.

- Drink adequate amounts of water throughout the day (½ to ⅔ oz for each pound of body weight).

- Check for candidiasis; if present, it must be treated before respiratory symptoms will improve.

- Nutritional supplements: beta carotene, vitamins B₆, C (polyascorbate or ester C), and E, a multivitamin complex, calcium (citrate or hydroxyapatite), chromium picolinate, magnesium (citrate, aspartate, or glycinate), selenium, zinc, proanthocyanidins (grape seed extract), grapefruit seed extract, and flaxseed oil or omega-3 fatty acids.

- Helpful herbs include echinacea, goldenseal, and mullein.

- Twenty minutes of aerobic exercise 3–5 times per week.

- Practice nasal irrigation and use a steam inhaler when experiencing respiratory symptoms.

- Explore the link between your habitual thoughts, attitudes, and beliefs, as well as repressed or improperly expressed emotions (especially anger, fear, and guilt) and your health problems. If necessary, seek professional guidance for resolving them and also deepen your social and spiritual connections.

Self-Care

The following therapies can be undertaken at home under appropriate professional supervision:

HAY FEVER

Biofeedback Training and Neurotherapy / Guided Imagery / Yoga

ACUPRESSURE: To relieve hay fever, place the thumb and index finger of one hand on the upper ridge of the eye socket, near the bridge of the nose. Press upward into the slight indentations in your eye socket. Spread the index and middle fingers of your other hand to press up underneath your cheekbones directly beneath your eyes. Hold these points for one minute with your eyes closed as you breathe deeply.

AROMATHERAPY: Lavender, eucalyptus, chamomile, melissa, rose.

AYURVEDA: • Basil tea with honey (especially basil from India or *Tulsi*) • *Calamus*, gotu kola, ginger, cloves, ephedra, bayberry • Apply essential oils such as eucalyptus, menthol, or camphor (or ginger paste) to temple and root of nose.

JUICE THERAPY: • Carrot, celery juice • Carrot, beet, cucumber • Carrot, celery, spinach, parsley

ASTHMA

Biofeedback Training and Neurotherapy / Flower Essences / Guided Imagery / Mind/Body Medicine / Qigong and Tai Chi / Yoga

AROMATHERAPY: • During an attack, inhale bergamot, camphor, eucalyptus, lavender, hyssop, or marjoram. • Try frankincense for calming.

AYURVEDA: • Make a tea from ½ teaspoon each of licorice and ginger in one cup of water. • To relieve congestion and cough and alleviate breathlessness, try ¼ cup of onion juice with a teaspoon of honey and ⅛ teaspoon black pepper. • Between attacks, fortify the body with tonics such as *ashwagandha, shatavari,* gotu kola, licorice, and *triphala.*

HOMEOPATHY: *Antimonium tart., Nux vomica.*

JUICE THERAPY: • Periodic fasting on juice or distilled water and lemon juice may be helpful. • Carrot and

spinach • Carrot and celery • Carrot and radish • Radish, lemon, garlic, comfrey, and horseradish mixed with carrots and beets • Lemon juice and water first thing in morning • Grapefruit

BRONCHITIS

Acupressure / Fasting / Qigong and Tai Chi / Reflexology / Yoga

AROMATHERAPY: • Steam inhalation with bergamot, camphor, eucalyptus, lavender, pine, sandalwood. • Clear mucus using bergamot, sandalwood, and thyme.

AYURVEDA: An herbal mixture of *sitopaladi* (500 mg), *punarnava* (300 mg), *trikatu* (100 mg), and *mahasudarshan* (300 mg); ¼ teaspoon of this mixture generally taken twice a day after lunch and dinner, with honey.

HOMEOPATHY: *Aconite, Bryonia, Phosphorus, Ferr phos., Sulfur, Arsen alb., Lymphomyosot, Calc. sulph.*

JUICE THERAPY: • Carrot and radish juice • Wheatgrass juice • Carrot, beet, and cucumber • Carrot and spinach • Carrot and celery • Carrot, beet, and cucumber

PNEUMONIA

Reflexology / Yoga

AROMATHERAPY: Camphor, eucalyptus, tea tree, pine, lavender, lemon

AYURVEDA: An herbal mixture of *sitopaladi* (500 mg), *punarnava* (300 mg), *pippali* (200 mg), and *abhrak bhasma* (100 mg); ¼ teaspoon taken with one teaspoon of *chyavanprash* three times a day or twice a day after lunch and dinner.

JUICE THERAPY: Carrot, spinach, parsley juice; add garlic, cumin

SINUSITIS

Qigong and Tai Chi

DIET: Avoid milk and dairy products, since the proteins they contain, especially in cow's milk, can increase and thicken mucus secretions.

EMPHYSEMA

Acupressure / Biofeedback Training and Neurotherapy / Guided Imagery / Qigong and Tai Chi / Reflexology / Yoga

AROMATHERAPY: Eucalyptus, pine

HOMEOPATHY: • *Aspidosperma* • *Carbo vegetabilis* when there is a feeling of being hungry for air and desire to be fanned.

JUICE THERAPY: • Carrot, spinach, celery, wheatgrass, watercress, potatoes, barley juices. Add a little garlic to juices. • Grape, orange, lemon, black currant

Professional Care

The following therapies should only be provided by a qualified health professional:

HAY FEVER

Acupuncture / Applied Kinesiology / Chelation Therapy / Chiropractic / Craniosacral Therapy / Hypnotherapy / Osteopathic Medicine

BODYWORK: Acupressure, reflexology, Rolfing

ASTHMA

Acupuncture / Chelation Therapy / Chiropractic / Craniosacral Therapy / Environmental Medicine / Hypnotherapy / Light Therapy / Magnetic Field Therapy

BODYWORK: Alexander Technique, Feldenkrais, Hellerwork, massage, shiatsu • Rolfing helps to free the rib cage and thereby promote better breathing, but cannot cure asthma.

TRADITIONAL CHINESE MEDICINE: Ginseng is used in traditional formulas to treat asthma.

OXYGEN THERAPIES: Ozone

BRONCHITIS

Applied Kinesiology / Biofeedback Training and Neurotherapy / Environmental Medicine / Enzyme Therapy / Magnetic Field Therapy / Naturopathic Medicine / Osteopathic Medicine / Yoga

DETOXIFICATION THERAPY: Often indicated if the person is strong enough and has other congestive conditions.

OXYGEN THERAPIES: • Hydrogen peroxide therapy • Ozone therapy—extremely low concentrations of ozone/oxygen are anecdotally said to be helpful in healing. • Hyperbaric oxygen therapy

TRADITIONAL CHINESE MEDICINE: Treats bronchitis with fresh lotus root to strengthen the lungs and pears to help dry coughs.

BODYWORK: Rolfing helps to free the rib cage and promote better breathing but cannot cure bronchitis. • Many forms of massage are helpful in normalizing respiratory function.

PNEUMONIA

Acupuncture / Magnetic Field Therapy / Naturopathic Medicine / Osteopathic Medicine

BODYWORK: Rolfing

FASTING: According to Dr. Chaitow, fasting is useful in the early stages, if the patient is not too frail. He has fasted elderly patients with pneumonia for 48 hours with excellent results. He uses repetitive soft tissue manipulation methods to help breathing function, along with herbal and nutrient support.

SINUSITIS

Acupuncture / Biofeedback Training and Neurotherapy / Energy Medicine / Herbal Medicine / Homeopathy / Hydrotherapy / Mind/Body Medicine

EMPHYSEMA

Acupuncture / Chelation Therapy / Chiropractic / Magnetic Field Therapy / Osteopathic Medicine

BODYWORK: Shiatsu, reflexology, Rolfing

Where to Find Help

For information on respiratory conditions, or referrals to a qualified health-care practitioner, contact the following organizations.

American Association of Naturopathic Physicians
8201 Greensboro Drive, Suite 300
McLean, Virginia 22102
(703) 610-9037
Website: www.naturopathic.org

Provides a directory of naturopathic physicians and offers referrals to a nationwide network of accredited or licensed practitioners. Also publishes a quarterly newsletter, for both professionals and the general public, and offers a series of brochures and pamphlets on a variety of subjects.

American Association of Oriental Medicine
433 Front Street
Catasauqua, Pennsylvania 18032
(888) 500-7999
Website: www.aaom.org

The AAOM is a national professional organization of acupuncturists who meet acceptable standards of competency and can provide you with the names of local members.

National Center for Homeopathy
801 North Fairfax, Suite 306
Alexandria, Virginia 22314
(703) 548-7790
Website: www.homeopathic.org

Provides a referral list of practicing homeopaths and other information. Gives courses for laypeople and professionals and organizes study groups around the country.

Sinus Survival
(888) 434-0033
Website: www.sinussurvival.com

Provides information about Dr. Robert Ivker's Sinus Survival and Asthma Survival programs, as well as Dr. Ivker's books and other products.

Harry H. Philibert, M.D.
213 Live Oak
Metairie, Louisiana 70005
(504) 837-2727

Dr. Philibert has trained approximately 3,000 physicians in the I.R.R. treatment protocol and also periodically provides seminars on the I.R.R. Therapy.

Buteyko Asthma Management
P.O. Box 1458
Hastings, New Zealand 4215
(011) 646-878-0101
Website: www.buteyko.co.nz

For further information about the Buteyko Breathing Reconditioning Technique.

Rosalba Courtney, D.O., N.D., C.A.
Alive and Well, Institute of Conscious Bodywork
100 Shaw Drive
San Anselmo, California 94960
(888) 259-5951

For further information about the Buteyko Breathing Reconditioning Technique.

Recommended Reading

Asthma Free in 21 Days. Kathryn Shafer, Ph.D., and Fran Greenfield, M.A. San Francisco: HarperSanFrancisco, 2000.

Asthma Survival. Robert Ivker, M.D. New York: Tarcher/Putnam, 2001.

Dr. Braly's Food Allergy and Nutrition Revolution. James Braly, M.D. New Canaan, CT: Keats Publishing, 1992.

Encyclopedia of Natural Medicine. Michael Murray, N.D., and Joseph Pizzorno, N.D. Rocklin, CA: Prima Publishing, 1991.

Sinus Survival: The Holistic Medical Treatment for Sinusitis, Allergies, and Colds. Robert Ivker, M.D. New York: Tarcher/Putnam, 2000.

SEXUALLY TRANSMITTED DISEASES

Sexually transmitted diseases (STDs) are more varied and prevalent than ever before, with traditionally common STDs, such as gonorrhea and syphilis, being joined by chlamydia and human immunodeficiency virus (HIV). More than 20 STDs have been identified and affect as many as 13 million Americans every year, at a cost of $10 billion in health-care expenses.[1] While prevention is the ideal way to deal with STDs, many natural treatments such as herbs, homeopathy, and nutritional supplements are effective, depending on the specific condition and its severity.

VENEREAL DISEASES, or what are now called sexually transmitted diseases, can affect anyone. It is possible to have only one sexual partner and still acquire an STD. Even newborn babies are susceptible if the mother is infected. "Most sexually transmitted diseases are caused by either a virus or bacteria," says Tori Hudson, N.D., former Academic Dean of the National College of Naturopathic Medicine, in Portland, Oregon. For example, bacteria cause diseases such as chlamydia, gonorrhea, and syphilis, while viruses cause herpes simplex and HIV (the increasingly controversial causative agent of AIDS). Even the very common *E. coli* bacteria and other normal bowel flora can cause "honeymoon cystitis," a bladder infection, usually in women, that occurs shortly after encountering a new sexual partner (hence the designation "honeymoon").

As the name suggests, STDs are usually transmitted through intimate sexual contact involving a variety of body parts, such as the genitals, mouth, and anus, but they can also be transmitted nonsexually. For example, hepatitis B, often spread sexually, can be transmitted by sharing a hypodermic needle or through a human bite. The incidence of STDs is on the rise, partially due to young people becoming sexually active earlier and marrying later. Plus, since divorce is now more common, sexually active people are more likely to have more than one sex partner during their lives.[2] The prevalence of STDs is also affected by socioeconomic and cultural factors as well, such as general health and nutritional status, access to protective measures, and sexual practices.

The potential for contracting an STD depends on the disease type, the gender of both the carrier and the receiver, and the nature of the sexual contact. A person may experience no symptoms (particularly in women)

or only very mild symptoms for a short or extended period of time. During this phase, serious complications may result and the STD can be passed to a sexual partner or, in the case of a pregnant woman, to her unborn child. STDs can cause other health problems as well, such as cervical cancer, pelvic inflammatory disease, and genital warts. Because of the many variables and potential problems associated with an STD, a trained health professional should be consulted if infection is suspected.

 See AIDS, Men's Health, Women's Health.

 Because of the many variables and potential problems associated with an STD, a trained health professional should be consulted if infection is suspected.

Prevention

To avoid STDs, Dr. Hudson offers the following precautions:

- Take care when selecting a sex partner. Find out about your partner's health and sexual history before pursuing a sexual relationship. Have sex only if the person has no apparent signs of infection and is willing to assure your protection during sexual intimacy. Be prepared to talk and inquire about past experiences. Be direct and persistent. Make conversations about health a natural part of the sexual relationship.

- Limit your number of sex partners. The more sexual partners a person has, the more vulnerable he or she is to STDs. Although "safer sex" ("safe sex" may be a misnomer) is an essential form of protection for many STDs, open lesions can occur on parts of the

Male Reproductive System

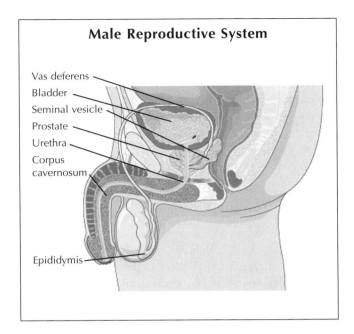

- Vas deferens
- Bladder
- Seminal vesicle
- Prostate
- Urethra
- Corpus cavernosum
- Epididymis

Female Reproductive System

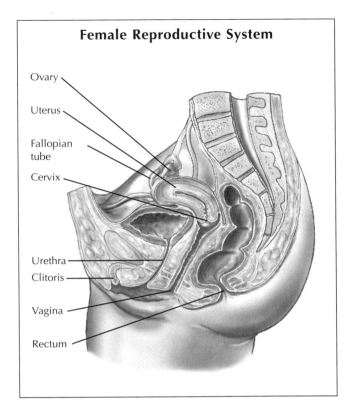

- Ovary
- Uterus
- Fallopian tube
- Cervix
- Urethra
- Clitoris
- Vagina
- Rectum

body that cannot be covered by a condom or other latex barrier.

- Use latex barriers. Except for people in long-term, monogamous relationships, a barrier-style contraceptive should always be used. Latex condoms give the best protection against STDs. Condoms made from natural products such as sheepskin are not as reliable as those made of latex and no condom can guarantee 100% protection. A latex dental dam—a device that, when inserted in the mouth, prevents secretions from being swallowed—is suitable for partners with genital warts or genital herpes. The female condom may help prevent the spread of STDs to and from the external genitals. Semen itself is an immune suppressant and should not be swallowed or left in the rectum, where irritation to the bowel can allow direct access to the bloodstream.

- Stay healthy. If you have sex with more than one person or if your partner does, have a checkup for STDs at least once a year. Pap smears should be considered an important part of a woman's exam. It is important that both women and men urinate after intercourse to help clear the urethra, thus preventing infection.

- If you may have been exposed to an STD, act responsibly. See your health-care practitioner immediately. Urge your partner to be examined and treated as well. Follow the treatment regimen exactly and do not have sex until you and your partner have been tested again or until you know how to ensure each other's protection.

 See Diet, Herbal Medicine, Nutritional Supplements.

CAUTION Because acute pelvic inflammatory disease (PID) can be severe or even life-threatening, proper diagnosis and medical care are essential. It is unwise to diagnose and treat PID without consulting a licensed health-care practitioner, particularly if a period has been missed after intercourse or when there is any pelvic pain or unusual vaginal, penile, scrotal, or rectal pain or discharge.

Common STDs and Their Treatment

From an alternative medicine approach, the key to treating any disease is stimulating the immune system. In the case of STDs, eliminate fatty foods, sugar, white flour, salt, and coffee from the diet, advises Dr. Hudson. The diet should be high in complex carbohydrates and contain an adequate amount of protein. However, the particular diet may depend on the individual's blood type and body type, as some people do better on high-protein and low-carbohydrate diets. The immune system can be protected by drinking pure, filtered water and eliminating alcohol, tobacco, and mood-altering drugs. Several nutrients, including vitamins A, C, and E and zinc, are necessary for optimal immune function and herbs such as echinacea and goldenseal fight off the offending organism while bolstering the immune system.

 See Diet.

NATURAL SOLUTIONS FOR URINARY TRACT INFECTIONS

Michael Gerber, M.D., H.M.D., of Reno, Nevada, makes the following recommendations for treating cystitis and other urinary tract infections:

- Uva ursi (bearberry) herb and tincture are helpful along with goldenrod *(Solidago virgaurea), Populus tremuloides,* and homeopathic *Cantharis.*

- Drinking plenty of pure water is very important as is the use of pancreatic enzymes and food-derived enzymes such as bromelain (from pineapple) and papain (from papaya), taken between meals to relieve inflammation.

- Buchu, juniper berry, licorice, willow, and birch all aid in diuresis (increasing the flow of urine) and in protecting the urinary tract.

- Acute urinary tract infections can benefit from alkalinizing the urine with baking soda (sodium bicarbonate), one teaspoon in a glass of water three times per day between meals, or a commercial antacid such as Alka Seltzer Gold (which contains sodium bicarbonate and potassium bicarbonate). The bacteria that cause infections do not thrive in an alkaline environment.

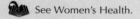 See Women's Health.

In the case of any STD, it is important to consult a physician who can evaluate the condition and determine if antibiotics or other pharmaceutical drugs are necessary or if natural remedies alone will be effective. Even where conventional medicine seems the best choice, one can always add natural therapies under the supervision of an alternative physician. For instance, with conditions for which antibiotics are necessary, the patient may take *Lactobacillus acidophilus* to counteract yeast overgrowth brought on by the drug and may also benefit greatly by utilizing cleansing herbs for the liver to help clear the drugs from the system. Additionally, having "friendly" bacteria (such as acidophilus) in the vagina helps to resist STD infections, although conventional doctors differ on how to increase vaginal *Lactobacillus* concentrations.

Chlamydia

Chlamydia are a group of microorganisms that cause primary lesions on the genitals and inflammation of the regional lymph nodes. Chlamydial infection is the most prevalent STD in the U.S., with 4-8 million new cases every year.[3] Chlamydia is a dangerous disease because it is often symptom free. This poses a particular threat for women and the children they bear. If chlamydia goes untreated or is not treated appropriately, it can cause tubal pregnancies and infertility in women and prematurity or death in newborns. *Chlamydia* have also been known to cause pneumonia as well as ear and eye infections in infants.

In women, *Chlamydia* can infect the cervix, urethra, eyes, and throat. Most commonly, though, *Chlamydia* strike the upper genital tract, including the fallopian tubes, endometrium (lining of the uterus), and pelvic peritoneum (lining of the pelvis), in pelvic inflammatory disease (PID). In fact, they are responsible for half of the one million cases of PID that occur yearly in the U.S. Symptoms, which can range from mild to intense, typically include vaginal discharge or bleeding, pelvic pain, pain with intercourse, changes in urination, and fever.[4]

Although the consequences are not as dire, men are also susceptible to chlamydial infection, especially in the urethra and epididymis (part of the excretory duct of the testes). In fact, urethritis, the most common STD seen in men, is frequently caused by *Chlamydia*. In these cases, it is called nongonococcal urethritis to differentiate it from urethritis caused by *Neisseria gonococcus*, another serious cause of STDs. As in women, this infection often has no symptoms and is thus difficult to prevent and treat. However, when detectable complaints include discharge from the penis, urethral itching, or changes in urination, medical care should be sought. An infection of the epididymis is characterized by one-sided pain in the scrotum as well as swelling and/or pain in that same region. Providing pain relief is an important part of the treatment of epididymitis, since pain can often be severe.

Treatment: According to Dr. Hudson, when using natural therapies for PID, urethritis, or any other genital chlamydial infections, the purpose is to increase circulation to the affected area. When this occurs, inflammation is reduced, healing occurs rapidly, the infection subsides, and the body's immunity is stimulated. There are several ways this can be accomplished.

If the infection is acute or pain is severe, a three-day water fast is beneficial in minimizing the pain, says Dr. Hudson. Digesting as little as possible allows the body's healing mechanisms to work more effectively. If a patient cannot tolerate a water fast for either medical or non-medical reasons, a fast using fruit and vegetable juices is an alternative. If the infected person is unable to undergo such a fast, or the condition is chronic, then a light diet of fresh fruits and vegetables for three to five days is another option.

Whether fasting or not, fluids should be increased. In addition to water, utilize the therapeutic effects of juices from watermelons, apples, nectarines, grapes, carrots, and green vegetables. Carrot juice, for example, is very high in beta carotene, the nontoxic precursor to vitamin A. According to Dr. Hudson, other juices, such as pomegranate, cranberry, celery, parsley, and cucumber, have been used for decades to treat urethritis. These foods are considered therapeutic because they promote urination.

When herbal preparations are used to treat epididymitis, it is best to consult a trained practitioner, says Dr. Hudson. Many old botanical texts recommend pulsatilla and podophyllum specifically for epididymal infections. However, both of these plants are potentially toxic and therefore must be administered by a knowledgeable professional in order to ensure a safe dose. "Given in medicinal doses," says Dr. Hudson, "these herbs have the ability to treat epididymitis with results comparable to conventional medicine."

Other herbs such as echinacea, goldenseal, horsetail, saw palmetto berries, cranberry extract, and chimaphilla are also recommended. Tom Kruzel, N.D., of Scottsdale, Arizona, who specializes in the treatment of male genital and urological infections, finds that saw palmetto is the most important herb in treating men for these infections. Berberine, an active constituent of goldenseal, has been shown to stimulate the immune system.[5] In India, berberine drops are used on patients with chlamydial eye infections. When this treatment was compared to the standard drug (sulfacetamide), it was found that the drug produced better initial results, but that only berberine killed the chlamydial parasite and only berberine-treated patients suffered no recurrences.[6]

Gonorrhea

Gonorrhea is caused by the gram-negative bacterium *Gonococcus neisseria*. Gonorrhea's presence is overshadowed by more common STDs, but in the U.S., gonorrhea is still a significant problem, with approximately 400,000 cases per year. Of the sexually transmitted diseases that American physicians are required to report to public health officials, gonorrhea is the most prevalent.[7]

In women, gonorrhea can infect the vagina, cervix, urethra, rectum, and throat, or it can migrate to the uterus, ovaries, or fallopian tubes and cause pelvic inflammatory disease. Men's reproductive organs, such as the penis and epididymis, are similarly infected by gonorrhea, as are the rectum and throat. When urethritis is caused by gonorrhea, it is called gonococcal urethritis.

A gonorrheal infection can cause redness and swelling in the affected area. The painful urination and pus-like discharge from the penis seen in nongonococcal urethritis (caused by *Chlamydia trachomatis*) are similar in gonococcal urethritis. Frequency of urination or

---

SUCCESS STORY: A CASE OF EPIDIDYMITIS

Tom Kruzel, N.D., of Scottsdale, Arizona, specializes in the treatment of male genital and urological infections. One of his cases involved Mario, 45, who visited his office following treatment for an itchy, red rash on his penis and scrotum. Mario's previous doctor had given him cortisone cream, which cleared up the rash, but three weeks later he developed right-sided epididymitis. When Dr. Kruzel examined Mario, the infection had progressed from a dull aching to a sharp pain accompanied by slight swelling.

Although Dr. Kruzel suspected the infection may have been due to *Chlamydia*, he did not confirm it with a culture because, he explains, "I rarely do a culture for *Chlamydia*, partially because it doesn't really alter my treatment plan that much and I'm not using antibiotics." Dr. Kruzel adds that it is often difficult, particularly with *Chlamydia*, to gather an adequate sample from a male patient and, when it is done, it is very painful. "What is most important to me is to have the symptoms delineated, because that way I can choose the botanical or homeopathic medicine that will work."

For this case, Dr. Kruzel chose saw palmetto and horsetail, both specific for the epididymis; pulsatilla, a good herb for swelling and pain seen in male genitourinary diseases; and homeopathic *Staphysagria*, for mental and emotional issues. A homeopathic constitutional remedy of *Lycopodium* was also prescribed.

At his three-week follow-up visit, Mario reported an 85% improvement of the pain, but the rash had returned, although with no itching. Without adjusting the medications, Dr. Kruzel told him to return in one month. "On the return visit, he was completely pain free and the skin rash was just about gone." The pain and rash completely disappeared within four months and there has been no recurrence.

---

an urgency to urinate may also occur. If the gonorrhea organism escapes from its original site of infection and enters the bloodstream, complications such as fever, skin rash, or joint pain can occur. While about 95% of men display some symptoms, only 50% to 75% of women do.[8] However, Dr. Hudson notes, "follow-up testing is critical in order to ascertain if there is a need for antibiotics." Frequently, antibiotics are needed in these cases.

Treatment: Natural therapies for gonorrhea, especially urethritis, epididymitis, and PID, are similar to those used for chlamydia.

Syphilis

Syphilis is caused by a bacterial microorganism. It usually leads to skin lesions in the early stages (that may involve any organ or tissue), but may not present any symptoms for many years. Syphilis should not be treated with natural therapies. According to Dr. Hudson, "Syphilis is a serious and potentially debilitating and life-threatening illness, and requires conventional treatment with penicillin or other antibiotics such as tetracycline. You would be putting yourself out on a limb to treat syphilis any other way."

However, Dr. Hudson says, homeopaths may use *Syphilinum* to stimulate the immune response and avoid long-term, more subtle problems from the disease. "Even though the organism is killed by penicillin, homeopaths believe there are alterations of the patient's vital force as a result of the disease. The disease leaves an imprint, which a parent can even pass along to a child," says Dr. Hudson. "Homeopathic remedies used in conjunction with other medicines can avert that process and help avoid long-term consequences."

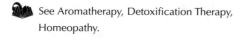 See Aromatherapy, Detoxification Therapy, Homeopathy.

Herpes

There are two main types of herpes. The first type, which also causes cold sores, is caused by herpes simplex virus type 1 (HSV1). Genital herpes, the most common type of genital ulceration, affects an estimated 60 million Americans and is caused by herpes simplex virus type 2 (HSV2). The first signs of an HSV2 infection can occur 4-7 days after sexual contact with an infected partner. Tingling, burning, or a persistent itch usually herald a herpes outbreak. A day or two later, small, pimple-like bumps appear over reddened skin. As the itching and tingling continue, the herpes pimples transform into painful blisters, which burst and exude blood and yellowish pus. Five to seven days after the first tingling sensation, scabs form and healing begins.

In women, blisters tend to accumulate on the external genital region, cervix, and around the anus. In men, lesions may occur on the glans (the bulbous end of the penis), the prepuce (the foreskin), and shaft of the penis, as well as around the anus. Herpes simplex virus can also cause nongonococcal urethritis infections in men.

Treatment: Treating herpes with natural medicines can significantly reduce the frequency and number of eruptions. Dr. Hudson reports that some patients suffering from chronic herpes are able to reduce their outbreaks from monthly to once or twice a year.

Recurrent herpes is clearly a stress-related illness. Anxiety is the greatest predictor of a herpes eruption, and thus stress reduction can help prevent herpes attacks.[9] Taking supplements to support the adrenal glands is especially important in times of stress. Adrenal glandular extract, vitamins A, B complex, B5, B6, and C, and zinc are recommended. A specific diet may also help—many HSV2 sufferers have decreased their herpes outbreaks by eating foods high in the amino acid lysine, such as seafood, chicken, turkey, eggs, dairy products, potatoes, and brewer's yeast, reports Dr. Hudson. Supplemental lysine can be taken as well.[10]

Anxiety is the greatest predictor of a herpes eruption, and thus stress reduction can help prevent herpes attacks.

A diet containing large amounts of arginine, another amino acid, appears to aggravate herpes. Foods to avoid include chocolate, nuts (specifically peanuts, almonds, cashews, walnuts), seeds (sunflower and sesame), and coconut. Foods containing a moderate amount of arginine should be eaten with discretion. These include wheat, soy, lentils, oats, corn, rice, barley, tomatoes, and squash. Those suffering from an outbreak should avoid these foods until the blisters have disappeared. Immunosuppressants such as drugs, alcohol, and tobacco should also be eliminated.

Aromatherapy uses essential oils that are believed to be effective in treating herpes simplex due to their strong antiviral properties. Combinations of oils such as lemon and geranium, or eucalyptus and bergamot, applied topically at the first sign of outbreak can lessen or prevent a full flare-up. Other essential oils that can be used are true rose oil or melissa oil, both of which have contributed, in some cases, to complete remission of herpes simplex lesions after one application.

Herbal remedies can also be used to treat herpes. "Herbs that strengthen the immune system and help the body resist infection can be taken internally. Tinctures of echinacea, Siberian ginseng, nettle, and goldenseal should be combined in equal parts and a half teaspoon taken three times a day," says David Hoffmann, B.Sc., M.N.I.M.H., an herbalist from Sebastopol, California, and past President of the American Herbalists Guild. Licorice and Indian gooseberry are also recommended.

When preventive measures do not stop herpes sores from appearing, there are several ways to diminish the discomfort and hasten recovery. Ice applied to the sores at the very beginning of an eruption can help. Cool compresses or baking soda compresses also soothe lesions. Aloe, goldenseal, lavender, and lycopodium can be applied directly to the herpes lesions in a salve. A popular topical ointment among naturopathic physicians contains licorice root. Researchers have discovered that glycyrrhizic acid, a constituent of licorice, inactivates HSV1-infected cell cultures.[11]

Vitamin C paste (made with powdered vitamin C and a little water) applied to the herpes lesions will dry them up very quickly, says Michael Gerber, M.D., H.M.D., of Reno, Nevada, although it causes an initial stinging sensation. Alternating vitamin C paste with vitamin E oil is also beneficial and more soothing. Lauric acid (also called monolaurin) is a good preventative treatment for herpes, as it stops viral replication in the cells of the body. The flavonoid quercetin taken orally has also been shown to inhibit the herpes virus.[12]

As with other STDs, herpes is most effectively controlled by halting its spread between partners. Herpes is potentially contagious from the first signs of tingling until the skin is healed. During an attack, the following precautions should be taken:

- Underwear should be worn to bed.
- Hands should be washed before and after touching any part of the body.
- No clothing, utensils, or other objects should be shared.
- Sexual contact should be avoided if lesions are on the genitals, as condoms will not guarantee safety.
- Kissing should be avoided if blisters are on the lips or in the mouth. If lesions are on an area that can be covered with a dressing, then intimate contact may be allowed.
- When being treated or examined by a health-care worker, notify that person if you have an active case so precautions can be taken.

Trichomonas

Although not as well-known as some STDs, *Trichomonas vaginalis*, a protozoa (single-cell parasite), is nonetheless a relatively frequent venereal condition. It is the third most common cause of vaginitis in women. Symptoms include a copious, odorous discharge from the vagina, intense itching and burning, and redness of the genital region. Although debated by some clinicians, *Trichomonas vaginalis* is also thought to infect men, leading to urethritis, prostatitis, epididymitis, and perhaps infertility.

SPECIAL CONSIDERATIONS FOR MEN

Men with untreated STDs, says Tom Kruzel, N.D., run the risk of infertility or impotence. Unfortunately, sometimes the only indications that an STD is present are mild symptoms, such as an aching in the hip or lower back or a mild pain in the testicles or scrotum. If it is a low-grade infection, the STD may persist for a long time, causing only fatigue, minimal fever, or malaise. Unaware of the consequences, many men will ignore these warning signs. A man also must remember to seek treatment if his partner is infected, even if he has no symptoms.

Treatment: Trichomonas can be difficult to treat with natural medicines. "As in other acute infections, it is beneficial to decrease sweets and refined carbohydrates," says Dr. Hudson. "Increase fresh fruits and vegetables, whole grains like brown rice, whole wheat flour, and oatmeal, and avoid coffee, rich foods, and junk foods." Dr. Hudson has also found that nutritional supplements are helpful, including vitamins A, C, and E, and zinc.

Supplementation with friendly bacteria (probiotics, which include *Lactobacillus acidophilus* and *Bifidobacteria bifidum*) is the most commonly recommended treatment for vaginitis. Probiotics help suppress the growth of yeast, improve digestion by increasing the production of some enzymes, produce acids that fight bacteria, and manufacture nutrients such as vitamins K, B_1, B_2, B_3, B_{12}, and folic acid.

When treating trichomonas, Jill E. Stansbury, N.D., of Battle Ground, Washington, mixes various herbs such as calendula, goldenseal, and echinacea, and prescribes them as a douche. She has patients douche with this formula once or twice a day or use the herbal douche in the morning and a plain yogurt douche at night. Other douche recommendations include: apple cider vinegar (two tablespoons to one quart water), acidophilus (two opened capsules to one quart water), or a solution of water and garlic from capsules or fresh juice.

Topical pau d'arco, black walnut, and tea tree oil (diluted) are also options and vitamin E cream may relieve itching. Betadine, or povidone iodine, is effective as a douche in several kinds of vaginitis, including yeast infections and *trichomonas*. The typically recommended mix is one part Betadine to 100 parts water, douching twice daily for two weeks.[13] A douche of grapefruit seed extract (10-20 drops in two cups of water) may also be used.

SPECIAL CONSIDERATIONS FOR WOMEN

STDs often affect each sex differently. Chlamydia, for example, may cause pelvic inflammatory disease in women, which can result in infertility. Natural health-care methods may not be enough for a woman in cases such as this, especially if she is considering having children in the future. She should always talk to her health-care practitioner about the possible use of antibiotics, along with natural remedies, because when a woman has an STD and does become pregnant, she runs the risk of passing the infection along to her baby.

It is now standard procedure among most obstetricians and midwives to screen women for STDs, often including HIV, during prenatal care. Mandatory treatment of HIV-positive women with anti-AIDS drugs can be especially draconian during pregnancy and can cause fetal deformities—seek competent legal and medical advice in such a situation.

If you are pregnant and have an STD, check with a health-care provider before taking any medications, including herbal preparations or nutritional supplements. Boric acid, for example, should not be used during pregnancy, though many herbal douches and suppositories are safe.

 It is vital that both sexual partners be treated at the same time if trichomonas is diagnosed, even if it is found in only one partner.

 See Candidiasis, Gastrointestinal Disorders.

Genital Warts

It is estimated that 40% to 80% of the U.S. population is infected with the human papilloma virus (HPV), the organism that causes genital warts. The reason this condition is so prevalent and the estimate of infection rate so wide is partly because HPV is difficult to detect. Not only are a quarter of HPV infections in regression and thus undetectable, but the life cycle of the virus is unpredictable. HPV can be transmitted from person to person in several ways. Any sexual contact, genital or oral, can spread HPV. This virus can also be picked up from inanimate objects that have been recently exposed to HPV and not properly cleaned (for example, toilet seats, medical equipment, underwear, tanning salon beds, and sexual aids or devices).

RESEARCH ON CERVICAL CANCER

Tori Hudson, N.D., spends much of her time conducting research on natural therapies for women's health conditions, including cervical cancer. Cervical dysplasia (abnormal changes in the tissues covering the cervix uteri) and cervical cancer are caused by the human papilloma virus,[14] a sexually transmitted virus, according to Dr. Hudson, but there are other significant factors in the development of the disease, including smoking, deficiencies of vitamins A and C and folic acid, and use of birth control pills.

Dr. Hudson examined the effect of a naturopathic protocol on various stages of dysplasia and cervical cancer in 43 women. Besides instructing her subjects to follow a healthy diet, take an herbal formula, and take various vitamins such as beta carotene, vitamin C, and folic acid, Dr. Hudson recommended that herbs and enzymes be applied locally and topically to the cervix. After six months, 38 patients following this protocol were disease free, three patients partially improved, and two patients showed no improvement. None of the patient's condition worsened during the naturopathic treatment.

While seeking proper medical evaluation and conventional or alternative treatment, the following aspects of Dr. Hudson's treatment can be applied:

Self-Treatment:

- Beta carotene: 150,000 IU daily
- Vitamin C: 2,000 mg daily (decrease this dosage if diarrhea occurs and consult a physician first if you have a history of kidney stones)
- Folic acid: 10 mg daily
- A diet of fresh fruits, fresh vegetables, and whole grains, along with the elimination of dairy products, meats, sugar, refined grains, junk food, coffee, and alcohol.

Methods of Prevention:

- Use condoms during intercourse and avoid unprotected sexual contact with anyone who has genital warts.
- Women should avoid smoking, which is the most significant co-factor in the development of cervical dysplasia and cervical cancer.

Most infected individuals exhibit no lesions or warts. A scant 2% to 3% have visible warts, while another 2% to 3% have flat warts that are not visible to the naked eye. Many times there are no symptoms associated with either the flat or visible warts. In other cases, burning, itching, and general irritation are felt and the affected skin may be red. This is especially true of flat warts. If a doctor suspects flat warts because of exposure or symptoms, this can be verified by applying white vinegar and then inspecting the area with a magnifying glass. Spots that turn white are often a positive indicator of warts.

Visible warts are usually small, raised, soft, moist bumps that are pink or red. They often resemble a tiny cauliflower. These cauliflower warts are easily spotted on a man's penis, at the opening to the urethra, or on his scrotum. Less detectable, although visible to the eye when found, are warts around a man's anus and in his rectum. Because a woman's genitals are less accessible, a closer inspection must be performed to locate warts on her vulva, vaginal wall, and cervix, as well as around the anus.

The flat wart is the most dangerous for women. The HPV virus can cause changes in the cervical cells, progressing to more severe cell abnormalities (called dysplasia) and possibly cancer. Typically, there are no symptoms to alert the woman of a problem. This is why an annual Pap smear, the most effective screening tool for detecting abnormalities, is vital.

Treatment: Conventional procedures for treating raised warts include local removal using electrocautery (burning the wart off), freezing the wart with liquid nitrogen, or applying acid or podophyllin, a prescription drug. Very aggressive chemotherapy is sometimes employed by gynecologists, which can cause pain, scarring, and narrowing of the vagina, making intercourse difficult and painful, according to Dr. Gerber. He recommends that less aggressive approaches be tried first. Many natural methods can be used alone or in addition to conventional treatment.

Dr. Hudson has developed an ointment of vitamin A and the herbs thuja and lomatium. When applied directly to the wart, this antiviral and immune-supportive mixture inhibits HPV. Lomatium and thuja can also be taken orally. *Thuja* is a common homeopathic remedy for warts as well. Deficiencies in vitamins A and C and folic acid can aggravate HPV infections and may be risk factors in cervical dysplasia and cancer. Smoking, which robs the body of vitamin C, is another risk factor.

Recommendations

- Find out about your partner's health and sexual history before pursuing a sexual relationship. Have sex only if the person has no apparent signs of infection and is willing to assure your protection during sexual intimacy.
- The more sexual partners a person has, the more vulnerable he or she is to STDs.
- Except for people in long-term, monogamous relationships, a barrier-style contraceptive should always be used. Latex condoms give the best protection against STDs.
- If you have sex with more than one person or if your partner does, have a checkup for STDs at least once a year.
- If you may have been exposed to an STD, act responsibly. See your health-care practitioner immediately. Urge your partner to be examined and treated as well.

Self-Care

The following therapies can be undertaken at home under appropriate professional supervision:

SYPHILIS

HERBAL MEDICINE: Add two tablespoons each of sarsaparilla and yellowdock root in one quart of boiling water. Simmer five minutes and add 3½ teaspoons dried thyme; cover and steep for one hour. Drink 1–3 cups per day. Women should also use often as a douche.

HYDROTHERAPY: Contrast sitz bath applied daily.

HERPES

Enzyme Therapy / Biofeedback Training and Neurotherapy

AROMATHERAPY: • Tea tree, bergamot, eucalyptus, lavender, chamomile, or palmarosa oils • True rose oil or melissa oil

AYURVEDA: An herbal mixture can be made of *shatavari* (500 mg), *guwel sattva* (200 mg), *kamadudha* (200 mg), and *neem* (300 mg). Take two teaspoons of this mixture twice a day after lunch and dinner. Also, tikta ghee can be applied locally or one teaspoon can be taken on an empty stomach.

HOMEOPATHY: *Rhus tox., Sepia, Natrum mur., Hepar sulph., Arsen alb., Caladium, Acidum nit.*

HYDROTHERAPY: • Hyperthermia (heat aggravates herpes infection, but may accelerate the healing process if tolerated) applied daily or every other day, followed by a short cold bath or sitz bath. • Apply contrast daily.

JUICE THERAPY: • Carrot, beet, celery juice • Avoid citrus, pineapple.

TOPICAL TREATMENT: • Glycyrrhizic acid (from licorice) applied to the skin lesions • Vitamin C paste • Squeeze a vitamin E capsule onto cotton and apply to lesion. • Zinc sulfate ointment • Calendula cream • Tea tree oil (one teaspoon diluted in one quart of water).

Professional Care

The following therapies should only be provided by a qualified health professional:

SYPHILIS

Magnetic Field Therapy / Naturopathic Medicine

HERPES

Energy Medicine / Detoxification Therapy / Environmental Medicine / Fasting / Magnetic Field Therapy / Naturopathic Medicine / Orthomolecular Medicine

OXYGEN THERAPIES: • Hydrogen peroxide therapy (IV) • Ozone (autohemotherapy) inactivates the genital herpes virus. Ozone therapy is potentiated by photoluminescence, exposing the blood to ultraviolet light during autohemotherapy.

Where to Find Help

For referrals and more information on, and treatment for, sexually transmitted diseases, contact:

American Association of Naturopathic Physicians

601 Valley Street, Suite 105
Seattle, Washington 98109
(206) 298-0126
Website: www.naturopathic.org

Provides a directory of naturopathic physicians and offers referrals to a nationwide network of accredited or licensed practitioners. Publishes a quarterly newsletter for both professionals and the general public. Also offers a series of brochures and pamphlets on a variety of subjects.

American College for Advancement in Medicine (ACAM)

23121 Verdugo Drive, Suite 204
Laguna Hills, California 92653
(800) 532-3688
Website: www.acam.org

ACAM provides referrals and information, including a directory of physicians worldwide trained in preventative medicine.

American Foundation for the Prevention of Venereal Disease

799 Broadway, Suite 638
New York, New York 10003
(212) 759-2069

The foundation provides educational material for the prevention of STDs and encourages responsible sexual relations.

American Holistic Medical Association

6728 Old McLean Village Drive
McLean, Virginia 22101
(703) 556-9728
Website: www.holisticmedicine.org

A professional organization for holistic practitioners, the AHMA offers information and services for its members. It also provides referrals for the public.

American Social Health Association

P.O. Box 13827
Research Triangle Park, North Carolina 27709
(919) 361-8400

A volunteer health agency dedicated to eliminating STDs as a social health problem.

Citizens Alliance for VD Awareness

P.O. Box 1073
Chicago, Illinois 60648
(312) 236-6339

The Citizens Alliance provides information to the public, especially high-risk groups, on symptoms, treatment, and prevention of STDs, including AIDS.

International Women's Health Coalition

24 East 21st Street
New York, New York 10010
(212) 979-8500
Website: www.iwhc.org

An organization that provides information to women, particularly about sexually transmitted diseases and other health concerns. Free pamphlets available upon request.

Recommended Reading

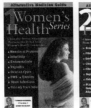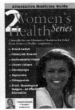

Alternative Medicine Guide to Women's Health 1 & 2. Burton Goldberg and the Editors of *Alternative Medicine.* Tiburon, CA: Future Medicine Publishing, 1998.

Color Atlas & Synopsis of Sexually Transmitted Diseases. H. Hunter Handsfield, M.D. New York: McGraw-Hill, 2000.

Encyclopedia of Natural Medicine. Michael Murray, N.D., and Joseph Pizzorno, N.D. Rocklin, CA: Prima Publishing, 1998.

Mind Your Body: A Sexual Health and Wellness Guide for Women. Beth Howard. New York: St. Martin's Press/Griffin, 1998.

The Sex Encyclopedia. Stephen Bechtel and the Editors of *Prevention* and *Men's Health* Magazines. New York: Fireside, 1993.

Sexually Transmitted Diseases. King K. Holmes et al., eds. New York: McGraw-Hill, 1999.

What Doctors Can't Heal. Bernard Jackson. Inglewood, CA: Strictly Honest, 1993.

SLEEP DISORDERS

Over 60 million Americans suffer from sleep disorders, including insomnia, excessive drowsiness, sleep apnea, and restless movement during sleep. For many of those with problems sleeping, the consequences are falling asleep on the job, inability to concentrate, and increased susceptibility to other illnesses because of an immune system compromised by lack of rest. According to many practitioners of alternative medicine, these disorders often are related to nutritional or behavioral factors and may be remedied by addressing the various causes and symptoms underlying the condition.

WE SPEND UP to a third of our lives asleep. Although some hard-driven people may view sleep as an inconvenience that curtails productivity and leisure activities, slumber is certainly no waste of time. In fact, sleep may play a more crucial role than diet or exercise in fostering optimal health. "Sleep is a natural restorative, an antidote to the damage done to our bodies during the course of the day. It allows the body to replenish its immune system, eliminate free radicals, and ward off heart disease and mood imbalances," says Herbert Ross, D.C., author of *Sleep Disorders: An Alternative Medicine Definitive Guide.* As an essential part of the daily human cycle, sleep is a determining factor in the state of a person's health.

A National Sleep Foundation Survey found millions of Americans are suffering from daytime sleepiness—43% of adults say that they are so sleepy during the day that it interferes with daily activity.[1] Drowsy driving causes at least 100,000 car accidents in the U.S. each year, according to the National Highway Traffic Safety Administration; 62% of adults reported driving while feeling drowsy. And 60% of children under the age of 18 complained of feeling tired during the day, while 15% admitted to falling asleep at school.

"The quantity and quality of sleep vary from person to person, but how well and how long one sleeps is ultimately the result of physical and psychological influences," says John Zimmerman, Ph.D., of the Mountain Medical

> *Sleep is a natural restorative, an antidote to the damage done to our bodies during the course of the day. It allows the body to replenish its immune system, eliminate free radicals, and ward off heart disease and mood imbalances.*
>
> —HERBERT ROSS, D.C.

Sleep Center, in Carson City, Nevada. Not only does stress, illness, and anxiety contribute to sleep disorders, but so can external circumstances, such as a noisy sleeping room, as well as disturbed biological rhythms due to night-shift work and jet lag. A shortened attention span, the loss of physical strength, and difficulty in responding to unfamiliar situations are all common symptoms of sleep disorders.

Altogether, Americans spend an estimated $16 billion each year on sleep-related medical care. Unfortunately, much of this money is poorly spent, because conventional sleeping aids—potentially addictive sedatives—ultimately create more sleep disturbances than they eliminate. Alternative medicine practitioners can make sure that finding the right treatment protocol doesn't turn into a nightmare. They realize that sleep disorders often arise from poor diet, toxic overload, disrupted circadian rhythms, geopathic, electromagnetic, and emotional stress, and hormonal and structural imbalances. Most people with sleep disorders will find relief by taking steps to promote overall health: improving diet, reducing stress, balancing hormones, and detoxifying the body, among others.

Types of Sleep Disorders

Sleep disorders are a particularly troublesome health concern. Not only can they be the result of other, often undetected ailments, but they also generate their own

THE CYCLES OF SLEEP

The phenomenon of sleep can be seen as a cycle consisting of two distinct states: rapid eye movement (REM), also known as dream sleep because almost all dreaming occurs in this state, and non-REM (NREM). Four stages of sleep take place during NREM, beginning when the person falling asleep passes from relaxed wakefulness (Stage 1) to an early stage of light sleep (Stage 2), and then to increasing degrees of deep sleep (Stages 3 and 4, also referred to as delta sleep). Most Stage 4 sleep (the deepest) occurs in the first several hours of sleep. A period of REM sleep normally follows each period of NREM sleep.

STAGE	DEGREE OF SLEEP	DURATION	LEVEL OF CONSCIOUSNESS	BRAIN WAVE ACTIVITY	PHYSIOLOGICAL PROCESSES
1	"Dozing," very light	30 seconds to 7 minutes	*Drifting in and out of sleep; awakened easily by all stimuli*	Irregular, rapid alpha waves	Muscles relax; smooth, even breathing; body temperature and heart rate begin to drop
2	Light	45-50 minutes in first cycle, decreasing to 25 minutes in last	*Awakened easily by sounds and movement*	Irregular theta waves, with intermittent rapid alpha activity and bursts of delta waves	Breathing, temperature, and heart rate continue to decrease; muscles relax further; eyes may roll slowly
3	Moderately deep	7-15 minutes in first 2 or 3 cycles, then disappears	*Difficult to awaken with stimuli*	Brain waves slow drastically, mostly large delta waves	Breathing and heart rate continue to drop but stabilize; very relaxed; may sweat
4	Very deep	12 minutes in first 2 or 3 cycles, then disappears	*Very difficult to awaken with stimuli*	Large, slow delta waves	Breathing and heart rate stable but slow; very relaxed; may sweat
REM	Dreaming	10 minutes at first increasing to 15-30 minutes as cycles continue	*May be awakened easier but difficult to adjust to reality*	Smaller, more regular alpha waves resembling those of Stage 1	Eyes roll back and forth; muscles freeze except for some twitching in face, toes, and fingers; breathing, heart rate irregular; penile erections in men

health complications. Sleep disorders fall into two categories, dyssomnias and parasomnias. Dyssomnias are conditions characterized by difficulty in falling asleep or maintaining sleep or by excessive sleepiness during the day. Insomnia, sleep apnea, narcolepsy, restless legs syndrome, periodic limb movements in sleep, hypersomnia, and delayed and advanced sleep phase syndromes are dyssomniac conditions. Parasomnias are behavioral abnormalities that occur during sleep, including sleepwalking, night terrors, and REM behavior disorder.

Insomnia

Insomnia, characterized by an inability either to fall asleep or to remain asleep during the course of the night, can be traced to a number of physical, mental, behavioral, and situational factors. Fifty-eight percent of U.S. adults report bouts of insomnia recurring at least a few times each week, with shift workers experiencing insomnia more frequently than regular day workers (66% compared to 55%).[2]

Insomnia has been classified in terms of the time of night that it affects. According to Dr. Zimmerman, there are three main types of insomnia: sleep-onset insomnia, sleep-maintenance insomnia, and early-morning-awakening insomnia. People who take hours to fall asleep but sleep relatively well throughout the remainder of the night have sleep-onset insomnia. Those who wake up several times in the middle of the night and have trouble falling back to sleep suffer from sleep-maintenance insomnia. Individuals who awaken too early have what is called early-morning-awakening insomnia.

Sleep Apnea

Sleep apnea refers to a serious condition in which there is intermittent cessation of breathing during sleep, which forces the individual to repeatedly wake up to take

CIRCADIAN RHYTHMS AND THE BODY'S CLOCKS

Sleeping during the night likely evolved to keep animals, including the human species, out of harm's way. Supporting this theory is the fact that most of us still follow the sun's cycles, sleeping when the sun is down and waking when it's up. In fact, we even possess innate cycles similar to those of the sun, called circadian rhythms. Scientists believe that these rhythms are guided partly by genes, which have evolved in many species, from fruit flies to humans.[3]

Circadian rhythms are regularly recurring, biological changes in our mental and physical behaviors over the course of a day. As indicated by the term *circadian* (Latin for "around a day"), these rhythms repeat approximately every 24 hours and are primarily controlled by the body's biological "clock." Circadian rhythms are most commonly linked to sleep/wake patterns and account for the fluctuations of alertness and drowsiness throughout the day. People with normal circadian rhythms are most alert during the morning and afternoon, but tend to get drowsy toward evening and feel the need for sleep at night. Research shows that circadian rhythms occur in other physiological processes as well, including blood pressure, body temperature, hormone levels, and the immune system.[4]

The body clock is actually part of the hypothalamus, an area of the brain just above the point where the optic nerves cross (about an inch behind the back of the bony eye sockets). Specifically, the clock is a cluster of hypothalamic nerve cells called the suprachiasmatic nuclei (SCN). In much the same way that a grandfather clock keeps time with the evenly spaced swings of a pendulum, the body clock tells time with the slow ebb and flow of

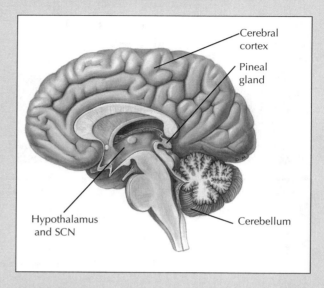

protein molecules in the SCN. In controlled conditions where test subjects are deprived of light and other time cues, a "day" by body clock standards is close to 25 hours. However, we do not exist in a dark vacuum. Light, from both the sun and artificial devices, as well as environmental cues such as alarm clocks, influence our circadian rhythms and set our body clocks to follow the 24-hour cycle of the sun.

How light manages to sway our internal timepieces also depends on the hypothalamus. The optic nerves relay information about external light levels to the SCN, which in turn sends the light signals to several regions of the brain, including the pea-sized pineal gland. The pineal gland is instrumental in sleep, because it secretes melatonin, the sleep-inducing hormone.

---

breaths of air. There are three types of sleep apnea, according to Dr. Zimmerman: central sleep apnea, obstructive sleep apnea, and a combination of the first two types called mixed-type sleep apnea. Central sleep apnea refers to a defect in the central nervous system that affects the diaphragm. It can result in poor quality sleep, frequent awakening during the night, and excessive fatigue throughout the day. Obstructive sleep apnea occurs when a blockage develops in the upper airway, preventing normal air flow.

In an episode of sleep apnea, the sleeper involuntary stops breathing for up to 60 seconds, resulting in decreased blood levels of oxygen and increased amounts of carbon dioxide. This change in blood gases alerts the brain to stimulate the breathing process. To do so, the brain must awaken the body from deep sleep. The sleeper

then resumes breathing, usually with a loud snort or gasp, and then quickly falls back to light sleep. People with obstructive sleep apnea usually snore heavily before and after the breathing pauses.

These apneic events can occur up to 30 times each hour, although the sleeper rarely realizes this because the awakenings are so brief. However, these constant arousals prevent the person from getting enough deep sleep and lead to excessive daytime sleepiness, morning headaches (from lack of oxygen), depression, irritability, sexual dysfunction, learning and memory difficulties, and falling asleep during daily activities. Sleep apnea has also been linked to irregular heartbeat, heart attack,[5] high blood pressure, and stroke, as well as sudden infant death syndrome (SIDS),[6] so it is prudent that people who suspect that they or their children suffer from this disorder get medical care.

Restless Legs Syndrome and Periodic Limb Movements

Restless legs syndrome (RLS) is an unpleasant sleep disorder in which sufferers often feel creeping, crawling, prickling, burning, itching, or tugging sensations in the legs while resting or sitting for extended periods of time. Sometimes the arms may be affected as well. At night, the sensations can be so bothersome that RLS patients feel the need to move the legs and often cannot get to sleep until the discomfort subsides.

Periodic limb movements in sleep (PLMS) is a disorder that often but not necessarily co-exists with restless legs syndrome. PLMS is characterized by sudden, involuntary, and repetitive leg jerking that occurs at the onset of sleep as well as during the course of sleep. These movements can happen every ten to 60 seconds, perhaps hundreds of times, usually in the first half of the night during NREM sleep.

Narcolepsy

Narcolepsy is a chronic sleep disorder in which patients experience daytime sleepiness so excessive that they fall asleep at inappropriate times for a few seconds up to 30 minutes. These sleep "attacks" can occur repeatedly in the course of normal daily activities—talking, eating, working, walking—even after a full night's sleep. Other classic symptoms of narcolepsy are cataplexy, an episodic disorder marked by the sudden loss of muscle function; sleep paralysis, in which the person is temporarily unable to talk or move when falling asleep or waking up; and hypnagogic hallucinations, often-frightening dreamlike experiences that sometimes occur in Stage 1 sleep. Of the estimated 200,000 Americans with narcolepsy, only 20% to 25% suffer from all four symptoms; the rest experience only sleep attacks or a combination of attacks and other symptoms.[7]

Other Dyssomniac Conditions

Delayed sleep phase syndrome (DSPS) is a condition in which people chronically stay up quite late, usually until 3-4 a.m., and then sleep all morning, getting up at 10-11 a.m. If DSPS sufferers must arise earlier in the morning, they do so with great difficulty and experience daytime drowsiness and impaired performance, but still cannot go to sleep until the early morning hours

Advanced sleep phase syndrome (ASPS) is the direct opposite of DSPS. In ASPS, a person tends to fall asleep very early in the evening, usually between 6 p.m. and 9 p.m., and wake up before dawn, sometimes as early as 1 a.m. Sufferers may fall asleep at dinner parties and other social functions, but may force themselves with great difficulty to stay awake in the evening.

Hypersomnia is a sleep disorder in which people sleep too much, either for prolonged periods at night or during the day. Some people normally sleep longer than others—ten or more hours a day—but this does not necessarily indicate a disorder.

Parasomnias

Parasomnias are abnormal physical behaviors that occur during sleep. Usually these conditions involve arousal during the slow-wave stages (3 and 4) of NREM sleep. Parasomniacs aren't actively conscious of their actions and, upon waking, often cannot recall what happened during the nocturnal episodes. Parasomnias tend to run in families and are more common in children.

Sleepwalking, or somnambulism, usually occurs in Stage 4, the deepest sleep stage, during the first third of the night. This parasomnia, as its name suggests, typically involves walking, sitting, or other repetitive, routine motions. Sleepers, however, are not acting out their dreams; each episode generally lasts between five and 15 minutes.[8] Sleepwalkers appear to be conscious during the episodes—their eyes are usually open and pupils dilated, and they're often able to safely navigate around obstacles, such as furniture. But they are not actively conscious of their actions and don't recall the episode upon waking. An estimated four million Americans have consulted doctors about their sleepwalking, according to the American Medical Association.[9] Approximately 10% to 15% of children between the ages of five and 12 have experienced sleepwalking,[10] but adults may also experience this parasomnia.

Night terrors (also called "sleep terrors") are frightening episodes for both sleepers and their housemates. People experiencing this parasomnia suddenly let out a piercing scream or cry, and may even jump out of bed, run out of the house, and do bodily harm to themselves or others. These actions are accompanied by heavy sweating and heart palpitations. Though the sleepers may appear conscious of their acts—their pupils are dilated—they may not awaken until after the episode. Night terrors are not nightmares, because patients have no dream recall; in fact, episodes occur during the deep, NREM (nondream) stages of sleep. As with sleepwalking and other parasomnias, young children tend to suffer more from night terrors; only 1% of adults experience this disorder.[11]

REM behavior disorder (RBD) is a potentially dangerous parasomnia. As indicated by its name, this disorder occurs during the REM (dream) stage of sleep. Normally, most of our muscles become paralyzed during the REM phase to prevent us from acting out our dreams. In RBD, however, it appears the brain does not properly signal the paralysis function and sleepers physically engage in their dreams without being actively conscious of their behavior. Rhythmic movement disorder (RMD) involves head-banging, head-rolling, body-rocking, body-rolling, or other repetitive movements of the head and neck during sleep. It typically occurs immediately prior to sleep onset and is sustained into light sleep (Stages 1 and 2).[12]

Causes of Sleep Disorders

Sleep disorders occur for many reasons: psychological (anxiety and stress), biochemical (neurotransmitter imbalances or the inappropriate use of sleeping pills or other drugs), or medical (the physiological problems often associated with sleep apnea, PLMS, or restless legs syndrome). Other factors include daily living activities (poor diet, food allergies, lack of exercise), an accumulation of toxins in the body (from dietary and environmental sources), biomechanical stress and imbalances, and hormonal imbalances. Any of these contributing factors may also disrupt the circadian rhythms, which could lead to insomnia and other sleep disturbances.

Diet

Diet is a primary factor when considering sleep disorders. Intolerance to certain foods, eating excessively, the consumption of caffeine and sugar, as well as the intake of drugs, nicotine, and alcohol are important concerns.

Caffeine: Konrad Kail, N.D., past President of the American Association of Naturopathic Physicians, notes that caffeine can have a pronounced effect on sleeping habits. "Even a few cups of coffee in the morning can interfere with the quality and quantity of sleep at night," says Dr. Kail, adding that caffeine consumption has been associated with insomnia, periodic limb movement syndrome, and restless legs. He points out that many over-the-counter medications such as cold and cough preparations that contain caffeine or caffeine-related substances, as well as nonherbal teas and soft drinks, can also increase sleep disorders.

Sugar: Much like caffeine, sugar is often consumed because it gives the body an immediate source of energy. As effective as caffeine for providing a short burst of energy, sugar's high is also short-lived. Once consumed, sugar creates uneven blood sugar levels that can disrupt sleep in the middle of the night as your body metabolizes the sugar and demands more. It induces hypoglycemia during the night, according to Kenneth Rifkin, N.D., of Lake Oswego, Oregon.[13] Hypoglycemia, or low blood sugar (glucose), is a condition often associated with diabetes. Symptoms of hypoglycemia include anxiety,

weakness, sweating, rapid heart rate, dizziness, headache, irritability, and poor or double vision, among others.

Drugs, Alcohol, and Nicotine: The sleeping process can be significantly disturbed by drug and alcohol intake. Drugs that may lead to insomnia include thyroid preparations, oral contraceptives, beta-blockers, and marijuana.[14] Alcohol can reduce overall sleep time, including both REM and non-REM sleep.[15] Because nicotine acts as a stimulant, many smokers have insomnia and other sleep problems.[16]

Food Intolerance: Katie Data, N.D., of Fife, Washington, first looks for intolerances to certain foods when treating patients with sleep disorders. She finds the most common food sensitivities are dairy products, wheat, corn, and chocolate. Sugars found in many foods create uneven blood sugar levels (hypoglycemia) that can disrupt sleep and could cause insulin rebound. During the rebound, the body is overwhelmed with an influx of simple sugars and releases excess insulin, which drops the blood sugar levels too low. This condition causes an emergency adrenal stress reaction in the body that prevents sleep and may also result in food addictions; these may develop into a vicious cycle—bingeing on sugary or caffeinated foods and the addictive foods—that keeps sleep patterns out of balance.

Herbert Rinkel, M.D., former Associate Instructor in Medicine at the University of Oklahoma School of Medicine, is considered one of the first to bring to light the issue of food sensitivities. While still a medical student, he discovered his own intolerance to eggs and began to research the field. Dr. Rinkel found that symptoms of tension and jitteriness, common to food-sensitive individuals, are apt to manifest in restlessness and inattentiveness by day and insomnia by night. He concluded that insomnia, as well as tossing about or crying out at night, are frequent manifestations of food intolerance.

Dr. Rinkel says that fatigue is often one of the first symptoms of food intolerance and is most troublesome early in the morning upon rising. This is particularly noticeable in children with food intolerances. People suffering from food intolerances are often irritable during the morning hours and may need a nap in the late afternoon. They frequently suffer from insomnia as well, according to Dr. Rinkel.[17]

According to Dr. Kail, intolerance to certain foods can cause histamine (a substance produced by the body during an allergic reaction) to be released in the brain, which in turn can disturb a person's biochemistry, and can, in some cases, lead to sleep disturbance. He explains that in the brain, histamine replaces neurotransmitters, but because it does not function like other neurotransmitters, it creates a dysfunction in the biochemical pathways of the brain (which are responsible for thinking, mood, and behavior). When these pathways are disrupted, the consequence is exhibited as symptoms, one of which is insomnia.

Environmental Factors

"Items that interfere with the body's electromagnetic field and create electromagnetic fields of their own can disrupt sleep," states Anthony Scott-Morley, D.S.C., Ph.D., M.D. (Alt. Med.), B.A., from Dorset, England. These include electric blankets, electrically heated waterbeds, electric clocks (at the head of the bed), and 60-cycle frequencies (household electric current), as well as power lines and generators.

Also, sleeping near or over geopathic stress zones seriously affects the sleep habits of sensitive individuals. Geopathic stress is defined as an abnormal energy field, often of an electromagnetic nature, created deep underground by large mineral deposits, water streams, or geological faults. Accumulated exposure to these discordant energies (usually due to the location of our homes or beds) can create illnesses, including cancer, migraines, depression, and disrupted sleep.

Dr. Zimmerman adds that sleep problems can sometimes be attributed to factors like ventilation, humidity, noise, or an uncomfortable mattress. Excessive light in the bedroom can also disrupt sleep.

 See Allergies, Environmental Medicine, Stress.

Mental/Emotional Factors

Numerous mental and emotional factors can precipitate sleep disorders, especially insomnia, according to Dr. Zimmerman. These include grief, depression, anxiety, fear, and excitement. Dr. Kail agrees. "Anxiety and depression are two common causes of insomnia. If the insomnia is simply due to a short-term reaction to a situation in one's life, the insomnia will normally disappear as soon as the situation changes." It is rare to see a patient who has a severe case of insomnia due to purely emotional factors, however, he adds. "It is normally a biochemical problem, and biochemical breakdown can take place in many ways. For example, if your digestive system is stressed and unable to digest protein, the amino acids that affect neurotransmission will not be available to your brain and you can become ill emotionally without having anything emotionally stressful going on in your life."

Stress and pent-up emotional issues can wreak havoc on the brain, deregulating brain chemicals and organs that are instrumental in procuring a good night's rest. Unmanaged daily stress can deplete your hormonal and nutrient reserves and create a vicious cycle of less sleep and more stress. Additionally, unresolved psychological issues, such as deep-seated internal fears or relationship conflicts, can disturb brain chemistry and hinder deep sleep.

Physiological Factors

John Hibbs, N.D., of Bastyr University, in Kenmore, Washington, points out that adrenal function can have a significant effect on sleep patterns. In particular, he notes that high nighttime levels of cortisone are associated with many sleep disorders. Cortisone is a hormone secreted by the adrenal glands in the morning or during periods of wakefulness and activity; it is converted in the body into the stress hormone cortisol.

Dr. Hibbs also points out that insomnia can result from any number of conditions that interrupt the sleeping process, including stomach problems or bladder ailments. Concerning periodic limb movements, Dr. Hibbs notes that it is sometimes triggered by a rheumatic disorder or nervous system illness, while sleep apnea may be linked to obesity, particularly if the patient also has heart disease or lung problems from chronic smoking.

While it may not seem readily apparent, the role of the liver and colon are important for establishing and maintaining regular, restful sleep. Both the colon and the liver remove externally acquired toxins and metabolic waste from the body. If either system is not working properly, the body can become dangerously toxic, resulting in conditions such as food allergies and bacterial overgrowth that have been shown to disturb sleep. Heavy metals such as mercury are particularly toxic to the body and can directly cause insomnia. Toxic load can also deplete vitamins and minerals essential to inducing a good night's sleep.

Hormonal imbalances in both men and women can disrupt sleep. While women undergo hormonal shifts in their lifetime such as menopause, it is now known that men undergo a similar shift, referred to as andropause. In both cases, primary sex hormones, such as estrogen and progesterone in women and testosterone in men, shift and decline, resulting in a host of emotional, psychological, and physical changes. Sleep is often disrupted during these transitions.

Sleep can be disrupted if you have structural imbalances, particularly in the spine. Such conditions block the flow of nerve impulses, either causing pain that keeps you awake at night or impinging on the nervous system's ability to send sleep signals. The lack of regular exercise can lead to sleep disorders as well, because it causes muscular tension and allows stress to build up in the body.

Treating Sleep Disorders

Treatments for sleep disorders vary, but effective cures include simple dietary changes, nutritional supplements,

ARE CONVENTIONAL TREATMENTS EFFECTIVE?

Each year, 13 million Americans receive prescriptions for sedatives (sleeping pills).[19] But many medications prescribed by conventional medical practitioners can hide the root cause of a sleep disorder and lead to more dangerous health risks and dependencies. According to Konrad Kail, N.D., over-the-counter or prescription sleeping pills can alter the brain-wave patterns of sleep, thereby preventing a normal cycle of sleep stages. All types of sleeping "aids" function by sedating or depressing the brain. Benzodiazepines slow the brain waves, antidepressants manipulate the levels of brain chemicals, and over-the-counter drugs block histamine and other chemical reactions in the brain and body. Most sleeping pills have a deleterious effect on your sleep cycle, increasing the time spent in light, Stage 2 sleep and diminishing the time spent in deep sleep and REM sleep.

Prescription hypnotics, such as benzodiazepines, can cause a number of side effects including dependence, withdrawal symptoms, a hangover effect, and alteration of the memory process, and may potentiate the effects of alcohol.[20] "Research that has investigated performance on mental tasks (such as learning and decision-making) and motor tasks (such as driving a car) on days after the use of sleeping pills finds that people usually do worse after taking a pill than they do after a night of insomnia," states sleep expert Russel J. Reiter.[21] Another serious side effect that can occur is rebound insomnia—upon discontinuation of the drug, sleep can actually worsen compared to pretreatment levels.[22]

natural hormone replacement therapy, behavioral treatments, herbal and homeopathic remedies, traditional Chinese medicine, and Ayurvedic medicine.

Diet

Diet is especially important when treating sleep disorders, and it is essential to rule out food intolerances as a cause. In one study of infants, sleeplessness was eliminated by removing cow's milk from the diet and then reproduced by its reintroduction.[18] Leon Chaitow, N.D., D.O., of London, England, and other alternative practitioners recommend a combination of nutritional adjustments to aid sleep, including:

- A marked reduction in alcohol consumption.

- Avoid caffeine in all forms (tea, coffee, cola, chocolate).

- Eat a protein-rich snack at bedtime (turkey is one example).

- Eat more raw vegetables and salad greens.

- Eat whole grains and high-fiber foods and avoid simple carbohydrates such as cereals, pastries, and white flour. Whole grains contain many B vitamins, which act as natural sedatives for calming irritability and tension that may hinder deep sleep.

- Eat more protein in the form of moderate amounts of meat, nuts, beans, and avocados. Protein is digested more slowly and doesn't cause an insulin spike, which may interfere with sleep.

- Eat a wide variety of foods to ensure that you are getting sufficient nutrition and consider eating foods on a four-day rotational basis.

- Be aware of the fat content of foods. More important than the total fat is the kind of fat you are eating. Incorporate "healthy fats" such as olive oil, flaxseed oil, walnut oil, and fish oils to be certain your metabolism is running smoothly.

- Take 1 g of niacinamide (vitamin B3) at bedtime (for those that sleep easily but awaken and cannot get back to sleep).

- Take at least 1 g of chlorella or other blue-green algae product at bedtime (as a source of tryptophan).

Nutritional Supplements

The following information highlights specific nutritional supplements known to aid sleep:

- Calcium, especially when contained in food, has a sedative effect on the body, says Dr. Hibbs, who notes that, for adults, doses of approximately 600 mg of liquid calcium have been shown to have a relaxing effect. Magnesium (in doses of approximately 250-500 mg) can also help induce sleep. Magnesium deficiency can cause anxiety, muscle tremors, confusion, irritability, and pain. Magnesium-rich foods include kelp, wheat bran, almonds, cashews, blackstrap molasses, and brewer's yeast.

- The B vitamins are known to have a sedative effect on the nerves. Vitamin B6 (pyridoxine) strongly influences the immune and nervous systems and is needed by the body for the conversion of the amino acid tryptophan to the brain neurotransmitter serotonin, which helps to control sleep. Vitamin B6 supplements of 50-100 mg daily can help to prevent insomnia. Dr. Hibbs notes that 1-2 tablespoons of nutritional yeast is an excellent source of B6 and can be stirred into a glass of juice. Vitamin B12 is another important supplement when treating insomnia, notes Dr. Hibbs, who adds that 25 mcg of vitamin B$_{12}$, supplemented with 100 mg of pantothenic acid (B$_5$), can serve as an effective anti-insomnia vitamin regimen. The best food sources of the B vitamins are liver, whole grains, wheat germ, tuna, walnuts, bananas, sunflower seeds, and blackstrap molasses.

- Vitamin E has been shown effective in treating restless legs syndrome, which may be caused by decreased circulation to the legs. In one study, a 78-year-old female with a history of restless legs found that, after two months of vitamin E supplementation (300 IU daily), she was completely cured.[23] Food sources include cold-pressed polyunsaturated vegetable oils (such as sunflower and safflower), leafy green vegetables, avocados, nuts and seeds, and whole grains. Typical recommended dose: 30 IU daily; for those suffering from restless legs syndrome, 800-1,200 IU of vitamin E should be taken per day. However, if hypertension is present, the dose should start at 40 IU and then be gradually increased while carefully monitoring blood pressure.

- Copper is important for normal function of the central nervous system. Deficiencies in copper have been linked to greater difficulties in getting to sleep and decreased quality of sleep. It may also help alleviate allergic reactions, particularly the levels of histamine. The body's absorption of copper is blocked by a diet high in refined foods or from taking high levels of vitamin C, zinc, and iron. Typical therapeutic dose is 2-5 mg. Copper toxicity is seen more often than copper deficiency, so use of supplements is recommended only after copper levels are measured through hair or urine analysis.

- Iron is essential to red blood cell synthesis, oxygen transport, and energy production. Supplementing with iron has produced significant relief of symptoms in restless legs syndrome.[24] Food sources include kelp, organ meats, egg yolk, blackstrap molasses, lecithin, certain nuts and seeds, millet, beets, parsley, and dark-green leafy vegetables.

- Chromium, available in liquid or capsule form, is often effective for someone with a blood sugar problem that is keeping them awake at night. Dr. Hibbs recommends brewer's yeast as a source or, alternatively, taking 200-500 mcg of chromium polynicotinate twice a day.

- Tryptophan is considered the best amino acid for sleeping problems. It is a precursor to serotonin, which is then converted into melatonin. The presence of melatonin allows the body to drop off into slumber. Tryptophan occurs naturally in certain foods, including turkey and other meats, milk and cheese, pumpkin seeds, and legumes. Unfortunately, L-tryptophan supplements are no longer readily available (except by prescription from custom-compounding pharmacies). There is, however, a substitute called 5-HTP, or 5-hydroxytryptophan, which is a form of tryptophan that is a metabolic step closer to serotonin. It has been shown to be effective in treating depression, fibromyalgia, headaches, and insomnia.[25] The typical recommended dosage of 5-HTP is 25-50 mg daily; it is more effective if taken with N-acetyl-L-carnitine.

- Phosphatidyl-serine, an amino acid that helps the hypothalamus regulate the amount of cortisone produced by the adrenals, is helpful for those who cannot sleep because of high cortisone levels, usually induced by stress. Cortisone is usually at high levels in the morning, for wakefulness, but in stressed individuals it may be high at night and prevent sleeping.

 See Bodywork, Chiropractic, Detoxification Therapy, Diet, Light Therapy, Natural Hormone Replacement Therapy, Nutritional Medicine.

Natural Hormone Therapy

Hormone levels can have a profound influence on sleep. One of the primary symptoms of menopause for women and andropause for men is disturbed sleep. Aging, stress, and an increasingly toxic environment are some of the main factors causing hormonal disruption. By rebalancing hormone levels through nutrition, herbs, and hormone replacement therapy, you can return to getting a good night's sleep.

John R. Lee, M.D., of Sebastopol, California, treats women who are having trouble sleeping with natural progesterone. Estrogen tends to cause brain cells to swell and causes the irritability and sleep disturbances associated with premenstrual syndrome (PMS) and menopause, according to Dr. Lee. Progesterone restores hormonal balance and its calming effect promotes sleep. A randomized, double-blind study involving 63 postmenopausal women over a seven-month period found that hormone therapy "improved sleep quality, facilitated falling asleep, and decreased nocturnal awakenings and restlessness."[26]

A man's testosterone levels start to slowly decrease beginning around age 30, then more rapidly around age 60. Usually by the time a man reaches his mid-fifties (although symptoms may appear earlier), indications of "male menopause" (andropause) are noticeable. Andropause symptoms include fatigue, lack of energy, obesity, a loss of sexual interest and possibly sexual dysfunction, depression or emotional malaise, panic attacks,

MELATONIN—RESETTING THE BIOLOGICAL CLOCK

Research repeatedly confirms the benefits of melatonin supplementation for various sleep/wake rhythm disturbances. Studies have found that melatonin supplements are nontoxic and safe for short-term use, with only mild side effects such as headaches and abdominal cramps in test subjects administered extremely large doses of melatonin (3,000-6,600 mg).

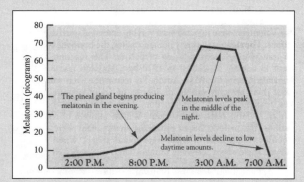

Melatonin effectively relieves insomnia (including cases associated with jet lag and shift work), sleep phase syndromes, and REM behavior disorders. Melatonin can decrease sleep-onset latency in Stages 1 and 2 (light sleep), a helpful boost for those suffering from sleep-onset insomnia.[29] Melatonin has been found to significantly increase deep sleep, REM sleep, and sleep efficiency (time spent in sound sleep), without the "hangover" or stupor effects common with over-the-counter and prescription sleeping pills. Melatonin also works quickly—people usually fall asleep within 30 minutes of taking the supplements.

If melatonin does have a down side, it is on two counts. First, researchers have not discovered the optimal dose of melatonin supplementation. Thus, people taking this hormone generally need to experiment with different dosages before finding the right one for their needs, usually starting with 0.5-2.0 mg per night at bedtime and gradually increasing the dose. Second, the long-term effects of melatonin supplementation are unknown. Also, there is a chance the pineal gland could stop producing its own melatonin if you are supplying it from an external source; this could cause the gland to atrophy. Hence, self-dosing melatonin supplements on a long-term basis is not recommended, without first consulting a health-care practitioner.

decrease in short-term memory, and insomnia. There appears to be a direct relationship between testosterone levels and REM sleep, according to a clinical study. Testosterone levels in four male subjects were measured at 10-20 minute intervals throughout the night. Researchers found a pattern of increases in testosterone concentrations just prior to the onset of periods of REM sleep.[27] Researchers on another study confirmed this finding, stating that there were "positive associations between sleep efficiency, decreased latency to onset of REM, and number of REM episodes, and circulating testosterone."[28] Thus, fluctuations in testosterone during male menopause could have a profound effect on sleep.

Behavioral Treatments

There are many behavioral self-help techniques that can be used for treating insomnia. Dr. Zimmerman offers the following suggestions for a better night's sleep:

1. Don't look at the clock during the sleep period: Few people realize this, but the awareness of how long you have been trying to fall asleep can be a major contributing cause of insomnia. Worrying about how late it is, or how much time is left before you have to get up in the morning, can only contribute to anxiety.

2. Do not spend too much time in bed trying to fall asleep: If you cannot fall asleep in a comfortable period of time, get out of bed and out of the bedroom. Sit or lie down comfortably in another area of the house and engage in some quiet, relaxing activity such as reading or listening to music. When you start to feel sleepy, then (and only then) go back to bed. Do not fall asleep on the sofa or in a chair, because it is important to reserve the sleepy feeling only for the bed. This will strengthen the association of being sleepy and being in bed. Repeat this process as often as necessary during the night and eventually you will break the psychological association of being in bed yet not feeling sleepy enough to fall asleep. In addition, avoid most nonsleeping behaviors in bed. Eliminate reading or watching television in bed.

3. Try sleep restriction therapy: This behavioral self-help measure is based on the observation that many insomniacs spend a great deal of time in bed when they are not actually sleeping. In order to get a good idea if you are spending too much time in bed without sleeping, compute your sleep efficiency index: divide the estimated total amount of sleep you get on a given night by the total amount of time you

spend in bed from the time you turn out the lights until you get up in the morning. If your total sleep time is six hours and your total time in bed is eight hours, your sleep efficiency index is 75%, a figure indicating that you could benefit from sleep restriction therapy. A normal sleep efficiency index is usually 85% or higher. In order to do sleep restriction therapy, compute your sleep efficiency index for one week. If it averages less than 90%, deliberately go to bed later (but preferably not later than 11 p.m.) and/or wake up earlier in the morning. By restricting your time in bed to be about equal to your typical total sleep time, you will increase your sleep efficiency. If you begin to feel sleepy during the day, reward yourself by going to bed earlier or waking up a little later until you have reached a total in-bed time that is not substantially longer than your total sleep time.

4. Exercise: Studies have shown that exercise in the late afternoon or early evening increases the amount of deep sleep that a person gets at night. Evening is a good time for light exercise such as walking. Most physicians recommend a program that elevates the heart rate by 50% to 75% for at least 20 minutes each day.[30] Be warned, however, that the timing of the exercise is important. Exercise done too close to bedtime has a counterproductive effect, since it raises the heart rate and gets the adrenaline going.

5. Spend some time in bright sunlight during the morning hours: Dr. Zimmerman states that few people realize what a powerful influence the bright early morning sunlight has upon circadian rhythm. Studies have shown that exposure to bright, early morning sunlight (between about 7 a.m. and 9 a.m.) for at least 15 minutes is perhaps the most powerful signal that sets the biological clock each morning and entrains it to the 24-hour light/dark cycle. Bright light in the morning has a beneficial effect upon winter depression or seasonal affective disorder (SAD) as well.

Bedtime Rituals

Meditating before going to bed may help to ease worry about falling asleep. If one is prone to insomnia caused by worrying, evenings are definitely not the time to balance a checkbook or to worry about the next day's business. Dr. Zimmerman recommends a warm bath before retiring to help increase circulation to the skin and relax the muscles, and adds that baking soda or Epsom salts (¼–½ cup) in bath water will soothe the nerves on the surface of the skin. A few drops of pine needle essence,

oil of eucalyptus, or mustard powder can also help to relax an individual. Massage, shiatsu, and reflexology are some of the best ways to relieve muscular tension before sleep. Also, breathing techniques can calm the body and promote sleep. Controlled breathing, such as yoga breathing, can help people fall asleep more quickly.

Herbal Medicine

Certain herbs have long been known to induce a peaceful and restful sleep. Chamomile tea and lime blossom tea with a pinch of skullcap are both soothing remedies. Valerian can also bring on a restful sleep. Studies have shown that valerian has an extremely beneficial effect among irregular sleepers (particularly women) and people with difficulty falling asleep.[31] In Germany, valerian root and its teas and extracts are approved as over-the-counter medicines for "states of excitation" and "difficulty in falling asleep owing to nervousness."[32] These herbs should be taken about 45 minutes before bedtime.[33]

For insomnia, David Hoffmann, B.Sc., M.N.I.M.H., of Sebastopol, California, past President of the American Herbalists Guild, recommends linden flowers, which are especially effective for people with blood pressure problems. Stronger remedies such as passionflower or hops can be very relaxing. Pharmacological studies indicate antispasmodic, sedative, anxiety-allaying, and hypotensive (blood pressure–lowering) activity of passionflower extracts.[34] European medicinal plant researchers have approved the use of hops for such conditions as nervous tension, excitability, restlessness, and sleep disturbances.

An extract of the kava-kava plant (a slow-growing bushy perennial) acts as a natural tranquilizer. In one study, when 29 patients diagnosed with anxiety (including panic disorder and general tension) took kava-kava (100 mg three times daily for four weeks) and were then evaluated using three standard psychological profiles of anxiety, all measures were significantly lower. No side effects or adverse reactions occurred and benefits were noted as early as the first and second weeks.[35] A typical recommended dose is 100 mg of kava extract (standardized to 70% kavalactones, the active ingredient) daily, divided into three equal doses.

The flower of the chamomile plant (German or wild, *Matricaria recutita*; Roman, *Anthemis nobilis*) produces a calming effect, easing anxiety and reducing tension.[36] It can thus be helpful with overall anxiety, sleep disorders, and muscle tension. Its calming property has a beneficial effect on the gastrointestinal system as well.

Hoffmann also suggests an herb bath before going to bed. Fill a muslin bag with chamomile, linden flowers, or lavender, and hang it from the faucet so that the hot water runs through it. He also recommends herbs such as Siberian ginseng and licorice, pantothenic acid

BIOFEEDBACK FOR INSOMNIA

Biofeedback training is a method of learning how to consciously regulate normally unconscious bodily functions (breathing, heart rate, and blood pressure) through the use of simple electronic or other monitoring devices. Learning relaxation techniques guided by biofeedback helps you reduce or eliminate sleep problems.

Sleep researcher Peter Hauri, Ph.D., says that people who have insomnia because of extreme muscle tension can be helped using biofeedback. In two experiments, Dr. Hauri found that biofeedback had a lasting effect on insomnia. In the first study, at Dartmouth Medical School, 45 insomniacs kept records of their sleep habits and then spent three nights in a sleep laboratory. They were given biofeedback training and then continued with biofeedback at home. They returned to the lab for checkups after several weeks and again after nine months. The study showed that insomniacs who were tense and anxious were helped by biofeedback, but it didn't help people who were relaxed muscularly but still couldn't sleep. In a second study, 16 subjects had suffered with chronic insomnia for at least two years. They were evaluated during three nights at the Dartmouth Sleep Disorders Center, then they participated in biofeedback training. Sleep improved for the 16 subjects after the biofeedback training, and again at the nine-month checkup. But Dr. Hauri again emphasizes that muscle-tension biofeedback works best for people who can't sleep because they are muscularly tense.[37]

"Biofeed-in" therapy may also be helpful. One of the most effective biofeed-in techniques for insomnia is auditory binaural sound therapy. In this therapy, earphones are placed on both ears and pulsing sounds are delivered at different rates in each ear. The sound difference between the ears is gradually decreased over a few minutes. This entrains the brain waves to slow down.

(vitamin B5), and exercise, all of which can help return the adrenal glands to normal functioning.

Homeopathy

For occasional, acute, or short-term insomnia, here are some basic remedies and their indicators. Take them in 30C dosage, one hour before going to bed for ten nights. Repeat the dose if you wake and cannot get to sleep again. For chronic insomnia, you will need to see a classical homeopathic practitioner (or one that is able to use that approach) to get a constitutional remedy.[38]

Aconite: Sleep problems worse after shock or panic; restlessness, nightmares, fear of dying.

Arsenicum album: Waking between midnight and 2 a.m., restless, worried, apprehensive, foreboding dreams of fire or danger.

Belladonna: Restlessness, irritability, overly sensitive to stimuli including light, noise, and touch; excited, angry and trouble falling asleep.

Chamomilla: Feeling wide awake and irritable during first part of night, especially if person is a child and wants to be carried around.

Coffea: Mind overactive as the result of good or bad news; inability to switch off.

Ignatia: Yawns a lot but can't sleep, dreads not being able to sleep, especially after emotional upset; when sleep comes, nightmares come too; grief is also an indication.

Lycopodium: Mind very active at bedtime, going over and over work done during the day; person aware of frequent dreaming, talks and laughs in sleep, wakes around 1 a.m.

Natrum muriaticum: Anxiety, anxious dreams, becoming ill after emotional trauma; sudden noise and heat bother the person.

Nux vomica: Sleeplessness due to great mental strain, overindulgence in food or alcohol, or withdrawal from alcohol or sleeping pills; wakes around 3 a.m. or 4 a.m., then falls asleep just as it is time to get up; nightmares, irritable during the day.

Pulsatilla: Restless in first sleep, feels too hot, throws covers off, then feels too cold and lies with arms above head; not thirsty, insomnia worse after rich food.

Rhus toxicodendron: Irritable, restless, walks about, can't sleep, especially if there is pain or discomfort.

Cocculus: Too tired to sleep, giddy.

Opium: Sharp senses, bed too hot.

In addition, Robert Milne, M.D., of Las Vegas, Nevada, traces many cases of insomnia to grief. For grieving individuals whose symptoms include irritability, sobbing, and muscle spasms, *Ignatia amara* is often used. Another remedy, *Muriaticum acidum*, is recommended for grief-stricken insomnia patients who are marked by extreme emotional sensitivity (another symptom may be an intolerance of sunlight).

Traditional Chinese Medicine

Traditional Chinese medicine views almost all sleep disorders as stemming from kidney problems or weakness. According to Roger Hirsh, O.M.D., of Santa Monica, California, the kidneys, like all the body's organs, store energy. When the kidney's ability to store energy is compromised, sleep disorders can result. Dr. Hirsh cites the example of people who get a surge of energy at 11 p.m., preventing them from falling asleep. The energy should go deep in the body, says Dr. Hirsh, but because there is kidney energy deficiency, the kidney is unable to hold the energy in, which keeps the person awake. Though the energy reserves of the kidney are depleted during the aging process, a person can help preserve or restore energy vital to the sleep process by tonifying the kidneys. This is done primarily with herbal remedies, such as a commonly available six-herb formula known as *liu wei di huang wan*. In addition, Qigong postures and exercises are beneficial to the kidneys and can help the sleep process.

Some Chinese doctors recommend that their patients with insomnia soak their feet in hot water before bedtime, then dry the feet and put on loose-fitting cotton socks, followed by loose wool socks over the other socks (but not pulled up as far). Alternatively, a hot water bottle against a pillow at the foot of the bed to warm the feet also relaxes the body.

Studies show that some insomnia may be due to a deficiency of endorphins and thus acupuncture is often a useful therapy. During acupuncture, patients tend to become drowsy or even fall asleep, possibly because of increased levels of endorphins.[39]

 See Acupuncture, Ayurvedic Medicine, Traditional Chinese Medicine.

Ayurvedic Medicine

The Ayurvedic approach to sleep disorders focuses on *vata*, the constitutional unit of the body that regulates breathing and circulation. According to Virender Sodhi, M.D. (Ayurveda), N.D., Founder of the Ayurvedic & Naturopathic Medical Clinic, in Bellevue, Washington, people with a *vata* imbalance frequently exhibit irritability, anxiety, and fear, making it difficult for them to rest or relax. "Our aim," says Dr. Sodhi, "is to calm down, relax, and pacify the excessive *vata* system."

TREATMENT GUIDELINES FOR SLEEP APNEA

- Use a CPAP—the continuous positive airway pressure (CPAP) device is a mask that forces air through the nose to keep the throat open.

- Lose weight—reduces fat in the throat and can open up the airway.

- Sew a tennis ball into the back of the person's pajama top—to prevent sleeping on the back.

- Stop smoking—cigarettes can cause nasal and throat swelling.

- Avoid alcohol, tranquilizers, sleeping pills, and antihistamines in the evening—these can relax throat muscles to the point of collapse.

- Use nasal tape—available over-the-counter, nasal strips pull the sides of the nose outward, holding the nasal passages open.

- Eliminate allergens in the home—dust, mold, or other allergens may cause nasal congestion.

- Raise the head of the bed or add pillows—sleeping with your head raised helps drain congestion and open your airways.

- Develop a consistent sleep schedule—regular sleeping may help keep breathing stable and decrease snoring.

- Wash out your sinuses—a process called pulsatile nasal irrigation uses a WaterPik with a special attachment to clear out thick secretions. Ask your health-care practitioner.

- Get a custom dental splint—good for people with large tongues, the dental splint holds the jaw forward so that the tongue can't fall back toward the throat and obstruct breathing.

A primary treatment for sleep disorders is the topical application of oil to the head and feet. Depending on an individual's body type, different kinds of oil are used at varying temperatures to relax the nervous system. These include coconut oil (*pitta* type, used at room temperature), sesame oil (*vata* type, applied warm), and mustard oil (*kapha* type, applied warm). Meditation is another form of treatment. Dr. Sodhi explains that by repeating soothing mantras, such as "I sleep properly," in the morning and evening, it is possible to alleviate the anxiety and fear that can interfere with normal sleeping habits. Other forms of meditation, including the use of visualization

FENG SHUI FOR AN ENERGY-FRIENDLY BEDROOM

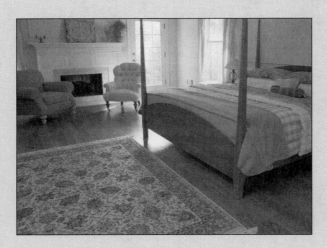

Feng shui is a method from traditional Chinese culture concerned with the proper ways to arrange furniture, rooms, houses, offices, churches, tombs, and other human-made structures with respect to maximizing the favorable energies. The term, which means "wind and water" (although popularly it is known as the art of placement), is drawn from the ancient Chinese philosophy of Taoism, which linked energies of the solar system and Earth with human habitation and activities. Feng shui documents the flow or impedance of basic life force energy, or *qi*, through environments, building structures, homes, and rooms for the benefit or detriment of their inhabitants. Here are some ways to make your bedroom a health-enhancing, not health-draining, environment, according to feng shui:

- Where you put the bed is very important in feng shui. Ideally, it should be diagonally across from the room

entrance, so that people in the bed have a full view of anyone coming in the door.[40] If you move your bed to straddle the corner, be sure to put a headboard or shelf behind it with plants, candles, stones, or other nurturing items. Corners are considered a place where *qi* can stagnate unless you add items that keep the *qi* flowing. If you can't place the bed catercorner to the entrance, add a mirror to reflect the entryway or place a wind chime between the entrance and the bed and keep the mirror opposite the entrance. Also, try to have the bed face the morning sunlight.

- Avoid placing your bed next to a window because you will lose too much vital energy *(qi)* out the window during the night. Also, the energy coming in the windows at night could disrupt your body's *yin* energies and prevent sleep. But allow as much air and sunlight into the bedroom during the day as possible to accumulate *qi* to help replenish the body during sleep.

- Pay attention to other details of *qi* flow in the bedroom. If you have a bathroom off the bedroom, be sure to buffer the *qi* of the bathroom with a curtain, mirror, or other divider. If you have a desk in the bedroom, have it screened off or away from the main flow of *qi*.

- Do not face sharp edges. The sharp edges from bookcases, dressers, and other furniture in the bedroom should not face where you lie in bed. Otherwise, the energy coming off the edges is sharp and this bombardment with energy rays can harm your health and create irritability.

and aromas (sandalwood, chamomile, jasmine, rose), can also be effective.

Addressing Electromagnetic Pollution and Geopathic Stress

To minimize the effects of electromagnetic pollution on sleep, Dr. Scott-Morley recommends that all electrical appliances such as radios, alarm clocks, televisions, and computers should be at least six feet from the bed. Electric blankets and electric heating pads should not be used and all appliances should be unplugged before sleeping (or the electricity breaker switch for the bedroom should be turned off). The bed frame should be made of wood with no long metal parts, and the mattress and box platform should not contain metal coils. Waterbeds should be avoided. Do not sleep directly over garages, fuel tanks, or steel girders.

"Because geopathic stresses are usually confined to a small area, moving the bed to another location may be sufficient to avoid these stresses," says Dr. Scott-Morley. "The best way to detect geopathic disturbance is with instruments such as the geomagnetometer, despite some limitations. If dowsing is employed, then at least two dowsers should independently survey the property to see if both obtain the same results."

Recommendations

- Reduce alcohol consumption and avoid caffeine in all its forms.

- Eat more protein in the form of moderate amounts of meat, nuts, beans, and avocados. Protein is digested more slowly and doesn't cause an insulin spike, which may interfere with sleep. Eat whole grains and high-fiber foods and avoid simple carbohydrates such as cereals, pastries, and white flour.

- Calcium, especially when contained in food, has a sedative effect on the body. Magnesium (in doses of approximately 250 mg) can also help induce sleep. Tryptophan is considered the best amino acid for sleeping problems (L-tryptophan is a precursor to serotonin, which is then converted into melatonin); 5-HTP is the readily available supplement form of tryptophan.

- Melatonin effectively relieves insomnia (including cases associated with jet lag and shift work), sleep phase syndromes, and REM behavior disorders.

- Hormone levels can have a profound influence on sleep. By rebalancing hormone levels through nutrition, herbs, and hormone therapy, you can return to getting a good night's sleep.

- Do not spend too much time in bed trying to fall asleep. If you cannot fall asleep in a comfortable period of time, get out of bed and out of the bedroom. Sit or lie down comfortably in another area of the house and engage in some quiet, relaxing activity such as reading or listening to music.

- Meditating before going to bed may help to ease worry about falling asleep.

- Chamomile tea and lime blossom tea with a pinch of skullcap are both soothing remedies. Valerian can also bring on a restful sleep. Stronger remedies such as passionflower, kava-kava, or hops can be very relaxing.

- To minimize the effects of electromagnetic pollution on sleep, all electrical appliances such as radios, alarm clocks, televisions, and computers should be at least six feet from the bed. Electric blankets and electric heaters should not be used and all appliances should be unplugged before sleeping.

- Having a professional dowser or baubiologist find the geopathic fields in the bedroom so that the bed can be moved away from these fields also helps sleep considerably.

Self-Care

The following therapies can be undertaken at home under appropriate professional supervision:

Biofeedback Training and Neurotherapy / Guided Imagery / Qigong and Tai Chi

HYDROTHERAPY: Immersion bath or wet sheet pack (neutral application as needed for sedation).

JUICE THERAPY: Carrot, spinach, lettuce, celery juice.

LIGHT THERAPY: Full-spectrum and bright-light therapies have been effective in treating sleep disorders and seasonal affective disorder. Researchers have found three hours of light therapy (2,500–3,000 lux) accompanied by intravenous vitamin B_{12} (5–6 mg daily) reset the circadian rhythms of melatonin secretion and can be effective in rectifying delayed sleep phase syndromes and other sleep/wake disturbances.[41]

Professional Care

The following therapies should only be provided by a qualified health professional:

Acupuncture / Ayurvedic Medicine / Chiropractic / Craniosacral Therapy / Detoxification Therapy / Magnetic Field Therapy / Osteopathic Medicine / Naturopathic Medicine / Traditional Chinese Medicine

Where to Find Help

For more information on sleep disorders, or referrals to a qualified health-care practitioner, contact the following organizations.

National Sleep Foundation
1522 K Street N.W., Suite 500
Washington, D.C. 20005
Website: www.sleepfoundation.org

The National Sleep Foundation (NSF) is an independent nonprofit organization dedicated to improving public health and safety by achieving public understanding of sleep and sleep disorders, and by supporting public education, sleep-related research, and advocacy.

American Sleep Apnea Association
1424 K Street N.W., Suite 302
Washington, D.C. 20005
(202) 293-3650
Website: www.sleepapnea.org

The American Sleep Apnea Association is dedicated to reducing injury, disability, and death from sleep apnea and to enhancing the well-being of those affected by this disorder. The ASAA promotes education and awareness, support groups, research, and improvement of care.

American Sleep Disorders Association (ASDA)
1610 14th Street N.W., Suite 300
Rochester, Minnesota 55901
(507) 287-6006

The ASDA can refer you to a sleep disorders center near you.

American Association of Oriental Medicine
433 Front Street
Catasauqua, Pennsylvania 18032
(888) 500-7999
Website: www.aaom.org

The AAOM is a national professional trade organization of acupuncturists who meet acceptable standards of competency and can provide you with the names and locations of local members.

American Association of Naturopathic Physicians
8201 Greensboro Drive, Suite 300
McLean, Virginia 22101
(703) 610-9037
Website: www.naturopathic.org

Provides a directory of naturopathic physicians and offers referrals to a nationwide network of accredited or licensed practitioners. Also publishes a quarterly newsletter, for both professionals and the general public, and offers a series of brochures and pamphlets on a variety of subjects.

Recommended Reading

The Complete Guide to Sleep. Dian Dincin Buchman, Ph.D. New Canaan, CT: Keats Publishing, 1997.

No More Sleepless Nights. Peter Hauri, Ph.D., and Shirley Linde, Ph.D. New York: John Wiley, 1990.

The Promise of Sleep. William C. Dement, M.D., Ph.D., with Christopher Vaughan. New York: Delacorte Press, 1999.

Sleep Disorders: An Alternative Medicine Definitive Guide. Herbert Ross, D.C., and Keri Brenner, L.Ac., with Burton Goldberg. Tiburon, CA: AlternativeMedicine.com Books, 2000.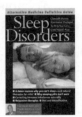

Sleep Right in Five Nights. James Perl, Ph.D. New York: William Morrow/Quill, 1993.

STRESS

Current estimates show that between 70% and 80% of all visits to physicians are for stress-related disorders.[1] Chronic stress directly affects the immune system and, if not effectively dealt with, can seriously compromise health. Alternative medicine offers many beneficial strategies for reducing stress and its effects, including acupuncture, biofeedback, meditation, guided imagery, and lifestyle counseling, as well as diet and nutritional programs, herbs, and exercise.

STRESS CAN BE defined as a reaction to any stimulus or challenge that upsets normal function and disturbs mental or physical health. It can be brought on by internal conditions such as illness, pain, or emotional conflict, or by external circumstances such as a death in the family or financial problems. Even a positive experience—a new marriage, a job promotion, or financial gain—can be a stress-provoking event.

Although a certain amount of stress is a normal part of our lives, prolonged bouts of stress can lead to exhaustion and illness, along with more serious health problems.

"Stress can also be caused by allergic reactions, poor diet, nutritional deficiencies, substance abuse, or biochemical imbalances in the body," according to Konrad Kail, N.D., past President of the American Association of Naturopathic Physicians. "These internal imbalances are a major contributing factor to stress. They help to set up a cycle in which a stressor causes a biochemical imbalance in the body; this, in turn, depletes the immune system, causing illness, which creates more stress for the person, and the cycle continues."

Although a certain amount of stress is a normal part of our lives, prolonged bouts of stress can lead to exhaustion and illness, along with more serious health problems. Eric Peper, Ph.D., Associate Director of the Institute of Holistic Healing Studies at San Francisco State University, states that up to 80% of the health problems in America today are considered stress-related. According to Dr. Kail, "Repeated incidences of stress can interfere with digestion, alter brain chemistry, increase heart rate and blood pressure, and affect metabolic and immune functioning."

He cites studies that show depressed immune function to be associated with many stress-inducing experiences and conditions, including bereavement, divorce, job loss, school or professional examinations, depression, loneliness, and sleep deprivation.[2] Stress is a pervasive problem among Americans, according to a poll of corporate executives. For example, 44% of employees polled said their work load is excessive compared to 37% in 1988; 43% are bothered by excessive job pressure; and 55% worry considerably about their company's future; 25% of both men and women feel stressed out at work every day, another 12% feel it almost every day, and another 38% feel it once to several days a week.[3]

Fortunately, stress and its effects can be reduced through exercise, relaxation therapies, diet and nutrition, acupuncture, and lifestyle changes. These therapeutic approaches can help restore normal function to the internal biochemical processes and help to reverse chronic stress.

Types of Stress

While some sources of stress are always harmful to the body (distress) and clearly to be avoided whenever possible, other sources of stress can produce a positive effect on the body (called positive stress, or eustress), depending upon the person, situation, and context. Some have said that the difference between positive stress and distress can be likened to a violin string—you want to have just the right amount of tension to make music, but not so much that the string snaps. Signs of distress are registered in the body as a headaches, heart palpitations, pain, constricted throat, clammy palms, weariness, nausea, or

927

Autonomic Nervous System

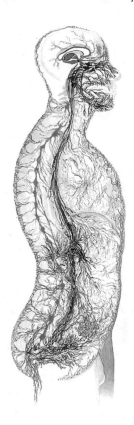

The autonomic nervous system (ANS) can be likened to your body's automatic pilot. It keeps you alive through breathing, heart rate, and digestion, without your being aware of it or participating in its activities. The ANS has two divisions: the sympathetic, which expends body energy, and the parasympathetic, which conserves energy. The sympathetic nervous system is associated with arousal and stress; it prepares us physically when we perceive a threat or challenge by increasing our heart rate, blood pressure, and muscle tension. The parasympathetic nervous system slows heart rate and increases intestinal and most gland activity.

diarrhea. Though the demands, or "stressors," that can provoke a bodily reaction are quite varied, they fall into four broad categories:

- Physical Stress—trauma (infection, injury, surgery); exercise (too much or too little); intense physical labor; environmental pollution (pesticides, herbicides, toxins, heavy metals, inadequate light, radiation, noise, geopathic stress, electromagnetic fields); childbirth; illness (viral, bacterial, or fungal agents); fatigue; inadequate supply of oxygen; hypoglycemia;

hormonal and biochemical imbalances; dietary stress (protein or fat excesses or deficiencies, sugar, hydrogenated oils, food allergens, nutritional deficiencies); dehydration; substance abuse; poor joint alignment; dental problems.

- Psychological Stress—emotional stress (resentment, fear, frustration, sadness, anger, or bereavement); mental stress (information overload, perfectionism, worry, guilt, shame, jealousy, self-criticism, anxiety, and a sense of loss of control); perceptual stress (beliefs, attitudes, world view).

- Psychosocial Stress—relationship difficulties (friends, neighbors, colleagues, employer, family); lack of social support; isolation.

- Psychospiritual Stress—crisis of values, meaning, and purpose; joyless striving versus meaningful work; misalignment with core beliefs.

How Stress Affects Health

Almost everyone experiences stress on a daily basis. Although stress itself is not a disease, it can aggravate numerous conditions, including allergies, arthritis, asthma, atherosclerosis, cancer, colitis, diabetes, emphysema, gastritis, hypertension, hypoglycemia, neuromuscular syndromes, speech problems, and ulcers, according to Dr. Kail. "Whatever the source or cause of the stress, human beings respond biochemically to stress in a very predictable manner," he adds. "Stress begets illness which increases stress, thereby aggravating the illness." Dr. Kail's review of the available research reveals the following recurrent themes associated with stress:

- High levels of stress increase susceptibility to illness.[4]

- Chronic stress results in a suppression of the immune system, which in turn creates increased susceptibility to illness, especially to immune-related disorders and cancer.[5]

- Emotional stress leads to hormonal imbalances (adrenal, pituitary, thyroid, and others) that further interfere with immune function.[6]

Pioneering stress researcher Hans Selye, M.D., noted a consistent pattern of response to stress in his studies and termed this the *General Adaptation Syndrome* (GAS). Outlined in three stages, it consists of the alarm reaction, the stage of resistance, and the stage of exhaustion.[7] Initially, the body's biochemistry tends to react to stress in an orderly fashion. Stimulation of the sympathetic nervous system (part of the autonomic nervous system) activates the secretion of hormones from endocrine glands and constricts both the blood vessels and the involuntary muscles of the body. When the endocrine glands are stimulated, heart rate, glucose metabolism, and oxygen consumption increase. The parasympathetic nervous system is also stimulated, which begins a process of relaxation. The pituitary gland responds by releasing a variety of hormones throughout the body, which influences the defensive and adaptive mechanisms. Endorphins, the body's own natural painkillers, are also released.[8]

The adrenal glands are responsible for the production of the hormones epinephrine (adrenaline) and norepinephrine (noradrenaline). These hormones are released in direct response to the sympathetic nervous system, which is responsible for the fight-or-flight response to stress or physical threats. The adrenal cortex, the outer layer, is responsible for the production of corticosteroids (also called adrenal steroids), including cortisol and cortisone. Under conditions of stress, high amounts of cortisol are released.

Dr. Selye points out, however, that chronic stress eventually depletes the body's resources and its ability to adapt. If stress continues and remains unattended for a long period, coping functions will be compromised and illness will result.

Stress-Related Anxiety

Stress is not always an unhealthy experience, and some people even seem to thrive on it. Dr. Kail explains, for example, that stress can help top-level executives control anxiety. Middle-management employees, by contrast, are far more susceptible to uncontrollable situations and, as it turns out, are at higher risk for cancer. "Any stress that allows an individual to defend against anxiety is anti-cancer," according to Frederick Levenson, Ph.D., who teaches at Hofstra University and the Center for Modern Psychoanalytic Studies, in New York City. "Any stress that places the individual in high performance anxiety situations in which the variables cannot be manipulated will produce high levels of internal carcinogens."[9]

In a 1997 study of 7,372 men and women, Michael Marmot, Ph.D., showed that the level of influence or control over one's work experiences affects the risk for heart disease. More specifically, the lower the amount of control employees had over their work, the higher the incidence of heart problems. This factor proved to be more important than sheer volume of work or income level.[10]

Everyone reacts differently to stress, and the amount of emotional stress a person experiences depends on the individual's coping functions. A person's temperament and learned experiences are important psychological mediators of stress and anxiety level. Most people are aware of the studies regarding people who exhibit either Type A or Type B behavior. Unlike their more relaxed,

noncompetitive, and philosophical Type B counterparts, Type As are typically portrayed as being impatient—they try to do many things at once as they strive toward a valued goal. This goal-oriented behavior and the tendency to be self-critical and short-tempered prevent them from experiencing a sense of joy in their achievements. Beginning in the 1960s, studies began to show that personality type has a profound influence on health. One study followed 3,000 middle-aged men over eight-and-a-half years and found that Type As were twice as likely to develop heart disease as Type Bs.[11] A recent study of air traffic controllers found that Type As had three-and-a-half times more job-related injuries and 38% more illnesses overall than Type Bs.[12]

Some common symptoms of anxiety include excessive or unwarranted worrying, a rising sense of panic, restlessness, insomnia, trembling or feeling shaky, muscle tension, fatigue, infections, shortness of breath, heart palpitations, sweaty or clammy hands, back pain, hot flashes or chills, dizziness, irritability, loss of memory, and difficulty concentrating.

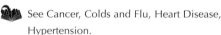 See Cancer, Colds and Flu, Heart Disease, Hypertension.

Increased Susceptibility to Infections

Of all the body's systems, stress damages immune function the most. It does so by overly activating the sympathetic part of the autonomic nervous system, which results in an increased secretion of adrenal hormones, especially cortisol and adrenaline. These hormones inhibit white blood cell function, decrease the production of lymphocytes, and cause the thymus gland, the master gland of the immune system, to shrink. The end result is that there is a significant reduction in immune system function and an increased susceptibility to infection and illness.

In an experiment on the relationship between stress and the probability of viral infection, 420 people were evaluated for occurrences of stress during the course of a year. These included such events as job loss, death in the family, moving, divorce, or feeling frightened, nervous, sad, angry, irritated, or unable to cope with current demands. They were then exposed to one of five cold viruses and tested one month later for antibodies. Ninety percent of those who were under the greatest stress became infected, compared to 74% of those who experienced the least amount of stress.[13] In another study of 100 subjects, those who experienced stress (particularly the type of stress associated with tension and anger) were four times more likely to develop a cold or bacterial infection.[14]

Researchers at New York's Mount Sinai Hospital found that men who lost their spouse experienced a significant drop in their immune function. The T cells and B lymphocytes, important to the immune system's surveillance mechanism, stopped doing their job. Interestingly enough, if these white blood cells were removed from the body and placed in a solution that is normally stimulating, they remained passive.[15]

Heart Problems

Stress may trigger arrhythmias or cause the bioelectrical system that controls the heartbeat to malfunction in some individuals, with potentially fatal results. Using nuclear imaging techniques, it has been shown that the blood supply to the heart in a stressful situation is actually diminished, even though more work is being demanded from it. Arteries constrict not only in our arms and legs but also in our hearts, leading to spasms in the heart muscle.[16]

Researchers at Duke University Medical Center studied 126 people for five years and found that 27% of those who responded adversely to mental stress, such as public speaking or tight deadlines, later suffered serious heart problems. Grief can also torment the mind and heart. A study of 1,236 men and 538 women found that within the first 24 hours following the death of a loved one, close friends and family members have a 14-fold increased risk of heart attack. The risk of heart attack remains eight times above normal on the second day; six times on the third day, and 2–4 times above normal for the next month.[17]

Allergies and Asthma

Dr. Kail reports that physicians are seeing increasing numbers of patients complaining of stress-related disorders such as allergies, candidiasis, and chronic fatigue syndrome. He explains that an allergic reaction is a stressor that can trigger a variety of symptoms, including irritability, aggressive behavior, depression, and anxiety. During an allergic reaction, the body releases histamine, a chemical that is present in cells throughout the body. Histamine causes inflammation, excess stomach acid, a narrowing of the air pathways in the lungs, and increased stress on other organs and glands. Dr. Kail also notes that because stress affects the immune and endocrine systems, leaving them in a weakened, susceptible state, chronic stress may actually precipitate the allergic reaction in the first place.

In one experiment, 130 adults with asthma documented (three times a day for three weeks) their stressors, frequency of asthma symptoms, peak flow readings (a measure of how much air the lungs can expel), and use of bronchodilators. Stress was positively correlated with lowered breathing ability and increased symptoms of asthma and use of bronchodilators.[18] "Allergies are significant stressors," says Dr. Kail. "Their proper diagnosis and treatment should be included in any medical checkup."

 See Allergies, Diabetes, Respiratory Conditions.

Treating and Reducing Stress

If stress contributes to illness, then stress reduction should promote healing. This theory for alleviating stress is the basis of numerous relaxation therapies, such as meditation, guided imagery, biofeedback, yoga, and Qigong. Other methods for treating stress include dietary changes, herbal medicine, exercise, Ayurvedic medicine, and traditional Chinese medicine.

Life experiences, beginning with infancy and childhood, shape behavior in significant ways. How these experiences are handled often affects our ability to deal with stress in the future. Therefore, it is important for both children and adults to learn effective coping skills (or "stress hardiness") when dealing with stressful stimuli and events. Failure to do so, says Dr. Kail, can result in emotional imbalance, which in turn affects the biochemistry of the body and can lead to serious psychological and physiological problems.

Relaxation Therapies

Meditation, biofeedback, guided imagery, yoga, and Qigong all have one thing in common—they facilitate deep relaxation and reduce stress. Herbert Benson, M.D., of Harvard Medical School, called this physiological mechanism "the relaxation response" and has applied its principles to the treatment of illness, using it to lower blood pressure and decrease gastric acid secretion.[20] Dean Ornish, M.D., of the University of California at San Francisco, has been able to reverse heart disease by employing a combination of meditation, stress-reduction exercises, psychotherapy, and a vegetarian diet.[21] Stress-reduction techniques often employ deep breathing and visualization in order to enhance the relaxation process.

MEDITATION

Meditation is a safe and simple way to balance a person's physical, emotional, and mental states. At the University of Massachusetts Medical School, Jon Kabat-Zinn, Ph.D., founded the Stress Reduction Clinic in 1979 to help people suffering from chronic pain, chronic diseases such as cancer and heart disease, as well as stress-related disorders such as abdominal pain, chronic diarrhea, and ulcers. According to Dr. Kabat-Zinn, these conditions are often the most difficult to treat and the patients have frequently tried more conventional forms of medicine without complete success. Dr. Kabat-Zinn's stress-reduction program was originally designed to test the value of using meditation to help patients develop effective coping strategies for stress, and to see whether meditation would have any effect on their chronic medical conditions. According to Dr. Kabat-Zinn, the majority of people improved in a number of ways.[22]

Meditation is so effective in reducing stress and tension that, in 1984, the National Institutes of Health recommended meditation over prescription drugs as the first treatment for mild hypertension.[23] In addition, Dr. Benson has documented that meditation has the beneficial physiological effect of slowing breathing rate, increasing oxygen utilization, creating a more relaxed brain-wave rhythm, and increasing blood flow.[24] Meditation has also been shown to have a positive effect on immune function and in strengthening the body's defenses against infectious disease.[25]

Transcendental Meditation (TM) is the most well-documented type of meditation regarding its physiological effects, with more than 500 clinical studies conducted to date.[26] Research shows that during TM practice, the body gains a deeper state of relaxation than during ordinary rest or sleep.[27] Changes in brain waves indicate a state of enhanced awareness and coherence and TM has been found to increase intelligence, creativity, and perceptual ability and reduce blood pressure and rates of illness by 50%.[28] TM also causes decreased blood levels of cortisol, a hormone responsible for many of the deleterious physiological changes seen with stress.[29]

BIOFEEDBACK TRAINING

Biofeedback training is another method for learning how to regulate body functions to reduce physical and psychological stress. It is often used in conjunction with other relaxation and stress-reduction techniques. Through the use of visual or auditory signals from a machine that records physiological responses, one can learn to voluntarily relax specific muscles, alter the brain's electrical activity, reduce heart rate and blood pressure, increase body warmth, and improve gastrointestinal function.[30]

Biofeedback devices give immediate "feedback" or information about the biological system of the person being monitored, so that he or she can learn to consciously influence that system. For example, a person seeking to regulate their heart rate would train with a biofeedback device set up to transmit one blinking light or one audible beep per heartbeat. Electrodes are placed on the patient's skin (a simple, painless process) and the person is then instructed to use various techniques, such

MIND/BODY MEDICINE AND STRESS

A basic premise in mind/body medicine is that chronic stress contributes to illness and that relaxation, positive ways of coping with stress, and restoration of integral physical and mental/emotional functioning will improve one's health. More important than the stressors themselves is the person's ability to cope with them. If there is a psychological process that is conducive to the development of chronic disease, as the science of psychoneuroimmunology suggests, then there is a corresponding psychological process for recovery. This process may include counseling, involvement in a therapeutic support group, and/or the conscious decision to alter one's lifestyle and behavior. Feelings of hope and renewed optimism not only improve one's psychological state, but also promote better immune function.

In a recent research review, Jeanne Achterberg, Ph.D., President of the Association for Transpersonal Psychology, cited numerous studies demonstrating that feelings of security, coupled with the ability to cope, counter the negative emotions that can interfere with healing, compromise the immune system, and encourage cardiovascular disease.[19] Pioneering stress researcher Hans Selye, M.D., pointed out that overly ambitious goals and personal objectives that exceed one's experience and skills commonly increase stress. He suggested that a person measure the benefit of performing a stressful task to determine if it is worth the involvement. He also recommended that people avoid unnecessary stress and try to limit stress or stressful situations to more manageable scheduled times whenever possible.

as meditation, relaxation, and visualization, to effect the desired response (muscle relaxation, lowered heart rate). The biofeedback device reports the person's progress by a change in the speed of the beeps or flashes. By learning to alter the rate of the flashes or beeps, the person would be subtly programmed to control heart rate.

Neurotherapy, an extension of biofeedback, reprograms a person's dominant brain wave patterns (beta, alpha, theta, delta), bringing them into an optimal state of harmony and dynamic functioning. The result of this reprogramming is that, once it takes hold, lasting change occurs that is entirely independent of the conscious self-regulation skills gained via biofeedback. Optimizing brain wave function in turn optimizes the nervous system,

LISTEN TO YOUR HEART

It's no secret that the heart is directly involved in our experience of emotions. Most people are aware that fright, anxiety, and stress, among other feelings, increase the heart rate—a pounding heart is a common sign of strong emotions. Indeed, scientists have found that even the slightest emotional change immediately shifts heart rate variability (HRV), the measurement of beat-to-beat changes in the heart rate; it is also called heart rhythm. Contrary to some commonly held beliefs, a healthy heart does not beat at steady intervals throughout the day. In fact, the intervals between heartbeats vary even while we're asleep. Scientists at the Institute of HeartMath, in Boulder Creek, California, have found that HRV serves as a communication tool among the heart, brain, and body. A sudden, rapid, erratic heartbeat pattern signals the brain and body via the nervous system that an emotionally charged situation is at hand.

Learning to modulate heart rate variability can effectively reduce negative responses to stressful situations and improve your health. The Institute of HeartMath has developed three techniques that are clinically proven to turn off the stress response and lower cortisol release,[31] improve cognitive performance and mood,[32] and reduce hypertension and the risk of dying from congestive heart failure and heart disease.[33] These techniques employ strategies similar to cognitive therapy, biofeedback, visualization, Transcendental Meditation, and other established mind/body protocols.

One technique, called Freeze-Frame, is an effective strategy for dealing with daily stresses. It enables patients to arrest the stress response to difficult situations by replacing negative perceptions with positive feelings, such as feelings of appreciation, love, or enjoyment. These feelings restore calm and control to the heart rate. Here are the five steps of Freeze-Frame, as developed by the Institute of HeartMath and included in the book *The Heart-Math Solution.* [34]

1. Recognize the stressful feeling and "Freeze-Frame" it. Take a time-out.

2. Make a sincere effort to shift your focus away from the racing mind or disturbed emotions to the area around your heart. Pretend you're breathing through your heart to help focus your energy in this area. Keep your focus there for ten seconds or more.

3. Recall a positive, enjoyable feeling or memory you've had in life and try to re-experience it.

4. Using your intuition, common sense, and sincerity, ask your heart, "What would be a more efficient response to the situation, one that would minimize future stress?"

5. Listen to what your heart says in answer to your question. It's an effective way to put your reactive mind and emotions in check and find a source of common sense as the solution.

---

which improves the functioning of all the other body systems.

 See Diet, Environmental Medicine, Flower Essences, Guided Imagery, Herbal Medicine, Light Therapy, Mind/Body Medicine, Naturopathic Medicine, Nutritional Medicine, Qigong and Tai Chi, Yoga.

GUIDED IMAGERY AND VISUALIZATION

Many people find guided imagery to be an easy way to learn to relax, as the active nature of this practice makes it comfortable and enjoyable. A typical application, as described by Martin L. Rossman, M.D., of the Academy for Guided Imagery, in Mill Valley, California, is to close your eyes, take a few deep, easy breaths, and recall a time and place when you felt relaxed and peaceful. You should then imagine being there, noticing in detail the sights, sounds, and smells of this place, focusing especially on

the specific feelings of peacefulness and relaxation. This simple practice can be used in combination with other relaxation techniques or alone as a quick stress reducer.

Guided imagery can also be used to accomplish specific objectives besides relaxation and stress reduction, such as increasing immune response, reducing susceptibility to disease, controlling pain, losing weight, or dealing with anxiety or depression. The relaxation–imagery process can also serve as a method of evaluating current belief systems and altering those beliefs. Alterations in the symbols and pictures that one uses can dramatically change beliefs to ones more compatible with optimizing health.

YOGA AND QIGONG

Yoga has long been associated with reducing stress. The physical postures, meditation, and breathing exercises that are part of the practice of yoga can have a healing and relaxing effect on both body and mind. In fact, the concept behind the study of yoga is the integration of mind and body, explained by the observation that when the mind is restless and agitated, the health of the body will be adversely affected, and that when the body is ill, mental functioning will be compromised.

Since the early 1970s, more than 1,000 studies of yoga and meditation have demonstrated their effectiveness in reducing stress and anxiety, lowering blood pressure and heart rate, alleviating pain, providing relief from addictions, heightening visual and auditory perceptions, and improving memory, intelligence, and motor skills, as well as metabolic and respiratory function.[35] Yoga has also been shown to markedly reduce blood pressure in adults suffering from hypertension, thereby decreasing the need for drug therapy.[36]

According to recent medical studies in both China and the U.S., Qigong can also reduce stress. This ancient Chinese exercise combines graceful movements and rhythmic breathing, and if practiced regularly can improve muscular strength and flexibility and reverse damage caused by prior injuries and disease. Research has shown that Qigong also initiates the "relaxation response," leading to decreased heart rate, lowered blood pressure, stress reduction, and increased energy and tissue regeneration.[37]

Diet and Nutritional Supplements

"Often, symptoms of stress such as anxiety, depression, allergic-like reactions, food and chemical intolerances, and hyperactivity can be explained by a careful examination of diet, as well as vitamin, mineral, enzyme, and other nutrient levels," according to Dr. Kail. He suggests that those suffering from stress avoid caffeine and food additives and stick to a fresh, whole foods diet that is high in complex carbohydrates, moderate in protein, and low in fat. Less than 2% of the diet should consist of simple sugars, and those should come from fruit, not fruit juice.

Stress also tends to increase the likelihood of faulty digestion and malabsorption and, because of this, many individuals may have vitamin deficiencies, says Dr. Kail. For example, he notes that vitamin B6 is rapidly depleted during times of stress and needs to be replenished on a regular basis. His nutritional program includes supplements of multivitamins and minerals, particularly B-complex vitamins and vitamins A, C, and E, as well as calcium and trace elements. He finds these deficient in most people. Dr. Kail also strongly encourages his patients to use stress-reduction techniques and plenty of exercise in conjunction with his nutritional program.

Hypoglycemia (low blood sugar) is one stress-related disorder that can be directly addressed by diet. Harvey Ross, M.D., an orthomolecular psychiatrist in Los Angeles, California, notes that people with hypoglycemia are

---

PROGRESSIVE RELAXATION EXERCISE

Find a quiet place with soft lighting. Sit in a comfortable chair, feet flat on the floor, eyes closed.

- Become aware of your breathing. Take in a few deep breaths and mentally say, as you let out each breath, "Relax."

- Concentrate on your face, feeling any tension in your face and eyes. Make a mental picture of this tension—such as a rope tied in a knot or a clenched fist—and then mentally picture it being untied or relaxing and becoming comfortable, lying limp, like a relaxed rubber band.

- Experience the feeling of your face and eyes becoming relaxed. As they relax, feel a wave of relaxation spreading throughout your body.

- Tense your eyes and face, squeezing tightly, then relax and again feel the relaxation spreading throughout your body.

- Apply the previous instructions to other parts of your body. Move slowly down your body—jaw, neck, shoulders, back, upper and lower arms, hands, chest, abdomen, thighs, calves, ankles, feet, toes—until every part of your body is relaxed. Mentally picture the tension in each part of the body, then picture the tension melting away; tense the area and then relax it.

When you have relaxed each part of your body, rest quietly in this comfortable state for two to five minutes. Now let the muscles in your eyelids lighten up and prepare to open your eyes and become aware of the room. Finally, let your eyes open. You are ready to continue with the day's activities, refreshed and relaxed.

---

particularly vulnerable to stress because they have low energy and often their thinking and concentration are impaired. "Their mood is usually depressed. When life's little stresses—or big stresses—come up, they just don't have the tools to deal with them." He believes a person is genetically predisposed to hypoglycemia and a poor diet—usually high in refined carbohydrates—and stress set off the symptoms. "If a person has poor energy and depression not directly related to life's events and is anxious and irritable, yet his doctor says everything is normal, he should start thinking about a nutritional cause for these problems—particularly hypoglycemia."

SUCCESS STORY: A NATUROPATHIC PHYSICIAN'S APPROACH TO STRESS

Konrad Kail, N.D., recalls the case of June, a 30-year-old sales representative and mother of two, who came to him with a two-year history of stress-related disorders. "Her symptoms included recurrent episodes of fatigue, difficulty concentrating, confusion, dizziness, emotional swings, body aches, gastrointestinal upset, night sweats, recurrent low-grade fevers, swollen glands, and severe premenstrual symptoms," says Dr. Kail. "To her advantage, she did not smoke or drink and tried to eat a wholesome diet, but she consumed two cups of coffee and three glasses of black tea daily." Recently, she had become more susceptible to minor illnesses such as colds and flu. Her history included mononucleosis and frequent childhood ear infections.

A symptom survey showed findings compatible with digestive disturbance, liver-gallbladder dysfunction, and inadequately functioning endocrine glands. The physical examination was fairly normal except for findings of rhinitis and other signs of allergy and a few tender lymph nodes in the neck. June's spleen and thyroid were marginally enlarged and her neck and shoulder muscles were tight. Also, anxiety and depression scores were in the mild to moderate range, according to Dr. Kail.

Laboratory tests ordered by Dr. Kail suggested poor protein digestion, mild bowel toxicity, possible hydrochloric acid deficiency, adrenal fatigue, and a severe vitamin C deficiency. Further tests revealed allergy/sensitivity, candidiasis, and chronic Epstein-Barr virus infection. "These stressors were interfering with her body's ability to defend against minor illness," says Dr. Kail. "Also, her average body temperature was very low, suggesting thyroid dysfunction, and transit time in her digestive system was 32 hours, indicating constipation."

Dr. Kail reported his findings to June, explaining that her systems were having trouble maintaining a state of balance, most likely caused by a combination of physical and mental/emotional stressors. For treatment, he prescribed digestive aids in the form of plant enzymes taken before meals. Adrenal and thyroid supplements were also recommended, as were the herbs black radish and dandelion to stimulate liver function and to regulate her hormones. Additionally, June was given a multivitamin/mineral supplement to replace any nutritional deficiencies. Dr. Kail used acupressure to treat her allergies and an herbal preparation of *Urtica dioica* (which inhibits histamine, the chemical mediator of allergic reactions) to treat the chronic fatigue syndrome. The yeast infection was treated with grapefruit seed extract.

Finally, Dr. Kail asked June to exercise strenuously and to spend 30 minutes a day practicing a variety of relaxation and visualization techniques. According to Dr. Kail, over the course of a year June was able to attain 90% of her previous energy and strength capabilities and her symptoms were reduced greatly.

In treating hypoglycemia, Dr. Ross uses an individualized program that includes a strict diet and the addition of nutritional supplementation with multivitamins, chromium (100-200 mg daily), and glutamine (1,000 mg, three times a day, 30 minutes before meals). He recommends a high-protein, low-carbohydrate diet and, instead of three meals daily, the patient eats smaller meals five times a day, with frequent high-protein snacks. After the first four months, patients are introduced to a maintenance diet that includes no more than three servings of fruit a day. Ideally, patients will refrain from processed foods and sugars, but they may occasionally have a small amount of sugar. However, in times of increased stress, they may need to return to the stricter dietary program, cautions Dr. Ross.

Exercise

Physical exercise is commonly regarded as an effective means of reducing stress. But while a good workout can have beneficial effects, over-exercising can wear on the body's resources and contribute to stress. It is important, therefore, to devise an exercise routine appropriate to the needs of the individual. "I don't think there's a single thing in life that is as therapeutic as the right kind of exercise program applied over time," says John Hibbs, N.D., of Bastyr University, in Kenmore, Washington. "But misapplied, it can be just another stressor."

Dr. Hibbs cites the example of Type A individuals, whose lives are defined by a constant drive to achieve. "Turn them loose in the gym and what are they inclined to do? The same thing: work really hard, pump, pump, pump. There are studies now showing that such exercise does not decrease your chance of heart disease and stroke, it might even increase it." Instead, Dr. Hibbs recommends what he calls "tissue aerobic exercise"—relaxing exercise that allows blood flow to continue to the tissues. The heart rate should increase and you should sweat, but you don't need to get your heart rate up to 140, according to Dr. Hibbs.

Exercise results in increased energy, improved self-image, and reduced anxiety and depression. Exercise also helps alleviate other physiological stressors, such as chronic constipation, by toning the abdominal muscles and stimulating the peristaltic action of the colon. Walking, lifting weights, rowing, and jogging are effective stress-reducing activities (except for those with chronic fatigue). Stretching exercises also help relax tense muscles.

Herbal Medicine

One of the most universal methods of relaxing is drinking a cup of hot tea. Many herbalists suggest brewing certain herbs known for their stress-relieving properties.

Daniel O. Gagnon, a medical herbalist affiliated with the Botanical Research and Educational Institute, in Santa Fe, New Mexico, recommends chamomile (German or wild, *Matricaria recutita*; Roman, *Anthemis nobilis*) to help promote relaxation. Chamomile tea is used daily by millions of people worldwide to decrease their stress level. The flower of the chamomile plant produces a calming effect, easing anxiety and reducing tension.[38] It can thus be helpful with overall anxiety, sleep disorders, and muscle tension. Gagnon has found it to be one of the best herbal remedies for treating acute and chronic gastritis and gastric ulcers, which are often caused by an inability to deal with stress.

Another effective herbal treatment is passionflower *(Passiflora incarnata)*. It may be used safely during the day, as it will not cause drowsiness. Pharmacological studies indicate antispasmodic, sedative, anxiety-allaying, and hypotensive (blood pressure–lowering) activities of passionflower extracts.[39] Passionflower is said to help in quieting worry and giving a feeling of well-being.

To keep the central nervous system from being overwhelmed, Gagnon suggests valerian *(Valeriana officinalis)*, which is especially useful when dealing with high emotional stress. The odorous root of valerian has been used in European traditional medicine as a natural tranquillizer for centuries. In Germany, valerian root and its extracts are approved as over-the-counter medicines for "states of excitation" and "difficulty in falling asleep owing to nervousness."[40]

He also recommends American ginseng *(Panax quinquefolius)* to help support the entire body during stressful times. American ginseng can help protect against the effects of emotional, mental, and physical stress because of its ability to work as an adaptogen, a substance that

14 STEPS TO LESS STRESS

Although stressful situations are unavoidable, the following guidelines can help you avoid the emotional strain of stress.

- Plan regular diversions and cultivate interests outside of work.

- Get enough sleep. Establish a regular bedtime hour. Avoid sleeping pills.

- Do exercises that you enjoy, appropriate for your age and physical condition, on a daily basis.

- Avoid hurry and worry. These are learned behaviors that can interfere with eating, sleeping, working, and recreation. They can be unlearned.

- Don't be afraid of compromise. In a stressful situation, you can fight, back off, or compromise. Seldom are the ideal circumstances available.

- Love more. Learn to use things and love people rather than vice versa.

- Identify your fears. You can even list them. Fears add to emotional paralysis.

- Make a decision, right or wrong, and then act on it. Anxiety results when you sit in the middle, allowing your fears to tug at you from opposite directions.

- Laugh more. Laughter is a good tension breaker.

- Try to remain calm in the face of stressful situations. After unavoidable upsets, re-establish serenity.

- Avoid self-pity.

- Avoid loneliness. Reach out and take the initiative in developing friendship.

- Avoid coping solutions that involve alcohol or drugs. This also applies to stimulants such as tobacco, caffeine, sugar, over-eating, gambling, etc.

- Consider alleviating stress and achieving a state of relaxed awareness through techniques such as meditation, deep diaphragmatic breathing, yoga, Qigong, biofeedback, or self-hypnosis.

helps the body be more prepared and more resistant to everyday stresses, according to Gagnon.[41]

Flower Essences

Many people who have difficulty coping with stress find flower essences to be helpful. Flower essences (or remedies) were originally developed in the 1930s by Edward Bach, a British physician interested in the link between

LAUGH FOR THE HEALTH OF IT

Scientific research in the mind/body discipline of psychoneuroimmunology (PNI) has verified the presence of interrelated pathways connecting the brain and immune system. So it's of little surprise that genuinely felt laughter has been shown to dampen stress, reduce the production of stress-related hormones, and enhance immune system function. Humor provides an individual with what psychologists call "cognitive control"—although events in our external world are often beyond our control, we can influence our emotional response by shifting the perspective from which we view them. Laughter does that.

"Finding humor in a situation and laughing freely with others can be a powerful antidote to stress," says Patty Wooten, R.N. "Our sense of humor gives us the ability to find delight, experience joy, and to release tension." Laughter can be an effective self-care tool. An ability to laugh at a situation, problem, or even ourselves gives us a feeling of power, according to Wooten. Humor and laughter can foster a positive and hopeful attitude. We are less likely to succumb to feelings of depression and helplessness if we are able to laugh at what is troubling us. Some tips for staying on the lighter side of life:

- Laughter is much more effective when it is spontaneous.

- Increase your exposure to humorous materials; they are plentiful.

- Build a library of humorous cartoons, movies, or television episodes so that they are available when needed.

- Focus on the type of humor that's right for you.

- Learn to stay in touch with your "inner clown," that playful, childlike nature that often gets lost as we meet the challenges of daily life.[43]

emotions and physical illness. He began to investigate the healing potential of the wildflowers native to the English countryside and found that the essences distilled from 38 flowering plants and trees had a profound effect on the underlying psychological and emotional states that influence physical illness. These remedies became known as the Bach® Flower Remedies. Today, there are numerous flower remedies available to address the specific psychological and emotional factors involved in many stress-related conditions.[42]

"Flower essences precisely address the interface between body and mind," says Patricia Kaminski, of the Flower Essence Society, in Nevada City, California. "Their impact is not weak but subtle, and when you take them they prompt a shift in view from within, engendering recognition of feelings that exist below the level of our ordinary awareness." Flower essences can help alleviate emotions such as apprehension, worry, loneliness, depression, and fear. They can also act as a catalyst for calmness and mental clarity. Usually flower remedies prove effective in removing the emotional blocks within one to 12 weeks. However, in some instances of deeply rooted psychological patterns, it may take longer. Once an individual's emotional state has improved, however, the remedies no longer need to be taken.

Traditional Chinese Medicine

According to traditional Chinese medicine (TCM), stress may be a factor in the development of many diseases. Treatment of stress in TCM includes acupuncture and herbs to help balance the body's energies and relieve the tension that constricts the functioning of a particular part of the body. Maoshing Ni, D.O.M., Ph.D., L.Ac., President of Yo San University of Traditional Chinese Medicine, in Marina del Rey, California, says that stress is a nervous response of the body to external or internal irritants. According to TCM, the liver is affected first, and continued stress then impacts other organs. Dr. Ni treats stress with a combination of acupuncture and herbs such as astragalus, ligustra, and ginseng. He also prescribes visualization and breathing exercises through the practice of Qigong and Tai Chi.

One of Dr. Ni's patients, a 52-year-old lawyer who worked 80 hours a week, came to him complaining of headaches, neck and low-back pain, insomnia, high blood pressure, and impotence of six months' duration. Dr. Ni treated the patient with acupuncture and herbs, and gave him some Qigong exercises that he could do at work. After weekly treatment for six weeks, his pain became minimal, his blood pressure returned to normal, he was no longer impotent, and he only occasionally suffered from insomnia. Dr. Ni points out that such patients need to be treated on a continuing basis to maintain the positive effects.

 See Acupuncture, Ayurvedic Medicine, Traditional Chinese Medicine.

Ayurvedic Medicine

"In treating stress through Ayurveda, we look at four areas: consciousness, physiology, behavior, and environment," says Hari Sharma, M.D., President of the Maharishi Ayurveda Medical Association. Exact treatment varies according to body type, according to Dr. Sharma, but the same four areas are addressed. Mental stress is relieved by Transcendental Meditation. Physiology is addressed by dietary changes that include avoiding stimulants and eating a whole foods diet, along with daily massages with sesame oil. Behavior modification involves adhering to a daily routine, with regular hours of work, sleep, and meals, and a more organized lifestyle. The patient's environment is improved through music and aromatherapy, and a cleaner, more restful living space (for example, one should keep the bedroom a soothing and pleasing place to rest, devoid of work materials and clutter). If these four areas of life are attended to, stress should be relieved within a few days, according to Dr. Sharma. The most important factor, he says, is to keep the regular daily schedule as stress free as possible.

Recommendations

- Avoid caffeine and food additives, and stick to a fresh, whole foods diet that is high in complex carbohydrates, moderate in protein, and low in fat.

- Since stress contributes to illness, stress reduction should promote healing. This is the basis of numerous relaxation therapies, such as meditation, guided imagery, biofeedback, yoga, and Qigong.

- Walking, lifting weights, rowing, or jogging are effective stress-reducing activities. Stretching exercises help relax tense muscles.

- Herbs that help relieve stress include chamomile, passionflower, valerian, and American ginseng.

- Flower essences can help alleviate emotions such as apprehension, worry, loneliness, depression, and fear. They can also act as a catalyst for calmness and mental clarity.

- Get enough sleep. Establish a regular bedtime hour and avoid sleeping pills.

- Love more. Learn to use things and love people rather than vice versa.

- Avoid hurry and worry. These are learned behaviors that can interfere with eating, sleeping, working, and recreation. They can be unlearned.

- Laugh more. Laughter is a good tension breaker.

Self-Care

The following therapies can be undertaken at home under appropriate professional supervision:

AROMATHERAPY: For anxiety, use bergamot, chamomile, camphor, cedarwood, clary sage, cypress, frankincense, geranium, hyssop, jasmine, juniper, lavender, lemon, marjoram, melissa, neroli, rose, sandalwood, or ylang ylang.

HYDROTHERAPY: Constitutional hydrotherapy, immersion bath or wet sheet pack (apply two to five times weekly); neutral application as needed for sedation. Leon Chaitow, N.D., D.O., of London, England, reports that the neutral bath, where one is immersed in 95° F water for two hours, has a sedative effect and can be helpful in achieving complete relaxation in anyone who is suffering from severe anxiety, agitation, irritability, exhaustion, chronic pain, or insomnia.

Professional Care

The following therapies should only be provided by a qualified health professional:

Acupuncture / Biofeedback Training and Neurotherapy / Craniosacral Therapy / Magnetic Field Therapy / Orthomolecular Medicine / Osteopathic Medicine / Traditional Chinese Medicine

BODYWORK: • Massage with essential oils. • Acupressure, reflexology, shiatsu, Alexander Technique, Feldenkrais Method • Rolfing can be helpful in conjunction with psychotherapy.

Where to Find Help

For additional information and referrals for treatment of stress, contact the following organizations.

Academy for Guided Imagery
P.O. Box 2070
Mill Valley, California 94942
(800) 726-2070 or (415) 389-9325
Website: www.healthy.net/agi

For information on guided imagery.

American Association for Therapeutic Humor
222 Meramec, Suite 303
St. Louis, Missouri 63105
(314) 863-6232

For more information on humor therapy.

American Association of Naturopathic Physicians
8201 Greensboro Drive, Suite 300
McLean, Virginia 22101
(703) 610-9037
Website: www.naturopathic.org

Provides a directory of naturopathic physicians and offers referrals to a nationwide network of accredited or licensed practitioners. Also publishes a quarterly newsletter and offers brochures and pamphlets on a variety of subjects.

Association for Applied Physiopsychology and Biofeedback
10200 West 44th Avenue, Suite 304
Wheat Ridge, Colorado 80033
(303) 422-8436
Website: www.aapb.org

For more information on biofeedback or for referrals to practitioners.

Institute of HeartMath
14700 West Park Avenue
Boulder Creek, California 95056
(831) 338-8500
Website: www.heartmath.org

For more about HeartMath techniques and seminars.

Mind-Body Medical Institute
Beth Israel Deaconess Medical Center
110 Francis Street, Suite 1A
Boston, Massachusetts 02215
(617) 632-9530
Website: www.mindbody.harvard.edu

A treatment program at a medical center where the relaxation response can be learned. The clinic uses yoga, meditation, and stress reduction as part of its program.

Stress Reduction Clinic
University of Massachusetts Medical Center
55 Lake Avenue North
Worcester, Massachusetts 01655
(508) 856-2656
Website: www.umassmed.edu/cfm

The Stress Reduction Clinic is a training program to teach meditative-type awareness.

Recommended Reading

25 Natural Ways to Manage Stress and Avoid Burnout. James Scala. Los Angeles: Keats, 2000.

Creating Wholeness: A Self-Healing Workbook Using Dynamic Relaxation, Images and Thoughts. Erik Peper. New York: Plenum, 1993.

Don't Sweat the Small Stuff—And It's All Small Stuff. Richard Carlson. New York: Hyperion, 1997.

Full Catastrophe Living. Jon Kabat-Zinn, Ph.D. New York: Delta, 1990.

Mind/Body Medicine: How to Use Your Mind for Better Health. Daniel P. Goleman and Joel Gurin. New York: Consumer Reports Books, 1995.

Minding the Body/Mending the Mind. Joan Borysenko. New York: Bantam Doubleday Dell, 1993.

The Relaxation Response. Herbert Benson, M.D., with Miriam Z. Klipper. New York: Wholecare, 2000.

Stress and Natural Healing: Herbal Medicines and Natural Therapies. Christopher Hobbs. Santa Cruz, CA: Botanica Press, 1997.

Stress Management. James S. Gordon, M.D. New York: Chelsea House, 2000.

Stress Without Distress. Hans Selye, M.D. New York: New American Library, 1991.

Why Zebras Don't Get Ulcers: An Updated Guide to Stress, Stress-Related Diseases, and Coping. Robert M. Sapolsky. New York: W.H. Freeman, 1998.

VISION DISORDERS

Nearly 60% of Americans require vision correction by the time they reach adulthood, but standard treatments such as corrective lenses or surgery may in fact contribute to further visual impairment. Fortunately, many vision problems can be prevented or treated through the use of nutrition, eye exercises, behavioral optometry, biofeedback, Ayurvedic medicine, and traditional Chinese medicine.

MANY PEOPLE grow accustomed to their vision problems, assuming that their eyes are deteriorating as a result of aging. However, poor diet and nutrition, physical, mental, and emotional stress, poor visual skills, and side effects of pharmaceutical drugs are the causes of many vision problems, which are often unrelated to eye disease or dysfunction of the visual system.

"The proper functioning of our visual system has far-reaching effects on our general health, beyond an ability to see clearly," says Glen Swartwout, O.D., of Hilo, Hawaii. "Information processed by the eyes helps to regulate functions such as biological rhythms, as well as the nervous, endocrine, and immune systems. It also provides the dominant source of information for human perception, thinking, and coordination of movement."

The ability to process visual information depends on highly refined eye/brain communication. As light strikes the retina (the innermost layer of the eye, which receives images), chemical changes convert the light energy to a visual nerve impulse, which is then processed by the brain. According to Dr. Swartwout, when eye/brain communication is disrupted, related problems include blurred vision, altered depth perception, loss of central or peripheral vision, double vision, sensitivity to light, and changes in color perception. If not treated, impaired vision can lead to any number of physiological or psychological problems, including lack of coordination, spatial disorientation, or reading, writing, and learning difficulties.

Types of Vision Disorders

Conditions that can impair vision range from relatively minor problems, such as myopia (nearsightedness), to more serious illnesses, like glaucoma (increased pressure in the eye) and cataracts.

Poor Eyesight

Poor eyesight, including nearsightedness, farsightedness, and astigmatism, is a condition that usually results from a refractive error (deflection of a light ray from a straight path as it moves through the eye).

Nearsightedness occurs when the visual image falls in front of the retina, preventing proper focusing on distant objects. Causes stem from a longer than normal eye, a steeply curved cornea, or the inability of the lens of the eye to sufficiently relax.

Farsightedness (hyperopia) occurs when the visual image focuses behind the retina, preventing proper vision of nearby objects. Causes stem from the eye being shorter than normal, the cornea too flat, lack of muscle tone in the ciliary muscle that controls the lens, or a combination of these factors.

Astigmatism is a condition in which the shape of the cornea is more oval than round, causing the eye to focus on two points instead of one. Blurring, fatigue, and headaches are often the result.

Cataracts

Defined as a partial or complete clouding of the lens of the eye, cataracts are the leading cause of impaired vision and blindness in the United States.[1] Though one can develop cataracts at any age, it occurs most frequently in older adults. Dr. Swartwout notes that in addition to the aging process, risk factors include extensive exposure to radiation or infrared light, certain medications such as steroids, injuries, and diseases. He adds that cataracts have also been linked to vitamin, mineral, and protein imbalances.

Conjunctivitis

Also known as pink eye, conjunctivitis is an irritating inflammation of the conjunctiva, the mucous membrane

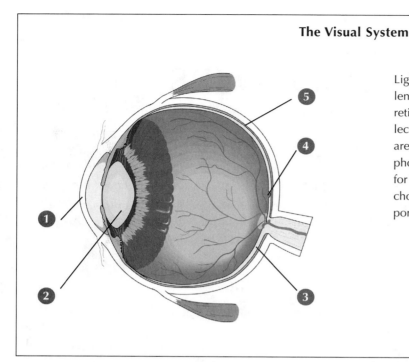

The Visual System

Light rays enter the eye through the cornea (1) to the lens (2) where light is focused as it travels to the retina (3). The retina, an extension of the brain, collects light through photo- or light-sensitive cells. The area of the retina with the highest concentration of photosensitive cells is the macula (4), responsible for central vision. Surrounding the retina is the choroid (5), which is filled with capillaries transporting nutrients to the eye.

that lines the eye and eyelid. Symptoms include discharge from the eye (often containing pus), pain, swelling, and redness, as well as itching and discomfort with bright lights. Eyelids may stick together upon awakening. Causes of conjunctivitis include infections, allergies, stress, and poor nutrient levels.

Glaucoma

Glaucoma is a group of several diseases generally characterized by loss of peripheral vision, accompanied in many cases by an increase in fluid pressure within the eyeball. It is frequently asymptomatic in the early stages and often goes undetected. Today, there are two million cases of glaucoma in the U.S., making it a leading cause of blindness among older adults.[2] And although aging is a factor, other causes include serious eye injuries, eye surgery, certain medications including steroids, and eye tumors. Glaucoma may also be linked to nutritional deficiency in the retina and optic nerve and to excess toxins and metabolic wastes. In addition, the risk of developing glaucoma significantly increases among women who experience early menopause, as shown by a recent study of over 3,000 women conducted at the Netherlands Opththalmic Research Institute. Women who entered menopause before age 45 were more than twice as likely to develop glaucoma as women who were at least 50 years old when they became menopausal. The study indicates that female hormones may play a protective role against glaucoma.[3]

Lazy Eye

Usually beginning in childhood, lazy eye, or amblyopia, results when one eye begins to function below capacity. It occurs when the brain receives dissimilar information from each eye (for example, one eye is myopic and the other astigmatic) and favors one eye in order to focus on a single image. The affected eye then becomes accustomed to being ignored and the result is diminished overall vision.

Macular Degeneration

Macular degeneration is a condition in which the macula (the central area of the retina) deteriorates, resulting in the loss of sharp vision. It is the leading cause of severe visual loss in both the U.S. and Europe for those 55 years or older and is the third leading cause of impaired vision among those over 65.[4] In addition to aging, risk factors include atherosclerosis and hypertension. Macular degeneration may also be linked to nutritional deficiencies, chemical exposure, and cigarette smoking.[5]

Night Blindness

Night blindness is often a symptom of retinitis pigmentosa, a disease that causes deterioration of the rods (cells that distinguish light and dark) in the retina and progressive loss of sight. Vitamin A and zinc deficiencies can also lead to night blindness.

Retinal Detachment

Retinal detachment, a peeling away of the retina from the back of the eye, can result in blindness. It occurs when a hole or tear in the retina permits fluid to collect between it and the back of the eye. Injuries to the eyes are the leading, but not exclusive, cause of retinal detachment.

Retinopathy

Retinopathy is a serious visual disorder characterized by hemorrhages of the retinal blood vessels. It is usually associated with either hypertension or diabetes and is a major cause of blindness among diabetics.

Causes of Vision Disorders

Dr. Swartwout notes that a great many factors can contribute to visual problems, including nutritional deficiency, alcohol, drugs, physical strain, dental problems, poor posture, environmental pollution, harmful lighting, and emotional stress. If these problems go untreated, vision disorders and eye disease can occur. "Drugs and surgery do not correct or eliminate the causes of eye disease, which are often individual and multifactorial," he adds.

Drugs and surgery do not correct or eliminate the causes of eye disease, which are often individual and multifactorial.

—GLEN SWARTWOUT, O.D.

Poor Diet and Nutrition

Many eye ailments can be traced in part to poor dietary and nutritional habits. According to Dr. Swartwout, cataracts, glaucoma, and macular degeneration have been linked to vitamin and mineral deficiencies, while the muscles that control eye movement (and thus visual performance) are affected by nutritional imbalances. In his experience, specific foods that often contribute to eye disease and vision impairment include sugar, eggs, dairy products, fats, fried and processed foods, wheat, alcohol, tobacco, and coffee.

Dr. Swartwout also notes that imbalances in the metabolic system also interfere with vision. "If the blood pH (acid-base balance) becomes too acidic, muscle tone increases, turning the eyes inward, while an alkaline pH will interfere with normal muscle tone, leaving the eyes posturing outward and generally fatigued." Blindness and cataracts are linked to diabetes and reduced night vision is often linked to impaired liver function. Gastrointestinal disorders such as *Candida* overgrowth and parasites contribute to vision problems because they interfere with the normal assimilation of nutrients.

Pharmaceutical Drugs

According to Leonard Levine, Ph.D., certain prescription drugs can impair the health of the visual system.[6] For example, the *Physicians' Desk Reference* lists 94 medications that can cause glaucoma, including antihypertensives, steroids, and antidepressants. A partial list of drugs that adversely affect the eyes includes the following:

- Antihistamines—anti-allergy drugs that increase pressure in the eye
- Chlorothiazide and furosemide—diuretics that can cause blurred vision and dryness in the eyes
- Chlorpromazine—a drug used to treat mental disorders that can cause blurred vision
- Digoxin—a heart medication that can cause distorted or blurred vision
- Ethambutol—a drug used to treat tuberculosis that can cause severe loss of vision and altered color perception
- Gold—a drug used to treat arthritis and lupus that can cause corneal inflammation and blurred vision
- Haloperidol—a drug used to treat mental disorders that can temporarily paralyze the eye muscles and cause blurred vision
- Hydroxychloroquine sulfate—a drug used to treat arthritis, lupus, and malaria that can reduce the ability to see red and distort central vision
- Oral contraceptives—birth control drugs that can cause blurred vision and a variety of other problems
- Steroids—anti-inflammatory drugs that can cause cataracts, glaucoma, and other problems
- Tetracycline—an antibiotic that can reduce visual acuity and alter color vision[7]

Dr. Levine adds that, of the ten most frequently prescribed drugs, many hamper the optometric examination or cause erroneous findings such as cataracts and decreased accommodation (the inability of the eye to properly adjust to various distances) and may result in misdiagnosis or inappropriate treatment.

Environmental Factors

"Fluorescent lighting, electromagnetic stress, computer monitors, lack of sunlight, and poorly lit work and school environments are all potential hazards for the eyes," says

THE LINK BETWEEN NEARSIGHTEDNESS AND "NEAR-WORK" ACTIVITIES

Recent research conducted in Singapore has found that myopia, or nearsightedness, more commonly occurs among people who are highly educated and students who are high academic achievers. This finding suggests that myopia, which has rapidly increased in Asian countries and other developed nations during the past 100 years, may be due as much to "near-work" activities (such as reading, working at a computer, graphic design, and drawing) as to heredity or other factors. Among the findings of researchers was that myopia increased by nearly 400% among Singapore soldiers who had taken accelerated education programs in school. A similar fourfold increase in myopia was found among students who finished two years of pre-college courses.[8]

Dr. Swartwout. In one study involving 160,000 Texas schoolchildren, 98% of the students entered kindergarten without major eye disorders, but at the close of sixth grade over 50% had developed vision problems. When researchers redesigned the classrooms to allow for optimal visual performance, the incidence of chronic disorders decreased significantly.[9]

Mental/Emotional Factors

According to Dr. Swartwout, when the eyes are not functioning properly, psychological capacities can be significantly impaired. Conversely, mental disorders can cause vision problems. For example, emotional disturbances in a child's life, such as divorce or other severe stress and abuse, can lead to eye turns (an eye that turns inward or wanders outward) and lazy eye, while school-related stress often triggers nearsightedness and astigmatism.

"Each time there is a change in the cognitive demand of our visual activity or a change in our emotional state, our focus changes," Dr. Swartwout points out. "Stress heightens the demand on the near-focusing response, requiring increased precision and muscular response."

Physical Factors

Any tension in the neck, shoulders, or face interferes with the flexibility a person needs to smoothly and accurately track objects and judge distance and depth. The performance of many skills depends on vision, especially driving and sports-related activities. Excess physical tension also promotes fatigue, which interferes with information processing, such as reading.

Treating Vision Disorders

A new generation of optometrists is investing postgraduate years mastering programs designed to prevent and eliminate vision impairment and improve visual performance. People with poor vision can reduce their dependency on prescription lenses and, in some cases, eliminate the need altogether. A combination of approaches including diet and nutrition, behavioral optometry, syntonic optometry, biofeedback training, light therapy, the Bates method, herbal remedies, traditional Chinese medicine, and Ayurvedic medicine can not only enhance visual performance but also play an important role in improving movement, coordination, and learning abilities.

 See Biofeedback Training and Neurotherapy, Chelation Therapy, Diet, Energy Medicine, Flower Essences, Homeopathy, Nutritional Medicine, Oxygen Therapies, Traditional Chinese Medicine.

Diet and Nutritional Supplements

Diet and nutrition play a central role in the proper functioning of the eyes. Vision disorders, including cataracts, glaucoma, and macular degeneration, can be traced in part to nutritional deficiencies and a number of physicians have developed nutritional therapy programs to treat and prevent specific vision ailments.

Dr. Swartwout reports that cataracts can result from a nutritional disorder and are further aggravated by smoking, drinking alcohol, and the use of some prescription drugs (especially cortisone and other steroids). In a study conducted by Dr. Swartwout, two-thirds of his patients showed improved vision within four weeks of making changes in diet, health habits, and nutritional supplementation.[10] These findings are supported by the individual research of other doctors, including Gary Todd, M.D., an ophthalmologist from North Carolina, and Stuart Kemeny, M.D., an ophthalmologist from California. In a two-year study of 50 patients, Dr. Todd found that nutritional supplementation eliminated the need for cataract surgery in over 50% of his patients and 88% showed improved vision. In two studies conducted by Dr. Kemeny at the International Cataract Clinic, in Mexico, subjects were prescribed nutritional supplements, ultraviolet light–absorbing glasses, and special eye drops. Vision improved in 54% of his patients in the first study and 85% in the second.[11]

When treating cataracts and glaucoma, Dr. Swartwout stresses the relationship between nutrition and vision. For prevention of both disorders, he recommends a diet consisting of unrefined, natural foods, in addition to vitamin and nutritional supplements. Conversely,

SUCCESS STORY: HEALING SUDDEN-ONSET BLINDNESS

"When Todd first came to me, he was clinically blind," reports Corazon Ibarra-Ilarina, M.D., H.M.D., of Reno, Nevada. "Using a cane, he had to be assisted into the examination room by his father." Todd's ordeal had begun two months earlier, when he awoke one morning, looked in a mirror, and saw a small spot in front of his eyes. By the afternoon, the spot had grown larger, prompting Todd to see an eye doctor, who found that his left eye tested normal, but his right eye showed a vision loss of 25%. Further examination revealed that the retina was not detached or torn, but by the next day Todd's vision loss was 30% and continued to degenerate.

One month later, his vision was 60%, despite having consulted with several M.D.s, two neural ophthalmologists, a rheumatology specialist, and a retina surgeon. All of his tests came back negative, except for an antinuclear antibody blood test, which revealed that his immune function was abnormal. As a result, he was placed on high doses of the steroid solumedrol in the hope that it would boost his immune system. Two weeks later, Todd was 96% blind in his right eye and, two weeks after that, the vision in his left eye had deteriorated by 75%.

Todd turned to Dr. Ibarra-Ilarina, who conducted a series of standard medical tests, along with traditional Chinese medicine (TCM) diagnosis and electrodermal screening (EDS), which indicated a state of severe toxicity throughout Todd's body. "Conventional drugs did not help him and probably contributed to the spread of blindness to his left eye, which developed about a month after he had massive doses of corticosteroids," Dr. Ibarra-Ilarina says. "Todd's degree of toxicity is increasingly common. We call it 'biotoxicosis,' a potentially lethal poisoning of the entire biological system. In Todd's case, there were environmen-

tal, emotional, and drug-related factors, plus imbalances in his nervous, immune, and endocrine systems."

According to TCM diagnosis, Todd had a pathological energy cycle involving his liver, spleen, and kidneys. "This is a condition that is notoriously difficult to treat," Dr. Ibarra-Ilarina says. His treatment was divided into several phases, beginning with dietary and exercise counseling, along with bath therapy (using seaweed extracts, apple cider vinegar, and Epsom salts) and homeopathic drainage therapy to help him detoxify and stimulate the liver. This was followed with chelation therapy and intravenous infusions of vitamins and minerals, including high doses of vitamin C, followed by intravenous hydrogen peroxide. Todd's liver was then further detoxified using a combination of herbs, homeopathic remedies, and electrodermal therapy.

Next, Dr. Ibarra-Ilarina supported the imbalanced and deficient energy in Todd's liver and balanced his neuro-endocrine-immune dysfunction with additional nutritional supplements, homeopathic remedies, Chinese herbs, and adrenal glandular therapy. Finally, she worked on Todd's emotional, mental, and spiritual disturbances using Anthroposophical medicines and flower essences. "We also sought to engage Todd in affirmations, meditation, and prayer," Dr. Ibarra-Ilarina says.

Todd's improvement was slow but steady. In all, Todd spent a month at Dr. Ibarra-Ilarina's Bio Medical Health Center, where he received daily treatments. When he left, the vision in his left eye was restored to nearly 100%, and he had 60% visual capacity in his right eye. The remaining 40% may not return on account of possible nerve damage to the eye, Dr. Ibarra-Ilarina speculates. Nonetheless, Todd says, "Because of Dr. Ibarra-Ilarina's treatments, I can live my life again as normally as any fully sighted person."

refined, processed, and junk foods may contribute to the development of cataracts and glaucoma, along with stress, alcohol, caffeine, sugar, and smoking, all of which deplete essential nutrients.

Like cataracts and glaucoma, macular degeneration can be linked to nutritional deficiencies, especially among older individuals. Jonathan Wright, M.D., Director of the Tahoma Clinic, in Kent, Washington, and Alan Gaby, M.D., of Seattle, Washington, point out that there is a large body of clinical evidence suggesting that nutrient supplementation, particularly with antioxidants, may

retard the aging process. According to Drs. Wright and Gaby, "With advancing age, nutritional status tends to decline because of reduced gastrointestinal absorption and impaired uptake of nutrients. The sensory organs appear to be especially vulnerable to the effects of nutritional deficiency and the purposes of supplementation are to delay the process of cellular degeneration and enhance the function of those cells."[14]

Drs. Wright and Gaby have reviewed the role of nutritional factors in cataracts and macular degeneration and found the following nutrients to be beneficial:[15]

ARE CONVENTIONAL TREATMENTS FOR VISION DISORDERS EFFECTIVE?

It is often thought that once vision is impaired, it can only be restored through corrective lenses, drugs, or surgery. Glen Swartwout, O.D., of Hilo, Hawaii, points out that not only is this untrue, these remedies may contribute to further visual impairment.

Corrective Lenses—As a person's eyes grow progressively weaker, doctors often prescribe stronger corrective lenses. But prescription eyeglasses can contribute to the progression of nearsightedness and astigmatism, because they make the image smaller, leading to insufficient movement of the extraocular eye muscles (muscles that control eye movement and coordination). Corrective lenses also contribute to the progressive worsening of farsightedness by forcing the ciliary muscle (muscle that facilitates near vision) to relax its tone, thus losing its ability to compensate for farsightedness without glasses.

Long-term dependency on corrective lenses can lead to reduced flexibility of the eye muscles, sensitivity to artificial light, and a loss of depth perception, according to Dr. Swartwout. He points out that some optometrists now recommend using progressively weaker lenses to help strengthen the eyes. In the case of myopia (often triggered by a spasm of the ciliary muscle), which is usually corrected with negative (concave) lenses, Dr. Swartwout uses a positive (convex) lens, which helps the ciliary muscles relax and thus vision is improved. Contact lenses may pose their own problems. For instance, an article in *The Lancet* revealed a 65% higher incidence of microbial keratitis (inflammation of the cornea due to infection) in contact lens wearers.[12] Extended-wear soft contacts carry the highest risk, but any foreign object worn in the eye is a potential danger, says Dr. Swartwout.

Prescription Drugs—Drugs are commonly used in the treatment of glaucoma and certain retinal disorders. But while medications may prove effective in halting the progress of a vision disorder, they can also prevent its cure. For instance, Dr. Swartwout notes that eye drops are widely prescribed to reduce pressure in the eyes due to glaucoma. This elevated pressure, however, is generally a response to some imbalance and drugs can complicate the body's effort to eliminate this imbalance. "It is essential to be able to identify and remove the cause of a problem," says Dr. Swartwout. "The danger of drugs is that they only partially control the symptoms of a disease and very often their effectiveness wanes, requiring stronger doses, new medications, or more radical measures. Side effects of drugs pose yet another hazard."

Surgery—Surgery is used for a wide variety of eye ailments, from nearsightedness and crossed eyes to cataracts, glaucoma, and retinal detachment. But because the visual mechanism is extraordinarily delicate, complications from surgical treatment for chronic eye problems are common and even a "successful" operation can disrupt the subtle functions of the eyes. Depending on the nature of the procedure and the circumstances of the case, the hazards range from vision distortions to partial or total loss of eyesight.

Dr. Swartwout believes that surgery to correct refractive errors (nearsightedness, farsightedness, astigmatism) is generally unwarranted. He points out that radial keratotomy, a common operation used to remedy myopia, requires the surgeon to cut 90% of the way through the cornea. In some cases, the cornea has been completely penetrated resulting in blindness. And because of scar tissue, the eye is weak and cannot withstand the pressures generated by subsequent injury. Radial keratotomy can also lead to less severe problems, such as vision distortion and fluctuation, and nighttime glare. A more natural alternative for treating myopia is a process called orthokeratology, which safely reshapes the cornea using special gas-permeable contact lenses.

Eye muscle surgery, used to treat such conditions as crossed eyes and walleye (an eye that wanders outward), also carries significant risks and for the most part can be avoided in favor of nonsurgical techniques. In the case of severe disorders such as cataracts and glaucoma, the dangers of the condition sometimes outweigh those of the surgery. Yet, as Dr. Swartwout says, "If we can treat them preventively at an earlier stage, then we can prevent the need for most eye surgeries."

LASIK (laser in situ keratomileusis) is a more recent laser surgical procedure used to correct myopia, hyperopia, and astigmatism. The procedure involves the use of a thin blade that creates a flap near the apex of the cornea. A laser then vaporizes some of the cornea and the corneal flap is reattached. Another procedure, known as PRK (photorefrac-

ARE CONVENTIONAL TREATMENTS FOR VISION DISORDERS EFFECTIVE? continued

tive keratectomy), also uses laser surgery to reshape the cornea, but without the corneal flap. Typically, however, it results in more short-term discomfort and a longer time period before vision improves. While LASIK and PRK have become popular for improving vision disorders, neither is risk-free. According to Jay B. Lavine, author of *The Eye Care Sourcebook*, potential complications include:

- The creation of free radicals by the laser, which destroy keratocytes that help maintain the cornea's structural integrity and lead to thinning of the cornea and other corneal damage.

- "Dry Eye Syndrome" caused by diminished tear secretion.

- Halos around lights or a starburst appearance of lights at night.

- Loss of visual acuity.

- Damage to the vitreous (located between the lens and retina), retinal tears and detachment, and macular holes and pucker, especially among patients who are highly myopic.

- Optic nerve damage and destruction, presumably caused by the high intraocular pressure that occurs during surgery.[13]

- Zinc: Necessary for normal visual function and adaptation to the dark; zinc deficiency may lead to cataracts and supplementation reduces visual loss in macular degeneration.

- Selenium: Antioxidant that may help prevent cataracts; can improve visual acuity in patients with macular degeneration when combined with vitamin E.

- Taurine: May protect cells from harmful effects of ultraviolet light.

- Vitamin C (ascorbic acid): One of the most important antioxidants for the eye; supplementation can improve vision in those with cataracts.

- Vitamin E: A deficiency of this antioxidant may lead to cataracts; large doses can prevent macular degeneration.

- Vitamin A: Necessary for maintenance of healthy rods and cones in the retina.

- Riboflavin: Necessary co-factor for the antioxidant enzyme glutathione reductase; riboflavin deficiency leads to cataracts.

- N-acetyl-cysteine: Antioxidant that may prevent cataracts and other degenerative changes in the eye.

- *Ginkgo biloba:* Antioxidant that improves arterial blood flow and enhances cellular metabolism; may prevent degenerative changes in the eye.

- Flavonoids: A group of compounds found in plants that have antioxidant and anti-inflammatory effects; improves night vision and adaptation to the dark, visual acuity, and capillary integrity to reduce hemorrhage in diabetic retinopathy; found in high concentrations in blueberries and grapes.

It is often thought that once vision is impaired, it can only be restored through corrective lenses, drugs, or surgery. Not only is this untrue, but these remedies may contribute to further visual impairment.

Other useful nutrients for ensuring vision health are the carotenoids lutein, lycopene, and zeaxanthin. Food sources of lutein: kale, collard and mustard greens, spinach, Swiss chard, red peppers, parsley, romaine lettuce, dill, celery, carrots, corn, tomatoes, potatoes, and red, blue, and purple fruits. Food sources of lycopene: tomatoes, tomato juice and catsup, watermelon, guava, pink grapefruit, green peppers, dried apricot, and carrots. Food sources of zeaxanthin: kale, spinach, collard and mustard greens, Swiss chard, red peppers, paprika, corn, okra, parsley, dill, romaine lettuce, and red, blue and purple fruits.[16]

One patient of Dr. Wright's, a woman in her early seventies, came to him with rapidly deteriorating central vision in both eyes (20/100 in the right eye, 20/80 in the left eye). He recommended a program combining zinc, selenium, vitamin E, and taurine (an amino acid). To ensure proper absorption, the zinc and selenium were administered intravenously; the vitamin E and taurine were taken orally, along with additional supplements of zinc and selenium. According to Dr. Wright, the patient responded well to the treatment, with significant improvement in both eyes (20/40 in the right eye, 20/30 in the left). She was able to discontinue the IVs after 13 months, but found it necessary to maintain the oral supplements.

Behavioral Optometry

Defined as the art and science of developing visual abilities to achieve optimal visual performance and comfort, behavioral optometry is based on the work of the late A.M. Skeffington, O.D., D.O.S., who believed that vision is learned and can be enhanced through education, training, and corrective lenses.[17] Behavioral optometry helps patients recognize old behaviors that interfere with vision-related activities and teaches them new, more efficient behaviors by developing the following skills:

- Eye movement (ocular motility)
- Eye focus
- Eye teaming (binocularity)
- Peripheral vision
- Eye-hand coordination
- Visual perception and memory
- Information processing
- Visualization

Problems in visual tracking and acuity contribute to reading, speaking, and writing difficulties.[18] Therefore, when visual skills are improved, learning becomes easier. According to Harold Solan, O.D., Director of the Learning Disabilities Unit at the State University of New York, the proper development of visual perception skills is essential for the formation of reading comprehension and arithmetic skills in the elementary grades. Through the use of appropriate visual testing and training, behavioral optometrists can help children whose problems in reading and math relate to poor visual functioning.[19]

Ray Gottlieb, O.D., Ph.D., a behavioral optometrist in Madison, New Jersey, cites the case of a first-grader named Eric. When Eric began working with Dr. Gottlieb, he was lagging far behind his classmates in all subjects. He suffered from poor memory, a short attention span, and a lack of athletic ability. He spent much of the time daydreaming aimlessly with his head flopped backward, his eyes upturned, and his mouth gaping open.

Dr. Gottlieb's visual examination of Eric revealed poor eye movement skills, faulty eye posturing, and inadequate focusing. After six weeks of working with Dr. Gottlieb, Eric's vision problems began improving. His teachers reported significant progress in both his learning skills and physical appearance and his athletic ability improved to the point that, in six months, he was playing on both the soccer and basketball teams.

Behavioral optometrists address learning-related visual problems and difficulties with motor coordination, sensory integration, environmental sensitivity, and educational dysfunctions as they relate to perception. The effects of emotional and psychological factors upon vision are also considered and, with proper training, significant changes in academic, athletic, and social/emotional behavior can occur.

Syntonic Optometry

In recent years, researchers have found that full-spectrum light (sunlight or an artificial source containing the full spectrum) improves the functioning of the nervous, endocrine, and immune systems. Syntonic optometry, or colored light therapy, selects specific bands of frequencies (seen as colored lights) within this full spectrum to improve visual ability and treat some eye ailments, including peripheral vision problems, color and night blindness, crossed eyes, and lazy eye. Many optometrists are also discouraging the use of standard incandescent and fluorescent lights, which do not contain the full spectrum of light and therefore can contribute to vision problems.

An instrument called the Lumatron Light Stimulator® is utilized by syntonic optometrists to help alleviate peripheral vision problems, night blindness, light sensitivity, and color blindness. Developed by John Downing, O.D., Ph.D., Director of the Light Therapy Institute, in Santa Rosa, California, the Lumatron emits 11 wave bands of color, ranging from red through violet, at a rate of zero to 60 cycles a second. Patients sit underneath a hood at the front of the instrument and look at the light, which restimulates the neural/visual system.

According to Dr. Downing, "The visual field significantly expands after stimulation, which is an indication that more photocurrent is traveling from the eye to the visual cortex." A typical treatment consists of 25–30 sessions over four to six weeks. The Lumatron is currently being used in 20 countries by hundreds of physicians.

Biofeedback Training

Biofeedback is used to measure and regulate various bodily functions and can be used to treat refractive errors, lazy eye, crossed eyes, macular degeneration, and glaucoma. Joseph Trachtman, O.D., Ph.D., a New York-based optometric physician, is the inventor of the Accommotrac Vision Trainer®, an instrument that measures the retina for clarity of image. As the patient's focusing changes, the Accommotrac converts the visual image into sound so that very small changes can be detected and then controlled. The treatment consists of weekly, hour-long sessions in which patients learn how to refine control over the eye muscle, thus allowing both nearsighted and farsighted individuals to significantly improve their vision.

According to Dr. Trachtman, "We're able to take people who have extremely poor vision and either elimi-

A MULTIFACETED PROGRAM FOR MACULAR DEGENERATION

Conventional medicine considers macular degeneration incurable. However, scientific studies have demonstrated that retinal tissue does have regenerative capabilities. "No one alternative therapy has emerged that can be considered a panacea," says Grace Halloran, Ph.D., of Integrated Visual Healing (IVH), in San Leandro, California. "Using a multifaceted approach, educating individuals and training them to be their own therapist as an ongoing commitment, we consistently see the cessation of degeneration, dramatic improvement, and even cases of complete reversal."

Dr. Halloran's protocol grew out of her own loss of vision from macular degeneration at the age of 24. Her frustration with conventional approaches led her to educate herself about the alternative treatments available. "The experience of hundreds of individuals, myself included, has proven that when alternative methods are employed, eye health and visual function are often improved," says Dr. Halloran. "Individuals facing sight loss from serious eye disorders need to aggressively explore lifestyle changes to improve overall health and reject the victim mentality that so often accompanies the conventional medical diagnosis of conditions that cause sight to fail."

Dr. Halloran took everything she had experienced and learned from alternative medicine and put together the IVH program. IVH incorporates ancient and modern therapies, increasing overall health with special focus on the eyes.

- Diet and Nutrition: IVH begins with the basics—eating organic, whole, fresh, minimally processed foods. Nutritional supplementation is also considered essential for individuals at risk or who have serious eye disorders. Nutrition education is a critical component in the IVH program.

- Acupressure: This is a form of acupuncture, employing the same points, that stimulates energy flow with finger pressure instead of needles. Visual health can be enhanced by massaging points on the head, ears, hands, and feet to stimulate the energy flow to the eyes.

- Micro-Current Therapy: This is a high-tech, noninvasive acupuncture technique. One device, called the MicroStim, is suitable for both clinical and home use.

- Color Therapy: Ancient Egyptian texts allude to this form of healing, which is inexpensive and suitable for self-application at home. For instance, magenta stimulates the macular region, blue-green seems to increase lymph flow in the eyes, and the green-yellow range improves field of vision and night sight.

- Massage: "We teach a version of Touch for Health, a system developed by Dr. John Thie, which combines applied kinesiology (muscle testing and movement) with lymphatic massage therapy," says Dr. Halloran. It is useful for on-going home therapy.

- Stress Management: Over time, chronic stress reduces the blood supply to the eyes, which can result in severe degeneration. Under stress, even normal-sighted people tend to lose side vision and focusing ability. Since sight loss itself creates stress, training in stress management is vital.

- Eye Exercises: Poor posture and chronic muscle tension impair circulation to and from the head. Nerve, lymph, and blood circulation are all affected by the level of tension in the upper torso. Participants in the IVH program are taught a series of exercises specifically designed to stimulate right/left brain function, coupled with yoga-like stretches to elongate and tone the upper torso to improve circulation.

nate or reduce the need for their eyeglasses." He recalls one patient who, after six months of treatment, showed an improvement in vision from 20/400 to about 20/30. When Dr. Trachtman saw the patient a couple of years after the treatment, he found that the patient had maintained most of the improvement.

The Accommotrac is sensitive to eye position and can be used to treat crossed eyes, lazy eye, and a condi-

tion called nystagmus, characterized by oscillating eye movement. Dr. Trachtman has also helped patients suffering from macular degeneration by training them to use a part of the eye other than the deteriorating macula.

Steve Fahrion, Ph.D., founding member of Life Sciences Institute of Mind–Body Health, in Topeka, Kansas, says that the use of biofeedback to relax the forehead muscles can reduce pressure in the eyeball and therefore can be used to treat glaucoma. This technique involves placing electrodes on the forehead in order to get an auditory tone that indicates the level of stress. By increasing relaxation, the pressure in the eye area can be reduced. According to Dr. Fahrion, one of his colleagues has used this approach successfully to control his glaucoma for several years.

The Bates Method

Pioneering New York ophthalmologist William Bates, M.D., was the first to discover that chronic eye problems were frequently stress-related. He demonstrated the correlation between various vision disorders and tension unconsciously placed on the muscles that control the eyes. From this, Dr. Bates developed a set of eye exercises to reduce eye stress and correct eye and vision-related disorders. Dr. Bates explained that "perfect sight is a product of perfectly relaxed organs, unconsciously controlled," and that vision improves naturally when people stop interfering with it.[20] Under relaxed conditions, refractive errors tend to be self-correcting.

Perfect sight is a product of perfectly relaxed organs, unconsciously controlled.

—WILLIAM BATES, M.D.

Paul Anderson, a Bates method practitioner in Kirkland, Washington, succeeded in correcting his own vision from 20/300 to 20/20 and advocates natural vision-improvement techniques be included in schools and workplaces. "Putting on glasses to correct an image distorted by mental strain will not, in the long run, prove beneficial to the child or to society," he says.[21]

Herbal Remedies

David Hoffmann, B.Sc., M.N.I.M.H., of Sebastopol, California, past President of the American Herbalists Guild, treats cataracts with an eyewash consisting of an infusion of eyebright. A stronger mix can be made with equal parts eyebright and goldenseal. In treating macular degeneration, European research shows that *Ginkgo biloba* and bilberry can be beneficial.[22] In addition to ginkgo, Hoffman recommends taking milk thistle (100 mg) and bilberry (100 mg) three times a day. Hoffman also notes that Siberian ginseng may be helpful in treating some forms of color blindness.[23]

For macular degeneration, glaucoma, and cataracts, bilberry and grapeseed extract may be helpful. Pine bark extract (pycnogenol) and curcumin are useful herbal remedies for cataracts.[24] For conjunctivitis, a simple home remedy suggested by Joseph Pizzorno, N.D., President Emeritus of Bastyr University, in Kenmore, Washington, is made by adding goldenseal root powder (1 tbsp), salt (1 tsp), and vitamin C (250 mg) to a quart of water. After letting the solution settle, the clear liquid is used to thoroughly wash out the eye several times a day.

Traditional Chinese Medicine

Traditional Chinese medicine traces most vision ailments to liver function. Treatment often combines acupuncture, herbs, and dietary changes. According to Maoshing Ni, D.O.M., Ph.D., L.Ac., President of Yo San University of Traditional Chinese Medicine, in Marina del Rey, California, acupuncture is effective in balancing and readjusting tension in the eye muscles, thereby improving the shape of the eye and its ability to function properly. For nearsightedness and farsightedness, a typical course of treatment involves ten acupuncture sessions. Eye exercises are often recommended to help maintain the improvement.

With more serious disorders such as cataracts and glaucoma, treatment involves the use of herbs and dietary changes. Dr. Ni cites the example of a man who underwent treatment for glaucoma for three months, which included weekly acupuncture sessions, herbal treatments, and dietary changes. By the end of treatment, the patient's eye pressure had returned to normal, allowing him to discontinue his medication and postpone surgery indefinitely. Upon discharge, Dr. Ni provided stress-management techniques and instructed the man to maintain his modified diet. A similar approach can sometimes stop or even reverse the growth of a cataract, according to Dr. Ni.

Ayurvedic Medicine

Ayurvedic medicine generally considers vision disorders to be caused by digestive problems. Ayurvedic techniques attempt to improve metabolic function and eye exercises are used to strengthen ailing vision and prevent healthy eyes from deteriorating. Herbal remedies and nutritional supplements are the basis of Ayurvedic treatment for vision problems. Herbs such as *amla, triphala,* and licorice, along with substances rich in beta carotene, such as carrots and spinach, are prescribed to stimulate the digestive system and strengthen the eyes.

Virender Sodhi, M.D. (Ayurveda), N.D., Director of the Ayurvedic & Naturopathic Medical Clinic, in Bellevue, Washington, recalls treating his mother, who was suffering from retinal hemorrhages and had been declared legally blind. A previous physician had prescribed heavy doses of cortisone, which had no effect on her vision but caused her to gain nearly 60 pounds and develop high blood pressure. Dr. Sodhi treated her using *amla* tablets combined with a series of eye exercises. As a result, her vision improved substantially, allowing her to regain the ability to read and write.

 Any effective prevention-oriented regimen includes annual visits to an optometrist. If you are feeling a persistent irritation in your eyes, however, or if objects begin to look markedly different to you, seek immediate professional attention. Early detection of potentially serious conditions increases the likelihood that minimal treatment will be required to restore your eyes to their natural state.

In another case, Dr. Sodhi treated a 9-year-old girl suffering from severe corneal ulcers in one eye. The patient's ophthalmologist, observing that the eye was badly scarred, recommended corneal transplant surgery, which has a 50% chance of failure. But when Dr. Sodhi discovered an allergy to chocolate was causing blurred vision and severe headaches, he instituted a three-month dietary treatment combined with herbs. To strengthen the musculature of the eye and increase the pliability of the cornea, eye exercises were also prescribed, plus eye rinses with *triphala*. At the end of treatment, the ulcers were gone and there was no trace of scarring.

Craniosacral Therapy

According to John Upledger, D.O., Medical Director of the Upledger Institute, in Palm Beach Gardens, Florida, visual motor disturbances can occur if the membranes attached to the temporal bone put pressure on the nerves to the eye. He uses craniosacral therapy to relieve the pressure and help restore motor control of the eyes.

Other structural problems can also interfere with vision, according to Dr. Upledger. He recalls one patient whose vision improved from 20/200 to 20/40 within a matter of minutes after treating her cervical vertebrae (spinal neck vertebrae). "In addition, manipulation of the bones of the occipital region [base of the skull] can release pressure on the lobes of the brain and improve vision by allowing the correct messages to get through to these areas," says Dr. Upledger.

EYE EXERCISES FOR VISUAL FITNESS

One of the easiest treatments for improving visual fitness and efficiency is to give your eyes frequent breaks throughout the day. Here are a few exercises for relaxing the eyes:

- Every 30-60 minutes, give your eyes a five-minute rest from concentrated work. Look up from your work, relax your gaze, and let your eyes wander across the room or simply stare off into space.

- The eyes need oxygen and will function better when the body is rested and circulation is improved. Breathe deeply for several minutes, then stretch your neck and shoulders. Roll your head around in a circle, side to side and up and down. Touch your ear to your shoulder and repeat for the other side. Yawn and stretch the muscles of your face, which often hold a lot of tension.

- Blink regularly to reduce eyestrain. Blinking also increases the amount of concentrated work your eyes can accomplish comfortably.

- Palming is easy to practice and offers effective eye relief. Sit comfortably in a relaxed position and breathe deeply as you gently cover your eyes with your palms. Yoga teachers suggest that you first rub your hands together vigorously to create some penetrating warmth and energy, which will provide additional comfort to your eyes.

The process of accommodation—which means switching one's focus between near and distant objects without losing clarity—becomes more difficult as the lenses of the eyes grow less flexible with age. To enhance flexibility, try each of these procedures daily for 15-20 seconds, with prescription lenses removed:

- Perform rapid switches from close-up to long-range focus in a smooth and effortless manner by pretending to follow an imaginary ping-pong game.

- Tack some reading material to the wall and read it from a comfortable distance, then increase the distance a little bit each day. Eventually, you'll be able to read the material from across the room. Near vision can also be improved by getting closer to the material each day.

Recommendations

- Emphasize a diet rich in carotenoids and other antioxidants, especially dark, leafy green vegetables and red, blue, and purple fruits.

- Helpful nutritional supplements include vitamins A, C, and E, flavonoids, N-acetyl-cysteine, riboflavin, selenium, taurine, and zinc.

- Herbal remedies include bilberry, *Ginkgo biloba*, grape seed extract, pine bark (pycnogenol), and Siberian ginseng.

- Frequent or regular "near-work" activities (such as reading, working at a computer, and drawing) can lead to myopia (nearsightedness). If you engage in such activities, take breaks from your work throughout the day, practice eye exercises, and avoid a buildup of chronic tension, especially in the face, neck, and shoulders.

- Expose yourself frequently to sunlight.

- Avoid exposure to chemicals, environmental pollutants, and cigarette smoke. Also, avoid or minimize exposure to fluorescent lightning, computer monitors, and electromagnetic pollution, and avoid working in poorly lit environments.

Self-Care
The following therapies can be undertaken at home under appropriate professional supervision:

Qigong and Tai Chi / Yoga

JUICE THERAPY: Fresh carrot juice, or combine carrot with celery, parsley, spinach, or cucumber.

TOPICAL TREATMENT: • For eyestrain or pressure on the eyeball, use a raw-potato eye pack. Grate organic, unsprayed white potatoes (peel and pulp) and place a small spoonful on the eyelid and over entire eye. Cover with a piece of gauze and leave in place for one or two hours. • For eye infections or irritations, use fresh cucumber juice. Wash hands thoroughly, then cut off a chunk of cucumber, peel, and grate. Put grated cucumber in a large sterile gauze pad or boiled cheesecloth. Squeeze a few drops of cucumber juice directly into eye. Be sure to use fresh cucumber and gauze each time.

Professional Care
The following therapies should only be provided by a qualified health professional:

Chelation Therapy / Chiropractic / Detoxification Therapy / Magnetic Field Therapy / Naturopathic Medicine / Osteopathic Medicine

BODYWORK: • Acupressure, reflexology, and shiatsu massage can relieve accompanying muscular tension. • Rolfing, Feldenkrais Method, and Alexander Technique can help reduce vision-affecting physical and emotional stress.

ENVIRONMENTAL MEDICINE: Environmental medicine takes into consideration chemical or food sensitivities, electromagnetic pollution, and geopathic stress, all environmental hazards to which the retina is particularly sensitive.

Where to Find Help

Vision-improvement practitioners may be listed in the Yellow Pages under "Eyesight Training." They may or may not be licensed. A licensed eye doctor can help you find alternative care or you can contact the following organizations.

American Academy of Ophthalmology
P.O. Box 7424
San Francisco, California 94210
(415) 561-8500
Website: www.aao.org

Provides information on various eye conditions and vision disorders.

American Association of Oriental Medicine
433 Front Street
Catasauqua, Pennsylvania 18032
(888) 500-7999
Website: www.aaom.org

The AAOM is a national professional organization of acupuncturists who meet acceptable standards of competency and can provide you with the names and locations of local members.

Ayurvedic and Naturopathic Medical Clinic
2115 112th Avenue N.E.
Bellevue, Washington 98004
(425) 453-8022
Website: www.ayurvedicscience.com

Dr. Virender Sodhi's clinic provides medical training for physicians and health-care practitioners, as well as individual courses for laypeople.

National Eye Research Foundation
910 Skokie Boulevard, Suite 207A
Northbrook, Illinois 60062
(800) 621-2258
Website: www.nerf.org

Provides education and referrals for preventative and thera-peutic eye care. They have information on contact lens safety, the use of color fields to uncover systemic diseases, and alter-natives to surgical intervention for crossed eyes.

Integrated Visual Healing
655 Lewelling Blvd. #214
San Leandro, California 94579
(510) 357-0477

Provides information and training on the IVH protocol devel-oped by Grace Halloran, Ph.D., as well as a directory of prac-titioners.

Behavioral Optometry
College of Optometrists in Vision Development
243 N. Lindbergh Boulevard, Suite 310
St. Louis, Missouri 63141
(888) 268-3770
Website: www.covd.org

The College of Optometrists in Vision Development is an international certifying organization for optometrists who spe-cialize in vision therapy. Provides referrals upon request.

Optometric Extension Program Foundation
1921 E. Carnegie Avenue, Suite 3-L
Santa Ana, California 92705
(949) 250-8070
Website: www.oep.org

Offers continuing education in behavioral optometry for con-sumers and optometrists. Provides referrals upon request.

Syntonic Optometry
College of Syntonic Optometry
15 Western Avenue
Augusta, Maine 04330
(866) 486-0190
Website: www.syntonicphototherapy.com

A society of optometrists who practice phototherapy. They offer courses on the optometric application of phototherapy and a nationwide directory of practitioners trained in its use.

Recommended Reading

The Bates Method for Better Eyesight Without Glasses. W.H. Bates. New York: Henry Holt/Owl Books, 1981.

Greater Vision: A Comprehensive Program for Physical, Emo-tional, and Spiritual Clarity. Marc Grossman and Vinton McCabe. Los Angeles: Keats Publishing, 2001.

Light, Medicine of the Future. Jacob Liberman, O.D., Ph.D. Santa Fe, NM: Bear & Company, 1991.

Natural Eye Care: An Encyclopedia. Marc Grossman and Glen Swartwout. New Canaan, CT: Keats Publishing, 1999.

Seeing Beyond 20/20: Improve the Quality of Your Vision and Your Life. Michael R. Kaplan, M.D. Hillsboro, OR: Beyond Words Publishing, 1987.

The Eye Care Sourcebook. Jay B. Lavine. Chicago: Con-temporary Books, 2001.

WOMEN'S HEALTH

Women's health care focuses on helping a woman maintain optimal health as her reproductive system develops and matures. Alternative medicine helps to educate women in a variety of preventative steps to maintain overall health, as well as providing natural treatments for symptoms and diseases related to hormonal and physiological imbalances.

CONVENTIONAL APPROACHES to women's health have often used surgery and other invasive medical procedures to deal with common physiological functions, such as the hormonal imbalances experienced during menopause. Alternative medicine offers a variety of therapeutic approaches such as diet, nutritional supplementation, herbal medicine, homeopathy, naturopathic medicine, traditional Chinese medicine, and Ayurvedic medicine, which can be safely used to address the diverse symptoms of premenstrual syndrome and menopause, as well as diseases of the uterus, vagina, bladder, and breasts.

In turn, women need to make informed choices about diet, exercise, and stress management when taking care of their bodies, according to Susan M. Lark, M.D., of Los Altos, California. "These changes alone can produce great results. I've been very impressed in my own practice by how much women can really modify their health problems just by modifying their lifestyle."

Life Cycles

Throughout her life, a woman's reproductive system follows rhythmic patterns of change, monthly cycles, and the completion of those cycles with menopause. By becoming acquainted with the needs, characteristics, and problems of each phase, a woman can make informed choices about lifestyle and health care.

Menstruation

The reproductive organs mature during puberty, the stage during which a girl becomes a woman and menstruation begins. A woman menstruates an average of 500 times during her life. Yet there are many misconceptions about menstruation, and some have been repeated so often that they are considered fact. Most notable is the assumption that the average menstrual cycle is 28 days, neatly paralleling the cycles of the moon. While women's bodies do have an observable rhythm, the menstrual cycle actually has a wide range of lengths that can be considered normal. "The 28-day cycle is a complete myth," says Toni Weschler, M.P.H., of Seattle, Washington. "Cycles vary anywhere from about 24 days to 37 days. If a woman uses the 28-day cycle as a point of reference and her cycle is different, she may think there's something wrong with her."

While two or three generations ago women began to menstruate at around 15 or 16 years of age, today puberty begins at 12 or 13. Menstruation begins when body estrogen reaches a certain level, and Christiane Northrup, M.D., of Yarmouth, Maine, past President of the American Holistic Medical Association, cites several factors that may prematurely increase the body's supply. "High-fat diets help the body produce more estrogen," she says. "Then there are the hormones in beef and chicken, used to speed up their growth process, which we eventually consume. Antibiotics in meat (50% of the antibiotics in this country are fed to livestock) can change intestinal flora and slow proper elimination. Some estrogen, instead of being excreted, simply recycles."

The result of this hormone onslaught is a relative excess of estrogen, meaning there is too much estrogen in relation to the level of progesterone, the other primary female hormone. Also known as estrogen dominance, this condition is a primary cause in almost all female health conditions, including PMS, mood swings, excessive bleeding, endometriosis, fibroids, infertility, ovarian cysts, and fibrocystic breast disease.

The monthly menstrual cycle results from coordinated hormonal interplay among the hypothalamus, the pituitary gland, and the ovaries. Each month, at the start of the cycle, estrogen is secreted by the 10–20 eggs

Hormone Levels During the Menstrual Cycle

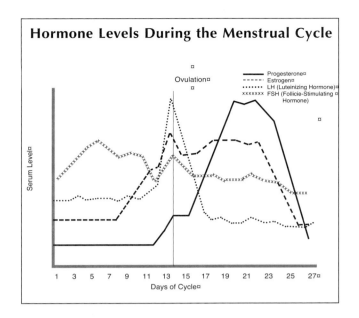

Female Reproductive System

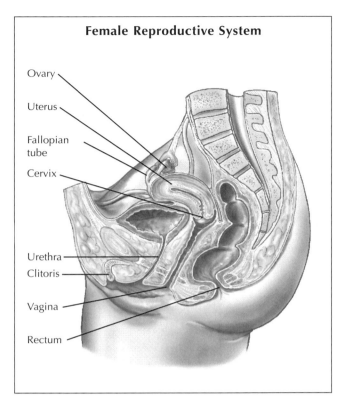

growing in the ovaries. The estrogen triggers the thickening of the lining of the uterus (the endometrium) with blood vessels, glands, and cells in anticipation of new life. It also causes the production of a cervical fluid that facilitates the passage of sperm through the cervical opening and enhances its survival. Once the mature egg has left the ovaries, it can be fertilized in the fallopian tubes.

Next, estrogen production subsides and progesterone production increases. This second hormone forms a thick cervical mucus plug in the cervix to prevent sperm or bacteria from entering, and maintains the endometrium in a nutritious, blood-rich stage in anticipation of the egg's fertilization by the sperm, i.e., conception. If conception does not occur, all hormone levels drop, some of the endometrial layer is released, or "shed," and this is called menstruation. The cycle then starts over. If fertilization does occur, progesterone secretion continues to increase, maintaining the uterine lining and pregnancy until the placenta takes over secreting progesterone and other hormones at about three months' gestation.

While women's bodies do have an observable rhythm, the menstrual cycle actually has a wide range of lengths that can be considered normal.

Getting to Know Your Cycle: It is important for each woman to become familiar with the individual pat-

terns of her monthly cycle. Dr. Northrup advises that, premenstrually, "a woman needs to take a little retreat time, moving slower and even resting her mind." When a woman is aware of her cycle, she might be able to plan her days accordingly.

The monthly cycle can also be used as a guide in maintaining general health, because, as research is now suggesting, a woman's immune system peaks before ovulation and decreases afterward.[1] One piece of evidence is the higher incidence of vaginal yeast and chlamydial infections just before menstrual periods.[2] There is a reason for this oscillation in immunity: the dip at this time is necessary so that the "foreign" sperm and the fertilized egg will be accepted by the woman's body, and an immune boost prior to ovulation cleanses the body of germs before possible pregnancy.[3]

Suzannah Doyle, a certified fertility educator from Corvallis, Oregon, says research now shows that vaccinations, surgery, and prescription drugs have fewer harmful effects when used on a woman before ovulation. Women are even more easily affected by alcohol consumed premenstrually versus during the fertile time. "In the future, a woman's own observed fertility signs will enable doctors to actually adjust drug dosages for their patients," Doyle adds. "Fertility signs are already being used by some health-care providers to increase the effectiveness and accuracy of surgeries, drug therapies, and procedures such as PAP smears and diaphragm fittings."

A WOMAN'S HORMONE GLOSSARY

Estrogen is one of the female "sex" hormones, produced mainly in the ovaries (some in the fat cells), that regulates the menstrual cycle. Estrogen is important for adolescent sexual development, prepares the uterus for receiving the fertilized egg by stimulating the uterine lining to grow, and affects all the body's cells; its levels decline after menopause. For the first 10-14 days in a woman's cycle, the uterus is mainly under the influence of estrogen. Estrogen levels begin to climb right before menstruation, from about days seven to 14, and peak at ovulation. There are three natural types of estrogen: estradiol (produced in the ovaries), estrone (produced from estradiol), and estriol (formed in smaller amounts in the ovaries). Estradiol is the most potent of the three. Estrogen slows down bone loss and it can help reduce the incidence of heart attacks; estrogen also improves skin tone, reduces vaginal dryness, influences mood, and can act as an antiaging factor.

Luteinizing hormone (LH), produced by the pituitary gland in the brain, is primarily responsible for ovulation in women. Its name comes from lutein, the yellowish fluid that fills the corpus luteum. This is a hormone-secreting body of endocrine tissues that forms the follicle or sac containing a developing egg. The corpus luteum controls the production of the key female hormones estrogen and progesterone during the second half of the menstrual cycle (called the luteal phase). Approaching mid-cycle, the ovary secretes increasing amounts of estrogen, and a sudden drop in estrogen levels just before mid-cycle triggers a dramatic surge of LH and follicle-stimulating hormone (FSH). This usually occurs between days 12 and 16 of the cycle, with ovulation (the release of the egg) at day 14. The sudden

increase in LH/FSH causes the corpus luteum (also called the follicular cyst) to burst, allowing the mature egg to travel down into the fallopian tubes. Following ovulation, the corpus luteum gradually shrinks, producing less estrogen and progesterone. The steady decline of these hormones ends in the shedding of the uterine lining (menstruation) and the beginning of a new cycle.

Follicle-stimulating hormone (FSH), produced by the pituitary gland in the brain, regulates the development and release of a mature egg from its follicle, or protective sac, in the ovary. Approaching mid-cycle, the ovary secretes more estrogen, which sensitizes the pituitary cells that produce FSH and LH. This results in a dramatic surge in LH and FSH at mid-cycle, when the estrogen level starts to drop and the hypothalamus secretes releasing hormones.

Progesterone is a hormone (produced in the corpus luteum of the ovaries) that prepares the uterus for a fertilized egg and then stops the cell proliferation in the uterus if pregnancy does not occur. When estrogen is high, during days seven to 14 of a woman's cycle, the level of progesterone is at its lowest. Its levels climb to a peak around days 14 to 24 and then dramatically drop off again just before the start of menstruation. When the cells stop producing progesterone, it is a signal to the uterus to let go of all the new cells produced during the month and to start afresh. In a sense, menstruation is progesterone withdrawal. Starting at age 35, a woman's progesterone production begins to decline.

Menopause

Strictly defined, menopause is the end of all menstrual bleeding. Generally, women experience menopause between the ages of 48 and 52, but some women cease menstruating as early as their late thirties and early forties while others stop in their mid-fifties. According to the U.S. Census Bureau, the number of menopausal women, 45 to 54 years old, numbers 13 million and is expected to grow by 73% by 2010. The aging "Baby Boom" population means that 3,500 American women enter the "menopausal years" every day. Yet, because women are healthier now, menopause no longer indicates the onset of old age, and women can expect to live a third of their adult lives after menopause.[4]

Menopause commences when the ovaries stop producing estrogen. Perimenopause is the period commonly thought of as the five to ten years before menopause (approximately between the ages of 35 and 50). It is characterized by several years of irregular cycles with no ovulation since the ovaries are at the end of their egg supply. Without an egg's presence, progesterone is no longer produced and therefore perimenopause is frequently characterized by estrogen dominance, with side effects ranging from water retention, weight gain, and mood swings, to fibrocystic breasts, breast cancer, fibroids, or endometrial cancer.

With the onset of menopause, however, estrogen levels do not drop to zero. Some estrogen is still produced in fat cells, the supporting tissue around the ovaries, and in the intestinal tract using precursors produced by the adrenals. Weight gain after menopause can be the body's attempt to take advantage of this situation. Estrogen is also made through other chemical pathways in the body.[5] It is this reserve of estrogen that many natural therapies draw on for their effectiveness.

Potential Menstrual Problems and Treatments

In the early years following puberty, it is common for menstrual periods to be irregular due to hormonal imbalances. Irregular bleeding, spotting, bleeding too much, clots, or a total absence of blood are all signs that a woman's reproductive system needs attention. Women may also experience symptoms such as cramping, headaches, and mood changes. Changes in diet and lifestyle, as well as professional treatment, can significantly relieve these conditions, and a variety of alternative therapies have long traditions of treating the range of women's health problems, both chronic and acute. Conditions addressed include those related to the menstrual cycle and menopause, as well as diseases of the, vagina, bladder, uterus and breasts.

Menstrual Cramps (Dysmenorrhea)

As many as 30% to 50% of all women suffer from pain during their menstrual period,[11] though until recently the medical community has considered this a "minor" complaint, with the implication that it was "all in a woman's head." New thinking takes menstrual cramps seriously and, in terms of hormones, proposes that primary dysmenorrhea is caused by excess production of prostaglandins (hormone-like fatty acids) by the endometrium following a decline in progesterone levels.[12]

At least 10% of younger women have dysmenorrhea symptoms so severe that they cannot participate in their normal activities.[13] Besides lower abdominal pain, cramp sufferers may also experience backache, pinching and pain sensations in the inner thighs, and many of the symptoms of premenstrual syndrome. According to Dr. Lark, primary spasmodic dysmenorrhea is the type most commonly found in women in their early teens to late twenties. "This is characterized by sharp, viselike pains that are caused by a constriction and tightening of the uterine muscle," she explains. "Blood circulation and oxygenation of uterine muscles and blood vessels are diminished and waste products of metabolism, such as carbon dioxide and lactic acid, build up and the pain and discomfort are intensified."

In contrast, primary congestive dysmenorrhea produces a dull aching in the low-back and pelvic regions, often accompanied by bloating, weight gain, breast tenderness, headaches, and irritability. "Unlike spasmodic cramping, these symptoms don't improve with age," says Dr. Lark. "Some of the worst symptoms are seen in women in their thirties and forties. Excessive amounts of estrogen can worsen these symptoms, since estrogen increases fluid and salt retention in the body."[14]

Diet: Dr. Lark recommends eating whole grains, legumes, fruits and vegetables, and seeds and nuts (such as ground, raw flaxseed, and pumpkin seed), while avoiding dairy products, saturated fats, salt, alcohol, sugar, and caffeine. For spasmodic symptoms specifically, choose fish such as trout, mackerel, and salmon, and avoid meat, poultry, dairy products, and eggs. For congestive symptoms, avoid sugar, alcohol, salt, dairy foods, and wheat.

Nutritional Supplements: Dr. Lark recommends vitamins B_3, B_6, and C, calcium, magnesium, potassium, zinc, and essential fatty acids, especially omega-3 oils such as eicosapentaenoic acid (EPA).

Herbal Medicine: According to David L. Hoffmann, B.Sc., M.N.I.M.H., past President of the American Herbalists Guild, painful cramps associated with menstruation or ovulation can be eased by combining the tinctures of skullcap, blackhaw (*Bumelia lanuginosa*), and black cohosh in equal parts and taking 1-2 teaspoons of this mixture as needed. For water retention, Hoffmann recommends dandelion leaf. "This is a rich source of potassium and, though this herb promotes excretion of urine, which also causes potassium loss, this herb simultaneously replaces the mineral. Take one teaspoon of the tincture three times a day, or an infusion of the fresh leaves three to five times a day." Dr. Lark also recommends ginger, *Ginkgo biloba*, white willow bark, red raspberry leaf, crampbark, chamomile, hops, and chastetree berry.

Homeopathy: According to Lauri Aesoph, N.D., an educator from Sioux Falls, South Dakota, *Sepia* and *Lachesis* are common treatments for cramps, and she adds that the cramps that are relieved by a hot water bottle or heating pad can also be helped by *Chamomilla*.

Traditional Chinese Medicine: According to Honora Lee Wolfe, Dipl.Ac., of Boulder, Colorado, "Menstrual cramps are due usually to either *qi* stagnation (when the vital energy is unable to move freely through the body) in the lower abdomen, or blood stasis, or a combination of both." Treatment can involve the use of both acupuncture and herbs according to the individual's needs.

Absence of Menstruation (Amenorrhea)

Just as some women are troubled by too much menstrual blood, others find that their menstrual periods just stop

NATURAL BIRTH CONTROL

Understanding a woman's menstrual cycle is instrumental in using natural birth control effectively. Contrary to popular belief, several methods of natural contraception are useful and safe, although some purported forms are unreliable, such as douching and withdrawal. The most notorious of these is the rhythm method, which involves predicting when the fertile phase "should" occur and abstaining from intercourse during this time. But, as Toni Weschler, M.P.H., of Seattle, Washington, states, "The rhythm method is based on women having regular cycles, which is why it does not work. The only way to determine when a woman is fertile and when she is not is to identify her fertility signs on a daily basis: basal body temperature, cervical fluid, and cervical position."

There are two natural birth control methods that employ observation of one's fertility signs. Natural family planning (NFP), says Weschler, "assumes a couple is abstinent during the woman's fertile time" and barrier methods are not used. Fertility awareness method (FAM) gives a couple the option of using barrier methods during fertile periods. The difference between NFP and FAM is philosophical, notes Weschler.

Fertility observation is used in the ovulation or Billings method, which relies specifically on checking cervical mucus rather than the cervix itself, and in the symptothermal method, which employs all three available fertility signals. Both of these methods must be carefully learned in order to be effective; however, when used scrupulously, the failure rates can be as low as 2% to 3%.[6]

Breast-feeding, which may suppress ovulation, has received mixed reports on its effectiveness as a contraceptive. Its reliability depends on how often a baby nurses and whether it is supplemented with other liquids or foods.[7] If a woman wants to use lactation to control fertility, NFP or FAM can be used as a backup method.

Natural barrier methods include the diaphragm, the male condom, the female condom, and the cervical cap (a small latex dome placed over the cervix). Some may not consider diaphragms natural because of the spermicide jelly or cream that should be used with them. Like the diaphragm, the cervical cap must be professionally fitted. Advantages of the cap include no spermicide use and the ability to leave it in the vagina longer than the diaphragm.

Another option in birth control is the female condom, which lines the vagina, protecting against transfer of virus and bacteria as well as sperm. This barrier device consists of a soft, thin, polyurethane sheath with two flexible rings. One ring lies inside the closed upper end of the sheath and holds the condom in place after insertion, while the other, on the opposite, open end, remains outside the vagina. This outer portion covers the labia and the base of the penis during intercourse. Among the objections to the female condom is the aesthetic issue of having part of the condom hanging outside the vagina during intercourse, but the advantages of the condom may override this objection. For one thing, the protection provided by the female condom places a woman in greater control of her own sexual health.

Although the female condom has been approved by the U.S. Food and Drug Administration, clinical trials have not demonstrated a high efficacy rate, especially in comparison to male condoms. In the U.S., 12.2% of the participating women became pregnant.[8] Male condoms can be used alone or with any of these female barriers to increase contraceptive success. When condoms are used properly, their effectiveness increases dramatically. Another advantage of barrier methods in general is that they may help protect against some sexually transmitted diseases and somewhat against AIDS. Latex condoms should be used rather than lambskin, which permit a high percentage of virus leakage because the material is so porous;[9] however, there is also some risk with latex condoms.[10]

(for a reason other than pregnancy or menopause). In this condition, called amenorrhea, a woman does not have a period for three or more months; a teenage girl who is age 16 and has not started menstruating yet is also judged to have this condition, as is a woman whose periods stop when she stops taking birth control pills.

Amenorrhea is mainly caused by temporary failure of the ovaries and pituitary gland, according to Ralph Golan, M.D., of Seattle, Washington. An underactive thy-

roid gland is also frequently a factor. Malfunctions in any of these organs lead to hormonal imbalance and lack of menstruation can be the manifestation of the disturbance. As with other reproductive health disorders with similar causality, restoring the function of the organs involved and rebalancing the hormones is essential for a successful treatment outcome.

Other causes of amenorrhea include nutritional deficiencies (often as the result of excess dieting or weight loss), poor adrenal function, and intense, extended exercise, as in marathon training.[15] Diet has a strong influence on menstrual regularity. An insufficient amount of "good" fats (unsaturated fats and essential fatty acids), a lack of protein, and an excess of carotene in the blood are all associated with amenorrhea.[16] Extreme emotional stress or tension can also result in a cessation of menstrual periods.

There are many types of amenorrhea, but one in particular, which is experienced by some young athletes, is often misunderstood, according to Dr. Northrup. "It is a common assumption that regular strenuous exercise can cause a young woman to miss her period. But these women are also restricting caloric intake and are, in fact, anorexic, just like every other woman who is addicted to a cultural ideal that is impossible for 90% of women to achieve. The nutritional needs for supporting the metabolic demands of the exercise are simply not being met. In my practice, I have found that if amenorrheic women eat at least 500 calories more per day, their periods become reestablished."

Herbal Medicine: According to David Hoffmann, herbs for amenorrhea include chasteberry, false unicorn root, blue cohosh, rue *(Ruta graveolens),* pennyroyal, and tansy.

Homeopathy: Australian homeopath Paul Callinan suggests using low-potency homeopathic remedies when the period has stopped (for reasons other than pregnancy or menopause). Take the selected remedy three times daily for one month, he says. If positive results are not obtained, he advises consulting a professional homeopath for a deeper analysis and more precise prescription. Here are Dr. Callinan's recommendations:[17]

- *Ferrum phosphoricum* 6X—when the menstrual flow is suppressed, accompanied by depressed spirits, debility, lethargy, constant dull headache, and irritability
- *Calcarea carbonica* 6C—when menstruation is absent, accompanied by chills, tiredness, swollen breasts, painful heavy legs, and being overweight
- *Kali sulphuricum* 6X—when the period is scanty or suppressed, with a sensation of weight and fullness in the abdomen
- *Aconitum napellus* 6C—when periods stop abruptly due to exposure to dry cold or sudden shock
- *Natrum muriaticum* 6X—when periods are absent, accompanied by headaches, constipation, and/or irritability
- *Sepia* 6C—when periods are missing, accompanied by tearfulness, irritability, the fear of losing control, and the loss of one's sexual interest

Excessive Menstruation (Menorrhagia)

Abnormally profuse menstrual flow is called menorrhagia, whether excessively long periods or heavy periods or both. A common cause of menorrhagia is, again, estrogen dominance. Abnormalities of the endometrium, iron and vitamin A deficiencies, hypothyroidism, and intrauterine devices are all considered possible causes.[18]

Diet: You can regulate your hormonal environment through diet, says Dr. Northrup. If you are a carbohydrate-sensitive woman (you crave sugar, chips, or other starches, are overweight, or have type O blood), reduce your consumption of these foods. They increase insulin levels in the blood and can lead to excess body fat; this is associated with excess circulating estrogen. If necessary, limit carbohydrate intake to once daily and make sure they are complex, not simple, carbohydrates, she says. Specifically, Dr. Northrup recommends soyfoods (miso, tofu, tempeh, soy sauce) and certain green vegetables (broccoli, kale, collard greens, Brussels sprouts).

Nutritional Supplements: Vitamin C with flavonoids, some forms of iron, and vitamin A may be beneficial. For bleeding between periods, mixed bioflavonoids may be helpful.[19]

Herbal Medicine: To treat excessive bleeding, Silena Heron, R.N., N.D., of Sedona, Arizona, uses astringent herbs such as partridge berry (squaw vine), yarrow, and lady's mantle *(Alchemilla).*

Homeopathy: French homeopathic physician Jacques Jouanny, M.D., and his colleagues suggest a series of symptomatic remedies for heavy bleeding, meaning they provide immediate relief of symptoms, but do not effect healing on the constitutional level as in classical homeopathy.[20]

- *Sabina* 5C—When periods are early, heavy, and last a long time; the blood is bright red, may contain blackish clots, and is aggravated by minor physical movements; there is also pain radiating from the sacrum to the pubic bone. (Dosage: five pellets hourly, until improvement)
- *Crocus sativus* 5C—When the period is overlong and black blood and long stringy clots are passed. (Dosage: five pellets, 3-4 times daily)
- *China* 9C—When there is black blood, pallor, low blood pressure, weakness, ear ringing, visual disorders, or sweating during or after menstruation. (Dosage: five pellets, 3-4 times daily)
- *Secale cornutum* 5C—When there is much black blood, the period lasts a long time and is followed by a blackish discharge for a few days or until the next menstruation. There may also be false labor pains. (Dosage: five pellets, 2-4 times daily)

CASTOR OIL PACKS TO BALANCE HORMONES

Castor oil benefits the lymph system and liver and may help balance hormone levels. Christiane Northrup, M.D., suggests applying a castor oil pack to the lower abdomen for one hour, three times per week. While the packs can be used at any time during your menstrual cycle, they work most effectively during the two weeks before your period, says Dr. Northrup. To prepare a castor oil pack, lightly heat enough castor oil to thoroughly wet but not soak a 10" x 12" flannel cloth. Immerse the flannel in the hot oil, then fold it to make three to four layers and place against the skin. (The oil helps to draw out toxins, release tension, and improve blood circulation, especially in the lower abdomen.) Wrap a non-electric heating pad or hot water bottle in a towel and place this over the castor oil pack, then cover the pack and bottle with another towel to retain heat. Keep in place for one to two hours. Following the treatment, the oil-soaked flannel may be wrapped in plastic and stored in a refrigerator for later use. After the flannel has been used 20 times, discard it.

Natural Hormone Therapy: Dr. Northrup advises using natural progesterone to restore hormonal balance. She usually recommends applying ½ teaspoon of the cream to your palms or other soft skin two times daily, beginning 2-3 weeks before menstruation. Stop at the onset of your period and then begin again one to two weeks later. Results should be apparent within three months, she says. If a stronger dose is required to counteract the estrogen, micronized oral progesterone tablets (by prescription) can be helpful when taken at 100 mg twice daily for the two weeks before menstruation, says Dr. Northrup. Two weeks after the period is finished, resume at this dosage, she adds.

Premenstrual Syndrome (PMS)

One of the most common hormone-related conditions of otherwise healthy women is premenstrual syndrome (PMS). For 10-14 days before menses, women may experience a wide variety of symptoms, including mood swings, headaches, abdominal bloating, depression, sugar craving, cramps, irritability, and weight gain. These will last through two to three days of menstruation, sometimes longer. "Sixty percent of women have enough symptoms due to PMS to suffer," according to Dr. Northrup. "This is far too many women suffering from a normal physiological function."

Theories on the causes of PMS vary, but hormonal, nutritional, and psychological factors are all possibilities, as are the stresses of Western culture.[21] Dr. Northrup contends that the underlying cause of PMS is that "we have all been socialized into thinking that menstruation is one of the most awful things women have to put up with. Given the unity of the mind and body, if you have been brought up to believe this, it doesn't take a scholar to figure out why so many women suffer from a normal body function."

Dr. Lark delineates four basic types of PMS. Type A is characterized by anxiety, irritability, and mood swings; Type C by sugar cravings, fatigue, and headaches; Type H by bloating, weight gain, and breast tenderness; and Type D by depression, confusion, and memory loss. She defines two other common subgroups: Acne, characterized by pimples and oily skin and hair, and Dysmenorrhea, with cramps, low-back pain, and nausea (she notes that many doctors do not consider dysmenorrhea part of PMS).[22]

Diet: According to Tori Hudson, N.D., Academic Dean at the National College of Naturopathic Medicine, in Portland, Oregon, a good diet for PMS includes fresh fruits, vegetables, whole grains, legumes, nuts and seeds, and fish, while foods to be avoided include refined sugars, high amounts of protein, dairy products, fats, salt, caffeine, and tobacco. Eating three small meals and three snacks between meals each day can greatly reduce PMS symptoms. When you don't eat for several hours, your blood sugar can drop, causing your body to produce more adrenaline. The increase in adrenaline tends to produce feelings of tension and aggression, making PMS symptoms more severe.

> *A good diet for PMS includes fresh fruits, vegetables, whole grains, legumes, nuts, seeds, and fish.*
>
> —TORI HUDSON, N.D.

Nutritional Supplements: Vitamin A has diuretic and anti-estrogen properties. Vitamin B complex with extra B₆ is helpful in combating depression and acting as a diuretic. In one study of 70 women with PMS who took vitamin B₆, 60% of those who had reported depression with their PMS said they were cured or markedly improved. Among those with headaches, 81% said they felt better; for bloating and swelling, 60%; for irritability, 56%; lethargy, 52%; and breast tenderness, 52%.[23]

Increasing calcium and magnesium intake to 500 mg two to three times a day alleviates spasmodic and congestive discomfort.[24] Vitamin E and zinc have been shown to be effective in alleviating the symptoms of PMS.[25] In one study, evening primrose oil (a source for the omega-6 oil gamma-linolenic acid or GLA) was shown to decrease irritability, swelling, breast tenderness, and tiredness.[26] Some clinicians find that evening primrose is more effective in reducing these PMS symptoms if fish or a supplement of eicosapentaenoic acid (EPA) is also consumed.

Exercise: Research suggests that even moderate exercise can benefit PMS sufferers. During exercise, the body releases endorphins, substances that reduce tension and anxiety. Exercise also increases circulation and alleviates bloating and breast tenderness. Walking briskly for 30 minutes three days a week can significantly decrease PMS symptoms. To further reduce stress, exercise in a pleasant place such as an outdoor park.

Herbal Medicine: David Hoffmann recommends chasteberry for general, long-term treatment of PMS. For specific short-term complaints, he suggests skullcap for irritability/anxiety symptoms, dandelion for water retention, and cramp bark for cramping.

Homeopathy: "Since the causes of women's health problems are often multisystemic, homeopathy is particularly suitable as a treatment because it addresses the physical, mental, and emotional origins of disease," says Jennifer Jacobs, M.D., M.P.H., Director of the Evergreen Center for Homeopathic Medicine and a member of the NIH Panel on Alternative Medicine. "We treat a range of these deep constitutional imbalances and give less attention to the ways these manifest in body or mind."

Traditional Chinese Medicine: In Chinese medicine, PMS is considered a blood stagnation problem. Nailini Chilkov, Lic.Ac., O.M.D., of Santa Monica, California, explains how Chinese medicine views irregular periods. "If you are less than 21 days, that is because you have too much heat in your system, you are bleeding too much. If your periods are stretched out, 33 to 35 days, then we say your system is too cold." Acupuncture and herbs are given to correct these conditions.

Ayurvedic Medicine: Ayurveda's approach to treating PMS relies on basic principles that, once understood, can also shed light on other women's health disorders. "All female disorders are caused by imbalances that fall into three categories of diagnosis: the balance of the *doshas* (or bodily humors)—*vata* (responsible for movement), *pitta* (for metabolism), and *kapha* (for structure); biological rhythm; and purification," explains Nancy Lonsdorf, M.D., Medical Director of the Maharishi Ayurveda Medical Association of Washington, D.C. "All treatments address these three areas of body health." In Ayurveda, the individual can do much for herself through dietary and lifestyle changes. In turn, the practitioner provides the diagnosis and sets the direction of self-care and can provide herbs to balance the interaction of the *doshas*. Dr. Lonsdorf provides the following guidelines for Ayurvedic self-care based on predominant symptoms:

- Balance of the *doshas*: *Vata* energy is responsible in menstruation for the flow of blood and the endometrial lining. An imbalance manifests as mood swings, a tendency to cry, insomnia, anxiety, and constipation. To correct an imbalance, establish regular daily routines, reduce your workload, increase rest and sleep, meditate, and add to the diet a little more oil, sweet-tasting foods (but not refined sugars), salt, and cooked warm foods such as cereal and stews. *Pitta* energy is responsible in menstruation for hormonal changes. An imbalance manifests as anger, irritability, skin rashes, and diarrhea. To correct an imbalance, reduce "Type A" behaviors (overactivity and overperformance), establish regular daily routines, meditate, and avoid spicy foods, greasy foods, artificial ingredients, chocolate, caffeine, and alcohol. *Kapha* energy is responsible in menstruation for the contents of the menstrual flow. An imbalance manifests as fluid retention, swollen breasts, weight gain, and lethargy. To correct an imbalance, increase exercise, avoid sour and sweet foods, and increase spicy foods and legumes.

- Biological rhythm: Dr. Lonsdorf recommends as a general good habit going to bed at 10 p.m. and rising at 6 a.m., hours at which the earth's energy enhances human energy.

- Purification: This is used to remove *ama* (waste and impurity) from the body. Dr. Lonsdorf sees a parallel in the notion of removing *ama* and the effects of facilitating menstrual flow since iron, eliminated with the blood, is now being linked to heart disease when in excess in the body.[27] Dietary procedures to improve digestion and elimination include drinking plenty of warm to hot water and avoiding meat, cheese, caffeine, and alcohol. On day 14 or 15 of the cycle, Dr. Lonsdorf suggests the use of a laxative, 4-5 teaspoons of castor oil or senna tea, followed by a light diet for the rest of the day.

Natural Hormone Replacement Therapy: The symptoms women often experience for 5-10 days before the onset of their menstrual periods—emotional ups and downs, headaches, depression, irritability, and weight gain—are typically caused by an insufficient production of progesterone (due to stress and poor diet) to balance the increased estrogen being produced, according to John R. Lee, M.D., of Sebastopol, California. "Unbalanced

AROMATHERAPY BATHS FOR PMS

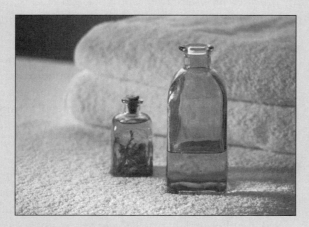

The following essential oil baths can help relieve PMS, according to aromatherapy educator Erich Keller.[28] Put drops (as directed below) into an empty, one-quart container; fill with warm water. For complete dispersion of oil particles in the bath, dribble the mixture slowly into the bath water as it pours from the tap. Remain in the bath for at least 20 minutes.

- Menstrual cramps and pain: 4 drops clary sage, 3 marjoram, 2 peppermint
- Muscle tension: 4 drops rosemary, 2 marjoram, 3 lavender
- Shock: 4 drops clary sage, 2 marjoram, 2 rose, 2 ylang-ylang
- Toxicity: 2 drops geranium, 2 rosemary, 2 juniper or 3 drops thyme, 2 rosemary, 1 lavender, 1 peppermint
- Insomnia: 4 drops neroli, 2 Roman chamomile
- Mental confusion: 6 drops lemon, 2 lemongrass, 2 lavender
- Fatigue: 6 drops rosemary, 2 bergamot
- Stress: 6 drops frankincense, 4 patchouli, 2 bergamot, 3 lavender
- Irritability: 1/8 ounce jojoba oil, 4 drops lavender, 3 chamomile, 2 clary sage, 1 frankincense. Wear this as a body fragrance, inhale directly from the container, or mix in your next bath.

estrogen will cause cellular edema (swelling), depression, loss of libido, irritability, and weight gain. Treatment with natural progesterone, given the ten days before menses, has been found to be successful.

"It is important that natural progesterone be used," cautions Dr. Lee. "Progestins, synthetic or chemically altered progesterone, have a long list of side effects such as abnormal menstrual flow, fluid retention, nausea, insomnia, jaundice, fever, the development of masculine characteristics, and allergies. But with natural progesterone, side effects are extremely rare." He has found only two minor problems related to its use. First, at higher dosages it may cause a feeling of euphoria. Second, in some individuals, it might slightly alter the timing of their menstrual cycle. Although conditions other than premenstrual syndrome can cause nervousness, depression, and irritability, the diagnosis of PMS can be established by serial blood tests for progesterone prior to therapy, adds Dr. Lee.

 See Aromatherapy, Ayurvedic Medicine, Herbal Medicine, Homeopathy, Mind/Body Medicine, Natural Hormone Replacement Therapy, Traditional Chinese Medicine.

Problems Related to Menopause

At the time of menopause, the hormonal output, instead of reducing gradually, alternately stops and starts. This general readjusting of the body's endocrine balance leads to many of the symptoms of menopause. The estrogen supply eventually regulates itself and reaches a plateau, where it remains until around age 70. Though doctors now know that the body still makes some estrogen, a common misconception is that menopause happens when a woman "runs out of estrogen." It was this generalization that led to the conclusion that simple estrogen replacement would remedy menopause, which was seen as a deficiency disease.

The symptoms of menopause are caused by estrogen dominance in the body as progesterone production declines in the years leading up to this change in a woman's body. Women may experience water retention, weight gain, memory loss, irritability, and depression. During menopause, decreased estrogen levels may cause bladder and vaginal atrophy, with the vaginal walls becoming drier and thinner, and a woman may have less interest in sex or slower arousal time. The hormonal changes also disrupt the delicate acid/alkaline balance of the vagina, which can lead to increased susceptibility to yeast and bacterial infections. Women may develop fibrocystic breasts, breast cancer, fibroids, or endometrial cancer.

However, no symptom is inevitable. During this time many women also experience increased energy, greater focus on their life goals, and a renewed interest in sex since pregnancy cannot result. Further, many women in other cultures do not have the side effects of menopause that are common to American women: Japanese and Indonesian women report far fewer hot flashes than do women from Western societies, and Mayan women in Mexico report no symptoms at all at menopause other than menstrual cycle irregularity.[29]

A wide variety of alternative therapies are effective in treating menopause. Western science so far has provided women with little data on care strategies for menopause that would make personal health decisions easier. As a result, menopausal women may turn to other avenues of treatment, learning to take care of their health care in general. As Fredi Kronenberg, Ph.D., at Columbia University Department of Rehabilitation Medicine, College of Physicians and Surgeons, in New York City, notes, "I think that in all the lectures and workshops I have given, the question that's asked of me most often is, 'What else can I take besides estrogen?' We are seeing increasing interest in alternative approaches because women who are asking these questions are part of the generation that is outspoken about wanting things to change."

I think that in all the lectures and workshops I have given, the question that's asked of me most often is, 'What else can I take besides estrogen?'

—FREDI KRONENBERG, PH.D.

There are various approaches to treating the symptoms of menopause, some as simple as walking for 30 minutes at the same time each day to stimulate the body's energies and to establish a calming regularity to life. Other approaches include dietary changes, herbs, homeopathy, and the disciplines of Chinese and Ayurvedic medicine. There are also treatments for specific problems of menopause—hot flashes, mood changes, vaginal atrophy—which are becoming word-of-mouth home remedies. A list of these treatments is provided for quick reference.

For Symptoms of Menopause

Menopause can trigger a wide variety of symptoms, some commonly associated with the condition—such as hot flashes—and others that are more subtle and may seem like actual behavioral changes—such as anxiety and depression. Before a woman assumes that she is having a profound personality change, she should become familiar with all the symptoms of menopause and begin a plan to treat them.

Hot Flashes: According to Dr. Kronenberg, "hot flashes are defined subjectively as recurrent, transient periods of flushing, sweating, and a sensation of heat, often accompanied by palpitations and a feeling of anxiety, and sometimes followed by chills. There is no evidence that the physiology of nocturnal hot flashes (night sweats) is different from that of daytime hot flashes."[30] According to Dr. Lark, 85% of women in the U.S. have hot flashes and 40% have symptoms severe enough to seek medical help.

Foods high in phytoestrogens (chemical compounds that the body can convert into usable estrogens) are thought to reduce the frequency of hot flashes. Japanese women have far fewer hot flashes than American women, and researchers have correlated this with the traditional Japanese diet that includes many soybean foods, which are high in natural phytoestrogens.[31] Dr. Lark emphasizes avoiding caffeine and alcohol and taking nutritional supplements of vitamin E and bioflavonoids. "Herbs to treat hot flashes," says David Hoffmann, "include dong quai, ginseng, gotu kola, and motherwort to help with palpitations that accompany hot flashes."

Ayurveda recommends treating for a *pitta* imbalance (see section on Premenstrual Syndrome). Traditional Chinese medicine may use dong quai and ginseng but, according to Honora Wolfe, each patient needs a specific formula that only a doctor can give based on diagnosis.

Homeopathy uses *Sepia*, *Lachesis*, and *Pulsatilla*, according to Dr. Jacobs, but she emphasizes that if hot flashes have become chronic, a woman should seek a more specific formula prescribed by a professional.

"Estrogen has been found to be very effective in treating hot flashes, but considering the potential side effects of estrogen replacement therapy, it is wise to attempt alternative treatment with vitamin E, a good diet, exercise, and simple perseverance, for they will eventually subside," says Dr. Lee. "If estrogen is chosen, however, it is especially important to include natural progesterone in the therapeutic plan."

Vaginal Dryness: Dr. Lark recommends low-dose estrogen vaginal cream for vaginal dryness, but she suggests supplementing it with vitamin E, taken orally and also applied directly to vaginal tissue. According to Dr. Lee, the use of natural progesterone alone, used transdermally, is sufficient to treat vaginal atrophy. David Hoffmann suggests calendula flowers for vaginal dryness. There are also new lubricating jellies sold over the counter for this specific purpose.

Anxiety: According to David Hoffmann, skullcap eases anxiety associated with menopause. He recommends taking ½ teaspoon with chasteberry. Herbs such as passionflower and valerian root are often prescribed by Dr. Lark for their calming properties. Other herbal remedies she recommends include chamomile, catnip, and peppermint tea.

Depression: For menopausal depression and its accompanying fatigue, stimulatory herbs such as oat straw *(Avena sativa),* ginger, cayenne pepper, dandelion root, blessed thistle, and Siberian ginseng improve vitality, partly due to the high levels of essential nutrients contained in these herbs, notes Dr. Lark. "St. John's wort can also lessen any depression that might occur," adds Hoffmann.

Perimenopause

During perimenopause, says Dr. Lark, "estrogen levels swing between highly elevated and deficient with many side effects. The triumvirate of issues—PMS, bleeding, and fibroids—is very common. Often women who've had no PMS or very mild symptoms will begin noticing more irritability or touchiness or classic PMS symptoms, such as food cravings, more tendency toward fluid retention, bloating, and breast tenderness. Combined with the more irregular menstrual cycle (the bleeding and even early onset of hot flashes), women can feel pretty awful during this transition time."

"The standard treatments are fairly draconian," notes Dr. Lark. These can include hormonal therapies, D & C (dilation and curettage, in which a doctor dilates the cervix and inserts a small, spoon-shaped instrument, a curette, to remove pieces of the uterus lining), the use of medication to control the symptoms, and even hysterectomy. "My goal is to get my patients through this vulnerable period with their uterus intact," continues Dr. Lark, "because once they've actually gone into menopause, these symptoms will subside and they will move into more of a simple estrogen-deficiency state; the fibroids will shrink, the PMS will go away, and the bleeding will stop."

Diet: Dr. Lark's outline for self-care includes a low-fat, high-fiber, vegetarian-based diet with whole grains, legumes, raw seeds and nuts, fruits, and vegetables making up the core of the diet. She advises avoiding salt, sugar, dairy products, alcohol, and caffeine (coffee, teas, colas, and chocolate).

Nutritional Supplements: Dr. Lark recommends vitamin B complex, vitamins B$_6$, C, and E, bioflavonoids, magnesium, and either evening primrose oil or borage oil.

Vitamin C and bioflavonoids should be taken together; the combination has been shown to reduce heavy bleeding.[32] Bioflavonoids are available as supple-ments, but they are also prevalent in soy products, buckwheat, grape skins and cherry skins, and the inner peel and pulp of citrus fruits. The bioflavonoids are also weakly estrogenic and help balance estrogen levels when needed, reducing the body's synthesis of estrogen or binding with estrogen receptor sites to increase the body's estrogen when low.[33] "Asian and African cultures, which feature bioflavonoid-containing foods, have lower rates of breast cancer, very few menopause symptoms, and do not tend to have these transition problems either," Dr. Lark points out. "The modulating effect of bioflavonoids also makes them beneficial for menopause."

Natural Hormone Replacement Therapy: Dr. Lee recommends supplementation with natural progesterone to correct any hormone imbalance during perimenopause, if a woman is suffering from symptoms due to estrogen dominance, such as water retention, loss of libido, weight gain, moodiness and irritability, depression, as well as fibrocystic breasts, breast cancer, or endometrial cancer.

General Recommendations for Menopause

The goal of any menopausal health program should be twofold: to eliminate the bothersome symptoms of menopause and to prevent the degenerative ailments—osteoporosis and heart disease—that are associated with the postmenopausal period. Hormone replacement therapy reduces the risk of these diseases, but not without potential side effects. "If a woman already has these diseases or is at unavoidable risk, these are reasons for taking hormones," says Kate O'Hanlan, M.D., co-author of *Natural Menopause: The Complete Guide.* In the case of osteoporosis, diet and exercise can also adequately prevent bone loss.[34]

Dr. Lark opposes an either/or approach to hormone replacement therapy. "In an ideal world, one would make use of all the options available to women," she says. "You need to individualize a program for each woman, using a mix of lifestyle changes, hormonal therapy, or whatever else is needed."

Diet: Dr. Lark recommends the same type of diet suggested for perimenopause, and notes that these guidelines are also appropriate for the prevention of heart disease and osteoporosis.

In various societies, older women traditionally eat certain foods to remedy menopausal side effects. In the South Seas, for example, women of menopausal age eat papaya, which contains phytoestrogens, once a day. Studies are beginning to show that these plant compounds can be helpful in menopause.[35] Traditional diets in Japan also are rich in phytoestrogens.[36] Studies of Japanese women with traditional Japanese diets show that these women's bodies contain levels of plant estrogens up to 1,000 times the level found in Western women, according to Dr. Kronenberg. "It may be that the reason these women don't have hot flashes is that they are eating a lot of weakly estrogenic substances all the time. These women also have a lower incidence of breast cancer, and one of the reasons suggested for this is that there are other things in the plant foods that are anticarcinogenic." In these studies, the higher estrogen levels were associated with intake of soybeans, soy products such as tofu and miso, and boiled beans.[37]

"As much as 50% of the Japanese diet contains phytoestrogenic foods, whereas Westerners eat 10% or less," Dr. Lark points out. "We really have very little dietary support as far as suppression of hot flashes and other menopausal symptoms." Foods in the Western diet that do contain phytoestrogens are apples, carrots, yams, green beans, peas, potatoes, red beans, brown rice, whole wheat, rye, and sesame seeds. Though these foods may contain 1/400th or less estrogen than a single dose of hormone supplement, "the metabolism of a stronger dose may not be well incorporated into the body's system," suggests Jing-Nuan Wu, L.Ac., O.M.D., Director of the Taoist Center, in Washington, D.C. "If you have a steady drumbeat instead of a thunderclap, it may actually do much more for the body."

Legumes are excellent sources of minerals needed by postmenopausal women, including calcium, magnesium, and potassium. They are also high in iron and vitamin B complex, nutrients important for the health of the liver, which plays a role in the metabolism of estrogen. Seeds and nuts are also good sources of calcium, magnesium, and potassium, and seeds such as flaxseed are mildly estrogenic. Seeds are also high in essential fatty acids, important because a deficiency of these oils may be responsible, in part, for the drying of the skin, hair, vaginal tissues, and other mucous membranes that occur with menopause; good sources are flaxseeds and pumpkin seeds. According to Dr. Lark, "The average healthy adult requires only four teaspoons per day of the essential oils in her diet, but menopausal women with extremely dry skin may need two to three tablespoons per day until the symptoms improve."[38]

Foods to avoid include most dairy products because of their high protein and fat content, caffeine because it can lead to hot flashes and mood swings, and alcohol because it can also cause hot flashes.

Lifestyle: According to Dr. O'Hanlan, "When the data from the Framingham study of heart disease was first analyzed, it looked like women who worked had more heart disease. Suzanne G. Haynes, Ph.D., Chief of the NCI's Health Education Division, reanalyzed the data

and found that actually it was the secretarial workers who had twice the rate of heart disease of housewives. The lowest risk was among working women who felt rewarded by their work. The stressor was jobs in which a woman had no autonomy or control of the environment, low recognition and sense of accomplishment, and low pay."[39]

Nutritional Supplements: According to Dr. Lark, "Clinical studies have shown the remarkable ability of bioflavonoids to control hot flashes.[40] Unlike estrogen therapy, no harmful side effects have been noted with bioflavonoid therapy." She also recommends that women taking hormone therapy supplement with vitamin B6 since they might become deficient in the vitamin. Dr. Lark also recommends vitamin E, calcium, magnesium, and potassium. Flaxseed oil and evening primrose oil are good sources of essential fatty acids.

Natural Hormone Replacement Therapy: "The most significant biologic consequence of menopause is the observed acceleration of osteoporosis. Due to anovulatory periods [not involving ovulation], poor diet, and lack of exercise, many women arrive at menopause with 25% to 30% loss of bone mass," reports Dr. Lee. "Any acceleration of osteoporosis at this time greatly increases their risk of fracture."

Healthy bone tissue is continually being made, reabsorbed, and made anew, Dr. Lee continues. "This is accomplished by two sets of bone cells, osteoblasts and osteoclasts. New bone is made by osteoblasts and old bone is reabsorbed by osteoclasts. In this regard, the role of estrogen is to partially suppress osteoclast-mediated bone reabsorption, and the role of progesterone is to stimulate osteoblast-mediated new bone formation. Thus, the role of progesterone is of prime importance." Effective treatment of postmenopausal osteoporosis requires supplementation with progesterone. Various synthetic progestins have some positive bone-building effects, according to Dr. Lee, but none are as effective as natural progesterone, which also is devoid of the adverse side effects of the progestins.

"There is no reason to assume that menopause signals the end of an active, healthy life," adds Dr. Lee. "Most women enjoy the absence of monthly menses. Most find to their surprise that their libido is unaffected. Their main concern is the aging they see in their female colleagues—the dryness and wrinkle lines that show in their face and body parts, the loss of fullness of their breasts, vaginal dryness, fracture proclivity, and the gray they see in their hair. Hormone replacement therapy promises many years of healthy life, though not the prevention of aging."

Hormone replacement should consist of progesterone and, if hot flashes or vaginal dryness (signs of estrogen deficiency) occur, estrogen supplements. With

ESTROGEN REPLACEMENT THERAPY

Perhaps the biggest debate today concerning women's health is the question of whether or not to supplement with hormones. Estrogen replacement therapy (ERT) is currently prescribed for osteoporosis and to relieve the symptoms of menopause. Some physicians recommend ERT when symptoms are "bothersome" while others use it only when symptoms become "disabling." Caution is used because estrogen has side effects, including stroke, gallbladder disease, liver tumors, fluid retention and weight gain, headaches, endometrial cancer, breast cancer, and uterine fibroids. Estrogen is not recommended for patients with uterine or breast cancer, a family history of breast cancer, obesity, phlebitis, varicose veins, diabetes, hypertension, edema, uterine fibroids, or fibrocystic breasts.

progesterone, good diet, and exercise, the bones remain strong and vigor for life also remains strong. Menopause is not the dreaded turning point of life as once was thought.

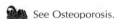 See Osteoporosis.

Herbal Medicine: David Hoffmann offers a simple formula using chasteberry as the base, combined with a choice of other herbs used for specific symptoms. He recommends combining ½ teaspoon of chasteberry with ½ teaspoon of tincture of each added herb. Hoffmann states, "Chasteberry will ease the unfoldment of the natural process of menopause." The optional herbs include St. John's wort for depression, motherwort for palpitations accompanying hot flashes, and skullcap for anxiety.

Dr. Heron uses individualized formulas for her patients, but finds that a general formula works for most women. She prescribes herbs in liquid preparation, taken throughout the month, one teaspoon of tincture formula three times a day. As she states, "This is because menopause is not pathological (disease-causing) and these herbs are not drugs, just tonics to the female reproductive system." In developing an individual formula she selects from the following herbs: chasteberry for its hormone-balancing effect; motherwort for its assistance in anxiety; false unicorn for hormonal and digestive benefit; dong quai, licorice, and alfalfa for estrogen enhancement; cramp bark or black haw bark because they both allay spasticity, which can promote hot flashes; and black cohosh as an antispasmodic and estrogen enhancer. Black cohosh was compared in a clinical study with estrogen replacement as a treatment for menopausal symptoms

after hysterectomy (with intact ovaries); it was shown to be as effective as synthetic hormones.[41]

Dr. Hudson reports, "I have been using an herbal formula for eight years and it does relieve the symptoms of menopause in most women. It has two parts licorice, two parts burdock root, two parts dong quai, one part wild yam, and one part motherwort. We powder the herbs and put them in capsules. The higher dose is two capsules three times a day, reducing it as needed."

Homeopathy: *Pulsatilla* is often suggested for a woman whose mood is changeable and is frequently weepy. When hot flushes extend all the way to the palms of the hands and soles of the feet, *Sulphur* is appropriate. *Bryonia* can help with a dry and thinning vagina.

Traditional Chinese Medicine: Traditional Chinese medicine offers both herbs and acupuncture for the treatment of menopause, and assesses a woman's menopausal status in terms of various body organs and substances, such as *qi* and blood in terms of *yin* and *yang*. As Honora Wolfe explains, "Symptoms of menopause result when hormonal fluctuations are causing *yin* and *yang* to come out of balance and be unstable for a time while the body readjusts its metabolism. The variations on this are quite complex. It is almost impossible to list herbs that work for menopause because the herbs are never given singly and because each person's diagnosis is very specific. However, there is one formula that is the most famous for menopause and this is the 'Two Immortals Decoction.'"

Traditional Chinese medicine does, however, have a generalized diet recommended for menopause, which focuses on keeping the spleen and stomach strong. Wolfe says, "If the digestion is strong, then all the other symptoms are easier to treat or prevent. The diet is just a basic grounded, balanced diet that is easy to digest. It consists of cooked foods, a little bit of animal protein, which helps to keep the blood strong, some eggs, which are very good for the kidney energy, lots of fresh and lightly cooked vegetables, and fruits in season but not eaten cold or necessarily refrigerated. It's also important to go easy on the alcohol, caffeine, sugar, salt, and fat."

Wolfe also recommends as much moderate exercise as a woman has time for or feels comfortable with. "Exercise keeps the *qi* and blood from stagnating. As we age, more problems are due to stagnation, so movement of any kind is healthful. Stretching is good because it keeps ligaments and joints supple."

Ayurvedic Medicine: According to Dr. Lonsdorf, "Menopause is a natural transition time that shouldn't be creating disease if we are in balance. Basically, it is a *vata* imbalance."

Cystitis and Vaginal Infections

Every year in the U.S., an estimated two million people, the majority of whom are women, suffer from bladder infection, also known as cystitis or, more generally, as urinary tract infection (UTI). Cystitis refers to irritations or bacterial infections that occur anywhere from the urethra (where the urine comes out from the bladder) to the lining of the bladder. These infections can occur in a single episode or recurrent episodes, or can exist as chronic conditions. Cystitis is common in sexually active women and menopausal women have a tendency to develop cystitis because, as estrogen levels decline, bacteria are more prone to adhere to the bladder lining and vaginal tissue.

Symptoms include burning and pain on urination, increased urinary urgency and frequency, pain over the pubic area or lower back, and increased urination throughout the night. In women, as severity increases, blood may color the urine red. Signs that the kidneys have also become involved are fever, chills, nausea, vomiting, and severe mid-back and/or loin pain. When this occurs, a doctor should be seen.

Larrian Gillespie, M.D., Director of the Pelvic Pain Treatment Center and the Women's Clinic for Interstitial Cystitis, in Beverly Hills, California, specializes in the treatment of cystitis. "A urinary tract infection is not a problem of bacteria getting into the bladder, it is a problem of bacteria not getting out," says Dr. Gillespie. "A study was done in which stool was placed directly into the bladder of medical students. By the second voiding, there were no more bacteria. So, an infection is directly the result of the bladder not efficiently evacuating the urine. It has nothing to do with the female anatomy being different from the male's—that is, 'too short.' If you can move 'dirt on the sidewalk' with your stream, instead of 'tinkling' drops out, you will not get a bladder infection."

There are a number of things a woman can do to avoid recurrent cystitis. First of all, do not urinate after intercourse until you feel the need to void, as squeezing out a few drops will not efficiently clean the bladder and the vagina. Second, an overly large fitted diaphragm will obstruct the bladder neck and prevent you from emptying your bladder after intercourse. The contraceptive sponge may also cause the same effect in women, so it is best to use either a cervical cap or have your diaphragm reduced in size, usually to a 65-70 millimeter size.

Some women, however, may develop symptoms of an infection when none exists. This hypersensitivity is often the result of changes in blood flow to the bladder.

It can be caused by endometriosis, lower back problems, and hormone problems. The symptoms of pressure or burning relieved by urination are characteristic of the painful bladder syndrome, interstitial cystitis. New research by Dr. Gillespie shows that the bladder is rarely the cause of this problem. "Hypersensitive bladder symptoms, such as those related to interstitial cystitis, can be caused by a stretch on the nerves that control blood flow into the bladder, bowel, and pelvic floor. By looking into the injury, we can switch the signals causing the bladder to lose oxygen and thereby improve circulation. This can be done through back stabilization exercises and acupressure."

In Dr. Gillespie's experience, many patients have unsuspected endometriosis, and it is necessary to perform microsurgery through a tiny incision in the belly button. "It is important to first check your urine for the presence of nitrites," says Dr. Gillespie. These compounds are formed by nitrifying bacteria. You can purchase a dip test from a pharmacy. If it is positive, contact your health practitioner for a single dose of antibiotics, according to Dr. Gillespie.

Diet: Intake of plenty of fluids along with a diet that avoids urine-acidifying foods and emphasizes urine-alkalinizing foods are recommended for both the elimination and prevention of UTIs. Joseph E. Pizzorno, Jr., N.D., President Emeritus of Bastyr University, in Kenmore, Washington, recommends a diet in which you restrict calorie intake, avoid all simple sugars, refined carbohydrates (white breads and pasta), and full-strength fruit juices, and eat generous amounts of garlic and onions. Dr. Pizzorno also recommends drinking at least 64 ounces of pure water or unsweetened liquid daily. This can include up to 16 ounces of unsweetened cranberry or blueberry juice daily.[42] Cranberries and blueberries have a high content of mannose, which is a sugar that binds to urinary cells and prevents bacteria from binding to those same cells.

The refined carbohydrate restrictions are also part of the anti-yeast diet recommended by William G. Crook, M.D., author of *The Yeast Connection and the Woman*. In addition to eliminating simple sugars, soft drinks, ready-to-eat cereals, corn syrup, pastries, white bread, and other white flour products, Dr. Crook advises avoiding hydrogenated and yeast-feeding foods and beverages, including dried fruits, mushrooms, condiments, alcohol, juices (except for freshly squeezed), leavened breads, bagels, pasta, pretzels, and pizza. Instead, eat vegetables and grain alternatives (such as amaranth and quinoa) and use unrefined oils such as flaxseed, walnut, sunflower, and olive.[43]

"If you have an infection, taking cranberry juice, which contains hippuric acid, makes as much sense as putting out a fire with gasoline," states Dr. Gillespie. "It only adds more acid to the urine, which in turn, increases the burning sensation. Cranberry juice may be helpful if you want to prevent an infection, but if you already have one, it only makes matters worse. Rather, try ¼ teaspoon of baking soda in water. You should feel the relief in 20 minutes." Corn silk tea contains silica, which also acts as a soothing coating to inflamed bladder tissue, if no allergy to corn is present. A half teaspoon of mannose powder in water swallowed every 1-2 hours can also improve a urinary infection.

Support for cranberry juice as a cystitis preventative comes from a study published in the *Journal of the American Medical Association*. The study tracked 153 women—all chronic UTI sufferers—over the course of six months; one group drank ten ounces daily of a commercially available cranberry juice, while a control group drank a non-cranberry beverage. At the end of the study, the cranberry juice drinkers had reduced their chances of developing a urinary tract infection by 73%, as compared with the non-cranberry drinkers.[44]

Foods that are high in the amino acids phenylalanine, tryptophan, tyrosine, and tyramine can irritate the bladder of patients with hypersensitive symptoms, adds Dr. Gillespie. Try avoiding bananas, pineapple, avocados, aspartame, figs, yogurt, chocolate, and citrus fruits. Wines that do not undergo malolactic fermentation will not increase your pain, according to Dr. Gillespie.

Nutritional Supplements: Dr. Pizzorno typically recommends the following supplements in the event of a cystitis outbreak: vitamin C (500 mg, preferably as the mineral ascorbate form, every two hours); vitamin A (50,000 IU daily); zinc (30 mg daily); uva ursi, also known as bearberry or upland cranberry (½ tsp fluid extract or 1½ tsp tincture); and goldenseal (*Hydrastis canadensis*, ½ tsp fluid extract or 1½ tsp tincture). *Lactobacillus acidophilus* and other friendly bacteria are also useful oral or vaginal supplements. They can help restore the bacterial balance in the urinary tract and vagina, which can help drive out the infectious bacteria causing the UTI.

Herbal Medicine: According to Hoffmann, herbs containing volatile oils that are excreted from the body via the kidneys produce good results in such infections. For an infection accompanied with pain and burning, he suggests combining tinctures of corn silk, bearberry (uva ursi), and buchu in equal parts and taking one teaspoon of this mixture three times a day. Hot infusions often ease the symptoms. He also recommends combining equal parts of dried marshmallow leaf, corn silk, couch grass, and bearberry and drinking a cup of the infusion four to five times a day.

Fresh parsley, eaten raw or brewed as a tea, is "a time-honored remedy for cystitis," say Julian and Susan Scott in *Natural Medicine for Women*. They recommend eating fresh parsley chopped or grated as a garnish; dried parsley is less effective.[45] Parsley tea, which is a diuretic and thus flushes out the urinary system, can be made by steeping a bunch of fresh parsley in several quarts of boiling water for about 20 minutes, then removing the parsley and drinking the tea hot or cold.

Homeopathy: In using homeopathy to permanently eliminate your cystitis, you will need to consult a classical homeopath who can prescribe a constitutional remedy, which is one that corrects imbalances in all aspects. However, for relief of acute cystitis, try the following remedies recommended by homeopaths Andrew Lockie, M.D., and Nicola Geddes, M.D. Take them in the 30C potency every 30 minutes for up to ten dosages:[46]

- For cystitis symptoms that are worse before menstrual periods, with fluid retention and joint pain—*Pulsatilla*
- For cystitis symptoms that are worse before menstrual periods—*Sepia, Lycopodium*
- For cystitis symptoms and weakness that are worse before menstrual periods—*Calcarea*
- For cystitis symptoms and weakness, fluid retention, and chilliness—*Arsenicum*
- For cystitis symptoms and fluid retention with joint pains—*Nux vomica*
- For cystitis symptoms and fluid retention—*Mercurius, Belladonna*
- For cystitis symptoms and weakness—*Causticum, Conium*
- For cystitis symptoms that are worse with heat and better with cold—*Apis*

Hydrotherapy: Contrast sitz baths (pelvic immersion in shallow tubs of alternating hot and cold water) can relieve cystitis pain and improve circulation in the pelvic area, states Dr. Hudson. To prepare the baths, find two basins or tubs that you can sit in comfortably (you need to be able to immerse your pelvis in water). Fill one with hot water to about the level of your navel and the other with cold water to the same level. Soak first in the hot bath for three to five minutes; then in the cold water for 30 seconds. Repeat three times, finishing with cold water. (Hot and cold compresses can be substituted if you don't have the tubs). Perform this treatment once or twice daily.[47]

Vaginal Infections (Vaginitis)

Vaginal infections account for nearly 7% of all visits to gynecologists.[48] Hormonal vaginitis is primarily a problem of postmenopausal women, as the vaginal tissue becomes thin and susceptible to irritation. There may also be vaginal discharge. Infectious vaginitis may be sexually transmitted or may arise from a disturbance to the delicate ecology of the healthy vagina.

A variety of causal factors contribute to vaginal infections. Bacterial vaginosis, for example, is caused by harmful bacteria such as *Neisseria gonorrhea* and *Chlamydia trachomatis*, while vaginal candidiasis (also called candidal vaginitis) results from an overgrowth of the yeast *Candida albicans*. About 90% of vaginitis is caused by such infectious organisms, particularly bacteria, *Candida*, and the parasitic protozoan *Trichomonas vaginalis*.[49] Other factors include local irritants (such as tight clothing or nylon pantyhose), hormonal changes, and emotional or psychological issues, among others.

In the past 20 years, yeast infection caused by *Candida* has increased 2½ times due to several factors, chief among them the increased use of antibiotics. The primary symptoms of candidal vaginitis are vulvar itching, which can be quite severe, and a thick, curdy discharge.[50] "If a yeast infection is recurrent, it is important to go to a doctor to be diagnosed," advises Dr. Hudson. "Sometimes there are systemic health problems that cause it—diabetes, for instance—and more worrisome these days is that chronic yeast vaginitis is the primary presenting symptom of women who are HIV-positive." Self-care for this condition includes diet and using suppositories for vaginal itching. One should also test for food, chemical, and environmental sensitivities.

Prevention: The following are simple steps you can take to help eliminate vaginitis and prevent its recurrence.[51]

- Shower daily to keep vulval area clean.
- Wipe from front to back after a bowel movement.
- Keep vaginal area dry.
- Wear cotton underwear and avoid nylon pantyhose.
- Avoid using perfumed chemical douches or other perfumed or chemical products in the vaginal area.
- Use condoms during sexual intercourse to reduce transmittal of infection.

Diet: A basic diet for vaginitis is low in fats, sugars, and refined foods.[52] For candidiasis, Dr. Hudson recommends that a woman follow a yeast-free diet, avoiding fermented foods and sugar, which may feed yeast growth, and also increase her intake of acidophilus-containing yogurt and garlic, both effective antifungals. According to an Israeli study, eating as little as a half cup of yogurt (enriched with *Lactobacillus acidophilus* or "active" bacterial cultures) daily may help prevent recurring episodes of vaginitis. Researchers noted that eating *Lactobacillus*-containing yogurt resulted in a clear increase in beneficial bacteria in the vagina and rectum, and therefore a significant decrease in the form of bacteria that causes vaginosis.[53] If a woman has an allergy to cow's milk products, goat milk yogurt may be a good alternative.

Nutritional Supplements: Vitamins and minerals that boost immune function and promote healthy tissues help strengthen the vaginal mucosa so that these delicate tissues can shield themselves against infiltration by infectious organisms. Vaginal infections have been known to respond to vitamins A, B complex, C, and E, beta carotene, certain bioflavonoids, zinc, lysine, lithium, and acidophilus. Iodine as a topical douche or boric acid or gentian violet vaginally are other options.[54]

Herbal Medicine: A tincture of herbal extracts consisting of two parts goldenseal *(Hydrastis canadensis)*, two parts echinacea *(Echinacea augustifolia)*, and one part phytolacca *(Phytolacca americana)*, taken at a dosage of 20-60 drops by mouth every two to four hours, can help relieve vaginitis. Goldenseal acts as an antifungal, echinacea builds immune strength, and phytolacca helps draw toxins from the body. This tincture can also be taken as a tea (1 tsp of the mixture in one cup of hot water). Drink one cup of the tea every two to four hours until symptoms are relieved.[55]

For candidal vaginitis, one herbal remedy is to swab the vagina with an extract of gentian violet *(Gentiana macrophylla)*. Paul Reilly. M.D., considers this plant, which has fungicidal properties, to be "as close to a specific treatment for *Candida*" as can be found in herbal medicine.

Topical Treatment: For vaginal infections, Dr. Heron recommends a douche of antiseptic herbs such as St. John's wort, goldenseal, echinacea, fresh plantain *(Plantago major)*, garlic, and calendula along with demulcent herbs like comfrey leaves and self-heal to soothe the membranes. Calendula is both antiseptic and reparative. This douche is alternated with one of acidophilus. A suppository prescribed by Dr. Hudson consists of powdered boric acid mixed with three herbs—berberis, goldenseal, and calendula (all antifungals)—prepared in capsule form. "This works so well," says Dr. Hudson, "that I no longer prescribe douches for this condition."

Other douches include apple cider vinegar (two tablespoons to one quart water), acidophilus (two opened capsules to one quart water), or a solution of water and garlic from capsules or fresh juice. Topical pau d'arco, black walnut, and diluted tea tree oil are also options and vitamin E cream may relieve itching.

Homeopathy: Drs. Lockie and Geddes typically suggest the following homeopathic remedies as emergency, short-term treatment for vaginal yeast *(Candida)* infections (6C potency, to be taken six times daily for up to five days):[56]

- For yeast infection with dryness of the vagina—*Aconite, Arsenicum, Belladonna, Berberis, Ferrum, Graphites, Lycopodium, Natrum muriaticum, Sepia*

- For yeast infection with intense itching in the vagina—*Caladium, Kreosotum, Lilium*

- For yeast infection with creamy vaginal discharge—*Calcarea phosphorica, Natrum phosphoricum, Pulsatilla, Secale*

- For yeast infection with burning pains in the vagina—*Belladonna, Berberis, Calcarea phosphorica, Cantharis, Chamomilla, Chelidonium, Graphites, Kali bichrom, Kreosotum, Mercurius, Natrum muriaticum, Nitricum acidum, Petroleum, Pulsatilla, Sulphur, Thuja*

- For yeast infection with burning pain in the vagina during intercourse—*Kreosotum, Lycopodium, Sulphur*

Problems with the Uterus and Ovaries

The health of the uterus and ovaries is an integral part of the health of the entire reproductive system. In recent years, problems with the uterus and ovaries have been on the rise, because of lifestyle and environmental changes, according to Dr. Lark. Common conditions affecting the uterus are fibroids, ovarian cysts, and endometriosis.

Fibroids

A fibroid is a tumor that arises from uterine muscle and connective tissue. Almost all cases are benign (not malignant). Since fibroids develop following the onset of menstruation, enlarge during pregnancy, and decrease after menopause, fibroids are thought to be estrogen dependent. One in five women in the U.S. has at least some evidence of fibroids, with most occurring in women in their thirties and forties.[57] Fibroids are much more common among black women, although the reason for this difference is not known.[58]

Fibroids are usually firm, spherical lumps that often occur in groups. They are of varying sizes, usually described in terms of vegetables and fruit—pea, lemon, apple, cantaloupe, etc. They can grow near the outer surface of the uterus, where they are easily detected during a pelvic examination, as well as near the inner lining of the uterus, where they may need ultrasound for detection. Fibroids normally shrink in size after menopause.

Most women have no symptoms at all, but there may be lower abdominal pain, a feeling of fullness and pressure in the lower abdomen, and frequent urination caused by tumor pressure on the bladder, plus heavy menstrual periods, bleeding between periods, and increased menstrual cramps. If a fibroid grows rapidly, it may outstrip its nutritional supply from nearby blood vessels, resulting in the degeneration and death of the oxygen-deprived tissue; severe abdominal pain may result. Rapid growth is common in pregnancy, when high estrogen levels stimulate tumor growth.

Birth control pills, with high levels of estrogen, and estrogen-replacement medication for menopause symptoms can also accelerate tumor growth. As Dr. Lark explains, "Fibroids are caused by periods of high estrogen production, and our strategy is to level these out so that the fibroids don't grow. We use a conservative approach, controlling estrogen production through nutrition and lifestyle and, if needed, reducing the bleeding in the same way. My issue with fibroids is that too many women have hysterectomies. A fibroid the size of a 13-week fetus (the size at which Western medicine begins discussing the need for a hysterectomy) and larger can be successfully treated by this approach. I've seen fibroid tumors shrink in women following a conservative approach."

Diet: Dr. Lark uses anti-estrogenic substances, focusing on flavonoids found in fruits and vegetables. "The flavonoids have 1/400th to 1/50,000th the estrogenic effect that synthetic estrogen does and therefore these flavonoids contribute very little to the total body supply," she explains. Dr. Lark recommends a whole foods diet with fresh vegetables and fruits, nuts and seeds, and whole grains. Foods to avoid include dairy products, red meat, fried fat, sugar, salt, caffeine, and alcohol.

Nutritional Supplements: Dr. Lark suggests the following supplements in treating fibroids.[59]

- Beta carotene (vitamin A precursor from vegetable sources): at least 20,000 IU daily

- Vitamin B complex: 50-100 mg daily, with additional B6 (up to 300 mg daily)

- Vitamin C: 1,000-4,000 mg daily, plus bioflavonoids (from grape skins, cherries, blackberries, blueberries, pulp and white rind of citrus fruits)

- Vitamin E (from wheat germ, walnut, or soybean oil): 400-2,000 IU daily

- Calcium: minimum of 800 mg daily during menstruation

- Magnesium: at least 400 mg daily

- Potassium: 99 mg, 1-3 times daily for one week preceding onset of menstruation

- Iron (the "heme" type from meat sources such as liver): 27 mg daily

Herbal Medicine: Hoffmann recommends a basic mixture of the tinctures of chasteberry, blue cohosh, wild yam, and cranesbill *(Geranium)* in equal amounts; ½ teaspoon three times a day. If there is much cramping pain, he advises taking ½ teaspoon of cramp bark tincture in addition to the basic mixture.

Herbalist Susun Weed, of Woodstock, New York, advises that to stop heavy bleeding caused by fibroids take ½ cup of an infusion (strong tea made from dried herbs) of cotton root bark *(Gossypium)* every half hour, or a dropperful every 5-10 minutes, until the bleeding stops.

For a brew to balance the effects of estrogen excess, mix equal parts of tinctures of the following herbs: black currant buds or leaves *(Ribes nigrum),* gromwell herb or seeds *(Lithospermum officinalis),* lady's mantle *(Alchemilla vulgaris),* and wild pansy flowers *(Viola tricolor).* Take one teaspoon of the tincture first thing in the morning and you can expect noticeable results in two to four months, says Weed.[60]

Magnet Therapy: Therapeutic-quality magnets, worn over the uterus at night while sleeping, can shrink a fibroid tumor over a period of months, according to William H. Philpott, M.D., of Choctaw, Oklahoma, author of *Magnet Therapy: An Alternative Medicine Definitive Guide.* Magnetic fields can stimulate metabolism and increase the amount of oxygen available to cells, which will decrease inflammation, he explains. It could take several months of magnet application before the fibroid starts shrinking and up to a year to eliminate it. However, the magnet will immediately stop the tumor growth process, states Dr. Philpott.

For treatment, he often recommends wearing a magnet over the lower abdomen/pubic area (to cover the uterus) every night while sleeping; specifically a 5″ by 12″ multi-magnet flexible mat, with a 4″ by 6″ by ½″ ceramic block booster magnet attached in the center of the mat with Velcro. The mat and booster are kept in place on the body by a wrap cloth. The most important thing to remember about magnetic therapy is that the negative pole is the side that faces the body.

Lifestyle: Regular aerobic exercise, slowly performed, at least three times weekly, bouncing on a rebounder (mini-trampoline), or Hatha yoga exercises can help reduce pelvic congestion, improve blood circulation, and relax uterine muscles. Stress reduction techniques such as meditation, deep-breathing exercises, counseling, psychotherapy, and emotional support from friends and family can ease stressful situations.[61]

Ovarian Cysts

The ovaries can develop various kinds of cysts and, of these, 75% to 85% are benign and do not require surgery. There are cysts that occur on the egg follicle and are the result of normal ovarian functions, follicular cysts

that happen when a normal egg follicle ruptures as it releases an egg, and corpus luteum cysts, which can be a signal to check for ectopic or uterine pregnancy. A sign of a follicular cyst can be a sudden onset of pain on one side of the abdomen lasting a few hours and occurring halfway between monthly periods. The sign of a corpus luteum cyst may be abnormal or slight bleeding. According to Dr. Hudson, a diagnosis must encompass the patient's history, a physical examination, pelvic ultrasound, in some cases laparoscopy, and in even fewer cases, laparotomy (surgical opening of abdomen) to rule out malignancy. Acute problems from this condition can be pain and bleeding.

In treating ovarian cysts, Dr. Hudson focuses on possible liver toxicity and designs treatments to maintain healthy liver function. She recommends a vegetarian diet using organic foods and nourishing the liver with beets, carrots, and lemons. Avoid fried foods, coffee, cigarettes, medications, alcohol, and sugar. She recommends as supplements vitamins A, E, and C, beta carotene, and zinc, as well as black currant oil or evening primrose oil.

Dr. Hudson suggests several steps to be taken for self-care: avoid chilling of the extremities, which can cause internal congestion; avoid wearing high heels, which can block pelvic circulation; heal all the emotional wounds of past sexual or physical insults or abuses; and make an effort to express creativity.

Endometriosis

In endometriosis, endometrial cells from the lining of the uterus migrate to locations where they are not normally found—in the uterine myometrium and outside the uterus on the ovaries, bladder, and gastrointestinal tract. It is estimated that 10% to 20% of all women in the U.S. have endometriosis. The probability of contracting the condition increases until age 44 and then declines.[62] The condition is stimulated by excess estrogen production, but the exact cause is unknown. One theory is that the endometrial cells are carried upward through the fallopian tubes (called retrograde menstruation), enabling them to implant in the abdomen, where they grow to form endometriosis patches. Delayed first pregnancy and menstruation at an earlier age, both more common today than two or three generations ago, have also been linked to endometriosis. In the past, a woman might have had fewer than 40 menstrual cycles before pregnancy, while now there might be 12 years of monthly periods before a woman decides to have a child.

The primary symptom of endometriosis is dysmenorrhea with dull, aching pain in the pelvis, lower abdomen, and back. "Once the endometrial cells are transplanted, they still respond to the monthly hormonal (estrogen) messages just as they would if remaining within the uterus, by filling with blood which is then released at the time of menses," explains Dr. Lee. "The drops of blood, however, have nowhere to go and can become a focus of excruciating pain and inflammation. Despite their small size (some no larger than a pinhead), pelvic pain that results can be disabling." Symptoms tend to increase gradually over the years as the endometriosis areas slowly increase in size. There are no specific laboratory tests that will detect endometriosis, but a biopsy can be performed in the office by a doctor.

For endometriosis, Dr. Lark follows the same protocol she does for fibroids—using weak estrogenic flavonoids to block the body's own production of estrogen—but she adds anti-inflammatory agents, since scarring and infection often accompany endometriosis. She advises, "The patient needs to include good sources of essential fatty acids because the body manufactures prostaglandins from these, some of which are anti-inflammatory agents. These EFAs are plentiful in fish such as salmon and in seeds and nuts. It is also equally important to reduce or eliminate meat, eggs, and especially dairy, because these foods are sources of arachidonic acid, which promotes inflammation."

Herbal Medicine: Dr. Heron treats endometriosis with a range of herbs meant to, as she explains, "increase circulation in the pelvis, thereby promoting drainage, discouraging adhesions, and facilitating removal of inflammatory substances. In addition, hormonal balance is reestablished, decreasing premenstrual syndrome." The herbs are intended to act as hormonal precursors and balancers and also to improve liver function and digestion, all components of the disease. "The result is usually symptom relief as a result of treating the underlying cause," says Dr. Heron. Patients consistently report a marked decrease in dysmenorrhea, dyspareunia (pain with intercourse), digestive symptoms, menorrhagia, and ovulation pain, along with an improvement in mental outlook and decrease of lassitude.

Dr. Heron develops formulas of herbs fine-tuned for the individual. She uses a polypharmacy approach, combining various herbs for an enhanced effect. She uses three of her own formulas, one for each phase of the cycle: during menses itself, between menses and ovulation (approximately day 14 or later), and from ovulation to the beginning of menses. The herbs used include dandelion, Oregon grape root, pasqueflower, chasteberry, false unicorn, cramp bark or black haw bark, black cohosh, motherwort, vervain, yarrow, hops, valerian, and borage.[63]

Nutritional Supplements: Supplement the diet with vitamin C, vitamin B6, folic acid, calcium, magnesium, and essential fatty acids, such linoleic acid and evening primrose oil.[64]

Natural Hormone Replacement Therapy: Natural progesterone can reverse endometriosis by helping to restore proper hormone balance, without side effects, says Dr. Lee. Natural progesterone can stop the spread of endometrial cells by blocking the activity of estrogen that otherwise stimulates the growth of the aberrant cells. Dr. Lee suggests using natural progesterone cream from days six to 26 of the monthly cycle, stopping just before menstruation begins. After four to six months of this treatment, the monthly pains and bleeding due to endometriosis will usually subside. Dr. Lee prefers transdermal (absorbed through the skin) natural progesterone in cream or oil formulation, because it is absorbed more efficiently and the effect lasts longer, without the emotional highs and lows from oral drops. A woman addressing endometriosis will probably need to use $\frac{1}{8}$ to $\frac{1}{2}$ teaspoon of cream per day or three to ten drops of oil per day, says Dr. Lee. The cream may be applied to the palms, face, neck, upper chest, breasts, inside of the arms, or behind the knees.

Traditional Chinese Medicine: According to Honora Lee Wolfe, "This condition may be due to blood stasis, *qi* stagnation, phlegm and dampness, damp heat, or some combination of these, but in turn this can be based on some organs being empty or not strong enough. It's almost always a combination of patterns, a concurrent insufficiency, or vacuity."

Ayurvedic Medicine: "This condition is a *vata* imbalance," explains Dr. Lonsdorf. "We treat this as we would any *vata* imbalance [see Premenstrual Syndrome section]. For prevention, we advise that a woman reduce her activities as much as possible for the first three days of her period each month, though this might be an unpopular suggestion to most busy women today. For exercise, we recommend a gentle walk rather than jarring aerobics classes at this time."

Breast Problems

Breast disorders can be hereditary and can also result from such environmental and lifestyle factors as diet, breast implants, and birth control pills. Since early detection of such problems—especially where cancer is concerned—is currently one of the primary strategies for prevention and successful treatment, it is important for women to examine their own breasts regularly. This must be done each month at the same time in a woman's cycle, in the same physical position, and using the same sequence of steps. Some lumps are easier to find when lying down and others are more apparent when sitting or standing, so you may want to use multiple positions. (See "How to Peform a Breast Self-Exam.") Some women draw a

HOW TO PERFORM A BREAST SELF-EXAM

This exam should be conducted once a month (for pre-menopausal women, just after your period). Start by standing in front of a mirror and looking carefully at each breast and the chest muscle area above it. (1) Look for anything out of the ordinary, such as puckering, dimpling, or scaling skin, nipple discharge or retraction, lumps, or asymmetry of breasts. (2) Raise your arms or clasp them behind your head and check for the same in this position. (3) Do the same check with your hands on your waist, pulling your shoulders and elbows slightly forward. (4) Feel for lumps in the lymph node area, from your breast into your armpit. (5) Squeeze each nipple to check for discharge. (6) Some women prefer to do this stage of the breast exam standing up, perhaps in the shower using soapy water so the fingers will glide more easily. With your right arm behind your head, examine your right breast with the fingers of your left hand. Using the pads of three or four fingers to press firmly into the breast, feel for lumps and cover the entire breast by following the patterns shown here. Some women prefer the radiating pattern (6a), thoroughly examining the breast by moving outward from the nipple in straight lines. Others prefer the circular pattern (6b), starting from the nipple and moving outward around the breast or vice versa. Repeat on the left breast. If you notice anything abnormal or something you're not sure about at any point in the exam, consult your physician.

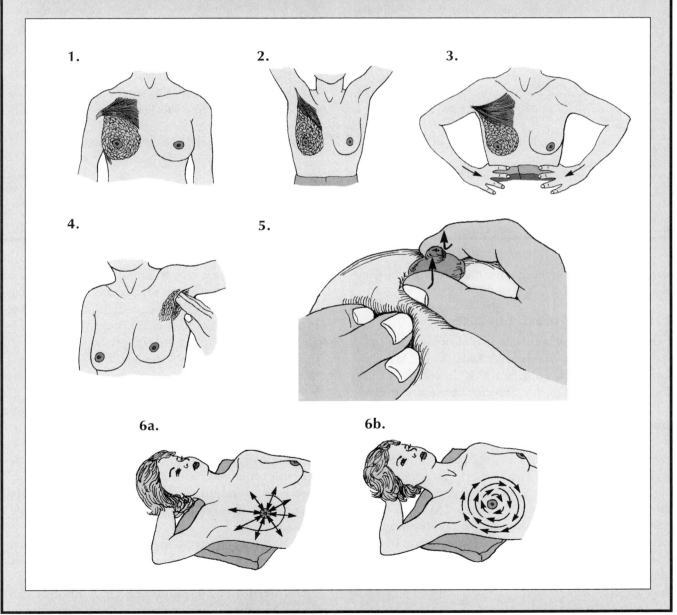

MAMMOGRAMS AND BREAST CANCER

There is an information gap on the causes, monitoring, and prevention of breast cancer because so little conclusive research has been done on the subject. However, it is known that 75% of patients survive breast cancer, and most breast cancers are present for 8-10 years before they can be detected as a lump or on a mammogram, according to Susan M. Love, M.D., Associate Professor of Clinical Surgery at the University of California at Los Angeles. "The problem of the prevention and treatment of breast cancer is the fact that 80% of women who get breast cancer don't have [the traditional] risk factors," says Dr. Love. "A low-fat diet may be preventative, but we won't have the results from studies for five to ten years." Recent studies, however, have disputed the long-standing belief that an additional risk factor is breast cancer in one's mother or sister. These studies state that although the risk of breast cancer is doubled among women whose mother had breast cancer before the age of 40 or whose sister had breast cancer, the risk associated with a mother or sister history is much smaller than thought. The study indicated that within middle-aged women, only 2.5% of breast cancer cases were attributable to family history.[67]

The benefit of mammography is still a subject of debate. According to John R. Gofman, M.D., Ph.D., and others, low-level radiation used in the test can cause cancer.[68]

Equivocal mammogram results lead to unnecessary surgery, and the accuracy rate of mammograms is poor. According to the National Cancer Institute (NCI), in women ages 40-49, there is a high rate of "missed tumors," resulting in 40% false-negative mammogram results. Breast tissue in younger women is denser, which makes it more difficult to detect tumors, and tumors grow more quickly in younger women, so cancer may develop between screenings.

Because there is no reduction in mortality from breast cancer as a direct result of early mammograms, it is recommended that women under 50 avoid screening mammograms,[69] although the American Cancer Society is still recommending a mammogram every two years for women ages 40-49. The NCI recommends that, after age 35, women perform monthly breast self-exams. For women over 50, many doctors still advocate mammograms. However, breast self-exams and safer, more accurate technologies such as thermography should be strongly considered as options to mammography. Early detection is currently one of the primary strategies for prevention and successful treatment, which is why the breast self-examination is so important.

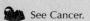 See Cancer.

---

sketch each time to record what they feel and compare to previous sketches.

Fibrocystic Breast Disease

Fibrocystic breast disease occurs in 80% of premenopausal women, according to Susan M. Love, M.D., Associate Professor of Clinical Surgery at the University of California at Los Angeles, and Director of the Breast Center. Common symptoms of this condition include pain and tenderness, and the texture of the breast changing, with small lumps detectable to the touch. This is usually a component of premenstrual syndrome and is considered a low risk factor for breast cancer. Fibrocystic breasts are apparently caused by an increased estrogen-to-progesterone ratio.[65] Caroline M. Shreeve, M.D., says that benign disorders of the breast are common among women whose diets include a high proportion of saturated animal fat and rare among those who eat little saturated animal fat but take in a high proportion of essential fatty acids.[66]

Any breast lump that is painful is likely to be a cyst rather than a tumor, which usually is not tender. Diagnosis can be aided by thermography, ultrasound mammogram (see "Mammograms and Breast Cancer"), or by aspiration biopsy (a needle is inserted into the lump under local anesthetic and the cyst fluid is withdrawn). When fluid is withdrawn and the lump disappears, it is good evidence that the lump was not a tumor.

Jonathan Wright, M.D., Director of the Tahoma Clinic, in Kent, Washington, reports success in eliminating breast cysts using a treatment of iodine (painted on intravaginally) and magnesium (administered intravenously) combined with a regimen of nutritional supplements including organic iodine tablets, chelated magnesium, vitamins B complex, B6, and E, and essential fatty acids.

Diet: Dr. Wright recommends a primarily vegetarian, high-fiber, low-fat, dairy-free diet for patients with fibrocystic breast disease.

Nutritional Supplements: Dr. Hudson recommends vitamin E, beta carotene, evening primrose oil, iodine, choline, flaxseed oil, vitamin B complex, and methionine.

Herbal Medicine: David Hoffmann says fibrocystic breasts can be treated with echinacea, goldenseal, herbal squaw vine, mullein, pau d'arco, poke root, and red clover. For long-term care, he recommends evening primrose oil and chasteberry. Dandelion is used for breast sores, tumors, and cysts, and parsley for swollen breasts.

Natural Hormone Replacement Therapy: Dr. Lee often recommends applying natural progesterone cream directly to the skin, allowing it to be absorbed transdermally. "Using progesterone transdermally from day 15 of the monthly cycle to day 25 will usually cause breast cysts to disappear," he states.

Other treatment options include:

- TENS (Transcutaneous Electric Nerve Stimulation) unit, preferably a micro-current type, applied to breasts to improve energy circulation

- Balancing movement and bodywork such as yoga, *Tai Chi*, *Qigong*, acupuncture, chiropractic, massage

- Mini-trampoline (rebounder) for lymphatic drainage and to improve circulation

- Colonics (using ozonated water) to help remove toxins and excess estrogen from the intestines

- Castor oil packs used in the pre-ovulatory phase (first two weeks) of the cycle to draw out toxins and excess estrogen, improve circulation in the breasts and chest (to further aid in the elimination of estrogen), and reduce inflammation

 Since early detection of such problems—especially where cancer is concerned—is currently one of the primary strategies for prevention and successful treatment, it is important for women to examine their own breasts regularly.

Silicone Implant Disease

Since breast implants gained acceptance in the 1970s, at least two million women have had their breasts enlarged with silicone implants. While the surgery may help women achieve what they think is an ideal body, it comes at a high cost—their health. Researchers estimate that 95% of women who get silicone implants will experience implant rupturing or silicone leakage within 20 years after their surgeries, some within the first few months.

Silicone implant disease (also called human adjuvant disease or silicone-induced illness) is a new illness category developed by physicians now treating women with implants. Typically the disease, which has been linked to autoimmune dysfunction, produces a cluster of symptoms, including any of the following: severe weight loss, hair loss, liver dysfunction, lymph node swelling, fatigue, weakness, granulomas, breast and nipple inflammation, skin shedding, circulation problems, arthritic pain, and chronic muscle pain and stiffness.

Most women, regardless of the type of breast implant they have in place, will probably eventually develop health problems as a result, states W. Lee Cowden, M.D., of Fort Worth, Texas. Disputing many doctors who attribute adverse symptoms solely to the effects of silicone leakage into the body, Dr. Cowden says that the health problems can stem from white blood cells breaking down the implant coating. In the case of saline implants, the body's white blood cells "chew off" little pieces of the silicone casing of the saline implant, then carry these into a distant tissue where that white blood cell finally dies. But this releases the foreign material into the tissues. The same sequence happens with silicone-filled implants, but to a larger degree, says Dr. Cowden. The important point, he says, is that all implants release silicone into the tissues even if the capsule has not ruptured, and that release is estimated at about five grams per year.

Silicone is a sensitizing agent, which means it initiates an autoimmune or hyperimmune process, which in turn can cause white blood cells to attack the nervous system, muscles, skin, joints, and vital organs. Then it manifests as symptoms typical of chronic fatigue, multiple sclerosis, or lupus. But it can also produce symptoms such as memory loss, poor concentration, arthritic pain, and even a multiple sclerosis–like syndrome.

If you're experiencing symptoms associated with silicone toxicity, "get explanted before you do anything else," urges Walter Crinnion, N.D., in Kirkland, Washington. Even after the silicone implants have been removed, silicone molecules that have migrated throughout the body remain in the tissues and must be removed from the body. Otherwise, they may continue supporting the negative symptoms, says Dr. Crinnion. His silicone detoxification program typically takes 4-8 weeks, requiring seven hours a day, five days a week. This aggressive detoxification program should only be done with close supervision by a competent health practitioner.

- Moderate exercise, 15-25 minutes daily, using a mini-trampoline or rebounder and exercise bicycle. This increases body temperature and stimulates the fatty tissues to release their stored toxins.

- Low-heat sauna (120°-130° F) in three one-hour sessions daily, with a 15-minute cooling off period between each session.

- Spring water plus electrolyte tablets consumed during the sauna (to replace electrolytes lost to perspiration) and herbal teas taken to generate more sweating.

- Hydrotherapy for 45 minutes: alternately, hot and cold towels are placed on the patient's abdomen, then back; mild electrical stimulation is applied to the skin on both sides of the body, one side at a time. This phase increases the amount of blood (carrying collected toxins) flowing through the liver for detoxification.

- Colonic irrigation for 45 minutes at the end of the day; this helps flush the toxins, dumped into the intestines by the liver, out of the body through the colon.

- Nutritional support (dosages vary with the individual): vitamin C (6,000-12,000 mg daily), liquid selenium (up to 600 mcg daily), magnesium (900 mg daily), vitamin A (30,000 IU daily, in divided doses), N-acetyl-cysteine (500-700 mg, three times daily, with meals), vitamin E (800-1,200 IU daily), taurine (an amino acid, 500-1,000 mg daily), milk thistle (three capsules daily), psyllium husk powder (3-5 capsules, evenings), and enzymes and hydrochloric acid (as needed for better digestion).

Recommendations

- Dysmenorrhea: Eat whole grains, legumes, fruits and vegetables, and seeds and nuts such as ground, raw flaxseed and pumpkin seed, while avoiding dairy products, saturated fats, salt, alcohol, sugar, and caffeine. Helpful supplements include vitamins B3, B6, and C, calcium, magnesium, potassium, zinc, and essential fatty acids. Painful cramps associated with menstruation or ovulation can be eased by combining the tinctures of skullcap, black haw, and black cohosh

- Amenorrhea: Herbs for amenorrhea include chasteberry, false unicorn root, blue cohosh, rue, pennyroyal, and tansy. Use low-potency homeopathic remedies when the period has stopped (for reasons other than pregnancy or menopause), such as *Ferrum phosphoricum* 6X, *Calcarea carbonica* 6C, *Kali sulphuricum* 6X, *Aconitum napellus* 6C, *Natrum muriaticum* 6X, or *Sepia* 6C.

- Menorrhagia: Recommended foods include soyfoods (miso, tofu, tempeh, soy sauce) and certain green vegetables (broccoli, kale, collard greens, Brussels sprouts). Iron, vitamin C with flavonoids, and vitamin A may be beneficial. To treat excessive bleeding, use astringent herbs such as partridge berry (squaw vine), yarrow, and lady's mantle. Natural progesterone can help restore hormonal balance.

- PMS: A good diet for PMS includes fresh fruits, vegetables, whole grains, legumes, nuts, seeds, and fish, while foods to be avoided include refined sugars, high amounts of protein, dairy products, fats, salt, caffeine, and tobacco. Increasing calcium and magnesium intake to 500 mg two to three times a day alleviates spasmodic and congestive discomfort. Vitamin E and zinc have been shown to be effective in alleviating the symptoms of PMS. Research suggests that even moderate exercise can benefit PMS sufferers. The herb chasteberry is recommended for general, long-term treatment of PMS. Natural progesterone can help restore hormonal balance.

- Menopause: Eat more foods containing phytoestrogens, such as apples, carrots, yams, green beans, peas, potatoes, red beans, brown rice, whole wheat, rye, and sesame seeds. Legumes are excellent sources of minerals needed by postmenopausal women. Vitamin E, calcium, magnesium, and potassium are recommended. Evening primrose oil is a good source of essential fatty acids. Natural progesterone can help restore hormonal balance. Traditional Chinese medicine offers both herbs and acupuncture for the treatment of menopause.

- Cystitis: Drinking plenty of fluids along with a diet that avoids urine-acidifying foods and emphasizes urine-alkalinizing foods are recommended for both the elimination and prevention of cystitis. Cranberry juice may be helpful if you want to prevent an infection. In the event of a cystitis outbreak, take vitamin C (500 mg, the mineral ascorbate form, every two hours), vitamin A (50,000 IU daily), zinc (30 mg daily), uva ursi (½ tsp fluid extract), and goldenseal (½ tsp fluid extract). *Lactobacillus acidophilus* and other friendly bacteria are also useful supplements.

- Vaginitis: The following are simple steps to help eliminate vaginitis and prevent its recurrence: shower daily to keep vulval area clean; wipe from front to back after a bowel movement; keep vaginal area dry; wear cotton underwear and avoid nylon pantyhose; avoid using perfumed chemical douches or other perfumed or chemical products in the vaginal area; and use condoms during sexual intercourse to reduce transmittal of infection.

- Fibroids: The following supplements may be helpful in treating fibroids: beta carotene (at least 20,000 IU daily); vitamin B complex (50-100 mg daily); additional vitamin B6 (up to 300 mg daily); vitamin C (1,000-4,000 mg daily) plus bioflavonoids; vitamin E (400-2,000 IU daily); calcium (minimum of 800 mg daily during menstruation); magnesium (at least 400 mg daily); potassium (99 mg, 1-3 times daily for one week preceding onset of menstruation); and iron

(27 mg daily, from liver, beets, or dark green, leafy vegetables).

- Ovarian Cysts: A vegetarian diet using organic foods and nourishing the liver with beets, carrots, and lemons.

- Endometriosis: Helpful herbs include dandelion, Oregon grape root, pasque flower, chasteberry, false unicorn, cramp bark or black haw bark, black cohosh, motherwort, vervain, yarrow, hops, valerian, and borage. Natural progesterone can reverse endometriosis by helping to restore proper hormone balance, without side effects.

- Fibrocystic Breast Disease: A primarily vegetarian, high-fiber, low-fat, dairy-free diet. Vitamin E, beta carotene, evening primrose oil, iodine, choline, flaxseed oil, vitamin B complex, and methionine may be helpful. Herbs include echinacea, goldenseal, squaw vine, mullein, pau d'arco, poke root, and red clover. Balancing movement and bodywork such as yoga, *Tai Chi, Qigong,* acupuncture, chiropractic, and massage.

- Silicone Implant Disease: Get explanted immediately, then detoxify the body.

Self–Care
The following therapies can be undertaken at home under appropriate professional supervision:

EXCESSIVE MENSTRUATION (MENORRHAGIA)
Yoga

AYURVEDA: Red raspberry or *manjistha.* Or try *shatavari* and *manjistha* in equal proportions.

MENSTRUAL CRAMPS (DYSMENORRHEA)
Qigong and Tai Chi / Yoga

HERBS: Mild diuretics may help relieve fluid retention.

JUICE THERAPY: One glass of blueberry and huckleberry juice daily.

PREMENSTRUAL SYNDROME (PMS)
Mind/Body Medicine / Yoga

MENOPAUSE
Mind/Body Medicine / Yoga

AROMATHERAPY: Clary sage

JUICE THERAPY: Carrot, celery, parsley, and spinach

CYSTITIS
Qigong and Tai Chi

AROMATHERAPY: Massage or bath with bergamot, lavender, eucalyptus, sandalwood, chamomile, juniper.

HOMEOPATHY: *Cantharis, Apis mel., Berberis*

JUICE THERAPY: • Carrot and apple juice • Cranberry juice • Watermelon juice • Garlic or onion juice may be added to carrot, beet, cucumber, or spinach juices. • Carrot, celery, spinach, and parsley

TOPICAL TREATMENT: Half a teaspoon of yogurt around vaginal opening after intercourse.

VAGINAL INFECTIONS
Yoga

HOMEOPATHY: *Cactus, Belladonna, Sepia*

ENDOMETRIOSIS
AROMATHERAPY: Cypress

HYDROTHERAPY: For bleeding between periods, use vaginal douches.

Professional Care
The following therapies can only be provided by a qualified health professional:

DYSMENORRHEA
BODYWORK: Acupressure, massage

DETOXIFICATION THERAPY: Many women's health conditions can be caused or exacerbated by the buildup of toxins in the body. In such cases, detoxification is necessary for complete healing to occur.

MENORRHAGIA
Acupuncture / Biofeedback Training and Neurotherapy / Chiropractic / Detoxification Therapy / Guided Imagery / Hypnotherapy / Light Therapy

BODYWORK: Acupressure, reflexology, shiatsu, massage

PREMENSTRUAL SYNDROME (PMS)
Acupuncture / Biofeedback Training and Neurotherapy / Guided Imagery / Hypnotherapy / Mind/Body Medicine / Yoga

BODYWORK: • Massage and hot baths relax the body and help release toxins. • Acupressure, shiatsu, reflexology, Feldenkrais Method, Rolfing

DETOXIFICATION THERAPY: Many women's health conditions involve the buildup of toxins in the body. Detoxification may be necessary for complete healing to occur.

MENOPAUSE
Acupressure / Detoxification Therapy / Natural Hormone Replacement Therapy

CYSTITIS
Acupuncture / Chiropractic / Detoxification Therapy / Environmental Medicine / Enzyme Therapy / Magnetic Field Therapy / Naturopathic Medicine / Osteopathic Medicine / Oxygen Therapies / Reflexology / Traditional Chinese Medicine

ENDOMETRIOSIS

Chiropractic / Detoxification Therapy / Guided Imagery

FIBROCYSTIC BREAST DISEASE

Biofeedback Training and Neurotherapy / Hypnotherapy / Mind/Body Medicine

DETOXIFICATION THERAPY: Many women's health conditions can be caused or exacerbated by the buildup of toxins in the body. In such cases, detoxification is necessary for complete healing to occur.

Where to Find Help

For information on women's health conditions or referrals to a qualified health-care practitioner, contact the following organizations.

National Women's Health Network

514 10th Street N.W., Suite 400
Washington, D.C. 20004
(202) 628-7814

A clearinghouse of publications and information packets on all women's health issues.

Office on Women's Health (OWH)

Department of Health and Human Services
200 Independence Avenue S.W., Room 730B
Washington, D.C. 20201
(202) 690-7650

The OWH publishes fact sheets, resource papers, meeting summaries, and articles on a variety of issues concerning women's health.

National Women's Health Resource Center, Inc. (NWHRC)

120 Albany Street, Suite 820
New Brunswick, New Jersey 08901
(877) 986-9472

The NWHRC is a nonprofit organization dedicated to helping women make informed decisions about their health and encourages women to embrace healthy lifestyles to promote wellness and prevent disease.

Recommended Reading

Alternative Medicine Guide to Women's Health 1 & 2. Burton Goldberg and the Editors of *Alternative Medicine.* Tiburon, CA: Future Medicine Publishing, 1998.

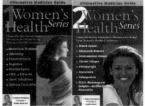

Our Bodies, Ourselves for the New Century. The Boston Women's Health Book Collective. New York: Simon & Schuster, 1998.

Straight Talk with Your Gynecologist: How to Get Answers That Will Save Your Life. Eddie C. Sollie, M.D. Hillsborough, OR: Beyond Words Publishing, 1992.

Women's Bodies, Women's Wisdom: Creating Physical and Emotional Health and Healing. Christiane Northrup. New York: Bantam Doubleday, 1998.

Women's Encyclopedia of Natural Medicine: Alternative Therapies and Integrative Medicine. Tori Hudson and Christiane Northrup. Los Angeles: Lowell House, 1999.

Fertility and Birth Control

The Fertility Awareness Handbook. Barbara Kass-Annese, R.N., C.N.P., and Hal Danzer, M.D. Alameda, CA: Hunter House, 1992.

The New No Pill, No Risk Birth Control Guide. Nona Aguilar. New York: Rawson Associates, 1986.

Your Fertility Signals. Merryl Winstein. St. Louis, MO: Smooth Stone Press, 1989.

Menstruation and PMS

Exclusively Female: A Nutrition Guide for Better Menstrual Health. Linda Ojeda. San Bernardino, CA: Borgo Press, 1985.

Dr. Susan Lark's Menstrual Cramps Self-Help Book. Susan Lark. Berkeley, CA: Celestial Arts, 1995.

Menopause

Dr. Susan Lark's Menopause Self-Help Book. Susan Lark, M.D. Berkeley, CA: Celestial Arts, 1990.

Hormone Replacement Therapy, Yes or No. Betty Kamen, Ph.D. Novato, CA: Nutrition Encounter, 1995.

Menopausal Years. Susun S. Weed. Woodstock, NY: Ash Tree Publishing, 1992.

Managing Menopause Naturally with Chinese Medicine. Honora Lee Wolfe. Boulder, CO: Blue Poppy Press, 1998.

Menopause Without Medicine. Linda Ojeda, Ph.D. Alameda, CA: Hunter House, 2000.

Natural Menopause: The Complete Guide. Susan Perry and Kate O'Hanlan, M.D. Reading, MA: Addison-Wesley, 1997.

Newsletters

Breast Cancer Action. Available from: 55 New Montgomery Street, Suite 323, San Francisco, CA 94105; (415) 243-9301; website: www.bcaction.org.

Health Wisdom for Women. For information, call: (207) 846-3626 or (800) 804-0935.

Don't ask the doctor, ask the patient.
—YIDDISH PROVERB

Quick Reference

A-Z Section of
Additional Health Conditions

HOW TO USE THIS SECTION

THIS QUICK Reference A-Z Section covers over 100 additional health conditions. Each condition is briefly described and information is supplied concerning its causes and symptoms. A self-care/professional care section cross-references each condition with the alternative therapies most appropriate for its treatment.

Self-care refers to treatments that can be undertaken in your own home, under the guidance of your physician. Professional care means you must see a qualified practitioner of this therapy for this condition. (Each of the health condition chapters in Part Three also contains a self-care/professional care section, at the end of the main text, which follows the same guidelines.)

Self-care modalities are not only cost-effective, but help you begin to take your health into your own hands. Self-care therapies include diet, nutritional supplementation, juice therapy, flower essences, meditation, yoga and Qigong, self-acupressure, and reflexology, and, in some cases, herbs, hydrotherapy, aromatherapy, and fasting. Ayurvedic medicine, naturopathic medicine, herbal medicine, homeopathy, hypnotherapy, detoxification therapies, guided imagery, and biofeedback all have self-care practices that can be used at home under the guidance of a physician, as well as more sophisticated applications for which you will need to see a professional.

Therapies generally requiring direct professional care include the following:

- Acupuncture
- Applied Kinesiology
- Biological Dentistry
- Bodywork (acupressure, Alexander Technique, Aston-Patterning, Feldenkrais Method, Hellerwork, massage, myotherapy, reflexology, Rolfing, shiatsu, Therapeutic Touch, Trager Approach)
- Cell Therapy
- Chelation Therapy
- Chiropractic
- Colon Therapy

- Craniosacral Therapy
- Environmental Medicine
- Enzyme Therapy
- Fasting
- Flower Essences
- Guided Imagery
- Herbal Medicine
- Hyperthermia
- Hypnotherapy
- Light Therapy
- Magnetic Field Therapy
- Mind/Body Medicine
- Natural Hormone Replacement Therapy
- Naturopathic Medicine
- Neural Therapy
- Orthomolecular Medicine
- Osteopathic Medicine
- Oxygen Therapies
- Prolotherapy
- Traditional Chinese Medicine

Regardless of whether you choose primarily self-care approaches or those involving professional services, it is recommended that you find an open-minded and trusted physician or health-care professional who can help you create an effective health-maintenance program.

Choosing Alternative Therapies for Health Conditions

Look up the health condition you are interested in under its alphabetical listing. Choose the alternative therapies listed for the health condition you want to investigate. In order to read about a particular therapy in greater detail, refer back to its chapter in Part Two. If you have further questions about the therapies, contact the professional organizations listed there for more information, as well as for referrals to physicians or other health professionals in your area who offer this service.

The possible contributing factors discussed under special notes give you and your physician more information (particularly if they are a specialist) concerning what underlying factors may be contributing to your health condition. One crucial concept to keep in mind is that no single treatment method is effective for everyone with a particular condition. Healing is complex because individuals are biochemically unique. What works for someone else may not work for you.

It is important to find a therapy that works for you and has the least long-lasting negative effects on your body, while at the same time building long-term positive effects on your overall lifestyle. The intention of this book is not to promote one therapy over another, but to help inform you about all of the therapies available so that you can decide which therapy best suits you. By making use of the information this book provides, you will be able to make intelligent, informed choices and take charge of your own health, in cooperation with your primary health-care practitioner.

When examining the alternative therapies listed in this Quick Reference guide, remember the following facts:

- Each section is intended to expose you to these alternatives. If you have questions or if you have symptoms that do not respond as they should, ask a qualified practitioner for guidance and answers. See the Where to Find Help section in the specific chapters in Part Two: Alternative Therapies.

- Diet and nutritional supplements are recommended for virtually every condition. Be sure to check with your physician before undertaking a dietary or nutritional program.

Instructions for Self-Care

Acupressure

Refer to the accompanying acupressure charts to locate points referred to in the Quick Reference A-Z and self-care sections of health condition chapters.

Aromatherapy

See the Aromatherapy chapter for instructions on the use of essential oils listed under each condition. (See the

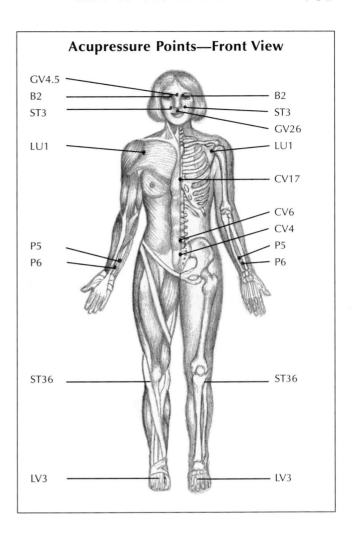

Acupressure Points—Front View

Where to Find Help section at the end of the Aromatherapy chapter for organizations that can refer you to a qualified aromatherapist.)

Ayurveda

Simple dietary, herbal, and topical treatments are provided that you can employ at home. You may want to read the chapter on Ayurvedic Medicine to see if you would like to consult an Ayurvedic physician. (See the Where to Find Help section at the end of the Ayurvedic Medicine chapter for organizations that can refer you to a qualified Ayurvedic physician.)

Diet

Diet plays an enormous role in health. General dietary guidelines are normally provided for each condition, such as a whole foods diet, vegetarian diet, low-fat diet, or raw foods diet. Pay particular attention to the foods that are beneficial to the condition and those that should be avoided. If you are ill or considering a major dietary change, please consult a health-care professional trained in nutritional medicine. (See the Where to Find Help

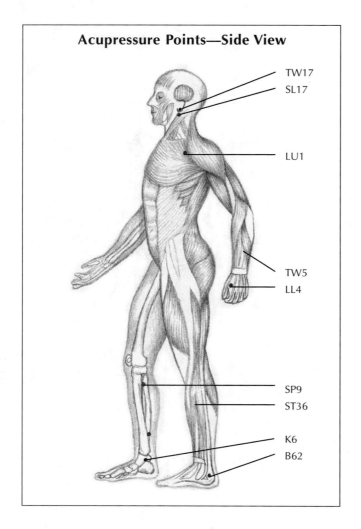

Acupressure Points—Side View

TW17
SL17
LU1
TW5
LL4
SP9
ST36
K6
B62

Acupressure Points—Back View

GB20   GV16
        GB20
GB21   GB21
B36   B36
B47   B47
B23   B23
TW5   TW5
LL4   LL4
B48   B48
B60   B60

section in the Diet chapter for organizations that can provide referrals for nutritional counseling.)

Flower Essences or Remedies

See the Flower Essences chapter for instructions on the use of flower remedies listed under each condition. (See the Where to Find Help section at the end of the Flower Essences chapter for organizations that can refer you to a qualified therapist.)

Herbs

Many herbs can be prepared as teas, although in some cases it is suggested to make a decoction, infusion, or other preparation. Certain herbs may be used in baths, steam inhalations, and in compresses to be applied topically to the body. In all cases please refer to the chapter on Herbal Medicine. It is recommended that you start with the herbal extracts or tinctures, as they can be much simpler to use than the fresh herbs and are more reliable in determining potency. If you are attempting to treat a health condition, please check with a qualified herbalist, practitioner of traditional Chinese medicine, or a naturopathic physician. (See the Where to Find Help section

in the Herbal Medicine chapter to find organizations that can refer you to health practitioners who are specialists in herbal medicine.)

Homeopathy

Remedies listed on the accompanying chart may be used individually or in combination with other remedies. Trevor Cook, Ph.D., D.I.Hom., President of the United Kingdom Homeopathic Medical Association, has created a simple system to make your own combination homeopathic remedies from the single remedies associated with particular symptoms of a health condition. According to Dr. Cook, nearly every combination prescription can be made from these 48 individual remedies. These remedies may be purchased separately or as a special combination kit consisting of each of the remedies in their liquid or pellet form.

How to Prepare the Homeopathic Remedies: The kit may also include a number of empty dropper bottles for combining the remedies. All potencies in kits are normally 12X potency (a low potency which is considered safe for most people). To prepare a combination treatment, add ten drops of each remedy indicated for a

HOMEOPATHIC REMEDIES IN QUICK REFERENCE A-Z SECTION

FULL NAME	ABBREVIATION	COMMON NAME
Aconitum napellus	*Aconite*	monkshood
Apis mellefica	*Apis mel.*	honey bee
Argentum nitricum	*Argen nit.*	silver nitrate
Arnica montana	*Arnica*	leopard's bane
Arsenicum album	*Arsen alb.*	arsenious oxide
Atropa belladonna	*Belladonna*	deadly nightshade
Berberis vulgaris	*Berberis*	barberry
Bryonia alba	*Bryonia*	wild bryony
Calcarea carbonica	*Calc carb.*	calcium carbonate
Calcarea fluorica	*Calc fluor.*	calcium fluoride
Calcarea phosphorica	*Calc phos.*	calcium phosphate
Calendula officinalis	*Calendula*	marigold
Cantharis vesicatoria	*Cantharis*	blister beetle
Carbo vegetabilis	*Carbo veg.*	vegetable charcoal
Chamomilla	*Chamomilla*	wild chamomile
Chelidonium majus	*Chelidonium*	celandine
Colchicum autumnale	*Colchicum*	autumn crocus
Cuprum metallicum	*Cuprum met.*	copper metal
Drosera rotundifolia	*Drosera*	sundew
Euphrasia officinalis	*Euphrasia*	eyebright
Ferrum phosphoricum	*Ferrum phos.*	iron phosphate
Gelsemium sempervirens	*Gelsemium*	yellow jasmine
Graphites	*Graphites*	black lead
Hamamelis virginiana	*Hamamelis*	witch hazel
Hepar sulfuris	*Hepar sulf.*	calcium sulfide
Hydrastis canadensis	*Hydrastis*	goldenseal
Hypericum perforatum	*Hypericum*	St. John's wort
Ignatia amara	*Ignatia*	St. Ignatius bean
Ipecacuanha	*Ipecac*	ipecacuanha
Kalium bichromicum	*Kali bich.*	potassium bichromate
Kalium phosphoricum	*Kali phos.*	potassium phosphate
Lachesis mutus	*Lachesis*	bushmaster snake venom
Ledum palustre	*Ledum*	wild rosemary
Lycopodium clavatum	*Lycopodium*	club moss
Magnesium phosphorica	*Mag phos.*	magnesium phosphate
Mercurius solubilis	*Merc sol.*	soluble mercury
Natrum muriaticum	*Nat mur.*	sodium chloride (salt)
Nux vomica	*Nux vom.*	poison nut
Phosphorus	*Phosphorus*	
Pulsatilla nigricans	*Pulsatilla*	windflower
Rhus toxicodendron	*Rhus tox.*	poison ivy
Ruta graveolens	*Ruta grav.*	bitterwort
Sepia officinalis	*Sepia*	juice of cuttlefish
Silicea	*Silicea*	
Sulfur	*Sulfur*	
Symphytum officinalis	*Symphytum*	comfrey
Thuja occidentalis	*Thuja*	tree of life
Urtica urens	*Urtica*	stinging nettle

Foot reflexology chart

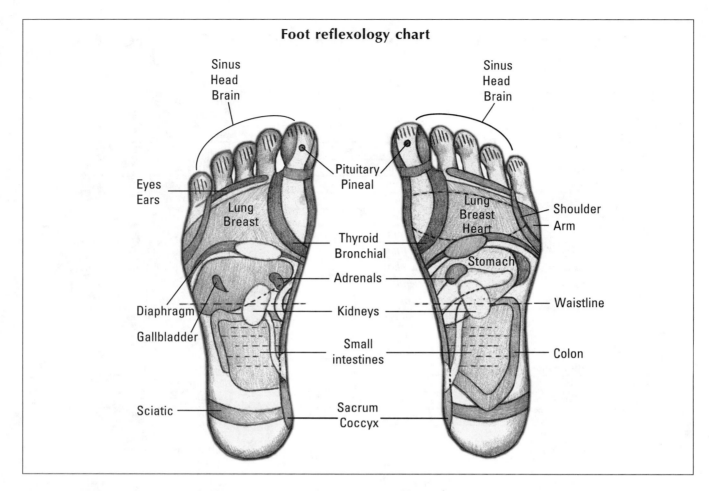

Sinus
Head
Brain

Sinus
Head
Brain

Eyes
Ears

Pituitary
Pineal

Lung
Breast

Lung
Breast
Heart

Shoulder
Arm

Thyroid
Bronchial

Stomach

Adrenals

Diaphragm

Kidneys

Waistline

Gallbladder

Small
intestines

Colon

Sciatic

Sacrum
Coccyx

particular condition to an empty bottle. Mix well, lightly tapping a firm, resilient surface about ten times and label the dropper bottle clearly. The standard dose for a combination remedy is ten drops taken in a clean mouth under the tongue. For a more in-depth discussion of homeopathy, refer to the Homeopathy chapter. (See the Where to Find Help section in the Homeopathy chapter to find organizations that can refer you to a qualified homeopathic physician.)

Hydrotherapy

There are many water therapy treatments that you can easily do in your own home for little or no cost. Please consult the Hydrotherapy chapter for complete instructions on how to perform the following hydrotherapy procedures:

- Cold compress
- Cold friction rub
- Constitutional hydrotherapy
- Contrast applications
- Enema/colon irrigation
- Hot packs
- Heating compress

- Hyperthermia
- Hot blanket pack
- Ice packs
- Immersion baths
- Sitz bath
- Sprays/showers
- Steam/sauna
- Wet sheet pack

(See the Where to Find Help section in the Hydrotherapy chapter for organizations that can refer you to a physical therapist or naturopathic physician who is knowledgeable of hydrotherapy procedures.)

Juice Therapy

Unless otherwise indicated, the raw juices in this section can be either used for a short three-day juice fast or incorporated into your daily diet. Check with your physician before undertaking a fast.

Meditation

Meditation, described in the Mind/Body Medicine chapter, may be beneficial for a variety of health conditions.

Although meditation can be practiced at home, it is helpful if you first receive proper instruction from a qualified instructor. (See the Where to Find Help section in the Mind/Body Medicine chapter for organizations that can refer you to a qualified teacher.)

Nutritional Supplements

This section gives you the most important nutritional supplements (vitamins, minerals, amino acids, enzymes, glandulars, and antioxidants) for helping to deal with each health condition. Before going on a new regime of supplementation, it is important to consult with a qualified health-care professional or call an organization listed in the Where to Find Help section in the Nutritional Medicine chapter that can refer you to a physician specializing in nutritional medicine.

Qigong and Tai Chi

Qigong and Tai Chi exercises that may be helpful for various health conditions. They are described and illustrated in the Qigong and Tai Chi chapter in Part Two. Although Qigong can be practiced at home, it is advised that you first receive proper instruction from a qualified instructor. (See the Where to Find Help section in the Qigong and Tai Chi chapter for organizations that can refer you to a qualified teacher or therapist.)

Reflexology

Use the accompanying chart to locate the reflex areas described in the Quick Reference A-Z and the self-care sections of the health condition chapters.

Yoga

The yoga postures described and illustrated in the Yoga chapter may be beneficial for a variety of health conditions. Although yoga can be practiced at home, it is advised that you first receive proper instruction from a qualified yoga instructor or yoga therapist. (See the Where to Find Help section in the Yoga chapter for organizations that can refer you to a qualified teacher or therapist.)

ABSCESS

Accumulation of pus, usually caused by bacterial infection (or viral, parasitic, fungal), in almost any body part (most common on the face, armpit, extremities, rectum, and female breast during lactation).

SYMPTOMS: Heat, swelling, tenderness, or redness over the infected area, which increase with severity. A severe abscess may cause fever, cellulitis (inflammation of cellular tissue, usually with associated pus formation), fatigue, weight loss, chills, abnormal functioning depending on the area affected or, at worst, blood infection and rupture.

CONSIDER: Boils, allergic infections, poor immune response, poor diet, and nutrient deficiencies. Chronic or recurrent abscesses may suggest food, environmental, or chemical allergies.

SPECIAL NOTES: *Mild:* External abscesses may respond to gentle heat from warm water soaks and to improved nutrition. Most abscesses, however, need to be treated with antibiotics or herbs. This requires acidophilus, B vitamins, and an increase in fluids. Need for specific treatment such as drainage, compression bandage, or surgery should be assessed by a doctor. *Moderate to severe:* May require bed rest, increased fluids, local ice packs, or hot baths. Incomplete drainage may result in fibrous wall with calcium accumulation resulting in a hardened mass. May be caused or worsened by decreased immune functioning.

An abscess should start to clear up in several days. A failure to clear up or bouts of reoccurrences may indicate problems with immune function and overall health and require professional care. Assess lifestyle to reduce stress or problems that may be contributing to a decrease in general health and immune functioning, and get plenty of rest.

Alternative Treatments

Refer to alternative therapy chapters for more information before evaluating or applying any treatment. Some conditions, including yours, may require a physician's care.

DIET: Increase liquids such as filtered water, fresh vegetable and fruit juices, and immune enhancer herbal teas like astragalus or nettle (8–10 glasses per day). Avoid all stressor foods, especially refined sugars, and alcohol for at least two weeks. Avoid cow's milk dairy products and processed foods. Drink water and juice of one fresh lemon on rising and before bed. If chronic, eat plenty of berries (fresh or frozen) or drink berry leaf teas.

NUTRITIONAL THERAPY: • Vitamin A (50,000 IU for two weeks) • Beta carotene (100,000 IU for two weeks) • Zinc (60 mg daily for two weeks) • Vitamin C (5–10 g daily) • Liquid chlorophyll • *Lactobacillus acidophilus* and *Bifidobacteria* (several times per day) • Proteolytic enzymes (on an empty stomach) • B complex vitamins • Pantothenic acid • Garlic capsules • If recurrent, consider an imbalance in the system and need for bowel cleanse and rejuvenation.

Self–Care

The following therapies can be undertaken at home under appropriate professional supervision.

AROMATHERAPY: • Lavender • Hot compress of bergamot, tea tree, lavender, chamomile, garlic

FASTING: Leon Chaitow N.D., D.O., suggests a short (48-hour) water or juice fast to encourage more rapid detoxification and healing.

FLOWER ESSENCES: Rescue Remedy Cream® may be applied to the area of healthy skin around the abscess, but not on top of or in the abscessed area, at least four times a day.

HERBS: Burdock root, cayenne, dandelion root, echinacea, goldenseal, red clover, yarrow, and yellowdock root.

HOMEOPATHY: *Belladonna, Merc sol., Hepar sulph., Silicea, Bryonia*

HYDROTHERAPY: Contrast application (apply daily).

JUICE THERAPY: • Carrot, beet, and celery juice • Cucumber • Wheat grass • Spinach • Also can add a small amount of yellowdock leaf juice (5% of total juice).

NATUROPATHIC MEDICINE: Use a paste of goldenseal root powder and calendula succus (the juice of the marigold flower). Place the paste over the abscess and leave it on 12–14 hours. It will often draw out the infection, while stimulating regeneration of the damaged tissues.

TOPICAL TREATMENT: • Calendula ointment • Apply mixture of zinc oxide cream one vitamin A capsule (10,000 IU), and liquid chlorophyll locally on external abscess, three times daily. If all three are not available, use whichever you can obtain. • Apply raw, unprocessed honey to infected area.

Professional Care

The following therapies should only be provided by a qualified health professional.

Craniosacral Therapy / Detoxification Therapy / Environmental Medicine / Guided Imagery / Light Therapy / Naturopathic Medicine / Osteopathic Medicine / Traditional Chinese Medicine

OXYGEN THERAPY: • Hydrogen peroxide therapy (IV) • Hyperbaric oxygen therapy.

ACNE

Inflammation of the skin because a sebaceous gland, located at the bottom of each hair follicle, becomes trapped with natural oils, causing bacterial buildup and inflammation. This condition may be worsened at adolescence, premenstrually, or mid-menstrual cycle due to hormonal action, and when under stress, eating a poor diet, or on contraceptives.

SYMPTOMS: Inflamed spots or elevations either on or under the skin. Blackheads form when the oil combines with skin pigments and gets trapped. Blackheads may suggest the need for better hygiene, or magnesium and vitamin A. Chronic, numerous whiteheads may suggest vitamin B₁ deficiency or absorption problems. Consistent raised spots on the outside of the arms and sometimes even the thighs, resembling "chicken skin," may suggest need for magnesium, vitamin A, or essential fatty acids or the need to avoid foods that inhibit the absorption of these nutrients, such as trans-fatty acids found in margarine and hydrogenated oils, (cottonseed oil and palm kernel oil).

CONSIDER: Food allergies, allergies to facial creams, soaps, shampoos, makeup, excess intake of refined sugars. Certain foods may aggravate (chocolate, fruit juices, carbonated beverages, caffeinated beverages, milk products). Excessive long-term intake of seafood or other high- iodine foods may also bring on acne bouts in some people.

SPECIAL NOTES: Vitamin B₆ may help for premenstrual or mid-menstrual cycle acne. Coexisting gum problems suggest the need for folic acid. A separate acne condition may occur in women 30-40 years old due to exercising or working all day with face makeup, lowered resistance due to stress, or hyper-response to bacteria or hormone problems. Another acne problem, acne rosacea (reddish spots in a pattern over nose and cheeks), may be a sign of low B vitamins or low hydrochloric acid in the stomach.

It may take up to one year to eliminate skin problems. They are some of the slowest conditions to respond to natural therapies, but the response is often more complete than with drugs.

Alternative Treatments

Refer to alternative therapy chapters for more information before applying any treatment. Some conditions, including yours, may require a physician's care.

DIET: Whole foods diet with special emphasis on vegetables (four to five servings per day, try to eat half of servings raw) and whole fruits (one to three times per day). The more severe the acne, the more you should reduce fats. Reduce especially animal fats (saturated) and also cut down on vegetable fats. Some people get acne in response to stressor foods such as caffeine, refined sugars, and alcohol. Processed foods such as colas, candies, and frozen and processed foods may also be a problem. Increase intake of pure water.

Increase fiber. Mono-cleansing diets for one to two days per week for several months may be helpful in people who are not hypoglycemic (low blood sugar), debilitated, or require food to keep up strength for working. Examples are steamed vegetables and brown rice without any animal products. Fasting one day a week is helpful for some: fresh vegetable juices, filtered water, lemon and honey, or water from wheatberries soaked for 12 hours.

NUTRITIONAL THERAPY: • Vitamin A (10,000 IU daily for two weeks); some orthomolecular physicians recommend higher initial doses • Beta carotene (50,000 IU for one month, then reduce to 25,000 IU) • Vitamin B complex (two to three times daily) • Vitamin B₆ • Thiamin (vitamin B₁) • Vitamin C (1,000 mg three times daily) • Vitamin E (800 IU daily) • Zinc helps prevent acne by regulating the oil glands[1] (80 mg daily unless it causes nausea; if so, reduce by 20 mg) • Essential fatty acids (one to two daily for one year); acne may be a symptom of an omega-3 fatty acid deficiency • Brewer's yeast • Chlorophyll • Pancreatin enzyme with meals (three times daily)

See Women's Health and Natural Hormone Replacement Therapy chapters if this is hormonally related.

Self-Care

The following therapies can be undertaken at home under appropriate professional supervision.

Fasting / Guided Imagery / Hypnotherapy / Meditation / Yoga

AROMATHERAPY: • Bergamot, lavender, rosemary, rosewood, thyme-linalol, tea tree oil • Massage with bergamot, camphor, geranium, juniper, lavender, neroli.

AYURVEDA: • Apply turmeric and sandalwood paste externally (½ teaspoon of each and enough water to make a paste) • Drink ½ cup aloe vera juice twice daily until acne clears.

BODYWORK: • Massage, acupressure, shiatsu, and reflexology are often recommended for skin problems. • Lymphatic drainage massage

FLOWER ESSENCES: • Crab Apple, for detox and purification and for not feeling attractive • Rescue Remedy®, if feeling stressed.

HERBS: When used with appropriate nutritional support, herbs may be helpful in the treatment of acne. Combine the tinctures of sarsaparilla, burdock, and cleavers in equal parts and take ½ teaspoonful of this mixture three times a day. An infusion of nettle can also be drunk two or three times a day. • An infusion of calendula mixed with equal parts of distilled witch hazel may be applied topically as a cleansing wash. • Forsythia works against bacteria by removing skin toxins. • Try a steam sauna for face with red clover, lavender, and strawberry leaves. Chamomile flowers are another option.

HOMEOPATHY: *Pulsatilla, Silicea, Berberis, Ledum, Sulfur, Arsen alb., Belladonna, Carbo veg.*

HYDROTHERAPY: • Contrast application: apply daily. • Hot Epsom salts baths two to three times a week.

JUICE THERAPY: • Two glasses raw juice daily • Carrot, beet, and celery juice • Any combination of carrot, cucumber, lettuce (not iceberg), and spinach, with carrot predominating.

NATUROPATHIC MEDICINE: While long-term improvement for acne requires treating the lifestyle and metabolic causes, improvement may be hastened by a proper facial hygiene. Washing the face three times a day with a soap made with the herb *Calendula officinalis* (marigold flowers) can be very effective in keeping the face clean and the cyst-forming infections minimized.

PRACTICAL HEALTH HINTS: Expose whole body to sun and air but take caution not to sunburn. Fresh air and daily exercise are very important. Be sure to get sufficient relaxation and sleep. Do not squeeze pimples or whiteheads, as this may lead to infection. Use non-oil-based makeup and wash off thoroughly each night. Avoid cosmetic products containing lanolin, isopropyl myristate, sodium laurel sulfate, laureth-4, and D and C red dyes, as they may be too rich for the skin and cause blackheads. Drink eight glasses of water a day. Use 100% cotton clothing and bed linen.

REFLEXOLOGY: Liver, adrenals, all glands, kidneys, intestines, thyroid, diaphragm.

STRESS REDUCTION: A study of teenagers taught methods of relaxation, including biofeedback, showed a marked reduction in acne outbreaks in severely affected individuals. Those who continued to practice at home maintained the progress they had made.[2]

TOPICAL TREATMENT: • Wipe face in the morning and evening with vitamin A-E emulsion, liquid chlorophyll, and aloe vera gel, or with cider vinegar and a dash of cayenne pepper. • Wipe three times daily with tea made from alfalfa, burdock root, echinacea, a teaspoon of apple cider vinegar, and a dash of cayenne pepper. • Vitamin A and tea tree oil can be used topically to decrease skin outbreaks.

Facial cleansing—Gently wash face with mild soap and water two to four times daily. Alternatives to soap are milk, diluted lemon juice, or a solution of one part rubbing alcohol to ten parts water. Rinse face with warm water and pat dry. Try to keep skin free of oil and use water-based products. Eric Jones, N.D., instructor of dermatology at Bastyr University, in Kenmore, Washington, recommends the use of soaps containing the herb calendula to help clean the pores without irritating the skin.

Facial masks—The following foods may be applied to the cleansed skin as a masque for 30 minutes before rinsing off with warm water: cooked and mashed carrots (let cool first), grated cucumber or sliced cucumber soaked in rum, whisked egg yolk, and oatmeal, cooked in milk until thick and then cooled. Or apply baking soda and water mixture to face, rinse immediately with water, and then rinse or spray with apple cider vinegar, plus do a final rinse with filtered water. • A bentonite clay mask, left on the skin for 15-20 minutes to help draw out inflammatory by-products of acne. • Rub oil from a vitamin E capsule over freshly washed and dried skin. Let remain for 30 minutes, then apply a coating of whisked egg whites over the vitamin E and leave for another 30 minutes. Rinse with filtered water. •

Apply a poultice made from chaparral, dandelion, and yellowdock root to affected area. • Or try a compress of goldenseal tea. • Overnight mask for drying the skin: diluted liquid hand soap or shampoo patted on a cleansed and dried face.

Professional Care

The following therapies should only be provided by a qualified health professional.

Environmental Medicine / Enzyme Therapy / Magnetic Field Therapy / Natural Hormone Replacement Therapy / Naturopathic Medicine / Orthomolecular Medicine / Osteopathic Medicine / Traditional Chinese Medicine

DETOXIFICATION THERAPY: Detoxification may be indicated, especially of the colon.

OXYGEN THERAPY: Hydrogen peroxide therapy (IV).

ANKYLOSING SPONDYLITIS

A rare rheumatologic condition that causes stiffness and inflammation of the spine and sacroiliac joints. Characterized by "bent forward" posture. May have genetic risk.

SYMPTOMS: *Mild and early:* Recurrent low back pain, pain along sciatic nerve that can go from buttocks to the leg and foot, and stiffness on rising in the morning. *Progresses:* Pain spreads from low back up to middle and/or higher in the neck. Pain in arms and legs. Fatigue, muscle rigidity and more stiffness, anemia, weight loss.

OCCURRENCE: 90% occurs in males from 20-40 years old.

CONSIDER: Test for identifying gastrointestinal problems, stool sample and scraping to identify amoebic, bacterial, fungal, or other parasitic problems. Test for food allergies and assess need for digestive enzymes.

Alternative Treatments

Refer to alternative therapy chapters for more information before evaluating or applying any treatment. Some conditions, including yours, may require a physician's care.

DIET: Whole foods diet with emphasis on variety and ruling out food allergies. Alan R. Gaby, M.D., has treated ankylosing spondylitis successfully by identifying allergenic foods and recommending avoidance and food allergy nutrients. Gut health may be related and bowel program may be useful. Two cups of vegetable broth daily. Researchers at King's College Hospital, in London, have found a link between ankylosing spondylitis and bowel dysbiosis (incursion or overgrowth by undesirable bacteria, in this case *Klebsiella*). They discovered that the majority of patients placed on a low-starch diet had the disease process halted.[3]

Leon Chaitow, N.D., D.O., of London, England, feels that an overgrowth of *Candida albicans* (a naturally occuring fungus in the body) is also involved in creating the damage to the gastrointestinal tract, which allows the *Klebsiella* bacteria to enter the bloodstream. He recommends further measures, including the use of friendly bacteria such as *Lactobacillus acidophilus* and *L. bulgaricus* to reestablish a normal bowel flora, and an anti-*Candida* approach, which includes a low-fat diet. He believes that the results of the low-fat diet in the King's College Hospital study may have been due to controlling both the *Klebsiella* bacteria and the *Candida*.

NUTRITIONAL THERAPY: Vitamin C to bowel tolerance. (See Orthomolecular Medicine chapter.)

Self-Care

The following therapies can be undertaken at home under appropriate professional supervision.

Fasting / Yoga

HERBS: Many anti-inflammatory and alterative herbs can be used to alleviate the symptoms of this condition. The following mixture has been used over long periods of time: a combination of the tinctures of meadowsweet, willow bark, black cohosh, prickly ash, celery seed, and nettle in equal parts, ½ teaspoonful of this mixture taken three times a day. In cases of rheumatoid arthritis, add wild yam and valerian to the mixture and take one teaspoonful of this mixture three times a day.

HYDROTHERAPY: Constitutional hydrotherapy (apply two to five times weekly). Or contrast application, applied daily as needed for relief of inflammation.

JUICE THERAPY: Carrot, beet celery, parsley, potato, alfalfa

Professional Care

The following therapies should only be provided by a qualified health professional.

Applied Kinesiology / Cell Therapy / Chelation Therapy / Chiropractic / Craniosacral Therapy / Environmental Medicine / Enzyme Therapy / Magnetic Field Therapy / Natural Hormone Replacement Therapy / Naturopathic Medicine / Neural Therapy / Osteopathic Medicine / Prolotherapy

ACUPUNCTURE: For chronic condition: moxa stick used up and down the spine for five to ten minutes a day along with herbs.

BODYWORK: • Feldenkrais • Rolfing can sometimes ease the pain and stiffness associated with ankylosing spondylitis, but cannot cure it.

OXYGEN THERAPY: Hydrogen peroxide therapy (IV).

ANOREXIA NERVOSA

An eating disorder where weight loss becomes an obsession and starvation begins to affect thinking patterns and personality.

SYMPTOMS: Physical symptoms include wasting of the body, including the muscle tissue, arrest of sexual development and cessation of menstruation, drying and yellowing of the skin, loss of texture of the hair, pain to the touch, lowered blood pressure and metabolic weight, anemia, and severe sleep disturbances. Mentally, the patient still sees herself as fat, may have a preoccupation with death, and often exercises frantically to keep physically fit. She often is manipulative, trying always to be the center of attention, and may become socially isolated.

OCCURRENCE: Predominantly in teenage females and is a problem only in developed countries.

SPECIAL NOTES: In both anorexia nervosa and bulimia nervosa, the underlying causative factors are believed to be solely due to an obsession with body fat, a fear of being (or becoming) fat, or overconcern with perfectionism. Although all of these factors are important, recent studies also show that, in most cases, an underlying zinc deficiency may contribute to the maintenance of the disorder.

Alternative Treatments

Refer to alternative therapy chapters for more information before evaluating or applying any treatment. Some conditions, including yours, may require a physician's care.

DIET: A well-balanced diet, high in fiber, should be followed when a regular eating pattern is being established. Avoid sugar and white flour products.

NUTRITIONAL THERAPY: Zinc deficiency can be a major contributing factor in anorexia; zinc supplementation has proven successful in overcoming dietary deficiencies and in helping anorexics regain their appetite and weight.[4] Ten years of study indicate that a liquid form of zinc sulfate heptahydrate supplement is beneficial in the diagnosis and treatment of anorexia nervosa. According to Alexander Schauss, Ph.D., a Certified Eating Disorder Specialist, the inability to taste a tablespoon of this supplement in the mouth may be indicative of inadequate zinc status. He recommends 100–120 ml per day of the zinc solution until symptoms improve, which may take two weeks.

Vitamin B$_{12}$, D, and E levels in the blood are often low in anorexia nervosa.

Intravenous feeding may be necessary in acute cases to replace lost calories and reverse protein deficiency. Psychological counseling by trained specialists, combined with nutritional therapy, is highly recommended.

Self-Care

The following therapies can be undertaken at home under appropriate professional supervision.

Biofeedback Training and Neurotherapy / Meditation / Yoga

AROMATHERAPY: As antidepressants, take bergamot, basil, chamomile, clary sage, lavender, neroli, and ylang ylang.

AYURVEDA: Cardamom, fennel, and fresh ginger to help regulate digestion and stop vomiting. Follow a bland diet and avoid coffee, tea, and other stimulants. For calming effect, valerian, nutmeg, *ashwagandha,* and sandalwood. Massage head and feet with sesame oil.

FLOWER ESSENCES: • Various essences to address underlying emotional and mental states of imbalance and negativity, such as fears, perfectionism, manipulative behavior, depression, and anxiety. • Crab Apple for obsessive habits relating to body image.

HERBS: To stimulate appetite, take ginger root, ginseng, gotu kola, peppermint. Gentian root helps stimulate the appetite and has been useful in helping anorexics regain their appetite.[5]

HYDROTHERAPY: Constitutional hydrotherapy (apply two to five times weekly).

HYPNOTHERAPY: Self-hypnosis to reinforce positive affirmations.

Professional Care

The following therapies should only be provided by a qualified health professional.

Hypnotherapy / Magnetic Field Therapy / Natural Hormone Replacement Therapy / Traditional Chinese Medicine

ANXIETY

Anxiety is a sense of fear and, in some cases, a feeling of impending doom. The term anxiety disorder *refers to a category of disturbances that includes generalized anxiety, post-traumatic stress disorder, phobias, and obsessive-compulsive disorders. A panic attack is an acute anxiety episode that may be accompanied by sweating, shortness of breath, hot or cold flashes, heart palpitations, and other forms of discomfort. Anxiety disorders occur in people of all ages, but appear to be more common among women. The exact cause is complex, involving constitutional factors, emotional stress, biochemical imbalances, and environmental triggers.*

SYMPTOMS: The occurrence of a panic attack is often unpredictable, but it may be associated with certain situations such as driving a car. Anxiety is an emotion that may feature excessive worry, sleep disturbances, shakiness, ritualistic behavior, fear of being alone or in public places, impatience, easy distraction, and great apprehension concerning the welfare of loved ones. Associated physical symptoms include racing pulse, heart palpitations, shortness or rapidity of breath, sweating, dry mouth, numbness and tingling of the hands and feet or cold/clammy hands, lightheadedness or dizziness, fatigue, trembling, indigestion, and diarrhea.[6]

Alternative Treatments

Refer to alternative therapy chapters for more information before evaluating or applying any treatment. Some conditions, including yours, may require a physician's care.

DIET: Assess diet for excessive consumption of stressor foods such as refined sugars, honey, maple syrup, or cow's milk products. Consume vegetable soups, broths, and a wide variety of green and yellow vegetables. Add more complex carbohydrates such as whole grains, beans, seeds, and nuts.

NUTRITIONAL THERAPY: • Calcium • Magnesium • Vitamin B complex • Pantothenic acid • Adrenal glandulars • Kidney glandulars • 5-HTP (5-hydroxytryptophan).

Stabilium, a product containing *Garum Armoricum* (a fish, salt, and herb preparation dating to the Roman Empire and traditionally used for its high nutritive value), is an adaptogen that can also help balance mood, improve sleep, and increase energy and stamina.[7] GABA (gamma-aminobutyric acid), an amino acid, can also affect mood by increasing levels of the brain neurotransmitter serotonin (a mood regulator).

Self-Care

The following therapies can be undertaken at home under appropriate professional supervision.

Acupressure / Biofeedback Training and Neurotherapy / Fasting / Guided Imagery / Qigong and Tai Chi / Yoga

FLOWER ESSENCES: Flower essences may prove helpful. Aspen is for apprehension, foreboding, and fear of unknown origin, while mimulus is for fear of known things, shyness, and timidity. Red chestnut is used for excessive anxiety and over caring for others. Rescue Remedy® for general stress from anxiety; Rock Rose for terror and panic from known fear.

HERBS: • *Panax ginseng* has a nutritive or tonic effect on the adrenal glands, improving blood flow to the brain and reducing the stress associated with mental/emotional issues.[8] • Valerian root, an herbal tranquilizer and muscle relaxant, is a good agent for calming the nervous system.[9] It helps balance mood swings and is not habit forming. Valerian-hops combination formulas are good daytime sedatives because they don't interfere with reflex actions. • Passionflower is another mild sedative that helps reduce anxiety, high blood pressure, nervous tension, and muscle tension, and encourages deep, restful sleep. • Extract of the kava-kava plant, an herbal tranquilizer native to Polynesia, can lower anxiety levels and alleviate panic disorder and general tension in as quickly as a week.[10] • St. John's wort, a highly popular remedy for depression, has proven effective for anxiety and mood swings as well.

HOMEOPATHY: *Aconite, Actaea rac., Drosera, Calc carb., Sulfur*

HYDROTHERAPY: Constitutional hydrotherapy, immersion bath, or wet sheet pack (apply two to five times weekly); neutral application as needed for sedation.

HYPNOTHERAPY: Self-hypnosis to impart to the mind imagery designed to bring about deep levels of relaxation.

MEDITATION: Develops the mind's ability to stop anxiety at its source.

Professional Care

The following therapies should only be provided by a qualified health professional.

Environmental Medicine / Light Therapy / Magnetic Field Therapy / Naturopathic Medicine / Orthomolecular Medicine / Traditional Chinese Medicine

BODYWORK: Rolfing may be very helpful if used in conjunction with psychotherapy.

DETOXIFICATION THERAPY: Not usually indicated, unless the person's condition warrants treatment.

ATHLETE'S FOOT

Athlete's foot is the most common fungal infection of the skin, characterized by fungal growth on the skin of the foot. The infectious fungal species thrives in warmth and dampness and is prevalent in gym locker rooms and around indoor swimming pools.

SYMPTOMS: Itching, burning, and stinging sensations, as well as scaling, cracking, and inflammation of the skin between the toes and on the soles of the feet. In some cases, the infection may involve the toenails.[11]

Alternative Treatments

Refer to alternative therapy chapters for more information before evaluating or applying any treatment. Some conditions, including yours, may require a physician's care.

DIET: Whole foods diet with emphasis on raw foods, less dairy products. Avoid foods high in yeast, such as beer and breads with yeast. Avoid sugar of all sorts (including honey and fruit juices) for some weeks while antifungal methods are being used. See Candidiasis chapter.

NUTRITIONAL THERAPY: • Acidophilus • *Bifidobacteria* and *L. bulgaricus* • Garlic capsules • Vitamin B complex • Pantothenic acid • Vitamin C to bowel tolerance (see Orthomolecular Medicine chapter) • Vitamin E • Vitamin A • Zinc

Self-Care

The following therapies can be undertaken at home under appropriate professional supervision.

Fasting

AROMATHERAPY: Tea tree oil, patchouli, geranium

FLOWER ESSENCES: Rescue Remedy Cream®; Crab Apple.

HERBS: Fungicidal herbs are an effective topical treatment for athlete's foot. Examples are myrrh, tea tree, and garlic. Tea tree oil can be applied directly or diluted with calendula oil for application to sensitive skin.

HOMEOPATHY: *Calendula, Chamomilla, Belladonna, Merc sol., Sulfur*

JUICE THERAPY: • Avoid fruit juices or dilute with water in a 2:1 ratio • Add garlic to vegetable juice.

TOPICAL TREATMENT: To the affected area, apply some of the following: tea tree oil, citrus seed extract, honey and crushed garlic, pau d'arco tea by wetting tea bag for ten minutes and then leave the bag itself on the area or use gauze or cotton soaked in tea if area is too large.

Professional Care

The following therapies should only be provided by a qualified health professional.

Environmental Medicine / Magnetic Field Therapy / Naturopathic Medicine / Traditional Chinese Medicine

DETOXIFICATION THERAPY: May be indicated, depending on the condition of the person.

OXYGEN THERAPY: • Hydrogen peroxide therapy (IV) • Hyperbaric oxygen therapy • Ozone/oxygen mixture may work as an effective antifungal agent and may easily be applied externally.

BAD BREATH

Bad breath, or halitosis, is an unpleasant odor emanating from the mouth, usually caused by some health problem in the mouth, teeth, gums, throat, or gastrointestinal tract. Other contributing factors may be smoking, liver disease, and poor protein digestion. The mouth is one window into the body. If there is a bad odor, it is a general sign that there is some underlying cause and imbalance that needs to be treated.

SYMPTOMS: Bad odor coming from the mouth that is usually not detectable by the person affected. Astute health practitioners smell the breath and examine carefully the tongue and mouth of all patients.

SPECIAL NOTES: Certain smells are associated with specific disease; for example, a metallic smell may represent diabetes or an active metabolism undergoing rapid weight loss; sour smells may represent stomach problems or tumors. Orthodox physicians do not agree that halitosis may represent intestinal problems, but anecdotal evidence by many alternative practitioners finds differently. Bad breath may also be caused by chronically infected sinuses, tonsils, or lungs.

Alternative Treatments

Refer to alternative therapy chapters for more information before evaluating or applying any treatment. Some conditions, including yours, may require a physician's care.

DIET: Whole foods diet with plenty of raw foods. Water with juice of fresh lemon and/or one teaspoon chlorophyll on rising and before bed. Include fiber in diet (oat bran, rice bran). Chew food well, don't overeat, and drink lots of liquids. See Diet chapter for information on the role antioxidants play in relieving bad breath.

NUTRITIONAL THERAPY: • If needed, bowel cleanse and rejuvenation • Proteolytic enzymes (two between meals, three times daily, and two with each meal) • Vitamin B complex (100 mg two times daily) •Vitamin C •Thiamin (vitamin B₁) • Niacin (vitamin B₃) •Vitamin B₆ • Garlic capsules • PABA (para-aminobenzoic acid) •Vitamin A • Beta carotene • Acidophilus • Digestive enzymes • Magnesium • Zinc • Charcoal

Fiber (psyllium or pectin fiber) helps remove toxins from the colon and thereby decreases bad breath. Chlorophyll products (wheat grass juice, chlorella, alfalfa tablets, barley juice) act as a blood purifier and can be effective in reducing and preventing bad breath, taken both with food and on an empty stomach.

Self–Care

The following therapies can be undertaken at home under appropriate professional supervision.

Fasting / Yoga

AROMATHERAPY: Peppermint, lavender, cardamom

AYURVEDA: *Triphala,* ½ teaspoon with warm water, 30 minutes before bedtime. Chew roasted cumin, fennel, and coriander seeds after each meal.

FLOWER ESSENCES: For negative feelings surrounding the problem, such as Crab Apple for low self-esteem or feeling toxic.

HERBS: • Chewing seeds of fennel or anise as needed will mask the odor and have a mild local antimicrobial effect. Alternatively, chew cardamom seeds, parsley leaves, or other chlorophyll–rich herbs such as basil and cilantro. • Peppermint or bergamot tea. • Attention must be given to underlying causes, such as tooth and gum disease or digestive illness.

HOMEOPATHY: *Arnica, Merc sol., Nux vom., Kali phos., Chelidonium*

HYDROTHERAPY: Constitutional hydrotherapy (apply two to five times weekly).

JUICE THERAPY: • Carrot and celery with parsley, spinach, watercress, alfalfa, comfrey, or beet tops • Wheat grass juice • Green juice • Carrot, spinach, and cucumber • Half a lemon in warm water each morning.

NATUROPATHIC MEDICINE: According to Joseph Pizzorno, N.D., bad breath is far more often due to maldigestion and a toxic bowel than to poor oral hygiene. People who experience bad breath, abdominal bloating and gas, and tiredness after meals may be deficient in stomach acid.

Professional Care

The following therapies should only be provided by a qualified health professional.

Applied Kinesiology / Environmental Medicine / Naturopathic Medicine

DETOXIFICATION THERAPY: Bad breath is often related to gastrointestinal toxicity, suggesting a need for intestinal cleansing with diet change.

OXYGEN THERAPY: Use of ozonated water gargle may be effective.

TRADITIONAL CHINESE MEDICINE: As this is considered a symptom of "stomach heat," it is most important to address the deeper cause of the digestive problem.

BED SORES

Ulcers of the skin formed by prolonged bed rest, which causes sustained pressure over bony areas of the body, such as the buttocks, hips, sacrum, and shoulder blades.

SYMPTOMS: Areas of redness, deep ulceration, and pain.

SPECIAL NOTES: Patients need to be moved frequently, and also require fresh air and light bed clothes. Daily baths with gentle soaps containing vitamin E and aloe vera, and sufficient natural light, may be helpful.

OCCURRENCE: In physically restricted patients, such as the disabled, comatose, and bedridden elderly.

TIME: Should start to heal within one week and may take up to six weeks, depending on severity of situation.

Alternative Treatments

Refer to alternative therapy chapters for more information before evaluating or applying any treatment. Some conditions, including yours, may require a physician's care.

DIET: Drink plenty of liquids (distilled water, herbal teas, fresh juices). Include plenty of fiber in the diet to keep the colon clean; oat bran and guar gum are both excellent. (If bowels do not move, use an enema.) Five to seven vegetables and fruits a day is optimal.

NUTRITIONAL THERAPY: • Oral vitamin E • Zinc •Vitamin A • Beta carotene •Vitamin C •Vitamin B complex • Zinc with copper • Vitamin D • Protein supplement (free-form amino acids) • Garlic capsules • If not responding to the above, pancreatic enzymes between meals (6–12 per day for one week along with bioflavonoids and vitamin C) may be helpful.

Vitamin C to bowel tolerance (see Orthomolecular Medicine chapter).

Self–Care

The following therapies can be undertaken at home under appropriate professional supervision.

Guided Imagery

FLOWER ESSENCES: Rescue Remedy Cream® can be applied (minimum four times a day) on unbroken skin around, but not directly on, sores or ulcers. Single flower essences are helpful to ease emotional discomfort and stress from physical condition.

HERBS: Comfrey root powder, echinacea powder, goldenseal, myrrh gum, pau d'arco, slippery elm powder, suma

HOMEOPATHY: *Calendula, Hypericum, Merc sol., Chamomilla, Phosphorus, Hamamelis, Silicea, Belladonna*

HYDROTHERAPY: • Contrast application: apply several times daily to promote healing. • Periodic cold compresses to stimulate sore areas

JUICE THERAPY: Carrot, beet, cantaloupe, currant, red grapes

NATUROPATHIC MEDICINE: A standard naturopathic approach is to wash the open wound with *Calendula succus* (juice of the marigold flower) and then cover it with zinc oxide.

TOPICAL TREATMENT: Application of a paste of goldenseal powder, vitamin E squeezed from capsule, along with zinc oxide applied topically. Also enzyme cream, vitamin E cream, aloe vera gel, comfrey ointment, calendula cream.

Leon Chaitow, N.D., D.O., suggests the "safest and oldest approach—application of raw honey or granulated sugar paste to open ulcers from bed-pressure sores—which has now been well-researched medically and shown to be at least as effective as medicated creams."

Professional Care

The following therapies should only be provided by a qualified health professional.

Acupuncture / Chelation Therapy / Magnetic Field Therapy / Naturopathic Medicine

OXYGEN THERAPIES: • Ozone therapy is useful applied externally in a fitted plastic bag. • Hyperbaric oxygen therapy.

BED-WETTING

Involuntary wetting of the bed in the middle of night during childhood. Usually spontaneously stops by teenage years. Often a general sign that there is some underlying problem.

CONSIDER: Hypoglycemia, diabetes, food allergies, and urinary tract infections.

SPECIAL NOTES: Cause of bed-wetting is unknown and controversial. Low blood sugar is one nutritional theory. Others are emotional stress, small and weak bladders that cannot hold urine all night, excessive consumption of liquid beverages, sleeping too soundly, food allergies, heredity, and behavioral problems.

TIME: Improvement may take up to several months, but some improvement may be seen within the first two weeks.

Alternative Treatments

Refer to alternative therapy chapters for more information before evaluating or applying any treatment. Some conditions, including yours, may require a physician's care.

DIET: Eat more frequent and smaller meals, up to five or six, throughout the day. Consume slow-release complex carbohydrates such as potatoes, yams, whole grains, breads, and beans. Avoid liquids around bedtime. Avoid drinking very sweet beverages such as fruit juice or cola more than one time per day. Take two teaspoons of raw honey at bedtime. Eat a small amount of protein from chicken, fish, soy, goat cheese, or nut butter, before bed.

NUTRITIONAL THERAPY: • Mixed amino acid supplements (two capsules, two or three times daily, ten minutes before meals) • Magnesium (100 mg two times daily) • Calcium (250 mg with dinner and before bed) •Vitamin B complex (one with breakfast and lunch) • Multivitamin (two to three daily)

Self-Care

The following therapies can be undertaken at home under appropriate professional supervision.

AROMATHERAPY: Before bedtime rub the child's abdomen with olive oil and 3%-5% cypress essence.

FLOWER ESSENCES: For emotional states as appropriate.

HERBS: If bed-wetting occurs because of lack of nervous control of the bladder, use an infusion of one part each of horsetail, St. John's wort, cornsilk, and lemon balm. Half a cup given three times a day, with the last dose well over an hour before bedtime.

HOMEOPATHY: *Berberis*

HYDROTHERAPY: A cool sitz bath for five minutes.

NATUROPATHIC MEDICINE: According to Joseph Pizzorno, N.D., supplemental magnesium has helped several children with this problem.

REFLEXOLOGY: Kidneys, diaphragm, ureters, adrenals, lower spine

Professional Care

The following therapies should only be provided by a qualified health professional.

Acupuncture / Biofeedback Training and Neurotherapy / Chiropractic / Hypnotherapy / Magnetic Field Therapy

BODYWORK: Shiatsu

ENVIRONMENTAL MEDICINE: Allergies can be a major cause of bed-wetting. Allergic reactions to food or environmental factors can cause sudden and violent contractions in the muscles of the bladder.

BERIBERI

A deficiency of thiamin (vitamin B1) causing neurologic, mental, and cardiovascular problems.

SYMPTOMS: *Mild:* fatigue, irritation, slow learning and confusion, poor cold tolerance, nausea, vomiting, whiteheads on face or upper torso. *Severe:* memory loss, heart pain, weight loss, abdominal and heart discomfort, poor digestion, gas, diarrhea, constipation, extreme fatigue, mood swings, mental confusion, tachycardia (rapid heart rate), heart failure, death.

CONSIDER: Parasites, gastrointestinal or liver disease, food allergies, severe stress.

SPECIAL NOTES: *Primary beriberi:* Occurs due to inadequate intake of vitamin B1 through food. This is found especially in people eating highly refined diets, as B1 is lost in the milling process. Especially prevalent in people subsisting on polished (white) rice. However, boiling before milling disperses the B₁ from the husk throughout the kernel and less B₁ is lost through this processing.

Secondary beriberi: Occurs due to loss of B1 by poor utilization, such as in liver disease, gastrointestinal problems, or alcoholism and drug addiction; through increased requirements, such as pregnancy, hyperthyroidism (overactive thyroid), breast-feeding, fever, stress (emotional and physical), genetic need for more than the average amount; and impaired absorption, such as with diarrhea, parasites, gastrointestinal loss of friendly bacteria, damage to the lining of the gastrointestinal tract by drugs, alcohol, stress, parasites, food allergies, celiac disease (wheat intolerance), or other gut problems.

TIME: Response should start within a few days to one week depending on severity of deficiency and symptoms.

Alternative Treatments

Refer to alternative therapy chapters for more information before evaluating or applying any treatment. Some conditions, including yours, may require a physician's care.

DIET: Eat foods rich in thiamin and other B vitamins such as brown rice, whole grains, raw fruits and vegetables, especially green leafy vegetables, legumes, seeds, nuts, and yogurt. Drinking excessive liquids (more than one glass) with meals may wash out thiamin and other B vitamins. Avoid raw fish.

NUTRITIONAL THERAPY: *Mild deficiency:* • Thiamin (30 mg a day in divided doses) *Severe:* Thiamin (30-100 mg per day in divided doses) •Vitamin B complex • Multivitamin and mineral complex •Vitamin C

With severe cardiac and mental symptoms such as in cardiovascular beriberi or Wernicke-Korsakoff syndrome (marked reduction of blood flow to the head with dramatic symptoms), B₁ needs to be given by injection, 50-100 mg two times daily.

Self-Care

The following therapies can be undertaken at home under appropriate professional supervision.

FLOWER ESSENCES: Rescue Remedy® for generalized stress (four drops in a half-glass of water). Sip frequently, then repeat. Single flower essences are helpful to ease emotional discomfort and stress from physical condition.

HOMEOPATHY: *Sulfur*

Professional Care

The following therapies should only be provided by a qualified health professional.

Naturopathic Medicine / Orthomolecular Medicine / Traditional Chinese Medicine

BLOOD CLOTS

Clots (thrombi) of blood formed inside major blood vessels, which are the major cause of many heart attacks, strokes, and other cardiovascular disorders.

SYMPTOMS: Usually none.

SPECIAL NOTES: Blood solidification, or clotting, usually occurs as a healthy response within minutes after the skin is cut or there is trauma that causes bleeding. A clot helps seal the damage. However, blood clotting can be dangerous if it is inside healthy blood vessels. Unhealthy clotting can occur from platelets that get "activated" to clump together. This occurs when platelets come in contact with damaged arterial walls (see Heart Disease chapter) or due to nutrient deficiencies, poor dietary habits, or genetics. Once platelets get sticky, their shape changes and they easily mesh or clump together, causing a clot. Another factor is the production of fibrin, which helps bind the clump of platelets together. Fibrin is the end product of a cascade of coagulation (clumping) factors that occurs with the activation of just one molecule, which can lead to the explosion of up to 30,000 molecules of fibrin at the site of injury on the arterial wall.

Factors that may cause a buildup of platelet stickiness and fibrin are: birth control pills, late stages of pregnancy, nutrient deficiencies, smoking, free radicals (inadequate antioxidant nutrients), a high-cholesterol diet, low essential fatty acids, genetics, a diet high in saturated fat and low in vegetables and fish, and liver disease.

Some doctors and medical researchers have found that prolonged sitting on long airline flights, especially in cramped conditions, puts a person at risk for developing pulmonary thrombosis.[12] Blood clots forming in the legs or another part of the body break loose and then block one of the arteries to the lungs. Some practical preventive measures include: getting up and walking the aisle every hour, wearing loose, comfortable clothing, periodically stretching the legs and tightening and loosening the muscles of the abdomen and buttocks, and taking some slow, deep breaths.

In studies done at Duke University, Salvatore V. Pizzo, M.D., showed that moderate exercise may help protect against heart attacks and strokes by enhancing the body's natural mechanism for dissolving blood clots. In addition, Dr. Pizzo found that the higher risk of blood clotting in women taking oral contraceptives can be significantly reduced by exercise.[13]

Alternative Treatments

Refer to alternative therapy chapters for more information before evaluating or applying any treatment. Some conditions, including yours, may require a physician's care.

DIET: Foods that act to decrease platelet stickiness and fibrin formation are garlic, ginger, onions, and hot peppers (capsicum), which protect against heart attack and stroke. Use granulated garlic on food as a regular spice. Fish oils help to reduce clotting of blood. Increase consumption of cold-water fish to at least three times per week.

Decrease sucrose consumption as sugar intake increases platelet stickiness.[14]

NUTRITIONAL THERAPY: • Vitamin B$_6$ • Garlic capsules • Niacin (vitamin B$_3$) • Lipotropic factors (nutrients useful for liver metabolism of fat) • Omega-3 and omega-6 fatty acids • Bromelain • Vitamin E may be useful in helping to dissolve blood clots • Vitamin C • Zinc • Magnesium • Manganese

If you are on aspirin as daily preventive therapy, you may want to begin a gut rejuvenation program to stimulate healing and proper gastrointestinal wall functioning, in order to offset aspirin's traumatization of the gut wall when taken on daily basis. It is a good idea to do a bowel cleanse and rejuvenation several times a year when on daily aspirin (consult your physician for guidance).

Self-Care

The following therapies can be undertaken at home under appropriate professional supervision.

Fasting

HERBS: Hawthorn berry

HOMEOPATHY: *Hamamelis*

HYDROTHERAPY: Contrast application (apply several times daily).

JUICE THERAPY: Garlic, carrot, parsley, spinach, celery, beet

Professional Care

The following therapies should only be provided by a qualified health professional.

Environmental Medicine / Osteopathic Medicine / Naturopathic Medicine

OXYGEN THERAPIES: • Ozone autohemotherapy (treatment by reinjection of the individual's own blood) • Hydrogen peroxide therapy (IV).

BODY ODOR

The most common cause of unpleasant smells coming off the body is poor hygiene and uncleanliness. Sweat has no odor but, if left on the skin for a few hours, bacteria decompose the sweat and can cause odor. The next most common cause is sweat containing a high level of garlic, curry, or other spicy food. However, when a person is very healthy, usually the foods can be eaten without lasting odor effects. The other causes for body odor that are not often appreciated are nutrient deficiencies (usually zinc), underlying health problems (usually liver disease or diabetes), or gastrointestinal problems (such as parasites or chronic constipation).

CONSIDER: Recommendation is to wash effectively once a day. Feet are most affected due to warm, airless environment, so check condition of feet and shoes. Consider

excessive caffeine consumption or emotional stress, which can influence body odors.

SPECIAL NOTES: The more wholesome the diet and the balance of nutrient biochemistry in the body, the less there are unpleasant odors emanating from the body.

Alternative Treatments

Refer to alternative therapy chapters for more information before evaluating or applying any treatment. Some conditions, including yours, may require a physician's care.

DIET: Whole foods diet with at least ⅓ to ½ raw foods. Increase fluids and pure water (seven to eight glasses per day). On rising and before bedtime, one glass of water with the juice of a fresh lemon and one teaspoon of chlorophyll.

NUTRITIONAL THERAPY: • Bowel cleanse and rejuvenation program several times a year • Vitamin B$_1$ (50 mg two times daily while problem exists and then 20–30 mg one time daily several times a week for one year) • Vitamin B complex • If not on a gut rejuvenation program, take vitamin A (25,000 IU daily for a few weeks) • Vitamin C (increase amount and frequency under periods of stress) • Vitamin B$_6$ (pyridoxine) • Chlorophyll • Magnesium • Zinc • PABA (para-aminobenzoic acid) • Liver glandulars and liver cleanse may be helpful.

Self-Care

The following therapies can be undertaken at home under appropriate professional supervision.

Fasting

AROMATHERAPY: Sage

FLOWER ESSENCES: Flower essences for negative feelings surrounding the problem, such as Crab Apple for low self-esteem, negative body image, or feeling toxic.

JUICE THERAPY: Fresh vegetable juices

HOMEOPATHY: *Hepar sulph., Sulfur*

HYDROTHERAPY: Immersion bath, wet sheet pack, or steam/sauna. Apply daily to produce sweating and elimination.

NATUROPATHIC MEDICINE: Leon Chaitow, N.D., D.O., suggests skin brushing daily—a natural bristle brush is gently used to scrub the skin of the entire body in gentle circular motions to encourage removal of dead skin, improved local circulation, elimination through the skin, and enhanced skin function generally. This should ideally be followed by a bath in which essential oils are used.

TOPICAL TREATMENT: Apply baking soda under arms and between toes. Avoid aluminum-based antiperspirants.

Professional Care

The following therapies should only be provided by a qualified health professional.

Applied Kinesiology / Environmental Medicine / Naturopathic Medicine / Traditional Chinese Medicine

DETOXIFICATION THERAPY: Detoxification may be indicated, depending on the person's condition.

BOILS

A pus-filled, inflamed area of the skin that can occur anywhere on the body, usually at an infected hair follicle. Most common sites are low back, thighs, buttocks, back of neck, and armpits. The infection is usually due to the bacteria Staphylococcus aureus.

SYMPTOMS: Starts as a very painful, slightly red bump. It then becomes more swollen, more painful, redder, filled with pus, gets a yellowish-white tip, and will keep draining or causing pain until the "core," a sac surrounding the pus, is expelled.

SPECIAL NOTES: Recurrent boils may occur in people with decreased immune function, diabetes, chronic gastrointestinal problems, underactive thyroid, lowered resistance due to borderline nutrient deficiencies, and chronic emotional stress. Bursting a boil can spread it, leaves scars, and does no good until the core is expelled.

Alternative Treatments

Refer to alternative therapy chapters for more information before evaluating or applying any treatment. Some conditions, including yours, may require a physician's care.

DIET: Lots of green, orange, and yellow vegetables, which are cleansing (try to have at least four different types of vegetables a day, keep this up for at least six months). Increase fluids, drink water throughout the day, and drink water with juice of fresh lemon and one teaspoon of chlorophyll on rising and before bed. A cleansing fast may be helpful in some people but not others, especially if the immune system is not fortified afterward. Check for nutritional deficiencies, particularly overconsumption of white sugar and white flour products.

A drink made by mixing greens (parsley, spinach, celery) in a blender with pineapple juice may be used to help purify the blood. According to Leon Chaitow, N.D., D.O., fresh or bottled beet root juice is traditionally used in Europe as a blood purifying drink.

NUTRITIONAL THERAPY: • Garlic capsules • Chlorophyll • Proteolytic (pancreatic) enzymes taken on empty stomach two to three times daily away from meals • Vitamin E emulsion • Coenzyme Q10 • Raw thymus glandular • Kelp • Zinc • Beta carotene • Vitamin A

Emphasize the role of building up the immune system and liver functioning, and in reducing chronic emotional stress, in the case of chronic boils. Thus, consider thymus glandular, vitamin B5 (1 g four times daily), vitamin C (1 g every hour), adrenal glandulars, blueberry leaf tea, liver programs, and bowel programs.

TOPICAL TREATMENT: Direct application of mixture of honey, oil from vitamins E and A, and some zinc oxide, several times a day up to once per hour, may be helpful.

Self-Care

The following therapies can be undertaken at home under appropriate professional supervision.

Fasting / Guided Imagery

AROMATHERAPY: Draw out the boil with bergamot, lavender, chamomile, clary sage.

AYURVEDA: To bring boil to a head, apply a poultice of cooked onions. Wrap in cloth and do not apply onion directly to boils. Application of a paste of ½ teaspoon each of turmeric and ginger powder directly to boil.

BODYWORK: Acupressure, reflexology, Shiatsu.

FLOWER ESSENCES: Rescue Remedy Cream® can be applied (minimum four times a day) on unbroken skin around, but not directly on, boils. Flower essences for negative feelings surrounding the problem, such as Rescue Remedy® to help alleviate stress or Crab Apple for low self-esteem, negative body image, and feeling toxic.

HERBS: A blend of the tinctures of echinacea, cleavers, and yellowdock in equal parts, one teaspoon three times a day. Additionally, drink a cup of an infusion of nettle, preferably fresh herb, twice a day.

HOMEOPATHY: *Bellis, Belladonna, Hepar sulph., Arnica, Silicea, Apis mel., Arsen alb., Lachesis • Phytolacca* must be taken alone, not in combination with other remedies.

HYDROTHERAPY: • Contrast application (apply daily) • Warm Epsom salts baths

JUICE THERAPY: • Wheat grass juice • Carrot, beet, and celery juice • Carrot, beet, and cucumber • Carrot, spinach • Carrot, lettuce, spinach and yellowdock (5%)

TOPICAL TREATMENT: • Poultice of goldenseal root powder paste • Hot Epsom salt pack (two tablespoons in one cup water) • Tea tree oil • One part sesame oil and one part lime juice mixed and applied externally.

Professional Care

The following therapies should only be provided by a qualified health professional.

Environmental Medicine / Magnetic Field Therapy / Naturopathic Medicine / Osteopathic Medicine / Traditional Chinese Medicine

DETOXIFICATION THERAPY: Detoxification is indicated after controlling the infection.

OXYGEN THERAPIES: • Ozone autohemotherapy (treatment by reinjection of the individual's own blood) • Hydrogen peroxide therapy (IV).

BRUISES

A darkish black and blue mark on the skin, usually formed without a cut, due to blood that leaks out of capillaries, generally after an injury, and collects just beneath the surface of the skin.

SYMPTOMS: First discolorations are black and blue. Then, when the hemoglobin of the blood breaks down, the color turns to yellow. Often associated with some swelling and surrounding redness of the tissues.

OCCURRENCE: More common in children from accidents. More frequently in women than men, may be due to estrogen demands of vitamin C on the body.

SPECIAL NOTES: Bruises that do not fade after a week, or are recurrent without cause, may be signs of bleeding disorders or vitamin C and bioflavonoid deficiencies, or signs of underlying stresses on the body that continually deplete the vitamin C stores. See a physician.

Alternative Treatments

Refer to alternative therapy chapters for more information before evaluating or applying any treatment. Some conditions, including yours, may require a physician's care.

DIET: Whole foods diet with emphasis on foods rich in vitamin C and bioflavonoids such as fresh fruits, green leafy vegetables, and buckwheat.

NUTRITIONAL THERAPY: •Vitamin C with bioflavonoids and rutin • Alfalfa tablets •Vitamin B6 • Folic acid •Vitamin E • Iron

Nutritional biochemist Jeffrey Bland, Ph.D., reports that higher doses of some bioflavonoids (especially rutin) increase blood vessel elasticity and so help to prevent rupturing of small blood vessels and easy bruising. When the bruises are not responsive to high dosages of vitamin C, increase the bioflavonoids to 2 g several times a day along with adrenal support (pantothenic acid up to 3-4 g per day, adrenal glandulars, blueberry leaf tea).

Self–Care

The following therapies can be undertaken at home under appropriate professional supervision.

Fasting / Guided Imagery

AROMATHERAPY: • Camphor, fennel, hyssop, lavender • Put a few drops of lavender oil on gauze compress and place on bruise.

FLOWER ESSENCES: Rescue Remedy Cream® can be applied on bruises (minimum four times a day).

HERBS: • Liberal applications of arnica salve on the effected area. Alternatively, application of a compress made with oil of hyssop or a mixture of turmeric and honey to bruise. • See Herbal Medicine chapter for the use of St. John's wort for bruises.

HOMEOPATHY: • *Arnica, Ruta grav., Hypericum, Hamamelis, Symphytum.* Do not apply *Arnica* cream to open wounds.

HYDROTHERAPY: Contrast application, apply several times daily as needed.

JUICE THERAPY: Carrot, beet, high-bioflavonoid sources

TOPICAL TREATMENT: • Mashed yerba santa leaves soaked in hot water, applied to the bruise and covered with a clean cloth. • Compress of chilled infusion of comfrey or sage. Remove when dry and apply comfrey ointment or calendula ointment. • Apply slice of raw onion to

bruise. • Witch hazel—Soak one ounce of witch hazel leaves and twigs in two cups of 151-proof alcohol for two weeks. Shake the mixture daily. Strain and use directly on bruise. (Or use commercial witch hazel solution.)

Leon Chaitow, N.D., D.O., suggests hot and cold applications (ring out towels in appropriate temperature water) applied locally in a sequence of 20 seconds hot, then ten seconds cold, for several minutes every hour to reduce the congestion of bruising. The sooner after the injury this is done, the better.

Professional Care

The following therapies should only be provided by a qualified health professional.

Applied Kinesiology / Environmental Medicine / Naturopathic Medicine / Traditional Chinese Medicine / Orthomolecular Medicine / Osteopathic Medicine

OXYGEN THERAPY: Hyperbaric oxygen therapy may be useful for extensive bruising (crash injuries).

BULIMIA

An eating disorder characterized by bouts of extreme overeating (bingeing) followed by self-induced vomiting. Often, but not always, associated with anorexia, in which bingeing and dieting are both carried out to extremes.

SYMPTOMS: Bulimics may be thin, normal, or slightly underweight. If anorexia is part of the eating disorder, there will be extreme loss of body weight. Bingeing and vomiting may occur several times a day, after most meals, or less frequently. Gastric symptoms, loss of menstruation, swollen face and neck especially after coming out of bathroom after eating meals, fatigue, dizziness, irritability, poor cold tolerance, severe food cravings, excessive exercise habits, poor stress coping skills, depression, and even suicidal tendencies may manifest. Vomiting exposes the teeth to gastric juice and there may be dental erosion. Using the hand to force vomiting may cause calluses on the back of the hands where the skin hits the teeth during the procedure.

OCCURRENCE: This disorder is often performed in secret, so that the rate of occurrence is not fully established. However, it is much more prevalent in women between the ages of 12 and 30.

CONSIDER: Nutrient deficiencies (especially zinc), food allergies, amino acid imbalances.

SPECIAL NOTES: In both anorexia nervosa and bulimia nervosa, the underlying causative factors believed to be solely due to an obsession with body fat, a fear of being (or becoming) fat, or overconcern with perfectionism. Although all of these factors are important, recent studies also show that in most cases, an underlying zinc deficiency may contribute to the disorder.

Alternative Treatments

Refer to alternative therapy chapters for more information before evaluating or applying any treatment. Some conditions, including yours, may require a physician's care.

DIET: A whole foods diet with regular eating patterns is paramount. Avoid all products containing sugar and white flour. Identification and avoidance of allergenic foods. Sufficient protein sources to adequately nourish the body.

NUTRITIONAL THERAPY: Liquid ionic multimineral complex and multivitamin complex supplements help overcome the extreme vitamin and mineral deficiencies associated with binge and purge eating and overuse of laxatives. Complex amino acids assist in balancing blood sugar levels, which helps reduce food cravings.

Self-Care

The following therapies can be undertaken at home under appropriate professional supervision.

Qigong and Tai Chi

FLOWER ESSENCES: Various essences to address underlying emotional and mental states of imbalance and negativity such as fears, perfectionism, manipulative behavior, depression, and anxiety. Crab Apple for obsessive habits relating to body image.

HOMEOPATHY: *Calc carb., Ipecac., Graphites*

HYDROTHERAPY: Constitutional hydrotherapy (apply two to five times weekly).

NATUROPATHIC MEDICINE: When associated with anorexia, bulimia seems to respond well to supplemental zinc.

Professional Care

The following therapies should only be provided by a qualified health professional.

Biofeedback Training and Neurotherapy / Hypnotherapy / Light Therapy / Natural Hormone Replacement Therapy / Naturopathic Medicine / Traditional Chinese Medicine

BUNIONS

Enlarged area of the inner part of the big toe associated with a fluid-filled pad (bursa) underneath the often hardened outer skin. This is caused by a swelling of the bursa of the metatarsophalangeal joint (joining toe to foot) of the big toe, which forces the toe to point inward as the joint itself protrudes outward.

SYMPTOMS: Large toe moves inward. Can become inflamed and create mild to extreme pain.

OCCURRENCE: More frequently in women from wearing pointed and tight-fitting shoes. According to Jonathan Wright, M.D., bunions are often hereditary.

SPECIAL NOTES: Bunions need to be treated or will get worse. Mild bunions can be treated mechanically, though larger ones may require surgery.

Alternative Treatments

Refer to alternative therapy chapters for more information before evaluating or applying any treatment. Some conditions, including yours, may require a physician's care.

NUTRITIONAL THERAPY: • DL-phenylalanine • Niacinamide • Magnesium • This is palliative, may improve symptoms of pain and inflammation, but is not curative and will not get rid of the causes. Thus, these need to be taken on a regular basis several times per day to keep blood levels elevated; improvement usually takes up to one month and will subside a short time after these nutrients are no longer taken.

Self-Care

The following therapies can be undertaken at home under appropriate professional supervision.

HERBS: Aloe vera juice, parsley tea, calendula

HINTS: Walk barefoot whenever possible. Exercise foot, rolling back and forth, from heel to toe, over a bottle.

HOMEOPATHY: • *Ruta grav., Silicea, Arnica* • *Benz ac.* must be taken alone, not in combination with other remedies.

HYDROTHERAPY: • Contrast application (apply daily) • Hot Epsom salts foot baths; to aid circulation use a whirlpool bath.

REFLEXOLOGY: Work around and directly on bunion.

TOPICAL TREATMENT: Apply aloe vera gel.

Professional Care

The following therapies should only be provided by a qualified health professional.

Acupuncture / Chiropractic / Magnetic Field Therapy / Naturopathic Medicine / Osteopathic Medicine / Prolotherapy

BODYWORK: • Alexander Technique • Foot massage • Manipulation of joint of big toe

According to Leon Chaitow, N.D., D.O., to correct or improve a bunion, structural and functional correction is needed of the postural and mechanical (weight-bearing) factors that led to its development. Fallen arches, postural muscle imbalance in the legs and pelvic area, problems involving low back and pelvic joint mechanics, as well as habits of use (running, walking, and standing postures relating to work, sport, and general function) all need attention from skilled practitioners using manipulation and rehabilitation methods, including physical therapists, chiropractors, and osteopaths.

BURNS

Heating of the skin, anything over 120° F, so that damage occurs.

SYMPTOMS: *First degree burns:* Skin reddens, as only the top layer of the skin (epidermis) is affected. Skin may peel away in several days and heals quickly. *Second degree burns:* Blisters are created due to damage to the deeper layer of the skin. Usually heal without scarring. *Third degree burns:* The full thickness of the skin is damaged by the heat. Area looks charred or white, and tissues below (bones and muscles) may be exposed. Requires burn specialist to treat properly.

SPECIAL NOTES: Immediately run cold water over the burn. According to Leon Chaitow, N.D., D.O., if possible and practical, run cold water over the area for as long as possible (hours if necessary); cover. This will also help prevent blisters.

On second degree burns place mixture of baking soda, olive oil, zinc ointment, and pure vitamin E to promote healing and prevent scarring. Do not break blisters. Elevate area of burn higher than heart, if possible, to alleviate swelling. To remove substances melted on skin such as plastic or tar, use ice-cold water.

Copper and zinc are lost through wound seepage. Loss of these minerals may significantly increase the need for supplementation during burns.

Alternative Treatments

Refer to alternative therapy chapters for more information before evaluating or applying any treatment. Some conditions, including yours, may require a physician's care.

DIET: High-protein diet for second and third degree burns to promote repair of damaged tissue. Increase intake of fluids. Increase high-zinc foods such as pumpkin seeds and oysters.

NUTRITIONAL THERAPY: • Vitamin E • Vitamin C with bioflavonoids • Zinc • Protein supplement (free-form amino acids) • Vitamin A • Vitamin B complex • Pantothenic acid (B5) • Spray burned area with vitamin C solution • Vitamin E can have a dramatic effect on burns of all kinds: fire, chemical, electrical, and sunburn. • Apply 100% solution of dimethylsulfoxide (DMSO) to minimize scarring and prevent loss of skin.

Self–Care

The following therapies can be undertaken at home under appropriate professional supervision.

Fasting / Guided Imagery

AROMATHERAPY: • Lavender, geranium, camphor • To prevent blistering, apply two to three drops of lavender oil. The discovery of the healing properties of lavender oil on burns was actually the basis for research into and development of the field of aromatherapy by French chemist René-Maurice Gattefossé (see Aromatherapy chapter).

AYURVEDA: Application of a paste made of fresh aloe vera gel or plain ghee, coconut oil, licorice ghee, or tikta ghee.

FLOWER ESSENCES: Rescue Remedy Cream® can be applied (minimum four times a day) on unbroken skin above burn or on healthy skin surrounding—but not on top of—an open wound resulting from burn. Rescue

Remedy® liquid can be used to calm the stressful feelings due to the burn. • Other essences to address negative thoughts and feelings surrounding injury.

HERBS: If a mild burn, apply a poultice, salve, or juice of plantain to the burn. Cool aloe vera gel may also be applied. Severe burns require immediate professional attention. For sunburn, cool aloe vera gel applied liberally to the burnt area may be helpful. If badly burned, a salve made with St. John's wort and calendula flowers may be helpful.

HOMEOPATHY: First degree: *Calendula, Hypericum, Arnica* (for shock), *Urtica urens, Belladonna.* Second degree: *Arnica* (for shock), *Cantharis, Belladonna.* Third degree: consult a physician. Sunburn: *Nat mur.* (as a preventative), *Urtica urens, Rhus tox.*

HYDROTHERAPY: Cold compress (apply immediately and as needed to control pain).

JUICE THERAPY: Carrot, cantaloupe, currants (add garlic to juice).

NATUROPATHIC MEDICINE: Gel from the freshly cut aloe vera leaf.

TOPICAL TREATMENT: Ice and vinegar

Professional Care

The following therapies should only be provided by a qualified health professional.

Cell Therapy / Light Therapy / Naturopathic Medicine / Orthomolecular Medicine

SPECIAL NOTES: Studies indicate up to 95% of burned tissue can be healed with minimal scarring using negative ion therapy. This method is also greatly helpful for pain reduction.[15]

MAGNETIC FIELD THERAPY: Magnetic treatments pioneered in the former Soviet Union have been demonstrated to be effective in healing burns.[16]

OXYGEN THERAPY: • Hydrogen peroxide therapy (IV) • Hyperbaric oxygen therapy • Ozone therapy: In infected burns, especially if not too extensive and relatively dry, ozone therapy has healing value. In wet burns, too much ozone may be absorbed.

TRADITIONAL CHINESE MEDICINE: A salve made with Lithospermum root *(zi cao)* and black sesame oil has been used for burns. Ginger juice has been applied fresh topically in traditional Chinese medicine.

BURSITIS

Inflammation of bursa, sac-like cavities filled with lubricating (synovial) fluid, at areas where friction is likely to occur, such as where muscles or tendons pass over bony places. Inflammation may be acute or chronic.

SYMPTOMS: Localized pain and tenderness, sometimes swelling and redness, may be associated with loss of normal range of motion of that joint, and sometimes becomes reddish colored and warm.

CONSIDER: Trauma, malposition of specific joint or joints above and below, chronic overuse, acute or chronic infection, calcium deposits secondary to calcium malabsorption, magnesium deficiency, localized trauma, allergies (especially airborne or food), vitamin B12 malabsorption, inflammatory arthritis, gout, rheumatoid arthritis, infective organisms (especially *Staphylococcus aureus*), and, rarely, tuberculosis organisms.

SPECIAL NOTES: Most commonly affected joints are shoulder, elbow, and hip, which are often referred to as "frozen" due to the loss of normal range of motion.

TIME: Improvement should start within ten days and not take longer than two months. Splinting and rest are helpful for acute bouts but much less for chronic.

Alternative Treatments

Refer to alternative therapy chapters for more information before evaluating or applying any treatment. Some conditions, including yours, may require a physician's care.

DIET: Identify and avoid food allergies. Eat foods high in magnesium: dark leafy green and many different green and yellow vegetables. Drink filtered water, apple cider vinegar, and honey on rising, before bed, and several times throughout the day. Avoid foods from the nightshade family: tomatoes, potatoes, eggplant. Take one tablespoon cod liver oil one to two hours before meals.

NUTRITIONAL THERAPY: • Vitamin B12 (intra-muscular injection) repeated on a daily basis • Calcium • Magnesium • Proteolytic enzymes between meals • Vitamin C and bioflavonoids

Self-Care

The following therapies can be undertaken at home under appropriate professional supervision.

Fasting / Guided Imagery

AROMATHERAPY: Juniper, chamomile, cypress

FLOWER ESSENCES: Rescue Remedy Cream® can be applied (minimum four times a day).

HERBS: Combine the tinctures of meadowsweet, horsetail, and willow bark in equal parts and take one teaspoon three times a day. Topically, gently rub into the affected area a mixture of equal parts tincture of lobelia and cramp bark. Drink strong chamomile tea, particularly at bedtime, to help relieve pain. Aloe vera gel may be helpful.

HOMEOPATHY: *Belladonna, Arnica, Ruta grav., Silicea*

HYDROTHERAPY: • Contrast application (apply one to three times daily). If acute, use an ice pack apply 20 minutes out of each hour for the first 24–36 hours. According to Leon Chaitow, N.D., D.O., any hot treatment (or bath) should finish with the area being chilled by a compress or spray (shower). • Baths using a pound or more of Epsom salts per bath. Soak for 25–30 minutes. Rinse and rub down with hot olive oil. Do once a week. • Also, try rosemary soaks for hands and feet or a bath for the whole body. Soak for 10–15 minutes, two to three times

a day. • Ice packs: Place one above and one below the joint for 20 minutes three times a day for one month (six ice cubes to a quart of cold water, or mix two-thirds water and one-third alcohol and freeze until slushy).

JUICE THERAPY: Equal parts carrot, celery, cucumber, beet.

LIFESTYLE: At the onset of inflammation, rest the affected area for a few days. Otherwise the problem may last for weeks.

REFLEXOLOGY: Reflex to affected area, adrenals, referral area to affected part.

TOPICAL TREATMENT: Mullein hot packs—boil three to four fresh mullein leaves in water for three minutes. Place over joint. Wrap with hot moist towel, then dry towel. Leave for 20 minutes three times a day.

Professional Care

The following therapies should only be provided by a qualified health professional.

Acupuncture / Applied Kinesiology / Chiropractic / Craniosacral Therapy / Environmental Medicine / Magnetic Field Therapy / Naturopathic Medicine / Neural Therapy / Osteopathic Medicine / Prolotherapy / Traditional Chinese Medicine

BODYWORK: Reflexology, acupressure, Feldenkrais, Rolfing.

DETOXIFICATION THERAPY: Detoxification may be indicated, depending on the condition of the person.

OXYGEN THERAPY: • Hydrogen peroxide therapy (IV) • Hyperbaric oxygen therapy.

ULTRASOUND: To break up calcium deposits and adhesions.

ENERGY MEDICINE: Electro-Acuscope, Light Beam Generator

LIGHT THERAPY: Cold (soft) laser photo stimulation therapy.

CANKER SORES

Painful ulcers on the mucous membrane surface of the mouth, cheek, or tongue that occur singly or in groups.

SYMPTOMS: *Mild:* Less than one centimeter in diameter, last ten days to two weeks, and heal without scarring. *Severe:* More than one centimeter, last several weeks to several months, leave scarring. Recurring attacks are common with several to many ulcers. Ulcers have whitish centers surrounded by redness.

OCCURRENCE: Women more than men.

CONSIDER: Bowel flora imbalances due to parasites, poor digestion, food sensitivities, chronic constipation or diarrhea, Crohn's disease.

SPECIAL NOTES: Stress, extreme heat such as associated with physical exertion, hot weather, extreme fatigue, fever, localized trauma such as after dental work, and nutrient deficiencies such as lysine, iron, vitamin B12, and folic acid. These may be contagious if they result from an infectious agent.

Alternative Treatments

Refer to alternative therapy chapters for more information before evaluating or applying any treatment. Some conditions, including yours, may require a physician's care.

DIET: Vary grains and add a variety of beans, seeds, and nuts. Mono-wheat diets contribute to canker sores. Avoid foods and substances that may irritate the ulcers such as coffee, alcohol, refined sugar, citrus fruits, spicy foods, mouthwashes, and smoking. *Severe:* Cut down on acid-forming foods such as animal products, grains, beans, and seeds, in relation to amount of vegetables and fruits.

According to Leon Chaitow, N.D., D.O., some cases develop from food sensitivity, with the most common culprits being milk, cheese, wheat, tomato, vinegar, lemon, pineapple, and mustard.

NUTRITIONAL THERAPY: • Vitamin C • Lysine (4 g for first four days, then 500 mg three times daily, on an empty stomach and apart from meals) • Vitamin B complex (two to three daily with meals, along with folic acid and vitamin B12) • Iron • Zinc gluconate lozenges • Acidophilus • Pantothenic acid

Self-Care

The following therapies can be undertaken at home under appropriate professional supervision.

Fasting / Guided Imagery

FLOWER ESSENCES: Rescue Remedy® liquid to help alleviate stress related to condition.

HERBS: For symptomatic relief, use a mouthwash made with sage and chamomile. Combine equal amounts and then infuse. Use as a gargle as often as needed. Internally, take a combination of equal parts tincture of echinacea and cleavers, ½ teaspoon three times a day.

JUICE THERAPY: Carrot, celery, cantaloupe. Avoid high acid fruits (pineapple, citrus).

NATUROPATHIC MEDICINE: While many local therapies exist, naturopathic physicians believe that the basic cause is most likely an allergy to wheat and possibly other grains. Local relief of pain can be achieved using a paste made up of echinacea tincture and myrrh gum.

TOPICAL TREATMENT: Using a cotton swab, dab each sore with an 8% solution of zinc chloride (from your pharmacist).

Professional Care

The following therapies should only be provided by a qualified health professional.

Environmental Medicine / Magnetic Field Therapy / Naturopathic Medicine

TRADITIONAL CHINESE MEDICINE: Watermelon frost powder

DETOXIFICATION THERAPY: Detoxification may be indicated, depending on the condition of the person.

OXYGEN THERAPY: • Hydrogen peroxide therapy (IV) • Ozone therapy.

CARBUNCLES

A cluster of interconnecting boils with the infection spreading underneath the skin. Great amount of pus, slow healing, and often associated with scarring (see Boils). Infective organism is usually Staphylococcus aureus.

SYMPTOMS: These develop more slowly than boils, are localized over a larger area, are extremely painful, swollen, and red, and may be accompanied by general feelings of fatigue, debilitation, and fever.

OCCURRENCE: More frequently in men, at the nape of the neck, buttocks, or thighs. Even though they can occur in very healthy people, they are often associated with diseases that are debilitating, diabetes mellitus, and found in the elderly. Carbuncles are very contagious.

SPECIAL NOTES: Carbuncles should be cultured to identify the infective organism and antibiotics used if needed. Carbuncles or boils in the nose require antibiotics as the infection can easily spread to the brain.

Alternative Treatments

Refer to alternative therapy chapters for more information before evaluating or applying any treatment. Some conditions, including yours, may require a physician's care.

DIET: Drink plenty of filtered water. Whole foods with lots of green, leafy vegetables, and grains such as buckwheat. (See Boils.)

NUTRITIONAL THERAPY: • Vitamin A • Vitamin C • Chlorophyll • Garlic • Proteolytic enzymes (on an empty stomach away from meals) • Acidophilus (see Boils.)

Self-Care

The following therapies can be undertaken at home under appropriate professional supervision.

Fasting / Guided Imagery

FLOWER ESSENCES: Rescue Remedy Cream® can be applied (minimum four times a day) on unbroken skin around, but not directly on, carbuncles. Flower Essences for negative feelings surrounding the problem, such as Rescue Remedy® to help alleviate stress or Crab Apple for low self-esteem, negative body image, and feeling toxic.

HERBS: Refer to section on boils.

HOMEOPATHY: *Ledum, Belladonna, Arsen alb., Lachesis.*

HYDROTHERAPY: Contrast application (apply daily).

JUICE THERAPY: • Carrot, beet, and celery juice, garlic • Wheat grass juice • Cucumber

TOPICAL TREATMENT: Refer to section on boils.

Professional Care

The following therapies should only be provided by a qualified health professional.

Magnetic Field Therapy / Naturopathic Medicine / Osteopathic Medicine / Traditional Chinese Medicine

DETOXIFICATION THERAPY: May be indicated, depending on the condition of the person.

OXYGEN THERAPY: External ozone/oxygen applications.

CARPAL TUNNEL SYNDROME

Compression of a nerve (median) in the wrist that produces numbness, tingling, and sometimes pain. Weakness and tingling of the first three fingers and thumb may also occur.

SYMPTOMS: Tingling of palm surface of hands, first three fingers, often worse at night or with driving. Can also be associated with tingling, burning, and pain of entire arm, neck and hip, and thigh. May be on one or both sides.

OCCURRENCE: More common in women after the age of 35.

CONSIDER: Conditions that can create swelling or fluid shifts (contribute to pressure on nerve) such as pregnancy, low thyroid, occupations that require forceful or repetitive wrist movements, vitamin B6 deficiencies, nerve disorders, or compression of the nerve root of the sixth cervical vertebra due to misalignment of the neck, muscular spasm, osteoarthritis, disk disease, or tumor. May be secondary to other wrist conditions.

SPECIAL NOTES: Treatment varies, symptoms may improve in one week or take several months. Often carpal tunnel can be successfully treated without surgery, although sometimes surgery is necessary. According to Steven Bailey, N.D., of Portland, Oregon, carpal tunnel is often a misdiagnosis of thoracic outlet compression syndrome, in which pressure to lower cervical and upper thoracic nerves results in dysfunction of the tissues and nerves associated with the brachial nerves.

Alternative Treatments

Refer to alternative therapy chapters for more information before evaluating or applying any treatment. Some conditions, including yours, may require a physician's care.

DIET: Whole foods diet. Limit protein intake. Eliminate foods high in yellow dyes. Good foods to focus on are whole grains, seeds, and nuts, soybeans, fresh salmon, brewer's yeast, molasses, liver, wheat bran and germ, and cod. Avoid stressor foods that deplete the body's level of B6 such as excessive consumption of sugars, caffeine, and processed grains and corn.

NUTRITIONAL THERAPY: • Vitamin B6 • Vitamin B complex • Magnesium • Essential fatty acids • Folic acid • Bromelain • Coenzyme Q10 • Kelp • Manganese • Pro-

tease enzyme formula • Pycnogenol • Zinc • Thyroid hormone

People with carpal tunnel syndrome often have a large deficiency of vitamin B6, or have lifestyle factors that inhibit B6 metabolism such as stress, or ingesting Yellow Dye No. 5 and tartrazine derivatives. It may also be that a deficiency of B6 (pyridoxine) may cause a pyridoxine-responsive neuropathy (nerve disorder). Treatment with B6 may relieve the symptoms in many cases, eliminating the need for surgery. Daily dosage ranges from 25-300 mg, depending on the person's biochemistry. Caution: Pyridoxine supplementation may create a nerve disorder (sensory neuropathy) in dosages as low as 300 mg, if taken daily for long periods. Most of the cases of vitamin B6 toxicity have been reported with dosages from 2-5 g per day.

Self-Care

The following therapies can be undertaken at home under appropriate professional supervision.

Biofeedback Training and Neurotherapy / Fasting / Qigong and Tai Chi

ACUPRESSURE: To relieve carpal tunnel wrist pain, firmly press P6 and TW5 (for an illustration of these points, see the acupressure chart in the introduction to this section) on the affected hand for two minutes. Position the fingertips between the bones of the forearm, two fingerwidths below the wrist crease. Grasp these points firmly to strengthen the wrist joint and relieve the carpal tunnel pain. Repeat three times daily for a month.

AROMATHERAPY: Marjoram, lavender, eucalyptus

FLOWER ESSENCES: Rescue Remedy® to help alleviate stress.

HERBS: Anti-inflammatory herbs effectively support the broader treatment. A simple approach involves combining equal parts of meadowsweet and willow bark tinctures and taking one teaspoon of this mixture three times a day. Other useful herbs include aloe vera, butcher's broom, corn silk, devil's claw, cayenne (capsicum), ginkgo, gravel root, marshmallow, skullcap, turmeric (curcumin), wintergreen oil, yarrow, yucca.

HOMEOPATHY: *Aconite, Arsen alb., Ignatia, Nat mur., Chamomilla, Colchicum.* Homeopathic treatment tends to be constitutional in nature and is therefore normally long-term, but usually successful.

HYDROTHERAPY: Contrast application (apply one to three times daily).

LIFESTYLE: Avoid repetitive wrist movement. Monoamine oxidase inhibitor antidepressant drugs can create a deficiency in vitamin B6 and should be avoided if possible.

NATUROPATHIC MEDICINE: Vitamin B6 is believed to be highly effective, but patience is necessary—most people don't respond for at least six weeks.

Professional Care

The following therapies should only be provided by a qualified health professional.

Applied Kinesiology / Chiropractic / Craniosacral Therapy / Light Therapy / Naturopathic Medicine / Orthomolecular Medicine / Osteopathic Medicine / Prolotherapy

ACUPUNCTURE: Acupuncture treatments have proved effective in giving substantial relief from pain and discomfort.

BODYWORK: Acupressure, Feldenkrais Method, Hellerwork, Rolfing

DETOXIFICATION THERAPY: May be indicated, depending on the condition of the person.

ENERGY MEDICINE: • Electro-Acuscope • A recent study found that the TENS (Transcutaneous Electrical Nerve Stimulator) unit and low-level laser acupuncture significantly reduced pain in carpal tunnel syndrome.[17]

NEURAL THERAPY: According to Deitrich Klinghardt, M.D., many cases can be traced to interference fields in the arm, shoulders, or neck, often caused by vaccination scars. Dr. Klinghardt reports great success using neural therapy to alleviate the problem.

OXYGEN THERAPY: Hyperbaric oxygen therapy.

CELLULITE

This is really not a condition, but a lay term for unsightly looking dimples in various parts of the body, especially the thighs, knees, buttocks, stomach, and arms.

SYMPTOMS: Loose, dimpled skin.

OCCURRENCE: More frequently in women.

SPECIAL NOTES: In general, this condition is considered to be due to an increased ratio of fat cells to lean body mass. Based on this assumption, reducing body fat content and building up muscle mass is imperative. Spot reducing, aimed at fat reduction at specific body sites, is extremely difficult. Most experts say that it is not possible.

Cellulite is formed by fibroid masses of protein that have accumulated in the spaces between the cells due to faulty elimination through the lymph system. Some alternative practitioners have had success in the elimination of this condition using lymphatic therapy. Since gravity is the primary force that creates cellulite, the following exercise is beneficial: First, gently jump on a mini-trampoline or rebounder (if available) to create pumping action in the lymph system. Then, using gravity to drain the lymph system, place your legs up against a wall or over a chair and massage, very lightly, the crease formed by the legs and the abdomen in order to open the deep inguinal lymph nodes, which is where the accumulation that forms the cellulite must pass to be eliminated from the body.

Alternative Treatments

Refer to alternative therapy chapters for more information before evaluating or applying any treatment. Some conditions, including yours, may require a physician's care.

DIET: Whole foods diet with less complex carbohydrates and sugars than is usually recommended for the average person. Large amounts of filtered water. Decrease fats to below 20% of the total diet and avoid as much as possible animal fats and processed fats. Also, do not eat protein at night as unused protein in the body puts a greater load on the lymph system.

Self-Care

The following therapies can be undertaken at home under appropriate professional supervision.

Fasting / Hydrotherapy

AROMATHERAPY: Juniper, rosemary, lavender, lemon, geranium

BODYWORK: Self-massage—massage affected area regularly.

FLOWER ESSENCES: Crab Apple if negative body image, two drops four times a day, continued until restoration of positive body image.

HERBS: Combine equal parts of horse chestnut bark and gotu kola tinctures and take ½ teaspoon three times a day. Topically apply a compress made with white birch oil, morning and evening, or apply an ointment or lotion made from horse chestnut twice a day.

JUICE THERAPY: Beet, carrot

TOPICAL TREATMENT: Aloe vera extract

Professional Care

The following therapies should only be provided by a qualified health professional.

Magnetic Field Therapy / Natural Hormone Replacement Therapy / Naturopathic Medicine

DETOXIFICATION THERAPY: May be indicated, depending on the condition of the person.

ENERGY MEDICINE: Light Beam Generator.

CEREBRAL PALSY

A general classification for a number of congenital (present at birth) conditions that are lifelong and are characterized by impairment in voluntary muscular movements (motor handicaps). Cerebral palsy is incurable, but much can be done to optimize patients' capabilities, through lifelong and complex therapies and a variety of interventions.

SYMPTOMS: 70% of cases are spastic (abnormal stiffness of muscles). The spasticity may be mild or severe. Hemiplegia characterizes both limbs involved on one side; the arm is usually more severe. Paraplegia means both legs are involved and the arms may not be or may be very mildly involved. Quadriplegia means that all four limbs are involved to some degree. Affected limbs are usually poorly developed, sometimes rigid due to excessive muscle tone, weakness, with a tendency to spasm and contracture (severe spasm that may lead to bone deformity unless there is some intervention).

Sometimes the first symptoms are "floppy baby syndrome," where the baby's muscles have too little tone and the baby flops around when held. The parents may recognize that something "seems wrong," but are not sure exactly what it is.

SPECIAL NOTES: Diagnosis may take up to the second year due to moving through certain developmental patterns.

The Peto Institute, in Hungary and the United Kingdom, provides an intensive physical therapy and exercise program called conductive education, which has for 40 years treated children with cerebral palsy with sometimes dramatic success in terms of improved function and speech.

Alternative Treatments

Refer to alternative therapy chapters for more information before evaluating or applying any treatment. Some conditions, including yours, may require a physician's care.

DIET: Marshall Mandell, M.D., of Norwalk, Connecticut, reports that those with cerebral palsy may have sensitivities or allergies to certain foods or elements they breathe or come in contact with, which may cause an increased reaction or intensified symptoms. He refers to this as a sort of "hay fever of the brain" and explains how food is passed through the digestive tract into the bloodstream and eventually to the brain, where the allergy triggers exaggerated symptoms. In some patients he has identified intermittent, unpredictable flare-ups of allergies, aggravating what he calls "biological weak spots," areas that may have healed to a degree but are still supersensitive to outside irritation.

NUTRITIONAL THERAPY: Identification and avoidance of food allergies may improve muscle tone or decrease the higher percentage of health problems associated with this condition (usually due to decreased immune system functioning because of loss of normal range of movement and muscle tone). Certain nutrients may help muscle tone: magnesium, vitamins B_1, B_6, and C, and bioflavonoids.

Professional Care

The following therapies should only be provided by a qualified health professional.

Acupuncture / Biofeedback Training and Neurotherapy / Craniosacral Therapy / Fasting / Magnetic Field Therapy / Naturopathic Medicine / Traditional Chinese Medicine

BODYWORK: Reflexology, Feldenkrais Method, and Rolfing can be helpful with less severe cases.

ENVIRONMENTAL MEDICINE: Dr. Mandell has found that many cases of cerebral palsy are exacerbated by brain allergies. Treating the brain allergies can often stabilize and improve cerebral palsy.

OSTEOPATHY: According to Leon Chaitow, N.D., D.O., osteopathy is the first choice, but only if cranial osteopathy (craniosacral therapy) is used. Cranial osteopathy, if provided by a fully qualified practitioner within hours or days of birth, can prevent much of the subsequent damage caused by a difficult labor or forceps delivery (which may have caused cranial distortion impeding normal function of the brain and nervous system). In older infants, results will often be less dramatic, but nevertheless substantial.

OXYGEN THERAPY: • Hydrogen peroxide therapy (IV) • Hyperbaric oxygen therapy

VISION THERAPY: Vision therapy may improve cerebral palsy with prism therapy, in which prisms manipulate posture and perception to awaken and alter brain function.

CHEMICAL POISONING

(See Detoxification Therapy chapter.)
Overexposure to chemicals that have harmful effects on the body, such as damage to the liver.

SYMPTOMS: Can be anything from skin conditions, such as rashes and boils, to organ damage, such as kidney or liver failure.

OCCURRENCE: Most often occurs in the home from household chemicals or in people who are exposed to chemicals on the job.

SPECIAL NOTES: Poisons may enter from topical exposure to skin, breathing in poison, chronic poisoning from gradual exposure on the job, accidental poisoning in the home (most often young children who swallow prescription drugs or household chemicals), or by a suicide attempt.

Leon Chaitow, N.D., D.O., states that anyone living in an industrial, urban, or even rural setting is likely to be somewhat affected over the long term by toxicity from chemicals. He adds that there is now evidence that everyone on the planet carries (in fatty tissues) residues of dioxin and DDT, and that lead burdens are now 200 times that present in skeletal remains of people living 1,000 years ago—and rising. Everyone can benefit from reducing this load.

In severe, acute cases, seek emergency help.

Alternative Treatments

Refer to alternative therapy chapters for more information before evaluating or applying any treatment. Some conditions, including yours, may require a physician's care.

DIET: Eat organically grown foods as much as possible. Short, periodic fasts are recommended to reduce toxicity. Eat a high-fiber diet to help cleanse the system. Recommended foods include brown rice, beans, barley, lentils, oatmeal, beets, carrots, spinach, garlic, onions, almonds, brazil nuts, bananas, lemons, grapes, dates, yogurt, fish.

NUTRITIONAL THERAPY: • According to Jonathan Wright, M.D., in emergency situations, a very high dose of vitamin C and glutathione given intravenously can be helpful. • Vitamin B complex with choline and inositol • Vitamin C with bioflavonoids • Vitamin E • Superoxide dismutase (SOD) • Raw liver extract • Protein supplements (free-form amino acids) • Selenium • L-cysteine and L-methionine • Garlic capsules • Coenzyme Q10

Self-Care

The following therapies can be undertaken at home under appropriate professional supervision.

Fasting

FLOWER ESSENCES: Crab Apple for detoxification. Star of Bethlehem for emotional shock or trauma, if poisoning caused by accident.

HERBS: Herbs that help the regeneration of liver cells are helpful, combined with ones that facilitate elimination of waste from the body. Specific details depend upon the chemicals involved, but one general practice is to combine the tinctures of milk thistle, licorice, and dandelion leaf in equal parts and take one teaspoon of this mixture three times a day.

HYDROTHERAPY: The late Hazel Parcells, N.D., D.C., Ph.D., reported excellent success with the following bath for pesticide and carbon monoxide poisoning. Pesticides: one cup household bleach in a full bath of water as hot as you can comfortably bear. Stay in until it cools to body temperature. The therapeutic value is in the exchange of fluids between tissues. The heat brings the toxins to the surface. As it cools, the toxins are drawn out of the body and into the water. Carbon monoxide poisoning: Add five drops of household bleach to a glass of water. Saunas may also be effective in helping chemical poisoning. Dr. Chaitow suggests regular Epsom salt baths and skin brushing to encourage skin function.

W. Lee Cowden, M.D., recommends the following protocol (under a physician's care): essential fatty acids like flaxseed, canola, safflower, or sunflower oil (two to three tablespoons to as much as ⅛ cup); co-enzymated B complex; vitamin C plus lecithin. Take all immediately before a light exercise session or a light, dry sauna. Immediately after exercise or sauna, take a cool shower with a good quality soap. Dr. Cowden suggests that people who are very ill from the toxins should take homeopathic detoxification remedies and work into the exercise and sauna program very slowly.

NATUROPATHIC MEDICINE: In addition to the appropriate specific therapy to neutralize the chemical poison, the liver is treated to help it detoxify the chemical and minimize damage to the liver cells. Considerable research and clinical experience has shown that the herb *Silybum marianum* (milk thistle) is very effective in assisting the liver when exposed to chemical toxins.

Professional Care

The following therapies should only be provided by a qualified health professional.

Homeopathy / Naturopathic Medicine

OXYGEN THERAPY: • Hydrogen peroxide therapy (IV) • Hyperbaric oxygen therapy may be useful for cyanide, carbon monoxide, and smoke inhalation.

CHILLS

An attack of feeling very cold that results in shivering, chattering of teeth, and paleness.

CONSIDER: Poor cold tolerance, which means that one gets cold very easily and has difficulty getting and staying warm. This can be a sign of decreased health due to many conditions; most common are thyroid dysfunction, adrenal disorder, poor digestion, and chronic respiratory disorders. The most common first sign of nutrient deficiencies (especially the B vitamins) or borderline nutrient deficiencies is poor cold tolerance.

According to Leon Chaitow, N.D., D.O., people who are easily chilled can have their circulatory and temperature regulatory mechanisms normalized by a slow progressive exposure to cold over a period of six months. During this time the individual should, on a daily basis, start the day in a warm bathroom standing feet only (moving the feet up and down as if marching on the spot) in cold water for 10-20 seconds. Week by week this increases to the point where, after a month, the individual is standing up to the mid-calf for a minute or so in cold water. At this point, they should end the process by sitting in the water (up to the waist) for ten seconds. Progressively, the person should reach a point where they can, after some months, lie in the bath for several minutes each morning. By this time, the circulatory and heat control mechanisms will be trained and hardened and chills will be a thing of the past, says Dr. Chaitow.

SPECIAL NOTES: This is frequently associated with a fever, especially one caused by an infection.

Alternative Treatments

Refer to alternative therapy chapters for more information before evaluating or applying any treatment. Some conditions, including yours, may require a physician's care.

NUTRITIONAL THERAPY: • Vitamin B complex (two to three times daily with meals) • Vitamin C • Niacin or vitamin B₃ (this helps some people and some it makes worse) • Vitamin B₁₂ and mixed amino acids (two capsules, ten minutes before meals, three times daily) • Thyroid support

Self-Care

The following therapies can be undertaken at home under appropriate professional supervision.

Fasting / Meditation / Yoga

FLOWER ESSENCES: Flower essences for accompanying emotional/mental states.

HERBS: Teas of chamomile, boneset, ginger, pennyroyal, or yarrow.

HOMEOPATHY: *Aconite* (sudden onset), *Euphrasia, Nat mur., Arsen alb., Sulfur, Pulsatilla*

Professional Care

The following therapies should only be provided by a qualified health professional.

Acupuncture / Applied Kinesiology / Detoxification Therapy / Environmental Medicine / Hypnotherapy / Naturopathic Medicine

CIRRHOSIS

A group of chronic liver diseases associated with abnormal changes in the normal microscopic architecture (interstitial cells) of the liver, which cause hardening and inflammation of the liver itself. (Sometimes the term cirrhosis is used to refer to any organ that has chronic interstitial inflammation.) The liver becomes damaged and cannot perform its many functions: storage and filtering of blood, production of bile (which helps digest fat and fat-soluble vitamins), and many metabolic actions like the conversion of sugar into glycogen (the form in which carbohydrates are stored in the body for energy; thus, another classic symptom of liver disease is extreme fatigue).

SYMPTOMS: Cirrhosis of the liver usually has a very long period of latency, meaning no overt symptoms. Some signs of mild liver disease may be fatigue, itching, rashes of unknown causes, constipation or diarrhea, alternating color of the stools, fever, and indigestion. Suddenly at onset, there is abdominal swelling, pain, vomiting of blood, swelling of the body in general, and jaundice (yellowing of the skin). Advanced stages lead to severe symptoms that may lead to coma and death.

SPECIAL NOTES: Biliary cirrhosis first affects the bile ducts, then moves into the liver, and is a disease of unknown causes. It is most frequent in women 35-60 years of age; 30% have no symptoms but the condition is discovered through abnormal blood tests; 50% have itching, rash, and fatigue as the initial signs that may occur months or even years before the actual disease is identified. Fifty percent of people at time of diagnosis have enlarged, excessively firm but nontender livers and enlarged spleens. Ten percent of people have patches of darkness on the skin and less then 10% have jaundice. Other possible signs are clubbing of nails, yellow stools, and kidney, bone, and nerve disease.

Alternative Treatments

Refer to alternative therapy chapters for more information before evaluating or applying any treatment. Some conditions, including yours, may require a physician's care.

DIET: Whole foods diet including seeds, nuts, whole grains, beans, and milks from soy, rice, and goat. According to Jonathan Wright, M.D., the current and best diet recommendations for cirrhosis are for a low-protein diet. Avoid processed fats such as margarine, hydrogenated oils, and foods with these oils added, rancid oils, and hardened vegetable fats. Use cold-processed oils.

Use nitrogen-packed nuts. Increase consumption of foods high in amino acids and potassium such as nuts, seeds, bananas, raisins, rice, wheat bran, kelp, dulse, brewer's yeast, and molasses. Drink plenty of filtered water. Avoid animal protein as well as raw or undercooked fish. Limit overall intake of fish. Strictly avoid alcohol.

Avoid stressors on the liver: overeating, drugs of any kind, a highly processed diet, especially with processed fats, additives, and foods high in animal protein, and accumulation of toxins from chemicals that have to be processed by the liver such as alcohol, drugs, acetaminophen, insecticides, chemicals from rancid and processed oils, possibly toxins from *Candida* yeast organisms within the body, possibly contraceptives, and preservatives.

NUTRITIONAL THERAPY: • Lipotropic factors • Vitamin B complex • Vitamin B_{12} • Folic acid • Niacin (B_3—in small doses such as 10-30 mg three times) • Liver glandulars • Vitamin C • Digestive enzymes with hydrochloric acid (HCl) and ox bile extract • Amino acids L-methionine, L-carnitine, L-cysteine, L-glutathione, L-arginine

According to Dr. Wright, anything that helps support the remaining liver function is very important. These include vitamin C, vitamin E, silymarin, lipoic acid, and raw liver tablets.

With liver disease, do not use more than 10,000 IU of vitamin A daily and avoid cod liver oil entirely.

The liver is further stressed by a toxic bowel. Bowel cleansing and rejuvenation techniques may be very important. Eat a whole foods diet for two weeks, then do a bowel cleanse and follow with bowel rejuvenation. Repeat the bowel cleanse once a month as needed and stay on bowel nutrients for up to one year depending on the severity of condition and response to treatment.

Self-Care

The following therapies can be undertaken at home under appropriate professional supervision.

Fasting / Flower Essences / Qigong and Tai Chi

AROMATHERAPY: Juniper, rosemary, rose

AYURVEDA: An herbal mixture of *kutki* (200 mg), *shanka pushpi* (500 mg), and *guduchi* (300 mg); ¼ teaspoon of this mixture generally taken twice a day, after lunch and dinner, with aloe vera juice.

HERBS: • Milk thistle may contribute to the treatment of cirrhosis as it helps liver cells regenerate. It may be taken in the form of tablets or the nonalcohol extract called a glycerate. The dose is based upon the content of silymarin (the active ingredient of milk thistle) and so standardized extracts are preferable. The typical dosage range is 70-200 mg of silymarin daily. • The herb *Picrorhiza kurroa* is not as well-known as milk thistle, but may have similar effects.[18] • Licorice.

HYDROTHERAPY: • Constitutional hydrotherapy (if illness is severe, apply two to seven times weekly). • Contrast application or cold friction to stimulate liver function (apply daily).

JUICE THERAPY: • Beet and carrot juice • Wheat grass juice • Add raw flaxseed oil and garlic as tolerated.

REFLEXOLOGY: Liver, pancreas, all glands

Professional Care

The following therapies should only be provided by a qualified health professional.

Cell Therapy / Magnetic Field Therapy / Natural Hormone Replacement Therapy / Naturopathic Medicine

DETOXIFICATION THERAPY: Detoxification may be indicated, depending on the condition of the person. Stay off alcohol, chemicals, and fats.

TRADITIONAL CHINESE MEDICINE: The Chinese herb Bupleurum *(chai-hu)* may be helpful.

COLD SORES (HERPES SIMPLEX)

Small fever blisters, often recurrent, found anywhere around the mouth, caused by the herpes simplex virus 1 (HSV1). Groupings of these blisters are called a cluster.

SYMPTOMS: The first bout may be accompanied by flu-like symptoms, with fever, neck pain, lymph node enlargement, and fatigue, or it may go unnoticed. After the first attack, the virus remains dormant in nerve cells, but can be reactivated by stress, colds, hot weather, anxiety, nutrient deficiencies, or other illnesses, especially ones with accompanying fever. Prolonged bouts may occur in people with immune suppression or in healthy people under high stress. Recurrent attacks start with a burning sensation that soon is followed by blisters that can be very sore and itch. Within a few days to several weeks, they burst, dry, encrust, and disappear.

OCCURRENCE: 90% of people have this infection at least one time during their lives.

CONSIDER: Herpes zoster, Coxsackie virus, low thyroid, health problems depressing immune function.

SPECIAL NOTES: These sores are very contagious. Oral sex can spread HSV1 from the mouth to the genitalia. The drug acyclovir is prescribed orally and topically. However, it may cause an increase in symptoms on cessation of the drug. Also, antiviral drugs are very strong to be able to penetrate the well-protected viruses, so they are hard on the body and especially the liver.

Alternative Treatments

Refer to alternative therapy chapters for more information before evaluating or applying any treatment. Some conditions, including yours, may require a physician's care.

DIET: Whole foods diet with more raw vegetables and cultured products such as yogurt and sauerkraut.

NUTRITIONAL THERAPY: • L-lysine cream applied directly on blisters • Lysine (4 g daily for the first four days, then 500 mg three times daily for two weeks). Do not take daily on a maintenance basis as it may create an imbalance among other amino acids. If continual daily lysine is the only way for you to prevent recurrent attacks, then decrease wheat and add other grains to diet and take lysine in small dosages with amino acid blends and consider amino-acid testing. • Vitamin B complex • Zinc gluconate • Vitamin C with bioflavonoids • Thymus extract • Acidophilus • Vitamin E • The flavonoid quercetin has been shown to inhibit the herpes virus.[19]

According to Jonathan Wright, M.D., the two amino acids that appear to be important in herpes infections are lysine and arginine. Arginine induces the growth and reproduction of the herpes simplex virus, while lysine inhibits the virus. What's important is the ratio of arginine to lysine. The higher the arginine to lysine ratio, the more herpes virus is likely to grow. Conversely, if lysine is high with respect to arginine, the growth is inhibited. Chocolate, peanuts, most cereal grains, nuts, and seeds have more arginine than lysine.

Self-Care

The following therapies can be undertaken at home under appropriate professional supervision.

Biofeedback Training and Neurotherapy / Fasting / Guided Imagery

AROMATHERAPY: Geranium, lemon, chamomile, tea tree, lavender.

FLOWER ESSENCES: Flower essences for accompanying emotional/mental states. Rescue Remedy Cream®. Crab Apple. Rescue Remedy® if feeling stressed.

HERBS: Herbs that boost resistance and strengthen the immune response should be taken. Combine the tinctures of echinacea, Siberian ginseng, nettle, and goldenseal in equal parts and take ½ teaspoon of this mixture three times a day. Externally apply dilute tincture of myrrh or calendula. Research has demonstrated the antiviral effects of licorice root and its specific application to inactivating herpes simplex particles and inhibiting the growth of the virus.[20]

HYDROTHERAPY: During early stages, use an ice application (on ten minutes, off five minutes).

JUICE THERAPY: Avoid citrus, pineapple.

TOPICAL TREATMENT: Vitamin E ointment or saturate gauze with vitamin E oil and apply for 15 minutes.

Professional Care

The following therapies should only be provided by a qualified health professional.

Environmental Medicine / Homeopathy / Magnetic Field Therapy / Naturopathic Medicine / Orthomolecular Medicine / Traditional Chinese Medicine

OXYGEN THERAPY: • Hydrogen peroxide therapy (IV) • Ozone therapy inactivates herpes and promotes skin healing.

CONVULSIONS

(Seek medical attention promptly. See Epilepsy.)
A variety of nonvoluntary contractions (single or series) of the voluntary muscles, from mild to severe, due to sudden uncontrolled changes in the electrical activity of the brain.

SYMPTOMS: May be mild, only slight muscle twitches and tingling, all the way to violent, jerking whole-body movements, sometimes associated with intense feelings of fear, familiarity, possible hallucinations, and sometimes a lapse of consciousness (a grand mal seizure). Seizures that reoccur are called epilepsy.

SPECIAL NOTES: Convulsions or seizures may be caused by many medical problems such as stroke, brain tumor, withdrawal from alcohol and drugs, metabolic disturbances, neurological disorders, and trauma from head injury. Febrile seizures (twitching, jerking convulsion associated with loss of consciousness in a child with a rapidly rising fever and often due to infections such as middle ear or tonsillitis) are common in children between six months and five years old and tend to run in families. They are usually not serious, even though they are frightening and occur in one out of 20 children.

Alternative Treatments

Refer to alternative therapy chapters for more information before evaluating or applying any treatment. Some conditions, including yours, may require a physician's care.

DIET: According to Melvyn Werbach, M.D., epileptics should have normal, well-balanced meals at regular intervals and children should not be allowed to take large meals as these predispose toward seizures. Alcohol is totally contraindicated as is caffeine (cola drinks, coffee, tea, chocolate). Aspartame (NutraSweet™) has been implicated in some cases of seizure.

NUTRITIONAL THERAPY: • Taurine • Magnesium • Vitamin B6 • Manganese • Have an amino acid blood screen. Working with a qualified practitioner is important. Supplementation with the amino acids taurine, dimethyl glycine, and/or DL-glutamic acid has been shown to be beneficial.

There are multiple nutritional deficiencies associated with seizures, including folic acid, niacin (vitamin B3), thiamin (B1), vitamin B6, vitamin D, copper, magnesium, manganese, and selenium. Some of these deficiencies may relate to anticonvulsant medication, while others may be related to the cause of the seizures. Any supplementation should be with the awareness of the medical practitioner responsible for the care of the individual. Omega-6 fatty acid supplementation may trigger or exacerbate temporal lobe epilepsy.

Self–Care

The following therapies can be undertaken at home under appropriate professional supervision.

Guided Imagery

ACUPRESSURE: A hospital study in Germany found that when a seizure occurred while nurses were preparing medication for injection, in almost all cases (over 100 were evaluated) very firm stimulation of the center of the nasal philtrum (the depression above the upper lip below the center of the nose) caused consciousness to be restored in an average of under 30 seconds.[21] This was long before the medication was ready (therefore making its use unnecessary). This point is Governor Vessel point 26 in traditional Chinese medicine. The only side effect noted was slight bruising of the lip area; no comparable study has been done on adults.

AROMATHERAPY: Chamomile, clary sage, lavender, neroli.

FLOWER ESSENCES: Flower essences for accompanying emotional/mental states. Rescue Remedy® after seizure.

HERBS: Asafetida, mugwort, skullcap, valerian root

HYDROTHERAPY: Constitutional hydrotherapy (apply two to five times weekly).

HOMEOPATHY: *Cuprum met., Belladonna, Cicuta*

Professional Care

The following therapies should only be provided by a qualified health professional.

Chiropractic / Environmental Medicine / Fasting / Light Therapy / Magnetic Field Therapy / Naturopathic Medicine / Osteopathic Medicine / Traditional Chinese Medicine

DETOXIFICATION THERAPY: Not indicated unless the condition is due to specific toxicity.

CORNS

A painful, hardened, cone-shaped area of increased growth of the corneous layer of the skin, found mainly over the toe joints and between the toes on the foot.

SYMPTOMS: Mostly pea-sized or slightly larger hardened areas on the feet, occurring where bony protuberances occur. Corns may only hurt in response to pressure or may hurt spontaneously.

CONSIDER: Calluses, warts, localized injury and inflammation, infection, or poor circulation. Corns, when pared away with a sharp instrument, have a clearly outlined translucent core.

SPECIAL NOTES: The harder corns occur mainly on the toes, while the "soft" corns occur mainly between the toes. Prevention is the most important cure, and this is accomplished by eliminating undue pressure at certain sites of the foot. Thus, assessment by a podiatrist, osteopath, or chiropractor who can evaluate foot gait, the role of other joints such as the pelvis in foot pressure problems, shoes, and the need for orthotics, pad, moleskins, etc., is very important in prevention as well as treatment.

Treatment also involves better fitting shoes. Corns do disappear when the inappropriate pressure is eliminated. Podiatrists can pare the corn away, but the cause still needs to be assessed. Patients with recurring corns and calluses need ongoing treatment by a podiatrist. Patients with poor circulation from serious diseases such as diabetes mellitus require special and regular care.

Alternative Treatments

Refer to alternative therapy chapters for more information before evaluating or applying any treatment. Some conditions, including yours, may require a physician's care.

DIET: A whole foods diet is recommended.

NUTRITIONAL THERAPY: • Vitamin A and vitamin E topically and orally • Essential fatty acids

Self–Care

The following therapies can be undertaken at home under appropriate professional supervision.

AROMATHERAPY: Lemon, verucas

FLOWER ESSENCES: Rescue Remedy Cream®

HERBS: Apply a salve made from calendula petals two to three times a day. This will soon soften the tissue and acts as an anti-inflammatory.

HOMEOPATHY: *Graphites, Silicea, Antim crud.*

HYDROTHERAPY: • Contrast application (apply daily) • Hot Epsom salts foot bath, then rub corns with fresh lemon juice

REFLEXOLOGY: Around and directly on the corns.

TOPICAL TREATMENT: • Aloe vera gel • Rub castor oil on corn twice daily.

Professional Care

The following therapies should only be provided by a qualified health professional.

Magnetic Field Therapy / Naturopathic Medicine

COUGHS

Sudden, explosive expulsion of air from the lungs, usually in order to expel something from the air passages. Productive cough-ing brings up mucus (referred to as sputum or phlegm) and an unproductive, dry cough does not.

SYMPTOMS: Different cough sound characteristics may signal different problems. A qualified practitioner should be able to evaluate.

EXAMPLES: Constant, severe coughing with thick mucus production may signal chronic bronchitis (bronchitis often associated with smoking or passive smoke exposure). A very dry cough with profound symptoms of fever and fatigue may signal an approaching severe bout of acute bronchitis. Viral bronchitis usually has a persistent cough that disturbs sleep.

Dry coughs that are usually worse at night may signal bronchospasm (temporary narrowing of the bronchi, the larger tubes of airways) that can be associated with asthma, infection, or allergies. Allergic coughs may occur along with runny nose and wheezing, or begin after certain foods are consumed or at different times of the year. Coughing associated with changes of posture suggest lung abscess or other severe diseases. Coughs associated with eating may suggest serious swallowing or trachea problems. Coughs due to exercise or cold air may signal asthma. In young children with inflammation of the respiratory tract, the airways can narrow so much that it produces a hoarse metallic cough called the croup. Persistent short, mild, dry coughs in the spring may signal hay fever. Rattles of secretions associated with a dry, barking cough may signal an infection of the trachea.

Pneumonia (lung inflammation secondary to infection) usually has painful coughing associated with flecks of blood. Cancers of the airways may produce a mild cough at first that gets worse and then produces mucus that is blood-flecked. Some coughing is a nervous manifestation, especially in children.

Sputum (expectorated matter) produced with the cough signals the following: changes (white to yellowish, green, or brown) mean that an infection is involved; blood streaking means infection is getting worse, must definitely see a doctor; gritty material in sputum may mean a serious condition of the lungs called broncholithiasis—inflammation or obstruction caused by calculi (stones, usually formed by mineral salts) in the bronchi. Cough sputum up for observation by a practitioner.

CONSIDER: Coughing may be due to a simple illness, like upper respiratory infection or the common cold, or may signal a more serious illness, such as cancer. May also be due to irritation from environment (smoke, dust, pollens), mucus dripping in back of the throat, a sign of nervousness, or a symptom of an underlying health disorder.

SPECIAL NOTES: Important questions about coughing: How long has it occurred? Did it start suddenly? Has it changed recently? What factors make it worse? What time of day? Is the cough associated with production of mucus? What color is the mucus? Are there any other pains or symptoms? Is the cough associated with work or exercise? Treatment of the cough depends entirely on the underlying cause.

Coughing up blood (hemoptysis): Blood appears in sputum due to a rupturing of blood vessels in airways, lungs, nose, or throat secondary to causes that may be mild or serious and need to be evaluated. May appear as bright red or rusty-brown streaks, pinkish froth, or bright red pure blood. May need a chest X ray. If X rays show abnormalities, if person is over 40, a smoker, or has coughed up blood before, may need bronchoscopy, a procedure that allows direct viewing of the lungs by insertion of a soft, flexible tube. One-third of people undergoing this procedure are found to have no underlying serious problem.

Alternative Treatments

Refer to alternative therapy chapters for more information before evaluating or applying any treatment. Some conditions, including yours, may require a physician's care.

DIET: • Eat whole foods including lots of raw fruits and vegetables. • Avoid mucus-producing foods: sugar, salty foods, dairy products, starches. • For dry cough, umeiboshi plum paste

According to George Sarantakos, Ph.D., a cough syrup can be made from eight ounces of warm pineapple juice and two teaspoons of honey. The bromelain in the pineapple juice is activated by the honey. Cough medicine to keep on hand: Mix juice of one lemon with two tablespoons glycerine, then add 12 teaspoons honey and stir. Stir before each use. Take one teaspoon every 30 minutes, reducing as needed. (Do not refrigerate.)

NUTRITIONAL THERAPY: • Zinc lozenges • Vitamin A • Folic acid • Vitamin C and bioflavonoids • Vitamin E

Self-Care

The following therapies can be undertaken at home under appropriate professional supervision.

Fasting / Guided Imagery / Yoga

AROMATHERAPY: Steam inhalation with thyme, benzoin, eucalyptus, frankincense, peppermint, sandalwood, chamomile, juniper. Also try myrrh.

AYURVEDA: • Take equal parts lemon juice and honey in teaspoon doses. • For cough with mucus: make a tea of ½ teaspoon ginger powder, a pinch of clove, and a pinch of cinnamon powder in one cup of water. • Gargle: add one pinch of salt and two pinches of turmeric powder to glass of water. • For chronic coughs: a confection of one part sesame seeds (black seeds if possible), ½ part *shatavari*. Add ginger and raw sugar to taste and take one ounce daily. Or try an herbal mixture of *sitopaladi* (500 mg), *yasti madhu* (300 mg), *punarnava* (300 mg), *kant kari* (200 mg), and *vasaka* (300 mg); ¼ teaspoon of this mixture generally taken twice a day after lunch and dinner.

FLOWER ESSENCES: Flower essences for accompanying emotional/mental states. Crab Apple if cough is due to infection.

HERBS: A cough is an important diagnostic signal from the body and should not be simply suppressed. Any longstanding or intransigent coughing should receive professional attention. Home treatment is safe and effective for minor coughs of short duration or associated with mild infections, but if in doubt seek skilled advice. Coltsfoot and mullein have been found to be safe and effective for children and adults. Use as an infusion at least three times a day while the symptoms remain. For a dry irritating cough, use an infusion of marshmallow leaves. Mullein and horehound are appropriate for adult coughs.

There are many effective kitchen remedies for coughs. Slice an onion into a deep bowl and cover in honey, let stand overnight. Strain the mixture of juice and honey. This makes a simple cough elixir. Take one teaspoon four or five times a day.

HOMEOPATHY: • For dry coughs, *Belladonna, Aconite, Drosera, Bryonia, Phosphorus.* • *Hyoscyamus, Rumex,* and *Spongia* must be taken alone, not in combination with other remedies. • For loose coughs, *Ipecac, Merc sol., Pulsatilla, Kali bich., Kali carb.*

HYDROTHERAPY: • Hot pack (apply to chest as needed to aid in expectoration). • Benzoin steam inhalation

JUICE THERAPY: • Fresh fruit and vegetable juices • Hot pear juice with cinnamon stick; can add cardamom, cumin to juices.

Professional Care

The following therapies should only be provided by a qualified health professional.

Applied Kinesiology / Chiropractic / Environmental Medicine / Magnetic Field Therapy / Naturopathic Medicine / Neural Therapy / Osteopathic Medicine / Traditional Chinese Medicine

BODYWORK: Acupressure, reflexology, shiatsu

DETOXIFICATION THERAPY: Detoxification may be helpful, depending on the condition of the person. (If due to infection—maybe; if due to allergies—yes.)

CUTS

Breaking of skin that causes bleeding and may be mild or severe. The more severe it is and the more underlying tissues involved, the longer it may take to heal and may require therapeutic stitching to assist in the healing.

Alternative Treatments

Refer to alternative therapy chapters for more information before evaluating or applying any treatment. Some conditions, including yours, may require a physician's care.

NUTRITIONAL THERAPY: • *If mild:* after cleaning the wound, cover with a mixture of zinc oxide cream and vitamin E oil. When healing has begun, and signs of inflammation, infection, and redness are gone, use topical aloe vera. • *If the laceration is severe, and thus referred to*

as a wound: apply pressure until the bleeding stops. Keep covered with a bandage that creates some pressure. Ascertain if stitches are necessary (outside help such as sutures will be needed to stop bleeding and keep structures together for healing). If stitches are necessary, go immediately to an emergency room. If stitches are not necessary, treat as mentioned above. • Vitamin C • Zinc • Vitamin A • Pantothenic acid

Problems with healing: increase vitamin C (three to six times daily), add proteolytic enzymes (three to four times daily, on empty stomach, until healing gets well underway). The amino acid arginine improves both the speed and quality of wound healing (it stimulates production by the body of growth hormone, which is involved in any new tissue growth).

Self-Care

The following therapies can be undertaken at home under appropriate professional supervision.

Guided Imagery

AYURVEDA: For minor cuts, use aloe vera gel with turmeric applied locally, or tikta ghee.

FASTING: If infection is a component, fasting may be beneficial.

FLOWER ESSENCES: Rescue Remedy Cream®

HERBS: Clean the cut and then apply comfrey leaf as an ointment or compress. Do not use comfrey for puncture wounds as the skin will heal before the deeper tissue. An alternative is calendula.

HOMEOPATHY: *Calendula, Hepar sulph., Ledum, Hypericum, Arnica* ointment.

HYDROTHERAPY: Ice pack (apply to the arterial trunk that supplies the area).

TOPICAL TREATMENT: Green clay, found in health food stores, is very effective for healing when made into a paste and applied topically to cuts. Tea tree oil is an effective antibacterial, antiviral, and antifungal agent.

Professional Care

The following therapies should only be provided by a qualified health professional.

Acupuncture / Naturopathic Medicine

OXYGEN THERAPY: Hyperbaric oxygen therapy and/or external ozone applications for accelerated wound healing.

DANDRUFF

A common scalp condition in which the dead skin is shed, producing irritating white flakes. Dandruff frequently accompanies scalp disease and is a primary cause of baldness and general hair loss. Its character is that of an unspecified seborrheal dermatitis, a mild scalp inflammation with excessive fatty secretions, and is frequently due to digestive disturbances. It is highly dependent on the general health of the whole body.

SYMPTOMS: White flakes appear on the hair and fall onto the shoulders and clothes. There may be itching, scaling, and redness of the scalp, and may also occur on other skin surfaces such as the face, chest, and back. Yellow crusting may appear.

SPECIAL NOTES: The most common cause of dandruff is seborrheic dermatitis. This is a skin condition that usually starts as dry or greasy scaling of the skin, but may progress to yellow-red scaling bumps along hairline, behind the ears, in the ear canals, on the eyebrows, on the bridge of the nose, in the folds around the nose, or on the breastbone. Don't pick or scratch scalp.

When infants get this condition, it is called cradle cap. According to Leon Chaitow, N.D., D.O., cradle cap is a yeast problem and many skin experts in Europe find that dandruff in adults is also a yeast problem. The problem should then be treated as for candidiasis.

Alternative Treatments

Refer to alternative therapy chapters for more information before evaluating or applying any treatment. Some conditions, including yours, may require a physician's care.

DIET: Increase raw foods within a whole foods diet. Eat more salads and green vegetables. Avoid fried foods. Reduce intake of fats, sugar, dairy products, chocolate, seafood, nuts.

NUTRITIONAL THERAPY: • Vitamin B6 • Vitamin A • Vitamin B complex • Essential fatty acids (particularly omega-6) • Vitamin C • Vitamin E • Beta carotene • Kelp tablets • Zinc

Self-Care

The following therapies can be undertaken at home under appropriate professional supervision.

Detoxification

AROMATHERAPY: Patchouli, rosemary, tea tree oil

FLOWER ESSENCES: Crab Apple

HERBS: Rinse the hair and scalp with a strong infusion of nettle, sage, and rosemary. Drink a cup of nettle tea and take evening primrose oil (three capsules) daily.

HOMEOPATHY: *Arsen alb., Graphites, Lycopodium, Thuja, Sepia, Sulfur, Cantharis*

HYDROTHERAPY: Contrast application (apply daily to scalp).

TOPICAL TREATMENT: • Pour warm apple cider vinegar over head and wrap head in a towel. After one hour, wash hair. • Apply vitamin E oil to scalp nightly for three weeks. • Tea tree oil shampoo.

According to Dr. Chaitow, selenium-based shampoos are effective because the selenium acts as an antifungal agent. Massage cold-pressed linseed oil into the scalp at night and wash it off in the morning (sleep on an old pillowcase). This is often successful in restoring scalp health.

Professional Care

The following therapies should only be provided by a qualified health professional.

Environmental Medicine / Natural Hormone Replacement Therapy / Naturopathic Medicine / Traditional Chinese Medicine

DETOXIFICATION THERAPY: May be indicated, depending on the condition of the person.

OXYGEN THERAPY: External ozone applications to control fungal growth.

DERMATITIS

Several forms of inflammation of the most superficial portion of the skin, most frequently caused by food allergies, contact allergies (makeup, nickel and other metals in jewelry, perfumes, creams), or toxic plant allergies such as poison ivy or poison oak. Many medical sources use the terms dermatisis and eczema interchangeably.

SYMPTOMS: Itching, flaking, color oozing, crusting, scaling, and thickening of the skin.

SPECIAL NOTES: If allergic cause is not removed and/or it is excessively scratched, the dermatitis may spread and become very severe. There are many types of dermatitis. Contact dermatitis is an inflammation produced by substances that touch the skin, from direct irritants, to allergic substances, to exposure to light. Atopic dermatitis is a severe, chronic, itching and inflammation of the skin in individuals with a family history of allergic disorders such as asthma, hay fever, and milk allergies. Seborrheic dermatitis is an inflammation of skin usually on the scalp, face, and, rarely, on the sternum (breastbone). Nummular dermatitis produces coin-shaped red bumps that itch severely and is seen in middle-aged people under stress and more often in the winter. There can also be chronic dermatitis of the hands and feet or a generalized dermatitis that affects wide areas of the skin with extreme scaling.

Alternative Treatments

Refer to alternative therapy chapters for more information before evaluating or applying any treatment. Some conditions, including yours, may require a physician's care.

DIET: Identify and avoid food allergies and other allergenic substances. Try a gluten-free diet with no wheat, oats, rye, barley. According to Leon Chaitow, N.D., D.O., in Europe the most likely allergy would be dairy foods, especially cow's milk as many studies have shown this to be the likeliest culprit food, followed by wheat. Eat lots of yogurt, sauerkraut, and naturally fermented foods.

NUTRITIONAL THERAPY: •Vitamin B6 •Vitamin B complex • Evening primrose oil or omega-6 fatty acids from other sources • Acidophilus • Zinc • Magnesium • Assess need for digestive enzymes or gastrointestinal problems such as parasites.

Self-Care

The following therapies can be undertaken at home under appropriate professional supervision.

Fasting / Hypnotherapy / Mind/Body Therapy / Reflexology / Yoga

AROMATHERAPY: Benzoin, chamomile, lavender, bergamot, geranium

FLOWER ESSENCES: Flower essences for accompanying emotional/mental states. Rescue Remedy Cream®. Crab Apple.

HERBS: Combine the tinctures of nettle, red clover, and cleavers in equal parts and take ½ teaspoon of this mixture three times a day. Drink an infusion of fresh nettle or cleavers twice a day. To alleviate itching, bathe the area with lukewarm or cold chickweed infusion. For cracked, dry, or painful skin, use a salve made from calendula flowers and St. John's wort leaves.

HOMEOPATHY: *Pulsatilla, Arsen alb., Lycopodium, Graphites, Petroleum, Sulfur, Thuja, Sepia*

HYDROTHERAPY: Cold compress (apply as needed to control pain or itching).

JUICE THERAPY: • Carrot, beet, cucumber, celery • Carrot, celery, apple • Cantaloupe

TOPICAL TREATMENT: • Aloe vera gel • Pyridoxine ointment • For itching, mix vitamin E, vitamin A, unflavored yogurt, a little honey, and zinc oxide, and place onto skin. • Evening primrose oil applied directly to cracks and sore areas of the skin (folds such as elbows and behind the knee, for example) can be very helpful in promoting healing.

Professional Care

The following therapies should only be provided by a qualified health professional.

Acupuncture / Environmental Medicine / Magnetic Field Therapy / Naturopathic Medicine / Osteopathic Medicine

DETOXIFICATION THERAPY: May be indicated, depending on the condition of the person.

OXYGEN THERAPY: Hydrogen peroxide therapy (IV).

DIZZINESS

Can be very mild: defined as dizziness, a short-lived sensation of faintness, unsteadiness with lightheadedness. May be more severe: defined as vertigo, either as subjective vertigo (individual has impression he or she is spinning) or objective vertigo (impression that objects are spinning around the individual). True vertigo has to do with a problem somewhere within the equilibratory system: middle ear, eighth (acoustic) cranial nerve, the brain stem, or the eyes. Unlike dizziness, vertigo is usually associated with nausea, vomiting, and severe sweating.

CONSIDER: True vertigo is never a sign of anxiety, but lightheadedness, giddiness, and fear of losing one's balance may be a sign of depression or anxiety.

SPECIAL NOTES: True dizziness is usually caused by a sudden drop of blood pressure in the brain from standing up too quickly (postural hypotension), fatigue, stress, low blood sugar (hypoglycemia), temporary blockage of blood to the brain as in a transient ischemic attack, low blood oxygenation, low blood iron, and certain drugs. Vertigo is mainly caused by labyrinthitis (usually viral infection of fluid filled canals of inner ear) and Meniere's disease, characterized by bouts of severe nausea, vomiting, ringing in the ears (tinnitus), hearing loss, and vertigo that can persist for days and weeks.

With any dizziness, first take a few deep breaths and sit down to rest. Severe or prolonged dizziness needs to be evaluated by an exam and blood tests.

According to Leon Chaitow, N.D., D.O., dizziness when standing after sitting or lying down can be an indication of adrenal exhaustion. The individual should take action to restore adrenal health by stopping the use of stimulants (caffeine, tobacco, alcohol) and via rest and normalization of lifestyle and nutritional balance.

When you feel this sensation upon standing, it helps if you can immediately squat down or cross your legs (strongly pressing them against each other), as this forces circulation up from the lower body/limbs to the trunk and head.

Alternative Treatments

Refer to alternative therapy chapters for more information before evaluating or applying any treatment. Some conditions, including yours, may require a physician's care.

DIET: Whole foods diet. If hypoglycemic, eat smaller meals throughout the day and restrict refined sugars, caffeinated beverages, and alcohol. If anemic, consume green drinks, chicken, dark green vegetables, and raw seeds.

NUTRITIONAL THERAPY: • Vitamin B complex • Niacin (B₃) • Vitamin E • Iron

Specific nutritional support for adrenal exhaustion) involves supplementation with vitamin C (3–5 g daily) and vitamin B₅ (500–1,000 mg daily of pantothenic acid/calcium pantothenate).

Self–Care

The following therapies can be undertaken at home under appropriate professional supervision.

Fasting / Guided Imagery

ACUPRESSURE: To relieve dizziness, firmly press GV26 (for an illustration of this point, see the acupressure chart in the introduction to this section) two-thirds of the way up from the upper lip to the nose using your index fingertip. Press deeply, applying firm pressure into the center of your upper gum for one minute.

BODYWORK: Acupressure, shiatsu, massage, Alexander Technique

FLOWER ESSENCES: Flower essences for accompanying emotional/mental states. Rescue Remedy® for accompanying stress.

HERBS: Ginger, ginkgo leaf extract
HOMEOPATHY: *Gelsemium, Phosphorus, Cocculus, Convallaria, Granatum*
HYDROTHERAPY: Hot foot bath
REFLEXOLOGY: Side of neck, ear reflex, cervicals

Professional Care

The following therapies should only be provided by a qualified health professional.

Chiropractic / Craniosacral Therapy / Environmental Medicine / Hypnotherapy / Magnetic Field Therapy / Naturopathic Medicine / Osteopathic Medicine / Traditional Chinese Medicine

BIOLOGICAL DENTISTRY: Check for mercury toxicity from amalgams.

DETOXIFICATION THERAPY: If allergies are present, detoxification is possibly helpful.

DYSENTERY

(Amoebiasis—See Parasitic Infections Chapter.)
An infection of the intestines, caused by either a group of bacteria called shigella *(thus, dysentery is called shigellosis) or by protozoan (single-celled) parasites called* Entamoeba *(this is called amebic dysentery).*

SYMPTOMS: *Shigellosis:* Sudden diarrhea that is very watery and sometimes bacterial contamination of the blood (toxemia) occurs. In severe cases, shigellosis may lead to bacteremic shock or cardiovascular collapse. *Amebic dysentery:* More gradual development of diarrhea. Diarrhea can become mixed with blood, pus, and mucus, and straining bowel movements may result in only scarce amounts of blood-stained, watery mucus. Dehydration may occur and fluids must be replenished in the body. Possible complications of amebic dysentery include amebic cysts in liver, brain, and other organs.

SPECIAL NOTES: If you are suffering from shigella or *Entamoeba histolytica,* you should seek medical help. Antibiotics may be necessary.

Alternative Treatments

Refer to alternative therapy chapters for more information before evaluating or applying any treatment. Some conditions, including yours, may require a physician's care.

DIET: Clove of garlic morning and evening, followed by hot tea with lemon (unsugared). Lots of unflavored yogurt. Avoid refined sugars and alcohol during attacks and for a week after episode.

NUTRITIONAL THERAPY: During and several weeks after episode: • Acidophilus • *Bifidobacteria* and *Lactobacillus bulgaricus* • Vitamin A • Citrus seed extract

Self-Care

The following therapies can be undertaken at home under appropriate professional supervision.

Fasting / Yoga

AROMATHERAPY: Chamomile, black pepper, cypress, eucalyptus, lemon, melissa

FLOWER ESSENCES: Flower essences for accompanying emotional/mental states. Rescue Remedy® for accompanying stress; Crab Apple if feeling contaminated; Olive for exhaustion.

HERBS: Use a decoction of oak bark to reduce the diarrhea and fluid loss. Drink an infusion of meadowsweet and chamomile to ease abdominal discomfort. Eat a clove of raw garlic morning and evening. Take electrolyte replacement if needed, made by dissolving one teaspoon of salt and four teaspoons of sugar (which helps intestines absorb both) in one quart of water. Be accurate with salt or this may create more dehydration.

HYDROTHERAPY: Constitutional hydrotherapy unless otherwise indicated (apply two to five times weekly).

Professional Care

The following therapies should only be provided by a qualified health professional.

Applied Kinesiology / Detoxification Therapy / Magnetic Field Therapy / Naturopathic Medicine / Osteopathic Medicine / Traditional Chinese Medicine

OXYGEN THERAPY: Ozone colon therapy.

ECZEMA

Inflammation of the skin, usually associated with blisters, red bumps, swelling, oozing, scaling, crusting, and itching. Eczema is often called dermatitis.

CONSIDER: There are different types of eczema depending on their causes and where they occur on the body. Eczema can be due to allergies, allergies secondary to digestive disorders such as hydrochloric acid deficiency, rashes secondary to immune diseases, genetic metabolic disorders, or nutritional deficiencies such as B vitamins, especially niacin (B3) and B6.

SPECIAL NOTES: There are various types of eczema. *Contact eczema or dermatitis:* Sharp demarcations where substances contact the skin and create a rash (may be due to direct irritants, allergic substances, from exposure to light, or certain chemicals and perfumes). *Atopic dermatitis or eczema:* Occurs in people with family histories of allergy, vitamin B12 problems, asthma, and allergic respiratory problems such as hay fever. In infants 2-18 months old, this causes weeping, crusty, red spots on face, scalp, and extremities, and in older children and adults it may be more localized and chronic. May subside by three to four years and may reoccur in adolescence or adulthood. *Seborrheic dermatitis or eczema:* Of scalp, face, and chest.

Nummular dermatitis or eczema: Coin-shaped chronic red spots with crusting and scaling. Normally occurs after the age of 35 and often associated with emotional stress and, in winter, with dry skin. *Chronic eczema:* Occurs in hands or feet, which can get very severe. *Generalized eczema:* Inflammation that is widespread over much of the skin. *Stasis eczema:* In lower legs, associated with poor venous return of the blood and tendency toward skin to turn brownish. *Localized scratch dermatitis or eczema:* Occurring in specific patches, often with whitish areas well demarcated by areas of increased pigmentation or color, such as arms, legs, ankles, around the genitals, and made worse by stress and scratching. Much more frequent in women between 20 and 50 years old.

Avoid irritating substances, wear natural nonirritating materials, use soothing ointments, and assess if diet, nutrients, and allergic components need to be considered.

Alternative Treatments

Refer to alternative therapy chapters for more information before evaluating or applying any treatment. Some conditions, including yours, may require a physician's care.

DIET: Whole foods diet with identification and avoidance of allergenic foods especially wheat and cow's milk products. Lemon juice mixed with equal parts olive or almond oil applied externally and taken internally. Excess consumption of fruit, especially citrus and sour, may aggravate symptoms. Eczema may be a symptom of an omega-3 fatty acid deficiency.

If there is a family history of asthma, hay fever, and food allergies, it may be helpful to delay solid food introduction to infants as a preventative measure. A ten-year study in New Zealand involving 1,265 children showed that children who were introduced to four or more types of solid foods before the age of four months were 2.9 times more likely to develop recurrent eczema than children not exposed to early solid feeding.[22]

NUTRITIONAL THERAPY: • Zinc • Vitamin A and GLA (gamma-linolenic acid), an omega-6 essential fatty acid found in high quantities in evening primrose oil, have been shown to improve the symptoms of eczema.[23] • Vitamin E • Vitamin B complex • Vitamin B6 • Magnesium

Self-Care

The following therapies can be undertaken at home under appropriate professional supervision.

Fasting / Yoga

AROMATHERAPY: Bergamot, chamomile, lavender, melissa, neroli, eucalyptus, geranium, juniper.

AYURVEDA: An herbal mixture of *kutki* (200 mg), *manjista* (300 mg), turmeric (200 mg), and *neem* (200 mg); one teaspoon of this mixture generally taken twice a day after lunch and dinner. Externally apply *neem* oil. Do not eat salt, sugar, or yogurt.

BODYWORK: Acupressure, shiatsu, reflexology.

FLOWER ESSENCES: Flower essences for accompanying emotional/mental states. Rescue Remedy® for accompanying stress. Crab Apple.

HERBS: Eczema is best treated internally, as the cause is usually a constitutional one. Alternative remedies such as cleavers, nettle, yellowdock, or red clover may be very effective. They are often combined with relaxing herbs such as chamomile, linden flowers, or skullcap. One combination would be equal parts of cleavers, nettle, and chamomile drunk as an infusion three times a day. A stronger mixture combines the tinctures of figwort, burdock, and cleavers in equal parts; take one teaspoon of this mixture three times a day. To alleviate itching, bathe the area with lukewarm or cold chickweed infusion. For cracked, dry, or painful skin, use a salve made from calendula flowers and St. John's wort leaves. Goldenseal applied externally may be helpful.

HOMEOPATHY: • *Dulcamara, Rhus tox., Sulfur, Arsen alb., Graphites* • *Petroleum* and *Psorinum* must be taken alone, not in combination with other remedies.

HYDROTHERAPY: Heating compress (apply once daily).

JUICE THERAPY: • Black currant, red grapes • Carrot, beet, spinach, cucumber, parsley • Green juices • Wheat grass

NATUROPATHIC MEDICINE: While not a cure, applying zinc oxide locally often helps relieve the severe itchiness of eczema.

REFLEXOLOGY: Diaphragm, liver, kidneys, intestines, adrenals, all glands, thyroid

MIND/BODY THERAPY: Biofeedback, guided imagery, relaxation

TOPICAL TREATMENT: • Evening primrose oil applied directly to cracks and sore areas of the skin (folds such as elbows and behind the knee, for example) may be very helpful in promoting healing. • Ginkgo and licorice root extract (applied topically) have been shown to improve the symptoms of eczema.[24]

Professional Care

The following therapies should only be provided by a qualified health professional.

Acupuncture / Environmental Medicine / Hypnotherapy / Magnetic Field Therapy / Naturopathic Medicine / Orthomolecular Medicine / Osteopathic Medicine

DETOXIFICATION THERAPY: Detoxification is indicated unless the person is weakened or deficient.

OXYGEN THERAPY: Hydrogen peroxide therapy (IV).

EDEMA

Abnormal amounts of excessive fluid (commonly water and sodium), usually in subcutaneous spaces (intercellular spaces, between the cells) in the body.

SYMPTOMS: Bloating and swelling of the face, fingers, hands, legs, and, in later stages, the abdomen. May be very slight, causing rings on fingers to feel tight or the face to feel puffy, or may be severe enough to cause stretching and shininess of skin and overall weight gain. If fluid accumulation creates such stretching and bagginess of the skin that pressure into it creates a "pit," called pitting edema, a doctor should be consulted immediately as this may be a sign of a very serious problem.

CONSIDER: Allergies, poor kidney excretion or secondary kidney problems related to protein absorption, vitamin B deficiencies, heart failure, or other liver and kidney disorders.

SPECIAL NOTES: Usually seen in extremities, but may even occur (in very slight amounts) in the brain associated with allergies that cause the brain to swell and manifest as headaches, memory problems, learning disorders, or behavioral changes. Flying in airplanes, traveling to a new climate, or stress can aggravate symptoms.

Small amounts of fluid buildup can occur anywhere in the body, such as in the spine (causing low back pain), in the lungs (mimicking asthma/bronchitis), and in the knees (mimicking arthritis), and should be a consideration in a wide variety of health problems that do not respond to the normal treatments.

Alternative Treatments

Refer to alternative therapy chapters for more information before evaluating or applying any treatment. Some conditions, including yours, may require a physician's care.

DIET: Whole foods diet with avoidance of foods that tend to worsen edema: caffeine, alcohol, salt, fried foods, cow's milk products, animal protein, sugar, white flour, chocolate, olives, pickles, tobacco, and soy sauce. Eating a diet of mainly processed grains and rice may lead to a vitamin B deficiency that can aggravate edema. Thus, focus on whole grains and watery fruits and vegetables, such as cucumbers, apples, potatoes, grapes, beets, onions, cabbage, and citrus.

NUTRITIONAL THERAPY: • Vitamin B complex • Vitamin B6 • Protein supplement (free-form amino acids) • Potassium (potassium may be used with any herbal diuretic, especially when taken with cornsilk tea) • Vitamin C • Pantothenic acid • Alfalfa tablets

Self-Care

The following therapies can be undertaken at home under appropriate professional supervision.

Fasting / Qigong and Tai Chi

AROMATHERAPY: Juniper, rosemary, geranium, fennel

AYURVEDA: For a chronic condition, include diuretic foods in the diet such as celery, carrot, parsley, cilantro, cranberries, pomegranate, corn, barley, rye, and adzuki beans. *Punarnava guggulu* (200 mg), generally taken twice a day after lunch and dinner.

HERBS: Competent diagnosis of the cause of water retention is essential, but diuretic herbs will address the symptoms. One effective diuretic herb is dandelion leaf, also a rich source of potassium. Stimulating kidney function can remove potassium from the body, impacting a range of functions but most crucial is electrolyte balance in the heart muscle. If the diuretic is treating edema associated with congestive heart failure, any reduction in potassium will aggravate the heart symptoms. Dandelion replaces all the potassium that is flushed from the body via diuresis. Take one teaspoon of the tincture three times a day, or an infusion of the fresh leaves three to five times a day. • Horse chestnut seed extract.

HYDROTHERAPY: Contrast application (apply daily, repeat hot/cold, change six to eight times during treatment).

JUICE THERAPY: • Pears, pineapple, watermelon, cranberries • Green juices (add a bit of dandelion juice) • Cucumber, parsley, celery, carrot

REFLEXOLOGY: Lymph system, kidneys, adrenals.

Professional Care

The following therapies should only be provided by a qualified health professional.

Chiropractic / Craniosacral Therapy / Environmental Medicine / Magnetic Field Therapy / Natural Hormone Replacement Therapy / Naturopathic Medicine / Osteopathic Medicine / Traditional Chinese Medicine

BODYWORK: Acupressure, reflexology, shiatsu, massage

DETOXIFICATION THERAPY: Depending on the condition of the person.

HYDROTHERAPY: Leon Chaitow, N.D., D.O., reports that the neutral bath (patient immersed in water at body temperature for two hours) has been effective in moving fluid from swollen tissues in cases of mild heart problems, swollen joints of rheumatoid patients, and fluid retention from cirrhosis of the liver.

OXYGEN THERAPY: Hyperbaric oxygen therapy.

EPILEPSY

Recurrent episodes of disturbances in brain electrical activity that manifest as sudden brief attacks of altered consciousness, sometimes loss of consciousness, involuntary and abnormal motor function and sensation, and alterations of the nervous system.

CONSIDER: Nutrient deficiencies, thyroid disorders, stress management strategies.

SPECIAL NOTES: The most common form of epilepsy is convulsive, in which the attack starts with loss of consciousness and motor control, and then the individual has extreme jerking muscular movements. The true cause of epilepsy is unknown. Based on clinical exam and brain studies, there are four types: grand mal epilepsy—major episodes associated with loss of consciousness; petit mal epilepsy—milder forms usually without loss of consciousness; psychomotor epilepsy—with different types of abnormal movements; autonomic epilepsy—associated with flushing, whiteness of skin, rapid heartbeat, high blood pressure, abdominal symptoms, and sweating.

Emergency techniques for someone having a seizure: Remain calm and move sharp objects away, do not put anything in the mouth, and loosen their clothing; if possible, put the person on the floor or bed and stay at the individual's side.

Alternative Treatments

Refer to alternative therapy chapters for more information before evaluating or applying any treatment. Some conditions, including yours, may require a physician's care.

DIET: Low-fat, low-carbohydrate diet. Eliminate fried foods, salt, sugar, meat, milk, and alcohol. For long-term care, follow a hypoglycemic diet (see Hypoglycemia). Avoid artificial sweeteners, excessive refined carbohydrates, and caffeine, and make sure the bowels move adequately (two to three times per day).

NUTRITIONAL THERAPY: • L-taurine and L-tyrosine amino acids (500 mg three times daily) along with an amino acid blend (two times daily) •Vitamin B complex • Vitamin B_6 • Magnesium • Folic acid (folic acid supplementation can cause a decrease in B_{12} levels and, in rare cases, may aggravate epilepsy) • Niacin (vitamin B_3) • Vitamin B_5 •Vitamin B_{12} • Manganese • Zinc • Calcium • Choline (start with 4 g daily and increase to 10-12 g within three months) • Dimethylglycine (100 mg two times daily) • Intramuscular B complex may be helpful.

Sometimes essential fatty acids can aggravate symptoms.

Self-Care

The following therapies can be undertaken at home under appropriate professional supervision.

Fasting

ACUPRESSURE: (See Convulsions.)

AYURVEDA: An herbal mixture of *saraswati churna* (200 mg), *brahmi* (300 mg), *jatamansi* (200 mg), and *punarnava* (300 mg), ¼ teaspoon of this mixture generally taken twice a day after lunch and dinner.

BODYWORK: Massage of abdomen after applying castor oil packs.

HERBS: For petit mal epilepsy, take one teaspoon of skullcap tincture three times a day.

HYDROTHERAPY: • Constitutional hydrotherapy (apply two to five times weekly) • Epsom salts bath twice weekly.

JUICE THERAPY: Celery, carrot, and lettuce juice (three glasses daily).

MIND/BODY THERAPY: Biofeedback, hypnotherapy, meditation

REFLEXOLOGY: Diaphragm, colon, ileocecal, whole spine, neck, all glands

YOGA: Increased circulation to the brain from breathing exercises and physical exercise is very important.

Professional Care

The following therapies should only be provided by a qualified health professional.

Cell Therapy / Chiropractic / Craniosacral Therapy / Environmental Medicine / Magnetic Field Therapy / Naturopathic Medicine / Osteopathic Medicine / Traditional Chinese Medicine

BIOLOGICAL DENTISTRY: Hal Huggins, D.D.S., reports the improvement or disappearance of certain motor problems, such as epilepsy and multiple sclerosis, after removing toxic dental amalgams.

BODYWORK: Acupressure, Feldenkrais Method, reflexology, Rolfing, shiatsu

DETOXIFICATION THERAPY: May be indicated, depending on other functions.

FAINTING

(See a physician immediately.)
A sudden and brief loss of consciousness, usually due to decreased flow of blood to the brain. Secondary to decreased heart output, usually due to arrhythmia (abnormal change in the beating of the heart). May also be due to heat exhaustion associated with excessive fluid loss, weakness, fatigue, anxiety, drenching sweats, and fainting.

CONSIDER: Low blood sugar, low blood pressure (hypotension), allergies, anemia, and nutrient deficiencies such as magnesium and iron.

PRACTICAL HINTS: If you feel faint, sit down and put your head between your knees until you feel better. Be sure there is plenty of fresh air.

Alternative Treatments

Refer to alternative therapy chapters for more information before evaluating or applying any treatment. Some conditions, including yours, may require a physician's care.

DIET: Whole foods diet with adequate protein foods and fluids.

NUTRITIONAL THERAPY: • Magnesium • Iron • Vitamin B complex • Pantothenic acid

Self-Care

The following therapies can be undertaken at home under appropriate professional supervision.

AROMATHERAPY: Peppermint, neroli, basil, lavender, rosemary, or black pepper (hold under nose).

FLOWER ESSENCES: For emotional states as appropriate. Rescue Remedy®: topically rub four drops on pulse points or lips as often as every three minutes.

HOMEOPATHY: *Ignatia, Aconite, Arsen alb.*

HYDROTHERAPY: Constitutional hydrotherapy (apply two to five times weekly).

REFLEXOLOGY: Pituitary

TRADITIONAL CHINESE MEDICINE: Massage just under the nose to bring a person out of a faint.

Professional Care

The following therapies should only be provided by a qualified health professional.

Environmental Medicine / Natural Hormone Replacement Therapy / Naturopathic Medicine / Oxygen Therapies

BODYWORK: Acupressure, reflexology, shiatsu

FASTING: Under a doctor's supervision.

FLATULENCE

Buildup and expulsion of flatus (intestinal gas) formed by fermentation, inappropriate digestion of most common carbohydrates and sometimes other foodstuffs, or swallowing of air. Released by burping (eructation) through the mouth or by relieving gas through the anus.

SYMPTOMS: Distention of abdomen, discomfort in abdomen that may be mild or severe, chest pains that may be mild and feel like slight pressure or may be severe enough to mimic a heart attack.

CONSIDER: Overeating, eating too quickly, excessive consumption of refined carbohydrates, excessive consumption of artificial sweeteners, food allergies, intestinal or stomach disorders, gallbladder disorders, deficiencies of B vitamins, excessive consumption of alcohol, parasites, emotional stress, and misalignment or spasm of the associated spinal vertebrae.

Alternative Treatments

Refer to alternative therapy chapters for more information before evaluating or applying any treatment. Some conditions, including yours, may require a physician's care.

DIET: Do not overeat. Overconsumption, even of healthy food, is the most common cause of flatulence. Eat simpler meals, meaning fewer different food items at one sitting. Chew food more slowly and thoroughly. Consume more high-fiber foods. Identify and avoid allergenic foods. You may try avoiding protein and carbohydrates eaten together at meals. Try chewing a sprig of parsley after meals. If eating beans, soaking them overnight in a quart of water containing six drops of iodine may help reduce gas.

Asafoetida powder is a powerful digestive agent. It dispels intestinal gas and, when used as a spice with beans, helps to decrease gas. Try sipping lemon juice or apple cider vinegar in water with meals. Add more fermented products such as yogurt, kefir, and buttermilk to the general diet.

Leon Chaitow, N.D., D.O., suggests the European method of using super-fine white, green, or yellow French clay (similar to bentonite). A teaspoon or two is dissolved in spring water and drunk, at least once a day away from mealtimes, to reduce the tendency to flatulence. The clay absorbs the impurities and gas and there are no reported side effects.

NUTRITIONAL THERAPY: • Vitamin B complex • Digestive enzymes such as hydrochloric acid or pancreatin • Acidophilus • Charcoal tablets • Several drops of peppermint oil in water sipped throughout the meal • Vitamin B₁ • Aloe vera juice or gel • Niacin (vitamin B₃) • Lipotropic factors (promotes the processing of dietary fat).

Self-Care

The following therapies can be undertaken at home under appropriate professional supervision.

Biofeedback Training and Neurotherapy / Fasting / Qigong and Tai Chi / Yoga

AROMATHERAPY: Bergamot, chamomile, fennel, juniper, lavender, peppermint, rosemary, coriander, anise

BODYWORK: Rub abdomen in a clockwise direction.

HERBS: Try anise water, made by steeping one teaspoon of anise seeds in one cup of water for ten minutes. It can be taken as a tea or strained and taken as needed by the tablespoon.

HOMEOPATHY: • *Carbo veg., Lycopodium, Argen nit., Chamomilla* • *Nux mosch.* and *Cinchona*

HYDROTHERAPY: • Constitutional hydrotherapy unless otherwise indicated (apply two to five times weekly) • Short cold sitz baths

JUICE THERAPY: • One tablespoon of garlic or yellow onion juice, or mix with carrot, parsley, beet, and celery juice • Papaya juice

NATUROPATHIC MEDICINE: Flatulence is almost always a sign of either maldigestion or food intolerance. When combined with bad breath and tiredness after meals, inadequate stomach acid is the typical cause.

REFLEXOLOGY: Intestines, stomach, liver, gallbladder, pancreas

Professional Care

The following therapies should only be provided by a qualified health professional.

Applied Kinesiology / Chiropractic / Environmental Medicine / Light Therapy / Magnetic Field Therapy / Naturopathic Medicine / Osteopathic Medicine / Traditional Chinese Medicine

DETOXIFICATION THERAPY: Colon and gastrointestinal detoxification.

FOOD POISONING

Any health problem that is characterized by abdominal pain associated with diarrhea, vomiting, sweating, and weakness, usually within 48 hours of eating a food contaminated with a virus or bacteria.

SYMPTOMS: Symptoms vary greatly. Onset may be 30 minutes to one hour with chemical poisoning; up to 12 hours with bacterial poisoning; 12 to 48 hours from viral or salmonella poisoning. Stomach pain, nausea, diarrhea, and, in very severe cases, collapse and shock.

OCCURRENCE: Many cases of diarrhea each year are probably due to food poisoning. Many go unreported as the cause is not known and is usually attributed to the stomach flu.

CONSIDER: Flu, gastrointestinal disorders, digestive enzyme deficiencies, drug interactions, stress, and nutrient deficiencies or excess (too much magnesium can cause loose stools and abdominal cramps). In infants, can also be due to intolerance to honey.

SPECIAL NOTES: Usually suspect food poisoning when a number of people who ate the same food get similar symptoms. Most common forms of food poisoning are infective types such as salmonella, found usually in farm animals or passed on by food handling or flies from contaminated fecal material. Food products most likely to cause problems are poultry such as chicken, duck, or geese, raw or partly cooked eggs, or raw fish such as clams, oysters, or sushi. Frozen poultry that is not completely thawed before being cooked is a common cause of this problem. Other organisms such as staphylococcal bacteria can be passed from food handlers through hands, coughing, sneezing, or breathing onto the food. Botulism is associated with food preserved at home.

Viruses can contaminate shellfish and are often due to contaminated waters. Foods that remain at room temperature too long, such as large portions of meat prepared for restaurants and allowed to sit out at room temperature, can encourage *Clostridium* to grow, often referred to as the "cafeteria germ." Other infective organisms can be *Giardia* and *Campylobacter*, which may take up to one week to show symptoms. Noninfective food poisoning is caused by poisonous mushrooms, toadstools, and fresh vegetables and fruits that have been contaminated accidentally with too many chemicals and insecticides, by being stored in inappropriate containers, or leakage of metals from the containers into the food.

If severe vomiting and diarrhea occur, emergency medical intervention must be sought. Keep samples of food for testing, if possible. If due to chemical or bacterial toxins, treatment may require pumping the stomach (gastric lavage). Milder cases can be home treated. Usually improves within three days unless due to botulism, chemical poisoning, or mushroom poisoning.

One covert problem with infective organisms is that sometimes they do not have identifiable initial symptoms but linger in the body and may cause long-term health problems that are difficult to diagnose. May also cause constipation in addition to diarrhea.

Alternative Treatments

Refer to alternative therapy chapters for more information before evaluating or applying any treatment. Some conditions, including yours, may require a physician's care.

DIET: Stop eating all solid food, drink plenty of fluids. Immediately, take six charcoal tablets, *Lactobacillus acidophilus, Bifidobacteria, L. bulgaricus,* and citrus seed extract. Take electrolyte replacement, if needed, made by dissolving one teaspoon of salt and four teaspoons of sugar (which helps the intestines absorb both) in one quart of water. Be accurate with salt amount or it may create more dehydration. If you are traveling in areas where food poisoning is common, try eating more hot, spicy foods to encourage more gastric secretions; avoid all drinking water except bottled water and any raw vegetables. Add high-fiber foods, and garlic.

NUTRITIONAL THERAPY: • Acidophilus • Charcoal tablets • Citrus seed extract • Garlic capsules • Vitamin C with bioflavonoids • Kelp

Unlike other antioxidants that are limited to attacking specific free radicals, lipoic acid is nonspecific and can perform the jobs of other antioxidants (such as vitamins C and E) when their supplies are low. Lipoic acid can also protect the liver from a damaging free-radical attack caused by ingesting poisonous mushrooms.

Self-Care

The following therapies can be undertaken at home under appropriate professional supervision.

Fasting

AYURVEDA: For general mild food poisoning, fast and drink cumin, coriander, fennel tea.

HOMEOPATHY: *Arsen alb., Chamomilla, Ipecac., Apis mel., Nux vom., Colchicum.*

HYDROTHERAPY: Constitutional hydrotherapy (apply two to five times weekly).

JUICE THERAPY: Carrot, beet, garlic.

Professional Care

The following therapies should only be provided by a qualified health professional.

Naturopathic Medicine

OXYGEN THERAPY: Ozone intestinal insufflation.

FRACTURES

A break in a bone.

SYMPTOMS: There may be almost no symptoms, or mild ones such as slight swelling and tenderness with only mild aching. Or there may be severe symptoms with intense pain, discoloration, breakage of skin, severe swelling and throbbing, with possible bleeding from surrounding ruptured tissues and loss of normal movement.

SPECIAL NOTES: There are two main types of fractures, closed (broken pieces remain beneath skin surface and there is little surrounding tissue disruption or damage) and open (one or both of the bone ends break through the skin). Fractures may also be classified as to the type of break: simple (broken bone does not pierce the skin),

compound (skin is pierced and exposed to organisms in the air), transverse (bone breaks all the way through), greenstick (only outer bone is broken and the break is not all the way through), and comminuted fracture (bone is shattered into smaller pieces).

X rays are required to verify break. A doctor needs to properly set the fracture and then the following treatments can be done to help optimize healing. Rehabilitative exercise and manual therapy for localized and associated areas should be considered.

Alternative Treatments

Refer to alternative therapy chapters for more information before evaluating or applying any treatment. Some conditions, including yours, may require a physician's care.

DIET: Diets high in calcium from dark leafy greens, dairy products, and raw seeds and nuts. Avoid excessive consumption of caffeine, red meat, and colas with phosphoric acid (which contributes to bone loss). Highly processed foods also have a high phosphorus content that may lead to bone loss.

NUTRITIONAL THERAPY: • Calcium • Magnesium • Vitamin C with bioflavonoids • Vitamin D • Zinc • Silicon • Vitamin K • Protein supplement (free-form amino acids)

Self-Care

The following therapies can be undertaken at home under appropriate professional supervision.

Biofeedback Training and Neurotherapy / Fasting / Guided Imagery

BODYWORK: Acupressure, shiatsu, massage

FLOWER ESSENCES: Rescue Remedy; Rescue Remedy Cream®. Flower essences for accompanying emotional/mental states.

HERBS: • Drink an infusion of equal parts comfrey leaf and horsetail to speed the healing once the fracture has been set. • Teas: comfrey, horsetail, Solomon's seal

HOMEOPATHY: *Calc phos., Symphytum, Ruta grav., Arnica, Aconite*

HYDROTHERAPY: • Contrast application (apply daily) • Apply ice to fracture to control internal bleeding • For arm and wrist fractures, alternate hot arm bath (three minutes) and cold arm bath (30 seconds).

JUICE THERAPY: Add watercress to beet and carrot juice.

REFLEXOLOGY: Reflex to affected area on foot, also referral area.

TOPICAL TREATMENT: • Poultice of turmeric paste mixed with a little hot water may be helpful with fractures and helps reduce swelling • Poultice of fresh mullein leaves

Professional Care

The following therapies should only be provided by a qualified health professional.

Cell Therapy / Magnetic Field Therapy / Naturopathic Medicine / Prolotherapy

ACUPUNCTURE: Electro-acupuncture to help facilitate healing.

CHIROPRACTIC: For fractures not requiring setting.

HYPNOTHERAPY: A randomized controlled study showed that hypnosis may be capable of enhancing both anatomical and functional fracture healing.[25]

OXYGEN THERAPY: Hyperbaric oxygen therapy is useful for refractory bone fractures.

FROSTBITE

Excessive exposure to damp cold (temperatures around freezing) causes frostnip and immersion (trench) foot. Exposure to dry cold (temperatures that are well below freezing) causes frostbite and accidental hypothermia.

SYMPTOMS: *Frostnip:* Hardened and whitened areas on face, ears, fingers, and extremities. Peeling of skin may occur within 24 to 72 hours and recurrent bouts of milder cold sensitivity may last for life.

Immersion foot: Feet swell, get pale, cold, clammy, and numb or tingling. Infection may occur later. Swelling and pain may persist for years.

Frostbite: Area becomes extremely cold, hard, white, and difficult to feel. Upon warming up, area gets very itchy, red, swollen, blotchy, and painful.

Hypothermia: Lethargy, poor coordination, mental confusion and irritability, hallucinations, slowed respiration and heart rate, and death.

CONSIDER: Conditions that increase risk to cold injury include anemia, drug or alcohol excess, exhaustion and hunger, and impaired circulation secondary to other diseases. The very young and the elderly are more at risk.

SPECIAL NOTES: Hypothermia occurs when the body cannot maintain its normal temperature. As soon as possible, warm the affected areas, the hands, feet, and abdomen. Rub the area vigorously to stimulate circulation. You may even snuggle and hug the person to increase warmth.

Alternative Treatments

Refer to alternative therapy chapters for more information before evaluating or applying any treatment. Some conditions, including yours, may require a physician's care.

NUTRITIONAL THERAPY: • Warm beverages • Vitamin B complex

Self-Care

The following therapies can be undertaken at home under appropriate professional supervision.

Fasting / Qigong and Tai Chi

FLOWER ESSENCES: Flower essences for accompanying emotional/mental states. Rescue Remedy®

HERBS: To stimulate circulation, drink hot ginger tea.

HYDROTHERAPY: Immersion bath (neutral application to warm slowly).

TOPICAL TREATMENT: Gel from a freshly cut aloe vera leaf.

Professional Care

The following therapies should only be provided by a qualified health professional.

Naturopathic Medicine

ACUPUNCTURE: To prevent permanent nerve damage.

OXYGEN THERAPY: • Hyperbaric oxygen therapy • External ozone application as a bactericidal and to enhance circulation.

TRADITIONAL CHINESE MEDICINE: *Dong quai* and peony formulas are effective.

FUNGAL INFECTION

(See also Infection, Viral Infections, Candidiasis chapter.)
A disease, usually of the skin, but may be of other organs, that is due to fungal organisms (simple parasitic life forms including molds, mildew, and yeast), sometimes called mycoses.

SYMPTOMS: May be mild, such as discoloration and swelling of the nail beds, moist, reddened patches over various parts of the body, cheesy and smelly discharge from the vagina. May be severe, infecting and disrupting normal organ functioning.

SPECIAL NOTES: May be more common and/or severe in people taking long-term antibiotic medication, corticosteroids, immunosuppressant drugs (used to inhibit normal immune functioning), contraceptives, and in people with conditions such as obesity, AIDS, and diabetes mellitus.

Alternative Treatments

Refer to alternative therapy chapters for more information before evaluating or applying any treatment. Some conditions, including yours, may require a physician's care.

DIET: Whole foods diet with emphasis on raw food less dairy products. Avoid foods high in yeast such as beer and breads with yeast. Avoid sugar of all sorts (including honey and fruit juices) for some weeks while antifungal methods are being used. (See Candidiasis chapter.)

NUTRITIONAL THERAPY: • Acidophilus • *Bifidobacteria* and *L. bulgaricus* • Garlic capsules • Vitamin B complex • Pantothenic acid • Vitamin C to bowel tolerance (see Orthomolecular Medicine chapter) • Vitamin E • Vitamin A • Zinc • Thymus glandular

Essential fatty acids (black currant, evening primrose, and salmon oils) can help maintain cellular integrity, protecting cells from fungal infection.

Leon Chaitow, N.D., D.O., suggests taking caprylic acid capsules (extract of coconut plant) as an antifungal agent, while acidophilus and other probiotics are being taken to repopulate sites where fungi had colonized. Grapefruit seed extract may also be an effective remedy.

Self-Care

The following therapies can be undertaken at home under appropriate professional supervision.

Fasting

AROMATHERAPY: Tea tree oil, patchouli, geranium

FLOWER ESSENCES: Rescue Remedy Cream®. Crab Apple.

HERBS: Fungicidal herbs are an effective topical treatment for skin infections. Examples are myrrh, tea tree, and garlic. Tea tree oil can be applied directly or diluted with calendula oil for application to sensitive skin. Oregano oil or capsules and products containing pau d'arco are good antifungals.

HOMEOPATHY: *Calendula, Chamomilla, Belladonna, Merc sol., Sulfur*

JUICE THERAPY: • Avoid fruit juices or dilute with water in a 2:1 ratio • Add garlic to vegetable juice.

NATUROPATHIC MEDICINE: Fungal infection of the nails is difficult to treat and requires patience. One therapy is to swab the infected area with tea tree or thuja oil twice a day.

TOPICAL TREATMENT: To the affected area, apply some of the following: tea tree oil or gel, citrus seed extract, honey and crushed garlic, pau d'arco tea by wetting tea bag for ten minutes and then leave the bag itself on the area or use gauze or cotton soaked in tea if area is large.

Professional Care

The following therapies should only be provided by a qualified health professional.

Environmental Medicine / Magnetic Field Therapy / Naturopathic Medicine / Traditional Chinese Medicine

DETOXIFICATION THERAPY: May be indicated, depending on the condition of the person.

OXYGEN THERAPY: • Hydrogen peroxide therapy (IV) • Hyperbaric oxygen therapy • Ozone/oxygen mixture may work as an effective antifungal agent and may easily be applied externally. Methods of internal application depend upon the clinical situation.

GALLBLADDER DISORDERS

The gallbladder is a small sac-like organ underneath the liver that receives, stores, and concentrates bile made in the liver. The liver sends the bile to the gallbladder through a small tube called the cystic duct. During digestion, the gallbladder contracts and delivers bile to the intestines (duodenum) to help break down (emulsify) fat that is contained in the food. The most common problem associated with the gallbladder is gallstones. Gallstones are round-shaped combinations of cholesterol, bile, pigments, and lecithin.

SYMPTOMS: Only 20% of people who have gallstones get symptoms (many people have gallstones that never bother them and are called "silent"). A major symptom of gallstones is usually right-sided pain in the abdomen that may be associated with right-sided shoulder pain. The shoulder pain may occur by itself without the abdominal pain.

There also may be centrally located upper abdominal pain over the breastbone. The pain, in general, wherever it manifests, is constant and progresses slowly, rising to a plateau, and then gradually decreases, usually within several hours after a meal and especially after meals containing large amounts of fat. Sometimes nausea, fullness, belching, heartburn, flatulence, and vomiting are present.

If the abdomen gets extremely painful, even to the touch, and a fever starts, this may be a symptom of acute cholecystitis, an irritation and infection in the gallbladder usually due to a gallstone becoming trapped. Recurrent attacks of this are called chronic cholecystitis.

OCCURRENCE: Women over 40 years old, fair-skinned, and overweight are more prone to gallstones. Women get gallstones four times as frequently as men. Twenty percent of adults over 65 years of age get gallstones that create problems and pain. Over half a million surgeries are performed each year to remove gallbladders due to gallbladder disorders, the most common being gallstones.

CONSIDER: Food allergies (especially to milk products and eggs), digestive disorders (especially caused by a deficiency of hydrochloric acid), intestinal diseases, excessively low-fiber diet, food intolerance, parasites, rapid weight loss, and stress. Constipation may also be connected to gallstones.

SPECIAL NOTES: Rarely does the gallbladder get inflamed without the presence of stones. Gallbladder cancer can occur, but is extremely rare (three cases per 100,000 people per year). This cancer usually causes jaundice (yellowing of skin), pain in the upper-right abdominal area, and is sometimes present with no symptoms at all.

Ultrasound may be needed for accurate diagnosis. New surgical methods use lasers, do not need to cut into the abdomen, and heal much more quickly. Jonathan Wright, M.D., states that most gallbladder surgeries could be easily avoided through nutritional and natural intervention, with emphasis on identification, avoidance, and treatment of food allergies.

Rule out dental implications. (See Biological Dentistry chapter.)

Alternative Treatments

Refer to alternative therapy chapters for more information before evaluating or applying any treatment. Some conditions, including yours, may require a physician's care.

DIET: Identify and avoid food allergies, especially eggs and/or cow's milk products. Cut down fat in the diet, below 20% of total foods. Do not, however, cut out fat completely—studies say that up to half of the people who try to lose weight by cutting out fat (eating less than 600 calories and three grams of fat per day) develop gallstones.[26] Especially avoid processed fats and hydrogenated oils and include monounsaturated fats. Eat less, as overeating is very stressful on the gallbladder. Eat regular meals, especially make sure to eat breakfast. It is hard on the gallbladder to go many hours without food and then suddenly have to deal with a large meal. Increase dietary fiber and decrease refined carbohydrates, which are a risk factor for gallstone formation.[27] Eat less animal foods and move toward a vegetarian-oriented diet. If you are overweight, lose the weight, but slowly and sensibly.

Fasting may be helpful during acute stages. Avoid animal products as much as possible during acute problems and eat small frequent meals. Black cherries, pears, beets (raw and cooked), fresh beet tops steamed with spinach leaves, or kale and yogurt are good. Increase dietary fiber and avoid refined carbohydrates. Eat more raw foods.

First gallbladder flush: Continue to eat mostly a whole foods diet with almost no animal products or processed foods. Drink plenty of raw, fresh apple juice or eat apples as much as possible, between meals, for six days. On the morning of seventh day, have ½ cup of olive oil mixed with ⅓ cup of fresh lemon juice. Drink all at once.

Second gallbladder flush: Upon rising, take three tablespoons of olive oil with three times the amount of fresh lemon juice. Or mix ⅛ ounce each of grapefruit juice and olive oil and take prior to meals.

NUTRITIONAL THERAPY: • Multi-enzymes with bile (bile is contraindicated if ulcers coexist) • Vitamin C • Vitamin B complex • Choline and inositol • Lipotropic factors • Alfalfa tablets • Lecithin • Unsaturated fatty acids • Acidophilus • L-taurine • Peppermint oil sipped in water throughout the meal may be helpful when having symptoms.

Self–Care

The following therapies can be undertaken at home under appropriate professional supervision.

Fasting / Yoga

HERBS: In conjunction with dietary and lifestyle advice. Combine the tinctures of wild yam, fringetree bark, milk thistle, and balmony in equal parts and take one teaspoon of this mixture three times a day. An infusion of chamomile or lemon balm may be drunk regularly throughout the day.

HYDROTHERAPY: Constitutional hydrotherapy (apply two to five times weekly). • Hot pack to abdomen and low back: apply 10-15 minutes several times daily for relief of colic pain, follow each hot application with a short period of cold application.

JUICE THERAPY: • Carrot, beet, cucumber (add a little garlic, radish, or fresh dandelion roots) • Grape, pear, grapefruit, lemon

TOPICAL TREATMENT: Castor oil packs on gallbladder.

Professional Care

The following therapies should only be provided by a qualified health professional.

Environmental Medicine / Magnetic Field Therapy / Naturopathic Medicine / Neural Therapy / Osteopathic Medicine

ACUPUNCTURE: For inflammation. Acupuncture may also be effective for the expulsion of gallstones.[28]

DETOXIFICATION THERAPY: Detoxification is indicated, unless the person is in a weakened state.

HAIR LOSS

Partial or complete loss of hair, called alopecia, which usually occurs on the scalp, but can occur anywhere on the body, such as the extremities and even eyebrows; hair can fall out or disappear in various patterns.

The most common pattern of hair loss is called male pattern baldness or hereditary alopecia. In this condition, hair is lost from the crown and temples and is often replaced by a more fine, downy type of hair. This pattern of hair loss is also called androgenic alopecia, meaning it is more common in males and is usually inherited. It may also affect women (female-pattern baldness) and occurs especially after menopause.

Alopecia areata is a sudden loss of very circumscribed areas of hair for no apparent reason or secondary to systemic disease. Alopecia universallis is loss of hair over the entire body and has a poor reversal rate if it occurs during childhood; it usually corrects itself, but is prone to recurrences if it begins in adulthood. Trichotillomania (hair pulling) is a neurotic disorder that usually occurs in children, may correct itself, and may be secondary to psychological problems or even physical ones such as heavy metal toxicity. Scarring alopecia is hair loss secondary to scarring due to localized trauma such as burns, physical injury, or X rays, and often the hair cannot regrow through the scarred tissue.

SYMPTOMS: Loss of hair in various patterns.

OCCURRENCE: More common in men but can occur in women and is on the rise in women.

CONSIDER: Low thyroid functioning, poor digestion, parasites, nutrient deficiencies such as iron or biotin, hormonal problems, aging, secondary to trauma, post-pregnancy, skin disease, diabetes, chemotherapy, and stress.

SPECIAL NOTES: If large amounts of hair are lost, it is important to see a doctor to rule out an underlying disease.

Circulation to the scalp is important. Increase exercise, scalp massage, and try lying on a slant board for 15 minutes a day.

Alternative Treatments

Refer to alternative therapy chapters for more information before evaluating or applying any treatment. Some conditions, including yours, may require a physician's care.

DIET: Whole foods diet high in the outer coverings of plants such as potato skins, green and red peppers, sprouts, and cucumbers. These are high in silicon, which gives strength to hair and nails. Foods high in iron, such as some lean meats and raisins, are also important. Sea vegetables such as kelp are good for the hair and thyroid. Drink goat's milk instead of cow's milk.

NUTRITIONAL THERAPY: • Flaxseed oil • Biotin • Zinc • Amino acid blends • Vitamin B complex • Iron • Trace minerals

Folic acid, biotin, vitamin B5, PABA (para-aminobenzoic acid), and silica help maintain the color and thickness of the hair. Kelp is a good source of the trace minerals needed for metabolism and supports the maintenance of hair, nails, and skin. The amino acid cysteine supplies sulfur, which is essential for healthy hair and nails. Inositol and zinc regulate the oil content in hair and are necessary for hair growth.

For dull, lifeless hair, use evening primrose oil, flaxseed oil, and vitamin E.

For lost hair color, try PABA, pantothenic acid, biotin, iodine or thyroid glandular, desiccated liver. Poor liver functioning may play a role; consider liver supplementation. High levels of copper can lead to brittle hair and split ends, and low copper levels can result in hair loss.

Self-Care

The following therapies can be undertaken at home under appropriate professional supervision.

Fasting / Yoga

AROMATHERAPY: For temporary or severe hair loss, use lavender, rosemary, thyme, sage.

AYURVEDA: The Ayurvedic herbs *ashwagandha* and *amla* are reputed to stimulate hair growth. Apply warm *bhringaraj* oil or *brahmi* oil to the scalp regularly.

FLOWER ESSENCES: Flower essences for accompanying emotional/mental states. Crab Apple.

HERBS: Massage the scalp nightly with an oil made of one part rosemary oil and two parts almond oil. Internal treatment will depend upon the cause of the hair loss.

HOMEOPATHY: *Sepia, Arnica, Acidum nit.*

JUICE THERAPY: Carrot, beet, spinach, nettle, alfalfa. Add a little onion juice to the vegetable juices.

TOPICAL TREATMENT: • Massage scalp with fingers daily. • Use double-strength herbal sage tea as a hair rinse or apply to scalp every day as a tonic. • Rub vitamin E oil into scalp nightly. • For two nights, rub castor oil into the scalp for ten minutes, then apply a hot damp towel for 30 minutes. Put a plastic shower cap on overnight and wash out the following morning. The next two nights use olive oil, then use wheat germ oil for two nights. Rest one night and repeat seven-day cycle. • Apple cider vinegar used as a hair rinse may stimulate hair growth.

Professional Care

The following therapies should only be provided by a qualified health professional.

Acupuncture / Cell Therapy / Magnetic Field Therapy / Natural Hormone Replacement Therapy / Naturopathic Medicine

TRADITIONAL CHINESE MEDICINE: Kidney tonics.

HANGOVER

Feelings of discomfort the morning after drinking alcohol in excess the preceding night.

Alternative Treatments

Refer to alternative therapy chapters for more information before evaluating or applying any treatment. Some conditions, including yours, may require a physician's care.

DIET: Avoid bingeing on alcoholic beverages. Eat a piece of dry whole grain bread before drinking or as a remedy afterward. Drink a glass of orange juice or tomato juice the next morning. Since excessive consumption of alcohol tends to cause dehydration, drink several glasses of water before bed and on rising, and preferably with lemon juice, if available.

NUTRITIONAL THERAPY: Before bed, after drinking to excess: • Vitamin B complex • Vitamin C (one gram) • Lipotropic formula (that contains, among other elements, cysteine and folic acid for liver detoxification, and an optional aspirin). If possible, take the formula before bed and repeat first thing in morning.

According to Leon Chaitow, N.D., D.O., supplementation with the amino acid glutamine dramatically reduced the craving for alcohol in nine out of ten patients (2 g daily in divided doses, away from mealtimes).

Self-Care

The following therapies can be undertaken at home under appropriate professional supervision.

Acupressure / Fasting

AROMATHERAPY: Rosemary, rose, fennel

FLOWER ESSENCES: Flower essences for accompanying emotional/mental states. Rescue Remedy® for accompanying stress; Olive for exhaustion, Hornbeam for mental tiredness. Crab Apple.

HERBS: Many commercially available mixtures of bitter herbs may help clear a hangover if taken first thing in the morning or last thing the night before; take ¼ teaspoon of a tincture combination of digestive bitters. Alternatively, combine gentian, mugwort, and dandelion root tinctures and take ¼ teaspoon. An infusion is preferable but extremely bitter. Refer to Addictions chapter for more suggestions.

HOMEOPATHY: *Nux vom., Arsen alb., Aconite, Sulfur, Lachesis*

HYDROTHERAPY: Hot spray/shower followed by cold rinse. Also, since alcohol causes dehydration, drink one quart of water.

Professional Care

The following therapies should only be provided by a qualified health professional.

Environmental Medicine / Magnetic Field Therapy / Naturopathic Medicine / Traditional Chinese Medicine

BODYWORK: Reflexology, Rolfing, shiatsu

OXYGEN THERAPY: Hyperbaric oxygen therapy is anecdotally very effective, but has no scientific proof of its usefulness.

HEAVY METAL TOXICITY

Metals that have no safe amount in the human system, may accumulate within the body (fat cells, central nervous system, bones, glands, and hair), and may have negative health effects. Any level of these toxic metals is not normal. The levels usually need to rise above the established safety ranges to actually manifest in health problems. However, there is individual variation and high normal levels may aggravate one person and not another.

SYMPTOMS: Wide variety of possible symptoms. In general, a harmful (above safety index range) amount of any toxic metal is a stress on the entire body and can manifest in a wide array of seemingly confusing symptoms or in the individual's weakest physical link. Symptoms that manifest depend on the type of metal toxicity, the age of the individual (children are more susceptible to toxic metal damage), the extent of the exposure, and the presence of antagonist/protective elements that inhibit absorption, binding, and effects of the toxic metals. For example, calcium deficiency aggravates lead toxicity, and the more normal levels of calcium in the body act to protect the system against lead toxicity.

The most common heavy metal toxicities are lead, cadmium, mercury, and nickel. Aluminum is not a heavy metal and is absorbed and removed from the body by different mechanisms. All may be associated with a metallic taste in the mouth.

POSSIBLE SIDE EFFECTS OF EACH ARE THE FOLLOWING:

Lead: Poor bone growth and development, learning disabilities, fatigue, poor task performance, irritability, anxiety, high blood pressure, weight loss, increased susceptibility to infection, ringing in the ears, decreased cognitive functioning and concentration and spelling skills, headaches, gastrointestinal problems, constipation, muscle and joint pain, tremors, and overall general decreased immune functioning.

Cadmium: Fatigue, irritability, headaches, high blood pressure, benign (noncancerous) enlargement of the prostate gland, increased risk for cancer, hair loss, learning disabilities, kidney and liver disorders, skin disorders, painful joints, and decreased immune functioning.

Mercury: Cognitive and memory problems, irritability, fatigue, insomnia, gastrointestinal disorders, decreased immune response, irrational behavior, numbness, tingling, muscular weakness, impaired vision and hearing, allergic conditions, asthma, and multiple sclerosis related to dental amalgams.

Nickel: Fatigue, respiratory illnesses, heart conditions, skin rashes, psoriasis, fatigue, and headaches.

Aluminum: Headaches, cognitive problems, learning disabilities, poor bone density (osteoporosis), ringing in the ears, gastrointestinal disorders, colic, hyperactivity in children, and ataxia (an abnormal walking pattern). Its possible role in poor memory or Alzheimer's disease is speculative at this time but also worth noting.

POSSIBLE ROUTES OF EXPOSURE TO AND CONTAMINATION FROM THE ABOVE METALS:

Lead: Cigarette smoke, eating paint that is lead-based (in children, especially in poor housing or older housing), eating and cooking foods in ceramic glazes that are lead-based, leaded gasoline, eating liver that may be contaminated with lead, living in the inner city that may have elevated lead air levels, contaminated water, canned foods (especially fruit in which the lead-soldered cans may leach into the food), certain bone meal supplements, and insecticides.

Cadmium: Cigarette and pipe smoke, instant coffee and tea, nickel-cadmium batteries, contaminated water, some soft drinks, refined grains, fungicides, pesticides, and some plastics.

Mercury: Mercury-based dental amalgam fillings, laxatives that contain calomel, some hemorrhoidal suppositories, inks used by some printers and tattooers, some paints, some cosmetics, and many products that may contain small amounts of mercury such as fabric softeners, wood preservatives, solvents, drugs, and some plastics and contaminated fish.

Nickel: Many pieces of jewelry contain nickel and wearing them next to skin creates some absorption. Some metal cooking utensils have nickel added to them, even stainless steel, which is mostly a problem when cooking acidic foods. Cigarette smoke, hydrogenated fats (as nickel is the catalyst for the reaction to create them), some refined foods, and fertilizers.

Aluminum: Aluminum-containing antacids, many over-the-counter drugs and douches that contain aluminum, aluminum cookware and aluminum foil (especially when preparing and storing acidic foods), antiperspirants, most commercial baking powders, and contaminated water.

ANTAGONIST/PROTECTIVE MINERALS FOR EACH TOXIC METAL:

Lead: Calcium, vitamin C, amino acids (L-lysine, L-cysteine, and L-cystine), iron, zinc

Cadmium: Zinc,[29] vitamin C, amino acids (L-methionine, L-cysteine, and L-lysine)

Mercury: Selenium,[30] vitamin C, amino acids (L-glutathione, L-methionine, L-cysteine, and L-cystine)

Nickel: Iron, zinc, vitamin C

Aluminum: Calcium, magnesium, vitamin B complex, vitamin C

Alternative Treatments

Refer to alternative therapy chapters for more information before evaluating or applying any treatment. Some conditions, including yours, may require a physician's care.

DIET: Whole foods diet with emphasis on apples, applesauce, garlic, onions, beans, seeds, whole grains other than wheat, fresh fruits and vegetables, and lots of filtered water, at least eight glasses a day, throughout the detoxifying process. Fermented products such as yogurt and kefir are also very good.

W. Lee Cowden, M.D., recommends a diet of organic vegetables, fruits, seeds, grains, and nuts. He adds that a small percentage of the population whose ancestors lived in the very northern latitudes cannot tolerate this diet. Symptoms of intolerance would be fatigue, sometimes muscle weakness, difficulty with memory and concentration, and feeling low-grade flu-like symtpoms. If these symptoms occur as a result of the dietary changes, test for urine pH (acid–base balance). If urine is too alkaline, add some organic meats and/or dairy products, if no allergies to dairy are present.

NUTRITIONAL THERAPY: • Detoxification program with vitamin C to bowel tolerance; detox products should contain the amino acids mentioned above • Folic acid • Liver glandular • Protective nutrients as mentioned in previous paragraphs per metal in question • Vitamin B complex • Multivitamin

If metal toxicity and symptoms are severe, detoxification can occur with an intravenous chelation program under a doctor's supervision along with this oral program.

Self-Care

The following therapies can be undertaken at home under appropriate professional supervision.

Fasting

AYURVEDA: *Pancha karma* for seven days, *dashamoola basti*, *yasti madhu vaman, brahmi ghee nasya, shatavari rasayana*,

aloe vera gel (two tablespoons three times a day), *tikta ghee* (½ teaspoon three times a day on an empty stomach).

FLOWER ESSENCES: Flower essences for accompanying emotional/mental states. Rescue Remedy® for accompanying stress; Crab Apple.

JUICE THERAPY: To support liver, kidneys, and skin, use carrot, celery, burdock, beet, garlic, and flaxseed or currant oils.

Professional Care

The following therapies should only be provided by a qualified health professional.

Homeopathy / Naturopathic Medicine / Orthomolecular Medicine / Traditional Chinese Medicine

CHELATION THERAPY: Chelation therapy can be an effective way of clearing the system of accumulated metals. DMSA (dimercaptosuccinic acid) has been shown to be a safe and effective chelating compound for heavy metals.[31]

OXYGEN THERAPY: Ozone therapy in conjunction with intravenous chelation therapy has proven to be effective in treating heavy metal toxicity.

HEMORRHOIDS

Veins in the lining of the anus that have become distended. Internal hemorrhoids are near the beginning of the anus and external hemorrhoids are at the opening of the anus; when they protrude outside the anus they are called prolapsing hemorrhoids.

SYMPTOMS: Bleeding (usually bright red fresh blood that shows up on the toilet paper after wiping), protrusion of tissues, sometimes itching, mucus, discomfort and pain upon evacuating fecal material and sometimes even sitting. Any bleeding should be checked to rule out more serious conditions. Proctoscopy (examination of the rectum through a tube) is needed to rule out cancer or polyps (small growths).

OCCURRENCE: The frequency of hemorrhoid occurrences in both children and adults leads some doctors to consider them normal.

Regular toilet habits of sitting at the same time each day to try to evacuate bowels and to avoid straining is very helpful.

Alternative Treatments

Refer to alternative therapy chapters for more information before evaluating or applying any treatment. Some conditions, including yours, may require a physician's care.

DIET: Whole foods diet with emphasis on high-fiber foods, citrus fruits (including the inner whitish rind), drinking plenty of fluids. Especially good are whole grains such as buckwheat and millet. One tablespoon of cold-processed vegetable oil a day, on food or taken alone. For bleeding hemorrhoids, eat foods rich in vitamin K: alfalfa, kale, dark-green leafy vegetables.

NUTRITIONAL THERAPY: • Vitamin C with bioflavonoids (3-6 g daily of each) and rutin (1 g daily) • Vitamin A (10,000-25,000 IU daily) • Folic acid (400-800 mcg daily) • Vitamin B complex (two times daily) • Essential fatty acids (three to four on empty stomach, on rising and before bed) • Magnesium • Potassium • Zinc, beta carotene, and linseed oil to soften stools.

Consider a bowel cleanse and rejuvenation program, as the anus is the last portion of the intestinal tract, which acts as a barometer of inner health.

Self-Care

The following therapies can be undertaken at home under appropriate professional supervision.

Fasting / Guided Imagery / Qigong and Tai Chi / Yoga

AROMATHERAPY: Cypress, juniper, frankincense, niaouli.

AYURVEDA: • Drink ½ cup of aloe vera juice three times daily until condition has cleared. • The Ayurvedic compound *triphala* is recommended for hemorrhoids. • A confection of one part sesame seeds (black seeds if possible), ½ part *shatavari* (if available); add ginger and raw sugar to taste. Take one ounce daily. • *Triphala guggulu* (200 mg), generally taken twice a day after lunch and dinner. Local application of castor oil for *vata* type, *tikta ghee* for *pitta* type.

FLOWER ESSENCES: Rescue Remedy® for accompanying stress. Rescue Remedy Cream® for external hemorrhoids, at least four times a day. Crab Apple.

HERBS: In Europe, there is nothing to match the aptly named pilewort. The North American equivalent is collinsonia. Combine the tinctures of collinsonia, cranesbill, and ginkgo in equal parts and take one teaspoon of this mixture three times a day. A topical application is used to alleviate the symptoms and compliment the internal treatment. Mix 10 ml of collinsonia tincture with 80 ml of distilled witch hazel and apply this combination after every bowel motion and as needed. Salves may also be used containing herbs such as calendula, St. John's wort, aloe, or plantain. Other useful herbs include bilberry, buckthorn bark, butcher's broom, comfrey root (poultice), gotu kola, horse chestnut (topical), parsley, passionflower, and stone root.

HOMEOPATHY: *Aloe, Hamamelis, Nux vom., Berberis, Acidum fluor., Thuja*

HYDROTHERAPY: Warm sitz bath applied daily, follow with a short cold bath.

JUICE THERAPY: • Carrot, parsley • Carrot, spinach • Carrot, spinach, celery, parsley • Carrot, watercress • Beets, if they don't speed up the gastrointestinal tract.

TOPICAL TREATMENT: • Epsom salts packs • Apply a combination of zinc oxide, vitamin E, and aloe vera gel or olive oil to affected area. • Apply witch hazel frequently to hemorrhoids to shrink blood vessels. • Calendula oint-

ment for pain and itching • Use a peeled garlic clove as a suppository for hemorrhoids.

REFLEXOLOGY: Diaphragm, adrenals, rectum, sigmoid, lower spine; also chronic area up the back of the heel.

Professional Care

The following therapies should only be provided by a qualified health professional.

Acupuncture / Applied Kinesiology / Light Therapy / Magnetic Field Therapy / Naturopathic Medicine / Osteopathic Medicine / Prolotherapy

BODY WORK: Myotherapy

DETOXIFICATION THERAPY: May be indicated, as hemorrhoids are usually caused by a congestive disorder—constipation, liver problems, etc.

OXYGEN THERAPY: • Ozone intestinal insufflation • Ozonated olive oil.

HEPATITIS

Inflammation of the liver that is associated with damage or death of liver cells. There is acute hepatitis (attack that eventually heals) or chronic (ongoing liver problems).

SYMPTOMS: In early stages, there is usually loss of appetite, fatigue, weight loss, fever, nausea, and vomiting. Extreme fatigue is a key sign. Rashes and pain in the joints may occur. In three to ten days, dark urine may manifest, and this may be followed by the skin turning yellow (jaundice). Jaundice usually takes one to two weeks to build up and then two to four weeks to fade. The liver is usually enlarged and tender to the touch. However, symptoms can range from mild flu-like symptoms to severe liver failure and brain coma.

OCCURRENCE: Twenty to 30 cases per 100,000 people in the United States.

SPECIAL NOTES: The most common cause is contamination with a virus, Type A or Type B, non-A or non-B. There can be other causes that lead to hepatitis, such as excessive alcohol consumption, drug abuse (including pharmaceuticals, such as acetaminophen), overexposure to certain chemicals (such as dry-cleaning fluids), and as a rare reaction to normal levels of therapeutic drugs.

The American Liver Foundation identifies five different viruses (termed A, B, C, D, and E) that cause hepatitis. Type C is a frequent cause of post-transfusion hepatitis. Recently, a test has been developed that can identify individuals infected with the hepatitis C virus. In general, individuals with the hepatitis C virus are identified either because they have abnormal liver tests or because a hepatitis C antibody test was obtained when they went to donate blood.

A positive test does not mean that you have a serious form of liver disease. Individuals infected with the hepatitis C may have no liver disease, a mild form of hepatitis (chronic persistent), or a more serious form of hepatitis (chronic active) that may progress over a number of years to cirrhosis. The usual indications for treatment are a positive antibody test for the hepatitis C virus, abnormal liver tests for more than six to 12 months, and a liver biopsy that shows chronic active hepatitis. Estimates are that approximately 20% of patients chronically infected with the hepatitis C virus will go on to develop cirrhosis.

Infectious hepatitis can spread easily the two weeks before and one week after jaundice appears. The feces contains the virus and so very strict toilet hygiene and hand and cloth washing should be observed during this time.

Alternative Treatments

Refer to alternative therapy chapters for more information before evaluating or applying any treatment. Some conditions, including yours, may require a physician's care.

DIET: Jonathan Wright, M.D., recommends a diet low in protein to minimize stress on the liver. Whole foods diet that follows a hypoglycemic regime and consisting of small meals throughout the day, avoiding stressor foods such as refined sugars, alcohol, and caffeine. Consume plenty of filtered water. Drinking fresh lemon juice in water every morning and evening, followed by vegetable juice, is therapeutic for the liver. Do this consistently for two to four weeks and then several mornings a week for several months and whenever liver symptoms reoccur. Have lots of vegetables each day, at least one salad and one meal of steamed or lightly sauteed vegetables per day. Grains that are easily digestible, such as millet, buckwheat, and quinoa, are very good.

NUTRITIONAL THERAPY: • Vitamin C (up to bowel tolerance to support the liver) • Beta carotene (100,000 IU daily for two weeks, then reduce to 25,000-50,000 IU) • Liver glandulars (three to four times daily) • Milk thistle extract • Vitamin B complex • Adrenal glandulars • Lipotropic factors • Pantothenic acid • Protein (free-form amino acids) • Betaine hydrochloric acid (HCl) • Multi-enzymes • If needed, multiminerals • Evening primrose oil

Self-Care

The following therapies can be undertaken at home under appropriate professional supervision.

Fasting / Guided Imagery / Qigong and Tai Chi

AROMATHERAPY: Rosemary

AYURVEDA: *Acute hepatitis:* Avoid hot, sour, spicy, and salty foods, meat, fish, cheese, oils, fried foods, and concentrated sweets. Try a mono-diet of mung beans for one week to strengthen the liver. Add basmati rice and liver-cleansing spices such as coriander and turmeric. Rest completely and avoid vigorous exercise. *Chronic hepatitis:* Take tonics such as aloe gel, *shatavari,* and the formula *Chyavan prash. Hepatitis B:* An herbal mixture of *kutki* (200 mg), *guduchi* (300 mg), and *shanka pushpi* (400 mg), generally taken twice a day after lunch and dinner. For

all types, fresh sugarcane juice, one cup three times a day. One-half cup fresh homemade yogurt with a pinch of baking soda twice a day and *brahmi ghee nasya.*

ENEMAS: • Three warm enemas daily • Chlorophyll enema (one pint for 15 minutes)

HERBS: As a range of pathologies are potentially present, competent diagnosis is essential. The liver-cell regenerative properties of herbs such as milk thistle and licorice can be helpful. Combine the glycerates of milk thistle, dandelion root, licorice, and wahoo in equal parts and take ½ teaspoon of this mixture three times a day. The wahoo can be replaced by fringetree bark. Refer to Cirrhosis for more dosage information on milk thistle.

Encouraging results were found in a preliminary study in which carriers of hepatitis B virus were treated with a preparation from the plant *Phyllanthus amarus* for 30 days. Fifty-nine percent of those treated had lost the hepatitis B antigen when tested 15-20 days after treatment and few or no toxic side effects were reported. *Phyllanthus amarus* has centuries of documented use in Ayurveda and may be a breakthrough in treatment of hepatitis B when used in conjunction with turmeric and milk thistle.[32]

HYDROTHERAPY: Constitutional hydrotherapy (apply two to five times weekly). For acute infectious hepatitis, alternate hot compress (one minute) and cold compress (five minutes) over the liver for one hour; repeat three times a day. For chronic hepatitis, place a cold compress on the liver every night for a few weeks; then, reduce to one week per month for six months.

JUICE THERAPY: • Short juice fast using beet, carrot, and wheat grass juices • Garlic, burdock, flax, black currants

Professional Care

The following therapies should only be provided by a qualified health professional.

Cell Therapy / Magnetic Field Therapy / Naturopathic Medicine

OXYGEN THERAPY: Ozone autohemotherapy (treatment by reinjection of the individual's own blood) has been shown to reduce viral load and normalize liver enzymes in hepatitis B and C.

DETOXIFICATION THERAPY: Depending on the condition of the person.

HIATAL HERNIA

Hiatal hernia is a disorder caused when the opening in the diaphragm where the stomach and esophagus meet becomes stretched, allowing the upper end of the stomach to push up into the chest cavity. The esophageal sphincter, which normally acts as a one-way valve to allow food to travel down into the stomach, is unable to prevent the contents of the stomach, including gastric acids, from traveling upward.

SYMPTOMS: Most people have no symptoms. Sometimes there is chest pain or heartburn. The heartburn can be worse on bending over, especially after eating, worse at night, or worse when lying down. Sometimes the pain of hiatal hernia can mimic other health problems such as stomach ulcers or heart attacks.

OCCURRENCE: More frequently in people who are over-weight or who smoke, and sometimes occurs in new-borns.

SPECIAL NOTES: Sometimes in association with a hiatal hernia there is some material from the stomach that gets pushed upward into the esophagus. This is called esophageal reflux and may cause the heartburn.

According to Leon Chaitow, N.D., D.O., there is a mechanical aspect to hiatal hernia, which can involve extreme tension in two large muscles that merge with the diaphragm—the psoas and quadratus lumborum. If either of these is chronically tense (very common), a stress will be imposed on the diaphragm that can result in the hernia. Osteopathic techniques can be applied to nor-malize these muscles.

Alternative Treatments

Refer to alternative therapy chapters for more information before evaluating or applying any treatment. Some conditions, includ-ing yours, may require a physician's care.

DIET: Strictly avoid overeating. Observe eating the fol-lowing to see if they aggravate the problem and, if so, avoid: spicy foods, fried foods, coffee, tea, carbonated drinks, citrus juices, alcohol, whipped cream, milk shakes, peppermint, green and red peppers, and onion. Avoid eating large meals and then lying down or bending over. Avoid drinking too much with meals or after dinner-time. Eat numerous small meals throughout the day. Try to reduce stress by eating in pleasant, relaxing settings. Avoid eating foods or food combinations that cause excess gas formation. Eat sufficient fiber.

NUTRITIONAL THERAPY: • Digestive enzymes if needed (pancreatin and hydrochloric acid) • Vitamin B complex (one teaspoon of liquid chlorophyll at dinner for two weeks) • Aloe vera juice • Multivitamin/mineral formula

Self-Care

The following therapies can be undertaken at home under appro-priate professional supervision.

Biofeedback Training and Neurotherapy / Fasting

BREATHING EXERCISES: Deep breathing exercises to strengthen the muscles of the diaphragm and to expand the lungs. According to Dr. Chaitow, many people with hiatal hernia have breathing restrictions and have a habit of swallowing air more frequently than the average. This leads to excessive air reaching the stomach, putting great stress on the diaphragmatic aperture through which the esophagus passes, exacerbating hiatal hernia problems. Breathing retraining and behavior modification meth-ods can be used to help slow down the rate of swallow-ing air to more normal levels.

EXERCISES AND LIFESTYLE HINTS: • Sit in an armchair and breathe in and hold your breath. Lift legs up toward your chest, lower, and then exhale. Repeat several times. For shortness of breath or food lodged in the esophagus, drink two 8-ounce glasses of water and bounce on your heels 12 times. • Sleep with your upper body in an ele-vated position to keep the chest cavity above the stom-ach. This will prevent the stomach from rising into the chest cavity. Put blocks under the head of the bed (four to eight inches high) or sleep with a wedge-shaped bolster.

HERBS: The main herbal goal is to reduce the inflam-mation and symptoms of reflux. Make an infusion with equal parts of comfrey root, marshmallow root, and meadowsweet and drink this often during the day. Have a cup last thing at night, keeping some by the bed to sip, if needed.

HOMEOPATHY: *Calc carb., Hepar sulph., Ferrum phos.*

HYDROTHERAPY: Contrast application (apply to abdomen daily).

REFLEXOLOGY: Diaphragm, stomach, adrenals

Professional Care

The following therapies should only be provided by a qualified health professional.

Applied Kinesiology / Chiropractic / Magnetic Field Therapy / Naturopathic Medicine / Traditional Chinese Medicine

DETOXIFICATION THERAPY: May be indicated, includ-ing diet changes and cleansing programs.

OSTEOPATHY: Osteopathic muscle energy techniques to normalize tight postural muscles if these are involved.

HICCUPS

A sound, sometimes called a hiccough, made by the vocal cords closing in response to the diaphragm suddenly contracting. A cluster of these is called an attack of the hiccups. This is extremely common and not serious.

SYMPTOMS: Hiccup sounds vary from person to person.

SPECIAL NOTES: Prolonged hiccup attacks that do not go away are very rare and require medication or surgery as they cause severe exhaustion.

There are numerous folk remedies to "cure" hiccups and their effectiveness varies from person to person.

Alternative Treatments

Refer to alternative therapy chapters for more information before evaluating or applying any treatment. Some conditions, includ-ing yours, may require a physician's care.

DIET: Chew a piece of dry or charred toast, very slowly. Sip a glass of water while walking slowly but continu-ously, until hiccups stop.

NUTRITION: Chew charcoal tablets or chewable papaya enzymes. Continue chewing tablets at least once an hour or, in extreme cases, continuously.

Self–Care

The following therapies can be undertaken at home under appropriate professional supervision.

Biofeedback Training and Neurotherapy / Fasting

ACUPRESSURE: Place your middle and index fingers behind each earlobe. Apply light to firm pressure on these tender points, TW17 and SI17 (for an illustration of these points see the acupressure chart in the introduction to this section), for two minutes as you concentrate on breathing slowly and deeply.

AYURVEDA: • Mix honey (two parts) and castor oil (one part); take one teaspoon. • A pinch of *mayur chandrika bhasma* with ½ teaspoon honey. Alternate nostril breathing with inner retention (see Yoga chapter).

BODYWORK: Massage any painful areas around vertebrae at level of diaphragm.

FLOWER ESSENCES: Rescue Remedy® for accompanying stress. Flower essences for accompanying emotional/mental states.

HERBS: Combine the tinctures of black cohosh, skullcap, and vervain and take ten drops of this mixture in a little hot water. Alternatively, sip a warm infusion of chamomile tea.

HOMEOPATHY: *Nux vom., Mag phos., Ignatia, Lycopodium, Ginseng, Acidum sulf.*

JUICE THERAPY: Remember to chew your juices (swish around before swallowing).

REFLEXOLOGY: Diaphragm, stomach

Professional Care

The following therapies should only be provided by a qualified health professional.

Chiropractic / Environmental Medicine / Hypnotherapy / Magnetic Field Therapy / Naturopathic Medicine / Osteopathic Medicine

BODYWORK: Reflexology

TRADITIONAL CHINESE MEDICINE: Especially effective if the hiccups have lasted for days.

HIVES (URTICARIA)

A skin condition characterized by itchy wheals (raised white bumps surrounded by a reddish area).

SYMPTOMS: Rashes of wheals typically appear on the arms, legs, or trunk, but can appear anywhere on the body. Wheals usually last for several hours.

SPECIAL NOTES: Most common cause is a histamine reaction due to allergies, especially to certain foods, such as strawberries, shellfish, peanuts, milk, and eggs, and some-times to drugs such as penicillin or to chemicals such as laundry soap.

Alternative Treatments

Refer to alternative therapy chapters for more information before evaluating or applying any treatment. Some conditions, including yours, may require a physician's care.

DIET: Identify allergenic foods and avoid. Most common offending foods are berries, fish (sometimes even just the fumes are sufficient to create an allergic episode), soy, beef, citrus, and peanuts. Usually, if there are some foods that cause this allergic reaction, there are other foods that constantly "stress" the system but with more subtle and confusing symptoms. Eat a varied diet without repeating foods in excess, especially any food suspected of causing an allergic reaction.

Hydrochloric acid secretions in the stomach are found to be low in most people with hives, which seems to relate to the B complex vitamin deficiency also commonly observed in these patients.

NUTRITIONAL THERAPY: • Pancreatic enzymes (four times daily on empty stomach during initial attack) • Bromelain and vitamin C taken away from meals (three to four times per day) • Vitamin B complex (two to four times daily with lots of water, then reduce to two times daily within two to three days)

Sometimes two bicarbonate tablets (such as Alka-Seltzer Gold) in water sipped every 15 minutes for one to two hours is also helpful.

After an attack, on daily prevention basis take: • Bioflavonoids and pantothenic acid (1-2 g) • Vitamin B complex • Essential fatty acids • Vitamin B6 • Practice a varied whole foods diet.

Alan R. Gaby, M.D., has found that acute or chronic hives respond well to an intravenous injection of a "cocktail" composed of magnesium chloride hexahydrate, calcium glycerophosphate, hydroxocobalamin, pyridoxine hydrochloride, dexpanthenol, B complex, and vitamin C. This is a modification of the nutrient cocktail popularized by John Meyers, M.D.

TOPICAL TREATMENT: Apply a mix of calamine lotion with beta carotene liquid. Or a vitamin A capsule squeezed together with some zinc oxide ointment can be placed over the affected area. If you do not have calamine liquid, try using unflavored yogurt.

Self–Care

The following therapies can be undertaken at home under appropriate professional supervision.

Biofeedback Training and Neurotherapy / Enemas / Fasting / Guided Imagery / Qigong and Tai Chi

AROMATHERAPY: Chamomile, tagetes

FLOWER ESSENCES: Flower essences for accompanying emotional/mental states. Rescue Remedy Cream®

HERBS: Parsley, peppermint oil

HOMEOPATHY: *Apis mel., Nat mur., Urtica urens*

HYDROTHERAPY: Add oatmeal to bath.

LIGHT THERAPY: For chronic urticaria, ultraviolet light therapy.

TOPICAL TREATMENT: Fresh coriander juice applied externally for itch and inflammation.

Professional Care

The following therapies should only be provided by a qualified health professional.

Acupuncture / Applied Kinesiology / Environmental Medicine / Light Therapy / Magnetic Field Therapy / Natural Hormone Replacement Therapy / Naturopathic Medicine / Neural Therapy / Orthomolecular Medicine / Osteopathic Medicine / Traditional Chinese Medicine

DETOXIFICATION THERAPY: Not indicated, unless to control the allergic state.

OXYGEN THERAPY: Hydrogen peroxide therapy (IV).

HYPERTHYROIDISM

Overproduction of thyroid hormone by the thyroid gland.

SYMPTOMS: Rapid heartbeat, enlarged thyroid (goiter), moist skin, trembling (tremors), widened pulse pressure (lower- and higher-end numbers), fatigue, anxiety, weight loss, bulging eyes, excessive sweating, increased appetite, extremely low tolerance to heat, diarrhea, chest pain, and gastrointestinal disturbances. In older persons with this condition, the symptoms may be the opposite.

OCCURRENCE: Much more rare than underactive thyroid (hypothyroidism).

SPECIAL NOTES: Hyperthyroidism may be associated with and often is called Graves' disease (toxic diffuse goiter)—hyperthyroidism combined with enlarged thyroid, eyes that bulge, rash and swelling in front of the lower leg that may appear before or after the condition, or thyrotoxicosis.

The thyroid is a "master" gland, meaning that it is influential on the overall health of the body. The thyroid gland sits at the base of the neck and consists of two lobes, one on each side of the windpipe (trachea). It combines and concentrates iodine with tyrosine into active thyroid hormone. These reactions are controlled and influenced by the pituitary gland. The thyroid gland has many physiologic effects on all the cells of the body. The two major ones are to help form protein RNA (building blocks of life) for every cell and to increase oxygen consumption by most cells. Thus, the thyroid greatly affects overall body metabolism.

Alternative Treatments

Refer to alternative therapy chapters for more information before evaluating or applying any treatment. Some conditions, including yours, may require a physician's care.

DIET: Whole foods diet. Eat foods that naturally and gently suppress thyroid hormone production (broccoli, Brussels sprouts, cabbage, cauliflower, kale, mustard greens, rutabagas, spinach, turnips, soybeans, peaches, and pears). Avoid dairy products, excessive and repetitive consumption of wheat products, coffee, tea, and caffeinated soft drinks.

NUTRITIONAL THERAPY: • Must see a qualified practitioner or orthomolecular physician. • High dosages of vitamin A and choline (under a doctor's supervision) • Vitamin B complex with extra thiamin (vitamin B_1) and amino acid supplements, three times daily as increased metabolism raises demand • Multivitamin/mineral complex • Vitamin C • Iodine or kelp • Calcium • Magnesium

Self-Care

The following therapies can be undertaken at home under appropriate professional supervision.

Biofeedback Training and Neurotherapy / Qigong and Tai Chi

HYDROTHERAPY: Ice packs (apply repeatedly as needed to reduce thyroid function).

JUICE THERAPY: • Carrot, celery, spinach, parsley • Cabbage, watercress, and spinach

Professional Care

The following therapies should only be provided by a qualified health professional.

Magnetic Field Therapy / Naturopathic Medicine / Traditional Chinese Medicine

HOMEOPATHY: *Thyroidinum.*

HYPOGLYCEMIA

An abnormally low level of blood sugar (glucose) or abnormal fluctuations of blood sugar levels, secondary to an oversecretion of insulin by the pancreas (insulin helps clear blood of glucose).

SYMPTOMS: Symptoms may vary from mild to severe, from occasional to after almost every meal. They include anxiety, weakness, sweating, rapid heart rate, extreme hunger, dizziness, poor or double vision, headache, irritability, irrational behavior, problems with memory, cognitive focus, and learning, and digestive problems. Most common time for symptoms to occur is in the afternoon, around 2 p.m. to 3 p.m. The symptoms of hypoglycemia mimic many other health problems. It may be that the symptoms are only similar but unrelated; however, it may be that hypoglycemia is coexisting with these other conditions or is occurring secondary to these other health problems.

OCCURRENCE: Classic hypoglycemia, the only type recognized by allopathic medicine, occurs in people with insulin-dependent diabetes mellitus. However, in the alternative and orthomolecular fields, hypoglycemia is considered a well-established condition that occurs during the early stages of adrenal stress and blood sugar imbalance problems. It is associated with many other conditions than diabetes, can exist by itself, and may be the early stages of pancreatic and diabetic problems.

CONSIDER: Excess consumption of simple sugars and refined carbohydrates, food allergies, low thyroid function, nutrient deficiencies (especially those that increase insulin sensitivity, such as vitamin B6, chromium, zinc, essential fatty acids, and amino acids such as alanine), excessive exercise, stress, missing meals or irregular eating habits, excessive alcohol, drug, or cigarette consumption, poor protein digestion, insufficient protein, poor digestion due to other factors, low digestive enzymes, and an excessively refined and processed diet.

SPECIAL NOTES: Causes of hypoglycemia may be abnormal fluctuations of glucose and insulin and perhaps even abnormal reaction to normal fluctuations of glucose and insulin. These fluctuations or reactions may be secondary to many other factors, such as food allergies, lifestyle influences, nutrient levels, hereditary predisposition, etc. There is much controversy as to exactly what causes hypoglycemia, what it is, who gets it, why they get it, and what to do.

Cigarette smoking greatly aggravates the stability of blood sugar. So does skipping breakfast, drinking more caffeinated beverages in the morning than is healthy for the body's pancreatic and adrenal response, and eating a diet low in fiber and high in sugar. All these morning activities may create periods of low blood sugar in the mid-to-late afternoon and are the most common cause of fatigue, poor concentration, and irritability at this time.

Alternative Treatments

Refer to alternative therapy chapters for more information before evaluating or applying any treatment. Some conditions, including yours, may require a physician's care.

DIET: Smaller, more frequent meals (five to six) throughout the day to help keep blood glucose levels up and to help heal the pancreas and adrenals. Whole foods diet low in stressor foods such as caffeine, refined sugars, and alcohol. Focus on whole grains, seeds, nuts, fermented dairy products, and lean meats and fish. If you cannot eat frequently enough, carry around raw seeds and nuts mixed with dried fruits (or roasted tamarind nuts for flavor) and munch these. Or try carrying some nut butter to eat on crackers. Identify and avoid food allergies. Avoid processed foods, dehydrated powders, and white flour products.

Eating high amounts of fiber helps stabilize the possible fluctuations in the blood sugar. Thus, if you are having a hypoglycemic attack, take some high-fiber food with a small glass of fruit juice immediately. Eating some fiber, such as a whole grain cracker or a few bites of brown rice, 30 minutes before meals with a few amino acid tablets will often calm down reactions that tend to occur after eating.

NUTRITION: • Chromium is vital in glucose metabolism (100 mcg three times daily) • Niacinamide • Pantothenic acid • Adrenal glandular •Vitamin C with bioflavonoids • Vitamin B complex • Vitamin B6 • Amino acids • Calcium and magnesium • Multiple trace minerals • Zinc is necessary for the proper production and utilization of insulin; copper and zinc levels must be maintained in relationship, because an excess of one produces a deficiency of the other.

If due to malabsorption, take hydrochloric acid (HCl) and/or digestive enzymes. •Vitamin B injections may be helpful; see an orthomolecular physician.

Self-Care

The following therapies can be undertaken at home under appropriate professional supervision.

Biofeedback Training and Neurotherapy / Qigong and Tai Chi

HERBS: Licorice, burdock, dandelion

HYDROTHERAPY: Constitutional hydrotherapy (apply two to five times weekly).

JUICE THERAPY: If reactive, then dilute all juices—carrot, beet with burdock, Jerusalem artichoke, garlic.

REFLEXOLOGY: Pancreas, all glands, liver

Professional Care

The following therapies should only be provided by a qualified health professional.

Applied Kinesiology / Chiropractic / Magnetic Field Therapy / Natural Hormone Replacement Therapy / Naturopathic Medicine / Orthomolecular Medicine / Traditional Chinese Medicine

ENVIRONMENTAL MEDICINE: According to Marshall Mandell, M.D., hypoglycemia is a commonly made misdiagnosis that can be applied to addictive food allergies. The withdrawal symptoms from a recent exposure to an addicting food are relieved by eating that particular food. On the surface, it would seem that the relieving food has caused an increased level of blood sugar, but this is not so. The prompt relief is actually the result of an exposure to an addicting substance that relieves the withdrawal symptoms it was causing.

It takes 45-60 minutes for a protein food, such as chicken, beef, nuts, or cheese, to be broken down into amino acids, with the remaining portion converted into liver starch (glycogen). The glycogen is then broken down and released from the liver as blood sugar or glucose. The fact that protein foods can very rapidly give relief of "hypoglycemic" symptoms within 5-10 minutes suggests that the mere introduction of these proteins into the body will eliminate symptoms that cannot be related to blood sugar levels, because there simply isn't enough time for the conversion to have taken place.

FASTING: In this condition, the transition phase from beginning a fast to a state of health could be rougher than in other conditions. If juice fasting, dilute juices; if water fasting, see a physician.

OSTEOPATHY: According to Michael Lesser, N.D., D.O., chronic muscular tensions brought about by stress throughout the body, particularly in the spinal regions, are a prime cause of hypoglycemia. When tense, these tissues are burning fuel at a high rate, creating a constant requirement for glucose, which the person may try to meet through sugar-rich snacks and stimulants.[33]

HYPOTHYROIDISM

Insufficient thyroid hormone, either by decreased production or increased breakdown.

SYMPTOMS: Fatigue, weight gain, slowed heart rate, constipation, irritability, sensitivity to cold, mental depression, slowness or slurring of speech, drooping and swollen eyes, swollen face, recurrent infections, increase in allergic reactions, headaches, hair loss, brittleness of hair, female problems (such as heavy menstrual flow, painful periods, and premenstrual tension), decreased immune functioning, and calcium metabolism problems. In childhood, hypothyroidism can cause a retardation of normal growth and development.

OCCURRENCE: This is a very common health problem. Hypothyroidism is recognized by medical doctors. However, unusual cases of hypothyroidism, such as borderline cases of underactive thyroid or individuals who have normal laboratory levels of thyroid hormone but in their case respond best and function optimally when supplemented with thyroid nutrients, are often unrecognized. Thus, they often go untreated. Undiagnosed thyroid problems can be the underlying cause in many reoccurring or nonresponsive health problems.

CONSIDER: Food allergies, deficiencies of B vitamins, iron, or digestive enzymes, liver disease, hormone imbalances, or parasites.

SPECIAL NOTES: In Hashimoto's disease, the body becomes allergic to its thyroid gland and forms antibodies against it, causing low thyroid.

Home thyroid test: Keep a thermometer by the bedside. In the morning before arising, lie still and put the thermometer under the armpit and hold it there for 15 minutes. A temperature below 97.5° F may indicate a problem with the thyroid gland. Take the temperature in this manner for three days, except for the first few days of the menstrual cycle and the middle day of the cycle, and calculate the average temperature. If it is consistently low, low thyroid may be a problem. The lower the temperature, the greater the degree of hypothyroidism.

Alternative Treatments

Refer to alternative therapy chapters for more information before evaluating or applying any treatment. Some conditions, including yours, may require a physician's care.

DIET: Consume foods that are naturally high in iodine such as fish, kelp, vegetables, and root vegetables (such as potatoes). Avoid foods that naturally slow the functioning of the thyroid such as cabbage, Brussels sprouts, mustard greens, broccoli, turnips, kale, spinach, peaches, and pears. Avoid sulfa drugs and antihistamines, which aggravate this problem. If you are on thyroid medication, increase calcium supplementation, as studies show that the drug increases bone loss significantly. Also, increase daily consumption of foods high in vitamin B complex, such as whole grains and raw nuts and seeds, and foods rich in vitamin A, such as dark green and yellow vegetables, avoiding repetitive consumption of the ones mentioned above.

NUTRITIONAL THERAPY: • An organic thyroid glandular extract, given under the supervision of a doctor, can help restore normal thyroid function. • Tyrosine (an amino acid) • Iodine • Vitamin B • Calcium/magnesium • Essential fatty acids • Vitamin A • Zinc • Kelp is one of the best natural sources of iodine.

Self-Care

The following therapies can be undertaken at home under appropriate professional supervision.

Biofeedback Training and Neurotherapy / Fasting / Qigong and Tai Chi / Yoga

HERBS: Mild cases sometimes respond to herbal bitters such as gentian or mugwort. Kelp has been used in the past, but is only specifically helpful where an iodine deficiency is present. Associated constipation may be alleviated with yellowdock, butternut, or cascara sagrada. The antidepressant herb St. John's wort can be helpful.

HOMEOPATHY: *Calc carb.* 1M is effective in treating hypothyroidism and improving thyroid function.

HYDROTHERAPY: Contrast application (apply daily to stimulate thyroid function).

JUICE THERAPY: Never juice raw cabbage, broccoli, kale, cauliflower.

LIFESTYLE: Aerobic exercise is important.

NATUROPATHIC MEDICINE: A commonly unrecognized cause of hypothyroidism is excessive consumption of foods from the brassica (cabbage) family. A component of the cabbage binds to iodine, making it unavailable to the thyroid gland for thyroid hormone production. Half a head of cabbage or the equivalent amount of broccoli, Brussels sprouts, etc., can be as effective in binding iodine as the medical drug thiouracil used to treat hyperthyroidism, according to Joseph Pizzorno, N.D.

Professional Care

The following therapies should only be provided by a qualified health professional.

Acupuncture / Cell Therapy / Magnetic Field Therapy / Naturopathic Medicine / Osteopathic Medicine / Traditional Chinese Medicine

DETOXIFICATION THERAPY: Helping the liver to detoxify toxins and excess hormones promotes thyroid hormonal balance.

ENVIRONMENTAL MEDICINE: According to Marshall Mandell, M.D., hypothyroidism has been associated with the presence of allergies and correcting the underactive thyroid has been helpful to varying degrees.

HOMEOPATHY: *Iodum.* Consult a physician.

INFECTION

Growth of disease-causing organisms (bacteria, viruses, fungi) anywhere in the body. The organisms grow in colonies that are invasive and multiply. They can damage cells through a variety of routes, such as directly, through release of toxins, or through allergic reaction. Many of the symptoms of the infection are usually a result of the immune system mounting a response to these foreign colonies.

SYMPTOMS: Redness, inflammation, pain, swelling, and formation of a pus-filled pocket (abscess) at the site of the infection. If fever and painful joints occur, this may be a sign of an infectious disease that is spreading throughout the body and a doctor must be seen at once.

Alternative Treatments

Refer to alternative therapy chapters for more information before evaluating or applying any treatment. Some conditions, including yours, may require a physician's care.

DIET: Increase dietary garlic and unflavored yogurt. Increase diluted orange juice, apples and apple juice, grapes and grape juice, cranberries, blueberries, strawberries, raspberries, peaches, plums, figs, cabbage, onion, kelp, and raw honey. During infection and recovery time, avoid refined sugar as this may depress natural immune response. Drink plenty of filtered water.

NUTRITIONAL THERAPY: According to Garry Gordon, M.D., the following can be effectively used as an antibiotic replacement, particularly if used at the first sign of any cold or flu or other infectious process: vitamin A (400,000 IU daily for five days), liquid garlic extract (up to two 4-ounce bottles a day) or the equivalent in high-quality garlic in capsules or tablets, and vitamin C to bowel tolerance (see Orthomolecular Medicine chapter). This protocol is to be used only under a physician's guidance. The dosages are for an average 175-pound adult and should be scaled down proportionately according to weight. The vitamin A should be taken for a period of at least three days, but no more than five days. Caution: Vitamin A at such high doses can cause headaches in about 1% of those using it. Should this occur, either decrease the dose or use a natural remedy like feverfew or a homeopathic remedy for headaches.

Essential fatty acids (EFAs) found in the oil of linseed, evening primrose, and certain fish, among other sources, also have antibacterial properties. Bromelain, an enzyme compound found in the pineapple plant, is an anti-inflammatory and has been shown to be as effective as antibiotics in treating pneumonia, bronchitis, kidney infection, and staph infection of the skin, among other infections.[34]

Alan R. Gaby, M.D., has found that acute infections respond well to an intravenous injection of a "cocktail" composed of magnesium chloride hexahydrate, calcium glycerophosphate, hydroxocobalamin, pyridoxine hydrochloride (vitamin B6), dexpanthenol, B complex, and vitamin C. This is a modification of the nutrient cocktail popularized by John Meyers, M.D.

Self-Care

The following therapies can be undertaken at home under appropriate professional supervision.

Guided Imagery

AROMATHERAPY: For fungicidal infections, use cedarwood. For infected wounds, use frankincense, tea tree, patchouli.

FASTING: Leon Chaitow, N.D., D.O., suggests a water-only fast for 24-36 hours at the onset of any infection, as it has a dramatic effect on the immune system, enhancing natural killer cells and other defensive immune activity. This is only true if the fast is a water-only regime. Caution: This is not appropriate for the very frail or very

---

BE CAREFUL WITH ANTIBIOTICS

When used appropriately, antibiotics are effective for serious or life-threatening bacterial infections. Their indiscriminate use, however, is ill-advised. First, although they are often prescribed for such conditions, antibiotics do not work against viruses or inflammatory conditions. Second, they kill not only harmful bacteria, but also beneficial bacteria in the gastrointestinal tract, which can lead to digestive and intestinal problems (notably *Candida albicans* yeast overgrowth) if not remedied. Third, indiscriminate use of antibiotics has produced multiple-drug-resistant bacterial strains and is in danger of rendering antibiotics ineffective against life-threatening infections.

If you suspect you have a bacterial infection, ask your doctor to take a culture of saliva or tissues and fluids from the infected area. If it is a bacterial infection, samples of different antibiotics can be placed in the growing cultures to determine which will be the most effective in killing that specific bacteria; this is called a sensitivity test. If you do take antibiotics, be sure to supplement with acidophilus during and after the course of treatment.

young unless supervised by an expert in these methods, such as a naturopathic or alternative physician.

FLOWER ESSENCES: Flower essences for accompanying emotional/mental states. Crab Apple; Rescue Remedy®. Rescue Remedy Cream® on unbroken skin.

HERBS: Herbs such as echinacea, goldenseal, and garlic can prevent and treat infection. In small amounts taken regularly, they boost resistance; larger doses combat specific infections. Berberine, an alkaloid component of certain plants, notably goldenseal, Oregon grape, and barberry, is a strong antimicrobial.[35] Goldenseal is one of nature's most potent antibiotics that also stimulates immune response. Its effects have been demonstrated against *Staphylococcus*, *Streptococcus*, *E. coli*, and *Mycobacterium tuberculosis*, among others.[36]

Echinacea can be taken internally as a tea or used externally as a poultice or wash on infectious sores. Echinacea has a broad spectrum of beneficial effects on the immune system, and has proven effective in treating infections in general, including colds, flu, upper respiratory infections, and urinary tract and genital infections.[37]

Stress must be treated as it has a direct impact on immunity. In addition to working with a stress management program, use adaptogenic herbs such as Siberian ginseng. Also, select the appropriate herb(s) most suited for the particular site of infection: garlic for the lungs, bearberry for bladder infections, myrrh topically for the skin.

Grapefruit seed extract is a multipurpose antibiotic for bacterial infections and can be applied topically or taken orally.[38] Olive leaf extract has antibacterial and antiviral properties; useful for a range of infections.[39] Tea tree oil is an antiseptic that assists in fighting a broad range of infectious microorganisms and is one of the best skin disinfectants, helpful for acne and other skin infections.[40]

HYDROTHERAPY: Constitutional hydrotherapy (apply one to two times daily, depending on severity of infection).

JUICE THERAPY: Carrot, celery, beet, cantaloupe

NATUROPATHIC MEDICINE: In general, goldenseal is the most useful herb for bacterial infections and licorice root is the most useful herb for viral infections.

REFLEXOLOGY: Adrenals, lymph system, region or area affected.

Professional Care

The following therapies should only be provided by a qualified health professional.

Craniosacral Therapy / Environmental Medicine / Magnetic Field Therapy / Naturopathic Medicine / Traditional Chinese Medicine

DETOXIFICATION THERAPY: May be indicated, depending on the person's condition. Control the infection first.

OXYGEN THERAPY: • Hydrogen peroxide therapy (IV) • Hyperbaric oxygen therapy has powerful antibiotic properties. • Ozone is a wide spectrum antibacterial, antivi-

ral, and antifungal agent at concentrations that spare normal tissues.

INFLAMMATION

Redness, swelling, pain, and heat in localized areas of the body, due to tissue injury secondary to disease process or trauma from physical, infectious, or chemical insult.

SYMPTOMS: Any part of the body can be affected, internal or external.

SPECIAL NOTES: Elevate and, if necessary, splint the affected area. Apply alternating heat and ice, or herbal poultices, take necessary antibiotics if due to a bacterial infection, consume a whole foods diet with emphasis on raw foods, plenty of fresh juices, and filtered water, and rest, if the inflammation is severe.

According to Leon Chaitow, N.D., D.O., inflammation is a natural and potentially beneficial response of the body to factors that are irritating or damaging it. The use of anti-inflammatory drugs against arthritis has shown that, over a period of years, people using these medications have worse damage to their joints than people not receiving any treatment. This is because, unpleasant as it may be, the inflammation of the joints in arthritis actually precedes a degree of normalization of the damaged surface.

When inflammation is excessive or chronic, it is useful to modify it, but always by methods that cause no further problems and always in the knowledge that the inflammation can be a useful and natural response to whatever is causing damage to the body.

Alternative Treatments

Refer to alternative therapy chapters for more information before evaluating or applying any treatment. Some conditions, including yours, may require a physician's care.

DIET: Whole foods diet or 75% raw foods diet. If there is chronic inflammation, you may consider a simple mono-diet for two to four days, eating fresh fruits and vegetables and whole grains only, with lots of filtered water. Cut down or avoid sugar, white flour, junk foods, colas. Increase dietary garlic and yogurt. Drink plenty of fluids. Drink a glass of water with one teaspoon of fresh lemon juice and one teaspoon of liquid chlorophyll on rising and before bed. At least one glass of fresh vegetable juice or green drink a day with lots of homemade soups containing many vegetables and potatoes. One teaspoon of honey taken once a day, and even applied locally, is excellent as it has antiseptic, antimicrobial, and antibiotic characteristics (use only raw honey for this purpose). Noni fruit is an anti-inflammatory.

NUTRITION: • Vitamin C with bioflavonoids (3 g the first hour, then 1 g every two hours for first few days, up to bowel tolerance; then keep to 3-6 g per day), zinc (30-60 mg daily), beta carotene (100,000 IU first three days, then reduce to 25,000 IU for several weeks), evening primrose oil, garlic capsules, vitamin A and E emulsion, silica, mineral complex with calcium. • S-adenosyl-L-methionine (SAMe) is an amino acid compound found to be an effective anti-inflammatory and pain reliever.[41]

Proteolytic enzymes are often effective for severe or chronic inflammation and may be taken even if antibiotics are used (four capsules, four times daily for several days to one week, taken away from meals). If proteolytic enzymes bother the gastrointestinal tract, try bromelain in large dosages (1 g), but still take on an empty stomach away from meals.

Dr. Chaitow's nutritional strategy is as follows: Inflammation as a phenomenon depends upon the presence of substances called leukotrienes, which the body manufactures from arachidonic acid (an essential fatty acid). The vast majority of arachidonic acid in the body derives from animal proteins and fats, and a simple nutritional strategy that reduces or eliminates these from the diet can markedly reduce inflammation when it is excessive or chronic. Another way of helping this take place is to eat oily fish (mackerel, herring, salmon) and/or to take supplemental eicosapentaenoic acid (EPA) capsules derived from such fish. EPA reduces the production of leukotrienes.[42]

Cutting out red meat and poultry skin, as well as full-fat dairy products, and eating fish can improve the levels of inflammation being experienced.

Self-Care

The following therapies can be undertaken at home under appropriate professional supervision.

Fasting / Guided Imagery / Reflexology

AROMATHERAPY: Chamomile, lavender, frankincense, myrrh

FLOWER ESSENCES: Rescue Remedy®. Rescue Remedy Cream® for skin inflammation, if used on unbroken skin.

HERBS: A range of anti-inflammatory herbs are available and should be selected depending upon the site of the inflammation. For example, in the lining of the digestive system, use herbs such as chamomile, lemon balm, licorice, or meadowsweet. For the skin, use calendula, St. John's wort, or plantain. For rheumatic or arthritic problems, use willow bark, meadowsweet, or wild yam. • Sea cucumber (bêche-de-mer) has specific anti-inflammatory compounds found to be effective with arthritic and joint conditions. • Yarrow is an anti-arthritic and anti-spasmodic herb that has a long tradition of use for arthritis and other joint diseases.[43] • The Ayurvedic herb *Boswellia serrata* is effective in reducing inflammation in arthritis.[44]

HOMEOPATHY: *Aconite, Belladonna, Ferrum phos., Sulfur*

HYDROTHERAPY: • Contrast application (apply daily). In the early stages of inflammation, place an ice bag over inflamed area or immerse in ice water.

JUICE THERAPY: • Currants, red grapes, flaxseed oil added to combined vegetable juices • Pineapple

Professional Care

The following therapies should only be provided by a qualified health professional.

Cell Therapy / Craniosacral Therapy / Enzyme Therapy / Light Therapy / Naturopathic Medicine

ACUPUNCTURE: Increases endorphin levels in joints and other regions of the body, and therefore may be highly effective in treating inflammatory disease conditions.[45]

DETOXIFICATION THERAPY: Inflammation is usually a congested condition, but detoxification depends on the specifics of the situation.

LIGHT THERAPY: Cold (soft) laser photo stimulation therapy.

MAGNETIC FIELD THERAPY: Exposure to a negative magnetic field may help reduce inflammation.

OXYGEN THERAPY: • Hydrogen peroxide therapy • Hyperbaric oxygen may be helpful in some cases.

INSECT BITES

Allergic reactions to stings from insects. The most common sting problems are from yellow jackets and honeybees. Other insects causing reactions are hornets, bumblebees, wasps, ants, and spiders.

SYMPTOMS: Swelling, redness, pain, dizziness, loss of breath, anxiety.

SPECIAL NOTES: Though it takes the venom of 100 bees to create a fatal dose for most adults, one bee sting may cause a fatal allergic reaction in a hypersensitive individual. In the United States, there are three to four times more deaths from bee stings than snake bites. The venom in these cases causes the heart to collapse. People with known hypersensitivities should carry a kit containing antihistamine and epinephrine when in areas likely to hold risk.

If you are experiencing symptoms such as flushing, generalized hives, swelling around the neck or tongue, difficulty breathing, faintness, or loss of consciousness or diarrhea, immediately consult your physician or go to the emergency room, as this may indicate a severe reaction to the sting.

Desensitization can be carried out under qualified supervision in a manner very similar to other allergic desensitization techniques.

Alternative Treatments

Refer to alternative therapy chapters for more information before evaluating or applying any treatment. Some conditions, including yours, may require a physician's care.

NUTRITIONAL THERAPY: • Vitamin C as soon as possible (5 g) with vitamin B$_5$ (1 g). Continue to take 1 g of vitamin C and 500 mg of B$_5$ every hour until pain and swelling subside. • Vitamin E (apply oil to sting)

Self-Care

The following therapies can be undertaken at home under appropriate professional supervision.

AROMATHERAPY: According to Jean Valnet, M.D., basil, cinnamon, garlic, lavender, lemon, onion, sage, savory, and thyme are effective due to their antitoxic and antivenomous properties. Lavender may be effective in treating itching from stings.

AYURVEDA: • Drink cilantro juice. • Apply sandalwood paste to sting.

FLOWER ESSENCES: Rescue Remedy®. Rescue Remedy Cream®

HERBS: Apply the fresh bruised leaf or juice of plantain to the sting. Aloe gel can also be applied.

HOMEOPATHY: Immediately use *Aconite, Lachesis, Apis mel., Hypericum, Urtica urens.* For insect bites, use *Ledum, Hypericum, Calendula.* For wasp stings, use *Apis mel., Calendula.*

HYDROTHERAPY: Cold compress as needed to reduce pain and swelling.

PRACTICAL HINTS: If you have a severe allergy to insect stings, you should take preventive measures when outdoors. Wear slacks, footwear, and gloves while gardening and avoid cosmetics, perfumes, and hairsprays if you are going to be outdoors.

TOPICAL TREATMENT: According to Leon Chaitow, N.D., D.O., apply vinegar or lemon juice or a paste made of bicarbonate of soda as soon as possible to neutralize the venom. The pulped heads and buds of marigolds (calendula) in a tincture (preserved in alcohol) may be applied to stings and other surface injuries. The pulped fresh (marigold) flower may also be applied directly to a sting and bandaged in place. • Crush a charcoal tablet on a cotton ball, place over sting, and cover with a bandage to reduce pain and swelling. • Use ice packs to relieve pain and swelling and to keep the poison from spreading. • For wasp stings, apply vinegar immediately. • To remove a bee stinger, try to scrape and lift it out with the dull edge of a knife or tweezers. After removing stinger, treat with a strong, cold solution of three parts baking soda and one part water. If there is no access to any of the above listed items, mud applied to the sting will help draw out toxins as it dries.

Professional Care

The following therapies should only be provided by a qualified health professional.

Environmental Medicine / Light Therapy / Naturopathic Medicine / Orthomolecular Therapy

JAUNDICE

Yellowing of the skin, the whites of the eyes (sclerae), and other tissues, which is not a disease itself but usually a major signal of disease within the liver and biliary (gallbladder) system.

SYMPTOMS: Sometimes jaundice is the only sign. Other symptoms may accompany yellowing, such as darkening of the urine, nausea, vomiting, abdominal pain, pale-colored feces, retaining fluid in the trunk of the body, digestive problems, generalized rashes, and severe fatigue. All of these symptoms mean a doctor must be seen immediately.

SPECIAL NOTES: The yellowing is due to increased circulation of bilirubin in the blood. This is a yellow-brown pigment, thus the color. Normally, bilirubin should be cleared from the blood by the liver and excreted in the feces as bile, which partly gives feces the dark brownish color. When this process is not happening normally, the brownish bilirubin builds up in the blood and decreases in the stools.

Jaundice usually signals the following disorders: hepatitis, cirrhosis of the liver, breakdown of blood (hemolysis), problems in the gallbladder or bile ducts (due to stones, inflammation, tumor, or infection), and pernicious anemia (secondary to vitamin B$_{12}$ deficiency). Neonatal jaundice (at birth) is common and usually is not a serious health problem.

With any of the above symptoms, blood tests need to be run immediately. Other tests may also be needed, such as liver biopsy or ultrasound scanning of the liver.

Alternative Treatments

Refer to alternative therapy chapters for more information before evaluating or applying any treatment. Some conditions, including yours, may require a physician's care.

DIET: Diluted raw vegetable juice fasting or consuming mainly raw foods may be beneficial during acute stage (first several weeks). Continue to consume a largely raw food diet with lots of fruits and vegetables for one month after this. To help the liver and biliary system (bile-conveying structures), upon arising take a glass of warm water with juice of ½ lemon. Eat plenty of raw apples and pears or grate together with yogurt and raw seeds or seed and nut butter. Consume plenty of raw green vegetables and sprouts to help cleanse the blood. Try drinking barley water throughout day (to make barley water, place one cup of barley in three quarts of water, then simmer for three hours). Avoid all hydrogenated and processed fats and deep-fried foods.

NUTRITIONAL THERAPY: • Lipotropic formula • Liver glandular • Digestive enzymes with bile if stools are pale • Vitamin C • Vitamin B complex • Protein supplements • Essential fatty acids

NEONATAL: Apply vitamin E oil to breast nipple at least three times a day.

Self-Care

The following therapies can be undertaken at home under appropriate professional supervision.

Fasting / Qigong and Tai Chi

AROMATHERAPY: Geranium, rosemary, lemon

AYURVEDA: *Acute hepatitis:* Avoid hot, sour, spicy, and salty foods, meat, fish, cheese, oils, fried foods, and concentrated sweets. Try a mono-diet of mung beans for one week to strengthen liver. Add basmati rice and liver-cleansing spices such as coriander and turmeric. Rest and avoid vigorous exercise. *Chronic hepatitis:* Take tonics such as aloe gel, *shatavari*, and the formula *chyavan prash*. Take an herbal mixture of *kutki* (200 mg), *guduchi* (300 mg), and *shanka pushpi* (400 mg), generally twice a day after lunch and dinner. For all types, fresh sugarcane juice, one cup three times a day, ½ cup fresh homemade yogurt with a pinch of baking soda twice a day, and *brahmi ghee nasya*.

ENEMAS: Alternate coffee and water enemas daily.

HERBS: • Jaundice can be a symptom of different conditions and so these suggestions do not replace competent diagnosis. Combine the glycerites (herb mixed in a glycerin solution) of milk thistle, dandelion root, fringetree bark, and boldo in equal parts and take ½ teaspoon of this mixture three times a day. • An infusion of chickweed or distilled witch hazel applied topically will reduce itching. • Aloe vera gel, barberry, chamomile, dandelion, gentian root, goldenseal, parsley, rose hips, yellowdock

HOMEOPATHY: *Bryonia, Cinchona, Merc sol., Chelidonium, Nat phos., Kali bich., Chamomilla (babies), Phosphorus, Nux vom.*

HYDROTHERAPY: • Constitutional hydrotherapy (apply daily) • Foot and hand baths with a handful each of celandine leaves, artichoke leaves, dog's tooth roots, and a half-handful each of chicory leaves and dandelion flowers in two quarts water.

JUICE THERAPY: • Carrot and beet juice with a little radish and/or dandelion root juice added • Grapes, pear, lemon • Carrot, celery, parsley • Carrot, beet, cucumber

REFLEXOLOGY: Liver points

Professional Care

The following therapies should only be provided by a qualified health professional.

Cell Therapy / Magnetic Field Therapy / Naturopathic Medicine / Osteopathic Medicine / Traditional Chinese Medicine

DETOXIFICATION THERAPY: Not indicated. Evaluate the state of the body and the cause of the jaundice, and then detoxification may be helpful.

LIGHT THERAPY: Neonatal jaundice may be treated with exposure to full-spectrum light or blue light.

KIDNEY STONES

Stones anywhere in the urinary tract. Kidney, bladder, the ducts in-between, or the ureters may become blocked with stones (renal or urinary calculi).

SYMPTOMS: May have no symptoms (called "silent") or have a variety of symptoms, depending on where the stone is located and its size. Possible symptoms include sudden severe and excruciating back pain that may come and go (intermittent), and often radiates from the back across the abdomen and into the genital area or inner thighs. This pain may be associated with nausea, vomiting, abdominal bloating, possible blood in the urine, pain on urination, and chills and fever. Stones in the urinary tract can be one of the most painful conditions, similar to the pain of childbirth.

OCCURRENCE: One in every 1,000 adults per year is hospitalized for urinary tract stones. One percent of autopsies reveals urinary stones. Stones tend to reoccur: about 60% of those who form stones will have another stone episode within seven years.

SPECIAL NOTES: The stones are formed from a number of mineral salt solutions in the urine. In the U.S., the most common component (70%) of stones is calcium (oxalate) and/or phosphate that has come out of solution. Higher-than-normal levels of oxalate in the urine, related to a high dietary intake of oxalic containing foods, such as rhubarb, spinach, leafy vegetables, and coffee, may promote stone formation. Stones that are high in calcium may be one of the first signals that there is a condition called hyperparathyroidism (excessive secretion of parathyroid hormone).

Research shows that soft drinks containing phosphoric acid encourage the recurrence of kidney stones in some people.[46]

CONSIDER: Stones are more common during the summer. This may be due to concentrated urine secondary to increased sweating and insufficient fluids to make up for this deficiency. Mild chronic dehydration may play a role in the development of stones. High levels of dietary refined carbohydrates may also encourage stone formation as the sugar stimulates the pancreatic release of insulin. This stimulates, in turn, increased calcium excretion through the urine. Other factors that cause increased calcium excretion in the urine (hypercalciuria) and may promote stone formation are increased dietary levels of coffee, colas, acid-forming diets (such as high protein and grains with insufficient alkalinizing vegetables and fruits), insufficient fluids such as water, excessive salt consumption, stress, and insufficient amounts of magnesium (which helps keep calcium in solution).

Diet alone cannot get rid of the stones. You must see a doctor. This condition may be genetically influenced. If one parent was a stone former, there is an increased risk in the children. Cadmium toxicity may also play a role in stone formation and needs to be assessed.

Alternative Treatments

Refer to alternative therapy chapters for more information before evaluating or applying any treatment. Some conditions, including yours, may require a physician's care.

DIET: The most important dietary actions are to increase fluids, increase fiber and green vegetables, and reduce refined sugar consumption. Must increase pure water to at least eight glasses or more per day, to the point where two to three quarts of urine are produced daily. Increase green vegetables, which are high in magnesium. Vegetarian-oriented diets may be helpful to prevent recurrences. Studies have shown that vegetarians have a 40%-60% decreased risk of stones and that meat intake is correlated with calcium oxalate stone formation.[47] Foods that are helpful in decreasing stone formation are cranberries, black cherries, rice bran, kombucha tea. It is helpful to reduce salt, sugar, dairy products, caffeine, alcohol, refined carbohydrates, nuts, chocolate, pepper. Limit protein intake.

Many experts believe that if stones are primarily composed of calcium, then dairy, produce, and other rich sources of calcium should be reduced. New research shows that this may not be necessary and that normal dietary levels of calcium do not by themselves encourage stones, and may actually be protective.[48] A safe strategy would be to keep calcium intake at normal levels (any supplementation should be of citrate, gluconate, lactate, or carbonate forms, which alkalize the urine reducing calcium secretion), while dealing with the other factors that are known to encourage stone formation—reducing meat intake, high sugar consumption, and making sure of adequate levels of magnesium in the diet, along with optimal fluid intake and increasing potassium-rich foods such as fruit and vegetables.

If, however, you are a stone former and have consumed large amounts of dairy products, consider limiting dairy products and boiling water for ten minutes before drinking as this lowers calcium content by precipitating calcium carbonate.

If the stones are high in oxalates, avoid foods containing or producing oxalic acid such as spinach, beets, parsley, Swiss chard, cabbage, rhubarb, and coffee. Also avoid vitamin C over 6 g per day, which may increase oxalate excretion. Asparagus contains asparagine, which helps in breaking up oxalate crystals. Option: Take one teaspoon of lemon juice each half hour for two days to help take the "rough edge" off kidney stones and flush them out.

NUTRITIONAL THERAPY: • Magnesium (200 mg two times daily) •Vitamin B₆ (50 mg three times daily) •Vitamin C (over 6 g per day may be harmful for this condition by increasing oxalate formation) • Vitamin A • Proteolytic enzymes (away from meals) • Raw kidney glandular • Fat-soluble chlorophyll • Lysine (deficiency may increase calcium excretion in the urine) • Methionine • Lipoic acid • Glutamic acid

Self-Care

The following therapies can be undertaken at home under appropriate professional supervision.

Fasting

AROMATHERAPY: Hyssop, juniper.

AYURVEDA: • Drink well-cooked barley soup with a pinch of *dugdapachan bhasma* or ¼ teaspoon of *gokshura*

and two pinches *mutral churna* or ¼ teaspoon of *punarnava*; generally taken one cup three times a day. • For general kidney disorders, an herbal mixture of *punarnava* (500 mg), *gokshura* (300 mg), *kamadudha* (200 mg), and *jatamansi* (200 mg), generally taken twice a day after lunch and dinner. *Punarnava guggulu* (200 mg) or *gokshura guggulu* (200 mg), generally taken two times a day after lunch and dinner. Cumin, coriander, fennel tea, generally taken one cup three times a day.

HERBS: • Combine the tinctures of gravel root, cornsilk, wild yam, blackhaw in equal parts and take one teaspoon of this mixture three times a day. • Drink one cup of an infusion of nettle three times a day. • Uva ursi and horsetail have diuretic (urine-increasing) and astringent properties, helpful for urinary "gravel" and inflammation, as well as bladder infections (cystitis), bladder cramps, and kidney stones. • Horsetail, a rich source of dietary silica, is specifically indicated for bladder and kidney irritation involving "scalding" or burning urine. • Dandelion root or extract helps the kidney eliminate its waste products.[49]

HOMEOPATHY: *Berberis, Sarsaparilla*

HYDROTHERAPY: Constitutional hydrotherapy (apply two to five times weekly) or hot pack to abdomen and low back (apply 10-15 minutes several times daily for relief of colicky pain).

JUICE THERAPY: • Lemon juice • Carrot, beet, and cucumber juice (add some garlic and/or horseradish to carrot) • Cranberry, watermelon

MIND/BODY THERAPY: Relaxation

REFLEXOLOGY: Ureter tubes, kidneys, bladder, diaphragm, parathyroid

Professional Care

The following therapies should only be provided by a qualified health professional.

DETOXIFICATION THERAPY: Usually the person is congestive, so detoxification may be indicated. Take fluids and control mineral balance.

NON-SURGICAL ALTERNATIVES: Lithotripsy therapy—in this treatment, kidney stones are shattered by ultra-short sound waves, allowing the fragments to be passed in the urine.

LARYNGITIS

Inflammation of the larynx or the voice box, the upper part of the windpipe, below the root of tongue (pharynx) and at top of trachea (windpipe).

SYMPTOMS: Hoarseness of the voice, loss of voice, rawness, constant urge to clear throat, tickling sensation at the back of the throat, pain, possible fatigue, difficulty swallowing, and fever.

CONSIDER: Viral, yeast (candidiasis), and bacterial infections (viral is most common and is not helped by antibiotics), excessive use of voice, screaming, rage, allergies or low-grade chronic allergies, inhalation of irritating substances, and secondary to illnesses such as flu, bronchitis, measles, diphtheria, and pneumonia.

Alternative Treatments

Refer to alternative therapy chapters for more information before evaluating or applying any treatment. Some conditions, including yours, may require a physician's care.

DIET: Whole foods diet with plenty of fluids, raw fruits, and vegetables. Decrease or avoid intake of refined carbohydrates.

NUTRITIONAL THERAPY: • Vitamin A (100,000 IU for first three days) • Vitamin C • Garlic capsules • Zinc lozenges • Use acidophilus if taking antibiotics.

Self-Care

The following therapies can be undertaken at home under appropriate professional supervision.

Guided Imagery

AROMATHERAPY: Inhalations with benzoin, lavender, frankincense, thyme, and sandalwood.

HERBS: A gargle made from an infusion of red sage and yarrow will alleviate the discomfort. Do not swallow. Alternative herbs would be chamomile or cranesbill. Internally, take 30 drops of echinacea tincture every hour for two days. • Gargle with bayberry or sage tea.

HYDROTHERAPY: Contrast application (apply one to two times daily to neck and throat) or heating compress (apply one to two times daily to neck and throat).

HOMEOPATHY: *Aconite, Hepar sulph., Phosphorus, Spongia, Causticum, Belladonna, Kali bich., Drosera, Carbo veg.*

JUICE THERAPY: • Carrot, pineapple • Carrot, apple • Carrot, celery • Carrot, beet, cucumber, ginger

NATUROPATHIC MEDICINE: Gargle with a tea made from licorice *(Glycyrrhiza glabra)* root.

REFLEXOLOGY: Throat, chest/lung, diaphragm, lymph system, all toes

TOPICAL TREATMENT: Cold compress on throat

Professional Care

The following therapies should only be provided by a qualified health professional.

Acupuncture / Environmental Medicine / Light Therapy / Magnetic Field Therapy / Naturopathic Medicine / Osteopathic Medicine / Traditional Chinese Medicine

DETOXIFICATION THERAPY: May be indicated, depending on the condition of the person. Acute infections will not be helped. Evaluate the cause.

OXYGEN THERAPY: • Hydrogen peroxide therapy (IV) • Ozonated water gargles may be helpful.

LUPUS

A chronic, inflammatory, autoimmune (the body attacking itself) disease that affects connective tissue (tissue that binds and supports various structures of the body and also includes the blood). Discoid lupus erythematosus (DLE) is a less serious type, affecting exposed areas of the skin and sometimes the joints. Systemic lupus erythematosus (SLE) is more serious, potentially fatal, and affects more organs of the body.

SYMPTOMS: Symptoms vary according to the severity of the illness and which organs are affected. SLE may occur very abruptly with a fever and mimic an acute infection or it may occur very slowly over months and years with only several episodes of fever and fatigue. Most people with SLE complain of pain in various joints that mimics arthritis, or in children simulates growing pains. In adults, there is often a history of growing pains. Over time, muscular contraction may deform the joints.

Many patients have rashes on the face or other areas, such as the neck, upper chest, and elbows. In DLE, the rash starts as red, circular thickened areas that leave scars, most often affecting the face and scalp, and may cause permanent hair loss. In SLE, there is a characteristic "butterfly-shaped" rash that occurs on the cheeks and over the bridge of the nose. Rashes in SLE patients do not scar and do not cause permanent hair loss.

Ulcers on mucous membranes such as the mouth and nose are common. Rashes and swelling of the hands and fingers may occur. Sensitivity to light (photophobia) occurs in 40% of people with SLE. Other problems may be kidney disorders, repetitive episodes of pleurisy (inflammation of the lining of the lungs), pericarditis (inflammation of the membrane surrounding the heart), iron deficiency anemia, and pulmonary hypertension (high blood pressure). Swelling of lymph nodes is common, especially in children.

SLE is classified as mild if the symptoms are mainly fever, joint pain, rash, headaches, pleurisy, and pericarditis. It is considered severe if it is associated with life-threatening diseases. Mild SLE may respond well to natural therapies. Aspirin may be useful, but in high dosages in people with SLE may cause liver toxicity. Anti-malarials (used to treat malaria) may help where joint and rash symptoms are predominant. Severe SLE requires immediate corticosteroid therapy.

OCCURRENCE: Occurs mostly in young women (90% of cases) and in young children.

CONSIDER: Rule out food allergies, rheumatoid arthritis, other connective tissue diseases, parasites, candidiasis, bowel problems, and digestive enzyme deficiencies, which may create symptoms that mimic SLE or worsen SLE. Rule out migraines, epilepsy, and psychoses.

SPECIAL NOTES: SLE is often chronic, with periods of improvement and relapse over many years. Sometimes there are years of remission between periods of symptoms.

Blood tests for antinuclear antibodies (ANA) and sometimes skin biopsies are diagnostic for this condition. According to the American Rheumatoid Association, there must be four of the following eight symptoms present for lupus to be diagnosed: ANA antibodies in the blood, low white blood cell or platelet count or hemolytic anemia, joint pain in a number of joints (arthritis), butterfly rash on cheeks, abnormal cells in the urine, light sensitivity, mouth sores, and seizure or psychosis.

Some drugs give a false positive test (looks like SLE): hydralazine, procainamide, and beta blockers. Sometimes these drugs produce a lupus-like condition that disappears when the drug is stopped. Birth control pills may cause flare-ups of lupus.

Treatments are aimed at decreasing symptoms. Allopathic medicine does not consider there to be a cure for lupus, but naturally oriented physicians report "cures" of lupus by eliminating causes and treating the body as a whole.

Alternative Treatments

Refer to alternative therapy chapters for more information before evaluating or applying any treatment. Some conditions, including yours, may require a physician's care.

DIET: Whole foods diet. Avoid overeating (more frequent, smaller meals are suggested), limit cow's milk and beef products, increase vegetables (especially green, yellow, and orange), and consume fish several times a week. Avoid alfalfa sprouts or tablets that contain L-canavanine sulfate, a substance that may aggravate lupus. Assess and treat for food and chemical allergies.

According to Leon Chaitow, N.D., D.O., hydrochloric acid deficiency is common in people with lupus. Supplementation with meals can help or stimulation of natural production can be achieved by careful use of specific herbs such as the "Swedish bitters" combination.

NUTRITIONAL THERAPY: • Vitamin C and bioflavonoids • Proteolytic enzymes (away from meals on an empty stomach) • Digestive enzymes with meals, if necessary • Calcium • Magnesium • Zinc • Essential fatty acids • Amino acids L-cysteine, L-methionine, L-cystine • Beta carotene and vitamin A for DLE • Vitamin E (1,500 IU daily) • Garlic capsules • Vitamin B complex • Vitamin B5 • Vitamin B12 (intramuscular injection of 1,000 mcg two times weekly) • Selenium

Avoid L-tryptophan supplementation, which may produce substances in the body that may promote the autoimmune process.

According to Jonathan Wright, M.D.:

1. Vitamin B6 in high doses (500 mg three times daily) can be useful in reducing symptoms.

2. Over 80% of SLE patients are severely hypochlorhydric (diminished secretion of hydrochloric acid in the stomach).

3. All SLE patients have food allergies and improve with appropriate identification and treatment.

4. Over 50% of women with SLE have levels of testosterone and DHEA lower than other women (not men) and improve with appropriate treatment.

Self-Care

The following therapies can be undertaken at home under appropriate professional supervision.

Biofeedback Training and Neurotherapy / Fasting / Guided Imagery / Qigong and Tai Chi

HERBS: • Mix equal parts of the tinctures of the Chinese herbs *Bupleurum falcatum*, licorice, and wild yam. Take one teaspoon of this mixture three times a day. • Drink an infusion of nettle twice a day. • In addition, as this autoimmune condition can manifest with a range of symptoms, these should be treated with the relevant herbs as they arise. • Echinacea, goldenseal, pau d'arco, red clover

HYDROTHERAPY: Constitutional hydrotherapy (apply two to five times weekly).

JUICE THERAPY: Carrot, celery, can add flaxseed oil, black currant oil, garlic

REFLEXOLOGY: All glands, intestines, liver, whole spine

TOPICAL TREATMENT: PABA (para-aminobenzoic acid) cream.

Professional Care

The following therapies should only be provided by a qualified health professional.

Cell Therapy / Chelation Therapy / Environmental Medicine / Enzyme Therapy / Magnetic Field Therapy / Naturopathic Medicine / Traditional Chinese Medicine

BODYWORK: Rolfing

DETOXIFICATION THERAPY: May be indicated, depending on the condition of the person.

LIGHT THERAPY: PUVA (Psoralen UV-A) therapy

OXYGEN THERAPY: • Hydrogen peroxide therapy (IV) • Hyperbaric oxygen therapy.

LYME DISEASE

Lyme disease was first recognized in the U.S. in 1975, after a mysterious outbreak of arthritis near Lyme, Connecticut. It was not until 1982 that the spirochete that causes Lyme, Borrelia burgdorferi (Bb), *was identified. Lyme disease is a multisystem inflammatory disease, at first affecting the skin in characteristic "bull's-eye" rashes (only 30% to 40% of adult patients exhibit these, however, and less than 10% of infected children), then spreading to the joints and nervous system. Many physicians now regard the disease not as a simple infection, but rather as a complex illness that often consists of other co-infections.*

SYMPTOMS: Variable, including skin lesions or rashes, flu-like symptoms, sleeping difficulties, muscle pains and weakness, headaches, back pain, fever, chills, nausea or vomiting, facial paralysis, enlargement of the lymph glands or spleen, irregular heartbeat, seizures, blurry vision, moodiness, memory loss, dementia, and joint pains (similar to arthritis). One hallmark of Lyme disease is fatigue unrelieved by rest.

CONSIDER: Lyme is sometimes called "the Great Imposter" because it is often misdiagnosed as other diseases, leading a patient (and often the physician) to believe the problem is chronic fatigue syndrome (CFS), borderline thyroid gland dysfunction, fibromyalgia, multiple sclerosis (MS), Lou Gehrig's disease (ALS), and other debilitating conditions. Joanne Whitaker, M.D., of Palm Harbor, Florida, believes that Lyme is at the base of most cases of CFS. If you have symptoms associated with CFS or these other illnesses, it is prudent to consider a Lyme disease diagnosis.

Lyme disease can also be a cause of or contributing co-factor to a variety of other degenerative diseases, including ALS, Alzheimer's, fibromyalgia, and MS. It can cause or play a role in neuropsychiatric problems, such as "brain fog" and bipolar disorder (manic depression), vision disorders, neurological problems, headaches, and even heart disease (Lyme carditis). Many people who are thought to have such conditions are actually misdiagnosed and have Lyme disease instead, according to Charles Ray Jones, M.D., of New Haven, Connecticut. Katrina Tang, M.D., H.M.D., of Reno, Nevada, adds, "Lyme disease eludes many doctors because it can mimic many other diseases. This poses a public health risk, because doctors may treat the wrong disease or not find the true cause, delaying treatment."

SPECIAL NOTES: Conventional wisdom holds that Lyme disease is relatively rare and only transmitted by ticks. In actuality, Lyme disease is epidemic and, in addition to ticks, can also be spread by other insects, including fleas, mosquitoes, and mites, and by human–to–human contact (including via breast-feeding). Transmission may also occur via blood transfusion, according to Dr. Tang. "If it weren't for AIDS," states researcher Nick Harris, Ph.D., Director of the International Lyme and Associated Diseases Society (ILADS), "Lyme would be the number one infectious disease in the U.S. and Western Europe." Although the U.S. Centers for Disease Control and Prevention (CDC) reports that there have been fewer than 160,000 confirmed cases of Lyme disease since 1980, Dr. Harris says that "Lyme is grossly underreported. In the U.S., we probably have about 200,000 cases per year."

Lyme disease is not a simple infection, but a complex illness that can consist of other infectious co-factors, especially the parasitic pathogens *Babesia* and *Ehrlichia*. When diagnosed at a very early stage, Lyme disease can be cured by a course of antibiotics. Delaying treatment, however, can be disastrous, since in its later stages "Lyme also includes collateral conditions that result from being ill with multiple pathogens, each of which can have a profound impact on the person's overall health," says Joseph J. Burrascano, M.D., of East Hamp-

ton, New York. "Together, damage to virtually all bodily systems can result."

Marylynn S. Barkley, Ph.D., M.D., Associate Professor of Neurobiology, Physiology, and Behavior at the University of California, at Davis, notes that approximately 15% of Lyme patients develop serious problems. For such patients, chronic debilitation and extreme pain can change their lives dramatically and, in some cases, has even led to suicide, Dr. Barkley notes.

TESTING: Most of the standard tests used to detect Lyme disease are notoriously unreliable. "The initial thing patients usually get is a Western Blot antibody test," explains Dr. Harris. "This test is not positive immediately after Bb exposure and only 60% or 70% of people ever show antibodies to Bb." Growing numbers of alternative physicians prefer using tests developed by Dr. Whitaker or Lida Mattman, Ph.D., of Warren, Michigan, although neither test has yet been awarded approval from the U.S. Food and Drug Administration (FDA) for diagnostic use. Dr. Whitaker's test, known as the Rapid Identification of Bb (RIBb), employs a highly purified fluorescent antibody stain specific for Bb, which is used to detect the organism. "RIBb provides results in 20-30 minutes, a key to getting the right treatment started quickly," Dr. Whitaker says.

Dr. Mattman's culture test also employs a fluorescent antibody staining technique, which allows her to study live cultures under a fluorescent microscope. "When a person is sick," Dr. Mattman explains, "antibodies get tied up in the tissues, in what is called an immune complex, and are not detected in the patient's blood. So it's not that the antibody isn't there or hasn't been produced, it just isn't detectable. Thus, the tests that are based on detecting antibodies give false negatives." Both the RIBb and Dr. Mattman's test do not look for antibodies to Bb but for the organism itself, in the same way that tuberculosis is diagnosed.

Compounding the problem of accurate detection is the fact that Lyme disease is pleomorphic, meaning it can radically change form. "We have examined blood samples from over 800 patients with clinically diagnosed Lyme disease with the RIBb test and have rarely seen Bb in anything but a cell wall–deficient (CWD) form. The problem is that a CWD organism doesn't have a fixed exterior membrane presenting information that would allow the immune system or drugs to attack it, or allow most current tests to detect it," says Dr. Whitaker.

As a CWD organism, Dr. Mattman notes, Bb is extremely diverse in its appearance, activity, and vulnerability. In addition, according to W. Lee Cowden, M.D., of Fort Worth, Texas, "Because Bb is pleomorphic, you can't expect any one antibiotic to be effective. Also, bacteria share genetic material with one another, so the offspring of the next bug can have a new genetic sequence that can resist the antibiotic."

In addition to the tests developed by Drs. Whitaker and Mattman, alternative physicians may examine a patient's medical history, genetic tendencies, metabolism, and nutritional and micronutritional status in searching for Lyme disease. They may also conduct a blood analysis using darkfield microscopy, employ muscle testing (kinesiology), and use electrodermal screening (EDS). Dr. Barkley has found that testing women around the time of menses increases the probability of detecting Bb, since women with Lyme disease have an exacerbation of their menstrual symptoms. Dr. Burrascano also employs a weighted list of diagnostic criteria and an exhaustive symptom checklist that he developed.

PREVENTION: In April 1998, the U.S. Department of Health and Human Services released the following guidelines for preventing Lyme disease caused by infection from ticks and other insects:

- Avoid tick-infested areas, especially in May, June, and July.

- Wear light-colored clothing so ticks are clearly visible.

- Wear long-sleeved shirts, pants, and a hat, and closed shoes and socks. Be sure to tuck pant legs into socks or boots, and tuck shirt into pants.

- Apply insect repellent to pants, socks, shoes, and exposed skin.

- Walk in the center of nature trails to avoid overgrown grass and brush.

- After being outdoors in tick-infested areas, remove, wash, and dry clothing.

- Inspect your body thoroughly and carefully remove any attached ticks. Also check pets for ticks.

- If you find a tick, tug gently but firmly with blunt tweezers near the head of the tick until it releases its hold on the skin. To reduce the risk of infection, try not to crush the tick's body or handle the tick with bare fingers.

- Swab the bite area thoroughly with an antiseptic to prevent bacterial infection.

Alternative Treatments

Refer to alternative therapy chapters for more information before evaluating or applying any treatment. Some conditions, including yours, may require a physician's care.

Alternative physicians agree that antibiotics are the primary treatment for Lyme disease, but that the accepted "standard" antibiotic therapies (of a duration and type acceptable to insurance carriers, HMOs, and conventional M.D.s) is insufficient. "Short-term oral antibiotics are effective for treating localized Lyme, but with disseminated Lyme [symptoms involving the entire body, especially the skin and nervous, musculoskeletal, and circulatory systems], the requirement for either intravenously administered antibiotics or long-term oral antibiotics becomes common," Dr. Barkley says. Most physicians recommend an immediate short course of antibiotics for anyone bitten by a deer tick or exhibiting symptoms that do not improve within 3-5 days. "Treatment duration varies with each individual," Dr. Jones says. "If one stops antibiotics prematurely, a more resilient infection will develop that will cause more brain and body injury."

DIET: Avoid alcohol and all sugars, because they feed the bacteria associated with Lyme disease. Dr. Cowden advises that "it is important to balance saliva pH between 6.7 and 7.0. Sufficient dietary minerals bring pH up if low." Increasing your intake of alkaline foods (most green vegetables, complex grains, almonds, yams, lentils, squash) also helps maintain proper pH balance. Dr. Cowden recommends identifying your metabolic type and eating accordingly, and identifying and eliminating foods to which you are allergic. Dr. Burrascano recommends daily yogurt, along with acidophilus preparations (two with each meal), to replenish the gastrointestinal tract with healthy intestinal flora, which are killed by antibiotics.

NUTRITIONAL THERAPY: Proper nutritional supplementation can help bolster immune function, which Lyme disease impairs and which can be further compromised by the use of antibiotics. Steven J. Bock, M.D., Medical Director of the Center for Progressive Medicine, in Albany, New York, recommends anti-inflammatory fatty acids such as fish oil and borage oil, a high-potency multivitamin/mineral formula, coenzyme Q10 (to shore up cellular energy levels), calcium pantothenate (500 mg three times daily), vitamin B_1, biotin, and inositol (650 mg of each, 2-3 times daily), and the amino acid L-carnitine (for cognitive enhancement). Magnesium is also useful for the headaches, tremors, twitches, cramps, muscle soreness, general weakness, and heart strain caused by Lyme.

To further boost immunity, Dr. Cowden recommends transfer factor, Thymic Protein A, glyconutrients (Ambrotose), and the immune-enhancing polysaccharide arabinogalactan (Larix). He cautions that vitamin C and grapeseed extract, as well as certain other substances, can interfere with the tissue uptake of antibiotics, making them less effective.

Probiotics should be used to maintain a healthy balance of intestinal flora and overall gastrointestinal health. Digestive enzymes may also help.

Self-Care

The following therapies can be undertaken at home under appropriate professional supervision.

HERBS: Herbal medicine is best administered under the guidance of a professional trained in their use. The following herbs can be used safely as a self-care protocol, however. Dr. Bock recommends astragalus, ginseng, and maitake and reishi mushrooms for general immune support. Cordyceps, a well-known medicinal herb from Tibet, is recommended by Dr. Burrascano to improve stamina, fatigue, and energy and to enhance lung and antioxidant function.

STRESS REDUCTION: Because stress diminishes immunity and energy levels, it is essential that people with Lyme disease effectively manage stress levels. Dr. Whitaker advises regular periods of rest and warns that parents of children with the disease not succumb to feelings of guilt. "I emphasize that it's not a parent's fault," she says. "You can't protect your child from Lyme exposure." Dr. Bock advises patients to use relaxation techniques, guided imagery and visualization, and biofeedback, and to join a group for emotional support. Breathwork can also help relieve stress.

Professional Care

The following therapies should only be provided by a qualified health professional.

Biofeedback Training and Neurotherapy / Detoxification Therapy / Environmental Medicine / Naturopathic Medicine / Orthomolecular Medicine

ACUPUNCTURE: Acupuncture combined with physical therapy can reduce the pain associated with Lyme disease.

BODYWORK: Bowen Therapy, due to its ability to balance and restore proper functioning of the autonomic nervous system, can be very effective in relieving the symptoms of Lyme disease.

OXYGEN THERAPY: Oxidative therapy (ozone) and hydrogen peroxide therapy (IV) can both be useful, reports Dr. Bock. He also employs photo-ox therapy, a combination of IV hydrogen peroxide or ozone and ultraviolet blood irradiation (UVB). "UVB appears to be highly effective in treating persistent viruses and antibiotic-resistant bacteria," he says.

MEMORY AND COGNITION PROBLEMS

Inability to focus mentally and utilize one's mental capabilities successfully and on demand.

SYMPTOMS: Poor mental focus, poor learning, poor memory, difficulty following information, conversation, or train of thought.

CONSIDER: Allergies, candidiasis, thyroid disorders, stroke or poor circulation to brain, amino acid imbalance, low blood sugar, poor mental habits and laziness requiring tutoring in learning techniques. (It is possible that coping strategies taught one to forget and not to think rather than to be able to concentrate.)

Alternative Treatments

Refer to alternative therapy chapters for more information before evaluating or applying any treatment. Some conditions, including yours, may require a physician's care.

DIET: Whole foods diet including fish and adequate protein. Avoidance of food allergies or other allergies that may cause cerebral allergies, contributing to poor concentration. Consider a diet associated with hypoglycemia as low blood sugar problems may be a contributing factor. Lots of pure water daily.

NUTRITIONAL THERAPY: • Supercholine • If low blood sugar, take chromium • Protein supplements or amino acids (identification of amino acid imbalance may be helpful) • Pantothenic acid • Vitamin B complex (deficiency of the B vitamins can result in numerous conditions related to the brain and nervous system, including memory loss or impairment, disorientation or confusion, irritability, mood swings, fatigue, or depression).[50] • Numerous observational studies have found insufficiencies of vitamin B6 (pyridoxine) in many elderly Americans. Pyridoxine supports the digestive, immune, and nervous systems and normal brain function.

Phosphatidyl-choline, found in lecithin, is the nutrient precursor to acetylcholine, an important brain chemical (neurotransmitter) involved in both memory and thought. DMAE (dimethylamine ethanol) also promotes the production of acetylcholine and has been shown to increase memory.[51] Phosphatidyl-serine (PS) supports and revitalizes nerve cells and has been shown in numerous studies to slow or reverse cognitive losses attributed to aging. PS also helps brain cells communicate and improves both memory and the ability to concentrate.[52]

Self-Care

The following therapies can be undertaken at home under appropriate professional supervision.

Fasting / Flower Essences / Qigong and Tai Chi / Yoga

HERBS: • *Ginkgo biloba* helps to improve the circulation of blood and oxygen to the entire body and the brain. Standardized extracts of ginkgo have been shown in numerous double-blind studies to greatly improve the supply of blood and oxygen to the brain (cerebral vascular insufficiency) and improve brain function.[53] • Ginseng has the ability to improve mental function and stamina as well as physical stamina. Siberian ginseng is most often recommended to improve mental function.[54] • Vinpocetine, an extract found in the periwinkle plant (*Vinca minor*), is a vasodilator and cerebral metabolic enhancer.[55]

Pycnogenol extract derived from grape seeds or pine bark provides antioxidant protection to the brain and central nervous system. It strengthens blood vessel and capillary walls and helps prevent and reverse ischemia (lack of oxygen due to poor blood flow) in brain tissue, which in turn helps reduce mental deterioration.[56]

Other herbs known to support brain function and longevity include *ashwagandha* and *Bacopa monniera* (Ayurvedic), bilberry, capsicum, fo-ti tieng (Chinese), garlic, ginseng, green tea, kelp, peppermint leaf, rosemary, sarsaparilla, and wood betony. • Mix one teaspoon each of skullcap and gotu kola with hot water for improved awareness.

HOMEOPATHY: *Argen nit., Arsen alb.*

HYDROTHERAPY: • Cold compress (apply as needed to the face and hands). • Constitutional hydrotherapy (apply two to five times weekly).

MIND/BODY THERAPY: • Guided imagery, biofeedback (attention deficit disorders), meditation. • Belly breathing for enhanced relaxation and concentration. Lie on your back with your knees bent and feet on the floor at hip's width, with your hands at your side. As you breathe, focus on your belly. As you inhale, imagine it expanding in all directions like a big balloon. As you exhale, feel it contract. Allow your exhalation to eventually become twice as long as your inhalation.

Professional Care

The following therapies should only be provided by a qualified health professional.

Applied Kinesiology / Cell Therapy / Chelation Therapy / Environmental Medicine / Hypnotherapy / Light Therapy / Magnetic Field Therapy / Natural Hormone Replacement Therapy / Naturopathic Medicine / Orthomolecular Therapy / Traditional Chinese Medicine

BODYWORK: Feldenkrais Method, Alexander Technique.

DETOXIFICATION THERAPY: Detoxification is not indicated unless the condition is part of a congestive disorder. May need colon cleansing, yeast treatment, or heavy metal detoxification.

VISION THERAPY: Vision therapy may be an effective method for improving mental focus. Accuracy of aiming, speed of movement, and quality of single, clear sight are often enhanced through vision therapy even in older individuals. Increases in attention, memory, and the ability to sustain focus are often the result.

MONONUCLEOSIS

An acute infectious, viral disease caused usually by the Epstein-Barr virus and sometimes by the cytomegalovirus. Both of these viruses belong to the herpes group. The disease is often referred to as "mono," "sleeping sickness," or the "kissing sickness," since it is very contagious and may be transmitted by kissing, and the cardinal symptom is severe tiredness. Mono affects the lymph tissue, the respiratory system, and sometimes other organs such as the liver, spleen, and, rarely, the heart and kidneys. It presents with an increase of abnormal white blood cells and development of persistent antibodies to the Epstein-Barr virus and short-lived antibodies to beef, horse, and sheep red blood cells.

SYMPTOMS: Symptoms occur four to seven weeks after exposure with severe incapacitating fatigue, headache, sometimes chills, often shortly followed by a very high fever, sore throat, with enlargement of different lymph nodes, especially the ones in the neck. It is possible for the symptoms to be varied and confusing, because the mono viruses can affect different organs such as the spleen, liver (sometimes a mild jaundice occurs for a short period of time), eyelids, and sometimes the heart. Ten percent of individuals develop rashes or sometimes darkened bruise-like areas in the mouth.

OCCURRENCE: Occurs most commonly at the age when the immune system is at its peak functioning (15-17 years old). The disease only occurs in individuals who have never had these viral antibodies before.

CONSIDER: Mono's symptoms are very similar to the flu, so that a severe flu bout must be ruled out.

SPECIAL NOTES: Almost all cases improve without drugs within four to six weeks. Antibiotics do nothing for mono unless there is an associated bacterial infection. Ampicillin, an antibiotic, will often make mono worse, may cause a rash, and should be avoided. Avoid aspirin as it may create complications in rare cases. The oral antiviral medication acyclovir is sometimes used in uncomplicated cases, but natural treatments may fair as well in some responsive individuals.

Any treatment in the early stages of this disease must emphasize appropriate bed rest (for at least one month or while fever and fatigue are still present). If there is enlargement of the spleen or liver, the rest may need to be prolonged and strenuous exercise must be avoided until these organs return to normal size.

Many mono patients suffer from ongoing fatigue, depression, and varied symptoms for months to follow, but those on natural treatments seem to avoid this pitfall or recover from these recurrences more quickly.

Alternative Treatments

Refer to alternative therapy chapters for more information before evaluating or applying any treatment. Some conditions, including yours, may require a physician's care.

DIET: Drink plenty of pure water, avoid excessive animal proteins, take amino acid blends or vegetable protein drinks several times per day between meals or for a snack to help build up the organs involved and maintain better blood sugar balance. Eat four to six smaller meals throughout the day and avoid overeating at each meal, eat as much raw foods as possible with emphasis on sprouts, seeds, and nuts, and consume wholesome soups made from a wide variety of vegetables and roots, such as potatoes, turnips, yams, and beets. Avoid processed foods, soft drinks, sugar, caffeine, white flour products, and fried foods.

Before retiring, take several bites of some complex carbohydrates (crackers, potatoes, pasta, etc.) along with several bites of a protein (nut butter, yogurt, cheese, seeds, etc.), along with the last B complex for the day, some vitamin C, and a large glass of pure water or warm herbal tea.

NUTRITIONAL THERAPY: • Vitamin C to bowel tolerance (see Orthomolecular Medicine chapter) • Free-form amino acids (¼ -½ teaspoon ten minutes before meals, three to four times daily) • Vitamin A (50,000 IU daily for two months) • Vitamin E emulsion (400-600 IU daily) • Vitamin B complex (low dose, three to four times daily) •

Acidophilus • Glandular tissue of organs involved (liver, spleen, or lymph/thymus) • Chlorophyll • Multivitamin/mineral supplement

Self-Care

The following therapies can be undertaken at home under appropriate professional supervision.

Biofeedback Training and Neurotherapy / Fasting / Qigong and Tai Chi

HERBS: Combine the tinctures of myrrh, echinacea, wormwood, cleavers, and calendula in equal parts and take ½ teaspoon of this mixture four times a day.

HOMEOPATHY: *Belladonna, Merc iod., Phytolacca*

HYDROTHERAPY: • Constitutional hydrotherapy (apply two to five times weekly). • Hyperthermia (apply one to two times weekly).

JUICE THERAPY: • Carrot, beet, tomato, green pepper (add a little garlic and onion) • Lemon, orange, pineapple • Wheat grass juice or other fresh green juices

Professional Care

The following therapies should only be provided by a qualified health professional.

Acupuncture / Cell Therapy / Magnetic Field Therapy / Naturopathic Medicine / Osteopathic Medicine / Traditional Chinese Medicine

ENVIRONMENTAL MEDICINE: According to Marshall Mandell, M.D., there have been mono-like reactions in allergic people who do not have the mono infection caused by the Epstein-Barr virus.

OXYGEN THERAPY: Ozone autohemotherapy (treatment by reinjection of the individual's own blood) has been shown effective against the Epstein-Barr virus.

MOTION SICKNESS

A disorder that manifests in some individuals experiencing motion, usually while traveling by car, train, sea, and air, or acceleration and deceleration by other means.

SYMPTOMS: Mild symptoms may be uneasiness and headache and may also include nausea. Severe symptoms may include vomiting, dizziness, excessive yawning, fatigue, weakness, inability to concentrate, excessive sweating and salivation, pallor (turning white), and severe distress. Prolonged motion sickness, such as on a long sea voyage or airplane flight, may produce depression, low blood pressure, dehydration, or worsen the condition of people who are already ill due to other factors.

SPECIAL NOTES: It is caused by movement on the organ of balance in the inner ear. Other factors that may play a role are genetics, anxiety, movement immediately after eating or eating too much, and poor ventilation. There is a great variation in susceptibility of different people.

Treatment is difficult compared to prevention. Susceptible people should position themselves where there is minimal motion, focus on a point on the horizon, and try to be in a well-ventilated area. If travel is short, avoid drinking or eating, move as little as possible, take preventive substances (see Nutritional Therapy) two hours before travel.

Alternative Treatments

Refer to alternative therapy chapters for more information before evaluating or applying any treatment. Some conditions, including yours, may require a physician's care.

DIET: On short trips, avoid eating and drinking at all. On longer trips, try sipping small amounts of fresh lemon or lime juice, strong green tea, or ginger tea.

NUTRITIONAL THERAPY: • Ginger (four capsules, taken two hours before travel and one per hour during the first few hours of travel) • Vitamin B complex • Vitamin B$_6$ (50 mg) • Magnesium (100 mg) • Charcoal tablets (four, taken several hours before travel) may be helpful if ginger capsules have not proven helpful in the past.

Self-Care

The following therapies can be undertaken at home under appropriate professional supervision.

Biofeedback Training and Neurotherapy / Fasting

ACUPRESSURE: Research has shown that the nausea associated with travel sickness eases dramatically following strong direct thumb pressure to acupressure point P6 (see acupressure chart in the introduction to this section), which lies on the palm side of the wrist, two thumb widths above the main wrist crease, between the tendons, on each arm. A minute of firm pressure to this point on one arm, followed by the same to the other, usually relieves motion sickness nausea for hours at a time.

AROMATHERAPY: A drop of peppermint oil on the tongue.

FLOWER ESSENCES: Flower essences for accompanying emotional/mental states. Rescue Remedy®; Scleranthus.

HERBS: Numerous clinical trials have shown ginger to be effective in preventing the symptoms of motion sickness.[57] It may be taken as a cup of fresh infusion, eaten as candied ginger, or as capsules of the powder. For people who do not like the taste of ginger, the capsules are ideal (usual dosage is two to four, as needed).

HOMEOPATHY: • *Ipecac., Colchicum, Nux vom., Ignatia, Belladonna* • *Cocculus* must be taken alone, not in combination with other remedies.

JUICE THERAPY: Ginger.

NATUROPATHIC MEDICINE: A simple, readily available therapy for nausea due to motion is to drink ginger tea. This is made by simply putting a teaspoon of ground culinary ginger into a cup of boiling water and drinking as often as needed.

REFLEXOLOGY: Ear reflex, diaphragm, neck, spine

Professional Care

The following therapies should only be provided by a qualified health professional.

Acupuncture / Hypnotherapy / Naturopathic Medicine / Osteopathic Medicine

ENVIRONMENTAL MEDICINE: According to Marshall Mandell, M.D., motion sickness is often a sensitivity reaction to the traffic fumes a person is exposed to while driving.

TRADITIONAL CHINESE MEDICINE: Roasted ginger in capsules two to three times a day, two days before traveling.

MUSCULAR CRAMPS

Muscles are bundles of specialized cells that are able to contract and relax, creating movement. There are three types of muscles: skeletal, smooth, and cardiac (heart). Skeletal muscle has a certain level of constant contraction called muscle tone. However, excessive tone or abnormal tone can create spasms, cramps, and twitches.

SYMPTOMS: Tightness, discomfort, pain, and sometimes tingling and burning are associated with areas in which the muscle tone has become excessive and/or the muscles are impinging on the associated tissues or nerves.

OCCURRENCE: Everyone experiences muscle cramping at some time. People more susceptible to this condition usually are sedentary (sit most of the day), do not exercise regularly, and eat too few green vegetables (magnesium-rich foods) or consume foods that reduce calcium availability to the body (acid diets higher in animal foods and grains and meats, or higher in commercial colas, caffeinated beverages, refined sugars, and processed foods high in phosphates).

CONSIDER: Insufficient exercise, low thyroid function, deficiency in iron (anemia), magnesium, calcium, vitamin E, folic acid, dietary imbalance, excessive coffee consumption, maladjustment of the spine or local area, residue from past injury to the area or corresponding one, stress, poor circulation secondary to heart problems, problems secondary to disease such as diabetes or arthritis, or fatigue in general.

SPECIAL NOTES: The healthier the metabolism and tone of muscles (in a well-exercised and nourished individual), the less the tendency toward cramps, spasms, and twitches. The healthy individual will be less prone to injury from trauma and will heal more quickly once injured, or will have fewer symptoms from small repetitive motions that may create problems in less-toned individuals. Poor posture, poor or inadequate circulation, sitting habits at work, shoes, and not taking intermittent rest or exercise/stretching periods throughout the day, especially at a job that requires sustained positions, all contribute toward susceptibility to spasms.

Diuretic medication aggravates loss of minerals, particularly potassium, calcium, and magnesium, and may worsen muscle spasms. Also, check for food sensitivities.

Alternative Treatments

Refer to alternative therapy chapters for more information before evaluating or applying any treatment. Some conditions, including yours, may require a physician's care.

DIET: Whole foods diet high in calcium-rich and magnesium-rich foods: leafy green vegetables, fruits (particularly apricots), yogurt, kefir, millet, sesame seeds. Also excellent are kelp, brewer's yeast, cornmeal, alfalfa, and honey. Avoid excessive consumption of citrus, meat, liver, and excess grains. The idea is to eat an alkaline diet (high in fresh vegetables and fruits) so that the overall metabolism of the body is not acidic, causing the loss or imbalance of calcium. Vitamin E deficiency may also aggravate normal metabolism of muscles. Vitamin E is found in raw seeds and nuts and whole grains. Reduce phosphorus in diet, which is usually accomplished by avoiding processed foods and eating five to seven servings of vegetables and fruits per day.

NUTRITIONAL THERAPY: • Magnesium (magnesium aspartate is excellent, but any magnesium should be helpful; may be taken hourly if needed, but it may create loose stools, which will stop once magnesium is reduced) • Calcium • Vitamin E (400 IU three times daily) • Vitamin B complex with extra niacin (B_3) and thiamin (B_1) • Potassium • Vitamin C • Silicon • Niacinamide • Chlorophyll • Multimineral and trace element formula • Folic acid (500 mcg three times daily)

Some cases of muscular spasm that do not respond to the above are responsive to higher-than-normal dosages of folic acid, which may help improve microvascular circulation.

Alan R. Gaby, M.D., has found that acute or chronic muscle spasms respond well to an intravenous injection of a "cocktail" composed of magnesium chloride hexahydrate, calcium glycerophosphate, hydroxocobalamin, pyridoxine hydrochloride (vitamin B_6), dexpanthenol, B complex, and vitamin C. This is a modification of the nutrient cocktail popularized by John Meyers, M.D.

If cramps are determined to be of a biochemical origin (disruption in electrolyte and trace element balance), mineral therapy with magnesium/calcium/potassium aminoethanol phosphate (AEP) may be effective.

There are many possible causes for muscular cramps, some simple, some complex. Cramps may occur in the calves due to a deficiency of sodium in the blood. Calf cramps brought on by neuralgia can also be a symptom of diabetes. Cramps may occur after long hikes, due to a slipped disk, or due to venous congestion and venous thrombosis, as during pregnancy.

Self-Care

The following therapies can be undertaken at home under appropriate professional supervision.

Biofeedback Training and Neurotherapy / Fasting / Guided Imagery

AROMATHERAPY: Rosemary, lavender, marjoram, chamomile, clary sage

BODYWORK: • Acupressure, shiatsu, reflexology, massage, Rolfing, Feldenkrais Method, Hellerwork • Massage painful muscles with a mixture of grated ginger juice and equal parts olive or sesame oil. • For nighttime leg cramps, soak in a warm bath before going to bed, then stretch your legs. • Regular stretching using yoga reduces the likelihood of cramps, especially in main trouble areas such as the hamstring and calf muscles.

FLOWER ESSENCES: Rescue Remedy® Cream. Rescue Remedy® for accompanying stress.

HERBS: • Drink a strong decoction of cramp bark tea as needed or take ½ teaspoon of cramp bark tincture four times a day. • For temporary relief, apply a mixture of equal parts tincture of lobelia and cramp bark to the affected muscles.

HYDROTHERAPY: • Hot pack, immersion, or sitz bath (apply as needed to relieve pain) • Take a full, hot bath for 20-60 minutes.

JUICE THERAPY: • Carrot, beet, celery, cucumber • Sweet fruit juices

NATUROPATHIC MEDICINE: Quite possibly the most commonly deficient mineral, especially in men, is magnesium. As a first line of treatment for muscle cramps, supplement the diet with magnesium and apply local Epsom salt packs.

REFLEXOLOGY: Hip/knee, hip/sciatic, lower spine, parathyroid, adrenals

TOPICAL TREATMENT: Apply mixture of essential oils (evening primrose or flaxseed oil), vitamin A, and zinc oxide locally over the area (three times daily for the first few days).

Professional Care

The following therapies should only be provided by a qualified health professional.

Acupuncture / Applied Kinesiology / Chiropractic / Environmental Medicine / Light Therapy / Magnetic Field Therapy / Natural Hormone Replacement Therapy / Naturopathic Medicine / Orthomolecular Medicine / Osteopathic Medicine

DETOXIFICATION THERAPY: May be indicated, depending on the condition of the person.

HYPNOTHERAPY: To promote muscular relaxation.

NAIL PROBLEMS

Nail changes, unless due to localized trauma (usually crushing or pressure), fungus (often associated with acrylic nails for cosmetic purposes), or bacteria (tinea and candidiasis), are usually signs of metabolic and nutritional changes within the body. Nails may also be affected by skin disease or general illness.

SYMPTOMS: Thickened and curved nails (onychogryposis) most often affect the big toe of elderly individuals and may signify poor circulation, a vascular system that is beginning to degenerate, or thyroid disease. Pitting may signify alopecia areata (hair loss or tendency toward hair loss during stress) or anemia. Pitting together with onycholysis (separation of the nail from its normal attachment to the nail bed) may be seen in psoriasis. Brittle, ridged, and curved nails may be seen in anemia secondary to iron deficiency. Brittle nails may be seen in thyroid problems, iron deficiency, kidney disorders, and poor circulation or be a symptom of an omega-3 fatty acid deficiency. Vertical lines in nails may suggest poor nutrient absorption, iron deficiency, or decreased general health or poor protein metabolism. Horizontal lines may occur with severe stress on the body, either emotionally or from disease and/or infection. Flat nails may suggest poor circulation from Raynaud's disease, while nail beading (bumps) may be arthritis. Nails that chip, crack, peel, and break suggest poor mineral levels often secondary to low digestive enzymes or food allergies.

Red skin around the cuticles may suggest poor essential fatty acid metabolism, cuticle biting and nervousness, or connective tissue disorders, such as lupus. Nails that appear thin and brassy in color, often ridged, suggest tendency to lose hair. Nails that are very square and wide may suggest tendency toward hormonal disorders. Black splinter-like marks under the nail bed may come from bleeding disorders or heart disease. Greenish color may be bacterial disease. Whitish nails may suggest anemia or kidney disorders. Whitish nails with pink color near the tips may suggest liver disease such as cirrhosis. Yellowish color or elevation of the ends of the nails may suggest bronchial, lung, or lymphatic disease, or may be secondary to continual nail polish wear or nicotine staining from smoking. Bluish color may be iron deficiency, heart problems, or respiratory disease or heavy metal poisoning. Darkening of the overall nail bed may suggest vitamin B_{12} deficiency. White spots on nails may signify zinc deficiency. These are sometimes called "Yom Kippur" spots, as fasting for one day on the Jewish holiday of Yom Kippur is enough, in some borderline individuals, to create a zinc deficiency that shows up as transient white spots on the fingernails.

Genetics may play a role in producing poorly formed or easily injured nails that suggest joint and connective tissue problems or may just not be significant at all. The whole person must be assessed to judge significance. Diagnosis should not be made on nail condition alone.

Alternative Treatments

Refer to alternative therapy chapters for more information before evaluating or applying any treatment. Some conditions, including yours, may require a physician's care.

DIET: Fresh carrot juice is excellent for strengthening the nails (by providing calcium and phosphorus). Problems with nails can be due to numerous dietary factors including excess salt intake, improper protein/calcium balance, and excess intake of citrus, lemon juice, and vinegar. In particular, assess and then consume, if appropriate, foods high in iron, quality sources of protein, whole grains, and seeds and nuts. Eat consistently, chew well, and decrease stressful life circumstances and stressor foods.

NUTRITIONAL THERAPY: • Silicon • Protein (free-form amino acids) • Calcium • Iron • Vitamin B complex • Biotin (a B vitamin)[58] • Gelatin • Zinc

According to Jonathan Wright, M.D., more than 90% of the people with poor fingernails tested in his laboratory don't have enough stomach acid.

Self–Care

The following therapies can be undertaken at home under appropriate professional supervision.

Fasting

AROMATHERAPY: Lemon

AYURVEDA: *Fungal infection:* local application of ½ teaspoon aloe vera gel and ¼ teaspoon of turmeric. *Brittle nails:* an herbal mixture of *prawal panchamrit* (200 mg) and *shatavari* (500 mg) with goat's milk, generally taken twice a day after lunch and dinner. The minerals calcium, magnesium, and zinc are also beneficial. *Infected cuticles and nails:* apply *neem* oil locally.

HERBS: Drink an infusion made from equal parts of nettle and horsetail three times a day.

HOMEOPATHY: *Calc phos., Graphites, Sulfur, Nat mur., Ferrum phos.*

JUICE THERAPY: Carrot, beet, celery blend

Professional Care

The following therapies should only be provided by a qualified health professional.

Magnetic Field Therapy / Natural Hormone Replacement Therapy / Naturopathic Medicine

OXYGEN THERAPY: When due to fungal infection, ozone may be effective.

TRADITIONAL CHINESE MEDICINE: Detoxifies the liver.

NAUSEA

Unpleasant sensation that usually occurs in the higher abdominal area and may proceed on to vomiting. It is not an illness itself but secondary to other factors such as pregnancy, inner ear disorders, overindulgence of food or alcohol, flu, or parasites.

SPECIAL NOTES: If there is a deficiency of digestive enzymes, bowel cleansing is recommended. Toxic stress in the liver or associated biliary system can also create a tendency to nausea. Anxiety and emotional stress in general may cause nausea in some individuals.

Alternative Treatments

Refer to alternative therapy chapters for more information before evaluating or applying any treatment. Some conditions, including yours, may require a physician's care.

DIET: Eat smaller, more frequent meals, avoid fats and especially processed fats, nibble on whole-grain crackers, sip liquids such as lemon water and fresh juices. Avoid aspartame (NutraSweet™) and monosodium glutamate (MSG).

NUTRITIONAL THERAPY: • Vitamin B complex • Vitamin B6 • Magnesium

Excessive intake of zinc in particular, or too many vitamins and minerals at one time, may cause nausea.

Self–Care

The following therapies can be undertaken at home under appropriate professional supervision.

Biofeedback Training and Neurotherapy / Fasting / Guided Imagery / Qigong and Tai Chi

ACUPRESSURE: To relieve nausea, firmly press P6 (for an illustration of this point number, see the acupressure chart in the introduction to this section) in the middle of the inner side of the forearm, two thumb widths above the wrist crease. Sit comfortably as you firmly hold this point for two minutes, taking long deep breaths, making sure that the exhalation should take longer than inhalation to achieve a sense of ease and calm. Then get some fresh air and walk around, swinging your hands freely by your sides. According to Leon Chaitow, N.D., D.O., research at Queens University, Belfast, has shown this to be effective in treating morning sickness nausea as well as the nausea associated with administration of chemotherapy and anesthesia.

AROMATHERAPY: • Peppermint, rosewood • Put a drop of peppermint oil on the tongue.

FLOWER ESSENCES: Rescue Remedy®

HERBS: The treatment depends upon the cause. An infusion of ginger or peppermint can be very settling.

HOMEOPATHY: *Ipecac., Nux vom., Pulsatilla, Calc fluor., Colchicum, Arsen alb.*

HYDROTHERAPY: Constitutional hydrotherapy (apply two to five times weekly).

MIND/BODY MEDICINE: Meditation has reduced anticipatory nausea associated with chemotherapy.

NATUROPATHIC MEDICINE: A simple, readily available therapy for nausea due to motion or other causes (e.g., early in pregnancy) is to drink ginger tea. This is made by simply putting a teaspoon of ground culinary ginger into a cup of boiling water and drinking as often as needed.

REFLEXOLOGY: Liver, gallbladder, stomach, diaphragm

Professional Care

The following therapies should only be provided by a qualified health professional.

Acupuncture / Craniosacral Therapy / Detoxification Therapy / Environmental Medicine / Hypnotherapy / Magnetic Field Therapy / Naturopathic Medicine / Neural Therapy / Osteopathic Medicine

BODYWORK: Therapeutic Touch, shiatsu.

NEURALGIA, NEURO-PATHY, NEURITIS

Neuralgia: Spasms of pain that extend along the course of a nerve. There are many types of neuralgias, according to the nerve or body part affected or to the cause (such as the disease—gouty, anemic, diabetic, syphilitic). The most common neuralgias are Bell's palsy and trigeminal neuralgia.

Neuropathy: Disturbances and pathologies in the peripheral nervous system (nerves outside of the spine), often noninflammatory in nature, and may be secondary to diseases such as diabetes, pressure from nerve entrapment in carpal tunnel syndrome, disk lesions, or due to unknown causes (usually nutritional deficiencies). When several peripheral nerves are involved, it is called polyneuropathies.

Neuritis: Inflammation of a nerve or group of nerves. Symptoms are similar to above, except more often include burning and may manifest with swelling and fever and, in some severe cases, episodes of convulsions. Can occur anywhere in body, such as sciatic nerve (buttocks or down the leg) or the optic nerve (eye).

SYMPTOMS: Mild or severe pain, constant or intermittent pain, burning, tingling, or stabbing forms of discomfort or pain.

CONSIDER: Associated diseases such as diabetes, thyroid disease, pressure from a tumor, nutrient deficiency, metabolic imbalance, infection, gout, leukemia, alcohol abuse, heavy metal toxicity, or direct trauma. Assessment of a possible underlying disease must be made by a doctor.

Alternative Treatments

Refer to alternative therapy chapters for more information before evaluating or applying any treatment. Some conditions, including yours, may require a physician's care.

DIET: Whole foods diet, increase fluid intake, and avoid stressor and stimulating foods, such as caffeinated beverages, refined sugars, cigarettes, and commercial carbonated beverages.

NUTRITIONAL THERAPY: • Thiamin (vitamin B$_1$, 100 mg two to three times daily) • Folic acid (500 mcg two times daily) • Niacin (vitamin B$_3$) • Vitamin B complex • Vitamin B$_{12}$ (intramuscular injections are best in acute conditions) • Vitamin C and bioflavonoids • Vitamin B$_6$ • Pantothenic acid • Brewer's yeast • Calcium • Magnesium • Lecithin • Sometimes proteolytic enzymes on an empty stomach away from meals is helpful especially in neuritis; take with vitamin C and bioflavonoids.

Self-Care

The following therapies can be undertaken at home under appropriate professional supervision.

Biofeedback Training and Neurotherapy / Fasting / Yoga

AROMATHERAPY: Chamomile, eucalyptus, cedarwood, juniper, lavender

HERBS: Combine equal parts of the tinctures of St. John's wort, skullcap, oat, and Siberian ginseng. Take one teaspoon of this mixture three times a day. This may be made stronger, if there is much pain, by the addition of valerian or Jamaican dogwood. Externally, peppermint oil can be applied as a mild local anesthetic.

HOMEOPATHY: *Belladonna, Aconite, Mag phos., Phytolacca, Chelidonium, Lycopodium, Arsen alb.*

HYDROTHERAPY: Contrast application (apply daily).

JUICE THERAPY: Parsley, celery, carrot blend

TOPICAL TREATMENT: Epsom salt packs

Professional Care

The following therapies should only be provided by a qualified health professional.

Acupuncture / Cell Therapy / Chiropractic / Craniosacral Therapy / Environmental Medicine / Light Therapy / Magnetic Field Therapy / Naturopathic Medicine / Neural Therapy / Osteopathic Medicine / Traditional Chinese Medicine

DETOXIFICATION THERAPY: May be indicated, depending on the condition of the person.

OXYGEN THERAPY: Hyperbaric oxygen therapy may be useful for acute conditions of neuralgia. Hydrogen peroxide therapy may be useful for neuritis.

NOSEBLEEDS

Bleeding or loss of blood from the mucous membrane that lines the nose, usually from only one nostril.

OCCURRENCE: Most commonly occur in childhood and usually are not serious.

CONSIDER: In adults, most nosebleeds are secondary to trauma to the nose (external blows, blowing nose too strongly and rupturing membranes, or to scratches from the fingernails), from irritating crust formations secondary to colds, infections, or the flu, very dry conditions such as high altitudes or desert areas, sudden changes in atmospheric pressure, and from nutrient deficiencies, most commonly vitamin C and/or bioflavonoids. In adults, recurrent nosebleeds may signify underlying disease such as high blood pressure (hypertension), a tumor in the nose or sinuses, or a bleeding disorder.

What to do immediately: If nose starts to bleed immediately after a traumatic blow to the head, this may signify a fracture in the skull and individual must proceed to a hospital immediately.

In other instances, when there is not a danger of skull fracture, do the following: Sit, lean forward, blow all blood and clots out of both nostrils, open mouth and breathe through the mouth (avoiding blood clots obstructing air passages). Pinch lower part of nose for 20 minutes, then slowly release pressure and avoid any contact or pressure with the nose. If bleeding continues after the first 20 minutes of pressure, pack nose with gauze and apply crushed ice within a cloth against the nose and cheek. Lie back, once nose is packed and ice is applied, and refrain from any motion or activity for several hours. If bleeding continues after 20 minutes, notify a doctor. May need to cauterize (therapeutic application of heat) or, in very rare and severe cases, may require surgery.

Once bleeding has stopped: Squeeze contents of vitamin E and vitamin A capsules into lining of nose. May also use zinc oxide, aloe vera gel, comfrey, or calendula ointment, and then place small gauze piece against the gel.

Blood thinners such as Coumadin or aspirin may cause nosebleeds. If this happens, notify your doctor, who may alter dosage of blood thinners.

Alternative Treatments

Refer to alternative therapy chapters for more information before evaluating or applying any treatment. Some conditions, including yours, may require a physician's care.

DIET: Vitamin K is essential for blood clotting and is found in watercress, dark green leafy vegetables, kale, and alfalfa.

NUTRITIONAL THERAPY: • Vitamin C (3 g at start of bleeding and 1 g every hour if bleeding continues) • Rutin and other bioflavonoids

Self-Care

The following therapies can be undertaken at home under appropriate professional supervision.

Fasting / Flower Essences

AROMATHERAPY: Lemon, lavender, cypress, frankincense

BODYWORK: Acupressure, shiatsu, reflexology

HERBS: Use a snuff made from finely ground oak bark. If the nosebleed is related to hypertension, refer to that chapter.

HOMEOPATHY: *Hyoscyamus, Chamomilla, Rhus tox., Ipecac., Belladonna, Hamamelis*

HYDROTHERAPY: Ice pack (apply over nose and to back of neck to stop bleeding).

JUICE THERAPY: Carrot, beet, with ginger or cayenne

PRACTICAL HINTS: Sit down with head tipped forward. Stay in a cool room.

Professional Care

The following therapies should only be provided by a qualified health professional.

Acupuncture / Environmental Medicine / Naturopathic Medicine / Osteopathic Medicine / Traditional Chinese Medicine

PANCREATITIS

Inflammation of the pancreas, which may be either acute (short-lived episode that heals completely) or chronic (irreversible, degenerative cellular changes within the pancreas that continue and progress even after the cause, usually alcohol, is removed).

SYMPTOMS: Half of individuals with an acute pancreatitis attack, which usually lasts about 48 hours, have severe abdominal pain that radiates straight into the back. Pain usually begins suddenly, reaches a severe and maximum intensity within several minutes, and persists for hours or days. Pain is slightly relieved by sitting and worse with movement. The pain is often accompanied by nausea, vomiting, sweating, increased heart rate, dizziness, pallor, and feeling very ill. During the attack, pancreatic enzymes are released into the bloodstream and diagnosis of acute pancreatitis is made by assessment of the blood levels of these enzymes.

Chronic pancreatitis has similar symptoms, although the attacks usually last longer and are recurrent, becoming more severe as the disease progresses. Chronic pancreatitis is often related to gallbladder disorders or stones. In some individuals, the only sign of pancreatitis is either malabsorption (manifesting as pale-colored, bulky, and greasy stools, as the injured pancreas does not release adequate pancreatin enzymes) or diabetes (as the injured pancreas does not make enough insulin).

Recurrences may be prevented by treating the cause, such as avoiding alcohol, treating the liver and gallbladder, losing weight, improving nutrition, and avoiding drugs. Chronic pancreatitis may need insulin, or nutritional and natural programs to balance blood sugar and support the pancreas, and nutrients or even drugs to reduce the pain. Rarely, after other options have been tried and failed, surgery is necessary to remove the pancreas or gallstones that are creating obstructions.

Alternative Treatments

Refer to alternative therapy chapters for more information before evaluating or applying any treatment. Some conditions, including yours, may require a physician's care.

DIET: In acute state, fasting from all fluids and foods may be advised as presence of food in intestines stimulates the pancreas and makes the symptoms worse. Intravenous solutions given by doctors and other therapeutic interventions may be necessary. Once abdominal pain is gone, the blood levels of pancreatic enzymes are normal, and appetite and feeling of well-being returns, foods can be reintroduced. Diet should follow diabetic protocol (see Diabetes chapter).

Refined sugars, caffeine, and alcohol should be strictly avoided. Small, frequent meals with emphasis on complex carbohydrates, vegetables, and small amounts of fruits should be consumed. Exercise is also important to stabilize blood sugar.

NUTRITIONAL THERAPY: • Chromium (300 mcg daily) • Pancreatin enzymes with meals • Pancreas glandular • Lipotropic factors •Vitamin B complex with extra niacin and pantothenic acid •Vitamin C (buffered) • Try L-phenylalanine for pain reduction in chronic pancreatitis. • Acidophilus • Magnesium • Multimineral • Liquid chlorophyll

Self-Care

The following therapies can be undertaken at home under appropriate professional supervision.

Fasting / Flower Essences / Qigong and Tai Chi

AROMATHERAPY: For weakness, marjoram, lemon

HERBS: Combine equal parts of the glycerates of fringe-tree bark, balmony, and milk thistle. Take one teaspoon three times a day.

HYDROTHERAPY: Constitutional hydrotherapy (apply two to five times weekly).

JUICE THERAPY: Carrot, Jerusalem artichoke (minimum protein intake), beet and garlic (diluted 50/50).

Professional Care

The following therapies should only be provided by a qualified health professional.

Cell Therapy / Enzyme Therapy / Homeopathy / Magnetic Field Therapy / Naturopathic Medicine / Osteopathic Medicine / Traditional Chinese Medicine

DETOXIFICATION THERAPY: Detoxification is probably indicated, unless condition may be chronic and/or due to undernourishment.

OXYGEN THERAPY: Hydrogen peroxide therapy (IV).

PARALYSIS

Total loss or partial impairment of motor function (voluntary movement of a part of the body) because one or more muscles cannot be properly contracted. Paralysis is usually classified according to the cause or to the nerve, muscle, or body part involved. It can involve a wide range of muscles and can be permanent or temporary.

SYMPTOMS: The affected body part manifests loss of controlled motion, either rigid or spastic muscle, or possibly flaccid (soft and floppy) muscle. When all four limbs and the trunk of the body are paralyzed, it is called quadriplegia. Paraplegia is when both legs and possibly part of the trunk is involved. Hemiplegia is when half of the body is paralyzed.

SPECIAL NOTES: Paralysis may be caused by spinal cord problems, brain disorders, congenital defects affecting the spine and brain, traumatic injury to the spine and brain, diseases that affect these organs, peripheral nerve disorders, and muscle diseases.

Alternative Treatments

Refer to alternative therapy chapters for more information before evaluating or applying any treatment. Some conditions, including yours, may require a physician's care.

DIET: Whole foods diet high in foods rich in magnesium, which is a natural muscle relaxant. Such foods are dark leafy greens and green drinks (blended greens plus pineapple juice). Avoid foods that tend to make the blood sugar rise and drop rapidly and thus may contribute to muscular weakness or spasticity, such as excessive consumption of refined sugars, caffeinated beverages, and nutrient-poor meals, which lower the body levels of minerals and trace minerals.

NUTRITIONAL THERAPY: • Vitamin B$_6$ • Magnesium • Niacinamide •Vitamin B complex •Vitamin C • Free-form amino acids

Vitamin-mineral injections may be helpful in some individuals. Consult an orthomolecular physician.

Self-Care

The following therapies can be undertaken at home under appropriate professional supervision.

Biofeedback Training and Neurotherapy / Fasting / Yoga

AYURVEDA: *Yogaraj guggulu* (200 mg) for *vata* types, *kaishore guggulu* (200 mg) for *pitta* types, or *punarnava guggulu* (200 mg) for *kapha* types, generally taken twice a day after lunch and dinner. For all doshas, take *triphala*, ½ teaspoon with warm water and *netra basti*.

REFLEXOLOGY: Whole spine, brain, related reflex area.

Professional Care

The following therapies should only be provided by a qualified health professional.

Acupuncture / Chiropractic / Craniosacral Therapy / Environmental Medicine / Magnetic Field Therapy / Naturopathic Medicine / Neural Therapy / Osteopathic Medicine

HOMEOPATHY: *Aconite, Arsen alb., Ignatia, Chamomilla, Colchicum, Conium mac.* Consult a physician.

OXYGEN THERAPY: Hyperbaric oxygen therapy may be useful for paralysis due to brain damage.

PARKINSON'S DISEASE

A slow, progressive disorder of the central nervous system.

SYMPTOMS: The four major symptoms are slowness of movement, muscular rigidity, resting tremor (trembling at rest or when not moving), and postural instability (shuffling, unbalanced walk that progresses into uncontrollable tiny, running steps to keep from falling). This disease usually begins as a slight tremor in one hand, arm, or leg. The tremor is at its peak during rest, improves with movement, and is completely absent during sleep. The tremor gets worse with fatigue and stress. In 50% to 80% of individuals with Parkinson's disease, the tremor starts in one hand and resembles trying to roll a pill between the fingers; thus, it is called a "pill-rolling tremor." The jaw, tongue, forehead, and eyelids may also tremble, but the voice is not shaky. Another early sign is a severe decrease in blinking of the eyes. As the disease progresses, there is more stiffness, weakness, and both sides of the body become involved, and the initial tremors may become less prominent. There may develop a shaking of the head, a mask-like expression on the face in which the eyes do not blink, and a rigid, bent-over posture that is permanent. Speech becomes difficult and slow, handwriting becomes small. Depression and dementia may occur. All daily activities become difficult.

OCCURRENCE: 50,000 cases a year in the geriatric population in the United States, or one in 200 elderly. Men are more susceptible than women.

SPECIAL NOTES: If untreated, the disease progresses over 15 years to severe incapacitation. Modern treatment with complicated drug combinations, mobility exercises, and support groups has reduced the severity of this disease. The cause is unknown. However, an imbalance of two brain chemicals, dopamine and acetylcholine, seems to be involved. A deficiency of dopamine in the brain may be due to underlying nutritional deficiencies, cerebral vascular disease (blockage of blood vessels in brain), side effects of anti-psychotic drugs, carbon monoxide poisoning, abuse of certain designer drugs, and a rare infection (encephalitis lethargica).

Levodopa is the most commonly used drug and cannot be taken with vitamin B_6. Using vitamin B_6 alone may be just as effective in some individuals. This drug should be taken away from protein meals, which decrease its effectiveness.

Alternative Treatments

Refer to alternative therapy chapters for more information before evaluating or applying any treatment. Some conditions, including yours, may require a physician's care.

DIET: Whole foods diet with emphasis on lots of fluids, raw foods (50% to 75% of the diet), and sprouts. Also good are green leafy vegetables, rutabagas, sesame seeds, and sesame butter.

If on the drug levodopa, must decrease the foods that are rich in vitamin B_6—whole grains (especially oats), raw nuts (especially peanuts), bananas, potatoes, liver, and fish. According to Jonathan Wright, M.D., most drug treatment for Parkinson's is done with Sinemet (trade name for a combination of levadopa and carbidopa), for which one doesn't need to avoid vitamin B_6.

NUTRITIONAL THERAPY: Assessment of individual amino acids is important. Consult an orthomolecular doctor. If unable to do so, take GABA (gamma-aminobutyric acid—500 mg once daily), along with a mixed amount of free-form amino acids, calcium, and magnesium. If on

levodopa, take B vitamins separately, all of them without vitamin B_6 (injectable form is optimal, but high oral intake of each at about 50 mg two times daily is good). If not on levodopa, take vitamin B complex (100 mg three times daily), along with vitamin B_6 (300 mg three times daily), lecithin (one teaspoon three times daily), vitamin C, evening primrose oil, multivitamin/mineral complex, and DHEA (a steroid hormone produced by the adrenal glands). Consult with your doctor.

Researchers from Hahnemann University, in Philadelphia, report that monkeys suffering from neurological damage regained their ability to walk and climb after receiving injections of GM1 ganglioside, a substance that occurs naturally in nerve cells. The researchers speculate that GM1 ganglioside may stimulate dopamine production and stabilize injured neurons, offering hope of it becoming an effective treatment for people with Parkinson's disease.[59]

Vitamin C may help "on-off attacks" (two to five years on levadopa results in shortened positive response time to treatment) and other side effects of levadopa. Long-term vitamin E (1,000 IU daily) supplementation may also slow the progression of Parkinson's disease.

The coenzyme nicotinamide adenine dinucleotide (NADH) in a therapeutic dose of 25-50 mg a day produces a beneficial effect in patients with Parkinson's, with the most noticeable results occurring after intravenous rather than after intramuscular administration.[60]

A study with four patients with Parkinson's disease who were given injections of 100 mg of neotrophin-1 (complex glycoproteins, in this case derived from snake venom) resulted in dramatic improvement after a period of six to eight weeks.[61]

Self-Care

The following therapies can be undertaken at home under appropriate professional supervision.

Fasting / Flower Essences / Yoga

HERBS: • Passionflower works synergistically with the drug L-dopa (levodopa). The reduction in passive tremor produced by using both L-dopa and passionflower is usually greater than the L-dopa by itself. Passionflower has only a minimal effect if used alone. Take ½ teaspoon of passionflower tincture three times a day. • Levodopa occurs naturally in the Ayurvedic herb *Mucuna pruriens*, found to be effective in the treatment of Parkinson's.[62]

HYDROTHERAPY: Constitutional hydrotherapy (apply two to five times weekly).

JUICE THERAPY: • Carrot and spinach juice or carrot, beet, radish, garlic, and cucumber daily • Seasonal raw fruits and vegetables

ORTHOMOLECULAR MEDICINE: Abram Hoffer, M.D., Ph.D., F.R.C.P., recommends large quantities of vitamin B_3, either niacin or niacinamide, to protect people against the tendency of L-dopa to cause psychosis. However, the vitamins in these quantities do not have much effect on the tremor.

REFLEXOLOGY: Whole spine, all glands, diaphragm, chest/lung

Professional Care

The following therapies should only be provided by a qualified health professional.

Cell Therapy / Chelation Therapy / Craniosacral Therapy / Light Therapy / Magnetic Field Therapy / Natural Hormone Replacement Therapy / Naturopathic Medicine / Traditional Chinese Medicine

BODYWORK: Feldenkrais Method

DETOXIFICATION THERAPY: May be indicated, depending on the condition of the person.

HYPNOTHERAPY: To promote muscular relaxation and increase the mind's capacity to tolerate tremors.

PELLAGRA

Severe deficiency of niacin. Primary deficiencies usually occur in areas where maize (Indian corn) is the major constituent of the diet. Maize has a bound form of niacin that is not digestible unless it is pretreated with alkali such as in the preparation of tortillas. It also is low in tryptophan, which further helps the body assimilate niacin. Secondary deficiencies are associated with certain disorders that promote nutrient deficiencies, including severe diarrhea, parasites, cirrhosis of the liver, post-surgical nutrient deficiencies, stress, increased need due to genetics, and overconsumption of junk food (very low in B vitamins and high in refined sugars that use up B vitamins in their assimilation).

SYMPTOMS: Diarrhea, dementia, and dermatitis; in other words, symptoms of the skin and mucous membranes, the central nervous system, and the gastrointestinal tract. Other symptoms may be redness and swelling of the tongue and lips, burning of the mouth, pharynx, esophagus, abdominal distention and pain or discomfort, poor digestion, vomiting, diarrhea that is possibly bloody, weakness, weight loss, poor stress-coping skills, irritability, poor cold tolerance, confusion, memory impairment, and paranoia. In chronic cases, the skin that is exposed and manifests symptoms may turn dark, become thicker, rougher, and very dry. Symptoms may appear in any combination or singly.

OCCURRENCE: Mainly in rural and poor communities in India and South Africa, where people subsist mainly on maize, in alcoholics, or individuals who live on junk food diets.

CONSIDER: Rule out tongue and lip redness and swelling due to other vitamin deficiencies or diseases, diarrhea, and skin and central nervous system disorders due to other diseases.

SPECIAL NOTES: Multiple deficiencies of all the B vitamins and protein often occur together. Therefore, supplementation and dietary nutrient intervention should be balanced.

Alternative Treatments

Refer to alternative therapy chapters for more information before evaluating or applying any treatment. Some conditions, including yours, may require a physician's care.

DIET: Eat foods rich in niacin, B vitamins, protein, and the amino acid tryptophan: whole grains, bananas, raw seeds and nuts, peanuts, liver, avocados, broccoli, potatoes, tomatoes, legumes, collard greens, enriched breads and cereals, salmon, halibut, tuna, swordfish, skinless breast of chicken, and turkey. Strictly avoid refined sugars for the first several weeks of therapy. Brewer's yeast is a good natural source of the B vitamins if there is no candidiasis.

NUTRITIONAL THERAPY: • Niacinamide (300–1,000 mg in divided doses three times daily, depending on severity of symptoms). This is preferable and more commonly used instead of niacin, which usually creates uncomfortable flushing and chills and sometimes stomach pains. (If oral therapy cannot be taken, 100-250 mg injectable two to three times daily.) •Vitamin B complex (100 mg three times daily) • Protein supplements

Professional Care

The following therapies should only be provided by a qualified health professional.

Magnetic Field Therapy / Naturopathic Medicine / Orthomolecular Medicine / Traditional Chinese Medicine

PERIODONTAL (GUM) DISEASE

Inflammation or degeneration of the tissue that surrounds and supports the teeth—the periodontium made up of the gingiva (gums), the bone the teeth are "set" in (alveolar bone), the supporting ligaments (periodontal ligament), and tissue that connects these structures (cementum). The most common and often initial form of periodontal disease is inflammation of the gums, called gingivitis, which can be acute (short-lived episode), chronic (ongoing), or recurrent. Untreated gingivitis proceeds further with increasing inflammation and involvement of more tissues, such as the membranes around the base of the teeth and possible erosion of the underlying bone. This is then called periodontitis and is the major cause of bone loss in adults.

SYMPTOMS: Red, inflamed gum tissue that bleeds easily when exposed to very minimal injury such as with flossing or brushing the teeth, or eating hard foods such as raw apples. There is usually no pain.

OCCURRENCE: High in individuals with poor oral hygiene—poor habits of oral brushing and flossing with a characteristic buildup of bacterial plaque (sticky deposits made up of mucus and microorganisms that grow and adhere to carbohydrate residues left on the teeth due to insufficient cleaning habits). Increased during pregnancy and puberty, which may be secondary to hormonal factors or due to increased physiologic need for folic acid and B vitamins during these periods.

CONSIDER: Other risk factors for periodontal disease include problems with the biting surface (malocclusion), breathing through the mouth, food impaction, nutrient deficiencies (especially folic acid and vitamin B complex), decreased local tissue circulation secondary to plaque buildup or consistently eating low–fiber foods and insufficient flossing, and buildup of calculus (tartar or calcified plaque mixed with saliva).

Gingivitis may be one of the first signs that there is an underlying systemic problem or debilitating disease such as diabetes or leukemia, heavy metal toxicity, lowered resistance, allergies, or vitamin deficiencies. Periodontal disease may be aggravated and/or caused by hydrochloric acid deficiency, insufficient calcium in the diet or stressor foods that rob it from the system, and imbalances in the body with other minerals such as magnesium and zinc.

SPECIAL NOTES: Birth control pills tend to increase the body's requirement for folic acid and, if this is not met, there may be an increased risk of gingivitis. Smokers are two to four times more likely to suffer periodontal disease than nonsmokers.

The best treatment is prevention with daily removal of plaque through brushing and flossing, routine cleaning by a dentist every six months (more often if the disease is already occurring) not only to prevent but to monitor progress and condition of gums and supporting tissues, and eating a diet high in whole foods and fiber and avoiding excessive consumption of refined carbohydrates. Any underlying systemic problems must also be treated.

Alternative Treatments

Refer to alternative therapy chapters for more information before evaluating or applying any treatment. Some conditions, including yours, may require a physician's care.

DIET: Whole foods diet with emphasis on as many fresh fruits and vegetables as possible (five to seven servings daily), high–fiber foods, avoidance of refined sugars and carbohydrates, and sufficient pure water (especially first thing in the morning and last thing in the evening) to help cleanse the mouth. Foods to emphasize are blueberries, hawthorne berries, grapes.

NUTRITIONAL THERAPY: • Floss one to two times daily and then rinse mouth (for one minute) with several mouthfuls of liquid folic acid (0.1% solution) and then swallow. In one study, 60 individuals with gingivitis rinsed for one minute two times daily and had beneficial results.[63] If you cannot find liquid folic acid, buy folic acid crystals in 800 mcg capsules, empty two capsules in water and use this to gargle. • Take folic acid orally (500 mcg to 1 mg daily depending on severity of condition) •Vitamin C (1-3 g daily) with bioflavonoids •Vitamin A (25,000 IU daily for several months) • Calcium (650-1,500 mg daily) •

Vitamin B complex • Beta carotene •Vitamin E •Vitamin K • Magnesium • Zinc

"Pink toothbrush" is a syndrome caused by mild gum bleeding that causes the toothbrush to appear pink and is treated by the above. According to Jonathan Wright, M.D., coenzyme Q10 is widely recommended in Japan for periodontal disease.

Gum infection: Vitamin A (large dosages for first three days and then slowly reduce to maintenance dose over one to two weeks) with vitamin E and zinc. Or use oil from vitamin A and E capsules along with zinc oxide cream. May add aloe vera gel when the infection is gone and gums are in last stages of healing.

If gums do not respond within several weeks of adherence to flossing and nutrient program, see a dentist and/or physician. It is a good idea to get regular hygienic check-ups to assess the levels of infective pockets, monitor progress, and avoid periodontal disease that has gone into the bone and must be dealt with immediately to prevent further bone loss and more serious problems.

Self–Care

The following therapies can be undertaken at home under appropriate professional supervision.

Fasting

AYURVEDA: Bleeding gums: drink lemon water (juice of ½ lemon in one cup water). • Massage gums with coconut oil or goldenseal, bayberry, or myrrh. • Take 5 g of *amla* powder in one cup water daily. • Swish a mouthful of warm sesame oil for two minutes and then massage the gums and brush the teeth with *catechu* and *neem* powder paste.

HERBS: Used both internally and topically, herbs may be most helpful. Combine equal parts of the tinctures of myrrh and echinacea and apply small amounts to the gums three times a day using a very fine paintbrush. Use a mouthwash made from an infusion of sage or chamomile; do not swallow. For internal use, combine the tinctures of echinacea, cleavers, and prickly ash in equal parts and take one teaspoon twice a day.

HYDROTHERAPY: Contrast application (apply daily to face over involved areas).

JUICE THERAPY: Juices high in beta carotene, such as carrot or cantaloupe.

TOPICAL TREATMENT: • Toothpaste or other oral hygienic products that contain vitamin C, tea tree oil, citrus seed extract, or baking soda promote the health of the mouth, gums, and teeth. • Brush teeth with mixture of baking soda and hydrogen peroxide. • Brush tongue if coated in morning. • Massage gums with fingers. • For bleeding gums and pyorrhea (discharge of pus), use one teaspoon apple cider vinegar in a cup of water, morning and evening, as mouthwash and drink remainder. •Applying chlorophyll directly to the gums, rinsing with diluted hydrogen peroxide, or using a toothpaste containing tea tree oil, citrus seed extract, or hydrogen peroxide can aid in reversing gingivitis.

Professional Care

The following therapies should only be provided by a qualified health professional.

Acupuncture / Environmental Medicine / Magnetic Field Therapy / Naturopathic Medicine / Traditional Chinese Medicine

DETOXIFICATION THERAPY: May be indicated, depending on the condition of the person.

OXYGEN THERAPY: • Hyperbaric oxygen therapy • Ozonated water.

PLEURISY

Inflammation of the pleura, the membranes lining the lungs and thoracic cavity, which are constantly moist to facilitate lung movement within the chest. The inflammation is usually caused by a lung infection, but in more unusual circumstances may be caused by lung cancer, rheumatoid arthritis, and pulmonary embolism (blockage of a pulmonary artery by foreign matter).

SYMPTOMS: The symptoms of this disease come on very suddenly, with the primary characteristic being pain associated with inhaling and/or coughing. The pain may vary from vague discomfort to a severe and stabbing sensation. The pain may refer (travel) toward the shoulder of the involved side. Breathing usually becomes more rapid and shallow than usual. Motion on the side of the trunk that is involved may become limited.

SPECIAL NOTES: Treatment of the underlying lung condition is paramount, along with natural analgesics for the pain and anti-inflammatories for the inflammation.

Alternative Treatments

Refer to alternative therapy chapters for more information before evaluating or applying any treatment. Some conditions, including yours, may require a physician's care.

DIET: Emphasize fresh fruits and vegetables, hearty soups, organic citrus fruits (nibbling on the insides of the rinds), and using the spice turmeric very generously.

NUTRITIONAL THERAPY: • Vitamin A (200,000 IU first three days, reduce to 100,000 next three days, and then 50,000 IU for next two weeks) • Lung glandular (three to four tablets, 3-4 times daily before meals) • Vitamin C with bioflavonoids to bowel tolerance (see Orthomolecular Medicine chapter) • Essential fatty acids (six capsules, two times daily on empty stomach, before each meal containing some fat) • Proteolytic enzymes (four to six tablets, two to four times daily on an empty stomach) • Bromelain (100-200 mg daily, away from mealtimes, to reduce inflammatory process without side effects)

Self-Care

The following therapies can be undertaken at home under appropriate professional supervision.

Fasting / Qigong and Tai Chi / Yoga

HERBS: Mix equal parts of dried mullein and pleurisy root and drink as a hot infusion several times a day. In addition, combine the tinctures of pleurisy root, elecampane, and echinacea in equal parts and take one teaspoon of this mixture three times a day. Also, take either a clove of raw garlic or three capsules of garlic oil daily with each meal.

HOMEOPATHY: *Aconite, Bryonia, Apis mel., Cantharis, Kali carb., Sulfur, Arsen alb., Phosphorus*

HYDROTHERAPY: Constitutional hydrotherapy (apply daily) • Leon Chaitow, N.D., D.O., suggests alternating hot and cold applications to the rib cage many times a day to improve circulation and drainage (30 seconds to a minute hot, followed by ten seconds cold). Repeat the alternations three to five times, finishing with cold.

JUICE THERAPY: • Carrot, celery, parsley • Carrot, celery • Carrot, pineapple • Carrot, beet, cucumber • Garlic

REFLEXOLOGY: Lymph system, adrenals, diaphragm, chest/lung

Professional Care

The following therapies should only be provided by a qualified health professional.

Acupuncture / Environmental Medicine / Magnetic Field Therapy / Naturopathic Medicine

BODYWORK: • Osteopathic Medicine • Rolfing (Osteopathy and Rolfing both help to free the rib cage and thereby may promote better breathing, but cannot cure pleurisy.)

DETOXIFICATION THERAPY: May be indicated, depending on the condition of the person.

POISON OAK/IVY

Plants such as poison oak, ivy, sumac, ragweed, and primrose may cause a severe allergic reaction (contact dermatitis) when the oils from the leaves, bark, stems, flowers, and fruit come in contact with the skin or are inhaled. Certain species of plants are also poisonous when eaten.

SYMPTOMS: Contact dermatitis or allergic symptoms vary greatly and usually start with burning and itching. The skin then starts to swell, a rash spreads, and blisters form that may ooze. In severe cases, systemic symptoms may manifest, such as feeling ill in general, lethargy (fatigue), sleep disorders, and general discomfort.

Symptoms of internal poisoning from eating plants are varied and depend on the plant. There are hundreds of poisonous plants, the most common being the nightshades, belladonna (which produces rash, confusion, difficulty swallowing, blurred vision, and coma), foxglove (erratic heartbeat, irritation of the mouth, abdominal symptoms such as pain and diarrhea), and black berries eaten from nightshades or red holly berries (abdominal pain, vomiting, flushing, hyperactivity, delirium, and coma).

Eating poisonous plants must be treated by pumping the stomach (gastric lavage). Death from eating poisonous plants is extremely rare. The plants are the most poisonous in the spring and early summer but are even a problem when they are dried at other times of the year.

OCCURRENCE: Poison ivy accounts for 350,000 cases of contact dermatitis per year. Young children are the most commonly affected, from playing in patches of poisonous plants or being attracted to eating the colorful berries. Children should be taught not to eat wild plants and how to distinguish poisonous ones. Poison oak, ivy, and sumac grow as vines or bushes, and the leaves have three leaflets (ivy and oak) or a row of paired leaflets (sumac).

SPECIAL NOTES: Wash any clothing that has come in contact with the plants. Sometimes cases that do not go away are due to repeated exposure through contaminated clothing. The best treatment is prevention, so if walking in areas where poisonous plants are common, know how to identify them and wear protective clothing. Some sensitive individuals may react or continue to be exposed from petting animals that have run through patches of the plants or by inhaling smoke from burning plants. In rare cases, if the reaction seems so severe that there is difficulty breathing, you may need to contact a physician and take corticosteroids. Very hot water as from showering tends to spread the rash and increase itching afterward.

Alternative Treatments

Refer to alternative therapy chapters for more information before evaluating or applying any treatment. Some conditions, including yours, may require a physician's care.

NUTRITIONAL THERAPY: • Vitamin C (3 g first hour, then 1 g per hour, for first few days if reaction is severe) • Vitamin A (100,000 IU first two days in severe reaction and 50,000 IU if it is less severe, then reduce to 25,000 IU for next several days) • Vitamin E (1,000 IU first several days) • Zinc (50 mg first few days) • Vitamin B complex (100 mg of each two to three times daily for the first few days) • May add zinc oxide or unflavored yogurt to any of the topical treatments mentioned below.

Self-Care

The following therapies can be undertaken at home under appropriate professional supervision.

Fasting / Guided Imagery

FLOWER ESSENCES: Rescue Remedy Cream®; Crab Apple.

HERBS: Apply a poultice or tincture combination of equal parts of witch hazel, mugwort, white oak bark, and plantain.

HYDROTHERAPY: Cold compress (apply as needed to control itching and pain).

TOPICAL TREATMENT: • Rinse affected area with apple cider vinegar and goldenseal. • Frequent warm baths with apple cider vinegar or cornstarch. • Apply one of the following: aloe vera gel, witch hazel, paste of baking soda and witch hazel, paste of activated charcoal powder.

Professional Care

The following therapies should only be provided by a qualified health professional.

Applied Kinesiology / Chelation Therapy / Environmental Medicine / Magnetic Field Therapy / Naturopathic Medicine / Traditional Chinese Medicine

DETOXIFICATION THERAPY: May be indicated, depending on the condition of the person.

OXYGEN THERAPY: Hyperbaric oxygen therapy.

POLIO

A childhood viral infection, with a wide range of manifestations from general mild illness to paralysis.

SYMPTOMS: Symptoms may vary widely, but there are two major types. *"Minor illness":* 80% to 90% of poliomyelitis infections, usually in very young children, may have no symptoms or mild ones such as sore throat, fatigue, fever, headache, and vomiting. Symptoms occur three to five days after exposure and last for 24–72 hours. *"Major illness":* In older children and adults, the two most characteristic symptoms are fever and muscular paralysis. Central nervous system symptoms occur such as deep muscle pain, tingling and hypersensitivities of skin, meningitis (inflammation of the outer coverings of spinal cord and brain), severe stiff neck and backache, fever, severe headache, generalized muscle aches, and possibly widespread muscle twitching. These symptoms may occur very rapidly, culminating in severe weakness or muscular paralysis within a few hours from onset. The lower limbs are the most commonly affected. If the infection spreads to the brain, there may also be difficulty in swallowing and in respiration.

SPECIAL NOTES: Recovery from the minor illness, nonparalytic polio, is total. Recovery from the major illness, paralytic polio, occurs in half the individuals. Twenty-five percent suffer from minor residual muscle weaknesses and one in ten dies. Less than 25% are left with severe muscular disabilities. Years later, even patients who have totally recovered, it appears that some individuals have a relapse called a "post-polio" episode, in which there is a recurrence of muscular weakness and pain.

Alternative Treatments

Refer to alternative therapy chapters for more information before evaluating or applying any treatment. Some conditions, including yours, may require a physician's care.

DIET: Whole foods diet with emphasis on foods rich in magnesium, such as dark-green leafy vegetables.

NUTRITIONAL THERAPY: • Magnesium (100-800 mg daily). First, increase dosage up to the amount that creates very soft stools, then reduce by 100-200 mg and this will be your daily dose. Sometimes, one form of magnesium will irritate a particular individual and every dose will seem to create softer stools. You may need to explore different types of magnesium. • Niacinamide (taken four times daily to keep blood levels high, to increase muscular strength and motion, and to decrease pain). If not taken regularly, it will not help.

Self-Care

The following therapies can be undertaken at home under appropriate professional supervision.

Biofeedback Training and Neurotherapy / Yoga

JUICE THERAPY: Carrot, beet, radish, celery

HYDROTHERAPY: Constitutional hydrotherapy (apply two to five times weekly) or heating compress • Cold socks treatment several times daily, for head or chest congestion; replace socks when dry. • Whirlpool baths may improve circulation.

Professional Care

The following therapies should only be provided by a qualified health professional.

Environmental Medicine / Magnetic Field Therapy / Prolotherapy / Traditional Chinese Medicine

BODYWORK: Feldenkrais Method (for treatment of post-polio syndrome).

FASTING: Under a doctor's supervision.

HYPNOTHERAPY: Valuable in increasing motivation for rehabilitation.

PRE- AND POSTOPERATIVE COMPLICATIONS

Nutrients and natural products taken before and after a surgical procedure may decrease healing time and pain, reduce complications, and increase quality of life during this period. Use for several weeks prior and several months to one year after surgery that requires invasion into the body, usually under a general anesthetic.

Preoperative Alternative Treatments

Refer to alternative therapy chapters for more information before evaluating or applying any treatment. Some conditions, including yours, may require a physician's care.

DIET: Whole foods diet with avoidance of excess refined sugars, colas, and processed foods. In particular, try to eat five to seven helpings of vegetables and fruits per day with unprocessed oils. Try to have at least one glass of fresh vegetable juice per day. Vary vegetables used in the juice.

Do not try to follow a weight-loss program before surgery, as this may cause a deficiency in amino acids, which are critical for wound healing.

NUTRITIONAL THERAPY: • Zinc • Pantothenic acid • Vitamin B complex • Vitamin C • Multivitamin/mineral complex • Vitamin E • Essential fatty acids (omega-3 fatty acids) • Magnesium will help the body hold on to its potassium • Potassium (50-100 mcg) • Beta carotene (100,000 IU per day a few days before surgery; you may notice an orange or yellow skin tone) • Alpha-ketoglutarate immediately before surgery • For cardiovascular surgery, take coenzyme Q10 (200 mg).

Two weeks before surgery, start building up the immune and body defense systems by taking a daily high-potency multivitamin/mineral complex, additional vitamin C, bioflavonoids, the herb echinacea, and antioxidants such as pycnogenol (pine bark or grape seed extract). Do not attempt any detoxification or cleansing program (except under special circumstances). Forty-eight hours before surgery, take anti-inflammatory nutrients such as protease or bromelain (pineapple enzymes), which will reduce the swelling, inflammation, and pain of surgery. Continue taking liquid ionic trace minerals until the post-surgical healing is complete. Many vital body processes depend on the movement of ions (ionic minerals) across the cell membranes. Minerals in the liquid ionic form can be readily absorbed by the body through the small intestine, providing key nutrients to those areas in need of repair after surgery.

To prevent blood pressure irregularities during surgery: • Vitamin C (10 g) • Magnesium sulfate (3 g) • Vitamin B_6 (500 mg) • Zinc sulfate (50 mg)

Self-Care

The following therapies can be undertaken at home under appropriate professional supervision.

Fasting / Qigong and Tai Chi

FLOWER ESSENCES: Rescue Remedy®

HERBS: See Postoperative section. According to W. Lee Cowden, M.D., for preoperative anemia, use yellowdock, mustard greens, turnip greens, spinach, kale. Yellowdock capsules are most effective when taken with vitamin C.

HOMEOPATHY: *Arnica*

HYDROTHERAPY: Constitutional hydrotherapy (apply two to five times weekly).

Professional Care

The following therapies should only be provided by a qualified health professional.

OXYGEN THERAPY: Hyperbaric oxygen therapy.

Postoperative Alternative Treatments

Refer to alternative therapy chapters for more information before evaluating or applying any treatment. Some conditions, including yours, may require a physician's care.

DIET: Same as preoperative recommendations except, initially, consume lighter foods such as soups, juices, broths, and pureed vegetables and fruits. Avoid refined sugars and excess consumption of fruit juices.

NUTRITIONAL THERAPY: Same as preoperative nutrients, except add free-form amino acids, glutamine, and extra vitamin B6. If there is difficulty in healing or a history of difficulty in healing, taking proteolytic enzymes (on an empty stomach and between meals) may hasten the healing process. • Alpha-ketoglutarate immediately after surgery. • Sublingual coenzymated B complex once or twice a day will help to speed healing. • Arginine in a very high dose. • Chromium (200-400 mcg a day) • Selenium (50 mcg per day) • Give aloe vera juice as soon as the patient is able to drink.

Severe trauma to the body, such as surgery, suppresses immune function. Supplementation with vitamins A and C following surgery has been shown to boost immunity. Vitamin C also aids in the healing of surgical incisions, as does the amino acid arginine.[64] It is also important to support the adrenal glands in handling the stress of surgery; take adaptogenic herbs such as ginseng or adaptogenic formulas.

To reduce the inflammation caused by surgery, continue to take protease or bromelain; omega-3 essential fatty acids (fish and flaxseed oils) are also anti-inflammatory. • Vitamin E and GLA can be given postoperatively by putting a teaspoon or two of flaxseed oil (for GLA) and 400 IU of vitamin E (puncture capsule and squirt onto skin along with flaxseed oil) onto the skin away from the incision once a day.

According to Alan R. Gaby, M.D., glutamine (250 mg per pound of body weight a day) reduces postoperative decrease in muscle protein synthesis and improves nitrogen balance. Glutamine requirements seem to increase after surgery to a level that isn't met by endogenous (coming from within) synthesis.

If antibiotic therapy is used before or after surgery, take acidophilus or a probiotic (beneficial intestinal bacteria) combination during and after the course of antibiotics. This recolonizes the good bacteria killed by the antibiotics and helps prevents an overgrowth of harmful microorganisms normally kept in check by the beneficial flora.

Self-Care

The following therapies can be undertaken at home under appropriate professional supervision.

FLOWER ESSENCES: Rescue Remedy®

HERBS: To facilitate postoperative healing, combine herbs that help the body deal with the physiological stress of the surgery and support the healing process in the tissue, organs, and systems that experience the most trauma during the operation. A generalization can be made for all surgery as follows: combine an adaptogen with herbs to support liver detoxification, cerebral oxygen availability, and general wound healing. Combine Siberian ginseng, ginkgo, milk thistle, and hawthorn tinctures in equal amounts; take ½ teaspoon of this mixture three times a day in the week leading up to surgery and for two weeks after. • Externally apply vitamin E oil with a calendula salve to optimize healing. Aloe vera gel can also be used topically.

HOMEOPATHY: *Arnica*

HYDROTHERAPY: Constitutional hydrotherapy (apply two to five times weekly).

Professional Care

The following therapies should only be provided by a qualified health professional.

Enzyme Therapy

PSORIASIS

Common, chronic skin condition that is prone to recurrences.

SYMPTOMS: Patches of skin that may be thickened and reddened and covered with silvery scales. It usually does not itch, but does cause discomfort and cosmetic embarrassment. Areas most commonly affected are the arms, elbows, behind the ears, scalp, back, legs, and knees.

According to Helmut Christ, M.D., of West Germany, "It has now been established that psoriasis is not a skin disorder, strictly speaking, but instead an inherited metabolic disturbance, which is triggered by environmental or stressful conditions, like faults in the diet, flu-like conditions, the administration of penicillin, death of a family member, surgery, etc."[65]

OCCURRENCE: Two percent of people in the United States and Europe. It occurs equally in men and women, and less in blacks and Asians. Psoriasis usually occurs between the ages of 15 and 30, although it can manifest at any time. It does reoccur, so once it has been contracted it can always potentially return. Patients with psoriasis have a higher incidence of rheumatoid diseases.

CONSIDER: Food allergies, essential fatty acid deficiencies, low digestive enzymes and hydrochloric acid, vitamin B complex deficiencies, and emotional stress.

SPECIAL NOTES: Psoriatic attacks can be stimulated by anxiety, illness, drugs (such as beta-blockers, lithium, and chloroquine), poison ivy or oak, skin damage (such as cuts, lacerations, surgery, and sunburn), food allergies, nutrient deficiencies, and several infections, bacterial or viral in origin. The true cause is unknown, but the physiological mechanism is that the new skin is being produced ten times faster than the old skin is being shed.

This creates an accumulation of the new skin, which forms thickened patches with the characteristic psoriatic scales.

Mild cases of psoriasis may be helped by moderate sunlight or ultraviolet light.

Alternative Treatments

Refer to alternative therapy chapters for more information before evaluating or applying any treatment. Some conditions, including yours, may require a physician's care.

DIET: Assess and treat for food allergies. Eat a varied diet, rotating foods, and eliminate wheat and associated wheat products for several months to assess benefit. Whole foods diet as much as possible. Consume seafood high in omega-3 fatty acids, such as salmon, sardines, mackerel, herring. Orally each day on a rotating basis, take one tablespoon of a natural oil, such as olive and flaxseed. Increase intake of pure water. Citrus foods may aggravate psoriasis in some individuals.

A good rule of thumb is that, if you itch today, then you ate something yesterday that your skin cannot tolerate.

Dr. Christ recommends avoiding all alcohol, nuts (except almonds), and aromatic spices (mustard, pepper, curry, etc.). He recommends eating fish, beef, venison, poultry, all kinds of fruits and vegetables, pasta, olives, olive oil, saffron, garlic, onion, herbs, and parsley. He highly recommends fresh hand-pressed fruit juices, beet juice, carrot juice, yogurt, curd, sauerkraut, and pickles without pepper.

NUTRITIONAL THERAPY: • Unsaturated fatty acids, particularly evening primrose oil (six capsules, two times daily) • Supplementing with fish oil; an omega-3 essential fatty acid, can help heal the skin lesions of psoriasis.[66] • Vitamin A (75,000 IU daily for first two weeks, then reduce to 50,000 IU daily for two to three months, then 25,000 daily) • Folic acid (100-500 mcg daily) • Vitamin B complex • Vitamin B6 • Vitamin C with bioflavonoids • Zinc • Lecithin (one tablespoon with two meals a day for the first month) • Assess for hydrochloric acid deficiency. • Multimineral supplement • Vitamin B12 (by injection) may be helpful in some individuals.

Copper toxicity and low levels of zinc are characteristic of psoriasis, eczema, and acne.

European fumaric acid treatment: Dr. Christ reports success in treating psoriasis with fumaric acid monoethyl ester and fumaric acid dimethyl ester (not fumaric acid alone). He feels that psoriasis results from a metabolic error, possibly from defective fumaric acid metabolism. Fumaric acid enters into the citric acid cycle, which is the center for energy production on the cellular level. Results from clinical investigation of fumaric acid in Switzerland, West Germany, the Netherlands, and Japan are promising. Fumaric acid tablets, ointment, lotion, and scalp lotions are used in the treatment.[67] The complete fumaric acid treatment protocol for psoriasis may be obtained from the Rheumatoid Disease Foundation.[68]

Fumaric acid may be obtained from Cardiovascular Research.[69]

Self–Care

The following therapies can be undertaken at home under appropriate professional supervision.

Biofeedback Training and Neurotherapy / Fasting / Guided Imagery / Yoga

AROMATHERAPY: Bergamot (to help heal skin plaques), lavender (to reduce excessive itching), melissa (for irritated skin), jasmine (for dry sensitive skin), geranium (for dry irritating skin), and sandalwood mysore (for dehydrated, inflamed, and sensitive skin).

BODYWORK: • Reflexology • Massage the area with two drops calendula oil and one drop lavender oil in two tablespoons of almond oil.

FLOWER ESSENCES: Flower essences for accompanying emotional/mental states. Rescue Remedy Cream®; Crab Apple

HERBS: • This intransigent skin condition can respond to herbs, but it often takes time. Herbs such as sarsaparilla are used as the core of any treatment.[70] Additional herbs can be added for associated anxiety, etc. • Combine equal parts of burdock, sarsaparilla, and cleavers tinctures and take one teaspoon three times a day. • Drink an infusion of fresh nettle or cleavers, two or three times a day. • Silymarin is beneficial for psoriasis due to its positive effects on liver function.[71]

HOMEOPATHY: *Psorinum, Sulfur, Graphites, Cuprum met., Arsen alb.*

HYDROTHERAPY: • Heating compress (apply daily to affected areas). • According to Leon Chaitow, N.D., D.O., treatment of psoriasis in the Dead Sea region of Israel has a long history of success and has led to salt and mud from that region being marketed for home use. Dead Sea products can be used regularly on the skin or in baths to help promote healing of psoriatic lesions, as part of a comprehensive approach that also tackles dietary and allergy issues. Dr. Chaitow recommends a neutral bath (at body temperature for profound relaxation effect) in which a pound or more of sea salt has been dissolved. Soak for 45 minutes every day (pat dry) during acute phases.

JUICE THERAPY: • Apple and carrot • Beet, cucumber, and grape • No citrus • Beet, carrot, burdock, yellowdock (two to three leaves per quart), garlic

LIFESTYLE: Frequent exercise, such as jogging, is recommended, in order to work up a good sweat.

MIND/BODY THERAPY: Deep breathing exercises, stress reduction.

REFLEXOLOGY: Thyroid, adrenals, liver, diaphragm, kidneys, intestines, all glands.

TOPICAL TREATMENT: • Apply seawater to skin with cotton several times daily. • Linseed or avocado oil • Topical capsaicin cream can reduce the scaling, thickness, redness, and itching. • Aloe vera gel

Professional Care

The following therapies should only be provided by a qualified health professional.

Acupuncture / Chelation Therapy / Environmental Medicine / Hypnotherapy / Light Therapy / Magnetic Field Therapy / Naturopathic Medicine / Orthomolecular Medicine / Osteopathic Medicine

DETOXIFICATION THERAPY: May be indicated, unless person is weak or deficient.

OXYGEN THERAPY: Hydrogen peroxide therapy (IV).

RASHES

A skin reaction that is usually temporary.

SYMPTOMS: Most often consists of eruptions, a group of spots, or areas of redness and inflammation.

OCCURRENCE: Everybody has rashes at some time.

SPECIAL NOTES: Most rashes are not a sign of a serious problem and rashes are an element of most childhood illnesses. Skin disorders occur with rashes (allergic reactions, dermatitis, eczema, psoriasis) and certain health disorders occur with rashes, such as liver and gallbladder problems, lupus, bleeding disorders, deficiencies of vitamins B and C or omega-3 fatty acids, and autoimmune diseases. If rashes continue, if they form a "butterfly" shape over the cheeks, or if associated with a high fever and joint pains, see a doctor to rule out more serious illnesses.

Alternative Treatments

Refer to alternative therapy chapters for more information before evaluating or applying any treatment. Some conditions, including yours, may require a physician's care.

DIET: Assess and treat for food allergies. Drink plenty of pure, filtered water. Avoid suspicious foods, the most common being citrus, berries, peanuts, shellfish, and dairy products. It is possible to suddenly develop skin reactions to foods or products (such as soaps, perfumes, jewelry) that were not reactive before. Check exposure to new products (fabric softeners, aftershaves, new clothing, etc.). Eat plenty of green, leafy vegetables and yellow vegetables such as carrots, pumpkin, sweet potatoes, and winter squash. The most important emphasis is to eat a wide variety of foods and rotate them as much as possible. Avoid aspartame (NutraSweet™).

NUTRITIONAL THERAPY: • Vitamin A (orally and topically) • Vitamin C • Vitamin E (orally and topically) • Sometimes allergic reactions can be neutralized by taking ½ teaspoon of baking soda (or two Alka-Seltzer Gold tablets) in water every 15 minutes three times and then every several hours, until the rash or reaction subsides. Do not continue this for more than a few days at a time. • Flaxseed oil or eicosapentaenoic acid (EPA) and gamma-linolenic acid (GLA) taken regularly may, over time, prevent more recurrences.

Self-Care

The following therapies can be undertaken at home under appropriate professional supervision.

Fasting

AYURVEDA: • Apply the pulp of cilantro leaf to the rash. • Drink coriander tea (one teaspoon of coriander seeds to one cup water), ½ teaspoon of *ghee* with a pinch of black pepper orally. *Neem* oil locally. Drink fresh cilantro, two tablespoons, three times a day.

FLOWER ESSENCES: Rescue Remedy Cream®

HERBS: • Burdock root, gentian root • Fresh juice of coriander is good taken internally for allergies, hay fever, and skin rashes. • Take fresh aloe vera juice or gel.

HOMEOPATHY: *Belladonna, Sulfur, Graphites, Calc carb.*

HYDROTHERAPY: • Cold compress (apply as needed to control pain and/or itching). • According to Leon Chaitow, N.D., D.O., to relieve the irritation of most forms of skin rashes, 20–30 minutes in a warm (just above body heat) alkaline bath containing bicarbonate of soda (one cup) is useful (for urticaria, eczema, shingles pain, heat rash, allergic reactions to chemicals or plants, poison ivy or insect stings, sunburn). • For the same skin conditions as the alkaline bath, an oatmeal bath can be used. Water can be fairly warm (but not very hot). Add a few tablespoons of finely ground uncooked oatmeal powder to the bath and tie into a cloth at least a pound of coarse uncooked oatmeal. Hang this from the tap so that the water runs through it. When the bath is full, remove cloth and use it as a sponge to gently pat areas of particular irritation. Thirty minutes in the oatmeal bath followed by patting the skin dry is indicated daily while skin is irritated.

JUICE THERAPY: • Drink fresh vegetable and fruit juices, especially carrot, beet, radish, and garlic. • Wheat grass juice

NATUROPATHIC MEDICINE: According to Dr. Chaitow, from a naturopathic perspective, skin rashes usually represent evidence of elimination of toxic wastes through the skin, or of an active immune reaction to an invading organism. Suppression of such a rash can lead to chronic disease states, and the most that should be done for the majority of rashes is to observe them and moderate any irritation they may be causing, while avoiding any treatment that "makes" the rash go away.

Professional Care

The following therapies should only be provided by a qualified health professional.

Acupuncture / Naturopathic Medicine / Osteopathic Medicine / Traditional Chinese Medicine

DETOXIFICATION THERAPY: May be indicated, depending on the condition of the person.

OXYGEN THERAPY: Hydrogen peroxide therapy.

RAYNAUD'S DISEASE

Constriction and spasm of the smaller vascular system (arterioles) that most commonly occur in the fingers and occasionally in the nose, tongue, and feet.

SYMPTOMS: Initially, symptoms occur in response to cold and emotionally stressful situations. The fingers become white or bluish; sometimes they also turn reddish. Tingling sensations are common. Rarely, the walls of the arteries thicken and the blood flow is permanently obstructed so that ulcers, infections, and even gangrene (death of tissue) may form around the nails.

OCCURRENCE: More common in young women.

CONSIDER: Rule out nutrient deficiencies, since this causes poor cold tolerance and decreased circulation.

SPECIAL NOTES: A common cause is smoking, which constricts the arterioles and creates poor circulation. Anything that increases circulation is helpful, such as deep breathing and biofeedback techniques. When these symptoms develop without any known cause, this condition is labeled Raynaud's disease. When these same symptoms occur secondary to other health problems, this is then called Raynaud's phenomenon and is usually more serious.

Some drugs produce these symptoms as a side effect; for example, the beta-blockers used in blood pressure treatment as well as ergotamine used in migraine treatment may trigger Raynaud's symptoms.

Keep hands and feet as warm as possible. Exercise, stopping smoking, massage, bodywork, and manipulation are all helpful.

Alternative Treatments

Refer to alternative therapy chapters for more information before evaluating or applying any treatment. Some conditions, including yours, may require a physician's care.

DIET: Consume foods high in vitamin E such as raw seeds and nuts. Hot vegetable soups, vegetable purees, and many vegetables and fruits that are high in minerals are excellent. According to Jonathan Wright, M.D., foods high in magnesium are recommended, as Raynaud's disease is a vasospastic condition and magnesium is a nutritional vasodilator. Leon Chaitow, N.D., D.O., recommends avoiding coffee, as this constricts blood vessels.

NUTRITIONAL THERAPY: • Vitamin E (1,000–1,500 IU daily) • Magnesium (200 mg three times daily) • Iron (if anemic) • Vitamin B complex • Niacin (vitamin B$_3$) • Digestive enzymes, if necessary • Folic acid (1 g daily) • Evening primrose oil (1,000 mg) • Take eicosapentaenoic acid (EPA) capsules (three to six daily) for at least three months, as these may decrease the viscosity of blood, allowing better circulation.

Self-Care

The following therapies can be undertaken at home under appropriate professional supervision.

Biofeedback Training and Neurotherapy / Fasting / Guided Imagery / Qigong and Tai Chi

EXERCISE: Rapid arm movement exercise can force blood through the tiny capillaries. Stand with arms at your side and swing them strongly round and round (like a windmill) forward and up, back and down, and forward and up, as high as you can and as fast as you can (60–80 swings a minute). This often relieves hand symptoms in a minute or two.

HERBS: Combine equal parts of the tinctures of ginkgo, prickly ash, and ginger and take ½ teaspoon of this mixture three times a day.

HOMEOPATHY: *Arsen alb., Secale*

HYDROTHERAPY: • Constitutional hydrotherapy (apply two to five times weekly, begin with narrow contrast). • According to Dr. Chaitow, a method by which you can condition your circulatory system is recommended by some experts and has had success in large trials. Place two bowls with warm water in different environments. One in a warm room and one in a cold room (or outside in the cold). Dress as for indoors (lightly) and immerse the hands in the warm water indoors for 2–4 minutes. Go to the outside (or cold room) and do the same, but this time for 8–10 minutes. Go to the warm room and repeat the first immersion. This triple immersion (warm room, cold room, warm room) should be done not less than four and ideally six times a day, every other day, until the symptoms of Raynaud's syndrome markedly improve. The conditioning process involves your body getting used to having warm hands in a cool atmosphere.

JUICE THERAPY: Fresh fruit and vegetable juices.

Professional Care

The following therapies should only be provided by a qualified health professional.

Acupuncture / Chelation Therapy / Environmental Medicine / Enzyme Therapy / Magnetic Field Therapy / Natural Hormone Replacement Therapy / Naturopathic Medicine / Neural Therapy / Orthomolecular Medicine

BIOFEEDBACK: • According to Dr. Chaitow, one of the most useful measures for anyone with Raynaud's syndrome is application of biofeedback methods, which focus on circulatory markers (temperature of the hands, etc.). • Autogenic training focuses on warmth of hands and feet as part of its methodology and may be very useful in helping to develop control over these states.

CHIROPRACTIC AND OSTEOPATHY: • Osteopaths and chiropractors claim success in treating this condition by working on the neck and upper spinal structures to improve nerve and circulation supply. • Massage on a regular basis can assist in normalizing circulatory flow and relaxing tense structures in the neck and shoulder area.

OXYGEN THERAPY: • Hydrogen peroxide therapy • Hyperbaric oxygen therapy

TRADITIONAL CHINESE MEDICINE: *Dong quai* and peony formula are effective.

RINGWORM

Infections caused by fungi that invade "dead" tissues (from skin, hair, nails, groin, feet, and trunk).

SYMPTOMS: The name occurs as the condition creates ring-shaped, reddish, patches that may also be scaly or blistered, which spread uniformly outward leaving a circular patch of normal skin within the ring.

Alternative Treatments

Refer to alternative therapy chapters for more information before evaluating or applying any treatment. Some conditions, including yours, may require a physician's care.

DIET: According to Leon Chaitow, N.D., D.O., if ringworm is a frequent occurrence, there may be benefit in treating fungi systemically as well as topically. A course involving a low-sugar diet and supplementation with garlic and probiotic substances such as *Lactobacillus acidophilus* and *Bifidobacteria* for several months may clear the tendency. (See Candidiasis chapter.)

NUTRITIONAL THERAPY: • Vitamin A (orally and topically) • Vitamin B complex • Vitamin C with bioflavonoids • Citrus seed extract • Vitamin E (orally and topically) • Evening primrose oil • Bee pollen

Self-Care

The following therapies can be undertaken at home under appropriate professional supervision.

Fasting / Reflexology

AROMATHERAPY: Rosemary, tea tree, lavender, geranium, peppermint, thyme

HERBS: Apply a paste made of equal parts myrrh powder and goldenseal powder mixed with a little water.

HOMEOPATHY: *Sepia, Arsen alb., Graphites*

JUICE THERAPY: Strawberry and date juice (use fresh dates).

NATUROPATHIC MEDICINE: Local applications of tea tree, thuja, or thyme oils may be effective.

TOPICAL TREATMENT: • Dr. Chaitow suggests that a thin slice of garlic bandaged directly over the skin lesion and left for several days has a powerful antifungal effect, and has been shown in clinical practice often to be more effective than orthodox skin creams. • Apply a poultice of strong goldenseal root tea to area. Dry and dust with goldenseal root powder.

Professional Care

The following therapies should only be provided by a qualified health professional.

Magnetic Field Therapy / Naturopathic Medicine / Traditional Chinese Medicine

OXYGEN THERAPY: • Externally applied ozone therapy is an antifungal agent. • Ozonated olive oil.

SCIATICA

A condition that manifests as radiating pain from the back either into the buttock and/or the lower extremity (leg), usually on the back (posterior) and outward (lateral) side. It represents pain referred somewhere along the path of the sciatic nerve.

SYMPTOMS: Discomfort, pain, burning, tingling, stabbing, aching anywhere along the path of the sciatic nerve (from the buttock, down the leg, into the foot, although the most commonly affected areas are the buttock and thigh). In severe cases, the pain may be associated with weakness. Pain can be very severe and recurrent, unless the cause is found and treated.

According to Leon Chaitow, N.D., D.O., there needs to be a clear distinction between sciatic neuralgia and sciatic neuritis. Neuritis is an active inflammatory process whereas neuralgia is an irritation of the nerve often resulting from outside mechanisms (disk, bone, muscle, distant trigger point activity). The advice given below regarding diet, nutrients, and herbs can help neuritis more than neuralgia. Manipulative and exercise methods are more helpful for neuralgia resulting from mechanical dysfunction. Sometimes neuralgia and neuritis coincide and both approaches are found useful.

CONSIDER: Sometimes chronic musculoskeletal pain may be secondary to low thyroid conditions, nutrient deficiencies, old injuries in associated joints that never healed completely or correctly, referred pain from problems in internal organs, or emotional stress.

SPECIAL NOTES: Treatment must include removing the pressure on the sciatic nerve (misalignment of lumbar spine), prolapsed (herniated) intervertebral disk, spasm of the buttock muscles (usually the piriformis), abnormal stresses on associated joints, or secondary to injuries of the foot, knee, hip, or back that alter the walking gait and put abnormal and asymmetrical strain on the muscles. Insufficient exercise and muscles that have become excessively weak and/or tense can create imbalances, which are the most underappreciated causes of chronic musculoskeletal problems.

Alternative Treatments

Refer to alternative therapy chapters for more information before evaluating or applying any treatment. Some conditions, including yours, may require a physician's care.

DIET: Since thiamin (vitamin B1) and magnesium act as natural muscle relaxants, eat foods that are high in these nutrients : dark leafy green vegetables, yellow vegetables, whole grains, and raw seeds and nuts. Avoid excess consumption of foods that drain the body of these nutrients, such as caffeinated beverages, chocolate, and refined sugars.

NUTRITIONAL THERAPY: • Magnesium • Thiamin (vitamin B₁) • Vitamin B complex • Vitamin B₁₂ (injections may be helpful in some cases that are chronic and unresponsive to any other treatment) • Vitamin E • Calcium • Manganese sulfate

Self-Care

The following therapies can be undertaken at home under appropriate professional supervision.

Fasting / Guided Imagery / Yoga

ACUPRESSURE: To relieve sciatica, lie down on your back with your legs bent, feet flat on the floor. Place your hands underneath your buttocks (palms down) beside the base of your spine. Close your eyes and take long, deep breaths and rock your knees from side to side for two minutes to press acupressure point B48 (for an illustration of this point, see the acupressure chart in the introduction to this section) in the buttocks. Reposition your hands for comfort and to enable different parts of the buttocks muscles to be pressed. Also, try swaying your legs from side to side with your knees pulled into your abdomen and your feet off the floor.

AROMATHERAPY: Apply a cold press and lightly massage with chamomile, lavender, or birch.

AYURVEDA: *Triphala guggulu* (200 mg), ¼ teaspoon generally taken with warm water twice a day after lunch and dinner. *Dashamoola tea basti, mahanarayan* oil massage, and bathe with ⅓ cup of ginger powder and ⅓ cup baking soda.

HERBS: • Mix equal parts willow bark and St. John's wort tincture and take ½ teaspoon three times a day. • Massage with warm St. John's wort oil will help alleviate pain. • Black cohosh, chamomile, fenugreek, juniper berries, mugwort, parsley, rosemary, skullcap

HOMEOPATHY: *Colocynth, Viscum album, Lachesis, Rhus tox., Aconite, Arsen alb., Lycopodium, Mag phos., Ruta grav.* Dr. Chaitow recommends *Atropa belladonna* 6X for neuralgia.

HYDROTHERAPY: • Contrast application (apply daily). • According to Dr. Chaitow, a neutral bath (body temperature) has a profoundly calming effect.

REFLEXOLOGY: Hip/sciatic, hip/knee, lower spine, shoulder, chronic sciatic area.

ENERGY MEDICINE: The Transcutaneous Electrical Nerve Stimulator (TENS), which applies an electrical current to affected nerves, is invaluable for relief of most but not all nerve pains.

TOPICAL TREATMENT: According to Dr. Chaitow, for neuralgic type pain, apply moist or dry heat to the affected leg(s) for one hour, four times a day. This is only valid for neuralgic type pain where heat acts to relax muscles. If there is inflammation (neuritis), heat will inflame the area further. Use hot and cold alternating applications, finishing with cold.

Professional Care

The following therapies should only be provided by a qualified health professional.

Applied Kinesiology / Cell Therapy / Chiropractic / Craniosacral Therapy / Detoxification Therapy / Environmental Medicine / Enzyme Therapy / Magnetic Field Therapy / Naturopathic Medicine / Neural Therapy / Osteopathic Medicine / Prolotherapy

BODYWORK: Acupressure, reflexology, shiatsu, massage, Alexander Technique, Feldenkrais Method, Trager Approach, Rolfing, Hellerwork.

TRADITIONAL CHINESE MEDICINE: Combination of acupuncture and herbal formulas depending upon cause of particular symptom.

SHINGLES (HERPES ZOSTER)

An acute viral (varicella-zoster virus, which also causes chicken pox) infection of the central nervous system that affects certain areas of the skin.

SYMPTOMS: Several days (three to four) before the skin outbreaks occur, there is usually fatigue, fever, chills, and sometimes gastrointestinal upset. On the third to fourth day, the skin area becomes excessively sensitive. On the fourth or fifth day, characteristic small blisters erupt that crust and hurt along the path of a nerve so that the reddened outbreak affects a strip of skin, forming a line. This usually occurs over the ribs in the thoracic area and is usually limited to one side. Rarely, it can affect the lower part of the body or the face. The affected area is very sensitive and the pain may be severe. The eruptions heal about five days later. Most people heal without any further problems except occasional scarring along the path of the nerve. In some individuals (about 30%), especially the elderly, pain may persist for long periods of time, months to years later, and sometimes be recurrent (2%). The older the individual and the longer the rash lasts, the more likely a lingering problem with pain will persist. One attack of herpes zoster usually gives immunity for life.

OCCURRENCE: Can occur in any age group, but is most common after 50 years of age. Several hundred cases per 100,000 people occur each year in the United States. It is a fairly common viral infection, but especially in those individuals whose immune systems have been severely compromised (cancer, HIV, severe trauma).

CONSIDER: Chicken pox (in children), pleurisy, Bell's palsy, herpes simplex, appendicitis, colic, gallstones, colitis, trigeminal neuralgia, or contact dermatitis.

SPECIAL NOTES: If the eruptions last longer than two weeks, rule out possible underlying immune problems or cancer (particularly Hodgkin's disease). During a childhood bout of chicken pox, not all of the viral organisms are destroyed. Some lie dormant in sensory (skin) nerves for many years. When events occur that decrease immune function, such as severe emotional stress, severe illness, or long-term usage of corticosteroids, the immune system cannot suppress the dormant organisms any longer and they become active again, causing infection along the pathway of the nerve.

See an ophthalmologist immediately if herpes zoster occurs near the eyes or on the forehead, as it can cause blindness.

Alternative Treatments

Refer to alternative therapy chapters for more information before evaluating or applying any treatment. Some conditions, including yours, may require a physician's care.

DIET: Whole foods diet and avoid of excessive consumption of refined carbohydrates.

NUTRITIONAL THERAPY: • Vitamin B12 injections combined with adenosine monophosphate (AMP), which is usually administered by an orthomolecular physician. Also, place plain yogurt mixed with zinc oxide, if available, along the path of the nerve two to three times daily; this often clears up herpes zoster in 24-48 hours, if the regime is started at the first sign of the outbreak. • L-lysine (4-5 g initially, then 500 mg two times daily for several weeks only) • Vitamin B12 (orally every hour first day) • Vitamin B complex • High doses of vitamin C plus bioflavonoids. Use Dr. Cathcart's vitamin C bowel tolerance technique (see Orthomolecular Medicine chapter). • Calcium

Self–Care

The following therapies can be undertaken at home under appropriate professional supervision.

Biofeedback Training and Neurotherapy / Fasting / Qigong and Tai Chi

AROMATHERAPY: Lemon, geranium, bergamot, eucalyptus, tea tree, lavender, chamomile. (See Aromatherapy chapter.)

FLOWER ESSENCES: Rescue Remedy® for accompanying stress. Crab Apple.

HERBS: • Combine equal parts of oat straw, St. John's wort, and skullcap tinctures and take one teaspoon of this mixture four times a day. • Peppermint oil applied topically may reduce the pain through a mild local numbing effect. Do not attempt this if the skin is extremely sensitive. • Colloidal oatmeal powder may be dusted on the affected skin to act as a dry lubricant, hopefully reducing pain from contact with clothes.

HOMEOPATHY: *Arsen alb., Rhus tox., Sepia, Natrum mur., Hepar sulph., Caladium, Acidum nit.*

HYDROTHERAPY: According to Leon Chaitow, N.D., D.O., the most calming and stress-reducing bath is the neutral bath (body temperature), in which the individual soaks for 30-60 minutes. Someone needs to keep heat at body temperature, using a bath thermometer to check every few minutes.

JUICE THERAPY: • Carrot and celery juice with one tablespoon of parsley juice • Spinach, beet

NATUROPATHIC MEDICINE: A gel made from licorice root appears to be an excellent topical application. Joseph Pizzorno, N.D., has seen serious pain and inflammation totally clear in just three days after application.

REFLEXOLOGY: Diaphragm, all glands, whole spine

ENERGY MEDICINE: According to Dr. Chaitow, the Transcutaneous Electrical Nerve Stimulator (TENS), which applies an electrical current to affected nerves, is invaluable for relief of most but not all nerve pains. This method is well worth a try to see if the often intractable burning pain can be calmed in this safe manner.

TOPICAL TREATMENT: • Vitamin E oil • Apply apple cider vinegar to rash.

Professional Care

The following therapies should only be provided by a qualified health professional.

Acupuncture / Magnetic Field Therapy / Naturopathic Medicine / Neural Therapy / Orthomolecular Medicine

ENERGY MEDICINE: Light Beam Generator

DETOXIFICATION THERAPY: May be indicated, depending on the condition of the person.

ENVIRONMENTAL MEDICINE: Treatment with weak dilutions of influenza vaccine can give relief to shingles.

OXYGEN THERAPY: Hydrogen peroxide therapy • Ozone may inactivate the herpes viruses. May be applied externally to lesions and/or internally as in autohemotherapy (withdrawal and intramuscular injection of patient's own blood).

SORE THROAT

Inflammation in the pharynx (throat).

SYMPTOMS: Associated with varying amounts of pain (often experienced as rawness), usually with swallowing or speaking, accompanied by dryness, feelings of constantly needing to clear throat, and congestion of mucous membranes. Postnasal drip, enlargement of lymph nodes in the neck, and fever may also be present. Slight loss of normal voice, or hoarseness, often accompanies a sore throat and is usually not serious.

CONSIDER: Usually caused by viral infections, but may also be caused by bacterial infections, tonsillitis (secondary to inflammation of the tonsils), overuse of the voice, irritating substances such as smoking, allergic reactions, infections within the mouth, bacterial exposure, or associated with many illnesses as part of the symptom picture.

SPECIAL NOTES: Viral infections do not respond to antibiotics while bacterial infections do respond. It is difficult to differentiate between the two merely by observation.

Sore throats are rarely serious, but often are the first symptom of many other health problems, such as the flu, herpes simplex, mononucleosis, and many childhood illnesses. Rarely, a sore throat occurs before the manifesting of a serious medical problem. If the sore throat does not resolve within two weeks, see a doctor. If any sore throat occurs with a rash, see a doctor. Waking up with a chronic tickle in the throat may be a sign of food allergies or environmental irritants or allergies.

A sore throat caused by a *Streptococcus* infection (often called strep throat) must be identified and treated, or else it could create rheumatic fever or acute glomerulonephritis (disease of the glomerulus, a network of blood capillaries of the kidney).

Alternative Treatments

Refer to alternative therapy chapters for more information before evaluating or applying any treatment. Some conditions, including yours, may require a physician's care.

DIET: Increase fluid intake, including lots of pure water, hot herbal teas, diluted fruit juices, and broths. Especially good is sipping warm water mixed with powdered vitamin C plus lemon and honey. Avoid refined sugars.

NUTRITIONAL THERAPY: • Vitamin C with bioflavonoids • Vitamin A (a high dose for the first few days) • Beta carotene (high dose for the first few days) • Zinc lozenges (one every two hours unless nausea occurs, in which case decrease dosage). Lozenges or liquid throat formulas containing zinc, vitamin C, and slippery elm bark are effective for relieving the pain of a sore throat.

Self–Care

The following therapies can be undertaken at home under appropriate professional supervision.

Fasting / Guided Imagery / Yoga

AROMATHERAPY: Inhalations with benzoin, lavender, thyme, eucalyptus, geranium, clary sage, sandalwood.

AYURVEDA: • Gargle with a mixture of hot water and ¼ teaspoon of turmeric powder and a pinch of salt. • Gargle with other astringent herbs such as alum, sumac, sage, and bayberry.

FLOWER ESSENCES: Rescue Remedy® for accompanying stress. Crab Apple.

HERBS: • If due to an infection, chew a small piece of osha root *(Ligusticum porteri)* as needed to alleviate the symptoms. Alternatively, gargle with an infusion of sage or licorice. • For a sore throat due to smoke or pollution irritation, gargle with an infusion of lavender or hyssop. • Ginger, slippery elm, or mouseroot teas are used for sore throats. • Echinacea and goldenseal are also sore throat remedies. Use a gargle made from tincture of goldenseal root or sage. • Tea tree oil, an ingredient in some throat lozenges, is a powerful antiseptic and assists in fighting a broad range of infectious agents. • Take ⅛ teaspoon ground black pepper mixed with one teaspoon of honey.

HOMEOPATHY: *Lachesis, Ignatia, Arnica, Aconite, Hydrastis, Gelsemium, Merc sol., Phytolacca*

HYDROTHERAPY: • Contrast application (apply one to two times daily to neck and throat). • Heating compress (apply one to two times daily to neck and throat).

JUICE THERAPY: • Juice of red potato • Pineapple

REFLEXOLOGY: Lymph system, all toes, adrenals, cervicals

TOPICAL TREATMENT: Gargle several times a day with either apple cider vinegar, hot water, and one teaspoon of salt, or hot water with a teaspoon each of lemon juice and honey.

Professional Care

The following therapies should only be provided by a qualified health professional.

Acupuncture / Environmental Medicine / Enzyme Therapy / Magnetic Field Therapy / Naturopathic Medicine / Neural Therapy / Traditional Chinese Medicine

DETOXIFICATION THERAPY: May be indicated, depending on the condition of the person. Detoxification may be helpful with chronic low-grade infection or allergies.

ENERGY MEDICINE: Light Beam Generator

LIGHT THERAPY: Monochromatic red light therapy.

SPORTS INJURIES

Any type of injury that occurs while performing sports or during general exercise. The most common injuries are soft tissue ones, such as strains (exercise to a harmful degree, over exertion or stretching of muscles, ligaments, and tendons), sprains (injury to joint so that some of the soft tissues are actually torn or ruptured but the overall continuity of the joint itself is still intact), and other muscular injuries. Also common are joint dislocations, fractures, and head injuries, all of which need to be seen by a doctor.

SYMPTOMS: A wide variety of symptoms depending on the sport, the body parts and joints involved, and the degree of injury to that part.

OCCURRENCE: Widespread. On the increase as exercise is on the rise.

SPECIAL NOTES: The better overall shape muscles are in, the more adequate the stretch and warm-up time, the better the overall nutrient status of the individual, the less emotionally stressed the individual is, the better the equipment that is utilized, the less the likelihood of injuries.

Equally important is cool down time after activity, in which the muscles are allowed to slowly return to a neutral nonactive state. This helps circulation and removes acidic products that result from exertion, preventing subsequent stiffness. Both warm-up and cool down can effectively be helped by what is called "performance" massage, which anyone can learn to apply to themselves or their friends, but which is best applied by a licensed massage therapist with certification in sports massage.

It is very important to approach sports activities and exercise with common sense and information. Re-injuries are even more difficult to heal and may create more stubborn residual problems. Thus, it is important to contact a sports medicine practitioner, an exercise physiologist, or a personal trainer when embarking on a new program. Even if it is only for a one-time consultation to make sure you are on a safe path with a sensible program, it is worth it to avoid injuries down the road. Often, when you are unknowingly doing something that makes you vulnerable to injury, it will not show up or occur for several weeks to several months, until enough repetition has occurred. Thus, prevention and education is the paramount guideline when exercising or starting new sports.

Alternative Treatments

Refer to alternative therapy chapters for more information before evaluating or applying any treatment. Some conditions, including yours, may require a physician's care.

DIET: Whole foods diet especially adequate in complex carbohydrates (60% to 70% of diet) and quality non-processed fats (no more than 20% to 25% of diet). Especially important to limit fat intake and excessive calories of any kind, as both can contribute to excess body fat. Excess fat will infiltrate muscles and cause them to be metabolically "out of shape" and more prone to injury. If there is inadequate complex carbohydrates, especially in the face of increased demand due to sports activities, the body will go into its protein reserves and burn muscle, defeating the purpose of the exercise and making the individual actually weaker. Thus, it is not realistic to increase protein consumption because of increased exercise output. It is more important to increase quality carbohydrates, such as fresh fruits and vegetables, whole grains, potatoes, and other root vegetables.

Don't eat solid foods immediately before exercising, limit it to 1½ to two hours before or after exercise, unless you already have a habit of doing this and it does not seem to disagree with you. After all, there are no set rules except the ones that work best for each person. Also, if you are only lightly or moderately exercising, the rules for food and exercise are not as important as if you are heavily exercising or performing in competition. However, if you are prone toward allergic food reactions, especially avoid eating any allergenic foods around times of athletic performance as exercise may enhance allergic reactions substantially.

Magnesium is one of the most important minerals for quality soft tissue tone. Green leafy vegetables are the best source. Foods that tend to "rob" the body of magnesium should be avoided. They are caffeinated beverages, commercial sodas, excess refined sugars, and diets too high in animal protein and acid foods and too low in fresh fruits and vegetables.

Drink adequate fluids an hour or so before heavy exercising, even if you do not feel thirsty. Dehydration is a stress on the body and decreases performance capabilities.

NUTRITIONAL THERAPY: *Prevention:* • Vitamin E (orally and topically) may help protect against muscle damage from exercise. • Vitamin C levels in the body may help heal micro and macro injuries. • Magnesium keeps muscles flexible but toned and less susceptible to injury. • Free-form amino acids.

Acute injury: • Calcium • Magnesium and valerian root may help reduce pain and muscle spasm. Take magnesium and calcium for first two days when injured. • Manganese sulfate may help repair ligaments and must be taken every hour with vitamin C. • Proteolytic enzymes on an empty stomach, six every hour for the first three hours, then four times daily between meals for several days. If prone to injury, taking three capsules, three times daily between meals, for one week before competition may reduce injury rate and speed up healing time if injured. • Free-form amino acids.

Bone fracture: • Microcrystalline hydroxyapatite • Vitamin B6 • Vitamin B complex • Essential fatty acids • Zinc

Branched-chain amino acids (BCAAs), which include leucine, isoleucine, and valine, are important for energy production and the formation and repair of muscles. Whey protein (derived from dairy) is a good source of BCAAs. There are nondairy formulas containing BCAAs available for people who do not eat dairy products.

Recent studies reveal that antioxidant vitamins (A, C, E) offer protection against exercise-induced muscle injury in athletes.[72] Other antioxidants include selenium, the amino acids cysteine and glutathione, coenzyme Q10, ginkgo, ginseng, chlorella, spirulina, and green tea. Coenzyme Q10, dimethylglycine (DMG), and germanium sesquoxide support oxygen delivery to the cells and tissues of the body, which is an essential component of athletic endurance and performance.

Plant-based digestive enzymes, taken between meals, help reduce the pain and inflammation in muscles, tendons, ligaments, and other soft tissue, caused by sports injuries such as a sprained ankle or pulled muscle. Papain, trypsin, and SOD (superoxide dismutase) are other anti-inflammatory enzymes. Pycnogenol (pine park or grape seed extract), bromelain (enzyme compound from pineapple), vitamin E, and evening primrose oil also help reduce inflammation.

According to Leon Chaitow, N.D., D.O., healing following injury is speeded up when the amino acids arginine and glycine are supplemented (away from meals).

Self-Care

The following therapies can be undertaken at home under appropriate professional supervision.

Fasting / Biofeedback Training and Neurotherapy / Guided Imagery / Qigong and Tai Chi

AROMATHERAPY: Everlast

BODYWORK: Massage

FLOWER ESSENCES: Rescue Remedy Cream®

HERBS: • Valerian root, a sedative and tranquilizer, is a muscle relaxant, effective for cramps and spasm. Topical application of lobelia extract helps reduce these muscle afflictions. Passionflower, another sedative and nervine (supports the nervous system), can also aid in easing muscle spasms. • White willow bark, which is high in salicylates (the active ingredient in aspirin), possesses anti-inflammatory and analgesic (pain-relieving) properties. Feverfew also reduces both pain and inflammation. Turmeric and boswellia decrease inflammation and boswellia additionally improves blood supply to the joints.[73] • For muscle and connective tissue injuries, comfrey root is both soothing and stimulates tissue repair.[74] When used topically, comfrey root soothes and stimulates repair of injured muscles and connective tissues. Comfrey should be used internally only under the supervision of a qualified health-care professional.

HOMEOPATHY: *Arnica* ointment for overuse, tendinitis, and post-traumatic inflammation. *Arnica* in an oral form may be useful until the acute inflammatory phase has passed.

HYDROTHERAPY: If acute, use an ice pack (apply 20 minutes out of each hour for the first 24-36 hours.

JUICE THERAPY: Raw fresh vegetable juices.

NATUROPATHIC MEDICINE: A combination of bromelain and curcumin (from the spice turmeric) makes a very good oral anti-inflammatory therapy for sports injuries

TOPICAL TREATMENT: According to Jonathan Wright, M.D., dimethylsulfoxide (DMSO) used topically is often useful.

Professional Care

The following therapies should only be provided by a qualified health professional.

Acupuncture / Applied Kinesiology / Chiropractic / Enzyme Therapy / Magnetic Field Therapy / Natural Hormone Replacement Therapy / Naturopathic Medicine / Neural Therapy / Osteopathic Medicine / Traditional Chinese Medicine

BODYWORK: • Feldenkrais Method, Rolfing • Skilled sports massage therapy to injuries is important to help prevent fibrosis and scar tissue from developing at injury sites. It is also effective in reducing the chances of injury.

ENERGY MEDICINE: Electro-Acuscope, Light Beam Generator

LIGHT THERAPY: • Monochromatic red light therapy • Cold (soft) laser photo stimulation therapy

OXYGEN THERAPY: • Hydrogen peroxide therapy (IV) • Hyperbaric oxygen therapy

PROLOTHERAPY: William J. Faber, D.O., reports that relief for tennis elbow, wrist pain, chronic shoulder dislocation, rotator cuff tears, pain after severe injury, ankle weakness, and chronic and acute knee problems can be provided through prolotherapy.

SPRAINS

When a joint is stretched or injured beyond its normal capacity, the ligaments that connect bone to muscle may be injured without tearing or may tear partially or completely. The capsule that surrounds the joint, made up of fibrous tissue, may also be injured.

SYMPTOMS: *Grade 1:* Mild, minimal sprain, without any ligamentous tearing, with possible mild tenderness and swelling of the area. *Grade 2:* Partial tearing of ligament with very obvious swelling, bruising (black, blue, and yellow), and difficulty trying to use the joint normally, such as in weight bearing. *Grade 3:* A complete tear with much swelling, extreme bruising with hemorrhaging under the skin, joint instability, and inability to use the joint at all.

Muscle spasms (muscle contractions that are not voluntary) may be associated with all grades of sprains, either primary as part of the injury or secondary due to the compensatory use of associated muscles because of the injury. Pain due to sprains usually increases when attempts are made to move the involved joint.

SPECIAL NOTES: *Grade 1:* Require supportive elastic bandages, tape, or therapeutic splinting to create immobilization, elevation, followed by very gentle exercise. Consider optional assessment by a manual practitioner. *Grade 2:* Requires immobilization for three weeks. Needs manual medicine and rehabilitation. *Grade 3:* Requires casting or, rarely, surgery. Requires manual medicine and rehabilitation. X rays are usually necessary to rule out fractures.

Initially, for all sprains, ice for 20 minutes (optimal is to alternate ice and moist heat, 20 minutes each, starting and ending with ice), elevate joint, immobilize, and take something for swelling, pain, and healing. When joint no longer hurts after use, and all swelling, bruising, and associated spasm is gone, gentle mobilization exercises should be initiated.

Alternative Treatments

Refer to alternative therapy chapters for more information before evaluating or applying any treatment. Some conditions, including yours, may require a physician's care.

DIET: Whole foods diet with plenty of fresh fruits, vegetables, nuts, seeds, and whole grains.

NUTRITIONAL THERAPY: • Take proteolytic enzymes (such as bromelain from pineapple) away from meals on an empty stomach. *Grade 1:* Six initially, then 3, three times daily. *Grade 2:* Six initially, then 4, four times daily. *Grade 3:* Six initially, then contnuing with six, four times daily for longer periods of time. Take until joint swelling is gone and pain is almost gone; decrease dosage as healing improves. • Take enzymes with vitamin C and bioflavonoids. Increase bioflavonoids depending on amount of bruising. Initially, take with one buffered aspirin to help with reduction of pain and swelling. • Increase calcium, magnesium, and valerian with more muscle spasm involved. • According to Leon Chaitow, N.D., D.O., healing following injury is speeded up when the amino acids arginine and glycine are supplemented (away from meals).

Self–Care

The following therapies can be undertaken at home under appropriate professional supervision.

Biofeedback Training and Neurotherapy / Fasting / Guided Imagery

AROMATHERAPY: Make a cold compress with camphor, lavender, chamomile, eucalyptus, or rosemary.

HERBS: • Combine equal parts of the tinctures of horsetail, nettle, and willow bark and take one teaspoon of this mixture three times a day. • Apply comfrey to the affected area.

HOMEOPATHY: *Ruta grav.*

HYDROTHERAPY: • Contrast application (apply daily, if acute). • Ice pack (apply 20 minutes out of each hour for the first 24–36 hours). • Ice and contrast

JUICE THERAPY: Raw fresh vegetable juices, including beet, radish, garlic (can dilute with comfrey tea).

REFLEXOLOGY: Work reflex area on foot, referral area to sprained joint.

TOPICAL TREATMENT: According to Jonathan Wright, M.D., dimethyl sulfoxide (DMSO) used topically is often useful.

Professional Care

The following therapies should only be provided by a qualified health professional.

Acupuncture / Applied Kinesiology / Chiropractic / Craniosacral Therapy / Energy Medicine / Magnetic Field Therapy / Naturopathic Medicine / Neural Therapy / Osteopathic Medicine / Prolotherapy

BODYWORK: Feldenkrais Method, massage, Rolfing.

STIES

An acute pus-filled infection (abscess), usually due to Staphylococci, of one or more glands of the eye, normally located near the eye lashes.

SYMPTOMS: Initially pain and redness occur, followed by a small, swollen, roundish area on the margin of the eyelid. A small yellowish spot in the center indicates pus. When the abscess breaks open and the pus is discharged, the pain is relieved. Swelling can occur around the whole area.

SPECIAL NOTES: Do not attempt to squeeze the lump with your fingers, as this may spread the infection into

the bloodstream and can become extremely serious. Sties tend to recur.

Alternative Treatments

Refer to alternative therapy chapters for more information before evaluating or applying any treatment. Some conditions, including yours, may require a physician's care.

DIET: Whole foods diet high in garlic. Avoid refined sugars.

NUTRITIONAL THERAPY: • Vitamin A (100,000 IU first two days, then reduce to 50,000 IU the next two days, and then 25,000 IU daily for next week) • Vitamin C • Beta carotene (50,000 IU daily for first few days)

Self–Care

The following therapies can be undertaken at home under appropriate professional supervision.

Fasting

DETOXIFICATION THERAPY: According to Leon Chaitow, N.D., D.O., if sties are recurrent, consider a detoxification program (including periodic short fasts), followed by remodelling of lifestyle and dietary habits.

HERBS: • Use an eyewash made with a fresh and well-filtered infusion of eyebright and goldenseal. • Red raspberry tea

HOMEOPATHY: *Pulsatilla, Hepar sulph., Sulfur, Graphites*

HYDROTHERAPY: • Contrast application (apply daily over the face and eyes). • Hot compresses should be applied for ten minutes, two to four times daily.

REFLEXOLOGY: Eye reflex, neck area, all toes

TOPICAL TREATMENT: Eyebath of chamomile (use flower tops) or red raspberry tea.

Professional Care

The following therapies should only be provided by a qualified health professional.

Applied Kinesiology / Light Therapy / Naturopathic Medicine / Traditional Chinese Medicine

STROKE

A sudden and severe episode in which there is some kind of blockage of blood to the brain, resulting in damage to part of the brain. When the symptoms from a stroke last for 24 hours or less, followed by full recovery of lost functions, the episode is called a transient ischemic attack (TIA).

In case of stroke, get the individual to a hospital immediately.

SYMPTOMS: Stroke symptoms may develop within a few minutes to over several days. Symptoms are loss and/or impairment of movement, sensation, and specific functions controlled by the part of the brain that is damaged, not necessarily the specific artery that is affected. For example, damage to the speech center of the brain results in loss or slurring of speech. Also associated are headaches, dizziness, confusion, difficulty swallowing, and visual problems.

About 30% of cases of stroke are fatal, about 30% result in partial loss of function, and about 30% completely recover. Many people who become paralyzed by a stroke learn to walk again. However, loss of intellectual functioning tends to not recover as well. TIAs usually last only several minutes and are warning signals.

OCCURRENCE: Two hundred cases per 100,000 people in the United States per year. Higher incidence in the elderly and in males.

SPECIAL NOTES: Strokes are the most common cause of neurological damage in the industrialized world and are a leading cause of death in these countries. The most common causes of strokes are arteriosclerosis (thickening of lining of arteries), high blood pressure (hypertension), or both. Other risk factors are old age, smoking, a recent heart attack, elevated blood fats (hyperlipidemia), diabetes, blood platelet stickiness associated with raised levels of red cells (polycythemia) or low levels of nutrients that prevent stickiness such as vitamin B6, irregular heart beat (atrial fibrillation), oral contraceptives in women under 50 years of age, and history of a damaged heart valve.

IMPORTANT: According to David Hughes, Ph.D., hyperbaric oxygen therapy done within the first six hours of a stroke may significantly improve the stroke victim's condition.

Alternative Treatments

Refer to alternative therapy chapters for more information before evaluating or applying any treatment. Some conditions, including yours, may require a physician's care.

DIET: A whole foods diet with emphasis on garlic, onions, vitamin B6 (all three tend to prevent platelets from sticking together), and unprocessed fats. Limit fats to 10% to 15% of total diet, avoid deep-fried foods, animal fats, and semi-solid fats, and concentrate on fresh fruits and vegetables. Especially good are raw nuts and seeds, whole grains, fresh vegetables such as broccoli, sprouts, and kelp. Limit foods that are natural plant sources of estrogens, such as soybeans and peanuts. Avoid alcoholic beverages and especially alcoholic binges (four drinks or more in a short period of time). Consume more fish, especially fresh-water varieties.

NUTRITIONAL THERAPY: • Vitamin E (high dosages) • Omega-3 fatty acids (fish oils) • Vitamin B6 • Vitamin B complex • Magnesium • Vitamin C to bowel tolerance (see Orthomolecular Medicine chapter) • *Ginkgo biloba* • Superoxide dismutase (SOD) • According to Leon Chaitow, N.D., D.O., well-researched studies show that taking garlic (raw or as a deodorized oil capsule) dramatically reduces platelet adhesiveness allowing improved circulatory function.

Self-Care

The following therapies can be undertaken at home under appropriate professional supervision.

Biofeedback Training and Neurotherapy / Flower Essences / Guided Imagery / Meditation / Qigong and Tai Chi / Yoga

BODYWORK: Massage

AROMATHERAPY: *For muscular paralysis:* • Lavender • Rub spinal column and paralyzed part with mixture of one quart of rubbing alcohol and one ounce each of essence of lavender, essence of rosemary, and essence of basil.

HERBS: • To improve circulation to extremities, use elder flowers, hyssop, rosemary, yarrow. • To nourish nervous system, use damiana, lavender, rosemary, Siberian ginseng. Consult a trained herbalist.

HYDROTHERAPY: • Constitutional hydrotherapy (apply two to five times weekly) • Swimming exercise to restore strength.

REFLEXOLOGY: Tip of big toe (opposite side from paralysis), other toes, reflexes to affected areas.

Professional Care

The following therapies should only be provided by a qualified health professional.

Chelation Therapy / Hypnotherapy / Light Therapy / Magnetic Field Therapy / Naturopathic Medicine / Osteopathic Medicine / Sound Therapy / Traditional Chinese Medicine

BODYWORK: Feldenkrais Method.

PROLOTHERAPY: For pain after a stroke.

VISION THERAPY: Vision therapy may be an important ingredient in rehabilitation. Victims suffer aim, focus, and eye movement impairment as well as visual field and perceptual defects. Without evaluation by a behavioral optometrist, these can be overlooked and recovery hindered. Therapy includes awareness training, visual/motor exercises, and lenses and prisms. Gross and fine movement control, hand-eye coordination, attention, memory, and learning skills improve dramatically.

SUNBURN

Overexposure of the skin to ultraviolet radiation (sunlight), causing inflammation and burns of the skin. Occurs more in fair-skinned individuals.

SYMPTOMS: Symptoms appear up to 24 hours after exposure. The symptoms peak at 72 hours, unless the burning is severe. The affected skin turns anywhere from mildly reddish to severely red and darker. Symptoms range from skin becoming mildly tender to severe pain and swelling. Blisters may appear, which then open and the outer layer of the skin peels away. Sunburn on the lower extremities is usually more painful and takes longer to heal. If a large enough portion of the skin is affected, systemic symptoms may occur, such as chills, fever, weakness, and shock. Secondary infections may follow once the skin has peeled. The new skin may be very sensitive to touch and to further sunlight for several weeks.

Burns are classified into three degrees. First degree burns merely redden the skin. Second degree burns cause swelling and more pain and blisters that fill with water. Third degree burns result in more severe damage to the skin, are more prone to infection, and must be seen by a doctor.

SPECIAL NOTES: The best treatment is prevention. Initial summer exposure should not exceed 30 minutes in the midday sun, even in persons with darker skin. The best time for sun exposure is before 11 a.m. and after 3 p.m. Cloudy summer days and foggy winter days, especially at higher altitudes, have a greater danger of sunburn as they appear to be safer but have almost the same amount of ultraviolet exposure. Reflections off of water, metal, snow, sand, and silvery objects may increase the amount of rays absorbed. In the 1950s and 1960s, sun worshippers used aluminum foil reflectors to increase the suntanning effect. This may have resulted in many cases of skin cancer. Repeated overexposure to the sun and sunburns increases aging of the skin and increases risk of skin cancers.

Research suggests that sunscreens themselves may be instrumental in causing melanoma (skin cancer).[75] In a controversial study, Cedric Garland, Dr.P.H., and Frank Garland, Ph.D., of San Diego, California, report that by using a sunscreen, one prevents the skin from producing vitamin D, which interferes with melanoma growth and that of other cancers. According to this study, there is no evidence that sunscreens prevent cancer in humans. They only prevent sunburn, the body's natural method of warning that the skin has received too much sun. The Garlands also state that the rise in melanoma rates have been directly proportionate to the sales rates of sunscreens. Queensland, Australia, has the highest rate of melanoma in the world and was also the place where sunscreens were first and most strongly recommended by the medical community.

SUNSCREENS: If you should choose to use a sunscreen, they are rated by the FDA's Sun Protection Factors (SPF) by numbers. One is the least protective and 15 is the most protective. In some foreign countries, their 10 is equal to 15 in the United States. Effective sunblocker formulas contain 5% para-aminobenzoic acid (PABA). Put on 30 minutes before going out into sun, as it takes at least this length of time to bind to the skin. Use the highest protection sunscreens at first. Once a tan is achieved, the lower protection numbers may be used. Reapply when going in and out of the water or with prolonged sun exposure and sweating. Sometimes PABA produces allergic reactions, so those sensitive individuals should use benzophenone sunscreens. Opaque formulas that contain zinc oxide or titanium dioxide block the sun physically by reflecting it off the skin. Some suntanning oils and creams do not contain sunscreen and do not offer any protection against the sun.

Patients taking drugs that react when in sunlight (photosensitivity usually demonstrated by rash when in the sun) should not regard sunscreens as protection against these reactions. Also occurs in individuals with lupus erythematosus. Avoid further sun, apply cold compresses, and avoid creams that contain local anesthetics such as benzocaine, which may actually aggravate the symptoms.

Alternative Treatments

Refer to alternative therapy chapters for more information before evaluating or applying any treatment. Some conditions, including yours, may require a physician's care.

NUTRITIONAL THERAPY: • Vitamin E (orally and topically) • Vitamin A depending on severity of burn (for mild cases, 50,000 IU daily for several days; for more severe cases, 100,000 IU for first three days, then reduce to 50,000 IU daily for several weeks). • Vitamin C (amounts of all the antioxidants depend on degree of severity) • Potassium (100 mg daily for one to two weeks) • Mix together vitamins A, E, essential fatty acids, zinc oxide, and aloe gel, and place on skin. • Calcium • Magnesium

Self–Care

The following therapies can be undertaken at home under appropriate professional supervision.

Fasting

AROMATHERAPY: • Spray or rub with lavender and chamomile. • To prevent blistering, apply two to three drops of lavender oil.

FLOWER ESSENCES: Rescue Remedy Cream®

HERBS: Apply cool aloe vera gel liberally to the burnt area. If badly burnt, apply a salve made with St. John's wort and calendula flowers.

HOMEOPATHY: *Natrum mur.* (as preventative); *Urtica urens, Rhus tox.*

HYDROTHERAPY: • Cold compress (apply immediately and as needed to control pain) • Bathe with apple cider vinegar or colloidal oatmeal.

JUICE THERAPY: Carrot juice

NATUROPATHIC MEDICINE: The gel from the freshly cut aloe vera leaf applied to sunburn combined with large oral doses of vitamin E.

TOPICAL TREATMENT: • Mixture of apple cider vinegar (two parts) and olive oil (one part) • PABA cream

Professional Care

The following therapies should only be provided by a qualified health professional.

Naturopathic Medicine

OXYGEN THERAPY: External ozone therapy to decrease inflammation and prevent infection.

TRADITIONAL CHINESE MEDICINE: Apply Chinese black tea externally.

SWELLING

Enlargement of a localized area, usually secondary to infection, injury, or holding and shifting of bodily fluids.

Alternative Treatments

Refer to alternative therapy chapters for more information before evaluating or applying any treatment. Some conditions, including yours, may require a physician's care.

DIET: Whole foods diet with a decrease in salt, commercial sodas, and refined sugars and an emphasis on increasing pure water and herbal teas but avoiding excess caffeinated beverages and undiluted fruit juices.

NUTRITIONAL THERAPY: • Proteolytic enzymes (on empty stomach) • Bromelain (on empty stomach) • Vitamin C and bioflavonoids • Vitamin B complex • Vitamin B6

Self–Care

The following therapies can be undertaken at home under appropriate professional supervision.

Fasting

AYURVEDA: • Drink barley water (boil four parts water with one part barley and strain). • For external swelling, apply mixture of turmeric (two parts) and salt (one part) to affected area. • *Punarnava guggulu* (200 mg) generally taken twice a day after lunch and dinner.

HERBS: Make a fomentation (hot pack) of ginger root. Increases circulation to an area of swelling, pain, or stiff joints.

HOMEOPATHY: *Belladonna, Aconite, Ferrum phos., Sulfur*

HYDROTHERAPY: Contrast application (apply repeatedly as needed to reduce swelling). According to Leon Chaitow, N.D., D.O., alternating immersion of the swollen area, or applications of hot and cold (damp towels will do nicely) to the area, reduces swelling by speeding up drainage of lymph (the clear fluid that is the medium for waste disposal following injury or inflammation) and flushing the area with fresh blood. Alternatively, ice massage can be useful if the swelling relates to an acute problem.

JUICE THERAPY: • Fresh pineapple juice • Carrot, celery, cucumber

Professional Care

The following therapies should only be provided by a qualified health professional.

Acupuncture / Environmental Medicine / Magnetic Field Therapy / Naturopathic Medicine / Traditional Chinese Medicine

BODYWORK: According to Dr. Chaitow, lymphatic drainage massage and other massage techniques may help to remove swelling by opening the drainage (lymphatic) channels, which might be overloaded. This may be especially useful for chronic swelling.

OSTEOPATHY: Cranial and other osteopathic techniques are aimed precisely at enhancing drainage and lymphatic flow.

TENDINITIS

A tendon is a fibrous cord that attaches a muscle to a bone or a muscle to another muscle. Inflammation can occur to the tendon itself (tendinitis) or to the lining of the tendon called the tendinous sheath (tenosynovitis). Inflammation usually occurs to both simultaneously. If the muscle that attaches to the tendon is chronically overloaded through overuse or abuse (trauma), the tendon attachment to the bone becomes irritated, causing what is called a periosteal pain point. If this condition continues, the tendon itself becomes inflamed.

SYMPTOMS: The tendons that are involved are usually very painful and tender to the touch and are painful on motion of the involved joint. Often the joint motion becomes restricted because of the pain and the abnormal changes to the tendons themselves that affect movement. The pain can become severe depending on the degree of inflammation. Very severe pain may radiate to the joints above and below this joint. The pain may affect daily life and make sleep difficult when the joint is moved during movements while sleeping. The involved tendons often have a "creaking" quality to them due to "friction rubs" from the inflammation itself, and may become swollen because of the inflammation or due to fluid accumulation. Sometimes, calcium becomes deposited in the area, or the swollen tendon sheath puts extra pressure on where it inserts into the bone, so that the bone enlarges at that site in response to this chronic pressure.

OCCURRENCE: Very common in many individuals. More common in middle-aged and older individuals due to decreased circulation in the tendons associated with repeated microtrauma. The most common cause of tendinitis is repeated or extreme trauma, excessive (not usual) exercise, and strain. Certain systemic diseases have a higher incidence of tendinitis, such as rheumatoid arthritis, autoimmune disorders, gout, Reiter's syndrome (an inflammatory syndrome), when blood cholesterol levels are excessively high (hyperlipoproteinemia, Type 11), and in younger women with certain sexually transmitted diseases.

SPECIAL NOTES: The most common areas to get tendinitis are the shoulder capsule (subdeltoid bursitis), the tendons of the big thumb (de Quervain's disease), and the hip capsule (trochanteric bursitis). Tendinitis and bursitis are really interchangeable terms as bursa are located near tendons.

Treatment needs to involve immobilization (splinting of the involved part), compresses with cold or heat (whatever seems to help, which varies between individuals), agents to reduce pain locally and systemically (orally and topically), and therapeutic exercise, which should increase as joint becomes better and is able to tolerate increased movement.

Alternative Treatments

Refer to alternative therapy chapters for more information before evaluating or applying any treatment. Some conditions, including yours, may require a physician's care.

DIET: Avoidance of the nightshade family of plants (white potato, tomato, eggplant, all peppers except black, and tobacco); if restricted for a long time, over years, this may be effective. Assessment and treatment of food allergies is imperative, as inflammation may be aggravated by food allergies in many people.

NUTRITIONAL THERAPY: • Vitamin B6 • Vitamin B complex • Vitamin C with bioflavonoids • Copper orally (2-4 mg daily) and/or wear a copper bracelet. Copper is absorbed topically through the skin and may decrease chronic joint pains.[76] • Manganese • Bromelain • Essential fatty acids • Cod liver oil (one tablespoon, one to two hours before meals) • DL-phenylalanine and/or calcium/magnesium may help with pain • Vitamin E • Selenium

Self-Care

The following therapies can be undertaken at home under appropriate professional supervision.

Acupressure / Biofeedback Training and Neurotherapy / Fasting / Guided Imagery

BODYWORK: Massage, shiatsu

FLOWER ESSENCES: Rescue Remedy Cream®

HERBS: Combine equal parts of the tinctures of willow bark, cramp bark, and prickly ash and take one teaspoon of this mixture three times a day.

HOMEOPATHY: *Aconite, Thuja, Ruta grav., Belladonna, Apis mel.*

HYDROTHERAPY: • Contrast application (apply one to three times daily) • If acute, use an ice pack (apply 20 minutes out of each hour for the first 24-36 hours) • Epsom salt bath (several tablespoons of Epsom salts per bath; soak for 25-30 minutes, then rinse and rub down with hot olive oil; once a week).

OSTEOPATHY: According to Leon Chaitow, N.D., D.O., if the tendinitis relates to chronic overload or misuse of muscles, then relaxing and stretching these muscles reduces the stress on the tendon. Osteopathic muscle energy methods can usually be safely used at home in a way that achieves this goal. The most successful method uses yoga-type stretches following mild painless contractions of the involved muscle.

TOPICAL TREATMENT: • Rest the injured area and elevate above the level of the heart. • Salt and vinegar therapy for stiff joints, sprains, inflammation. Soak several layers of gauze or muslin with apple cider vinegar, then place coarse, kosher salt thickly on the gauze and wrap around affected area. • To loosen tight tendons and joints rub iodized salt moistened with apple cider vinegar on affected area twice a week. Be sure it is not too liquid. • Mullein hot packs. Boil three to four fresh mullein leaves in water for three minutes. Place over joint, wrap with a hot moist towel, then dry towel. Leave in place for 20 minutes, three times a day.

Professional Care

The following therapies should only be provided by a qualified health professional.

Acupuncture / Cell Therapy / Chiropractic / Craniosacral Therapy / Energy Medicine / Magnetic Field Therapy / Naturopathic Medicine / Neural Therapy / Osteopathic Medicine / Prolotherapy

BODYWORK: Feldenkrais Method, Rolfing

DETOXIFICATION THERAPY: Detoxification is indicated. Treat inflammation locally.

LIGHT THERAPY: • Monochromatic red light therapy • Cold (soft) laser photo stimulation therapy

OXYGEN THERAPY: • Hydrogen peroxide therapy (IV) • Hyperbaric oxygen therapy.

TONSILLITIS

Acute (short-lived) infection of the tonsils, usually caused by streptococcal organisms and less commonly viral.

SYMPTOMS: Swelling and pain in the neck, pain in the throat, particularly painful on swallowing, and often the pain radiates to the ears. In very young children, the main symptom may be refusal to eat and they may not complain of sore throat. Other symptoms may be high fever, abscesses on the tonsils, temporary hearing loss, headache, hoarseness, coughing, vomiting, and general ill feelings and fatigue.

OCCURRENCE: This is mainly a childhood condition, occurring most frequently in children under nine years of age. Most children experience at least one episode. It can occur in older individuals, but it is more rare.

SPECIAL NOTES: Throat cultures (must see a doctor) are necessary to rule out strep throat and family members need to be tested at first, as they may be carriers and need to be treated along with the infected individual.

According to the German system of homotoxicology, the tonsils are organs of excretion for toxins, and detoxification processes as well as inflammatory reactions take place in the tonsils. One theory is that many cases of chronic and recurring tonsillitis are due to the fact that the acute stage of the inflammation was quickly suppressed by powerful pharmaceutical drugs and the detoxification process was not able to occur. In treating tonsillitis, one should attempt to both destroy the pathogen and also aid in the discharge of toxins.

Treatment needs to include bed rest, lots of fluids, agents to reduce pain, and antibiotics if the infective organism is strep.

Alternative Treatments

Refer to alternative therapy chapters for more information before evaluating or applying any treatment. Some conditions, including yours, may require a physician's care.

DIET: Lots of fluids, especially diluted fresh fruit juices, warm broths, and light soups. To relieve pain, take two tablespoons each of honey and glycerine with one squeeze of lemon juice; warm and sip slowly. If on antibiotics, consume yogurt with live cultures.

NUTRITIONAL THERAPY: • Vitamin A (100,000 IU first three days, then 25,000 IU for the next week) • Zinc lozenges (slowly dissolve in mouth every two to four hours) • Vitamin B complex • Vitamin C • If on antibiotics, take *Lactobacillus acidophilus* and *Bifidobacteria.* • Garlic capsules • Ginger packs and zinc oxide should be applied externally to reduce pain.

Self-Care

The following therapies can be undertaken at home under appropriate professional supervision.

Guided Imagery / Relaxation / Yoga

AROMATHERAPY: Inhalations with bergamot, thyme, lavender and benzoin, tea tree, geranium, lemon (use as a gargle as well).

FASTING: According to Leon Chaitow, N.D., D.O., there is no better approach than a pure water or diluted juice fast for the first 48 hours, followed by broths, etc., as recommended.

FLOWER ESSENCES: Rescue Remedy® for accompanying stress. Crab Apple.

HERBS: Combine the tinctures of cleavers and echinacea in equal parts and take one teaspoon three times a day. Drink a hot infusion made from equal parts of dried elder flower, yarrow, and peppermint throughout the day.

HOMEOPATHY: *Belladonna, Merc sol., Phytolacca, Lachesis, Aconite*

HYDROTHERAPY: • Contrast application (apply one to two times daily to neck and throat) • Heating compress (apply one to two times daily to neck and throat) • Gargle with hot water.

JUICE THERAPY: • Carrot, beet and tomato • Carrot, pineapple • Carrot, orange • Carrot, apple • Carrot, celery • Ginger

REFLEXOLOGY: Lymph system, all toes, adrenals, cervical

Professional Care

The following therapies should only be provided by a qualified health professional.

Acupuncture / Magnetic Field Therapy / Naturopathic Medicine / Neural Therapy / Osteopathic Medicine / Traditional Chinese Medicine

DETOXIFICATION THERAPY: May be indicated, depending on the condition of the person.

OXYGEN THERAPY: Hyperbaric oxygen therapy may be useful as an antibiotic.

TUBERCULOSIS

An infection, often referred to as TB, either acute or chronic, which occurs as pulmonary tuberculosis (in the lungs) or extrapulmonary tuberculosis (other bodily sites) and is also classified when it occurs in childhood or adulthood. It is caused by the bacterium Mycobacterium tuberculosis.

SYMPTOMS: TB most commonly affects the lungs and is often asymptomatic (no symptoms) until the lung lesions (where the TB is growing on the lungs) become large enough to be seen on X ray or to create problems. The earliest symptoms are usually coughing (often first demonstrates as early morning cough) and flu-like symptoms. Other symptoms are chest pain, difficulty breathing, coughing up blood, decreased appetite, fever, sweats (worse at night), and weight loss. Complications can occur, such as collecting fluid between the lung and the chest wall (pleural effusion), collecting air in the same space (pneumothorax), or even death. Sometimes symptoms do not occur for up to two years following initial infection. The speed of the symptoms varies widely from individual to individual.

OCCURRENCE: In the United States, TB is responsible for 1,800 deaths per year and 20,000 new cases are reported per year; 15% of these cases are extrapulmonary TB. Most at risk are older nonwhite males (African-Americans, Hispanics, and Asians), especially if they have a history of being in physical contact with active cases (any person in a household with an active individual, especially a child, should be given an antituberculosis antibiotic drug as prevention) or people who were not appropriately treated with drugs, and in individuals from Central and South America, Africa, and Southeast Asia. People with illnesses that decrease immune competence (alcoholics, malnourished, diabetics, and HIV-positive) are more at risk. The major risk of catching TB from another active individual is before diagnosis is made. When individuals are on appropriate treatment, within ten to 14 days they become noninfectious, even though the sputum (material coughed up) still has the active TB laboratory markers.

SPECIAL NOTES: Prevention is the key and this has historically been done through vaccinations—Bacillus Calmette-Guérin (BCG) vaccination in high-risk groups or contact tracing performed on relatives and friends of TB patients through skin testing and X ray to rule out early stages. Vaccinations are useful where TB is still a problem. Recently, TB was so well controlled in the United States that vaccines were rarely used. However, there is now an increase in certain areas, such as California and New York City. Ask your doctor for advice in this matter according to where you reside. Diagnosis must include a chest X ray and skin and sputum tests.

Drugs that act as immune suppressants, such as corticosteroids, can retrigger tuberculosis.

Treatment must include drugs. Two or more drugs should be used to avoid bacterial resistance to one drug. The drugs used are hard on the liver, thus laboratory tests monitoring liver functions must be run regularly.

Alternative Treatments

Refer to alternative therapy chapters for more information before evaluating or applying any treatment. Some conditions, including yours, may require a physician's care.

DIET: Whole foods diet with plenty of raw foods, fluids, and lots of pears, pear juice, and pear sauce, as pears may hasten healing of the lungs. Other foods that may be helpful are fenugreek and alfalfa sprouts, garlic, pomegranate, and all forms of fermented milk such as yogurt and kefir. Make a puree of steamed asparagus using a blender; keep refrigerated, then take four tablespoons at breakfast and dinner for a few months.

NUTRITIONAL THERAPY: • Vitamin A (300,000 IU for first three days, then 200,000 IU next two days, then 50,000 IU daily for several weeks) • Beta carotene (25,000-50,000 IU) • Vitamin E (increase up to 1,000 IU daily, unless a premenopausal woman with many PMS) • Lipotropic formula (one daily) • Deglycyrrihizinated licorice • Citrus seed extract • Vitamin C • Lung glandular • Essential fatty acids • Vitamin B complex • Multiminerals • Zinc

Self-Care

The following therapies can be undertaken at home under appropriate professional supervision.

Qigong and Tai Chi

HERBS: • Combine the tinctures of echinacea, elecampane, and mullein in equal parts and take one teaspoon three times a day. • Take three capsules of garlic three times a day.

HINTS: Get plenty of fresh air, rest, light, exercise, and relaxation.

HYDROTHERAPY: Constitutional hydrotherapy (apply two to five times weekly).

JUICE THERAPY: Raw potato juice. After juicing, allow the starch to settle and pour off the juice. Combine with an equal part of carrot juice, add one teaspoon of olive or almond oil, one teaspoon of honey, and beat until it foams. Drink three glasses daily.

TOPICAL TREATMENT: • Eucalyptus oil packs • Grape packs • Alcohol (grain) packs

Professional Care

The following therapies should only be provided by a qualified health professional.

Magnetic Field Therapy / Traditional Chinese Medicine

FASTING: Fasting may be indicated under a doctor's supervision.

LIGHT THERAPY: • Red light • Sunlight

URINARY PROBLEMS

(See also Women's Health chapter and Bed-Wetting)
The urinary tract is that part of the body involved in formation, concentration, and excretion of urine. The urinary tract system includes the kidneys, which make urine out of the blood and are associated with their own blood and nerve supplies, the ureters, which are tubes taking urine from the kidneys to the bladder, and the urethras, which are tubes taking urine from the bladder out of the body (excretion). Urinary problems may vary widely. They usually involve a problem anywhere along the entire urinary tract, including the kidneys.

SYMPTOMS: Most people urinate four to six times a day, usually all during the daytime. It is not typical to get up in the middle of the night to urinate, especially two times or more, on a somewhat regular basis (unless there have been much more liquids consumed during the day). This is called nocturia (urination during the night) and is often suggestive of early diabetes or of kidney, heart, or liver disease. Also, it may not be associated with a serious disease, but may be secondary to other non-serious bladder problems, such as obstruction.

Straining, nocturia, changes in force of stream of the urine, and hesitancy are usually signs of bladder obstruction and are more common in middle-aged to older men, often secondary to an enlarged prostate due to a variety of problems, but most often not serious. Pain or burning on urination (dysuria) suggests inflammation or irritation of the bladder or the urethra and is usually due to an infection from bacteria. Incontinence (loss of urine without warning, often after sneezing, laughing, running, or coughing) is associated with many conditions, such as bladder dysfunctions, cystocele (abnormal pocket formed by lax tissue) as a result of stretching or aging of muscles of the pelvic floor, injuries from childbirth, fibroids on the uterus that push down on the bladder, and may now be successfully treated with simple surgical procedures if the problem becomes severe enough and decreases quality of life.

Normal urine is usually clear or slightly yellowish. Certain vitamins make the urine bright yellow and have a strong odor. This is not a sign that something is wrong, but rather a normal metabolic process of vitamin ingestion. This colormetric characteristic of urine while taking vitamins is often used as a milepost to help elderly patients remember to take their vitamins ("keep taking enough to keep your urine bright yellow"). Presence of other color pigments in urine usually means the following: red (foods such as beets, this is normal), brown, black, blue, green, or red (from certain drugs), and colors other than normal such as brownish or black may suggest the presence of diseases or blood in the urine and must be investigated by a doctor. Cloudy urine most often is a normal precipitate of phosphate salts in alkaline urine, but may suggest pus from a urinary tract infection.

Pain anywhere in the urinary tract may refer to different areas of the body and may be the only symptom of a problem in the urinary tract and thus be confusing. Pain from kidney disease is often referred to the low back, or between the twelfth rib and the iliac crest (hip), and sometimes to the sternum (chest bone). Bladder infections may refer pain to just above the pubic area and along the urethra. Urinary problems and/or reproductive problems may create a feeling of abdominal fullness in both men and women.

OCCURRENCE: Family history of problems in this area, especially kidney disease, may suggest a heredity predisposition. If urinary problems occur with ear and eye disorders, this may indicate congenital (tendency towards or presence of at birth) urinary/kidney problems. Recent infections of the respiratory tract, the heart, or skin may be causes for later problems in the urinary tract and kidneys. History of past kidney problems, trauma (such as accidents or injuries), or other conditions such as high blood pressure or drugs, or history of past kidney stones or stones in a primary relative (in one's personal family), all may be important information to figure out what problem an individual is having in this area.

Alternative Treatments

Refer to alternative therapy chapters for more information before evaluating or applying any treatment. Some conditions, including yours, may require a physician's care.

DIET: For urinary infections, laboratory studies have shown that cranberry juice may inhibit bacteria from sticking to the lining cells of the bladder and causing urinary tract infections, explaining its long history as a folk remedy.[77] Caffeine has been linked to urinary incontinence. Research shows that, in people with weak bladder muscles, caffeine causes the muscles around the bladder to contract and exert additional pressure.[78] The following foods and additives are known to irritate the bladder: coffee, tea, artificial sweeteners, carbonated beverages, tomato-based foods. Elimination of these from the diet can often result in complete relief of symptoms.

NUTRITIONAL THERAPY: • Vitamin C • Pain and burning (acute) may be helped by cranberry juice along with vitamin C. However, in chronic cases, vitamin C may aggravate some individuals, in dosages over 1-2 grams. Instead, try alkalinizing the body by taking baking soda (½ teaspoon) or two Alka-Seltzer Gold tablets. • Vitamin B₁ (30-50 mg two to three times per day between meals

for no more than one week, to help reduce pain, burning, and irritation) • Add mineral ascorbates with meals three times daily. • In men, if the urinary problem is secondary to prostate problems, the prostate must be treated accordingly (see Men's Health chapter).

Problems secondary to pelvic muscle atrophy or stretching may respond to mixed amino acids (two to three times daily, 10-15 minutes before meals, for at least six months), along with a Kegel exercise program both for women and men (squeezing together of all the musculature around the urinary and reproductive areas, accomplished by trying to squeeze everything below up towards the belly button). Repeat 50 times morning and evening as a regular part of the day, not to be discontinued once symptoms improve or go away. In other words, like other exercises, these must be kept up daily.

Self-Care
The following therapies can be undertaken at home under appropriate professional supervision.

Yoga

ACUPRESSURE: Rub the acupressure points SP6 and ST36 (see acupressure chart in the introduction to this section) vigorously in a circular motion for 20-30 seconds. Do it several times a day and before bedtime.

AROMATHERAPY: • Tea tree oil • For infections, use sandalwood, bergamot, juniper.

BIOFEEDBACK TRAINING: May be effective in treating incontinence.

HERBS: • For mild water retention and possibly mild cystitis symptoms, make an infusion of equal parts of bearberry, dandelion leaf, and nettle. Drink hot three times a day or as needed. • For blood in urine, use comfrey. • Difficult or burning urination: fennel, horsetail, jasmine flowers, licorice. • Cystitis, painful urination: hibiscus. • Urinary tract infections: buchu, burdock, coriander, cornsilk, echinacea, goldenrod, juniper berries, marshmallow root, shave grass. • Urinary incontinence: skullcap.

HOMEOPATHY: Urethritis: *Aconite, Apis mel., Cantharis*

HYDROTHERAPY: • For incontinence, use a sitz bath (apply daily with emphasis on cold). • For urethritis, apply contrast sitz bath daily.

JUICE THERAPY: • Carrot, parsley, celery, cucumber • Cranberry

LIFESTYLE: For incontinence, use pelvic exercises (100-200 contractions of the bladder muscles daily can greatly improve bladder control).

Professional Care
The following therapies should only be provided by a qualified health professional.

Acupuncture / Magnetic Field Therapy / Naturopathic Medicine / Osteopathic Medicine

VARICOSE VEINS

Valves in the veins prevent blood from draining back into certain areas, especially the legs. When these valves are absent from birth or become incompetent, pooling of blood occurs in superficial (not deep) veins. This pooling of blood encourages the veins to become enlarged (dilated and swollen), elongated, and twisted and bent more than normal (tortuous). When this happens, the veins are called varicose.

SYMPTOMS: At first, the veins become more tense and stiff and this can be felt but not seen. Then they become more enlarged and twisted and may be seen easily as bluish, blackish prominent tubular elevations from the rest of the surrounding skin. Symptoms are not directly related to the size or degree of the varicosities. For example, very severe varicose veins may have no symptoms at all while patients with tiny varicosities may complain of aching, leg fatigue, itching, burning, or heat that seems relieved by elevating the legs or wearing stockings that compress the legs. Most commonly, symptoms seem to increase during the premenstrual cycle (anywhere from mid-cycle to onset of the period). The most common sites for varicose veins are the back of lower leg (the calves) and along the inside of the lower and upper legs.

OCCURRENCE: Varicose veins are very common and affect more women than men. Overall, varicose veins affect about 15% of adults in the United States. Varicosities do occur in families.

SPECIAL NOTES: Varicosities in other parts of the body are varicocele (varicose veins in the scrotum), hemorrhoids (varicose veins in the anus), and esophageal varices (varicose veins in the esophagus). Risk factors for varicosities are sedentary lifestyle, obesity, smoking, standing for very long periods at a time, and hormonal changes at pregnancy or menopause.

If the problem of blood backsliding and pooling becomes severe enough that tissues do not get adequate nutrients and oxygen, the skin around the varicosities may become very thin, discolored, hardened, and prone to deep sores (ulcers). These need to be treated by cleaning, keeping covered, and improving the circulation and return of blood to the heart by leg compresses, elevating legs, exercise program, and nutrients and warm foods that increase circulation. If a large varicosity is traumatized, such as bumping the leg or straining at the stool and bruising or lacerating a hemorrhoid, it may cause severe bleeding. Apply moderate pressure, lie down, elevate the legs, and contact a physician.

Wear support stockings. Contact an exercise physiologist or trainer and start a sensible overall exercise program (daily walking and swimming are excellent). Walking barefoot as much as possible is also excellent, along with walking on grass first thing in the morning when there is still dew on it (avoid in the colder climates during winter). Massage the area every night with almond oil, with drops of myrrh oil and vitamin C crys-

tals added, even over hemorrhoids. If there is some burning, discontinue or try eliminating the vitamin C.

Alternative Treatments

Refer to alternative therapy chapters for more information before evaluating or applying any treatment. Some conditions, including yours, may require a physician's care.

DIET: Ideally, start with a bowel-cleansing program or at least a few days on just fruits, vegetables, and whole grains with lots of pure water to start cleansing the system. Whole foods diet with emphasis on the following foods: fresh fruits, including berries and cherries, organic citrus fruits (making sure to nibble on the inside of the rinds), whole grains especially buckwheat (whole grain and noodles) and millet, garlic, onions, ginger, and cayenne pepper. Eat plenty of fish and cut down on red meat as much as possible. Moderately restrict fats and refined carbohydrates in diet. Foods to avoid: sugar, salt, alcohol, fried foods, processed and refined foods, animal protein, cheeses (goat is okay), and ice cream.

NUTRITIONAL THERAPY: • Rutin (1 g per day for up to one year) and bioflavonoids (1 g daily for same time). Some people may have to stay on rutin and bioflavonoids permanently, as their metabolism requires these to prevent recurrence. • Vitamin C (take throughout the day every several hours) • Vitamin B complex • Vitamin B₆ or pyridoxine (30-100 mg daily for several months) • Vitamin E (400 IU).

For leg cramps: • Vitamin E • Calcium • Magnesium • Folic acid (1 g daily for several months) • Lecithin • Vitamin D (500 mg daily for two months)

For ulcers accompanying varicosities: • Vitamin E (orally and topically) • Zinc (orally and topically as zinc oxide cream) • Essential fatty acids (orally and topically: squeeze one capsule on area two times daily). If ulcers do not heal, try adding proteolytic enzymes (four to six, between meals, three times daily for two weeks).

Self-Care

The following therapies can be undertaken at home under appropriate professional supervision.

Fasting / Yoga

AROMATHERAPY: Cypress as bath oil. Lavender, juniper, rosemary (do not massage directly on top of vein), lemon

BODYWORK: Acupressure, reflexology, massage.

HERBS: • Combine equal parts of the tinctures of hawthorn, ginkgo, prickly ash, and yarrow and take one teaspoon of this mixture three times a day. • A lotion for external use can be made with ten parts distilled witch hazel and one part tincture of horse chestnut.[79] This may be applied often to help ease any discomfort.

HOMEOPATHY: *Calc fluor., Hamamelis, Pulsatilla, Calc carb., Carbo veg.*

HYDROTHERAPY: Cold compress or sprays/showers (apply cold application daily to affected veins, using a gentle spray).

JUICE THERAPY: • Carrot, celery, and parsley • Carrot, spinach, and turnip • Carrot, beet, cucumber • Carrot, celery, spinach • Watercress

REFLEXOLOGY: Colon, liver, adrenals, referral area on the arm.

Professional Care

The following therapies should only be provided by a qualified health professional.

Acupuncture / Chelation Therapy / Enzyme Therapy / Magnetic Field Therapy / Naturopathic Medicine / Prolotherapy / Traditional Chinese Medicine

OXYGEN THERAPY: Ozone.

VERTIGO

A subjective impression of losing one's equilibrium (feeling off-balance), due to a sensation that the individual is moving around in space (subjective vertigo) or the room and objects in it are moving around the individual (objective vertigo).

True vertigo is an organic disturbance within the equilibratory system (ears, inner ear canals, the eighth cranial nerves servicing the ears, the associated brain parts, and the eyes) that may be caused by mild disturbances or secondary to specific health disorders such as middle ear infections, herpes zoster viral infection, inflammation of the semicircular ear canals (labyrinthitis), obstruction in an ear tube, tumor, or nerve inflammation. True vertigo is contrasted to false vertigo or episodes of dizziness, faintness, or lightheadedness, which are common complaints and most often not a sign of any serious underlying problem.

SYMPTOMS: True vertigo usually comes on very suddenly and is accompanied by difficulty in walking steadily and feeling dizzy or faint. There may also be nausea, a generally ill sensation, and pallor (losing color, turning white).

OCCURRENCE: May occur in healthy people in specific situations such as on a roller coaster or other amusement-type rides, sailing, looking out the window of a car, or watching a fast-paced movie. True vertigo associated with underlying disorders often occurs with vomiting and severe unsteadiness of gait. However, not all vertigos accompanied with these symptoms are due to underlying illness. Some people get this way by sitting on a sailboat.

CONSIDER: Sudden attacks of vertigo, tinnitus (ringing in the ears), and hearing loss, often associated with nausea and vomiting, are symptoms of Meniere's disease (see Hearing and Ear Disorders chapter). According to Jonathan Wright, M.D., some vertigo is set off by allergies. Vertigo can be a sign of many other problems and a severe attack of it warrants a thorough examination of the ears, eyes, and nervous system by a doctor.

SPECIAL NOTES: True vertigo is not necessarily a sign of a psychological problem. However, obsessive fear of losing one's balance or inappropriate giddiness may be a sign of depression or anxiety neurosis. According to Leon Chaitow, N.D., D.O., anxiety itself is often the end result of hyperventilation (inappropriate breathing patterns), which is commonly associated with vertigo. Breath retraining and appropriate manual (osteopathic, chiropractic, soft tissue manipulation) attention to spinal and thoracic restrictions, as well as postural reintegration and stress reduction, are often needed to normalize such problems.

Stay still. Avoid rapid body movements, especially of the head. Preventative measures: reduce stress, get bodywork, especially reflexology or chiropractic, and practice routine and adequate sleep habits.

Alternative Treatments

Refer to alternative therapy chapters for more information before evaluating or applying any treatment. Some conditions, including yours, may require a physician's care.

DIET: Avoid caffeine, especially espresso and chocolates, salt, fried foods, nicotine, drugs and alcohol, and aspartame (NutraSweet™).

NUTRITIONAL THERAPY: • Vitamin B complex (two times daily) • Vitamin B_6 (100 mg daily) • Niacin or vitamin B_3 (30 mg three times daily) • Vitamin C plus bioflavonoids and rutin • *Ginkgo biloba* extract (120 mg daily) • Ginger capsules. For prevention of acute attack, take six tablets several hours before suspected episode. During an attack, take 3-6, two to three times daily on empty stomach. For prevention in general in a prone individual, take two tablets, twice daily on an empty stomach, not to be taken for more than one month. Consult an orthomolecular physician before taking ginger if there is a history of female problems or estrogen-related tumors. • Choline (500 mg two times daily) • Calcium • Adrenal glandulars • Vitamin E

Self-Care

The following therapies can be undertaken at home under appropriate professional supervision.

Fasting / Qigong and Tai Chi

AYURVEDA: • Mix sesame oil with small amounts of camphor, cardamom, and cinnamon and apply to head. • The Ayurvedic herb *amla* is used for vertigo. • An herbal mixture of *shatavari* (500 mg), *kamadudha* (200 mg), ginger (100 mg), and *brahmi* (300 mg), generally taken twice a day after lunch and dinner. • *Brahmi ghee nasya*

FLOWER ESSENCES: Rescue Remedy® for accompanying stress. Scleranthus.

HERBS: Ginkgo[80] and ginger[81] may help with the symptoms of vertigo, but competent diagnosis is essential. Take one 40 mg tablet of ginkgo or two capsules of ginger three times a day.

HOMEOPATHY: *Gelsemium, Phosphorus, Cocculus, Aconite, Nat. mur., Sulfur, Silicea, Lycopodium, Belladonna.*

REFLEXOLOGY: Ear reflex, neck, cervicals, big toes.

Professional Care

The following therapies should only be provided by a qualified health professional.

Chiropractic / Craniosacral Therapy / Environmental Medicine / Hypnotherapy / Magnetic Field Therapy / Natural Hormone Replacement Therapy / Naturopathic Medicine / Osteopathic Medicine / Traditional Chinese Medicine

VIRAL INFECTIONS

Infection by a virus. A virus is a minute infectious agent, consisting of a nucleic acid core (either DNA or RNA, which is the basic infectious material), with a protein shell (capsid), which is often multilayered with fats. It is this capsid that is very difficult for many drugs to penetrate, thus requiring antiviral drugs to be very aggressive.

SYMPTOMS: Viral infections classically demonstrate fever, generalized aches, chills, fatigue, and symptoms that are specific for that virus. For example, the cold virus usually produces mucus in the nose and throat, the mononucleosis virus produces severe fatigue and sometimes liver enlargement, and the polio virus produces paralysis.

OCCURRENCE: Viruses that occur mainly in humans are spread most commonly through respiratory routes and physiologic fluids (such as blood and semen). There are several hundred viruses that may potentially infect humans. Many are just being recognized and new ones may form or mutate, so that their physiologic expression, their interrelationships, their symptoms and assessments, and their prevention and treatment are not fully known. Some viruses do not produce overt symptoms or disease. Others do and are important to understand for the health and longevity of the human race.

Viruses vary tremendously in their effects on the body. The common cold is an acute (short-lived) viral infection. Some viruses cause cancer and terminal diseases. Some viruses incubate over a long period before any expression of the physiologic problems. These are called "slow" viruses, meaning they have a prolonged incubation period, such as the HTLV-III virus, which has been linked to AIDS. Exposure to it may take one year before it shows up in the blood and many years before symptoms appear in the individual.

SPECIAL NOTES: A virus is the smallest of parasites, as it is totally dependent on cells (plant, animal, or bacterial) for reproduction. Viruses stimulate host antibody production. Thus, identification of infection by a virus is often performed in the laboratory by measuring the blood level of antibodies to that virus.

Viruses do not respond to antibiotics. However, viral infections may cause individuals that are susceptible to bacterial infections to become infected with both; thus, sometimes antibiotics are given for some viral infections to prevent complications. This is a controversial treatment regime and overuse of antibiotics is not beneficial for most individuals. Viruses may be controlled and the symptoms may be reversed but, up until now, viruses have not been successfully eradicated from the body. Modern medicine is trying to change this.

Alternative Treatments

Refer to alternative therapy chapters for more information before evaluating or applying any treatment. Some conditions, including yours, may require a physician's care.

DIET: Whole foods diet with as few stressor foods as possible.

NUTRITIONAL THERAPY: • Vitamin C to bowel tolerance. According to Robert Cathcart, M.D., this is an effective way to deal with viral problems, but the protocol must be strictly followed (see Orthomolecular Medicine chapter). • Zinc • Proteolytic enzymes (4–6, three times daily on an empty stomach, between meals) • Acidophilus • Vitamin A • Raw thymus glandular • Vitamin B complex • Pantothenic acid (1–3 g two to three times daily) • Garlic capsules • Lysine • L-cysteine (an amino acid screen assessment by an orthomolecular physician may be beneficial). • Olive leaf extract is antibacterial and antiviral, effective against numerous viruses, including herpes, influenza, and Coxsackie virus.[82] • Quercetin is an antiviral flavonoid (antioxidant plant pigment) that appears to inhibit both the ability of viruses to infect and to replicate.[83] • Larch arabinogalactan, a complex sugar, enhances the function of the immune system in fighting viral infections.[84]

Self-Care

The following therapies can be undertaken at home under appropriate professional supervision.

Fasting / Guided Imagery

HERBS: • Combine equal parts of the tinctures of echinacea, goldenseal, and myrrh and take one teaspoon of this mixture three times a day. • Astragalus strengthens the body's ability to resist infection and reduces the frequency and length of colds and other viral conditions. • Garlic helps in fighting infectious agents, including viruses.

HOMEOPATHY: *Calendula, Chamomilla, Belladonna, Merc sol., Sulfur*

HYDROTHERAPY: • Constitutional hydrotherapy (apply two to five times weekly). • Hyperthermia (apply one to two times weekly).

JUICE THERAPY: Carrot, celery, beet, garlic

Professional Care

The following therapies should only be provided by a qualified health professional.

Environmental Medicine / Enzyme Therapy / Magnetic Field Therapy / Naturopathic Medicine

DETOXIFICATION THERAPY: Detoxification may be indicated unless the person is weak or deficient. Lighter diet is often recommended.

OXYGEN THERAPY: • Hydrogen peroxide therapy (IV) • Hyperbaric oxygen therapy • Ozone inactivates lipid-enveloped viruses (herpes, mumps, measles, retroviruses like HIV, hepatitis, polio, echo virus, Coxsackie virus).

VOMITING

The forceful and involuntary (unless it is self-induced as in eating disorders) expulsion of contents of the stomach out through the mouth.

SYMPTOMS: Upset stomach, nausea, sweating, turning white, and general ill feelings all usually precede the desire or urgency to vomit. Sometimes vomiting brings a sensation of relief. The dry heaves occur when vomiting continues even after being unable to expel any more food, so that the stomach is empty and what is brought up is liquid, whitish and sour, and nausea continues.

OCCURRENCE: Most people vomit several times throughout their lives. It rarely means anything serious unless it continues without a good reason. Some examples of normal events that may produce vomiting are: pregnancy, eating "tainted" food, emotional disgust, an alcoholic binge, after anesthesia, and exercising excessively after eating too much food. Vomiting also needs to be induced in some cases of poisoning.

CONSIDER: Nausea and vomiting may be symptoms of gastric disease (ulcers or inflammation), appendicitis, reaction to microbial toxins, drugs (chemotherapy, hormones such as estrogens), minerals (most commonly zinc and iron), radiation, motion sickness, obstruction somewhere in the gastrointestinal tract, or a metabolic disorder such as diabetes or liver disease. It may also be symptomatic of psychological disorders such as eating disorders, and bulimia (self-induced vomiting).

Vomiting blood (hematemesis) means that there is bleeding somewhere in the digestive tract, and a physician must be contacted at once. Depending on the cause of the blood, the extent of bleeding, and how much it is mixed together with the contents of the stomach, the vomited blood may appear as coffee grounds (mixed with stomach acid), streaked, totally bloody, dark red, brown, or black.

SPECIAL NOTES: Vomiting is a well-orchestrated physiologic phenomenon. Vomiting occurs when the center in the brain for vomiting is activated. Once this occurs, messages are sent to the diaphragm (muscular sheet separating the abdomen from the chest) to strongly press downward on the stomach, for the top of the stomach and esophagus (food pipe) to relax, and for the lower valve of the stomach that connects it to the rest of the intestine to strongly close. This acts like a device to extract food forcibly out of the stomach, up through the mouth, and out of the body. The brain also sends messages at the same time to close off the valve to the windpipe so that the food is not at risk of entering the lungs and causing suffocation.

Alternative Treatments

Refer to alternative therapy chapters for more information before evaluating or applying any treatment. Some conditions, including yours, may require a physician's care.

DIET: Continue to drink fluids, but avoid solid food and especially dairy. After vomiting has subsided, start with a light vegetable broth and toasted whole-grain bread. If digestion occurs, move to yogurt, potatoes, soups, brown rice, and steamed vegetables. After two to three days, resume a normal diet.

NUTRITIONAL THERAPY: Wait one day after the vomiting has stopped to take supplements and take very light supplements for the first few days. • Folic acid (400-500 mcg two to three times daily) • Vitamin A (10,000 IU) • Deglycyrrihizinated licorice • Acidophilus • Vitamin B_1 (50 mg) • In a few days, you may add more of your regular supplements.

Self-Care

The following therapies can be undertaken at home under appropriate professional supervision.

Fasting / Relaxation / Yoga

ACUPRESSURE: According to Leon Chaitow, N.D., D.O., if vomiting is associated with nausea resulting from travel or motion sickness, from pregnancy (morning sickness), or due to anesthesia or medication (chemotherapy), then strong thumb pressure on the point on the inner surface of the forearm, two thumb widths above the wrist crease, in the center between the tendons, will usually reduce or eliminate vomiting (P6, see acupressure chart in the introduction to this section).

AROMATHERAPY: Massage or place compress (black pepper, chamomile, fennel, camphor, lavender, peppermint, rose) over stomach.

FLOWER ESSENCES: Rescue Remedy® for accompanying stress; Crab Apple; Olive, for exhaustion.

HERBS: Treatment depends upon the cause. (Please refer to Motion Sickness.) An infusion of ginger or peppermint can be very settling.

HOMEOPATHY: *Ipecac., Phosphorus, Arsen alb., Nux vom.*

HYDROTHERAPY: Constitutional hydrotherapy (apply two to five times weekly).

JUICE THERAPY: Any vegetable juice with added ginger.

Professional Care

The following therapies should only be provided by a qualified health professional.

Acupuncture / Craniosacral Therapy / Environmental Medicine / Hypnotherapy / Magnetic Field Therapy / Naturopathic Medicine / Osteopathic Medicine / Therapeutic Touch / Traditional Chinese Medicine

DETOXIFICATION THERAPY: May be indicated to handle the problem.

WARTS

Warts are very common, contagious skin tumors (benign or noncancerous), "bumps," or "growths" that are caused by any of at least 35 viruses (human papillomavirus). Some warts can turn into cancerous tumors. However, the term wart *is loosely used for many benign, "wart-like" skin structures that are not caused by a virus, such as a raised, darkened skin tumor, common in the elderly, called a senile wart or verrucae, that is actually nonviral and more related to aging.*

SYMPTOMS: Warts may occur singly or in clusters. Their appearance and size varies tremendously depending on where they erupt on the body and the degree of irritation or trauma they receive through daily wear of the skin. The most common wart *(Verrucae vulgaris)* is a well-defined, rough-surfaced, roundish or irregular growth that may be light gray, brown, grayish-black, or yellow, and is usually firm to the touch. This wart most commonly appears on the knees, elbows, fingers, face, and scalp.

Periungual warts occur around the nail beds. Plantar warts occur on the sole of the foot, are very common, and often appear flattened due to the pressure of walking on them. They are distinguished from other foot growths (corns, calluses) by the fact that when they are scratched they "pinpoint" bleed. They may be incredibly painful but this does not necessarily indicate something serious. When there are several plantar warts close together, they form a plague-like appearance called mosaic warts. Warts that appear on a stalk (pedunculated) are common with age, particularly around the neck, chest, face, scalp, and armpits. Warts that are common on the face (eyelids, lips, neck) may appear as yellowish long, narrow, small growths.

Warts usually disappear on their own, without any treatment, within several months. However, in some individuals, they may continue for years or reoccur at the same or different parts of the body.

OCCURRENCE: The most common wart *(Verruca vulgaris)* is universal, occurs in almost everyone, and is usually not serious. Warts in general are more common in older children and usually do not occur in elderly individuals. However, the elderly are prone to other nonviral skin growths, such as aging spots and moles.

SPECIAL NOTES: *Mole* is a term applied to almost any pigmented skin blemish or growth that is not viral in origin and may be congenital (from birth) or not. Moles are usually not serious unless irritated constantly or change color, turn darker, or start to bleed. Moles are not warts and should not be treated as such. It is possible that immune functioning has something to do with healing and immunity to future warts, since immunosuppressed (poor immune function, secondary to serious illness such as diabetes or AIDS) individuals are much more susceptible to a wide variety of viral infections, such as warts.

Natural healing of warts may require one to two months of care, with the wart disappearing suddenly in one to three days.

Alternative Treatments

Refer to alternative therapy chapters for more information before evaluating or applying any treatment. Some conditions, including yours, may require a physician's care.

DIET: Diet is mainly an issue here if warts reoccur or do not regress, indicating the immune system may be slightly compromised. The more whole foods that are consumed, the better the possible enhancement of immune function. Thus, avoid stressor foods as much as possible. Foods to emphasize are those high in vitamin A, such as dark green and yellow vegetables, cold-water fish, and eggs. Sulfur-containing foods such as onions, garlic, Brussels sprouts, cabbage, and broccoli are also excellent. Consume adequate fermented milk products such as yogurt. Excess protein and fats may be discharged in the form of warts, moles, callouses, acne, and boils.

NUTRITIONAL THERAPY: • Vitamin A (100,000 IU for five days, then reduce to 25,000 IU for one month) • Beta carotene (50,000 IU for several weeks) • Vitamin C • L-cysteine (500 mg two times daily for one month, with an amino acid blend one time daily) • Vitamin B complex. • Zinc • Vitamin E

Apply two times daily for ten days a mixture of: garlic oil, vitamin E, castor oil, vitamin A (squeeze these oils from capsules onto the skin) with a drop of zinc oxide cream and paste from one crushed garlic clove. Be careful not to get onto surrounding areas and cover well after applying. If surrounding skin gets irritated, then try eliminating the fresh garlic paste.

Self-Care

The following therapies can be undertaken at home under appropriate professional supervision.

Fasting / Guided Imagery

AROMATHERAPY: Lemon

HERBS: Apply the milky latex from the stem of dandelions to the wart morning and night.

HOMEOPATHY: *Thuja, Causticum, Calc carb., Ruta grav., Graphites*

NATUROPATHIC MEDICINE: Persistent local application of thuja oil is often an effective way of removing warts. However, equally effective is the belief that the remedies will work.

Professional Care

The following therapies should only be provided by a qualified health professional.

Naturopathic Medicine

HYPNOTHERAPY: The worst case of warts reported by Joseph Pizzorno, N.D.—over 100 on hands, face, and arms—did not respond to either thuja oil or the standard medical approach of removal with liquid nitrogen. However, after only two sessions with a hypnotherapist, the warts were gone within a month and never returned.

TRADITIONAL CHINESE MEDICINE: Direct moxibustion.

WHOOPING COUGH

An acute bacterial disease (Bordetella pertussis) *that is distinguished by a spasmodic cough that ends in a specific long, high-pitched "crowing" sound (on inhalation it sounds like a "whoop," thus its name). It is highly contagious.*

SYMPTOMS: The bacteria invade the body and take one to three weeks to start producing symptoms. The whole respiratory tract may be affected. The entire symptom stage takes about six weeks, but may extend to three months. Initially, catarrh (mucus) is produced, along with fatigue, sneezing, coughing (starts first at night with a hacking sound without the whooping component and then begins to occur all day long), tearing of the eyes, and poor appetite. Usually, there is no accompanying fever. The second stage, 10-14 days after symptoms start to appear, produces a spasmodic cough consisting of about five to sometimes over 15 rapid coughs, followed by a "characteristic whooping" sound produced on the last several inhalations. Large amounts of mucus are produced. Gagging and even vomiting may occur after the whooping sounds. Infants may tend to "choke" rather than whoop. The last stage (convalescent) starts at around four weeks with all the symptoms decreasing while the individual is generally starting to feel improved. The spasmodic coughing may return at different times for a period following the disease, especially if the upper respiratory tract is irritated or reinfected, even by a cold.

CONSIDER: Bronchitis, pneumonia, flu, smoker's cough, and inhalant allergies.

Alternative Treatments

Refer to alternative therapy chapters for more information before evaluating or applying any treatment. Some conditions, including yours, may require a physician's care.

DIET: Drink plenty of liquids. Especially good is a combination of one to two tablespoons honey, one tablespoon apple cider vinegar, one tablespoon fresh lemon juice, one teaspoon each of horehound and licorice extracts, 1/8 teaspoon cayenne pepper, and vitamin C powder; add warm water and sip all day long, drinking three to six cups per day. Light foods can be taken between fits of coughing. During acute stage, particularly avoid all dairy products. Eat fruits, vegetables, brown rice, clear vegetable soups, potatoes, and whole grain toast.

Add one clove of finely sliced garlic to four ounces of raw honey, then cover and let sit overnight. Add one teaspoon of mixture per cup of warm water. Sip throughout the day.

NUTRITIONAL THERAPY: • Zinc lozenges (every two hours unless it causes nausea) • Vitamin C (in divided doses every hour, up to bowel tolerance) • Vitamin A (200,000 IU first three days, 100,000 IU next three days, then 25,000 IU for several months) • Beta carotene (50,000 IU daily for one month, then reduce to 25,000 IU daily) • Lung glandulars • Garlic capsules • Acidophilus

Self-Care

The following therapies can be undertaken at home under appropriate professional supervision.

AROMATHERAPY: Steam inhalation with tea tree, basil, chamomile, camphor, eucalyptus, peppermint, rose, lavender, thyme.

FLOWER ESSENCES: Rescue Remedy® for accompanying stress; Crab Apple; Olive, for exhaustion.

HERBS: The herbal tradition proposes a number of herbs as possible remedies, but they are not dramatically effective. These herbs include the antimicrobial and antispasmodic remedies sundew, thyme, butterbur, and wild cherry bark. One approach is to combine dried sundew, wild cherry bark, and anise in equal parts and make an infusion with one teaspoon in a cup of water. This should be consumed several times a day.

HOMEOPATHY: *Drosera, Pertussinum, Cuprum met., Mag phos.*

HYDROTHERAPY: • Constitutional hydrotherapy (apply two to five times weekly) or heating compress. • Cold socks treatment several times daily for head or chest congestion; replace socks when dry.

JUICE THERAPY: • Orange, lemon • Carrot, watercress.

Professional Care

The following therapies should only be provided by a qualified health professional.

Light Therapy / Magnetic Field Therapy / Naturopathic Medicine / Neural Therapy / Traditional Chinese Medicine

OSTEOPATHY: According to Leon Chaitow, N.D., D.O., osteopathic manipulative attention can reduce the severity of the cough dramatically and make the patient far more comfortable.

OXYGEN THERAPY: Hydrogen peroxide therapy (IV).

WORMS

Worms are parasites that may commonly invade the intestinal tract and uncommonly invade other parts of the body. There are many types of worms such as tapeworms, roundworms, hookworms, pinworms, whipworms, and flukeworms.

SYMPTOMS: Symptoms may vary depending on the worm. Pinworms *(Enterobius vermicularis)* are characterized by itching around the anus, but sometimes there are no symptoms at all. However, symptoms may include abdominal pain, joint pain, insomnia, convulsions, and many other widely varying signs. The whipworm *(Trichiura)* may not cause symptoms or, if there is a heavy infection, it may cause mild to severe abdominal pain and diarrhea, along with weight loss, anemia, appendicitis, and rectal prolapse in women and children. Tapeworm may cause mild to severe abdominal symptoms, such as cramping, up to abdominal obstruction. Systemic symptoms may be fever, coughing, wheezing, and, if the worms enter the lungs (they may travel through the lymphatic system), there may also be severe lung problems. Adult worms may even create problems in the appendix, liver, gallbladder, or pancreas. Hookworms are usually asymptomatic (no symptoms), but may cause a rash at the site where they invaded the body, may migrate to the lungs and cause pulmonary problems, or may cause severe stomach pains or anemia. Severe blood loss may create other problems such as heart failure.

In general, worms may be associated with overall fatigue, flu-like symptoms, and vitamin and mineral deficiencies. Often there are intestinal symptoms, digestive symptoms such as gas and burping, fatigue, joint pains, lowered resistance, and even mood changes and depression.

INCIDENCE: Universal

CONSIDER: Low digestive enzymes, food allergies, nutrient deficiencies, fungal infections, or severe stress reactions.

SPECIAL NOTES: Prevention measures include proper hygiene proper elimination of waste. Avoid walking barefoot on soil that may be contaminated and avoid eating improperly cooked meat.

Worms may actually come out of the anus at night, when in bed, due to the warmth. Thus, children especially may be checked while sleeping. Worms are very contagious. Check all members of household if one has been diagnosed. Be very careful with personal hygiene. Keep toilet seats cleaned after every use for several days at beginning of treatment.

For severe infections, use bowel-cleansing programs with high colonics or home enemas for the first few weeks.

Alternative Treatments

Refer to alternative therapy chapters for more information before evaluating or applying any treatment. Some conditions, including yours, may require a physician's care.

DIET: Fasting under a doctor's supervision can be helpful. (Adults, on fresh juice or a mono diet of one fruit or brown rice and vegetables for four days; children for only one day). While fasting or just eating a whole foods diet, do the following for the first four days: four times daily, chew small amounts of a mixture of pumpkin seeds, papaya seeds, papaya pulp, unsweetened yogurt, one tablespoon wormwood tea, one tablespoon chaparral tea, and one tablespoon peppermint tea. Take with filtered water and two garlic capsules. On the fifth day, mix four cups of a mixture of senna and peppermint teas, plus two tablespoons castor oil, and drink all at once, with eight garlic capsules and six charcoal capsules taken all together. Continue to consume a small amount of the original mixture one time daily for two weeks. Do not be scared if you see and remove the worms from your anus.

Other alternatives: Fig juice may kill roundworms. Before meals, try pepsin and glycerine in hot water. Upon arising and at bedtime, try one clove of peeled garlic followed by a glass of hot tea with lemon, no sweetener. Children with pinworms may try a heavily salted diet for one to two weeks. Tapeworms may respond to fasting on raw pineapple for three days (bromelain in pineapple kills the worms).

NUTRITIONAL THERAPY: • Garlic capsules •Vitamin C • Zinc •Vitamin A • Beta carotene • Deglycyrrihizinated licorice (two to three times daily on an empty stomach) • Aloe vera juice or gel (two times daily on an empty stomach) • Acidophilus

Self–Care

The following therapies can be undertaken at home under appropriate professional supervision.

Fasting

AROMATHERAPY: • Bergamot, chamomile, camphor, lavender, peppermint, melissa • For ringworm, tea tree, thyme

AYURVEDA: • *Neem* may be effective in eliminating ringworm and parasites. • *Pippali* or Indian long pepper *(Piper longum)* is often used for worms. • As a broad spectrum antibiotic, use an herbal mixture of *vidanga* (300 mg), *trikatu* (300 mg), *chitrak* (200 mg), and *kutki* (200 mg), generally taken twice a day after lunch and dinner. *Triphala* ½ teaspoon with warm water 30 minutes before sleep at night.

FLOWER ESSENCES: Rescue Remedy® for accompanying stress; Crab Apple. Olive; for exhaustion.

HERBS: Make an infusion of fresh pumpkin seeds, one ounce of crushed seeds to a pint of boiling water. Drink a cup three times a day, six days a week, for three weeks. Eat one ounce of pumpkin seeds a day as well. Other herbs are specific for certain worms, but can be toxic (see a qualified practitioner).

Professional Care

The following therapies should only be provided by a qualified health professional.

Acupuncture / Magnetic Field Therapy / Naturopathic Medicine

DETOXIFICATION THERAPY: May be indicated, depending on the condition of the person.

OXYGEN THERAPY: Hyperbaric oxygen therapy.

WOUNDS

Any interruption of the skin or underlying tissue caused by damage. There are many types of wounds: superficial paper cuts, surgical wounds, pressure sores, diabetic ulcers, or effects of trauma. Any type of injury to the skin poses a threat due to the risk for infection or further damage if the wound becomes complicated.

SYMPTOMS: For wounds, ulcers, and burns, there are differences in both symptoms and healing. Acute wounds (caused by trauma or surgery) can be as simple as a laceration requiring limited local care, or as complicated as a wound requiring surgical closure or even greater care. Chronic wounds (such as arterial, venous, or diabetic ulcers) may involve greater time for complete healing. Due to the lack of blood supply and loss of tissue in these chronic wounds, the symptom of pain will have to be addressed. Burns (superficial, partial thickness, and full thickness) require even greater attention to pain control as well as rates of secondary infection, and pose a heightened importance to healing for cosmetic purposes.

SPECIAL NOTES: There are many different types of wound therapies; however, the best therapy is prevention. Adequate nutrition and appropriate prosthetics aid the body in maintaining a healthy and normal skin and tissue environment. Systemic illnesses such as diabetes, cancer, kidney failure, or leukemia require careful evaluation and control to maintain skin integrity.

When prevention fails, it is important to remember to apply evidence-based standards in healing regimens whenever possible. Alternative therapies promote safe and effective means to heal wounds and maintain healthy bodies.

Alternative Treatments

Refer to alternative therapy chapters for more information before evaluating or applying any treatment. Some conditions, including yours, may require a physician's care.

DIET: Diet and nutrition are paramount in maintaining healthy skin and healing skin that has been wounded or injured. A diet rich in vitamin A and zinc enhances wound healing. Foods high in these nutrients include green and yellow vegetables, raw seeds and nuts, eggs, and cold-water fish. Vitamin C is also excellent for wound healing and may be found in fresh fruits and vegetables. Avoiding excess saturated and processed fats, as well as refined sugars, caffeine, tobacco, and alcohol, is a critical adjunctive measure to effective wound healing.

NUTRITIONAL THERAPY: Nutritional goals to enhance skin integrity and wound healing involve quantity and quality of food, as well as appropriate nutrients to achieve overall wellness. Individuals at risk for skin breakdown or suffering from tissue damage should maintain a well-balanced diet that includes foods from the four basic food groups. • Vitamin A (50,000 IU daily for several weeks) aids in collagen synthesis and epithelialization • Zinc (30-60 mg) aids in cell proliferation, acts as a co-factor for enzymes, and enhances utilization of vitamin A • Pantothenic acid (B5; 500 mg twice daily) acts as a coenzyme • Vitamin C acts as an antioxidant and sustains cell membrane integrity • Vitamin B complex stimulates cell repair and nerve regeneration • Noni fruit *(Morinda citrifolia)* improves immune function, stimulates cell regeneration, and fights pain and inflammation.

Self-Care

The following therapies can be undertaken at home under appropriate professional supervision.

AROMATHERAPY: Lavender, myrrh, bergamot, chamomile, tea tree, eucalyptus, juniper, and rosemar.

AYURVEDA: • *Ashwagandha* is an excellent rejuvenating herb that enhances complexion and immunity. • Aloe vera gel exerts anti-inflammatory activity and works well on minor cuts and abrasions.

HERBS: • Calendula: a 5% calendula ointment combination with allantoin has been shown to speed wound healing and has anti-inflammatory and antimicrobial properties. • Echinacea ointment • Goldenseal (in salve form) may increase the rate of healing. • Distilled witch hazel promotes healing.

JUICE THERAPY: • Beet: the greens are rich in beta carotene, vitamins C and E, and magnesium; the root is rich in potassium, folic acid, and the antioxidant glutathione. • Carrot: excellent source of beta carotene, potassium, trace minerals, and antioxidants. • Celery: rich in potassium, sodium, and antioxidants.

HOMEOPATHY: *Calendula, Hypericum, Ledum*

TOPICAL TREATMENT: Unprocessed honey may help to disinfect wounds, sores, and actively promote wound healing.

Professional Care

The following therapies should only be provided by a qualified health professional.

Magnetic Field Therapy / Neural Therapy / Naturopathic Medicine

OXYGEN THERAPY: Hyperbaric oxygen therapy creates a supersaturated oxygenated environment to promote healing.

ENERGY MEDICINE: Studies indicate that wounds treated with positive electrical stimulation heal faster than wounds not treated in this manner. Negative pressure wound therapy has been utilized to accelerate healing for both chronic and acute wounds.

LIGHT THERAPY: Photon energy improves nutrition in injured tissues and also accelerates the proliferation of cells to aid in the production of new tissue.

TRADITIONAL CHINESE MEDICINE: Pseudo-ginseng *(yun nan pai yao)* externally.

Appendices

APPENDIX A

LIFE-SAVING TESTS YOUR DOCTOR MAY NOT KNOW ABOUT

TO DEVELOP an effective and personalized health maintenance program, it is important to gather data on your present health status. Laboratory testing is a part of medicine familiar to us all. Most of us have had fingers pricked for blood samples or been asked to provide a urine sample for analysis. These traditional tests are often useful but, from the vantage point of alternative medicine, are limited in scope. They may be able to provide basic information on your cholesterol levels or determine if your white blood cell count is abnormally high or indicate whether an organ, such as a kidney or liver, is diseased, but they are of limited value since organs and glands have a reserve capacity that masks dysfunction. In other words, abnormal function begins long before conventional medicine reveals the problem. Conventional tests are not sensitive enough to signal impending problems. The tests listed here make it possible to assess the health status of your immune, endocrine, and cardiovascular systems, so that imbalances are detected earlier, before a disease fully manifests.

The complete blood count, biological terrain assessment, electrodermal screening, and darkfield analysis can help you get a picture of your overall health status. Digestive function can be assessed using a stool or urine analysis (these tests are also valuable for getting information on general health). Specific tests are available to assess how well individual body systems are working, including the immune system, the endocrine glands, and the brain. Other tests look for possible nutritional deficiencies or excesses of toxins and stress in the body.

Complete Blood Count as a Guide to Therapy

General blood chemistry offers an overall snapshot of a person's health status. But the limitation of the test is the one-dimensional aspect of blood chemistry reporting. Traditionally, blood tests report on just a handful of the thousands of substances found in the blood, focusing on those that identify disease once it's full-blown. As a result, blood chemistry analysis in its present form is an untapped reservoir of highly detailed information. A new method has now been developed for making practical use of information revealed by the standard blood test. Carbon Based Corporation's Blood Test Report offers practitioners and clients a user-friendly formulation of the information, opening a therapeutic window to one's unique biochemistry.

The test's Basic Status Report alphabetically lists the amounts detected of about 44 substances normally found in the blood. It also ranks these items, such as cholesterol, lymphocytes, sodium, and bilirubin, according to their relative deviation from the mean or average value. This ranking demonstrates by what percentage a person's readings are higher or lower than a statistical norm. The idea is to provide a statistical context for the test results.

The test's Panel Report groups the results according to 14 key biochemical functions, including electrolytes, enzymes, pH, fatty acids, and proteins. Data in the report that are irregular may thus indicate possible problem areas. In the Disease Indicators Report, over 140 diseases are tested for as an early warning indicator. Here, known disease patterns are correlated with the individual's results. The CBC Blood Test Report can depict a person's potential disease patterns; that is, whether abnormalities in their blood indicate a predisposition toward a certain disease.

The Drug Interactions Report identifies potential aggravating effects if the patient were to use any of hundreds of conventional drugs. Finally, the Biochemical Pharmacology Report suggests which supplements are indicated for the abnormal blood chemistry.

Biological Terrain Assessment (BTA)

French biologist Louis Claude Vincent, Ph.D., discovered that the key to healing was not the use of powerful drugs, but rather knowing the patient's biochemistry and the optimal conditions or "terrain" for body function. In 1958, Dr. Vincent was hired by the French government to determine why people living in certain regions of France had high cancer rates. This assignment led him to examine the relationship between the external environment—molded by a person's emotional and physical stress exposure, dietary choices, and other lifestyle habits—and the internal environment of the body. Dr. Vincent concluded that the components of the blood, urine, and saliva afford insight into the way the body functions. By monitoring biochemical changes in these fluids and by making appropriate changes in diet, lifestyle, and medical treatment, health can be reestablished and disease processes retarded or possibly reversed.

Biological terrain is a phrase used to describe the conditions, general health, and activity level of cells. This includes the status of microorganisms at the cellular level: some are beneficial to life and health, others are not. Each type of bacterium, fungus, or virus thrives in a precise biochemical medium. Viruses require a fairly alkaline environment to function, whereas fungi favor a more acidic environment; bacteria can thrive under various conditions, but their growth is best stimulated in high-sugar conditions. An excess of toxins in one's diet and environment tends to increase the production of acid within cells, forcing the body to compensate by producing a strong alkaline chemical reaction in the blood, which, in turn, tends to favor the growth of fungi.

The BTA tests for pH (acid/alkaline balance), resistivity (mineral "competency" or amounts), and redox (oxidation-reduction) values. The results help doctors determine the factors causing malabsorption and maldigestion, including bacterial overgrowth, parasitic infection, and enzymatic depletion. The test analyzes biochemical factors in the blood, saliva, and urine. The reason for using all three bodily fluids is because urine is a good indicator of the body's secretory ability and toxic load on cells; blood is a good indicator of toxicity and oxygen balance; and saliva offers insight into a person's digestive capacities.

 See Detoxification Therapy, Enzyme Therapy.

Electrodermal Screening

Electrodermal screening (EDS) is a quick method to identify most underlying conditions, especially ones involving toxic or allergic substances. A blunt, noninvasive electric probe is placed at specific points on the hands, face, or feet, corresponding to acupuncture points at the beginning or end of energy meridians. Minute electrical discharges from these points serve as informa-

tion signals about the condition of the body's organs and systems, useful for the physician in evaluation and developing a treatment plan.

The waiting period of laboratory analysis is avoided by the immediate feedback of computerized testing of the body's organs and systems via acupuncture points. As a cross-reference, specific blood, urine, and stool analyses can then be ordered to serve as confirmation of electrodermal results. By quickly pinpointing problems, EDS can save unnecessary, guesswork testing. For example, if EDS indicates that a person has a specific type of parasite, running a stool analysis for that parasite eliminates the trial-and-error testing to see if parasites, in general, are a problem. EDS can also be helpful in determining the body's tolerance to medications or remedies that may be prescribed.

The key idea with EDS is that it is a "data acquisition process" in which the trained practitioner conducts an "interview" with the patient's organs and tissues, gathering information about the basic functional status of those systems and their energy pathways. As such, EDS is an investigational, not diagnostic, device because it requires the physician's knowledge of acupuncture, physiology, and therapeutic substances to interpret the energy imbalances, establish their precise focus, and select the most appropriate therapeutic response.

 See Energy Medicine.

Darkfield Microscopy: Looking at Live Blood Cells

Darkfield microscopy is a way of studying living whole blood cells under a specially adapted microscope that projects the dynamic image onto a video screen. In this way, the skilled practitioner can detect early stages of illness in the form of known disease-producing microorganisms. Also, the amount of time the blood cell stays viable indicates the overall health of the individual. Darkfield microscopy provides fundamental information on what is happening in the blood. For example, the health of a white blood cell can be determined by whether the cell wall is smooth or ragged or leaking cytoplasm. It can also tell if a cell has been damaged by free radicals.

Darkfield microscopy is a useful early detection tool that also allows patients to monitor the effectiveness of a particular therapy. Darkfield microscopy has been used to detect:

• Vitamin and mineral deficiencies
• Toxicity

- Degree of oxygenation
- Liver function
- Abnormal blood clotting
- Arteriosclerosis
- Allergic reactions
- Immune system function

Digestive Function Tests

The health of the digestive system is of paramount importance. Imbalances in the digestive system have far-reaching effects on the body and contribute to the development of serious illness. Chronic gastrointestinal problems (irritable bowel syndrome, gas, bloating, diarrhea, or indigestion) frequently lead to intestinal permeability, or leaky gut syndrome, in which the intestinal mucosa (lining) breaks down. This allows undigested food matter and other toxins access to the bloodstream. Once in the bloodstream, toxins initiate a cascade effect that can ultimately weaken the immune system and put stress on the liver.

 See Gastrointestinal Disorders.

Comprehensive Digestive Stool Analysis

The Great Smokies Diagnostic Laboratory in Asheville, North Carolina, offers the Comprehensive Digestive Stool Analysis, which consists of 18 tests. The test reviews the patient's overall gastrointestinal health by investigating the following areas:

Colon Environment—In the large intestine reside bacteria that help in digestion and the health of the colon. A delicate balance exists between the many colonies of "friendly" bacteria (probiotics). Specifically, these flora include *Lactobacillus acidophilus* and *Bifidobacteria bifidum*, bacteria that are involved in vitamin synthesis, the detoxification of pro-carcinogens (substances that become carcinogenic or cancer-causing), and they support the immune system. To give a better picture of the overall colonic environment, the stool analysis measures several indicators of dysbiosis, including pH, short-chain fatty acids, and the enzyme beta-glucuronidase.

Mycology—The intestinal tract normally contains small amounts of *Candida albicans*, a yeast-like fungus, and other species of yeast. In some cases, wide use of antibiotics, birth control pills, and a high carbohydrate diet may cause an overgrowth of *Candida*, causing a condition known as candidiasis.

Digestive Abnormalities—Maldigestion, or incomplete digestion, is a common problem for many Americans, especially people over 60. As people grow older or

succumb to an overgrowth of pathogenic bacteria, the production of HCl (hydrochloric acid) decreases, altering the stomach's pH and the release of digestive enzymes. Digestive acids are an important trigger for digestion of carbohydrates, fats, and proteins. Without this trigger, these nutrients pass through the gastrointestinal tract undigested. The stool analysis measures the presence of several markers to determine how well fats, carbohydrates, proteins, and other nutrients are being digested and absorbed.

Integrity of Immune System—The largest part of the immune system is located just outside of the intestinal wall. Known as the secretory IgA, this part of the immune system acts as sentry against escaping food particles or other inappropriate substances. A stool analysis can determine the levels at which the secretory IgA is functioning.

Urine Analysis

Many alternative health-care professionals rely on low-cost urine analysis (or urinalysis) to assess their patients' digestive function and enzyme status. The urinalysis provides information on what a person cannot digest, absorb, or assimilate, along with any nutritional problems one might have. A urinalysis can also reveal the degrees of kidney function, bowel toxicity, and pH (acid/alkaline balance), and show how the body is handling proteins, fats, carbohydrates, vitamin C, and other essential nutrients. An individual's total urine output over a 24-hour period must be collected, not just periodic samples. This enables a physician to see how the concentrations of various substances in the urine change over time. The fluctuations are then averaged to give a complete picture of digestive problems.

Gastric Analysis

Many people are deficient in digestive factors (hydrochloric acid and pancreatic enzymes) needed to adequately break down food so that cells can absorb important nutrients. When digestion is incomplete or inadequate, food molecules can be inappropriately absorbed into the bloodstream, contributing to the onset of many diseases. Inside the stomach, a very low pH (acid level) is needed to break down food. To maintain the optimal pH (around 2, which is very acidic), the stomach secretes hydrochloric acid (HCl). With age and in some health conditions, HCl levels tend to decline, leading to impaired digestion.

In order to determine HCl levels, physicians use the Heidelberg Gastric Analysis. After a 12-hour fast, the patient swallows a Heidelberg capsule, a device about the size of a vitamin that has a pH meter and radio transmitter inside. Once the capsule is swallowed, the patient drinks a solution of bicarbonate of soda, which stimulates the stomach to secrete hydrochloric acid. The capsule measures and transmits the changing pH levels to a receiver placed over the patient's stomach, indicating whether or not they are producing adequate HCl. The capsule can easily pass through the gastrointestinal tract for excretion.

Another, less expensive gastric test is called the string test, in which a capsule is supplied with a string inside it. Patients come in exactly 25 minutes after finishing a fairly large protein meal. They swallow the capsule while holding on to the end of the string. The capsule goes down into the stomach and dissolves, leaving the end of the string in the stomach contents. After 10 minutes the string is pulled out, and the end that was in the stomach is painted with a chemical that changes color in acid. A color guide shows the pH of the stomach contents.

Intestinal Permeability Test

The Intestinal Impermeability Test, or lactulose and mannitol test, requires a person to fast overnight and then drink a solution containing the sugars mannitol and lactulose, both of which are naturally found in fruits and other foods. Urine is collected over the next several hours and brought to the laboratory for analysis. Ordinarily, mannitol is easily absorbed; therefore a good bit should be present in the urine. Lactulose, on the other hand, is not easily absorbed and should pass out of the body with a bowel movement rather than through the urine. An indicator of a leaky gut is if the lactulose has managed to become absorbed and both sugars are found in the urine. On the other hand, if neither sugar is found in the urine in their expected ratios, digestive malabsorption may be an issue.

Tests to Assess Nutritional Deficiencies

Are you presently getting all the vitamins, minerals, amino acids, enzymes, and antioxidants your body needs to stay healthy? Thorough testing can detect deficiencies and help you implement a program of supplementation. Among the laboratory tests for nutrient status, those discussed below are relatively inexpensive and provide detailed, practical information on the status of enzymes, vitamins, minerals, and other essential nutrients.

Pantox Antioxidant Profile: Using a small blood sample, this diagnostic screen measures the status of more than 20 nutritional factors as a way of determining the body's antioxidant defense system. Specifically, the screen reports on lipoproteins (cholesterol, triglycerides), fat-soluble antioxidants (vitamins A, E, carotenoids, coenzyme Q10), water-soluble antioxidants (vitamin C, uric acid, bilirubin), and iron balance. It then compares the results against a database of 7,000 healthy profiles to determine if the patient is getting the right antioxidants in the correct amounts.

Functional Intracellular Analysis (FIA): The functional intracellular analysis is a group of tests that measures the cellular function of key vitamins, minerals, antioxidants, amino acids, fatty acids, and metabolites (choline, inositol). Rather than simply measuring these levels of micronutrients in the blood (which may or may not provide useful information about actual cell metabolism), the FIA test measures how these micronutrients are actually functioning within the activities of living white blood cells. More specifically, FIA assesses the amount of cell growth for metabolically active lymphocytes, a type of white blood cell, as a way of identifying micronutrient deficiencies that are known to interfere with growth or immune function in the cell. These tests also assess the status of carbohydrate metabolism in terms of insulin function and fructose intolerance.

Nutricheck USA: The Nutricheck USA test helps to identify specific nutrient imbalances. The patient fills out a questionnaire, which includes 110 questions indicative of various nutritional deficiencies. The results are returned with a bar-graph printout indicating probable nutritional deficiencies. Along with other diagnostic assessments, it is an invaluable tool in putting together an accurate and appropriate nutrition and supplementation protocol for the patient. The questions address physical, psychological, and emotional parameters, which give further insight into the patient.

Cell Membrane Lipid Profile: This blood test screens the patient for adequate levels of essential fatty acids by analyzing red blood cell membranes. The correct formation of cell membranes is dependent upon essential fatty acids. The test measures levels of omega-3 and omega-6 fatty acids that inhibit inflammation as well as toxic pro-inflammatory fatty acids. Correct fatty-acid content in the body is extremely important in arthritis and other inflammatory processes. Dietary supplementation to correct fatty acid imbalances can be accurately monitored through this profile.

Organic Acid Analysis: The levels at which organic acids (intermediate compounds of metabolism) appear in the blood or urine help determine how well energy production, enzyme reactions, and other chemical operations are functioning. Organic acid analysis allows the practitioner to peer into the energy cycles of the cell (also called the Krebs cycle) and pinpoint nutritional deficiencies as well as the presence of toxic chemicals. Low or high levels of a particular organic acid suggest a deficiency in a specific amino acid, vitamin, or mineral needed to "start" its corresponding biochemical reaction. This information can assist doctors in developing therapeutic programs of avoidance and nutritional support.

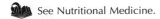 See Nutritional Medicine.

Testing for Stress Levels

The adrenal glands play a central role in maintaining the body's energy levels. When a person is subject to stress, whether physical, psychological, or emotional, the adrenals release the hormones adrenaline, cortisol, and DHEA to prepare the body for flight or fight. Constant stress exhausts the adrenals. When these glands are functioning poorly, the result can be fatigue, a signal that you may need your adrenal hormones tested. Normal antibody production is also dependent upon healthy adrenal glands. The following tests measure specific hormone levels in the blood and provide guidelines for supplementation should you find your measures out of the normal range.

 See Stress.

Aeron LifeCycles Saliva Assay Report

The Aeron LifeCycles saliva assay report, which can be ordered by both patients and physicians, provides graphs of individual hormone levels. Changing levels can be plotted over time on the same graph if supplementation or subsequent testing is done. Although hormones are present in saliva only in fractional amounts compared to the blood, "clinically relevant and highly accurate levels of hormones can be determined in saliva," says John Kells, President of Aeron LifeCycles, in San Leandro, California, a laboratory that offers the saliva-based test for measuring levels of eight different hormones. "Saliva testing provides a means to establish whether or not your hormone levels are within the expected normal range for your age." The saliva assay has several advantages over traditional blood testing for hormones. It is painless and noninvasive, and tests can be performed simply at any time or place. As the test is less expensive than blood testing, you can do frequent testing to monitor changes (brought on by interventions such as diet, exercise, herbs, stress reduction, allergy desensitization, or acupuncture) and to adjust dosages of over-the-counter hormones such as DHEA or melatonin.

Adrenal Stress Index (ASI)

This simple, noninvasive saliva test, can pinpoint whether an imbalance in the adrenal glands might be contributing to your allergies or allergy-related condition. The adrenal glands do not secrete their hormones at a constant level throughout the day; instead, hormones are released in a cycle, with the highest volume in the morning and the lowest at night. This 24-hour cycle, known as circadian rhythm, can influence a variety of body functions, from immune response to quality of sleep. The ASI saliva test evaluates how well your adrenal glands are functioning by tracking the 24-hour cycle. Four saliva samples taken at intervals throughout the day are used to reconstruct the adrenal rhythm in the laboratory and determine if the three main stress hormones, cortisol, adrenaline, and DHEA, are being secreted in proper proportion to each other, and at the right times. Based on the results, a physician can prescribe the appropriate treatment to restore the balance of hormones and correct the circadian rhythm.

DHEA Challenge Test

While many people taking DHEA report improvement in allergies, sleeping patterns, energy level, and ability to cope with stress, some people actually experience the opposite effect. Depending upon a person's genetic makeup, a certain amount of DHEA from a supplement may be converted by the body into the hormones testosterone and estradiol, a type of estrogen. If you are one of those people who are genetically predisposed to convert DHEA, you may experience unwanted side effects with supplementation as a result of increased amounts of testosterone and estradiol. These side effects can include fatigue, insomnia, irritability, acne, oily skin, deepening of the voice, and an increase in body hair. Through a simple saliva sample, the DHEA Challenge Test determines whether, in your particular case, DHEA supplements will improve—or worsen—your health. The test works by measuring levels of the two hormones (testosterone and estradiol) in the saliva both before and after a five- to seven-day treatment with the DHEA hormone (15 mg for women, 25 mg for men). If your testosterone and estradiol levels are too high following the "challenge" to the system, continuing to take DHEA supplements is probably not advisable.

Testing for Toxicity

The average adult carries up to 100 identifiable toxic substances in various tissues. Evidence continues to mount that toxins from the food we eat, air we breathe, and water we drink are compromising our health status. Toxins—substances the body cannot digest, assimilate, and use—place a burden on our body, depleting levels of essential nutrients that are required by the immune system to function optimally. Toxins also divert energy and resources required for repair and maintenance, and upset the delicate balance required to regulate the immune, endocrine, and cardiovascular systems for health and longevity.

Chronic low-level exposure to toxic heavy metals, in particular, can cause or exacerbate allergies and other diseases. One of the most insidious heavy metals is mercury, a common component of "silver" fillings or amalgams. Mercury suppresses the immune system and interferes with enzyme function, thus impairing DNA repair as well as the body's ability to form the hormone insulin.

 See Biological Dentistry, Environmental Medicine.

Testing can identify which metals are present and in what amounts. On the basis of this information, a physician is able to develop an individualized detoxification and nutritional program.

Hair Analysis: Hair trace-mineral analysis allows physicians to measure critical mineral and toxic metal levels in the body's tissues. Hair is a soft tissue of the body; testing the hair is obtaining the equivalent of a soft-tissue biopsy, without any surgery. Although hair is technically dead, the minerals present in the hair cell during its formation are locked within the hair structure. Minerals as well as toxic metals in the hair are in a higher concentration than in the blood, making these elements easier to measure through hair analysis.

Hair analysis is an average reading over a several-month period; it gives a picture over time of the body's metabolic changes. A one-gram sample of hair (hair cannot be dyed, permed, bleached, or treated; pubic hair can be substituted) is cut and sent to the laboratory by the health-care practitioner. The laboratory then burns the hair and the elements are viewed and quantified via atomic spectroscopy. The results are then returned to the practitioner for interpretation. Hair analysis and its diagnostic value were once considered controversial but due to stricter standards within the industry and better handling of samples, accuracy and reliability are now excellent.

ToxMet Screen: The ToxMet screen provides an inexpensive but detailed analysis of the levels of specific heavy metals in a patient's system, based on a urine sample. ToxMet tests for levels of four highly toxic heavy metals, including arsenic, cadmium, lead, and mercury; it also reports on levels for ten potentially toxic elements, such as aluminum, bismuth, boron, nickel, and strontium. Finally, information is gathered on a patient's status regarding 14 essential metals and minerals, such as copper, calcium, chromium, molybdenum, selenium, and vanadium.

EDTA Lead Versonate 24-Hour Urine Collection Test: In this test, a physician intravenously administers EDTA (ethylenediaminetetraacetic acid), a

---

DETOXIFICATION FUNCTION TESTS

Even if your body isn't overwhelmed by heavy metals, your health problems may still be caused by toxic overload if your body's detoxification system (organ processes that eliminate toxins from the body) isn't working properly. Here are two laboratory tests that can help your physician determine how efficiently your body detoxifies itself.

Functional Liver Detoxification Profile—If your liver is unable to adequately detoxify your body's store of toxins and waste products, this situation may contribute significantly to the emergence and continuation of illness. Excess free radicals and by-products of incomplete metabolism resulting from poor detoxification can create problems in the cells. The Detoxification Profile helps to identify places where your system is impaired in its ability to detoxify. It looks at the liver's ability to convert potentially dangerous toxins into harmless substances that can then be eliminated by the body; this conversion process occurs in two major chemical reactions referred to as Phase I and Phase II. During Phase I, the liver converts toxic compounds into intermediate toxins. In Phase II, the liver converts these intermediate toxins into substances that can be eliminated from the body, delivering them to the colon (via the gallbladder) or bladder for excretion. The Detoxification Profile determines the presence of enzymes needed to start the conversion process and the rate at which Phase I and II detoxification are operating.

Oxidative Stress Profile—When your ability to detoxify is impaired and/or you are deficient in antioxidants, free radicals run unchallenged throughout the body, damaging cells. They tend to affect the immune, endocrine, and nervous systems, damaging mitochondria, interrupting communication among cells, and depleting key nutrients and antioxidants. This is called oxidative stress. The Oxidative Stress Profile assesses the degree of free-radical damage in the body and it measures the body's levels of L-glutathione, an amino acid complex central to detoxification.

---

chemical that chelates or binds with heavy metals. EDTA pulls heavy metals out of the patient's system, which are excreted in the urine. The urine is then collected over a 24-hour period and analyzed by a laboratory for proportions of heavy metals.

DMPS Challenge Test: This test is similar to the EDTA test, but it uses the chemical DMPS (2,3-dimercaptopropane-1-sulfonate) intravenously, instead of EDTA. DMPA is orally administered and has been found to be more precise in measuring heavy metal toxicity because it can bind heavy metals lodged in hard-to-access tissues. One of DMPA's strength is its ability to cross the blood-brain barrier. Many substances diffuse poorly from the blood into the brain. Those that do not easily pass into the nervous tissue require the use of a protein carrier to get into the brain to chelate and remove any heavy metals found in the brain tissue.

Candidiasis Test

In addition to causing leaky gut syndrome, an overgrowth of the *Candida albicans* fungus has been shown to confuse the immune regulatory system. The Comprehensive Digestive Stool Analysis can usually detect candidiasis, but there is another test that may assist your physician in pinpointing this imbalance. The *Candida* Antibody Titer Blood Test tests for the body's reaction to the presence of *Candida* as indicated by the levels of antibodies IgA, IgM, and IgG, rather than measuring the level of *Candida* directly. The test is useful, but not totally reliable. If positive, it can indicate past or present *Candida* infection somewhere in the body, but it may not indicate intestinal overgrowth. If negative, it may mean that although *Candida* is present, the body's immune mechanisms did not react appropriately to create the antibodies against *Candida*. This occurs in individuals with a compromised immune system.

 See Candidiasis, Parasitic Infections.

Parasitic Infection Tests

Parasitic infection can be difficult to diagnose. One of the main problems with parasitic infections and their link to systemic illness is that many parasitology laboratories fail to find the majority of intestinal parasites in stool specimens submitted to them. David Casemore, M.D., of the Public Health Laboratories in Bodewuddan, Rhyl, Great Britain, adds that parasitic infection "is almost certainly underdetected, possibly by a factor of ten or more."[1] While the Comprehensive Digestive Stool Analysis can detect biochemical abnormalities indicating parasitic infection, doctors frequently overlook these clues.

According to Martin Lee, Ph.D., Director of Great Smokies Diagnostic Laboratory, in Asheville, North Carolina, many doctors, hospitals, and laboratories fail to diagnose parasitic infection because they rarely allow the time for careful analysis or multiple procedures using stool specimens collected over several days. Dr. Lee suggests that if you suspect an intestinal parasite, or just want to be tested as a preventive measure, make sure your physician, hospital, or lab follows the guidelines set by

the U.S. Centers for Disease Control and Prevention and the *Manual of Clinical Microbiology*. You can also ask your health-care practitioner to try one of these tests:

- Indirect Fluorescent Antibody (IFA): In this type of immunofluorescent testing, technicians tag special immune cells with fluorescent dyes, which make them highly visible under a darkfield microscope. As these cells specifically attack parasites, they will only show up where there is a parasitic presence.

- Electrodermal Screening (EDS): EDS can use a computerized list or vials containing specimens of various parasites to test the meridians of the patient; if parasites are a factor, there will be a corresponding weakened EDS reading.

Immune System Tests

The immune system has responsibility for an enormous number of functions related to body maintenance and tissue repair. Measuring the activity of the immune system is a vital component in determining the level of function and possible disease states and to provide benchmarks for immune enhancement strategies. Certain levels of T and B immune cells (white blood cells) can point to chronic disease. For example, individuals with chronic fatigue syndrome may have increased T-cell activity, abnormal levels and impaired function of natural killer cells (foreign protein destroyers), and the presence of autoantibodies.

Jesse Stoff, M.D., of Tucson, Arizona, relies on standard blood tests to establish the state of a patient's biochemistry and immune function and provide the information needed to design an individualized treatment program targeting the specific deficiencies or areas of weakness. The tests most frequently used are a T and B Cell Panel, natural killer (NK) cell function, and nitrogen balance.

- T and B Cell Panel—This test, Dr. Stoff says, gives information about 25 immune system components and the structural status of an individual's immune system. Some viruses and other infections are also detected by this test. The T and B Cell Panel and the blood test for NK cell function are relatively inexpensive standard laboratory tests that any physician can order. Through these tests, the clinician can see where the hole exists in the person's immune system defense and whether the deficiency is in T, B, or NK cells. Then you can determine which immunomodulators (substances that can regulate, or modulate, the activities of the immune system) will work best to plug the hole.

- Sedimentation Rate—Another common measure of immune system activity is the sedimentation rate (SED rate), a non-specific indicator of inflammation in the body's tissues. Technically speaking, it counts the rate at which red blood cells settle in a given volume of blood within one hour. Good health and a lack of infections are indicated by low numbers. The number rises when there are more proteins than normal in the bloodstream, providing evidence of infection, inflammation, immune disorders, or cancer.

- Stool Analysis—A stool analysis can serve as a "window" into not only digestive inadequacies but also immune system function. For example, fecal secretory IgA is a specialized antibody protein involved in the immune system's defense response to foreign substances. Fecal sIgA serves as the first line of defense against invading pathogens, toxins, and food allergens in the intestines. Low levels mean an increased susceptibility to infection and food allergies. Stool analysis is also useful to generally assess the health status of the intestines and their function, especially regarding intestinal parasites and the population of numerous bacteria, both helpful and pathogenic.

Testing for Allergies

Allergies place a significant burden upon the immune system and should be identified and eliminated. There are numerous tests to identify allergens (allergy-causing substances), including provocative neutralization, Nambudripad's Allergy Elimination Technique, electrodermal screening, the ELISA test, and the elimination diet.

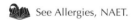 See Allergies, NAET.

Provocative Neutralization (P/N)

This method of testing uses extracts administered sublingually. It can be used to detect food and chemical sensitivities and takes into account a variety of patient responses, not just skin inflammation. In fact, patient complaints such as headaches or spaciness are often reproduced in a matter of minutes after receiving the extract; thus, symptoms can be linked directly to the specific allergen. Conventional allergists do not use this testing method, but alternative physicians find it to be both a highly accurate test for allergy triggers and remarkably effective treatment for symptomatic relief.

P/N is performed by introducing extracts of the suspected allergens either into the skin with an injection or as a drop of liquid under the tongue. The same substance is then given in weaker and weaker dilutions every ten minutes, starting with a 1:5 ratio and decreasing by a multiple of five each time, until a "neutralization" dose is reached. (Neutralization is determined when the symptoms disappear.) If a reaction is to occur, it most likely will do so at the strongest doses. In addition to measuring the size of a wheal's increase, a physician using P/N looks for changes in the patient's appearance, physical and mental function, pulse rate, breathing, and behavior.

Electrodermal Screening (EDS)

In an EDS session, a trained practitioner places a blunt, noninvasive electric probe at acupuncture points on the patients hands or feet, correspond to specific internal functions. The EDS device emits a microcurrent that carries information (the electromagnetic spectrum of the allergen being tested) into the acupuncture point via the probe. If the patient's energy response (conductance) drops or does not reach a normal peak, then that response is interpreted as "positive," indicating a sensitivity or allergy to the allergen.

Few clinical studies have tested the effectiveness of EDS as a tool for identifying allergy triggers. A 1997 double-blind, controlled study used EDS testing with 41 polysymptomatic allergy patients. In the first group of 17 patients, EDS correctly differentiated 82% of the time between house dust mite or histamine (allergens) and saline or water (non-allergens). In the second group of 24 patients, EDS discriminated 96% of the time between allergenic and non-allergenic substances, leading the researchers to state that EDS is a reliable method for detecting allergy triggers.[2]

Although EDS findings are accurate in diagnosis and in identifying food, environmental, and chemical allergy triggers, the physician should order additional blood, urine, or stool tests to confirm the EDS results in all cases.

Nambudripad's Allergy Elimination Technique (NAET)

Developed by Devi S. Nambudripad, D.C., L.Ac., R.N., Ph.D., of Buena Park, California, NAET not only makes it easier to determine the allergens that may be playing a hidden role in disease, but also enables practitioners to reprogram patients' brains and nervous systems so that they no longer react to the substances. NAET practitioners employ kinesiology to detect offending allergens. Patients hold the suspected substance while the practitioner tests the strength of certain muscles. If an allergy to the substance exists, the muscles will exhibit weakness that improves once the patient is no longer in contact with it.

Once the allergens have been determined, the next step is to eliminate the allergic reaction. This is accomplished by having patients again hold the allergenic substance while they are treated with acupuncture. "Because your energy pathways are unblocked while you are holding the substance during the acupuncture treatment, your body stops reacting to it," Dr. Nambudripad says. "This leads your brain to stop viewing it as harmful." Once the treatment is complete, patients are then instructed to avoid exposure to the substance for 25-30 hours, after which time they should no longer experience allergic reactions to it.

ELISA Test

Many alternative medicine practitioners consider the ELISA (enzyme-linked immunoserological assay) to be among the most sensitive and useful blood tests in detecting food allergies. The ELISA requires a small blood sample to be taken from the patient, then sent within 72 hours to any one of several specialized laboratories. At the lab, technicians process the sample to collect the IgG antibodies, which are involved in delayed allergic reactions. A drop of this serum is placed in tiny holding containers or "wells," each containing a single potentially allergenic food or food component, such as gluten from wheat. A computer then analyzes the samples.

The assay specifically looks for evidence of every IgG-mediated food allergy, including antibodies for IgG's subsets (components): IgG1, IgG2, IgG3, and IgG4. Each IgG subset is responsible for attacking specific kinds of invading protein molecules. It's important to note that any allergen, not just food, can prompt a reaction by any IgG subset or IgE. Hence, allergists using the ELISA make sure to test for all types of allergic responses.

Elimination-and-Challenge Diet

There are several variations of this diet developed by Albert H. Rowe, M.D., of Oakland, California, but the main idea in all of them is to abstain for four to seven days from eating foods that may be causing a delayed allergic reaction. It takes an average of four days for the delayed allergic reaction to a food to dissipate. Once the body is cleared of the test foods, and the patient's symptoms have disappeared, they are ready to proceed with the "challenge" phase.

Reintroduce the test foods separately, as single-item meals. If you experience symptoms such as aches, pains, digestive difficulty, fatigue, an inability to think clearly, or increase in any symptom within a few hours (although it may take up to 72 hours), it may be due to allergy. Ideally, one food is tested each day, and only organic foods are consumed to avoid mistaking a reaction to pesticide residue for a reaction to the food itself.[3]

Testing Hormone Levels

As an individual ages, there is a measurable decline in hormones needed for proper cell activity and proteins

vital to tissue repair. Most of the key hormones at play in a man's or woman's body—estrogen, testosterone, DHEA—decline as we age, leaving us more susceptible to reduced physiological functioning and possibly disease. Thyroid function is also critical to a number of metabolic processes in the body. Monitoring hormone levels is vital to maintaining health and preventing illness.

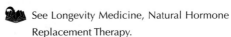 See Longevity Medicine, Natural Hormone Replacement Therapy.

Aeron LifeCycles Saliva Assay Report

There are age-associated optimal levels of progesterone, estradiol, estriol, estrogen, and cortisol. Aeron LifeCycles uses these as a reference point in the saliva assay. These target values can then be used as a dosage guideline for supplementation. The Aeron LifeCycles saliva assay report provides graphs of individual hormone levels. Changing levels can be plotted over time on the same graph if supplementation or subsequent testing is done.

Thyroid Testing

The thyroid gland plays an important role in many cellular activities. When it is not functioning properly, the thyroid can contribute to obesity, low energy, depression, and a constellation of other health and metabolic problems. Sub-optimal thyroid function can contribute to heart disease, due to a reduced ability of the body to process cholesterol. Also, the excess adrenaline produced in hypothyroidism appears to cause chronic degeneration of the aorta (the main arterial trunk). Many patients fall through the cracks of medicine's obliviousness to thyroid function or, if they're fortunate enough to have a thyroid test, they may get "normal" results because most standard tests are not sensitive enough to identify hypothyroidism.

The TRH (thyrotropin-releasing hormone) test is a far more sensitive laboratory measure than routine thyroid blood tests and can show conclusively that a patient is suffering from an underactive thyroid, explains Raphael Kellman, M.D., a New York City physician who specializes in thyroid-related cases and uses the test regularly in his clinical practice. "In patients I've seen with three or more typical symptoms of hypothyroidism, 35% to 40% have tested "normal" in standard tests, while TRH tests show they have an underactive thyroid."

First, through a simple blood test, the physician measures the patient's level of TSH (thyroid-stimulating hormone), then gives an injection of TRH (a harmless synthetic hormone modeled after the TRH secreted by the hypothalamus gland), and finally draws blood 25 minutes later to remeasure the TSH. The TRH injection stimulates the pituitary gland, which produces thyroid-stimulating hormone; if the thyroid is underfunctioning, the pituitary gland will secrete excess TSH upon stimulation. If the second TSH blood test measures are high, the thyroid is underactive.

Testing Brain Function

With age, some individuals experience periods of forgetfulness, difficulty learning new information, or the inability to think clearly. While Alzheimer's disease is a common form of senile dementia, afflicting approximately 10% of those over the age of 65 and almost 50% of those over the age of 85, it is just one of several causes of poor mental function. Impaired blood flow and oxygen to the brain, low glucose levels, low thyroid hormone levels, high stress hormone production, depression, imbalances in brain chemicals such as serotonin and dopamine, parasites, and brain inflammation are other possible causes. Pesticides, fertilizers, heavy metals (such as lead, mercury and aluminum), and other chemicals that find their way into the body can significantly reduce brain functions to levels as low as 50% of original capacity.

 See Alzheimer's Disease and Senile Dementia, Mental Health.

Many nutrients, such as the B vitamins, are critical to proper brain function. Fatty acid deprivation works against optimal brainpower. Docosahexaenoic acid (DHA) is a long-chain fatty acid found in fish, egg yolks, and marine algae, and is the predominant omega-3 fatty acid in brain tissue. As the brain is dependent on dietary fatty acids, reductions in DHA content of the diet may contribute to degenerative changes in the nervous system. The delicate balance of electrolytes also controls the electrical activity within the brain. For this reason, many of the tests previously mentioned relating to nutrition, toxic load, and stress have relevance when attempting to better understand sub-optimal brain function.

According to Eric Braverman, M.D., of the New York University Medical Center, in New York City, the aging brain slows down in terms of its electrical voltage and frequency or speed. The voltage output of the brain is easily measured using a standard electroencephalograph (EEG). This measure provides a good indication of the level of brain function and the relative age and health status of the brain. Also declining with age is the level of alpha functioning. Alpha is the dominant rhythm of the brain and has been associated with creative ability. A healthy 20-year-old might have alpha rhythms of 8-10 beats per second, while a 70-year-old might register at

A SIMPLE THYROID TEST

Broda O. Barnes, M.D., Ph.D., a pioneer in thyroid research and author of *Hypothyroidism: An Unsuspected Illness*, was the first to use resting body temperature, called basal temperature, as an indicator of thyroid function. Based on more than four decades of research, Dr. Barnes found that consistently low basal temperature is a dependable indicator of problems with thyroid function. His simple test, known as the basal temperature test, involves taking underarm temperatures on consecutive mornings.

To take the basal temperature test, place a thermometer under your armpit before getting out of bed in the morning. You can use either a traditional mercury or a digital thermometer. A digital thermometer will record your temperature in a few seconds while a mercury thermometer should be left under your arm for ten minutes. It is important to lie still and relax while recording the temperature. Perform the test and record your temperature for two consecutive days. The temperature for normal thyroid function is 97.8° F to 98.2° F. Dr. Barnes indicates that a reading below 97.8° F strongly suggests hypothyroidism.

7.5 per second. Decreases in alpha functioning indicate a reduced energy state.

Voltage and speed both decline with age. While a 30-year-old may have a processing speed of 330 milliseconds for a required task, a person with Alzheimer's might take 440 milliseconds. According to Dr. Braverman, the most fundamental cause of deteriorating brain function is the loss of dopamine receptors, which most commonly occurs with psychiatric disorders such as anxiety and depression. All forms of mental illness produce slower processing speed times and lower voltage output, a condition Dr. Braverman refers to as "electropause."

Dr. Braverman has developed a testing protocol that makes use of the following measures as a way of assessing brain function:

- Standard psychological tests.
- Neuro-psychological tests, such as IQ, memory, and physical dysfunction.
- Biochemical measures of health status.
- BEAM (Brain Electrical Activity Map) Test—The BEAM test relies upon both EEG and spectral analysis of EEG to determine brain function. This test

identifies subtleties in brain function and brain deterioration that cannot be revealed through traditional tests such as MRI scans. Dr. Braverman challenges an individual's brain function through the use of various images and sounds, and a test that requires an individual to perform a variety of mental tasks. Meanwhile, the voltage output of the brain is measured with the aid of a standard EEG device. It is this measure that Dr. Braverman says provides a good indication of the level of brain function.

- Brain nutrient decline, such as levels of amino acids (specifically trytophan and tyrosine), the B vitamin choline, and phosphatidyl-serine.

- Altered blood flow to the brain.

- Hormone deficiencies, particularly DHEA, calcitonin, estrogen and progesterone, testosterone, growth hormone, and melatonin.

Additional Tests for Identifying Brain-Related Problems

Electroencephalography (EEG) makes use of two electrodes to record the brain's electrical activity in both the right and left hemispheres. Changes in voltage in specific areas of the brain help doctors identify problem areas and assess brain function for the extent of degeneration that may occur with Alzheimer's or other diseases. Strokes also produce a slowed EEG.

Magnetic Resonance Imaging (MRI) employs a large magnetic field that is subjected to a specific radio frequency. The absorption of this radio signal is converted into a visual image. It offers greater detail than a CAT scan in identifying brain lesions and stroke and the general condition of brain tissue. It is a preferred testing procedure, since it doesn't involve surgery or subject a person to radiation.

Positron Emission Photography (PET) produces a multi-colored picture of the brain, which indicates brain activity. This test is used extensively as an assessment tool for possible Alzheimer's disease. A PET scan does expose an individual to radiation—equivalent to an X ray—though not as much as a CAT scan.

Where to Find Help

The following organizations can provide information and answer questions about the various tests mentioned here.

For information about the CBC Blood Test Report, contact:

Carbon Based Corporation
153 Country Club Drive
Incline Village, Nevada 89445
(702) 832-8485

For information about the BTA test, contact:

Biological Technologies International
P.O. Box 560
Payson, Arizona 85547
(520) 474-4181

To find a practitioner skilled in electrodermal screening (EDS), contact:

American Association of Acupuncture and Bio-Energetic Medicine
2512 Manoa Road
Honolulu, Hawaii 96822
(808) 946-2069

For more information about EDS devices and seminars, contact:

Biosource, Inc.
1388 West Center Street
Orem, Utah 84057
(801) 226-1117

Digital Health, Inc.
1770 East Fort Union Blvd., No. 101
Salt Lake City, Utah 84121
(801) 944-4070

Computronix Electro-Medical Systems
145 Canyon Oaks Drive
Argyle, Texas 76226
(817) 241-2768

EDMED
1223 Wilshire Blvd. #321
Santa Monica, California 90403
(310) 394-6497

To order a Comprehensive Digestive Stool Analysis, contact:

Great Smokies Diagnostic Laboratory
63 Zillicoa Street
Asheville, North Carolina 28801
(800) 522-4762 or (704) 253-0621
Website: www.gsdl.com

For information about urine analysis, contact:

21st Century Nutrition
6421 Enterprise Lane
Madison, Wisconsin 53719
(800) 662-2630
Website: www.loomisenzymes.com

For more about the Heidelberg Gastric Analysis, contact:

Heidelberg International, Inc.
933 Beasley Street
Blairsville, Georgia 30512
(706) 745-9698

For more about the string test, contact:

Diagnos-techs
6620 South 192nd Place, #J104
Kent, Washington 98032
(425) 251-0596

For more information about Intestinal Permeability Test, contact:

Great Smokies Diagnostic Laboratory
63 Zillicoa Street
Asheville, North Carolina 28801
(800) 522-4762 or (704) 253-0621
Website: www.gsdl.com

For more information on the Pantox Antioxidant Profile (available only through a licensed health-care practitioner), contact:

Pantox Laboratories
4622 Sante Fe Street
San Diego, California 92109
(888) 726-8698 or (619) 272-3885

For the Functional Intracellular Analysis, contact:

SpectraCell
515 Post Oak Blvd., Suite 830
Houston, Texas 77027
(800) 227-5227 or (713) 621-3101

For more on Nutricheck USA, contact:

Nutricheck USA
11312 200th Street East
Graham, Washington 98338
(800) 771-7926

For the Cell Membrane Lipid Profile, contact:

MetaMetrix Medical Laboratory
5000 Peachtree Blvd., Suite 110
Norcross, Georgia 30071
(800) 221-4640 or (770) 446-5483

For more information about the Aeron LifeCycles Saliva Assay Report, contact:

Aeron LifeCycles
1933 Davis Street, Suite 310
San Leandro, California 94577
(800) 631-7900 or (510) 729-0375

For the DHEA Challenge Test, contact:

Diagnos-techs
6620 South 192nd Place, #J104
Kent, Washington 98032
(425) 251-0596

For more on hair analysis, contact:

Analytical Research Labs, Inc.
8650 North 22nd Avenue, P.O. Box 37964
Phoenix, Arizona 85069
(602) 995-1580

For more on the ToxMet Screen, contact:

MetaMetrix Medical Laboratory
5000 Peachtree Blvd., Suite 110
Norcross, Georgia 30071
(800) 221-4640 or (770) 446-5483

To find a physician in your area who can perform the EDTA Lead Versonate 24-Hour Urine Collection and DMPS Challenge Test, contact:

American College for Advancement in Medicine
23121 Verdugo Drive, Suite 204
Laguna Hills, California 92653
(800) 532-3688 or (714) 583-7666
Website: www.acam.org

For information about the Functional Liver Detoxification and Oxidative Stress Profiles, contact:

Great Smokies Diagnostic Laboratory
63 Zillicoa Street
Asheville, North Carolina 28801
(800) 522-4762 or (704) 253-0621
Website: www.gsdl.com

For more information about Candida Antibody Titer Blood Test, contact:

Great Smokies Diagnostic Laboratory
63 Zillicoa Street
Asheville, North Carolina 28801
(800) 522-4762 or (704) 253-0621
Website: www.gsdl.com

To locate a physician skilled in provocative neutralization, contact:

American Academy of Environmental Medicine
P.O. Box CN1001-8001
New Hope, Pennsylvania 18938
(215) 862-4544

For further information about NAET, and for referrals, contact:
Devi S. Nambudripad Pain Clinic
6714 Beach Blvd.
Buena Park, California 90621
(714) 523-8900
Website: www.naet.com

For ELISA tests, contact:

Immuno Laboratories, Inc.
1620 West Oakland Park Blvd.
Fort Lauderdale, Florida 33311
(800) 231-9197 or (954) 486-4500
Website: www.immunolabs.com

Meridian Valley Laboratory
515 West Harrison Street, Suite 9
Kent, Washington 98042
(253) 859-8700
Website: www.meridianvalleylab.com

MetaMetrix Medical Laboratory
5000 Peachtree Blvd., Suite 110
Norcross, Georgia 30071
(800) 221-4640 or (770) 446-5483

Great Smokies Diagnostic Laboratory
63 Zillicoa Street
Asheville, North Carolina 28801
(800) 522-4762 or (704) 253-0621
Website: www.gsdl.com

For a Complete Thyroid Panel (must be ordered by a physician), contact:

Meridian Valley Laboratory
515 West Harrison Street, Suite 9
Kent, Washington 98042
(253) 859-8700
Website: www.meridianvalleylab.com

The Broda O. Barnes Research Foundation is a nonprofit information and education organization dedicated to improving endocrine function. For more information, contact:

Broda O. Barnes Research Foundation
P.O. Box 98
Trumbull, Connecticut 06611
(203) 261-2101

For more information on assessing brain function, contact:

PATH (Place for Achieving Total Health)
274 Madison Avenue, 4th Floor, Room 402
New York, New York 10016
(212) 213-6155

APPENDIX B

VACCINATIONS

VACCINATION, ONCE a commonly accepted medical practice, has over the past decade become embroiled in controversy. Accumulating evidence indicates there may be many more risks than previously thought regarding once trusted vaccines. At the same time, advances in the fields of preventive medicine, nutrition, and immunology suggest unnatural ways of boosting immunity may be completely unnecessary. The one thing upon which everyone seems to agree is that we should become more informed on both sides of this question.

The U.S. government and most conventional physicians pressure parents to start childhood vaccinations as early as two months of age. The first vaccines given are hepatitis B, DPT (diphtheria, pertussis, tetanus), influenza type B, and polio. In total, an average American child is vaccinated against ten childhood diseases and receives up to 21 shots over the first 15 months of life. During the 1990s, vaccination campaigns to help prevent infectious diseases, administered by governments and the pharmaceutical industry, were stymied by myriad scientific and media claims. The impressive disappearance of once rampant epidemics like polio and smallpox, generally attributed to vaccines, critics argued, pale in comparison to new vaccine induced pandemics.

Parents learned that unvaccinated children pose less of a social threat than vaccinated children, particularly with polio.[1] Physicians learned that the mercury-derivative thimerosal, used in certain vaccines, can cause brain and nerve damage in their patients.[2] Scientists learned that vaccines, commonly prepared in animal cells, often carry animal viruses linked to human diseases.[3] Lawyers learned that class action lawsuits on behalf of victims with

A report by the Centers for Disease Control and Prevention, based on a five-year study during the 1990s, projected more than 800,000 serious vaccine injuries may be overlooked every year in America due to "gross underreporting" of vaccine side effects.

cancer and brain damage can proceed against vaccine makers who suppressed such risks.[4] Politicians learned that skyrocketing rates of autism among America's youth, commonly thought to be caused by genetic aberrations, may be more correctly attributed to vaccine-induced brain injuries.[5] A shocking report issued by the U.S. Centers for Disease Control and Prevention (CDC), based on a five-year study during the early 1990s, projected more than 800,000 serious vaccine injuries may be overlooked every year in America due to "gross underreporting" of vaccine side effects.[6]

"Due to this acknowledged deficiency of injury reporting, the litmus test for the public health practice of vaccination has not been, and cannot be, conducted," states Leonard G. Horowitz, D.M.D., M.A., M.P.H., an expert in public health education. "This is one glaring flaw with vaccination policies. The fundamental tenant upon which the entire field of public health rests has not been met. In medicine, it is pledged to 'above all do no harm.' In public health, however, some harm might be done in an effort to help larger populations, but everyone agrees that benefits should outweigh risks. To determine this, scientific 'risk/benefit' analyses are supposed to be conducted. Unfortunately, due to the acknowledged deficiency of injury reporting, not one study has ever been conducted in this regard. In essence, authorities do not know this basic truth about vaccines—vaccinations may be killing and maiming more people than they are helping and saving."

A disturbing example of this was published in May 2001 in *Medical Hypotheses*. HIV/AIDS researchers learned that the first AIDS cases that occurred during the late 1970s, simultaneously in New York City and central Africa, were most likely triggered by a 1974 experimental hepatitis B vaccine, given to gay men in New York City and central African women. That vaccine had been partially prepared in contaminated chimpanzees shipped from Africa to New York by a major biological weapons contractor.[7]

"Probably 20% of American children, one in five, suffers from 'development disability'," according to Harris Coulter, Ph.D., Founder and Director of the Center for Empirical Medicine, in Washington, D.C. "This is a stupefying figure and we have inflicted it on ourselves. 'Development disabilities' are nearly always generated by encephalitis. And the primary cause of encephalitis in the U.S. and other industrialized countries is the childhood vaccination program. To be specific, a large proportion of the millions of U.S. children and adults suffering from autism, seizures, mental retardation, hyperactivity, dyslexia, and other branches of the hydra-headed entity called 'development disabilities' owe their disorders to one of the vaccines against childhood diseases."[8]

A large proportion of the millions of U.S. children and adults suffering from autism, seizures, mental retardation, hyperactivity, dyslexia, and other branches of the hydra-headed entity called 'development disabilities' owe their disorders to one of the vaccines against childhood diseases.

—HARRIS COULTER, PH.D.

The U.S. government has finally begun to recognize the problems associated with vaccinations. Congress adopted the Vaccine Adverse Effect Reporting System (VAERS) and the National Vaccine Injury Compensation Program (NVICP). The purpose of VAERS, monitored by the Food and Drug Administration and the CDC, is to gather information from physicians regarding adverse reactions to vaccinations. Over 33,000 reactions were reported between 1992 and 1996. Compensation is provided for families with well-founded complaints.[9] The NVICP has paid out over $1.2 billion to parents of children injured or killed by vaccines.

All of the above begs the question, "Are there any safe vaccines?"

Vaccine Ingredients

All vaccines contain active ingredients, stabilizers, and sterilizers. The active ingredients mostly include protein particles, DNA, and RNA from bacteria and viruses. These active agents are grown in a variety of animal and human mediums, including bovine fetal serum, monkey kidney cells, chicken embryos, yeast cell cultures, and human fetal tissues. These growth mediums can become contaminated with extraneous viruses, bacteria, fungi, foreign genetic materials, and undesirable protein particles, any of which may enter the final vaccine formulas. "As a result, vaccine production has been historically plagued by such contaminations and in this way, some health authorities argue, vaccinations have become quite harmful, if not deadly," Dr. Horowitz says. The stabilizers and sterilizers in vaccines include aluminum derivatives, mercury-based products (through the 1990s), antibiotics, and formaldehyde (effectively used to preserve corpses).

"Most of these components challenge the human immune system, leaving people at greater risk of infections," Dr. Horowitz explains. "Vaccine proteins have been implicated in making people more sensitive to environmental allergens, such as dust and pollens, that would typically be ignored by stimulated white blood cells. In fact, one of the leading scientific theories advanced to explain autoimmune diseases, such as rheumatoid arthritis, chronic fatigue immune dysfunction, multiple sclerosis, and Guillain-Barré syndrome, refers to this very process."

When vaccines inject foreign RNA, DNA, and proteins into the bloodstream, these elements, called antigens, attach to various cells and tissues throughout the body. Scientists refer to the ensuing combination of foreign particle and host proteins as "antigenic complexes." White blood cells are then stimulated to seek and destroy more than the foreign agents. Sensitized in this way, people's own immune systems become self-defeating. Nerves, connective tissues, and joints often end up inflamed—under attack by one's own immune system.[10]

Types of Vaccines

Here is an overview of some of the most common vaccines and the risks associated with them.

Polio

Most people have forgotten that during the great polio epidemics of the early 1900s, the natural polio virus produced no serious injuries in over 90% of those infected.[17] There have been no cases of wild polio in the U.S. since the 1970s. Polio vaccines have been largely credited for this, but nutrition and hygiene experts more often credit these factors above vaccinations. Many alternative medical professionals are also concerned that every case of polio since the 1970s was caused by the oral polio vaccine.[18] This risky vaccine was finally terminated in 1999 by U.S. government officials.[19] They favored another one thought to be safer. "Unfortunately, given the deficiency of risk/benefit studies, this is essentially speculation," says Dr. Horowitz. "Time will tell whether this new polio vaccine, called IPOL, results in fewer childhood injuries, including paralytic diseases and meningitis associated with poliomyelitis." This killed polio vaccine has been shown to cause elevated temperatures in up to 38% of those receiving it, sleepiness, fussiness, crying, decreased appetite, vomiting, possibly Guillain-Barré syndrome, and allergic reactions in those allergic to neomycin, polymyxin B, and streptomycin. Precautions were also urged for pregnant women and others.

Reactions to Albert Sabin's live (attenuated) viral vaccine, recommended through the 1990s, included contraction of polio by those who had received the vaccine and by those who came in contact with body fluids and wastes of others who were immunized. The live virus in this vaccine is reportedly shed for up to eight weeks after inoculation. For this reason, remaining stocks of this vaccine are not recommended for use in households where someone has a compromised immune system. Guillain-Barré syndrome has also occurred in many people given this vaccine.[20]

Like every polio vaccine manufactured since the 1950s, IPOL® includes viruses grown on monkey kidney cells, which have historically been contaminated with extraneous viruses. This occurred despite repeated authoritative safety assurances. The monkey kidney cells are grown in a culture supplemented with newborn calf serum, which adds an additional risk of bovine contaminations. After sterilizing and stabilizing the solution, the manufacturer admits calf protein contamination (genetic material included) remains at the level of approximately one part per million.[21] "This is equal to the amount of fluoride officials add to drinking water to produce profound changes in cellular function in teeth," Dr. Horowitz adds. "So that is certainly enough to cause genetic mutations of cells and increased cancer risks within the vaccinated population."

Recently, it was determined that monkey kidney cells in which polio virus was grown were contaminated with the monkey cancer virus SV40 resistant to formaldehyde deactivation, during earlier production periods (1950s and 1960s). Also, monkey retroviruses that function similarly to HIV, the AIDS virus, contaminated these cultures. The SV40 virus has been found in tumor cells of children whose parents were vaccinated against polio using the earlier contaminated vaccines.[22]

Hemophilus Influenzae B (HiB)

This disease typically strikes infants up to 15 months of age and is fatal in 3%-6% of mostly immune-compromised children who contract it. Incidence of this disease today is low. The vaccine is said to help reduce this risk even more and to help prevent meningitis and subacute bacterial endocarditis. The HiB vaccine, however, does not protect children from other forms of meningitis caused by *Pneumococcus* and *Meningococcus* viruses and fungi. It has also been shown to be ineffective in 41% of cases, according to some studies.[23] Moreover, alternative treatments are available for HiB.

HiB vaccine has been known, on occasion, to cause pneumonia and infections of the blood, joints, bone, and soft tissue. It is often combined with the DPT vaccine. This combination has the highest reaction rate of any vaccine available today. Reactions range from localized pain and swelling at the injection site to severe diseases. Some individuals contract HiB from the vaccine. Reactions occurred in up to 30% of patients. When administered in conjunction with DPT, reactions occurred in up to 77.9% of patients. Many reactions were severe, including seizures, kidney failure, Guillain-Barré syndrome, and death.[24] The HiB vaccine contains yeast, thimerosal (a mercury derivative phased out after 2000), and diphtheria toxoid when given alone.[25]

Pertussis (Whooping Cough)

Caused by the bacteria *Bordetella pertussis*, whooping cough is a disease that is rarely fatal, with a 99.8% recovery rate. It is most serious and life-threatening in children under six months of age, but there are many excellent alternative methods of treatment available.[26] The vaccine is most often given in conjunction with diphtheria and tetanus (DPT). This vaccine may cause whooping cough, pneumonia, convulsions, inflammation of the brain, and death associated with pertussis. Additional side effects include fever, pain, swelling, diarrhea, projectile vomiting, excessive sleepiness, high-pitched screaming, inconsolable crying bouts, seizures, convulsions, collapse, shock, breathing problems, brain damage, and sudden infant death syndrome (SIDS).

One in 600 suffered a severe reaction in one study.[27] Another study found one in 875 suffered shock-collapse and convulsions.[28] This group was only tracked for the first 48 hours following vaccination. A more recent study indicates that one in 100 react with convulsions, collapse, or high-pitched screaming and one in three of those cases sustained permanent brain damage.[29] In a study of 103 children who died of SIDS, 70% died within three weeks

DO VACCINES IMPAIR IMMUNE FUNCTION?

A healthy immune system provides the ability to resist or subdue infection, allergy, and degenerative disease. As we mature and age, the immune foundation we develop during our first years of life will remain vitally important. At birth, certain immune defense mechanisms are already in place. Although newborns aren't able to produce all the antibodies and other immune defenses they will need, they are already capable of recognizing more than a million identifying characteristics of foreign substances, or antigens. Infants who are breast-fed receive maternal antibodies and immune cell–stimulating substances from breast milk. For the first few months of life, these maternal antibodies can provide passive immunity against many specific infections.

During the first year of life, babies develop their own antibodies. Other immune defenses also continue to develop as body cells mature and as the child is exposed to numerous bacteria, viruses, and fungi in the environment, which stimulate long-term or even lifelong immune-cell memory. The subsequent resistance to a specific antigen is called natural immunity.

By contrast, artificial immunity—as conferred by vaccination against diseases such as polio and pertussis—is quite different. Vaccinated immunity relies only on antibody response to inoculation with specific antigen strains. The hope is that the immune system will be sufficiently stimulated and produce enough antibodies to create immunity to the vaccine antigen. But there are intrinsic problems with vaccination theory. The immune system is not a one-truck fire station: antibodies aren't the only way to snuff out invading disease agents. There are many immune defense mechanisms (including biological response modifiers such as interferon) and different biochemical messengers (including hormones and neurotransmitters). All are involved in maintaining strong natural immunity.

A larger problem with vaccination, however, is that it appears to have an adverse effect on immune function. In the case of childhood vaccination, it is thought that current vaccines cause serious defects in immune development and function. While the assumption has always been that we can have both vaccinated immunity and a healthy immune system, this is apparently not true. When an immune system, especially a developing one, is bombarded with "inactivated" antigens suspended in solutions of toxic additives, contaminants, and solvents, immune function can become impaired.

Randall Neustaedter, O.M.D., L.Ac., C.C.H., of Redwood City, California, author of *The Vaccine Guide: Making an Informed Choice*, believes that vaccines can disable the immune system. Observing that illnesses tend to begin when babies are 3-4 months old—the point at which maternal antibodies are beginning to wear out, leaving babies susceptible to environmental microbes—Dr. Neustaedter asks, "Why aren't these babies developing their own antibodies in response to the initial viral or bacterial infections? What prevents their immune systems from mounting a vigorous response?"

Dr. Neustaedter thinks that researchers need to spend more time investigating immune system reactions to vaccines. Dr. Neustaedter says that investigations thus far have produced the same conclusion—vaccines can trigger immune suppression.

- A 1996 study in the *New England Journal of Medicine* revealed that tetanus vaccine disables the immune system in HIV patients. Tetanus vaccination produced a drop in T cells, a classic marker of immune deficiency, in 10 of 13 patients, along with a rise in viral replication.[11]

- Dr. Neustaedter notes that the immune-destructive effect of vaccines can persist over a long period of time. In one study, published in the *Journal of Infectious Diseases*, the measles vaccine produced a long-term depressive effect on interferon production. The vaccination of one-year-olds with measles vaccine caused a precipitous drop in their level of alpha-interferon production. This decline persisted one year following vaccination, when the study was terminated.[12]

- A study at the Karolinska Institute and Hospital, in Stockholm, Sweden, found that children who had not received the full spectrum of vaccinations had a lower incidence of allergies than children who had been fully vaccinated.[13]

- Other researchers are saying that vaccines are disabling the body's ability to react normally to disease, thereby creating autoimmune conditions. In 1994, a committee of investigators at the Institutes of Medicine directly associated vaccines with the rising occurrence of autoimmune diseases, such as multiple sclerosis, that attack and destroy the myelin sheath (tubular

DO VACCINES IMPAIR IMMUNE FUNCTION? continued

insulation) of nerves. They said it is "plausible that injection of an inactivated virus, bacterium, or live attenuated virus might induce in the susceptible host an autoimmune response by deregulation of the immune response or by autoimmunity triggered by similarities of proteins in the vaccine to host proteins such as those of myelin."[14]

- A study published in the *New Zealand Medical Journal* in 1996 revealed that an epidemic of diabetes followed a massive campaign to vaccinate children against hepatitis B. The study showed a 60% increase in childhood insulin-dependent diabetes, an autoimmune disease, occurring in the years following the vaccination program.[15]

These are just a few studies amidst the growing proof, according to Dr. Neustaedter, that tampering with the immune system can cause devastating disease.[16]

of the DPT vaccine and 37% of those died within the first week.[30] Government and industry officials minimize such risks. They claim the rate of severe injury is less than or equal to 1%. "Multiply this by more than 20 recommended or mandated, childhood vaccinations and the risks escalate dramatically," Dr. Horowitz points out.

The DaPT vaccine is recommended as a safer option for pertussis. But side effects of the DaPT were tracked for only 72 hours and included tenderness, erythema, induration, fever, drowsiness, fretfulness, vomiting, upper respiratory infection, diarrhea, rash, febrile seizures, persistent or unusual crying, lethargy, anaphylactic shock, convulsions, brain damage, and death.[31] This vaccine is not recommended for children under 15 months old or for those who have not had three injections of DPT. Both forms of the vaccine contained thimerosal (a mercury derivative) until recently. They still contain formaldehyde and aluminum phosphate. Aluminum has been linked to Alzheimer's dementia.[32]

Diphtheria

The diphtheria component of the DPT or DaPT vaccines includes the same side effects and reactions as those listed for pertussis. There have only been about five cases of diphtheria reported annually since 1980. It is rarely fatal and can be successfully treated with antibiotics and bed rest.[33]

Tetanus

The incidence of tetanus is very low, though the death rate may be as high as 20%.[34] Contracting tetanus, caused by *Clostridium tetani* bacteria contaminating soils and excreta, does not provide life-long immunity. But neither does the vaccine. Moreover, there is an antitoxin for people who decline this vaccine. To prevent severe reactions from this vaccine, the tetanus component has been significantly diluted to the point of being clinically ineffective, according to Dr. Isaac Golden, author of *Vaccination? A Review of Risks and Alternatives.*

Side effects of the tetanus vaccine are many and can be severe.[35] Tetanus given in the DPT or DaPT shot includes the same side effects and reactions as those listed for pertussis.

Rubeola (Measles)

Measles has been known to cause pneumonia, encephalitis (inflammation of the brain), and degenerative diseases of the nervous system with convulsions. However, the death rate for measles is very low (3 in 10,000,000).[36] Since 1984, more than 55% of confirmed cases of measles occurred in fully immunized persons.[37]

The measles vaccine is a live viral vaccine and carries the risk that it may actually cause measles, according to Dr. Horowitz. "Another problem with this vaccine is the great risk of pushing the incidence of this disease into the late teens and adulthood. Then it can cause more adverse and long-lasting effects and is more often fatal," he says. Many other adverse reactions to the measles vaccine have been reported in the scientific literature. Parents should check the *Physicians' Desk Reference (PDR)* in local libraries for the full range of reactions.[38]

The measles vaccine is most often given as a part of the MMR (measles, mumps, rubella) vaccine, which may cause many more problems, ranging from flu-like symptoms and dizziness to brain damage.[39] Measles vaccine contains chick embryo cells, neomycin, sorbitol, and hydrolyzed gelatin, as does the MMR vaccine.[40]

Mumps

Though mumps is rarely fatal, it can cause children to develop inflammation of the testicles, joints, kidneys, or thyroid, and hearing impairment. Most of these risks occur when mumps is contracted in adolescence or adulthood.[41] Mumps vaccine risks vary from mild to severe. When it is combined in the MMR vaccine, the adverse reactions seem to be compounded. Mumps vaccine contains live viruses and should not be given to pregnant women.[42]

Rubella (German Measles)

German measles can cause children to develop inflammation of the brain or joints. In infants born to mothers who contracted rubella during pregnancy, there is a risk of birth defects. The greatest risk with rubella is to those who contract it not as a child but later in life. If children contract rubella during childhood, they remain immune for life. Prior to the vaccine, 85% of the U.S. population was immune.[43] Up to 80% of individuals who contract rubella have been immunized against it.[44]

Adverse reactions from the rubella vaccine occur in 5%-10% of teenage girls and 30% of adult women.[45] Problems include contracting rubella from the live virus in the vaccine. As with all other vaccines, the *PDR* provides a long list of side effects, ranging from fever and skin rashes to optic neuritis, encephalitis, and autoimmune diseases such as chronic fatigue syndrome.[46] This poses serious questions regarding the vaccine's safety and efficacy.

Rubella is most often administered in the MMR vaccine, with heightened risks due to the combined challenge to the immune system. In addition, it is cultured on the tissue of an aborted fetus.[47]

Hepatitis B (HepB)

The hepatitis B viral infection can cause chronic inflammation of the liver leading to cirrhosis, liver cancer, and possibly death. According to the CDC, more than 4,500 high-risk persons die annually in the U.S. due to HepB. Individuals at high risk for this infection include the sexually promiscuous, injected drug users, and health-care and emergency personnel exposed to blood or body fluids. The childhood risk of developing HepB is extremely low if parents are not infected. Approximately 98% of infected people develop life-long immunity, never become seriously ill or injured, and never transmit the disease to others.[48]

The HepB vaccine is not effective against hepatitis A, C, D, E, F, or G and, according to the *PDR*, the vaccine has been linked to numerous side effects.[49] Despite this fact, all published clinical trials of HepB vaccine only followed experimental subjects for less than a week post-vaccination. Most of the vaccine side effects occur beyond this brief period.

During the administration of President Bill Clinton, a HepB vaccine "mandate" was issued for all newborns. Nationwide, 12-hour-old infants with immature immune systems were subjected to the first of three HepB injections over six months. The predicted results were devastating. Vaccination critics, including doctors representing the Association of American Physicians and Surgeons (AAPS), tallied that almost 25,000 people had been seriously harmed in 1996 alone. The AAPS noted that there were 440 deaths, 7,726 emergency room visits, and 2,549 hospital stays in 24,772 reported cases. "Stunningly, these numbers reflected approximately 10% of actual injuries due to, as the CDC put it, 'gross underreporting'," Dr, Horowitz says. This means almost a quarter million people—mostly infants, children, and teens—were likely injured annually during the late 1990s due to this one vaccine.[50] Following these reports, government officials were forced to rescind the mandate.

Until recently, the most commonly used HepB vaccines also contained toxic mercury-based thimerosal. The vaccine still contains aluminum hydroxide, yeast protein, and phosphate buffers.[51]

Varicella (Chicken Pox)

Aside from parental inconvenience, chicken pox is a generally benign childhood illness. Rarely does the disease result in pneumonia, secondary skin lesions, or generalized infections. Childhood illness confers life-long immunity. This is not the case for those vaccinated against the disease, however. "Once immunity wears off during adulthood, the disease can have more severe effects," Dr. Horowitz says. "This risk detracts from this vaccine's basic rationale. When chicken pox is contracted during pregnancy, birth defects may result. Chicken pox in adults often manifests as shingles, a chronic and painful condition. Contracting chicken pox later in life may also increase the risk of herpes simplex infections."

Side effects and adverse reactions for the chicken pox vaccine are extensive and may be severe, including contracting chicken pox from the live vaccine (in 27% of cases).[52] Varicella vaccine is cultured on cells from aborted fetuses and guinea pig cell cultures. It contains live virus, monosodium glutamate (MSG), sucrose, phosphate, processed gelatin, neomycin, fetal calf serum, and foreign RNA and DNA.[53]

Hepatitis A

Hepatitis A infections potentially result in prolonged or relapsed hepatitis, but rarely result in chronic liver disease.[54] Hepatitis A usually causes a mild "flu-like" illness, jaundice, severe stomach pains and diarrhea; in rare cases, it may result in death. Infection confers lifelong immunity.[55] The CDC urges good personal hygiene (hand washing) and proper sanitation to prevent Hepatitis A infections.[56] This is because it is spread by contaminated water or food, infected food handlers, unsanitary conditions following natural disasters, ingestion of raw or undercooked shellfish, institutionalized individuals, children not yet toilet trained, blood transfusions, or sharing needles with infected people. Transmission is most likely to occur in developing countries where sanitation is poor

MAKING INFORMED DECISIONS

The National Vaccine Information Center (NVIC), founded by parents of vaccine-injured children, is dedicated to the prevention of vaccine injuries and deaths through public education. This nonprofit organization has a wealth of information on its website and an online registry for reporting adverse vaccine reactions. NVIC co-founder Barbara Loe Fisher has devoted nearly 20 years to educating the public about vaccine risks and lobbying for vaccine safety. She has written extensively, including co-authorship (with Harris Coulter, Ph.D.) of the well-known book *A Shot in the Dark: Why the P in the DPT Vaccination May Be Hazardous to Your Child's Health*. For those trying to make vaccination decisions, says Fisher, begin with this checklist:

- Become familiar with diseases and their vaccines, even while pregnant. The first vaccine is given within 12 hours of birth.

- Interview the baby's doctor ahead of time about your vaccine concerns and be a part of the decision-making process. Give the doctor a detailed family history, including any autoimmune and neurological problems in the family. If these are part of your family history, children could be at greater risk of reacting to vaccines.

- Consider the medical evaluation and history for each child. If it is evident that certain vaccines are contraindicated—such as the pertussis vaccine because of a family history of neurological problems—then you're on a different decision-making path than someone for whom the risks aren't as defined.

- Stay informed of new vaccine developments, including recalls and new formulations. For example, vaccines that are free of mercury-based preservative are now available in single-dose vials.

- Know your state law, including which vaccines are mandated. Every state offers a medical exemption to vaccination. All states except West Virginia and Mississippi offer a religious exemption and 17 states have a philosophical or personal belief exemption.

- If you're going to vaccinate, ask to see the vial, the expiration date, and the lot number.

- Keep in mind that "not all the diseases we vaccinate for are killer diseases for most children," says Fisher. "Ask yourself, is it better to protect children against infectious diseases early in life through temporary immunity from a vaccine or are they better off contracting certain contagious infections and attaining permanent immunity? We have to weigh whether vaccine complications cause more injury and death than the diseases do."

- If a child does have an adverse reaction to a vaccine, report it. (The NVIC will help you to make an official report to the U.S. Food and Drug Administration. Go to the NVIC website. Your privacy will be respected.) Doctors are required by law to report any injury, hospitalization, or death within 30 days of vaccination, but many do not. As a parent, the law allows you to report the reaction.

and the infection rate of children under 5 years old is 90%.

Fatalities from Hepatitis A infections are low—less than 0.6% overall—and 70% of these infections occur in people over 49 years of age. Many of these victims had underlying liver disease.[57] Others at-risk include those people using blood-clotting factor concentrates.[58] As with other vaccines, a spectrum of side effects and adverse reactions have been noted.[59] Aborted fetal tissue is an ingredient in the Havrix® Hep A vaccine, as is formaldehyde, aluminum hydroxide, and 2-phenozyethanol.[60]

Pneumococcal Disease

Pneumococcal disease can result in meningitis, blood infection, pneumonia, or ear infections. Studies indicate that the pneumococcal vaccine may only decrease ear infections by 9%. A 20% reduction in chronic ear infections, and ear tube insertions, among vaccinated individuals was shown in another study. Children have a 7.5 in 5,000 chance of developing this disease if under age 2, and a one in 5,000 chance of developing it if over age 2. Risk factors for developing this disease are immunoglobulin deficiency, nephrotic syndrome, Hodgkin's disease, congenital or acquired immunodeficiency, some upper respiratory infections, spleen dysfunction, and splenectomy or organ transplant. This vaccine (PCV) was originally marketed for immunocompromised children. It is contraindicated for children with thrombocytopenia, coagulation disorders, or sensitivity to diphtheria toxoid.[61]

Possible side effects and complications from the vaccine vary from mild to anaphylaxis and death. Vaccine recipients were followed for three days and almost 10% of the subjects made a visit to the emergency room in the follow-up period. There were eight cases of SIDS among the 17,066 subjects involved in this trial. Children in the control group received another experimental vaccine, so there have been no studies done with children who received no vaccine.[62]

Prevnar vaccine contains aluminum sulfate, protein polysaccharides from seven strains of *Streptococcus pneumoniae* bacteria, diphtheria toxin, and yeast extract. Studies indicate that this vaccine may interfere with the safety and efficacy of other vaccines.[63]

Vaccination Exemptions and Summary

"A grave political concern is that vaccine makers provide economic incentives to myriad public health, medical, and academic organizations and officials to promote a rapidly expanding vaccine industry," Dr. Horowitz warns. "As a result of conflicting interests in pharmaceutical industry–directed science and medical education, the vast majority of physicians, nurses, and school administrators who encourage vaccination, along with political officials, never learn the full scope of vaccination side effects." This may be deadly to society and is the main reason why such conflicting interests have been harshly criticized by leading medical academics and organizations on behalf of the public's trust.[64]

Parents need to research for themselves all sides of the vaccine issue. Only then can a fully informed choice be made regarding this critical health and safety concern. For parents who decide to forego vaccinations for themselves and their children, there are religious and philosophical waivers available in most states. Parents are infrequently told about these exemptions, because schools get a stipend from the federal government (as advanced by pharmaceutical lobbyists) to promote optimal compliance with vaccination recommendations.[65]

The best way to prevent dreaded infectious diseases, particularly in infants and children, is by naturally boosting immunity.[66] From breast-feeding to proper nutrition and a lot of love, children, along with adults, typically thrive and survive biological attacks. This seems to be the growing consensus among alternative medical experts.

Where to Find Help

Much has been written on the benefits of vaccinations. To make a truly informed choice, however, educating yourself about the possible adverse effects of vaccinations may be life-saving for you and your loved ones. The following is a resource list for further investigation of this topic.

National Vaccine Information Center
512 W. Maple Avenue, Suite 206
Vienna, Virginia 22180
(800) 909-7468 or (703) 938-3783
Website: www.909shot.com

The National Vaccine Information Center (NVIC), operated by Dissatisfied Parents Together (DPT), is a national, non-profit, educational organization dedicated to preventing vaccine injuries and deaths through public education. NVIC/DPT represents vaccine consumers and health-care providers, including parents whose children suffered illness or died following vaccination. NVIC/DPT supports the right of vaccine consumers to have access to the safest and most effective vaccines as well as the right to make informed, independent vaccination decisions.

Vaccination Liberation
2101 Pallets Court
Virginia Beach, Virginia 23454
(757) 486-3129

Provides books, resources, and community outreach to help informed decision-making regarding vaccinations.

Vaccination Risk Awareness Network
P.O. Box 169
Winlaw, B.C. V0G 2J0, Canada
(250) 355-2525
Website: www.vran.org

Canada's leading resource concerned with vaccination risks and alternative health-care practices for prevention of infectious diseases.

Vaccine Information and Awareness (VIA)
12799 La Tortola
San Diego, California 92129
(858) 484-3197
Website: www.access1.net/via

An excellent resource for alternative information regarding vaccinations.

Vaccine Policy Institute
251 W. Ridgeway Drive
Dayton, Ohio 45459
(937) 435-4750

Provides legislative support and political education regarding vaccines and their adverse affects on public health.

Tetrahedron Publishing Group

P.O. Box 2033
Sandpoint, Idaho 83864
(888) 508-4787
Website: www.tetrahedron.org

Contact them for vaccine awareness resources, vaccination exemption materials, and information on alternatives for preventing infectious diseases.

Internet Resource

www.vaccinewebsite.com

A comprehensive online resource providing extensive information about the health risks of vaccinations. Also includes links to organizations that can assist parents in making informed choices about vaccinations for their children.

Recommended Reading

Emerging Viruses: AIDS & Ebola—Nature, Accident or Intentional? Leonard Horowitz and W. John Martin. Sandpoint, ID: Tetrahedron Publishing Group, 1998.

Immunization: The Reality Behind the Myth. W. James and R. Mendelsohn. Westport, CT: Bergin & Garvey, 1995.

Safer Medicine: Towards Clinical, Scientific, Evidence Based Medicine. M. Eisenstein. Chicago: CMI Press, 2000.

A Shot in the Dark. Harris Coulter, Ph.D., and Barbara Fisher. Garden City Park, NY: Avery Penguin Putnam, 1991.

The Vaccine Guide: Making an Informed Choice. R. Neustaedter. Berkeley, CA: North Atlantic Books, 1996.

Vaccination and Immunization: Dangers, Delusions, and Alternatives. Leon Chaitow. London: Beekman, 1996.

Vaccines: Are They Really Safe and Effective? N. Miller. Santa Fe, NM: New Atlantean Press, 1996.

APPENDIX C

ANTIBIOTICS

THE DISCOVERY of penicillin in 1928 ushered in one of the greatest changes in modern medical history—the antibiotic era. The miracles brought about by this new drug, and those that followed, thoroughly convinced physicians that infectious diseases might some day be wiped out. Indeed, antibiotics were dubbed "magic bullets" because of their seemingly precise action on the bacterial invaders that contributed to so much disease. But realities of the human condition coupled with the tenacity of the microbes have tempered such enthusiasm. The promise of antibiotics is fading as problems surface on a variety of fronts. Resistant bacteria, immune suppression, yeast colonization, superinfection, overuse and misapplication of antibiotics (including antibiotics ingested through meat and poultry), and the reemergence of diseases such as tuberculosis (once nearly eradicated from industrialized countries) have caused doctors to take a new look at these miracle drugs.

CAUTION If you suspect you have a bacterial infection, ask your doctor to take a culture of saliva, tissues, or fluids from the infected area. If testing confirms that a bacterial infection exists, a sensitivity test, in which samples of different antibiotics are placed in the growing bacteria, can determine which antibiotic will be most effective in treating that specific bacteria. If you do take antibiotics, be sure to supplement with acidophilus during and after the course of treatment.

Problems Associated with the Inappropriate Use of Antibiotics

"While antibiotics are very useful when the body's immune system is overwhelmed, their excessive use causes many problems," states Joseph Pizzorno, N.D., President Emeritus of Bastyr University, in Kenmore, Washington, and author of *Total Wellness*. Dr. Pizzorno

cautions against using antibiotics indiscriminately, adding that they provide little, if any, benefit for conditions such as acne, recurrent bladder infections, nonbacterial sore throats, and chronic cases of bronchitis, ear infections, and sinusitis. "Relying on antibiotics in the treatment of these conditions does not make sense," he says. "The antibiotics rarely provide benefit and these conditions are effectively treated with natural measures."[1] In addition, although they are often prescribed for such conditions, antibiotics are not effective against viruses or inflammatory conditions. The following are the main problems associated with indiscriminate antibiotic use.

Destruction of Friendly Bacteria

The human body is home to trillions of bacteria, many of which are vital for optimum health. It is a delicately balanced ecosystem much like the rain forests of this planet. *Bifidobacteria* in the large intestine and acidophilus in the small intestine and vagina protect against infection by yeast and harmful bacteria. Likewise, "friendly" bacteria found on the skin protect against bacterial, yeast, and fungal infections. Overuse of antibiotics, especially broad-spectrum antibiotics, as well as steroid drugs (such as "the pill") can seriously disrupt the normal ecology of the body and render anyone more susceptible to subsequent bacterial, yeast, viral, and parasitic infection.

Yeast Overgrowth

Yeast overgrowth is a common side effect of antibiotic use. Women who use antibiotics often develop bowel and vaginal yeast infections. Children treated repeatedly with antibiotics for ear infections often develop yeast and fungal infections of the middle ear.[2]

Nutrient Loss

Antibiotics can contribute to nutrient loss. By disrupting the population of beneficial bacteria in the gut, antibiotics can adversely influence the availability of vitamins A, B_1, B_2, B_3, B_6, and B_{12}, and folic acid. Zinc and magnesium can also be lost. When antibiotics cause diarrhea, the loss of these nutrients can be significant.

Immune Suppression

Antibiotics can, in some cases, hinder the immune response. For example, children given amoxicillin for chronic earaches suffer 2-6 times the rate of recurrent middle-ear effusion than children who took a placebo.[3] According to Carol Jessop, M.D., a clinical professor at the University of California at San Francisco, 80% of her patients who suffer from chronic fatigue syndrome had a history of recurrent antibiotic treatment.[4]

Dr. Pizzorno reports that chronic exposure to antibiotics can also cause certain forms of bacteria and fungi to develop into forms capable of functioning without cell walls. "Most antibiotics work by inhibiting the synthesis of bacterial cell walls," he explains. "This is normally quite effective and results in the death of virtually all bacteria. However, some bacteria continue to survive with either no or only partially developed cell walls. Unfortunately, by losing their cell walls, they become essentially invisible to the immune system. That is because the body recognizes an invader by the foreign proteins in its cell wall."[5]

Able to avoid detection by the immune system, cell wall–deficient bacteria are able to spread throughout the body becoming, in effect, "stealth pathogens." According to Dr. Pizzorno, stealth pathogens may be involved in a variety of chronic health problems, including septicemia (blood infection), urinary tract infections, meningitis, heart valve infection, rheumatic fever, Crohn's disease, ulcerative colitis, and blinding inflammation of the eye.[6]

 See Gastrointestinal Disorders, Heart Disease, Vision Disorders, Women's Health.

Development of Food Allergies or Intolerance

Antibiotics can contribute to the development of food intolerance. According to Leo Galland, M.D., "It is no accident that the most allergic generation in history has been raised on antibiotics. Several times a week, I see a new patient whose allergies appeared or became much worse after a course of antibiotics."[7]

 See Allergies, Candidiasis.

Antibiotic-Resistant Bacteria

Bacteria resistant to antibiotics are a rapidly emerging problem with potentially disastrous consequences. In 1941, only 40,000 units per day of penicillin for four days were required to cure pneumococcal pneumonia. Today, a patient could receive 24 million units of penicillin a day and still die of pneumococcal meningitis.[8] Strains of *Streptococcus pneumoniae* that are resistant to penicillin (about 30%) also have decreased susceptibility to broad-spectrum cephalosporin antibiotics.[9]

A similar situation exists with regard to other antibiotics. Let's survey the extent of multiple drug-resistant bacteria:

- Three bacterial species (*E. faecalis, M. tuberculosis,* and *P. aeruginosa*) capable of generating life-threatening illnesses, including tuberculosis, are now resistant to over 100 different antibiotics.[10]

- 90% of *Staphylococcus aureus* strains (which cause blood poisoning, wound infections, and pneumonia) are resistant to penicillin and other similar drugs.[11]

- 40% of *Pneumococcus* strains (which cause pneumonia) are partly or completely resistant to numerous antibiotics in several regions of the U.S. In a recent outbreak of pneumococcal pneumonia in a day-care center, carriers of a penicillin-resistant strain of the bacterium were more likely to have previously received preventive antibiotics for recurrent ear infections.[12]

- In October 2001, the *New England Journal of Medicine* reported that urinary tract infections among women are becoming more difficult to treat because of the increasing prevalence (in one of the groups in the study, 39%) of antibiotic-resistant strains of *E. coli.*[13]

- An increasing number of bacteria (including a strain of *S. aureus,* paradoxically named for its resistance to an older antibiotic) are evolving resistance to vancomycin, considered the potent antibiotic of last resort (or resistance).[14]

- *Haemophilus influenzae* is a bacterium responsible for ear infections, sinusitis, epiglottitis, and meningitis. Recent studies have shown that roughly 32% of the strains of this bacterium are resistant to ampicillin, the drug most commonly used against it.[15]

Overuse and inappropriate use of antibiotics have led to the current crisis. The U.S. Centers for Disease Control and Prevention (CDC) estimates that 33% (50 million out of 150 million) of antibiotic prescriptions given each year in the U.S. are not needed.[16] A study published in the *Journal of the American Medical Association* demonstrated that 21% of all adult antibiotic prescriptions—about 12 million—are useless, given for virally caused colds and respiratory tract infections. Antibiotics only kill bacteria.

Add to this the prolific use of antibiotics in livestock production—traces of which may be ingested by people

NATURAL SUBSTANCES WITH
PROVEN ANTIBACTERIAL PROPERTIES[28]

SUBSTANCE	ACTIVITY	NOTES	DOSAGE
Garlic (freshly cut cloves, garlic capsules with certified allicin content)	Broad-spectrum antibiotic	*Numerous studies show garlic to be at least as potent a bactericide as many of the pharmaceutical antibiotics: 1 mg of allicin has the antibiotic activity of 15 units of penicillin.*	Two or more cloves daily (can mince and drink in flavored tea) or enough capsules to provide 5-10 mg of allicin
Sulfur-bearing antioxidants (alpha-lipoic acid, N-acetyl-cysteine, taurine)	Elevates levels of glutathione, the cell's "master" detoxifier	*Studies have shown that sulfur-bearing antioxidants elevate levels of glutathione. These should be taken with vitamin C (ascorbate powder preferred) and bioflavonoids.*	Follow label directions for maximum dosage
Melatonin	Boosts glutathione levels during sleep	*Melatonin has anti-aging, antioxidant, and immune-stimulating effects.*	5-10 mg taken at bedtime
Phytic acid (IP-6)	Natural iron chelator with strong antibiotic and antioxidant actions	*Many pathogens need iron to grow. Studies have shown that iron removal affects their activity.*	Take 2,000-4,000 mg with pure water (not juice), between meals
Oil of oregano (as a liquid or powder; must come from wild, whole-leaf oregano)	Natural antibiotic	*A study in the* Journal of Food Protection *(July 2001) showed that oregano completely inhibited the growth of 25 germs. Wild oregano, entirely different from the "kitchen" variety, has over 50 antibacterial compounds.*	Follow label directions for maximum dosages
Essential oils: Ravensara (*Ravensara aromatica*); MQV ("Niaouli" or *Melaleuca quinquenervia viridiflora*); Thyme (*Thymus vulgaris*, linalool type)	These oils show powerful antibacterial activity	*Essential oils must be organic and therapeutic grade. Avoid "bargain" products. Test first by putting a drop on the elbow to check for irritation (except for thyme, which can irritate skin).*	Bring water to boil in a pot, turn off heat, add 2-5 drops of oil to the water, cover head and pot with a towel, and breathe deeply for five minutes. Keep your eyes closed; can repeat up to three times daily.

eating meat produced using such methods—and you start to better understand why bacteria are increasingly resistant to drugs. A 2001 study found that in meat samples contaminated with salmonella, 84% of the salmonella strains were resistant to at least one antibiotic and 53% were resistant to at least three antibiotics.[17]

According to Mitchell L. Cohen of the CDC, "Unless currently effective antimicrobial agents can be successfully preserved and the transmission of drug-resistant organisms curtailed, the post–antibiotic era may be rapidly approaching, in which infectious disease wards housing untreatable conditions will again be seen."[18] What is needed is a reduced employment of these often life-saving drugs so that they work when one really needs them. This more selective use of antibiotics will also help stem the explosion of resistant organisms now appearing worldwide.

Enhancing Immune Function

Reducing antibiotic usage is both sensible and recommended by many health experts, including the World Health Organization (WHO), in order to avoid the rise of antibiotic-resistant infectious diseases for which treatment may be nearly impossible.[19] But is there an effective alternative outside the loop of antibiotic use and antibiotic-resistant bacteria? The answer lies in alternative medicine, which works with the body and its complex microbiological ecology to restore homeostasis and immunity. Help the body rebalance its biochemistry—cellular terrain—and the proper balance of friendly and unfriendly bacteria will emerge.

The immune system is a barometer of health and any return to a healthy state should involve immune enhancement. There are many ways to improve immune function so that the need for antibiotics can be reduced. By addressing diet, nutritional status, lifestyle, hygiene, genetic uniqueness, environmental factors, and psychological factors such as mood and stress, one can improve resistance to disease and minimize the chance that invading microbes will gain a foothold.

Diet and Nutrition

In 1991, 104 children with chronic ear infections were tested for allergies to foods: 78% tested positive for one or more foods. After removing the offending foods for eleven weeks, 70 of the 81 children experienced significant improvement.[20] Children with severe measles are susceptible to complications such as pneumonia, ear infections, croup, diarrhea (all commonly treated with antibiotics), and death. When such children were supplemented with vitamin A, the rate of complications was cut in half.[21]

Environment

Exposure to foreign chemicals can also diminish resistance to infection. In one study, 92 pregnant women had their amniotic fluid analyzed for toxic metals. A toxicity risk score was calculated based on the number and amount of metals present. When the children were assessed at age three, those with the highest toxic risk scores were found to have experienced more infections (of the ear, nose, throat, and other areas) and more illness in general than those with low scores.[22] In another study, mercury amalgam fillings were found to trigger the development of bacterial resistance to several common antibiotics.[23]

 See Diet, Environmental Medicine, Mind/Body Medicine, Nutritional Medicine, Orthomolecular Medicine, Stress.

Heredity

Certain genetic conditions predispose a person to infection. There is now evidence that nutrition may play a role in reversing this to some extent. For example, children with Down syndrome are highly susceptible to ear and upper respiratory infection by the bacteria *S. pneumoniae*

and *H. influenzae*. In one study, when children with Down syndrome were given the trace element selenium, the production of antibodies against these bacteria increased and the rates of infectious illness went down.[24]

Lifestyle

Those who lead a sedentary life are often predisposed to respiratory infection. When sedentary women with a history of respiratory infection simply began walking for 45 minutes each day, their rate of respiratory infection dropped dramatically.[25]

Mood, Mind, and Stress

Psychological factors have a significant impact on resistance to disease. Those who write about their deepest feelings or past traumas, or who share them with another person, experience an upsurge in immune function. Those who "confess" regularly in this way suffer fewer infections and make fewer trips to the doctor.[26] A study conducted at Harvard Medical School found that, in people who harbored the strep bacteria in their throats, half of those under high stress actually became sick compared with only 20% of those under low stress.[27]

By addressing these and other primary factors about the way people live, doctors could sharply curtail their reliance upon antibiotics while simultaneously achieving their goal—to build immunity and direct their patients back toward health.

Alternatives to Antibiotics

Practitioners of alternative medicine already possess an arsenal of methods and substances that are helpful in promoting healing from infection.[29]

- Herbal Medicine: There are numerous herbs useful in the care of infections. Some are directly antibacterial or antiviral while others are immune potentiators. Some herbs do both. Examples include goldenseal, licorice, astragalus, garlic, *Panax ginseng*, reishi and shiitake mushrooms, slippery elm, and echinacea. Of these, echinacea and garlic are among the most widely used, extensively researched, and effective of all immune-building plants.

- Essential Oils: Essential plant oils useful during various types of infectious illness include tea tree oil, thyme, savory, eucalyptus, lavender, geranium, and citrus seed extract.

- Homeopathic Medicine: Homeopathy initially gained notice in the U.S. because of its effectiveness against epidemic infectious diseases. Medicines commonly used during infection include *Apis mellefica*,

Arsenicum album, Belladonna, Rhus toxicodendron, Mercurius iod., Hepar sulphuris, Lachesis mutus, and others.

- Vitamins and Minerals: Numerous vitamins and minerals are known to be important in immune function. Among those commonly used to potentiate immune function or promote healing during infection are zinc, selenium, vitamins A, B, C, and E, beta carotene, and coenzyme Q10.

- Probiotics: Supplements such as acidophilus can be used to enhance digestion and reverse many of the negative intestinal effects of prolonged antibiotic therapy. Many doctors also prescribe acidophilus (for the small intestine) and *Bifidobacteria* (for the large intestine) concurrently whenever antibiotics must be prescribed.

 See Aromatherapy, Herbal Medicine, Holistic Self-Care, Homeopathy, Nutritional Medicine.

Recommended Reading

Beyond Antibiotics: Healthier Options for Families. M.A. Schmidt, L.H. Smith, and K.W. Sehnert. Berkeley, CA: North Atlantic Books, 1992.

Nature's Virus Killers. Mark Stengler with Arden Moore. New York: M. Evans, 2000.

Total Wellness. Joseph Pizzorno. Rocklin, CA: Prima Publishing, 1996.

APPENDIX D

KEY TO PROFESSIONAL TITLES

Ac.Phys.	Acupuncture Physician
B.M.	Bachelor of Medicine
B.M.E.D.	Bachelor of Music Education
B.Sc.	Bachelor of Science
B.S.N.	Bachelor of Science in Nursing
C.A.	Certified Acupuncturist
C.C.N.	Certified Clinical Nutritionist
Ch.B.	Bachelor of Surgery
C.Ht.	Certified Hypnotherapist
C.N.	Certified Nutritionist
D.Ac.	Diplomate of Acupuncture
D.C.	Doctor of Chiropractic
D.D.S.	Doctor of Dental Surgery
D.H.A.N.P.	Diplomate of Homeopathic Academy of Naturopathic Physicians
D.Hom.(Med)	Diplomate of Homeopathic Medicine
D.I.B.A.K.	Diplomate of the International Board of Applied Kinesiology
D.I.Hom.	Diplomate of the Institute of Homeopathy
Dipl.Ac.	Diplomate of Acupuncture (NCCA)
Dipl. C.H.	Diplomate of Chinese Herbs
D.M.D.	Doctor of Dental Medicine
D.O.	Doctor of Osteopathy
D.O.M.	Doctor of Oriental Medicine
D.Sc.	Doctor of Science
D.V.M.	Doctor of Veterinary Medicine
F.A.A.E.M.	Fellow of the American Academy of Environmental Medicine
F.A.A.F.P.	Fellow of the American Academy of Family Practice
F.A.A.P.	Fellow of the American Academy of Pediatrics
F.A.A.P.M.	Fellow of the American Academy of Physical Medicine
F.A.C.A.	Fellow of the American College of Allergists
F.Ac.A.	Fellow of the Acupuncture Association (British)
F.A.C.A.I.	Fellow of the American College of Allergy and Immunology
F.A.C.N.	Fellow of the American College of Nutrition
F.A.C.S.	Fellow of the American College of Surgeons
F.A.C.O.G.	Fellow of the American College of Obstetricians and Gynecologists
F.A.G.D.	Fellow of the Academy of General Dentistry
F.A.O.A.S.	Fellow of the American Osteopathic Academy of Sclerotherapy
F.I.A.C.A.	Fellow of the International Academy of Certified Acupuncturists
F.I.A.O.M.T.	Fellow of the International Academy of Oral Medicine and Toxicology
F.I.C.A.N.	Fellow of the International College of Applied Nutrition

F.I.C.C.	Fellow of the International College of Chiropractors
F.I.C.S.	Fellow of the International College of Surgeons
F.N.A.A.O.M.	Fellow of the National Academy of Acupuncture and Oriental Medicine
F.N.T.O.S.	Fellow of the Natural Therapeutic and Osteopathic Society
F.R.C.Psy.	Fellow of the Royal College of Psychiatry
H.M.D.	Homeopathic Medical Doctor
L.Ac.	Licensed Acupuncturist
L.C.S.W.	Licensed Clinical Social Worker
Lic.Ac.	Licensed Acupuncturist
L.M.T.	Licensed Massage Therapist
M.A.	Master of Arts
M.Ac.O.M.	Master of Acupuncture and Oriental Medicine
M.D.	Medical Doctor
M.F.Hom.	Member of the Faculty Homeopathy (British)
M.N.I.M.H.	Member of the National Institutes of Medical Herbalist (British)
M.P.H.	Master of Public Health
M.R.C.G.P.	Member of the Royal College of General Practitioners (British)
M.R.C.P.	Member of the Royal College of Physicians (British)
M.S.	Master of Science
NCCA	National Commission for the Certification of Acupuncturists
N.D.	Doctor of Naturopathy
N.M.D.	Naturopathic Medical Doctor
O.M.D.	Oriental Medical Doctor
O.M.M.	Osteopath Manipulative Medicine
P.H.N.	Public Health Nurse
R.C.O.G.	Royal College of Obstetricians and Gynecologists
R.D.	Registered Dietician
rer. nat.	Rerum Naturalium
R.M.T.	Registered Music Therapist
R.N.	Registered Nurse

ENDNOTES

Part One: Medicine for the 21st Century

UNDERSTANDING ALTERNATIVE MEDICINE

1 D.M. Eisenberg et al. "Unconventional Medicine in the United States: Prevalence, Costs, and Patterns of Use." *New England Journal of Medicine* 328 (January 1993), 246-252.

2 A nationwide telephone survey of 1,000 Americans conducted by the Stanford Center for Research in Disease Prevention at Stanford University in Palo Alto, California. Angus Reid Group, Inc., #610-160 Bloor Street East, Toronto, Ontario, Canada M4W 1B9; (416) 324-2900.

3 Larry Trivieri, Jr. *The American Holistic Medical Association Guide to Holistic Health* (New York: John Wiley & Sons, 2001), viii.

4 R.A. Cooper and S. Stoflet. "Trends in the Education and Practice of Alternative Medicine Clinicians." *Health Affairs* 15:3 (Fall 1996), 226-238.

5 Larry Trivieri, Jr. *The American Holistic Medical Association Guide to Holistic Health* (New York: John Wiley & Sons, 2001), 273.

6 Ibid., 13.

7 Ibid.

8 Ibid., 4-5.

9 Ibid., 4.

10 Ibid., 5-11.

11 P. Bergner and K. Kail. "The U.S. Health Care Costs Crisis: A Crisis of Chronic Disease." American Association of Naturopathic Physicians (September 1992).

12 Ibid.

13 U.S. Centers for Disease Control and Prevention, Public Health Service (1975).

14 Larry Trivieri, Jr. *The American Holistic Medical Association Guide to Holistic Health* (New York: John Wiley & Sons, 2001), vii.

15 W.G. Crook. *Chronic Fatigue Syndrome and the Yeast Connection* (Jackson, TN: Professional Books, 1984, 1992).

16 L. Alvin et al. "Electric and Magnetic Fields: Measurements and Possible Effects on Human Health from Appliances, Powerlines, and Other Common Sources: What We Know, What We Don't Know in 1990." Special Epidemiological Studies Program, California Department of Health Services.

17 L. Sinclair. "Entrepreneurs Tackle Electromagnetic Fields." *Business* (March/April 1993), 34-35.

18 R. Williams. *Biochemical Individuality* (Austin, TX: University of Texas Press, 1980).

HOW THE BODY WORKS

1 Joseph Pizzorno. *Total Wellness* (Rocklin, CA: Prima Publishing, 1996), 39.

2 L. Trivieri. "The Lymphatic System: The Overlooked Key to Vibrant Health—An Interview with Samuel West, D.N., N.D." *The Healthy Edge Letter* 1:2 (April 1998), 5.

3 Ibid., 8.

4 Joseph Pizzorno. *Total Wellness* (Rocklin, CA: Prima Publishing, 1996), 90-100.

5 Robert S. Ivker, Robert A. Anderson, and Larry Trivieri, Jr. *The Complete Self-Care Guide to Holistic Medicine* (New York: Tarcher/Putnam, 1999), 103.

6 Ibid., 104.

7 Ibid., 106-121.

8 A. Kalo-Klein and S.S. Witkin. "*Candida Albicans*: Cellular Immune System Interactions During Different Stages of the Menstrual Cycle." *American Journal of Obstetrics and Gynecology* 161:5 (November 1989), 1132-1136.

9 P. Braus. "Facing Menopause." *American Demographics* 15:3 (March 1993), 44-49.

10 A.H. Follingstad. "Estriol, the Forgotten Estrogen?" *Journal of the American Medical Association* 239:l (January 1978), 29-30.

HOLISTIC SELF-CARE

1 Fereydoon Batmanghelidj, M.D. *Your Body's Many Cries for Water* (Falls Church, VA: Global Health Solutions, 1992).

2 Larry Trivieri, Jr. *The American Holistic Medical Association Guide to Holistic Health* (New York: John Wiley & Sons, 2001), 22-23.

3 L. Alm et al. "Effect of Fermentation on B Vitamin Content of Milk in Sweden." *Journal of Dairy Science* 65 (1982), 353-359.

4 G. Perdigon et al. "Enhancement of Immune Response in Mice Fed with *Streptococcus thermophilus* and *Lactobacillus acidophilus*." *Journal of Dairy Science* 70:5 (1987), 919-926. H. Link-Amster et al. "Modulation of a Specific Humoral Immune Response and Changes in Intestinal Flora Mediated Through Fermented Milk Intake." *FEMS Immunology and Medical Microbiology* 10:1 (1994), 55-63.

5 L. Alm. *Journal of Dairy Science* 64:4 (1981), 509-514.

6 M.F. Bernet et al. "*Lactobacillus acidophilus* LA-1 Binds to Cultured Human Intestinal Cell Lines and Inhibits Attachment and Cell Invasion by Enterovirulent Bacteria." *Gut* 35:4 (1994), 483-489. S.J. Bhatia et al. "*Lactobacillus acidophilus* Inhibits Growth of *Campylobacter pylori in Vitro*." *Journal of Clinical Microbiology* 27:10 (1989), 2328-2330.

7 B. Friend and K. Shahani. "Nutritional and Therapeutic Aspects of *Lactobacilli*." *Journal of Applied Nutrition* 36, 125-153. I. Hamdan. "Acidolin: An Antibiotic Produced by *Lactobacillus acidophilus*." *Journal of Antibiotics* 27:8 (1974), 631-636.

8 G. Reddy. "Antitumour Activity of Yogurt Components." *Journal of Food Protection* 46 (1983), 8-11. T. Mizutani and T. Mitsuoka. "Inhibitory Effect of Some Intestinal Bacteria on Liver Tumorigenesis in Gnotobiotic C3H/He Male Mice." *Cancer Letters* 11:2 (1980), 89-95.

9 K. Shehani. "Role of Dietary *Lactobacilli* in Gastrointestinal Microecology." *American Journal of Clinical Nutrition* 33 (1980), 2248-2257.

10 G. Mott et al. "Lowering of Serum Cholesterol by Intestinal Bacteria in Cholesterol-Fed Piglets." *Lipids* 8:7 (1973), 428-431. M. Fukushima and M. Nakano. "Effects of a Mixture of Organisms, *Lactobacillus acidophilus* or *Streptococcus faecalis* on Cholesterol Metabolism in Rats Fed on a Fat- and Cholesterol-Enriched Diet." *British Journal of Nutrition* 76:6 (1996), 857-867.

11 P.S. Moshchich et al. "Prevention of Dysbacteriosis in the Early Neonatal Period Using a Pure Culture of Acidophilic Bacteria." *Pediatriia* (1989), 25-30.

12 J. Rasic. *Bifidobacteria and Their Role* (Boston: Birkhauser Verlag, 1983).

13 M. Speck. "Interactions Among *Lactobacilli* and Man." *Journal of Dairy Science* 59 (1976), 338-343.

14 L. Chaitow and N. Trenev. *Probiotics* (New York: HarperCollins, 1990).

15 R. Giannella et al. "Gastric Acid Barrier to Ingested Microorganisms in Man: Studies *in Vivo* and *in Vitro*." *Gut* 13:4 (1972), 251-256. D. Hentges et al. "Effect of a High-Beef Diet on the Fecal Bacterial Flora of Humans." *Cancer Research* 37:2 (1977), 568-571.

16 S. Finegold. "Effect of Broad Spectrum Antibiotics on Normal Bowel Flora." *Annals of New York Academy of Sciences* 145, 269-281.

17 J.T. Salonen et al. "Physical Activity and Risk of Myocardial Infarction, Cerebral Stroke, and Death: A Longitudinal Study in Eastern Finland." *American Journal of Epidemiology* 115:4 (1982), 526-537.

18 L. Trivieri. "Understanding Your Body's Healing Systems: An Interview with Joseph Pizzorno, N.D." *The Healthy Edge Letter* 1:5 (December 1998), 8.

19 Larry Trivieri, Jr. *The American Holistic Medical Association Guide to Holistic Health* (New York: John Wiley & Sons, 2001), 27.

20 Ibid.

21 Ibid., 28.

22 Ibid., 34.

23 Ibid.

24 Ibid., 36.

25 Robert S. Ivker, Robert A. Anderson, and Larry Trivieri, Jr. *The Complete Self-Care Guide to Holistic Medicine* (New York: Tarcher/Putnam, 1999), 76.

26 Ibid., 77.

MEDICAL FREEDOM

1 U.S. Department of Health and Human Services, Public Health Service, Publication No. 88-50210 (1988).

2 Barry Siegel. "Faith Lost, A Doctor Turns Bitter." *The Los Angeles Times* 112 (September 12, 1993), A1.

3 U.S. price information collected from pharmacies in Los Angeles, California (June 1993). Price information for Mexico supplied by Farmacia Paris, in Tijuana, Mexico.

4 B. Lynes. *The Healing of Cancer* (Wilmington, MA: Marcus Books, 1992).

5 *Physicians' Desk Reference* (Oradell, NJ: Medical Economics, 1993).

6 J. Whitaker. "Act Now to Protect Your Health." *Health & Healing* (September 1993).

7 M.S. Wilkes, M.D., et al. "Pharmaceutical Advertisements in Leading Medical Journals: Expert's Assessments." *Annals of Internal Medicine* 116 (1992), 912-919.

8 U.S. Food and Drug Administration, Department of Health and Human Services, Public Health Service. *Dietary Supplements Task Force Final Report* (May 1992), 2.

9 H.T. Stelfox et al. "Conflict of Interest in the Debate Over Calcium-Channel Antagonists." *New England Journal of Medicine* 338:2 (January 8, 1998), 101-106.

10 S. Krimsky et al. "Financial Interests of Authors in Scientific Journals: A Pilot Study of 14 Publications." *Science and Engineering Ethics* 2:4 (1996), 395-410.

11 Harris Coulter, Ph.D. *The Controlled Clinical Trial: An Analysis* (Washington, DC: The Center for Empirical Medicine, 1991). Available as a free, downloadable e-book on the Internet: www.empiricaltherapies.com/bookcatalog.html.

12 Ibid.

13 Ibid.

14 Ibid.

15 R. Moss. *Cancer Therapy* (New York: Equinox Press, 1992), 319.

16 J. Kamen. "Hope, Heartbreak and Horror." *Omni* 15:11 (September 1993), insert. A. Liversridge. "Heresy: Three Modern Galileos." *Omni* 15:8 (June 1993), 43.

17 W.G. Rothstein. *American Medical Schools and the Practice of Medicine: A History* (New York: Oxford University Press, 1987), 143-144.

Part Two: Alternative Therapies

ACUPUNCTURE

1 R. Gerber, M.D. *Vibrational Medicine* (Santa Fe, NM: Bear & Company, 1988).

2 P. De Vernejoul et al. "Study of Acupuncture Meridians Using Radioactive Tracers." *Bulletin de L'Academie Nationale de Medicine* (October 22, 1985), 1071-1075.

3 C.D. Lytle. *An Overview of Acupuncture* (Washington, DC: United States Department of Health and Human Services, Health Sciences Branch, Division of Life Sciences, Office of Science and Technology, Center for Devices and Radiological Health, Food and Drug Administration, 1993).

4 Zhu Zong-xiang. "Research Advances in the Electrical Specificity of Meridians and Acupuncture Points." *American Journal of Acupuncture* 9:3 (July-September 1981), 203-215.

5 R.O. Becker, M.D. *Cross Currents: The Promise of Electro-Medicine, The Perils of Electropollution* (Los Angeles: Jeremy P. Tarcher, 1990).

6 R.O. Becker, M.D., and G. Selden. *The Body Electric: Electromagnetism and the Foundation of Life* (New York: William Morrow, 1985), 235.

7 World Health Organization. *Viewpoint on Acupuncture* (Geneva, Switzerland: World Health Organization, 1979).

8 P. Huard and M. Wong. *Chinese Medicine* (New York: World University Library, McGraw-Hill, 1968).

9 D.M. Hau. "Effects of Electroacupuncture on Leukocytes and Plasma Protein in the X-Irradiated Rats." *American Journal of Chinese Medicine* (1980), 354-366.

10 K.B. Chatfield. "The Treatment of Pesticide Poisoning with Traditional Acupuncture." *American Journal of Acupuncture* 13 (1985), 339-345.

11 K.B. Chatfield. "The Scientific Basis of Acupuncture." In: Joseph E. Pizzorno and Michael T. Murray, eds. *The Textbook of Natural Medicine* (Seattle, WA: John Bastyr College Publications, 1988).

12 D. Eisenberg, M.D., and T.L. Wright. *Encounters with Qi: Exploring Chinese Medicine* (New York: Penguin, 1987), 77.

13 G.T. Lewith and D. Machin. "On the Evaluation of the Clinical Effects of Acupuncture." *Pain* 16 (June 1983), 111-127.

14 V.N. Tsibuliak, A.P. Alisov, and V.P. Shatrova. "Acupuncture Analgesia and Analgesic Transcutaneous Electroneurostimulation in the Early Postoperative Period." *Anesthesiology and Reanimatology* 2 (1995), 93-98.

15 L. Lao et al. "Efficacy of Chinese Acupuncture on Postoperative Oral Surgery Pain." *Oral Surgery, Oral Medicine, Oral Pathology* 79:4 (1995), 423-428.

16 *British Medical Journal* 322 (2001), 1574-1578.

17 B. Millman. "Acupuncture: Context and Critique." *Annual Review of Medicine* 28 (1977), 223-236.

18 J. Cheung. "Effect of Electroacupuncture on Chronic Painful Conditions in General Medical Practice—A Four-Years' Study." *American Journal of Chinese Medicine* 13 (1985), 33-38.

19 J. Sodipo. "Therapeutic Acupuncture for Chronic Pain." *Pain* 7 (1979), 359-365.

20 J.S. Han. "Acupuncture Activates Endogenous Systems of Analgesia." National Institutes of Health Consensus Conference on Acupuncture, Program & Abstracts, Bethesda, Maryland (November 3-5, 1997).

21 E. Susman. "Brain Scans Show Acupuncture Dulls Pain." *Excite News* (December 1, 1999).

22 M.L. Bullock, P.D. Culliton, and R.T. Oleander. "Controlled Trial of Acupuncture for Severe Recidivist Alcoholism." *The Lancet* 1:8652 (June 1989), 1435-1439.

23 NADA Newsletter Committee. *National Acupuncture Detoxification Association Newsletter* (December 1, 1992), 1-6.

24 A.H. Wen and S.Y. Cheung. "How Acupuncture Can Help Addicts." *Drugs and Society* 2 (1973), 18-20.

25 Jay Holder, M.D. "New Auricular Therapy Formula to Increase Retention of the Chemically Dependent in Residential Treatment." Research study funded by the State of Florida, Department of Health and Rehabilitative Services (1991).

26 NADA Newsletter Committee. *National Acupuncture Detoxification Association Newsletter* (December 1, 1992), 1-6.

27 D. Eisenberg, M.D., and T.L. Wright. *Encounters with Qi: Exploring Chinese Medicine* (New York: Penguin, 1987), 68-74.

28 P. Huard and M. Wong. *Chinese Medicine* (New York: World University Library, McGraw-Hill, 1968).

29 NADA Newsletter Committee. *National Acupuncture Detoxification Association Newsletter* (December 1, 1992), 1-6.

30 Lombardo N. Emerson et al. "Acupuncture to Treat Anxiety and Depression in Alzheimer's Disease and Vascular Dementia: A Pilot Feasibility and Effectiveness Trial." H. Kao et al. "Acupuncture Enhancement in Clinical Symptoms and Cognitive-Motor Abilities of Alzheimer's Disease Patients." Papers presented at the World Alzheimer's Conference, Washington, D.C. (July 9-18, 2000).

31 N. Sonenklar. "Acupuncture and Attention Deficit Hyperactivity Disorder." National Institutes of Health, Office of Alternative Medicine Research Grant #R21-RR09463 (1993).

32 NADA Newsletter Committee. *National Acupuncture Detoxification Association Newsletter* (December 1, 1992), 1-6.

33 K.D. Phillips and W.D. Skelton. "Effects of Individualized Acupuncture on Sleep Quality in HIV Disease." *J Assoc Nurses AIDS Care* 12:1 (January-February 2001), 27-39.

34 S. Siterman et al. "Does Acupuncture Treatment Affect Sperm Density in Males with Very Low Sperm Count? A Pilot Study." *Andrologia* 32:1 (January 2000), 31-39.

35 J. Shen et al. "Electroacupuncture for Control of Myeloablative Chemotherapy-Induced Emesis: A Randomized Controlled Trial." *Journal of the American Medical Association* 284:21 (December 6, 2000), 2755-2756.

36 Larry Trivieri. *The American Holistic Medical Association Guide to Holistic Health* (New York: John Wiley & Sons, 2001), 355.

37 R.O. Becker, M.D. *Cross Currents: The Promise of Electromedicine, The Perils of Electropollution* (Los Angeles: Jeremy P. Tarcher, 1990).

APPLIED KINESIOLOGY

1 G. Leisman, P. Shambaugh, and A.H. Ferentz. "Somatosensory Evoked Potential Changes During Muscle Testing." *International Journal of Neuroscience* 45:1-2 (March 1989), 143-151.

2 G. Leisman et al. "Electromyographic Effects of Fatigue and Task Replication on the Validity of Estimates of Strong and Weak Muscles in Applied Kinesiology Muscle-Testing Procedures." *Perceptual and Motor Skills* 80 (1995), 963-977.

3 W. Schmitt and G. Leisman. "Correlation of Applied Kinesiology Muscle Testing Findings with Serum Immunoglobin Levels for Food Allergies." *International Journal of Neuroscience* 96:3-4 (1998), 237-244.

AROMATHERAPY

1 H. Wagner and L. Sprinkmeier. "Uber die Pharmakologischen Wirkungen von Melissengeist." *Deutsche Apotheker Zeitung* 113 (1973), 1159.

2 P. Franchomme and D. Penoel. *Aromatherapie Exactement* (Limoges: Roger Jollois, 1990).

3 E.F. Pena. "*Melaeuca alternifolia* Oil: Its Use for Trichomonal Vaginitis and Other Vaginal Infections." *Obstetrics and Gynecology* 19:6 (1962), 793.

4 R.H. Wolbling and R. Milbradt. "Klinik und Therapie des Herpes Simplex." *Therapiewoche* 34 (1984), 1193-1200.

5 Robert B. Tisserand. *The Art of Aromatherapy* (Rochester, VT: Healing Arts Press, 1977).

6 G.H. Dodd. "Receptor Events in Perfumery." In: S. van Toller and G. H. Dodd, eds. *Perfumery: The Psychology and Biology of Fragrance* (London: Chapman and Hall, 1988).

7 J. Steele. "Brain Research and Essential Oils." *Aromatherapy Quarterly* 3 (Spring 1984), 5.

8 T.S. Lorig et al. "The Effects of Low Concentration Odors on EEG Activity and Behavior." *Journal of Psychophysiology* 5 (1991), 69-77.

9 R.B. Tisserand. *The Art of Aromatherapy* (Rochester, VT: Healing Arts Press, 1977).

10 P. Belaiche. *Traite de Phytotherapie et Diaromatherapie Tome I-Liaromatogramme* (Paris: Maloine S.A., 1979).

11 A. Woolfson. "Intensive Aromacare." *International Journal of Aromatherapy* 4:2 (1992), 12-13. Jane Buckle, R.N. "Aromatherapy in Nursing." *Alternative Medicine* 27 (December 1998/January 1999), 36-40.

12 C. Horrigan. "Complementing Cancer Care." *International Journal of Aromatherapy* 3:4 (1991), 15-17.

13 W. Keller and W. Kober. "Moglickeiten der Verwendung Atherischer Âle zur Raundesinfektion I." *Arzneimittelforschung* 5 (1955), 224. W. Keller and W. Kober. "Moglickeiten der Verwendung Atherischer Âle zur Raundesinfektion II." *Arzneimittelforschung* 6 (1955), 768.

14 J.C. Maruzella. "The *In Vitro* Antibacterial Activity of Essential Oils and Oil Combinations." *Journal of the American Pharmaceutical Association: Scientific Edition* 47 (1958), 294. J.C. Maruzella. "Antibacterial Activity of Essential Oil Vapors." *Journal of the American Pharmaceutical Association: Scientific Edition* 49 (1960), 692. J.C. Maruzella. "Effects of Vapors of Aromatic Chemicals on Fungi." *Journal of Pharmaceutical Science* 50 (1961), 655.

15 H. Wagner and L. Sprinkmeier. "Uber die Pharmakologischen Wirkungen von Melissengeist." *Deutsche Apotheker Zeitung* 113 (1973), 1159.

16 R.B. Tisserand. *The Essential Oil Safety Data Manual* (Hove: The Tisserand Aromatherapy Institute, 1988).

17 R. Deininger. "The Spectrum of Activity of Plant Drugs Containing Essential Oils (Especially Their Antibacterial, Antifungal and Antiviral Activity)." In: K. Schnaubelt, ed. Proceedings of the First Wholistic Scientific Aromatherapy Conference, Pacific Institute of Aromatherapy, San Rafael, California (1995), 15-43.

18 Kurt Schnaubelt. *Medical Aromatherapy: Healing with Essential Oils* (Berkeley, CA: Frog Ltd., 1999), 98, 243-244.

19 A. Lembke and R. Deininger. "Wirkung van Bestandteilen Etherischer Ole auf Bakterien, Pilze und Viren." In: *Phytotherapie 1 Phytotherapie Kongress, Koln 1987* (Stuttgart: Hippokratos Verlag, 1988).

20 J. Valnet, M.D. *The Practice of Aromatherapy* (Rochester, VT: Healing Arts Press, 1980).

21 Kurt Schnaubelt. *Advanced Aromatherapy: The Science of Essential Oil Therapy* (Rochester, VT: Healing Arts Press, 1998), 102.

22 F.C. Czygan. "Essential Oils—Aspects of History of Civilization." In: K.H. Kubeczka, ed. *Atherische Âle, Analytik, Physiologie, Zusammensetzung* (Stuttgart: Georg Thieme Verlag, 1982).

23 J. Valnet, M.D. *The Practice of Aromatherapy* (Rochester, VT: Healing Arts Press, 1980).

24 W. Brandt. "Spasmolytische Wirkung Atherischer Ole." *Zeitschrift fur Phytotherapy* 9:2 (1988), 33-39.

25 H. Wagner. "Zum Wirknachweis Antiphlogistisch Wirksamer Arzneidrogen." *Zeitschrift fur Phytotherapie* 8:5 (1987), 135-141. H. Wagner. "Phlanzeninhaltsstoffe mit Wirkung aus das Komplementsystem." *Zeitschrift fur Phytotherapie* 8:5 (1987), 148-149.

26 Kurt Schnaubelt. *Medical Aromatherapy: Healing with Essential Oils* (Berkeley, CA: Frog Ltd, 1999), 93-97.

27 Ibid.

28 Ibid.

29 Ibid., 226-255.

30 G. Buchbauer and M. Hafner. "Aroma Therapy." *Pharmazie in Unserer Zeit* 14:1 (1985), 8-18.

31 J.C. Maruzella. "The *In Vitro* Antibacterial Activity of Essential Oils and Oil Combinations." *Journal of the American Pharmaceutical Association: Scientific Edition* 47 (1958), 294. J.C. Maruzella. "Antibacterial Activity of Essential Oil Vapors." *Journal of the American Pharmaceutical Association: Scientific Edition* 49 (1960), 692. J.C. Maruzella. "Effects of Vapors of Aromatic Chemicals on Fungi." *Journal of Pharmaceutical Science* 50 (1961), 655.

32 D. Gumbel. *Wie Neugeboren Durch Heilkrauter-Essenzen* (Munich: Grafe und Unzer, 1990).

33 Ibid.

34 P. Franchomme and D. Penoel. In: Roger Jollois, ed. *Aromatherapie Exactement* (Limoges, 1990).

35 "Aromatherapy on the Wards: Lavender Beats Benzodiazepines." *International Journal of Aromatherapy* 1:2 (1988), 1.

36 W.D. Rees, B.K. Evans, and J. Rhodes. "Treating Irritable Bowel Syndrome with Peppermint Oil." *British Medical Journal* 2:6194 (October 1979), 835-836.

AYURVEDIC MEDICINE

1 Larry Trivieri, Jr. *The American Holistic Medical Association Guide to Holistic Health* (New York: John Wiley & Sons, 2001).

2 R. Gupta et al. "Antioxidant and Hypercholesterolaemic Effects of *Terminalia arjuna* Tree-bark Powder: A Randomised Placebo-Controlled Trial." *J Assoc Physicians India* 49 (February 2001), 231-235.

3 A. Puri et al. "Immunostimulant Activity of Dry Fruits and Plant Materials Used in Indian Traditional Medical System for Mothers After Childbirth and Invalids." *Journal of Ethnopharmacology* 71:1-2 (July 2000), 89-92.

4 J.N. Dhuley. "Adaptogenic and Cardioprotective Action of *Ashwagandha* in Rats and Frogs." *Journal of Ethnopharmacology* 70:1 (April 2000), 57-63.

5 P.U. Devi. "*Withania somnifera Dunal (Ashwagandha)*: Potential Plant Source of a Promising Drug for Cancer Chemotherapy and Radiosensitization." *Indian Journal of Experimental Biology* 34:10 (October 1996), 927-932.

6 I. Gupta et al. "Effects of *Boswellia serrata* Gum Resin in Patients with Bronchial Asthma: Results of a Double-Blind, Placebo-Controlled 6-Week Clinical Study." *European Journal of Medical Research* 3:11 (November 17, 1998), 511-514.

7 S. Agnihotri and A.D. Vaidya. "A Novel Approach to Study Antibacterial Properties of Volatile Components of Selected Indian Medicinal Herbs." *Indian Journal of Experimental Biology* 34:7 (1996), 712-715.

8 T. Mustafa and K.C. Srivastava. "Ginger *(Zingiber officinale)* in Migraine Headache." *Journal of Ethnopharmacology* 29:3 (July 1990), 267-273.

9 A.K. Azad Khan, S. Akhtar, and H. Mahtab. "*Coccinia indica* in the Treatment of Patients with Diabetes Mellitus." *Bangladesh Med Res Counc Bull* 5:2 (December 1979), 60-66.

10 J.T. Piper et al. "Mechanisms of Anticarcinogenic Properties of Curcumin: The Effect of Curcumin on Glutathione Linked Detoxification Enzymes in Rat Liver." *Int J Biochem Cell Biol* 30:4 (April 1998), 445-456.

11 Swami Sada Shiva Tirtha. *The Ayurveda Encyclopedia* (Bayville, NY: Ayurveda Holistic Center Press, 1998), 45-46.

12 I. Gupta et al. "Effects of *Boswellia serrata* Gum Resin in Patients with Bronchial Asthma: Results of a Double-Blind, Placebo-Controlled, 6-Week Clinical Study." *European Journal of Medical Research* 3:11 (November 17, 1998), 511-514. A. Jacob et al. "Effect of Indian Gooseberry *(Amla)* on Serum Cholesterol Levels in Men Aged 35-55 Years." *European Journal of Clinical Nutrition* 42 (1988), 939-944. A. Kanase et al. "Curative Effects of *Mandur Bhasma* on Liver and Kidney of Albino Rats After Induction of Acute Hepatitis by CCl(4)." *Indian Journal of Experimental Biology* 35:7 (July 1997), 754-64. N.R. Biswas et al. "Comparative Double-Blind Multicentric Randomised Placebo-Controlled Clinical Trial of an Herbal Preparation of Eye Drops in Some Ocular Ailments." *Journal of the Indian Medical Association* 94:3 (March 1996), 101-102.

13 R.H. Bannerman, J. Burton, and C. Wen-Chieh, eds. *Traditional Medicine and Health Care Coverage* (Geneva, Switzerland: World Health Organization, 1983). H.M. Sharma, B.D. Triguna, and D. Chopra. "Maharishi Ayur-veda: Modern Insights into Ancient Medicine." *Journal of the American Medical Association* 266:13 (1991), 2633-2637.

14 V. Sodhi. "Ayurveda: The Science of Life and Mother of the Healing Arts." In: J.E. Pizzorno and M.T. Murray, eds. *A Textbook of Natural Medicine* (Seattle, WA: John Bastyr College Publications, 1989).

15 H.M. Sharma, B.D. Triguna, and D. Chopra. "Maharishi Ayur-veda: Modern Insights into Ancient Medicine." *Journal of the American Medical Association* 266:13 (1991), 2633-2637. Letters to the Editor. "Maharishi Ayur-veda." *Journal of the American Medical Association* 266:13 (1991), 1769-1774.

BIOFEEDBACK TRAINING AND NEUROTHERAPY

1 S.L. Fahrion. "Autogenic Biofeedback Treatment for Migraine." *Research and Clinical Studies in Headache* 5 (1978), 47-71.

2 E.B. Blanchard and F. Andrasik. "Biofeedback Treatment of Vascular Headache." In: John P. Hatch, Johnnie G. Fisher, and John D. Rugh, eds. *Biofeedback* (New York: Plenum Publishing, 1987).

3 E. Peper and V. Tibbetts. "Fifteen-Month Follow-up with Asthmatics Utilizing EMG/Incentive

Inspirometer Feedback." *Biofeedback and Self-Regulation* 17:2 (June l992), 143-151.

4 S.L. Fahrion. "Hypertension and Biofeedback." *Primary Care: Clinics in Office Practice* 3 (September 1991), 663-682.

5 C.B. Yucha et al. "The Effect of Biofeedback in Hypertension." *Applied Nursing Research* 14:1 (February 2001), 29-35.

6 S.R. Brown et al. "Biofeedback Avoids Surgery in Patients with Slow-Transit Constipation: Report of Four Cases." *Diseases of the Colon and Rectum* 44:5 (May 2001), 737-740.

7 Deputy Surgeon General Faye G. Abdellah, quoted in: N.E. Miller. "RX: Biofeedback." *Psychology Today* 19:2 (February 1985), 54-59.

8 B. Dworkin et al. "A Behavioral Method for the Treatment of Idiopathic Scoliosis." *Proceedings of the National Academy of Sciences* 82 (April 1985), 2493-2497.

9 Deputy Surgeon General Faye G. Abdellah, quoted in: N.E. Miller. "RX: Biofeedback." *Psychology Today* 19:2 (February 1985), 54-59.

10 Urinary Incontinence Guideline Panel. *Urinary Incontinence in Adults: Clinical Practice Guideline* AHCPR Pub. No. 92-0038 (Rockville, MD: Agency for Health Care Policy and Research, Public Health Service, U.S. Department of Health and Human Services, 1992).

11 D.B. Smith et al. "A Self-Directed Home Biofeedback System for Women with Symptoms of Stress, Urge, and Mixed Incontinence." *Journal of Wounds, Ostomy, and Continence Nursing* 27:4 (July 2001), 240-246.

12 M.R. Werbach, M.D. *Third Line Medicine: Modern Treatment for Persistent Symptoms* (Los Angeles: Third Line Press, 1986).

13 P. Norris and G. Porter. *Why Me? Harnessing the Healing Power of the Human Spirit* (Walpole, NH: Stillpoint Publishing, 1985).

14 L. Trivieri. "Brain Wave Therapy: A Breakthrough Addiction Therapy." *The Healthy Edge Letter* 1:2 (April 1998), 3-4.

15 K. Thornton. "Improvement/Rehabilitation of Memory Functioning with Neurotherapy/ QEEG Biofeedback." *Journal of Head Trauma Rehabilitation* 15:6 (December 2000), 1285-1296.

16 L. Trivieri. "Brain Wave Therapy: A Breakthrough Addiction Therapy." *The Healthy Edge Letter* 1:2 (April 1998), 1-2.

17 Ibid., 4.

BIOLOGICAL DENTISTRY

1 O. Neuner. "The Diagnosis and Therapy of Focal and Field Disorders." *Raum & Zeit* 2:4 (1991), 38-42.

2 W.A. Price. *Dental Infections Volume 1: Oral and Systemic* (Cleveland, OH: Benton Publishing, 1973).

3 F.G. Strauss and D.W. Eggleston. "IgA Nephropathy Associated with Dental Nickel Alloy Sensitization." *American Journal of Nephrology* 5 (1985), 395-397.

4 "Dental Mercury Hygiene: Summary of Recommendations in 1990." *Journal of the American Dental Association* 122 (August 1991), 112.

5 Final Report of the Subcommittee on Risk Management of the Committee to Coordinate Environmental Health and Related Programs. *Dental Amalgam: A Scientific Review and Recommended Public Health Service Strategy for Research, Education and Regulation* (Washington, DC: Public Health Service, 1993).

6 "Dental Mercury Hygiene: Summary of Recom-

mendations in 1990." *Journal of the American Dental Association* 122 (August 1991), 112.

7 W. Melillo. "How Safe is Mercury in Dentistry?" *The Washington Post Weekly Journal of Medicine, Science and Society* (September 1991), 4.

8 World Health Organization. *Environmental Health Criteria for Inorganic Mercury 118* (Geneva: World Health Organization, 1991).

9 P. Grandjean, M.D., et al. "Reference Intervals for Trace Elements in Blood: Significance of Risk Factors." *Scandinavian Journal of Clinical and Laboratory Investigation* 2 (June 1992), 321-337.

10 R. Schiele et al. "Studies on the Mercury Content in Brain and Kidney Related to Number and Condition of Amalgam Fillings." Paper presented at the Institution of Occupational and Social Medicine, University Erlangen, Nurnberg, West Germany (March 12, 1984).

11 Final Report of the Subcommittee on Risk Management of the Committee to Coordinate Environmental Health and Related Programs. *Dental Amalgam: A Scientific Review and Recommended Public Health Service Strategy for Research, Education and Regulation* (Washington, DC: Public Health Service, 1993).

12 "Socialstyrelsen (Swedish Social Welfare and Health Administration) Stops Amalgam Use." *Svenska Dagbladet* (May 1987), 1.

13 Agency for Toxic Substances and Disease Registry 1993. Division of Toxicology, Chart.

14 J. Taylor. *The Complete Guide to Mercury Toxicity from Dental Fillings* (San Diego: Scripps Publishing, 1988).

15 S. Ziff. "Consolidated Symptom Analysis of 1,569 Patients." *Bio-Probe Newsletter* 9:2 (March 1993), 7-8.

16 H.A. Huggins. *It's All in Your Head: The Link Between Mercury Amalgams and Illness* (New York: Avery/Penguin Putnam, 1993), 103.

17 L.J. Hahn et al. "Dental 'Silver' Tooth Fillings: A Source of Mercury Exposure Revealed by Whole-Body Image Scan and Tissue Analysis." *FASEB Journal* 3 (1989), 2641-2646. L.J. Hahn et al. "Whole-Body Imaging of the Distribution of Mercury Released from Dental Fillings into Monkey Tissues." *FASEB Journal* 4 (1990), 3256-3260.

18 M.J. Vimy, Y. Takahashi, and F.L. Lorscheider. "Maternal-Fetal Distribution of Mercury Released from Dental Amalgam Fillings." *American Physiological Society* 258 (1990), R939-R945.

19 P. Grandjean, M.D. "Reference Intervals for Trace Elements in Blood: Significance of Risk Factors." *Scandinavian Journal of Clinical and Laboratory Investigation* 2 (June 1992), 321-337. R. Schiele et al. "Studies on the Mercury Content in Brain and Kidney Related to Number and Condition of Amalgam Fillings." Paper presented at the Institution of Occupational and Social Medicine, University Erlangen, Nurnberg, West Germany (March 12, 1984). M.J. Vimy et al. "Glomerular Filtration Impairment by Mercury from Dental 'Silver' Fillings in Sheep." *The Physiologist* 33 (August 1990), A94. N.D. Boyd et al. "Mercury from Dental 'Silver' Tooth Fillings Impairs Sheep Kidney Function." *American Physiological Society* 261 (1991), R1010-R1014.

20 International Labour Office. *Encyclopedia of Occupational Health and Safety* (New York: McGraw-Hill, 1972).

21 United States Environmental Protection Agency, Office of Health and Environmental Assessment. *EPA Mercury Health Effects Update Health Issue*

Assessment Final Report EPA-600/8.84.019F (Washington, DC: U.S. Environmental Protection Agency, 1984).

22 W.A. Price. *Nutrition and Physical Degeneration* (La Mesa, CA: The Price-Pottinger Nutrition Foundation, 1970).

23 J.A. Yiamouyiannis. *Fluoride: The Aging Factor* (Delaware, OH: Health Action Press, 1986), 74-75.

24 R.N. Mukherjee and F.H. Sobels. "The Effect of Sodium Fluoride and Iodoacetamide on Mutation Induction by X-Irradiation in Mature Spermatozoic of Drosophila." *Mutation Research* 6:2 (1968), 217-225.

25 D. Black. *Fluoridation: How Wise is It?* (Springville, UT: Tapestry Press, 1990), 1.

26 C. Kopf. "Doctor Who Advocated Fluoridation Now Calls It a Fraud." *The Forum Health Freedom News* 11:6 (July/August 1992), 28.

27 C. Danielson et al. "Hip Fractures and Fluoridation in Utah's Elderly Population." *Journal of the American Medical Association* 268:6 (August 1992), 746-748.

28 J.A. Yiamouyiannis and D. Burk. "Fluoridation and Cancer Age-Dependence of Cancer Mortality Related to Artificial Fluoridation." *Fluoride* 10:3 (1977), 102-123.

29 D. Pendrys. "Risk of Fluorosis in a Fluoridated Population: Implications for the Dentist and Hygienist." *Journal of the American Dental Association* 126:12 (1995), 1617-1624.

30 Ibid.

31 K. Wang. "A Report of 22 Cases of Temporomandibular Joint Dysfunction Syndrome Treated with Acupuncture and Laser Radiation." *Journal of Traditional Chinese Medicine* 12:2 (June 1992), 116-118.

32 P. Grandjean, M.D. "Reference Intervals for Trace Elements in Blood: Significance of Risk Factors." *Scandinavian Journal of Clinical and Laboratory Investigation* 2 (June 1992), 321-337. R. Schiele et al. "Studies on the Mercury Content in Brain and Kidney Related to Number and Condition of Amalgam Fillings." Paper presented at the Institution of Occupational and Social Medicine, University Erlangen, Nurnberg, West Germany (March 12, 1984). N.D. Boyd et al. "Mercury from Dental 'Silver' Tooth Fillings Impairs Sheep Kidney Function." *American Physiological Society* 261 (1991), R1010-R1014.

BODYWORK

1 The Bodywork KnowledgeBase is an abstracted collection of the world literature on massage compiled by Richard Van Why, available from the American Massage Therapy Association.

2 J. Yates. *A Physician's Guide to Therapeutic Massage* (Canada: Massage Therapists Association of British Columbia, 1990).

3 The Bodywork KnowledgeBase is an abstracted collection of the world literature on massage compiled by Richard Van Why, available from the American Massage Therapy Association.

4 American Massage Therapy Association. "Massage Therapy: Facts for Physicians." *American Massage Therapy Association (AMTA) Fact Sheet* (1999). Available from: AMTA, 820 Davis Street, Suite 100, Evanston, IL 60201.

5 Quebec Task Force on Spinal Disorders. "Scientific Approach to the Assessment and Management of Activity-Related Spinal Disorders: A Monograph for Clinicians." *Spine* 12:7 Suppl (September 1987), S1-59.

6 Larry Trivieri, Jr. *The American Holistic Medical Association Guide to Holistic Health* (New York: John Wiley & Sons, 2001), 219.

7 American Massage Therapy Association. "Massage Therapy: Facts for Physicians." *American Massage Therapy Association (AMTA) Fact Sheet* (1999). Available from: AMTA, 820 Davis Street, Suite 100, Evanston, IL 60201.

8 G. Beard. *Beard's Massage* (Philadelphia: W.B. Saunders, 1981).

9 W. Barlow. *The Alexander Technique* (New York: Alfred A. Knopf, 1973).

10 F.P. Jones. "Body Awareness in Action." In: M. Murphy. *The Future of the Body* (Los Angeles: Jeremy P. Tarcher, 1992).

11 R.J. Dennis. "Functional Reach Improvement in Normal Older Women After Alexander Touch Instruction." *Journal of Gerontology: Medical Sciences* 54:1 (January 1999), M8-11.

12 C. Stallibrass. "An Evaluation of the Alexander Technique for the Management of Disability in Parkinson's Disease—A Preliminary Study." *Clinical Rehabilitation* 11:1 (February 1997), 8-12.

13 O. Elkayam et al. "Multidisciplinary Approach to Chronic Back Pain: Prognostic Elements of the Outcome." *Clinical and Experimental Rheumatology* 14:3 (May-June 1996), 281-288.

14 M. Feldenkrais. *Awareness Through Movement* (New York: Harper & Row, 1977).

15 Ibid.

16 S.K. Johnson et al. "A Controlled Investigation of Bodywork in Multiple Sclerosis." *Journal of Alternative and Complementary Medicine* 5:3 (June 1999), 237-243.

17 Trager® and Mentastics® are registered service marks of the Trager Institute.

18 D. Juhan. "The Trager Approach." *The Trager Journal* 2 (Fall 1987), 1-3.

19 D. Juhan. "Multiple Sclerosis and the Trager Approach." (February 1, 1993). Available on the Internet: www.trager.com.

20 R. Feitis. *Ida Rolf Talks About Rolfing and Physical Reality* (Boulder, CO: Rolf Institute, 1978).

21 I.P. Rolf. *Structural Integration: Gravity, An Unexplored Factor in a More Human Use of Human Beings* (San Francisco: Guild for Structural Integration, 1962).

22 I. Rolf. *Rolfing: The Integration of Human Structures* (New York: Harper and Row, 1977).

23 L. Connolly. "Ida Rolf." *Human Behavior* 6:5 (May 1977), 17-23.

24 J. Cottingham, S. Porges, and K. Richmond. "Shifts in Pelvic Inclination Angle and Parasympathetic Tone Produced by Rolfing Soft Tissue Manipulation." *Physical Therapy* 68:9 (September 1988), 1364-1370.

25 N. Franklin. "My Favorite Bodywork." *Medical Self-Care* 24 (Spring 1984), 53.

26 N. Richardson. "Aston-Patterning." *Physical Therapy Forum* 6:43 (1987), 1-3.

27 Hellerwork Pearlsoft Research Study (October 1982-March 1983). Conducted by Body of Knowledge, Inc., 406 Berry Street, Mt. Shasta, CA 96067.

28 C.F. Fan et al. "Acupressure Treatment for Prevention of Postoperative Nausea and Vomiting." *Anesthesiology Analg* 84:4 (April 1997), 821-825.

29 D.C. Byers. *Better Health with Foot Reflexology: The Original Ingham Method* (St. Petersburg, FL: Ingham Publishing, 1983).

30 B. Flocco. "Reflexology and Premenstrual Syndrome Research Study." A paper presented at the International Council of Reflexologists Conference, Virginia Beach, Virginia (1991).

31 N.L. Stephenson et al. "The Effects of Foot Reflexology on Anxiety and Pain in Patients with Breast and Lung Cancer." *Oncology Nursing Forum* 27:1 (January-February 2000), 67-72.

32 L. Launso et al. "An Exploratory Study of Reflexological Treatment for Headache." *Alternative Therapies in Health and Medicine* 5:3 (May 1999), 57-65.

33 B. Prudden. *Pain Erasure* (New York: Ballantine Books, 1980).

34 Elaine R. Ferguson. "The Healing Touch: Fact or Fiction?" *Alternative Medicine* 34 (March 2000), 77.

35 Larry Trivieri. "Therapeutic Touch and the Dimensions of Healing: An Interview with Dr. Dolores Krieger." *The Healthy Edge Letter* 1:3 (April 1998), 5-9.

36 P. Heidt. "Effect of Therapeutic Touch in Anxiety Levels of Hospitalized Patients." *Nursing Research* 30 (1981), 32. J.F. Quinn. "Therapeutic Touch as Energy Exchange: Testing the Theory." *Advances in Nursing Science* 2 (January 1984), 42-49. D. Krieger. *The Therapeutic Touch* (Englewood Cliff, NJ: Prentice-Hall, 1979). N. Samerel. "The Experience of Receiving Therapeutic Touch." *Journal of Advances in Nursing* 17:6 (1992), 651-657.

37 M.J. Smith. "Enzymes are Activated by the Laying-On of Hands." *Human Dimensions* (February 1973), 46-48. D. Wirth. "The Effect of Non-Contact Therapeutic Touch on the Healing of Full Thickness Dermal Wounds." *Subtle Energies* 1 (1990), 1-20.

38 M. Bogusalawski. "The Use of Therapeutic Touch in Nursing." *Journal of Continuing Education in Nursing* (October 1979), 9-15. M.S. Glick. "Caring Touch and Anxiety in Myocardial Infarction Patients in the Intermediate Cardiac Care Unit." *Intensive Care Nursing* 2:2 (1986), 61-66.

39 V. Bzdek and E. Keller. "Effects of Therapeutic Touch on Tension Headache Pain." *Nursing Research* 35 (1986), 101-106.

40 D. Krieger. *Accepting Your Power to Heal* (Santa Fe, NM: Bear and Company, 1993). D. Krieger. *The Personal Practice of Therapeutic Touch* (Santa Fe, NM: Bear and Company, 1993). D. Krieger. *The Therapeutic Touch* (Englewood Cliff, NJ: Prentice-Hall, 1979).

41 D. Krieger. "Therapeutic Touch During Childbirth Preparation by the Lamaze Method and Its Relation to Marital Satisfaction and State of Anxiety in the Married Couple." Nursing Research Emphasis Grant for Doctoral Programs, U.S. Public Health Service #NU-00833-02. *Proceedings of the Research Day of Sigma Theta Tau, Epsilon Chapter* (New York: New York University, 1984).

42 Healing Touch International, Inc. "Healing Touch Fact Sheet." Available on the Internet: www.healingtouch.net.

43 K. Olson and J. Hanson. "Using Reiki to Manage Pain: A Preliminary Report." *Cancer Prevention and Control* 1:2 (June 1997), 108-113.

44 M. Murphy. *The Future of the Body* (Los Angeles: Jeremy P. Tarcher, 1992).

CELL THERAPY

1 Darryl See, M.D. Personal communication (2000).

2 Diane Krause et al. *Cell* (May 4, 2001). Miriam Falco. "Placenta Source of Stem Cells, Researchers Say." *CNN.com/Health* (April 12, 2001). Marc Hedrick et al. *Tissue Engineering* (April 201).

3 A. Kment. "Die Verteilung Trittium Markierung Herz, Leber, Nieren und Zellen bei alten Ratten." *Die Therapiewoche* (1955), 152. F. Schmid and J. Stein. *Zelifroschunguno Zell Therapy* (Bern and Stutgard: Hans Huber Verlag, 1963).

4 National Institutes of Health. "Stem Cells: A Primer." Available on the Internet: www.nih.gov/news/stemcell/primer.htm.

5 F.H. Valone et al. "Immunotherapy of Multiple Myeloma Using Idiotype-Loaded Dendritic Cells (APC8020)." Abstracts of the American Society of Clinical Oncology 36th Annual Meeting, New Orleans, Louisiana (May 20-23, 2000), 1776. M.B. Faries et al. "Effective Immunization to Melanoma Antigens by Intranodal Injection of Mature, CD8+ Dendritic Cells." Abstracts of the American Society of Clinical Oncology 36th Annual Meeting, New Orleans, Louisiana (May 20-23, 2000), 1778. R.J. Amato et al. "Patients with Renal Cell Carcinoma (RCC) Using Autologous Tumor-Derived Heat Shock Protein-Peptide Vomplex (HSPPC-96) With or Without Interleukin-2 (IL-2)." Abstracts of the American Society of Clinical Oncology 36th Annual Meeting, New Orleans, Louisiana (May 20-23, 2000), 1782. J.W. Smith II et al. "Vaccination of Breast Cancer Patients with a Tumor Cell Vaccine Genetically Modified to Express the Co-Stimulatory Molecule, CD80." Abstracts of the American Society of Clinical Oncology 36th Annual Meeting, New Orleans, Louisiana (May 20-23, 2000), 1783.

6 N.N. Aksenova et al. "Effect of Ribonuclease on Anti-Tumor Activity of Ribonuclease Acid from Normal Tissues." *Nature* 207:3 (July 1965), 40-42. P. Alexander et al. "Effect of Nucleic Acids from Immune Lymphocytes on Rat Sarcomata." *Nature* 213 (February 1967), 569-572.

7 E.M. Molnar. *Forever Young* (West Hartford, CT: Witkower Press, 1985).

8 F. Schmid. *Cell Therapy: A New Dimension of Medicine* (Thoune, Switzerland: Ott Publishers, 1983).

9 Ibid.

10 Ibid.

11 D.D. Spencer, M.D., et al. "Unilateral Transplantation of Human Fetal Mesencephalic Tissue into the Caudate Nucleus of Patients with Parkinson's Disease." *New England Journal of Medicine* 327 (November 1992), 1541-1548.

12 C.R. Freed et al. "Transplantation of Embryonic Dopamine Neurons for Severe Parkinson's Disease." *New England Journal of Medicine* 344:10 (2001), 710-719.

13 Helen Hodges et al. Paper presented at the annual conference of the British Neuroscience Association (April 9, 2001). T. Veizovic et al. "Resolution of Stroke Deficits Following Contralateral Grafts of Conditionally Immortal Neuroepithelial Stem Cells." *Stroke* 32:4 (2001), 1012-1019.

14 D. Orlic et al. "Bone Marrow Cells Regenerate Infarcted Myocardium." *Nature* 410:6829 (2001), 701-705. See also: A.A. Kocher et al. "Neovascularization of Ischemic Myocardium by Human Bone-Marrow-Derived Angioblasts Prevents Cardiomyocyte Apoptosis, Reduces Remodeling and Improves Cardiac Function." *Nature Medicine* 7:4 (2001), 430-436.

CHELATION THERAPY

1 G.F. Gordon. "Chelation Therapy for Health and Longevity: What Everyone Needs to Know to Live as Long as Possible." *Clinical Practice of Alternative Medicine* 1:3 (2000).

2 American College for Advancement in Medicine.

"Position Paper on EDTA Chelation Therapy." Available on the Internet: www.acam.org/chelationtherapy/information.php.

3 E.M. Cranton, M.D. "Protocol of the American College of Advancement in Medicine for the Safe and Effective Administration of Intravenous EDTA Chelation Therapy." In: E.M. Cranton, M.D., ed. *A Textbook on EDTA Chelation Therapy* (New York: Human Sciences Press, 1989), 269-305.

4 C.H. Farr, M.D., R. White, and M. Schachter, M.D. "Chronological History of EDTA Chelation Therapy." Paper presented to the American College of Advancement in Medicine, Houston, Texas (May 1993).

5 M. Walker and G. Gordon. *The Chelation Answer: How to Prevent Hardening of the Arteries and Rejuvenate Your Cardiovascular System* (New York: M. Evans, 1982).

6 Available on the American Heart Association website: www.amhrt.org/hs96/has.html.

7 Z. Strauts, M.D. "Correspondence Re: *Berkeley Wellness Letter* and Chelation Therapy." *Townsend Letter for Doctors* 106 (May 1992), 382-383.

8 T.L. Chappel, M.D. "Preliminary Findings From the Meta-Analysis Study of EDTA Chelation Therapy." Paper presented at the American College of Advancement in Medicine meeting, Houston, Texas (May 5-9, 1993).

9 M. Walker and G. Gordon. *The Chelation Answer: How to Prevent Hardening of the Arteries and Rejuvenate Your Cardiovascular System* (New York: M. Evans, 1982), 175.

10 E. Olszewer, M.D., and J.P. Carter, M.D. "EDTA Chelation Therapy: A Retrospective Study of 2,870 Patients." In: E.M. Cranton, M.D., ed. *A Textbook on EDTA Chelation Therapy* (New York: Human Sciences Press, 1989), 183.

11 M. Walker. *Chelation Therapy* (Stamford, CT: New Way of Life, 1984).

12 E. Olszewer, M.D., and J.P. Carter, M.D. "EDTA Chelation Therapy: A Retrospective Study of 2,870 Patients." In: E.M. Cranton, M.D., ed. *A Textbook on EDTA Chelation Therapy* (New York: Human Sciences Press, 1989), 197-211.

13 Ibid.

14 E.W. McDonagh, C.J. Rudolph, and E. Cheraskin, M.D. "An Oculocerebro-vasculometric Analysis of the Improvement in Arterial Stenosis Following EDTA Chelation Therapy." In: E.M. Cranton, M.D., ed. *A Textbook on EDTA Chelation Therapy* (New York: Human Sciences Press, 1989), 155-166.

15 C. Hancke and K. Flytie. "Benefits of EDTA Chelation Therapy in Arteriosclerosis: A Retrospective Study of 470 Patients." *Journal of Advancement in Medicine* 6:3 (1993), 161.

16 H.R. Alsleben, M.D., and W.E. Shute, M.D. *How to Survive the New Health Catastrophes* (Anaheim, CA: Survival Publications, 1973).

17 E.W. McDonagh, C.J. Rudolph, and E. Cheraskin, M.D. "An Oculocerebro-vasculometric Analysis of the Improvement in Arterial Stenosis Following EDTA Chelation Therapy." In: E.M. Cranton, M.D., ed. *A Textbook on EDTA Chelation Therapy* (New York: Human Sciences Press, 1989), 155-166.

18 H.R. Casdorph, M.D. "EDTA Chelation Therapy: Efficacy in Brain Disorders." In: E.M. Cranton, M.D., ed. *A Textbook on EDTA Chelation Therapy* (New York: Human Sciences Press, 1989), 131-153.

19 H.R. Alsleben, M.D., and W.E. Shute, M.D. *How to Survive the New Health Catastrophes* (Anaheim, CA: Survival Publications, 1973).

20 W. Blumer, M.D., and E.M. Cranton, M.D. "Ninety Percent Reduction in Cancer Mortality After Chelation Therapy with EDTA." In: E.M. Cranton, M.D., ed. *A Textbook on EDTA Chelation Therapy* (New York: Human Sciences Press, 1989), 1989, 183.

21 H.R. Alsleben, M.D., and W.E. Shute, M.D. *How to Survive the New Health Catastrophes* (Anaheim, CA: Survival Publications, 1973).

22 Ibid.

23 H.R. Casdorph. "EDTA Chelation Therapy: Efficacy in Brain Disorder." *Journal Advancement in Medicine* 2:1/2 (1989), 131-153. E.W. McDonagh et al. "The Effect of EDTA Chelation Therapy Plus Supportive Multivitamin-Trace Mineral Supplementation Upon Renal Function: A Study in Blood Urea Nitrogen." *Journal of Holistic Medicine* 5 (1983), 163-171.

24 M.T. Grier and D.G. Meyers. "So Much Writing, So Little Science: A Review of 37 Years of Literature on Edetate Sodium Chelation Therapy." *Annals of Pharmacotherapy* 27 (1993), 1504-1509.

25 R.S. Scharffenberg. *EDTA Chelation Literature: Subject Index* (North Hollywood, CA: American Academy of Medical Preventics, 1976).

26 J. Heimbach et al. "Safety Assessement of Iron EDTA [Sodium Iron (Fe3+) Ethylenediaminetetracaetic Acid]: Summary of Toxicological Fortification and Exposure Data." *Food and Chemical Toxicology* 38 (2000), 99-111.

27 W. Blumer, M.D., and E.M. Cranton, M.D. "Ninety Percent Reduction in Cancer Mortality after Chelation Therapy with EDTA." In: E.M. Cranton, M.D., ed. *A Textbook on EDTA Chelation Therapy* (New York: Human Sciences Press, 1989), 183-188.

28 J.P. Trowbridge, M.D., and M. Walker. *The Healing Powers of Chelation Therapy* (Stamford, CT: New Way of Life, 1992).

CHIROPRACTIC

1 N. Altman. *Everybody's Guide to Chiropractic Health Care* (Los Angeles: Jeremy P. Tarcher, 1990).

2 T. Rondberg. *Chiropractic First* (Chandler, AZ: Chiropractic Journal, 1996), 104.

3 P. Manga et al. *A Study to Examine the Effectiveness and Cost Effectiveness of Chiropractic Management of Low-Back Pain* (Richmond Hill, Ontario: Kenilworth Publishing, 1993).

4 *Chiropractic in New Zealand: Report of the Commission of Inquiry* (Wellington, New Zealand: P.D. Hasselberg, Government Printer, 1979).

5 "Safety in Chiropractic Practice, Part I: The Occurrence of Cerebrovascular Accidents After Manipulation to the Neck in Denmark from 1978-1988." *Journal of Manipulative and Physiological Therapeutics* 19 (1996), 371-377.

6 M. Stano. "The Economic Role of Chiropractic: Further Analysis of Relative Insurance Costs for Low Back Care." *Journal of the Neuromusculoskeletal System* 3:3 (Fall 1995), 139-144.

7 K.B. Jarvis et al. "Cost Per Case Comparison of Back Injury Claims: Chiropractic versus Medical Management for Conditions with Identical Diagnosis Codes." *Journal of Occupational Medicine* 33:8 (August 1991), 847-852.

8 T.W. Meade et al. "Low Back Pain of Mechanical Origin: Randomised Comparison of Chiropractic and Hospital Outpatient Treatment." *British Medical Journal* 300:6737 (June 1999), 1431-1437.

9 Rand Corporation. "The Appropriateness of Spinal Manipulation for Low Back Pain: Indications and Ratings by a Multidisciplinary Expert Panel." Rand Corporation Study (1991).

10 *The Art of Healthy Living: The Consumer's Guide to Chiropractic Care* (1998). Available from: American Chiropractic Association, 1701 Clarendon Blvd., Arlington, VA 22209.

11 N. Altman. *Everybody's Guide to Chiropractic Health Care* (Los Angeles: Jeremy P. Tarcher, 1990).

12 K. Wood. "Resolution of Spasmodic Dysphonia via Chiropractic Manipulative Management." *Journal of Manipulative and Physiological Therapeutics* 14:6 (July-August 1991), 376-378.

13 D.L. Berkson. "Osteoarthritis, Chiropractic, and Nutrition: Osteoarthritis Considered as a Natural Part of a Three-Stage Subluxation Complex: Its Reversibility, Its Relevance and Treatability by Chiropractic and Nutritional Correlates." *Medical Hypotheses* 36 (1991), 356-367.

14 I. Coulter et al. "Chiropractic Patients in a Comprehensive Home-Based Geriatric Assessment, Follow-up and Health Promotion." *Topics in Clinical Chiropractic* 3:2 (1996), 46-55.

15 T. Warner and S. Warner. "Communicating Easily." *The Chiropractic Journal* 12:7 (April 1998), 36.

16 R.M. Froehle. "Ear Infection: A Retrospective Study Examining Improvement from Chiropractic Care and Analyzing the Influencing Factors." *Journal of Manipulative and Physiological Therapeutics* 19:3 (1996), 169.

17 P.N. Fysh. "Chronic Recurrent Otitis Media: Case Series of Five Patients with Recommendations for Case Management." *Journal of Clinical Chiropractic Pediatrics* 1:2 (1996), 66.

18 R.L. Graham and R.A. Pistolese. "An Impairment Rating Analysis of Asthmatic Children Under Chiropractic Care." *Journal of Vertebral Subluxation Research* 1:4 (1997), 41.

CRANIOSACRAL THERAPY

1 V.M. Fryman. "A Study of the Rhythmic Motions of the Living Cranium." *Journal of the American Osteopathic Association* 70 (May 1971), 928-945. D.K. Michael and E.W. Retzlaff. "A Preliminary Study of Cranial Bone Movement in the Squirrel Monkey." *Journal of the American Osteopathic Association* 74 (May 1975), 866-869. E.W. Retzlaff, D.K. Michael, and R.M. Roppel. "Cranial Bone Mobility." *Journal of the American Osteopathic Association* 74 (May 1975), 869-873.

2 "Common Problems." Available from: The Cranial Academy, 8202 Clearvista Parkway, Suite 9-D, Indianapolis, IN 46256; website: www.cranialacademy.com/cmpr.html.

3 J.E. Upledger. *Your Inner Physician and You: Craniosacral Therapy SomatoEmotional Release* (Berkeley, CA: North Atlantic, 1992).

4 Andrew Weil, M.D. *Natural Health, Natural Medicine* (Boston: Houghton Mifflin, 1990).

5 J.E. Upledger. *Your Inner Physician and You: Craniosacral Therapy SomatoEmotional Release* (Berkeley, CA: North Atlantic, 1992).

6 Ibid.

DETOXIFICATION THERAPY

1 Environmental Protection Agency. "EPA Data Show Steady Progress in Cleaning Nation's Air." *Environmental News* (October 1992). As reported in: "Did You Know." *Our Toxic Times* 3:12 (December 1992), 5.

2 Environmental Protection Agency. "130 Cities Exceed Lead Levels for Drinking Water." *Environmental News* (October 1992). As reported in: "Did You Know." *Our Toxic Times* 3:12 (December 1992), 3.

3 P. Saifer, M.D. *Detox* (Los Angeles: Jeremy P. Tarcher, 1984).

4 D.W. Schnare. *The Unpolluting of Man* (Los Angeles: Foundation Essay Series, Foundation for Advancements in Science and Education video).

5 J. Carper. *The Food Pharmacy* (New York: Bantam, 1988).

6 I. Ofek et al. "Anti–*Escherichia Coli* Adhesin Activity of Cranberry and Blueberry Juices." *New England Journal of Medicine* 324 (May 1991), 1599.

7 G. Cheney. "Anti-Peptic Ulcer Dietary Factor (Vitamin U) in Treatment of Peptic Ulcer." *Journal of the American Dietetic Association* 26 (September 1950), 668-672.

8 R. Altman et al. "Identification of Platelet Inhibitor Present in the Melon (*Cucurbitacea Cucumis Melo*)." *Thrombosis and Haemostatis* 53:3 (June 1985), 312-313.

9 M.A. Adetumbi and B.H. Lau. "*Allium sativum* (Garlic): A Natural Antibiotic." *Medical Hypotheses* 12:3 (November 1983), 227-237. B.H. Lau. "Anticoagulant and Lipid Regulating Effects of Garlic (*Allium sativum*)." In: G. A. Spiller and J. Scala, eds. *New Protective Roles for Selected Nutrients* (New York: Alan R. Liss, 1989).

10 K.C. Srivastava and T. Mustafa. "Ginger (*Zingiber officinale*) and Rheumatic Disorders." *Medical Hypotheses* 29:1 (May 1989), 25-28. M.A. Al-Yahya et al. "Gastroprotective Activity of Ginger (*Zingiber officinale Rosc.*) in Albino Rats." *American Journal of Chinese Medicine* 17:1-2 (1989), 51-56.

11 T. Mustafa and K.C. Srivastava. "Ginger in Migraine Headache." *Journal of Ethnopharmacology* 29:3 (July 1990), 267-273. A. Grontved and E. Hentzer. "Vertigo-Reducing Effect of Ginger Root." *Journal of Oto-Rhino-Laryngology and Its Related Specialties* 48:5 (1986), 282-286.

12 M.T. Murray and J.E. Pizzorno. *Encyclopedia of Natural Medicine* (Rocklin, CA: Prima Publishing, 1990). S.J. Taussig. "The Mechanism of the Physiological Action of Bromelain." *Medical Hypotheses* 6:1 (January 1980), 99-104.

13 Additional recipes can be found in: Elson Haas, M.D. *The Detox Diet* (Berkeley, CA: Celestial Arts, 1998).

14 Christopher Hobbs, L.Ac. *Foundations of Health: Healing With Herbs & Foods* (Loveland, CO: Botanica Press, 1994).

15 W. John Diamond, M.D., and W. Lee Cowden, M.D., with Burton Goldberg. *Alternative Medicine Definitive Guide to Cancer* (Tiburon, CA: Future Medicine Publishing, 1997), 101-102.

16 D.W. Schnare et al. "Evaluation of a Detoxification Regimen for Fat Stored Xenobiotics." *Medical Hypotheses* 9:3 (1982), 265-282.

17 M. Walker and G. Gordon. *The Chelation Answer: How to Prevent Hardening of the Arteries and Rejuvenate Your Cardiovascular System* (New York: M. Evans, 1982).

18 D.W. Schnare et al. "Evaluation of a Detoxification Regimen for Fat Stored Xenobiotics." *Medical Hypotheses* 9:3 (1982), 265-282.

19 J.W. Shields M.D. "Lymph, Lymph Glands, and Homeostasis." *Lymphology* 25:4 (December 1992), 147-153.

20 D.W. Schnare et al. "Evaluation of a Detoxification Regimen for Fat Stored Xenobiotics." *Medical Hypotheses* 9:3 (1982), 265-282.

21 Z. Gard, M.D., and E. Brown. "Literature Review and Comparison Studies of Sauna/Hyperthermia in Detoxification." *Townsend Letter for Doctors* 107 (June 1992), 470-478.

DIET

1 Hazel Parcells, N.D., D.C., Ph.D. "The Challenge to Stay Healthy." *Parcells Letter* 1:2 (February 1996), 1-2.

2 Paul Bergner. *The Healing Power of Minerals: Special Nutrients and Trace Minerals* (Rocklin, CA: Prima Publishing, 1997), 68-75.

3 Melvyn Werbach, M.D. *Nutritional Influences on Illness* (Tarzana, CA: Third Line Press, 1993), 124.

4 James Braly, M.D. *Food Allergy and Nutrition Revolution* (New Canaan, CT: Keats Publishing, 1992), 242.

5 Jon D. Kaiser. *Immune Power* (New York: St. Martin's Press, 1993), 29.

6 P.J. Geiselman and D. Novin. "Sugar Infusion Can Enhance Feeling." *Science* 218:4571 (October 1982), 490-491.

7 D. Steinman. *Diet for a Poisoned Planet* (New York: Ballantine Books, 1990), 11.

8 R. Winter. *A Consumer's Dictionary of Food Additives* (New York: Crown Publishing, 1989).

9 June M. Chan et al. "Plasma Insulin-Like Growth Factor 1 and Prostate Cancer Risk: A Prospective Study." *Science* 3:7 (July 1994), 1089-1097. "Breast Cancer, rBGH and Milk." *Rachel's Environment & Health Weekly* 598 (May 8, 1998).

10 R. Winter. *A Consumer's Dictionary of Food Additives* (New York: Crown Publishing, 1989).

11 Ibid.

12 C.P. Weinstock. "Doubt Prisoners' Calm Behavior Linked to Diet Sans Sugar and Bread." *Medical Tribune* (January 1985), 32.

13 J.D. Weissman. *Choose to Live* (New York: Grove Press, 1988).

14 S. Schoenthaler, W. Doraz, and J. Wakefield, Jr. "The Impact of a Low Food Additive and Sucrose Diet on Academic Performance in 803 New York City Public Schools." *International Journal of Biosocial Medical Research* 8:2 (1986), 185-195. S. Schoenthaler, W. Doraz, and J. Wakefield, Jr. "Testing of Various Hypotheses as Explanations for the Gains in National Standardized Academic Test Scores in the 1978-83 New York City Nutrition Policy Modification Project." *International Journal of Biosocial Medical Research* 8:2 (1986), 196-203.

15 Donald W. Thayer, U.S.D.A. Eastern Regional Research Center. "Report on Wholesomeness Studies of Chicken." (March 19, 1984).

16 M. Friedman, ed. *Nutritional and Toxicological Consequences of Food Processing* (New York: Plenum Press, 1991).

17 Ibid.

18 Brian Tokar. "Exchange." *Safe Food News* (Fall 1993), 6. (Now called *Food and Water Journal*. Available from: Food & Water, Inc., R.R. 1, Box 68D, West Danville, VT 05873.)

19 B. Liebman. "Crying Over Milk." *Nutrition Action* (December 1992), 1, 6-7.

20 Ibid.

21 G. Ursin et al. "Milk Consumption and Cancer Incidence: A Norwegian Prospective Study." *British Journal of Cancer* 61:3 (March 1990), 456-459.

22 B. Liebman. "Crying Over Milk." *Nutrition Action* (December 1992), 1, 6-7.

23 *The Surgeon General's Report on Nutrition and Health*

DHH(PHS) Publication No. 88-50210 (Washington, DC: U.S. Department of Health and Human Services, Public Health Service, 1988).

24 E.L. Wynder et al. "Nutrition and Metabolic Epidemiology of Cancers of the Oral Cavity, Esophagus, Colon, Breast, Prostate, and Stomach." In: G.R. Newell and N.M. Ellison, eds. *Nutrition and Cancer: Etiology and Treatment* (New York: Raven, 1981), 11-48.

25 D. Steinman. *Diet for a Poisoned Planet* (New York: Ballantine Books, 1990), 74.

26 Laura DeFrancesco. "Quickening the Diagnosis of Mad Cow Disease: New Tests for Prions Shorten Time Frame for Detection." *The Scientist* 15:12 (June 11, 2001), 22.

27 Sandra Blakeslee. "Stringent Steps Taken by U.S. on Cow Illness." *The New York Times* (January 14, 2001).

28 Ibid.

29 Tosha Sweitzer. "Bovine Spongiform Encephalopathy: Is It a Threat?" Available on the Internet: www.purefood.org/madcow/threat61201.cfm.

30 *Humane Farming Association Special Report* XII:4 (1996). Jean C. Buzby et al. "USDA Modernizes Meat and Poultry Inspection." *Food Review* (January-April 1997), 14-17. *Humane Farming Association Special Report* XIII:3 (1997). Philip Cohen. "Mad Cows in Disguise." *New Scientist* (July 12, 1997), 6. Kieran Mulvaney. "Mad Cows and the Colonies: It Can't Happen Here?" *E Magazine* (July 17, 1996). Jeffrey Kluger. "U.S. Beef: Could Mad Cow Disease Strike Here?" *Time* (January 27, 1997). Michael W. Fox. *Eating With Conscience: The Bioethics of Food* (Troutdale, OR: NewSage Press, 1997).

31 G.G. Fein et al. "Prenatal Exposure to Polychlorinated Biphenyls: Effects on Birth Size and Gestational Age." *Journal of Pediatrics* 105:2 (August 1984), 315-320.

32 P. Toniolo et al. *American Journal of Epidemiology* 153 (2001), 1142-1147.

33 D. Ornish. *Stress, Diet and Your Heart* (New York: Holt, Rinehart, and Winston, 1982, 1983).

34 "Position of the American Dietetic Association: Vegetarian Diets." *Journal of the American Dietetic Association: ADA Reports* 88:3 (March 1988), 351-355.

35 Earl R. Mindell, Ph.D. *Earl Mindell's Food as Medicine* (New York: Simon & Schuster, 1994), 176.

36 Lita Lee, Ph.D., and Lisa Turner, with Burton Goldberg. *The Enzyme Cure* (Tiburon, CA: Future Medicine Publishing, 1998).

37 Earl R. Mindell, Ph.D. *Earl Mindell's Food as Medicine* (New York: Simon & Schuster, 1994), 171-172.

38 Burton Goldberg and the Editors of *Alternative Medicine Digest*. *Alternative Medicine Guide to Heart Disease* (Tiburon, CA: Future Medicine Publishing, 1998), 205.

39 Ibid.

40 Earl R. Mindell, Ph.D. *Earl Mindell's Food as Medicine* (New York: Simon & Schuster, 1994), 306

41 R.L. Walford, S.B. Harris, and M.W. Gunion. "The Calorically Restricted Low-Fat Nutrient-Dense Diet in Biosphere 2 Significantly Lowers Blood Glucose, Total Leukocyte Count, Cholesterol, and Blood Pressure in Humans." *Proceedings of the National Academy of Sciences* 89:23 (December 1992), 11533-11537.

42 R.L. Walford and M. Crew. "How Dietary Restriction Retards Aging: An Integrative

Hypothesis." *Growth, Development, and Aging* 53:4 (Winter 1989), 139-140.

43 Lita Lee, Ph.D., and Lisa Turner, with Burton Goldberg. *The Enzyme Cure* (Tiburon, CA: Future Medicine Publishing, 1998).

44 Earl R. Mindell, Ph.D. *Earl Mindell's Food as Medicine* (New York: Simon & Schuster, 1994), 20, 27-28.

45 R.S. Jope and G.V. Johnson. "Neurotoxic Effects of Dietary Aluminum." *Ciba Foundation Symposium* 169 (1992), 254-267.

46 H. Liukkonen-Lilja and S. Piepponen. "Leaching of Aluminum from Aluminum Dishes and Packages." *Food Additives and Contaminants* 9:3 (May/June 1992), 213-223.

47 B.J. Miller, S.M. Billedeau, and D.W. Miller. "Formation of N-nitrosamines in Microwaved Versus Skillet-Fried Bacon Containing Nitrite." *Food and Chemical Toxicology* 27:5 (May 1989), 295-299.

48 R. Quan, M.D., et al. "Effects of Microwave Radiation on Anti-Infective Factors in Human Milk." *Pediatrics* 89:4 (April 1992), 667-669.

49 G. Lubec, C. Wolf, and B. Bartosch. "Amino Acid Isomerisation and Microwave Exposure." *The Lancet* 2:8676 (December 1989), 1392-1393.

50 Environmental Protection Agency. "819 Cities Exceed Lead Level for Drinking Water." *EPA Environmental News* (May 11, 1993), R110.

51 D. Steinman. *Diet for a Poisoned Planet* (New York: Ballantine Books, 1990), 203.

52 J.H. Woltgens, E.J. Etty, and W.M. Nieuwland. "Prevalence of Mottled Enamel in Permanent Dentition of Children Participating in a Fluoride Programme at the Amsterdam Dental School." *Journal de Biologie Buccale* 17:1 (March 1989), 15-20. C. Danielson et al. "Hip Fractures and Fluoridation in Utah's Elderly Population." *Journal of the American Medical Association* 268:6 (August 1992), 746-748.

ENERGY MEDICINE

1 James L. Oschman and Nora H. Oschman. "How Healing Energy Works." *Convergence* 6:3 (Summer 1993), 24-30.

2 C. Norman Shealy. *Sacred Healing* (Boston: Element Books, 1999), 135.

3 Elaine R. Ferguson. "The Healing Touch: Fact or Fiction?" *Alternative Medicine* 34 (March 2000), 77.

4 Ibid.

5 Larry Trivieri. "Therapeutic Touch and the Dimensions of Healing: An Interview with Dr. Dolores Krieger." *The Healthy Edge Letter* 1:3 (April 1998), 5-9.

6 Healing Touch International, Inc. "Healing Touch Fact Sheet." Available on their website: www.healingtouch.net.

7 K. Olson and J. Hanson. "Using Reiki to Manage Pain: A Preliminary Report." *Cancer Prevention and Control* 1:2 (June 1997), 108-113.

8 Elaine R. Ferguson. "The Healing Touch: Fact or Fiction?" *Alternative Medicine* 34 (March 2000), 74-77.

9 Ibid.

10 Ibid.

11 J.A. Simington and G.P. Lain. "Effects of Therapeutic Touch on Anxiety in the Institutionalized Elderly." *Clinical Nursing Research* 2:4 (November 1993), 438-450.

12 E. Keller and V.M. Bzdek. "Effects of Therapeutic Touch on Tension Headache Pain." *Nursing Research* 35:2 (March-April 1986), 101-106.

13 P. Heidt. "Effect of Therapeutic Touch in Anxiety Levels of Hospitalized Patients." *Nursing Research* 30 (1981), 32. J.F. Quinn. "Therapeutic Touch as Energy Exchange: Testing the Theory." *Advances in Nursing Science* 2 (January 1984), 42-49. N. Samerel. "The Experience of Receiving Therapeutic Touch." *Journal of Advances in Nursing* 17:6 (1992), 651-657. D. Wirth. "The Effect of Noncontact Therapeutic Touch on the Healing of Full Thickness Dermal Wounds." *Subtle Energies* 1 (1990), 1-20. D. Krieger. *Accepting Your Power to Heal* (Santa Fe, NM: Bear and Company, 1993).

14 Zhu Zong-xiang. "Research Advances in the Electrical Specificity of Meridians and Acupuncture Points." *American Journal of Acupuncture* 9:3 (July/September 1981), 203-215.

15 D. Tucker. Position paper on Electroacupuncture Biofeedback ratified by the California Acupuncture Association, included in the California Acupuncture Association Completed Scope of Practice (March 14, 1993).

16 Ibid.

17 C.W. Smith and S. Best. *Electromagnetic Man: Health and Hazard in the Electrical Environment* (London: J.M. Dent and Sons, 1989), 88.

18 J.A. Zacharski. *Therapeutic Connection Between Cervical Problems and TMJ Dysfunction* (Self-Published Pamphlet, 1985).

19 K.M. Lucero. "The Electro-Acuscope/Myopulse System." *Rehab Management: The Journal of Therapy and Rehabilitation* 4:3 (April/May 1991).

20 Ibid.

21 G. Rein. "Effect of Non-Hertzian Scalar Waves on the Immune System." *U.S. Psychotronics Association Journal* (1989).

22 T.M. Srinivasan. "Machines with Promise." *Bridges* 8:4 (Winter 1997), 1.

23 J.J. Tsuei et al. "Study on Bioenergy in Diabetic Mellitus Patients." *American Journal of Acupuncture* 17:1 (1989), 31-38.

24 J.J. Tsuei et al. "Food Allergy Study Utilizing the EAV Acupuncture Technique." *American Journal of Acupuncture* 12:2 (June 1984), 105-116.

25 S.G. Sullivan. "Evoked Electrical Conductivity on Lung Acupuncture Points in Healthy Persons and Lung Cancer Patients." *American Journal of Acupuncture* 13:3 (1985), 261.

26 P. Madill. "Electroacupuncture: A True and Legitimate Preventive Medicine." *American Journal of Acupuncture* 7:4 (December 1979), 279-292.

ENVIRONMENTAL MEDICINE

1 T.G. Randolph. *Human Ecology and Susceptibility to the Chemical Environment* (Springfield, IL: C.C. Thomas, 1981).

2 Larry Trivieri, Jr. *The American Holistic Medical Association Guide to Holistic Health* (New York: John Wiley & Sons, 2001).

3 W. Crook. "Food Allergy: The Great Masquerader." *Pediatric Clinics of North America* 22:1 (February 1975), 227-238.

4 Bioecologic medicine incorporates the differences in individual's nutritional needs due to metabolic variations.

5 William J. Rea, M.D. *Chemical Sensitivity, Vol. 3* (Boca Raton, FL: C.R.C. Lewis, 1996), 1555-1579.

6 American Academy of Anti-Aging Medicine Program Guide (1997).

7 Michael Hodgson, M.D., M.P.H. "The Medical Evaluation" and "The Sick Building Syndrome" in "Effects of the Indoor Environment on Health."

Cited in: *Occupational Medicine: State of the Art Reviews* 10:1 (January-March 1995), 167-194.

8 Will Block and John Morgenthaler. "Food Allergies More Common Than You Think: Interview with Michael Rosenbaum, M.D." *Life Enhancement* 34 (June 1997), 3-7.

9 J.B. Miller, M.D. "Intradermal Provocative/Neutralizing Food Testing and Subcutaneous Food Extract Injection Therapy." In: J. Brostoff and S. Challacombe, eds. *Food Allergy and Intolerance* (London: Bailliere Tindall Publishers, 1987), 932-947.

10 L. Dickey. "History and Documentation of Coseasonal Antigen Therapy: Intracutaneous Serial Dilution Titration, Optimal Dosage, and Provocative Testing." *Clinical Ecology* (Springfield, IL: Charles C. Thomas, 1976), 18-25.

11 J. Krop et al. "A Double-Blind, Randomized, Controlled Investigation of Electrodermal Testing in the Diagnosis of Allergies." *Journal of Alternative and Complementary Medicine* 3:3 (Fall 1997), 241-248.

12 Larry Trivieri, Jr. *The American Holistic Medical Association Guide to Holistic Health* (New York: John Wiley & Sons, 2001).

13 R.L. Bergmann et al. "Allergen Avoidance Should Be First Line Treatment for Asthma." *European Respiratory Review* 8:53 (1998), 161-163. See also: David J. Hill et al. "The Melbourne House Dust Mite Study: Eliminating House Dust Mites in the Domestic Environment." *Journal of Allergy and Clinical Immunology* 99 (March 1999), 323-329.

14 Larry Trivieri, Jr. *The American Holistic Medical Association Guide to Holistic Health* (New York: John Wiley & Sons, 2001).

15 J. Egger et al. "A Controlled Trial of Oligoantigenic Diet Treatment in the Hyperkinetic Syndrome." *The Lancet* 1:8428 (1985), 540-545.

16 J. Egger et al. "A Controlled Trial of Hyposensitisation in Children with Food-Induced Hyperkinetic Syndrome." *The Lancet* 339:8802 (1992), 1150-1153.

17 S. Schoenthaler et al. "The Impact of a Low Food Additive and Sucrose Diet on Academic Performance in 803 New York City Public Schools." *International Journal of Biosocial Research* 8:2 (1986), 185-195.

18 W. Rea et al. "Elimination of Oral Food Challenge Reaction by Injection of Food Extracts: A Double-Blind Evaluation." *Archives of Otolaryngology* 110:14 (April 1984), 248-252. See also: G.K. Scadding and J. Brostoff. "Low-Dose Sublingual Therapy in Patients with Allergic Rhinitis Due to House Dust Mite." *Clinical Allergy* 16:5 (September 1986), 483-491. Several other studies have confirmed the same results found by Drs. Rea and Brostoff.

19 N.A. Ashford and C.S. Miller. *Chemical Exposures: Low Levels and High Stakes* (New York: Van Nostrand Reinhold, 1990).

20 "Pesticides and Groundwater: A Health Concern for the Midwest." Proceedings of the Freshwater Foundation Conference, Navarre, Minnesota (October 16-17, 1986).

21 N.A. Ashford and C.S. Miller. *Chemical Exposures: Low Levels and High Stakes* (New York: Van Nostrand Reinhold, 1990).

22 D. Steinman and S. Epstein, M.D. *The Safe Shopper's Bible* (New York: Macmillan, 1994).

23 D.W. Schnare et al. "Body Burden Reductions of PCBs, PBBs and Chlorinated Pesticides in Human Subjects." *Ambio: A Journal of the Human Environment* 13:5-6 (1984), 378-380. D.W.

Schnare. *The Unpolluting of Men* videotape (Los Angeles: Foundation Essay Series, Foundation for Advancements in Science and Education). P. Saifer, M.D., and M. Zellerbach. *Detox* (Los Angeles: Jeremy P. Tarcher, 1984).

24 United States Environmental Protection Agency. *Chemicals Identified in Human Biological Media: A Database* EPA 560/13-80-036B (Washington, DC: U.S. EPA, 1980).

25 W. Rea et al. "Pesticides and Brain Function Changes in a Controlled Environment." *Clinical Ecology* 2:3 (Summer 1984), 145-150. E.L. Baker, T.J. Smith, and P.J. Landrigan. "The Neurotoxicity of Industrial Solvents: A Review of the Literature." *American Journal of Industrial Medicine* 8:3 (1985), 207-217. R. Feldman, R. Mayer, and A. Taub. "Evidence for Peripheral Neurotoxic Effect of Trichloroethylene." *Neurology* 20:6 (1970), 599-606. P. Gregersen et al. "Neurotoxic Effects of Organic Solvents in Exposed Workers: An Occupational, Neuropsychological and Neurological Investigation." *American Journal of Industrial Medicine* 5:3 (1984), 201-225. J.E. Karlsson et al. "Effects of Low-Dose Inhalation of Three Chlorinated Aliphatic Organic Solvents on Deoxyribonucleic Acid in Gerbil Brain." *Scandinavian Journal of Work, Environment and Health* 13:5 (October 1987), 453-458. A.M. Seppalainen. "Neurophysiology Aspects of the Toxicity of Organic Solvents." *Scandinavian Journal of Work and Environmental Health* 11:Suppl. 1 (1985), 61-64. D.J. Ecobichon and R.M. Joy, eds. *Pesticides and Neurological Diseases* (Boca Raton, FL: CRC Press, 1982). R. Saracci et al. "Cancer Mortality in Workers Exposed to Chlorophenoxy Herbicides and Chlorophenols." *The Lancet* 338:8774 (October 1991), 1027-1032.

26 L. Darlington et al. "Placebo-Controlled, Blind Study of Dietary Manipulation Therapy in Rheumatoid Arthritis." *The Lancet* 1:8475 (February 1986), 236-238.

27 Larry Trivieri, Jr. *The American Holistic Medical Association Guide to Holistic Health* (New York: John Wiley & Sons, 2001).

ENZYME THERAPY

1 E. Howell, M.D. *Food Enzymes for Health and Longevity* (Woodstock Valley, CT: Omangod Press, 1980).

2 E. Howell, M.D. *Food Enzymes for Health and Longevity* (Woodstock Valley, CT: Omangod Press, 1980). E. Howell, M.D. *Enzyme Nutrition: The Food Enzyme Concept* (Wayne, NJ: Avery Publishing Group, 1987).

3 E. Howell, M.D. *Food Enzymes for Health and Longevity* (Woodstock Valley, CT: Omangod Press, 1980).

4 A.C. Guyton, M.D. *Textbook of Medical Physiology* (Philadelphia: W.B. Saunders, 1987). E. Howell, M.D. *Food Enzymes for Health and Longevity* (Woodstock Valley, CT: Omangod Press, 1980).

5 E. Howell, M.D. *Food Enzymes for Health and Longevity* (Woodstock Valley, CT: Omangod Press, 1980).

6 A. Immerman. "Evidence for Intestinal Toxemia— An Inescapable Clinical Phenomenon." *The American Chiropractic Association Journal of Chiropractic* 13 (April 1979), S25.

7 M. Wolf and K. Ransberger. *Enzyme Therapy* (New York: Vantage Press, 1972).

8 Ibid.

9 J.E. Morley, M.B. Sterman, and J.H. Walsh, eds. *Nutritional Modulation of Neural Function: UCLA Forum in Medical Sciences 28* (San Diego, CA: Academic Press, 1988).

10 C.B. Jaeger et al. "Polymer Encapsulated Dopaminergic Cell Lines as 'Alternative Neural Grafts'." *Progress in Brain Research* 82 (1990), 41-46.

11 M. Wolf and K. Ransberger. *Enzyme Therapy* (New York: Vantage Press, 1972).

12 Kilmer S. McCully, M.D. "Homocysteine Theory: Development and Current Status." *Atherosclerosis Review* 11 (1983), 157-246. Kilmer S. McCully, M.D. *The Homocysteine Revolution: Medicine for the New Millennium* (New Canaan, CT: Keats Publishing, 1997).

13 Garry F. Gordon, M.D. "Bypassing Heart Surgery." *Alternative Medicine* 30 (July 1999), 30-38.

14 S. Gupta. "Chronic Infection in the Aetiology of Atherosclerosis: Focus on *Chlamydia Pneumoniae*." *Atherosclerosis* 143:1 (1999), 1-6. T. Gura. "Chlamydia Protein Linked to Heart Disease." *Science* 283:5406 (1999), 1238-1239.

15 M.K. Dasgupta et al. "Circulating Immune Complexes in Multiple Sclerosis: Relation with Disease Activity." *Neurology* 32:9 (1982), 1000-1004.

16 M. Wolf and K. Ransberger. *Enzyme Therapy* (Los Angeles: Regent House, 1972), 156-166, 193-194.

17 H.E. Solorzano del Rio, M.D. Unpublished Paper (1992), 11.

18 Ibid.

19 A.J. Cichoke. "The Effect of Systemic Enzyme Therapy on Cancer Cells and the Immune System." *Townsend Letter for Doctors & Patients* (November 1995), 30-32.

20 M. Wolf and K. Ransberger. *Enzyme Therapy* (New York: Vantage Press, 1972).

21 N.J. Gonzalez and L.L. Isaacs. "Evaluation of Pancreatic Proteolytic Enzyme Treatment of Adenocarcinoma of the Pancreas, with Nutrition and Detoxification Support." *Nutrition and Cancer* 33:2 (1999), 115-116.

22 John Boik. *Cancer & Natural Medicine* (Princeton, MN: Oregon Medical Press, 1995).

FLOWER ESSENCES

1 E. Bach and F.J. Wheeler. *The Bach Flower Remedies* (New Canaan, CT: Keats Publishing, 1977). Originally published by C.W. Daniel, Saffron Walden, Essex, England, in 1933.

2 Ibid.

3 Ibid.

4 Ibid.

5 L.J. Kaslof. *The Bach Remedies: A Self-Help Guide* (New Canaan, CT: Keats Publishing, 1988), 3.

6 R.A. Van Haselen. "The Relationship Between Homeopathy and the Dr. Bach System of Flower Remedies: A Critical Appraisal." *British Homeopath Journal* 88:3 (July 1999), 121-127.

7 L.J. Kaslof. *The Bach Remedies: A Self-Help Guide* (New Canaan, CT: Keats Publishing, 1988), 22.

8 Ibid., 9.

9 G. Vlamis, ed. *Bach Flower Remedies to the Rescue* (Rochester, VT: Healing Arts Press, 1990).

10 L.J. Kaslof. *The Bach Remedies: A Self-Help Guide* (New Canaan, CT: Keats Publishing, 1988).

11 Ibid.

12 Copyright ©2001 Alicia Sirkin and Elisabeth Wiley. Used with permission.

GUIDED IMAGERY

1 A.A. Sheikh, P. Richardson, and L.M. Moleski. "Psychosomatics and Mental Imagery." In: A.A. Sheikh and J.T. Shaffer, eds. *The Potential of Fantasy and Imagination* (New York: Brandon, 1979). T.X. Barber. "Physiologic Effects of 'Hypnotic Suggestions': A Critical Review of Recent Research, (1960-1964)." *Psychological Bulletin* 63 (April 1965), 201-222. H. Benson. *The Relaxation Response* (New York: William Morrow, 1975). E. Jacobsen. *You Must Relax: A Practical Method of Reducing the Strains of Modern Living* (New York: McGraw-Hill, 1934). R. Jevning, R.K. Wallace, and M. Beidebach. "The Physiology of Meditation: A Review. A Wakeful Hypometabolic Integrated Response." *Neuroscience & BioBehavioral Reviews* 16:3 (Fall 1992), 415-424. J. Schultz, and W. Luthe. *Autogenic Training: A Psychophysiologic Approach in Psychotherapy* (New York: Grune and Stratton, 1959). K. Pelletier. *Mind as Healer, Mind as Slayer: A Holistic Approach to Preventing Stress Disorders* (New York: Delacorte Press/St. Lawrence, 1977). J. Levine, N.C. Gordon, and H.L. Fields. "The Mechanism of Placebo Analgesia." *The Lancet* 2:8091 (September 1978), 654-657.

2 G. Rosen, A. Kleinman, W. and Katon. "Somatization in Family Practice: A Biopsychosocial Approach." *Journal of Family Practice* 14:3 (March 1982), 493-502. J.D. Stoeckle, I.K. Zola, and G.E. Davidson. "The Quantity and Significance of Psychological Distress in Medical Patients: Some Preliminary Observations about the Decision to Seek Medical Aid." *Journal of Chronic Disease* 17 (October 1964), 959-970.

3 C. Simonton and S. Matthews. *Getting Well Again* (Los Angeles: Jeremy P. Tarcher, 1978).

4 Ibid.

5 P. Norris and G. Porter. *Why Me? Harnessing the Healing Power of the Human Spirit* (Walpole NH: Stillpoint Publishing, 1985).

6 K. Kolcaba and C. Fox. "The Effects of Guided Imagery on Comfort of Women with Early Stage Breast Cancer Undergoing Radiation Therapy." *Oncology Nurses Forum* 26:1 (January-February 1999), 67-72.

7 E.G. Walker et al. "Psychological, Clinical and Pathological Effects of Relaxation Training and Guided Imagery During Primary Chemotherapy." *British Journal of Cancer* 80:1-2 (April 1999), 262-268.

8 D.L. Tusek et al. "Guided Imagery: A Significant Advance in the Care of Patients Undergoing Elective Colorectal Surgery." *Diseases of the Colon and Rectum* 40:2 (February 1997), 172-178.

9 M. Castes et al. "Immunological Changes Associated with Clinical Improvement of Asthmatic Children Subjected to Psychological Intervention." *Brain Behav Immun* 13:1 (March 1999), 1-13.

10 H.C. Wichowski and S.M. Kubsch. "Increasing Diabetic Self-Care Through Guided Imagery." *Complement Ther Nurs Midwifery* 5:6 (December 1999), 159-163.

11 S.K. Avants and A. Margolin. "'Self' and Addiction: The Role of Imagery in Self-Regulation." *Journal of Alternative and Complementary Medicine* 1:4 (Winter 1995), 339-345.

12 M.J. Esplen et al. "A Randomized Controlled Trial of Guided Imagery in Bulimia Nervosa." *Psychol Med* 28:6 (November 1998), 1347-1357.

13 R. Zachariae et al. "Effects of Psychologic Intervention on Psoriasis: A Preliminary Report." *Journal of the American Academy of Dermatology* 34:6 (June 1996), 1008-1015.

14 J. Achterberg. *Imagery in Healing: Shamanism and Modern Medicine* (New York: Random House, 1985).

1124

15 B. Turkoski and B. Lance. "The Use of Guided Imagery with Anticipatory Grief." *Home Healthcare Nurse* 14:11 (November 1996), 878-888.

HERBAL MEDICINE

1 N.R. Farnsworth et al. "Medicinal Plants in Therapy." *Bulletin of the World Health Organization* 63:6 (1985). 965-981.

2 Ibid.

3 Herb Trade Association. "Definition of 'Herb'." (Austin, TX: Herb Trade Association, 1977).

4 M. Blumenthal. "Focus on Rain Forest Remedies." *HerbalGram* 27 (1992), 8-10. R. Eisner. "Botanists Ply Trade in Tropics, Seeking Plant-Based Medicinals." *The Scientist* 4 (June 1991), 1, 4, 5, 25.

5 Andrew Weil, M.D. "A New Look at Botanical Medicine." *Whole Earth Review* 64 (1989), 3-8.

6 N.R. Farnsworth et al. "Medicinal Plants in Therapy." *Bulletin of the World Health Organization* 63:6 (1985). 965-981. O. Akerele. "Summary of WHO Guidelines for the Assessment of Herbal Medicines." *HerbalGram* 28 (1992), 13-16.

7 O. Akerele. "Summary of WHO Guidelines for the Assessment of Herbal Medicines." *HerbalGram* 28 (1992), 13-16. O. Akerele. "Guidelines for the Assessment of Herbal Medicines." *HerbalGram* 28 (1992), 17-20.

8 M. Blumenthal. "FDA Declares 258 OTC Ingredients Ineffective: Many Herbs Included." *HerbalGram* 23 (1990), 32-35.

9 British Herbal Medicine Association. *British Herbal Pharmacopoeia, Vol. 1* (Bournemouth, Dorset, England: British Herbal Medicine Association, 1990).

10 M. Blumenthal. "German MDs Required to Pass Herb Exam." *HerbalGram* 26 (1992), 45.

11 M. Blumenthal. "European Scientific Cooperative for Phytotherapy Symposium: European Harmony in Phytotherapy." *HerbalGram* 24 (1990), 41-45.

12 M.T. Murray and J.E. Pizzorno. *Encyclopedia of Natural Medicine* (Rocklin, CA: Prima Publishing, 1991), 83.

13 D. Hoffmann. *The New Holistic Herbal* (Rockport, MA: Element, 1991), 28.

14 R.H. Davis et al. "Wound Healing: Oral and Topical Activity of Aloe Vera." *Journal of the American Podiatric Medical Association* 79:11 (1989), 559-562. V. Visuthikosol et al. "Effect of *Aloe vera* Gel to Healing of Burn Wound: A Clinical and Histologic Study." *Journal of the Medical Association of Thailand* 78:8 (1995), 403-409.

15 M. Blumenthal et al., eds. *Complete German Commission E Monographs—Therapeutic Guide to Herbal Medicines* (Austin, TX: American Botanical Council, Integrative Medicine Communications, 1998).

16 M. Blumenthal et al., eds. *Health Professionals Guide to Popular Herbs* (Austin, TX: American Botanical Council, 2001).

17 C.J. Henry and B. Emery. "Effect of Spiced Food on Metabolic Rate." *Human Nutrition, Clinical Nutrition* 40:2 (March 1986), 165-168.

18 H. Glatzel. "Treatment of Dyspeptic Disorders with Spice Extracts." *Hippokrates* 40:23 (December 1969), 916-919.

19 H. Glatzel. "Blood Circulation Effectiveness of Natural Spices." *Med Klin* 62:51 (December 1967), 1987-1989.

20 G. Buzzanca and S. Laterza. "Clinical Trial with an Antirheumatic Ointment." *Clin Ter* 83:1 (October 1977), 71-83.

21 M. Blumenthal et al., eds. *Complete German Commission E Monographs—Therapeutic Guide to Herbal Medicines* (Austin, TX: American Botanical Council, Integrative Medicine Communications, 1998).

22 German Ministry of Health. *Chamomile Flowers* Commission E Monographs for Phytomedicines (Bonn, Germany: German Ministry of Health, 1984).

23 F. Brantner. "Sexual Hormones from Plants in Female Medicine." *Ehk* 28 (1979), 413.

24 G. Hahn et al. "Monk's Pepper." *Notabene Medici* 16 (1986), 233, 236, 297-301.

25 H. Attelmann et al. "Investigation of the Treatment of Female Imbalances with Agnolyt." *Geriatrie* 2 (1972), 239.

26 H.W. Kayser and S. Istanbulluoglu. "Treatment of PMS Without Hormones." *Hippokrates* 25:25 (1954), 717.

27 R. Schellenberg. "Treatment of the Premenstrual Syndrome with *Agnus Castus* Fruit Extract: Prospective, Randomized, Placebo-Controlled Study." *British Medical Journal* 322 (2001), 134-137.

28 W. Amann. "Improvement of Acne Vulgaris with *Agnus Castus* (Agnolyt)." *Therapie der Gegenwart* 106 (1967), 124-126.

29 T. Wegner. "Devil's Claw: From African Traditional Remedy to Modern Analgesic and Anti-inflammatory." *HerbalGram* 50 (2000), 47-54.

30 P. Chantre et al. "Efficacy and Tolerance of *Harpagophytum procumbens* versus Diacerhein in Treatment of Osteoarthritis." *Phytomedicine* 7 (2000), 177-183.

31 M. Blumenthal et al., eds. *Complete German Commission E Monographs—Therapeutic Guide to Herbal Medicines* (Austin, TX: American Botanical Council, Integrative Medicine Communications, 1998).

32 S. Foster. *Echinacea: The Purple Coneflower* Botanical Series 301 (Austin, TX: American Botanical Council, 1991).

33 German Ministry of Health. *Echinacea Purpurea Leaf* Commission E Monographs for Phytomedicines (Bonn, Germany: German Ministry of Health, 1989).

34 B. Barrett et al. "Echinacea for Upper Respiratory Tract Infection." *Journal of Family Practice* 48:8 (1999), 628-635.

35 V.V. Berdyshev. "Effect of the Long-Term Intake of *Eleutherococcus* on the Adaptation of Sailors in the Tropics." *Voenno Meditsinskii Zhurnal* 5 (May 1981), 57-58.

36 V.I. Kupin and E.B. Polevaia. "Stimulation of the Immunological Reactivity of Cancer Patients by *Eleutherococcus* Extract." *Voprosy Onkologii* 32:7 (1986), 21-26.

37 P.J. Medon, P.W. Ferguson, and C.F. Watson. "Effects of *Eleutherococcus Senticosus* Extracts on Hexobarbital Metabolism *In Vivo* and *In Vitro*." *Journal of Ethnopharmacology* 10:2 (April 1984), 235-241.

38 General Accounting Office (GAO). *Dietary Supplements: Uncertainties in Analyses Underlying FDA's Proposed Rule on Ephedrine Alkaloids* (Washington, DC: United States General Accounting Office, 1999).

39 British Herbal Medicine Association. *British Herbal Pharmacopoeia* (Bournemouth, Dorset, England: British Herbal Medicine Association, 1983, 1992).

40 C. Hobbs. "Valerian: A Literature Review." *HerbalGram* 21 (1989), 19-34.

41 S. Foster. *Feverfew* Botanical Series 310 (Austin, TX: American Botanical Council, 1991). C. Hobbs. "Valerian: A Literature Review." *HerbalGram* 21 (1989), 19-34.

42 D.V.C. Awang. "The Pharmacological Activity of Commercial Plant Products." Presentation at the Annual Spring Meeting of the Nonprescription Drug Manufacturers Association of Canada, Ottawa, Canada (1992). D.V.C. Awang et al. "Parthenolide Content of Feverfew *(Tanacetum parthenium)* Assessed by HPLC and H-NMR Spectroscopy." *Journal of Natural Products* 54:6 (November-December 1991), 1516-1521.

43 D.V.C. Awang. "Feverfew Feedback." *HerbalGram* 22 (1990), 2-4, 42.

44 M. Blumenthal, A. Goldberg, and J. Brinckmann. *Herbal Medicine: Expanded Commission E Monographs* (Newton, MA: Integrative Medicine Communications, 2000).

45 S. Foster. *Garlic* Botanical Series 311 (Austin, TX: American Botanical Council, 1991).

46 R. McCaleb. "Anticancer Effects of Garlic—More Proof." *HerbalGram* 27 (1992), 22-23. W.C. You et al. "Allium Vegetables and Reduced Risk of Stomach Cancer." *Journal of the National Cancer Institute* 81:2 (January 1989), 162-164.

47 E. Block. "Antithrombotic Agent of Garlic: A Lesson from 5,000 Years of Folk Medicine." In: R.P. Steiner, ed. *Folk Medicine: The Art and the Science* (Washington, DC: The American Chemical Society, 1986).

48 J. Koscielny et al. "The Antiatherosclerotic Effect of *Allium sativum*." *Atherosclerosis* 144 (1999), 237-249.

49 S. Foster. *Garlic* Botanical Series 311 (Austin, TX: American Botanical Council, 1991).

50 Ibid.

51 M. Blumenthal et al., eds. *Complete German Commission E Monographs—Therapeutic Guide to Herbal Medicines* (Austin, TX: American Botanical Council, Integrative Medicine Communications, 1998).

52 S. Warshafsky, R. Kamer, and S. Sivak. "Effect of Garlic on Total Serum Cholesterol: A Meta-Analysis." *Annals of Internal Medicine* 119:7 Part 1 (1993), 599-605. C. Stevinson, M. Pittler, and E. Ernst. "Garlic for Treating Hypercholesterolemia." *Annals of Internal Medicine* 133 (2000), 420-429.

53 A. Grontved et al. "Ginger Root Against Seasickness. A Controlled Trial on the Open Sea." *Acta Oto-Laryngologica* 105:1-2 (January-February 1988), 45-49.

54 M.E. Bone et al. "Ginger Root—A New Antiemetic: The Effect of Ginger Root on Postoperative Nausea and Vomiting After Major Gynaecological Surgery." *Anaesthesia* 45:8 (August 1990), 669-671. W. Fischer-Rasmussen et al. "Ginger Treatment of Hyperemesis Gravidarum." *European Journal of Obstetrics & Gynecology and Reproductive Biology* 38:1 (January 1991), 19-24.

55 Vutyavanich et al. "Ginger for Nausea and Vomiting in Pregnancy: Randomized, Double-Masked, Placebo-Controlled Trial." *Obstetrics and Gynecology* 97:4 (April 2001), 577-582.

56 N. Shoji et al. "Cardiotonic Principles of Ginger (*Zingiber officinale Roscoe*)." *Journal of Pharmaceutical Sciences* 71:10 (October 1982), 1174-1175.

57 T. Mustafa and K.C. Srivastava. "Ginger (*Zingiber officinale*) in Migraine Headache." *Journal of Ethnopharmacology* 29:3 (July 1990), 267-273.

58 A.Y. Leung. "Fresh Ginger Juice in Treatment of Kitchen Burns." *HerbalGram* 16 (1989), 6.

59 S. Foster. *Ginkgo* Botanical Series 304 (Austin, TX: American Botanical Council, 1991).

60 P.L. Le Bars et al. "A Placebo-Controlled, Double-Blind, Randomized Trial of an Extract of *Ginkgo biloba* for Dementia. North American EGb

Study Group." *Journal of the American Medical Association* 278:16 (1997), 1327-1332.

61 J. Kleijnen and P. Knipschild. "*Ginkgo biloba*." *The Lancet* 340:8828 (November 1992), 1136-1139. M.H. Pittler and E. Ernst. "*Ginkgo biloba* Extract for the Treatment of Intermittent Claudication: A Meta-Analysis of Randomized Trials." *American Journal of Medicine* 108 (2000), 276-281.

62 P. Braquet, ed. *Ginkgolides: Chemistry, Biology, Pharmacology and Clinical Perspectives, Vol. 1* (Barcelona, Spain: J. Prous Science Publishers, 1988). P. Braquet, ed. *Ginkgolides: Chemistry, Biology, Pharmacology and Clinical Perspectives, Vol. 2* (Barcelona, Spain: J. Prous Science Publishers, 1989). E.W. Fungfeld, ed. Rokan: *Ginkgo biloba* (New York: Springer-Verlag, 1988).

63 S. Shibata et al. "Chemistry and Pharmacology of *Panax*." *Economic and Medicinal Plant Research* 1 (1985), 217-284.

64 I.I. Brekhman and I.V. Dardymov. "Pharmacological Investigation of Glycosides from Ginseng and *Eleutherococcus*." *Lloydia* 32 (1969), 46-51. E. Bombardelli, A. Cirstoni, and A. Lietti. "The Effect of Acute and Chronic *(Panax)* Ginseng Saponins Treatment on Adrenal Function; Biochemical and Pharmacological." *Proceedings 3rd International Ginseng Symposium* 1 (1980), 9-16. S.J. Fulder. "Ginseng and the Hypothalamic-Pituitary Control of Stress." *American Journal of Chinese Medicine* 9 (1981), 112-118.

65 L.M. Feng, H.Z. Pan, and W.W. Li. "Anti-Oxidant Action of *Panax Ginseng*." *Chung Hsi I Chieh Ho Tsa Chih* 7:5 (May 1987), 262, 288-290. H. Hikino et al. "Antihepatotoxic Actions of Ginsenosides from *Panax Ginseng* Roots." *Planta Medica* 52 (1985), 62-64. T.B. Ng and H.W. Yeung. "Hypoglycemic Constituents of *Panax Ginseng*." *General Pharmacology* 6 (1985), 549-552.

66 Y.S. Huo. "Anti-Senility Action of Saponin in *Panax Ginseng* Fruit in 327 Cases." *Chung Hsi I Chieh Ho Tsa Chih* 4:10 (October 1984), 578, 593-596.

67 C.N. Joo. 'The Preventative Effect of Korean *(P. ginseng)* Saponins on Aortic Atheroma Formation in Prolonged Cholesterol-Fed Rabbits." *Proceedings of the 3rd International Ginseng Symposium* (1980), 27-36. F. Scaglione et al. "Immunomodulatory Effects of Two Extracts of *Panax Ginseng* C.A. Meyer." *Drugs Under Experimental Clinical Research* 16:10 (1990), 537-542. M. Yamamoto and T. Uemura. "Endocrinological and Metabolic Actions of *P. Ginseng* Principles." *Proceeding 3rd International Ginseng Symposium* (1980), 115-119.

68 V. Vuksan et al. "American Ginseng *(Panax quinquefolius)* Reduces Postprandial Glycemia in Non-diabetic Subjects and Subjects with Type 2 Diabetes Mellitus." *Archives of Internal Medicine* 160 (2000), 1609-1613. V. Vuksan, J.L. Sievenpiper, and J. Wong. "American Ginseng *(Panax quinquefolius L.)* Attenuates Postprandial Glycemia in a Time-Dependent but Not Dose-Dependent Manner in Healthy Individuals." *American Journal of Clinical Nutrition* 73:4 (April 2001), 753-758.

69 D. Hoffmann. *The New Holistic Herbal* (Rockport, MA: Element, 1991), 204.

70 F.E. Hahn and J. Ciak. "Berberine." *Antibiotics and Chemotherapy* 3 (1976), 577-588.

71 V.P. Choudhry, M. Sabir, and V.N. Bhide. "Berberine in Giardiasis." *Indian Pediatrics* 9:3 (March 1972), 143-146.

72 Y. Kumazawa et al. "Activation of Peritoneal Macrophages by Berberine-Alkaloids in Terms of Induction of Cytostatic Activity." *International Journal of Immunopharmacology* 6 (1984), 587-592.

73 D. Hoffmann. *The New Holistic Herbal* (Rockport, MA: Element, 1991), 204.

74 C. Hobbs. "Hawthorn: A Literature Review." *HerbalGram* 21 (1990), 19-33.

75 M. Blumenthal and R. Upton, eds. *Hawthorn Leaf with Flower Extract*—Crataegus spp. (Soquel, CA: American Herbal Pharmacopoeia and Therapeutic Compendium, 1999).

76 M. Blumenthal et al. *Complete German Commission E Monographs—Therapeutic Guide to Herbal Medicines* (Austin, TX: American Botanical Council, Integrative Medicine Communications, 1998).

77 Ibid.

78 M. Blumenthal et al. *Complete German Commission E Monographs—Therapeutic Guide to Herbal Medicines* (Austin, TX: American Botanical Council, Integrative Medicine Communications, 1998). A. Fussel et al. "Effect of a Fixed Valerian-Hop Extract Combination (Ze 9109) on Sleep Polygraphy in Patients with Non-Organic Insomnia: A Pilot Study." *Eur J Med Res* 5 (2000), 385-390. M.J. Lataster and A. Brattstrom. "The Treatment of Patients with Sleep Disorders: Efficacy of Tolerance of Valerian-Hop Tablets." *Notabene Medici* 4 (1996), 182-185. B. Vonderheid-Guth et al. "Pharmacodynamic Effects of Valerian and Hops Extract Combination (Ze 9109) on the Quantitative-Topographical EEG in Healthy Volunteers." *Eur J Med Res* 5 (2000), 139-144.

79 M.H. Pittler and E. Ernst. "Horse-Chestnut Seed Extract for Chronic Venous Insufficiency: A Criteria-Based Systematic Review." *Archives of Dermatology* 134:11 (1998), 1356-1360.

80 M. Blumenthal et al. *Complete German Commission E Monographs—Therapeutic Guide to Herbal Medicines* (Austin, TX: American Botanical Council, Integrative Medicine Communications, 1998).

81 M.H. Pittler and E. Ernst. "Efficacy of Kava Extract for Treating Anxiety: A Systematic Review and Meta-Analysis." *Journal of Clinical Psychopharmacology* 20 (2000), 84-89.

82 D. Armanini et al. "Affinity of Licorice Derivatives for Mineralocorticoid and Glucocorticoid Receptors." *Clinical Endocrinology* 19 (November 1983), 609-612.

83 H. Hikino and Y. Kiso. "Natural Products for Liver Diseases." In: H. Wagner, H. Hikino, and N.R. Farnsworth, eds. *Economic and Medicinal Plant Research, Vol. 2* (London: Academic Press, 1988).

84 R. Pompei et al. "Antiviral Activity of Glycrrhizic Acid." *Experientia* 36 (March 1980), 304-305.

85 G. Vogel. "Natural Substances with Effects on the Liver." In: H. Wagner and P. Wolff, eds. *New Natural Products and Plant Drugs with Pharmacological, Biological or Therapeutic Activity* (Heidelberg, Germany: Springer-Verlag, 1977).

86 H. Hikino and Y. Kiso. "Natural Products for Liver Diseases." In: H. Wagner, H. Hikino, and N.R. Farnsworth, eds. *Economic and Medicinal Plant Research, Vol. 2* (London: Academic Press, 1988).

87 V. Fintelmann. "Modern Phytotherapy and Its Uses in Gastrointestinal Conditions." *Planta Medica* 57:7 (1991), S48-S52.

88 R.F. Weiss. *Herbal Medicine* (Beaconsfield, England: Beaconsfield Publishers, 1988), 261.

89 H. Wagner, F. Willer, and B. Kreher. "Biologically Active Compounds from the Aqueous Extract of *Urtica dioica*." *Planta Medica* 55:5 (October 1989), 452-454.

90 P. Mittman. "Randomized, Double-Blind Study of Freeze-Dried *Urtica dioica* in the Treatment of Allergic Rhinitis." *Planta Medica* 56:1 (February 1990), 44-47.

91 D. Hoffmann. *The New Holistic Herbal* (Rockport, MA: Element, 1991), 218.

92 H. Wagner et al. "Search for the Antiprostatic Principle of Stinging Nettle *(Urtica dioica)* Roots." *Phytomedicine* 1 (1994), 213-224. M. Blumenthal et al. *Complete German Commission E Monographs—Therapeutic Guide to Herbal Medicines* (Austin, TX: American Botanical Council, Integrative Medicine Communications, 1998).

93 German Ministry of Health. *Passion Flower Leaves* Commission E Monographs for Phytomedicines (Bonn, Germany: German Ministry of Health, 1985).

94 S. Foster. *Passion Flower* Botanical Series 314 (Austin, TX: American Botanical Council, 1993).

95 S. Foster. *Peppermint* Botanical Series 306 (Austin, TX: American Botanical Council, 1991).

96 German Ministry of Health. *Peppermint Oil* Commission E Monographs for Phytomedicines (Bonn, Germany: German Ministry of Health, 1986).

97 M.H. Pittler and E. Ernst. "Peppermint Oil for Irritable Bowel Syndrome: A Critical Review and Meta-Analysis." *American Journal of Gastroenterology* 93:7 (1998), 1131-1135.

98 M. Blumenthal et al. *Complete German Commission E Monographs—Therapeutic Guide to Herbal Medicines* (Austin, TX: American Botanical Council, Integrative Medicine Communications, 1998).

99 ESCOP, European Scientific Cooperative for Phytotherapy. *Peppermint Oil* (Meppel, The Netherlands: European Scientific Cooperative for Phytotherapy, 1992).

100 E. Bombardelli and P. Morazzoni. "*Prunus africana* (Hook. f.) Kalkm." *Fitoterapia* LXVIII:3 (1997), 205-218.

101 C. Chatelain, W. Autet, and F. Brackman. "Comparison of Once and Twice Daily Dosage Forms of *Pygeum africanum* Extract in Patients with Benign Prostatic Hyperplasia: A Randomized, Double-Blind Study, with Long-Term Open Label Extension." *Urology* 54 (1999), 473-478.

102 D. Hoffmann. *The New Holistic Herbal* (Rockport, MA: Element, 1991), 234.

103 I. Matei, E. Gafitanu, and V. Dorneanu. "Value of *Hypericum Perforatum* Oil in Dermatological Preparations." *Revista Medico-Chirurgicala Societatii de Medici Si Naturalisti Gin Iasi* 81:1 (January-March 1977), 73-74.

104 R. Melzer, U. Fricke, and J. Holzl. "Vasoactive Properties of Procyanidins from *Hypericum Perforatum L.* in Isolated Porcine Coronary Arteries." *Arzneimittelforschung* 41:5 (May 1991), 481-483.

105 O. Suzuki et al. "Inhibition of Monoamine Oxidase by Hypericin." *Planta Medica* 50 (1984), 272-274. H. Muldner and M. Zoller. "Antidepressive Effect of a Hypericum Extract Standardized to an Active Hypericine Complex: Biochemical and Clinical Studies." *Arzneimittelforschung* 34:8 (1984), 918-920.

106 G. Champault, J.C. Patel, and A.M. Bonnard. "A Double-Blind Trial of an Extract of the Plant *Serenoa Repens* in Benign Prostatic Hyperplasia." *British Journal of Clinical Pharmacology* 18 (1984), 461-462. C. Boccafoschi and S. Annoscia. "Comparison of *Serenoa Repens* Extract with Placebo by Controlled Clinical Trial in Patients with Prostatic Adenomatosis." *Urologia* 50 (1983), 1257-1268.

107 T.J. Wilt et al. "Saw Palmetto Extracts for Treatment of Benign Prostatic Hyperplasia." *Journal of the American Medical Association* 280:18 (1998), 1604-1609.

108 L.S. Marks, D.L. Hess, and F.J. Dorey. "Tissue Effects of Saw Palmetto and Finasteride: Use of Biopsy Cores for *In Situ* Quantification of Prostatic Androgens." *Urology* 57 (2001), 999–1005.

109 L.S. Marks et al. "Effects of a Saw Palmetto Herbal Blend in Men with Symptomatic Benign Prostatic Hyperplasia." *Journal of Urology* 163:5 (May 2000), 1451–1456.

110 ESCOP, European Scientific Cooperative for Phytotherapy. *Valerian Root* (Meppel, The Netherlands: European Scientific Cooperative for Phytotherapy, 1990). German Ministry of Health. *Senna Commission E Monographs for Phytomedicines* (Bonn, Germany: German Ministry of Health, 1984–).

111 German Ministry of Health. *Valerian Commission E Monographs for Phytomedicines* (Bonn, Germany: German Ministry of Health, 1985).

112 ESCOP, European Scientific Cooperative for Phytotherapy. *Valerian Root* (Meppel, The Netherlands: European Scientific Cooperative for Phytotherapy, 1990).

113 C. Hobbs. "Valerian: A Literature Review." *HerbalGram* 21 (1989), 19–34.

114 A. Fussel et al. "Effect of a Fixed Valerian-Hop Extract Combination (Ze 9109) on Sleep Polygraphy in Patients with Non-Organic Insomnia: A Pilot Study." *Eur J Med Res* 5 (2000), 385–390. M.J. Lataster and A. Brattstrom. "The Treatment of Patients with Sleep Disorders: Efficacy of Tolerance of Valerian-Hop Tablets." *Notabene Medici* 4 (1996), 182–185. B. Vonderheid-Guth et al. "Pharmacodynamic Effects of Valerian and Hops Extract Combination (Ze 9109) on the Quantitative-Topographical EEG in Healthy Volunteers." *Eur J Med Res* 5 (2000), 139–144. M. Blumenthal et al. *Complete German Commission E Monographs—Therapeutic Guide to Herbal Medicines* (Austin, TX: American Botanical Council, Integrative Medicine Communications, 1998).

115 "Drug Therapy of Hemorrhoids: Proven Results of Therapy with a Hamamelis Containing Hemorrhoid Ointment—Results of a Meeting of Experts. Dresden, 30 August 1991." *Fortschritte der Medizin* 109:Suppl 116 (1991), 1–11.

116 P. Bernard et al. "Venitonic Pharmacodynamic Value of Galenic Preparations with a Base of Hamamelis Leaves." *Journal de Pharmacie de Belgique* 27:4 (July–August 1972), 505–512.

HOMEOPATHY

1 R.H. Bannerman, J. Burton, and C. Wen Chieh, eds. *Traditional Medicine and Health Care Coverage* (Geneva, Switzerland: World Health Organization, 1983).

2 D. Eskinazi. "Homeopathy Revisited: Is Homeopathy Compatible with Biomedical Observations?" *Archives of Internal Medicine* 159 (September 1999), 1981–1987.

3 A. Lange. "Homeopathy." In: J.E. Pizzorno and M.T. Murray, eds. *A Textbook of Natural Medicine* (Seattle WA: John Bastyr College Publications, 1989).

4 D. Eskinazi. "Homeopathy Revisited: Is Homeopathy Compatible with Biomedical Observations?" *Archives of Internal Medicine* 159 (September 1999), 1981–1987.

5 S. Hahnemann. Translated by W. Boericke, M.D. *Organon of Medicine* (New Dehli: B. Jain Publishing, 1992).

6 R.B. Smith, Jr., and G.W. Boericke. "Changes Caused by Succussion on N.M.R. Patterns and Bioassay of Bradykinin Triacetate (BKTA) Succussions and Dilution." *Journal of the American Institute of Homeopathy* 61 (November/December 1968), 197–212.

7 E. Del Giudice and G. Preparata. "Superradiance: A New Approach to Coherent Dynamical Behaviors of Condensed Matter." *Frontier Perspectives* 1:2 (Fall/Winter 1990).

8 B. Rubik. "Frontiers of Homeopathic Research." *Frontier Perspectives* 2:1 (Spring/Summer 1991).

9 R. Gerber, M.D. *Vibrational Medicine* (Santa Fe, NM: Bear & Company, 1988), 84.

10 D. Eskinazi. "Homeopathy Revisited: Is Homeopathy Compatible with Biomedical Observations?" *Archives of Internal Medicine* 159 (September 1999), 1981–1987.

11 R. Leviton. "Homeopathy." *Yoga Journal* 85 (March/April 1989), 42–51, 97–98, 100, 105.

12 C. Day. *The Homeopathic Treatment of Small Animals: Principles and Practice* (Essex, England: C.W. Daniel, 1990).

13 G. Vithoulkas. "Homeopathy." In: R.H. Bannerman, J. Burton, and C. Wen Chieh, eds. *Traditional Medicine and Health Care Coverage* (Geneva, Switzerland: World Health Organization, 1983).

14 J. Kleignen et al. "Clinical Trials of Homeopathy." *British Medical Journal* 302 (February 1991), 316–323.

15 R.G. Gibson et al. "Homeopathic Therapy in Rheumatoid Arthritis: Evaluation by Double-Blind Clinical Therapeutic Trial." *British Journal of Clinical Pharmacology* 9 (May 1980), 453–459. M. Shipley et al. "Controlled Trial of Homeopathic Treatment of Osteoarthritis." *The Lancet* 1 (1983), 97–98. A.M. Scofield. "Experimental Research in Homeopathy: A Critical Review." *British Homeopathic Journal* 73 (1984), 161–266.

16 J.P. Ferley et al. "A Controlled Evaluation of a Homeopathic Preparation in the Treatment of Influenza-Like Syndromes." *British Journal of Clinical Pharmacology* 27 (March 1989), 329–335.

17 R.A. Anderson. *The Scientific Basis for Homeopathic Medicine* (Lynwood, WA: American Health Press, 2000), 434.

18 Ibid.

19 P. Fisher et al. "Effect of Homeopathic Treatment on Fibrositis (Primary Fibromyalgia)." *British Medical Journal* 299 (1989), 365–366.

20 M.A. Taylor et al. "Randomised Controlled Trial of Homeopathy versus Placebo in Perennial Allergic Rhinitis with Overview of Four Trial Series." *British Medical Journal* 321 (August 19–26, 2000), 471–476.

21 R.A. Anderson. *The Scientific Basis for Homeopathic Medicine* (Lynwood, WA: American Health Press, 2000), 435.

22 K.H. Friese et al. "The Homeopathic Treatment of Otitis Media in Children: Comparisons with Conventional Therapy." *International Journal of Clinical Pharmacology and Therapeutics* 35:7 (July 1997), 296–301.

23 D.T. Reilly et al. "Is Homeopathy a Placebo Response: Controlled Trial of Homeopathic Potency, with Pollen in Hayfever as Model." *The Lancet* 2:8512 (October 1986), 881–886.

24 H. Albertini et al. "Homeopathic Treatment of Neuralgia Using *Arnica* and *Hypericum*: A Summary of 60 Observations." *Journal of the American Institute of Homeopathy* 78 (September 1985), 126–128.

25 W. Gerhard. "The Biological Treatment of Migraines, Based on Experience." *Biological Therapy* 5:3 (June 1988), 67–71.

26 S. Zenner and H. Metelmann. "Therapeutic Use of *Lymphomyosot*: Results of a Multicenter Use Observation Study on 3,512 Patients." *Biological Therapy* 8:3 (June 1990), 49. See also: *Biological Therapy* 8:4 (October 1990), 79.

27 H.L. Coulter. *Divided Legacy: A History of the Schism in Medical Thought, Vol. 2* (Washington, DC: Wehawken Book Company, 1973–1977).

28 D. Ullman. *Homeopathy: Medicine for the 21st Century* (Berkeley, CA: North Atlantic Books, 1988), 126. *Discovering Homeopathy: Medicine for the 21st Century* (Berkeley, CA: North Atlantic Books, 1991).

29 H.L. Coulter. *Divided Legacy: A History of the Schism in Medical Thought, Vol. 2* (Washington, DC: Wehawken Book Company, 1973–1977).

30 T. Cook. *Samuel Hahnemann: The Founder of Homeopathic Medicine* (Wellingborough, Northhamptonshire, England: Thorsons, 1981).

31 H.L. Coulter. *Divided Legacy: A History of the Schism in Medical Thought, Vol. 2* (Washington, DC: Wehawken Book Company, 1973–1977).

32 S. McAuliffe. "Homeopathy Goes Mainstream: New Treatments for Old Ills." *Longevity* 4:12 (November 1992), 62.

HYDROTHERAPY

1 L. Chaitow. *The Body/Mind Purification Program* (New York: Simon and Schuster, 1990).

2 W. Boyle and A. Saine. *Lectures in Naturopathic Hydrotherapy* (East Palestine, OH: Buckeye Naturopathic Press, 1991).

3 H. Weatherburn. "Hyperthermia and AIDS Treatment." *British Journal of Radiology* 61 (September 1988), 862–863.

4 L. Chaitow. *The Body/Mind Purification Program* (New York: Simon and Schuster, 1990).

5 P. Airola. *How to Get Well* (Sherwood, OR: Health Plus Publishers, 1990).

6 A. Thrash, M.D. *Home Remedies: Hydrotherapy, Massage, Charcoal, and Other Simple Treatments* (Groveland, CA: New Life Books, 1981).

7 D.D. Buchman. *The Complete Book of Water Therapy* (New York: Dutton, 1979).

8 P. Airola. *How to Get Well* (Sherwood, OR: Health Plus Publishers, 1990).

HYPERTHERMIA

1 D. Tyrrell, I. Barrow, and J. Arthur. "Local Hyperthermia Benefits Natural and Experimental Common Colds." *British Medical Journal* 298 (1989), 1280–1283.

2 B. Spire et al. "Inactivation of Lymphadenopathy-Associated Virus by Heat, Gamma Rays, and Ultraviolet Light." *The Lancet* 1:8422 (January 26, 1985), 188–189.

3 A. Thrash, M.D. *Home Remedies* (Groveland, CA: New Life Books, 1981).

4 L. Standish et al. "One Year Open Trial of Naturopathic Treatment of HIV Infection Class IV-A in Men." *Journal of Naturopathic Medicine* 3:1 (1992), 42–64.

5 H. Weatherburn. "Hyperthermia and AIDS Treatment." *British Journal of Radiology* 61:729 (September 1988), 862–863.

6 D. Tyrrell, I. Barrow, and J. Arthur. "Local Hyperthermia Benefits Natural and Experimental Common Colds." *British Medical Journal* 298 (1989), 1280–1283.

7 A.W.T. Konings. "Membranes as Targets for Hyperthermic Cell Killing." *Recent Results in Cancer Research* 109 (1988), 9-21. G. Toffoli et al. "Effect of Hyperthermia on Intracellular Drug Accumulation and Chemosensitivity in Drug-Sensitive and Drug-Resistant P388 Leukaemia Cell Lines." *International Journal of Hyperthermia* 5:2 (1989), 163-172.

8 M.M. Park et al. "The Effect of Whole Body Hyperthermia on the Immune Cell Activity of Cancer Patients." *Lymphokine Research* 9:2 (1990), 213-223.

9 A.J. Neville and D.N. Sauder. "Whole Body Hyperthermia (41(-42(C) Induces Interleukin-1 *in Vivo*." *Lymphokine Research* 7:3 (Fall 1988), 201-206.

10 A.C. Guyton, M.D. *Textbook of Medical Physiology* (Philadelphia: W.B. Saunders, 1986).

11 Summary of Abstracts, 22nd International Clinical Hyperthermia Society (September 23, 1999). Available on the Internet: www.hyperthermia-ichs.org. H. Ge and J. Huang. "Regional Hyperthermia in the Treatment of Primary Hepatic Carcinoma." *Journal of Surgical Oncology* 74:3 (July 2000), 193-195. M. Hiruma and A. Kawada. "Hyperthermic Treatment of Bowen's Disease with Disposable Chemical Pocket Warmers: A Report of 8 Cases." *Journal of the American Academy of Dermatology* 43:6 (December 2000), 1070-1075. H. Riess et al. "A Pilot Study of a New Therapeutic Approach in the Treatment of Locally Advanced Stages of Rectal Cancer: Neoadjuvant Radiation, Chemotherapy and Regional Hyperthermia." *European Journal of Cancer* 31A:7-8 (July-August 1995), 1356-1360.

12 Z.R. Gard, M.D., and E.J. Brown. "Literature Review and Comparison Studies of Sauna/Hyperthermia in Detoxification." *Townsend Letter for Doctors* 107 (June 1992), 470-478.

13 M.A. Harvey, M.M. McRorie, and D.W. Smith. "Suggested Limits to the Use of the Hot Tub and Sauna by Pregnant Women." *Canadian Medical Association Journal* 125 (July 1981), 50-53.

14 N.M. Sawtell and R.L. Thompson. "Rapid *in Vivo* Reactivation of Herpes Simplex Virus in Latently Infected Murine Ganglionic Neurons after Transient Hyperthermia." *Journal of Virology* 66:4 (April 1992), 2150-2156.

15 J.L. Skibba et al. "Oxidative Stress as a Precursor to the Irreversible Hepatocellular Injury Caused by Hyperthermia." *International Journal of Hyperthermia* 7:5 (September/October 1991), 749-761.

16 U.S. Centers for Disease Control. "Self-Induced Malaria Associated with Malariotherapy for Lyme Disease—Texas." *Journal of the American Medical Association* 266:16 (October 1991), 2199.

HYPNOTHERAPY

1 R.M. Hackman et al. "Hypnosis and Asthma: A Critical Review." *Journal of Asthma* 37:1 (2000), 1-15.

2 S. Findlay, D. Podolsky, and J. Silberner. "Wonder Cures from the Fringe." *U.S. News and World Report* 3:13 (September 23, 1991), 68-74.

3 R.H. Bannerman, J. Burton, and C. Wen Chieh, eds. *Traditional Medicine and Health Care Coverage* (Geneva, Switzerland: World Health Organization, 1983), Chapter 13.

4 K.G. Olsen. "Hypnosis and Hypnotherapy." *The Encyclopedia of Alternative Health Care* (New York: Pocket Books, 1989, 1990).

5 M.E. Faymonville et al. "Hypnosis and Its Application in Surgery." *Rev Med Liege* 53:7 (1998), 414-418. E.V. Lang et al. "Adjunctive Non-Pharmacological Analgesia for Invasive Medical Procedures: A Randomised Trial." *The Lancet* 355:9214 (2000), 1486-1490.

6 M.M. Tinterow, M.D. "Hypnotherapy for Chronic Pain." *Kansas Medicine* 88:6 (June 1987), 190-192, 204.

7 M.M. Tinterow, M.D. "The Use of Hypnotic Anesthesia for Major Surgical Procedure." *The American Surgeon* 26 (November 1960), 732-737.

8 M.M. Tinterow, M.D. "Hypnotherapy for Chronic Pain." *Kansas Medicine* 88:6 (June 1987), 190-192, 204.

9 A.A. Barrios. "Hypnotherapy: A Reappraisal." *Psychotherapy: Theory, Research and Practice* 7:1 (Spring 1970), 2-7.

10 G. Sunnen with B. DeBetz. "Miscellaneous Medical Applications of Hypnosis." In: *A Primer of Clinical Hypnosis* (Boston: PSG Publishing, 1985), 221-226.

11 Ibid.

12 G. Sunnen. "Hypnosis in Psychosomatic Medicine." Available on the Internet: www.trioc.com/sunnen/topics/psychosomatic.htm.

13 R.M. Hackman, et al. "Hypnosis and Asthma: A Critical Review." *Journal of Asthma* 37:1 (2000), 1-15.

14 R.J. Leventhal. "Management of Fibromyalgia." *Annals of Internal Medicine* 131:11 (1999), 850-858.

15 R.M. Houghton et al. "Gut-Focused Hypnotherapy Normalises Rectal Hypersensitivity in Patients with Irritable Bowel Syndrome (IBS)." Paper presented at the Annual Meeting of the American Gastroenterological Association, Orlando, Florida (May 16-19, 1999).

16 S.M. Sellick and C. Zaza. "Critical Review of 5 Nonpharmacologic Strategies for Managing Cancer Pain." *Cancer Prevention and Control* 2:1 (1998), 7-14.

17 C.S. Ginandes and D.I. Rosenthal. "Using Hypnosis to Accelerate the Healing of Bone Fractures: A Randomized Controlled Pilot Study." *Alternative Therapies in Health and Medicine* 5:2 (1999), 67-75.

18 G.J. Wood and H.H. Zadeh. "Potential Adjunctive Applications of Hypnosis in the Management of Periodontal Diseases." *American Journal of Clinical Hypnosis* 41:3 (1999), 212-225.

19 A. Vickers and C. Zollman. "Hypnosis and Relaxation Therapies." *British Medical Journal* 319:7221 (1999), 1346-1349.

20 K.I. Saichek. "Hypnotherapy." In: D.W. Novey, ed. *Clinician's Complete Reference to Complementary and Alternative Medicine* (St. Louis, MO: Mosby, 2000), 53-63.

21 G.J. Pratt, D.P. Wood, and B.M. Alman. *A Clinical Hypnosis Primer* (La Jolla, CA: Psychology and Consulting Associates Press, 1984).

LIGHT THERAPY

1 J. Ott. "Color and Light: Their Effects on Plants, Animals and People." *International Journal of Biosocial Research* 7-10 (1985-1988), 1-131.

2 P.A. Roos. "Light and Electromagnetic Waves: The Health Implications." *Journal of the Bio-Electro-Magnetics Institute* 3:2 (Summer 1991), 7-12.

3 J. Ott. *Health and Light* (Old Greenwich, CT: The Devin-Adair Company, 1973).

4 *National Institute of Health Report* (Washington, DC: United States Health Service, National Institutes of Health, 1978).

5 P.A. Roos. "Light and Electromagnetic Waves: The Health Implications." *Journal of the Bio-Electro Magnetics Institute* 3:2 (Summer 1991), 7-12.

6 A.R. Kennedy, M.A. Ritter, J.B. Little. "Fluorescent Light Induces Malignant Transformation in Mouse Embryo Cell Cultures." *Science* 207:4436 (1980), 1209-1211.

7 F.C. Garland et al. "Occupational Sunlight Exposure and Melanoma in the U.S. Navy." *Archives of Environmental Health* 45 (1990), 261-267.

8 V. Beral et al. "Malignant Melanoma and Exposure to Fluorescent Lighting at Work." *The Lancet* 2:8293 (August 7, 1982), 290-293.

9 "Excessive Sunlight Exposure, Skin Melanoma, Linked to Vitamin D." *International Journal of Biosocial and Medical Research* 13:1 (1991), 13-14.

10 J.N. Ott in an interview with J.S. Bland. *Preventive Medicine Update* (January 1991).

11 A.J. Lewy, T.A. Wehr, and F.K. Goodwin. "Light Suppresses Melatonin Secretion in Humans." *Science* (December 1980), 210.

12 J.W. Hyman. *The Light Book* (New York: Ballantine Books, 1991).

13 "Excessive Sunlight Exposure, Skin Melanoma, Linked to Vitamin D." *International Journal of Biosocial and Medical Research* 13:1 (1991), 13-14.

14 J. Ott. "The Effect of Color and Light: Part 3." *International Journal of Biosocial Research* 9 (1987), 71-107. W.P. London. "Full-Spectrum Classroom Light and Sickness in Pupils." *The Lancet* 2:8569 (November 21, 1987), 1205-1206.

15 F.C. Garland et al. "Occupational Sunlight Exposure and Melanoma in the U.S. Navy." *Archives of Environmental Health* 45 (1990), 261-267.

16 P. Recer. "Sun May Prevent Breast Cancer." *Seattle Post-Intelligencer* (November 4, 1997), A1, A4.

17 Z.R. Kime. *Sunlight* (Penryn, CA: World Health Publications, 1980).

18 "Winter Blues? Try a Little Morning Light." *Bioenergy Health Newsletter* (December 1987), 7.

19 G. Gutfeld. "The New Science of Rays and Rhythms: Cutting-Edge Light Therapies That Can Brighten Your Health." *Prevention* 45:2 (February 1993), 67-71, 116-123.

20 "Winter Blues? Try a Little Morning Light." *Bioenergy Health Newsletter* (December 1987), 7.

21 K.A. Laycock et al. "Characterization of a Murine Model of Recurrent Herpes Simplex Viral Keratitis Induced by Ultraviolet B Radiation." *Investigative Opthamology and Visual Science* 32:10 (September 1991), 2741-2746. H.R. Taylor. "Ultraviolet Radiation and the Eye: An Epidemiologic Study." *Transactions of the American Ophthalmological Society* 87 (1990), 802-853. H.R. Taylor. "The Biologic Effects of UV-B on the Eye." *Photochemistry and Photobiology* 50:4 (October 1989), 489-492.

22 M. Walker. *The Power of Color: The Art & Science of Making Colors Work for You* (Garden City Park, NY: Avery Publishing Group, 1991).

23 S.V. Kravkov. "Color, Vision and the Autonomic Nervous System." *Journal of the Optical Society of America* 31 (April 1944), 335-337.

24 H.J. Vreman et al. "Light-Emitting Diodes: A Novel Light Source for Phototherapy." *Pediatrics Research* 44:5 (1998), 804-809. A.M. Sazonov et al. "Low-Intensity Non-Coherent Red Light in the Comprehensive Treatment of Gastroduodenal Ulcers." *Soviet Medicine* 12 (1985), 42-46.

25 W.C. Symonds and B. Bremner. "A Ray of Hope for Cancer Patients: Photodynamic Therapy May Stop Early-Stage Tumors." *Business Week* (June 10, 1996), 104-106.

1128

26 Ibid.

27 J. Liberman. *Light: Medicine of the Future* (Santa Fe, NM: Bear and Company, 1991).

LONGEVITY MEDICINE

1 R.G. Cutler. "Evolution of Human Longevity: A Critical Overview." *Mech Ageing Dev* 9:3-4 (February 1979), 337-354. H. Markowe. "Health Trends in the Last 75 Years." *Health Trends* 26 (1994), 98-105. K.G. Manton and J.W. Vaupel. "Survival After the Age of 80 in the United States, Sweden, France, England and Japan." *New England Journal of Medicine* 333 (1995), 1232-1235.

2 J.R. Wilmoth et al. "Increase of Maximum Life Span in Sweden, 1861-1999." *Science* 289:5488 (2000), 2366-2368. J.R. Wilmoth. "Demography of Longevity: Past, Present, and Future Trends." *Experimental Gerontology* 35:9-10 (2000), 1111-1129.

3 Jeffrey S. Bland. *Improving Genetic Expression in the Prevention of the Diseases of Aging* (Monograph), 4.

4 "Telomeres: Beginning to Understand the End." *Science* 270:5242 (December 8, 1995), 1601-1607. W.E. Wright and J.W. Shay. "The Two-Stage Mechanism Controlling Cellular Senescence and Immortalization." *Experimental Gerontology* 27:4 (1992), 383-389.

5 "Positional Cloning of the Werners Syndrome Gene." *Science* 272:5259 (April 12, 1996), 258-262.

6 National Institutes of Health. *Biochemistry and Aging* (Washington, DC: National Institutes of Health, 1997).

7 "Good Habits Outweigh Genes as Key to a Healthy Old Age." *The New York Times* (February 28, 1996). Jeffrey S. Bland. *Improving Genetic Expression in the Prevention of the Diseases of Aging* (Monograph), 18-19.

8 Jeffrey S. Bland. *Improving Genetic Expression in the Prevention of the Diseases of Aging* (Monograph), 19.

9 R.G. Cutler. "Alterations with Age in the Informational Storage and Flow Systems of the Mammalian Cell." *Birth Defects* 14:1 (1978), 463-498. U.T. Brunk, C.B. Jones, and R.S. Sohal. "A Novel Hypothesis of Lipofuscinogenesis and Cellular Aging Based on Interactions Between Oxidative Stress and Autophagocytosis." *Mutation Research* 275:3-6 (1992), 395-403.

10 A.M. McCormick and J. Campisi. "Cellular Aging and Senescence." *Current Opinion in Cell Biology* 3 (1991), 230-234.

11 E. Lonn et al. "Effects of Oxygen Free Radicals and Scavengers on the Cardiac Extracellular Collagen Matrix During Ischemia-Reperfusion." *Canadian Journal of Cardiology* 10:2 (1994), 203-213.

12 Jeffrey S. Bland. *Improving Genetic Expression in the Prevention of the Diseases of Aging* (Monograph), 27-28.

13 Jeffrey S. Bland. *Improving Genetic Expression in the Prevention of the Diseases of Aging* (Monograph), 72. A.T. Lee and A. Cerami. "Role of Glycation in Aging." *Annals of the New York Academy of Sciences* 663:1 (1992), 63-70.

14 Jeffrey S. Bland. *Improving Genetic Expression in the Prevention of the Diseases of Aging* (Monograph), 107.

15 Ibid., 79-80.

16 *British Medical Journal* 315 (1997), 1-10.

17 A. Whittemore et al. "Diet, Physical Activity and Colorectal Cancer Among Chinese in North America and China." *Journal of the National Cancer Institute* 82 (1990), 915-926. J. Barone et al. "Dietary Fat and Natural Killer Cell Activity." *American Journal of Clinical Nutrition* 50 (1989), 861-867.

18 British Medical Association. "Diet, Nutrition and Health." *BMA Report* 4:11 (1986), 49.

19 Position statement of the American Dietetic Association. "Vegetarian Diets" (1997).

20 Dharma Singh Khalsa, M.D. *Brain Longevity* (New York: Warner Books, 1997), 267.

21 Ibid., 262.

22 Ibid., 251.

23 Melvyn R. Werbach, M.D. and Michael T. Murray, N.D. *Botanical Influences on Illness* (Tarzana, CA: Third Line Press, 1998), 119.

24 R.C. Wren, F.L.S. *Potter's New Cyclopaedia of Botanical Drugs and Preparations* (London: Saffron Walden/C.W. Daniel Company, 1994), 128-129.

25 Jack Masquelier. "Recent Advances in the Therapeutic Activity of Procyanidins, Natural Products as Medicinal Agents." In: J.L. Beal and E. Reinhard, eds. Supplement of *Plant Medica, Journal of Medicinal Plant Research*, and *Journal of Natural Products* (July 1980), 244-255.

26 Dharma Singh Khalsa, M.D. *Brain Longevity* (New York: Warner Books, 1997), 51.

27 H. Baker et al. "Vitamin Profiles in Elderly Persons Living at Home or in Nursing Homes, Versus Profiles in Healthy Subjects." *Journal of the American Geriatric Society* 27 (1979), 444.

28 James F. Balch, M.D., and Phyllis A. Balch, C.N.C. *Prescription for Nutritional Healing* (Garden City Park, NY: Avery Publishing Group, 1997), 15.

29 Ibid., 16-17, 51.

30 Alex Schauss. *Minerals and Human Health* (Hurricane, UT: Life Sciences Press, 1995), 1-3.

31 M. Scofield. *Work Site Health Promotion* (Philadelphia: Hanley & Belfus, 1990), 459.

32 Hans Selye, M.D. *Stress Without Distress* (New York: J.B. Lippincott, 1974), 93-94.

33 Kenneth Bock, M.D., and Nellie Sabin. *The Road to Immunity* (New York: Simon & Schuster, 1997), 77-87.

34 M.R. Werbach, M.D. *Nutritional Influences on Illness* (New Canaan, CT: Keats Publishing, 1988).

35 R.F. Weiss. *Herbal Medicine* (Gothenburg, Sweden: A.B. Arcanum, 1988).

36 Dharma Singh Khalsa, M.D. *Brain Longevity* (New York: Warner Books, 1997).

37 Darryl See, M.D. Personal communication (2000).

MAGNETIC FIELD THERAPY

1 R.O. Becker, M.D. *Cross Currents: The Promise of Electromedicine, The Perils of Electropollution* (Los Angeles: Jeremy P. Tarcher, 1990).

2 A.R. Davis and W.C. Rawls. *Magnetism and Its Effects on the Living System* (New York: Exposition Press, 1974).

3 R.O. Becker, M.D. *Cross Currents: The Promise of Electromedicine, The Perils of Electropollution* (Los Angeles: Jeremy P. Tarcher, 1990), 187.

4 R.O. Becker and A.A. Marino. *Electromagnetism & Life* (Albany, NY: State University of New York Press, 1982). R.O. Becker and G. Seldon. *The Body Electric: Electromagnetism & the Foundation of Life* (New York: William Morrow, 1986).

5 *New Encyclopedia, Vol. 24* (Chicago: Encyclopedia Britannica, 1986), 200.

6 K. Nakagawa, M.D. "Magnetic Field Deficiency Syndrome and Magnetic Treatment." *Japanese Medical Journal* 2745 (December 1976).

7 N. Wertheimer and E. Leeper. "Electrical Wiring Configurations and Childhood Cancer." *American Journal of Epidemiology* 109 (1979), 273-284.

8 J. Wolpay. *Biological Effects of Power Line Fields* (New York State Power-Lines Project Scientific Advisory Panel, 1987).

9 M. Speers, J. Dobbins, and V. Miller. "Occupational Exposures and Brain Cancer Mortality: A Preliminary Study of East Texas Residents." *American Journal of Industrial Medicine* 13 (1988), 629-638.

10 M. Feychting and A. Ahlbom. "Childhood Leukemia and Residential Exposure to Weak Extremely Low Frequency Magnetic Fields." *Environmental Health Perspectives* Suppl 2 (1995), 59-62. See also: D.A. Savitz. "Overview of Epidemiologic Research on Electric and Magnetic Fields and Cancer." *American Ind Hyg Association Journal* 54:4 (1993), 197-204.

11 R.O. Becker, M.D. *Cross Currents: The Promise of Electromedicine, The Perils of Electropollution* (Los Angeles: Jeremy P. Tarcher, 1990), 208.

12 C. Smith and S. Best. *Electromagnetic Man: Health and Hazard in the Electrical Environment* (London: J.M. Dent and Sons, 1989).

13 J.C. Murphy et al. "International Commission for Protection Against Environmental Mutagens and Carcinogens. Power Frequency Electric and Magnetic Fields: A Review of Genetic Toxicology." *Mutation Research* 296:3 (March 1993), 221-240.

14 R.O. Becker, M.D. *Cross Currents: The Promise of Electromedicine, The Perils of Electropollution* (Los Angeles: Jeremy P. Tarcher, 1990), 210.

15 J. Fontenot and S.A. Levine. "Melatonin Deficiency: Its Role in Oncogenesis and Age-Relative Pathology." *Journal of Orthomolecular Medicine* 5:1 (1990), 22-24.

16 Ron Lawrence, M.D., Ph.D., Paul J. Rosch, M.D., F.A.C.P., and Judith Plowden. *Magnet Therapy: The Pain Cure Alternative* (Rocklin, CA: Prima Health, 1998), 38.

17 R.O. Becker and G. Seldon. *The Body Electric: ElectroMagnetism and the Foundation of Life* (New York: William Morrow, 1986).

18 Ron Lawrence, M.D., Ph.D., and Paul J. Rosch, M.D., F.A.C.P. *Magnet Therapy: The Pain Cure Alternative* (Rocklin, CA: Prima Publishing, 1998), 117.

19 W. Philpott and S. Taplin. *Biomagnetic Handbook* (Choctaw, OK: Enviro-Tech Products, 1990).

20 D. Man et al. "Effect of Permanent Magnetic Field on Postoperative Pain and Wound Healing in Plastic Surgery." Paper presented at the Second World Congress for Electricity and Magnetism in Biology and Medicine, Bologna, Italy (June 8-13, 1997). J. Jerabek and W. Pawluk. *Magnetic Therapy in Eastern Europe: A Review of 30 Years of Research* (Chicago: William Pawluk, M.D., 1998), 53, 65, 67.

21 J.C. Mulier and F. Spaas. "Out-Patient Treatment of Surgically Resistant Non-Unions Induced Pulsing Current—Clinical Results." *Arch Orthop Trauma Surg* 97:4 (1980), 293-297.

22 R. Sandyk. "Alzheimer's Disease: Improvement of Visual Memory and Visuoconstructive Performance Treatment with Picotesla Range Magnetic Fields." *International Journal of Neuroscience* 76:3-4 (June 1994), 185-225.

23 R. Sandyk. "Magnetic Fields in the Therapy of Parkinsonism." *International Journal of Neuroscience* 66:3-4 (October 1992), 209-235. R. Sandyk. "A Drug Naïve Parkinsonian Patient Successfully

Treated with Weak Electromagnetic Fields." *International Journal of Neuroscience* 79:1-2 (1994), 99-110. R. Sandyk and K. Derpapas. "The Effects of External Picotesla Range Magnetic Fields on the EEG in Parkinson's Disease." *International Journal of Neuroscience* 70:1-2 (1993), 85-96.

24 Y. Omote. "An Experimental Attempt to Potentiate Therapeutic Effects of Combined Use of Pulsing Magnetic Fields and Antitumor Agents." *Nippon Geka Gakkai Zasshi* 89:8 (August 1988), 1155-1166.

25 M. Riviere et al. "Test with Lymphosarcoma on Mice." *Comptes Rendus de'l'Academie des Sciences* (March 1, 1965).

26 I. Troeng. Commenting on the study's results. Laholm, Sweden (July 1984). See: M. Riviere et al. "Test with Lymphosarcoma on Mice." *Comptes Rendus de'l'Academie des Sciences* (March 1, 1965).

27 B. Pasche et al. "Effects of Low Energy Emission Therapy in Chronic Psychophysiological Insomnia." *Sleep* 19:4 (1996), 327-336.

28 T. Zyss. "Deep Magnetic Brain Stimulation—The End of Psychiatric Electroshock Therapy?" *Medical Hypotheses* 43:2 (1994), 69-74.

MIND/BODY MEDICINE

1 E.L. Idler, S.V. Kasl, and J.H. Lemke. "Self-Evaluated Health and Mortality Among the Elderly in New Haven, Connecticut, and Iowa and Washington Counties, Iowa, 1982-1986." *American Journal of Epidemiology* 131:1 (January 1990), 91-103.

2 M.H. Antoni et al. "Cognitive-Behavioral Stress Management Intervention Buffers Distress Responses and Immunologic Changes Following Notification of HIV-1 Seropositivity." *Journal of Consulting and Clinical Psychology* 59:6 (December 1991), 906-915. M.H. Antoni et al. "Psychological and Neuroendocrine Measures Related to Functional Immune Changes in Anticipation of HIV-1 Serostatus Notification." *Psychosomatic Medicine* 52:5 (September-October 1990), 496-510. H. Benson et al. "Decreased Blood Pressure in Borderline Hypertensive Subjects Who Practiced Meditation." *Journal of Chronic Diseases* 27:3 (March 1974), 163-169. M.A. Chesney et al. "Nonpharmacologic Approaches to the Treatment of Hypertension." *Circulation* 76:1 Part 2 (July 1987), I104-I109. M. Caudill et al. "Decreased Clinic Use by Chronic Pain Patients: Response to Behavioral Medicine Intervention." *Clinical Journal of Pain* 7:4 (December 1991), 305-310.

3 D.L. Healy et al. "The Thymus-Adrenal Connection: Thymosin has Corticotropin-Releasing Activity in Primates." *Science* 222:4630 (1983), 1353-1355.

4 R. Ader and N. Cohen. "Behaviorally Conditioned Immunosuppression." *Psychosomatic Medicine* 37:4 (July-August 1975), 333-340. V.K. Ghanta et al. "Neural and Environmental Influence on Neoplasia and Conditioning of NK Activity." *Journal of Immunology* 135:2 Suppl (August 1985), 848S-852S.

5 B. Moyers. *Healing and the Mind* (New York: Doubleday, 1993).

6 J. Borysenko. *Minding the Body/Mending the Mind* (New York: Bantam Books, 1988).

7 J.V. Basmajian. "Learned Control of Single Motor Units." In: G. Schwartz and J. Beatty, eds. *Biofeedback: Theory and Research* (New York: Academic Press, 1977), 415-431.

8 M. Murphy. *The Future of the Body* (Los Angeles: Jeremy P. Tarcher, 1992).

9 E. Green, M.D., and A. Green. *The Ins and Outs of Mind-Body Energy, Science Year, 1974* (Chicago: World Book Science Annual Field Enterprises Educational Corp., 1973), 137-147.

10 B. Moyers. *Healing and the Mind* (New York: Doubleday, 1993), 200-201.

11 Ibid., 206-207.

12 D. Chopra. *Quantum Healing: Exploring the Frontiers of Mind/Body Medicine* (New York: Bantam Books, 1989). L. Dossey. *Space, Time, & Medicine* (Boulder, CO: Shambhala, 1982). D. Kunz. *The Personal Aura* (Wheaton, IL: Theosophical Publishing House, 1991).

13 R.J. Williams. *Nutrition Against Disease: Environmental Prevention* (New York: Bantam Books, 1972).

14 H. Selye, M.D. *Stress Without Distress* (New York: Penguin, 1975).

15 D. Seedhouse and A. Cribb, eds. *Changing Ideas in Health Care* (New York: John Wiley & Sons, 1990).

16 H. Benson, M.D. *The Relaxation Response* (New York: William Morrow, 1975).

17 M. Talbot. *The Holographic Universe* (New York: Harper Collins, 1991), 98-99.

18 L. LeShan. *Cancer as a Turning Point: A Handbook for People with Cancer, Their Families and Health Professionals* (New York: Plume, 1990).

19 M.E. Seligman. *Learned Optimism* (New York: Alfred A. Knopf, 1991).

20 M.A. Visintainer, J.R. Volpicelli, and M.E. Seligman. "Tumor Rejection in Rats After Inescapable or Escapable Shock." *Science* 216:4544 (April 1982), 437-439.

21 J. Achterberg. *Imagery in Healing: Shamanism and Modern Medicine* (Boston: Shambhala, 1985).

22 N. Cousins. *Head First: The Biology of Hope and the Healing Power of the Human Spirit* (New York: Penguin Books, 1989).

23 R.O. Becker, M.D., and D.G. Murray. "The Electrical Control System Regulating Fracture Healing in Amphibians." *Clinical Orthopedics and Related Research* 73 (November-December 1970), 169-198. R.O. Becker, M.D., and G. Selden. *The Body Electric: Electromagnetism and the Foundation of Life* (New York: William Morrow, 1985). R.O. Becker, M.D. *Cross Currents: The Promise of Electromedicine, The Perils of Electropollution* (Los Angeles: Jeremy P. Tarcher, 1990).

24 D.E. Woolridge. *The Machinery of the Brain* (New York: McGraw-Hill, 1963).

25 D. Krieger. *Accepting Your Power to Heal: The Personal Practice of Therapeutic Touch* (Santa Fe, NM: Bear & Co., 1993).

26 J.F. Quinn. "Therapeutic Touch as Energy Exchange: Testing the Theory." *Advances in Nursing Science* 6:2 (January 1984), 42-49.

27 D. Krieger. *The Therapeutic Touch: How to Use Your Hands to Help or Heal* (Englewood Cliffs, NJ: Prentice-Hall, 1979).

28 N. Samarel. "The Experience of Receiving Therapeutic Touch." *Advanced Nursing* 17:6 (June 1992), 651-657.

29 A. Montagu. *Touching: The Human Significance of the Skin* (New York: Harper and Row, 1978).

30 O. Weininger. "Physiological Damage Under Emotional Stress as a Function of Early Experience." *Science* 119 (February 1954), 285-286.

31 D. Ornish, M.D. *Dr. Dean Ornish's Program for Reversing Heart Disease* (New York: Random House, 1990).

32 S.C. Kobasa, S.R. Maddi, and S. Kahn. "Hardiness and Health: A Prospective Study." *Journal of Personality and Social Psychology* 42:1 (January 1982), 168-177.

33 D. Spiegel et al. "Effect of Psychosocial Treatment on Survival of Patients with Metastatic Breast Cancer." *The Lancet* 2:8668 (October 1989), 888-891.

34 L.F. Berkman and S.L. Syme. "Social Networks, Host Resistance, and Mortality: A Nine-Year Follow-Up Study of Alameda County Residents." *American Journal of Epidemiology* 109:2 (February 1979), 186-204.

35 J. Achterberg. "Ritual: The Foundation for Transpersonal Medicine." *ReVision* 14:3 (1992), 158-164.

36 R. Kellner et al. "Changes in Chronic Nightmares After One Session of Desensitization or Rehearsal Instructions." *American Journal of Psychiatry* 149:5 (May 1992), 659-663.

37 J.S. House, K.R. Landis, and D. Umberson. "Social Relationships and Health." *Science* 241:4865 (July 1988), 540-545.

38 J. Achterberg. *Imagery in Healing: Shamanism and Modern Medicine* (Boston: Shambhala, 1985).

39 C. Norman Shealy. *90 Days to Self-Health* (New York: Dial Press, 1977).

40 J. van Dixhoorn et al. "Cardiac Events After Myocardial Infarction: Possible Effects of Relaxation Therapy." *European Heart Journal* 8:11 (November 1987), 1210-1214.

41 E. Peper and V. Tibbetts. "Fifteen-Month Follow-Up with Asthmatics Utilizing EMG/Incentive Inspirometer Feedback." *Biofeedback and Self Regulation* 17:2 (June 1992), 143-151.

42 Phillip Montrose and Jane Montrose. *Getting Thru to Your Emotions with EFT* (Sacramento, CA: Holistic Communications, 2000), 18.

43 Larry Trivieri, Jr. *The American Holistic Medical Association Guide to Holistic Health* (New York: John Wiley & Sons, 2001), 136.

44 F.P. Gallo. "Energy Psychology and Psychotherapy." Available on the Internet: www.energypsych.com/frames/front.html.

45 Ibid.

46 Larry Trivieri, Jr. *The American Holistic Medical Association Guide to Holistic Health* (New York: John Wiley & Sons, 2001), 112.

47 D.H. Shapiro and R.N. Walsh. *Meditation: Classic and Contemporary Perspectives* (New York: Aldine, 1984).

48 Dharma Singh Khalsa and Cameron Stauth. *Meditation as Medicine: Activate the Power of Your Natural Healing Force* (New York: Pocket Books, 2001), 33-49.

49 R. Dilts, T. Halbom, and S. Smith. *Beliefs: Pathways to Health and Well-Being* (Portland, OR: Metamorphous Press, 1990), 1-2.

NAET

1 Devi Nambudripad. *Say Goodbye to Illness* (Buena Park, CA: Delta Publishing, 1993), iii-vi.

2 Larry Trivieri. "NAET: A Revolutionary Approach for Eliminating Allergies." *The Healthy Edge Letter* 1:1 (January 1998), 3-4.

NATURAL HORMONE REPLACEMENT THERAPY

1 John R. Lee, M.D., with Virginia Hopkins. *What Your Doctor May Not Tell You About Menopause* (New York: Warner Books, 1996), 300.

2 Michael Murray, N.D., and Joseph Pizzorno, N.D. *Encyclopedia of Natural Medicine* (Rocklin, CA: Prima, 1998), 636.

1130

3 Graham A. Colditz et al. "The Use of Estrogens and Progestins and the Risk of Breast Cancer in Postmenopausal Women." *New England Journal of Medicine* 332 (1995), 1589-1593.

4 "Aging Men Lose Testosterone, But It Isn't Male Menopause." *The Wall Street Journal* (February 2, 1998), B1.

5 A.W. Meikle et al. "Effects of Fat-Containing Meal on Sex Hormones in Men." *Metabolism* 39:9 (1990), 943-946.

6 C.D. Hunt et al. "Effects of Dietary Zinc Depletion on Seminal Volume and Zinc Loss: Serum Testosterone Concentrations and Sperm Morphology in Young Men." *American Journal of Clinical Nutrition* 55:1 (1992), 148-157.

7 Joseph Pizzorno. *Total Wellness* (Rocklin, CA: Prima Publishing, 1996), 244.

8 Eugene Shippen and William Fryer. *The Testosterone Syndrome* (New York: M. Evans, 1998), 49.

9 S.J. Brown. "Environmental Doctors Take Up Pollution Prevention Cause." *Family Practice News* (January 1, 1995), 6.

10 J. Yeh and A.J. Friedman. "Nicotine and Cotinine Inhibit Rat Testis Androgen Biosynthesis *in Vitro*." *Journal of Steroid Biochemistry* 33:4A (1989), 627-630.

11 Joseph Pizzorno. *Total Wellness* (Rocklin, CA: Prima Publishing, 1996), 242.

12 Lita Lee. "Hypothyroidism: A Modern Epidemic." *Earthletter* (Spring 1994), 1.

13 Tom Valentine. "If You Eat Soy, Watch Your Thyroid Function: New Study." *True Health* (Autumn 1997), 1-3. R.L. Divi et al. "Anti-Thyroid Isoflavones from Soybean: Isolation, Characterization, and Mechanisms of Action." *Biochemical Pharmacology* 54:10 (November 15, 1997), 1087-1096. Stephen E. Langer. *Solved: The Riddle of Illness* (New Canaan, CT: Keats Publishing, 1995).

14 Stephen E. Langer. *Solved: The Riddle of Weight Loss* (Rochester, VT: Healing Arts Press, 1989), 15-17.

15 Lynne McTaggert and Harold Gaier. "Thyroid Disease: Overactive Medicine." *What Your Doctors Don't Tell You* 7:7 (October 1996), 2-5.

16 Lita Lee. "Hypothyroidism: A Modern Epidemic." *Earthletter* (Spring 1994), 2.

17 W. Pierpoli. "Melatonin Extends Rats' Lives." *Brain/Mind Bulletin* 13:9 (June 1988), 1, 8.

18 M. Kato. "Biological Influences of Electromagnetic Fields." *Hokkaido Igaku Zasshi* 70:4 (July 1995), 551-560.

19 M.L. Roa et al. "Blood Serotonin, Serum Melatonin and Light Therapy in Healthy Subjects and in Patients with Nonseasonal Depression." *Acta Psychiatrica Scandinavica* 86 (1992), 127-132.

20 D.J. Kennaway et al. "Phase Delay of the Rhythm of 6-Sulphatoxy Melatonin Excretion by Artificial Light." *Journal of Pineal Research* 4:3 (1987), 315-320. A.J. Lewy et al. "Light Suppresses Melatonin Secretion in Humans." *Science* (December 1980), 210.

21 O. Van Reeth et al. "Nocturnal Exercise Phase Delays Circadian Rhythms of Melatonin and Thyrotropin Secretion in Normal Men." *American Journal of Physiology* 266:6 Part 1 (June 1994), E964-E974.

22 P.J. Murphy et al. "Nonsteroidal Anti-Inflammatory Drugs Affect Normal Sleep Patterns in Humans." *Physiology and Behavior* 55:6 (June 1994), 1063-1066.

23 K.P. Wright, Jr., et al. "Caffeine and Light Effects on Nighttime Melatonin and Temperature Levels in Sleep-Deprived Humans." *Brain Research* 747 (1997), 78-84. S. Rojdmark et al. "Inhibition of Melatonin Secretion by Ethanol in Man." *Metabolism* 42:8 (August 1993), 1047-1051.

24 K. Honma et al. "Effects of Vitamin B12 on Plasma Melatonin Rhythm in Humans: Increased Light Sensitivity and Phase-Advances the Circadian Clock." *Experientia* 48 (1992), 716-720. H. Tioh et al. "Effects of Vitamin B12 and Bright Light on Circadian Rhythms." *Japanese Journal of Psychiatry and Neurology* 48:2 (1994), 502-505. D.J. Kanofsky. "Magnesium Deficiency in Chronic Schizophrenia." *International Journal of Neuroscience* 61 (1991), 87-90.

25 William Regelson, M.D., and Carol Colman. *The Superhormone Promise* (New York: Simon & Schuster, 1996).

26 Ibid.

27 Joseph Pizzorno. *Total Wellness* (Rocklin, CA: Prima Publishing, 1998), 236.

28 William Regelson, M.D., and Carol Colman. *The Superhormone Promise* (New York: Pocket Books, 1997), 155, 176.

29 Ibid., 117, 139-147.

30 R.J. Reiter et al. "Melatonin in Relation to Cellular Antioxidative Defense Mechanisms." *Hormonal and Metabolic Research* 29 (1997), 363-372.

31 R.J. Reiter. "Novel Intracellular Actions of Melatonin: Its Relation to Reactive Oxygen Species." *Frontiers of Hormone Research* 21 (1996), 160-166.

32 E. Reimund. "The Free Radical Flux Theory of Sleep." *Medical Hypotheses* 43 (1994), 231-233.

33 S.H. Kennedy et al. "Melatonin and Cortisol 'Switches' During Mania, Depression, Euthymia in a Drug-Free Bipolar Patient." *Journal of Nervous and Mental Disease* 177:5 (1989), 300-303. P. Monteleone et al. "Depressed Nocturnal Plasma Melatonin Levels in Drug-Free Paranoid Schizophrenics." *Schizophrenia Research* 7 (1992), 77-84.

34 G.J. Maestroni. "T-Helper-2 Lymphocytes as Peripheral Target of Melatonin Signaling." *Journal of Pineal Research* 18 (1995), 84-89.

35 R.J. Reiter et al. "The Role of Melatonin in the Pathophysiology of Oxygen Radical Damage." In: M. Moller and P. Pevet, ed. *Advances in Pineal Research 8* (London: John Libbey, 1994), 278.

36 D. Mueller-Wieland et al. "Melatonin Inhibits LDL Receptor Activity and Cholesterol Synthesis in Freshly Isolated Human Mononuclear Leukocytes." *Biochemical and Biophysical Research Communications* 203:1 (1994), 416-421. N. Birau et al. "Hypertensive Effect of Melatonin in Essential Hypertension." *ICRS Medical Science* 9 (1981), 906.

37 E. Barret-Connor et al. "A Prospective Study of Dehydroepiandrosterone Sulfate, Mortality and Cardiovascular Disease." *New England Journal of Medicine* 315:24 (1986), 1519-1524.

38 P. Ebeling and V.A. Kolvisto. "Physiological Importance of Dehydroepiandrosterone." *The Lancet* 343:8911 (1994), 1470-1481.

39 G. Ravaglia. "The Relationship of Dehydroepiandrosterone Sulfate (DHEA) to Endocrine-Metabolic Parameters and Functional Status in the Oldest-Old." *Journal of Clinical Endocrinology and Metabolism* 81 (1996), 1173-1178.

40 William Regelson, M.D., and Carol Colman. *The Superhormone Promise* (New York: Pocket Books, 1997), 109-113.

41 James Jamieson. *Growth Hormone* (East Canaan, CT: Safegoods Press, 1996), 14-15. Ron Klatz. *Grow Young with Human Growth Hormone* (New York: HarperCollins, 1997), 42.

NATUROPATHIC MEDICINE

1 From the preamble to the Constitution of the World Health Organization.

2 R.H. Banneman, J. Burton, and C. WenChieh. *Traditional Medicine and Health Care Coverage* (Geneva, Switzerland: World Health Organization, 1983).

NEURAL THERAPY

1 D.K. Klinghardt, M.D., and B. Wolfe, M.D. Advanced Neural Therapy Workshop, Santa Fe, New Mexico (December 5-6, 1992). J.P. Dosch, M.D. *Facts About Neural Therapy According to Huneke: Regulation Therapy—Brief Summary for Patients* (Portland, OR: Medicina Biologica, 1985).

2 J. Gleditsch, M.D., and F. Hopfer, M.D. *Neural Therapy, Reflex Zones and Somatopies* (Carmel Valley, CA: American Academy of Biological Dentistry).

3 D.K. Klinghardt, M.D., and B. Wolfe, M.D. Advanced Neural Therapy Workshop, Santa Fe, New Mexico (December 5-6, 1992).

4 Ibid.

5 J.P. Dosch, M.D. *Facts About Neural Therapy According to Huneke: Regulation Therapy—Brief Summary for Patients* (Portland, OR: Medicina Biologica, 1985).

6 R.G. Gibson et al. "Neural Therapy in the Treatment of Multiple Sclerosis." *Journal of Alternative and Complementary Medicine* 5:6 (December 1999), 543-552.

7 D. Klinghardt. "Neural Therapy and the Brain." Lecture presented at the American Academy of Neural Therapy, Seattle, Washington (December 1988). Available on the Internet: www.neuraltherapy.com.

8 A. Pischinger. *Matrix and Matrix Regulation: Basis for a Holistic Theory in Medicine* (Brussels: Haug International, 1991).

9 R.F. Kidd. "Results of Dental Removal and Mercury Detoxification Using DMPS and Neural Therapy." *Alternative Therapies in Health and Medicine* 6:4 (July 2000), 49-55.

10 J.P. Dosch, M.D. *Facts About Neural Therapy According to Huneke: Regulation Therapy—Brief Summary for Patients* (Portland, OR: Medicina Biologica, 1985).

NUTRITIONAL MEDICINE

1 E.M. Pao and S. Mickle. "Problem Nutrients in the United States." *Food Technology* (September 1981), 58-79.

2 "Dietary Intake Source Data: U.S. 1976-1980." Data from the National Health Survey, Series 11 #231, DHHS Publication PHS-8361 (March 1983).

3 M. Brin. "Erythrocyte as a Biopsy Tissue for Functional Evaluation of a Thiamine Adequacy." *Journal of the American Medical Association* 187 (1964), 762-766. M. Brin. "Example of Behavioral Changes in Marginal Vitamin Deficiency in the Rat and Man." In: *Behavioral Effects of Energy and Protein Deficits* NIH Publication No. 79-1906 (Washington, DC: National Institutes of Health, 1979), 272-277. M. Brin. "Drugs and Environmental Chemicals in Relation to Vitamin Needs." In: J. Hathcock, ed. *Nutrition and Drug Interrelations* (New York: Academic Press, 1978), 131-150.

4 L.J. Machlin and M. Brin. "Vitamin E." In: R. Alfin-Slater and D. Kritchevsky, eds. *Human Nutrition—A Comprehensive Treatise, Vol. 3* (New York: Plenum Press, 1980).

5 Ralph Golan, M.D. *Optimal Wellness* (New York: Ballantine, 1995), 120

6 D.F. Horrobin. "Fatty Acid Metabolism in Health and Disease." *American Journal of Clinical Nutrition* 57 Suppl (1993).

7 L.O. Simpson. "The Etiopathogenisis of Premenstrual Syndrome as a Consequence of Altered Blood Rheology: A New Hypothesis." *Medical Hypotheses* 25:4 (April 1988), 189-195.

8 N. Ishibashi et al. "*Bifidobacteria*: Research and Development in Japan." *Food Technology* 47:6 (1993), 126-134. See also: D.C. Hoover. "*Bifidobacteria*: Activity and Potential Benefit." *Food Technology* 47:6 (1993), 120-124.

9 R.L. Baehner and L.A. Boxer. "Role of Membrane Vitamin E and Cytoplasmic Glutathione in the Regulation of Phagocytic Functions of Neutrophils and Monocytes." *American Journal of Pediatric Hematology and Oncology* 1:1 (1979), 71-76.

10 D. Benton and G. Roberts. "Effect of Vitamin and Mineral Supplementation on Intelligence of a Sample of School Children." *The Lancet* 1:8578 (January 1988), 140-143.

11 D.M. Tucker et al. "Nutritional Status and Brain Function in Aging." *American Journal of Clinical Nutrition* 52 (1990), 93-102.

12 J.E. Enstrom, L.E. Kamin, and M.A. Klein. "Vitamin C Intake and Mortality Among a Sample of the United States Population." *Epidemiology* 3 (1992), 194-202.

13 R. Cathcart, M.D. "Vitamin C, Titrating to Bowel Tolerance, Anascorbemia, and Acute Induced Scurvy." *Medical Hypotheses* 7 (1981), 1359-1376.

14 H.B. Stahelin et al. "Beta Carotene and Cancer Prevention: The Basel Study." *American Journal of Clinical Nutrition* 53:Suppl 1 (January 1991), 265S-269S.

15 D.A. Street et al. "A Population-Based Case Control Study of the Association of Serum Antioxidants and Myocardial Infarction." *American Journal of Epidemiology* 131 (1991), 719-720.

16 Harvard Physicians Study (ongoing).

17 K.G. Berge and P.L. Canner. "Coronary Drug Project: Experience with Niacin. Coronary Drug Project Research Group." *European Journal of Clinical Pharmacology* 40:Suppl 1 (1991), S49-S51.

18 L. Packer. "Protective Role of Vitamin E in Biological Systems." *American Journal of Clinical Nutrition* 53:4 (April 1991), 1050S-1055S.

19 S.A. Factor. "Retrospective Evaluation of Vitamin E Therapy in Parkinson's Disease." Presented at: "Vitamin E: Biochemistry and Health Implications," New York Academy of Sciences Meeting, New York City (November 1988).

20 Garland et al. "Dietary Vitamin D and Calcium and Risk of Colorectal Cancer: A 19-Year Prospective Study in Men." *The Lancet* 1 (1985), 307.

21 N. Karanja et al. "Plasma Lipids and Hypertension: Response to Calcium Supplementation." *American Journal of Clinical Nutrition* 45:1 (January 1987), 60-65.

22 M. Simonoff et al. "Low Plasma Chromium in Patients with Coronary Artery and Heart Diseases." *Biological Trace Elements Research* 6:5 (October 1984), 431-439. H.A. Newman et al. "Serum Chromium and Angiographically Determined Coronary Artery Disease." *Clinical Chemistry* 24:4 (April 1978), 541-544.

23 D.A. Wood et al. "Adipose Tissue and Platelet Fatty Acids and Coronary Heart Disease in Scottish Men." *The Lancet* 2:8395 (July 1984), 117-121.

24 R. Kutsky. "Iodine." *Handbook of Vitamins, Minerals, and Hormones* (New York: Von Nostrand Reinhold, 1981), 125.

25 S.L. Meacham et al. "Effect of Boron Supplementation on Blood and Urinary Calcium, Magnesium, and Phosphorus, Urinary Boron in Athletic and Sedentary Women." *American Journal of Clinical Nutrition* 61 (1995), 341-345.

26 F.H. Nielsen. "Studies on the Relationship Between Boron and Magnesium, Which Possibly Affects the Formation and Maintenance of Bones." *Magnesium and Trace Elements* 9 (1990), 61-69.

27 J.T. Salonen et al. "Interactions of Serum Copper, Selenium and Low Density Lipoprotein Cholesterol in Atherogenesis." *British Medical Journal* 302:6779 (March 1991), 756-760.

28 N.W. Stead et al. "Effect of Selenium Supplementation on Selenium Balance in the Dependent Elderly." *American Journal of the Medical Sciences* 290:6 (December 1985), 228-233.

29 G.E. Shambaugh, Jr., M.D. "Zinc: The Neglected Nutrient." *American Journal of Otology* 10:2 (March 1989), 156-160.

30 E.R. Braverman, M.D., and C. Pfeiffer, M.D. *The Healing Nutrients Within: Facts, Findings, and New Research on Amino Acids* (New Canaan, CT: Keats Publishing, 1987).

31 R.B. Singh. "A Randomized, Double-Blind, Placebo-Controlled Trial of L-Carnitine in Suspected Acute Myocardial Infarction." *Postgraduate Medical Journal* (1995).

32 S. Lewin. *Vitamin C: Its Molecular Biology and Medical Potential* (New York: Van Nostrand Reinhold, 1973).

33 T. Fujioka et al. "Clinical Study of Cardiac Arrhythmias Using 24-Hour Continuous Electrocardiographic Recorder (5th Report): Antiarrhythmic Addiction of Coenzyme Q10 in Diabetics." *Tohoku Journal of Experimental Medicine* 141:Suppl (1983), 453-463.

34 M.E. Rosenbaum, M.D., and D. Bosco. *Super Fitness Beyond Vitamins: The Bible of Super Supplements* (New York: New American Library, 1987).

35 A.M. Preston. "Cigarette Smoking—Nutritional Implications." *Progress in Food and Nutrition Science* 15:4 (1991), 183-217.

36 D.D. Fulghum. "Ascorbic Acid Revisited." *Archives of Dermatology* 113:1 (1977), 91-92.

37 M.G. Mustafa. "Biochemical Basis of Ozone Toxicity." *Free Radical Biology and Medicine* 9:3 (1990), 245-265.

38 E.M. Haas, M.D. *Staying Healthy with Nutrition* (Berkeley, CA: Celestial Arts, 1992), 741.

39 "Survey for Nutritional Health Alliance 1992." *Whole Foods Magazine* 16:3 (March 1993), 55.

ORTHOMOLECULAR MEDICINE

1 R.A. Kunin, M.D. "Orthomolecular Psychiatry." In: R.P. Heumer, M.D., ed. *The Roots of Molecular Medicine: A Tribute to Linus Pauling* (New York: W.H. Freeman, 1986), 180-213.

2 R.A. Kunin, M.D. "Principles That Identify Orthomolecular Medicine: A Unique Medical Specialty." *Journal of Orthomolecular Medicine* 2:4 (1987), 203-206.

3 D.C. Loomis. "Which is Safer: Drugs or Vitamins?" *Townsend Letter for Doctors* 105 (April 1992), 219.

4 R.F. Cathcart. "The Method of Determining Proper Doses of Vitamin C for the Treatment of Disease by Titrating to Bowel Tolerance." *Orthomolecular Psychiatry* 10:2 (1981), 125-132.

5 J.R. Crouse III. "New Developments in the Use of Niacin for Treatment of Hyperlipidemia: New Considerations in the Use of an Old Drug." *Coronary Artery Disease* 7:4 (April 1996), 321-326.

6 H.B. Stahelin et al. "Beta Carotene and Cancer Prevention: The Basel Study." *American Journal of Clinical Nutrition* 53 (January 1991), 265S-269S.

7 MRC Vitamin Study Research Group. "Prevention of Neural Tube Defects: Results of the Medical Research Council Vitamin Study." *The Lancet* 338:8760 (July 1991), 131-137.

8 N. Whitehead, F. Reyner, and J. Lindenbaum. "Megaloblastic Changes in the Cervical Epithelium: Association with Oral Contraceptive Therapy and Reversal with Folic Acid." *Journal of the American Medical Association* 226:12 (December 1973), 1421-1424. D. Kitay and W.B. Wentz. "Cervical Cytology in Folic Acid Deficiency of Pregnancy." *American Journal of Obstetrics and Gynecology* 104:7 (August 1969), 931-938.

9 K. Woods et al. "Intravenous Magnesium Sulfate in Suspected Acute Myocardial Infarction: Results of the Second Leicester Intravenous Magnesium Intervention Trial (LIMIT-2)." *The Lancet* 339:8809 (June 1992), 1553-1558.

10 G.W. Evans. "The Effect of Chromium Picolinate on Insulin Controlled Parameters in Humans." *International Journal of Biosocial Medical Research* 11:2 (1989), 163-180.

11 R.A. Anderson et al. "Effects of Supplemental Chromium on Patients with Symptoms of Reactive Hypoglycemia." *Metabolism: Clinical and Experimental* 36:4 (April 1987), 351-355.

12 A. Leaf and P.C. Weber. "Cardiovascular Effects of n-3 Fatty Acids." *New England Journal of Medicine* 318:9 (March 1988), 549-557.

13 T. Kojima et al. "Long-Term Administration of Highly Purified Eicosapentaenoic Acid Provides Improvement of Psoriasis." *Dermatologica* 182:4 (1991), 225-230.

14 H. van der Tempel et al. "Effects of Fish Oil Supplementation in Rheumatoid Arthritis." *Annals of the Rheumatic Diseases* 49:2 (February 1990), 76-80.

15 J.V. Wright, M.D. *Dr. Wright's Guide to Healing with Nutrition* (New Canaan, CT: Keats Publishing, 1990).

OSTEOPATHIC MEDICINE

1 M. Lesser, M.D. *Nutrition and Vitamin Therapy* (New York: Bantam, 1981).

2 I.M. Korr. *Neurobiological Mechanisms in Manipulative Treatment* (New York: Plenum Press, 1979). I.M. Korr. "The Spinal Cord as Organizer of the Disease Processes: IV Axonal Transport and Neurotrophic Function in Relation to Somatic Dysfunction." *Journal of the American Osteopathic Association* 80:7 (March 1981), 451-459.

3 E. Ernst and M.H. Pittler. "Experts' Opinions on Complementary/Alternative Therapies for Low Back Pain." *Journal of Manipulative and Physiological Therapies* 22:2 (February 1999), 87-90.

4 F.M. Purse. "Clinical Evaluation of Osteopathic Manipulative Therapy in Measles." *Journal of the American Osteopathic Association* 61 (December 1961), 274-276.

5 F.M. Purse. "Manipulative Therapy of Upper Respiratory Infections in Children." *Journal of the American Osteopathic Association* 65:9 (May 1966), 964-972.

6 Larry Trivieri. *The American Holistic Medical Association Guide to Holistic Health* (New York: John Wiley & Sons, 2001), 157-162.

1132

7 H.H. Fryett. *Principles of Osteopathic Technique* (Carmel, CA: American Academy of Osteopathy, 1970).

8 A.T. Still. *Philosophy of Osteopathy* (Colorado Springs, CO: American Academy of Osteopathy, 1975).

OXYGEN THERAPIES

1 O. Warburg. "The Prime Cause and Prevention of Cancer." Revised lecture at the meeting of the Nobel Laureates, National Cancer Institute, Bethesda, Maryland (June 30, 1966).

2 C.H. Farr. Presented at the Fourth International Conference on Bio-Oxidative Medicine, Reston, Virginia (April 1-4, 1993).

3 C.H. Farr. *Workbook on Free-Radical Chemistry and Hydrogen Peroxide Metabolism, Including Protocol for the Intravenous Administration of Hydrogen Peroxide* (1992). Contains 32 citations with references in the workbook and 123 citations in the Protocol. Available from: International Bio-Oxidative Medicine Foundation, P.O. Box 13205, Oklahoma City, OK 73189.

4 D. Perrin. Unpublished study (Great Britain, 1993).

5 Richard Leviton. "Healing AIDS, Cancer, and Multiple Sclerosis with Oxygen." *Alternative Medicine* 23 (April/May 1998), 62-66.

6 Ibid.

7 R. Neubauer and M. Hall-Dickenson, with V. Neubauer. "New Hope for Kids with Cerebral Palsy and Brain Injuries." *Alternative Medicine* 33 (January 2000), 44-50.

8 Richard Leviton. "Healing AIDS, Cancer, and Multiple Sclerosis with Oxygen." *Alternative Medicine* 23 (April/May 1998), 62-66.

9 K.H. Wells et al. "Inactivation of Human Immunodeficiency Virus Type I by Ozone *in Vitro*." *Blood* 78:7 (1991), 1882-1890.

10 F. Sweet, M. Ka, and S. Lee. "Ozone Selectively Inhibits Growth of Human Cancer Cells." *Science* 2009:72 (1990), 931.

11 Ibid.

12 K.S. Zanker. "*In Vitro* Synergistic Activity of 5-Fluorouracil with Low-dose Ozone against Chemoresistant Tumor Cell Line and Fresh Human Cells." *International Journal of Experimental and Clinical Chemotherapy* 36 (1990).

13 J. Varro. "Ozone Applications in Cancer Cases." In: J. LaRaus, ed. *Medical Applications of Ozone* (Norwalk, CT: International Ozone Association Pan American Committee, 1983), 97-98.

14 W. Forest. "AIDS, Cancer Cured by Hyperbaric Oxygenation." *Townsend Letter for Doctors* 105 (April 1992), 231-238.

15 "Immunomodulating Effect of Great Masses of Ozone Among Patients Presenting and Acquired Dysimmunity of Viral Origin." *Proceedings of the Ninth Ozone World Congress, Vol. 3* (New York: International Ozone Association, 1989).

16 The off-the-record source states, "When medical ozone use is discontinued, T-cell counts can drop quickly and steeply. Therefore, a person should have another way of supporting T-cell levels before he stops ozone."

17 S. Schulz. "Effekte von Ozon/O2 bei der Clindamycin-Induzierten Enterocolitis beim Sibirischem Zweghamster." *OzoNachrichten* 3 (1984), 2-16.

18 S.L. Helfland et al. "Oxygen Intermediaries are Required for Interferon Activation of NK Cells." *Journal of Interferon Research* 3:2 (1983), 143-151.

19 W. John Diamond, M.D., and W. Lee Cowden,

M.D., with Burton Goldberg. *Alternative Medicine Definitive Guide to Cancer* (Tiburon, CA: Future Medicine Publishing, 1997), 919.

20 C.H. Farr. *The Therapeutic Use of Intravenous Hydrogen Peroxide* (Oklahoma City, OK: Genesis Medical Center, 1987).

21 C.H. Farr. *Workbook on Free-Radical Chemistry and Hydrogen Peroxide Metabolism, Including Protocol for the Intravenous Administration of Hydrogen Peroxide* (1992). Contains 32 citations with references in the workbook and 123 citations in the Protocol. Available from: International Bio-Oxidative Medicine Foundation, P.O. Box 13205, Oklahoma City, OK, 73189.

22 C.H. Farr. *The Use of Dilute Hydrogen Peroxide to Inject Trigger Points, Soft Tissue Injuries and Inflamed Joints* (Oklahoma City, OK: International Bio-Oxidative Medicine Foundation, 1992).

23 C.H. Farr. "Rapid Recovery from Type A/Shanghai Influenza Treated with Intravenous Hydrogen Peroxide." (Oklahoma City, OK: Genesis Medical Center).

24 R. Haskell. "Case History: Multiple Sclerosis Patient." Proceedings of the First International Conference on Bio-Oxidative Medicine, Dallas, Texas (February 17-19, 1989), 13.

25 J. Mealey. "Regional Infusion of Vinblastine and Hydrogen Peroxide in Tumor-Bearing Rats." *Cancer Research* 25 (1965), 1839-1843.

26 N.T. Kaibara et al. "Experimental Studies on Enhancing the Therapeutic Effect of Mitomycin-C with Hydrogen Peroxide." *Japanese Journal of Experimental Medicine* 41 (1971), 323-329.

27 C.H. Farr. *Protocol for Intravenous Administration of Hydrogen Peroxide* (Oklahoma City, OK: International Bio-Oxidative Medicine Foundation, 1993), 32.

28 Nathaniel Altman. "Hydrogen Peroxide in Medicine." *Oxygen Healing Therapies* (Rochester, VT: Healing Arts Press, 1995), 42-43.

PROLOTHERAPY

1 G. Hackett. *Ligament and Tendon Relaxation (Skeletal Disability) Treated by Prolotherapy (Fibro-osseus Proliferation)* (Springfield, IL: Charles C. Thomas, 1958).

2 J. Maynard et al. "Morphological and Biochemical Effects of Sodium Morrhuate on Tendons." *Journal of Orthopaedic Research* 3:2 (1985), 236-248.

3 M.J. Ongley et al. "A New Approach to the Treatment of Chronic Low Back Pain." *The Lancet* 2:8551 (July 18, 1987), 143-146.

4 R.G. Klein et al. "A Randomized Double-Blind Trial of Dextrose-Glycerine-Phenol Injections for Chronic, Low Back Pain." *Journal of Spinal Disorders* 6:1 (February 1993), 23-33.

5 Y.K. Liu et al. "An *In Situ* Study of the Influence of a Sclerosing Solution in Rabbit Medial Collateral Ligaments and Its Junction Strength." *Connective Tissue Research* 11:2-3 (1983), 95-102.

6 K.D. Reeves and K. Hassanein. "Randomized Prospective Double-Blind Placebo-Controlled Study of Dextrose Prolotherapy for Knee Osteoarthritis With or Without ACL Laxity." *Alternative Therapies in Health and Medicine* 6:2 (2000), 37-46.

7 K.D. Reeves and K. Hassanein. "Randomized, Prospective, Placebo-Controlled, Double-Blind Study of Dextrose Prolotherapy for Osteoarthritic Thumbs and Finger (DIP, PIP and Trapeziometacarpal) Joints: Evidence of Clinical Efficacy." *Journal of Alternative and Complementary Medicine* 6:4 (2000), 311-320.

8 D.J. Fletcher. "Regaining the Ability to Heal." *Alternative Medicine* 35 (May 2000), 67.

QIGONG AND TAI CHI

1 F. Li-da. "The Effects of External *Qi* on Bacterial Growth Patterns." *China Qi Gong* 1 (1983), 36.

2 D. Eisenberg, M.D. *Encounters with Qi* (New York: W.W. Norton, 1985).

3 S. Chang, M.D. *The Complete System of Self-Healing: Internal Exercises* (San Francisco: Tao Publishing, 1986).

4 R.H. Lee, ed. *Scientific Investigations into Chinese Qi-Gong* (San Clemente, CA: China Healthways Institute, 1992).

5 Ibid.

6 Y. Hong, J.X. Li, and P.D. Robinson. "Balance Control, Flexibility, and Cardiorespiratory Fitness Among Older Tai Chi Practitioners." *British Journal of Sports Medicine* 34:1 (February 2000), 29-34.

7 N.G. Kutner et al. "Self-Reported Benefits of Tai Chi Practice by Older Adults." *J Gerontol B Psychol Sci Soc Sci* 52:5 (September 1997), 242-246.

8 C. Lan et al. "12-Month Tai Chi Training in the Elderly: Its Effect on Health Fitness." *Med Sci Sports Exerc* 30:3 (March 1998), 345-351.

9 C. Lan et al. "The Effect of Tai Chi on Cardiorespiratory Function in Patients with Coronary Artery Bypass Surgery." *Med Sci Sports Exerc* 31:5 (May 1999), 634-638.

10 W.H. Wu et al. "Effects of Qigong on Late Stage Complex Regional Pain Syndrome." *Alternative Therapies in Health and Medicine* 5:1 (January 1999), 45-54.

11 C.X. Wang and D.H. Xu. "Influence of Qigong Therapy Upon Serum HDL-C in Hypertensive Patients." *Zhong Xi Yi Jie He Za Zhi* 9:9 (September 1989), 516, 543-544.

12 H. Ryu et al. "Acute Effect of Qigong Training on Stress Hormonal Levels in Man." *American Journal of Chinese Medicine* 24:2 (1996), 193-198.

13 I. Reuther. "Qigong Yangshen as a Complimentary Therapy in the Management of Asthma: A Single Case Appraisal." *Alternative and Complementary Medicine* 4:2 (Summer 1998), 173-183.

14 M. Wao. "Effects of Qigong Walking on Diabetic Patients: A Pilot Study." *Journal of Alternative and Complementary Medicine* 5:4 (August 1999), 353-358.

15 R. Jahnke. *The Self-Applied Health Enhancement Methods* (Santa Barbara, CA: Health Action Books, 1991).

SOUND THERAPY

1 D. Soibelman. *Therapeutic and Industrial Uses of Music: A Review of the Literature* (New York: Columbia University Press, 1948).

2 T. Wigram. "The Physical Effects of Sound." *British Society for Musical Therapy Bulletin* 7 (Autumn 1989), 15.

3 D. Black. *Healing with Sound* (Springville, UT: Tapestry Press, 1991).

4 L. Glass and M.C. Mackey. *From Clocks to Chaos: The Rhythms of Life* (Princeton, NJ: Princeton University Press, 1988).

5 D. Black. *Healing with Sound* (Springville, UT: Tapestry Press, 1991).

6 Don Campbell, ed. *Music Physician for Times to Come: An Anthology* (Wheaton, IL: Quest Books, 1991).

7 R. Sprintge and R. Droh. "Towards Research Stan-

dards in Musicmedicine/Music Therapy: A Proposal for a Multimodal Approach." *MusicMedicine* (St. Louis: MMB Music, 1992), 345-349.

8 Don Campbell. *The Mozart Effect* (New York: Avon Books, 1997), 231.

9 M.D. Cassity and Kimberly A. Kaczor-Theobold. "Domestic Violence: Assessments and Treatments by Music Therapists." *Journal of Music Therapy* 27 (1990), 179-194.

10 R. Rebollo Pratt et al. "The Effects of Neurofeedback Training with Background Music on EGG Patterns of ADD and ADHD Children." *International Journal of Arts Medicine* 4 (1995), 24-31.

11 J.D. Cook. "Music as an Intervention in the Oncology Setting." *Cancer Nursing* (1986), 23-28. J.M. Frank. "The Effects of Music Therapy and Guided Visual Imagery on Chemotherapy Induced Nausea and Vomiting." *Oncology Nursing Forum* 12 (1985), 47-52.

12 Deforia Lane, with Rob Wilkins. *Music as Medicine* (Grand Rapids, MI: Zondervan, 1994), 194-195.

13 J.P. Scatelli. "The Effects of Sedative Music on Electromyographic Biofeedback Assisted Relaxation Training on Spastic Cerebral Palsied Adults." *Journal of Music Therapy* 19 (1982), 210-218.

14 M. Humpal. "The Effects of an Integrated Early Childhood Music Program on Social Interaction Among Children with Handicaps and Their Typical Peers." *Journal of Music Therapy* 28 (1991), 161-177.

15 E. Podolsky, ed. *Music Therapy* (New York: Philosophical Library, 1954).

16 Don Campbell. *The Mozart Effect* (New York: Avon Books, 1997), 248-249.

17 Paul Chance. "Music Hath Charms to Soothe a Throbbing Head." *Psychology Today* (February 1987), 14. D. Ingber et al. "Music Therapy: Tune-Up for Mind and Body." *Science Digest* (January 1982), 78.

18 Phyllis Updike. "Music Therapy Results for ICU Patients." *Applied Research* 9 (1990), 39-45.

19 Don Campbell. *The Mozart Effect* (New York: Avon Books, 1997), 273.

20 W.J. Gardner, J.C.R. Licklider, and A.Z. Weisz. "Suppression of Pain by Sound." *Science* 132 (July 1960), 32-33.

21 K.D. Kryter. *The Effects of Noise on Man* (New York: Academic Press, 1985), 449.

22 Don Campbell. *The Mozart Effect* (New York: Avon Books, 1997), 261.

23 K.M. Stevens. "My Room—Not Theirs! A Case Study of Music During Childbirth." *Journal of the Australian College of Midwives* 5:3 (September 1992), 27-30.

24 Don Campbell. *The Mozart Effect* (New York: Avon Books, 1997), 267.

25 Ibid., 271.

26 C.A. Prickett and R.S. Moore. "The Use of Music to Aid Memory of Alzheimer's Patients." *Journal of Music Therapy* 28 (1991), 101-110.

27 R.H. Lee, ed. *Scientific Investigations into Chinese Qi-Gong* (San Clemente, CA: China Healthways Institute, 1992), 18.

28 P.G. Manners. *Techniques and Theories for the Emerging Pattern of Current Research* (Monograph). Available from: Bretforton Hall Clinic, Bretforton, Vale of Worcestershire, WR11 5JH, England.

TRADITIONAL CHINESE MEDICINE

1 *A Proposed Standard International Acupuncture Nomenclature: Report of a World Health Organization Scientific Group* (Geneva, Switzerland: World Health Organization, 1991).

2 T.J. Kaptchuk. *The Web That Has No Weaver* (Chicago: Congdon & Weed, 1983).

3 *Journal of Alternative and Complementary Medicine* 3:4 (1993), 383-389.

4 Jason Elias and Katherine Ketcham. *Feminine Healing: A Woman's Guide to Healthy Body, Mind and Spirit* (New York: Warner Books, 1997), 241-255.

5 Jake Fratkin. *Chinese Herbal Patent Formulas* (Boulder, CO: Shya Publications, 1986), 133.

6 It would be impossible to cite every study that might be relevant. A sampling of a few articles includes: T. Tani. "Treatment of Type I Allergic Disease with Chinese Herbal formulas: Minor Blue Dragon Combination and Minor Bupleurum Combination." *International Journal of Oriental Medicine* 14:3 (September 1989), 155-166. A. Chen, M.D. "Effective Acupuncture Therapy for Migraine: Review and Comparison of Prescriptions with Recommendations for Improved Results." *American Journal of Acupuncture* 17:4 (1989), 305-316. G.S. Chen. "The Effect of Acupuncture Treatment on Carpal Tunnel Syndrome." *American Journal of Acupuncture* 18:1 (1990), 5-10. K. Chen and H. Liang. "Progress of Geriatrics Research in Chinese Medicine." *International Journal of Oriental Medicine* 14:1 (March 1989), 49-56. S. Siterman et al. "Does Acupuncture Treatment Affect Sperm Density in Males with Very Low Sperm Count? A Pilot Study." *Andrologia* 32:1 (January 2000), 31-39.

7 H. Zhuang et al. "Effects of *Radix Salviae Miltiorrhizae* Extract Injection on Survival of Allogenic Heart Transplantation." *Journal of Traditional Chinese Medicine* 10:4 (December 1990), 276-281. W. Lu. "Treatment of AIDS by TCM and Materia Medica." *Journal of Traditional Chinese Medicine* 11:4 (December 1991), 249-252. G. Di Concetto, M.D., and L. Sotte. "Treatment of Headaches by Acupuncture and Chinese Herbal Therapy: Conclusive Data Concerning 1,000 Patients." *Journal of Traditional Chinese Medicine* 2:3 (September 1991), 174-176.

8 F. Liu. "Application of Traditional Chinese Drugs in Comprehensive Treatment of Primary Liver Cancer." *Journal of Traditional Chinese Medicine* 10:1 (March 1990), 54-60. This study showed that TCM diagnosis could enhance the prognosticative accuracy of survival of patients with primary liver cancer and that Chinese herbal medicine allowed patients to recuperate to a point where they could successfully undergo surgery and complete regimens of chemotherapy, thus prolonging survival.

YOGA

1 Studies include: S. Telles and T. Desiraju. "Oxygen Consumption During Pranayamic Type of Very Slow-Rate Breathing." *Indian Journal of Medical Research* 94 (October 1991), 357-363. V. Singh et al. "Effect of Yoga Breathing Exercises *(Pranayama)* on Airway Reactivity in Subjects with Asthma." *The Lancet* 335:9702 (June 1990), 1381-1383.

2 D. Goleman. *The Meditative Mind* (Los Angeles: Jeremy P. Tarcher, 1988).

3 Ibid.

4 J. Borysenko. *Minding the Body/Mending the Mind* (New York: Bantam Books, 1988).

5 Studies include: K. Nespor. "Pain Management and Yoga." *International Journal of Psychosomatics* 38:1-

4 (1991), 76-81. A. Stancak, Jr., et al. "Observations on Respiratory and Cardiovascular Rhythmicities During Yogic High-Frequency Respiration." *Physiological Research* 40:3 (1991), 345-354. A.H. Brownstein and M.L. Dembert. "Treatment of Essential Hypertension with Yoga Relaxation Therapy in a USAF Aviator: A Case Report." *Aviation Space and Environmental Medicine* 60:7 (July 1989), 684-687.

6 H. Herzog et al. "Changed Pattern of Regional Glucose Metabolism During Yoga Meditative Relaxation." *Neuropsychobiology* 23:4 (1990-1991), 182-187.

7 Studies include: K. Nespor. "Pain Management and Yoga." *International Journal of Psychosomatics* 38:1-4 (1991), 76-81. A. Stancak, Jr., et al. "Observations on Respiratory and Cardiovascular Rhythmicities During Yogic High-Frequency Respiration." *Physiological Research* 40:3 (1991), 345-354. A.H. Brownstein and M.L. Dembert. "Treatment of Essential Hypertension with Yoga Relaxation Therapy in a USAF Aviator: A Case Report." *Aviation Space and Environmental Medicine* 60:7 (July 1989), 684-687.

8 J. Funderburk. *Science Studies Yoga: a Review of Physiological Data* (Honesdale, PA: Himalayan International Institute of Yoga Science & Philosophy of USA, 1977), 36-41.

9 Ibid., 93.

10 S.C. Manchanda et al. "Retardation of Coronary Atherosclerosis with Yoga Lifestyle Intervention." *J Assoc Physicians India* 48:7 (July 2000), 687-694.

11 J. Funderburk. *Science Studies Yoga: a Review of Physiological Data* (Honesdale, PA: Himalayan International Institute of Yoga Science & Philosophy of USA, 1977), 42, 47-72.

12 P.K. Vendanthan et al. "Clinical Study of Yoga Techniques in University Students with Asthma: A Controlled Study." *Allergy & Asthma Proceedings* 19:1 (January/February 1998), 3-9.

13 D. Behera. "Yoga Therapy in Chronic Bronchitis." *J Assoc Physicians India* 46:2 (February 1998), 207-208.

14 J. Funderburk. *Science Studies Yoga: a Review of Physiological Data* (Honesdale, PA: Himalayan International Institute of Yoga Science & Philosophy of USA, 1977), 45, 75.

15 S.C. Jain et al. "A Study of Response Pattern of Non-Insulin-Dependent Diabetics to Yoga Therapy." *Diabetes Res Clin Pract* 19:1 (January 1993), 69-74.

16 M.S. Garfinkel et al. "Yoga-Based Intervention for Carpal Tunnel Syndrome: A Randomized Trial." *Journal of the American Medical Association* 280:18 (November 11, 1998), 1601-1603.

17 J. Funderburk. *Science Studies Yoga: a Review of Physiological Data* (Honesdale, PA: Himalayan International Institute of Yoga Science & Philosophy of USA, 1977), 73-74.

18 D.S. Shannahoff-Khalsa and L.R. Beckett. "Clinical Case Report: Efficacy of Yogic Techniques in the Treatment of Obsessive Compulsive Disorders." *International Journal of Neuroscience* 85:1-2 (March 1996), 1-17.

19 J. Funderburk. *Science Studies Yoga: a Review of Physiological Data* (Honesdale, PA: Himalayan International Institute of Yoga Science & Philosophy of USA, 1977), 21.

20 K. Uma et al. "The Integrated Approach of Yoga: A Therapeutic Tool for Mentally Retarded Children: A One Year Controlled Study." *Journal of Mental Deficiency Research* 33:5 (October 1989), 415-421.

1134

Part Three: Health Conditions

ADDICTIONS

1 National Institute on Drug Abuse and the National Institute on Alcohol Abuse and Alcoholism. "Economic Costs of Alcohol and Drug Abuse Estimated at $246 Billion in the United States." U.S. National Institutes of Health press release (May 13, 1998).

2 Antoine Bechara et al. Neuropsychologia 39 (2001), 376-389.

3 Susan Brink. "Your Brain on Alcohol." U.S. News & World Report 130:18 (May 7, 2001), 50-57.

4 R.J. Wurtman. "Ways That Foods Can Affect the Brain." Nutrition Reviews 44:Suppl. (May 1986), 2-6.

5 J. Mathews Larson and B. Parker. "Alcoholism Treatment with Biochemical Restoration as a Major Component." Int J Biosocial Med Res 9 (1987), 92-100.

6 D. Stephen, M.D. Nutritional Medicine (London: Pan Books, 1987).

7 J. Mathews Larson and B. Parker. "Alcoholism Treatment with Biochemical Restoration as a Major Component." Int J Biosocial Med Res 9 (1987), 92-100.

8 J.E. Pizzorno and M.T. Murray. A Textbook of Natural Medicine (Seattle, WA: John Bastyr College Publications, 1985).

9 Journal of the American Medical Association (October 1994).

10 Barbara Crossette. "Agency Sees Risk in Drug to Temper Child Behavior." The New York Times (February 29, 1996). Erik L. Goldman. "Ritalin Wrongly Used to Diagnose Attention Deficit." Family Practice News (November 1, 1995), 33.

11 J.E. Pizzorno and M.T. Murray. A Textbook of Natural Medicine (Seattle, WA: John Bastyr College Publications, 1985).

12 N.R. DiLuzio. "A Mechanism of the Acute Ethanol-Induced Fatty Liver and the Modification of Liver Injury by Antioxidants." Lab Invest 15 (1966), 50-61.

13 I. Das, R.E. Burch, and H.K.J. Hahn. "Effects of Zinc Deficiency on Ethanol Metabolism and Alcohol and Aldehyde Dehydrogenase Activities." Journal of Laboratory and Clinical Medicine 104 (1984), 610-617. A.A. Yunice and R.D. Lindeman. "Effect of Ascorbic Acid and Zinc Sulphate on Ethanol Toxicity and Metabolism." Proceedings of the Society for Experimental Biology and Medicine 154 (1977), 146-150.

14 M.L. Bullock, P.D. Culliton, and R.T. Oleander. "Controlled Trial of Acupuncture for Severe Recidivist Alcoholism." The Lancet 1:8652 (June 1989), 1435-1439. NADA Newsletter Committee. National Acupuncture Detoxification Association Newsletter (December 1, 1992), 1-6.

15 S. Toteva and I. Milanov. "The Use of Body Acupuncture for Treatment of Alcohol Dependence and Withdrawal Syndrome: A Controlled Study." American Journal of Acupuncture 24 (1996), 19-24.

16 Daniel S.J. Choy, M.D., F.A.C.P. "Acupuncture and Smoking Cessation." Alternative & Complementary Therapies (November/December 1996), 399-404.

17 S.K. Avants et al. "A Randomized Controlled Trial of Auricular Acupuncture for Cocaine Dependence." Archives of Internal Medicine 160:15 (August 14-28, 2000), 2305-2312.

18 J. Holder, M.D. "New Auricular Therapy Formula to Increase Retention of the Chemically Dependent in Residential Treatment." Research study funded by the State of Florida, Department of Health and Rehabilitative Services (1991).

19 Patricia Kaminski and Richard Katz. Flower Essence Repertory (Nevada City, CA: Flower Essence Society, 1996).

20 Jay Holder, D.C. Molecular Psychiatry (February 2001).

21 L. Trivieri. "Brain Wave Therapy: A Breakthrough Addiction Therapy." The Healthy Edge Letter 1:2 (April 1998), 1-2.

22 J. Zand. "Natural Medicine for the Recovering Addict." Explore! 5 (1994), 37-38.

23 Editorial Staff. "Replacing Addiction with a Coping Skill." Health and Wellness 1:1 (December 1991).

AIDS

1 UNAIDS. "Report on the Global HIV/AIDS Epidemic: December 2000." UNAIDS. "Report on the Global HIV/AIDS Epidemic: June 2000." U.S. Centers for Disease Control and Prevention. "Guidelines for National Human Immunodeficiency Virus Case Surveillance, Including Monitoring for Human Immunodeficiency Virus Infection and Acquired Immunodeficiency Syndrome." Morbidity and Mortality Weekly Report 48:RR-13 (1999), 1-27, 29-31. U.S. Centers for Disease Control and Prevention. "HIV Prevention Strategic Plan Through 2005." Draft (September 2000). U.S. Centers for Disease Control and Prevention. HIV/AIDS Surveillance Report 12:1 (2000), 1-44. U.S. Centers for Disease Control and Prevention. HIV/AIDS Surveillance Report 11:2 (1999), 1-44. S.L. Murphy. "Deaths: Final Data for 1998." National Vital Statistics Reports 48:11 (1998).

2 A.J. France. "Changing Case-Definition for AIDS." The Lancet 340:8832 (December 1992), 1414. G.T. Stewart. "Changing Case-Definition for AIDS." The Lancet 340:8832 (December 1992), 1414.

3 P.H. Duesberg. "AIDS Acquired by Drug Consumption and Other Noncontagious Risk Factors." Pharmocological Therapy 55 (1992), 2101-2177.

4 Ibid., 2109.

5 E. Papadopulos-Eleopulos, V.F. Turner, and J.M. Papadimitriou. "Has Gallo Proven the Role of HIV in AIDS?" Emerg Med 5 (1993), 113-123.

6 C. Farber. "Fatal Distraction." SPIN Magazine 8:3 (May 1992), 36.

7 Gary Null. "HIV Equals AIDS and Other Myths of the AIDS War." Penthouse Magazine (November/December 1995).

8 C. Farber. "AIDS: Words from the Front." SPIN Magazine (June 1988), 73.

9 Gary Null. "HIV Equals AIDS and Other Myths of the AIDS War." Penthouse Magazine (November/December 1995).

10 C. Farber. "AIDS: Words from the Front." SPIN Magazine (June 1988), 4.

11 Ibid.

12 Ibid., 36.

13 B. Guccione. "Interview with Peter Duesberg." SPIN Magazine (September 1993).

14 C. Farber. "Fatal Distraction." SPIN Magazine 8:3 (May 1992), 36.

15 Reported by doctors Jorge Eichberg and Krishna Murthy of the Southwest Foundation for Biomedical Research.

16 Stefan Lanka. "HIV: Reality of Artefact?" Continuum Magazine 3:1 (April/May 1995), 4-9.

17 Christine Johnson. "Is HIV the Cause of AIDS?" Continuum Magazine 5:1 (1997).

18 Roberto A. Giraldo, M.D. "Everybody Reacts Positive on the ELISA Test for HIV." Continuum Magazine 5:5 (1999).

19 The Wall Street Journal (January 11, 1995), B8.

20 Christine Johnson. Continuum Magazine (April/May 1995). A.L. Mason et al. "Detection of Retroviral Antibodies in Primary Biliary Cirrhosis and Other Idiopathic Biliary Disorders." The Lancet 351 (1998), 1620-1624. E. Papadopulos-Eleopulos, V.F. Turner, and J.M. Papadimitriou. "HIV Antibodies: Further Questions and a Plea for Clarification." Current Medical Research and Opinion 13 (1997), 627-634.

21 Christine Maggiore. What If Everything You Thought You Knew About AIDS was Wrong? (Los Angeles: HEAL, 1996).

22 Valendar F. Turner. "Where Have We Gone Wrong?" Continuum Magazine 5:3 (1997).

23 "Report." General Practitioner 7 (September 1987).

24 L. Chaitow and S. Simon. A World Without AIDS (London: Thorsons, 1989).

25 E. Papadopulos-Eleopulos, V.F. Turner, and J.M. Papadimitriou. "Kaposi's Sarcoma and HIV." Medical Hypotheses 39 (1992), 22-29. V.D. Beral, R. Bull, and S. Darby. "Kaposi's Sarcoma and Sexual Practices Associated with Faecal Contact in Homosexual or Bisexual Men with AIDS." The Lancet 339 (1990), 632-636. V. Beral et al. "Kaposi's Sarcoma Among Persons with AIDS: A Sexually Transmitted Infection?" The Lancet 335 (1990), 123-128.

26 P.H. Duesberg. "AIDS Acquired by Drug Consumption and Other Noncontagious Risk Factors." Pharmocological Therapy 55 (1992), 201-277.

27 World Health Organization. "Acquired Immunodeficiency Syndrome (AIDS): WHO/CDC Case Definition for AIDS." Weekly Epidemic Record 61 (1986), 69-76.

28 Christine Maggiore. What If Everything You Thought You Knew About AIDS was Wrong? (Los Angeles: HEAL, 1996), 8.

29 E. Papadopulos-Eleopulos et al. "Factor VIII, HIV and AIDS in Haemophiliacs: An Analysis of Their Relationship." Genetica 95:1-3 (1995), 25-50. Christine Johnson. "Bad Blood or Bad Science: Are Haemophiliacs with AIDS Diagnoses Really Infected with HIV?" Continuum Magazine 5:4 (1997).

30 Gary Null. "HIV Equals AIDS and Other Myths of the AIDS War." Penthouse Magazine (November/December 1995).

31 J. Learmont et al. "Long-Term Symptomless HIV-1 Infection in Recipients of Blood Products From a Single Donor." The Lancet 340:8824 (October 1992), 863-867.

32 C. Farber. "Fatal Distraction." SPIN Magazine 8:3 (May 1992), 36. G. Kolata. "Doctors Stretch Rules on AIDS Drug: Some Give Possibly Toxic AZT Before Symptoms Develop." The New York Times 137 (December 21, 1987), A1. Dr. Douglas Dietrich, of the New York Medical Center, told Times reporter Gina Kolata, "I've followed patients who've had T-cell counts of less then 10 for a year, and nothing happened to them."

33 E. Papadopulos-Eleopulos et al. "A Critical Analysis of the HIV-T4 Cell-AIDS Hypothesis." Genetica 95:1-3 (1995), 5-24.

34 Valendar F. Turner and Andrew McIntyre. "The Yin and Yang of HIV." Nexus Magazine 6:4 (June-July 1999).

35 E. Papadopulos-Eleopulos. "A Mitotic Theory." *Journal of Theoretical Biology* 96 (1982), 741-758. E. Papadopulos-Eleopulos. "Reappraisal of AIDS: Is the Oxidation Caused by the Risk Factors the Primary Cause?" *Medical Hypotheses* 25 (1988), 151-162.

36 Gary Null. "HIV Equals AIDS and Other Myths of the AIDS War." *Penthouse Magazine* (November/December 1995).

37 S.S. Cohen. "Antiretroviral Therapy for AIDS." *New England Journal of Medicine* 317:10 (September 1987), 629. E. Dournon et al. "Effects of Zidovudine in 365 Consecutive Patients with AIDS and ARC." *The Lancet* 2:8623 (1988), 1297-1302. P. Duesberg. "AIDS Epidemiology." *Proceedings of the National Academy of Sciences* 88 (1991), 1575. P. Gill et al. "Azydomythmidine Associated with Bone Marrow Failure in Anti-Immune Deficiency Syndrome." *Annals of Internal Medicine* 107:4 (1987), 502-505. D. Richman et al. "Toxicity of AZT in Treating AIDS and ARC: The AZT Working Group." *New England Journal of Medicine* 317 (1987), 192. K. Smothers. "Pharmacology and Toxicology of AIDS Therapies." *The AIDS Reader* 1 (1991), 29. P. Volberding. "Zidovudine in Asymptomatic Human Immunodeficiency Virus Infection." *New England Journal of Medicine* 322 (1990), 941. R. Yarchoan et al. "Anti-Retroviral Therapy for AIDS." *New England Journal of Medicine* 317 (1987), 630.

38 D. Abrams. "Lecture to Medical Students." *Synapse* (1996).

39 S.P. Buchbinder et al. "Long-Term HIV-1 Infection Without Immunologic Progression." *AIDS* 8 (1994), 1123-1128. G. Pantaleo et al. "Studies in Subjects with Long-Term Nonprogressive Human Immunodeficiency Virus Infection." *New England Journal of Medicine* 332 (1995), 209-216.

40 L. Standish et al. "One Year Open Trial of Naturopathic Treatment of HIV Infection Class lV-A in Men." *Journal of Naturopathic Medicine* 3:1 (1992), 42-64.

41 M. Fischl et al. "Safety and Efficacy of AZT in Treatment of Subjects Mildly Symptomatic HIV Type-1 Infection." *Annals of Internal Medicine* 112 (1990), 727-737. P. Volberding et al. "AZT in Asymptomatic HIV Infection: A Controlled Trial in Patients with Fewer than 500 CD4-Positive Cells per Cubic Millimeter." *New England Journal of Medicine* 322 (1990), 941.

42 S.M. Blower et al. "Predicting the Unpredictable: Transmission of Drug-Resistant HIV." *Nature Medicine* 7:9 (2001), 1016-1020.

43 Bill Sardi. "Can Cancer-Fighting Natural Products Combat AIDS?" *Nutrition Science News* 2:3 (March 1997), 144-148.

44 L. Chaitow and S. Simon. *A World Without AIDS* (London: Thorsons, 1989), 91. D. Campbell. "Living Positively." *New Statesman* 29 (January 1989).

45 D. Campbell. "AIDS: The Race Against Time." *New Statesman* 6 (January 1989). B. Gavrzer. "Why Do Some People Survive AIDS." *Daily Breeze* (September 18, 1988). M.V. Elliott. "AIDS—The Unheard Voices." BBC Television, Meditel Productions (November 1987).

46 L. Standish et al. "One-Year Open Trial of Naturopathic Treatment of HIV Infection in Class lV-A in Men." *Journal of Naturopathic Medicine* 3:1 (1992), 42-64.

47 R. Brayton et al. "Effect of Alcohol and Various Diseases on Leukocyte Mobilization, Phagocytosis and Intracellular Bacterial Killing." *New England Journal of Medicine* 2:3 (1970), 123-128. A. Saxena et al. "Immunomodulating Effects of Caffeine in Rodents." *Indian Journal of Experimental Biology* 22:6 (1984), 293-301.

48 W. Crook. *The Yeast Connection* (Jackson, TN: Professional Books, 1984).

49 L. Chaitow and N. Trenev. *Probiotics* (New York: HarperCollins, 1990).

50 M.K. Baum et al. "High Risk of HIV-Related Mortality is Associated with Selenium Deficiency." *J Acquir Immune Defic Syndr Hum Retrovirol* 15:5 (August 15, 1997), 370-374.

51 E. Mantera-Tienza et al. "Low Vitamin B6 in HIV Infection." Fifth International Conference on AIDS (June 1989).

52 G. Harriman et al. "Vitamin B12 Malabsorption in AIDS." *Archives of Internal Medicine* 149:9 (1989), 2039-2041. M.K. Baum et al. "High Risk of HIV-Related Mortality is Associated with Selenium Deficiency." *J Acquir Immune Defic Syndr Hum Retrovirol* 15:5 (August 15, 1997), 370-374.

53 M.K. Baum et al. "High Risk of HIV-Related Mortality is Associated with Selenium Deficiency." *J Acquir Immune Defic Syndr Hum Retrovirol* 15:5 (August 15, 1997), 370-374. B. Dworkin et al. "Selenium Deficiency in AIDS." *Journal of Parenteral and Enteral Nutrition* 10:4 (1986), 405-407.

54 N. Fabris et al. "AIDS, Zinc Deficiency and Thymic Hormone Failure." *Journal of the American Medical Association* 259 (1988), 839-840.

55 T. Pulse et al. "A Significant Improvement in a Clinical Pilot Study Utilizing Nutritional Supplements, Essential Fatty Acids, and Stabilized Aloe Vera Juice in 29 HIV Seropositive, ARC and AIDS Patients." *Journal for the Advancement of Medicine* 3:4 (1990), 209-230.

56 D.A. Fryberg, R.J. Mark, and B.P. Griffith. "The Effect of Supplemental Beta Carotene on Immunologic Indices in Patients with AIDS: A Pilot Study." *Yale J Biol Med* 68 (1995), 19-23.

57 L.C. Robson, R.M. Schwartz, and W.D. Perkins. "The Effects of Vitamin B6 Deficiency on the Lymphoid System and Immune Responses." In: C.P. Tryfiates, ed. *Vitamin B6 Metabolism and Role in Growth* (Westport, CT: Food and Nutrition Press, 1980), 205-222. J. Tamura, K. Kubota, and H. Murakami. "Immunomodulation by Vitamin B12: Augmentation of CD8+ Lymphocytes and Natural Killer (NK) Cell Activity in Vitamin B12-Deficient Patients by Methyl-B12 Treatment." *Clinical and Experimental Immunology* 116 (1999), 28-32.

58 A. Tang et al. "Association Between Serum Vitamin A and E Levels and HIV-1 Disease Progression." *AIDS* 11:5 (April 1997), 613-620.

59 P. Guitierrez. "Influence of Ascorbic Acid on Free Radical Metabolism of Xenobiotics." *Drug Metabolism Review* 18:3-4 (1989), 319-343. J. Blakeslee et al. "Human T-Cell Leukaemia Virus: Inhibition by Retinoids, Ascorbic Acid and Vitamin E." *Cancer Research* 45 (1985), 3471-3476. P. Bouras et al. "Monocyte Locomotion: In Vivo Effect of Ascorbic Acid." *Immunopharmocology and Immunotoxicity* 11:1 (1989), 119-129.

60 R. Cathcart, M.D. "Vitamin C in the Treatment of AIDS." *Medical Hypotheses* 14 (1984), 432-433.

61 K.W. Beck. "Serum Trace Elements in HIV-Infected Subjects." *Biol Trace Elem Res* 25 (1990), 89-93.

62 Siro Passi. "Progressive Increase of Oxidative Stress in Advancing Human Immunodeficiency." *Continuum Magazine* 5:4 (1997).

63 P.A. Raju et al. "Glutathione Precursor and Antioxidant Activities of N-Acetylcysteine and Oxothiazolidine Carboxylate Compared in *In Vitro* Studies of HIV Replication." *AIDS Res Hum Retroviruses* 10:8 (August 1994), 961-967.

64 Y. Sun et al. "Preliminary Observation on the Effects of Chinese Herbs." *Journal of Biological Response Modifiers* 2 (1983), 227-237.

65 M. Walker. "Carnivora Therapy for Cancer and AIDS." *Explore!* 3:5 (1992), 10-15. M. Walker. "Carnivora and AIDS." *Townsend Letter for Doctors* (May 1992), 351-359.

66 M. Stimpel et al. "Macrophage Activation and Induction of Cytotoxicity by Purified Polysaccharide Fractions from *Echinacea purpurea*." *Infection and Immunity* 46 (1984), 845-849.

67 *Chemical and Pharmaceutical Bulletin* 36:6 (1988), 2090-2097. N. Abe et al. "Interferon Induction by Glycyrrhizin." *Microbiology and Immunology* 26:6 (1982), 535-539.

68 R. Sharma et al. "Berberine Tannate in Acute Diarrhea." *Indian Pediatrics Journal* 7 (1978). V. Choudray et al. "Berberine in Giardiasis." *Indian Pediatrics Journal* 9 (1979), 143-146. R. Sack et al. "Berberine Inhibits Intestinal Secretory Response in *Vibrio Cholerae*, *E. coli* Enterotoxins." *Infection and Immunity* 35:2 (1982), 471-475.

69 M. Adetumbi et al. "*Allium sativum*: A Natural Antibiotic." *Medical Hypotheses* 12 (1983), 227-237. S. Vahora et al. "Medicinal Use of Indian Vegetables." *Planta Medica* 23 (1973), 381-393. "Garlic in Cryptococcal Meningitis." *Chinese Medical Journal* 93 (1980), 123-126. R. Sharma et al. "Berberine Tannate in Acute Diarrhea." *Indian Pediatrics Journal* 7 (1978).

70 E. Brekhmann. *Man and Biologically Active Substances* (London: Pergamon Press, 1980). A. Takada et al. "Restoration of Radiation Injury by Ginseng." *Journal of Radiation* 22 (1981), 323-325.

71 D. Meruelo et al. "Therapeutic Agents with Dramatic Retroviral Activity." *Proceedings of the National Academy of Sciences* 85 (1988), 5230-5234. H. Someya. "Effect of a Constituent of Hypericum on Infection and Multiplication of Epstein-Barr Virus." *Journal of the Tokyo Medical College* 43:5 (1985), 815-826. C. Barbagallo et al. "Antimicrobial Activity of Three Hypericum Species." *Fitoteripia* LVIII:3 (1987), 175-177.

72 Michael Breckenridge. "Hyssop Provides Startling Results in HIV Treatment." *Well Being Journal* (September/October 1996), 12-16.

73 Jasbir B. Kahlon, Dr.PH., et al. "Inhibition of AIDS Virus Replication by Acemannan *in vitro*." *Molecular Biotherapy* 3 (1991), 127-135. T.L. Pulse, M.D., and Elizabeth Uhlig, RRA. "A Significant Improvement in a Clinical Pilot Study Utilizing Nutritional Supplements, Essential Fatty Acids, and Stabilized Aloe Vera Juice in 29 HIV Seropositive, ARC, and AIDS Patients." *Journal of Advancement in Medicine* 3:4 (1990), 209-230.

74 Q.C. Zhang. "Preliminary Report on the Use of *Momordica Charantia* Extract by HIV Patients." *Journal of Naturopathic Medicine* 3:1 (1992), 65-69. R. Baker. "MAP30: *Momordica* Anti-HIV Protein Research Notes." *BETA* (1991), 14. J. Hierholzer et al. "*In Vitro* Effects of Monolaurin Compounds on Enveloped RNA and DNA Viruses." *Journal of Food Safety* 4:1 (1982). J. Sands et al. "Extreme Sensitivity of Enveloped Viruses to Long Chained Unsaturated Monoglycerides and Alcohols." *Antimicrobial Agents and Chemotherapy* 15:1 (1979), 67-73. T. Aoki et al. "Antibodies to HTLV-1 and HTLV-III in Sera from Two Japanese Patients." *The Lancet* 20 (October 1984), 936-937.

75 S. Dharmananda. "Chinese Herbal Therapies for the Treatment of Immunodeficiency Syndromes."

Oriental Healing Arts International Bulletin 12:1 (January 1987), 24-38.

76 Q.C. Zhang. "Preliminary Report on the Use of *Momordica Charantia* Extract by HIV Patients." *Journal of Naturopathic Medicine* 3:1 (1992), 65-69.

77 D. Orman and D. Margetis. "Effectiveness of Acupuncture and Chinese Phytomedicinals in the Treatment of HIV and AIDS." *Journal of Naturopathic Medicine* 3:1 (1992), 80-82.

78 M. Smith, M.D., and N. Rabinowitz, M.D. "Acupuncture Treatment of AIDS." Lincoln Hospital Acupuncture Clinic, New York City (March 1985). M. Smith, M.D. "Research in Use of Acupuncture with AIDS." *American Journal of Acupuncture* 16:2 (April-June 1988).

79 L. Chaitow and S. Martin. *A World Without AIDS* (London: Thorsons, 1989), 131.

80 Barbara Brewitt, M.Div., Ph.D., Biomed Comm, Inc., 2 Nickerson Street, Suite 302 Seattle, WA 98109; (206) 284-3433; Website: www.biomedcomm.com.

81 B. Spire et al. "Inactivation of Lymphadenopathy-Associated Virus by Heat, Gamma Rays, and Ultraviolet Light." *The Lancet* 1:8422 (January 1985), 188-189. H. Weatherburn. "Hyperthermia and AIDS Treatment." *British Journal of Radiology* 61:729 (September 1988), 862.

82 L. Standish et al. "One-Year Open Trial of Naturopathic Treatment of HIV Infection Class IV-A in Men." *Journal of Naturopathic Medicine* 3:1 (1992), 42-64.

83 K. Nault. "AIDS, Cancer—An Answer (Ozone Therapy)." Reported in *Crosswinds* (December 1988), based on an Associated Press report (October 28, 1988).

84 K. Well et al. "Inactivation of Human Immunodeficiency Virus Type-1 by Ozone *in Vitro*." *Blood* 78 (1991), 1882-1890.

85 B. Vallancien and J.M. Winkler. "Immunomodulating Effect of Ozone Among Patients with AIDS." Conference Report, New York, New York (1989).

86 M.T. Carpendale, J. Freeberg, and J.M. Griffiss. "Does Ozone Alleviate AIDS Diarrhea?" *Journal of Clinical Gastroenterology* 17:2 (September 1993), 142-145.

87 Michelle Reillo, B.S.N., R.N., Lifeforce, Inc., 1006 Morton Street, Suite 100, Baltimore, MD 21201; (410) 528-0150.

88 "AIDS 1982-1992: Hope and Challenge of 10 Years of LSU AIDS Therapy with Ozone and a Multimodal Treatment Program." *Townsend Letter for Doctors* (August/September 1995), 52-61.

89 G. Soloman. "The Emerging Field of Psychoneuroimmunology." *Institutes for the Advancement of Health* 2:1 (1985), 6-19.

90 L. Chaitow and S. Martin. *A World Without AIDS* (London: Thorsons, 1989), 131.

91 L. Chaitow. *Soft Tissue Manipulation* (Rochester, VT: Healing Arts Press, 1989).

92 *Journal of Alternative and Complementary Medicine* (December 1992). G. Ironson et al. "Massage Therapy is Associated with Enhancement of the Immune System's Cytotoxic Capacity." *International Journal of Neuroscience* 84:1-4 (February 1996), 205-217.

ALLERGIES

1 American Academy of Allergy, Asthma & Immunology. *The Allergy Report 1* (Milwaukee, WI: American Academy of Allergy, Asthma & Immunology, 2000), 1.

2 Ibid., 2.

3 M. Lesser, M.D. *Nutrition and Vitamin Therapy* (Berkeley, CA: Parker House, 1982).

4 J. Mansfield, M.D. *Arthritis: The Allergy Connection* (San Francisco: Thorsons, 1990).

5 J.W. Gerrard et al. "The Familial Incidence of Allergy Disease." *Annals of Allergy* 36 (1976), 10.

6 F. Haschke et al. "Does Breast Feeding Protect from Atopic Diseases?" *Padiatrie und Padologie* 25:6 (1990), 415-420.

7 D. de Boissieu, C. Dupont, and J. Badoual. "Allergy to Nondairy Proteins in Mother's Milk as Assessed by Intestinal Permeability Tests." *Allergy* 49:10 (December 1994), 882-884.

8 K. Van Duren-Schmidt et al. "Prenatal Contact with Inhalant Allergens." *Pediatric Research* 41:1 (January 1997), 128-131.

9 William J. Rea, M.D. *Chemical Sensitivity, Vol. 3* (Boca Raton, FL: CRC Lewis, 1996), 1555-1579.

10 James Braly M.D. *Dr. Braly's Food Allergy & Nutrition Revolution* (New Canaan, CT: Keats Publishing, 1992), 61.

11 Ranjit Kumar Chandra. "Food Hypersensitivity and Allergic Disease: A Selective Review." *American Journal of Clinical Nutrition* 66 (1997), 526S-529S.

12 D.M. Fergussen, J.L. Horwood, and F.T. Shannon. "Early Solid Feeding and Recurrent Childhood Eczema: A 10-Year Longitudinal Study." *Pediatrics* 86:4 (October 1990), 541-546.

13 A. Custovic et al. "Indoor Allergens are a Primary Cause of Asthma." *European Respiratory Review* 8:532 (1998), 155-158.

14 R.F. Cathcart III, M.D. "The Vitamin C Treatment Of Allergy and the Normally Unprimed State of Antibodies." *Medical Hypotheses* 21:3 (November 1986), 307-332.

15 Jaqueline Krohn, M.D., Frances A. Taylor, M.A., and Erla Mae Larson, R.N. *The Whole Way to Allergy Relief & Prevention* (Vancouver, B.C.: Hartley & Marks Publishers, 1996), 55.

16 J. Krop et al. "A Double-Blind, Randomized, Controlled Investigation of Electrodermal Testing in the Diagnosis of Allergies." *Journal of Alternative and Complementary Medicine* 3:3 (Fall 1997), 241-248.

17 P. Yanick, Jr. "Immune Disorders-Allergy." *Townsend Letter for Doctors* 118 (May 1993), 498-500, 502.

18 E. Wolkenstein and F. Horak. "Protective Effect of Acupuncture on Allergen Provoked Rhinitis." *Wiener Medizinische Wochenschrift* 148:19 (1998), 450-453.

19 R.L Zhou and J.C. Zhang. "Desensitive Treatment with Positive Allergens in Acupoints of the Head for Allergic Rhinitis and Its Mechanism." *Chung Hsi I Chieh Ho Tsa Chih Chinese Journal of Modern Developments in Traditional Medicine* 11:12 (December 1991), 721-723.

ALZHEIMER'S DISEASE AND SENILE DEMENTIA

1 D.A. Evans, M.D. "Estimated Prevalence of Alzheimer's Disease in the United States." *Millbank Quarterly* 68:2 (1990), 267-289. P.H. St. George-Hyslop. "Piecing Together Alzheimer's." *Scientific American* 283:6 (2000), 76-83.

2 D.A. Evans, M.D., et al. "Prevalence of Alzheimer's Disease in a Community Population of Older Persons: Higher than Previously Reported." *Journal of the American Medical Association* 262:18 (November 1989), 2551-2556.

3 Richard Leviton. *Brain Builders* (Englewood Cliffs, NJ: Prentice Hall, 1995), 68-69.

4 Neil F. Bence, Roopal M. Sampat, and Ron R. Kopito. "Impairment of the Ubiquitin-Proteasome System by Protein Aggregation." *Science* (May 25, 2001), 1552-1555.

5 P.H. St. George-Hyslop. "Piecing Together Alzheimer's." *Scientific American* 283:6 (2000), 76-83.

6 Jerrold Maxmen, M.D. and Nicholas Ward, M.D. *Essential Psychopathology and Its Treatment* (New York: W.W. Norton, 1995), 125.

7 P.H. St. George-Hyslop. "Piecing Together Alzheimer's." *Scientific American* 283:6 (2000), 76-83.

8 D.M. Mann and M.M. Esiri. "The Pattern of Acquisition of Plaques and Tangles in the Brains of Patients Under 50 Years of Age with Down's Syndrome." *Journal of the Neurological Sciences* 89:2-3 (February 1989), 169-179.

9 Dharma Singh Khalsa, M.D. "Integrated Medicine and The Prevention and Reversal of Memory Loss." *Alternative Therapies* 4:6 (November 1998), 39-40.

10 M.R. Werbach, M.D. *Nutritional Influences on Mental Illness* (Tarzana, CA: Third Line Press, 1993). D.C. Martin. "B12 and Folate Deficiency Dementia." *Clinics in Geriatric Medicine* 4:4 (November 1988), 841-852. D.E. Thomas et al. "Tryptophan and Nutritional Status of Patients with Senile Dementia." *Psychological Medicine* 16:2 (May 1986), 297-305. A.M. Keatinge et al. "Vitamin B_1, B_2, B_6 and C Status in the Elderly." *Irish Medical Journal* 76 (December 1983), 488-490. G.E. Gibson et al. "Reduced Activities of Thiamine-Dependent Enzymes in the Brains and Peripheral Tissues of Patients with Alzheimer's Disease." *Archives of Neurology* 45:8 (August 1988), 836-840. M.G. Cole and J.F. Prchal. "Low Serum B_{12} in Alzheimer-Type Dementia." *Age and Ageing* 13:2 (March 1984), 101-105. A. Burns and T. Holland. "Vitamin E Deficiency." *The Lancet* 1:8484 (April 1986), 805-806. I.J. Deary et al. "Serum Calcium Levels in Alzheimer's Disease: A Finding and an Aetiological Hypothesis." *Personality and Individual Differences* 8:1 (1987), 75-80. K. Torizumi et al. "Relationship Between Parathyroid Hormone and Magnesium in Sera of Dementia Patients." *Radioisotopes* 37:4 (April 1988), 203-208. N.I. Ward and J.A. Mason. "Neutron Activation Analysis Techniques for Identifying Elemental Status in Alzheimer's Disease." *Journal of Radioanalytic Nuclear Chemistry* 113:2 (1987), 515-526.

11 *Physicians' Desk Reference* (Oradell, NJ: Medical Economics, 1993).

12 P. Zatta et al. "Alzheimer Dementia and the Aluminum Hypothesis." *Medical Hypotheses* 26 (1988), 139-142.

13 Editorial Staff. "Growing Evidence for Aluminum/Alzheimer's Link." *Clinical Psychiatry News* (December 1988), 2.

14 Thompson et al. Research study from the Sanders-Brown Center on Aging at the University of Kentucky Medical Center, Lexington, Kentucky, published in *Neurotoxicology* 9 (1988), 1.

15 R. Shiele et al. "Studies on the Mercury Content in Brain and Kidney Related to Number and Condition of Dental Fillings." Institution of Occupational and Social Medicine, University Erlangen, Nurnberg, West Germany (March 12, 1984).

16 Ward Dean, M.D. *Smart Drugs II* (Menlo Park, CA: Health Freedom Publications, 1993), 56-57.

International Journal of Neuroscience 59:4 (August 1991), 259-262. *Brain Research* 528:1 (September 24, 1990), 170-174. E. Souetre et al. "Abnormal Melatonin Response to 5-Methoxypsoralen in Dementia." *American Journal of Psychiatry* 146:8 (August 1989), 1037-1040. "Concentrations of Serotonin and Its Related Substances in the Cerebrospinal Fluid in Patients with Alzheimer-Type Dementia." *Neuroscience Letter* 141:1 (1992), 9-12.

17 Jerrold Maxmen, M.D., and Nicholas Ward, M.D. *Essential Psychopathology and Its Treatment* (New York: W.W. Norton, 1995), 119-120. Jeffrey S. Bland. *Improving Genetic Expression in the Prevention of the Diseases of Aging* (Monograph), 115-116. William Faloon. *The Life Extension Foundation Disease Prevention and Treatment Protocols* (Hollywood, FL: Life Extension Media, 1998), 5-6.

18 John Dommisse, M.D., F.R.C.P.(C). "A Nutritional-Metabolic Approach to Memory Loss: 18 Years' Experience." *The Science of Anti-Aging Medicine* (Chicago: American Academy of Anti-Aging Medicine, 1996), 119-128.

19 M. Imagawa et al. "Coenzyme Q10, Iron, and Vitamin B6 in Genetically Confirmed Alzheimer's Disease." *The Lancet* 340:8820 (September 1992), 671.

20 *Journal of Nutrition Research* 1, 259-266.

21 M. Imagawa et al. "Coenzyme Q10, Iron, and Vitamin B6 in Genetically Confirmed Alzheimer's Disease." *The Lancet* 340:8820 (September 1992), 671.

22 David J. Canty, Ph.D. "Lecithin and Choline in Human Health and Disease." *Nutrition Reviews* 52:10 (October 1994), 327-339.

23 M. Gautherie et al. "Vasodilator Effect of *Ginkgo biloba* Extract Determined by Skin Thermometry and Thermography." *Therapie* 27:5 (September-October 1972), 881-892. D.M. Warburton. "Clinical Psychopharmacology of *Ginkgo biloba* Extract." *Presse Medicale* 15:31 (September 1986), 1595-1604. M. Allard. "Treatment of the Disorders of Aging with *Ginkgo biloba* Extract: From Pharmacology to Clinical Medicine." *Presse Medicale* 15:31 (September 1986), 1540-1545.

24 S. Kanowski et al. "Proof of Efficacy of the *Ginkgo biloba* Special Extract EGb. 761 in Outpatients Suffering From Mild to Moderate Primary Degenerative Dementia of the Alzheimer-Type of Multi-Infarct Dementia." *Pharmacopsychiatry* 29 (1996): 47-56.

25 E. McDonagh, C. Rudolph, and E. Cheraskin. "An Oculocerebrovasculometric Analysis of the Improvement in Arterial Stenosis Following EDTA Chelation Therapy." In: E. Cranton, ed. *A Textbook on EDTA Chelation Therapy, Special Issue, Journal of Advancement in Medicine* 2:1-2 (New York: Human Sciences Press, 1989), 155. H.R. Casdorph. "EDTA Chelation Therapy: Efficacy in Brain Disorders." In: E. Cranton, ed. *A Textbook on EDTA Chelation Therapy, Special Issue, Journal of Advancement in Medicine* 2:1-2 (New York: Human Sciences Press, 1989), 131-153.

26 T. Warren. *Beating Alzheimer's* (Garden City Park, NY: Avery Publishing Group, 1991).

27 Dharma Singh Khalsa, M.D. "Integrated Medicine and the Prevention and Reversal of Memory Loss." *Alternative Therapies* 4:6 (November 1998), 39-40.

28 J. Suhr. "New Study: Alzheimer's Disease Patients May Benefit From Muscle Relaxation." Ohio University website: www.ohiou.edu/research-news.

ARTHRITIS

1 National Institutes of Health. *How to Cope with Arthritis* NIH Publication No. 82-1092 (Washington, DC: U.S. Department of Health and Human Services, Public Health Service, 1991).

2 Arthritis Foundation. "Arthritis Fact Sheet." Available from: Arthritis Foundation, 1330 West Peachtree Street, Atlanta, GA 30309; (404) 872-7100; website: www.arthritis.org. Michael T. Murray, N.D. *Arthritis* (Rocklin, CA: Prima Publishing, 1994), 3.

3 National Institutes of Health. *1993 Research Highlights: Arthritis, Rheumatic Diseases, and Related Disorders* NIH Publication No. 93-3413 (Washington, DC: U.S. Department of Health and Human Services, Public Health Service, 1993).

4 David S. Pisetsky, M.D., Ph.D., with Susan Flamholtz Trien. *Duke University Medical Center Book of Arthritis* (New York: Ballantine Books, 1995), 75-76.

5 "Briefing Paper for the Government Affair." Arthritis Foundation Agenda (March 19, 1993).

6 J.E. Pizzorno and M.T. Murray. *Encyclopedia of Natural Medicine* (Rocklin, CA: Prima Publishing, 1991).

7 Joseph Candel and David Sudderth. *The Arthritis Solution* (Rocklin, CA: Prima Publishing, 1997), 3.

8 J.L. Decker. "Arthritis." In: *Medicine for the Layman* NIH Publication No. 83-1945 (Washington, DC: U.S. Department of Health and Human Services, Public Health Service, 1982), 9-10.

9 A. di Fabio. *Gouty Arthritis* (Franklin, TN: The Rheumatoid Disease Foundation, 1989).

10 J.E. Pizzorno and M.T. Murray. *Encyclopedia of Natural Medicine* (Rocklin, CA: Prima Publishing, 1991).

11 R.F. Peat. "Hormone Balancing: Natural Treatment." *Journal of the Rheumatoid Disease Medical Association* 1:1 (1986).

12 C.O. Truss, M.D. *The Missing Diagnosis* (Birmingham, AL: C. Orion Truss, 1982). W.G. Crook, M.D. *The Yeast Connection* (Jackson, TN: Professional Books, 1986). W.G. Crook, M.D., and L. Stevens. *Solving the Puzzle of Your Hard-to-Raise Child* (Jackson, TN: Professional Books, 1987).

13 J.L. Decker. "Arthritis." In: *Medicine for the Layman* NIH Publication No. 83-1945 (Washington, DC: U.S. Department of Health and Human Services, Public Health Service, 1982), 11.

14 A. di Fabio. *Treatment and Prevention of Osteoarthritis, Parts I and II* (Franklin, TN: The Rheumatoid Disease Foundation, 1989).

15 James Balch, M.D., and Phyllis Balch. *Prescription for Nutritional Healing* (Garden City Park, NY: Avery Publishing, 1997), 138.

16 J.L. Decker. "Arthritis." In: *Medicine for the Layman* NIH Publication No. 83-1945 (Washington, DC: U.S. Department of Health and Human Services, Public Health Service, 1982), 11.

17 A. di Fabio. *The Art of Getting Well* (Franklin, TN: The Rheumatoid Disease Foundation, 1987). A. di Fabio. *Treatment and Prevention of Osteoarthritis, Parts I and II* (Franklin, TN: The Rheumatoid Disease Foundation, 1989).

18 This report is based solely on product labeling as published by PDR®. Copyright ©1993 by Medical Economics Data, a division of Medical Economics Company, Inc. All rights reserved.

19 Joseph Pizzorno, N.D., Michael T. Murray, N.D., and Patrick Donovan, R.N., N.D. "Bowel Toxemia, Permeability and Disease: New Informa-

tion to Support an Old Concept." *Textbook of Natural Medicine, IV: Bowel Toxemia* (Seattle, WA: Bastyr College Publications, 1985), 2.

20 J.E. Pizzorno and M.T. Murray. *Encyclopedia of Natural Medicine* (Rocklin, CA: Prima Publishing, 1991).

21 Ibid.

22 Ibid.

23 A. di Fabio. *Treatment and Prevention of Osteoarthritis, Parts I and II* (Franklin, TN: The Rheumatoid Disease Foundation, 1989).

24 Robert Garrison Jr., M.A., R.Ph., and Elizabeth Somer, M.A., R.D. *Nutrition Desk Reference* (New Canaan, CT: Keats Publishing, 1995), 242.

25 Susan E. Brown, Ph.D. *Better Bones, Better Body* (New Canaan, CT: Keats Publishing, 1996), 125.

26 J.E. Pizzorno and M.T. Murray. *Encyclopedia of Natural Medicine* (Rocklin, CA: Prima Publishing, 1991), 449.

27 T.H. Lee et al. "Effect of Dietary Enrichment with Eicosapentaenoic and Docosahexaenoic Acids on *In Vitro* Neutrophil and Monocyte Leukotriene Generation and Neutrophil Function." *New England Journal of Medicine* 312:19 (May 1985), 1217-1224.

28 J.E. Pizzorno and M.T. Murray. *Encyclopedia of Natural Medicine* (Rocklin, CA: Prima Publishing, 1991), 494.

29 J.E. Pizzorno and M.T. Murray. *A Textbook of Natural Medicine* (Seattle, WA: John Bastyr College Publications, 1989).

30 L.W. Blau. "Cherry Diet Control for Gout and Arthritis." *Texas Report on Biology and Medicine* 8 (1950), 309-311.

31 J.E. Pizzorno and M.T. Murray. *Encyclopedia of Natural Medicine* (Rocklin, CA: Prima Publishing, 1991), 337.

32 L. Pauling. *How to Live Longer and Feel Better* (New York: Avon Books, 1987). A. di Fabio. *The Art of Getting Well* (Franklin, TN: The Rheumatoid Disease Foundation, 1988).

33 G. Krystal, G.M. Morris, and L. Sokoloff. "Stimulation of DNA Synthesis by Ascorbate in Cultures of Articular Chondrocytes." *Arthritis and Rheumatism* 25 (1982), 318-325.

34 A. Mullen and C.W.M. Wilson. "The Metabolism of Ascorbic Acid in Rheumatoid Arthritis." *Proceedings of the Nutrition Society* 35 (1976), 8A-9A.

35 W. Kaufman, M.D. "The Use of Vitamin Therapy to Reverse Certain Concomitants of Aging." *Journal of the American Geriatrics Society* 3:11 (November 1955), 927-936. W. Kaufman, M.D. "Niacinamide: A Most Neglected Vitamin." *Journal of the International Academy of Preventive Medicine* 8:1 (Winter 1983). W. Kaufman, M.D. *The Common Form of Joint Dysfunction: Its Incidence and Treatment* (Brattleboro, VT: E.L. Hildreth, 1949).

36 H. Reichel, H.P. Koeffler, and A.W. Norman. "The Role of Vitamin-D Endocrine System in Health and Disease." *New England Journal of Medicine* 320 (1989), 980-981.

37 Jason Theodosakis, M.D., M.S., M.P.H., Brenda Adderly, M.H.A., and Barry Fox, Ph.D. *The Arthritis Cure* (New York: St. Martin's Griffin, 1997), 35-36.

38 R.L. Travers, G.C. Rennie, and R.E. Newnham. "Boron and Arthritis: The Results of a Double-Blind Pilot Study." *Journal of Nutrition in Medicine* 1 (1990), 127-132.

39 S.L. Meacham et al. "Effect of Boron Supplementation on Blood and Urinary Calcium, Magnesium, and Phosphorus, Urinary Boron in

Athletic and Sedentary Women." *American Journal of Clinical Nutrition* 61 (1995), 341-345.

40 F.H. Nielsen. "Studies on the Relationship Between Boron and Magnesium Which Possibly Affects the Formation and Maintenance of Bones." *Magnesium and Trace Elements* 9 (1990), 61-69.

41 C.L. Keen and S. Zidenberg-Cherr. "Manganese." In: M.L. Brown, ed. *Present Knowledge in Nutrition* 6th Ed. (Washington, DC: International Life Sciences Institute, 1990), 279-286.

42 John Anderson. "Quick-Acting Natural Arthritis Relief." *Alternative Medicine Digest* 20 (October/November 1997), 90.

43 D. Rothman et al. "Botanical Lipids: Effects in Inflammation, Immune Response, and Rheumatoid Arthritis." *Seminars in Arthritis and Rheumatism* (October 1995).

44 John Anderson. "S-Adenosyl-L-Methionine—Nutrient Duo Relieves Depression and Pain." *Alternative Medicine* 27 (December 1998/January 1999), 72.

45 H. Muller-Fassbender. "Double-Blind Clinical Trial of S-Adenosylmethionine Versus Ibuprofen in the Treatment of Osteoarthritis." *American Journal of Medicine* 83:Suppl 5A (1987), 81-83.

46 S. Glorioso et al. "Double-Blind Multicentre Study of the Activity of S-Adenosylmethionine in Hip and Knee Osteoarthritis." *International Journal of Clinical Pharmacology Research* 5 (1985), 39-49.

47 Julian Whitaker. *Health and Healing* (December 1995), 4-5.

48 I.W. Lane, Ph.D. "Shark Cartilage and the Pain of Arthritis." *Explore!* 3:6 (1992), 23.

49 J.E. Pizzorno and M.T. Murray. *Encyclopedia of Natural Medicine* (Rocklin, CA: Prima Publishing, 1991), 340.

50 John Anderson. "New Zealand's Green-Lipped Mussel for Arthritis Relief." *Alternative Medicine Digest* 21 (December 1997/January 1998), 74-77.

51 "Consumer Bulletin: Sea Cucumbers." *Whole Foods* (October 1994).

52 R.A. Hazelton. "A Cure in Rheumatoid Arthritis: A Six-Month Placebo-Controlled Study." University of Queensland, Australia, August 1992.

53 M. Walker. "Biochemical Components of Sea Cucumber for Human Benefit." *Explore!* 3 (1992), 12-17. M. Walker. "Chinese Seafood Eases Arthritis." *Natural Health* (March/April 1993).

54 R. Bingham, M.D. "Yucca Extract." *Journal of the Academy of Rheumatoid Diseases* 2:1 (1990), 20.

55 Elson M. Haas, M.D. *Staying Healthy with Nutrition* (Berkeley, CA: Celestial Arts, 1992), 272.

56 Kerry Bone. "Developments on Phytotherapy: *Boswellia serrata*." *The Modern Phytotherapist* 3:1 (Summer 1996). G.B. Singh et al. *Agents and Actions* 18 (1996), 407. M.L. Sharma et al. "Effect of Salai Guggal ex-*Boswellia serrata* on Cellular and Humoral Immune Responses and Leucocyte Migration." *Agents and Actions* 24:1-2 (1988), 161-164. M.L. Sharma et al. *International Journal of Immunopharmacology* 11 (1989), 647.

57 G. Kesava Reddy and S.C. Dhar. "Effect of a New Non-Steroidal Anti-inflammatory Agent on Lysosomal Stability in Adjuvant-Induced Arthritis." *Italian Journal of Biochemistry* 36:4 (1987), 205-217.

58 Kerry Bone, M.N.I.M.H. *Phytosynergistic Prescribing for Professional Prescribers* (Lake Oswego, OR: Communications Medicus, 1994), 23.

59 J.E. Pizzorno and M.T. Murray. *A Textbook of Natural Medicine* (Seattle, WA: John Bastyr College Publications, 1989).

60 J. Heimlich. *What Your Doctors Won't Tell You* (New York: Harper Perennial, 1990).

61 Ibid.

62 M.A. Van de Laar et al. "Food Intolerance in Rheumatoid Arthritis II: Clinical and Histological Aspects." *Annals of Rheumatic Disease* 51:3 (1992), 303-306.

63 A.M. Denman et al. "Joint Complaints and Food Allergic Disorders." *Annals of Allergy* 51:2 Part 2 (1983), 260-263.

64 I. Rolf. *Rolfing: The Integration of Human Structures* (New York: Harper & Row, 1977).

65 Michael Murray, N.D., Joseph Pizzorno, N.D., and Rick Kitaeff, N.D. *A Textbook of Natural Medicine: Non-Pharmacological Control of Pain IV* (Seattle, WA: Bastyr Publications, 1986), 2.

AUTISM

1 A. Knivsberg et al. "Dietary Intervention in Autistic Syndrome." *Brain Dysfunction* 3 (1990), 315-327.

2 J.L. Nanson. "Autism in Fetal Alcohol Syndrome: A Report of Six Cases." *Alcoholism, Clinical and Experimental Research* 16:3 (1992):558-565.

3 T. Hashimoto et al. "Reduced Brainstem Size in Children with Autism." *Brain and Development* 14:2 (1992), 94-97.

4 D.J. Cohen, W.T. Johnson, and B.K. Caparulo. "Pica and Elevated Blood Lead Level in Autistic and Atypical Children." *American Journal of Diseases of Children* 130:1 (January 1976), 47-48. M. Lesser. *Vitamin Therapy* (Berkeley, CA: Parker House, 1980). P. Accardo et al. "Autism and Plumbism: A Possible Association." *Clinical Pediatrics* 27:1 (January 1988), 41-44.

5 M.S. George et al. "Cerebral Blood Flow Abnormalities in Adults with Infantile Autism." *Journal of Nervous and Mental Disease* 180:7 (July 1992), 413-417.

6 P.I. Markowitz. "Autism in a Child with Congenital Cytomegalovirus Infection." *Journal of Autism and Developmental Disorders* 13:3 (September 1983), 249-253.

7 M.R. Werbach, M.D. *Nutritional Influences on Mental Illness* (Tarzana, CA: Third Line Press, 1991), 75.

8 H.L. Coulter. *Vaccination, Social Violence, and Criminality: The Medical Assault on the American Brain* (Berkeley, CA: North Atlantic Books, 1990).

9 Available on the California Department of Developmental Services website: www.dds.ca.gov /Autism/main/AutismReport.cfm.

10 A.J. Wakefield et al. "Ileal Lymphoid Nodular Hyperplasia, Non-Specific Colitis, and Regressive Developmental Disorder in Children." *The Lancet* 351 (1998), 637-641. B. Taylor et al. "Autism and Measles, Mumps, and Rubella Vaccine: No Epidemiological Evidence for a Causal Association." *The Lancet* 353 (1999), 2026-2029.

11 V. Singh and V. Yang. "Serological Association of Measles Virus and Human Herpes Virus-6 with Brain Autoantibodies in Autism." *Clinical Immunology and Immunopathology* 88:1 (1988), 105-108.

12 Defeat Autism Now! (DAN!). *Mercury Detoxification Consensus Group Position Paper* (San Diego, CA: Autism Research Institute, 2001).

13 Jeffrey Bland, Ph.D. *The 20-Day Rejuvenation Diet Program* (New Canaan, CT: Keats Publishing, 1997), 197.

14 K. Eto. "Pathology of Minamata Disease." *Toxicologic Pathology* 25:6 (1997), 614-623. Y. Korogi et al. "Representation of the Visual Field in the Stri-ate Cortex: Comparison of MR Findings with Visual Field Deficits in Organic Mercury Poisoning (Minamata Disease)." *American Journal of Neuroradiology* 18:6 (1997), 1127-1130. M.L. Queiroz and D.C. Dantas. "B Lymphocytes in Mercury-Exposed Workers." *Pharmacology & Toxicology* 81:3 (1997), 130-133. Sallie Bernard et al. "Autism: A Unique Type of Mercury Poisoning." Available from: ARC Research, 14 Commerce Drive, Cranford, NJ 07016; (201) 444-7306.

15 Defeat Autism Now! (DAN!). *Mercury Detoxification Consensus Group Position Paper* (San Diego, CA: Autism Research Institute, 2001).

16 R.J. McClelland et al. "Central Conduction Time in Childhood Autism." *British Journal of Psychiatry* 160 (May 1992), 659-663.

17 W.G. Crook, M.D., and L. Stevens. *Solving the Puzzle of Your Hard to Raise Child* (Jackson, TN: Professional Books, 1987).

18 J.J. McEachin, T. Smith, and O.I. Lovaas. "Long-Term Outcome for Children with Autism Who Received Early Intensive Behavioral Treatment." *Am J Ment Retard* 97:4 (1997), 359-372.

19 W.G. Crook, M.D., and L. Stevens. *Solving the Puzzle of Your Hard to Raise Child* (Jackson, TN: Professional Books, 1987).

20 L.C. Tollbert. "Ascorbic Acid: Therapeutic Trial in Autism." Presentation at the Autism Society of America Annual Conference, Indianapolis, Indiana (July 10-13, 1991).

21 J.R. Lightdale et al. "Evaluation of Gastrointestinal Symptoms in Autistic Children Before and Following Secretin Infusion." Paper presented at the World Congress of Pediatric Gastroenterology, Boston, Massachusetts (August 2000).

22 K. Horvath et al. "Gastrointestinal Abnormalities in Children with Autistic Disorder." *Journal of Pediatrics* 135:5 (1999), 559-563. K. Horvath et al. "Improved Social and Language Skills After Secretin Administration in Patients with Autistic Spectrum Disorders." *J Assoc Acad Minor Phys* 9:1 (1998), 9-15.

23 K. Horvath et al. "Secretin Improves Intestinal Permeability in Autistic Children." Paper presented at the World Congress of Pediatric Gastroenterology, Boston, Massachusetts (August 2000).

24 A. Knivsberg et al. "Dietary Intervention in Autistic Syndrome." *Brain Dysfunction* 3 (1990), 315-327.

25 W.G. Crook, M.D., and L. Stevens. *Solving the Puzzle of Your Hard to Raise Child* (Jackson, TN: Professional Books, 1987).

26 John E. Upledger, D.O., O.M.M. "Autism-Observations, Experiences and Concepts." Available on the Internet: www.upledger.com/clinic/ autism.htm.

27 J. Upledger. *Your Inner Physician and You: Craniosacral Therapy SomatoEmotional Release* (Berkeley, CA: North Atlantic, 1992).

28 John E. Upledger, D.O., O.M.M. "Autism-Observations, Experiences and Concepts." Available on the Internet: www.upledger.com/clinic/autism.htm.

BACK PAIN

1 J.N.A. Gibson, G. Waddell, and I.C. Grant. "Surgery for Degenerative Lumbar Spondylosis (Cochrane Review)." In: *The Cochrane Library 1* (Oxford: Update Software, 2001).

2 J.S. Saal, J.A. Saal, and E.F. Yurth. "Nonoperative Management of Herniated Cervical Intervertebral Disc with Radiculopathy." *Spine* 21:16 (August 15, 1996), 1877-1883.

3 M.P. Schatz, M.D. *Back Care Basics: A Doctor's Gentle Yoga Program for Back and Neck Pain Relief* (Berkeley, CA: Rodmell Press, 1992).

4 Ibid.

5 D.N. Foster and M.N. Fulton. "Back Pain and the Exercise Prescription." *Clinics in Sports Medicine* 10:1 (January 1991), 197-209.

6 M. Feldenkrais. *Body and Mature Behavior: A Study of Anxiety, Sex, Gravitation, and Learning* (New York: International Universities Press, 1970).

7 B.W. Koes et al. "Randomized Clinical Trial of Manipulative Therapy and Physiotherapy for Persistent Back and Neck Complaints: Results of One-Year Follow-Up." *British Medical Journal* 304:6827 (March 1992), 601-605.

8 T.W. Meade et al. "Low Back Pain of Mechanical Origin: Randomised Comparison of Chiropractic and Hospital Outpatient Treatment." *British Medical Journal* 300:6737 (June 1990), 1431-1437.

9 P. Shekelle et al. "Spinal Manipulation for Low Back Pain." *Annals of Internal Medicine* 117:7 (October 1992), 590-598.

10 K.B. Jarvis, R.B. Phillips, and E.K. Morris. "Cost per Case Comparison of Back Injury Claims: Chiropractic versus Medical Management for Conditions with Identical Diagnostic Codes." *Journal of Occupational Medicine* 33:8 (August 1991), 847-852.

11 M.P. Schatz, M.D. *Back Care Basics: A Doctor's Gentle Yoga Program for Back and Neck Pain Relief* (Berkeley, CA: Rodmell Press, 1992).

12 Jerome Schofferman, M.D., et al. "Childhood Psychological Trauma Correlates with Unsuccessful Spine Surgery." *Spine* 17:65 (June 1992), S138-S144.

13 Brian Nelson, M.D., and David Carpenter, M.S. "Can Spinal Surgery Be Prevented by Aggressive Strengthening Exercises? A Prospective Study of Cervical and Lumbar Patients." *Archives of Physical Medicine and Rehabilitation* 80 (January 1999), 20-25.

14 G. Crolle and E. D'este. "Glucosamine Sulfate for the Management of Arthrosis: A Controlled Clinical Investgation." *Current Medical Research and Opinion* 7 (1980), 104-109. A. Reichelt et al. "Efficacy and Safety of Intramuscular Glucosamine Sulfate in Osteoarthritis of the Knee: A Randomized, Placebo-Controlled, Double-Blind Study." *Arzneim Forsch* 44 (1994), 75-80.

CANCER

1 American Cancer Society. *Cancer Facts and Figures 1993* (Atlanta, GA: American Cancer Society, 1993).

2 S.S. Epstein. "Evaluation of the National Cancer Program and Proposed Reforms." *International Journal of Health Services* 23:1 (1983), 15-44.

3 J. Madeleine Nash. "The Enemy Within." *Time* (Fall 1996), 20.

4 American Cancer Society. *Facts About Cancer* (Atlanta, GA: American Cancer Society, 1996).

5 J.S. Bailar and E.M. Smith. "Progress Against Cancer?" *New England Journal of Medicine* 314 (1986), 1226.

6 B. Hankey, Chief of the Cancer Statistics Branch, National Cancer Institute. Personal communication (1994). The incidence of all cancers combined for the total population increased 13% from 1975 to 1989, from 332 per 100,000 to 376 per 100,000. The mortality rate rose 7%, from 162 deaths per 100,000 to 173 per 100,000.

7 National Cancer Institute. *Cancer Statistics Review, 1973-1989* (Washington, DC: National Institutes of Health, Office of Cancer Communications, 1992).

8 Tim Beardsley. "A War Not Won." *Scientific American* (January 1994), 130-138.

9 D. Kabelitz. "Modulation of Natural Killing by Tumor Promoters. The Regulatory Influence of Adherent Cells Varies with the Type of Target Cell." *Immunobiology* 169:4 (May 1985), 436-446.

10 J.E. Cleaver and D. Bootsma. "Xeroderma Pigmentosum: Biochemical and Genetic Characteristics." *Annual Review of Genetics* 9 (1975), 19-38. P.J. Fialkow. "Clonal Origin and Stem Cell Evolution of Human Tumors." In: J.J. Mulvihill, R.W. Miller, and J.F. Fraumeni, Jr., eds. *Genetics of Human Cancer* (New York: Raven Press, 1977), 439-453. A.G. Knudson. "Mutation and Human Cancer." *Advances in Cancer Research* 17 (1973), 317-352. A.G. Knudson. "Genetics and Etiology of Human Cancer." *Advances in Human Genetics* 8 (1977), 1-66.

11 H. Dreher. *Your Defense Against Cancer* (New York: Harper & Row, 1988), 18.

12 Ibid.

13 R.A. Zakour, T.A. Kunkel, and L.A. Loeb. "Metal-Induced Infidelity of DNA Synthesis." *Environmental Health Perspectives* 40 (August 1981), 197-205.

14 American Institute for Cancer Research. *The Cancer Process* (Washington, DC: American Institute for Cancer Research, 1991).

15 T.H. Mugh II. "Studies Stir Fears over Cancer Risks for Children." *The Los Angeles Times* 111 (November 8, 1992), A1.

16 B. Holmberg. "Magnetic Fields and Cancer: Animal and Cellular Evidence: An Overview." *Environmental Health Perspectives* 103:Suppl 2 (1995), 63-67.

17 U.S. Department of Health, Education, and Welfare. *Geomagnetism, Cancer, Weather, and Cosmic Radiation* (Salt Lake City, UT: U.S. Department of Health, Education, and Welfare, 1979).

18 D. Steinman. *Diet for a Poisoned Planet* (New York: Ballantine Books, 1992), 265.

19 C.B. Simone, M.D. *Cancer and Nutrition* (Garden City Park, NY: Avery Publishing Group, 1992), 20-21.

20 John W. Gofman, M.D., Ph.D., and Egan O'Connor. *X-Rays: Health Effects of Common Exams* (San Francisco: Sierra Club Books, 1985), 18.

21 M. Wasserman et al. "Organochlorine Compounds in Neoplastic and Adjacent Apparently Normal Breast Tissue." *Bulletin of Environmental Contaminants and Toxicology* 15 (1976), 478-484.

22 J. Westin and E. Richter. "Israeli Breast Cancer Anomaly." *Annals of the New York Academy of Sciences* 609 (1990), 269-279.

23 T.H. Maugh II. "Experts Downplay Cancer Risk of Chlorinated Water." *The Los Angeles Times* (July 2, 1992).

24 John Yiamouyiannis, Ph.D. *Fluoride: The Aging Factor* (Delaware, OH: Health Action Press, 1993), 61. Dr. Yiamouyiannis states, "It is quite clear that fluoride causes genetic damage.... Most evidence indicates that fluoride acts on the DNA repair enzyme system.... Furthermore, fluoride-induced genetic damage may also result form the general metabolic imbalance caused by fluoride selectively inhibiting certain enzymes."

25 D. Trichopoulos, F.P. Li, and D.J. Hunter. "What Causes Cancer?" *Scientific American* (September 1996), 80-87.

26 C.B. Simone. *Breast Health* (Garden City Park, NY: Avery Publishing Group, 1995), 134.

27 H. Dreher. *Your Defense Against Cancer* (New York: Harper & Row, 1988), 200.

28 C.B. Simone, M.D. *Cancer and Nutrition* (Garden City Park, NY: Avery Publishing Group, 1992), 15, 134.

29 A.L. Weinstein et al. "Breast Cancer Risk and Oral Contraceptive Use: Results from a Large Case-Control Study." *Epidemiology* 2:5 (September 1991), 353-358.

30 Joseph Pizzorno, N.D. *Total Wellness* (Rocklin, CA: Prima Publishing, 1996), 55.

31 M. Mayell. "Zapping Your Daily Diet: The Risks of Irradiated Foods." *EastWest* (February 1986), 36.

32 Ibid.

33 B. Rosenberg. "A Diner's Guide to Irradiation." *Science Digest* (September 1986), 30.

34 M.F. Jacobson. "Undoing Delaney: FDA Allows Free Use of Dangerous Additives." *Eating Clean: Overcoming Food Hazards* (Washington, DC: Center for the Study of Responsive Law, 1990), 48-49.

35 G.A. Strong. *Does Mercury from Dental Amalgam Contribute to Free Radical Pathology?* (Billings, MT: Strong Health Publications, 1995), 30-33.

36 Committee on Diet, Nutrition and Cancer, Assembly of Life Sciences, National Research Council. *Diet, Nutrition and Cancer* (Washington, DC: National Academy Press, 1982).

37 P. Toniolo et al. "Consumption of Meat, Animal Products, Protein and Fat and Risk of Breast Cancer: A Prospective Cohort Study in New York." *Epidemiology* 5:4 (1994), 391.

38 E. Giovannucci et al. "Intake of Fat, Meat and Fiber in Relation to Risk of Colon Cancer in Men." *Cancer Research* 54:9 (1994), 2390.

39 Committee on Diet, Nutrition and Cancer, Assembly of Life Sciences, National Research Council. *Diet, Nutrition and Cancer* (Washington, DC: National Academy Press, 1982).

40 Ibid.

41 C.B. Simone, M.D. *Cancer and Nutrition* (Garden City Park, NY: Avery Publishing Group, 1992), 15.

42 M.G. Enig et al. "Dietary Fat and Cancer Trends." *Federation Proceedings* 37 (1978), 2215-2220.

43 C.B. Simone. *Cancer and Nutrition* (Garden City Park, NY: Avery Publishing Group, 1992), 99.

44 J. Boik. "Humoral Factors that Affect Neoplasia: Eicosanoids." *Cancer and Natural Medicine* (Princeton, MN: Oregon Medical Press, 1995), 46-49.

45 P. Bougnoux et al. "Alpha-linolenic Acid Content of Adipose Breast Tissue: A Host Determinant of the Risk of Early Metastasis in Breast Cancer." *British Journal of Cancer* 70:2 (1994), 330-334.

46 J.B. Bristol. "Colorectol Cancer and Diet: A Case-Control Study with Special Reference to Dietary Fibre and Sugar." *Proceeding of the American Association of Cancer Research* 26 (March 1985), 206. See also: J.B. Bristol et al. "Sugar, Fat and the Risk of Colorectal Cancer." *British Medical Journal Clinical Research Edition* 291:6507 (November 1985), 1467-1470.

47 Joseph Pizzorno, N.D. *Total Wellness* (Rocklin, CA: Prima Publishing, 1996), 39-40.

48 A.W. Hsing et al. "Cancer Risk Following Primary Hemochromatosis: A Population-based Cohort Study in Denmark." *Journal of Cancer* (1995), 160-162.

49 P. Knekt et al. "Body Iron Stores and Risk of Cancer." *International Journal of Cancer* 56 (1994), 379-382. See also: R.G. Sevenes et al. "Moderate Elevation of Body Iron Level and Increased Risk of Cancer Occurrence and Death." *Journal of Cancer* 56 (1994), 364-369.

50 E. Giovannucci and W.C. Willett. "Dietary Lipids and Colon Cancer." *Principles Pract Oncol PPO Updates* 9:5 (1995), 1-12.

51 R.S. Sandler. "Diet and Cancer: Food Additives, Coffee, and Alcohol." *Nutrition and Cancer* 4:4 (1983), 273-278. See also: "Beer Drinking and the Risk of Rectal Cancer." *Nutrition Reviews* 42:7 (July 1984), 244-247. J.D. Potter and A.J. McMichael. "Alcohol, Beer and Lung Cancer: A Meaningful Relationship?" *International Journal of Epidemiology* 13:2 (June 1984), 240-242.

52 C.B. Simone. *Breast Health* (Garden City Park, NY: Avery Publishing Group, 1995), 143.

53 D. Simon et al. "Coffee Drinking and Cancer of the Lower Urinary Tract System." *Journal of the National Cancer Institute* 54:3 (1975), 587.

54 J. Mulvihill. "Caffeine as a Teratogen and Mutagen." *Teratology* 8:69 (1973). See also: D. Weinstein et al. "The Effects of Caffeine on Chromosomes of Human Lymphocytes." *Mutation Research* 16 (1972), 391.

55 R. Adler, ed. *Psychoneuroimmunology* (New York: Academic Press, 1981).

56 B.L. Bloom, S.J. Asher, and S.W. White. "Marital Disruption as a Stressor: A Review and Analysis." *Psychological Bulletin* 85:4 (1978), 867-894. L.L. LeShan. "An Emotional Life History Pattern Associated with Neoplastic Disease." *Annals of the New York Academy of Sciences* 125:3 (1966), 780-793. B.L. Ernster et al. "Cancer Incidence by Marital Status: U.S. Third National Cancer Survey." *Journal of the National Cancer Institute* 63:3 (1979), 567-585.

57 S. Greer and T. Morris. "Psychological Attributes of Women Who Develop Breast Cancer: A Controlled Study." *Journal of Psychosomatic Research* 19:2 (1975), 147-153.

58 H. Dreher. *Your Defense Against Cancer* (New York: Harper & Row, 1988), 246-247.

59 Christiane Northrup, M.D. *Women's Bodies, Women's Wisdom* (New York: Bantam Books, 1994), 35-40.

60 Ann Louise Gittleman. *Guess What Came to Dinner: Parasites and Your Health* (Garden City Park, NY: Avery Publishing Group, 1993).

61 D. Trichopoulos, F.P. Li, and D.J. Hunter. "What Causes Cancer?" *Scientific American* (September 1996), 82-83.

62 William Carlsen. "Rogue Virus in the Vaccine." *The San Francisco Chronicle* (July 15, 2001), A1.

63 Joseph Pizzorno, N.D. *Total Wellness* (Rocklin, CA: Prima Publishing, 1996), 93-94.

64 Quoted in: Robert A. Weinberg. *Racing to the Beginning of the Road: The Search for the Origin of Cancer* (New York: Harmony Books, 1996), 11.

65 R. Walters. "Enderlein Therapy: A Cancer Therapy That Promotes Gentle Self-Healing." *Raum & Zeit* 3:1 (1991), 24.

66 R.M. McAllister, M.D., S.T. Horowitz, Ph.D., and R.V. Gilden, Ph.D. *Cancer* (New York: Basic Books, 1993), 39, 43.

67 F.P. Perera. "Uncovering New Clues to Cancer Risk." *Scientific American* (May 1996), 54-62.

68 W. John Diamond, M.D., W. Lee Cowden, M.D., with Burton Goldberg. *Alternative Medicine Definitive Guide to Cancer* (Tiburon, CA: Future Medicine Publishing, 1997), 703.

69 Virginia L. Ernster et al. "Incidence of and Treatment for Ductal Carcinoma in Situ of the Breast." *Journal of the American Medical Association* 275 (March 27, 1996), 913-918.

70 C.J. Wright and C.B. Mueller. "Screening Mammography and Public Health Policy: The Need for Perspective." *The Lancet* 346 (July 1995), 29-32.

71 D. Plotkin. "Good News and Bad News About Breast Cancer." *The Atlantic Monthly* (June 1996), 82.

72 M.A. Helvie et al. "Mammographic Follow-up of Low-Suspicion Lesions: Compliance Rate and Diagnostic Yield." *Radiology* 178 (1991), 155-158.

73 National Women's Health Network. *Mammography in Women Before Menopause* (Washington, DC: National Women's Health Network, 1993).

74 Ibid.

75 G. Dardick. "Breast Self-Examine: A New Program Makes Early Detection Easier." *East West* (July/August 1991), 32-36.

76 S.S. Epstein and D. Steinman. *New Hope—Everything You Wanted to Know About Breast Cancer Prevention But the Cancer Establishment Never Told You: A Guide for Dramatically Reducing Your Risk* (New York: Macmillan, 1993.)

77 Committee on Diet, Nutrition, and Cancer, Assembly of Life Sciences, National Research Council. *Diet, Nutrition and Cancer* (Washington, DC: National Academy Press, 1982).

78 H. Dreher. *Your Defense Against Cancer* (New York: Harper & Row, 1988), 38.

79 Committee on Diet, Nutrition, and Cancer, Assembly of Life Sciences, National Research Council. *Diet, Nutrition and Cancer* (Washington, DC: National Academy Press, 1982).

80 B.R. Goldin et al. "Estrogen Excretion Patterns and Plasma Levels in Vegetarian and Omnivorous Women." *New England Journal of Medicine* 307 (1982), 1542-1547.

81 Committee on Diet, Nutrition, and Cancer, Assembly of Life Sciences, National Research Council. *Diet, Nutrition and Cancer* (Washington, DC: National Academy Press, 1982).

82 M.G. Enig et al. "Dietary Fat and Cancer Trends." *Federation Proceedings* 37 (1978), 2215-2220.

83 H. Dreher. *Your Defense Against Cancer* (New York: Harper & Row, 1988), 113.

84 J.B. Bristol. "Colorectal Cancer and Diet: A Case-Control Study with Special Reference to Dietary Fibre and Sugar." *Proceedings of the American Association of Cancer Research* 26 (March 1985), 206. J.B. Bristol et al. "Sugar, Fat and the Risk of Colorectal Cancer." *British Medical Journal* 291:6507 (November 1985), 1467-1470.

85 D. Simon, S. Yen, and P. Cole. "Coffee Drinking and Cancer of the Lower Urinary System." *Journal of the National Cancer Institute* 54:3 (March 1975), 587-591. J.J. Mulvehill. "Caffeine as Teratogen and Mutagen." *Teratology* 8:1 (August 1973), 69-72. D. Weinstein, I. Mauer, and H.M. Solomon. "The Effects of Caffeine on Chromosomes of Human Lymphocytes: In Vivo and In Vitro Studies." *Mutation Research* 16:4 (December 1972), 391-399.

86 R.S. Sandler. "Diet and Cancer: Food Additives, Coffee and Alcohol." *Nutrition and Cancer* 4:4 (1983), 273-279. Editorial Staff. "Beer Drinking and the Risk of Rectal Cancer." *Nutrition Reviews* 42:7 (July 1984), 244-247. J.D. Potter and A.J. McMichael. "Alcohol, Beer and Lung Cancer: A Meaningful Relationship?" *International Journal of Epidemiology* 13:2 (1984), 240-242.

87 B. Smith. "Organic Foods vs. Supermarket Foods: Element Level." *Journal of Applied Nutrition* 45:1 (1993), 35-39.

88 "Study Finds Vitamins Cut Cancer Deaths." *The Los Angeles Times* (September 15, 1993).

89 C. La Vecchia et al. "Dietary Vitamin A and the Risk of Invasive Cervical Cancer." *International Journal of Cancer* 34:3 (1984), 319-322.

90 M.S. Menkes et al. "Serum Beta Carotene, Vitamins A and, Selenium and the Risk of Lung Cancer." *New England Journal of Medicine* 315 (1986), 1250.

91 "Dietary Aspects of Carcinogenesis." (September 1983).

92 P. Ramaswany and R. Natarajan. "Vitamin B6 Status in Patients with Cancer of the Uterine Cervix." *Nutrition and Cancer* 6 (1984), 176-180.

93 K.A. Steinmetz and J.D. Potter. "Vegetables, Fruit, and Cancer II: Mechanisms." *Cancer Causes and Control* (1991), 427-442.

94 Michael T. Murray, N.D. *Encyclopedia of Nutritional Supplements* (Rocklin, CA: Prima Publishing, 1996).

95 H.B. Stahelin et al "Cancer, Vitamins, and Plasma Lipids: Prospective Basel Study." *Journal of the National Cancer Institute* 73 (1984), 1463-1468.

96 E.T. Cameron et al. "Ascorbic Acid and Cancer: A Review." *Cancer Research* 39 (1979), 663-681.

97 R.H. Yonemoto. "Vitamin C and Immunological Response in Normal Controls and Cancer Patients." *Medico Dialogo* 5 (1979), 23-30.

98 B.V. Siegel and J.I. Morton. "Vitamin C and the Immune Response." *Experientia* 33 (1977), 393-395.

99 R.A. Good et al. "Nutrition, Immnity and Cancer—A Review." *Clinical Bulletin* 9 (1979), 3-12, 63-75.

100 J. Boik. "Conducting Research on Natural Agents: Vitamin D Metabolites." *Cancer and Natural Medicine* (Princeton, MN: Oregon Medical Press, 1995), 181.

101 H.B. Stahelin et al "Cancer, Vitamins, and Plasma Lipids: Prospective Basel Study." *Journal of the National Cancer Institute* 73 (1984), 1463-1468.

102 C.E. Butterworth et al. "Improvement in Cervical Dysplasia Associated with Folic Acid Therapy in Users of Oral Contraceptives." *American Journal of Clinical Nutrition* 35:1 (1982), 73-82.

103 W.C. Willett and B. MacMahon. "Prediagnostic Serum Selenium and the Risk of Cancer." *The Lancet* 2:8342 (July 1983), 130-134.

104 M.L. Slattery, A.W. Sorenon, and M.H. Ford. "Dietary Calcium Intake as a Mitigating Factor in Colon Cancer." *American Journal of Epidemiology* 128:3 (1988), 504-514.

105 V.W. Stadel. "Dietary Iodine and the Risk of Breast, Endometrial, and Ovarian Cancer." *The Lancet* 1:7965 (1976), 890-891.

106 J.M. Blondell. "The Anticarcinogenic Effect of Magnesium." *Medical Hypotheses* 6:8 (1980), 863-871.

107 P. Whelen, B.E. Walker, and J. Kelleher. "Zinc, Vitamin A and Prostatic Cancer." *British Journal of Urology* 55:5 (1983), 525-528.

108 Emile Bliznakov and Gerald Hunt. *The Miracle Nutrient Coenzyme Q10* (New York: Bantam Books, 1987).

109 B. Leibovitz et al. "Dietary Supplements of Vitamin E, Beta-carotene, Coenzyme Q10, and Selenium Protect Tissues Against Lipid Peroxidation in Rat Tissue Slices." *Journal of Clinical Nutrition* 120 (1990), 97-104.

110 K. Folkers et al. "Survival of Cancer Patients on Therapy with CoQ10." *Biochemical and Biophysical Research Communications* 192:1 (1993), 241-245.

111 F. Kroning. "Garlic as an Inhibitor for Spontaneous Tumors in Mice." *Acta Unio Internationalis Contra Cancrum* 20:3 (1964), 855.

112 W.C. You et al. "Allium Vegetables and Reduced Risk of Stomach Cancer." *Journal of the National Cancer Institute* 81:2 (1989), 162-164.

113 Earl R. Mindell, Ph.D. *Earl Mindell's Food as Medicine* (New York: Simon & Schuster, 1994), 31.

114 E. Giovannucci et al. "Intake of Carotenoids and Retinol in Relation to Risk of Prostate Cancer." *Journal of the National Cancer Institute* 87:23 (December 6, 1995), 1767-1776. Martin M. Stevenson. "Tomato Sauce Helps Reduce the Risk of Prostate Cancer." *Modern Medicine* 64 (February 1, 1996), 17. S. Franceschi et al. "Tomatoes and Risk of Digestive-Tract Cancers." *International Journal of Cancer* 59:2 (October 15, 1994), 181-184.

115 Earl R. Mindell, Ph.D. *Earl Mindell's Food as Medicine* (New York: Simon & Schuster, 1994), 171-172.

116 S. Barnes et al. "Soybeans Inhibit Mammary Tumors in Models of Breast Cancer." In: M. Pariza, ed. *Mutagens and Carcinogens in the Diet* (New York: Alan R. Liss, 1990), 239-257.

117 M.J. Messina et al. "Soy Intake and Cancer Risk: A Review of the In Vitro and In Vivo Data." *Nutrition & Cancer* 21:2 (1994), 113-131.

118 E.L. Wynder et al. "Diet and Breast Cancer in Causation and Therapy." *Cancer* 58:8 Suppl (1986), 1804-1831.

119 P. Greenward and E. Lanze. "Dietary Fiber and Colon Cancer." *Contemporary Nutrition* 11:1 (1986).

120 "Risk Reduction Objectives." *Healthy People 2000* (Washington, DC: U.S. Public Health Service, U.S. Dept. of Health and Human Services, 1990), 425.

121 L. Chaitow and N. Trenev. "The *Lactobacilli* and *Bifidobacteria*." *Probiotics* (Prescott, AZ: Hohm Press, 1995), 24-25.

122 Y. Aso et al. "Preventive Effect of *Lactobacillus casei* Preparation on the Recurrence of Superficial Bladder Cancer in a Double-blind Trial." *European Urology* 27 (1995), 104-109.

123 I.G. Gogdanov et al. "Antitumor Glycopeptides from *Lactobacillus Bulgaricus* Cell Wall." *FEBS Letters* 57 (1975), 259-261. Cited by: R. Moss. *Cancer Therapy* (New York: Equinox Press, 1993), 239.

124 D. Steinman and S.S. Epstein. *The Safe Shopper's Bible* (New York: Macmillan, 1994).

125 Ibid.

126 L.F. Berkman and S.L. Syme. "Social Networks, Host Resistance, and Mortality: A Nine-Year Follow-Up Study of Alameda County Residents." *American Journal of Epidemiology* 109:2 (February 1979), 189-204.

127 D. Spiegel et al. "Effect of Psychosocial Treatment on Survival of Patients with Metastatic Breast Cancer." *The Lancet* 2:8668 (October 1989), 888-891.

128 B. Lynes. *The Healing of Cancer* (Queensville, Ontario, Canada: Marcus Books, 1989), 10.

129 J. Cairns, M.D. "The Treatment of Diseases and the War Against Cancer." *Scientific American* (November 1985).

130 B. Fisher et al. "Five-Year Results of a Randomized Clinical Trial Comparing Total Mastec-tomy and Segmental Mastectomy With or Without Radiation in the Treatment of Breast Cancer." *New England Journal of Medicine* 11 (March 1985), 312.

131 R.E. Curtis et al. "Risk of Leukemia Associated with the First Course of Cancer Treatment: an Analysis of the Surveillance, Epidemiology, and End Results Program Experience." *Journal of the National Cancer Institute* 72:3 (March 1984), 531-544.

132 J.D. Boice and L.B. Travis. "Body Wars: Effect of Friendly Fire (Cancer Therapy)." *Journal of the National Cancer Institute* 87:10 (1995), 732-741.

133 Joseph Neglia, M.D. Paper presented at the American Association for Cancer Research annual meeting, New Orleans, Louisiana (March 27, 2001).

134 Robert C. Atkins, M.D. *Dr. Atkins' Health Revolution: Cancer Therapy* (Boston: Houghton Mifflin, 1988), 324.

135 A. Brohult. "Effect of Alkoxyglycerols on the Frequency of Injuries Following Radiation Therapy for Carcinoma of the Uterine Cervix." *Acta Obstetrica et Gynecologica Scandinavica* 56:4 (1977), 441-448. See also: A. Brohult. "Effect of Alkoxyglycerols on the Frequency of Injuries Following Radiation Therapy." *Experientia* 29 (1973), 81-82.

136 B. Hallgren and S. Larsson. "The Glycerol Ethers in the Liver Oils of Elasmobranch Fish." *Lipid Research* 3 (1962), 31-38.

137 Ibid., 39-43.

138 W.E. Berdel et al. "Antitumor Action of Alkyl-lysophospholipids." *Anticancer Research* 1:6 (1981), 345-352.

139 L. Diamoede. "Increased Ether Lipid Cytotoxicity by Reducing Membrane Cholesterol Content." *International Journal of Cancer* 49:3 (1991), 409-413.

140 A. Brohult et al. "Regression of Tumor Growth after Administration of Alkoxyglycerols." *Acta Obstetrica et Gynecologica Scandinavica* 57 (1978), 79-83.

141 A. Brohult. "Alkoxyglycerols and Their Use in Radiation Treatment." *Acta Radiologica* 223 (1963), 7-99.

142 S. Burzynski, M.D. "Antineoplastons." From a lecture presented at the World Research Foundation Congress, Los Angeles, California (October 7, 1990).

143 S. Burzynski, M.D. "Synthetic Antineoplastons and Analogs." *Drugs of the Future* 11:8 (1986), 679.

144 S. Burzynski, M.D. "Antineoplastons." From a lecture presented at the World Research Foundation Congress, Los Angeles, California (October 7, 1990).

145 R. Pelton and L. Overholser. "Antineoplastons." *Alternatives in Cancer Therapy* (New York: Simon & Schuster, 1994), 192.

146 H. Tsuda et al. "The Inhibitor Effect of Antineoplaston A10 on Breast Cancer Transplanted to Athymic Mice and Human Hepatocellular Carcinoma Cell Lines." *Kurume Medical Journal* 37 (1990), 97-104.

147 F. Wiewel. "Burzynski's Antineoplastons Increase Activity of Tumor Suppressor Genes." *Options* 1:4 (1995), 2.

148 "Special Hearing on Alternative Medicine." Subcommittee of the Committee on Appropriations, United States Senate (June 24, 1993), 36-41.

149 G. Naessens. "Béchamp's Microzyma to the Somatid Theory: 714X, a Highly Promising Non-Toxic Treatment for Cancer and Other Immune Deficiencies." Symposium (unpublished manuscript), Quebec, Canada (1991).

150 G. Naessens. "Béchamp's Microzyma to the Somatid Theory: 714X, a Highly Promising Non-Toxic Treatment for Cancer and Other Immune Deficiencies." Symposium (unpublished manuscript), Quebec, Canada (1991).

151 M. Kuroda et al. "Decreased Serum Levels of Selenium and Glutathione Peroxidase Activity Associated with Aging, Malignancy and Chronic Hemodialysis." *Trace Elements in Medicine* 5:3 (1988), 97-103.

152 J. Boit. "Amino Acids." *Cancer and Natural Medicine: A Textbook of Basic Science and Clinical Research* (Princeton, MN: Oregon Medical Press, 1995), 139-140.

153 M.S. Palermo et al. "Immunomodulation Exerted by Cyclophosphamide is Not Interfered by N-Acetyl Cysteine." *International Journal of Immunopharmacology* 8:6 (1986), 651-655. See also: A. Schmitt-Graff and M.E. Scheulen. "Prevention of Adriamycin Cardiotoxicity by Niacin, Isocitrate or N-Acetyl-Cysteine in Mice. A Morphological Study." *Pathology Resident Practice* 181:2 (1986), 168-174. J.A. Kim et al. *Seminars in Oncology* 10:Suppl 1 (1983), 86.

154 V.A. Filov et al. "Results of Clinical Evaluation of Hydrazine Sulfate." *Voprosy Onkologii* 36:6 (1990), 721-726. See also: M.L. Gershanovich et al. "Results of Clinical Study of Antitumor Action of Hydrazine Sulfate." *Nutrition and Cancer* 3 (1981), 7-12.

155 R.T. Chlebowski et al. "Hydrazine Sulfate's Influence on Nutritional Status and Survival in Non-Small-Cell Lung Cancer." *Journal of Clinical Oncology* 8:1 (1990), 9-15. This was a randomized, placebo-controlled clinical trial—the gold standard of modern medical research.

156 V. Filov et al. "Results of Clinical Evaluation of Hydrazine Sulfate." *Voprosy Onkologii* 36 (1990), 721-726.

157 W.J. Adams and D.L. Morris. "Short-Course Cimetidine and Survival with Colorectal Surgery." *The Lancet* 344 (December 24/31, 1994), 1768-1769.

158 S. Matsumoto. "Cimetidine and Survival with Colorectal Cancer." *The Lancet* 346 (July 8, 1995), 115.

159 R. Hast et al. "Cimetidine as an Immune Response Modifier." *Medical Oncology and Tumor Pharmacotherapy* 6:1 (1989), 111-113.

160 N.H. Brockmeyer et al. "Cimetidine and the Immuno-Response in Healthy Volunteers." *Journal of Investigative Dermatology* 93 (1989), 757-761.

161 W.I. Lane and L. Cormac. *Sharks Don't Get Cancer* (Garden City Park, NY: Avery Publishing, 1992), 47.

162 T.H. Maugh II. "Angiogenesis Inhibitors Link Many Diseases." *Science* 212:4501 (June 1981), 1374-1375.

163 W.I. Lane and L. Cormac. *Sharks Don't Get Cancer* (Garden City Park, NY: Avery Publishing, 1992), 47.

164 I. William Lane. "Shark Cartilage Therapy Results and Research Today." Physician Information Package, Cartilage Consultants (Spring 1995). Contact Lane Labs at (201) 391-8601.

165 Gerald Batist, of McGill University, in a study presented at the American Association for Cancer Research annual meeting, New Orleans, Louisiana (March 26, 2001).

166 I.W. Lane. *Shark Cartilage Update Newsletter* 1:3 (1994), 1.

1142

167 T. Oikawa et al. "A Novel Angiogenic Inhibitor Derived from Japanese Shark Cartilage. Extraction and Estimation of Inhibitory Activities Toward Tumor and Embryonic Angiogenesis." *Cancer Letters* 51 (1990), 181-186.

168 L. Altman. "Tumor Growth is Controlled by Substance Found in Sharks." *The New York Times* (May 1, 1996).

169 H.W. Manner et al. "Amygdalin, Vitamin A and Enzyme Induced Regression of Murine Mammary Adenocarcinomas." *Journal of Manipulative and Physiological Therapeutics* 1:4 (December 1978), 246-248.

170 Ibid.

171 R. Ericson. *Cancer Treatment: Why So Many Failures?* (Memorial Park Ridge, IL: GE-PS Cancer Memorial, 1979), 68.

172 R.W. Moss. *The Cancer Industry: Unraveling the Politics* (New York: Paragon House, 1989).

173 D. Rubin. "Dosage Levels for Laetrile." *Choice* 3:6 (1977), 8-9.

174 J.W. Nowicky et al. "Ukrain as Both an Anticancer and Immunoregulatory Agent." *Drugs Under Experimental and Clinical Research* XVIII:Suppl (1992), 51-54.

175 A. Lohninger and F. Hamler. "Chelidonium Majus L. (Ukrain) in the Treatment of Cancer Patients." *Drugs Under Experimental and Clinical Research* XVIII:Suppl (1992), 73-77.

176 A. Staniszewski et al. "Lymphocyte Subsets in Patients with Lung Cancer Treated with Thiophosphoric Acid Alkaloid Derivatives from Chelidonium Majus L. (Ukrain)." *Drugs Under Experimental and Clinical Research* XVIII:Suppl (1992), 63-67. P. Pengsaa et al. "The Effect of Thiophosphoric Acid (Ukrain) on Cervical Cancer, Stage IB Bulky." *Drugs Under Experimental and Clinical Research* XVIII:Suppl (1992), 69-72.

177 J.W. Nowicky. "New Immuno-Stimulating Anticancer Preparation: Ukrain." Proceedings of the 13th International Congress of Chemotherapy, Vienna, Austria (August 28-September 2, 1983).

178 J. Nowicky. "Cancer Treatment Using Anticancer Preparation Alkaloid Derivative Ukrain." Fourth Mediterranean Congress of Chemotherapy. Rhodos, Greece (October 1984). *Chemioterapia* 4:Suppl 2 (1985), 1169-1171. See also: J. Nowicky et al. "Biological Activity of Ukrain In Vitro and In Vivo." Fifth Mediterranean Congress of Chemotherapy, Cairo, Egypt (January 26-November 1, 1986). *Chemioterapia* 6:Suppl 2 (1987), 683-685.

179 O. Hohenwarter et al. "Selective Inhibition of In Vitro Cell Growth by the Anti-Tumor Drug Ukrain." *Drugs Under Experimental and Clinical Research* 18:Suppl (1992), 1-4.

180 A. Liepins. "Ukrain as an Experimental Cytotoxic Agent." *Journal of Chemotherapy* 5:Suppl 1 (1992), 797-799.

181 J.W. Nowicky et al. "Macroscopic UV-marking Through Affinity." *Journal of Tumor Marker Oncology* 3:4 (1988), 463-465.

182 Ibid.

183 R. Walters. *Options: The Alternative Cancer Therapy Book* (Garden City Park, NY: Avery Publishing Group, 1993), 75.

184 V. Livingston-Wheeler, M.D. *The Conquest of Cancer* Transcript from a videotape program. (San Diego, CA: Waterside Productions, 1984), 25.

185 Ibid., 26, 29.

186 S. Duerksan. "Skeptical Scientists Test Alleged 'Cancer Vaccine'." *Townsend Letter for Doctors* 47 (May 1987).

187 G.F. Springer. "T and Tn General Carcinoma Autoantigens." *Science* 224 (1984), 1198-1206. See also: D.B. Avichezer et al. "Immunoreactivities of Polyclonal and Monoclonal Antibodies Specific for Human Thomsen-Friedenreich (T) and Tn Antigens with Human Carcinoma Cells." Abstract from the 25th Israel Immunological Society Meeting (1995).

188 G.F. Springer. "T/Tn Antigen: Two Decades of Experience in Early Immuno-detection and Therapy of Human Carcinoma." *Jung Foundation Proceedings* (Stuttgart, Germany: G. Thieme).

189 G.F. Springer et al. "T/Tn Pancarcinoma Autoantigens: Fundamental Diagnostic and Prognostic Aspects." *Cancer Detection and Prevention* 19 (1995), 173-182.

190 G.F. Springer. "T/Tn Antigen: Two Decades of Experience in Early Immuno-detection and Therapy of Human Carcinoma." *Jung Foundation Proceedings* (Stuttgart, Germany: G. Thieme). Note: 12 of the 26 patients were over age 50 at the time of the operation.

191 F. Wiewel. Personal communication with Charles Starnes (1995).

192 Patricia Spain Ward. "History of BCG Vaccine (Bacillus Calmette-Guerin)." *Townsend Letter for Doctors & Patients* (October 1996), 72-77.

193 E. Enby et al. "Hidden Killers: Causes of Cancer: A New Look." *The Revolutionary Medical Discoveries of Professor Gunther Enderlein* (Saratoga, CA: Sheehan Communications, 1990), 77.

194 Ibid.

195 R. Walters. "Enderlein Therapy: A Cancer Therapy that Promotes Gentle Self-healing." *Raum & Zeit* 3:1 (1991), 24-27.

196 W. James. "Nutrition and Cancer: The Gonzales Story." *World Research Foundation News* 3rd & 4th Quarter (1990), 5.

197 Ibid.

198 M. Gerson, M.D. *A Cancer Therapy: Results of Fifty Cases* (Bonita, CA: Gerson Institute, 1990).

199 G. Hildenbrand and S. Cavin. "Five-Year Survival Rates of Melanoma Patients Treated by Diet Therapy after the Manner of Gerson: A Retrospective Review." *Alternative Therapies in Health and Medicine* 1:4 (1995), 29-37.

200 M. Dewhirst, Professor of Radiation Oncology and Director of the Duke Hyperthermia Program at the Duke University Medical Center, Durham, North Carolina. Personal communication (1996).

201 Ibid.

202 *Cancer: A Healing Crisis* (Los Angeles: Cancer Resource Center, 1980), xiii.

203 Ibid.

204 "Special Hearing on Alternative Medicine." Subcommittee of the Committee on Appropriations, United States Senate (June 24, 1993), 65.

205 E. Pisha et al. "Discovery of Betulinic Acid as a Selective Inhibitor of Human Melanoma that Functions by Induction of Apoptosis." *Nature Medicine* 10 (1995), 1046-1051.

206 M. Centofanti. "Birch Bark Has Anticancer Bite." *Science News* 148 (1995), 231. Original report appeared in *Nature Medicine* (October 1995).

207 B. Cook. "Tree of Life Helps in Advanced Cancer." *International Journal of Alternative & Complementary Medicine* (January 1992), 23.

208 "Cancer Patients Should Eat Pineapples." *International Journal of Alternative & Complementary Medicine* (January 1992), 23. Original report appeared in *Planta Medica* 54:5 (1988), 377-378.

209 J.A. Duke. "Weeds? Or Wonder Drugs?" *Organic Gardening* (July/August 1994), 39.

210 L. Tenney. "Gotu kola." *Today's Herbal Health* (Provo, UT: Woodland Books, 1992), 78.

211 T.D. Babu et al. "Cytotoxic and Antitumor Properties of Certain Taxa of *Umbelliferae* with Special Reference to *Centella asiatica*." *Journal of Ethnopharmacology* 48 (1995), 53-57.

212 J.D. Haag et al. "Enhanced Inhibition of Protein Isoprenylation and Tumor Growth by Perillyl Alcohol, an Hydroxylated Analog of D-limonene." *Proceedings of the American Association of Cancer Research* 33 (1992), 524.

213 R. Brown. *Bee Hive Product Bible* (Garden City Park, NY: Avery Publishing, 1994), 47.

214 Ibid., 116-117.

215 Ibid., 49.

216 T. Johnson. "Herbs for Cancer." Personal communication (1996).

217 C. Lersch et al. "Simulation of Immunocompetent Cells in Patients with Gastrointestinal Tumors During an Experimental Therapy with Low-Dose Cyclophophamide, Thymostimulin, and *Echinacea purpurea* Extract (Echinacin)." *Tumordiagen Therapy* 13 (1992), 115-120. Cited in: M. Werbach and M. Murray. *Botanical Influences on Illness* (Tarzana, CA: Third Line Press, 1994), 94-95.

218 C. Lersch et al. "Stimulation of the Immune Response in Outpatients with Hepatocellular Carcinomas by Low Doses of Cyclophopsphamide (LDCY), *Echinacea purpurea* Extracts (Echinacin) and Thymostimulin." *Arch Geschhwulstforsch* 60:5 (1990), 379-383.

219 B. Luettig et al. "Macrophage Activation by the Polysaccharide Arabinogalactan Isolated from Plant Cell Cultures of *Echinacea purpurea*." *Journal of the National Cancer Institute* 81:9 (1989), 669-675.

220 R. Walters. "Essiac." *Options: The Alternative Cancer Therapy Book* (Garden City Park, NY: Avery Publishing, 1993), 110.

221 R. Thomas. *The Essiac Report* (Los Angeles: Alternative Treatment Information Network, 1993). R. Moss. "Essiac." *Cancer Therapy: The Independent Consumer's Guide* (New York: Equinox Press, 1992), 146-147. Moss reviews the technical cancer-related research on Essiac; many substances isolated from the herbs in Essiac show specific kinds of anticancer activity. Q.H. Chen et al. "Studies on Chinese Rhuabrb XII. Effect of Anthraquinone Derivatives on the Respiration and Glycolysis of Ehrlich Ascites Carcinoma Cells." *Acta Pharmaceutica Sinica* 15 (1980), 65-70. K. Kawai et al. "A Comparative Study on Cytotoxicities and Biochemical Properties of Anthraquinone Mycotoxins Emodin and Skyrin from *Penicillium Islandium Sopp*." *Toxicology Letters* 20 (1984), 155-160. M. Lu and Q.H. Chen. "Biochemical Study of Chinese Rhuabrb XXIX. Inhibitory Effects of Anthraquinone Derivatives on P338 Leukemia in Mice." *Journal of the China Pharmacology University* 20 (1989), 155-157. K. Morita et al. "A Desmutagenic Factor Insolated from Burdock (*Arctium lappa linne*)." *Mutation Research* 129 (1984), 25-31.

222 T. Chisaka et al. *Chemical and Pharmaceutical Bulletin* (1988). Cited in: J. Wilner. "Green Tea." *The Cancer Solution* (Boca Raton, FL: Peltec Publishing, 1994), 75. A. Bu-Abbas et al. "Marked Antimutagenic Potential of Aqueous Green Tea Extracts: Mechanism of Action." *Mutagenesis* 9 (1994), 325-331. H. Mukhtar et al. "Green Tea and Skin-Anticarcinogenic Effects." *Journal of*

Investigative Dermatology 102 (1994), 3-7. J.E. Klaunig. "Chemopreventive Effects of Green Tea Components on Hepatic Carcinogenesis." *Preventative Medicine* 21 (1992), 510-519. Y.T. Gao et al. "Reduced Risk of Esophageal Cancer Associated with Green Tea Consumption." *Journal of the National Cancer Institute* 86 (1994), 855-858.

223 Office of Technology Assessment. *Unconventional Cancer Treatments* (Washington, DC: U.S. Government Printing Office, 1990). M. Kazuyoshi et al. "A Desmutagenic Factor Isolated from Burdock. *Arctium lappa linne.*" *Mutation Research* 129 (1984), 25-31. B.N. Dhawan et al. "Screening of Indian Plants for Biological Activity: VI." *Indian Journal of Experimental Biology* 15 (1977), 208. A. Hoshi et al. "Anti-Tumor Activity of Berberine Derivatives." *Japanese Journal of Cancer Research* 67 (1976), 321-325.

224 M.J. Messina et al. "Soy Intake and Cancer Risk: A Review of *in Vitro* and *in Vivo* Data." *Nutrition and Cancer* 21:2 (1994), 113-131.

225 J. Boik. "Conducting Research on Natural Agents: A Summary of Effects of *Glycyrrhiza uralensis.*" *Cancer and Natural Medicine* (Princeton, MN: Oregon Medical Press, 1995), 179. H. Pierson. "Designer Foods and Cancer." World Congress on Cancer, Sydney, Australia (April 1994), 25.

226 S. Austin et al. "Long-Term Follow-Up of Cancer Patients Using Contreras, Hoxsey, and Gerson Therapies." *Journal of Naturopathic Medicine* 5:1 (1994), 74-76. Given the small size of this study, and the fact that many different cancers were involved, at different stages and with different treatments used for each cancer, it is impossible to draw statistically meaningful conclusions from this study. However, the results at least suggest a benefit for cancer patients receiving the Hoxsey formula. In no way should the reader assume that the Gerson or Contreras clinics are failing to help patients based on the results of this study. Remember, these were advanced-stage cancer patients, many of whom had undergone and failed to improve with conventional therapies first.

227 Office of Technology Assessment. *Unconventional Cancer Treatments* (Washington, DC: U.S. Government Printing Office, 1990), 83. Iscador with copper is used for primary tumors of the liver, gallbladder, stomach, and kidneys; Iscador with mercury is used to treat tumors of the intestines and lymphatic system; Iscador with silver is used to treat cancers of the breast and urogenital tract; and Iscador without any added metals is used to treat most other cancers. The OTA report notes that this form, *Viscum album*, differs markedly from mistletoe found in the U.S.

228 H. Kiene. "Clinical Studies on Mistletoe Therapy for Cancerous Diseases: A Review." *Therapeutikon* 3:6 (1989), 347-350.

229 T. Hajito and C. Lanzrein. "Natural Killer and Antibody-Dependent Cell-Mediated Cytotoxicity and Large Granular Lymphocyte Frequencies in *Viscum album*-Treated Breast Cancer Patients." *Oncology* 43:Suppl 1 (1986), 93-97. T. Hajito. "Immunomodulatory Effects of Iscador: A *Viscum album* Preparation." *Oncology* 43:Suppl 1 (1986), 51-65.

230 J. Nienhaus. "Tumor Inhibition and Thymus Stimulation with Mistletoe Preparations." *Elemente Naturowissenschaft* 13 (1970), 45-54. See also: G. Salzer and H. Muller. "Local Treatment of Malignant Pleural Effusions with Mistletoe Preparation Iscador." *Praxix Pneumologia* 32 (1978), 721-729. M. Linder. "Mistletoe Preparations Prevent

Changes in Copper Metabolism." American Association of Cancer Researchers annual meeting, Saint Louis, Missouri (1982).

231 R. Leroi. "Fundamentals of Mistletoe Therapy." *Krebsgeschehen* 5 (1979), 145-146. H. Kiene. "Clinical Studies on Mistletoe Therapy for Cancerous Diseases: A Review." *Therapeutikon* 3:6 (1989), 347-533.

232 Ronald Grossarth-Maticek et al. *Alternative Therapies in Health and Medicine* 7 (May 2001), 57-78.

233 Studies on clinical effects of Iscador were all cited in *Journal of Anthroposophical Medicine* 11:2 (1994), 20-26. See also: R. Heiligtag. *Anthroposophical Medicine and Therapies for Cancer* (Spring Valley, NY: Mercury Press, 1994).

234 R. Chang. Personal communication (1995). New York-based Raymond Chang, M.D., formerly at Memorial Sloan-Kettering Cancer Center, is an expert on medicinal mushrooms.

235 K. Adachi et al. "Potentiation of Host-Mediated Antitumor Activity in Mice by Beta-Glucan Obtained from *Grifola frondosa* (Maitake)." *Chemical & Pharmacological Bulletin* 35:1 (1987), 262-270.

236 H. Nanba. "Maitake Mushroom: Immune Therapy to Prevent Cancer Growth and Metastasis." *Explore!* 6:1 (1995), 17.

237 H. Nanba. "Antitumor Activity of Orally Administered 'D-fraction' from Maitake Mushroom (*Grifola frondosa*)." *Journal of Naturopathic Medicine* 1:4 (1993), 10-15.

CANDIDIASIS

1 W. Krause, H. Matheis, and K. Wulf. "Fungaemia and Funguria After Oral Administration of *Candida albicans*." *The Lancet* 1:7595 (1969), 598-599.

2 P. Sutton et al. "*In Vivo* Immunosuppressive Activity of Gliotoxin, a Metabolite Produced by Human Pathogenic Fungi." *Infection and Immunity* 62 (1994), 1192-1198. P. Waring and J. Beaver. "Gliotoxin and Related Epipolythiodioxopiperazines." *Gen Pharmacol* 27 (1996), 1311-1316. P. Waring et al. "Cellular Uptake and Release of the Immunomodulating Fungal Toxin Gliotoxin." *Toxicon* 32 (1994), 491-504. J.P. Beaver and P. Waring. "A Decrease in Intracellular Glutathione Concentration Precedes the Onset of Apoptosis in Murine Thymocytes." *European Journal of Cell Biology* 68 (1995), 47-54.

3 R. Marshall. "Resistant Polysystemic Candidiasis and Coincident Immuno-Suppressant Factors." *Journal of Alternative and Complementary Medicine* (May/June 1993).

4 Editorial Staff. "Contributions of Micro-Organisms to Foods and Nutrition." *Nutrition News* 38:4 (1975). M. Speck. "Natural Antibiotic Activity of *Lactobacillus Acidophilus* and *Bulgaricus*." *Cultured Dairy Products Journal* 18:2 (July 1983).

5 J. Bland, ed. *Medical Application of Clinical Nutrition* (New Canaan, CT: Keats Publishing, 1983).

6 Dennis W. Remington, M.D., and Barbara Higa Swasey, R.D. *Back To Health: Yeast Control* (Provo, UT: Vitality House International, 1989), 16

7 Orian C. Truss, M.D. *The Missing Diagnosis* (Birmingham, AL: The Missing Diagnosis, 1985), x, 3. Jack Tips, N.D., Ph.D. *Conquer Candida and Restore Your Immune System* (Austin, TX: Apple-A-Day Press, 1995), 126.

8 Jack Tips, N.D., Ph.D. *Conquer Candida and Restore Your Immune System* (Austin, TX: Apple-A-Day Press, 1995), 59-60.

9 C.O. Truss. *Journal of Orthomolecular Psychiatry* 13:2 (1984).

10 J.E. Pizzorno and M.T. Murray. *A Textbook of Natural Medicine* (Seattle, WA: John Bastyr College Publications, 1989).

11 K.W. Sehnert, M.D., and J. Mathews-Larson. *International Journal of Biosocial and Medical Research* 13:1 (1991), 67-76.

12 Ann Louise Gittleman, M.S. *Supernutrition for Women* (New York: Bantam, 1991), 79.

13 Jack Tips, N.D., Ph.D. *Conquer Candida and Restore Your Immune System* (Austin, TX: Apple-A-Day Press, 1995), 60-61.

14 Stephen Langer, M.D., with James F. Scheer. *Solved: The Riddle of Weight Loss* (Rochester, VT: Healing Arts Press, 1989), 24.

15 Simon Martin. *Candida: The Natural Way* (Boston, MA: Element Books, 1998), 10-11. This information is adapted from a *Candida* questionnaire developed by William Crook, M.D., and included in his book *The Yeast Connection Handbook* (Jackson, TN: Professional Books, 1996), 15-19.

16 Stephen Langer, M.D., with James F. Scheer. *Solved: The Riddle of Weight Loss* (Rochester, VT: Healing Arts Press, 1989), 24.

17 Jack Tips, N.D., Ph.D. *Conquer Candida and Restore Your Immune System* (Austin, TX: Apple-A-Day Press, 1995), 68-69.

18 Michael T. Murray, N.D. "Chronic Candidiasis: A Natural Approach." *American Journal of Natural Medicine* 4:4 (May 1997), 17-19.

19 M. Rosenbaum, M.D., and M. Susser, M.D. *Solving the Puzzle of Chronic Fatigue Syndrome* (Tacoma, WA: Life Sciences Press, 1992), 131.

20 Jacqueline Young. *Cystitis: The Natural Way* (Rockport, MA: Element Books, 1997), 68.

21 J. Trowbridge and M. Walker. *The Yeast Syndrome* (New York: Bantam Books, 1986).

22 J.E. Pizzorno and M.T. Murray. *A Textbook of Natural Medicine* (Seattle, WA: John Bastyr College Publications, 1989).

23 W.J. Crinnion. "Clinical Trial Results on Neesby's Capricin." (Unpublished manuscript, September 10, 1985). Available from: Probiologic, Inc., 1803 132nd Avenue NE, Bellevue, WA 98005.

24 I. Neuhauser. "Successful Treatment of Intestinal Moniliasis with Fatty Acid-Resin Complex." *Archives of Internal Medicine* 93 (1954), 53-60.

25 S. Ankri and D. Mirelman. "Antimicrobial Properties of Allicin from Garlic." *Microbes Infect* 1:2 (February 1999), 125-129.

26 J.E. Pizzorno and M.T. Murray. *A Textbook of Natural Medicine* (Seattle, WA: John Bastyr College Publications, 1989).

27 From research done by Luis E. Todd, M.D., at the Universidad Autonoma de Nuevo Leon, Monterrey, Mexico. An abstract is available on the Internet: www.sover.net/~samallen/nutri.htm.

28 L. Chaitow. *Post Viral Fatigue Syndrome* (London: Dent, 1989).

CHILDREN'S HEALTH

1 S.C. Dees and D. Lefkowitz III. "Secretory Otitis Media in Allergic Children." *American Journal of Diseases of Children* 124:3 (September 1972), 364-368.

2 J. Ruokonen, A. Paganus, and H. Lehti. "Elimination Diets in the Treatment of Secretory Otitis Media." *International Journal of Pediatric Otorhinolaryngology* 4:1 (March 1982), 39-46.

3 E.I. Cantekin, T.W. McGuire, and T.L. Griffith. "Antimicrobial Therapy for Otitis Media with Effusion." *Journal of the American Medical Association* 266:23 (December 18, 1991), 3309-3317.

4 M. Diamant and B. Diamant. "Abuse and Timing of Use of Antibiotics in Acute Otitis Media." *Archives of Otolaryngology* 100:3 (September 1974), 226-232.

5 H.L. Coulter and B.L. Fisher. *DPT—A Shot in the Dark* (San Diego, CA: Harcourt Brace Jovanovich, 1985). H.L. Coulter. *Vaccination, Social Violence, and Criminality: The Medical Assault on the American Brain* (Berkeley, CA: North Atlantic Books, 1990).

6 R. Berkow, M.D., and A.J. Fletcher, eds. *Merck Manual of Diagnosis and Therapy* (Rahway, NJ: Merck, 1992), 2167.

7 N.Z. Miller. *Vaccines: Are They Really Safe and Effective?* (Santa Fe, NM: New Atlantean Press, 1992).

8 U.S. Food and Drug Administration. "Adverse Events Associated with Childhood Vaccines: Evidence Bearing on Causality." Press release (September 1993).

9 Charlotte Sondergaard et al. *Pediatrics* 108 (2001), 342-346.

10 C.D. Bluestone, M.D. "Eustachian Tube Function and Allergy in Otitis Media." *Pediatrics* 61:5 (May 1978), 753-760.

11 U.M. Saarinen. "Prolonged Breast Feeding as Prophylaxis for Recurrent Otitis Media." *Acta Paediatrica Scandinavica* 71:4 (July 1982), 567-571. J. Backon. "Prolonged Breast Feeding as a Prophylaxis for Recurrent Otitis Media: Relevance of Prostaglandins." *Medical Hypotheses* 13:2 (February 1984), 161.

12 "Breast Feeding Prevents Otitis Media." *Nutrition Reviews* 41:8 (August 1983), 241-242.

13 K.H. Friese et al. "Otitis Media in Children: A Comparison of Conventional and Homeopathic Drugs." *HNO Head and Neck Otorhinolarynology* 44 (1996) 462-466.

14 J.H. Kellogg, M.D. *Rational Hydrotherapy* (Philadelphia: F.A. Davis Publishing, 1902).

15 Interview with Fred Baughman, M.D., on the PBS program *Frontline* (May 4, 2000).

16 Barbara Crossette. "Agency Sees Risk in Drug to Temper Child Behavior." *The New York Times* (February 29, 1996). Erik L. Goldman. "Ritalin Wrongly Used to Diagnose Attention Deficit." *Family Practice News* (November 1, 1995), 33.

17 T.W. Jones, et al. "Independent Effects of Youth and Poor Diabetes Control on Responses to Hypoglycemia in Children." *Diabetes* 40:3 (March 1991), 358-363.

18 L.J. Stevens et al. "Essential Fatty Acid Metabolism in Boys with Attention-Deficit Hyperactivity Disorder." *American Journal of Clinical Nutrition* 62:4 (1995), 7661-768. J.R. Burgess et al. "Long-Chain Polyunsaturated Fatty Acids in Children with Attention-Deficit Hyperactivity Disorder." *American Journal of Clinical Nutrition* 71:1 Suppl (2000), 327S-330S.

19 J.L. Rapoport. "Diet and Hyperactivity." *Nutrition Reviews* 44 Suppl (May 1986), 158-162.

20 U.S. Department of Health and Human Services, Public Health Service. *More Than You Ever Thought You Would Know About Food Additives* FDA Publication 82-2160 (Washington, DC: U.S. Department of Health and Human Services, 1982).

21 J. Egger et al. "Controlled Trial of Oligoantigenic Treatment in the Hyperkinetic Syndrome." *The Lancet* 1:8428 (March 1985), 540-545. J.P. Harley et al. "Hyperkinesis and Food Additives: Testing the Feingold Hypothesis." *Pediatrics* 61:6 (1978), 818-828.

22 Michael F. Jacobson, Ph.D., and David Schardt, M.S. *Diet, ADHD, and Behavior* (Washington, DC: Center for Science in the Public Interest, 1999). Available from: Center for Science in the Public Interest, 1875 Connecticut Avenue N.W. #300, Washington, D.C. 20009; (202) 332-9110; website: www.cspinet.org.

23 Diagnostic Classification Steering Committee. ed. Michael J. Thorpy. *The International Classification of Sleep Disorders: Diagnostic and Coding Manual* (Rochester, MN: American Sleep Disorders Association, 1990).

24 U.S. Dept. of Health and Human Services. *Sleep Disorders* HHS Publication No. (ADM) 87-1541 (Washington, DC: U.S. Government Printing Office, 1987).

25 W.L. Robson et al. "Enuresis in Children with Attention-Deficit Hyperactivity Disorder." *Southern Medical Journal* 90:5 (May 1993), 503-505.

26 J. Egger et al. "Effect of Diet Treatment on Enuresis in Children with Migraine or Hyperkinetic Behavior." *Clinical Pediatrics* 31:5 (May 1992), 302-307.

CHRONIC FATIGUE SYNDROME

1 L.A. Jason et al. "A Community-Based Study of Chronic Fatigue Syndrome." *Archives of Internal Medicine* 159:18 (1999), 2129-2137.

2 S. Straus, M.D. *Chronic Fatigue Syndrome* NIH Publication No. 90-3059 (Washington, DC: U.S. Department of Health and Human Services, Public Health Service, 1990), 5.

3 Ibid.

4 M. Rosenbaum, M.D., and M. Susser, M.D. *Solving the Puzzle of Chronic Fatigue Syndrome* (Tacoma, WA: Life Sciences Press, 1992).

5 L. Chaitow. *Post Viral Fatigue Syndrome* (London: Dent, 1989).

6 B.A. Cunha, M.D. *Infectious Disease News* 5:11 (November 1992), 8-9.

7 S. Straus, M.D. *Chronic Fatigue Syndrome* NIH Publication No. 90-3059 (Washington, DC: U.S. Department of Health and Human Services, Public Health Service, 1990), 5.

8 M. Rosenbaum, M.D., and M. Susser, M.D. *Solving the Puzzle of Chronic Fatigue Syndrome* (Tacoma, WA: Life Sciences Press, 1992), 22.

9 Editorial. "Depression, Stress and Immunity." *The Lancet* 1:8548 (June 1987), 1467-1488.

10 N. Hodgkinson. "'Yuppie Flu'—Is It All in the Mind Say Doctors." *Sunday Times London* (July 17, 1988).

11 "Diagnostic Blood Test for CFIDS?" *The CFIDS Treatment News* 2:1 (Spring 1991), 3. Alan Landay et al. "Chronic Fatigue Syndrome: Clinical Condition Associated with Immune Activation." *The Lancet* 338:8769 (September 21, 1991). Personal correspondence with Jay Levy, M.D., Division of Hematology and Oncology, Department of Medicine, University of California at San Francisco (October 1997).

12 Alan L. Landay et al. "Chronic Fatigue Syndrome: Clinical Condition Associated with Immune Activation." *The Lancet* 338:8769 (September 21, 1991), 707-712.

13 Michael Murray, N.D. *Chronic Fatigue Syndrome* (Rocklin, CA: Prima Publishing, 1994), 55.

14 L. Simpson. "M.E. and B12." *JRS Medicine* (October 1991), 633.

15 C.W. Lapp. "Chronic Fatigue Syndrome is a Real Disease." *North Carolina Family Physician* 443:1 (1992), 6-11.

16 I.M. Cox, M.J. Campbell, and D. Dowson. "Red Blood Cell Magnesium and Chronic Fatigue Syndrome." *The Lancet* 337:8744 (March 1991), 757-760.

17 W.D. Snively and R.L. Westerman. "The Clinician Views Potassium Deficit." *Minnesota Medicine* (June 1965), 713-719.

18 A.R. Gaby. "Aspartic Acid Salts and Fatigue." *Currents in Nutritional Therapeutics* (November 1982).

19 G.R. Faloona and S.A. Levine. "The Use of Organic Germanium in Chronic Epstein-Barr Virus Syndrome (CEBVS): An Example of Interferon Modulation of Herpes Reactivation." *Orthomolecular Medicine* 3:1 (1988), 29-31.

20 P.M. Kidd. "Germanium-132 (Ge-132): Homeostatic Normalizer and Immunostimulant: A Review of its Preventive and Therapeutic Efficacy." *Int Clinical Nutrition Review* 7:1 (1987), 11-20.

21 D.F. Horrobin. "Post-Viral Fatigue Syndrome, Viral Infections in Atopic Eczema, and Essential Fatty Acids." *Medical Hypotheses* 32:3 (1990), 211-217.

22 P.O. Behan et al. "Effect of High Doses of Essential Fatty Acids on the Post-Viral Fatigue Syndrome." *Acta Neurol Scand* 82:3 (1990), 209-216. P.O. Behan and W. Behan. "Essential Fatty Acids in the Treatment of Post-Viral Fatigue Syndrome." In: D.F. Horrobin, ed. *Omega-6 Essential Fatty Acids: Pathophysiology and Roles in Clinical Medicine* (New York: Alan R. Liss, 1990), 275-282.

23 Michael Murray N.D. *Encyclopedia of Nutritional Supplements* (Rocklin, CA: Prima Publishing, 1996), 438.

24 Kyle Roderick. "NADH Shows Promise in Study-FDA Trial a First for Nutritional Supplements." *The CFIDS Chronicle* (January/February 1998). Available on the Internet: www.cfids.org/chronicle/medical/nadh98.html.

25 This report is based solely on product labeling as published by PDR®. Copyright ©1993 by Medical Economics Data, a division of Medical Economics Company, Inc. All rights reserved.

26 C. DeVinci et al. "Lessons from a Pilot Study of Transfer Factor in Chronic Fatigue Syndrome." *Biotherapy* 9:1-3 (1996), 87-90.

CHRONIC PAIN

1 American Chronic Pain Association, P.O. Box 850, Rocklin, CA 95677; (916) 632-0922; website: www.theacpa.org.

2 R. Melzack and T. Scott. "The Effects of Early Experience on the Response to Pain." *Journal of Physiology and Comparative Psychology* 50 (1957), 971.

3 D. Bresler and R. Katz. "Chronic Pain: Alternative to Neural Blockade." In: M. Cousins and P. Bridenbaugh, eds. *Neural Blockade in Clinical Anesthesia and Management of Pain* (Philadelphia: Lippincott, 1980).

4 R. Sternbach. *Pain: A Psychophysiological Analysis* (New York: Academic Press, 1968).

5 M. Murphy. *The Future of the Body* (Los Angeles: Jeremy P. Tarcher, 1992).

6 D. Bresler and R. Katz. "Chronic Pain: Alternative to Neural Blockade." In: M. Cousins and P. Bridenbaugh, eds. *Neural Blockade in Clinical Anesthesia and Management of Pain* (Philadelphia: Lippincott, 1980).

7 E. Jellinek. "Clinical Tests on Comparative Effectiveness of Analgesic Drugs." *Biometrics Bulletin* 2 (1946), 87.

8 L. Lasagna et al. "A Study of the Placebo Response." *American Journal of Medicine* 16 (1954), 770.

9 R. Sternbach. *Pain: A Psychophysiological Analysis* (New York: Academic Press, 1968).

10 The following article summarizes this research: Stephen Birch, L.Ac., Richard Hammerschlag, Ph.D., and Brian M. Berman, M.D. "Acupuncture in the Treatment of Pain." *Journal of Alternative and Complementary Medicine* 2:1 (1996), 101-124.

11 L. Lao et al. "Efficacy of Chinese Acupuncture on Postoperative Oral Surgery Pain." *Oral Surgery, Oral Medicine, Oral Pathology* 79:4 (1995), 423-428.

12 B. Millman. "Acupuncture: Context and Critique." *Annual Review of Medicine* 28 (1977), 223-236.

13 J. Cheung. "Effect of Electroacupuncture on Chronic Painful Conditions in General Medical Practice—A Four-Years' Study." *American Journal of Chinese Medicine* 13 (1985), 33-38.

14 V.N. Tsibuliak, A.P. Alisov, and V.P. Shatrova. "Acupuncture Analgesia and Analgesic Transcutaneous Electroneurostimulation in the Early Postoperative Period." *Anesthesiology and Reanimatology* 2 (1995), 93-98.

15 D.K. Klinghardt, M.D., and B. Wolfe, M.D. Presentation at the Advanced Neural Therapy Workshop, Santa Fe, New Mexico (December 5-6, 1992).

16 J.P. Dosch, M.D. *Facts About Neural Therapy According to Huneke: Regulation Therapy—Brief Summary for Patients* (Portland, OR: Medicina Biologica, 1985).

17 T. Fried, R. Johnson, and W. McCracken. "Trancutaneous Electrical Nerve Stimulation: Its Role in the Control of Chronic Pain." *Arch Phys Med Rehabil* 65:5 (May 1984), 228-231.

18 K.M. Lucero. "The Electro-Acuscope/Myopulse System." *Rehab Management: Journal of Therapy and Rehabilitation* 4:3 (April/May 1991).

19 R.O. Becker. *The Body Electric: Electro-Magnetism and the Foundation of Life* (New York: William Morrow, 1986). R.O. Becker. *Cross Currents* (Los Angeles: Jeremy P. Tarcher, 1990).

20 H. Hannemann. *Magnet Therapy: Balancing Your Body's Energy Flow for Self-Healing* (New York: Sterling, 1990), 16. D. Foley-Nolan et al. "Pulsed High-Frequency (27 MHz) Electromagnetic Therapy for Persistent Neck Pain." *Orthopedics* 13:4 (1990), 445-451. A. Gill Taylor. "A Center to Test for Efficacy of Static Magnetic Fields and Other Selected Complementary and Alternative Therapies." Paper presented at the Fifth Annual Meeting of the North American Academy of Magnetic Therapy, Los Angeles, California (January 22-24, 1999).

COLDS AND FLU

1 E. Cheraskin, M.D. *Vitamin C: Who Needs It?* (Birmingham, AL: Arlington Press, 1993).

2 Ibid., 4.

3 Ibid.

4 J.E. Pizzorno and M.T. Murray. *A Textbook of Natural Medicine* (Seattle, WA: John Bastyr College Publications, 1989).

5 This report is based solely on product labeling as published by PDR®. Copyright ©1993 by Medical Economics Data, a division of Medical Economics Company, Inc. All rights reserved.

6 J.E. Pizzorno and M.T. Murray. *A Textbook of Natural Medicine* (Seattle, WA: John Bastyr College Publications, 1989).

7 S. Cohen, D.A.J. Tyrell, and A.P. Smith. "Psycho-logical Stress and Susceptibility to the Common Cold." *New England Journal of Medicine* 325:9 (August 1991), 606-612.

8 Ibid.

9 E. Cheraskin, M.D. *Vitamin C: Who Needs It?* (Birmingham, AL: Arlington Press, 1993), 2.

10 Ibid., 9.

11 J.E. Pizzorno and M.T. Murray. *A Textbook of Natural Medicine* (Seattle, WA: John Bastyr College Publications, 1989).

12 Ibid.

13 Robert C. Atkins, M.D. "Putting the Freeze on Colds." *Dr. Atkins' Health Revelations* (January 1995), 4-5.

14 Earl Mindell, R.Ph., Ph.D., and Virginia Hopkins, M.A. *Prescription Alternatives* (New Canaan, CT: Keats Publishing, 1998).

15 Ibid.

16 S. De Flora et al. "Attenuation of Influenza-Like Symptomatology and Improvement of Cell-Mediated Immunity With Long-Term N-Acetylcysteine Treatment." *European Respiratory Journal* 10 (1997), 1535-1541.

17 J.E. Pizzorno and M.T. Murray. *A Textbook of Natural Medicine* (Seattle, WA: John Bastyr College Publications, 1989). R.F. Weiss. *Herbal Medicine* (Beaconsfield, England: Beaconsfield Publishers, 1988).

18 Daniel Gagnon. "Herbal Care for Colds & Flu." *Herbs for Health* 1:2 (September/October 1996), 34-39.

19 Robert D. Willix, Jr., M.D. "How to Battle Colds and Flu the Natural Way." *Dr. Robert D. Willix Jr.'s Health & Longevity* 4:10 (October 1997), 1-6.

20 J.E. Pizzorno and M.T. Murray. *Encyclopedia of Natural Medicine* (Rocklin, CA: Prima Publishing, 1991), 228.

CONSTIPATION

1 M. Sweeney. "Constipation. Diagnosis and Treatment." *Home Care Provider* 2:5 (October 1997), 250-255.

2 G.J. Subak-Sharpe, M. Bogdonoff, R. Bressler, eds. *The Physicians' Manual for Patients* (New York: Times Books, 1984).

3 N. Petrakis and E. King. "Cytological Abnormalities in Nipple Aspirates of Breast Fluid from Women with Severe Constipation." *The Lancet* 2:8257 (Novembeer 1981), 1203-1204.

4 American Cancer Society. *Cancer Facts and Figures 1993* (Atlanta, GA: American Cancer Society, 1993).

5 R. Taylor. "Management of Constipation 1: High Fibre Diets Work." *British Medical Journal* 300:6731 (April 1990), 1063-1064.

6 J.E. Pizzorno and M.T. Murray, eds. *A Textbook of Natural Medicine* (Seattle, WA: John Bastyr College Publications, 1989).

7 Ibid.

8 This report is based solely on product labeling as published by PDR®. Copyright ©1993 by Medical Economics Data, a division of Medical Economics Company, Inc. All rights reserved.

9 J.E. Pizzorno and M.T. Murray, eds. *A Textbook of Natural Medicine* (Seattle, WA: John Bastyr College Publications, 1989).

10 J. Cummings et al. "Colonic Response to Dietary Fibre from Carrot, Cabbage, Apple, Bran." *The Lancet* 1:8054 (January 1978), 5.

11 Sujata Owens, LCEH (Bom), R.S. Hom. (NA). "A Case of Severe Constipation with Colic and Congenital Deformities." In: Stephen King, N.D., et al., eds. *Small Remedies & Interesting Cases VII, Proceedings of the 1995 Professional Case Conference* (Seattle, WA: International Foundation for Homeopathy, 1995).

12 Clare Maxwell-Hudson. *Massage: The Ultimate Illustrated Guide* (New York: DK Publishing, 1999), 148-149.

13 *Alternative Medicine Digest* 9 (November 1995), 13.

14 *Canadian Journal of Microbiology* 31 (1985), 50-53.

DIABETES

1 P.H. Forsham, M.D. "Treatment of Type I and Type II Diabetes." *Townsend Letter for Doctors* 53 (December 1987), 390-393.

2 L. Neergaard. "Study Proves Walking, Dropping Weight Cuts Diabetes Risk in Half." Associated Press report (August 9, 2001).

3 L. Neergaard. "Study Proves Walking, Dropping Weight Cuts Diabetes Risk in Half." Associated Press report (August 9, 2001). Jane Brody. "Personal Health." *The New York Times* (November 15, 1995).

4 *Diabetes in America* (Bethesda, MD: National Institutes of Health, 1985).

5 L. Jovanovic-Peterson and C.M. Peterson. "Is Exercise Safe or Useful for Gestational Diabetic Women?" *Diabetes* 40:Suppl 2 (December 1991), 179-181.

6 J.E. Pizzorno and M.T. Murray. *A Textbook of Natural Medicine* (Seattle, WA: John Bastyr College Publications, 1988).

7 W.H. Philpott. "Diabetes: A Reversible Disease." Unpublished paper available from: Philpott Medical Services, 17171 S.E. 29th Street, Choctaw, OK, 73020.

8 J. Karljalainen et al. "Bovine Albumin Peptide as a Possible Trigger of Insulin-Dependent Diabetes Mellitus." *New England Journal of Medicine* 327:5 (1992), 302-307.

9 J.E. Pizzorno and M.T. Murray. *A Textbook of Natural Medicine* (Seattle, WA: John Bastyr College Publications, 1988).

10 P.H. Forsham, M.D. "Treatment of Type I and Type II Diabetes." *Townsend Letter for Doctors* 53 (December 1987), 390-393.

11 P.Z. Zimmet. "Kelly West Lecture 1991—Challenges in Diabetes Epidemiology, from West to the Rest." *Diabetes Care* 15:2 (February 1992), 232-252.

12 D. Satter. "Diabetes Called Sure Fate for Obese People." *The Los Angeles Times* (February 13, 1972), Section C.

13 H. King and M. Rewers. "Diabetes in Notes is Now a Third World Problem." *Bulletin of the World Health Organization* 69:6 (1991), 643-648.

14 Editorial Staff. "The Prevention and Natural Treatment of Diabetes." *Prevention* 30:10 (October 1978), 108-113.

15 W.H. Philpott, M.D., and D.K. Kalita. *Victory Over Diabetes* (New Canaan, CT: Keats Publishing, 1983).

16 Andrew Weil. *Natural Health, Natural Medicine* (Boston: Houghton Mifflin, 1990), 279.

17 M.S. Chen et al. "Prevalence and Risk Factors of Diabetic Retinopathy Among Non-Insulin Dependent Diabetic Subjects." *American Journal of Ophthalmology* 114:6 (December 1992), 723-730. G. Marshall et al. "Factors Influencing the Onset and Progression of Diabetic Retinopathy in Subjects with Insulin-Dependent Diabetes

Mellitus." *Ophthalmology* 100:8 (August 1993), 1133-1139. L.J. Mandarino. "Current Hypotheses for the Biochemical Basis of Diabetic Retinopathy." *Diabetes Care* 15:12 (December 1992), 1892-1901.

18 Andrew Weil. *Natural Health, Natural Medicine* (Boston: Houghton Mifflin, 1990), 279.

19 T.H. Maugh III. "New Method to Fight Diabetes Found Effective." *The Los Angeles Times* (June 14, 1993), 1.

20 Ann Louise Gittleman, M.S. *Supernutrition for Women* (New York: Bantam, 1991), 68.

21 J.W. Anderson and B. Sieling. "High Fiber Diets for Diabetics: Unconventional but Effective." *Geriatrics* 36:5 (May 1981), 64-72.

22 Ibid.

23 S.M. Berger, M.D. *What Your Doctor Didn't Learn in Medical School & What You Can Do About It* (New York: Avon Books, 1989), 179-200.

24 Richard N. Podell, M.D., F.A.C.P., and William Proctor. *The G-Index Diet* (New York: Warner, 1993).

25 Dan Hurley. "Studies Confirm Diabetes Risk from Cow's Milk in Infants." *Medical Tribune* (February 2, 1995), 11.

26 W.H. Philpott and D.K. Kalita. *Victory Over Diabetes* (New Canaan, CT: Keats Publishing, 1983).

27 J. Potts. "Avoidance Protective Food Testing in Assessing Diabetes Responsiveness." *Journal of Diabetes* 26:Suppl 1 (1977). J. Potts. "Value of Specific Testing for Assessing Insulin Resistance." *Journal of Diabetes* 29:Suppl 2 (1980). J. Potts. "Blood Sugar-Insulin Responses to Specific Foods versus GTT." *Journal of Diabetes* 30:Suppl 1 (1981). J. Potts. "Insulin Resistance Related to Specific Food Sensitivity." *Journal of Diabetes* 35:Suppl 1 (1986).

28 R.L. Searcy, M.D. *Diagnostic Biochemistry* (New York: McGraw-Hill, 1969).

29 E. Albert, M.D. "Current Concepts in Diabetes Mellitus." *New York State Journal of Medicine* 53:22 (November 1953), 2607-2610.

30 J.M. Ellis, M.D. *Vitamin B6: The Doctor's Report* (New York: Harper & Row, 1973).

31 C.L. Jones and V. Gonzalez, M.D. "Pyroxidine Deficiency: A New Factor in Diabetic Neuropathy." *Journal of American Podiatry Association* 68:9 (September 1978), 646-653.

32 J.E. Pizzorno and M.T. Murray. *A Textbook of Natural Medicine* (Seattle WA: John Bastyr College Publications, 1988), 14.

33 D. Koutsikos, B. Agroyannis, and H. Tzanatos-Exarchou. "Biotin for Diabetic Peripheral Neuropathy." *Biomedicine and Pharmacotherapy* 44:10 (1990), 511-514.

34 P.S. Devamanoharan et al. "Prevention of Selenite Cataract by Vitamin C." *Experimental Eye Research* 52:5 (May 1991), 563-568.

35 W.H. Philpott, M.D., and D.K. Kalita. *Victory Over Diabetes* (New Canaan, CT: Keats Publishing, 1983).

36 W.E. Shute. *Vitamin E for Ailing and Healthy Hearts* (New York: Pyramid House, 1969).

37 C. Colette et al. "Platelet Function in Type I Diabetes: Effects of Supplementation with Large Doses of Vitamin E." *American Journal of Clinical Nutrition* 47:2 (February 1988), 256-261.

38 M.J. Stuart. "Vitamin E Deficiency: Its Effect on Platelet-Vascular Interaction in Various Pathological States." *Annals of the New York Academy of Sciences* 393 (1982), 277-288. J. Watanabe et al. "Effect of Vitamin E on Platelet Aggregation in

Diabetes Mellitus." *Thrombosis and Haemostasis* 51 (1984), 313-316.

39 Editorial Staff. "Chromium Enrichment of Foods Urged." *Medical World News* 15:7 (October 1974), 33-35.

40 E.W. Toepfer et al. "Chromium in Foods Related to Biological Activity." *Journal of Agricultural Food Chemistry* 21:1 (1973), 69-73.

41 Richard Anderson, Ph.D. "Beneficial Effect of Chromium for People with Type II Diabetes." *Diabetes* 45:Suppl 2 (1996), 124A/454.

42 W. Merz and K. Schwarz. "Relation of Glucose Tolerance Factor to Impaired Intravenous Glucose Tolerance of Rats on a Stock Diet." *American Journal of Physiology* 196:3 (1959), 614-618.

43 K.M. Hambidge. "Chromium Nutrition in Man." *American Journal of Clinical Nutrition* 27:5 (May 1974), 505-514.

44 A. Sjogren et al. "Magnesium, Potassium, and Zinc Deficiencies in Subjects with Type II Diabetes." *Acta Medica Scandinavica* 224 (1988), 461-463.

45 J. Sheehan. "Importance of Magnesium Chloride Repletion After Myocardial Infarction." *American Journal of Cardiology* 63:14 (April 1989), 35G-38G.

46 R.A. Reinhart. "Clinical Correlates of the Molecular and Cellular Actions of Magnesium on the Cardiovascular System." *American Heart Journal* 121:5 (May 1991), 1513-1521.

47 G. Norbiato et al. "Effects of Potassium Supplementation on Insulin Binding and Insulin Action in Human Obesity: Protein-Modified Fast and Refeeding." *European Journal of Clinical Investigation* 14:6 (December 1984), 414-419.

48 Reader's Digest. *Healing Power of Vitamins, Minerals, and Herbs* (Pleasantville, NY: Reader's Digest Association, 1999), 369.

49 E.J. Underwood, M.D. *Trace Elements in Human and Animal Nutrition* (Orlando, FL: Academic Press, 1986-1987).

50 K. Keeton. *Longevity: The Science of Staying Young* (New York: Viking, 1992).

51 Andrew Weil. *Natural Health, Natural Medicine* (Boston: Houghton Mifflin, 1990), 279.

52 "Abstracts: The Netherlands Society for the Study of Diabetes, March 17 and 23, 1984, Utrecht." *Netherlands Journal of Medicine* 29:2 (1986), 65-70. M.M. Kandgraf-Leurs et al. "Pilot Study on Omega-3 Fatty Acids in Type I Diabetes Mellitus." *Diabetes* 39:3 (March 1990), 369-375. G.A. Jamal et al. "Gamma-linolenic Acid in Diabetic Neuropathy." *The Lancet* 1 (1986), 1098.

53 W.H. Philpott, M.D., and D.K. Kalita. *Victory Over Diabetes* (New Canaan, CT: Keats Publishing, 1983).

54 G. Riccardi and A.A. Rivallese. "Effects of Dietary Fiber and Carbohydrate on Glucose and Lipoprotein Metabolism in Diabetes Patients." *Diabetes Care* 14 (December 1991), 1115-1125.

55 D. Williams. *DMSO: The Complete Up-to-Date Guidebook* (Ingram, TX: Mountain Home Publishing, 1987).

56 L. Neergaard. "Study Proves Walking, Dropping Weight Cuts Diabetes Risk in Half." Associated Press report (August 9, 2001).

57 Richard N. Podell, M.D., F.A.C.P., and William Proctor. *The G-Index Diet* (New York: Warner, 1993), 36.

58 M.D. Ivorra, M. Paya, and A. Villar. "A Review of Natural Products and Plants as Potential Anti-Diabetic Drugs." *Journal of Ethnopharmacology* 27:3 (December 1989), 243-275. Atta-ur-Rahman and K. Zaman. "Medical Plants with Hypoglycemic

Activity." *Journal of Ethnopharmacology* 26:1 (January 1989), 1-55.

59 Michael T. Murray, N.D. "Are Botanical Medicines Useful in Diabetes?" *American Journal of Natural Medicine* 1:3 (November 1994), 5-7.

60 Ibid.

61 A. Scharrer and M. Ober. "Anthocyanosides in the Treatment of Retinopathies." *Klin Monatsbl Augenheilkd* 178 (1981), 386-389. G. Lagrue et al. "Pathology of the Microcirculation in Diabetes and Alterations of the Biosynthesis of Intracellular Matrix Molecules." *Front Matrix Biol S. Karger* 7 (1979), 324-325.

62 P. Cutler, M.D. "Deferoxamine Therapy in High-Ferritin Diabetes." *Diabetes* 38 (October 1989), 1207-1210.

FIBROMYALGIA

1 Jacob Teitelbaum, M.D. *From Fatigued to Fantastic!* (Garden City Park, NY: Avery Publishing Group, 1996).

2 Leon Chaitow, N.D., D.O. "Fibromyalgia: The Muscle Pain Epidemic—Is ME by Another Name?" Available on the Internet: healthy.net/library/articles/chaitow/fibromy/fibro1.htm.

3 Don Goldenberg, M.D. Presentation to the 1994 American College of Rheumatology meeting. Dr. Goldenberg is Chief of Rheumatology at Newton-Wellesley Hospital, in Newton, MA, and Professor of Medicine at Tufts University School of Medicine, in Medford, MA.

4 Richard P. Van Why. *Fibromyalgia Syndrome and Massage Therapy: Issues and Opportunities* (Self-Published, 1994). Available from: Richard P. Van Why, 123 East 8th Street, Frederick, MD 21701. Devin Starlanyl, M.D., and Mary Ellen Copeland, M.S. M.A. *Fibromyalgia and Chronic Myofascial Pain Syndrome: A Survival Manual* (Oakland, CA: New Harbinger Publications, 1996), 8.

5 Allen Tyler, M.D. N.D., D.C. "Influenza A Virus: A Possible Precipitating Factor in Fibromyalgia?" *Alternative Medicine Review* 2:2 (1997), 82-86.

6 D. Buskila et al. "Fibromyalgia in Hepatitis C Virus Infection: Another Infectious Disease Relationship." *Archives of Internal Medicine* 157:21 (November 24, 1997), 2497-2500.

7 U.M. Anderberg et al. "Elevated Plasma Levels of Neuropeptide Y in Female Fibromyalgia Patients." *European Journal of Pain* 3:1 (March 1999), 19-30.

8 M.J. Schwarz et al. "Relationship of Substance P, 5-Hydroxyindole Acetic Acid and Tryptophan in Serum of Fibromyalgia Patients." *Neuroscience Letters* 259:3 (January 15, 1999), 196-198.

9 A. Leal-Cerro et al. "Growth Hormone (GH)-Releasing Hormone-GH-Insulin-Like Growth Factor-1 Axis in FM." *Journal of Clinical Endocrinology and Metabolism* 84:9 (September 1999) 3378-3381.

10 E.N. Griep, J.W. Boersma, and E.R. de Kloet. "Altered Reactivity of the Hypothalamic-Pituitary-Adrenal Axis in the Primary Fibromyalgia Syndrome." *Journal of Rheumatology* 20:3 (March 1993), 469-474. U.M. Anderberg. "Stress Can Induce Neuroendocrine Disorders and Pain." *Lakartidningen* 96:49 (December 8, 1999), 5497-5499. L.J. Crofford, N.C. Engleberg, and M.A. Demitrack. "Neurohormonal Perturbations in Fibromyalgia." *Baillieres Clin Rheumatol* 10:2 (May 1996), 365-378.

11 Nancy Stedman, M.S. *The SAM-e Handbook* (New York: Three Rivers Press, 2000), 109.

12 Leon Chaitow, N.D., D.O. "Fibromyalgia: The Muscle Pain Epidemic—Is It ME by Another

Name?" Available on the Internet: healthy.net/library/articles/chaitow/fibromy/fibro1.htm.

13 K. Kaartinen et al. "Vegan Diet Alleviates Fibromyalgia Symptoms." *Scandanavian Journal of Rheumatology* 29:5 (2000), 308-313.

14 Michael T. Murray, N.D. *Chronic Fatigue Syndrome* (Rocklin, CA: Prima Publishing, 1994), 55.

15 G. Abraham. "Management of Fibromyalgia: Rationale for the Use of Magnesium and Malic Acid." *Journal of Nutritional Medicine* 3 (1992), 49-59.

16 Chanchal Cabrera, M.N.I.M.H., Gaia Garden Herbal Dispensary, 2672 West Broadway, Vancouver, BC V6K 2G3, Canada; (604) 734-4372.

17 Chuck Cochran, D.C. *Cetyl Myristoleate* (New York: Healing Wisdom Publications, 1997).

18 John Anderson. "S-Adenosyl-L-Methionine-Nutrient Duo Relieves Depression and Pain." *Alternative Medicine* 27 (December 1998/January 1999), 72.

19 S. Glorioso et al. "Double-Blind Multicentre Study of the Activity of S-Adenosylmethionine in Hip and Knee Osteoarthritis." *International Journal of Clinical Pharmacology Research* 5 (1985), 39-49.

20 Chanchal Cabrera, M.N.I.M.H., Gaia Garden Herbal Dispensary, 2672 West Broadway, Vancouver, BC, V6K 2G3, Canada; (604) 734-4372.

21 C.J. Henry and B. Emery. "Effect of Spiced Food on Metabolic Rate." *Human Nutrition, Clinical Nutrition* 40:2 (March 1986), 165-168.

22 G. Buzzanca and S. Laterza. "Clinical Trial with an Antirheumatic Ointment." *Clin Ter* 83:1 (October 1977), 71-83.

23 Daniel J. McCarty et al. "Treatment of Pain Due to Fibromyalgia With Topical Capsaicin: A Pilot." *Seminars in Arthritis and Rheumatism* 23:6 Suppl 3, 41-47.

24 Simon Y. Mills, M.A. *Dictionary of Modern Herbalism* (Rochester, VT: Healing Arts Press, 1988), 58-59.

25 ESCOP, European Scientific Cooperative for Phytotherapy. *Valerian Root* (Meppel, The Netherlands: ESCOP, European Scientific Cooperative for Phytotherapy, 1990). S. Foster. *Chamomile* Botanical Series 307 (Austin, TX: American Botanical Council, 1991).

26 *British Homeopathic Journal* 75:3 (1986), 142-147.

27 *British Medical Journal* 299 (1989), 365-366.

28 D.J. Fletcher. "Regaining the Ability to Heal." *Alternative Medicine* 35 (May 2000), 67.

29 From the patient records of Ross A. Hauser, M.D. To contact Dr. Hauser: Caring Medical & Rehabilitation Services, S.C., 715 Lake Street, Suite 600, Oak Park, IL 60301; (708) 848-7789.

30 H. Sprott et al. *Wien Klin Wochenschr* 112:13 (July 7, 2000), 580-586.

31 *Scandinavian Journal of Rheumatology* 15:2 (1986), 174-178.

32 R.G. Gamber et al. "Treatment of Fibromyalgia with Osteopathic Manipulation and Self-Learned Techniques." 37th Annual American Osteopathic Association Research Conference Abstracts (1993).

33 Brian Berman, M.D. *The SAM-e Handbook* (New York: Three Rivers Press, 2000), 157.

GASTROINTESTINAL DISORDERS

1 J.E. Pizzorno and M.T. Murray. *Encyclopedia of Natural Medicine* (Rocklin, CA: Prima Publishing, 1991), 239.

2 Ibid., 240.

3 P. Young. *Asthma and Allergies: An Optimistic Future* NIH Publication No. 80-388 (Washington, DC: National Institutes of Health, 1980).

4 J.E. Pizzorno and M.T. Murray. *Encyclopedia of Natural Medicine* (Rocklin, CA: Prima Publishing, 1991), 239.

5 Robert S. Ivker, Robert O. Anderson, and Larry Trivieri. *The Complete Self-Care Guide to Holistic Medicine* (New York: Tarcher/Putnam 1999), 257.

6 Robert Crayhon. *Health Benefits of FOS* (New Canaan, CT: Keats Publishing, 1995).

7 M. Walker. "Soil-Based Organisms Support Immune System Functions from the Ground Up." *Townsend Letter for Doctors & Patients* 169 (August/September 1997), 85-92.

8 Elaine Gottschall. *Breaking the Vicious Cycle: Intestinal Health Through Diet* (Kirkton, Ontario, Canada: Kirkton Press, 1994).

9 This report is based solely on product labeling as published by PDR®. Copyright ©1993 by Medical Economics Data, a division of Medical Economics Company, Inc. All rights reserved.

10 Melvyn R. Werbach, M.D. *Nutritional Influences on Illness* (Tarzana, CA: Third Line Press, 1996).

11 Donald J. Brown, N.D. *Herbal Prescriptions for Better Health* (Rocklin, CA: Prima Publishing, 1996).

12 James A. Duke, Ph.D. *The Green Pharmacy* (Emmaus, PA: Rodale Press, 1997).

13 Robert Ullman, N.D., and Judyth Reichenberg-Ullman, N.D. *Homeopathic Self-Care* (Rocklin, CA: Prima Publishing, 1997).

14 "Heartburn and Ulcers: Natural Ways to Spell R-e-l-i-e-f." *Dr. Christiane Northrup's Health Wisdom for Women* (April 1997), 2-5. Patricia Kaminski and Richard Katz. *Flower Essence Repertory* (Nevada City, CA: Earth-Spirit, 1994).

15 J.E. Pizzorno and M.T. Murray. *Encyclopedia of Natural Medicine* (Rocklin, CA: Prima Publishing, 1991), 395.

16 Ibid., 399.

17 Ibid., 400.

18 Ibid., 289.

19 Ibid., 343.

20 Ibid., 344.

HEADACHES

1 J.E. Pizzorno and M.T. Murray, eds. *A Textbook of Natural Medicine* (Seattle, WA: John Bastyr College Publications, 1988-1989).

2 Robert Milne, M.D., and Blake More, with Burton Goldberg. *Alternative Medicine Definitive Guide to Headaches* (Tiburon, CA: Future Medicine Publishing, 1996), 51.

3 J. Egger et al. "Is Migraine Food Allergy? A Double-Blind Controlled Trial of Oligoantigenic Diet Treatment." *The Lancet* 2:8355 (October 1983), 865-869.

4 Defense Against Mercury Syndromes, DAMS, Inc., 6025 Osuna Blvd., N.E., Suite B, Albuquerque, NM 87109-2523.

5 C.J. Rudolph et al. "An Observation of the Effect of EDTA Chelation and Supportive Multivitamin Trace Mineral Supplementation of Blood Platelet Volume: A Brief Communication." *Journal of Advancement in Medicine* 3:3 (Fall 1990). E. Morgenstern and G. Stark. "Morphometric Analysis of Platelet Ultra-Structure in Normal and Experimental Conditions." *Platelets* (1975), 37-42.

6 E.S. Johnson et al. "Efficacy of Feverfew as Pro-

phylactic Treatment of Migraine." *British Medical Journal* 291:6495 (August 1985), 569-573.

HEARING AND EAR DISORDERS

1 D. Black. *Healing with Sound* (Springville, UT: Tapestry Press, 1991).

2 C.D. Bluestone. "Otitis Media in Children: To Treat or Not to Treat?" *New England Journal of Medicine* 306:23 (June 1982), 1399-1404.

3 J.E. Pizzorno and M.T. Murray. *A Textbook of Natural Medicine* (Seattle, WA: John Bastyr College Publications, 1988-1989).

4 U.M. Saarinen. "Prolonged Breast Feeding as Prophylaxis for Recurrent Otitis Media." *Acta Paediatrica Scandinavica* 71:4 (July 1982), 567-571.

5 R.J. Hagerman and A.R. Falkenstein. "An Association Between Recurrent Otitis Media in Infancy and Later Hyperactivity." *Clinical Pediatrics* 76:5 (May 1987), 253-257.

6 A. Toufexis. "Now Hear This—If You Can." *Time* 138:5 (August 1991), 50-51.

7 S.C. Dees and D. Lefkowitz III. "Secretory Otitis Media in Allergic Children." *American Journal of Diseases of Children* 124:3 (September 1972), 364-368.

8 J. Ruokonen, A. Paganus, and H. Lehti. "Elimination Diets in the Treatment of Secretory Otitis Media." *International Journal of Pediatric Otorhinolaryngology* 4:1 (March 1982), 39-46.

9 B.J. Asman and P. Fireman. "The Role of Allergies in the Development of Otitis Media with Effusion." *International Pediatrics* 3:3 (1988), 231-233. Editorial Staff. "Antibiotic Use: Adult Prescriptions Fall as Pediatric Prescriptions Soar." *Medical World News* 28:21 (November 1987), 8-10.

10 M. Diamant and B. Diamant. "Abuse and Timing of Use of Antibiotics in Acute Otitis Media." *Archives of Otolaryngology* 100:3 (September 1974), 226-232.

11 E.I. Cantekin, T.W. McGuire, and T.L. Griffith. "Antimicrobial Therapy for Otitis Media with Effusion (Secretory Otitis Media)." *Journal of the American Medical Association* 266:23 (December 1991), 3309-3317.

12 P. Adlington and W.K. Hooper. "Virus Studies in Secretory Otitis Media." *Journal of Laryngology and Otology* 94:2 (February 1980), 191-196. M. Arola, T. Ziegler, and O. Ruuskanen. "Respiratory Virus Infection as a Cause of Prolonged Symptoms in Acute Otitis Media." *Journal of Pediatrics* 116:5 (May 1990), 697-701.

13 S.R. Cohen and J.W. Thompson. "Otitic Candidiasis in Children: An Evaluation of the Problem an Effectiveness of Ketoconazole in 10 Patients." *Annals of Otology, Rhinology, and Laryngology* 99:6 Part 1 (June 1990), 427-431.

14 W.G. Crook, M.D. "Ear Infections: Is the Treatment Part of the Problem?" *Environmental Physician* (Winter 1992-1993).

15 F.L. van Buchen, J.H. Dunk, and M.A. van Hof. "Therapy of Acute Otitis Media: Myringotomy, Antibiotics, or Neither? A Double-Blind Study in Children." *The Lancet* 2:8252 (October 1981), 883-887.

16 M. Strome, P. Topf, and D.M. Vernick. "Hyperlipidemia in Association with Childhood Sensorineural Hearing Loss." *Laryngoscope* 98:2 (February 1988), 165-169.

17 J.T. Spencer, Jr. "Hyperlipoproteinemia, Hyperinsulinism and Meniere's Disease." *Southern Medical Journal* 74:10 (October 1981), 1194-1197.

18 M. Bondestam, T. Foucard, and M. Gebre-Med-

hin. "Subclinical Trace Element Deficiency in Children with Undue Susceptibility to Infections." *Acta Paediatrica Scandinavica* 74:4 (July 1985), 515-520. T.T. Jung. "Prostaglandins, Leukotrienes, and Other Arachidonic Acid Metabolites in the Pathogenesis of Otitis Media." *Laryngoscope* 98:9 (September 1988), 980-993.

19 M. Lewis et al. "Prenatal Exposure to Heavy Metals: Effects on Childhood Cognitive Skills and Health Status." *Pediatrics* 89:6 Part 1 (June 1992), 1010-1015.

20 F.A. Campos, H. Flores, and B.A. Underwood. "Effect of an Infection on Vitamin A Status of Children as Measured by the Relative Dose Response (RDR)." *American Journal of Clinical Nutrition* 46:1 (July 1987), 91-94. G.D. Hussey and M. Klein. "A Randomized, Controlled Trial of Vitamin A in Children with Severe Measles." *New England Journal of Medicine* 323:3 (July 1990), 160-164.

21 A. Bendich. "Vitamin E Status of U.S. Children." *Journal of the American College of Clinical Nutrition* 11:4 (August 1991), 441-444.

22 "Says Food Allergy Seems Important Cause of Otitis Media." *Family Practice News* 21:5 (1991), 14.

23 D.S. Hurst. "Allergy Management of Refractory Serous Otitis Media." *Otolaryngology and Head and Neck Surgery* 102:6 (January 1990), 664-669.

24 S.R. Cohen and J.W. Thompson. "Otitic Candidiasis in Children: an Evaluation of the Problem an Effectiveness of Ketoconazole in 10 Patients." *Annals of Otology, Rhinology, and Laryngology* 99:6 Part 1 (June 1990), 427-431.

25 A. Fiocchi et al. "A Double-Blind Clinical Trial for the Evaluation of the Therapeutical Effectiveness of a Calf Thymus Derivative (Thymomodulin) in Children with Recurrent Respiratory Infections." *Thymus* 8:6 (1986), 331-339. R. Genova and A. Guerra. "Thymomodulin in Management of Food Allergy in Children." *International Journal of Tissue Reactions* 8:3 (1986), 239-242. P. Cazzola, P. Mazzanti, and G. Bossi. "In Vivo Modulating Effect of a Calf Thymus Acid Lysate on Human T Lymphocyte Subsets and CD4+/CD8+ Ration in the Course of Different Diseases." *Current Therapeutic Research* 42:6 (December 1987), 1011-1017.

26 G. Romeo and M. Giorgetti. "Therapeutic Effects of Vitamin A Associated with Vitamin E in Perceptual Hearing Loss." *Acta Vitaminol Enzymol* 7:1-2 (1985), 139-143.

27 Earl L. Mindell. *The MSM Miracle* (New Canaan, CT: Keats Publishing, 1997).

28 K. Ehrenberger and R. Brix. "Glutamic Acid and Glutamic Acid Diethylester in Tinnitus Treatment." *Acta Otolaryngol* 95:5-6 (1983), 599-605.

29 Denise K. Houston et al. "Age-Related Hearing Loss, Vitamin B12 and Folate in Elderly Women." *American Journal of Clinical Nutrition* 69 (March 1999), 564-571.

30 J.E. Pizzorno and M.T. Murray, eds. *A Textbook of Natural Medicine* (Seattle, WA: John Bastyr College Publications, 1988-1989), 1-4.

31 A. Wacker and W. Hilbig. "Virus Inhibition by Echinacea purpurea." *Planta Medica* 33 (1978), 89-102.

32 *Tufts University Health and Nutrition Letter* (November 1997), 8.

33 B. Meyer. "A Multicenter Randomized Double-Blind Study of *Gingko biloba* Extract versus Placebo in the Treatment of Tinnitus." In: Funfgeld, ed. *Rokan (Ginkgo biloba)—Recent Results in Pharmacology and Clinic* (New York: Springer-Verlag, 1988), 245-250.

34 D.B. Mowrey, Ph.D. *The Scientific Validation of Herbal Medicine* (New Canaan, CT: Keats Publishing, 1986), 216-217.

35 K.H. Friese, M.D., et al. "Acute Otitis Media in Children: A Comparison of Conventional and Homeopathic Treatment." *Biomedical Therapy* XV:4 (October 1997), 113-116, 122.

HEART DISEASE

1 J.R. Privitera, M.D. "Clots: Life's Biggest Killer." Unpublished manuscript (1992).

2 R.G. Petersdorf et al. *Harrison's Principles of Internal Medicine* (New York: McGraw-Hill, 1983).

3 Ibid.

4 CASS Principal Investigators and Associates. "Myocardial Infarction and Mortality in the Coronary Artery Surgery Study (CASS) Randomized Trial." *New England Journal of Medicine* 310:12 (March 1984), 750-758.

5 Valentine Fuster, ed. *The Vulnerable Artherosclerotic Plaque: Understanding, Identification and Modification* American Heart Association Monograph Series (Futura Publishing, 1998).

6 Paul W. Ewald. *Plague Time: How Stealth Infections Cause Cancers, Heart Disease, and Other Deadly Ailments* (New York: Free Press, 2000), 109-110.

7 Ibid., 113.

8 American Heart Association (AHA). Available on the Internet: www.amhrt.org/hs96/has.html.

9 National Institutes of Health. *Stroke: Hope Through Research* NIH Publication No. 83-2222 (Washington, DC: U.S. Department of Health and Human Services, Public Health Services, National Institutes of Health, 1983).

10 National Institute of Neurological Disorders and Stroke. *Stroke Research Highlights* (Washington, DC: National Institutes of Health 1990).

11 National Institutes of Health. *Stroke: Hope Through Research* NIH Publication No. 83-2222 (Washington, DC: U.S. Department of Health and Human Services, Public Health Services, National Institutes of Health, 1983).

12 S.L. Robbins, R.S. Cotran, and V. Kumar, eds. *Pathological Basis of Disease* (New York: W.B. Saunders, 1984).

13 D. Jaffe et al. "Coronary Arteries in Newborn Children: Intimal Variations in Longitudinal Sections and Their Relationships to Clinical and Experimental Data." *Acta Paediatrica Scandinavica Supplement* 219 (1971), 3-28.

14 G.M. Kostner et al. "The Interaction of Human Plasma Low Density Lipoproteins with Glycosamino-Glycans: Influence of the Chemical Composition." *Lipids* 20:1 (January 1985), 24-28.

15 Richard Passwater. *Supernutrition for Healthy Hearts* (New York: Dial Press, 1977). T. Gordon et al. *American Journal of Medicine* 62 (1977), 707-714. P. Williams et al. *The Lancet* 1 (1979), 72-75.

16 R.D. Morris et al. "Chlorination, Chlorination Byproducts, and Cancer: A Meta-Analysis." *American Journal of Public Health* 82:7 (July 1992), 955-963.

17 R. Winslow. "Experts Worry That Side-Effect Fear Could Set Back Cholesterol Battle." *The Wall Street Journal* CCXXXVIII:37 (August 22, 2001), B1, B4.

18 This report is based solely on product labeling as published by PDR®. Copyright ©1993 by Medical Economics Data, a division of Medical Economics Company, Inc. All rights reserved.

19 T.M. Burton and G. Harris. "Note of Caution: Study Raises Specter of Cardiovascular Risk for Hot Arthritis Pills." *The Wall Street Journal* CCXXXVIII:37 (August 22, 2001), A1, A8.]

20 R.J. Morin and S.K. Peng. "The Role of Cholesterol Oxidation Products in the Pathogenesis of Atherosclerosis." *Annals of Clinical and Laboratory Science* 19:4 (July-August 1989), 225-237.

21 J.G. Hattersley. "Acquired Atherosclerosis: Theories of Causation, Novel Therapies." *Journal of Orthomolecular Medicine* 6:2 (1991), 83-98.

22 S.K. Peng and C.B. Taylor. "Cholesterol Autooxidation, Health and Arteriosclerosis." *World Reviews of Nutrition and Diet* 44 (1984), 117-154.

23 K.S. McCully. "Homocysteine Theory of Arteriosclerosis: Development and Current Status." *Atherosclerosis Reviews* 11 (1983), 157-246.

24 R.D. Morris et al. "Chlorination, Chlorination Byproducts, and Cancer: A Meta-Analysis." *American Journal of Public Health* 82:7 (July 1992), 955-963. J. Yiamouiannis. *Fluoride: The Aging Factor* (Delaware, OH: Health Action Press, 1986).

25 K.S. McCully. "Homocysteine Theory of Arteriosclerosis: Development and Current Status." *Atherosclerosis Reviews* 11 (1983), 157-246.

26 Robert S. Ivker, Robert A. Anderson, and Larry Trivieri. *The Complete Self-Care Guide to Holistic Medicine* (New York: Tarcher/Putnam, 1999), 326-327.

27 "C-Reactive Protein as a Heart Disease Risk Factor." *The Doctor's Prescription for Healthy Living* 4:1 (January 1999).

28 Ibid.

29 S. Tommasi et al. "High C-Reactive Protein Level May Be a Marker for Cardiac Events." *American Journal of Cardiology* 83 (June 15, 1999), 1595-1599.

30 S. Fichtlscherer et al. "Elevated C-Reactive Protein Levels and Impaired Endothelial Vasoreactivity in Patients with Coronary Artery Disease." *Circulation* 102:9 (2000), 1000.

31 Robert S. Ivker, Robert A. Anderson, and Larry Trivieri. *The Complete Self-Care Guide to Holistic Medicine* (New York: Tarcher/Putnam, 1999), 350.

32 Ibid., 327.

33 *Arteriosclerosis, Thrombosis, and Vascular Biology* 21 (August 2001), 1346-1352.

34 Broda Barnes and Lawrence Galton. *Hypothyroidism: The Unsuspected Illness* (New York: Harper & Row, 1976).

35 Eugenia Halsey. "Researchers Pinpoint Link between Smoking and Heart Disease." Internet: CNN Interactive Main Food & Heath Page (May 3, 1996).

36 Linda Ciampa. "Study: Passive Smoke and Even Greater Risk." Internet: CNN Interactive Heath Page (May 19, 1997).

37 H.L. Queen. *Chronic Mercury Toxicity: New Hope Against an Endemic Disease* (Colorado Springs, CO: Queen and Company, 1988).

38 J. McConnaughey. "Heart Risk Changes with Neighborhood, Research Finds." Associated Press report (July 12, 2001).

39 P. Stern. "Gum Disease Raises Stroke Risk." Reuters Health report (October 27, 2000).

40 Dean Ornish, M.D. *Dr. Dean Ornish's Program for Reversing Heart Disease* (New York: Ballantine, 1990).

41 Ibid.

42 *The Lancet* 344:8933 (November 1994), 1356.

43 M.G. Hertog et al. "Antioxidant Flavonols and

Coronary Heart Disease Risk." *The Lancet* 349:699 (1997).

44 Ilja C.W. Arts et al. *American Journal of Clinical Nutrition* 74 (August 2001), 227-232.

45 A.J. Olszewski and K.S. McCully. "Fish Oil Decreases Serum Homocysteine in Hyperlipidemic Men." *Coronary Artery Disease* 4 (1993), 53-60.

46 S. Renaud and A. Nordy. "'Small is Beautiful': Alpha-Linoleic Acid and Eicosapentaenoic Acid in Man." *The Lancet* 1:8334 (May 1983), 1169.

47 S. Rostler. "Fatty Acids Up Sudden Death Risk in Healthy Men." Reuters Health report (August 13, 2001).

48 S. Rostler. "Trans Fat Worse for Heart Than Saturated Fat." Reuters Health report (July 12, 2001).

49 D.A. Street et al. "A Population-Based Case Control Study of the Association of Serum Antioxidants and Myocardial Infarction." *American Journal of Epidemiology* 131 (1991), 719-720.

50 K.G. Berge and P.L. Canner. "Coronary Drug Project: Experience with Niacin. Coronary Drug Project Research Group." *European Journal of Clinical Pharmacology* 40:Suppl 1 (1991), S49-S51. M.H. Luria. "Effect of Low-Dose Niacin on High-Density Lipoprotein Cholesterol and Total Cholesterol/High-Density Lipoprotein Ratio." *Archives of Internal Medicine* 148:11 (November 1988), 2493-2495.

51 P.L. Canner et al. "Fifteen-Year Mortality in Coronary Drug Project Patients: Long-Term Benefit with Niacin." *Journal of the American College of Cardiology* 8:6 (December 1986), 1245-1255.

52 J.G. Hattersley. "Heart Attacks and Strokes." *Townsend Letter for Doctors* 104 (February/March 1992).

53 S.H. Mudd et al. "The Natural History of Homocystinuria Due to Cystathionine Beta-Synthose Deficiency." *American Journal of Human Genetics* 37:1 (January 1985), 1-31.

54 Editorial. "Is Vitamin B6 an Antithrombotic Agent?" *The Lancet* 1:8233 (June 1981), 1299-1300.

55 M.M. Suzman. "Effect of Pyridoxine and Low Animal Protein Diet in Coronary Artery Disease." Abstracts of the 46th Scientific Sessions. *Circulation* Suppl IV (October 1973), 254.

56 M.M. Suzman. "Effect of Pyridoxine and Low Animal Protein Diet in Coronary Artery Disease." Abstracts of the 46th Scientific Sessions. *Circulation* Suppl IV (October 1973), 254.

57 K.S. McCully. "Homocysteine Theory of Arteriosclerosis: Development and Current Status." *Atherosclerosis Reviews* 11 (1983), 157-246.

58 L. Brattstrom et al. "Higher Total Plasma Homocysteine Due to Cystathionine Beta-Synthase Deficiency." *Metabolism: Clinical and Experimental* 37:2 (February 1988), 175-178.

59 A.J. Olszewski et al. "Reduction of Plasma Lipid and Homocysteine Levels by Pyridoxine, Folate, Cobalamin, Choline, Riboflavin, and Troxerutin in Atherosclerosis." *Atherosclerosis* 75:1 (January 1989), 1-6.

60 L. Brattstrom et al. "Impaired Homocysteine Metabolism in Early-Onset Cerebral and Peripheral Occlusive Artery Disease. Effects of Pyridoxine and Folic Acid Treatment." *Atherosclerosis* 81:1 (1990), 51-60. A.J. Olszewski et al. "Reduction of Plasma Lipid and Homocysteine Levels by Pyridoxine, Folate, Cobalamin, Choline, Riboflavin, and Troxerutin in Atherosclerosis." *Atherosclerosis* 75:1 (January 1989), 1-6.

61 A.J. Olszewski et al. "Reduction of Plasma Lipid and Homocysteine Levels by Pyridoxine, Folate, Cobalamin, Choline, Riboflavin, and Troxerutin in Atherosclerosis." *Atherosclerosis* 75:1 (January 1989), 1-6.

62 I. Jialal and S.M. Grundy. "Effect of Dietary Supplementation with Alpha-Tocopherol on the Oxidative Modification of Low Density Lipoprotein." *Journal of Lipid Research* 33:6 (June 1992), 899-906. M. Steiner. "Influence of Vitamin E on Platelet Function in Humans." *Journal of the American College of Nutrition* 10:5 (October 1991), 466-473. D. Boscoboinik, A. Szewczyk, and A. Azzi. "Alpha-Tocopherol (Vitamin E) Regulates Vascular Smooth Muscle Cell Proliferation and Protein Kinase C Activity." *Archives of Biochemistry and Biophysics* 286:1 (April 1991), 264-269. B. Hennig et al. "Protective Effects of Vitamin E in Age-Related Endothelial Cell Injury." *International Journal of Vitamin and Nutrition Research* 59 (1989), 273-279.

63 E. Rimm et al. "Vitamin E Consumption and the Risk of Coronary Heart Disease in Men." *New England Journal of Medicine* 328:20 (May 1993), 1450-1456. M.J. Stampfer et al. "Vitamin E Consumption and the Risk of Coronary Heart Disease in Women." *New England Journal of Medicine* 328:20 (May 1993), 1444-1449.

64 M. Stampfer et al. "Vitamin E and Heart Disease Incidence in the Nurses Health Study." Presented at the American Heart Association Annual Meeting, New Orleans, Louisiana (November 18, 1992).

65 E. Rimm et al. "Vitamin E Consumption and the Risk of Coronary Heart Disease in Men." *New England Journal of Medicine* 328:20 (May 1993), 1450-1456. M.J. Stampfer et al. "Vitamin E Consumption and the Risk of Coronary Heart Disease in Women." *New England Journal of Medicine* 328:20 (May 1993), 1444-1449.

66 K.F. Gey et al. "Inverse Correlation Between Plasma Vitamin E and Mortality from Ischemic Heart Disease in Cross-Cultural Epidemiology." *American Journal of Clinical Nutrition* 53:Suppl. 1 (January 1991), 326S-334S.

67 K.S. McCully. "Homocysteine Metabolism in Scurvy, Growth, and Arteriosclerosis." *Nature* 231:5302 (June 1971), 391-392.

68 M. Rath and L. Pauling. "Hypothesis: Lipoprotein(a) is a Surrogate for Ascorbate." *Proceedings of the National Academy of Sciences* 87:16 (August 1990), 6204-6207.

69 M. Rath and L. Pauling. "Solution to the Puzzle of Human Cardiovascular Disease: Its Primary Cause is Ascorbate Deficiency Leading to the Deposition of Lipoprotein(a) and Fibrinogen/Fibrin in the Vascular Wall." *Journal of Orthomolecular Medicine* 6 (1991), 125-134.

70 E.R. Ginter et al. "Vitamin C in the Control of Mypercholesterolemia in Man." *International Journal for Vitamin and Nutrition Research* Suppl 23 (1982), 137-152.

71 M. Rath and L. Pauling. "Solution to the Puzzle of Human Cardiovascular Disease: Its Primary Cause is Ascorbate Deficiency Leading to the Deposition of Lipoprotein(a) and Fibrinogen/Fibrin in the Vascular Wall." *Journal of Orthomolecular Medicine* 6 (1991), 125-134.

72 M. Rath and L. Pauling. "Hypothesis: Lipoprotein(a) is a Surrogate for Ascorbate." *Proceedings of the National Academy of Sciences* 87:16 (August 1990), 6204-6207.

73 Y. Hanaki, S. Sugiyama, and T. Ozawa. "Ratio of Low-Density Lipoprotein Cholesterol to Ubiquinone as a Coronary Risk Factor." *New England Journal of Medicine* 325:11 (September 1991), 814-815. B. Frei, M.C. Kim, and B.N. Ames. "Ubiquinol-10 is an Effective Lipid-Soluble Antioxidant at Physiological Concentrations." *Proceedings of the National Academy of Sciences* 87:12 (1990), 4879-4883.

74 Richard A. Passwater and Chitan Kandaswami. *Pycnogenol: The Super "Protector" Nutrient* (New Canaan, CT: Keats Publishing, 1994), 79.

75 Ibid., 81.

76 J.T. Salonen et al. "Interactions of Serum Copper, Selenium and Low Density Lipoprotein Cholesterol in Atherogenesis." *British Medical Journal* 302:6779 (March 1991), 756-760.

77 N.W. Stead et al. "Effect of Selenium Supplementation on Selenium Balance in the Dependent Elderly." *American Journal of the Medical Sciences* 290:6 (December 1985), 228-233.

78 D.A. Wood et al. "Adipose Tissue and Platelet Fatty Acids and Coronary Heart Disease in Scottish Men." *The Lancet* 2:8395 (July 1984), 117-121.

79 M.S. Seelig and H.A. Heggtveit. "Magnesium Interrelationships in Ischemic Heart Disease: A Review." *American Journal of Clinical Nutrition* 27:1 (January 1974), 59-79. W.H. Davis et al. "Monotherapy with Magnesium Increases Abnormally Low Density Lipoprotein Cholesterol: A Clinical Assay." *Current Therapeutic Research* 36:2 (August 1984), 341.

80 N. Karanja et al. "Plasma Lipids and Hypertension: Response to Calcium Supplementation." *American Journal of Clinical Nutrition* 45:1 (January 1987), 60-65.

81 R.I. Press, J. Geller, and G.W. Evans. "The Effect of Chromium Picolinate on Serum Cholesterol and Apolipoprotein Fractions in Human Subjects." *Western Journal of Medicine* 152:1 (January 1990), 41-45.

82 M. Urberg, J. Benyi, and R. John. "Hypercholesterolemic Effects of Nicotinic Acid and Chromium Supplementation." *Journal of Family Practice* 27:6 (December 1988), 603-606.

83 M. Simonoff et al. "Low Plasma Chromium in Patients with Coronary Artery and Heart Diseases." *Biological Trace Elements Research* 6:5 (October 1984), 431-439. H.A. Newman et al. "Serum Chromium and Angiographically Determined Coronary Artery Disease." *Clinical Chemistry* 24:4 (April 1978), 541-544.

84 *Northeast Center for Environmental Medicine Health Letter* (Fall 1992).

85 Bella Koifman, M.D. "Improvement of Cardiac Performance by Intravenous Infusion of L-Arginine in Patients with Moderate Congestive Heart Failure." *Journal of the American College of Cardiology* 26:5 (November 1, 1995), 1251-1256.

86 R.B. Singh. "A Randomized, Double-Blind, Placebo-Controlled Trial of L-Carnitine in Suspected Acute Myocardial Infarction." *Postgraduate Medical Journal* (1995).

87 G.M. Kostner et al. "HMG CoA Reductase Inhibitors Lower LDL Cholesterol Without Reducing Lp(a) Levels." *Circulation* 80:5 (1989), 1313-1319.

88 T.E. Strandberg et al. "Long-Term Mortality After 5-year Multi-Factorial Primary Prevention of Cardiovascular Diseases in Middle-Aged Men." *Journal of the American Medical Association* 266:9 (September 1991), 1225-1229.

89 K. Folkers et al. "Lovastatin Decreases Coenzyme-Q Levels in Humans." *Proceedings of the National*

Academy of Sciences 87:22 (November 1990), 8931-8934.

90 T.L. Chappel. "Preliminary Findings From the Media Analysis Study of EDTA Chelation Therapy." Paper presented to the American College of Advancement in Medicine, Houston, Texas (May 5-9, 1993).

91 M. Walker and G. Gordon. *The Chelation Answer* (New York: M. Evans, 1982), 175.

92 Jack V. Tu et al. "Use of Cardiac Procedures and Outcomes in Elderly Patients with Myocardial Infarction in the United States and Canada." *New England Journal of Medicine* 336:21 (May 22, 1997).

93 D. Grady. "Mental Decline is Linked to Heart Bypass Surgery." *The New York Times* (February 8, 2001).

94 "Delaying Bypass Surgery May Cut Stroke Risk." Reuters Health report (July 16, 2001).

95 "Study Suggests Common Heart Test May Harm Patients." Available on the Internet: CNN Interactive Health Page (September 16, 1996).

96 Julian Whitaker. "Heart Surgery Does More Harm Than Good." *Dr. Julian Whitaker's Health & Healing* 7:5 (May 1997), 1-3.

97 T. Maugh. "Invasive Heart Attack Treatment Questioned." *The Los Angeles Times* (March 20, 1997).

98 R.F. Weiss. *Herbal Medicine* (Gothenburg, Sweden: A.B. Arcanum, 1988).

99 S.A. Barrie, J.V. Wright, M.D., and J.E. Pizzorno. "Effect of Garlic Oil on Platelet Aggregation, Serum Lipids and Blood Pressure in Humans." *Journal of Orthomolecular Medicine* 2:1 (1987), 15-21.

100 K.C. Srivastava. "Effects of Aqueous Extracts of Onion, Garlic and Ginger on Platelet Aggregation and Metabolism of Arachidonic Acid in the Blood Vascular System." *Prostaglandins, Leukotrienes and Medicine* 13 (1984), 227-235.

101 Morton Walker, D.P.M. "Antimicrobial Attributes of Olive Leaf Extract." *Townsend Letter for Doctors & Patients* (July 1996), 80-85. Harold E. Renis. "In Vitro Antiviral Activity of Calcium Elenolate." *Antimicrobial Agents and Chemotherapy-1969* (1970), 167-171. B. Juven et al. "Studies on the Mechanism of the Antimicrobial Action of Oleuropein." *Journal of Applied Bacteriology* 35 (1972), 559-567.

102 *New England Journal of Medicine* 312 (1985), 1250-1259.

103 *Atherosclerosis* 63 (1987), 137-143. *Hypertension* 4:Suppl III (1982), 34.

104 C.H. Farr, M.D., R. White, and M. Schachter, M.D. "Chronological History of EDTA Chelation Therapy." Presented to the American College of Advancement in Medicine, Houston, Texas (May 1993).

105 M. Walker and G. Gordon. *The Chelation Answer* (New York: M. Evans, 1982).

106 E. Olszewer, M.D., and J.P. Carter, M.D. "EDTA Chelation Therapy: A Retrospective Study of 2,870 Patients." *Journal of Advancement in Medicine* 2:1-2 (1989), 183.

107 David A. Steenblock, M.S., D.O. "Review of Hyperbaric Oxygen for Stroke Rehabilitation." *Explore!* 7:5 (1996/1997), 49-53.

108 C.H. Farr. "The Therapeutic Use of Intravenous Hydrogen Peroxide." Monograph. (Oklahoma City, OK: Genesis Medical Center, 1987). E. Baker. *The Unmedical Miracle—Oxygen* (Indianola, WA: Drelwood Communications, 1991).

109 M. Walker. "The Biological Therapies of Harvey Bigelsen, M.D." *Explore!* 4:2 (1993), 50-53.

110 C.H. Farr. "The Therapeutic Use of Intravenous Hydrogen Peroxide." Monograph. (Oklahoma City, OK: Genesis Medical Center, 1987).

111 D. Ornish, M.D., et al. "Can Lifestyle Changes Reverse Coronary Heart Disease? The Lifestyle Heart Trial." *The Lancet* 336:8708 (July 1990), 129-133.

112 *Health Psychology* (July 1999).

113 *American Journal of Epidemiology* 154 (August 1, 2001), 230-235. C.E. Huggins. "A Fiery Temper May Increase Heart Attack Risk." Reuters Health report (August 8, 2001).

114 P. Peck. "A New Way Hotheads May Be Hurting Their Hearts: For Men, Holding in Anger Can Make the Problem Worse." WebMD Medical News (May 5, 2000).

115 "Study: Anger Strains Kids' Hearts." Gannett News Service (April 27, 1999).

116 *Archives of Internal Medicine* 161 (July 23, 2001), 1725-1730. E. Edelson. "Hopelessness Begets Hypertension: More Evidence that Depression's a Matter of the Heart." *HealthSCOUT Reporter* (February 21, 2000).

117 Chung San i Hsueh Yuan. "Treatment of 103 Cases of Coronary Diseases with *Ilex pubescens*." *Am Chinese Medical Journal* 1 (1973), 64.

118 CASS Principal Investigators and Associates. "Myocardial Infarction and Mortality in the Coronary Artery Surgery Study (CASS) Randomized Trial." *New England Journal of Medicine* 310:12 (March 1984), 750-758.

119 J. Peltz. "Insurer to Reimburse Cost of Non-Surgical Heart Care." *The Los Angeles Times* (July 8, 1993), 1.

HYPERTENSION (HIGH BLOOD PRESSURE)

1 J.E. Pizzorno and M.T. Murray, eds. "Hypertension." *A Textbook of Natural Medicine* (Seattle, WA: John Bastyr Publications, 1988).

2 H.Y. Chow, J.C. Wang, and K.K. Cheng. "Cardiovascular Effects of Gardenia Florida L. (*Gardenise Fructus*) Extract." *American Journal of Chinese Medicine* 4:1 (1976). 47-51. G.J. Brewer. "Molecular Mechanisms of Zinc Action on Cells." *Agents and Actions* 8:Suppl (1981), 37-49. A.E. Bennett, R. Doll, and R.W. Howell. "Sugar Consumption and Cigarette Smoking." *The Lancet* 1 (May 1970), 1011-1014. A. Kershbaum et al. "Effects of Smoking and Nicotine on Adrenocortical Secretion." *Journal of the American Medical Association* 203:4 (January 1968), 275-278. S.P. Fortmann et al. "The Association of Blood Pressure and Dietary Alcohol: Differences by Age, Sex, and Estrogen Use." *American Journal of Epidemiology* 118:4 (October 1983), 497-507.

3 J.E. Pizzorno and M.T. Murray, eds. "Hypertension." *A Textbook of Natural Medicine* (Seattle, WA: John Bastyr Publications, 1988).

4 J. He et al. "Effect of Migration on Blood Pressure: the Yi People Study." *Epidemiology* 2:2 (March 1991), 88-97. N.R. Poulter et al. "The Kenyan Luo Migration Study: Observations on the Initiation of a Rise in Blood Pressure." *British Medical Journal* 300:6730 (April 1990), 967-972. C.E. Salmond, I.A. Prior, and A.F. Wessen. "Blood Pressure Patterns and Migration: A 14-Year Cohort Study of Adult Tokelauans." *American Journal of Epidemiology* 130:1 (July 1989), 37-52.

5 R.J. Havlik et al. "Weight and Hypertension." *Annals of Internal Medicine* 98:5 Part 2 (May 1983), 855-859.

6 H.W. Gruchow, K.A. Sobocinski, and J.J. Barboriak. "Alcohol, Nutrient Intake, and Hyperten-

sion in U.S. Adults." *Journal of the American Medical Association* 253:11 (March 1985), 1567-1570.

7 G.R. Meneely and H.D. Battarbee. "High Sodium-Low Potassium Environment and Hypertension." *American Journal of Cardiology* 38:6 (November 1976), 768-785. L.M. Resnick, R.K. Gupta, and J.H. Laragh. "Intracellular Free Magnesium in Erythrocytes of Essential Hypertension: Relationship to Blood Pressure and Serum Divalent Cations." *Proceedings of the National Academy of Sciences* 81:20 (October 1984), 6511-6515.

8 T. Lang et al. "Relation Between Coffee Drinking and Blood Pressure: Analysis of 6,321 Subjects in the Paris Region." *American Journal of Cardiology* 52:10 (December 1983), 1238-1242.

9 S.P. Fortmann et al. "The Association of Blood Pressure and Dietary Alcohol: Differences by Age, Sex and Estrogen Use." *American Journal of Epidemiology* 118:4 (October 1983), 497-507. H.W. Gruchow, K.A. Sobocinski, and J.J. Barboriak. "Alcohol, Nutrient Intake, and Hypertension in U.S. Adults." *Journal of the American Medical Association* 253:11 (March 1985), 1567-1570.

10 A.E. Bennett, R. Doll, and R.W. Howell. "Sugar Consumption and Cigarette Smoking." *The Lancet* 1 (May 1970), 1011-1014.

11 K.L. Schroeder and M.S. Chen, Jr. "Smokeless Tobacco and Blood Pressure." *New England Journal of Medicine* 312:14 (April 1985), 919. N.B. Hampson. "Smokeless is Not Saltless." *New England Journal of Medicine* 312:14 (April 1985), 919-920.

12 K.J. Egan et al. "The Impact of Psychological Distress on the Control of Hypertension." *Journal of Human Stress* 9:4 (December 1983), 4-10.

13 J.L. Pirkle et al. "The Relationship Between Blood Lead Levels and its Cardiovascular Risk Implications." *American Journal of Epidemiology* 121:2 (February 1985), 246-258. Howard Hu et al. "The Relationship of Bone and Blood Lead to Hypertension: The Normative Aging Study." *Journal of the American Medical Association* 275:15 (April 17, 1996), 1171-1176. A.D. Torres, A.N. Rai, and M.L. Hardiek. "Mercury Intoxication and Arterial Hypertension: Report of Two Patients and Review of the Literature." *Pediatrics* 105:3 (March 2000), E34.

14 *Journal of the American Medical Association* (April 1996).

15 *Science News* 148 (October 21, 1995), 268.

16 S.C. Glauser, C.T. Bello, and E.M. Gauser. "Blood-Cadmium Levels in Normotensive and Untreated Hypertensive Humans." *The Lancet* 1 (April 1976), 717-718.

17 D.B. Foushee, J. Ruffin, and U. Banerjee. "Garlic as a Natural Agent for the Treatment of Hypertension: A Preliminary Report." *Cytobios* 34:135-136 (1982), 145-152. V. Petkov. "Plants with Hypotensive, Antiatheromatous and Coronary Dilating Action." *American Journal of Chinese Medicine* 7:3 (1979), 197-236.

18 "Reducing Hypertension: Is Diet Better Than Drugs?" *Alternative & Complementary Therapies* 3:1 (February 1997), 3. William M. Vollmer et al. *New England Journal of Medicine* 336 (1997), 1117-1124.

19 *Hypertension* 22:3 (September 1993), 371-379.

20 Jiang He et al. "Oats and Buckwheat Intakes and Cardiovascular Disease Risk Factors in an Ethnic Minority of China." *American Journal of Clinical Nutrition* 61 (1995), 366-372.

21 P. Pietinen et al. "Intake of Dietary Fiber and Risk of Coronary Heart Disease in a Cohort of Finnish

Men." *Circulation* 94:11 (December 1996), 2720-2727.

22 F. Skrabal, J. Aubock, and H. Hortnagl. "Low Sodium/High Potassium Diet for Prevention of Hypertension: Probable Mechanisms of Action." *The Lancet* 2:8252 (October 1981), 895-900. Paul K. Whelton et al. "Effects of Oral Potassium on Blood Pressure." *Journal of the American Medical Association* 277 (1997), 1624-1632.

23 B. Armstrong et al. "Urinary Sodium and Blood Pressure in Vegetarians." *American Journal of Clinical Nutrition* 32:12 (December 1979), 2472-2476. I.L. Rouse et al. "Vegetarian Diet and Blood Pressure." *The Lancet* 2:8352 (1983), 742-743.

24 H.J. Henry et al. "Increasing Calcium Intake Lowers Blood Pressure. The Literature Reviewed." *Journal of the American Dietetic Association* 85:2 (February 1985), 182-185. J.M. Belizam et al. "Reduction of Blood Pressure with Calcium Supplementation in Young Adults." *Journal of the American Medical Association* 249:9 (March 1983), 1161-1165.

25 D.A. McCarron, C.D. Morris, and C. Cole. "Dietary Calcium in Human Hypertension." *Science* 217:4556 (1982), 267-269.

26 L.E. Griffith et al. "The Influence of Dietary and Nondietary Calcium Supplementation on Blood Pressure: An Updated Meta-Analysis of Randomized Controlled Trials." *American Journal of Hypertension* 12:1 Part 1 (January 1999), 84-92.

27 T. Dyckner and P.O. Wester. "Effect of Magnesium on Blood Pressure." *British Medical Journal* 286:6381 (January 1983), 1847-1849.

28 H.F. Galley et al. "Regulation of Nitric Oxide Synthase Activity in Cultured Human Endothelial Cells: Effect of Antioxidants." *Free Radicals in Biology and Medicine* 21 (1996), 97-101.

29 H.F. Galley et al. "Combination Oral Antioxidant Supplementation Reduces Blood Pressure." *Clinical Science* 92 (1997), 361-365.

30 K. Namba et al. "Effect of Taurine Concentration on Platelet Aggregation in Gestosis Patients with Edema, Proteinuria, and Hypertension." *Acta Medica Okayama* 46:4 (August 1992), 241-247. A. Ceriello et al. "Anti-Oxidants Show an Anti-Hypertensive Effect in Diabetic and Hypertensive Subjects." *Clinical Science* 81:6 (December 1991), 739-42. S.R. Maxwell. "Can Anti-Oxidants Prevent Ischemic Heart Disease?" *Journal of Clinical Pharmacy and Therapeutics* 18:2 (April 1993), 85-95.

31 N.F. Gordon and C.B. Scott. "Exercise and Mild Essential Hypertension." *Primary Care Clinics in Office Practice* 18:3 (September 1991), 683-694.

32 Richard H. Grimm, Jr., M.D., Ph.D., et al. *Journal of the American Medical Association* 275:20 (May 22/29, 1996), 1549-1556.

33 H. Tanaka et al. "Swimming Training Lowers the Resting Blood Pressure in Individuals with Hypertension." *Journal of Hypertension* 15:6 (1997), 651-657.

34 I.B. Goldstein et al. "Home Relaxation Techniques for Essential Hypertension." *Psychosomatic Medicine* 46:5 (September-October 1984), 398-414. C. Brassard and R.T. Couture. "Biofeedback and Relaxation for Patients with Hypertension." *Canadian Nurse* 89:1 (January 1993), 49-52. H.M. Whyte. "NHMRC Workshop on Non-Pharmacological Methods of Lowering Blood Pressure." *Medical Journal of Australia* 2:1 Suppl (July 1983), S13-S16. E.B. Blanchard et al. "Preliminary Results from a Controlled Evaluation of Thermal Biofeedback as a Treatment for Essential Hyper-

tension." *Biofeedback and Self Regulation* 9:4 (December 1984), 471-495. R. Murugesan, N. Govindarajulu, and T.K. Bera. "Effect of Selected Yogic Practices on the Management of Hypertension." *Indian J Physiol Pharmacol* 44:2 (April 2000), 207-210. M. Mayer. "Qigong and Hypertension: A Critique of Research." *Journal of Alternative and Complementary Medicine* 5:4 (August 1999), 371-382.

35 The 1988 Report of the Joint National Committee of the American Medical Association. "The Joint National Committee on Detection, Evaluation, and Treatment of High Blood Pressure." *Archives of Internal Medicine* 148 (1988), 1023-1038.

36 C.B. Yucha et al. "The Effect of Biofeedback in Hypertension." *Appl Nurs Res* 14:1 (February 2001), 29-35.

37 A. McGrady, P.A. Nadsady, and C. Schumann-Brzezinski. "Sustained Effects of Biofeedback-Assisted Relaxation Therapy in Essential Hypertension." *Biofeedback and Self-Regulation* 16:4 (December 1991), 399-411.

38 T.A. Aivazyan et al. "Efficacy of Relaxation Techniques in Hypertensive Patients." *Health Psychology* 7:Suppl (1988), 193-200.

39 Lee-Lan Yen. "Comparison of Relaxation Techniques, Routine Blood Pressure Measurements, and Self-Learning Packages in Hypertension Control." *Preventive Medicine* 25:3 (May/June 1996), 339-345.

40 V. Petkov. "Plants with Hypotensive, Antiatheromatous and Coronary Dilating Action." *American Journal of Chinese Medicine* 7:3 (1979), 197-236.

41 ESCOP, European Scientific Cooperative for Phytotherapy. *Garlic* (Meppel, The Netherlands: European Scientific Cooperative for Phytotherapy, 1992).

42 Paola Ficarra and Rit Ficarra. "HPLC Analysis of Oleuropein and Some Flavonoids in Leaf and Bud of *Olea Europea L.*" *Il Farmaco* 46:6 (1991), 803-815.

43 C. Hobbs. "Hawthorn: A Literature Review." *HerbalGram* 21 (1990), 19-33.

44 *Townsend Letter for Doctors* (May 1994), 432-434. *Explore!* 4:5 (1993), 17-19. M. Mayell. "Maitake Extracts and Their Therapeutic Potential." *Alternative Medicine Review* 6:1 (February 2001), 48-60.

45 H. Jin et al. "Treatment of Hypertension by Ling zhi Combined with Hypotensor and Its Effects on Arterial, Arteriolar, and Capillary Pressure and Microcirculation." In: H. Nimmi et al., eds. *Microcirculatory Approach to Asian Traditional Medicine* (New York: Elsevier Science, 1996), 131-138.

46 S.G. Ivanov et al. "The Magnetotherapy of Hypertension Patients." *Terapevticheskii Arkhiv* 62:9 (1990), 71-74.

MEN'S HEALTH

1 Robert O. Ivker, Robert Anderson, and Larry Trivieri, Jr. *The Complete Self-Care Guide to Holistic Medicine* (New York: Tarcher/Putnam, 1999), 245-246.

2 J.I. Silverstein, G.H. Badlani, and A.D. Smith. "Management of Benign Prostatic Hypertrophy: Alternatives to Standard Therapy." *Clinical Geriatric Medicine* 6:1 (1990), 69-84.

3 Robert O. Ivker, Robert Anderson, and Larry Trivieri, Jr. *The Complete Self-Care Guide to Holistic Medicine* (New York: Tarcher/Putnam, 1999), 238.

4 E.W. Hook III, M.D., and K.K. Holmes, M.D. "Gonococcal Infections." *Annals of Internal Med-

icine* 102:2 (February 1985), 229-243. W.E. Stamm, M.D., et al. "Chlamydia trachamotis Urethral Infections in Men: Prevalence, Risk Factors, and Clinical Manifestations." *Annals of Internal Medicine* 100:1 (January 1984): 47-51.

5 J.E. Pizzorno and M.T. Murray. *A Textbook of Natural Medicine* (Seattle, WA: John Bastyr College Publications, 1989).

6 Ibid. J. Dyerberg et al. "Eicosapentaenoic Acid and Prevention of Thrombosis and Atherosclerosis." *The Lancet* 2:8081 (July 1978), 117-119.

7 American Cancer Society. *Cancer Facts and Figures 1993* (Atlanta, GA: ACS, 1994).

8 Ibid.

9 J. Blaivas, M.D. "Prostatism and Prostatic Cancer." (Virginia Geriatric Education Center, 1990).

10 D.R. Smith, M.D. *General Urology* (Los Altos, CA: Lange Medical Publications, 1984). W.B. Abrams and R. Berkow, eds. *Merck Manual of Geriatrics* (Rahway, NJ: Merck, Sharp and Dohme Research Labs, 1990). J. Blaivas, M.D. "Prostatism and Prostatic Cancer." (Virginia Geriatric Education Center, 1990).

11 "Vasectomy Linked to Tripled Risk of Prostate Cancer." *Medical World News* (September 25, 1989).

12 G. Mavligit, M.D., et al. "Chronic Immune Stimulation by Sperm Alloantibodies-Support for the Hypothesis That Spermatozoa Induce Immune Dysregulation in Homosexual Males." *Journal of the American Medical Association* 251:2 (January 1984), 237-241.

13 D.R. Smith, M.D. *General Urology* (Los Altos, CA: Lange Medical Publications, 1984). T. Kruzel. "What is the Prostate and Why is it Doing This to Me?" *Health Review Newsletter* (August 1991).

14 Ibid.

15 This report is based solely on product labeling as published by PDR®. Copyright ©1993 by Medical Economics Data, a division of Medical Economics Company, Inc. All rights reserved.

16 Robert O. Ivker, Robert Anderson, and Larry Trivieri, Jr. *The Complete Self-Care Guide to Holistic Medicine* (New York: Tarcher/Putnam, 1999), 243-244.

17 D.R. Smith, M.D. *General Urology* (Los Altos, CA: Lange Medical Publications, 1984).

18 J. Dyerberg et al. "Eicosapentaenoic Acid and Prevention of Thrombosis and Atherosclerosis." *The Lancet* 2:8081 (July 1978), 117-119.

19 A.E. Lewis. "Glandular Therapy: Historical Background and Emerging Scientific Status." *PHP Technical Information Series* (February 1990).

20 A. Morales, D.H. Surridge, and P. Marshall. "Yohimbine for Treatment of Impotence in Diabetes." *New England Journal of Medicine* 305:20 (November 1981), 1221. K. Reid et al. "Double-Blind Trial of Yohimbine in Treatment of Psychogenic Impotence." *The Lancet* 2:8556 (August 1987), 421-423. A. Morales et al. "Nonhormonal Pharmacological Treatment of Organic Impotence." *Journal of Urology* 128:1 (July 1981), 45-47.

21 D.J. Brown. "Literature Review-Ginkgo Biloba; Phytotherapy Review & Commentary." *Townsend Letter for Doctors* (December 1991).

22 H.W. Felter, M.D. *The Eclectic Materia Medica, Pharmacology and Therapeutics* (Portland, OR: Eclectic Medical Publications, 1983).

23 T.A. Stamey et al. "Prostate Specific Antigen as a Serum Marker for Adenocarcinoma of the Prostate." *New England Journal of Medicine* 317:15

(October 1987), 909-916. F. Ellingwood, M.D. *American Materia Medica, Therapeutics and Pharmacognosy* (Portland, OR: Eclectic Medical Publications, 1983). F. Brinker. *An Introduction to the Toxicology of Common Botanical Medicinal Substances* (Portland, OR: NCNM Publications, 1983). E. Funk, M.D. *Potter's Therapeutics Materia Medica and Pharmacy* (Philadelphia: P. Blankiston's Son, 1917). J.M. Scudder, M.D. *Specific Medication and Specific Medicines* (Cincinnati, OH: J.M. Scudder, 1880).

24 N. Farnsworth et al. "*Eleuthrococcus senticosus*: Current Status as an Adaptogen." *Economic and Medicinal Plant Research* 1 (1985), 156-215. I.I. Brekhman and I.V. Dardymov. "Pharmacological Investigation of Glycosides from Ginseng and *Eleuthrococcus*." *Lloydia* 32:1 (March 1969), 46-51.

25 M. Walker. "*Serenoa Repens* Extract (Saw Palmetto) Relief for Benign Prostatic Hypertrophy." *Townsend Letter for Doctors* (February/March 1991). M. Murray. "Liposterolic Extract of *Serenoa Repens* in the Treatment of Benign Prostatic Hyperplasia." *Phyto-Pharmica Review* 1:5 (August 1988).

26 J. Lange and M. Bordeaux. "Clinical Experimentation with V1326 in Prostatic Disorders." *Bordeaux Medical* 3:11 (November 1970), 2807-2808. G. Viollet. "Clinical Experimentation of a New Treatment for Prostatic Adenoma." *Vie Medicale* 23 (1970), 3457. T. Kruzel. "What is the Prostate and Why is It Doing This to Me?" *Health Review Newsletter* (August 1991).

27 H.W. Felter, M.D. *The Eclectic Materia Medica, Pharmacology and Therapeutics* (Portland, OR: Eclectic Medical Publications, 1983).

28 H.W. Felter, M.D. *The Eclectic Materia Medica, Pharmacology and Therapeutics* (Portland, OR: Eclectic Medical Publications, 1983). F. Ellingwood, M.D. *American Materia Medica, Therapeutics and Pharmacognosy* (Portland, OR: Eclectic Medical Publications, 1983). D.M.R. Culbreth, M.D. *A Manual of Materia Medica and Pharmacology* (Portland, OR: Eclectic Medical Publications, 1983). E. Funk, M.D. *Potter's Therapeutics Materia Medica and Pharmacy* (Philadelphia: P. Blankiston's Son, 1917). F. Brinker. *An Introduction to the Toxicology of Common Botanical Medicinal Substances* (Portland, OR: NCNM Publications, 1983).

29 H.W. Felter, M.D. *The Eclectic Materia Medica, Pharmacology and Therapeutics* (Portland, OR: Eclectic Medical Publications, 1983). F. Ellingwood, M.D. *American Materia Medica, Therapeutics and Pharmacognosy* (Portland, OR: Eclectic Medical Publications, 1983). D.M.R. Culbreth, M.D. *A Manual of Materia Medica and Pharmacology* (Portland, OR: Eclectic Medical Publications, 1983). E. Funk, M.D. *Potter's Therapeutics Materia Medica and Pharmacy* (Philadelphia: P. Blankiston's Son, 1917).

30 N. Farnsworth et al. "*Eleuthrococcus senticosus*: Current Status as an Adaptogen." *Economic and Medicinal Plant Research* 1 (1985), 156-215. I.I. Brekhman and I.V. Dardymov. "Pharmacological Investigation of Glycosides from Ginseng and *Eleuthrococcus*." *Lloydia* 32:1 (March 1969), 46-51.

31 E. Funk, M.D. *Potter's Therapeutics Materia Medica and Pharmacy* (Philadelphia: P. Blankiston's Son, 1917). F. Brinker. *An Introduction to the Toxicology of Common Botanical Medicinal Substances* (Portland, OR: NCNM Publications, 1983). T.A. Khwaja et al. "Recent Studies on the Anticancer Activities of Mistletoe (*Viscum album*) and its Alkaloids." *Oncology* 43:Suppl. 1 (1986), 42-50. N. Bloksma et al. "Stimulation of Humoral and Cellular Immunity by Viscum Preparations." *Planta Medica* 46:4 (December 1982), 221-227. F. Ellingwood, M.D. *American Materia Medica, Therapeutics and Pharmacognosy* (Portland, OR: Eclectic Medical Publications, 1983). J.M. Scudder, M.D. *Specific Medication and Specific Medicines* (Cincinnati, OH: The Scudder Brothers, 1903). H.W. Felter, M.D. *The Eclectic Materia Medica, Pharmacology and Therapeutics* (Portland, OR: Eclectic Medical Publications, 1983). J. Mose. "Effect of Echinacin on Phagocytosis and Natural Killer Cells." *Medizinische Welt* 34:51-52 (December 1983), 1463-1467. A. Wacker and W. Hilbig. "Virus Inhibition by *Echinacea purpurea*." *Planta Medica* 33 (1978), 89-102. W. Martin. "Treatment of Prostate and Breast Cancer." *Townsend Letter for Doctors* (May 1990). F. Brinker. *An Introduction to the Toxicology of Common Botanical Medicinal Substances* (Portland, OR: NCNM Publications, 1983).

32 N. Farnsworth et al. "*Eleuthrococcus senticosus*: Current Status as an Adaptogen." *Economic and Medicinal Plant Research* 1 (1985), 156-215.

33 S. Dharmananda. *Your Nature, Your Health: Chinese Herbs in Constitutional Therapy* (Portland, OR: Institute for Traditional Medicine and Preservation of Health Care, 1986).

34 W. Martin. "Treatment of Prostate and Breast Cancer." *Townsend Letter for Doctors* (May 1990). R. Trattler. *Better Health Through Natural Healing* (New York: McGraw-Hill, 1985). R. Schmid. *Traditional Foods are Your Best Medicines* (Stratford, CT: Ocean View Publications, 1987).

35 R. Schmid. *Traditional Foods Are Your Best Medicines* (Stratford, CT: Ocean View Publications, 1987).

MENTAL HEALTH

1 D.A. Regier et al. "The De Facto U.S. Mental and Addictive Disorders Service System." *Archives of General Psychiatry* 50 (February 1993), 85.

2 C.B. Clayman, ed. *The American Medical Association Encyclopedia of Medicine* (New York: Random House, 1989).

3 P.R. Breggin. *Toxic Psychiatry: Why Therapy, Empathy and Love Must Replace the Drugs, Electroshock, and Biochemical Therapies of the "New Psychiatry"* (New York: St. Martin's Press, 1991).

4 Robert S. Ivker, Robert A. Anderson, and Larry Trivieri, Jr. *The Complete Self-Care Guide to Holistic Medicine* (New York: Tarcher/Putnam, 1999).

5 J.M. Zito et al. "Trends in the Prescribing of Psychotropic Medications to Preschoolers." *Journal of the American Medical Association* 283:8 (February 23, 2000), 1025-1030.

6 Jean West. "Children's Drug is More Potent Than Cocaine." *The London Observer* (September 9, 2001).

7 Kelly Patricia O'Meara. "New Research Indicts Ritalin." InsightMag.com (September 8, 2001). Available on the Internet: www.insightmag.com/archive/200110015.shtml.

8 P.A. Ahmann et al. "Placebo-Controlled Evaluation of Ritalin Side Effects." *Pediatrics* 91:6 (June 1993), 1101-1106.

9 Ibid.

10 J. Roberts. "Behavioural Disorders are Overdiagnosed in U.S." *British Medical Journal* 312 (March 16, 1996), 657.

11 Kelly Patricia O'Meara. "New Research Indicts Ritalin." InsightMag.com (September 8, 2001). Available on the Internet: www.insightmag.com/archive/200110015.shtml.

12 Joseph Glenmullen. *Prozac Backlash* (New York: Simon & Schuster, 2000).

13 Ibid.

14 Gary Greenberg. "The Serotonin Surprise." *Discover* 22:7 (July 2001).

15 C.K. Varley and J. McClellan. "Case Study: Two Additional Sudden Deaths with Tricyclic Antidepressants." *Journal of the American Academy of Childhood and Adolescent Psychiatry* 36:3 (March 1997), 390-394.

16 S.A. McDermid et al. "Adolescents on Neuroleptic Medication: Is This Population at Risk for Tardive Dyskinesia?" *Canadian Journal of Psychiatry* 43:6 (August 1998), 629-631. M.A. Richardson et al. "Neuroleptic Use, Parkinsonian Symptoms, Tardive Dyskinesia, and Associated Risk Factors in Child and Adolescent Psychiatric Patients." *American Journal of Psychiatry* 148:10 (October 1991), 1322-1328.

17 C. Kappagoda et al. "Clonidine Overdose in Childhood: Implications of Increased Prescribing." *J Paediatr Child Health* 34:6 (December 1998), 508-512. J.F. Wiley, 2nd, et al. "Clonidine Poisoning in Young Children." *Journal of Pediatrics* 116:4 (April 1990), 654-658. J.B. Prince et al. "Clonidine for Sleep Disturbances with Attention-Deficit Hyperactivity Disorder: A Systematic Chart Review of 62 Cases." *Journal of the American Academy of Childhood and Adolescent Psychiatry* 35:5 (May 1996), 599-605.

18 This report is based solely on product labeling as published by PDR®. Copyright ©1993 by Medical Economics Data, a division of Medical Economics Company, Inc. All rights reserved.

19 J.E. Pizzorno and M.T. Murray. *A Textbook of Natural Medicine* (Seattle, WA: John Bastyr College Publications, 1989).

20 B. Lozoff, E. Jimenez, and A. Wolf. "Long-Term Developmental Outcome of Infants with Iron Deficiency." *New England Journal of Medicine* 325 (September 1991), 687-694.

21 G. Schrauzer and K. Shrestha. "Lithium in Drinking Water and Incidences in Crimes, Suicides and Arrests Related to Drug Addictions." *Biological Trace Element Research* 25:2 (May 1990), 105-113. E. Wickham and J. Reed. "Lithium for the Control of Aggressive and Self-Mutilating Behavior." *International Clinical Psycho-Pharmacology* 2:3 (July 1987), 181-190.

22 S. Schoenthaler, W. Doraz, and J. Wakefield, Jr. "The Impact of a Low Food Additive and Sucrose Diet on Academic Performance in 803 New York City Public Schools." *International Journal of Biosocial Research* 8:2 (1986), 185-195.

23 C. Pfeiffer. *Mental and Elemental Nutrients: A Physician's Guide to Nutrition and Health Care* (New Canaan, CT: Keats Publishing, 1975).

24 B. Feingold. *Why Your Child is Hyperactive* (New York: Random House, 1975).

25 J.E. Pizzorno and M.T. Murray. *A Textbook of Natural Medicine* (Seattle, WA: John Bastyr College Publications, 1989).

26 K.S. Rowe. "Synthetic Food Colourings and 'Hyperactivity': A Double-Blind Crossover Study." *Austr Paediatr J* 24:2. (April 1988), 143-147.

27 C.M. Carter et al. "Effects of a Few Food Diet in Attention Deficit Disorder." *Arch Dis Child* 69:5 (November 1993), 564-568.

28 J. Breakey. "The Role of Diet and Behaviour in Childhood." *J Paediatr Child Health* 33:3 (June 1997), 190-194.

29 J. Egger et al. "Controlled Trial of Oligoantigenic Treatment in the Hyperkinetic Syndrome." *The Lancet* 1:8428 (March 1985), 540-545. J. O'Shea

and S. Porter. "Double-Blind Study of Children with Hyperkinetic Syndrome Treated with Multi-Allergen Extract Sublingually." *Journal of Learning Disabilities* 14:1 (April 1981), 189-191.

30 F. Perry et al. "Environmental Power-Frequency Magnetic Fields and Suicide." *Health Physics* 41:2 (August 1981), 267-277.

31 F. Perry and L. Pearl. "Health Effects of ELF Fields and Illness in Multistorey Blocks." *Public Health* 102:1 (January 1988), 11-18.

32 D.I. Dowson and G.T. Lewith. "Overhead High Voltage Cables and Recurrent Headache and Depressions." *The Practitioner* 232:1447 (April 1988), 435-436.

33 J.E. Pizzorno and M.T. Murray. *A Textbook of Natural Medicine* (Seattle, WA: John Bastyr College Publications, 1989).

34 W. Walsh. "Biochemical Treatment of Behavior, Learning & Mental Disorders." *Townsend Letter for Doctors* (August/September 1992), 299.

35 J.E. Pizzorno and M.T. Murray. *A Textbook of Natural Medicine* (Seattle, WA: John Bastyr College Publications, 1989).

36 J. Ott. "Color and Light: Their Effects on Plants, Animals and People." *International Journal of Biosocial Research* 7-10 (1985-1988), 1-131.

37 J. Ott. *Health and Light* (Old Greenwich, CT: Devin-Adair, 1973).

38 P.A. Roos. "Light and Electromagnetic Waves: The Health Implications." *Journal of the Bio-Electro-Magnetics Institute* 3:2 (Summer 1991), 7-12.

39 *Harvard Mental Health Letter* 8:7 (January 1992).

40 Ibid.

41 R.S. Lazarus and S. Folkman. *Stress, Appraisal, and Coping* (New York: Springer Publishing, 1984).

42 P.G. Nixon. "Human Functions and the Heart." In: D. Seedhouse and A. Cribb, eds. *Changing Ideas in Health Care* (New York: John Wiley & Sons, 1989).

43 J. Achterberg. "Ritual: The Foundation for Transpersonal Medicine." *ReVision* 14:3 (1992), 158-164.

44 C. Simonton and S. Matthews. *Getting Well Again* (Los Angeles: Jeremy P. Tarcher, 1978).

45 *Harvard Mental Health Letter* 8:8 (February 1992).

46 D. Spiegel et al. "Effect of Psychosocial Treatment on Survival of Patients with Metastatic Breast Cancer." *The Lancet* 2:8668 (October 1989), 888-891.

47 L.F. Berkman and S.L. Syme. "Social Networks, Host Resistance, and Mortality: A Nine-Year Follow-Up Study of Alameda County Residents." *American Journal of Epidemiology* 109:2 (February 1979), 186-204.

48 S. Cohen, A. Tyrrell, and A. Smith. "Psychological Stress and Susceptibility to the Common Cold." *New England Journal of Medicine* 325:9 (August 1991), 606-612.

49 *Harvard Mental Health Letter* 8:7 (January 1992).

50 D. Healy et al. "The Thymus-Adrenal Connection: Thymosin Has Corticotropin-Releasing Activity in Primates." *Science* 222:4630 (1983), 1353-1355.

51 B. Moyers. *Healing and the Mind* (New York: Doubleday, 1993).

52 Ibid.

53 M. Henderson. "Virus in DNA 'is Cause of Mental Illness'." *The London Times* (April 10, 2001). Available on the Internet: www.thetimes.co.uk/article/o,,2-112215,00.html.

54 V. Muldner and M. Zoller. "Antidepressive Effect of a Hypericum Extract Standardized to an Active Hypericine Complex: Biochemical and Clinical Studies." *Arzneimittel Forschung* 34:8 (1984), 918-920.

55 A. Hoffer, M.D., H. Osmond, and J. Smythies. "Schizophrenia: A New Approach II: Results of a Year's Research." *Journal of Mental Science* 100:418 (January 1954), 29-45.

56 A. Hoffer. "Chronic Schizophrenic Patient Treated Ten Years or More." *Journal of Orthomolecular Medicine* 8 (1993).

57 E. Johnstone et al. "Disabilities and Circumstance of Schizophrenic Patients—A Follow-Up Study." *The British Journal of Psychiatry* 159 Suppl 13 (1991), 3-46.

58 M.R. Werbach, M.D. *Nutritional Influences on Mental Illness* (Tarzana, CA: Third Line Press, 1991).

59 J.D. Beasley. *The Betrayal of Health: The Impact of Nutrition, Environment, and Lifestyle on Illness in America* (New York: Times Books, 1991).

60 W. Walsh. "Biochemical Treatment of Behavior, Learning and Mental Disorders." *Townsend Letter for Doctors* (August/September 1992), 299.

61 Ibid.

62 A. Knivsberg et al. "Dietary Intervention in Autistic Syndromes." *Brain Dysfunction* 3 (November/December 1990), 315-327.

63 L. Braud, M. Lupin, and W. Braud. "The Use of Electromyographic Biofeedback in the Control of Hyperactivity." *Journal of Learning Disabilities* 8:7 (1975). M. Lupin et al. "Children, Parents, and Relaxation Tapes." *Academic Therapy* 12:1 (1976).

64 L. Chaitow. *The Stress Protection Plan* (San Francisco: Harper, 1992).

65 R. Kellner et al. "Changes in Chronic Nightmares After One Session of Desensitization or Rehearsal Instructions." *American Journal of Psychiatry* 149:5 (May 1992), 659-663.

66 A. Berquier and R. Ashton. "Characteristics of the Frequent Nightmare Sufferer." *Journal of Abnormal Psychology* 101:2 (May 1992), 246-250.

67 Larry Trivieri. *The American Medical Association Guide to Holistic Health* (New York: John Wiley & Sons, 2001), 132-133.

68 Francine Shapiro and Margot Silk Forrest. *EMDR: The Breakthrough "Eye Movement" Therapy for Overcoming Anxiety, Stress, and Trauma* (New York: Basic Books, 1997), 5.

69 Fred P. Gallo and Harry Vincenzi. *Energy Tapping* (Oakland, CA: New Harbinger Publications, 2000), 9-14.

70 Mechthild Scheffer. *Bach Flower Therapy: Theory and Practice* (Rochester, VT: Healing Arts Press, 1988), 214.

71 W. Philpott and S. Taplin. *Biomagnetic Handbook* (Choctaw, OK: Enviro-Tech Products, 1990).

MULTIPLE SCLEROSIS

1 B.W. Agranoff and D. Goldberg. "Diet and the Geographical Distribution of Multiple Sclerosis." *The Lancet* 2:7888 (November 1974), 1061-1066.

2 E. Gusev et al. "Environmental Risk Factors in MS: A Case-Control Study in Moscow." *Acta Neurol Scand* 94:6 (December 1996), 386-394.

3 R.L. Swank. "Multiple Sclerosis: Chronicle of Its Incidence with Dietary Fat." *American Journal of Science* 220:2 (October 1950), 421-430. H.M. Sinclair. "Deficiency of Essential Fatty Acids and Atherosclerosis." *The Lancet* 270:1 (1956), 381-383. M. Alter, M. Yamoor, and M. Harshe. "Multiple Sclerosis and Nutrition." *Archives of Neurology* 31:4 (October 1974), 267-272. B.W. Agranoff and D.

Goldberg. "Diet and the Geographical Distribution of Multiple Sclerosis." *The Lancet* 2:7888 (November 1974), 1061-1066. M.A. Crawford, P. Budowski, and A.G. Hassam. "Dietary Management in Multiple Sclerosis." *Proceedings of the Nutrition Society* 38:3 (December 1979), 373-379.

4 A. Tokatli, T. Coskun, and I. Ozalp. "Biotinidase Deficiency with Neurological Features Resembling Multiple Sclerosis." *J Inherit Metab Dis* 20:5 (September 1997), 707-708.

5 D. Gay, G. Dick, and G. Upton. "Multiple Sclerosis Associated with Sinusitis: Case-Controlled Study in General Practice." *The Lancet* 1:8940 (April 1986), 815-819.

6 W.G. Crook, M.D. *The Yeast Connection* (Jackson, TN: Professional Books, 1984).

7 J. Bland, Ph.D. *The 20-Day Rejuvenation Diet Program* (New Canaan, CT: Keats Publishing, 1997), 127-128.

8 George Gillson, M.D., Ph.D., et al. "Transdermal Histamine in Multiple Sclerosis: Part One-Clinical Experience." *Alternative Medicine Review* 4:6 (1999), 424-428. George Gillson, M.D., Ph.D., et al. "Transdermal Histamine in Multiple Sclerosis: Part Two-A Proposed Theoretical Basis for Its Use." *Alternative Medicine Review* 5:3 (2000), 224-248.

9 International Labour Office. *Encyclopedia of Occupational Health and Safety* (New York: McGraw-Hill, 1972).

10 M.J. Vimy, Y. Takahashi, and F.L. Lorscheider. "Maternal-Fetal Distribution of Mercury Released from Dental Amalgam Fillings." *American Physiological Society* 258 (1990), R939-R945. F.L. Lorscheider et al. "Mercury from Amalgam Tooth Fillings: Its Tissue Distribution and Effects on Cell Functions." *The Toxicologist* 12 (1992), 1.

11 M.J. Vimy et al. "Glomerular Filtration Impairment by Mercury from Dental 'Silver' Fillings in Sheep." *The Physiologist* 33 (August 1990), A94. N.D. Boyd et al. "Mercury from Dental 'Silver' Tooth Fillings Impairs Sheep Kidney Function." *American Physiological Society* 261 (1991), R1010-R1014. B. Ahlrot-Westerlund, M.D. "Mercury in Cerebrospinal Fluid in Multiple Sclerosis." *Sweden Journal of Biological Medicine* 1 (March 1989), 6.

12 M. Kato. "Biological Influences of Electromagnetic Fields." *Hokkaido Igaku Zasshi* 70:4 (July 1995), 551-560.

13 L.L. Williams, D.M. Doody, and L.A. Horrocks. "Serum Fatty Acid Proportions are Altered During the Year Following Acute Epstein-Barr Virus Infection." *Lipids* 23:10 (October 1988), 981-988.

14 Lida H. Mattman, Ph.D. *Cell Wall Deficient Forms-Stealth Pathogens* (Boca Raton, FL: CRC Press, 1993).

15 J. Rose et al. "Genetic Susceptibility in Familial Multiple Sclerosis Not Linked to the Myelin Basic Protein Gene." *The Lancet* 341:8854 (May 1993), 1179-1181.

16 R.L. Swank and B.B. Dugan. "Effect of Low Saturated Fat Diet in Early and Late Cases of Multiple Sclerosis." *The Lancet* 336:8706 (July 1990), 37-39.

17 M. Mayer. "Essential Fatty Acids and Related Molecular and Cellular Mechanisms in Multiple Sclerosis: New Looks at Old Concepts." *Folia Biologica (Praha)* 45 (1999), 133-141.

18 J. Nieves, Ph.D., et al. "High Prevalence of Vitamin D Deficiency and Reduced Bone Mass in Multiple Sclerosis." *Neurology* 44 (September 1994), 1687.

1154

19 E.H. Reynolds, J.C. Linnell, and J.E. Faludy. "Multiple Sclerosis Associated with Vitamin B12 Deficiency." *Archives of Neurology* 48:8 (August 1991), 808-811.

20 T.Q. Nijist et al. "Vitamin B12 and Folate Concentrations in Serum and Cerebrospinal Fluid of Neurological Patients with Special Reference to Multiple Sclerosis and Dementia." *Journal of Neurology, Neurosurgery, and Psychiatry* 53:11 (November 1990), 951-954.

21 Masayuki Yasui et al. "Magnesium-Related Neurological Disorders." In: *Mineral and Metal Neurotoxicology* (Boca Raton, FL: CRC Press, 1997), 219-226.

22 D.F.L. Money. "Vitamin E and Selenium Deficiencies and Their Possible Aetological Role in Sudden Infant Death Syndrome." *New Zealand Medical Journal* 71 (1970), 32-34.

23 O. Andersen and J.B. Nielsen. "Effects of Simultaneous Low-Level Dietary Supplementation with Inorganic and Organic Selenium on Whole-Body, Blood, and Organ Levels of Toxic Metals in Mice." *Environmental Health Perspectives* 102:Suppl 3 (1994), 321-324.

24 M. Mutanen. "Bioavailability of Selenium." *Annals of Clinical Research* 18 (1986), 48-54.

25 K. Folkers and A. Wolaniuk. "Research on Coenzyme Q10 in Clinical Medicine and in Immunomodulation." *Drugs Exp Clin Res* 11:8 (1985), 539-545.

26 G. Ali Qureshi and Shahid M. Baig. "Role of Neurotransmitter Amino Acids in Multiple Sclerosis in Exacerbation, Remission and Chronic Progressive Course." *Biogenic Amines* 10:1 (1993), 39-48.

27 J. Clausen. "Mercury and Multiple Sclerosis." *Acta Neurol Scand* 87 (1993), 461-464. R. Siblerud. "A Comparison of Mental Health of Multiple Sclerosis Patients with Silver/Mercury Dental Fillings and Those with Fillings Removed." *Psychol Rep* 70 (1992), 1139-1151.

28 S.D. Somerfield et al. "Bee Venom Melittin Blocks Neutrophil O2-Production." *Inflammation* 10:2 (June 1986), 175-182.

29 C.J. Webster et al. "The Chief Scientist Reports...Hyperbaric Oxygen for Multiple Sclerosis." *Health Bulletin* 47:6 (November 1989), 320-331.

30 M.P. Barnes et al. "Hyperbaric Oxygen and Multiple Sclerosis: Short-Term Results of a Placebo-Controlled Double-Blind Trial." *The Lancet* 1:8424 (February 1985), 287-300. C.M. Wiles et al. "Hyperbaric Oxygen in Multiple Sclerosis: A Double-Blind Trial." *British Medical Journal* 292:6517 (February 1986), 367-371.

31 "Reversal of Alexia in Multiple Sclerosis by Weak Electromagnetic Fields." *International Journal of Neuroscience* 83 (1995), 69-79.

32 "Resolution of Partial Cataplexy in Multiple Sclerosis by Treatment with Weak Electromagnetic Fields." *International Journal of Neuroscience* 84 (1996), 157-164.

33 T.L. Richards et al. "Double-Blind Study of Pulsing Magnetic Effects on Multiple Sclerosis." *Journal of Alternative and Complementary Medicine* 3:1 (Spring 1997), 21-29. R. Sandyk. "Further Observations on the Effects of External Pico-Tesla Range Magnetic Fields on Visual Memory and Visuospatial Functions in Multiple Sclerosis." *International Journal of Neuroscience* 77:3-4 (August 1994), 203-227.

34 B.L. Maguire. "The Effects of Imagery on Attitudes and Moods in Multiple Sclerosis Patients." *Alternative Therapies in Health and Medicine* 2:5 (September 1996), 75-79.

35 H. Sutcher. "Hypnosis as Adjunctive Therapy for Multiple Sclerosis: A Progress Report." *Am J Clin Hypn* 39:4 (April 1997), 283-290.

36 C. Husted et al. "Improving Quality of Life for People with Chronic Conditions: The Example of T'ai Chi and Multiple Sclerosis." *Alternative Therapies in Health and Medicine* 5:5 (September 1999), 70-74.

37 Murat Emre, M.D., and Katherine De Decker. "Effects of Cigarette Smoking on Motor Functions in Patients with Multiple Sclerosis." *Archives of Neurology* 49 (December 1992), 1243-1247.

38 Jack H. Petajan, M.D., Ph.D., et al. "Impact of Aerobic Training on Fitness and Quality of Life in Multiple Sclerosis." *Annals of Neurology* 39:4 (April 1996), 432-441.

OBESITY AND WEIGHT LOSS

1 *Patient Care* (November 30, 2000).

2 Jeffrey Norris. "Weighing In On Obesity." *UCSF Magazine* (September 2000).

3 T.B. Van Itallie. "Health Implications of Overweight and Obesity in the United States." *Annals of Internal Medicine* 103:6 Part 2 (1985), 983-988.

4 K.M. Rexrode et al. "A Prospective Study of Body Mass Index, Weight Change, and Risk of Stroke in Women." *Journal of the American Medical Association* 277:19 (1997), 1539-1545.

5 J.E. Manson et al. "Body Weight and Mortality Among Women." *New England Journal of Medicine* 333:11 (1995), 677-685.

6 L. Garfinkel. "Overweight and Cancer." *Annals of Internal Medicine* 103:6 Part 2 (1985), 1034-1036. F.X. Pi-Sunyer. "Health Implications of Obesity." *American Journal of Clinical Nutrition* 53:6 Suppl (1991), 1595S-1603S.

7 *Patient Care* (November 30, 2000).

8 Editorial Staff. "Body Weight, Health and Longevity: Conclusions and Recommendations of the Workshop." *Nutrition Reviews* 43:2 (February 1985), 61-63. D. Ingram et al. "Obesity and Breast Disease: The Role of the Female Sex Hormones." *Cancer* 64:5 (September 1989). 1049-1053.

9 JoAnne E. Manson et al. "Body Weight and Mortality Among Women." *New England Journal of Medicine* 333:11 (1995), 677-685.

10 Jeffrey Norris. "Weighing In On Obesity." *UCSF Magazine* (September 2000).

11 Philip Elmer-DeWitt. "Fat Times." *Time* 145:3 (January 16, 1995).

12 Carol J.G. Ward. "Weighty Resolution: Be Wary of Fad Dieting." *The Arizona Republic* (January 4, 1999), D3.

13 "America's Weight Problem Continues." Calorie Control Council press release (May 11, 1998). For more information, contact the Calorie Control Council at (404) 252-3663.

14 Lisa Grunwald. "Discovery: Do I Look Fat to You? 28 Questions (and All the Answers) About Our National Obsession." *Life* (February 1, 1995), 58.

15 Gene-Jack Wang et al. "Brain Dopamine and Obesity." *The Lancet* 357:9253 (February 3, 2001), 354.

16 P.M. Warwick et al. Recent Advances in Obesity Research II: Proceedings of the International Conference on Obesity (London: Newman, 1978).

17 Stephen Langer, M.D., and James F. Scheer. *Solved: The Riddle of Illness* (New Canaan, CT: Keats Publishing, 1995), 185.

18 Ibid., 186-189.

19 Ibid., 188-189.

20 Daniel B. Mowrey, Ph.D. *Fat Management: The Thermogenic Factor* (Lehi, UT: Victory Publications, 1994), 173.

21 Stephen Langer, M.D., with James F. Scheer. *Solved: The Riddle of Weight Loss* (Rochester, VT: Healing Arts Press, 1989), 143.

22 E.P. Heleniak and B. Aston. "Prostaglandins, Brown Fat and Weight Loss." *Medical Hypotheses* 28:1 (January 1989), 13-33.

23 Ann Louise Gittleman, M.S. *Beyond Pritikin* (New York: Bantam, 1996), 30.

24 Jack Tips, N.D., Ph.D. *Your Liver...Your Lifeline* (Ogden, UT: Apple-A-Day Press, 1995), 90.

25 Bernard Jensen, D.C., Ph.D., and Sylvia Bell. *Tissue Cleansing Through Bowel Management* (Escondido, CA: Bernard Jensen International, 1981), 23.

26 Editorial Staff. "Alterations in Metabolic Rate after Weight Loss in Obese Humans." *Nutrition Reviews* 43:2 (February 1985), 41-42.

27 D. Porte, Jr., and S.C. Woods. "Regulation of Food Intake and Body Weight by Insulin." *Diabetologia* 20:Suppl (March 1981), 274-280.

28 Lisa Grunwald. "Discovery: Do I Look Fat to You? 28 Questions (and All the Answers) About Our National Obsession." *Life* (February 1, 1995), 58.

29 Ibid.

30 JoAnne E. Manson et al. "Body Weight and Mortality Among Women." *New England Journal of Medicine* 333:11 (1995), 677-685.

31 Editorial Staff. "Alterations in Metabolic Rate after Weight Loss in Obese Humans." *Nutrition Reviews* 43:2 (February 1985), 41-42.

32 "Controlling Weight No Longer Considered Dieting." Calorie Control Council press release (May 11, 1998). For more information, contact the Calorie Control Council at (404) 252-3663.

33 "Rating the Diets." *Consumer Reports* (June 1993), 353-357.

34 National Institute of Diabetes and Digestive and Kidney Diseases. *Understanding Adult Obesity* NIH Publication No. 94-3680 (Washington, DC: National Institutes of Health, 1998).

35 Susan McQuillan, M.S., R.D., with Edward Saltzman, M.D. *Complete Idiot's Guide to Losing Weight* (New York: Alpha Books, 1998), 29.

36 Elizabeth Somer, M.A., R.D. *Food and Mood* (New York: Henry Holt, 1995), 260.

37 Hara Estroff Marano. "Chemistry & Craving." *Psychology Today* (January/February 1993), 74.

38 Kathleen A. Pichola, Ph.D. "Preventing Eating Disorders: Promoting Healthy Body Image." Unpublished seminar materials. For more information, contact: Kathleen A. Pichola, Ph.D., 12429 Cedar Road, Suite 18, Cleveland Heights, OH 44106.

39 "Increasing Prevalence of Overweight Among U.S. Adults: The National Health and Nutrition Examination Surveys, 1960 to 1991." *Journal of the American Medical Association* 272 (1994), 205-207.

40 Daniel B. Mowrey, Ph.D. *Fat Management: The Thermogenic Factor* (Lehi, UT: Victory Publications, 1994), 40-41.

41 H. Trowell, D. Burkitt, and K. Heaton. *Dietary Fibre, Fibre-Depleted Foods and Disease* (New York: Academic Press, 1985).

42 M.H. Davidson et al. "The Hypo-Cholesterolemic Effects of Beta-Glucan in Oatmeal and

Oat Bran: A Dose-Controlled Study." *Journal of the American Medical Association* 265:14 (April 1991), 1833-1839. J.W. Anderson and C.A. Bryant. "Dietary Fiber: Diabetes and Obesity." *American Journal of Gastroenterology* 81:10 (October 1986), 898-906.

43 A. Kendall et al. "Weight Loss on a Low-Fat Diet: Consequence of the Imprecision of the Control of Food Intake in Humans." *American Journal of Clinical Nutrition* 53:5 (May 1991), 1124-1129.

44 Y. Schutz, J.P. Flatt, and E. Jequier. "Failure of Dietary Fat to Promote Fat Oxidation: A Factor Favoring the Development of Obesity." *American Journal of Clinical Nutrition* 50:2 (August 1989), 307-314.

45 J.P. Flatt. "Body Weight, Fat Storage, and Alcohol Metabolism." *Nutrition Reviews* 50:9 (September 1992), 267-270.

46 J.P. Flatt. "Body Weight, Fat Storage, and Alcohol Metabolism." *Nutrition Reviews* 50:9 (September 1992), 267-270. P.M. Suter, Y. Schutz, and E. Jequier. "The Effect of Ethanol on Fat Storage in Healthy Subjects." *New England Journal of Medicine* 326:15 (April 1992), 983-987.

47 Ralph Golan, M.D. *Optimal Wellness* (New York: Ballantine, 1995), 400.

48 Stephen E. Langer, .M.D., and James F. Scheer. *Solved: The Riddle of Illness* (New Canaan, CT: Keats Publishing, 1995), 31

49 M.R. Werbach, M.D. *Nutritional Influences on Illness* (Tarzana, CA: Third Line Press, 1993).

50 D.S. Gridley et al. "*In Vivo* and *In Vitro* Stimulation of Cell-mediated Immunity by Vitamin B₆." *Nutrition Research* 8:2 (1988), 201-207.

51 B.W. Morris et al. "The Trace Element Chromium—a Role in Glucose Homeostasis." *American Journal of Clinical Nutrition* 55:5 (May 1992), 989-991.

52 Mark Mayell. *Off-the-Shelf Natural Health* (New York: Bantam, 1995), 369.

53 Ralph Golan, M.D. *Optimal Wellness* (New York: Ballantine, 1995), 189-191. Kathleen DesMaisons, Ph.D. *Potatoes Not Prozac* (New York: Simon & Schuster, 1998), 95-136.

54 Richard N. Podell, M.D., F.A.C.P., and William Proctor. *The G-Index Diet* (New York: Warner, 1993).

55 Ralph Golan, M.D. *Optimal Wellness* (New York: Ballantine, 1995), 191-192.

56 Reader's Digest. *Healing Power of Vitamins, Minerals, and Herbs* (Pleasantville, NY: Reader's Digest Association, 1999), 369.

57 Michael Tierra, L.Ac., O.M.D. *The Way of Herbs* (New York: Pocket Books, 1998), 143-144. Maggie Greenwood-Robinson, Ph.D. *Natural Weight Loss Miracles* (New York: Perigee/Berkley Publishing Group, 199), 142-143.

58 Michael Tierra, L.Ac., O.M.D. *The Way of Herbs* (New York: Pocket Books, 1998), 196-197.

59 Lester A. Mitscher, Ph.D., and Victoria Dolby. *The Green Tea Book: China's Fountain of Youth* (Garden City Park, NY: Avery Publishing Group, 1998), 120-121.

60 D. van Dale and W.H. Saris. "Repetitive Weight Loss and Weight Regain: Effects on Weight Reduction, Resting Metabolic Rate, and Lipolytic Activity Before and After Exercise and/or Diet Treatment." *American Journal of Clinical Nutrition* 49:3 (March 1989), 409-416.

61 Ann Louise Gittleman, M.S. *Beyond Pritikin* (New York: Bantam, 1996), 30.

62 Maggie Greenwood-Robinson, Ph.D. *Natural Weight Loss Miracles* (New York: Perigee/Berkley Publishing, 1999), 89-90.

63 Robert Crayhon, M.S. *The Carnitine Miracle* (New York: M. Evans, 1998), 74, 213.

64 Stephen Fulder, Ph.D. *The Ginseng Book: Nature's Ancient Healer* (Garden City Park, NY: Avery, 1996), 65.

65 A.G. Dulloo and D.S. Miller. "The Thermogenic Properties of Ephedrine/Methylxanthine Mixtures: Animal Studies." *American Journal of Clinical Nutrition* 43:3 (March 1986), 388-394. A. Astrup et al. "The Effect of Chronic Ephedrine Treatment on Substrate Utilization, the Sympathoadrenal Activity and Energy Expenditure During Glucose-Induced Thermogenesis in Man." *Metabolism: Clinical and Experimental* 35:3 (March 1986), 260-265.

66 A.G. Dulloo and D.S. Miller. "The Thermogenic Properties of Ephedrine/Methylxanthine Mixtures: Animal Studies." *American Journal of Clinical Nutrition* 43:3 (March 1986), 388-394. A.G. Dulloo and D.S. Miller. "Aspirin as a Promoter of Ephedrine-Induced Thermogenesis: Potential Use in the Treatment of Obesity." *American Journal of Clinical Nutrition* 45:3 (March 1987), 564-569.

OSTEOPOROSIS

1 National Institute of Arthritis and Musculoskeletal and Skin Diseases. "Osteoporosis: Progress and Promise." Available on the Internet: www.nih.gov/niams/healthinfo/opbkgr.htm.

2 L.G. Tolstoi and R.M. Levin. "Osteoporosis: The Treatment Controversy." *Nutrition Today* (July/August 1992), 6-12.

3 M.E. Nelson et al. "A 1-Year Walking Program and Increased Dietary Calcium in the Postmenopausal Woman: Effects on Bone." *American Journal of Clinical Nutrition* 53:5 (May 1991), 1304-1311

4 U.S. Department of Health and Human Services, Public Health Service, National Institutes of Health. "Medicine for the Layman: Osteoporosis."

5 Ruth S. Jacobowitz. "Making Noise About the Silent Disease: Osteoporosis." *éternelle* (Summer 1995), 18.

6 Susan E. Brown, Ph.D. *Better Bones, Better Body* (New Canaan, CT: Keats Publishing, 1996), 42.

7 Ibid., 5, 32.

8 Ibid., 141.

9 Susan E. Brown, Ph.D. *Better Bones, Better Body* (New Canaan, CT: Keats Publishing, 1996), 198-199. Susan Lark, M.D. *The Menopause Self-Help Book* (Berkeley, CA: Celestial Arts, 1992), 11. Linda Ojeda, Ph.D. *Menopause Without Medicine* (Alameda, CA: Hunter House, 1995) 95-100. Eileen Hoffman, M.D. *Our Health, Our Lives* (New York: Pocket Books, 1995), 152. *The PDR Family Guide to Women's Health and Prescription Drugs* (Montvale, NJ: Medical Economics, 1994), 371-375.

10 C. Coats, M.D. "Negative Effects of a High-Protein Diet." *Family Practice Recertification* 12:12 (December 1990), 80-94.

11 A.G. Marsh et al. "Vegetarian Lifestyle and Bone Mineral Density." *American Journal of Clinical Nutrition* 48:Suppl. 3 (September 1988), 837-841.

12 S.M. Weed. *Menopausal Years* (New York: Ash Tree Publishing, 1992), 22.

13 J.A. Thom et al. "The Influence of Refined Carbohydrate on Urinary Calcium Excretion." *British Journal of Urology* 50:7 (December 1987), 459-464.

14 R.P. Heaney. "Calcium Bioavailability." *Boletin-Asociacion Medica del Puerto Rico* 79:1 (January 1987), 27-29. R.P. Heaney and R.R. Recker. "Effects of Nitrogen, Phosphorus and Caffeine on Calcium Balance in Women." *Journal of Laboratory and Clinical Medicine* 99:1 (January 1982), 46-55.

15 D.P. Kiel et al. "Caffeine and the Risks of Hip Fracture: the Framingham Study." *American Journal of Epidemiology* 132:4 (October 1990), 675- 684.

16 R.F. Klein. "Alcohol-Induced Bone Disease: Impact of Ethanol on Osteoblast Proliferation." *Alcoholism, Clinical and Experimental Research* 21:3 (May 1997), 392-399.

17 Alan Gaby, M.D. *Preventing and Reversing Osteoporosis* (Rocklin, CA: Prima Publishing, 1994), 18.

18 Susan E. Brown, Ph.D. *Better Bones, Better Body* (New Canaan, CT: Keats Publishing, 1996), 65-67.

19 Ibid.

20 J.C. Prior et al. "Spinal Bone Loss and Ovulatory Disturbances." *International Journal of Gynecology and Obstetrics* 34 (1990), 253-256.

21 C. Cooper et al. "Water Fluoridation and Hip Fracture." *Journal of the American Medical Association* 19:32 (July 1991), 513-514. M.F. Sowers et al. "A Prospective Study of Bone Mineral Content and Fracture in Communities with Differential Fluoride Exposure." *American Journal of Epidemiology* 133:7 (April 1991), 649-660.

22 Johannes Bijilsma. "Prevention of Glucocorticoid Induced Osteoporosis." *Annals of the Rheumatic Diseases* 56 (September 1997), 507-509.

23 "The Real 'Good News' for Osteoporosis Sufferers." *Bio/Tech News* Special Issue. Available from: Bio/Tech News, Box 30568, Parkrose Center, Portland, OR 97294.

24 Susan E. Brown, Ph.D. *Better Bones, Better Body* (New Canaan, CT: Keats Publishing, 1996), 48.

25 National Center for Health Statistics, Centers for Disease Control and Prevention, Hyattsville, Maryland. Eileen Hoffman, M.D. *Our Health, Our Lives* (New York: Pocket Books, 1995), 219. Vicki Hufnagel, M.D. *No More Hysterectomies* (New York: Plume/Penguin, 1989), 66.

26 Vicki Hufnagel, M.D. *No More Hysterectomies* (New York: Plume/Penguin, 1989), 108.

27 A.W.C. Kung and K.K. Pun. "Bone Mineral Density in Premenopausal Women Receiving Long-Term Physiological Doses of Levothyroxine." *Journal of the American Medical Association* 265:20 (1991), 2688-2691.

28 L.K. Bachrach et al. "Recovery from Osteopenia in Adolescent Girls with Anorexia Nervosa." *Journal of Clinical Endocrinology and Metabolism* 72:3 (March 1991), 602-606.

29 M.E. Nelson. "Hormone and Bone Mineral Status in Endurance-Trained and Sedentary Postmenopausal Women." *Journal of Clinical Endocrinology and Metabolism* 66:5 (May 1988), 927-933.

30 National Institutes of Health Consensus Conference: "Osteoporosis." *Journal of the American Medical Association* 252:6 (August 1984), 799-802.

31 S.M. Wolfe, M.D., and the Public Citizen Health Research Group. *Women's Health Alert* (Reading, MA: Addison-Wesley Publishing, 1991), 124.

32 T. Lohman et al. "Effects of Resistance Training on Regional and Total Bone Mineral Density in Premenopausal Woman: A Randomized Prospective Study." *Journal of Bone and Mineral Research* 10:7 (July 1995), 1015-1024.

33 Peter Pietschmann. "Exercise and Physical Therapy in the Prevention and Treatment of Osteoporosis." *Osteoporosis* 18 (1996), 265-270.

34 Lynne McTaggart. "Beating Osteoporosis Without Drugs." *What Doctors Don't Tell You* 6:12 (March 1996), 3.

35 Linda Ojeda, Ph.D. *Menopause Without Medicine* (Alameda, CA: Hunter House, 1995), 101.

36 Ibid.

37 M. Gambacciani et al. "Effects of Combined Low Dose of the Isoflavone Derivative Ipriflavone and Estrogen Replacement on Bone Mineral Density and Metabolism in Postmenopausal Women." *Maturitas* 28:1 (September 1997), 75-81. S. Adami et al. "Ipriflavone Prevents Radial Bone Loss in Postmenopausal Women with Low Bone Mass Over 2 Years." *Osteoporosis International* 7 (1997), 119-125. C. Gennari et al. "Effect of Chronic Treatment with Ipriflavone in Postmenopausal Women with Low Bone Mass." *Calcif Tissue Int* 61 (1997), S19-S22. D. Agnusdei et al. "A Double-Blind, Placebo-Controlled Trial of Ipriflavone for Prevention of Postmenopausal Spinal Bone Loss. *Calcif Tissue Int* 61 (1997), 142-147.

38 N. Appleton. *Healthy Bones: What You Should Do About Osteoporosis* (Garden City Park, NY: Avery Publishing Group, 1991), 61-62.

39 H.L. Wolfe. *Menopause: A Second Spring* (Boulder, CO: Blue Poppy Press, 1990), 151.

40 Susan E. Brown, Ph.D. *Better Bones, Better Body* (New Canaan, CT: Keats Publishing, 1996), 239.

41 J.R. Lee, M.D. "Significance of Molecular Configuration Specificity: The Case of Progesterone and Osteoporosis." *Townsend Letter for Doctors* 119 (June 1993), 558-562.

42 J.T. Hargrove et al. "Menopausal Hormone Replacement Therapy with Continuous Daily Oral Micronized Estradiol and Gynecology." *Obstetrics and Gynecology* 73:4 (April 1989), 606-612.

43 R. Lindsay et al. "Bone Response to Termination of Oestrogen Treatment." *The Lancet* 1:8078 (June 1978), 1325-1327.

44 S.M. Wolfe, M.D., and the Public Citizen Health Research Group. *Women's Health Alert* (Reading, MA: Addison-Wesley Publishing, 1991), 124.

45 L.A. Pruitt et al. "Weight-Training Effects on Bone Mineral Density in Early Postmenopausal Women." *Journal of Bone and Mineral Research* 7:2 (February 1992), 179-185.

46 Susun Weed. *Menopausal Years: The Wise Woman Way* (Woodstock, NY: Ash Tree Publishing, 1992), 159, 190.

47 Linda Ojeda, Ph.D. *Menopause Without Medicine* (Alameda, CA: Hunter House, 1995), 101.

PARASITIC INFECTIONS

1 W. Crewe and D.R.W. Haddock. *Parasites and Human Disease* (New York: Wiley Medical Publications, 1985).

2 Ann Louise Gittleman, M.S. *Guess What Came to Dinner: Parasites and Your Health* (Garden City Park, NY: Avery Publishing Group, 1993), 1, 9. J.M. Mansfield, ed. *Parasitic Diseases* (New York: Marcel Dekker, 1981).

3 R.B. Oxner et al. "Dientamoeba Fragilis: A Bowel Pathogen?" *New Zealand Medical Journal* 100:817 (1987), 64-65. S.S. Desser and Y.J. Yang. "Dientamoeba Fragilis in Idiopathic Gastrointestinal Disorders." *Canadian Medical Association Journal* 114:4 (1976), 290-293. J. Yang and T. Scholten. "Dientamoeba Fragilis: A Review with Notes on Its

Epidemiology, Pathogenicity, Mode of Transmission and Diagnosis." *American Journal of Tropical Medicine and Hygiene* 26:1 (1977), 16-22.

4 A.A. Mahmoud. "Parasitic Protozoa and Helminths: Biological and Immunological Challenges." *Science* 246:4933 (November 1989), 1015-1022.

5 M. Susser, M.D., and M. Rosenbaum, M.D. *Solving the Puzzle of Chronic Fatigue Syndrome* (Tacoma, WA: Life Sciences Press, 1992).

6 A. Hall et al. "Intensity of Reinfection with Ascaris Lumbricoides and Its Implications for Parasite Control." *The Lancet* 339:8804 (May 1992), 1253-1257.

7 R. Leventhal and R.F. Cheadle. *Medical Parasitology: A Self-Instructional Text* (Philadelphia: F.A. Davis, 1989).

8 Ibid.

9 M.J. Spencer et al. "Parasitic Infections in a Pediatric Population." *Pediatric Infectious Diseases* 2:2 (March/April 1983), 110-113.

10 Sheldon Margen, M.D., and Dale A. Ogar. "Is Meat Safe to Eat." *Your Health* 36:25 (December 9, 1997), 34.

11 K.O. Adams et al. "Intestinal Fluke Infestation as a Result of Eating Sushi." *American Journal of Clinical Pathology* 86:5 (1986), 688-689. T. Ishizuka and A. Ishizuka. "A Case of Diphyllobothriasis Due to Eating Masou-Sushi." *Medical Journal of Australia* 145:2 (1986), 114.

12 Hermann Bueno, M.D. *Uninvited Guests* (New Canaan, CT: Keats Publishing, 1996), 13.

13 Ann Louise Gittleman, M.S. *Guess What Came to Dinner: Parasites and Your Health* (Garden City Park, NY: Avery Publishing Group, 1993), 12.

14 Hermann Bueno, M.D. *Uninvited Guests* (New Canaan, CT: Keats Publishing, 1996), 12.

15 Ibid., 15.

16 Ann Louise Gittleman, M.S. *Guess What Came to Dinner: Parasites and Your Health* (Garden City Park, NY: Avery Publishing Group, 1993), 15-16. Hermann Bueno, M.D. *Uninvited Guests* (New Canaan, CT: Keats Publishing, 1996), 14.

17 Ann Louise Gittleman, M.S. *Guess What Came to Dinner: Parasites and Your Health* (Garden City Park, NY: Avery Publishing Group, 1993), 9-19.

18 D. Juranek. "Giardiasis." U.S. Centers for Disease Control, Division of Parasitic Infection, Atlanta, Georgia.

19 M.J. Spencer et al. "Parasitic Infections in a Pediatric Population." *Pediatric Infectious Diseases* 2:2 (March/April 1983), 110-113.

20 Ann Louise Gittleman, M.S. *Guess What Came to Dinner: Parasites and Your Health* (Garden City Park, NY: Avery Publishing Group, 1993), 37-56. Hermann Bueno, M.D. *Uninvited Guests* (New Canaan, CT: Keats Publishing, 1996), 20-32.

21 A.C. Chester et al. "Giardiasis as a Chronic Disease." *Digestive Diseases and Science* 30:3 (1985), 215-218.

22 J.J. Plorde. "Intestinal Nematodes." In: G.W. Thorne et al., eds. *Harrison's Principles of Internal Medicine* 8th Ed. (New York: McGraw-Hill, 1977).

23 L. Galland, M.D., et al. *Journal of Nutritional Medicine* 1 (1990), 27-31.

24 *New England Journal of Medicine* (July 21, 1986).

25 L. Galland, M.D. *Super-Immunity for Kids* (New York: Dell Publishing, 1989).

26 Ann Louise Gittleman, M.S. *Guess What Came to Dinner: Parasites and Your Health* (Garden City Park, NY: Avery Publishing Group, 1993), 80-86. Her-

mann Bueno, M.D. *Uninvited Guests* (New Canaan, CT: Keats Publishing, 1996), 33.

27 D. Casemore, M.D. "Foodborne Protozoal Infection." *The Lancet* 336:8728 (December 1990), 1427-1432.

28 Ann Louise Gittleman, M.S. *Guess What Came to Dinner: Parasites and Your Health* (Garden City Park, NY: Avery Publishing Group, 1993), 94-95. Gary Null, Ph.D. *The Woman's Encyclopedia of Natural Healing* (New York: Seven Stories, 1996), 285. Pavel I. Yutsis, M.D. "Intestinal Parasites at Large." *Explore!* 7:1 (1996), 27-31.

29 Ann Louise Gittleman, M.S. *Guess What Came to Dinner: Parasites and Your Health* (Garden City Park, NY: Avery Publishing Group, 1993), 97.

30 Ibid., 96.

31 Ibid., 108-114.

32 J. Bland. "Aloe Vera to Treat Gastrointestinal Problems." *Journal of Alternative Medicine* (1985).

33 V.P. Choudhry, M. Sabir, and V.N. Bhide. "Berberine in Giardiasis." *Indian Pediatrics* 9:3 (March 1972), 143-146.

PREGNANCY AND CHILDBIRTH

1 R.J. Williams. *Nutrition Against Disease, Environmental Protection* (New York: Bantam Books, 1971), 57.

2 B. Barnes and S.G. Bradley. *Planning for a Healthy Baby* (London: Ebury Press, 1990).

3 W.A. Price. *Nutrition and Physical Degeneration* (New Canaan, CT: Keats Publishing, 1989).

4 C. Hirson. "Coeliac Infertility-Folic Acid Therapy." *The Lancet* 1:643 (February 1970), 412. D.W. Dawson and A.H. Sawyers. "Infertility and Folate Deficiency: Case Reports." *British Journal of Obstetrics and Gynaecology* 89:8 (August 1982), 678-680. I. Jackson, W.B. Doig, and G. McDonald. "Pernicious Anaemia as a Cause of Infertility." *The Lancet* 2:527 (December 1967), 1159-1160. H. Pschera et al. "Fatty Acid Composition of Cervical Mucus, Lecithin and Primary Infertility." *Infertility* 2:1 (1988). 123-132.

5 M. Cimons. "U.S. Advises Folic Acid to Reduce Birth Defects." *The Los Angeles Times* (September 15, 1992), A1-A17. MRC Vitamin Study Research Group. "Prevention of Neural Tube Defects: Results of the Medical Research Council Vitamin Study." *The Lancet* 338:8760 (1991), 131-137.

6 A. Wilcox, C. Weinberg, and D. Baird. "Caffeinated Beverages and Decreased Fertility." *The Lancet* 2:8626/8627 (December 1988), 1453-1456.

7 P.M. Zavos. "Cigarette Smoking and Human Reproduction: Effects on Female and Male Fecundity." *Infertility* 12:1 (1989), 35-46.

8 W.R. Phipps et al. "The Association Between Smoking and Female Infertility as Influenced by Cause of the Infertility." *Fertility and Sterility* 48:3 (September 1987), 377-382.

9 B. Barnes and S.G. Bradley. *Planning for a Healthy Baby* (London: Ebury Press, 1990). M.A. Stenchever, T.J. Kunysz, and M.A. Allen. "Chromosome Breakage in Users of Marijuana." *American Journal of Obstetrics and Gynecology* 118:1 (January 1974), 106-113.

10 M.B. Bracken et al. "Association of Cocaine Use with Sperm Concentration, Motility, and Morphology." *Fertility and Sterility* 53:2 (February 1990), 315-322.

11 B. Barnes and S.G. Bradley. *Planning for a Healthy Baby* (London: Ebury Press, 1990).

12 M.C. Terreros, J.C. De Luca, and F.N. Dulout.

"The Effect of a Hypoproteic Diet and Ethanol Consumption on the Yield of Chromosomal Damage Detected in the Bone Marrow Cells of Mice." *Journal of Veterinary Medical Science* 55:2 (April 1993), 191-194.

13 F. De Rosis et al. "Female Reproductive Health in Two Lamp Factories: Effects of Exposure to Inorganic Mercury Vapour and Stress Factors." *British Journal of Industrial Medicine* 42:7 (July 1985), 488-494.

14 P.R. Sutton. "Acute Dental Caries, Mental Stress, Immunity and the Active Passage of Ions Through the Teeth." *Medical Hypotheses* 31:1 (January 1990), 17. S. Cohen, D.A.J. Tyrrell, and A.P. Smith. "Psychological Stress and Susceptibility to the Common Cold." *New England Journal of Medicine* 325:9 (August 1991), 606-612. K.L. Harrison, V.J. Callan, and J.F. Hennessey. "Stress and Semen Quality in an In Vitro Fertilization Program." *Fertility and Sterility* 48:4 (October 1987), 633-636.

15 M. Samuels, M.D., and N. Samuels. *The Well Pregnancy Book* (New York: Summit Books, 1986).

16 Editorial Staff. "Czechoslovakian Study: Unwanted Children Face Struggle." *Pregnancy and Child Birth: Brain/Mind Bulletin Collections* 15:02B (1991).

17 M. Samuels, M.D., and N. Samuels. *The Well Pregnancy Book* (New York: Summit Books, 1986).

18 Ibid.

19 J.W. Kardaun et al. "Testicular Cancer in Young Men and Parental Occupational Exposure." *American Journal of Industrial Medicine* 20:2 (1991), 219-227.

20 G.M. Al-Hachim. "Teratogenicity of Caffeine: A Review." *European Journal of Obstetrics & Gynecology and Reproductive Biology* 31:3 (June 1989), 237-247.

21 C.B. Ernhart et al. "Alcohol Teratogenicity in the Human: A Detailed Assessment of Specificity, Critical Period, and Threshold." *American Journal of Obstetrics and Gynecology* 156:1 (January 1987), 33-39.

22 K. Mulvihill. "Even Small Amounts of Alcohol in Pregnancy Harmful." Reuters Health report (August 7, 2000).

23 J.C. Peacock et al. "Cigarette Smoking and Birthweight: Type of Cigarette Smoked and a Possible Threshold Effect." *International Journal of Epidemiology* 20:2 (1991), 405-412.

24 "Smoking May Be Risk Factor for Infant Colic." Reuters Health report (August 6, 2001).

25 *British Journal of Obstetrics and Gynecology* 107 (July 2000), 935-938.

26 *Nutrition Reviews* 56 (August 1998), 236-244. *European Journal of Pediatric Surgery* Suppl 1 (December 6, 1996), 7-9.

27 *Epidemiology* 11 (July 2001), 439-446.

28 "Doctors Ignore Acne Drug Birth Defect Warnings." Available on the Internet: www.mercola.com/2001/aug29/accutane.htm.

29 *Journal of Family Practice* 50 (May 2001), 433-437.

30 Editorial Staff. "Aspirin-Pregnancy Link: Lowered I.Q.s." *Pregnancy and Child Birth: Brain/Mind Bulletin Collections* 13:9K (1991).

31 Editorial Staff. "Valium Inhibits Cell Fusion in Lab Tests." *Pregnancy and Child Birth: Brain/Mind Bulletin Collections* 12:13D (1991).

32 L.M. O'Leary et al. "Parental Occupational Exposures and Risk of Childhood Cancer: A Review." *American Journal of Industrial Medicine* 20:1 (1991), 17-35.

33 J.W. Kardaun et al. "Testicular Cancer in Young Men and Parental Occupational Exposure." *American Journal of Industrial Medicine* 20:2 (1991), 219-227.

34 *New England Journal of Medicine* 344:12 (March 22, 2001).

35 Alan Gaby. "Preventing Birth Defects and Treating Toxemia of Pregnancy: Commentary." *Dr. Jonathan Wright's Nutrition & Healing* 3:11 (November 1996), 10-11.

36 *Journal of Reproductive Medicine* 46 (May 2001), 209-212.

37 Alan Gaby. "Preventing Birth Defects and Treating Toxemia of Pregnancy: Commentary." *Dr. Jonathan Wright's Nutrition & Healing* 3:11 (November 1996), 10.

38 P. Simkin, J. Whalley, and A. Keppler. *Pregnancy, Childbirth and the Newborn: The Complete Guide* (New York: Meadowbrook Press, 1991).

39 D. Rush, Z. Stein, and M. Susser. "A Randomized Controlled Trial of Prenatal Nutritional Supplementation in New York City." *Pediatrics* 65:4 (April 1980), 683-697.

40 P. Simkin, J. Whalley, and A. Keppler. *Pregnancy, Childbirth and the Newborn: The Complete Guide* (New York: Meadowbrook Press, 1991).

41 D. Rush, Z. Stein, and M. Susser. "A Randomized Controlled Trial of Prenatal Nutritional Supplementation in New York City." *Pediatrics* 65:4 (April 1980), 683-697.

42 G. Baum et al. "Meclozine and Pyridoxine in Pregnancy Sickness." *Practitioner* 190:1136 (1963), 251-253.

43 N. Kawasaki et al. "Effect of Calcium Supplementation on the Vascular Sensitivity to Angiotensin II in Pregnant Women." *American Journal of Obstetrics and Gynecology* 153:5 (November 1985), 576-582.

44 MRC Vitamin Study Research Group. "Prevention of Neural Tube Defects: Results of the Medical Research Council Vitamin Study." *The Lancet* 338:8760 (July 1991), 131-137.

45 Editorial Staff. "Excessive Folic Acid." *American Family Physician* 32:4 (October 1985), 290-291.

46 K. Simmer, C. James, and R.P. Thompson. "Are Iron-Folate Supplements Harmful?" *American Journal of Clinical Nutrition* 45:1 (January 1987), 122-125.

47 J.M. Gertner et al. "Pregnancy as State of Physiologic Absorptive Hypercalciuria." *American Journal of Medicine* 81:3 (September 1986), 451-456.

48 P. Simkin, J. Whalley, and A. Keppler. *Pregnancy, Childbirth, and the Newborn: The Complete Guide* (New York: Meadowbrook Press, 1991).

49 E.W. Page and E.P. Page. "Leg Cramps in Pregnancy: Etiology and Treatment." *Obstetrics and Gynecology* 1 (1953), 94.

50 Editorial. "Vitamin A and Teratogenesis." *The Lancet* 1:8424 (February 1985), 319-320.

51 K.J. Rothman et al. "Teratogenicity of High Vitamin A Intake." *New England Journal of Medicine* 333 (1995), 1369-1373.

52 Alan Gaby. "Preventing Birth Defects and Treating Toxemia of Pregnancy: Commentary." *Dr. Jonathan Wright's Nutrition & Healing* 3:11 (November 1996), 10.

53 Carl Jones, H. Goer, and P. Simkin. *The Labor Support Guide-for Father, Family and Friends* (Seattle, WA: Pennypress, 1984).

54 A.D. Haverkamp et al. "The Evaluation of Continuous Fetal Heart Rate Monitoring in High-Risk Pregnancy." *American Journal of Obstetrics and Gynecology* 125:3 (June 1976), 310-320.

55 N.M. Lopez. "Why Natural Childbirth is Better Than Medicated Childbirth." *NAPSAC News* 14:1 (1989), 6-7.

56 "WHO Antenatal Care Randomised Trial for the Evaluation of a New Model of Routine Antenatal Care." *The Lancet* 357:9268 (May 19, 2001).

57 N.M. Lopez. "Why Natural Childbirth is Better Than Medicated Childbirth." *NAPSAC News* 14:1 (1989), 6-7.

58 S. Langendoerfer et al. "Pediatric Follow-Up of a Randomized Controlled Trial of Intrapartum Fetal Monitoring Techniques." *Journal of Pediatrics* 97:1 (July 1980), 103-107.

59 L. Righard and M.O. Alade. "Effect of Delivery Room Routines on Success of First Breast-Feed." *The Lancet* 336:8723 (November 1990), 1105-1107.

60 P. Walton and F. Reynolds. "Epidural Analgesia and Instrumental Delivery." *Anaesthesia* 39:3 (March 1984), 218-223. M.C. Klein et al. "Does Episiotomy Prevent Perineal Trauma and Pelvic Floor Relaxation?" *Online Journal of Current Clinical Trials* (July 1, 1992).

61 N.M. Lopez. "Why Natural Childbirth is Better Than Medicated Childbirth." *NAPSAC News* 14:1 (1989), 6-7.

62 M.C. Klein et al. "Does Episiotomy Prevent Perineal Trauma and Pelvic Floor Relaxation?" *Online Journal of Current Clinical Trials* (July 1, 1992).

63 D.S. Seidman et al. "Long-Term Effects of Vacuum and Forceps Deliveries." *The Lancet* 337:8757 (June 1991), 1583-1585. S. Nuijen and R. Housman. "Fatal Forceps." *Medicine, Science, and the Law* 23:4 (October 1983), 254-256.

64 Ibid.

65 S. Nuijen and R. Housman. "Fatal Forceps." *Medicine, Science, and the Law* 23:4 (October 1983), 254-256.

66 *British Journal of Obstetrics and Gynaecology* 108 (August 2001), 678-688.

67 R.S. Stafford. "Alternative Strategies for Controlling Rising Cesarean Section Rates." *Journal of the American Medical Association* 263:5 (February 1990), 683-687.

68 J.F. Barrett et al. "Inconsistencies in Clinical Decisions in Obstetrics." *The Lancet* 336:8714 (September 1990), 549-551.

69 "The Demise of Natural Childbirth." *The London Daily Mail* (June 13, 2001).

70 Ibid.

71 L.B. Richards. "Natural Birth Following Cesareans." *NAPSAC News* 14:1 (1989), 1-5.

72 Ibid.

73 J.C. Carroll et al. "The Influence of the High-Risk Care Environment on the Practice of Low-Risk Obstetrics." *Family Medicine* 23:3 (March/April 1991), 184-188.

74 Ibid.

75 Ibid.

76 Ibid.

77 Editorial Staff. "Home Birth Has Better Record in First Return." *Pregnancy and Child Birth: Brain/Mind Bulletin Collections* 2:7G (1991). P. Simkin, J. Whalley, and A. Keppler. *Pregnancy, Childbirth and the Newborn* (New York: Meadowbrook Press, 1991).

78 K.D. Scott et al. "A Comparison of Intermittent and Continuous Support During Labor: A Meta-Analysis." *American Journal of Obstetrics and Gynecology* 180:5 (May 1999), 1054-1059.

79 J. Kennell et al. "Continuous Emotional Support During Labor in a U.S. Hospital: A Randomized Controlled Trial." *Journal of the American Medical Association* 265:17 (May 1, 1991), 2197-2201.

80 P. Keenan. "Benefits of Massage Therapy and the Use of a Doula During Labor and Childbirth." *Alternative Therapies in Health and Medicine* 6 (January 2000), 66-74.

81 D. Wang et al. "Clinical Observation on Doula Delivery." *Chung Hua Fu Chan Ko Tsa Chih* 32:11 (November 1997), 659-661.

82 G. Manning-Orenstein. "A Birth Intervention: The Therapeutic Effects of Doula Support versus Lamaze Preparation on First-Time Mothers' Working Models of Caregiving." *Alternative Therapies in Health and Medicine* 4 (July 1998), 73-81.

83 J. Zhang et al. "Continuous Labor Support from Labor Attendant for Primiparous Women: A Meta-Analysis." *Obstetrics and Gynecology* 88:4 Part 2 (October 1996), 739-744.

84 E. Noble. *Childbirth with Insight* (Boston: Houghton Mifflin, 1983).

85 Ibid.

86 Ibid.

87 M.R. Odent. "Position in Delivery." *The Lancet* 335:8698 (May 1990), 1166. J.C. Carroll et al. "The Influence of the High-Risk Care Environment on the Practice of Low-Risk Obstetrics." *Family Medicine* 23:3 (March/April 1991), 184-188.

88 J.C. Carroll et al. "The Influence of the High-Risk Care Environment on the Practice of Low-Risk Obstetrics." *Family Medicine* 23:3 (March/April 1991), 184-188.

89 Ibid.

90 P. Simkin, J. Whalley, and A. Keppler. *Pregnancy, Childbirth and the Newborn* (New York: Meadowbrook Press, 1991).

91 J. Golding et al. "Childhood Cancer, Intramuscular Vitamin K, and Pethidine Given During Labour." *British Medical Journal* 305:6849 (August 1992), 341-346.

92 F.H. Lawler, R.S. Bisonni, and D.R. Holtgrave. "Circumcision: A Decision Analysis of Its Medical Value." *Family Medicine* 23:8 (November/December 1991), 587-593.

93 J. Jason. "Breast-Feeding in 1991." *New England Journal of Medicine* 325:14 (October 1991), 1036-1038.

94 B.S. Worthington-Roberts, J. Vermeersch, and S.R. Williams. *Nutrition in Pregnancy and Lactation* (St. Louis, MO: Times Mirror/Mosby College Publishing, 1985).

95 P.F. Hennart et al. "Lysozyme, Lactoferrin, and Secretory Immunoglobulin-A Content in Breast Milk: Influence of Duration of Lactation, Nutrition Status, Prolactin Status, and Parity of Mother." *American Journal of Clinical Nutrition* 53:1 (January 1991), 32-39.

96 M.J. Parmely, A.E. Beer, and R.E. Billingham. "*In Vitro* Studies on the T-lymphocyte Population of Human Milk." *Journal of Experimental Medicine* 144:2 (August 1976), 358-370.

97 J.W. Lawton and K.F. Shortridge. "Protective Factors in Human Breast Milk and Colostrum." *The Lancet* 1:8005 (January 1977), 253.

98 Ibid.

99 J. Jason. "Breast-Feeding in 1991." *New England Journal of Medicine* 325:14 (October 1991), 1036-1038.

100 J.W. Lawton and K.F. Shortridge. "Protective Factors in Human Breast Milk and Colostrum." *The Lancet* 1:8005 (January 1977), 253.

101 Editorial Staff. "Necrotizing Enterocolitis and Breast Milk." *American Family Physician* 43:5 (1991), 1788.

102 U.M. Saarinen. "Prolonged Breast Feeding as Prophylaxis for Recurrent Otitis Media." *Acta Paediatrica Scandinavica* 71:4 (July 1982), 567-571. L. Lothe and T. Lindberg. "Cow's Milk Whey Protein Elicits Symptoms of Infantile Colic in Colicky Formula-Fed Infants: A Double-Blind Crossover Study." *Pediatrics* 83:2 (February 1989), 262-266. S.R. Halpern et al. "Development of Childhood Allergy in Infants Fed Breast, Soy, or Cow Milk." *Journal of Allergy and Clinical Immunology* 51:3 (March 1973), 139-151. A. Lucas et al. "Breast Milk and Subsequent Intelligence Quotient in Children Born Preterm." *The Lancet* 339:8788 (February 1992), 261-264.

103 B.S. Worthington-Roberts, J. Vermeersch, and S.R. Williams. *Nutrition in Pregnancy and Lactation* (St. Louis: Times Mirror/Mosby College Publishing, 1985).

104 J. Jason. "Breast-Feeding in 1991." *New England Journal of Medicine* 325:14 (October 1991), 1036-1038.

105 B.S. Worthington-Roberts, J. Vermeersch, and S.R. Williams. *Nutrition in Pregnancy and Lactation* (St. Louis: Times Mirror/Mosby College Publishing, 1985).

106 Ibid.

107 J. Myrabo. *The First Days After Birth: Care of Mother and Baby* (Seattle, WA: Pennypress, 1983).

108 The National Institute of Child Health and Human Development. *Reduce the Risk of Sudden Infant Death Syndrome (SIDS)* (Bethesda, MD: The National Institute of Child Health and Human Development, The National Institutes of Health, 1999).

109 P. Simkin, J. Whalley, and A. Keppler. *Pregnancy, Childbirth and the Newborn* (New York: Meadowbrook Press, 1991). S. Kitzinger. *Sex After the Baby Comes* (Seattle, WA: Pennypress, 1980).

110 R.V. Short et al. "Contraceptive Effects of Extended Lactational Amenorrhoea: Beyond the Bellagio Consensus." *The Lancet* 337:8743 (March 1991), 715-717. S.L. Huffman et al. "Suckling Patterns and Post-Partum Amenorrhea in Bangladesh." *Journal of Biosocial Science* 19:2 (April 1987), 171-179.

RESPIRATORY CONDITIONS

1 R.M. Cherniack. *Respiration in Health and Disease* (Philadelphia: W.B. Saunders, 1983), 179.

2 L. Jaroff. "Allergies: Nothing to Sneeze At." *Time* (June 22, 1992), 54.

3 U.S. Centers for Disease Control and Prevention. *Vital and Health Statistics, Current Estimates from the National Health Interview Survey, 1994* DHHS Publication No. PHS96-1521 (Washington, DC: U.S. Department of Health and Human Services, Public Health Services, National Center for Health Statistics, 1995).

4 Claudia Glenn Dowling and Anne Hollister. "An Epidemic of Sneezing and Wheezing." *Life* (May 1997), 78-92.

5 E. Rubenstein and D.D. Felderman, eds. *Scientific American Medicine* (New York: Scientific American, 1982).

6 U.S. Centers for Disease Control and Prevention. *Vital and Health Statistics, Current Estimates from the National Health Interview Survey, 1994* DHHS Publication No. PHS96-1521 (Washington, DC: U.S. Department of Health and Human Services, Public Health Services, National Center for Health Statistics, 1995).

7 S. Quirce and J. Sastre. "Occupational Asthma." *Allergy* 53 (1998), 633-641.

8 U.S. Department of Health and Human Services. "Table 10: Number of Deaths from 72 Selected Causes, Human Immunodeficiency Virus Infection, and Alzheimer's Disease by Age, U.S., 1997." *National Vital Statistics Report* 47:19 (June 30, 1999).

9 American Academy of Allergy, Asthma & Immunology. *Asthma and Allergy Management News* (June 1997), 3.

10 American Academy of Allergy, Asthma & Immunology. *The Allergy Report 1* (Milwaukee, WI: American Academy of Allergy, Asthma & Immunology, 2000), 3.

11 Jonathan Corren, M.D. "The Impact of Allergic Rhinitis on Bronchial Asthma." *Journal of Allergy and Clinical Immunology* 101:2 Part 2 (February 1998), S352-S356.

12 E. Rubenstein and D.D. Feldman, eds. *Scientific American Medicine* (New York: Scientific American, 1982).

13 P. Austin. *Natural Remedies: A Manual* (Seale, AL: Yuchi Pines Institute, 1983).

14 S. Rietveld, I. Van Beest, and W. Everaerd. "Stress-Induced Breathlessness in Asthma." *Psychological Medicine* 29:6 (November 1999), 1359-1366.

15 "Stress Management Strategies Benefit Some Asthmatics." *Modern Medicine* 65 (December 1997), 42-43.

16 J. Chihara. "Stress and Immunoallergy." *Rinsho Byori—Japanese Journal of Clinical Pathology* 46:6 (June 1998), 587-592.

17 David A. Mrazek. "Psychological Aspects in Children and Adolescents." *Asthma* 148 (1997), 2177-2183.

18 R. Bussing, R.C. Burket, and E.T. Kelleher. "Prevalence of Anxiety Disorders in Clinic-Based Sample of Pediatric Asthma Patients." *Psychosomatics* 37:2 (March 1996), 108-115.

19 E. Rubenstein and D.D. Feldman, eds. *Scientific American Medicine* (New York: Scientific American, 1982).

20 R. Weiss. *Herbal Medicine* (Beaconsfield, England: Beaconsfield Publishers, 1988).

21 E. Rubenstein and D.D. Feldman, eds. *Scientific American Medicine* (New York: Scientific American, 1982).

22 Ibid.

23 R. Weiss. *Herbal Medicine* (Beaconsfield, England: Beaconsfield Publishers, 1988).

24 R. Abramson. "EPA Officially Links Passive Smoke to Cancer." *The Los Angeles Times* 112 (June 8, 1993), A27.

25 *Physicians' Desk Reference* (Oradell, NJ: Medical Economics, 1990).

26 C.C. Pfeiffer, M.D., and the Publications Committee of the BrainBio Center. *Mental and Elemental Nutrients: Physician's Guide to Nutrition and Health Care* (New Canaan, CT: Keats Publishing, 1975).

27 D. Babcock. "Whomever May Have Asthma." *Townsend Letter for Doctors*.

28 F. Gurkan et al. "Intravenous Magnesium Sulphate in the Management of Moderate to Severe Acute Asthmatic Children Nonresponding to Conventional Therapy." *European Journal of Emergency Medicine* 6:3 (September 1999), 201-205.

29 H. Mangat, G.A. D'Souza, and M.S. Jacob. "Neb-

ulized Magnesium Sulphate versus Nebulized Salbutamol in Acute Bronchial Asthma: A Clinical Asthma." *European Respiratory Journal* 12:2 (August 1998), 341-344.

30 H. Hill et al. "Investigation of the Effect of Short-Term Change in Dietary Magnesium Intake in Asthma." *European Respiratory Journal* 10:10 (October 1997), 2225-2229.

31 A.V. Emel'ianov and V.I. Trofimov. "Effects of Glucocorticoid Therapy on Mineral Metabolism Indicators in Patients with Bronchial Asthma." *Klinicheskaia Meditsina* 73:2 (1995), 23-25.

32 W. Zwolfer et al. "Beneficial Effect of Acupuncture on Adult Patients with Asthma Bronchiale." *American Journal of Chinese Medicine* 21:2 (1993), 113-117.

33 R.A. Aleksandrova et al. "Bronchial Nonspecific Reactivity in Patients with Bronchial Asthma and the Preasthmatic State and Its Alteration Under the Influence of Acupuncture." *Terapevticheskii Arkhiv* 67:8 (1995), 42-45.

34 W. Gruber et al. "Alternative Medicine and Bronchial Asthma—A Review From a Pediatric Perspective." *Monatsschrift Kinderheilkunde* 145 (1997), 786-796.

35 P.K. Vendanthan et al. "Clinical Study of Yoga Techniques in University Students with Asthma: A Controlled Study." *Allergy & Asthma Proceedings* 19:1 (January/February 1998), 3-9.

36 *What Doctors Don't Tell You* 7:2 (May 1996), 11.

37 *Biological Therapy—Journal of Natural Medicine* 13:1 (January 1995), 4-11.

38 P. Austin. *Natural Remedies: A Manual* (Seale, AL: Yuchi Pines Institute, 1983).

39 P. Airola. *How to Get Well* (Phoenix, AZ: Health Plus Publishers, 1974).

40 John Bastyr College. *Naturopathic Treatment Notebook* (Seattle, WA: NCNM Library Reprint, 1984).

41 R. Weiss. *Herbal Medicine* (Beaconsfield, England: Beaconsfield Publishers, 1988).

SEXUALLY TRANSMITTED DISEASES

1 National Institute of Allergy and Infectious Diseases. "Sexually Transmitted Diseases-NIAID Fact Sheet." Available on the Internet: www.niaid.nih.gov/factsheets/stdinfo.htm.

2 Ibid.

3 H.L. Zimmerman et al. "Epidemiologic Differences Between Chlamydia and Gonorrhea." *American Journal of Public Health* 80:11 (1990), 1338-1342.

4 J.F. Potts. "Chlamydial Infection: Screening and Management Update, 1992." *Postgraduate Medicine* 91:1 (1992), 120-126. U.S. Department of Health and Human Services. *Chlamydia Trachomatis Infections: Policy Guidelines for Prevention and Control* (Atlanta, GA: Centers for Disease Control, 1985).

5 Y. Kumazawa et al. "Activation of Peritoneal Macrophages by Berberine Alkaloids in Terms of Induction of Cytostatic Activity." *International Journal of Immunopharmacology* 6:6 (1984), 587-592.

6 O.P. Babbar et al. "Effect of Berberine Chloride Eye Drops on Clinically Positive Tracoma Patients." *Indian Journal of Medical Research* 76 Suppl (1982), 83-88.

7 M.A. Krupp, M.J. Chatton, and L.M. Tierney, eds. *Current Medical Diagnosis & Treatment* (Los Altos: Lange Medical Publications, 1986).

8 *STD Training: Gonorrhea Notes* (Seattle, WA: Harborview Medical Center, 1985).

9 R.J. Derman. "Counseling the Herpes Genitalis Patient." *Journal of Reproductive Medicine* 31:Suppl 5 (May 1986), 439-444.

10 D.E. Walsh et al. "Subjective Response to Lysine in the Therapy of Herpes Simplex." *Journal of Antimicrobial Chemother* 12:5 (November 1983), 489-496.

11 R. Pompei et al. "Glyccyrhizic Acid Inhibits Virus Growth and Inactivates Virus Particles." *Nature* 281:5733 (October 1979), 690. R. Pompei et al. "Antiviral Activity of Glycyrrhizic Acid." *Experientia* 36:3 (March 1980), 304.

12 T.N. Kaul et al. "Antiviral Effect of Flavonoids on Human Viruses." *Journal of Medical Virology* 15 (1985), 71-79.

13 Julian Whitaker, M.D. *Dr. Whitaker's Guide to Natural Healing* (Rocklin, CA: Prima Publishing, 1995), 353.

14 A.M. Sebbelov et al. "The Prevalence of Human Papillomavirus Type 16 and 18 DNA in Cervical Cancer in Different Age Groups: A Study on the Incidental Cases of Cervical Cancer in Norway in 1983." *Gynecologic Oncology* 41:2 (May 1991), 141-148. T. Kawana. "Human Papilloma Virus and Cervical Cancer" *Gan To Kagaku Ryoho Japanese Journal of Cancer and Chemotherapy* 17:4 Part 1 (April 1990), 615-619.

SLEEP DISORDERS

1 National Sleep Foundation. "2000 Omnibus Sleep in America Poll." Available from: National Sleep Foundation, 1522 K Street NW, Suite 500, Washington, DC 20005; website: www.sleepfoundation.org.

2 Ibid.

3 N. Ishida, M. Kaneko, and R. Allada. "Biological Clocks." *Proceedings of the National Academy of Sciences* 96:16 (August 3, 1996), 8819-8820.

4 N. Ishida, M. Kaneko, and R. Allada. "Biological Clocks." *Proceedings of the National Academy of Sciences* 96:16 (August 3, 1996), 8819-8820.

5 U. Koehler and H. Shäfer. "Is Obstructive Sleep Apnea (OSA) a Risk Factor for Myocardial Infarction and Cardiac Arrhythmias in Patients with Coronary Heart Disease?" *Sleep* 19:4 (1995), 283.

6 National Institutes of Health and National Heart, Lung, and Blood Institute. *Sleep Apnea* NIH Publication No. 95-379 (Washington, DC: U.S. Department of Health and Human Services, 1995).

7 National Institutes of Health and National Heart, Lung, and Blood Institute. *Narcolepsy* NIH Publication No. 96-3649 (Washington, DC: U.S. Department of Health and Human Services, 1996).

8 Roger Fritz, Ph.D. *Sleep Disorders: America's Hidden Nightmare* (Naperville, IL, National Sleep Alert, 1993), 106.

9 Michael S. Aldrich. *Sleep Medicine* (New York: Oxford University Press, 1999).

10 John F. Simonds and Humberto Parrago. "Prevalence of Sleep Disorders and Sleep Behaviors in Children and Adolescents." *Journal of the American Academy of Child Psychiatry* 21 (1982), 383-388.

11 Michael S. Aldrich. *Sleep Medicine* (New York: Oxford University Press, 1999).

12 Diagnostic Classification Steering Committee and Michael J. Thorpy. *The International Classification of Sleep Disorders: Diagnostic and Coding Manual* (Rochester, MN: American Sleep Disorders Association, 1990).

13 Kenneth Rifkin, N.D., R.Ac. Personal communication.

14 J.E. Pizzorno and M.T. Murray. *A Textbook of Natural Medicine* (Seattle, WA: John Bastyr University, 1989).

15 B.M. Stone. "Sleep and Low Doses of Alcohol." *Electroencephalography and Clinical Neurophysiology* 48:6 (1980), 706-709.

16 Dian Dincin Buchman, Ph.D. *The Complete Guide to Sleep* (New Canaan, CT: Keats Publishing, 1997), 45.

17 H.J. Rinkel, T.G. Randolph, and M. Zeller. *Food Allergy* (Springfield, IL: Charles C. Thomas, 1950).

18 A. Kahn et al. "Insomnia and Cow's Milk Allergy in Infants." *Pediatrics* 76:6 (December 1985), 880-884.

19 Martin Moore-Ede, M.D., Ph.D., and Suzanne LeVert. *Complete Idiot's Guide to Getting a Good Night's Sleep* (New York: Alpha Books, 1998), 118.

20 W.F. Tsoi. "Insomnia: Drug Treatment." *Annals of the Academy of Medicine, Singapore* 20:2 (March 1991), 269-272.

21 Russel J. Reiter, Ph.D., and Jo Robinson. *Melatonin, Your Body's Natural Wonder Drug* (New York: Bantam, 1995), 124.

22 M. Lader. "Rebound Insomnia and Newer Hypnotics." *Psychopharmacology* 108:3 (1992), 248-255.

23 L.M. Tierney, Jr., M.D., et al. *Current Medical Diagnosis & Treatment* (Norwalk, CT: Appleton & Lange, 1993).

24 S.T. O'Keefe, K. Gaavin, and J.N. Lavan. "Iron Status and Restless Legs Syndrome in the Elderly." *Age and Aging* 23 (1994), 200-203.

25 T.C. Birdsall. "5-Hydroxytryptophan: A Clinically Effective Serotonin Precursor." *Alternative Medicine Review* 3:4 (1998), 271-280.

26 P. Polo-Kentola et al. "When Does Estrogen Replacement Therapy Improve Sleep Quality?" *American Journal of Obstetrics and Gynecology* 178:5 (1998), 1002-1009.

27 H.P. Roffwarg et al. "Plasma Testosterone and Sleep: Relationship to Sleep Stage Variables." *Psychosomatic Medicine* 44:1 (1982), 73-84.

28 R.C. Schiavi, D. White, and J. Mandeli. "Pituitary-Gonadal Function During Sleep in Healthy Aging Men." *Psychoneuroendocrinology* 17:6 (1992), 599-609.

29 Kathryn Reid et al. "Day-Time Melatonin Administration: Effects on Core Temperature and Sleep Onset Latency." *Journal of Sleep Research* 5 (1996), 150-154.

30 J.E. Pizzorno and M.T. Murray. *A Textbook of Natural Medicine* (Seattle, WA: John Bastyr College Publications, 1989).

31 M. Lader. "Rebound Insomnia and Newer Hypnotics." *Psychopharmacology* 108:3 (1992), 248-255.

32 German Ministry of Health. *Valerian: Commission E Monographs for Phytomedicines* (Bonn, Germany: German Ministry of Health, 1985).

33 W. Mitchell. *Naturopathic Applications of the Botanical Remedies* (Seattle, WA: Mitchell, 1983), 66-67.

34 S. Foster. *Passion Flower Botanical Series* 314 (Austin, TX: American Botanical Council, 1993).

35 E. Lehmann et al. "Efficacy of a Special Kava Extract *(Piper methysticum)* in Patients with Anxiety, Tension, and Excitedness of Non-Mental Origin." *Phytomedicine* 3 (1996), 113-119.

36 Simon Y. Mills, M.A. *The Dictionary of Modern Herbalism* (Rochester, VT: Healing Arts Press, 1988), 58-59.

37 Peter Hauri, Ph.D., and Shirley Linde, Ph.D. *No*

More Sleepless Nights (New York: John Wiley & Sons, 1990-1991), 98.

38 Andrew Lockie, M.D., and Nicola Geddes, M.D. *The Women's Guide to Homeopathy* (New York: St. Martin's, 1994), 238.

39 Abstracts of the 4th International Symposium. "Mobilizations of Endorphins as the Basis for Effectiveness of Acupuncture Therapy." *Acupuncture and Electro-Therapeutics Research International Journal* 13:4 (1988), 201.

40 Glenda Cassutt. "Energize Your Home for Good Health." *Natural Health* (May/June 1995), 95.

41 Hiroshi Itoh et al. "Effects of Vitamin B12 and Circadian Rhythms." *Japanese Journal of Psychiatry and Neurology* 48:2 (1994), 502-505. See also: Satoko Hashimoto et al. "Vitamin B12 Enhances the Phase-Response of Circadian Melatonin Rhythms to a Single Bright Light Exposure in Humans." *Neuroscience Letters* 220 (1996), 129-132.

STRESS

1 M. Scofield. *Work Site Health Promotion* (Philadelphia: Hanley & Belfus, 1990), 459.

2 *Harvard Mental Health Letter* 8:7 (January 1992). T.H. Holmes and M. Masuda. "Life Changes and Illness Susceptibility." Paper presented at "Separation and Depression: Clinical and Research Aspects," a symposium in Chicago, Illinois (December 1970).

3 Timothy D. Schellhardt. "Company Memo to Stressed-Out Employees: 'Deal With It'." *The Wall Street Journal* (October 2, 1996).

4 G.F. Soloman. "Emotions, Stress, the Central Nervous System and Immunity." *Annals of the New York Academy of Sciences* 164:2 (October 1969), 335-343. A.F. Rasmussen, Jr. "Emotions and Immunity." *Annals of the New York Academy of Sciences* 164:2 (October 1969), 458-462.

5 C.B. Bahnson and M.B. Bahnson. "Cancer as an Alternative to Psychosis: A Theoretical Model of Somatic and Psychologic Regression." In: D.M. Kissen and L.L. LeShan, eds. *Psychosomatic Aspects of Neoplastic Disease* (Philadelphia: J.B. Lippincott, 1964), 184-202. F.B. Levenson. *The Causes and Prevention of Cancer* (New York: Stein and Day, 1985).

6 R.W. Bartrop et al. "Depressed Lymphocyte Function After Bereavement." *The Lancet* 1:8016 (April 1977), 834-836.

7 H. Selye. *Stress Without Distress* (New York: New American Library, 1975).

8 J.D. Beasley and J. Swift. *Kellog Report: The Impact of Nutrition, Environment, and Lifestyle on the Health of Americans* (Annandale-on-Hudson, NY: Institute of Health Policy and Practice, The Bard College Center, 1989).

9 F.B. Levenson. *The Causes and Prevention of Cancer* (New York: Stein and Day, 1985).

10 Michael Marmot, Ph.D. *The Lancet* (July 25, 1997).

11 Redford B. William, M.D. "Hostility and the Heart." In: Daniel Goleman, Ph.D., and Joel Gurin, eds. *Mind/Body Medicine* (Yonkers, NY: Consumer Reports Books, 1993), 66-67.

12 C. David Jenkins. "The Mind and the Body." *World Health* 47:2 (March/April 1994), 6-7.

13 S. Cohen, D.A. Tyrrell, and A.P. Smith. "Psychological Stress and Susceptibility to the Common Cold." *New England Journal of Medicine* 325 (August 1991), 606-612.

14 *Harvard Mental Health Letter* 8:7 (January 1992).

15 Larry Dossey. *Meaning and Medicine* (New York: Bantam, 1991), 93.

16 C. Muscari et al. "Role of Reactive Oxygen Species in Cardiovascular Aging." *Molecular and Cellular Biochemistry* 160-161 (July/August 1996), 159-166.

17 *Family Practice News* (April 15, 1996).

18 "Stress Management Strategies Benefit Some Asthmatics." *Modern Medicine* 65 (December 1997), 42-43.

19 J. Achterberg. "Ritual: The Foundation for Transpersonal Medicine." *ReVision* 14:3 (1992), 158-164.

20 H. Benson, M.D. *The Relaxation Response* (New York: William Morrow, 1975).

21 D. Ornish, M.D. *Dr. Dean Ornish's Program for Reversing Heart Disease* (New York: Ballantine, 1990).

22 J. Kabat-Zinn. *Full Catastrophe Living* (New York: Delacorte Press, 1990).

23 D. Goleman. *The Meditative Mind* (Los Angeles: Jeremy P. Tarcher, 1988), 168.

24 J.F. Beary and H. Benson. "A Simple Psychophysiologic Technique Which Elicits the Hypometabolic Changes of the Relaxation Response." *Psychosomatic Medicine* 36:2 (March/April 1974), 115-120. G.S. Everly, Jr., and H. Benson. "Disorders of Arousal and the Relaxation Response: Speculations on the Nature and Treatment of Stress-Related Diseases." *International Journal of Psychosomatics* 36:1-4 (1989), 15-21.

25 D. Goleman. *The Meditative Mind* (Los Angeles: Jeremy P. Tarcher, 1988), 168.

26 R.A. Chalmers et al., eds. *Scientific Research on Maharishi's Transcendental Meditation and TM-Sidih Program: Collected Papers, Vols. 2-4* (Vlodrop, Netherlands: Maharishi Vedic University Press, 1989).

27 R.K. Wallace et al. "Physiological Effects of Transcendental Meditation." *Science* 167 (1970), 1751-1754. M.C. Dillbeck et al. "Physiological Differences Between TM and Rest." *American Physiologist* 42 (1987), 879-881.

28 R.W. Cranson et al. "Transcendental Meditation and Improved Performance on Intelligence-Related Measures: A Longitudinal Study." *Personality and Individual Differences* 12 (1991), 1105-1116.

29 D.H. Shapiro and R.N. Walsh. *Meditation: Classic and Contemporary Perspectives* (New York: Aldine, 1984).

30 M. Murphy. *The Future of the Body* (Los Angeles: Jeremy P. Tarcher, 1992).

31 R. McCraty et al. "The Impact of a New Emotional Self-Management Program on Stress, Emotions, Heart Rate Variability, DHEA, and Cortisol." *Integrative Physiological and Behavioral Science* 33:2 (April-June 1998), 151-170.

32 R. McCraty et al. "The Impact of an Emotional Self-Management Skills Course on Psychosocial Functioning and Autonomic Recovery to Stress in Middle School Children." *Integrative Physiological and Behavioral Science* 34:4 (October-December 1999), 246-268.

33 R. McCraty et al. "The Effects of Emotions on Short-Term Power Spectrum of Heart Rate Variability." *American Journal of Cardiology* 76:14 (November 15, 1995), 1089-093.

34 Doc Childre and Howard Martin with Donna Beech. *The HeartMath Solution* (San Francisco: Harper San Francisco, 1999), 67.

35 M. Murphy. *The Future of the Body* (Los Angeles: Jeremy P. Tarcher, 1992).

36 J. Funderburk. *Science Studies Yoga: A Review of Physiological Data* (Honesdale, PA: Himalayan International Institute of Yoga Science & Philosophy of USA, 1977), 36-41.

37 R. Jahnke. "The Most Profound Medicine, Part II and Part III: Physiological Mechanisms Operating in the Human System During the Practice of Qigong and Yoga *Pranayama*." *Townsend Letter for Doctors* 91-92 (January-February 1991), 124-130, 281-285.

38 Simon Y. Mills, M.A. *The Dictionary of Modern Herbalism* (Rochester, VT: Healing Arts Press, 1988), 58-59.

39 S. Foster. *Passion Flower* Botanical Series 314 (Austin, TX: American Botanical Council, 1993).

40 German Ministry of Health. *Valerian: Commission E Monographs for Phytomedicines* (Bonn, Germany: German Ministry of Health, 1985).

41 D.O. Gagnon. *Healing Herbs for Your Nervous System* (Santa Fe, NM: Santa Fe Botanical Research & Educational Project, 1992).

42 E. Bach and F.J. Wheeler. *The Bach Flower Remedies* (New Canaan, CT: Keats Publishing, 1977).

43 P. Wooten. "Laughter as Therapy for Patient and Caregiver." In: J. Hodgkin, G. Connors, and C. Bell, eds. *Pulmonary Rehabilitation* (Philadelphia: Lippincott, 1993), 10.

VISION DISORDERS

1 M.A. Krupp, M.J. Chatton, and L.M. Tierney, eds. *Current Medical Diagnosis and Treatment* (Los Altos, CA: Lange Medical Publications, 1982), 77-84.

2 J.E. Pizzorno and M.T. Murray. *A Textbook of Natural Medicine* (Seattle, WA: John Bastyr College Publications), 1989.

3 *American Journal of Epidemiology* 154 (July 15, 2001), 138-144.

4 J.E. Pizzorno and M.T. Murray. *A Textbook of Natural Medicine* (Seattle, WA: John Bastyr College Publications), 1989.

5 L.G. Hyman et al. "Senile Macular Degeneration: A Case-Control Study." *American Journal of Epidemiology* 118 (1983), 213-227. M.E. Paetkau et al. "Senile Discform Macular Degeneration and Smoking." *Canadian Journal of Ophthalmology* 13 (1978), 67-71.

6 L. Levine. "Optometrically-Relevant Side Effects of the Systemic Drugs Most Frequently Prescribed in 1991." *Journal of Behavioral Optometry* 3:5 (1992), 115-119.

7 *Physicians' Desk Reference* 46th Ed. (Montvale, NJ: Medical Economics, 1992).

8 *British Journal of Ophthalmology* 85 (July 2001), 855-860.

9 J. Liberman. *Light: Medicine of the Future* (Santa Fe, NM: Bear & Company, 1991). D.B. Harman. *The Coordinated Classroom* (Grand Rapids, MI: American Seating, 1951).

10 G. Swartwout and J. Henahan. *Cataract Prevention: A Nutritional Approach* (Farmington Hills, MI: The Holistic Optometrist, 1986).

11 A. Duarte. *Cataract Breakthrough* (Huntington Beach, CA: International Institute of Natural Health Sciences, 1982).

12 J.K. Dart, F. Stapleton, and D. Minassian. "Contact Lenses and Other Risk Factors in Microbial Keratitis." *The Lancet* 338:8768 (September 1991), 650-653.

13 Jay B. Lavine. *The Eye Care Sourcebook* (Chicago: Contemporary Books, 2001), 54-56.

14 A.R. Gaby, M.D., and J.V. Wright, M.D. "Nutritional Factors in Degenerative Eye Disorders: Cataract and Macular Degeneration." *Journal of Advancement in Medicine* 6:1 (Spring 1993), 27-39.

15 Ibid.

16 Robert S. Ivker, Robert A. Anderson, and Larry Trivieri, Jr. *The Complete Self-Care Guide to Holistic Medicine* (New York: Tarcher/Putnam, 1999), 435.

17 G.T. Peachey. "Perspectives on Optometric Visual Training." *Journal of Behavioral Optometry* 1:3 (1990), 65-70.

18 J.N. Zaba and R.A. Johnson. "Literacy: The Vision, Learning, and Volunteer Connection." *Journal of Behavioral Optometry* 3:5 (1992), 128-130.

19 H.A. Solan. "Visual Perceptual Factors and Reading. Clinical Implications of Some Recent Optometric Research." *Journal of Behavioral Optometry* 1:3 (1990), 59-64.

20 W.H. Bates. *The Bates Method for Better Eyesight Without Glasses* (New York: Henry Holt/Owl Books, 1981).

21 *Townsend Letter for Doctors* (November 1989).

22 L. Lebuisson et al. "Treatment of Senile Macular Degeneration with *Ginkgo biloba* Extract: A Preliminary Double-Blind, Drug Versus Placebo Study." In: *Rokan (Ginkgo biloba): Recent Results in Pharmacology and Clinic* (New York: Springer-Verlag, 1988). A. Scharrer and M. Ober. "Anthocyanosides in the Treatment of Retinopathies." *Klinische Monatsblatter fur Augenheilkunde* 178:5 (May 1981), 386-389.

23 M.I. Bykova and T.L. Sosnova. "The Experience in Using *Eleutherococcus* for Raising the Level of Color Discrimination Function in Railroad Engineers." *Gigiena i Sanitariia* 6 (June 1976), 108-110.

24 Robert S. Ivker, Robert A. Anderson, and Larry Trivieri, Jr. *The Complete Self-Care Guide to Holistic Medicine* (New York: Tarcher/Putnam, 1999), 436.

WOMEN'S HEALTH

1 A. Kalo-Klein and S.S. Witkin. "Candida Albicans: Cellular Immune System Interactions During Different Stages of the Menstrual Cycle." *American Journal of Obstetrics and Gynecology* 161:5 (November 1989), 1132-1136.

2 A. Kalo-Klein and S.S. Witkin. "Candida Albicans: Cellular Immune System Interactions During Different Stages of the Menstrual Cycle." *American Journal of Obstetrics and Gynecology* 161:5 (November 1989), 1132-1136.

3 G.A. Edelstam et al. "Cyclic Variation of Major Histocompatibility Complex Class II Antigen Expression in the Human Fallopian Tube Epithelium." *Fertility and Sterility* 57:6 (June 1992), 1225-1229.

4 P. Braus. "Facing Menopause." *American Demographics* 15:3 (March 1993), 44-49.

5 A.H. Follingstad. "Estriol, the Forgotten Estrogen?" *Journal of the American Medical Association* 239:l (January 1978), 29-30.

6 The Boston Women's Health Book Collective. *The New Our Bodies, Ourselves: A Book by and for Women* (New York: Simon and Schuster, 1992), 278.

7 S.L. Huffman et al. "Suckling Patterns and Post-Partum Amenorrheoea in Bangladesh." *Journal of Biosocial Science* 19:2 (April 1987), 171-179.

8 K.I. Kennedy and C.M. Visness. "Contraceptive Efficiency of Lactational Amenorrhoea." *The Lancet* 339:8787 (January 1992), 227-230.

9 P. Campbell. "Efficacy of Female Condom." *The Lancet* 341:8853 (May 1993), 1155.

10 C.D. Lytle et al. "Virus Leakage Through Natural Membrane Condoms." *Sexually Transmitted Diseases* 17:2 (April-June 1990), 58-62.

11 M.Y. Dawood. "Current Concepts in the Etiology and Treatment of Primary Dysmenorrhea." *Acta Obstetricia et Gynecologica Scandinavica* 138 Suppl (1986), 7-10.

12 S.M. Lark, M.D. *Menstrual Cramps: A Self-Help Program* (Los Altos, CA: Westchester Publishing, 1993).

13 J.E. Pizzorno and M.T. Murray, eds. *A Textbook of Natural Medicine* (Seattle, WA: John Bastyr College Publications, 1988-1989).

14 S.M. Lark, M.D. *Menstrual Cramps: A Self-Help Program* (Los Altos, CA: Westchester Publishing, 1993).

15 Ralph Golan, M.D. *Optimal Wellness* (New York: Ballantine Books, 1995), 329.

16 Ibid.

17 Paul Callinan. *Family Homeopathy: A Practical Handbook for Home Treatment* (New Canaan, CT: Keats Publishing, 1995), 184-185.

18 M.L. Taymor et al. "The Etiological Role of Chronic Iron Deficiency in Production of Menorrhagia." *Journal of the American Medical Association* 187:5 (1964), 323-327.

19 J.D. Cohen, M.D., and H.W. Rubin, M.D. "Functional Menorrhagia: Treatment with Bioflavonoids and Vitamin C." *Current Therapeutic Research* 2:11 (November 1960), 539-542. D.M. Lithgow and W.M. Poltizer. "Vitamin A in the Treatment of Menorrhagia." *South African Medical Journal* 51:7 (February 1977), 191-193.

20 Jacques Jouanny, M.D., et al. *Homeopathic Therapeutics: Possibilities in Chronic Pathology* (France: Editions Boiron, 1994), 189-190.

21 G.E. Abraham and M.M. Lubran. "Serum and Red Cell Magnesium Levels in Patients with Premenstrual Tension." *American Journal of Clinical Nutrition* 34:11 (November 1981), 2364-2366. T.M. John. "Premenstrual Syndrome as a Western Culture-Specific Disorder." *Culture, Medicine and Psychiatry* 11:3 (September 1987), 337-356.

22 S.M. Lark, M.D. *PMS Self-Help Book: A Woman's Guide* (Berkeley, CA: Celestial Arts, 1984), 26-27.

23 Alan R. Gaby, M.D. *Nutrition and Healing* 1:3 (October 1994), 6.

24 G.E. Abraham and M.M. Lubran. "Serum and Red Cell Magnesium Levels in Patients with Premenstrual Tension." *American Journal of Clinical Nutrition* 34:11 (November 1981), 2364-2366.

25 A. Stewart. "Clinical and Biochemical Effects of Nutritional Supplementation on the Premenstrual Syndrome." *Journal of Reproductive Medicine* 32:6 (June 1987), 435-441.

26 B. Larsson, A. Jonasson, and S. Fianu. "Evening Primrose Oil in the Treatment of Premenstrual Syndrome." *Current Therapeutic Research* 46:1 (July 1989), 58-63.

27 J.T. Salonen et al. "High Stored Iron Levels are Associated with Excess Risk of Myocardial Infarction in Eastern Finnish Men." *Circulation* 86:3 (September 1992), 803-811. S. Hite. *The Hite Report* (New York: Macmillan, 1976), 351.

28 Erich Keller. *Complete Home Guide to Aromatherapy* (Tiburon, CA: H.J. Kramer, 1991).

29 F. Kronenberg. "Hot Flashes: Epidemiology and Physiology." *Annals of the New York Academy of Sciences* 592 (1990), 52-86, 123-133.

30 Ibid.

31 H. Adlercreutz et al. "Urinary Excretion of Lignans and Isoflavonoid Phytoestrogens in Japanese

Men and Women Consuming a Traditional Japanese Diet." *American Journal of Clinical Nutrition* 54:6 (1991), 1093-1100.

32 J.D. Cohen, M.D., and H.W. Rubin, M.D. "Functional Menorrhagia: Treatment with Bioflavonoids and Vitamin C." *Current Therapeutic Research* 2:11 (November 1960), 539-542.

33 J.B. Adam. "Human Breast Cancer: Concerted Role of Diet, Prolactin and Adrenal C19-Delta-5 Steroids in Tumorigenesis." *International Journal of Cancer* 50:6 (April 1992), 854-858.

34 R.L. Prince et al. "Prevention of Postmenopausal Osteoporosis. A Comparative Study of Exercise, Calicium Supplementation, and Hormone-Replacement Therapy." *New England Journal of Medicine* 325:17 (October 1991), 1189-1195.

35 G. Wilcox et al. "Oestrogenic Effects of Plant Foods in Postmenopausal Women." *British Medical Journal* 301:6757 (October 1990), 905-906.

36 H. Adlercreutz et al. "Dietary Phyto-Oestrogens and the Menopause in Japan." *The Lancet* 339:8803 (May 1992), 1233.

37 H. Adlercreutz et al. "Urinary Excretion of Lignans and Isoflavonoid Phytoestrogens in Japanese Men and Women Consuming a Traditional Japanese Diet." *American Journal of Clinical Nutrition* 54:6 (1991), 1093-1100.

38 S.M. Lark, M.D. *Dr. Susan Lark's Menopause Self-Help Book* (Berkeley, CA: Celestial Arts, 1990), 107.

39 S.G. Haynes and M. Feinleib. "Women, Work and Coronary Heart Disease: Prospective Findings from the Framingham Heart Study." *American Journal of Public Health* 70:2 (February 1980), 133-141.

40 S.M. Lark, M.D. *Dr. Susan Lark's Menopause Self-Help Book* (Berkeley, CA: Celestial Arts, 1990).

41 S. Heron. "Botanical Treatment of Infertility, Endometriosis and Symptoms of Menopause." Paper presented to the American Association of Naturopathic Physicians Convention, Botanical Pharmaceuticals, Sedona, Arizona (November 3, 1989).

42 Joseph E. Pizzorno, N.D. "Natural Medicine Approach to the Treatment of Cystitis." *Alternative & Complementary Therapies* (October 1994), 32-34.

43 William G. Crook, M.D. *The Yeast Connection and the Woman* (Jackson, TN: Professional Books, 1995), 85-86.

44 J. Avorn et al. "Reduction of Bacteriuria and Pyuria After Ingestion of Cranberry Juice." *Journal of the American Medical Association* 271 (1994), 751-754.

45 Julian Scott, M.A., Ph.D., and Susan Scott. *Natural Medicine for Women* (New York: Avon Books, 1991), 180.

46 Andrew Lockie, M.D., and Nicola Geddes, M.D. *The Women's Guide to Homeopathy* (New York: St. Martin's Press, 1994), 88-89.

47 Bill Gottlieb. *New Choices in Natural Healing* (Emmaus, PA: Rodale Press, 1995), 547.

48 D. Eschenbach. "Vaginal Infection." *Clinical Obstetrics and Gynecology* 26:1 (March 1983), 186-202.

49 Julian Whitaker, M.D. *Dr. Whitaker's Guide to Natural Healing* (Rocklin, CA: Prima Publishing, 1995), 353.

50 J.E. Pizzorno and M.T. Murray, eds. *A Textbook of Natural Medicine* (Seattle, WA: John Bastyr College Publications, 1988-1989).

51 Paul Reilly, M.D. "Vaginitis and Vulvovaginitis." In: Joseph E. Pizzorno Jr., N.D., and Michael T.

1162

Murray, N.D., eds. *A Textbook of Natural Medicine, Vol. 2* (Seattle, WA: John Bastyr College Publications, 1988), 1-8.

52 J.E. Pizzorno and M.T. Murray, eds. *A Textbook of Natural Medicine* (Seattle, WA: John Bastyr College Publications, 1988-1989).

53 Eliezer Shalev et al. "Ingestion of Yogurt Containing *Lactobacillus acidophilus* Compared with Pasteurized Yogurt as Prophylaxis for Recurrent Candidal Vaginitis and Bacterial Vaginosis." *Archives of Family Medicine* 5 (November/December 1996), 593-596.

54 J.E. Pizzorno and M.T. Murray, eds. *A Textbook of Natural Medicine* (Seattle, WA: John Bastyr College Publications, 1988-1989).

55 Paul Reilly, M.D. "Vaginitis and Vulvovaginitis." In: Joseph E. Pizzorno Jr., N.D., and Michael T. Murray, N.D., eds. *A Textbook of Natural Medicine, Vol. 2* (Seattle, WA: John Bastyr College Publications, 1988), 1-8.

56 Andrew Lockie, M.D., and Nicola Geddes, M.D. *Women's Guide to Homeopathy* (New York: St. Martin's Press, 1994), 84.

57 *What You Need to Know About Cancer of the Uterus* NIH Publication No. 93-1562 (Washington, DC: National Institutes of Health, National Cancer Institute, 1991).

58 F.H. Stuart. *My Body, My Health: the Concerned Woman's Book of Gynecology* (New York: John Wiley & Sons, 1979), 422.

59 Susan M. Lark, M.D. *Fibroid Tumors and Endometriosis Self-Help Book* (Berkeley, CA: Celestial Arts, 1995), 121-144.

60 Susun Weed. *Menopausal Years: The Wise Woman Way* (Woodstock, NY: Ash Tree Publishing, 1992), 12-13.

61 Susan M. Lark, M.D. *Fibroid Tumors and Endometriosis Self-Help Book* (Berkeley, CA: Celestial Arts, 1995), 121-144.

62 J.S. Bernstein et al. *Hysterectomy: A Literature Review and Rating of Appropriateness* (Santa Monica, CA: Rand Publications, 1992), 7-8.

63 S. Heron. "Botanical Treatment of Infertility, Endometriosis and Symptoms of Menopause." Paper presented to the American Association of Naturopathic Physicians Convention, Botanical Pharmaceuticals, Sedona, Arizona (November 3, 1989).

64 V.G. Hufnagel, M.D., and S.K. Golant. *No More Hysterectomies* (New York: Penguin Books, 1989).

65 J.E. Pizzorno and M.T. Murray, eds. *A Textbook of Natural Medicine* (Seattle, WA: John Bastyr College Publications, 1988-1989).

66 C.M. Shreeve, M.D. *The Alternative Dictionary of Symptoms and Cures* (London: Century Hutchinson Publishing, 1986).

67 G.A. Colditz et al. "Family History, Age, and the Risk of Breast Cancer. Prospective Data from the Nurses' Health Study." *Journal of the American Medical Association* 270:3 (July 1993), 338-343.

68 John W. Gofman. *Preventing Breast Cancer* (San Francisco: Committee for Nuclear Responsibility, 1995).

69 National Women's Health Network. *Mammography in Women Before Menopause* (Washington, DC: National Women's Health Network, April 1993).

Quick Reference A-Z Section of Additional Health Conditions

1 James F. Balch, M.D., and Phyllis A. Balch, C.N.C. *Prescription for Nutritional Healing* (Garden City Park, NY: Avery Publishing, 1997), 29.

2 H. Hughes et al. "Treatment of Acne Vulgaris by Biofeedback Relaxation and Cognitive Imagery." *Journal of Psychosomatic Research* 27:3 (1983), 185-191.

3 L. Chaitow. "British Research Connects Ankylosing Spondylitis to Bowel Dysbiosis." *Townsend Letter for Doctors* (July 1989), 364-365.

4 D. Bryce-Smith and R.I.D. Simpson. "Anorexia, Depression and Zinc Deficiency." *The Lancet* 2 (1984), 1162. R. Bakan. "The Role of Zinc in Anorexia Nervosa: Etiology and Treatment." *Medical Hypotheses* 5 (1979), 731-736.

5 H. Glatzel. "Treatment of Dyspeptic Disorders with Spice Extracts." *Hippokrates* 40:23 (1969), 916-919. R. Deininger. "Amarum-Bitter Herbs. Common Bitter Principle Remedies and Their Action." *Krankenplege* 29:3 (1975), 99-100.

6 Bruce Berkowsky, N.M.D., M.H., HMC. "21st Century Self-Care" (unpublished manuscript).

7 Personal report by Jeffry L. Anderson, M.D., of Corte Madera, California, based on his clinical use of Stabilium with patients. T. Dorman et al. "The Effectiveness of Garum Armoricum (Stabilium) in Reducing Anxiety in College Students." *Journal of Advancement in Medicine* 8:3 (Fall 1995), 193-200.

8 S.K. Bhattacharya and S.K. Mitra. "Anxiolytic Activity of *Panax ginseng* Roots: An Experimental Study." *Journal of Ethnopharmacology* 34 (1991), 87-92. C. Hallstrom et al. "Effect of Ginseng on the Performance of Nurses on Night Duty." *Comp Med East West* 6 (1982), 277-282. S.J. Fulder. "Ginseng and the Hypothalamic-Pituitary Control of Stress." *American Journal of Chinese Medicine* 9 (1981), 112-118.

9 D.B. Mowrey, Ph.D. *The Scientific Validation of Herbal Medicine* (New Canaan, CT: Keats Publishing, 1986), 12.

10 E. Lehmann et al. "Efficacy of a Special Kava Extract *(Piper methysticum)* in Patients with States of Anxiety, Tension, and Excitedness of Non-Mental Origin." *Phytomed* 3 (1996), 113-119.

11 Bruce Berkowsky, N.M.D., M.H., HMC. "21st Century Self-Care" (unpublished manuscript).

12 Editor. "Economy Class Syndrome: Blood Clots Can Form in Your Legs on Long-Distance Flights." *Mayo Clinic Health Letter* 7:7 (July 1989), 7.

13 R.S. Williams et al. "Physical Conditioning Augments the Fibrinolytic Response to Venous Occlusion in Healthy Adults." *New England Journal of Medicine* 302:18 (May 1, 1980), 987-991. N.A. Dreyer and S.V. Pizzo. "Blood Coagulation and Idiopathic Thromboembolism Among Fertile Women." *Contraception* 22:2 (August 1980), 123-135.

14 S. Szanto and J. Yudkin. "The Effect of Dietary Sucrose on Blood Lipids, Serum Insulin, Platelet Adhesiveness and Body Weight in Human Volunteers." *Postgraduate Medical Journal* 45 (September 1969), 602. S. Szanto, J. Yudkin, and V.V. Kakkar. "Sugar Intake, Serum Insulin and Platelet Adhesiveness in Men With and Without Peripheral Vascular Disease." *Postgraduate Medical Journal* 45 (September 1969), 608.

15 T.A. David, M.D., J.R. Minehart, M.D., and I.H.

16 V.I. Gaiduk, N.K. Skachkova, and E.A. Fedorovskaia. "Effect of a Flow-Frequency Alternating Magnetic Field on the Microflora and Healing of Burn Wounds." *Vestnik Khirurhii Imeni I.I. Grekova* 134:4 (April 1985), 69-74.

17 K. Branco and M.A. Naeser. "Carpal Tunnel Syndrome: Clinical Outcome After Low-Level Laser Acupuncture, Microamps Transcutaneous Electrical Nerve Stimulation, and Other Alternative Therapies—An Open Protocol Study." *Journal of Alternative and Complementary Medicine* 5:1 (1999), 5-26.

18 S. Luper. "A Review of Plants Used in the Treatment of Liver Disease: Part 1." *Alternative Medicine Review* 3:6 (1998), 410-421.

19 T.N. Kaul et al. "Antiviral Effect of Flavonoids on Human Viruses." *Journal of Medical Virology* 15 (1985), 71-79.

20 R. Pompei et al. "Glycyrrhizic Acid Inhibits Virus Growth and Inactivates Virus Particles." *Nature* 281:5733 (October 25, 1979), 689-690.

21 R. Pothmann and G. Schmitz. "Acupressure in the Acute Treatment of Cerebral Convulsions in Children." *Journal of Alternative Medicine* 1:1 (1985), 63-67.

22 D.M. Fergusson, L.J. Horwood, and F.T. Shannon. "Early Solid Feeding and Recurrent Childhood Eczema: A 10-Year Longitudinal Study." *Pediatrics* 86:4 (October 1990), 541-546.

23 A.V. Strosser and L.S. Nelson. "Synthetic Vitamin A in the Treatment of Eczema in Children." *Annals of Allergy* 10 (1952), 703-704. S. Wright and J.L. Burton. "Oral Evening-Primrose-Seed Oil Improves Atopic Eczema." *The Lancet* (November 20, 1982), 1120-1122. D.F. Horrobin. "Essential Fatty Acid Metabolism and Its Modification in Atopic Eczema." *American Journal of Clinical Nutrition* 71:1 Suppl (2000), 367S-372S.

24 A.C. Markey et al. "Platelet Activating Factor-Induced Clinical and Histopathologic Responses in Atopic Skin and Their Modification by the Platelet Activating Factor Antagonist BN52603." *Journal of the American Academy of Dermatology* 23:2 (1990), 263-268.

25 C.S. Ginandes and D.I. Rosenthal. "Using Hypnosis to Accelerate the Healing of Bone Fractures: A Randomized Controlled Pilot Study." *Alternative Therapies in Health and Medicine* 5:2 (1999), 67-75.

26 P.J. Skerrett. "Fat May Cut Gallstone Risk in Dieters." *Medical Tribune* 34:5 (March 11), 15.

27 G. Misciagna et al. "Diet, Physical Activity, and Gallstones—A Population-Based, Case-Control Study in Southern Italy." *American Journal of Clinical Nutrition* 69:1 (1999), 120-126.

28 D.L. Diehl. "Acupuncture for Gastrointestinal and Hepatobiliary Disorders." *Journal of Alternative and Complementary Medicine* 5:1 (1999), 27-45.

29 R.A. Goyer. "Nutrition and Metal Toxicity." *American Journal of Clinical Nutrition* 61:3 Suppl (1995), 646S-650S.

30 Ibid.

31 A.L. Miller. "Dimercaptosuccinic Acid (DMSA), a Non-Toxic, Water-Soluble Treatment for Heavy Metal Toxicity." *Alternative Medicine Review* 3:3 (1998), 199-207.

32 S.P. Thyagarajan et al. "Effect of *Phyllanthus amarus* on Chronic Carriers of Hepatitis B Virus." *The Lancet* 2:8614 (October 1, 1988), 764-766.

Kornblueh, M.D. "Polarized Air as an Adjunct in the Treatment of Burns." *American Journal of Physical Medicine* 39:3 (June 1960), 111-113.

33 M. Lesser, M.D. *Nutrition and Vitamin Therapy* (Berkeley, CA: Parker House, 1980).

34 R. Neubauer. "A Plant Protease for the Potentiation of and Possible Replacement of Antibiotics." *Exp Med Surg* 19 (1961), 143-160.

35 A.H. Amin et al. "Berberine Sulfate: Antimicrobial Activity, Bioassay, and Mode of Action." *Canadian Journal of Microbiology* 15:9 (1969), 1067-1076.

36 D.B. Mowrey, Ph.D. *The Scientific Validation of Herbal Medicine* (New Canaan, CT: Keats Publishing, 1986), 158.

37 R. Bauer and H. Wagner. "Echinacea Specieas as Potential Immunostimulatory Drugs." *Econ Med Plant Res* 5 (1991), 253-321.

38 Allan Sachs, D.C., C.C.N. *The Authoritative Guide to Grapefruit Seed Extract* (Mendocino, CA: Life Rhythm, 1997), 17-19.

39 Morton Walker, D.P.M. "Antimicrobial Attributes of Olive Leaf Extract." *Townsend Letter for Doctors and Patients* (July 1996), 80-85.

40 P.M. Altman. "Australian Tea Tree Oil." *Australian Journal of Pharmacy* 69 (1988), 276-278.

41 C. Di Padova. "S-Adenosylmethionine in the Treatment of Osteoarthritis: Review of the Clinical Studies." *American Journal of Medicine* 83:5A (1987), 60-65.

42 M.J. James, R.A. Gibson, and L.G. Cleland. "Dietary Polyunsaturated Fatty Acids and Inflammatory Mediator Production." *American Journal of Clinical Nutrition* 71:1 Suppl (2000), 343S-348S.

43 *British Herbal Pharmacopoeia* (West Yorks, England: British Herbal Medicine Association, 1983). R.F. Chandler et al. "Herbal Remedies of the Maritime Indians: Sterols and Triterpenes of *Achillea Millefolium L.* (Yarrow)." *Journal Pharm Sci* 71:6 (1982).

44 R.R. Kulkarni et al. "Treatment of Osteoarthritis with a Herbomineral Formulation: A Double-Blind, Placebo-Controlled, Cross-Over Study." *Journal of Ethnopharmacology* 33 (1991), 91-95. G.K. Reddy et al. "Urinary Excretion of Connective Tissue Metabolites Under the Influence of a New Non-Steroidal Anti-Inflammatory Agent in Adjuvant Induced Arthritis." *Agents and Actions* 22 (1987), 99-105. H.P.T. Ammon et al. "Mechansim of Anti-Inflammatory Actions of Curcumine and Boswellic Acids." *Journal of Ethnopharmacology* 38 (1993), 113-119.

45 S. Ehrenprets. "Mobilization of Endorphins as the Basis for Effectiveness of Acupuncture Therapy." *Acupuncture and Electro-Therapeutics Res Int J* 13:4 (1988), 201-203.

46 J. Shuster et al. "Soft Drink Consumption and Urinary Stone Recurrence: A Randomized Prevention Trial." *Journal of Clinical Epidemiology* 45:8 (August 1992), 911-916.

47 W.G. Robertson, M. Peacock, D.H. Marshall. "Prevalence of Urinary Stone Disease in Vegetarians." *European Urology* 8:6 (1982), 334-339.

48 G.C. Curhan et al. "A Prospective Study of Dietary Calcium and Other Nutrients and the Risk of Symptomatic Kidney Stones." *New England Journal of Medicine* 328:12 (March 25, 1993), 833-838.

49 James F. Balch, M.D., and Phyllis A. Balch, C.N.C. *Prescription for Nutritional Healing* (Garden City Park, NY: Avery Publishing, 1997), 358.

50 Dharma Singh Khalsa, M.D. *Brain Longevity* (New York: Warner Books, 1997), 51.

51 Ibid., 262.

52 P.M. Kidd. "A Review of Nutrients and Botanicals in the Integrative Management of Cognitive Dysfunction." *Alternative Medicine Review* 4:3 (1999), 144-161.

53 Melvyn R. Werbach, M.D. and Michael T. Murray, N.D. *Botanical Influences on Illness* (Tarzana, CA: Third Line Press, 2000), 119. J.A. Mix and W.D. Crews, Jr. "An Examination of the Efficacy of *Ginkgo biloba* Extract EGb761 on the Neuropsychologic Functioning of Cognitively Intact Older Adults." *Journal of Alternative and Complementary Medicine* 6:3 (2000), 219-229.

54 R.C. Wren, F.L.S. *Potter's New Cyclopaedia of Botanical Drugs and Preparations* (Saffron, Walden, England: C.W. Daniel), 128-129.

55 P.M. Kidd. "A Review of Nutrients and Botanicals in the Integrative Management of Cognitive Dysfunction." *Alternative Medicine Review* 4:3 (1999), 144-161.

56 Jack Masquelier. "Recent Advances in the Therapeutic Activity of Procyanidins, Natural Products as Medicinal Agents." In: J.L. Beal and E. Reinhard, eds. Supplement of *Plant Medica, Journal of Medicinal Plant Research*, and *Journal of Natural Products* (July 1980), 2443-2455.

57 D.B. Mowrey and D.E. Clayson. "Motion Sickness, Ginger, and Psychophysics." *The Lancet* 1:8273 (March 20, 1982), 655-657. S. Holtmann et al. "The Anti-Motion Sickness Mechanism of Ginger: A Comparative Study with Placebo and Dimenhydrinate." *Acta Oto-laryngology Stockholm* 108:3-4 (September/October 1989), 168-174. A. Grontved et al. "Ginger Root Against Seasickness: A Controlled Trial on the Open Sea." *Acta Oto-laryngology Stockholm* 105:1-2 (January/February 1988), 45-49.

58 L.G. Hochman et al. "Brittle Nails: Response to Daily Biotin Supplementation." *Cutis* 51 (1993), 303-307.

59 J.S. Schneider et. al. "Recovery from Experimental Parkinism in Primates with GM1 Ganglioside Treatment." *Science* 256:5058 (May 8, 1992). 843-846.

60 W. Birkmayer and G.J. Birkmayer. "Nicotinamidadenindinucleotide (NADH): The New Approach in the Therapy of Parkinson's Disease." *Annals of Clinical and Laboratory Science* 19:1 (January-February 1989), 38-43.

61 A.D. Ericsson, M.D., et al. "Neurotrophin 1: Treatment of Parkinson's Disease." *Explore!* 3:6 (1992), 19-22.

62 "An Alternative Medicine Treatment for Parkinson's Disease: Results of a Multicenter Clinical Trial, HP-200 in Parkinson's Disease Study Group." *Journal of Alternative and Complementary Medicine* 1:3 (1995), 249-255.

63 A.R. Pack. "Folate Mouthwash: Effects on Established Gingivitis in Periodontal Patients." *Journal of Clinical Periodontology* 11:9 (October 1984), 619-628.

64 B.E. Cohen et al. "Reversal of Postoperative Immunosuppression in Man by Vitamin A." *Surg Gynecol Obstet* 149:5 (November 1979), 658-662. W.M. Ringsdorf, Jr., and E. Cheraskin. "Vitamin C and Human Wound Healing." *Oral Surg Oral Med Oral Pathol* 53:3 (March 1982), 231-236. A. Barbul et al. "Wound Healing and Thymotropic Effects of Arginine: A Pituitary Mechanism of Action." *American Journal of Clinical Nutrition* 37 (1983), 786-794.

65 A. di Fabio. "The Surprising Psoriasis Treatment." *Art of Getting Well* (Franklin, TN: Rheumatoid Disease Foundation, 1989).

66 V.A. Ziboh et al. *Archives of Dermatology* (November 1986).

67 A. di Fabio. "The Surprising Psoriasis Treatment." *Art of Getting Well* (Franklin, TN: Rheumatoid Disease Foundation, 1989).

68 The complete fumaric acid treatment protocol for psoriasis may be obtained from: Rheumatoid Disease Foundation, 5106 Old Harding Road, Franklin, TN 37064; (615) 646-1030.

69 Cardiovascular Research, 1061-B Shary Circle, Concord, CA 94518; (800) 888-4585.

70 F.M. Thurman. "The Treatment of Psoriasis with Sarsaparilla Compound." *New England Journal of Medicine* 227:4 (July 1942), 128-133.

71 Melvyn R. Werbach, M.D., and Michael T. Murray, N.D. *Botanical Influences on Illness* (Tarzana, CA: Third Line Press, 1988), 290.

72 "Radical Protection for Athletes (Dietary Supplements' Effects)." *Science News* 141:24 (June 13, 1992), 398.

73 C.K. Reddy et al. "Studies on the Metabolism of Glycosaminoglycans Under the Influence of New Herbal Anti-Inflammatory Agents." *Biochemical Pharmacol* 20 (1989), 3527-3534.

74 Simon Mills. *The Dictionary of Modern Herbalism* (Rochester, NY: Healing Arts Press, 1988), 67.

75 C.F. Garland, Dr.P.H., F.A.C.E., F.C. Garland, Ph.D., F.A.C.E., and E.D. Gorham, M.P.H. "Could Sunscreens Increase Melanoma Risk?" *American Journal of Public Health* 82:4 (April 1992), 614-615.

76 W.R. Walker and D.M. Keats. "An Investigation of the Therapeutic Value of the 'Copper Bracelet': Dermal Assimilation of Copper in Arthritic/Rheumatoid Conditions." *Agents and Actions* 6:4 (1976), 454-459.

77 D. Zafriri et al. "Inhibitory Activity of Cranberry Juice on Adherence of Type 1 and Type P Fimbriated *Escherichia coli* to Eucaryotic Cells." *Anti-Microbial Agents and Chemotherapy* 33:1 (January 1989), 92-98.

78 S.M. Creighton and S.L. Stanton. "Caffeine: Does It Affect Your Bladder?" *British Journal of Urology* 66:6 (December 1990), 613-614.

79 L. Ronberger and J. Golles. "On the Prevention of Thrombosis with Aesculus Extract." *Medizinische Klinik* 64:26 (1969), 1207-1209.

80 D.M. Warburton. "Clinical Psycho-Pharmacology of *Ginkgo biloba* Extract." *Presse Medicale* 15:31 (September 25, 1986), 1595-1604.

81 A. Grontved and E. Hentzer. "Vertigo-Reducing Effect of Ginger Root: A Controlled Clinical Study." *Journal of Oto-rhinolaryngology and Its Related Specialties* 48:5 (1986), 282-286.

82 Morton Walker, D.P.M. "Antimicrobial Attributes of Olive Leaf Extract." *Townsend Letter for Doctors and Patients* (July 1996), 80-85.

83 I. Beladi et al. "*In Vitro* and *In Vivo* Antiviral Effects of Flavonoids." In: L. Farkas et al., eds. *Flavonoids and Bioflavonoids* (New York: Elsevier, 1982), 443-450.

84 G.S. Kelly. "Larch Arabinogalactan: Clinical Relevance of a Novel Immune-Enhancing Polysaccharide." *Alternative Medicine Review* 4:2 (1999), 96-103.

Appendices

APPENDIX A: LIFE-SAVING TESTS YOUR DOCTOR MAY NOT KNOW ABOUT

1 David Casemore, M.D. "Foodborne Protozoal Infection." *The Lancet* 336 (December 1990), 1427-1432.

2 J. Krop et al. "A Double-Blind, Randomized, Con-

trolled Investigation of Electrodermal Testing in the Diagnosis of Allergies." *Journal of Alternative and Complementary Medicine* 3:3 (Fall 1997), 241-248.

3 Will Block and John Morgenthaler. "Food Allergies More Common Than You Think: Interview with Michael Rosenbaum, M.D." *Life Enhancement* 34 (June 1997), 3-7.

APPENDIX B: VACCINATIONS

1 D. Bookchin and J. Schumacher. "The Virus and the Vaccine." *The Atlantic Monthly* (February 2000), 68-80.

2 Committee on Government Reform, Dan Burton, Chairman, 106th Congress of the United States. "Mercury in Medicine—Are We Taking Unnecessary Risks?" Hearings before the U.S. Congress (July 18, 2000).

3 L.G. Horowitz and W.J. Martin. *Emerging Viruses: AIDS & Ebola—Nature, Accident or Intentional?* (Sandpoint, ID: Tetrahedron Publishing Group, 1998).

4 Committee on Government Reform, U.S. House of Representatives. Conflicts of Interest in Vaccine Policy Making: Majority Staff Report (August 21, 2000).

5 S. Kaplan. "Autism-Vaccine Link Raised in Hearing: Psychologist Tells House Panel That Steep Rise in Disorder May Stem from Immunization Campaign, A Theory Hotly Contested by Other Experts." *The Los Angeles Times* (April 7, 2000), 3.

6 L.G. Horowitz. *Horowitz on Vaccines* (Sandpoint, ID: Tetrahedron Publishing Group, 1998).

7 L.G. Horowitz. "Polio, Hepatitis B and AIDS: An Integrative Theory on a Possible Vaccine-Induced Pandemic." *Medical Hypotheses* 56:5 (2001), 677-686.

8 U.S. Food and Drug Administration. "Adverse Events Associated with Childhood Vaccines: Evidence Bearing on Causality." Press release (September 1993).

9 J.E. Pope et al. "The Development of Rheumatoid Arthritis after Recombinant Hepatitis B Vaccination." *Journal of Rheumatology* 25:9 (1998), 1687-1693. "France Suspends Hepatitis B Inoculations: Worry About Link Between Vaccine, Multiple Sclerosis." Associated Press report (October 4, 1998).

10 S.K. Stanley et al. "Effect of Immunization with a Common Recall Antigen on Viral Expression in Patients Infected with Human Immunodeficiency Virus Type 1." *New England Journal of Medicine* 334:19 (1996), 1222-1230.

11 T. Nakayama et al. "Long-Term Regulation of Interferon Production by Lymphocytes from Children Inoculated with Live Measles Virus Vaccine." *Journal of Infectious Diseases* 158:6 (1988), 1386-1390.

12 J.S. Alm et al. "Atopy in Children of Families with an Anthroposophic Lifestyle." *The Lancet* 353:163 (May 1, 1999), 1485-1488.

13 Institute of Medicine. *Adverse Events Associated with Childhood Vaccines: Evidence Bearing on Causality* (Washington, DC: National Academy Press, 1994).

14 J.B. Classen. "Childhood Immunisation and Diabetes Mellitus." *New Zealand Medical Journal* 109:1022 (1996), 195.

15 Randall Neustaedter, O.M.D., L.Ac., Classical Medicine Center, 1779 Woodside Road, Suite 201C, Redwood City, CA 94061; (650) 299-9170; website: www.cure-guide.com.

16 M. Burnet and D. White. *The Natural History of Infectious Disease* (Cambridge, England: Cambridge University Press, 1972), 16.

17 L. Strebel et al. "Epidemology in the U.S. One Decade After the Last Reported Case of Indigenous Wild Virus Associated Disease." *Clinical Infectious Diseases* (February 1992), 568-579.

18 "Federal Health Panel Advises Switching to Polio Shots." Associated Press report (June 19, 1999).

19 *Physicians' Desk Reference (PDR)* 50th Ed. (Oradell, NJ: Medical Economics, 1996), 885-886, 891-892, 1388-1390.

20 Ibid.

21 J. Butel et al. "Molecular Evidence of Simian Virus 40 Infections in Children." *Journal of Infectious Diseases* 180 (September 1999), 884-887.

22 *Physicians' Desk Reference (PDR)* 50th Ed. (Oradell, NJ: Medical Economics, 1996), 872-875.

23 R. Moskowitz. "Immunizations: The Other Side." *Mothering* (Spring 1984), 34.

24 I. Golden. *Vaccination? A Review of Risks and Alternatives* (Geelong, Victoria, Australia: Arum Healing Center, 1991), 31.

25 R. Moskowitz. "Immunizations: The Other Side." *Mothering* (Spring 1984), 34.

26 U.S. Department of Health and Human Services. "Immunization: Survey of Recent Research." (April 1983), 76.

27 "Nature and Rates of Adverse Reactions Associated with DPT and DT Immunizations." *Pediatrics* 68:5 (1981).

28 W. James. *Immunization: The Reality Behind the Myth* (South Hadley, MA: Bergin & Garvey, 1988), 14.

29 W.C. Torch. "Diptheria-Pertussis-Tetanus (DPT) Immunization: A Potential Cause of Sudden Infant Death Syndrome (SIDS)." American Academy of Neurology, 34th Annual Meeting (April 25-May 1, 1982). *Neurology* 32:4 Part 2.

30 *Physicians' Desk Reference (PDR)* 50th Ed. (Oradell, NJ: Medical Economics, 1996), 875-879, 892-895.

31 Ibid.

32 R. Mendelsohn. *How to Raise a Healthy Child...In Spite of Your Doctor* (Chicago: Contemporary Books, 1984), 223.

33 R. Moskowitz. "Immunizations: The Other Side." *Mothering* (Spring 1984), 34.

34 I. Golden. *Vaccination? A Review of Risks and Alternatives* (Geelong, Victoria, Australia: Arum Healing Center, 1991), 31.

35 R. Mendelsohn. *How to Raise a Healthy Child...In Spite of Your Doctor* (Chicago: Contemporary Books, 1984), 223.

36 J. Frank, Jr., et al. "Measles Elimination: Final Impediments." 20th Immunization Conference Proceedings (May 6-9, 1985), 21.

37 *Physicians' Desk Reference (PDR)* 50th Ed. (Oradell, NJ: Medical Economics, 1996), 1610-1611; 1687-1689.

38 S. Solovitch. "Do Vaccines Spur Autism in Kids?" *San Jose Mercury News* (May 25, 1999).

39 *Physicians' Desk Reference (PDR)* 50th Ed. (Oradell, NJ: Medical Economics, 1996), 1610-1611, 1687-1689.

40 R. Moskowitz. "Immunizations: The Other Side." *Mothering* (Spring 1984), 34.

41 *Physicians' Desk Reference (PDR)* 50th Ed. (Oradell, NJ: Medical Economics, 1996), 1708-1709.

42 R. Mendelsohn. *How to Raise a Healthy Child...In Spite of Your Doctor* (Chicago: Contemporary Books, 1984), 218.

43 Beverley Allan. *Australian Nurses Journal* (May 1978).

44 Hannah Allen. *Don't Get Stuck: The Case Against Vaccinations* (Oldsmar, FL: Natural Hygiene Press, 1985), 144.

45 *Physicians' Desk Reference (PDR)* 50th Ed. (Oradell, NJ: Medical Economics, 1996), 1697-1699.

46 "Attenuation of RA 27/3 Rubella Virus in WI-38 Human Diploid Cells." *American Journal of Diseases of Children* (August 1969), 118. See also: "Studies of Immunization with Living Rubella Virus." *American Journal of Diseases of Children* (October 1965), 110.

47 J. Hanchette. "Safety of Controversial Hepatitis B Vaccine at Center of Debate." Gannett News Service report (May 18, 1999).

48 *Physicians' Desk Reference (PDR)* 50th Ed. (Oradell, NJ: Medical Economics, 1996), 1744-1747, 2482-2484.

49 L.G. Horowitz. "Vaccinations for Global Genocide." In: *Death in the Air: Globalism, Terrorism and Toxic Warfare* (Sandpoint, ID: Tetrahedron Publishing Group, 2001), 255-298.

50 L.G. Horowitz. *Horowitz on Vaccines* (Sandpoint, ID: Tetrahedron Publishing Group, 1998). *Physicians' Desk Reference (PDR)* 50th Ed. (Oradell, NJ: Medical Economics, 1996), 1744-1747, 2482-2484.

51 L.G. Horowitz. "Vaccinations for Global Genocide." In: *Death in the Air: Globalism, Terrorism and Toxic Warfare* (Sandpoint, ID: Tetrahedron Publishing Group, 2001), 1762-1765.

52 Ibid.

53 U.S. Centers for Disease Control and Prevention. "CDC Viral Hepatitis A Fact Sheet." (September 29, 2000). Available on the Internet: www.cdc.gov/ncidod/diseases/hepatitis/a/fact.htm.

54 U.S. Centers for Disease Control and Prevention. "CDC Hepatitis A Vaccine Information Statement." (August 25, 1998).

55 U.S. Centers for Disease Control and Prevention. "CDC Hepatitis A Facts." (November 16, 2000).

56 *Mosby's GenRX®* 10th Ed. (St. Louis, MO: Mosby, 1998). Hepatitis A vaccine (003158) as posted on MDConsult website: www.mdconsult.com.

57 U.S. Centers for Disease Control and Prevention. "CDC Hepatitis A Vaccine Information Statement." (August 25, 1998).

58 U.S. Centers for Disease Control and Prevention. "CDC Hepatitis A Facts." (November 16, 2000).

59 *Mosby's GenRX®* 10th Ed. (St. Louis, MO: Mosby, 1998). Hepatitis A vaccine (003158) as posted on MDConsult website: www.mdconsult.com.

60 M. Horwin. "Prevnar: A Critical Review of a New Childhood Vaccine." (September 19, 2000); Prevnar package insert, Wyeth Lederle (February 17, 2000).

61 M. Horwin. "Prevnar: A Critical Review of a New Childhood Vaccine." (September 19, 2000); Prevnar package insert, Wyeth Lederle (February 17, 2000). E. Erdem Cantekin. "Pneumococcal Vaccine and Otitis Media." The National Vaccine Information Center's 2nd International Public Conference (September 8, 2000).

62 M. Horwin. "Prevnar: A Critical Review of a New Childhood Vaccine." (September 19, 2000); Prevnar package insert, Wyeth Lederle (February 17, 2000).

63 Committee on Government Reform, U.S. House of Representatives. "Conflicts of Interest in Vaccine Policy Making: Majority Staff Report." (August 21, 2000). K.M. Severyn. "Profits, not Sci-

ence, Motivate Vaccine Mandates." *Well Being Journal* 10:2 (2001), 1, 24. L.G. Horowitz. "Vaccination: The Ungodly Practice." In: *Healing Celebrations: Miraculous Recoveries Through Ancient Scripture, Natural Medicine and Modern Science* (Sandpoint, ID: Tetrahedron Publishing Group, 2000), 185-191.

64 L.G. Horowitz. *Horowitz on Vaccines* (Sandpoint, ID: Tetrahedron Publishing Group, 1998). L.G. Horowitz. "Vaccinations for Global Genocide." In: *Death in the Air: Globalism, Terrorism and Toxic Warfare* (Sandpoint, ID: Tetrahedron Publishing Group, 2001), 255-298.

65 L.G. Horowitz. "Vaccination: The Ungodly Practice." In: *Healing Celebrations: Miraculous Recoveries Through Ancient Scripture, Natural Medicine and Modern Science* (Sandpoint, ID: Tetrahedron Publishing Group, 2000), 185-191.

APPENDIX C: ANTIBIOTICS

1 Joseph Pizzorno, N.D. *Total Wellness* (Rocklin, CA: Prima Publishing, 1996), 58. Michael Murray, N.D., and Joseph Pizzorno, N.D. *Encyclopedia of Natural Medicine* 2nd Ed. (Rocklin, CA: Prima Publishing, 1998), 8.

2 S.R. Cohen and J.W. Thompson. "Otitic Candidiasis in Children: An Evaluation of the Problem and Effectiveness of Ketpconazole in 10 Patients." *Annals of Otology, Rhinology, and Laryngology* 99 (1990), 427-431.

3 E.I. Cantekin, T.W. McGuire, and T.L. Griffith. "Antimicrobial Therapy for Otitis Media with Effusion (Secretory Otitis Media)." *Journal of the American Medical Association* 266:23 (1991), 3309-3317.

4 W.G. Crook. *Chronic Fatigue Syndrome and The Yeast Connection* (Jackson, TN: Professional Books, 1992), 339-340.

5 Joseph Pizzorno, N.D. *Total Wellness* (Rocklin, CA: Prima Publishing, 1996), 58.

6 Ibid.

7 L. Galland and D.D. Buchman. *Superimmunity for Kids* (New York: E.P. Dutton, 1988), 201.

8 H.C. Neu. "The Crisis in Antibiotic Resistance." *Science* 257 (1992), 1064-1073.

9 National Institute of Allergy and Infectious Diseases. "Antimicrobial Resistance Fact Sheet." Available on the Internet: www.niaid.nih.gov /factsheets/antimicro.htm.

10 Burton Goldberg. "Resisting Antibiotics." *Alternative Medicine* 26 (October/November 1998), 12-13.

11 National Institute of Allergy and Infectious Diseases. "Antimicrobial Resistance Fact Sheet." Available on the Internet: www.niaid.nih.gov /factsheets/antimicro.htm.

12 M. Reichler. In: *Abstracts of 91st Annual Meeting of the American Society for Microbiology Dallas, Texas, May 5-9, 1991* (Washington, DC: American Society for Microbiology, 1991), 404.

13 A.R. Manges et al. "Widespread Distribution of Urinary Tract Infections Caused by a Multidrug-Resistant *Escherichia coli* Clonal Group." *New England Journal of Medicine* 345:14 (2001), 1007-1013.

14 National Institute of Allergy and Infectious Diseases. "Antimicrobial Resistance Fact Sheet." Available on the Internet: www.niaid.nih.gov /factsheets/antimicro.htm.

15 J.D. Wenger et al. "Bacterial Meningitis in the United States, 1988: The Report of a Multi-State Surveillance Study, The Bacterial Study Group." *Journal of Infectious Diseases* 162:6 (December 1990), 1316-1323.

16 R. Gonzales, J.F. Steiner, and M.A. Sande. "Antibiotic Prescribing for Adults with Colds, Upper Respiratory Tract Infections, and Bronchitis by Ambulatory Care Physicians." *Journal of the American Medical Association* 278:11 (1997), 901-904.

17 David G. White et al. "The Isolation of Antibiotic-Resistant *Salmonella* from Retail Ground Meats." *New England Journal of Medicine* 345:16 (2001), 1147-1154.

18 M.L. Cohen. "Epidemiology of Drug Resistance: Implications for a Post-Antimicrobial Era." *Science* 257(1992), 1050-1055.

19 World Health Organization. *Fighting Disease, Fostering Development: Report of the Director General* (London: HMSO, 1966).

20 "Says Food Allergy Seems Important Cause of Otitis." *Family Practice News* 21:5 (1991), 14.

21 G.D. Hussey and M.A. Klein. "A Randomized, Controlled Trial of Vitamin A in Children with Severe Measles." *New England Journal of Medicine* 323 (1990).

22 M. Lewis et al. "Prenatal Exposure to Heavy Metals: Effect on Childhood Cognitive Skills and Health Status." *Pediatrics* 89 (1992), 1010-1015.

23 A.O. Summers et al. "Mercury Released from Dental 'Silver' Fillings Increases the Incidence of Multiply Resistant Bacteria in the Oral and Intestinal Normal Flora." In: *Abstracts of 91st Annual Meeting of the American Society for Microbiology Dallas, Texas, May 5-9, 1991* (Washington, DC: American Society for Microbiology, 1991).

24 G. Anneren, C.G.M. Magnusson, and S.L. Nordvall. "Increase in Serum Concentrations of IgG2 and IgG4 by Selenium Supplementation in Children with Down's Syndrome." *Archives of Diseases of Children* 65 (1990), 1353-1355.

25 D.C. Neiman et al. "The Effects of Moderate Exercise Training on Natural Killer Cells and Acute Upper Respiratory Tract Infections." *International Journal of Sports Medicine* 11:6 (1990).

26 M.E.P. Seligman. *Learned Optimism* (New York: Alfred A. Knopf, 1991), 167-184. J.W. Pennebaker. *Opening Up: The Healing Power of Confiding in Others* (New York: Avon, 1991).

27 R.J. Meyer and R.J. Haggerty. "Streptococcal Infections in Families." *Pediatrics* 4 (1962), 539-549.

28 This information was compiled by health journalist Bill Sardi (www.billsardi.com). The information on essential oils is from Anne Vermilye, President of essential-oil product manufacturer BioExcel (www.bioexcel.com).

29 M.A. Schmidt, L.H. Smith, and K.W. Sehnert. *Beyond Antibiotics: Healthier Options for Families* (Berkeley, CA: North Atlantic Books, 1992).

INDEX

ABOUT THE EDITORS

Burton Goldberg (President) rose to national prominence in 1994 with the first edition of *Alternative Medicine: The Definitive Guide*, produced by his own publishing company. As a result of the publication of the *Guide*, he has become a focal point for the field of alternative medicine. He has spent over 20 years researching every aspect of holistic medicine, from California to Israel, Mexico to Russia. He also started a magazine, *Alternative Medicine*, which has received critical acclaim as a unique, consumer-oriented guide to all aspects of alternative medicine, and published additional books. Mr. Goldberg tirelessly promotes alternative medicine through media appearances each year and has earned the reputation as "the voice of alternative medicine."

Larry Trivieri, Jr., is a leading lay expert in the health and wellness field who has been exploring holistic approaches to healing and personal transformation for nearly 30 years. He served as senior editor for the first edition of *Alternative Medicine: The Definitive Guide.* He is also the co-author of *The Complete Self-Care Guide to Holistic Medicine* (Tarcher/Putnam, 1999) and author of *The American Holistic Medical Association Guide to Holistic Health* (John Wiley & Sons, 2001), and serves as a contributing editor for *Alternative Medicine* magazine. He has written articles for a variety of magazines and newspapers and been a guest on radio and television talk shows nationwide. He resides in his hometown of Utica, New York.

John W. Anderson has written extensively in the field of alternative medicine for the last six years. He was the research editor and a writer for *Alternative Medicine* magazine, focusing primarily on natural products, holistic pet care, and healing foods. From 1999 to 2002, he was the editor-in-chief of AlternativeMedicine.com Books, overseeing the publication of the *Alternative Medicine Definitive Guide Series* of titles and serving as the primary writer on *Weight Loss: An Alternative Medicine Definitive Guide.* He resides in San Francisco, California.

NOTES

NOTES

NOTES

NOTES

NOTES

NOTES

NOTES

NOTES

NOTES

NOTES

NOTES

NOTES

NOTES

Books Your Health Depends On!

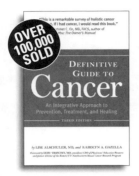

DEFINITIVE GUIDE TO CANCER, 3RD EDITION
AN INTEGRATIVE APPROACH TO PREVENTION, TREATMENT, AND HEALING

By Lise Alschuler, ND, and Karolyn A. Gazella

The single most important, lifesaving book on cancer ever published—proven, safe, nontoxic, and successful treatments from 37 top physicians for reversing cancer.

ISBN 978-1-58761-358-6 • $25.00

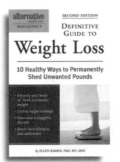

ALTERNATIVE MEDICINE MAGAZINE'S DEFINITIVE GUIDE TO WEIGHT LOSS, SECOND EDITION

By Ellen Kamhi, PhD, RN, HNC

Unlike any other weight loss book ever published, this book shows readers how to lose weight based on the workings of their individual biochemistry. Ellen Kamhi shows how to create a customized approach to weight loss—use supplements wisely, start exercising, resolve emotional issues, and correct underlying imbalances that may contribute to weight gain.

ISBN 978-1-58761-259-6 • $18.95

CANCER DIAGNOSIS: WHAT TO DO NEXT

By W. John Diamond, MD, and W. Lee Cowden, MD, with Burton Goldberg

Healing from cancer means learning as much as you can about your condition and the options available for treatment. While your doctor may or may not be open to alternative therapies, use this book as your guide on the road to recovery and to educate yourself about the wide range of safe, nontoxic, and effective alternative treatments for cancer.
• Early detection and prevention
• Choose the right alternative and conventional treatments

ISBN 978-1-88729-940-4 • $14.95

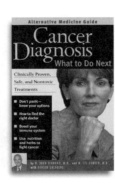

CHRONIC FATIGUE, FIBROMYALGIA & LYME DISEASE, SECOND EDITION: AN ALTERNATIVE MEDICINE DEFINITIVE GUIDE

By Burton Goldberg and Larry Trivieri, Jr.

Chronic fatigue, fibromyalgia, and environmental illness can be permanently reversed using nontoxic alternative medicine treatments. In this book, 26 leading physicians explain the techniques and natural substances that brought complete recovery to their patients.

ISBN 978-1-58761-191-9 • $18.95

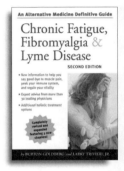

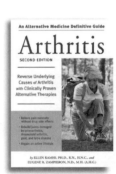

ARTHRITIS, 2ND EDITION: AN ALTERNATIVE MEDICINE DEFINITIVE GUIDE

By Eugene Zampieron, ND, AHG, and Ellen Kamhi, PhD, RN, HNC

Discover the underlying causes of arthritis and how proper nutrition, herbs, detoxification and other methods can put sufferers back on the move.

Dr. Eugene Zampieron specializes in autoimmune and rheumatic ailments. Ellen Kamhi holds a doctorate in nursing and public health and specializes in herbal and bioenergetic therapies.

ISBN 978-1-58761-258-9 • $18.95

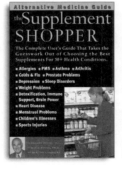

THE SUPPLEMENT SHOPPER

By Maile Pouls, PhD and Greg Pouls, DC, with Burton Goldberg

At last, a single book that explains everything you need to know about selecting nutritional supplements and how to match the best brand to your exact medical problem—over 100 conditions detailed.

"The brillant Pouls team provides a practical guide for using natural supplements to treat a variety of health problems."
—Elson M. Haas MD, author of *Staying Healthy with Nutrition.*

ISBN 978-1-88729-917-6 • $18.95

ALTERNATIVE MEDICINE GUIDE TO HEART DISEASE, STROKE & HIGH BLOOD PRESSURE

By Burton Goldberg and the Editors of *Alternative Medicine*

Save your heart from disease, attack, stroke, high blood pressure, and the dangers of angioplasty, bypass, and other invasive surgeries—12 top physicians explain their proven, safe, nontoxic and successful heart-saving treatments.

ISBN 978-1-88729-910-7 • $18.95

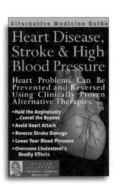

THE ENZYME CURE

By Lita Lee, PhD, and Lisa Turner, with Burton Goldberg

The complete self-help guide to using enzymes—the little known but powerful nutritional marvel of nature—to reverse 28 major health conditions, from one of the nation's leading enzyme therapists.

ISBN 978-1-88729-922-0 • $18.95

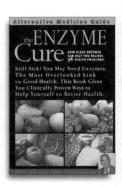

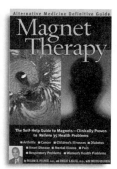
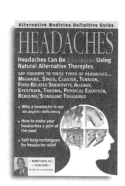
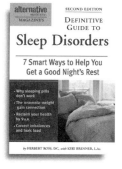
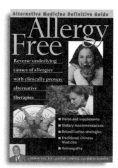
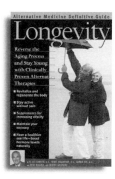
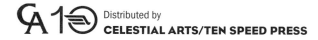